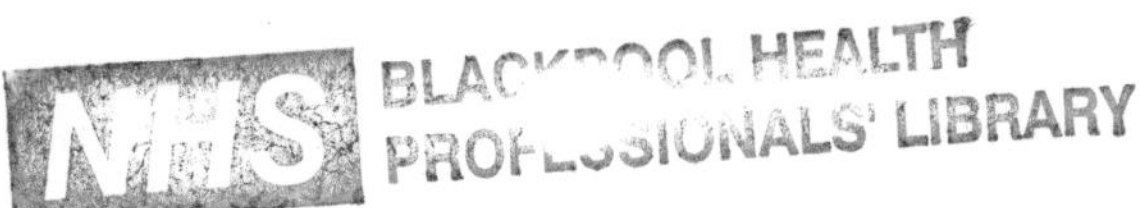

VOLUME TWO

Principles and Practice of ANESTHESIOLOGY

SECOND EDITION

David E. Longnecker, M.D.
Robert Dunning Dripps Professor
Chair, Department of Anesthesia
University of Pennsylvania Health System
Philadelphia, Pennsylvania

John H. Tinker, M.D.
Professor and Chairman
Department of Anesthesiology
University of Nebraska College of Medicine
Omaha, Nebraska

G. Edward Morgan, Jr., M.D.
Chief Medical Officer
Excellence in Medicine, LLC
Los Angeles, California

with 1448 *illustrations*

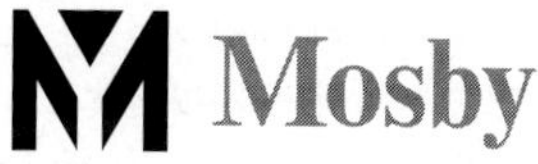

St. Louis Baltimore Boston Carlsbad Chicago Minneapolis New York Philadelphia Portland
London Milan Sydney Tokyo Toronto

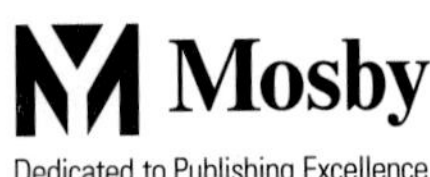

Senior Editor: Laurel Craven
Developmental Editor: Wendy Buckwalter
Project Manager: Chris Baumle
Project Specialist: David Orzechowski
Cover Designer: Nancy McDonald
Manufacturing Manager: William A. Winneberger, Jr.

Second Edition

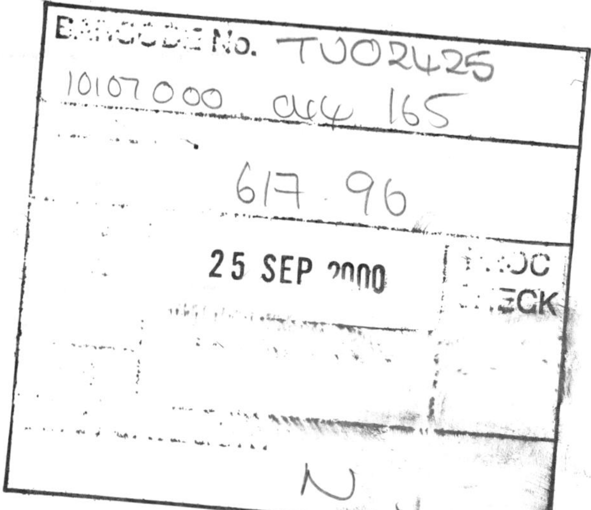

Printed in the United States of America
Composition by ATLIS Graphics & Design, Inc.
Printing/binding by Von Hoffman Press, Inc.

Mosby–Year Book, Inc.
11830 Westline Industrial Drive
St. Louis, Missouri 63146

Library of Congress Cataloging-in-Publication Data

Principles and practice of anesthesiology--2nd ed. / [edited by]
David E. Longnecker, John H. Tinker, G. Edward Morgan, Jr.
p. cm.
Includes bibliographical references and index.
ISBN 0-8151-5479-8
1. Anesthesiology. I. Longnecker, David E., 1939-
II. Tinker, John H. (John Heath), 1941- . III. Morgan, G. Edward.
[DNLM: 1. Anesthesia. 2. Anesthesiology–methods. WO 200
P957 1998]
RD81.P7427 1998
617.9′6--dc21
DNLM/DLC
for Library of Congress 97-24668
CIP

98 99 00 01 02/9 8 7 6 5 4 3 2 1

Contributors

Mark Abel, M.D.
Assistant Professor of Anesthesia
Department of Anesthesia
Mount Sinai Hospital
New York, New York

Christian M. Alexander, M.D.
Associate Professor of Anesthesiology
Jefferson Medical College of Thomas Jefferson University
Philadelphia, Pennsylvania

Hassan H. Ali, M.D.
Professor of Anesthesia and Anesthetist
Department of Anesthesia
Massachusetts General Hospital
Boston, Massachusetts

James K. Alifimoff, M.D.
Chairman, Anesthesia Section
Stormont Vail Regional Medical Center
Anesthesia Associates of Topeka
Topeka, Kansas

Stanley J. Aukburg, M.D.
Associate Professor of Anesthesia
University of Pennsylvania Health System
Philadelphia, Pennsylvania

Salvatore J. Basta, M.D.
Assistant Professor of Anaesthesia
Harvard Medical School
Associate Anesthetist
Massachusetts General Hospital
Boston, Massachusetts

Christopher D. Beatie, M.D.
Associate Professor of Clinical Anesthesiology
Department of Anesthesiology
UCLA School of Medicine
Attending Anesthesiologist
UCLA Medical Center
Los Angeles, California

Charles Beattie, M.D., Ph.D.
Professor and Chair
Anesthesiologist-in-Chief
Department of Anesthesiology
Vanderbilt University School of Medicine
Nashville, Tennessee

Robert F. Bedford, M.D.
Professor of Anesthesiology
University of South Florida School of Medicine
Chief, Anesthesiology Service
James A. Haley Veterans Hospital
Tampa, Florida

Ivor D. Berkowitz, M.B., B.Ch.
Associate Professor
Department of Anesthesiology and Critical Care Medicine
Associate Director
Pediatric Intensive Care Unit
The Johns Hopkins Medical Institutions
Baltimore, Maryland

Marina D. Bizzarri-Schmid, M.D.
Instructor in Anaesthesia
Harvard Medical School
Anesthesiologist
Brigham and Women's Hospital
Boston, Massachusetts

Denis L. Bourke, M.D.
Associate Professor of Anesthesiology
University of Maryland Medical School
Chief, Anesthesiology Service
Baltimore Veterans Affairs Medical Center
Baltimore, Maryland

Philip G. Boysen, M.D.
Chair, Department of Anesthesiology
Professor of Anesthesiology and Medicine
University of North Carolina School of Medicine
Chapel Hill, North Carolina

Michael J. Breslow, M.D., F.C.C.M.
Associate Professor of Anesthesiology, Medicine, and Surgery
Co-Director, Surgical Intensive Care Unit
The Johns Hopkins Medical Institutions
Baltimore, Maryland

David Bronheim, M.D.
Assistant Professor of Anesthesia
Mount Sinai School of Medicine
Director, Post Anesthesia Care
Mount Sinai Hospital
New York, New York

David H. Chestnut, M.D.
Alfred Habeeb Professor and Chair of Anesthesiology
Professor of Obstetrics and Gynecology
University of Alabama School of Medicine
Birmingham, Alabama

Albert T. Cheung, M.D.
Assistant Professor of Anesthesia
University of Pennsylvania Health System
Philadelphia, Pennsylvania

Rose Christopherson, M.D., Ph.D.
Associate Professor of Anesthesiology
Oregon Health Sciences University School of Medicine
Assistant Chief, Anesthesiology Service
Portland Veterans Administration Medical Center
Portland, Oregon

Pietro Colonna-Romano, M.D.
Associate Professor of Clinical Anesthesiology
Allegheny University, Hahnemann Division
Philadelphia, Pennsylvania

Mercedes Concepcion, M.D.
Assistant Professor of Anaesthesia
Harvard Medical School
Director of Orthopedic Anesthesia
Brigham and Women's Hospital
Boston, Massachusetts

Ray H. d'Amours, M.D.
Assistant Professor of Anesthesia
Director, Acute Pain Service
University of Pennsylvania Health System
Philadelphia, Pennsylvania

Mark Dershwitz, M.D., Ph.D.
Associate Professor of Anaesthesia
Harvard Medical School
Associate Anesthetist
Massachusetts General Hospital
Boston, Massachusetts

Dawn P. Desiderio, M.D.
Associate Professor of Anesthesiology
Cornell University Medical College
Associate Attending
Department of Anesthesiology and Critical Care Medicine
Memorial Sloan-Kettering Cancer Center
New York, New York

Clifford S. Deutschman, M.S., M.D., F.C.C.M.
Associate Professor of Anesthesia and Surgery
Attending Physician
Surgical Critical Care Service
University of Pennsylvania Health System
Philadelphia, Pennsylvania

Dennis D. Doblar, Ph.D., M.D.
Professor of Anesthesiology and Biomedical Engineering
Director of Clinical Research
University of Alabama School of Medicine
Birmingham, Alabama

Elana B. Doering, Ph.D., M.D.
Assistant Professor of Anesthesiology
Department of Anesthesiology
Columbia University College of Physicians and Surgeons
New York, New York

David L. Dull, M.D.
Clinical Assistant Professor
Department of Surgery
Division of Anesthesiology
Michigan State University College of Human Medicine
Grand Rapids, Michigan

John H. Eichhorn, M.D.
Professor and Chairman
Department of Anesthesiology
University of Mississippi School of Medicine
Chairman, Department of Anesthesiology
University of Mississippi Medical Center
Jackson, Mississippi

James B. Eisenkraft, M.D.
Professor of Anesthesiology
Mount Sinai School of Medicine of the City University of New York
Attending Anesthesiologist
Mount Sinai Medical Center
New York, New York

James J. Fehr, M.D.
Instructor
Department of Anesthesiology and Critical Care Medicine
The Johns Hopkins Medical Institutions
Baltimore, Maryland

F. Michael Ferrante, M.D.
Associate Professor of Anesthesia and Medicine
University of Pennsylvania Health System
Philadelphia, Pennsylvania

Hugh L. Flanagan, M.D.
Assistant Professor of Anaesthesia
Harvard Medical School
Department of Anesthesia
Brigham and Women's Hospital
Boston, Massachusetts

Robert B. Forbes, M.D., F.R.C.P.C.
Professor of Anesthesia
The University of Iowa College of Medicine
Chief, Division of Pediatric Anesthesia
The University of Iowa Hospitals and Clinics
Iowa City, Iowa

Steven M. Frank, M.D.
Associate Professor
Department of Anesthesiology and Critical Care Medicine
The Johns Hopkins Hospital
Baltimore, Maryland

Carlos D. Franco, M.D.
Assistant Professor of Anesthesiology
Rush-Presbyterian St. Luke's Medical Center
Attending Anesthesiologist
Department of Anesthesiology and Pain Management
Cook County Hospital
Chicago, Illinois

Kirk L. Fridrich, D.D.S., M.S.
Associate Professor, College of Dentistry
Graduate Program Director
Department of Oral and Maxillofacial Surgery
The University of Iowa Hospitals and Clinics
Iowa City, Iowa

Robert P. From, D.O.
Associate Professor of Anesthesia
Vice-Chair, Education
Department of Anesthesia
The University of Iowa College of Medicine
Iowa City, Iowa

William R. Furman, M.D.
Associate Professor
Department of Anesthesia and Critical Care Medicine
University of Chicago Pritzker School of Medicine
Chicago, Illinois

Robert R. Gaiser, M.D.
Assistant Professor of Anesthesia
University of Pennsylvania Health System
Philadelphia, Pennsylvania

Joseph M. Garfield, M.D.
Associate Professor of Anaesthesia
Harvard Medical School
Brigham and Women's Hospital
Boston, Massachusetts

Ralph T. Geer, M.D.
Associate Professor
Departments of Anesthesia and Internal Medicine
University of Pennsylvania Health System
Philadelphia, Pennsylvania

Simon Gelman, M.D., Ph.D.
Leroy D. Vandam/Benjamin G. Covino Professor of Anaesthesia
Harvard Medical School
Chairman, Department of Anesthesia
Brigham and Women's Hospital
Boston, Massachusetts

Peter S. A. Glass, M.B., Ch.B., F.F.A. (S.A.)
Associate Professor of Anesthesiology
Duke University School of Medicine
Director, Clinical Research
Department of Anesthesiology
Duke University Medical Center
Durham, North Carolina

Beth Glosten, M.D.
Associate Professor of Anesthesiology
University of Washington School of Medicine
Seattle, Washington

Lee Goldman, M.D.
Professor and Chairman
Department of Medicine
Associate Dean for Clinical Affairs
University of California, San Francisco, School of Medicine
San Francisco, California

Mark N. Gomez, M.D.
Associate Professor of Anesthesia
The University of Iowa College of Medicine
Iowa City, Iowa

Christopher M. Grande, M.D., M.P.H.
Executive Director
International Trauma Anesthesia and Critical Care Society (ITACCS)
Baltimore, Maryland

Vijay L. Gupta, F.R.C.A.
Clinical Pharmacology Research Fellow
Department of Anesthesiology
Duke University Medical Center
Durham, North Carolina

Theodore E. M. Hanley, M.D.
Clinical Assistant Professor of Anesthesia
Clinical Director of Anesthesia
Director of Ambulatory Surgery
State University of New York Health Science Center at Brooklyn College of Medicine
Brooklyn, New York

Kenneth L. Haspel, M.D.
Instructor of Anaesthesia
Harvard Medical School
Assistant Anesthetist
Medical Director, Post Anesthesia Care Unit
Massachusetts General Hospital
Boston, Massachusetts

Mark A. Helfaer, M.D.
Associate Professor
Departments of Anesthesiology and Critical Care Medicine and Pediatrics
The Johns Hopkins Medical Institutions
Baltimore, Maryland

William W. Hesson, J.D.
Adjunct Assistant Professor
The University of Iowa College of Medicine
Associate Director, External Relations and Legal Services
The University of Iowa Hospitals and Clinics
Iowa City, Iowa

Paul R. Hickey, M.D.
Professor of Anaesthesia
Harvard Medical School
Anesthesiologist-in-Chief
Children's Hospital
Boston, Massachusetts

Carol A. Hirshman, M.D.
Professor of Anesthesiology, Environmental Health Sciences, and Medicine
The Johns Hopkins Medical Institutions
Baltimore, Maryland

Robert S. Holzman, M.D.
Associate Professor of Anaesthesia
Harvard Medical School
Senior Associate in Anesthesia
Children's Hospital
Boston, Massachusetts

Atul R. Hulyalkar, M.D.
Cardiologist
North Ohio Heart Center
Elyria, Ohio

Mary M. Joseph, M.D.
Professor of Anesthesiology
University of Southern California School of Medicine
Los Angeles, California

Steven M. Karan, M.D.
Assistant Professor of Anesthesiology
Uniformed Services University of the Health Sciences
Bethesda, Maryland
Walter Reed Army Medical Center
Washington, DC

Jeffrey Katz, M.D.
Professor and Chair
Department of Anesthesiology
University of Texas Medical School at Houston
Chief of Anesthesiology
Hermann Hospital
Houston, Texas

Henrik Kehlet, Prof., M.D., Ph.D.
Professor of Surgery
Copenhagen University, Copenhagen
Division of Surgical Gastroenterology
Hvidovre University Hospital
Hvidovre, Denmark

Sean K. Kennedy, M.D.
Associate Professor of Anesthesia
Medical Director of the Operating Rooms
University of Pennsylvania Health System
Philadelphia, Pennsylvania

Mary A. Keyes, M.D.
Associate Professor of Clinical Anesthesia
UCLA School of Medicine
Los Angeles, California

Gerald Kirk, M.D.
Staff Anesthesiologist
St. Vincent Hospitals and Health Center
Indianapolis, Indiana

Jeffrey R. Kirsch, M.D.
Associate Professor
Vice Chairman, Education
Department of Anesthesiology and Critical Care Medicine
The Johns Hopkins Medical Institutions
Baltimore, Maryland

Vincent J. Kopp, M.D.
Assistant Professor of Anesthesiology and Pediatrics
Adjunct Assistant Professor of Social Medicine
University of North Carolina School of Medicine
Division Chief, Anesthesiology Consult Services
Medical Director, Preanesthesia Consult Clinic
University of North Carolina Hospitals
Chapel Hill, North Carolina

Ronald A. Kross, M.D.
Assistant Professor of Anesthesiology
Cornell University Medical College
Assistant Attending Anesthesiologist
Memorial Sloan-Kettering Cancer Center
New York, New York

Andrea J. Layman, M.D.
Staff Anesthesiologist
Heart and Lung Clinic
Bismarck, North Dakota

Thomas H. Lee, M.D., S.M.
Associate Professor of Medicine
Harvard Medical School
Medical Director
Partners Community HealthCare, Inc.
Boston, Massachusetts

Paul A. Leonard
Associate, Department of Anesthesia
The University of Iowa College of Medicine
Iowa City, Iowa

Thomas C. Lewis, M.D.
Assistant Professor of Anesthesiology
Vanderbilt University Hospital
Nashville, Tennessee

Edwin W. Lojeski, M.D.
Assistant Professor of Anesthesiology
Uniformed Services University of Health Sciences
Bethesda, Maryland
Attending Anesthesiologist
Walter Reed Army Medical Center
Washington, DC

David E. Longnecker, M.D.
Robert Dunning Dripps Professor
Chair, Department of Anesthesia
University of Pennsylvania Health System
Philadelphia, Pennsylvania

Mazen A. Maktabi, M.D.
Assistant Professor of Anesthesia
Director, Division of Neuroanesthesia
The University of Iowa College of Medicine
Iowa City, Iowa

Lynette J. Mark, M.D.
Assistant Professor
Department of Anesthesiology and Critical Care Medicine
The Johns Hopkins University School of Medicine
Baltimore, Maryland

Lynne G. Maxwell, M.D.
Associate Professor
Departments of Anesthesiology/Critical Care Medicine and Pediatrics
The Johns Hopkins University School of Medicine
Baltimore, Maryland

Robert W. McPherson, M.D., M.H.S.*
Professor
The Johns Hopkins Medical Institutions
Baltimore, Maryland

William T. Merritt, M.D.
Associate Professor
Department of Anesthesiology and Critical Care Medicine
Head, Liver Transplantation Anesthesiology
The Johns Hopkins Medical Institutions
Baltimore, Maryland

*Deceased

Paul S. Mesnick, M.D., M.J.
Assistant Professor of Anesthesiology
Northwestern University Medical School
Senior Attending Physician
Northwestern Memorial Hospitals
Chicago, Illinois

Ronald M. Meyer, M.D.
Assistant Professor of Anesthesiology
Northwestern University Medical School
Attending Anesthesiologist
Catholic Health Partners
Northwestern Memorial Hospital
Chicago, Illinois

Maged S. Mikhail, M.D.
Associate Professor of Anesthesiology
University of Southern California School of Medicine
Associate Director of Intensive Care
USC/Kenneth Norris Cancer Hospital
Los Angeles, California

Edward D. Miller, M.D.
Professor and Chairman
Department of Anesthesiology and Critical Care Medicine
Dean and Chief Executive Officer
The Johns Hopkins Medical Institutions
Baltimore, Maryland

Keith W. Miller, D. Phil.
Professor of Pharmacology
Department of Anaesthesia
Harvard Medical School
Boston, Massachusetts

Laurel E. Moore, M.D.
Assistant Professor
Department of Anesthesiology and Critical Care Medicine
The Johns Hopkins Medical Institutions
Attending Anesthesiologist
Johns Hopkins Bayview Medical Center
Baltimore, Maryland

G. Edward Morgan, Jr., M.D.
Chief Medical Officer
Excellence in Medicine, LLC
Los Angeles, California

Sheila M. Muldoon, M.D.
Professor of Anesthesiology
Uniformed Services University of the Health Sciences
Bethesda, Maryland

Michael F. Mulroy, M.D.
Staff Anesthesiologist
Virginia Mason Medical Center
Seattle, Washington

Frank L. Murphy, M.D.
Associate Professor of Anesthesia
University of Pennsylvania Health System
Philadelphia, Pennsylvania

David J. Murray, M.D.
Professor of Anesthesia
Washington University School of Medicine
Director, Clinical Simulation Center
Washington University
St. Louis, Missouri

Michael G. Muto, M.D.
Assistant Professor of Obstetrics, Gynecology, and Reproductive Biology
Harvard Medical School
Associate in Gynecologic Oncology
Division of Obstetrics and Gynecology
Brigham and Women's Hospital
Boston, Massachusetts

Gordon R. Neufeld, M.D.
Associate Professor of Anesthesiology
University of Pennsylvania Health System
Philadelphia, Pennsylvania

Charles W. Otto, M.D., F.C.C.M.
Professor of Anesthesiology
Associate Professor of Medicine
University of Arizona College of Medicine
Director, Critical Care Medicine
University Medical Center
Tucson, Arizona

Andranik Ovassapian, M.D.
Professor of Anesthesiology
Northwestern University Medical School
Chief, Anesthesia Service
VA Chicago Health Care System-Lakeside Division
Chicago, Illinois

Tanya L. Oyos, M.D.
Associate Professor of Clinical Anesthesia
Department of Anesthesia
Medical Director, PACU
The University of Iowa College of Medicine
Iowa City, Iowa

Sally C. Palmon, M.D.
Assistant Professor of Anesthesiology
Department of Anesthesiology and Critical Care Medicine
The Johns Hopkins Medical Institutions
Baltimore, Maryland

Arnold R. Parenteau, M.D.
Pain Management Fellow
Department of Anesthesia
The University of Iowa Hospitals and Clinics
Iowa City, Iowa

Winston C.V. Parris, M.D.
Professor of Anesthesiology
Vanderbilt University School of Medicine
Director, Pain Control Center
Vanderbilt University Medical Center
Nashville, Tennessee

L. Reuven Pasternak, M.D., M.P.H., M.B.A.
Associate Professor and Vice-Chairman
Department of Anesthesiology and Critical Care Medicine
The Johns Hopkins Medical Institutions
Chairman, Department of Anesthesiology
Johns Hopkins Bayview Medical Center
Baltimore, Maryland

Kent S. Pearson, M.D.
Associate Professor of Anesthesia
The University of Iowa College of Medicine
Associate Director, Surgical Intensive Care Unit
The University of Iowa Hospitals and Clinics
Iowa City, Iowa

Richard M. Pino, M.D., Ph.D.
Instructor of Anaesthesia
Harvard Medical School
Assistant in Anesthesia
Massachusetts General Hospital
Boston, Massachusetts

Burdett R. Porter, M.D.
Associate
Department of Anesthesia
The University of Iowa College of Medicine
Iowa City, Iowa

Francis X. Riegler, M.D.
Assistant Clinical Professor of Anesthesiology
University of California, Los Angeles, School of Medicine
Los Angeles, California

R. Gilbert Ritchie, Ph.D.
Assistant Professor of Anesthesiology
Administrative Director, Anesthesia Services
University of Alabama at Birmingham School of Medicine
Birmingham, Alabama

Henry Rosenberg, M.D.
Professor of Anesthesiology
Jefferson Medical College of Thomas Jefferson University
Philadelphia, Pennsylvania

Brian A. Rosenfeld, M.D., F.C.C.M.
Associate Professor
Departments of Anesthesiology, Medicine, and Surgery
The Johns Hopkins Medical Institutions
Baltimore, Maryland

Carl E. Rosow, M.D., Ph.D.
Associate Professor of Anaesthesia
Harvard Medical School
Anesthetist
Massachusetts General Hospital
Boston, Massachusetts

Alan F. Ross, M.D.
Associate Professor of Anesthesia
The University of Iowa College of Medicine
Director, Cardiothoracic Anesthesia
The University of Iowa Hospitals and Clinics
Iowa City, Iowa

Neal T. Sakima, M.D.
Assistant Professor
Department of Anesthesiology and Critical Care Medicine
The Johns Hopkins University School of Medicine
Baltimore, Maryland

Ivan S. Salgo, M.D.
Assistant Professor of Anesthesiology
University of Pennsylvania Health System
Philadelphia, Pennsylvania

Joseph S. Savino, M.D.
Associate Professor of Anesthesia
Section Chief
Cardiovascular Thoracic Anesthesia and Critical Care
University of Pennsylvania Health System
Philadelphia, Pennsylvania

Michael J. Sendak, M.D.
Assistant Professor
Department of Anesthesiology and Critical Care Medicine
The Johns Hopkins Medical Institutions
Chief, Department of Anesthesiology
Director, Perioperative Services
Maryland General Hospital
Baltimore, Maryland

Steven L. Shafer, M.D.
Associate Professor of Anesthesia
Stanford University School of Medicine
Staff Anesthesiologist
Palo Alto VA Health Care System
Palo Alto, California

Frederick E. Sieber, M.D.
Associate Professor
Department of Anesthesiology and Critical Care Medicine
Director, Neuroanesthesia
The Johns Hopkins Medical Institutions
Baltimore, Maryland

Neal W. Siex, D.O.
Assistant Professor of Anesthesiology
Vanderbilt University School of Medicine
Nashville, Tennessee

Raymond S. Sinatra, M.D., Ph.D.
Professor of Anesthesiology
Director, Acute Pain Service
Co-Director, Obstetrical Anesthesiology
Yale University School of Medicine
Attending Anesthesiologist
Yale-New Haven Hospital
New Haven, Connecticut

Charles E. Smith, M.D., F.R.C.P.C.
Associate Professor of Anesthesia
Case Western Reserve University
Director, Cardiothoracic Anesthesia
MetroHealth Medical Center
Cleveland, Ohio

Douglas S. Snyder, M.D.
Assistant Professor
Department of Anesthesiology and Critical Care Medicine
The Johns Hopkins Medical Institutions
Baltimore, Maryland

Martin D. Sokoll, M.D.
Professor of Anesthesia
The University of Iowa College of Medicine
Iowa City, Iowa

Richard J. Sperry, M.D., Ph.D.
Associate Professor of Anesthesiology
Associate Vice President for Health Sciences
University of Utah School of Medicine
Salt Lake City, Utah

Bruce D. Spiess, M.D.
Associate Professor of Anesthesiology
Chief, Division of Cardiothoracic Anesthesia
University of Washington School of Medicine
Seattle, Washington

Stanley W. Stead, M.D.
Associate Professor of Anesthesiology and Ophthalmology
University of California, Los Angeles, School of Medicine
Director, Ophthalmic Anesthesiology
Jules Stein Eye Institute
Los Angeles, California

John K. Stene, M.D., Ph.D.
Associate Professor of Anesthesia
Pennsylvania State University College of Medicine
Hershey, Pennsylvania

Robert H. Stiefel, M.S.
Instructor, Biomedical Engineering
Manager, Clinical Engineering Services
The Johns Hopkins Medical Institutions
Baltimore, Maryland

Judith L. Stiff, M.D., M.P.H.
Associate Professor
Department of Anesthesiology and Critical Care Medicine
The Johns Hopkins University School of Medicine
Attending Anesthesiologist
Johns Hopkins Bayview Medical Center
Baltimore, Maryland

Gary R. Strichartz, Ph.D.
Professor of Anaesthesia (Pharmacology)
Harvard Medical School
Vice Chairman for Research
Department of Anesthesia
Brigham and Women's Hospital
Boston, Massachusetts

Cephas P. Swamidoss, M.S., M.D.
Assistant Professor of Anesthesiology
Yale University School of Medicine
Attending Anesthesiologist
Yale-New Haven Hospital
New Haven, Connecticut

Duraiyah Thangathurai, M.D.
Professor of Anesthesiology, Surgery, and Urology
Vice Chairman, Department of Anesthesiology
University of Southern California School of Medicine
Director, Intensive Care and Anesthesia
USC/Kenneth Norris Cancer Hospital
Los Angeles, California

Daniel M. Thys, M.D.
Professor of Anesthesiology
Department of Anesthesiology
Columbia University College of Physicians and Surgeons
Director, Department of Anesthesiology
St. Luke's-Roosevelt Hospital Center
New York, New York

John H. Tinker, M.D.
Professor and Chairman
Department of Anesthesiology
University of Nebraska College of Medicine
Omaha, Nebraska

Mitchell D. Tobias, M.D.
Assistant Professor of Anesthesia
Head, Division of Hepatic Transplant Anesthesia
University of Pennsylvania Health System
Philadelphia, Pennsylvania

Michael M. Todd, M.D.
Professor of Anesthesia
Department of Anesthesia
The University of Iowa College of Medicine
Iowa City, Iowa

Rebecca S. Twersky, M.D.
Associate Professor of Anesthesiology
Vice Chair for Research
Medical Director, Ambulatory Surgery Unit
Director, Division of Ambulatory Anesthesia
State University of New York Health Science Center at Brooklyn College of Medicine
Brooklyn, New York

Leroy D. Vandam, Ph.B., M.D., M.A.
Professor of Anaesthesia, Emeritus
Harvard Medical School
Anesthesiologist
Brigham and Women's Hospital
Boston, Massachusetts

Garry V. Walker, M.D.
Assistant Professor of Anesthesiology
Vanderbilt University School of Medicine
PACU Coordinator and Staff Anesthesiologist
Veterans Affairs Medical Center
Nashville, Tennessee

David S. Warner, M.D.
Professor of Anesthesiology
Duke University Medical Center
Durham, North Carolina

Stuart J. Weiss, M.D., Ph.D.
Assistant Professor of Anesthesiology
University of Pennsylvania Health System
Philadelphia, Pennsylvania

Randall C. Wetzel, M.B., B.S., F.C.C.M., F.A.A.P.
Associate Professor
Departments of Anesthesiology/Critical Care Medicine and Pediatrics
Chief, Division of Pediatric Anesthesia
The Johns Hopkins Medical Institutions
Baltimore, Maryland

Tyrone B. Whitter, M.D., Ph.D.
Assistant Professor of Anesthesia
The University of Iowa College of Medicine
Iowa City, Iowa

Alon P. Winnie, M.D.
Professor of Anesthesiology
University of Illinois College of Medicine at Chicago
Chairman, Department of Anesthesiology and Pain Management
Cook County Hospital
Chicago, Illinois

Myron Yaster, M.D.
Associate Professor
Departments of Anesthesiology/Critical Care Medicine and Pediatrics
Director, Pediatric Pain Service
Children's Center
The Johns Hopkins Hospital
Baltimore, Maryland

Adolph J. Yates, Jr., M.D.
Assistant Professor of Orthopaedics and Rehabilitation
Oregon Health Sciences University
Chief of Orthopaedics
Portland Veterans Affairs Medical Center
Portland, Oregon

Helen M. Yates, M.B., B.Ch., B.A.O.
Staff Anesthesiologist
Portland Veterans Affairs Medical Center
Portland, Oregon

Preface

Principles and Practice of Anesthesiology is intended to serve novice and experienced practitioners who embrace the concept that modern anesthesiology includes the practices of perioperative medicine and pain medicine. We believe that anesthesiology has matured into a complete medical discipline that should focus on the patient and not on the procedure. As a result, this book is patient- and disease-oriented, in a manner similar to that found in textbooks of medicine, surgery, or pediatrics. There are other textbooks of anesthesiology that are complete and well written, but they focus on techniques (e.g., administration of drugs, mechanical procedures) rather than on the complete care of the patient. The organization of this book reflects our view of the anesthesiologist as a physician who makes important medical judgments about the care of surgical patients before, during, and after operation, and who provides care to nonsurgical patients as well. Whether practicing individually or as supervisor of an anesthesia care team, the anesthesiologist should possess a broad scope of medical knowledge that encompasses an understanding of coexisting diseases, of perioperative risks, and of perioperative management. We believe this view represents the foundation and future of anesthesia practice.

The practice of anesthesiology has grown increasingly complex. The sophistication needed to perform preoperative medical evaluations, to provide or supervise anesthesia care, to choose from a range of intraoperative techniques, and to manage postoperative care (especially postoperative pain management) has increased dramatically in recent years. Preoperative preparation of surgical patients now occupies a major role in anesthesia practice. Complex diagnostic techniques, such as intraoperative transesophageal echocardiography, are performed by anesthesiologists. The use of regional anesthesia and combined techniques has increased greatly, and the anesthesiologist is involved more frequently in the management of postoperative pain. Involvement in the treatment of patients with chronic pain or cancer-related pain has expanded. Sections of this book are devoted to these subspecialties because they are fully integrated into current anesthesia practice.

The editors, authors, and publisher of this textbook believe that modern texts should distill material and communicate information rather than simply present data. Therefore we have tried to illustrate important concepts in a way that helps the reader to understand, retain, and apply the information. It is our hope that the presentation and format of this book will allow the reader to use the material as a reference for practice and as a means of communicating complex information to other specialists or to those who are training in the specialty.

Finally, we acknowledge that the field of critical care medicine has grown dramatically from one that involved ventilatory support to a comprehensive subspecialty with several multiple-volume texts devoted exclusively to the subject. Attempting to cover all of critical care medicine in a few chapters seemed inconsistent with the scope of critical care practice and with principles on which this book was founded. Therefore we chose to emphasize and expand the coverage of regional anesthesia in the space traditionally reserved for an overview of critical care medicine, an approach that we believe represents a better educational investment for the majority of clinicians.

We hope that these philosophic approaches to the understanding and presentation of the principles of anesthesia practice will provide the reader with a fresh and innovative approach to the specialty. It is our goal that *Principles and Practice of Anesthesiology* represents a new way of looking at the dynamic nature of modern anesthesia practice.

The editors are grateful to Mark C. Rogers, M.D., M.B.A., and Benjamin G. Covino, Ph.D., M.D. (deceased), who were editors of the first edition. Their vision and wisdom contributed greatly to the philosophy that persists in the second edition of this textbook.

David E. Longnecker
John H. Tinker
G. Edward Morgan, Jr.

Contents

Section C
Inhalation Anesthesia

Section D
Intravenous Sedation and Analgesia

VOLUME TWO

Section E
Regional Anesthesia/Analgesia and Pain

Section F
Concurrent Drugs

PART III
SPECIALTY AREAS OF ANESTHETIC PRACTICE

CHAPTER 56

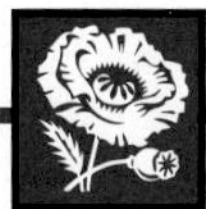

Mechanisms of Action of Local Anesthetic Agents

GARY R. STRICHARTZ

Local anesthetics produce their clinical effects by interfering with the electrical activity of the nervous system. Their primary action is to inhibit the propagation of nerve impulses in peripheral nerves and in the spinal cord. In addition, local anesthetics may act directly on sensory endings of nerves when applied topically and may inhibit synaptic transmission in the spinal cord when used for epidural or intrathecal blocks. These last two modes of action are poorly characterized at present. The central theme of this chapter is to explain how local anesthetics inhibit conduction of nerve impulses in axons.

ANATOMY OF PERIPHERAL NERVE

Ultrastructural Features

An appreciation of the action of local anesthetics on individual nerve fibers requires an understanding of the structure of peripheral nerves and of the kinetics of distribution of local anesthetics in nerves. Peripheral nerves are mixed nerves containing both myelinated and nonmyelinated fibers that conduct impulses to and from the central nervous system (CNS), subserving either sensory or motor functions. The schematized structure of a peripheral nerve is shown in Fig. 56-1. The entire nerve is surrounded by an epineurium, a loose covering of connective tissue. Within this structure, nerve fibers are collected in bundles by interior perineurial sheaths. These perineuria are formed by tightly joined epithelial cells,[1] which act as a major barrier to the diffusion of local anesthetics.[63,87] Between the fascicles runs a network of connective tissue epineurium that provides mechanical support and within which rests the intraneural blood vessels. Finally, each individual axon is intimately surrounded by nonneuronal glial cells that form the endoneurium.

Individual myelinated nerve fibers are each encased in a myelin sheath that extends, discontinuously, from the roots of the spinal cord to near the region of entry at the target organ. Each segment, or internode, of myelin is formed by one Schwann cell that wraps around the axon, forming an insulating cylinder of as many as several hundred bilayer

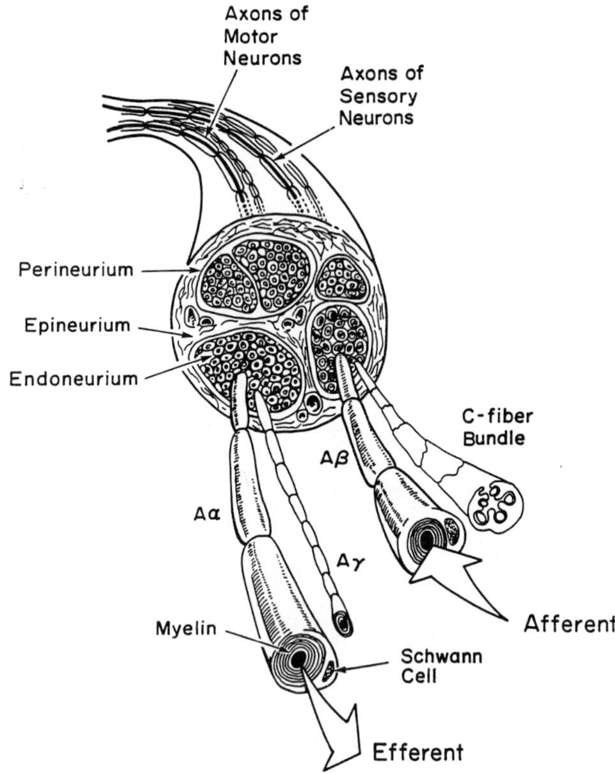

Fig. 56-1. Schematic cross-section of typical peripheral nerve branch shows ultrastructural details of myelinated and nonmyelinated nerve fibers. Different shapes of Schwann cells are detailed, forming myelin around one myelinated axon or encompassing several nonmyelinated C fibers.

membranes. The myelin sheath of peripheral fibers accounts for more than half the thickness of the fiber diameter. The length of each internode extends for about 100 times the fiber's outer diameter.[74]

Separating the myelinated regions are narrow zones, the nodes of Ranvier, that contain the structural elements essential for neuronal excitability (Fig. 56-2). These nodes are typically opposed by nonmyelinating fingers of Schwann cell and an astrocyte, structures that project to the surface of the axolemma and make several intimate contacts with the neuron surface while still permitting relatively free passage of drugs and ions to and from this region.[63,74] Between these extranodal glial cells and the axolemma lies the nodal-gap substance, composed of glycoprotein and other dense, negatively charged material. This substance may act as a "reservoir" to bind metal cations and basic drugs (e.g., local anesthetics) near the nodal membrane.[63] Thus, nowhere along the fiber is the axon membrane freely exposed to the surrounding medium.

In the peripheral nervous system (PNS) of mammals, all healthy fibers with a diameter greater than 1 μm are myelinated. (Neuropathologies from diseases, toxic insults, or nerve trauma often lead to local demyelination.) **Axons smaller than 1 μm are not myelinated but encased instead by a Schwann cell that forms an intimate cover around several (5 to 10) fibers** at once (Fig. 56-1). Cross-sectional electron micrographs of nonmyelinated nerves show that individual axons are located adjacent to the periphery of such a bundle, circumscribing the large nucleus of the Schwann cell. The Schwann cell's plasmalemma encloses each axon separately, folding the cytoplasm of the supporting cell around most of the axon's diameter.[74] Any one axon passes sequentially from one encasing Schwann cell to another with no apparent interruptions. The structural association between neuron and surrounding glia is maintained along the entire length of the fiber and may be functionally similar to that of the myelinated axon and its enclosing Schwann cell at each node of Ranvier. Glia not only provide a structural scaffold for nerve fibers, but also support neurons metabolically, remove accumulating ions (e.g., K^+), and may exchange lipids and proteins with their neuronal neighbors.

Both motor and sensory functions are subserved by myelinated and nonmyelinated fibers (Table 56-1). **The largest myelinated fibers include those that conduct efferent impulses to skeletal muscles (α axons) and others that carry afferent signals from muscle spindles (Ia axons) or from receptors sensitive to light touch of the skin (β axons). Smaller myelinated fibers conduct afferent impulses to control the lengths of the muscle spindles themselves (γ axons). Smaller myelinated fibers also efferently activate ganglia of the autonomic nervous system (B axons) or conduct afferent sensory information about joint position, skin cooling, or pain to the CNS (IB and δ axons). Among the nonmyelinated C fibers, the axons are either postganglionic elements of the efferent sympathetic nervous system or fibers conducting afferent sensory information about skin temperature or pain. This last modality, nociception, is coded by afferent impulses in both nonmyelinated C fibers and the smallest myelinated δ fibers.**

A common misconception among clinicians is to equate afferent impulse activity with sensation and efferent activity with motor functions, both somatic and visceral. However, afferent impulses are essential for posture, proprioception and coordinated motor performance, even though the information contained in such afferent discharges may be subliminal and not perceived as sensation. Efferent autonomic impulses may change peripheral conditions around cutaneous muscle, or joint endings of sensory fibers, for example by altering blood flow or by releasing substances that directly modify sensory endings, thereby modulating sensory signal processing.

A related error is the equation of small diameter fibers with "sensory" information and large diameter fibers with "motor" (somatic, skeletal muscle) activity. A simple reading of Table 56-1 will show how wrong this assumption is. These are important concepts in regional anesthesia, because the very desirable goal of a functionally selective nerve block will not be achieved simply by a differential blockade of impulses according to the size of fibers.

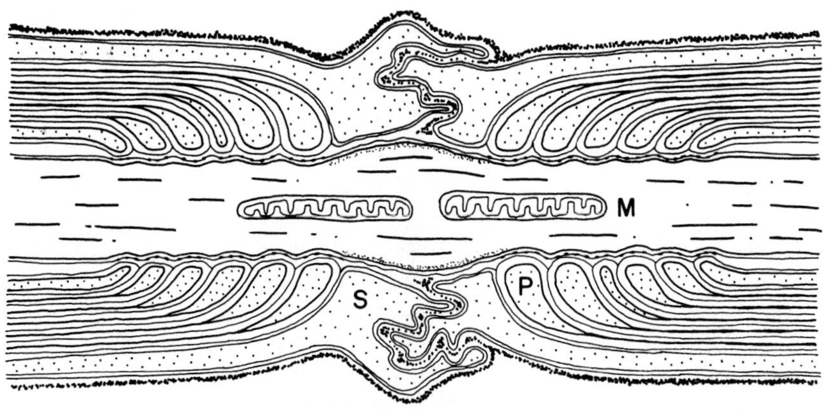

Fig. 56-2. Diagram of node of Ranvier shows mitochondria (M) in axoplasm, tight junctions of paranodal zone (P) where myelin abuts external axolemma, and Schwann cell (S) that surrounds axon, even at node. Hydrophilic pathways, filled with electron-dense nodal "gap substance," connect the perinodal space to bulk extracellular solution, providing a means for ions and polar drugs to reach node.

Table 56-1 Classification of axons in mammalian peripheral nerve

Fiber class	Subclass	Diameter (μ)	Myelin	Conduction velocity (m/s)	Location	Function
A	α	6–22	+	30–120	Efferent to muscles	Motor
I	a	10–22	+	50–100	Afferent from muscle spindles	Sensorimotor
A	β	6–22	+	30–120	Afferent from cutaneous joints	Tactile, proprioception
A	γ	3–6	+	15–35	Efferent to muscle spindles	Muscle tone
A	δ	1–4	+	5–25	Afferent sensory nerves	Pain, temperature, touch
B		< 3	+	3–15	Preganglionic autonomic	Various autonomic functions
C	sC	0.3–1.3	–	0.7–1.3	Postganglionic autonomic	Various autonomic functions
C	dC	0.4–1.2	–	0.1–2.0	Afferent sensory nerves	Pain, temperature

Despite the variety of anatomic structures and functional roles, the general electrophysiologic properties of individual axons derive from the same fundamental entities, the ion channels. These channels selectively permit the passage of different ions across the otherwise ion impermeable axolemma. Their behavior is described in detail in following sections, but at this point it is useful to note a key difference between myelinated and nonmyelinated axons. **The molecular properties of the ion channels are the same in each type of fiber, but their densities and spatial distributions differ. In mammalian myelinated fibers the sodium channels are restricted to the axon membrane at the node of Ranvier.** On the other hand, the voltage-sensitive potassium channels are present almost exclusively in the internodal regions of the axon, where they exert little influence on impulse propagation.[28,29,88] **In contrast, to the extent that they can be resolved spatially, both sodium and potassium channels are distributed uniformly along the axons of C fibers rather than being focused in particular locations.**[11] The structures of the surrounding cellular elements in peripheral nerves and the distributions of different ion channels influence both the rate of penetration and the overall impulse blocking action of local anesthetics.[117]

Bilayer Character of Nerve Membranes

The plasma membrane of nerve cells is a typical biologic membrane. Myelinated and nonmyelinated nerve fibers have axolemmae with the same general morphology, although the membrane has characteristic features in specialized regions, such as at sensory nerve endings, at nodes of Ranvier, and, notably, at the synapse.

The passive electrical properties of nerves arise directly from their intrinsic structure. First, all cell membranes are capacitors, electrical insulators between two conducting ionic solutions, and thus have the capability of storing electrical charge. The insulating portion of the membrane corresponds to the hydrocarbon "tails" of phospholipids that fill the core of the bilayer membrane. Charged and polar ends of the lipids at the membrane surfaces face the aqueous, ionic media. Capacitance is a function of both the width of the membranes and the dielectric constant of the material in the membrane interior. During a nerve impulse the capacitance varies by only 2%, providing evidence that the bilayer portion of the nerve membrane undergoes no major structural changes during nervous activity.

A second passive electrical property of nerves is the resting membrane ionic permeability. Resting ionic permeability is expressed in the unit of electrical conductance, the Sieman (S, which equals ohm^{-1}), and varies from nerve to nerve and also between different regions of the same nerve. The giant axon of the squid has a resting conductance of approximately 10^{-3} S · cm^{-2},[55] whereas the much smaller node of Ranvier in amphibian toad myelinated axons has 10-time greater resting conductance, 1 to 3 × 10^{-2} S · cm^{-2}.[29] In contrast, model bilayers formed only of phospholipids have much lower resting conductances, 10^{-8} to 10^{-7} S · cm^{-2}.[69–71] Lipids extracted from squid retinal axolemma can form bilayers of 10^{-7} S · cm^{-2} conductance, a value that is unchanged when the membrane potential varies from +120 to −120 mV.[126] The model bilayer values imply that neither resting nor active membrane conductance in nerves can be ascribed to pure phospholipid regions. When proteins are included in model phospholipid bilayers, the resting conductances greatly increase, from 10^{-8} S · cm^{-2} up to 10^{-3} to 10^{-5} S · cm^{-2}.[70,71] Proteins appear to account for almost all the membrane's ionic conductance, or permeability. Most ion channels are glycoproteins[19] with complex carbohydrates attached to the extracellular facing regions. Thus morphologic and electrical studies demonstrate that nerve membranes are mainly lipid bilayers encasing proteins, some of which permit ions to pass through a hydrocarbon interior of otherwise high resistance (Fig. 56-3).[105]

The lipid composition of the nerve membrane influences its structural and dynamic characteristics and modulates the activities of some of the intrinsic membrane channels and active transport and exchange "pumps." Membrane lipids may also regulate the rate of action and potency of various drugs, including local anesthetics.

Membranes are composed of phospholipids, other lipids (e.g., cerebrosides), cholesterol, proteins, and carbohydrates. Carbohydrates usually are conjugated to other compounds as proteins or lipids.[105] Protein accounts for more than 30% of the dry mass of nonmyelinated nerves, most of which is localized at the membrane surface and not within the hydrocarbon region. Cholesterol is interdigitated among the phospholipids and influences their behavior. Radiographic patterns of bilayers made only from phospholipids have been compared with those made from total lipid extract. The inclusion of cholesterol appears to increase the separation of polar lipid headgroups in the bilayer to that seen in the axolemma. Cholesterol also favors the parallel orientation of the fatty acid chains of phospholipids and increases the overall "degree of order" in the membrane, reducing the rotations of fatty acyl chains, particularly those of unsaturated lipids containing one or more double bond. The dynamics of lipids can effect the membrane partitioning

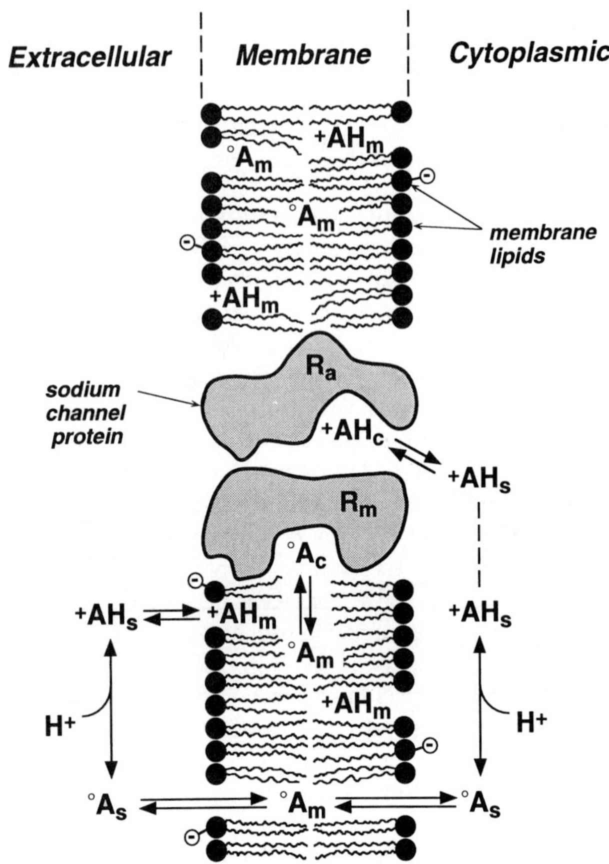

Fig. 56-3. Distribution of local anesthetics in nerve membrane. Anesthetics dissolved in extracellular and cytoplasmic aqueous solutions exist as neutral base (^0A_s) and protonated cations (^+AH_s). Both the charged form (^+AH_m) and the neutral form (^0A_m) partition into the membrane, but the latter accounts for almost all transmembrane diffusion of local anesthetic. Neutral anesthetic molecules may bind to sodium channels at a "membrane site" (R_m) via the membrane's hydrocarbon interior (^0A_c), whereas charged anesthetics may reach a site (R_a) in the polar pore of channel (^+AH_c). R_m and R_a may be the same site, or located closely to each other to permit rapid movement of anesthetic between them. Anesthetic molecules are adsorbed at the membrane-solution interface, where the protonated species (^+AH_m) can neutralize the charge on electrically negative phospholipids.

and permeability of local anesthetics as well as their access and orientation to target proteins within the membrane.

Despite their orderly alignment in the plane of the membrane, nerve lipids behave as fluid components within the membrane interior. "Fluidity" describes the rotational tumbling and the flexing of phospholipid fatty acyl groups, although there is also some lateral diffusion within the plane of the membrane and, at least in model membranes, transverse "flip-flop" of lipids from one side to the other. Phospholipid "tails" are most fluid and have the least orientation near the center of the hydrocarbon region. The fluidity decreases and orientation increases as the label is moved closer to the polar headgroup region of the lipids.[59] In other words, much more motion occurs in the center of a membrane than near the aqueous interface. This is of particular interest because local anesthetics appear to distribute in lipid bilayer membranes between the fatty acid core and the phospholipid headgroup region adjacent to extracellular and cytoplasmic solutions.[12]

PHYSIOLOGY OF PERIPHERAL NERVE

Ionic Basis of Impulse Propagation

Nerve impulses result from ion gradients and selective ionic permeability changes in nerve membranes. The gradients are literally "batteries" and the permeability changes are the "switches" that permit current to flow. A typical impulse, or action potential, in a nonmyelinated axon is shown in Fig. 56-4. **At rest, a membrane potential of approximately −60 mV exists, with the inside of the membrane being negative with respect to outside. During an action potential the inside of the nerve becomes less negative and for a brief period actually is more positive than the outside of the nerve. This depolarization is transient,** however, **and the membrane potential soon returns to the resting state.** In many nonmyelinated axons, including mammalian C fibers, a period of membrane hyperpolarization follows the impulse spike. During this period, which is often quite longer than the duration of the action potential, the membrane potential is more negative than at rest,[55] as shown in Fig. 56-4. In mammalian myelinated axons, however, this phase is small or absent, and the potential returns directly to the resting level from the peak depolarization.[29]

The shape of the action potential, the dynamic nature of threshold, and the refractory behavior of nerves can be explained in terms of the underlying changes in ionic permeability. As diagrammed in Fig. 56-4, the depolarization phase of the impulse is accompanied by an increase in Na^+ ion permeability (P_{Na}), whereas repolarization and the after-hyperpolarization are dominated by an increased K^+ permeability (P_K).[43] During the period of increased P_{Na}, Na^+ ions flow into the nerve, tending to depolarize it, and during increased P_K, potassium ions flow outward, tending to repolarize it. The net difference between the ionic currents carried by Na^+ and K^+ is a major factor that determines threshold behavior and impulse shape.

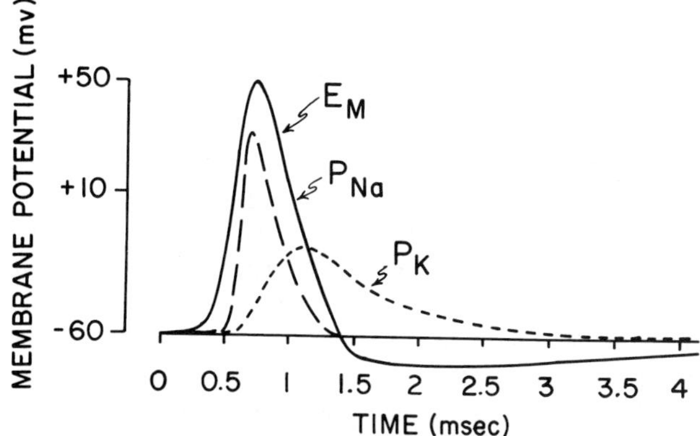

Fig. 56-4. Time course of membrane potential (E_m) and of potential-dependent sodium permeability (P_{Na}) and potassium permeability (P_K) changes during an action potential in the squid giant axon. (Modified from Hodgkin AL, Huxley AF: A quantitative description of membrane current and its application to conductance and excitation in nerve, *J Physiol (Lond)* 117:500, 1952)

Sodium Channels

The movement of ions through membranes requires the operation of discrete, pore-like structures, the ion channels (Fig. 56-3). The overall observed P_{Na} in a cell represents the summed opening and closing of many thousands of individual sodium channels. These sodium channels provide a selective pathway for passive ion transport of Na^+ down its electrochemical gradient. During one single impulse, however, very few Na^+ ions enter the nerve and the gradient of Na^+ concentration is changed little.

The term *channel* implies a structure that provides a defined pathway for ion transport when it is open. In contrast, an *ion carrier* shuttles back and forth carrying ions across the membrane. Sodium passes through the channels at rates of almost 10^7 ions per second, much faster than can be achieved by the fastest measured cation "carrier" molecules, which are limited to a few hundred crossings per second. The sodium channel may have several sites within its pore that interact with Na^+ ions during transport. The channel is not a long, water-filled tube through which hydrated ions diffuse as they would in free solution. Other monovalent cations can also permeate the Na^+ channel—Li^+ about as well as Na^+, K^+ about one tenth as well—but divalent cations such as Ca^{2+} and Mg^{2+} only permeate the channel about one hundredth as well or less. Associated with the surfaces of the channel molecules that interact with transported cations are various polar groups, at least two of which are negatively charged acidic groups. Low extracellular pH (e.g., 5.0) produces conditions that block Na^+ conductance by protonating these critical sites at the sodium channel pore.

Sodium channels have been solubilized from membranes, purified, and characterized biochemically. Channels from mammalian brain, peripheral nerve, and cardiac or skeletal muscle all appear to be composed of one large "alpha" glycoprotein with a molecular weight of 250,000 to 300,000 daltons,[7,24,46,68] which may or may not be conjugated to smaller "beta" subunit proteins with a molecular weight of 40,000 daltons.[71] The importance of the smaller subunit for mammalian tissue is unclear, because complete reconstruction of channel function can be accomplished with expression of the single, large polypeptide.[90,91] The smaller subunits do seem to be important for the efficient expression of functional channels in mammalian cells and, in many cases, actually modify the dynamics of channel closing during a depolarization.[94]

All sodium channels change configuration in response to membrane potential. Channels can exist in several different physical conformations broadly split into open (ion-conducting) or closed (nonconducting) states; the distribution between these states is a time-dependent function of the membrane potential. **Depolarizing potentials tend to open**

sodium channels, at least transiently, and hyperpolarizing potentials tend to close them.[56,102] This "voltage dependence" of membrane P_{Na} is the signal property on which regenerative action potentials depend.

The kinetics of transitions among different states of the sodium channels may be studied by holding the membrane at specified potentials (i.e., "voltage clamped"). When a typical nerve membrane is rapidly depolarized from the resting potential and held there, macroscopic sodium current (I_{Na}) follows the time course shown in Fig. 56-5*A*. An initial, rapid increase in I_{Na}, called activation, is followed by a slower, spontaneous decline, usually termed inactivation. If the size of the depolarizing test pulse is increased, both the peak I_{Na} and its rate of activation will increase as will its apparent rate of decline; thus its amplitude will increase but its overall duration will decrease. Finally, at large depolarizing potentials, P_{Na} reaches its maximal value and is not changed by larger depolarizing steps.

The molecular basis for this macroscopic permeability change is illustrated in Figure 56-5*B*.The membrane contains a finite number of sodium channels. When the channels open they each carry a constant inward current, implying that their unit permeability, or the equivalent "conductance," does not change its value during the open period.[101] Single channel kinetic behavior is described by three parameters: the time from depolarization to the first opening (the "activation" rate), the time during which the channel remains open (the "open time"), and the probability of opening more than once ("reactivation"). Both the probability of channel opening and the rate of opening, or activation rate, are greater for larger membrane depolarizations. However, for a sufficiently large depolarization, all the channels will be opened and the maximal P_{Na} will be reached in the shortest possible time. For some of the depolarizations shown in Fig. 56-5*B*, no channel opening occurs. This reflects the probabilistic nature of channel gating. Such nonopenings occur more frequently in membranes exposed to local anesthetics.

Sodium channels also have the ability to close sponta-

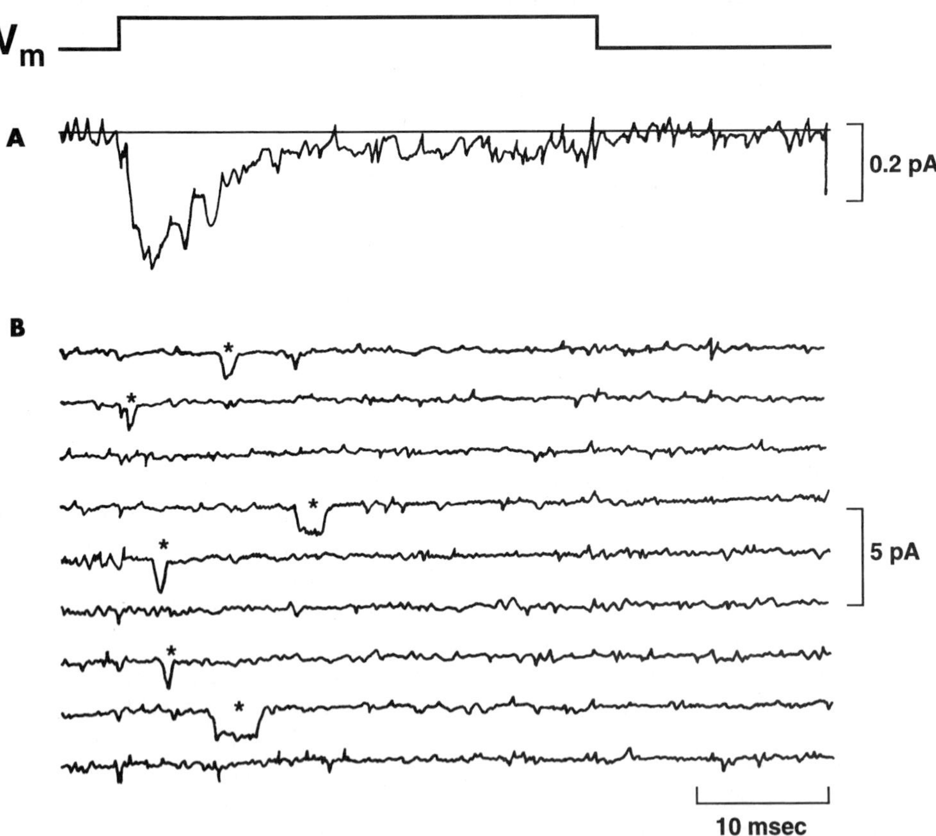

Fig. 56-5. The unitary basis for the transient rise in P_{Na} during membrane depolarization (V_m) to + 10 mV. A patch of skeletal muscle membrane containing one functional Na^+ channel was isolated by patch pipette and voltage clamped. **A,** The sum of the inward current through the Na^+ channel in the patch from 300 trial depolarizations (K^+ channels were blocked with tetraethylammonium and capacitive current was subtracted electronically). **B,** Nine individual trials from the set of 300 showing six individual Na^+ channel openings (asterisks). These data now show how the macroscopic Na^+ permeability change (see Fig. 56-4) is composed of the all-or-none opening and closing of individual Na^+ channels. (From Sigworth FJ, Neher E: Single Na^+ channel currents observed in cultured rat muscle cells, *Nature* 287:447, 1980.)

neously ("inactivate") during depolarization, resulting in only a transient increase in P_{Na} (Fig. 56-5*A*). At the single channel level, this means that channels rarely reactivate, particularly at membrane potentials less negative than −50 mV. The likelihood and rate of inactivation, however, depend on the metabolic state of the cell and are influenced by subunit interactions within the Na^+ channel, by phosphorylation of the alpha subunit, and by drugs, such as local anesthetics, as described below. Activation and inactivation processes represent sequential steps in the voltage-dependent opening of sodium channels and some of the early stages of activation must proceed before inactivation can occur.

A simple kinetic scheme is helpful in describing the time course of P_{Na} (Fig. 56-6). The states denoted by letters symbolize different conformations of the sodium channel macromolecule. At rest the channels are distributed almost exclusively between the two types of nonconducting states, R and I. The letter R denotes closed channels, favored by resting potentials and hyperpolarized membrane potentials; I denotes inactivated channels, in a conformation favored at depolarized membrane potentials. Upon depolarization, the channels proceed through several intermediate closed states (not drawn in Fig. 56-6) to O, the open, ion conducting state, then to I. This accounts for the transient nature of P_{Na}.

Changes in the distribution of channels among the various states occur in response to depolarization because the channel molecules have electrical charges or dipoles as part of their structure. Therefore these molecules move in response to the force from the membrane's electrical field, migrating from one surface to another and thereby opening the pathway for ion transport. At the resting potential the conformational steps that lead from R to O occur very infrequently. During depolarizations the steps occur more frequently, as the force of the membranes' electric field on the charged gating portion of the channel is great.

Another pathway between R and I is shown by the dashed line in Fig. 56-6. This line implies a reaction between closed and inactivated channels that can occur near the resting potential without passing through an open state. The equilibrium between R and I is dependent on the resting potential and also on channel phosphorylation; it is also susceptible to various drugs.

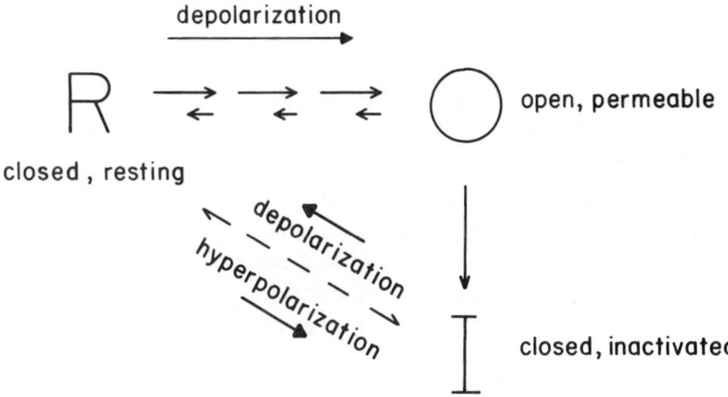

Fig. 56-6. A simple, three-state kinetic scheme for sodium channels that accounts for time course of P_{Na}. P_{Na} is proportional to number of open (O) channels; activation correspond to R → O transitions; inactivation to O → I transitions. Slow relaxations between R and I can also occur without channels entering the O state.

The molecular structures of many Na^+ channels are known, and the similarities among them and their relationship to other voltage-gated ion channels of known structure tells which parts of the alpha subunit can be assigned to different channel functions. Regions of the channel molecule located at some distance from the pore are responsible for sensing the membrane potential and activating and inactivating the channels. These regions contain highly charged or dipolar segments of amino acids that move in response to the electrical field in the membrane. Such activation gating corresponds to a translation of some of the charges all the way across the membrane as a channel becomes activated. The direct result of these molecular rearrangements is that a very small capacitative current flows.[2] Such gating current reflects the molecular conformational changes in sodium channels as they open during activation. The time course of the gating currents has been compared with that for the opening and the inactivation of channels in efforts to better understand the molecular steps for channel gating. Most charge moves during the latent period just following depolarization before the channel actually opens; it appears that several distinct closed states are populated before the final closed state is reached, and that there is no charge movement during the O to I transition. Further, inactivated channels can still contribute gating charge, but at a reduced level and, particularly, lacking the later components. It seems that the channel starts to activate in the normal way, but becomes stuck in an intermediate closed conformation.

Measurements of the currents flowing through single open sodium channels have shown that open channels have a single permeability value, which confirms the porelike mechanism.[56,101] A channel appears to have one or perhaps two open configurations and several closed and inactivated configurations. Inactivated states are favored by prolonged membrane depolarization. When a channel is inactivated, it cannot open in response to further depolarization. Because channels are either entirely open or entirely closed, the time course of P_{Na} (e.g., as shown in Fig. 56-5A) illustrates the fraction of sodium channels open during a prolonged depolarization and not a variable permeability of individual channels.

Biochemical analysis and site-directed mutagenesis have revealed a picture of the Na^+ channel as a complex, internally interactive macromolecule[22,24] (Fig. 56-7). **There are four similar domains (I to IV) of amino acids, each of which contains six alpha helical segments that span the width of the membrane plus a short, nonhelical loop that passes about halfway across and then returns.** By changing specific amino acids in the primary sequence, investigators have been able to deduce important relationships between these structures and the channel's functions.

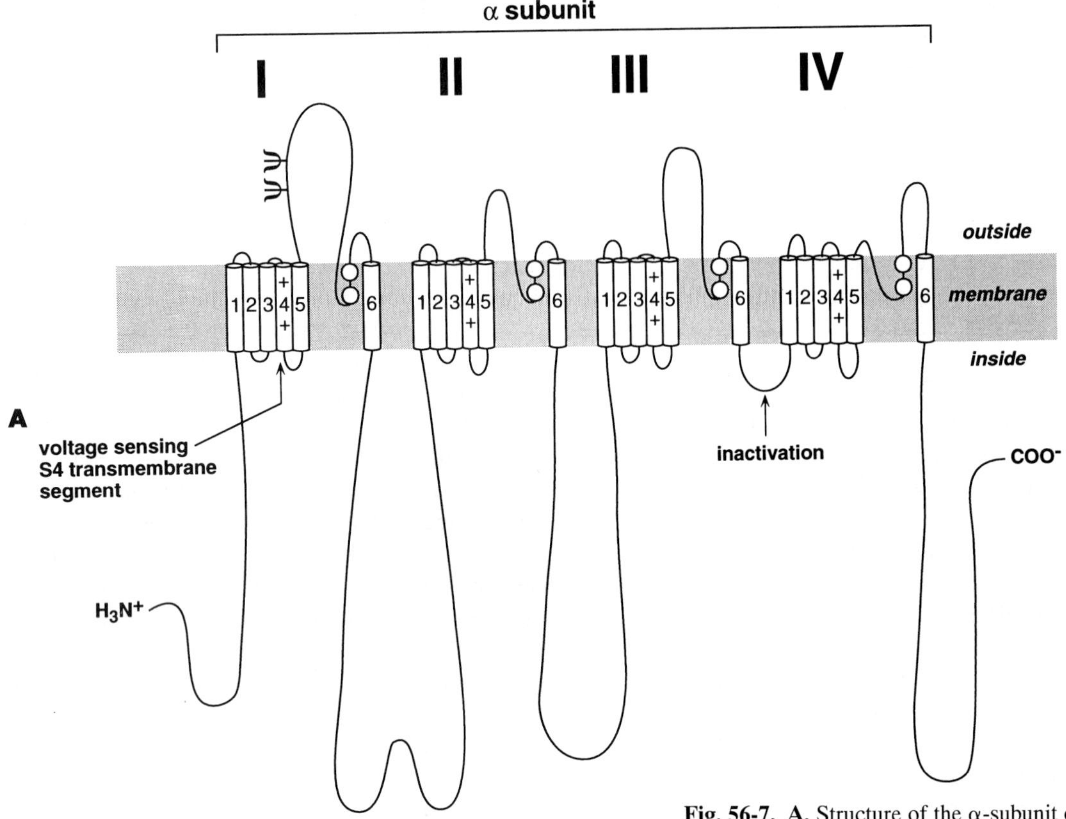

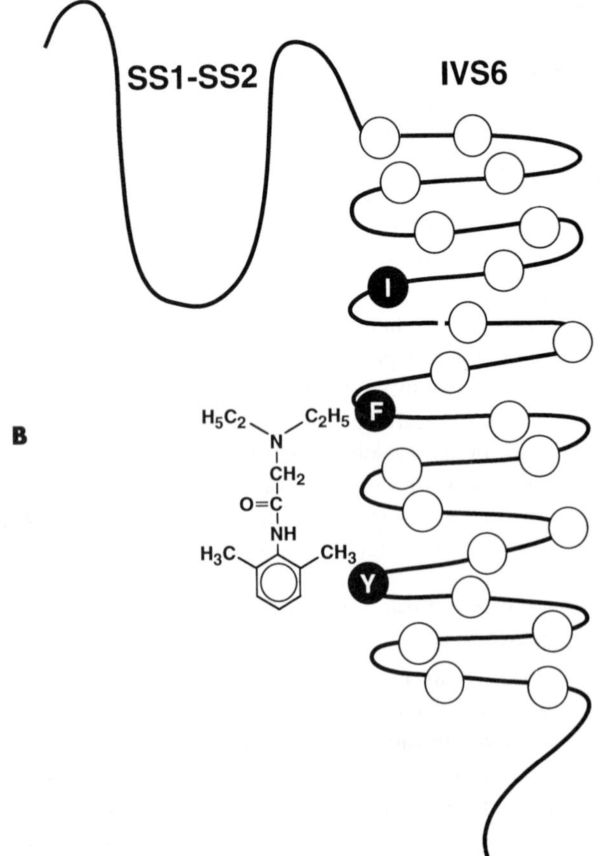

Fig. 56-7. A, Structure of the α-subunit of the sodium channel. The polypeptide chains are represented by continuous lines and the cylinders represent regions where the protein consists of transmembrane α helices. Ψ indicates sites of glycosylation by acidic sugars carrying negative charges. The repeated form and function of the four homologous domains (I through IV) of the α subunit is implied by their structural similarity. **Activation Gating.** The 4th transmembrane segments (S4) in each homologous domain act as voltage sensors. (+) symbols represent the positively charged amino acid residues within these segments. The membrane potential-associated electrical field exerts a force on these charged amino acid residues, pulling them toward the intracellular side of the membrane at rest and pushing them outwards at depolarizing potentials. **Pore.** The S5 and S6 transmembrane segments, of the four domains and the short membrane-associated loops between them (see panel B, segments SS1 and SS2), fold together to form the surface lining the pore of the channel. **Inactivation.** The short intracellular loop connecting homologous domains III and IV serves as the rapid inactivation gate of the Na^+ channel. It presumably folds into the intracellular mouth of the pore and occludes it after the channel opens. Activation gating does not proceed completely once inactivation has occurred. **B,** One part of the local anesthetic receptor site. Transmembrane segment S6 in domain IV (IVS6) is illustrated as an α helix, along with adjacent short segments SS1 and SS2 that contribute to formation of the channel's extracellular opening. Each circle represents an amino acid residue in segment IVS6. Three residues critical for local anesthetic binding are denoted by filled circles. The local anesthetic lidocaine is shown bound to two of these residues, phenylalanine (F) and tyrosine (Y). The third residue is isoleucine (I). Substitution by site-directed mutagenesis of a smaller alanine residue for isoleucine allows local anesthetics to reach their receptor site from outside the membrane. This residue therefore is assumed to form the outer boundary of the receptor site (see Ragsdale et al., 1994), which is normally not directly accessible from the extracellular solution.

One helical segment (S4) in each of the domains (four in all) carries many positive charges and appears to be the portion that senses depolarization[113] and moves across the membrane to activate channel opening.[67,128] A short cytoplasmic segment that connects domains III and IV is important for inactivation.[118] Apparently, it interacts with the channel when activation has occurred to prevent further conformational changes. The short nonhelical segment, or *P* region, of each domain forms a loop that extends part way into the membrane. When all four domains are circled into a cylindrical complex these *P* regions are at its center and together they act as the lining of the channel pore.

Parts of helical segments S5 and S6 appear to form an inner vestibule of the channel, a kind of funnel at the cytoplasmic approach to the narrow end of the pore. Changes in this region of the protein on domain IV yield dramatic changes in local anesthetic blockade (Fig. 56-7B), indicating its importance in the binding of these drugs,[78] as described below.

Several drugs and chemical reactions modify sodium channel inactivation. Treatment of the internal surface of the axon membrane by proteolytic enzymes or reagents prevents channel inactivation from occurring. Certain animal and plant toxins and some oxidizing chemicals applied to the outside of axon membranes also inhibit inactivation.[23,120–122] In addition, increasing external divalent cations (e.g., Ca^{2+}) modifies the voltage dependence of both the activation and the inactivation reactions. This occurs because the divalent cations associate with certain negative charges fixed to the outer surface and make the external interfacial potential less negative, as described later.[54]

Other drugs increase the probability of opening sodium channels. These include very lipophilic compounds, such as the frog neurotoxin batrachotoxin and the steroidal alkaloid veratridine, which are termed *activators.*[22,23,79,116] Another lipophilic compound, tetrahydrocannabinol, which is a psychoactive ingredient of marijuana, selectively inhibits activation.[107] These studies suggest that activation is altered by more hydrophobic compounds and inactivation by more hydrophilic compounds. This, in turn, implies that activation reactions correspond to structures deeper in the membrane's core, whereas inactivation reactions are more superficially located. However, this relationship is not perfect, because it has been shown that two structurally homologous polypeptide toxins isolated from scorpion venom, acting from the extracellular channel surface, modify gating in opposite ways; one specifically affects inactivation, whereas the other specifically alters activation.[108,123] The sodium channel macromolecule probably operates in an integrated manner with many regions changing during the different phases of the action potential.[24]

Resting Membrane Potential

An ionic pump coupled to Na^+-K^+ adenosine triphosphatase (ATPase) creates concentration gradients of Na^+ and K^+ ions. Ionic sodium is concentrated outside the cell and ionic potassium inside. Because of the selective permeability of the resting membrane to potassium, a very small number of positively charged K^+ ions diffuse out of the cell, leaving the inside electrically negative and making the outside electrically positive. Thus part of the resting potential results from K^+ ions diffusing down their concentration gradient.

If only K^+ ions were permeant, the resting potential would always equal the Nernst potential for K^+. However, other ions, including Na^+, also permeate the resting membrane, and the resting potential of nerves is usually 10 to 20 mV more positive than the K^+ Nernst potential. This nonequilibrium resting membrane potential is insufficient to prevent the diffusion of either ion, and as a result Na^+ enters and K^+ leaves the cell at rest. These processes occur much faster during impulse activity. Following membrane activation, the active transport of Na^+ and K^+, driven by the Na^+-K^+-ATPase pump, restores and maintains these ion gradients[85] (Fig. 56-8). This active transport requires energy, which is supplied as ATP. The rate of ion transport by the ATPase is determined largely by the intracellular Na^+ concentration. This concentration can increase significantly in axons, particularly those of small diameter, during a train of high-frequency impulses. Thus Na^+ ions act as substrates for transport and, by the same mechanism, catalyze the hydrolysis of ATP in the overall transport reaction.

Further, all Na^+-K^+-ATPases extrude more Na^+ ions than K^+ ions taken in for each ATP molecule hydrolyzed. This ionic imbalance means that during active transport of ions, a net ionic current flowing outward occurs across the cell membrane, a current that makes the resting membrane potential become more negative. Such a state persists until sufficient Na^+ is removed from the cell's interior to slow ion transport, reducing the associated pump current and the attendant hyperpolarization.[85] Thus, by activating electrogenic sodium-potassium transport, the impulse-dependent changes in ionic concentration slow or prevent further impulse activity. This provides an important mechanism for the maintenance of impulse transmission and for the control of firing frequencies during trains of action potentials, particularly in small-diameter nerve fibers.

Relationship of Ionic Currents to Membrane Action Potential

The concept of current flow through ion-selective, time-dependent, voltage-dependent channels explains the shape of the action potential. Once a depolarizing stimulus has opened sufficient sodium channels, the rate of membrane depolarization accelerates. During this rapid upswing the interplay among net inward current, depolarization, and the voltage-dependent P_{Na} constitutes a tightly coupled, positive feedback system. Near the peak of the action potential the rate of depolarization slows because of three reasons: (1)

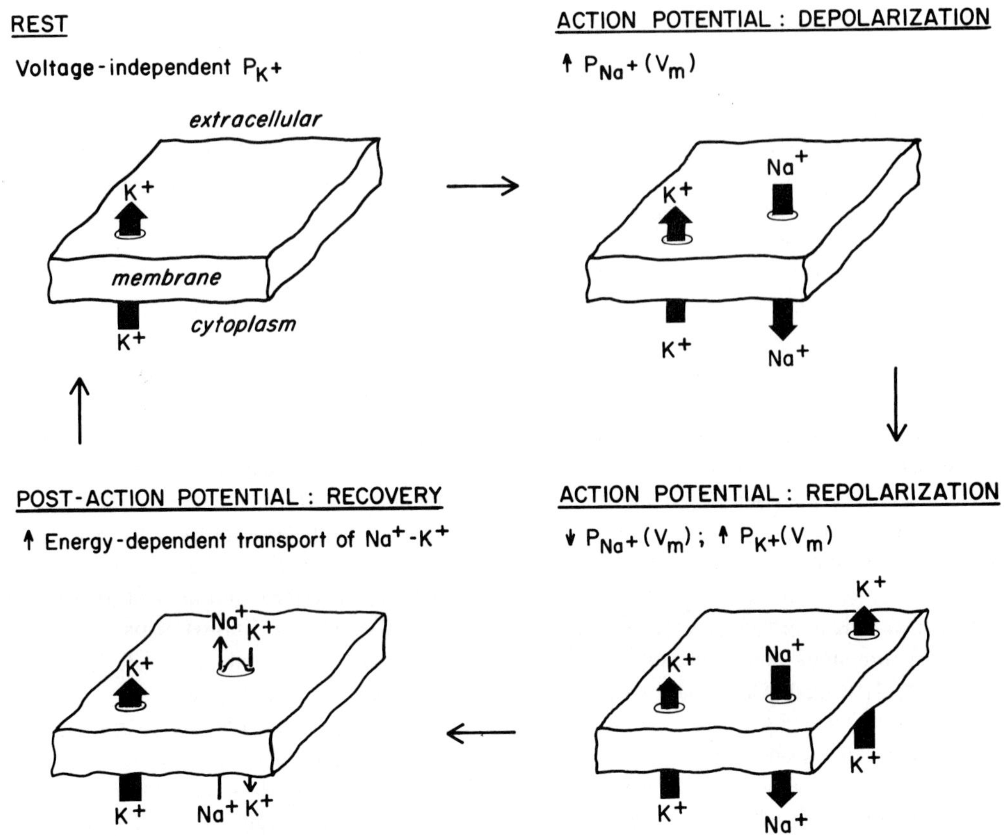

Fig. 56-8. Ionic currents during different phases of the nerve impulse. Clockwise, from upper left: at rest, selective permeability to K^+ accounts for negative resting membrane potential. Some Na^+ also enters cell, but basal activity of Na^+-K^+ pump counters the tendency of these fluxes to deplete ionic gradients. At the rising, depolarizing phase of the impulse, a large increase in voltage-dependent sodium permeability (P_{Na}) subserves an inrush of Na^+ ions. Repolarization of the action potential is accompanied by reduced P_{Na} and an increase in voltage-dependent potassium permeability (P_K), resulting in a net outflow of ionic current. Following the impulse, small increases in Na^+ and K^+ concentration inside and outside the membrane, respectively, stimulate the Na^+-K^+ pump, which thus accelerates pumping of ions to rapidly restore the conditions to those at rest.

the membrane potential approaches the Nernst potential for Na^+, so the electrochemical force driving inward Na^+ current is reduced; (2) the P_{Na} slowly inactivates, also reducing Na^+ current; and (3) the K^+ current grows, both because its electrochemical driving force increases, as the membrane potential moves away from the Nernst potential for K^+, and because the P_K slowly activates.

Eventually these factors lead to a reversal in the direction of the membrane current, from inward to outward, and the membrane repolarizes. The fast rate of repolarization (Fig. 56-4) corresponds to the largest outward current, as P_K reaches its maximal value. As the membrane repolarizes to its resting value or below (1) the effects of the action potential depolarization on activated and inactivated ion permeabilities are eventually reversed, (2) the Na^+-K^+-ATPase pump responds to the altered ion concentrations, and (3) the conditions initially present before the impulse are restored. Although impulse initiation is electrically complete within a few milliseconds, the restoration of initial ionic conditions may require minutes or even hours following long bursts of repetitive discharges.

Membrane Threshold

That point in the process of depolarization when continued stimulation is no longer needed and local processes can lead to a complete action potential is termed *threshold.* Achieving threshold leads to a state in which the balance of ionic current changes from being net outward to net inward. At rest the membrane is permeable to ions carrying leakage currents and to K^+ ions, but is almost impermeable to Na^+ ions. Small applied depolarizations, insufficient to produce an impulse, result both in a net outward current carried primarily by K^+ ions and in the activation of some sodium channels, which conduct a small inward current. However, the net membrane ionic current is outward, and the membrane will repolarize when the stimulus ceases. In contrast, when a sufficiently large stimulus is offered to the membrane, the inward Na^+ currents will exceed the sum of the outward K^+ and leakage currents, resulting in a net inward current that depolarizes the membrane. The point when the balance of stimulated ionic currents reverses from outward to inward, from those that repolarize to those that depolarizing, is the impulse firing threshold of the axon.

Threshold is not some constant value of the membrane potential but rather is a condition of the membrane. This is clear from the kinetics of P_{Na} and P_K. Both permeabilities require a finite time to activate, and, in addition, P_{Na} will slowly inactivate. For example, application of a large depolarizing stimulus to the nerve membrane for a period much briefer than the activation time for P_{Na} does not allow sufficient time for Na^+ channels to open; thus no net inward current would occur, and no impulse would be generated. On the other hand, if the membrane potential is changed very slowly to the same value, such that only a fraction of the Na^+ channels are open at any time (and these then inactivate) and K^+ channels activate and stay open, no net inward current will exist and no action potential will occur. This phenomenon is called *accommodation*. In contrast, if the rate and degree of the depolarizing stimulus are sufficient, often several impulses can be generated. Clearly the threshold for impulse firing depends on the shape of the stimulus and the history of membrane activity and is not equal to any constant, specified membrane potential.

The threshold can be modified by impulse activity and by drugs. Following a stimulus, the threshold changes because the P_{Na} and P_K are altered and require time to return to their resting states. P_K is initially increased, conducting a greater outward current than at rest. P_{Na} has a bimodal response to constant membrane depolarization. It is first rapidly activated but then becomes inactivated, being converted to a state from which further depolarization cannot activate it (Fig. 56-6).

Inactivation occurs more slowly than activation (see previous discussion and Fig. 56-5*B*). Immediately after an impulse many of the sodium channels are inactivated and a stimulated depolarization can produce little inward current. At these times, no membrane potential exists for which inward exceeds outward current, and the membrane is absolutely refractory to initiation of a second impulse. In a few milliseconds in the repolarized membrane, (1) the inactivation of sodium channels is somewhat reversed, (2) the elevated P_K falls toward its resting value, and (3) the membrane passes through a relative refractory period, with the membrane threshold returning to its previous resting value.

Further, during the very brief period immediately after one impulse (0.5 to 1 second), the threshold is actually lower than during the resting state (superexcitability), whereas sustained repetitive impulse activity leads to long periods of elevated threshold that persist for tens of minutes (depression).[80] Although the mechanisms responsible for these threshold changes are unknown, they are important factors in shaping axonal firing patterns. Importantly for this chapter, these patterns in turn modulate the effects of local anesthetics.

Impulse Propagation and Conduction Safety

A final consideration of axon electrophysiology is the propagation of impulses along the fiber. **The conservation of electrical charge requires that essentially all the ionic current entering a region of the nerve membrane must flow in a closed circuit back to its source. Thus the large inward current at a zone being depolarized by an impulse's rising phase must flow outward from the axon at other regions. The impulse sustains its own propagation because these local circuit currents act in the zone adjacent to the active membrane to lead a propagating wave of excitability** (Fig. 56-9).

Such a local circuit current provides sufficient charge to depolarize the adjacent, previously unexcited segment of membrane to threshold. This process occurs continuously along a nerve fiber. Even in a myelinated axon with far-spaced excitable membranes at the nodes of Ranvier, the current from one excited node spreads sufficiently to excite about five adjacent nodes. **The different phases of the action potential occur over a relatively long distance (about 10 cm) in the largest nerve fibers. The resulting local circuit current can bypass a length of inexcitable axon of several centimeters and still excite the membrane beyond, with impulse propagation reappearing beyond the inexcitable axon segment. For this reason a sufficient length of nerve must be exposed to local anesthetic agents in order to produce a blockade of propagated action potentials.**[32,82]

Normally, small reductions in current or permeability cannot prevent impulse propagation. For example, impulses still travel in a myelinated nerve that has more than half its sodium channels blocked, although the impulses are smaller and conducted more slowly.[95] However, some structural features of axons are associated with a lower margin of safety for impulse propagation. One notable example is the point where an axon branches and the total membrane area of the branches exceeds that of the parent axon. The local circuit current from an impulse traveling in the parent axon must divide at the branch point. If branches are unequal in size, the larger branch receives more of the local circuit current, because its resistance to entering current is lower. Sometimes the current partitioned to one of the axon branches is not sufficient to reach threshold, and the impulse only propagates along the other branch.[125] Bursts of high-frequency impulses may change the threshold properties of different branches in modest ways so that some impulses in the burst invade one axon, some the other axon, and some invade neither.[80]

Such processes may provide subtle forms of neuronal signal coding, an activity usually assigned to synaptic integration. Since branch points are often regions of lower con-

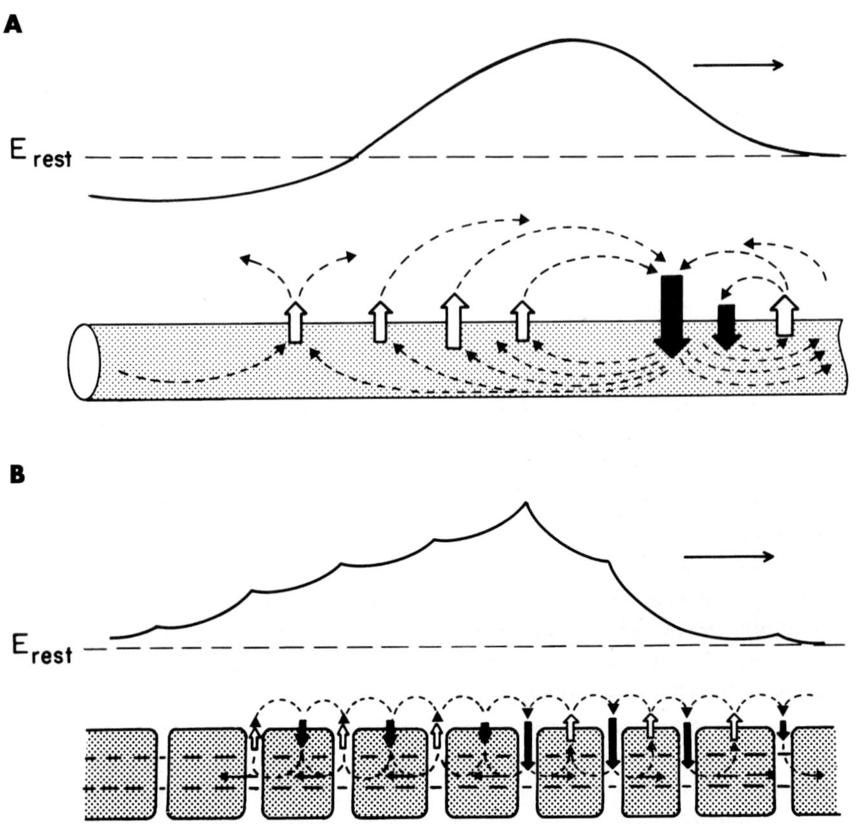

Fig. 56-9. Spatial distribution of membrane potential and corresponding membrane currents during propagation of action potential in a nonmyelinated (A) and a myelinated (B) axon. Filled arrows show net inward current, which depolarizes membrane from the resting potential (E_{rest}). Open arrows show net outward current, which repolarizes it. In nonmyelinated fiber, outward current after impulse is large enough to hyperpolarize membrane. Dashed lines indicate direction of longitudinal current carried by ions inside and outside axon. Note that active ionic current in myelinated nerve occurs only at nodes of Ranvier; current through myelinated internodes is capacitive in nature and not caused by ion translocation through membrane. Nevertheless, membrane potential changes continuously along entire fiber. Morphologic diagrams are not drawn to scale.

duction safety, they are more easily blocked pharmacologically than the unbranched extensions of axons.

MECHANISMS OF ACTION OF LOCAL ANESTHETICS

Various theories have been proposed to explain conduction blockade by local anesthetics. Original theories involved direct effects of local anesthetics on the membrane's lipid bilayer, either by an electrostatic interaction with negative electrical charges fixed on the surface of the nerve membrane (e.g., the Ca^{2+} displacement hypothesis[40]) or by causing an expansion of the bulk membrane, thereby interfering with normal channel functions (e.g., the membrane perturbation hypothesis[98]). These theories have found little experimental support over the past two decades. In recent years, most investigators have adopted on the hypothesis that local anesthetics exert a direct action on sodium channels.[114]

Effects of Local Anesthetics on Sodium Channels

Two general theories have been proposed to explain the action of local anesthetics on sodium channels: local anesthetics may cause a general perturbation of the bulk membrane structure, which results in a modulation of channel function,[64,98] or have a direct effect at specific binding sites ("receptors") in the sodium channel.[104] Most recent findings support the specific receptor hypothesis. Nevertheless, local membrane perturbation may provide part of the explanation for anesthetic actions. Also, it is doubtful that local anesthetic action can be accounted for solely in terms of an action at only one classic receptor site.[109]

Use-Dependent Inhibition

One aspect of local anesthetic action strongly suggests direct and specific interactions between anesthetic molecules and sodium channels. During brief membrane depolarizations repeated at high frequency (5 to 100 Hz), the degree of P_{Na} inhibition by local anesthetics increases. When the membrane is returned to the resting condition, the inhibition returns to its original level. This phenomenon, called *use-dependence,* is a characteristic feature of local anesthetics.[33,53]

Two separate features of local anesthetic action that underlie use-dependent block are evident from voltage-clamp experiments. First, channels are inhibited most effectively by charged anesthetics when the pattern of applied membrane potential sequentially opens and closes the sodium channel.[33,37,51,104,106] Once a channel opens, an anesthetic molecule appears to enter it and prevents the passage of Na^+ ions through it. The channel, however, can close with the anesthetic still bound within it. In this case a charged anesthetic dissociates only very slowly from the closed channel.[25] When the channel is reopened, the charged anesthetic may then leave more easily.[26,104]

Uncharged nonpolar anesthetic molecules may gain access to the receptor site even when the channel is closed.[51,52] Use-dependence is greatest when charged anesthetic molecules bind rapidly to sites accessible in open channels and dissociate slowly from these sites in closed channels. By contrast, uncharged, nonpolar anesthetics may rapidly leave closed channels, perhaps because their dissociation is not limited to the aqueous ion pathway of the channel. Because of this rapid unbinding, these molecules produce considerably less use-dependent blockade.[34,36,37,77] However, the potency of such hydrophobic drugs suggests that a portion of the channel separate from its ion permeation pathway may be one site that binds local anesthetics.[37,58,106]

The second feature of local anesthetic block that indicates a direct interaction with sodium channels is a change in the sodium inactivation process. When a membrane is exposed to local anesthetics, larger membrane hyperpolarizations are required to relieve the apparent inactivation. In other words, more energy is necessary to shift the channels from the I to the R state (Fig. 56-6).[51] This apparent shift in the R/I distribution at rest increases with increasing drug concentration as well as during use-dependent inhibition.[33,34] As with reduction of P_{Na}, the shift towards inactivation requires open channels for charged local anesthetics but occurs through closed channels when neutral drug molecules are present. The overall effect is complex when tertiary amine local anesthetics are used, as they are rapidly protonated and deprotonated between the charged and neutral forms of the molecule (see below). Local anesthetics induce a dynamic shift of sodium channels toward the inactivated state; the greater the binding of drug, the greater this shift.[4]

When Na^+ channels are partially digested by intracellular proteases, use-dependent block by many local anesthetics disappears.[17,130] Such treatment also removes inactivation, suggesting that local anesthetics bind to inactivated forms of the channel and thus stabilize those nonconducting configurations. If channel inactivation is prevented instead by agents that do not digest proteins, then use-dependent block persists.[20,111,124] Therefore, use-dependent inhibition requires the presence of a part of the channel that can be enzymatically degraded from the cytoplasmic surface. Modifications of inactivation by nondestructive methods do not modify this site. The tonic inhibition by local anesthetics of channels in resting membranes is minimally altered by either of these treatments. This suggests that block of resting channels is modulated by factors different than the ones involved in use-dependent block.[3,6,26,109,111]

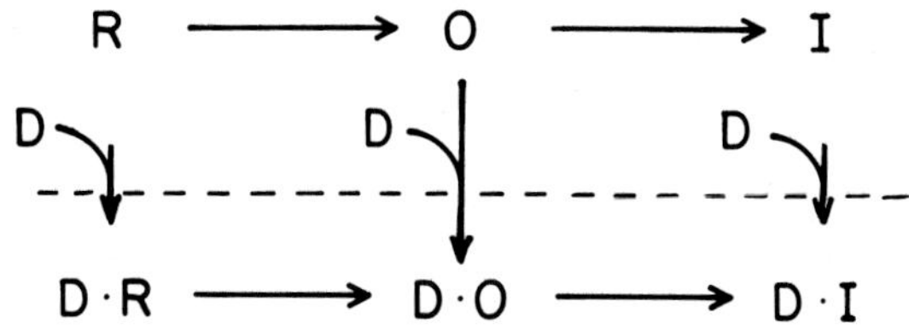

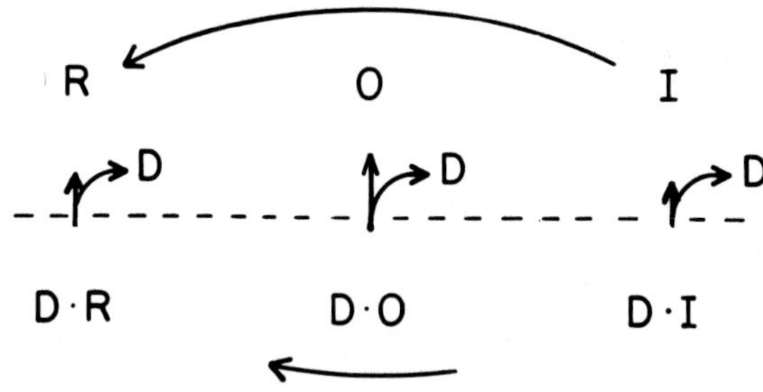

Fig. 56-10. Version of modulated receptor model explains both tonic and use-dependent block by local anesthetics. Normal channel gating is shown above dashed line (Fig. 56-7); gating of anesthetic-bound channels is shown below. **A,** Membrane depolarization induces formation of open (O) and inactivated (I) channel states that bind anesthetic molecules (D) more tightly than does resting state (R). **B,** During repolarization, drug dissociation is slow, as is conversion of inactivated to resting states in drug-bound channels. Repetitive depolarizations result in incremental accumulation of channels in D · I form, thus modeling use-dependent block. (Modified from Courtney KR: Mechanism of frequency-dependent inhibition of sodium currents in frog myelinated nerve by the lidocaine derivative GEA-968, *J Pharmacol Exp Ther* 195:225, 1975, and Hille B: Local anesthetics: hydrophilic and hydrophobic pathways for the drug-receptor reaction, *J Gen Physiol* 60:497, 1977.)

Modulated Receptor Hypothesis

All the observations just described have been integrated into a modulated receptor hypothesis.[16,51] This model of the sodium channel blockade incorporates a local anesthetic binding site with state-dependent affinity for the drug that can be altered indirectly by membrane potential. The latter process involves a voltage-dependent conformational change of the channel and may also include a direct effect of voltage on the binding reaction *per se*.[104] Channel gating is simplified by consideration of only three states: resting, open, and inactivated (Fig. 56-10). Anesthetic molecules, denoted by the letter D, bind with higher affinity to the O and the I state, populated by depolarization, than to the R state that is prevalent at rest. Reversal of this binding reaction during the period between depolarizing pulses is slower than the normal recovery from inactivation, leading to an accumulation of channels in the D · I or D · O states and thus simulating use-dependence.[25] Binding to O is faster than to I, but dissociation at the resting potential is equally fast, regardless of the state that originally bound the drug. Some binding of anesthetic molecules to resting channels does occur, however, and cannot be antagonized completely by membrane hyperpolarization, even though this usually completely relieves channel inactivation. The implication is that resting channels have a detectable affinity for local anesthetics.

Nature of the Local Anesthetic Binding Site

The structural and chemical features that favor the use-dependent inhibition by a drug differ from those favoring the resting, or tonic, inhibition.[37,129] Hydrophobic and neutral drugs are more potent in producing tonic block than are very polar or charged compounds.[9,97] Conversely, use-dependent inhibition is more readily produced by the polar and charged drugs.[16,34,52,99] At neutral or slightly acid extracellular pH, which favors the protonated drug species, the tertiary amine anesthetics produce a much larger use-dependent inhibition than when the extracellular pH is alkaline,[26,42] but have a lower tonic inhibition that occurs more slowly after the drug is added to the nerve.[52]

Two different explanations can account for these observations. The first proposes that a single, common receptor exists for both charged and neutral local anesthetics.[44,53] The receptor is only accessible to charged drug molecules that pass from the cytoplasm through the hydrophilic pore of the channel. However, the receptor can be reached by neutral molecules from either the cytoplasm or from the membrane lipid interior by a hydrophobic pathway (Fig. 56-3).[51] Because anesthetics at the binding site can be protonated from the external solution but not from the cytoplasmic solution, the receptor appears to be located near the outer end of the channel. Thus, lowering the extracellular pH protonates tertiary amine anesthetic molecules and locks them into the receptor site, limiting their dissociation route to the hydrophilic pathway. The hydrophilic pathway, designated for charged molecules, restricts drug diffusion and results in slow rates of anesthetic binding and dissociation and therefore in a significant use-dependence, even at low frequencies. In contrast, the hydrophobic pathway, accessible only to uncharged molecules, but equally available in closed and open channels, allows the anesthetic binding reaction to reverse rapidly between depolarizations and so sustains little use-dependent block.

The second explanation postulates that neutral and charged drugs have separate, distinct modes of action and separate corresponding binding sites.[16,65] For example, neutral drugs may distribute in the membrane interior and disrupt channel function through some generalized perturbation that does not require actual binding to the channel[47,64] and a specific, receptor-mediated action. Consequently, channels are less likely to open during a depolarization but can be recruited to an "activatable" closed state by large hyperpolarizations. In this regard, they behave like normal inactivated channels.[6,18,19] On the other hand, charged drugs may act at a specific site in the channel, where their binding produces changes that can be very similar to or quite different from those accompanying normal channel inactivation.[20]

These two models differ in detail, but they both contain a component in which channel gating leads to modified anesthetic binding and such binding acts reciprocally to modulate channel gating. This modulated receptor hypothesis is a concept of wide general application, extending to the actions of many drugs that affect ion channels.

Active Form of Local Anesthetics

The classic, lipid-soluble, tertiary amine anesthetics are distributed throughout all the separate phases of the nerve at equilibrium. Because they are weak bases with both hydrophobic and hydrophilic properties, anesthetic molecules are found as both protonated and neutral species in the aqueous interstitial and cytoplasmic compartments, and primarily as the uncharged base within the membrane lipid[12,38] (Fig. 56-3). The molecular distribution within the membrane further depends on both the lipid solubility of the anesthetic,[15] usually expressed in terms of the oil/water or octanol/water partition coefficient,[110] and on the molecule's polar regions and net charge.[93]

The presence of drug in both solutions and the membrane raises two fundamental questions regarding the active amine local anesthetics. Which is the pharmacologically active species, neutral base or charged cation, and at which side of the membrane does it act? Normally, the uncharged species of tertiary amine local anesthetics can pass relatively easily across biologic membranes.[72,73] However, it has been possible to restrict these molecules to only one side of the nerve membrane by using permanently charged quaternary amine derivatives. These derivatives are essentially membrane impermeant and thus remain on the side where they are applied. The results of many experiments on quaternary amine anesthetics show that sodium (and potassium) channels are blocked only by these drugs when they are present in the axoplasmic phase but not when they are added to the extracellular solution.[18,30,42,53,104] These findings agree with other experiments in which the intracellular pH and extracellular pH were varied in perfused giant axons and the sodium channel inhibition from externally applied tertiary amine anesthetics was measured.[72] Therefore **the cationic species of local anesthetics appears to be more potent than the neutral base and seems to inhibit channels from the cytoplasmic surface of the membrane.**[95,104]

However, neutral species of local anesthetic also have channel blocking activity.[27,72] In addition, uncharged local anesthetics such as benzocaine and its derivatives,[60,77,96] alcohols, barbiturates (weak acids), and other general anesthetics[47,75] also interfere with P_{Na}. Some features of the inhibition by tertiary and quaternary amine anesthetics also are similar to the actions of these neutral compounds.[33,47,52] The broad structural variety of agents showing local anesthetic action on sodium channels questions the assumption that a single, very specific receptor exists for mediating local anesthesia. This also provides support for the concept of more than one mechanism (or site) of action (Fig. 56-11).

Local Anesthetic Structure and Potency

The apparent potency of local anesthetics depends on the conditions of testing. For example, the value of the resting membrane potential, the internal and external pH, the nature of the buffer, the frequency (and duration) of depolarizing pulses, and the temperature of the preparation all affect the apparent potency.[10,13,21,35,37,127] It is thus essential to compare drugs under identical conditions to determine accurately their relative potencies. When the conditions are well controlled, consistent potency-structure relationships emerge from several different types of measurement.

Local anesthetic molecules with greater hydrophobicity are more potent blockers of resting, closed sodium channels.[9,102] Hydrophobicity, determined as the tendency of the drugs to selectively partition into apolar solvents (e.g., octanol) from aqueous solvents, can be increased by enlarging hydrocarbon substituents on the tertiary amine nitrogen and on the aromatic ring.[34,110] **Local anesthetics with greater lipid solubilities are more potent both because they are more concentrated in the interior of the nerve membrane and because they have easier access to the sodium channel receptor.**[8,10,73,102] However, the increased potency of lipophilic drugs cannot be ascribed simply to an increased uptake of anesthetic by the neuronal membrane lipid. This is because the inhibitory action can also be potentiated greatly when the nerve is cooled,[13,89,96,112] even though the measured membrane uptake of anesthetic is reduced.[13,89,93]

Potency of local anesthetics in blocking resting channels also depends on the nature of the covalent dipolar bond link-

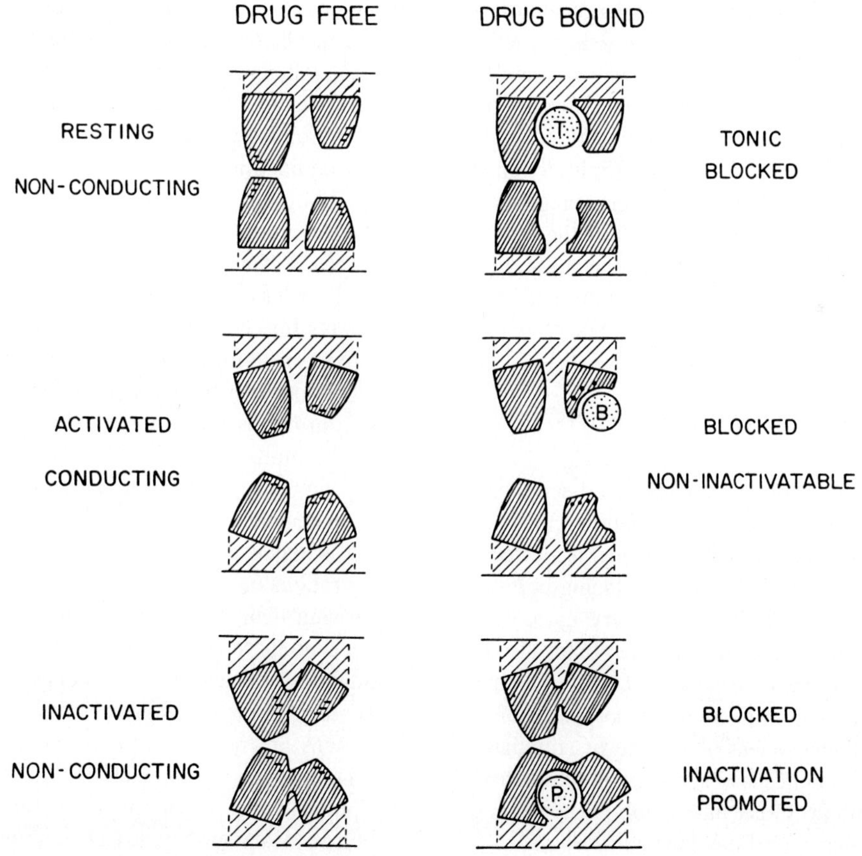

Fig. 56-11. Schematic drawing of three ways in which local anesthetics may interfere with normal operation of sodium channels. **A,** Column shows normal operation of drug-free channels. **B,** Column shows possible sites and modes of drug binding and action. *Top row* in column B: anesthetic molecule binds to resting channel and prevents it from assuming conducting state. *Middle row* in both columns: open channel is bound by anesthetic molecule that totally inhibits its permeability function and prevents normal inactivation from occurring. *Bottom row* in both columns: inactivated channel is bound by anesthetic, which stabilizes it in that conformation. (From Strichartz G: Interactions of local anesthetics with neuronal sodium channels. In Fozzard H, et al, editors: *Effects of anesthesia. Clinical Symposium Series,* Rockville, Md, 1985, American Physiological Society.)

ing the aromatic moiety to the tertiary amine group. Ester-bonded and ether-bonded molecules are most potent, linear amide-bonded molecules are less potent, and cyclic amide-bonded drugs are least potent.[34,36] This order represents increasing polarity among drug molecules and decreasing ability to act as hydrogen bond acceptors, either of which may be important in the bonding of local anesthetics to a resting channel site.[77] Both the polar and the lipophilic regions of a local anesthetic probably interact with the channel's binding site(s), which most likely includes part of the channel protein[78] and may also involve some of the membrane's lipid. The structural dependence of use-dependent block is similar but not identical. Ether-linked and ester-linked local anesthetics also give a larger use-dependent block than amide-linked drugs, but the largest use-dependent block corresponds to drugs of intermediate size and hydrophobicity.[9,34] Use-dependence requires the increased binding of drugs to depolarized channels and their slow dissociation from these channels in the repolarized membrane.[51] Intermediate-size drugs may accomplish this optimally; smaller lipophilic drugs reverse their binding too rapidly, and larger, more or less polar drugs bind too slowly to the transiently reactive channels to provide much additonal block during an impulse. Use-dependent block mirrors a dynamic relationship between channel and drug, not an equilibrium reaction. As the channel's conformation changes, so will the affinity for anesthetics and probably the contribution of different regions of the molecule to the total binding energy. Until the several possible binding regions for local anesthetics in the sodium channel are characterized, the detailed interpretation of structure-activity relationships at the molecular level remains somewhat speculative.

Location of Local Anesthetic Binding Site(s) in Sodium Channel

Functional regions of the sodium channel have been identified by their susceptibility to various biochemical, pharmacologic, and genetic manipulations. The channel is viewed as a large protein, glycosylated on its external-facing portions. When the channel is open, it provides a very narrow hydrophilic pathway for ions to traverse the membrane. Toxins such as tetrodotoxin and saxitoxin totally occlude the channel, seemingly by binding at or near the outer opening of the channel in a manner independent of voltage or stimulation frequency. No use-dependence is observed with tetrodotoxin on nerve channels, and no direct interaction exists between local anesthetics and this part of the channel.[49,50,119]

Conditions that decrease the passage of ions through the channel potentiate the block by charged anesthetics.[18,99] Quaternary anesthetic derivatives block channels as if they were binding within the membrane, not at the membrane's axoplasmic surface. Studies suggest that Na^+ ions in the channel's pore compete with charged local anesthetic molecules for a common binding site, but do not affect uncharged drug binding. However, the presence of ions in the channel pore may also prevent the binding of local anesthetics by some indirect, allosteric effect, not by direct competition.

Additional evidence suggests that anesthetic molecules are not simply plugging the pore. Certain agents, termed *activator drugs,* open sodium channels at rest and inhibit their subsequent inactivation, leading to long episodes of elevated P_{Na}. These activators include veratridine, aconitine, and batrachotoxin.[23,103] The permeability of batrachotoxin-modified channels has been examined by voltage-clamp and ion-flux studies.[22,61,76] Results of both experiments show an apparent competition between batrachotoxin and local anesthetics.[58,62,65,79] As noted before, the activator drugs are highly lipophilic molecules, and it is unlikely that they bind in the channel's polar pore. Therefore the apparent competition between batrachotoxin and local anesthetics requires either that the anesthetics bind to a site at the channel's hydrophilic regions, perhaps at the macromolecule's protein-lipid interface, or that the interaction is by some indirect, allosteric mechanism.

The second possibility could result from reciprocal, opposing effects of the drugs on sodium channel inactivation. Local anesthetics selectively stabilize an inactivated configuration, whereas batrachotoxin stabilizes an open, noninactivating channel. Thus the action of one drug could prevent or compromise that of the other without a requirement for direct competition. Indeed, local anesthetic molecules inhibit the binding of radiolabeled batrachotoxin to channels in the same order as their potency for blocking sodium conductance.[76] Kinetic analysis shows that this inhibition is caused, at least in part, by allosteric interactions. The rate constants for channel binding and for dissociation of batrachotoxin are both modified by local anesthetics; the latter can only occur if both drugs bind to the channel simultaneously, an impossible situation if there was direct, competitive inhibition.

In summary, local anesthetic molecules interact with sodium channels in more than one way. The drug's inhibitory effect is enhanced when channels respond to membrane depolarizations by undergoing certain conformational changes, increasing their affinity for local anesthetics.[115] The consequence of these molecular events is use-dependent block. Binding of local anesthetics occurs via a lipophilic site on the channel or in the membrane, but more than hydrophobic interactions are required to describe anesthetic actions. Ions passing through the channel, binding weakly as they go, and lipophilic activator drugs are both effective in modulating the action of local anesthetics. Calcium ions antagonize the inhibition by both charged and neutral local anesthetics, in part by mimicking the action of membrane hyperpolarization and thereby reducing the level of inactivation.

IMPULSE BLOCKADE BY LOCAL ANESTHETICS

The primary mechanism of action of local anesthetics is an inhibition of sodium conductance in peripheral

nerves. Ultimately, however, clinical local anesthesia is caused by a blockade of the excitation-conduction process in nerves. This section describes the inhibitory effect of local anesthetics on action potentials in nerve fibers and the relationship between these electrophysiologic actions and the effects on ionic channels.

Determinants of Potency

Potency for the blockade of action potentials in nerves by local anesthetics depends on more than the inhibition of sodium currents. Potassium currents are also reduced by local anesthetics,[5,43] an effect that can potentiate the drug's impulse blocking activity in two ways. First, inhibition of resting potassium channels[14] causes resting depolarization that favors blockade of Na^+ channels. Second, inhibition of the outward potassium currents flowing during the impulse broadens the action potential and gives more time for binding, less for dissociation during trains of impulses that drive use-dependent block.[39] Therefore a local anesthetic that blocks potassium currents as well as sodium currents is more potent in blocking impulses than an agent that inhibits sodium currents alone.

Impulses are blocked in a use-dependent, or phasic, mode by local anesthetics in the same manner as are sodium channels.[60] Sodium channel blockade is usually quantitated under voltage-clamp conditions. When the membrane is very rapidly repolarized by the voltage clamp, the anesthetic-free channels are quickly converted from the inactivated state to the resting, anesthetic-resistant conformation. However, at the falling phase of an impulse, repolarization occurs more gradually and to potentials that maintain significant channel inactivation. Compared with the response in voltage clamp, sodium channels during the impulse remain in the inactivated conformation longer. Thus, the binding of anesthetics during impulses is use-dependent, at relatively lower impulse frequencies.[60,106]

In all considerations of channel block versus impulse block, a relationship exists between the fraction of free sodium channels and the size of the action potential. However, neither the rate of depolarization nor the peak amplitude of an action potential in a single nerve fiber are directly proportional to the density of functional sodium channels.[31] For example, in large, rapidly conducting axons, the maximal rate of depolarization and the height of the action potential are reduced by only 20% to 25% or less when 50% of the sodium channels are blocked.[31] Complete inhibition of impulse formation and propagation requires the blockade of approximately 80% of the sodium channels. Therefore, the concentration of a local anesthetic required for blocking half the sodium current (IC50) is less than the IC50 for halving the action potential height. This latter IC50 is even less than the minimal concentration requirement (C_m) for impulse blockade in the same nerve. In large myelinated axons, the concentration to fully block impulses tonically is about 4 to 8 times the concentration to inhibit P_{Na} by half. This relationship is not known for smaller myelinated fibers or for nonmyelinated C fibers.

Other conditions that decrease the number of functional sodium channels enhance the impulse-blocking activity of local anesthetics and thereby affect their apparent potency.[100] As mentioned previously, brief depolarizing pulses reduce the C_m for impulse blockade by the conversion of sodium channels to a form (the inactivated state) with higher anesthetic affinity. A steady depolarization can also reduce the C_m of local anesthetics by decreasing the fraction of sodium channels available for activation to the open state, even if the binding of drugs were not state dependent.

Carbon dioxide potentiates the conduction blocking effect of local anesthetic agents. CO_2 increases the threshold for impulse firing,[10,81] perhaps by changing the extent of channel inactivation at rest. In addition, CO_2 acidifies the cytoplasm and thereby increases the concentration of the cationic form of local anesthetics inside the cell.[21,127] Nonionizable local anesthetics (e.g., benzocaine) are also potentiated by CO_2-bicarbonate buffers.[127] Potentiation of local anesthetic by CO_2-bicarbonate varies greatly among particular drugs, implying that the potentiation mechanism alters the local anesthetic binding site subtly at the molecular level.

Clinical Picture

In the clinical situation the onset, depth, and duration of local anesthesia depend on the amount of an injected anesthetic dose that reaches the site of action and how rapidly it arrives and is removed from the receptor site. As noted previously, several sheaths surrounding a nerve serve as barriers to the diffusion of local anesthetics (Fig. 56-1). The perineurium is the major barrier[1] that impedes the diffusion of local anesthetics to their site of action. Removal of the perineurium greatly accelerates the onset of anesthetic block.[87]

Within the nerve sheath, anesthetic molecules further distribute among the various compartments, depending on their hydrophobicity and pK_a as well as the polar or apolar nature[8] and pH of the compartments. The pK_a values and octanol-buffer partition coefficients of frequently used local anesthetics are listed in Table 56-2. Many uncharged anesthetic molecules are rapidly sequestered in the myelin sheath of myelinated nerves, but some also diffuse through the covering Schwann cell to the nodal membrane and into the axoplasm. The myelin may act as a depot for hydrophobic anesthetics and slow the block of myelinated fibers relative to their nonmyelinated neighbors.[45,70,86,92] In addition, highly lipophilic agents such as etidocaine may accumulate in myelin, which will function as a reservoir for anesthetic molecules, resulting in a greater degree of myelinated nerve blockade in nonequilibrium conditions, e.g., during drug washout. This may explain the prolonged motor block observed clinically with the exceptionally hydrophobic drug etidocaine.

Eventually, local anesthetic molecules are distributed in all the aqueous and membrane phases in the nerve. The rate

Table 56-2 Local anesthetic pK_a values, octanol-buffer* partition coefficients, and distribution coefficients at pH 7.4†

Drug	pK_a	Pc‡	Pn‡	$Q_{7.4}$§
Ester linked				
Procaine	8.9 ± 0.1	0.004 ± 0.01	100 ± 10	3.1
2-Chloroprocaine	9.1 ± 0.1	0.042 ± 0.010	810 ± 58	17.4
Tetracaine	8.4 ± 0.03	0.79 ± 0.05	5822 ± 325	541.0
Benzocaine	Not applicable	Not applicable	132	132
Amide linked				
Procainamide	9.4 ± 0.04‖	0.0021 ± 0.0005‖	7.3 ± 0.1‖	0.07‖
Mepivacaine	7.7 ± 0.1	0.15 ± 0.05	130 ± 15	42.0
Ropivacaine	8.2 ± 0.02‖	0.46 ± 0.03‖	775 ± 53‖	115.0‖
Bupivacaine	8.1 ± 0.02‖	2.0 ± 0.05	3420 ± 263	560.0
Lidocaine	7.8 ± 0.04	0.085 ± 0.01	366 ± 31	110.0
Prilocaine	8.0 ± 0.1‖	0.30 ± 0.02‖	129 ± 11‖	25.0‖
Etidocaine	7.9 ± 0.03	0.81 ± 0.05	7317 ± 523	1853.0

*150 mEq · l^{-1} NaCl and, 5 mm MES, 5 mm MOPS, 5 mm CAPS buffers.
†All measurements at 36° C, except as noted.
‡Partition coefficients expressed as relative concentrations (moles · l^{-1}) in octanol and buffer. *Pc* is the partition coefficient for the charged form, *Pn* for the neutral form.
§$Q_{7.4}$ = (Total drug · ml^{-1} octanol) ÷ (Total drug · ml^{-1} buffer) at pH 7.4.
‖At 25° C.
From Strichartz GR, Sanchez V, Arthur GR et al: Fundamental properties of local anesthetics. II. Measured octanol: buffer partition coefficients and pK_a values of clinically-used drugs, *Anesth Analg* 71:158, 1990.

of drug uptake and therefore the onset of conduction block depend on the pK_a of the anesthetic agent and the pH of the various compartments. **Because the uncharged form of the local anesthetic is more membrane permeant,[8] drugs with lesser pK_a values are taken up more rapidly and tend to have a shorter onset time for block.[73]** For example, the onset of action of lidocaine, which has a pK_a of 7.7 at 37° C, is significantly more rapid than the onset of a drug such as procaine, which has a pK_a of 8.9.[45] **The rate of removal of local anesthetics from nerve fibers and surrounding tissue, and therefore the duration of action, is also dependent on pK_a. For example, agents such as tetracaine and bupivacaine are highly tissue bound and produce a long duration of conduction block, whereas procaine is poorly tissue-bound and has a relatively short duration of action.** Dissociation of local anesthetics from sodium channels, as measured directly by electrophysiology takes only seconds, however.[3,52,117] Thus, the binding that correlates with duration of clinical blockade must be to other membranous or cytoplasmic regions of tissues and not to the Na^+ channel *per se.*

Length of Anesthetized Nerve

Anesthetic molecules diffuse from the site of injection not only transversely (through the nerve), but also longitudinally (along the axis), both within and outside the epineurium. Thus the drug concentration within the nerve is greatest near the site of injection and decreases as the nerve extends away in both directions. As a result, the extent of block is greatest at the site of drug application and less intense in areas distant from the injection point. Fibers may therefore be totally blocked along some region of their length but only partially blocked at adjacent regions.[83] **The length of blocked nerve must be sufficiently long to ensure that the local circuit currents that are necessary for continued impulse propagation are unable to activate the next adjacent excitable zone, leading to conduction blockade.[82] If an insufficient length of nerve is blocked, the impulse conduction will be slowed but complete conduction block will not occur.[32]**

Differential Blockade Among Fibers: Rejection of the Size Principle

Critical exposure length probably contributes to the phenomenon of differential nerve block by local anesthetics. Variations exist in critical lengths for nerve block of fibers of different types and size. In general, smaller nerve fibers have shorter critical lengths.[41,82,86,92] Additionally, the measured density of sodium channels appears to decrease as fiber diameter decreases, at least in nonmyelinated nerves, and this factor influences the critical length required for conduction block.[49] However, the relationship between size of myelinated and nonmyelinated axons and the critical length for conduction block is not so well defined. The sensitivity of large myelinated A fibers to local anesthetics may be related in part to the diameter of these fibers but also to the density of sodium channels clustered at the nodes of Ranvier. Thus at least two factors control the time course of conduction blockade in fibers of different types and size: the absolute sensitivity of the axon membrane to impulse inhibition by a drug, represented by the response of impulses at steady state to different anesthetic concentrations, and the critical length of the axon that must be blocked to prevent impulse propagation. Within a particular fiber type a correlation exists between fiber size and clinical signs of anesthesia. For example, sensory functions such as pain and temperature, which are mediated by afferent impulses in the smallest myelinated (Aδ) and in nonmyelinated C fibers, are the first to be blocked after administration of a local anesthetic.[66] Light touch and hair vibration sensations, which traverse larger myelinated Aβ fibers, disappear later and sometimes are not totally abolished. This order of sensory loss is consistent with the longitudinal spread of anesthetic molecules and the actual length required for conduction blockade in axons of various diameters. Restoration of function usually occurs in the reverse order.

No experimental support exists for the statement that smaller axons are more susceptible than larger axons to impulse blockade by local anesthetics. Many investigations of compound action potentials from many nerve fibers and of single axons, both *in vitro* and *in vivo*, have disproved this generalized "size principle."[16,48,57] Recent studies reveal an endogenous propensity for impulse failure distributed among peripheral axons according to sensory modality rather than size or morphology (i.e., myelinated versus nonmyelinated).[84] Whether the mechanisms of axons that govern this property can be exploited for the intentional control of sensory and motor function remains a challenge.

KEY POINTS

- Neuronal impulses are blocked by local anesthetic agents by inhibiting the increase in membrane sodium permeability. Anesthetic molecules interact directly with the sodium channels that span the nerve membrane as well as perturbing the lipid molecules in the membrane. The direct effect on sodium channels appears to be of primary importance for impulse inhibition. The contribution of membrane perturbation to conduction blockade by conventional local anesthetics is not clear.
- When a sodium channel is bound by a local anesthetic molecule, it takes on a conformation that cannot open in response to membrane depolarization. Changes in the conformation of the sodium channel that are induced by membrane depolarization lead to a tighter binding of local anesthetic molecules. This results in an incremental fall in the height of the action potential during repetitive stimulation, a phenomenon called use-dependent block.
- The physical location of the anesthetic binding site in the sodium channel is probably near the ion-conducting pore. Anesthetic actions are reduced (1) by ions entering the channel's pore from the extracellular opening, (2) by the resting potential of the membrane, (3) by extracellular Ca^{2+}, and (4) by other drugs that selectively bind to and stabilize the open channel conformation.
- The clinical potency of local anesthetics also depends on additional factors besides their affinity for sodium channels. Anesthetic molecules must penetrate the nerve sheath and distribute throughout the fascicles of fibers to reach all individual axons. Further, the anesthetic must diffuse longitudinally along a sufficient length of the nerve to prevent the local currents from generating impulses in drug-free, excitable areas of the nerve.
- The rate of diffusion of local anesthetics through the nerve sheath and membrane to the site of action in the sodium channel depends on many factors. These include the pK_a of the drug, the pH of the nerve compartments, the total amount of local anesthetic administered, and the vascular removal of the drug.
- Successful impulse blockade in individual fibers depends not only on a sufficient concentration of anesthetic within and along the axon, but also on the relative densities and anesthetic susceptibilities of sodium and potassium channels in the membrane. The diameter of a nerve fiber alone does not determine the relative sensitivity of different fibers to conduction blockade by local anesthetics. However, under clinical conditions the activities associated with smaller nerve axons are usually inhibited earlier than those associated with larger axons.

KEY REFERENCES

Butterworth JF, Strichartz GR: Molecular mechanisms of local anesthesia: a review, *Anesthesiology* 72:711, 1990.

Cahalan M: Local anesthetic block of sodium channels in normal and pronase-treated squid giant axons, *Biophys J* 23:285, 1978.

Catterall WA: The molecular basis of neuronal excitability, *Science* 223:653, 1985.

Gingrich KJ, Beardsly D, Yue DT: Ultra-deep blockade of Na^+ channels by a quaternary ammonium ion: Catalysis by a transition-intermediate state? *J Physiol* 471:319–341, 1993.

Hille B: *Ionic channels of excitable membranes,* ed 2, Sunderland, MA, 1991, Sinauer Associates.

Starmer CF, Grant AO, Strauss HC: Mechanism of use-dependent block of sodium channels in excitable membranes by local anesthetics, *Biophys J* 46:15–27, 1984.

REFERENCES

1. Akert K, Sandri C, Weibel R, Peper K, Moor N: The fine structure of the perineural endothelium, *Cell Tissue Res,* 165:281–295, 1976.
2. Almers W: Gating currents and chart movements in excitable membranes, *Rev Physiol Biochem Pharmacol* 82:96, 1978.
3. Almers W, Cahalan MD: Block of sodium channels by internally applied drugs: two receptors for tertiary and quaternary amine compounds? *Adv Physiol Sci* 4:67, 1981.
4. An RH, Bangalore R, Rosero S, Kass RS. Lidocaine effect on LQT3 mutant human sodium channels. *Circ Res* 79:103–108, 1996.
5. Arhem P, Frankenhaeuser B: Local anesthetics: effects on permeability properties of nodal membrane in myelinated nerve fibres from *Xenopus*. Potential clamp experiments, *Acta Physiol Scand* 91:11–21, 1974.
6. Armstrong CM, Croop RS: Simulation of Na channel inactivation by thiazine dyes, *J Gen Physiol* 80:641, 1982.
7. Barchi RL, Cohen SA, Murphy LE: Purification from rat sarcolemma of the saxitoxin binding component of the excitable membrane sodium channel, *Proc Natl Acad Sci U S A* 77:1306, 1980.
8. Bernards CM, Hill HF: Physical and chemical properties of drug molecules governing their diffusion through the spinal meninges, *Anesthesiology* 77:750–756, 1992.
9. Bokesch PM, Post C, Strichartz GR: Structure-activity relationship of lidocaine homologues on tonic and frequency dependent impulse blockade in nerve, *J Pharmacol Exp Ther* 237:773, 1986.
10. Bokesch PM, Raymond SA, Strichartz GR: Dependence of lidocaine potency on pH and PCO_2, *Anesth Analg* 66:9, 1987.
11. Bostock H, Sears TA: The internodal axon membrane: electrical excitability and continuous conduction in segmental demyelination, *J Physiol (Lond)* 280:273, 1978.
12. Boulanger Y, Schreier S, Leitch LC, et al: Multiple binding sites for local anesthetics in membranes: characterization of the sites and their equilibria by deuterium NMR of specifically deuterated procaine and tetracaine, *Can J Biochem* 58:986, 1980.
13. Bradley DJ, Richards CD: Temperature-dependence of the action of nerve blocking agents and its relationship to membrane-buffer partition coefficients: thermodynamic implications for the site of action of local anesthetics, *Br J Pharmacol* 81:161, 1983.
14. Bräu ME, Nau C, Hempelmann G, Vogel W: Local anesthetics potently block a potential insensitive potassium channel in myelinated nerve, *J Gen Physiol* 105:485–505, 1995.
15. Butterworth J, Moran JR, Whitesides GM, Strichartz GR: Limited nerve impulse blockade by "leashed" local anesthetics, *J Med Chem* 30:1295–1302, 1987.
16. Butterworth JF, Strichartz GR: Molecular mechanisms of local anesthesia: a review, *Anesthesiology* 72:711, 1990.
17. Cahalan M: Local anesthetic block of sodium channels in normal and pronase-treated squid giant axons, *Biophys J* 23: 285, 1978.
18. Cahalan MD, Almers W: Block of sodium conductance and gating current in squid giant axons poisoned with quaternary strychnine, *Biophys J* 27:57, 1979.
19. Cahalan MD, Almers W: Interactions between quaternary lidocaine, the sodium channel gates and tetrodotoxin, *Biophys J* 27:39, 1979.
20. Cahalan M, Shapiro BI, Almers W: Relationships between inactivation of sodium channels and block by quaternary derivatives of local anesthetics and their compounds. In Fink BR, editor: *Molecular mechanisms of anesthesia,* vol 2, New York, 1980, Raven Press.
21. Catchlove RFH: The influence of CO_2 and pH on local anesthetic action, *J Pharmacol Exp Ther* 181:298, 1972.
22. Catterall WA: Cooperative activation of action potential Na^+ ionophore by neurotoxins, *Proc Natl Acad Sci U S A* 72:1782, 1975.
23. Catterall WA: Neurotoxins that act on voltage-sensitive sodium channels in excitable membranes, *Annu Rev Pharmacol Toxicol* 20:15, 1981.
24. Catterall WA: The molecular basis of neuronal excitability, *Science* 223:653, 1985.
25. Chernoff DM: Kinetic analysis of phasic inhibition of neuronal sodium currents by lidocaine and bupivacaine, 58:53–68, 1990.
26. Chernoff DM, Strichartz GR: Kinetics of local anesthetic inhibition of neuronal sodium channels: pH- and hydrophobicity-dependence, *Biophys J* 58:69, 1990.
27. Chernoff DM, Strichartz GR: Tonic and phasic block of neuronal sodium currents by 5-hydroxyhexano-2′,6′-xylidide, a neutral lidocaine homologue, *J Gen Physiol* 93:1075, 1990.
28. Chiu SY, Ritchie JM: Potassium channels in nodal and internodal axonal membrane of mammalian myelinated fibres, *Nature* 284:170, 1980.
29. Chiu SY, Ritchie JM, Rogart RB, et al: A quantitative description of membrane current in rabbit myelinated nerve, *J Physiol (Lond)* 292:149, 1979.
30. Choi KL, Mossman C, Aube J, Yellen G: The internal quaternary ammonium receptor site of shaker potassium channels, *Neuron* 10:533–541, 1993.
31. Cohen I, Atwell D, and Strichartz G: The dependence of the maximum rate of rise of the action potential upstroke on membrane properties, *Proc R Soc Lond B Biol Sci* 214: 85, 1981.
32. Condouris GA, Goebel RH, Brady T: Computer simulation of local anesthetic effects using a mathematical model of myelinated nerve. *J Pharmacol Exp Ther,* 196: 737–745, 1976.
33. Courtney KR: Mechanism of frequency-dependent inhibition of sodium currents in frog myelinated nerve by the lidocaine derivative GEA-968, *J Pharmacol Exp Ther* 195:225, 1975.
34. Courtney KR: Structure-activity relation for frequency-dependent sodium channel block in nerve by local anesthetics, *J Pharmacol Exp Ther* 213:114, 1980.
35. Courtney KR: Significance of bicarbonate for antiarrhythmic drug action, *J Mol Cell Cardiol* 13:1031, 1981.
36. Courtney KR, Etter EF: Modulated anticonvulsant block of sodium channels in nerve and muscle, *Eur J Pharmacol* 88:1, 1983.
37. Courtney KR, Strichartz GR: Structural elements which determine local anesthetic activity. In Strichartz GR, editor: *Handbook of experimental pharmacology: local anesthetics,* New York, 1986, Springer-Verlag.
38. Desai S, Hadlock T, Messam C, Chafetz R, Strichartz GR: Ionization and adsorption of a series of local anesthetics in detergent micelles: studies in model membranes using in drug fluorescence, *J Pharmacol Exp Therap* 271:220–228; 1994
39. Drachman D, Strichartz GR: Potassium channel blockers potentiate impulse inhibition by local anesthetics, *Anesthesiology* 75:1051–1061, 1991.
40. Feinstein MB: Reaction of local anesthetics with phospholipids: a possible chemical basis for anesthesia, *J Gen Physiol* 48:357, 1964.
41. Franz DN, Perry RS: Mechanisms for differential block among single myelinated and non-myelinated axons by procaine, *J Physiol* 236:193, 1974.
42. Frazier DT, Narahashi T, Yamada M: The site of action and active form of local anesthetics. II. Experiments with quaternary compounds, *J Pharmacol Exp Ther* 171: 45, 1970.
43. Gilly WF, Armstrong CM: Gating current and potassium channels in the giant axon of the squid, *Biophys J* 29:485, 1980.
44. Gingrich KJ, Beardsly D, Yue DT: Ultra-deep blockade of Na^+ channels by a quaternary ammonium ion: catalysis by a transition-intermediate state? *J Physiol* 471: 319–341, 1993.
45. Gissen AJ, Covino BG, Gregus J: Differential sensitivity of fast and slow fibers in mammalian nerve: II. Margin of safety for nerve transmission, *Anesth Analg* 61:561, 1982.
46. Hartshorne RP, Catterall WA: Purification of the saxitoxin receptor of the sodium channel from rat brain, *Proc Natl Acad Sci U S A* 78:4620, 1981.
47. Haydon DA, Urban BW: The effects of some inhalation anaesthetics on the sodium current of the squid giant axon, *J Physiol (Lond)* 341:429, 1983.
48. Heavner JE, deJong R: Lidocaine blocking concentration for B- and C-nerve fibers. *Anesthesiology* 40:228, 1974.
49. Henderson R, Ritchie JM, Strichartz GR: The binding of labelled saxitoxin to the sodium channels in nerve membranes, *J Physiol (Lond)* 235:783, 1973.
50. Henderson R, Strichartz G: Ion fluxes through the sodium channels of garfish olfactory nerve membranes, *J Physiol (Lond)* 238:329, 1974.
51. Hille B: Local anesthetics: hydrophilic and

hydrophobic pathways for the drug-receptor reaction, *J Gen Physiol* 60:497, 1977.
52. Hille B: The pH-dependent rate of action of local anesthetics on the node of Ranvier, *J Gen Physiol* 69:475, 1977.
53. Hille B, Courtney K, Dum R: Rate and site of local anesthetics in myelinated nerve fibers. In Fink BR, editor: *Molecular mechanisms of anesthesia,* vol 1, New York, 1975, Raven Press.
54. Hille B, Woodhull AM, Shapiro B: Negative surface charge near sodium channels of nerve: divalent ions, monovalent ions, and pH, *Philos Trans R Soc Lond B Biol Sci* 270:301, 1975.
55. Hodgkin AL, Huxley AF: A quantitative description of membrane current and its application to conduction and excitation in nerve, *J Physiol (Lond)* 117:500, 1952.
56. Horn R, Patlak J: Single channel currents from excised patches of muscle membrane, *Proc Natl Acad Sci U S A* 77:6930, 1980.
57. Huang H, Thalhammer JG, Raymond SA, Strichartz GR. Effect of lidocaine on sciatic nerve conduction in rats: an *in vivo* single unit study, *Soc Neurosci,* 21:1411, 1995.
58. Huang LYM, Ehrenstein G, Catterall W: Interaction between batrachotoxin and yohimbine, *Biophys J* 23:219, 1978.
59. Hubbell WL, McConnell HM: Orientation and motion of amphiphilic spin labels in membranes, *Proc Natl Acad Sci U S A* 64: 20, 1969.
60. Kendig JJ, Courtney KR, Cohen EN: Anesthetics: molecular correlates of voltage- and frequency-dependent sodium channel block in nerve, *J Pharmacol Exp Ther* 210:446, 1979.
61. Khodorov BI: Chemicals as tools to study nerve fiber sodium channels: effects of batrachotoxin and some local anesthetics. In Tosteson DC, Ovchinniko YA, Latorre R, editors: *Membrane transport processes,* vol 2, New York, 1968, Raven Press.
62. Khodorov BI, Peganov E, Revenko S, Shishkova L: Sodium currents in voltage clamped nerve fiber of frog under the combined action of batrachotoxin and procaine, *Brain Res* 84:541–546, 1975.
63. Landon DN, Hall SM: The myelinated nerve fiber. In Landon DN, editor: *The peripheral nerve,* London, 1976, Chapman & Hall.
64. Lee AG: Model for action of local anesthetics, *Nature* 262:545, 1976.
65. LeeSon S, Wang GK, Concus A, Crill E, Strichartz GR: Stereoselecetive inhibition of neuronal sodium channels by local anesthetics: evidence for two sites of action? *Anesthesiology* 77:324–335, 1992.
66. Liu S, Kopacz DJ, Carpenter RL: Quantitative assessment of differential sensory nerve block after lidocaine spinal anesthesia, *Anesthesiology* 82:60–63, 1995.
67. Mannuzzu LM, Moronne MM, Isacoff EY: Direct physical measure of conformational rearrangement underlying potassium channel gating, *Science* 271:213–216, 1996.
68. Miller JA, Agnew WS, Levinson SR: Principal glycopeptide of the tetrodotoxin/ saxitoxin binding protein from *Electrophorus electricus:* isolation and partial chemical and physical characterization, *Biochemistry* 22:462–470, 1983.
69. Montal M, Mueller P: Formation of bimolecular membranes from lipid monolayers and a study of their electrical properties, *Proc Natl Acad Sci U S A* 69:3561, 1972.
70. Mueller P, Rudin DO: Induced excitability in reconstituted cell membrane, *J Theoret Biol* 4:268, 1963.
71. Mueller P, Rudin DO: Resting and action potentials in experimental bimolecular lipid membranes, *J Theoret Biol* 18:222, 1968.
72. Narahashi T, Frazier D, Yamada M: The site of action and active form of local anesthetics: I. Theory and pH experiments with tertiary compounds, *J Pharm Exp Ther* 171:32–44, 1970.
73. Ohki S: Permeability of axon membranes to local anesthetics, *Biochim Biophys Acta* 643:495, 1981.
74. Peters A, Palay SL, Webster HD: *The fine structure of the nervous system: the neurons and supporting cells,* Philadelphia, 1976, WB Saunders.
75. Post C, Butterworth JF, Strichartz GR, et al: Tachykinin antagonists have potent local anaesthetic-like actions, *Eur J Pharmacol* 117:347, 1985.
76. Postma SQ, Catterall WA: Inhibition of binding of ^{3}H-batrachotoxin A 20-α-benzoate to sodium channels by local anesthetics, *Mol Pharmacol* 25:219, 1984.
77. Quan C, Mok WM, Wang GK: Use-dependent inhibition of Na^+ currents by benzocaine homologs, *Biophys J* (in press).
78. Ragsdale DS, McPhee JC, Scheuer T, Catterall WA: Molecular determinants of state-dependent block of Na^+ channels by local anesthetics, *Science* 265:1724–1730, 1994.
79. Rando T, Wang, GK, Strichartz GR: The interaction of alkaloid neurotoxins, batrachotoxin and veratridine with the gating processes of neuronal sodium channels, *Mol Pharmacol* 29:467–477, 1986.
80. Raymond SA: Effects of nerve impulses on threshold of frog sciatic nerve fibres, *J Physiol (Lond)* 290:273, 1979.
81. Raymond SA, Roscoe RF: CO_2 as a local anaesthetic, *Reg Anesth* 9:43, 1984.
82. Raymond SA, Steffensen S, Gugino LD, Strichartz GR: The role of length of nerve exposed to local anesthetics in impulse blocking action, *Anesth Analg* 68:563, 1988.
83. Raymond SA, Strichartz GR: The long and short of differential block, *Anesthesiology* 70:725, 1989.
84. Raymond SA, Thalhammer JG, Popitz-Bergez F, et al: Changes in the axonal impulse conduction correlate with sensory modality in primary afferent fibers in the rat, *Brain Res* 526:318, 1990.
85. Ritchie JM: Electrogenic ion pumping in nervous tissue. In Sanadi R, editor: *Current topics in bioenergetics,* vol 4, New York, 1971, Academic Press.
86. Ritchie JM: On the relation between fibre diameter and conduction velocity in myelinated nerve fibres, *Proc R Soc Lond B Biol Sci* 217:29, 1982.
87. Ritchie JM, Ritchie B, Greengard P: The effect of the nerve sheath on the action of local anesthetics, *J Pharmacol Exp Ther* 150:160, 1965.
88. Ritchie JM, Rogart RB: Density of sodium channels in mammalian myelinated nerve fibers and nature of axonal membrane under the myelin sheath, *Proc Natl Acad Sci U S A* 74:211, 1977.
89. Rosenberg PH, Heavner JE: Temperature-dependent nerve blocking action of lidocaine and halothane, *Acta Anesth Scand* 24:314, 1980.
90. Rosenberg RL, Tomiko SA, Agnew WS: Single-channel properties of the reconstituted voltage-regulated Na channel isolated from the electroplax of *Electrophorus electricus, Proc Natl Acad Sci U S A* 81: 1239–1243, 1984.
91. Rosenberg RL, Tomiko DA, Agnew WS: Reconstitution of neurotoxin-modulated ion transport by the voltage-regulated sodium channel isolated from the electroplax of *Electorphorus electricus, Proc Natl Acad Sci U S A* 81:5594–5598, 1984.
92. Rushton WAH: A theory of the effects of fibre size in medullated nerve, *J Physiol (Lond)* 115:101, 1951.
93. Sanchez V, Ferrante FM, Cibotti N, Strichartz GR: Partitioning of tetracaine base and cation into phospholipid membranes: relevance to anesthetic potency, *Reg Anesth* 13(suppl):81, 1988.
94. Schreibmayer W, Wallner M, Lotan I: Mechanism of modulation of single sodium channels from skeletal muscle by the β_1-subunit from rat brain, *Pflugers Arch* 426(3–4):360–362, 1994.
95. Schwarz JR, Ulbricht W, Wagner HH: The rate of action of tetrodotoxin on myelinated nerve fibers of *Xenopus laevis* and *Rana esculenta, J Physiol (Lond)* 233:167, 1983.
96. Schwarz W: Temperature experiments on nerve and muscle membranes of frogs: indications for a phase transition, *Pflugers Arch* 383:27, 1979.
97. Schwarz W, Palade PT, Hille B: Local anesthetics: effect of pH on use-dependent block of sodium channels in frog muscle, *Biophys J* 20:343, 1977.
98. Seeman P: The membrane expansion theory of anesthesia. In Fink BR, editor: *Molecular mechanisms of anesthesia,* vol 1, New York, 1975, Raven Press.
99. Shapiro BI: Effects of strychnine on the sodium conductance of the frog node of Ranvier, *J Gen Physiol* 69:955, 1977.
100. Shin HC, Raymond SA, Strichartz GR. Potentiation by capsaicin of lidocaine's tonic impulse block in isolated rat sciatic nerve. *Neuroscience Letts* 174:14, 1994.
101. Sigworth FJ, Neher E: Single Na^+ channel currents observed in cultured rat muscle cells, *Nature* 287:447, 1980.
102. Skou JC: Local anesthetics: VI. Relation between blocking potency and penetration of a monomolecular layer of lipoids from nerves, *Acta Pharmacol Toxicol* 10:325–337, 1954.
103. Stallcup W: Comparative pharmacology of voltage-dependent sodium channels, *Brain Res* 135:37, 1977.
104. Strichartz GR: The inhibition of sodium currents in myelinated nerve by quaternary derivatives of lidocaine, *J Gen Physiol* 62:37, 1973.
105. Strichartz G: The composition and structure of excitable nerve membrane. In

Jamieson GA, Robinson DM, editors: *Mammalian cell membranes,* vol 3, London, 1977, Butterworths.

106. Strichartz G: Interactions of local anesthetics with neuronal sodium channels. In Fozzard H, et al, editors: *Effects of anesthesia. Clinical Symposium Series,* Rockville, MD, 1985, American Physiological Society.
107. Strichartz GR, Chiu SY, Ritchie JM: The effect of delta^{9}tetrahydrocannabinol on the activation of sodium conductance in the node of Ranvier, *J Pharmacol Exp Ther* 207:801, 1978.
108. Strichartz G, Rando T, Wang GK: An integrated view of the molecular toxinology of sodium channel gating in excitable cells, *Annu Rev Neurosci* 10:237, 1987.
109. Strichartz GR, Ritchie JM: The action of local anesthetics on ion channels of excitable tissues. In Strichartz GR, editor: *Handbook of experimental pharmacology: local anesthetics,* New York, 1986, Springer-Verlag.
110. Strichartz GR, Sanchez V, Arthur GR, et al: Fundamental properties of local anesthetics. II. Measured octanol: buffer partition coefficients and pKa values of clinically-used drugs, *Anesth Analg* 71:158, 1990.
111. Strichartz GR, Wang GK: The kinetic basis for phasic local anesthetic blockade of neuronal sodium channels. In Miller KW, Roth S, editors: *Molecular and cellular mechanism of anesthetics,* New York, 1986, Plenum Press.
112. Strichartz G, Zimmermann M: Selective conduction blockade among different fiber types in mammalian nerves by lidocaine combined with low temperature, *Annual Meeting Abstracts of the Society of Neuroscience,* 1983, p 675.
113. Stühmer W, Conti F, Harukazu S, Wang X, Noda M, Yahagi N. Kubo H, Numa S: Structural parts involved in activation and inactivation of the sodium channel, *Nature* 339:597–603, 1989.
114. Taylor RE: Effect of procaine on electrical properties of squid axon membrane, *Am J Physiol* 196:1071–1078, 1959.
115. Thomsen W, Hays SJ, Hicks JL, Schwarz RD, Catterall WA: Specific binding of the novel Na^+ channel blocker PD85,639 to the α subunit of rat brain Na^+ channels, *Mol Pharm* 43:955–964, 1993.
116. Ulbricht W: The effect of veratridine on excitable membranes of nerve and muscle, *Ergeb Physiol* 61:18, 1969.
117. Ulbricht W: Kinetics of drug action and equilibrium results at the node of Ranvier, *Physiol Rev* 61:785, 1981.
118. Vassilev PM, Scheurer T, Catterall WA: Identification of an intracellular peptide segment involved in sodium channel inactivation. *Science* 241:1658–1661, 1988.
119. Wagner HH, Ulbricht W: Saxitoxin and procaine act independently on separate sites of the sodium channel, *Pflugers Arch* 364:65, 1976.
120. Wang GK: Irreversible modification of sodium channel inactivation in toad myelinated nerve fibres by the oxidant chloramine-T, *J Physiol (Lond)* 346:127, 1984.
121. Wang GK, Brodwick MS, Eaton DC, Strichartz GR: Inhibition of sodium currents by local anesthetics in cloramine-T treated squid axons: the role of Na channel activation, *J Gen Physiol* 89:645–667, 1987.
122. Wang GK, Strichartz GR: Isolation of neurotoxins from *Centruroides* and *Leiurus* scorpion venoms and their action on sodium channels. In Chang DC, Tasaki I, Adelman WJ, editors: *Structure and function of excitable cells,* New York, 1982, Plenum Press.
123. Wang GK, Strichartz GR: Purification and physiological characterization of neurotoxins from venoms of the scorpions *Centruroides sculpturatus* and *Leiurus quinquestriatus, Mol Pharmacol* 23:519, 1983.
124. Wang GK, Strichartz GR: Local anesthetics produce phasic block of sodium channels during activation, *Biophys J* 45:286a, 1984.
125. Westerfield M, Joyner RW, Moore JW: Temperature-sensitive conduction failure at axon branch points, *J Neurophysiol* 41:1, 1978.
126. Wolff D, Canessa-Fisher M, Vargas F, et al: The molecular organization of nerve membranes: V. Properties of mono- and bimolecular films formed with lipids isolated from an axolemma-rich preparation from squid retinal axons, *J Membr Biol* 6:304, 1971.
127. Wong K, Strichartz GR, Raymond SA: On the mechanism of potentiation of local anesthetics by bicarbonate buffer: drug structure-activity studied on isolated peripheral nerve, *Anesth Analg* 76:131–143, 1993.
128. Yang N, George AL Jr, Horn R: Molecular basis of charge movement in voltage-gated sodium channels, *Neuron* 16:113–122, 1996.
129. Yeh JZ: Blockade of sodium channels by stereoisomers of local anesthetics. In Fink BR, editor: *Molecular mechanisms of anesthesia,* vol 2, New York, 1980, Raven Press.
130. Yeh JZ: Sodium inactivation mechanism modulates QX-314 block of sodium channels in squid axons, *Biophys J* 24:569, 1982.

CHAPTER 57

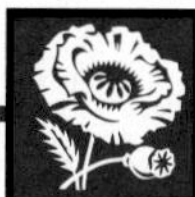

General Versus Regional Anesthesia

HENRIK KEHLET

Surgical trauma is a noxious stimulus to the body that produces a range of biologic alterations, including a complex series of neuroendocrine responses, alterations of immune functions, and modifications in other organ functions. These responses help the body heal tissue and adapt to injury. Responses to operation presumably evolved because they may confer an advantage to the patient, with survival acting as the final homeostatic defense mechanism.

The necessity for the stress response in modern anesthesiologic and surgical settings has been questioned.[10,11] Concern has arisen about the associated detrimental effects of operative procedures, such as myocardial infarction, pulmonary complications, and thromboembolism, which may not be directly related to imperfections in surgical technique. This has led to the hypothesis that the injury response may instead be a maladaptive response that erodes body mass and physiologic reserve.[10,11] An improved knowledge of the mechanisms underlying the metabolicresponses to surgery has been valuable in improving surgical outcome, primarily because of the development of rational supportive therapies and strategies for altering metabolic responses so that these features that are beneficial and promote recovery are stimulated. Other features, which may enhance catabolism and lead to organ dysfunction, are suppressed.

The choice of anesthetic technique, in addition to its specific effects on organ function and side effects, may have important implications for postoperative patient outcome. The response to surgical injury may be modified, particularly if the anesthetic is continued for postoperative pain relief.

This chapter updates knowledge on the differential effects of regional anesthetic techniques (epidural, intrathecal) versus general anesthesia on the surgical stress response and on postoperative outcome. For more detailed discussions on this topic, the reader is referred to recent reviews on the response to injury,[1] on anesthesia and surgical sequelae,[6,10,11,14] and on effects of regional anesthetic techniques for pain relief.[9,14]

METABOLIC RESPONSE TO SURGERY

The metabolic response to surgery is characterized by an increased secretion of catabolically acting hormones (cortisol, glucagon, catecholamines), whereas the anabolically acting hormones (insulin, testosterone, growth hormone) are inhibited. The resulting metabolic effect is hypermetabolism and release of substrate (glucose, amino acids, fat) from peripheral stores (muscle, fat tissue, liver). Concomitantly, changes in immune function take place; the general pattern is reductions in most components.[10,12,14,20]

Changes occur in coagulation and fibrinolysis,[10,14,17] resulting in a hypercoagulatory state. The release mechanisms responsible for these changes are primarily neural afferent stimuli and various humoral factors (arachidonic acid metabolites, complement activation, various cytokines).

The effect of general anesthesia on the metabolic response to surgery is summarized in Box 57-1. **In general, the choice of the specific general anesthetic should not depend on its effects on the surgical stress response. If present, these effects are slight and short-lived and have no inhibitory effect on postoperative catabolism. The exception is etomidate, which selectively inhibits two enzymes in adrenocorticosteroid synthesis, thereby inhibiting the cortisol and aldosterone response to surgery.** This has no effect on overall catabolism, despite an inhibitory effect extending for 4 to 16 hours after intraoperative use. **High-dose opioid anesthesia also effectively inhibits the classic catabolic hormone response to operation but has no important effect on the postoperative responses or total catabolism. Different opioids do not appear to have any important differential effects.** Experimental and some clinical studies have shown hypothermia to reduce the catabolic response and waste of nitrogen, but further data are needed for any conclusions to be made on clinical implications. The consequences of intraoperative heat loss may be an exaggerated stress response during postoperative rewarming.[3]

BOX 57-1
EFFECT OF GENERAL ANESTHESIA ON SURGICAL STRESS SYNDROME

General conclusion

No important or slight inhibitory effect on intraoperative responses; no effect on postoperative catabolism.

Exceptions

Etomidate: reduces adrenocortical responses; other hormonal and metabolic responses unaffected.

High-dose opioid anesthesia: reduces major part of intraoperative response, but without effects on postoperative catabolism; no important differences among various opioids.

Hypothermia: may inhibit catabolism, but more data are needed.

Note: Intraoperative heat loss and postoperative shivering increase catabolism.

Data from Carli F, MacDonald IA: Perioperative inadvertant hypothermia, *Br J Anaesth* 76:601, 1996; Kehlet H: Modification of responses to surgery by neural blockade: clinical implications. In Cousins MJ, Bridenbaugh PO, editors: *Neural blockade in clinical anesthesia and management of pain,* Philadelphia, 1997, JB Lippincott; and Liu SS, Carpenter RL, Neal JM: Epidural anesthesia and analgesia, *Anesthesiology* 82:1474, 1995.

In contrast to general anesthesia, the effect of regional anesthesia with local anesthetics on the surgical stress response is extensive (see Table 57-1).

Epidural or intrathecal local anesthetics block the surgical stress response by inhibition of the nociceptive signal from the surgical area to the central nervous system. In addition, blockade of reflexes involving efferent autonomic and somatic pathways may be effective. The modifying effect of regional anesthesia on the stress response (Table 57-1) is most pronounced with procedures involving the lower part of the body (gynecologic, urologic, orthopedic), whereas the effect is less with major abdominal and thoracic procedures. Reasons for this may include unblocked vagal afferents, unblocked phrenic afferents, insufficient afferent sympathetic blockade, insufficient afferent somatic blockade, unblocked pelvic afferents, or other mechanisms.[10,14,18] Probably the most important mechanism is insufficient afferent somatic and sympathetic blockade, which has most convincingly been shown by evoked-potential assessments that demonstrate little inhibition of fast-conducting neural pathways by conventional doses of thoracic epidural bupivacaine administration. In contrast, a pronounced inhibition is observed when bupivacaine is administered in large doses into the lumbar epidural space.[10]

A possible differential effect of intrathecal versus epidural local anesthetics on the stress response has not been shown in systematic comparative studies.[10] Unfortunately, no studies are available for intrathecal anesthesia during upper abdominal procedures. In addition, no data exist on the possible differential effects of various local anesthetics on the surgical stress response. Preliminary data suggest that combined intrathecal and epidural anesthesia may be more effective than either technique to block the stress response to abdominal surgery.[10]

The duration of neural blockade is important for the magnitude and duration of the modification of the postoperative stress response.[10] Thus, a single-dose neural blockade (intrathecal or epidural) has only a short (2 to 5 hours) inhibitory effect on the stress response.[10] Well-designed studies are needed to show the importance of continuing the blockade for 12 to 24 hours or longer, although the few studies available suggest that **effective neural block for 24 hours will have prolonged effects for 3 or 4 days on nitrogen balance, concentrations of free amino acids in skeletal muscle, and plasma creatinine phosphokinase.**[10] More data are needed for a firm conclusion on the optimal duration of regional anesthesia to inhibit the stress response. **Posttraumatic blockade has less inhibitory effect on the stress response than a block instituted before the surgical incision.**[10]

The effects of regional anesthesia on the stress response (summarized in Table 57-1) are derived mainly from studies using bupivacaine (0.5%) in large volumes (15 to 25 ml). Few data are available to draw conclusions on the differential inhibitory effects of various concentrations of bupivacaine or other local anesthetics when used postoperatively.

Table 57-1 Effects of regional anesthesia on surgical stress syndrome*

Type of response	Inhibition or improvement	No important effect	No data
Pituitary	β-Lipotrophin Adrenocorticotropin β-Endorphin Growth hormone Arginine vasopressin Thyroid-stimulating hormone Luteinizing hormone and follicle-stimulating hormone Prolactin	T3 and T4 Calcitonin gene-related peptide Coagulation and fibrinolysis Acute-phase proteins Water and sodium balance Granulocytosis and neutrophil function Liver enzymes and antipyrin clearance Hyperthermia	Gastrointestinal peptides Testosterone Estradiol Somatomedin Ca^{++}, Mg^{++}, Zn^{+}, and phosphate balance Macrophage-derived peptides (interleukins, tumor necrosis factor)
Adrenal and renal and nervous system	Cortisol Aldosterone Renin Epinephrine Norepinephrine		
Metabolic	Hyperglycemia and glucose tolerance Insulin resistance Lipolysis Muscle amino acids Nitrogen balance Hepatic urea production Oxygen consumption Urinary potassium excretion		
Immunologic	Complement activation (C3a, C5a) Lymphopenia Natural killer cell suppression		

*Lower abdominal (gynecologic) surgery, prostatectomy, and procedures on lower extremities; some results from abdominal procedures also included.
Data from Kehlet H: Modification of responses to surgery by neural blockade: clinical implications. In Cousins MJ, Bridenbaugh PO, editors: *Neural blockade in clinical anesthesia and management of pain,* Philadelphia, 1997, JB Lippincott; and Liu SS, Carpenter RL, Neal JM: Epidural anesthesia and analgesia, *Anesthesiology* 82:1474, 1995.

If a pronounced inhibition is warranted, large doses or high concentrations (0.25% or 0.5%) will probably be necessary. Unfortunately, this also may lead to muscle paralysis and urinary retention.

The effect of epidural or intrathecal anesthesia on the pituitary stress response is pronounced because all hormones are inhibited. Similarly, adrenocortical and medullary responses and norepinephrine are reduced by regional anesthesia. Subsequent metabolic functions (e.g., hyperglycemia, altered glucose and fat metabolism, changes in free concentrations of amino acids in muscle, hepatic nitrogen conversion, nitrogen balance) are maintained at near normal unstressed levels by regional anesthesia, although most of these metabolic effects are only seen with continuous epidural analgesia.

The effect of regional anesthesia on postoperative alterations in immune function generally is rather limited but may be more favorable than the effect of general anesthesia.[10,12,14,20] Regional anesthesia has no important effect on postoperative changes in thyroid hormones, acute-phase proteins, water and sodium balance, or on routine plasma liver enzymes and probably not on hypokalemia,[10] although more studies are needed on this parameter. The total effect on coagulation and fibrinolysis is moderate, because only a few individual parameters (thrombocyte aggregation, factor VIII-capacity, fibrinolysis inhibition activity) may be favorably influenced.[10,17] Unfortunately, no data are available on the effects on gastrointestinal hormones, sex hormones, somatomedin or other growth factors, mineral balance, or the metabolically important macrophage-derived peptides (e.g., interleukins, tumor necrosis factor).

Regional anesthesia has pronounced modulatory effects on most components of the surgical stress response compared with the negligible and short-lived effects of general anesthesia. The addition of general anesthetics to regional anesthesia does not obtund these effects.[10]

To obtain pronounced metabolic effects, the regional anesthetic technique should be continued postoperatively.

EFFECT OF POSTOPERATIVE PAIN RELIEF ON SURGICAL STRESS RESPONSE

Postoperative pain, if not adequately managed, may have adverse effects by enhancing the stress response. Reflex responses may be initiated that adversely affect respiratory function, increase cardiac demands, decrease intestinal motility, and initiate skeletal muscle spasm. An improved understanding of acute pain physiology has led to the use of various drugs in the epidural space for postoperative pain relief. Total postoperative pain relief cannot be achieved by a single agent or method without major expenditure on equipment and surveillance systems or without serious side effects, which has led to the development of improved pain-relieving techniques by combinations of agents (*balanced analgesia*).[9]

The effect of the different pain-relieving techniques on the surgical stress response is summarized in Table 57-2. **Epidural analgesia with local anesthetics appears to be the most efficient inhibitory technique. Pain relief by epidural opioids or clonidine seems less effective but probably is better than pain relief by systemic opioids, whether given by intermittent doses or by patient-controlled analgesia.** The various opioids appear to have no differential effects, although this has not been studied systematically. The use of combined analgesic regimens (balanced analgesia) for pain is relatively new, and it is too early to draw any conclusions regarding the effects on the stress response compared with other techniques. Combinations with other agents, such as nonsteroidal agents or glucocorticoids, may be promising and may further reduce some aspects of the response.[10]

Combinations of analgesic regimens will have a major role in the future treatment of patients with postoperative pain. Measures to provide concomitant modification of humoral-mediated responses and techniques to improve afferent neural blockade should be explored. Also, a modification of posttraumatic functional changes in the peripheral and central nervous systems associated with pain hypersensitivity requires evaluation to improve pain relief and perhaps the stress response.

Table 57-2 Effect of various postoperative pain-relieving techniques on surgical stress response

Technique	Surgical site*	Inhibitory effect†
Systemic opioids		↓
Epidural local	LB	↓↓↓↓
anesthetics	A/T	↓↓↓
Epidural opioids	LB	↓↓
	A/T	↓↓
Epidural clonidine	LB	↓↓
	A/T	?
Multimodal analgesia	LB	?
	A/T	

*LB — lower body; A/T — abdominal thoracic.
†↓ to ↓↓↓↓ indicates relative degree of efficiency.
Data from Kehlet H: Modification of responses to surgery by neural blockade: clinical implications. In Cousins MJ, Bridenbaugh PO, editors: *Neural blockade in clinical anesthesia and management of pain,* Philadelphia, 1997, JB Lippincott; and Liu SS, Carpenter RL, Neal JM: Epidural anesthesia and analgesia, *Anesthesiology* 82:1474, 1995.

EFFECTS ON POSTOPERATIVE MORBIDITY

The concept of "stress-free anesthesia and surgery" is based on the hypothesis that various aspects of postoperative morbidity may result from the increased demands on the body caused by the metabolic, endocrine, and immunologic responses to pain and stress.[10] Some aspects of this morbidity may be inhibited by effective pain management techniques. Among current techniques, regional anesthesia is the most effective method of reducing the stress response, especially in patients with surgical procedures involving the lower body.

This section reviews controlled clinical studies comparing organ function and postoperative complications in patients receiving epidural or intrathecal anesthesia versus general anesthesia. Single studies rarely have been conclusive because they usually report on small numbers of patients. To minimize these limitations and to obtain useful information for clinical practice, results of different trials have been combined. Unfortunately, the design of the studies and the quality of information preclude a proper metaanalysis of all the morbidity parameters. Overall, the complications from the epidural or intrathecal technique *per se* are rare compared with postoperative morbidity involving major operations in high-risk patients.

Blood Loss

Perioperative blood transfusion may lead to immunosuppression, increased risk of infectious complications, tumor recurrence (in cancer surgery), and the risk of transmission of infectious diseases. Therefore, techniques should be used to reduce operative blood loss.

More than 20 controlled studies have compared intraoperative blood loss and the subsequent need for blood transfusions in patients in whom surgery was performed during either regional anesthesia or general anesthesia.[10,14] **Most data were derived from studies involving elective hip surgery** (Fig. 57-1); **they show a reduction in intraoperative blood loss of approximately 30% in patients receiving regional anesthesia.** Similar results have been obtained in studies during prostatectomy, during lower limb vascular surgery, and during hysterectomy.[10] A similar trend, although statistically insignificant, has been observed during abdominal procedures.[10] The explanation for the reduced in-

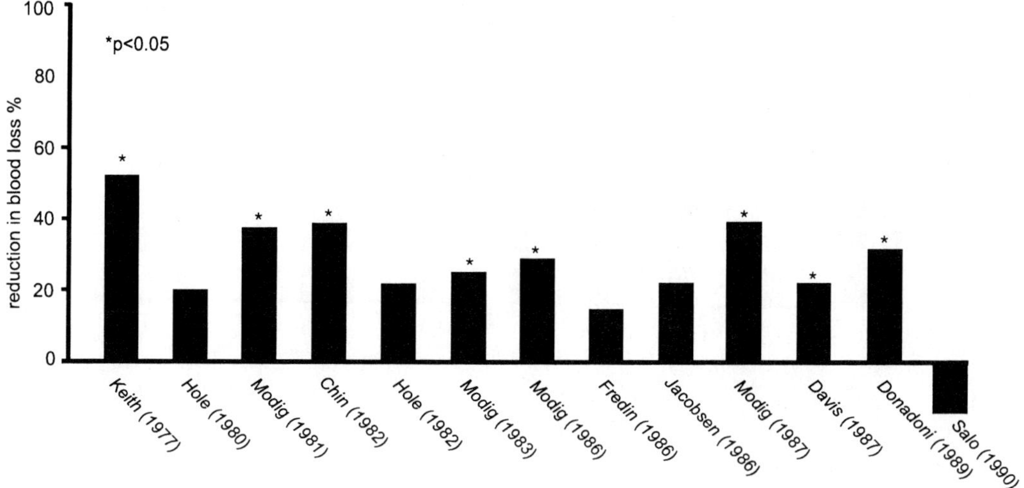

Fig. 57-1. Influence of regional anesthesia versus general anesthesia on intraoperative blood loss during hip replacement (controlled studies). * indicates a significant ($P < 0.05$) reduction of blood loss with regional anesthesia. Data from Kehlet M: Modification of responses to surgery by neural blockade: clinical implications. In Cousins MJ, Bridenbaugh PO, editors: *Neural blockade in clinical anesthesia and management of pain,* Philadelphia, 1997, JB Lippincott; and Liu SS, Carpenter RL, Neal JM: Epidural anesthesia and analgesia, *Anesthesiology* 82:1474, 1995.

traoperative blood loss is probably a combination of decreased mean arterial pressure, mean pulmonary arterial pressure, right atrial pressure, and peripheral venous pressure, leading to decreased venous oozing.[10] Continuous epidural analgesia has been reported to reduce postoperative blood loss through surgical drains also.[10] The available studies show no difference between the effects of epidural versus intrathecal anesthesia.

The magnitude of blood loss reduction during regional anesthesia compared with general anesthesia depends on the technique of general anesthesia. Blood loss is less in those with induced hypotension and in patients receiving spontaneous ventilation compared with those receiving intermittent positive-pressure ventilation, in whom venous pressure may be greater.[10]

Thromboembolic Complications

The pathogenesis of postoperative thromboembolism is probably related to unfavorable changes in the components of Virchow's triad. (Virchow's triad describes three components that lead to thrombosis: alteration of blood vessel walls or endothelium, stasis of blood flow, and hypercoagulability.) All three may be favorably altered to some extent by regional anesthetic techniques (Table 57-3).

Several controlled studies have shown that regional anesthesia reduces postoperative deep venous thromboembolism by approximately 50% (Fig. 57-2). In the six studies involving hip surgery, four used continuous epidural analgesia. **In the three studies using perfusion lung scans, the incidence of pulmonary embolism was dramatically less in patients receiving regional anesthesia compared with those receiving general anesthesia. The only study involving prostatectomy found a highly significant reduction in deep venous thrombosis when regional anesthesia was used.**

Table 57-3 Effect of regional anesthesia on pathogenic factors of postoperative thromboembolism (Virchow's triad)

Parameter	Result
Lower extremity blood flow	Increased by epidural or intrathecal local anesthetics
Thrombocyte aggregation	Reduced after epidural local anesthetics
Coagulation and fibrinolysis	Coagulation slightly reduced and fibrinolysis slightly improved after epidural local anesthetics

Data from Kehlet H: Modification of responses to surgery by neural blockade: clinical implications. In Cousins MJ, Bridenbaugh PO, editors: *Neural blockade in clinical anesthesia and management of pain,* Philadelphia, 1997, JB Lippincott; and Rosenfeld BA: Benefits of regional anesthesia on thromboembolic complications following surgery, *Reg Anesth* 21:6S:9, 1996.

In all orthopedic studies in Fig. 57-2, the control group (general anesthesia) did not receive prophylaxis for deep venous thrombosis except for aspirin in one study involving knee surgery.[22] In those undergoing peripheral vascular surgery, there was a reduction in graft thrombosis in accordance with the physiologic data showing increased lower ex-

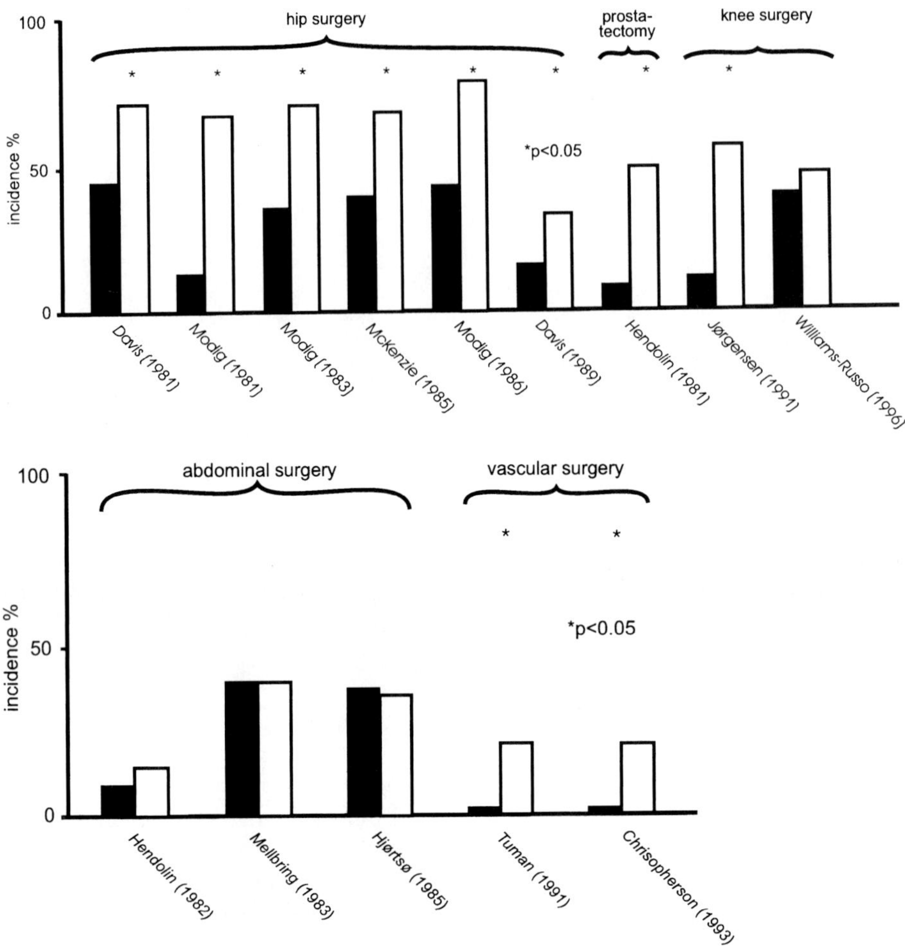

Fig. 57-2. Incidence of postoperative thromboembolism in patients receiving regional anesthesia (*dark bars*) versus general anesthesia (*light bars*) in controlled studies using phlebography or ^{125}I-fibrinogen scan. Data from Kehlet H: Modification of responses to surgery by neural blockade: clinical implications. In Cousins MJ, Bridenbaugh PO, editors: *Neural blockade in clinical anesthesia and management of pain,* Philadelphia, 1997, JB Lippincott; and Liu SS, Carpenter RL, Neal JM: Epidural anesthesia and analgesia, *Anesthesiology* 82:1474, 1995.

tremity and graft blood flow after regional anesthesia and a more favorable balance between coagulation and fibrinolysis.

The beneficial effect of continuous epidural analgesia on thromboembolism after abdominal surgery probably is less than with lower-extremity procedures (Fig. 57-2). The explanation may be that thoracic epidural analgesia (which may not provide all the positive alterations in Virchow's triad) was used in two of the studies, and in the third study, the control group received low-dose heparin. This suggests that continuous epidural analgesia is as effective as low-dose heparin in those undergoing abdominal surgery. The combination of regional anesthesia with other antithrombotic regimens has not been studied sufficiently, but additional heparin may further reduce thrombosis.[10,19]

Cerebral Function

Postoperative mental dysfunction is a well-recognized problem occurring within the first postoperative week and predominantly affecting elderly patients.[15] Unfortunately, the mechanism of postoperative mental deterioration is not known. The responses to injury, hypoxemia, and sleep deprivation may be important,[11] and these factors may all be positively influenced by regional anesthesia. In addition, preoperative use of various drugs, depression, and hospitalization may precipitate the patient's confusion.

Eighteen controlled studies have compared postoperative mental dysfunction in patients receiving regional or general anesthesia.[10,14] Most procedures involved major orthopedic surgery. In more than half the studies, an in-depth assessment of cerebral function was performed, often including a late postoperative follow-up evaluation. **The choice of anesthesia and the altered endocrine milieu do not appear to have a major effect on postoperative mental changes.** The data do not allow any analysis of intrathecal versus continuous epidural technique. Because most studies have used single-dose regional anesthesia, additional studies with continuous epidural analgesia are required to resolve the uncertainty.

Table 57-4 Effect of continuous epidural analgesia on pulmonary infection after major abdominal, vascular, and thoracic surgery

Reference	Postoperative analgesic techniques	Epidural analagesia	Systemic opioid
Rawal (1983)	○		
Hjortsø (1985)	○ ●		
Cushieri (1985)	●		
Yeager (1987)	○		
Hendolin (1987)	●		
Jayer (1988)	○		
Seeling (1990)	○ ●	118 complications in 593 patients	148 complications in 600 patients
Tuman (1991)	○ ●		
Ryan (1992)	●		
Kilbride (1992)	○	20%	25%
Davies (1993)	●		
Jayer (1993)	○ ●		
Garnett (1996)	○ ●	$P > 0.05$	

Data from Garnett RL, MacIntyre A, Lindsay P, et al: Perioperative ischaemia in aortic surgery, *Can J Anaesth* 43:769, 1996; Kehlet H: Modification of responses to surgery by neural blockade: clinical implications. In Cousins MJ, Bridenbaugh PO, editors: *Neural blockade in clinical anesthesia and management of pain,* Philadelphia, 1997, JB Lippincott; and Liu SS, Carpenter RL, Neal JM: Epidural anesthesia and analgesia, *Anesthesiology* 82:1474, 1995.
Compiled data from controlled studies including > 30 patients.
● — epidural local anesthetics; ○ — epidural opioid.

Available data suggest that regional anesthesia has either no effect or only a slight beneficial effect compared with general anesthesia on postoperative cerebral function. This finding suggests that mental dysfunction may be caused by factors other than the choice of anesthetic.[11,15]

Pulmonary Complications

Postoperative pulmonary infectious complications may be related to preoperative and postoperative lung dysfunction.[21] The anesthesia- and surgery-related factors contributing to this deterioration include pain, bronchospasm, muscle paralysis, microthromboembolism, blood transfusion, site of surgical incision, postoperative supine position and immobilization, general anesthesia, and distorted sleep patterns.[11,21] No technique has been able to normalize pulmonary function and totally ablate pain after major surgery, but continuous epidural analgesia with local anesthetics is the most effective technique and clearly more favorable than general anesthesia combined with postoperative systemic opioids.[5,10,14]

Despite the clinical importance of pulmonary complications, relative few studies have compared the incidence of pulmonary infections in patients receiving regional versus general anesthesia.[10,14] Several studies have reported that the incidence of postoperative pulmonary atelectasis is reduced with regional anesthesia, although the data include studies in which the complication was clinically relevant and not merely a radiologic diagnosis.

Eight studies have compared pulmonary complications after lower-body surgery in patients who were randomized to receive regional (predominantly single dose) or general anesthesia.[10,14] Most studies failed to show any statistically significant difference, but often reported a trend toward fewer complications in the group receiving regional anesthesia. Because of patient and procedure heterogenety, these results should be taken with caution and serve mainly as a stimulus for further large-volume, well-designed studies.

For major abdominal surgery, regional anesthesia most often is continued postoperatively with local anesthetics or opioids. Table 57-4 shows the results from the available studies. Overall, there was only a nonsignificant trend toward fewer pulmonary complications with continuous regional analgesia.

Insufficient data exist concerning the effect of regional versus general anesthesia on postoperative pulmonary infections. The available data only suggest a positive effect for regional anesthesia, which may be of clinical importance if confirmed in large-scale studies. Because no other measures have proved to be more effective in reducing pulmonary complications, regional anesthesia should be considered whenever the preoperative assessment suggests an increased risk. In particular, a continuous epidural technique should be considered for patients undergoing abdominal procedures. A more pronounced effect of epidural analgesia on pulmonary complications may be achieved if the postoperative pain relief is integrated into a multimodal re-

Table 57-5 Effect of continuous epidural analgesia on cardiac complications after major abdominal, vascular, and thoracic surgery

Reference	Postoperative epidural-analgesic techniques	Epidural analgesia		Systemic opioid
Hjortsø (1995)	● ○			
Yeager (1987)	○			
Seeling (1990)	● ○	91 complications in 337 patients		103 complications in 358 patients
Tuman (1991)	● ○			
Davies (1993)	○			
Beattie (1993)	●	27%		29%
Garnett (1996)	● ○		$P > 0.05$	

Data from Garnett RL, MacIntyre A, Lindsay P, et al: Perioperative ischaemia in aortic surgery, *Can J Anaesth* 43:769, 1996; Kehlet H: Modification of responses to surgery by neural blockade: clinical implications. In Cousins MJ, Bridenbaugh PO, editors: *Neural blockade in clinical anesthesia and management of pain,* Philadelphia, 1997, JB Lippincott; and Liu SS, Carpenter RL, Neal JM: Epidural anesthesia and analgesia, *Anesthesiology* 82:1474, 1995.
Compiled data from controlled studies including > 30 patients.
● — epidural local anesthetics; ○ — epidural opioid.

habilitation program with enforced mobilization and oral nutrition (to be discussed).

Cardiac Complications

The risk of postoperative myocardial infarction and dysrhythmias is related predominantly to (1) the surgical stimulus leading to increased demands on the heart, (2) intraoperative hypertension and hypotension, and (3) postoperative hypoxemia. Other factors (e.g., existing ischemic or other heart disease, hypertension) increase the risk of surgically related cardiac dysfunction. Apparently the choice of specific general anesthetics is less important than the changes induced by the surgical stimulus.

Because regional anesthesia may reduce or prevent reflex responses leading to hypertension or hypotension and increased demands on the heart,[8,10,14] this should have a beneficial effect on postoperative outcome. Cardiac complications may be induced from the cardiotoxicity of the local anesthetics (especially bupivacaine) or from the patient's compromised circulation during pronounced sympathetic blockade if bleeding and hypovolemia occur.

Several studies involving single-dose epidural analgesia or continuous epidural analgesia suggest a beneficial effect based on physiologic measurements of oxygen requirements, cardiac work, and hemodynamic alterations.[8,10,14] Other studies have shown epidural anesthesia to be beneficial in nonsurgical patients with or without angina pectoris and also to reduce exercise-induced myocardial ischemia.[10,14]

Despite the evidence from physiologic assessments that regional anesthesia may be advantageous in surgical patients, few well-designed, sufficiently large studies have investigated the effect of regional versus general anesthesia on cardiac complications. Single-dose regional anesthesia may not confer any advantage, even in lower body procedures,[2,10,14] wherein optimal stress-free conditions may be obtained with continuous regional analgesia. In major abdominal and thoracic procedures, continuous epidural analgesia has not been shown to reduce cardiac morbidity (Table 57-5). Additional data are required, probably with integration of the epidural analgesia into a postoperative rehabilitation program (to be discussed).[11]

Despite well-documented physiologic advantages of regional anesthesia,[8,10,14] the studies that evaluated clinically important cardiac complications did not convincingly show a beneficial effect in patients receiving regional anesthesia versus general anesthesia.

Gastrointestinal Function and Complications

Postoperative gastrointestinal paralysis continues to be a clinical problem, with relatively few improvements in the understanding of its pathogenesis and therapy. Although probably multifactorial, the most important factor leading to postoperative ileus is activation of sympathetic inhibitory reflexes.[4,10,14] Regional anesthesia would therefore be expected to have a beneficial effect on postoperative gastrointestinal paralysis.

The effects of epidural local anesthetics, epidural opioids, or combinations of local anesthetics and opioids, versus systemic or epidural opioids on postlaparotomy gastrointestinal motility are summarized in Fig. 57-3. A differential effect of various general anesthetics has not been studied systematically but is unlikely.[10] Addition of nitrous oxide (N_2O) probably has no important effect on postoperative nausea and ileus.[10] In studies with continuous epidural bupivacaine or low-dose epidural bupivacaine–opioid combinations, improved postoperative gastrointestinal motility was found compared with postoperative pain relief provided by systemic opioids or epidural opioids.[4,10,14] **Continuous epidural bupivacaine appears to be the most effective**

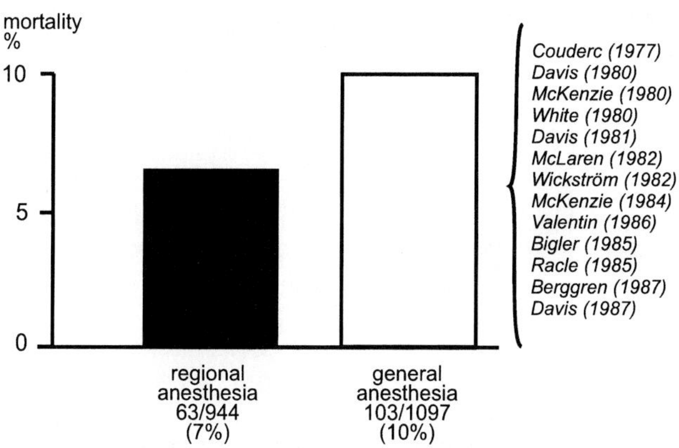

Fig. 57-3. Effect of continuous epidural analgesic techniques on postlaparotomy ileus (controlled studies). Data from Kehlet H: Modification of responses to surgery by neural blockade: clinical implications. In Cousins MJ, Bridenbaugh PO, editors: *Neural blockade in clinical anesthesia and management of pain,* Philadelphia, 1997, JB Lippincott; Liu SS, Carpenter RL, Mackey DC, et al: Effects of perioperative analgesic technique on recovery after colon surgery, *Anesthesiology* 83:757, 1995; and Liu SS, Carpenter RL, Neal JM: Epidural anesthesia and analgesia, *Anesthesiology* 82:1474, 1995.

measure to improve postoperative gastrointestinal ileus. Combined low-dose local anesthetic–opioid combinations may be equally effective.

The increased intraoperative and postoperative gastrointestinal motility in patients receiving continuous epidural bupivacaine has increased concern regarding the potential risk of anastomotic dehiscence, but data from controlled clinical studies have not supported this suspicion.[10] The few case reports of early dehiscence of a colonic anastomosis may represent an earlier presentation of a leak, resulting from imperfection of surgical technique.[10] In addition, epidural analgesia increases colonic blood flow,[4,10,14] which may be advantageous for healing of a gastrointestinal anastomosis.

Mortality

Improvements in perioperative care have reduced patient mortality, which makes documentation of the beneficial effects of new interventional regimens very difficult because of the need for large numbers of concurrent patients to be studied. This also applies to the effect of regional anesthesia versus general anesthesia on mortality. However, 12 controlled studies have compared early mortality (less than 30 days) after acute hip surgery for fracture, performed during either regional or general anesthesia (Fig. 57-4). Although only two studies were able to show a significant reduction in mortality rate using regional anesthesia, the general trend was toward lower mortality in most of the studies. The cumulative data show a significant reduction in mortality rate, from 10% to 7% (see Fig. 57-4). When patients were followed up for 2 months to 2 years, the initial difference in mortality disappeared.[10] No similar large-scale data are available from other surgical procedures, except for those undergoing peripheral vascular surgery in whom no difference in mortality could be shown between patients operated during intrathecal, epidural, or general anesthesia.[2]

Regional anesthesia (intrathecal or epidural) appears to reduce early postoperative mortality rate after acute hip surgery, although subsequent survival may depend on factors other than the choice of anesthetic.

Convalescence and Hospital Stay

The time until the patient can ambulate after major joint surgery performed was reported to be unaltered[10,16] or only slightly improved by continuous regional anesthesia.[10,22] No conclusive data exist on convalescence parameters such as postoperative fatigue, muscle performance, and return to work. On the basis of the apparent beneficial effects of regional anesthetic techniques on postoperative morbidity, a concomitant shortening of postoperative hospital stay should be expected. Available data suggest that hospital stay is unchanged in lower-body procedures or in abdominal and thoracic procedures performed with continuous regional versus general anesthesia (Table 57-6).

The explanation for these results in those undergoing upper abdominal or thoracic surgery has not been determined. One explanation may be the lack of important inhibitory effects of these techniques, primarily thoracic surgery using epidural analgesia, on the surgical stress response and postoperative organ dysfunction, as discussed previously. Another reason may be that the postoperative care program has not taken advantage of the analgesic and

Table 57-6 Effect of continuous epidural analgesia on postoperative hospital stay (days) after major abdominal, vascular, and thoracic surgery

Reference	Epidural analgesia	Systemic opioid
Rawal (1984) Yeager (1987) Seeling (1990) Bredtmann (1991) Tuman (1991) Ryan (1992) Davies (1993) Jayer (1993)	15 days	16 days
	$P > 0.05$	

Data from Kehlet H: Modification of responses to surgery by neural blockade: clinical implications. In Cousins MJ, Bridenbaugh PO, editors: *Neural blockade in clinical anesthesia and management of pain,* Philadelphia, 1997, JB Lippincott; and Liu SS, Carpenter RL, Neal JM: Epidural anesthesia and analgesia, *Anesthesiology* 82:1474, 1995.

Compiled data from controlled studies including > 30 patients (mean values).

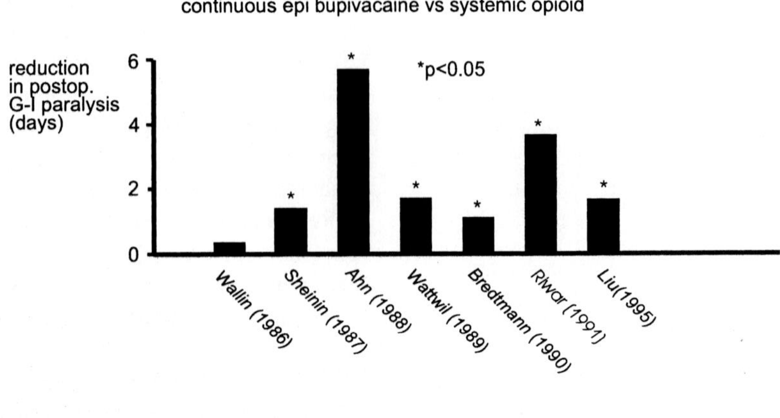

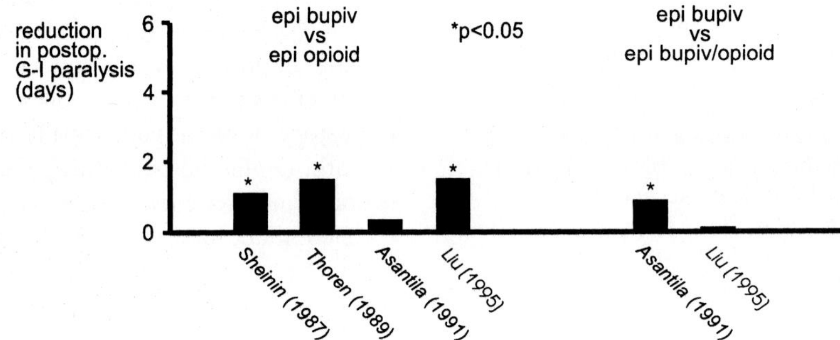

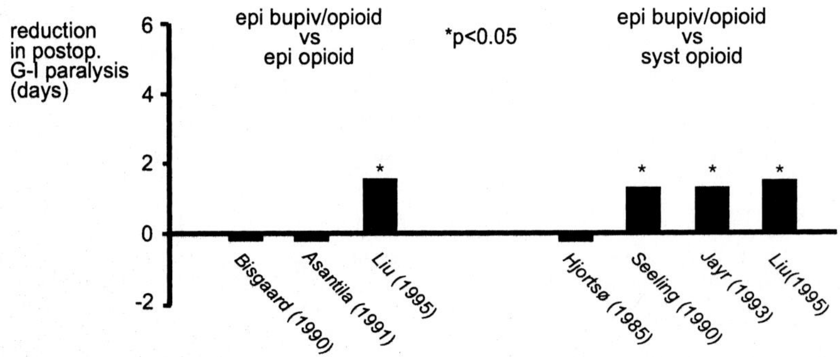

Fig. 57-4. Effect of regional versus general anesthesia on early (less than 30 days) mortality after acute surgery for hip fracture (controlled studies). Data from Kehlet H: Modification of responses to surgery by neural blockade: clinical implications. In Cousins MJ, Bridenbaugh PO, editors: *Neural blockade in clinical anesthesia and management of pain,* Philadelphia, 1997, JB Lippincott; and Liu SS, Carpenter RL, Neal JM: Epidural anesthesia and analgesia, *Anesthesiology* 82:1474, 1995.

physiological advantages of epidural analgesia with early mobilization and oral nutrition (to be discussed).[11]

MULTIMODAL APPROACH TO CONTROL POSTOPERATIVE PATHOPHYSIOLOGY AND REHABILITATION

Although effective functional postoperative pain relief with continuous epidural analgesia has a great potential to improve postoperative outcome, the available data have not conclusively demonstrated an important clinical effect. Because regional anesthetic and analgesic techniques may have favorable physiological effects compared with general anesthesia and systemic analgesic techniques, an analysis of factors other than pain that may contribute to postoperative morbidity is required.[11] Such factors may include the unnecessary routine use of nasogastric tubes or surgical drains, traditions limiting oral intake, a fixed postoperative "observation period," or protocols for immobilization. In addition, a postoperative rehabilitation program with enforced mobilization and oral nutrition, taking advantage of the provided functional pain relief, is required.[11] Preliminary uncontrolled observations in a variety of procedures, including herniotomy, colonic surgery, major joint replacements, coronary artery bypass grafting, mastectomy, cholecystectomy, and carotid endarterectomy[11] suggest that such an approach has major beneficial effects on postoperative outcome. Abbreviated postoperative hospital stay protocols should be developed as a multidisciplinary effort, with collaboration between anesthesiologists, surgeons, and surgical nurses and with integration of postoperative pain management (acute pain service) into a postoperative rehabilitation unit. Hopefully, such efforts will lead to a new series of well-designed studies to evaluate the effects of regional anesthetics and analgesic techniques on postoperative outcome.

CONCLUSION

Although long-term postoperative outcome is determined by many factors, the choice of anesthesia and postoperative pain relief is an important determinant of early outcome. Many controlled studies have shown that the surgical stress response is reduced by regional anesthetic techniques compared with intraoperative general anesthesia and postoperative pain relief with systemic opioids. In addition, several studies suggest that some postoperative morbidity parameters may be improved by regional anesthesia for procedures below the umbilicus, but the effects may be less or nonexistent in major upper abdominal and thoracic procedures. Finally, epidural analgesia is superior to other regimens in providing pain relief after major surgery.

Despite these beneficial data in favor of regional anesthetic techniques, more information is needed before definite indications and specific protocols can be recommended. This applies especially to the selection of patients and surgical procedures. The optimal anesthetic technique may then be chosen after weighing all available data as has been done for anesthesia during hip surgery in the elderly population, in whom regional anesthesia may be the preferred technique. The literature continues to report promising data supporting the theory that adequate inhibition of surgically induced nociceptive stimuli may improve postoperative outcome. It is hoped that such findings will continue to draw attention to this important area and increase the collaboration between anesthesiologists and surgeons for the overall management of the surgical patient.

KEY POINTS

- The metabolic response to surgery is characterized by an increased secretion of catabolically acting hormones (cortisol, glucagon, catecholamines), whereas the anabolically acting hormones (insulin, testosterone, growth hormones) are inhibited. The resulting metabolic effect is hypermetabolism and release of substrate (glucose, amino acids, fat) from peripheral stores (muscle, fat tissue, lever). Concomitantly, changes in immune function take place; the general pattern is reductions in most components.
- In general, the specific general anesthetic technique should not depend on its effects on the surgical stress response. If present, these effects are slight and short-lived and have no inhibitory effect on postoperative catabolism. The exception is etomidate, which selectively inhibits two enzymes in adrenocorticosteroid synthesis, thereby inhibiting the cortisol and aldosterone response to surgery.
- High-dose opioid anesthesia also effectively inhibits the classic catabolic hormone response to operation but has no important effect on the postoperative responses or on total catabolism. Different opioids do not appear to have any important differential effects.
- In contrast to general anesthesia, the effect of regional anesthesia with local anesthetics on the surgical stress response is extensive. Epidural or intrathecal local anesthetics block the surgical stress response by inhibition of the nociceptive signal from the surgical area to the central nervous system. In addition, blockade of reflexes involving efferent autonomic and somatic pathways may be effective.
- The duration of neural blockade is important for the magnitude and duration of the modification of the postoperative stress response.
- Effective neural block for 24 hours will have prolonged effects for 3 or 4 days on nitrogen balance, concentrations of free amino acids in skeletal muscle, and plasma creatinine phosphokinase.
- Posttraumatic blockade has less inhibitory effect on the stress response than a block instituted before the surgical incision.
- The effect of epidural or intrathecal anesthesia on the pituitary stress response is pronounced because all hormones are inhibited. Similarly, adrenocortical and medullary responses and norepinephrine are reduced by regional anesthesia. Subsequent metabolic functions (e.g., hyperglycemia, altered glucose and fat metabolism, changes in free concentrations of amino acids in muscle, hepatic nitrogen conversion, nitrogen balance) are maintained at near normal unstressed levels by regional anesthesia, although most of these metabolic effects are only seen with use of continuous epidural analgesia.
- Regional anesthesia has pronounced modulatory effects on most components of the surgical stress response compared with the negligible and short-lived effects of general anesthesia. The addition of general anesthetics to regional anesthesia does not obtund these effects. To obtain

pronounced metabolic effects, the regional anesthetic technique should be continued postoperatively.

- Epidural analgesia with local anesthetics appears to be the most efficient inhibitory technique. Pain relief by epidural opioids or clonidine seems less effective but probably is better than pain relief by systemic opioids, whether given by intermittent doses or by patient-controlled analgesia.
- Most data were derived from studies involving elective hip surgery and show a reduction in intraoperative blood loss of approximately 30% in patients receiving regional anesthesia.
- Several controlled studies have shown that regional anesthesia reduces postoperative deep venous thromboembolism by approximately 50%.
- In the three studies using perfusion lung scans, the incidence of pulmonary embolism was significantly less in patients receiving regional anesthesia compared with those receiving general anesthesia. The only study involving prostatectomy found a highly significant reduction in deep venous thrombosis when regional anesthesia was used.
- The beneficial effect of continuous epidural analgesia on thromboembolism after upper abdominal surgery is probably less than in lower-extremity procedures.
- Insufficient data exist concerning the effect of regional versus general anesthesia on postoperative pulmonary infections. The available data only suggest a positive effect for regional anesthesia.
- Despite well-documented physiologic advantages of regional anesthesia, the studies that have evaluated clinically important cardiac complications did not convincingly demonstrate a beneficial effect in patients receiving regional anesthesia versus general anesthesia.
- Continuous epidural bupivacaine appears to be the most effective measure to improve postoperative gastrointestinal ileus. Combined low-dose local anesthetic–opioid combinations may be equally effective.
- Regional anesthesia (intrathecal or epidural) appears to reduce early postoperative mortality after acute hip surgery, although long-term survival may depend on factors other than the choice of anesthetic.
- Available data suggest that hospital stay is unchanged in lower-body procedures or abdominal and thoracic procedures performed with continuous regional versus general anesthesia.

KEY REFERENCES

Liu S, Carpenter RL, Neal JM: Epidural anesthesia and analgesia. Their role in postoperative outcome, *Anesthesiology* 82:1474–1506, 1995.

Kehlet H: Modification of responses to surgery by neural blockade: clinical implications. In Cousins MJ, Bridenbaugh PO, editors: *Neural blockade in clinical anesthesia and management of pain,* Philadelphia, 1997, JB Lippincott.

Kehlet H: Multimodal approach to control postoperative pathophysiology and rehabilitation—a review, *Br J Anaesth* 78:606, 1997.

REFERENCES

1. Beal AL, Cerra FB: Multimodal organ failure syndrome in the 1990s. Systemic inflammatory response and organ dysfunction, *JAMA* 271:226, 1994.
2. Bode RH, Lewis KP, Zarich SW, et al: Cardiac outcome after peripheral vascular surgery. Comparison of general and regional anesthesia, *Anesthesiology* 84:3, 1996.
3. Carli F, MacDonald IA: Perioperative inadvertent hypothermia—what do we need to prevent? *Br J Anaesth* 76:601, 1996.
4. Carpenter RL: Gastrointestinal benefits of regional anesthesia/analgesia, *Reg Anesth* 21:6S:13, 1996.
5. Clerque, Aissa I, Holland J, et al: Respiratory benefits of regional anesthesia, *Reg Anesth* 21:6S:18, 1996.
6. Covino BG, Shires GT, editors: Influence of anaesthetic procedures on surgical sequelae, an update, *Acta Chir Scand Suppl* 550:1, 1988.
7. Garnett RL, MacIntyre A, Lindsay P, et al: Perioperative ischaemia in aortic surgery: combined epidural/general anesthesia and epidural analgesia vs. general anesthesia and i.v. analgesia, *Can J Anaesth* 43:769, 1996.
8. Hogan Q: Cardiovascular response to sympathetic block by regional anesthesia, *Reg Anesth* 21:6S:26, 1996.
9. Kehlet H, Dahl JB: The value of multimodal or balanced analgesia on postoperative pain relief, *Anesth Analg* 77:1048, 1993.
10. Kehlet H: Modification of responses to surgery by neural blockade: clinical implications. In: Cousins MJ, Bridenbaugh PO, editors: *Neural blockade in clinical anesthesia and management of pain,* Philadelphia, 1997, JB Lippincott.
11. Kehlet H: Multimodal approach to control postoperative pathophysiology and rehabilitation—a review, *Br J Anaesth* 78:606, 1997.
12. Leon-Cassasola OA: Immunomodulation and epidural anesthesia and analgesia, *Reg Anesth* 21:6S:24, 1996.
13. Liu SS, Carpenter RL, Mackey DC, et al: Effects of perioperative analgesic technique on recovery after colon surgery, *Anesthesiology* 83:757, 1995.
14. Liu SS, Carpenter RL, Neal JM: Epidural anesthesia and analgesia. Their role in postoperative outcome, *Anesthesiology* 82:1474, 1995.
15. Marcantonio ER, Goldman L, Mangione CM, et al: Clinical prediction rule for delirium after elective non-cardiac surgery, *JAMA* 271:134, 1994.

16. Møiniche S, Hjortsø N-C, Hansen BL, et al: The effect of balanced analgesia on early convalescence after major orthopedic surgery, *Acta Anaesthesiol Scand* 38:328, 1994.
17. Rosenfeld BA: Benefits of regional anesthesia on thromboembolic complications following surgery, *Reg Anesth* 21:6S:9, 1996.
18. Segawa H, Mori K, Kasai K, et al: The role of the phrenic nerves in stress response in upper abdominal surgery, *Anesth Analg* 82: 1215, 1996.
19. Sharrock NE, Brien W, Salvati EA, et al: The effect of intravenous fixed-dose heparin during total hip arthroplasty on the incidence of deep-vein thrombosis, *J Bone Joint Surg* 72A:1456, 1990.
20. Stevenson GW, Hall SC, Rudnick S: The effect of anesthetic agents on the human immune response, *Anesthesiology* 72:542, 1990.
21. Wahba RWM: Perioperative functional residual capacity, *Can J Anaesth* 38:384, 1991.
22. Williams-Russo P, Sharrock NE, Haas SB, et al: Randomized trial of epidural vs general anesthesia. Outcomes after primary total knee replacement, *Clin Orthop* 331: 199, 1996.

CHAPTER 58

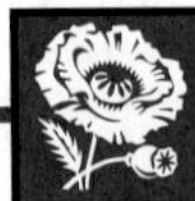

Pharmacology of Local Anesthetics

F. MICHAEL FERRANTE

THE PHYSIOLOGY OF NEURAL BLOCKADE AT THE ULTRASTRUCTURAL LEVEL

The Gating Model of Sodium Channel Kinetics

To begin to understand local anesthetic pharmacology and how local anesthetics produce neural blockade, the structure and function of the nerve membrane surrounding the axoplasm should first be examined (Fig. 58-1). The framework of the nerve membrane is composed of a double layer of phospholipid molecules. The polar phosphate heads of the phospholipid molecules face the extracellular fluid and the axoplasm. The hydrophobic lipid tails are oriented toward each other, forming a relatively impermeable ion barrier. Proteins are embedded within the lipid matrix and form channels through which ions may or may not pass. Voltage-driven configurational changes in the protein macromolecules of the channel cause it to open and close.

Ion channels exist for several discrete ions, but blockade of the sodium channel is responsible for production of local anesthesia. Ion selectivity of channels is determined by the presence of "filters" located at the pore aperture near the external entrance.

The sodium channel may exist in three separate states that determine transmembrane sodium flux (the gating model for sodium channel kinetics; Figs. 58-2 and 58-3). While the channel may be open or closed, three separate configurations of the channel (and therefore, conformations of channel protein macromolecules) are assumed to exist. With depolarization of the membrane, transient dimerization of abutting peptides occurs, opening the channel. During repolarization, the channel protein subunits assume a transitional configuration. Inactivation is a transitional phase between activated (open) and resting (closed) sodium channel protein conformations. The channel is still impermeable to sodium, but with further realignment of the protein subunits, the channel reverts to its resting (closed) state.[35,55,216]

Normal Impulse Generation and Propagation

The action potential

At rest, a negative electrical potential of 60 to 90 mV (the resting membrane potential) exists between the extracellular fluid and the axoplasm. **The resting membrane potential results from the greater proportion of potassium ions on the interior of the nerve membrane as compared with the extracellular fluid and because the membrane is permeable to potassium but impermeable to other cations in the resting state** (Fig. 58-4; the greater portion of sodium ions is found in the extracellular fluid as compared to the axoplasm). In the resting membrane state, the potassium channel is open with 30 times more potassium internal to the

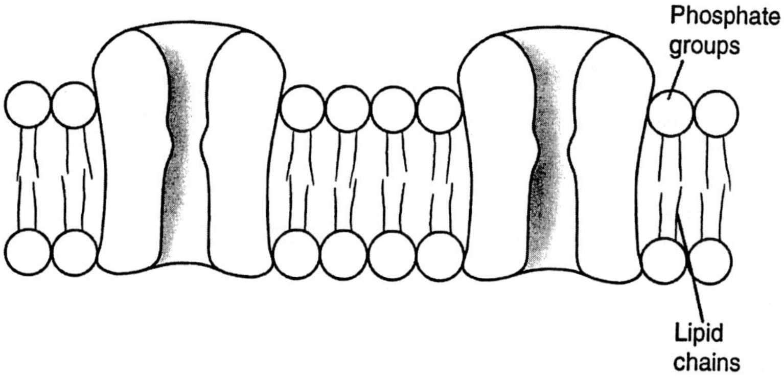

Fig. 58-1. Structure of the neuronal membrane. Ion channels are formed from protein macromolecules embedded within a lipid bilayer matrix. Voltage changes cause configurational realignment of protein macromolecules of the channel. Such changes of configuration allow the channel to open and close. Ion selectivity of the channel is determined by filters near the external pore aperture. (From de Jong RH: *Local anesthetics,* St. Louis, 1994, Mosby).

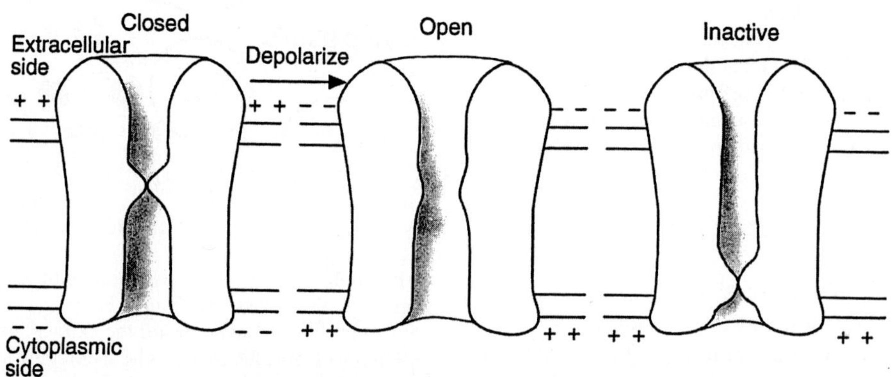

Fig. 58-2. The gating model of sodium channel kinetics. With depolarization, the axoplasmic side of the nerve membrane assumes a positive charge (*center*). Protein macromolecules of the channel undergo conformational changes from the resting state (closed) (*left*) to the ion-permeable state (open) (*center*). A transitional (inactive) state is formed when the channel proteins assume a different configuration, but the channel is still ion impermeable (closed) (*right*). With repolarization, the inactivated state reverts to the resting protein configuration (*left*). (From Siegelbaum SA, Koester J: Ion channels. In Kandel ER, editor: *Principles of neural science,* ed 3, Norwalk, CT, 1991, Appleton-Lange.)

membrane than in the extracellular fluid. A large outward diffusion gradient for potassium ions is established in the resting state. The axoplasmic side of the membrane is negatively charged because bulky, impermeable anions are left behind by permeable potassium ions.[55]

When nerve stimulation occurs, the electrical potential becomes progressively more positive (Fig. 58-5 and 58-6). **When reaching a potential of −55 mV, conformational changes occur in the proteins of the sodium channel,** which is referred to as the *firing threshold.* **At this point, sodium channels open to allow a massive (and passive) influx of sodium ions from the extracellular fluid through the channel to the axoplasm, which is driven by the electrochemical gradient.** This results in a reversal of the electrical potential so the axoplasmic surface of the membrane becomes more positively charged as compared with the external surface. At the peak of the action potential, the axoplasmic membrane has an electrical potential of 40 mV as compared with the external membrane surface. Shortly, the closing of sodium channels (deactivation) stops sodium influx. Potassium channels open to allow greater efflux of potassium ions down their concentration gradient. Deactivation coupled with the efflux of potassium ions reverses the positive electrical potential.

Deactivation is a distinct process from inactivation of sodium channels because it has a different gating mechanism. As sodium channels begin to open with depolariza-

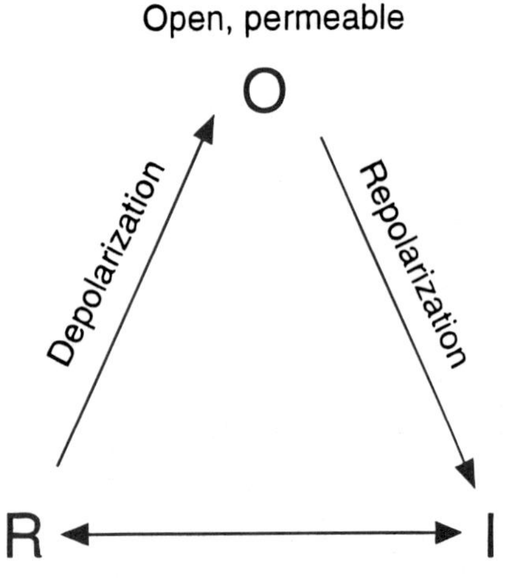

Fig. 58-3. The gating model for sodium channel kinetics. The channel can be permeable or impermeable to sodium ions, but the protein macromolecules of the channel exist in three conformations. With depolarization the channel moves from the closed, resting state (*R*) to the open, permeable state (*O*). During repolarization, the channel first assumes a transitional closed, inactivated state (*I*). With further realignment of the protein macromolecules of the channel, the resting state is reassumed. (From de Jong RH: *Local anesthetics,* St. Louis, 1994, Mosby.)

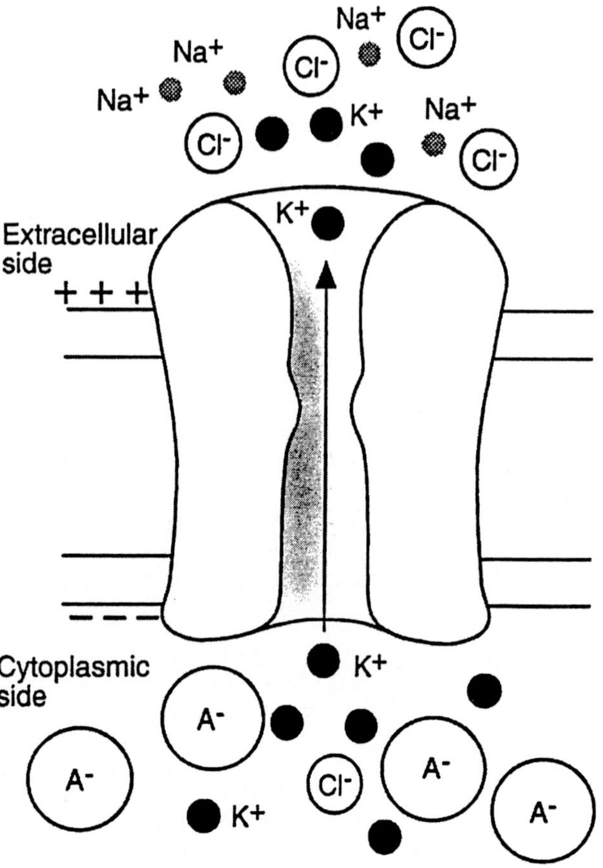

Fig. 58-4. Genesis of the resting membrane potential. In the resting state, the potassium channel is open with the diffusion gradient from the axoplasm toward the extracellular fluid. As potassium ions leave, the axoplasmic membrane surface becomes negatively charged as the channel is impermeable to negatively charged anions in the resting state. (From de Jong RH: *Local anesthetics,* St. Louis, 1994, Mosby.)

tion, other channels begin to close (deactivate) and enter the inactivated state. Deactivation and inactivation assist in repolarization of the membrane, although the closing of sodium channels and the efflux of potassium ions through open potassium channels are largely responsible for the return of the membrane to the resting membrane potential. Inactivation causes the nerve to be refractory to further stimulation. Thus, the action potential is propagated forward, preventing retrograde conduction of the action potential in the axon fiber.[55]

Classification of peripheral nerve fibers

Peripheral nerves contain axons of varying function, diameter, myelination, and conduction velocity (Table 58-1). Stimulation of a peripheral nerve (like the individual axon) results in a voltage response. This compound action potential (Fig. 58-7) is composed of several distinct peaks, each representing a group of nerve fibers of differing conduction velocities. Speed of conduction in the compound action potential is proportional to nerve diameter and the extent of myelination (Fig. 58-7).

In the earlier part of this century, Gasser and Erlanger[92] classified peripheral nerve fibers based on diameter, myelination, and conduction velocity (which is related to the extent of myelination because of saltatory conduction; to be discussed). This classification is still used today. By grouping nerves with respect to diameter and extent of myelination, we also are able to predict their functional roles with respect to proprioreception, autonomic function, sensation, and motor activity (Table 58-1).

Saltatory conduction

Depolarization in one segment of nerve results in depolarization in the adjacent segment because of the difference in electrical potential. Thus, once nerve stimulation has occurred, transmission of the impulse is self-sustaining and self-propagating, although conduction down an axon is different for myelinated and unmyelinated nerves.

The nerve membrane itself has high electrical capacitance. The largely aqueous axoplasm and extracellular fluid have low resistance. Therefore, current density is lost just a short distance from the site of initial depolarization. Thus, conduction is slow for unmyelinated nerves because of resistive and capacitative current losses. Threshold potential should be reached again and again for impulse propagation to occur.

The Schwann cells of myelinated nerves, in essence,

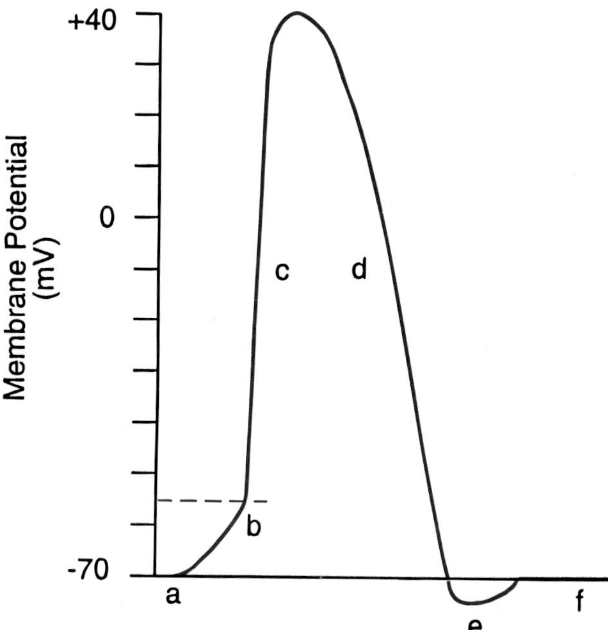

Fig. 58-5. The action potential. In the resting state **(A),** sodium channels are closed. Depolarization by an arriving impulse causes the membrane potential to reach the firing threshold *(dashed line at* **B**). At this point, there is massive sodium influx through open channels, which causes a steep increase in membrane potential **(C).** Deactivation (closing) of sodium channels occurs, and sodium influx halts. Potassium efflux increases, and the membrane potential becomes more negative **(D).** After hyperpolarization **(E),** the resting potential is restored **(F).** Local anesthetics lower the amplitude of the action potential, increase firing threshold **(B),** and slow the rate of depolarization **(C).** Neural blockade is achieved when these progressive changes make the firing threshold unattainable. (From de Jong RH: *Local anesthetics,* St. Louis, 1994, Mosby.)

wrap the nerve in an insulating substance, and current can travel farther before fading below threshold potential. **Impulse propagation can proceed by leaps from node of Ranvier to node of Ranvier before fading below threshold potential** (Fig. 58-8). **Such impulse transmission is referred to as saltatory conduction.**[50,55]

The Mechanism of Neural Blockade

Local anesthetics interdict impulse generation and propagation by blocking membrane permeability to sodium and interfering with the processes that generate the action potential (Figs. 58-5 and 58-6).[216] The nerve membrane itself and not the axoplasm or external neural supporting structures is the locus of impulse blockade.[35,159,255] Artificial lipid bilayer membranes[35,177] and isolated membranes filled with potassium-rich solution[159,255] behave like normal nerve and can be blocked by local anesthetics. Moreover, nerves stripped of their sheaths and Schwann cells undergo more rapid neural blockade.[82] Thus, only the membrane portion of a nerve participates in neural blockade. **Voltage-clamp experiments reveal that local anesthetics cause neural blockade by direct inhibition of transmembrane sodium flux.**[82,179]

Older theories underlying the mechanism of neural blockade localized the site of anesthetic binding to the external membrane surface.[37] Toxins such as tetrodotoxin and saxitoxin cause irreversible neural blockade and permanent cessation of transmembrane sodium ion flux by lodging on, in, or near the external pore of the sodium channel.[65,227]

The clinically useful local anesthetics bind to the internal membrane of the sodium channel itself. A local anesthetic receptor site has been recently defined in the pore of the sodium channel.[171] The binding site appears to be near the external pore of the sodium channel, because previous or re-

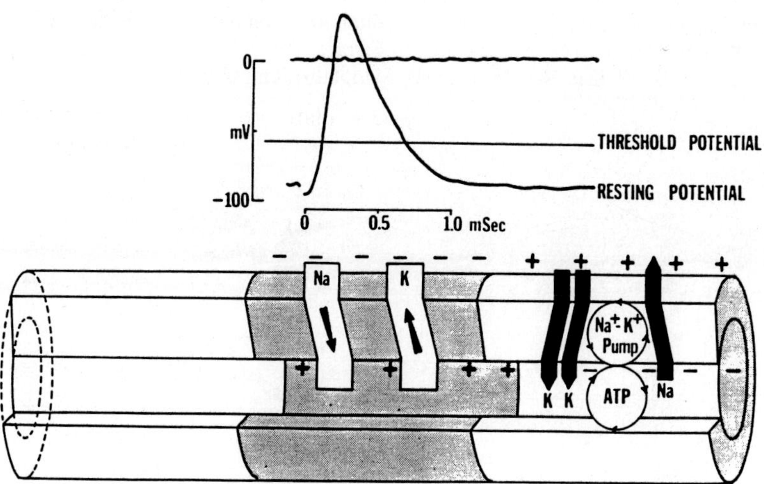

Fig. 58-6. Relationship between membrane action potential and ion flux across the neuronal membrane. (From Covino BG, Vassalo HG: *Local anesthetics: mechanism of action and clinical use,* New York, 1976, Grune & Stratton.)

Table 58-1 The Gasser and Erlanger classification of peripheral nerve fibers

Fiber type	Diameter	Myelination	Location	Physiologic function
Aα	Largest	(+)	Afferents and efferents, muscles and joints	Motor, propioreception
Aβ	↑	(+)	Afferents and efferents, muscles and joints	Motor, propioreception
Aγ		(+)	Efferents to muscle spindles	Muscle tone
Aδ		(+)	Sensory afferents	Pain, temperature, touch
B		(+)	Preganglionic sympathetic	Autonomic
C	Smallest	(−)	Sensory afferents	Pain, temperature, touch
C	Smallest	(−)	Postganglionic sympathetic	Autonomic

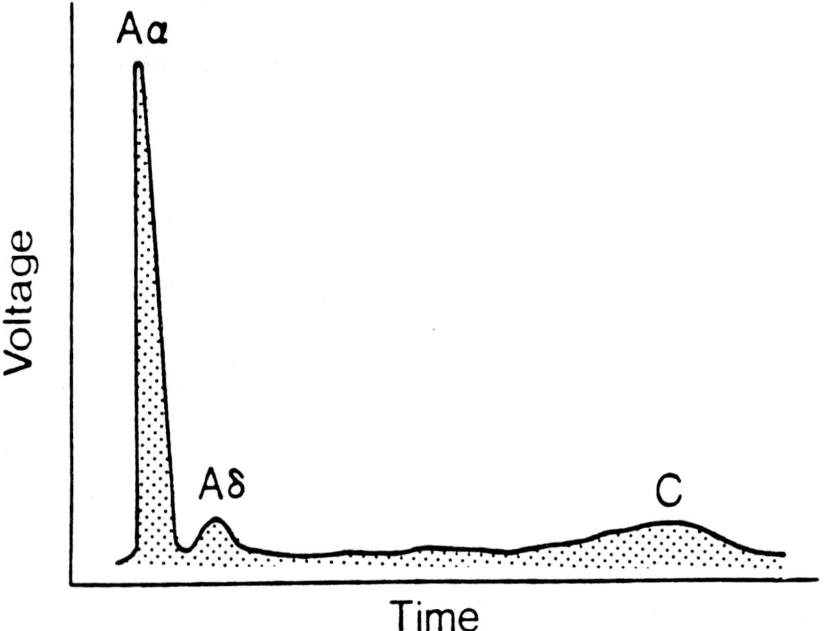

Fig. 58-7. The compound action potential. When a peripheral nerve is stimulated and the voltage is recorded at a distance from the site of stimulation, a compound action potential is generated. The compound action potential represents the summation of action potentials for discrete fiber types. (From Katz N, Ferrante FM: Nociception. In Ferrante FM, VadeBoncouer TR, editors: *Postoperative pain management,* New York, 1993, Churchill-Livingstone.)

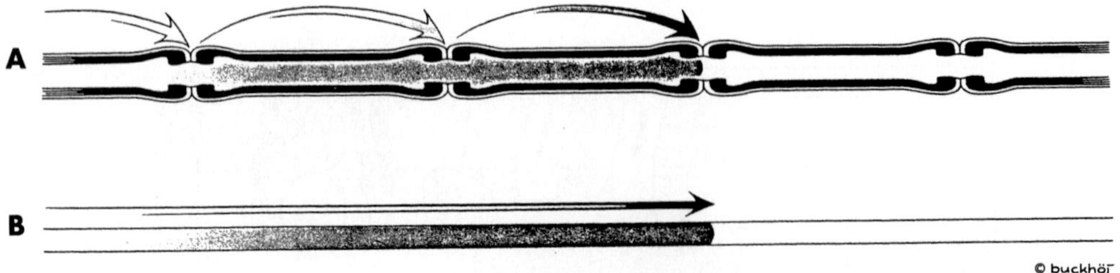

Fig. 58-8. Saltatory conduction. **(A)** In myelinated nerves, impulse propagation occurs by passage from node of Ranvier to node of Ranvier. **(B)** In unmyelinated nerves, impulse propagation occurs along the entire length of the nerve. (From Covino BG, Scott DB: *Handbook of epidural anaesthesia and analgesia,* Orlando, 1985, Grune & Stratton.)

peated stimulation (use- or frequency-dependent block[44]; Fig. 58-9) increases the intensity of neural blockade.[35,45,229]

Access to the receptor site (except for the notable exception of benzocaine; to be discussed) occurs by inward diffusion of uncharged local anesthetic base through the membrane to the axoplasmic side of the membrane. Here, dissociation creates a positively charged local anesthetic cationic moiety that diffuses back into the sodium channel. A cationic species is necessary for traversing the hydrophilic pathway of the pore to attach to the receptor site via electrostatic bonding (Fig. 58-10).[35,159,229]

Crucial to the mechanism of neural blockade by local anesthetics are mechanisms whereby conformational changes are elicited in the protein macromolecules of the channel. Local anesthetics preferentially bind to the receptor in the open and inactivated state of the sodium channel. They dissociate from the receptor site in the resting state.[228] These two events are not absolute but rather relative events because association and dissociation are linked. Rate constants for the two phenomena differ so that one kinetic state or the other is dominant.[115]

This has lead to two hypotheses for local anesthetic action, depending on alterations (or lack thereof) in affinity of local anesthetic for the receptor.[35,112,114,220] The modulated receptor hypothesis[112,114] assumes that affinity for the receptor changes as a function of the conformational state of pore protein macromolecules. Binding affinity is increased in the open and inactivated channel state, and decreased binding affinity is present in the resting channel state. The guarded receptor hypothesis[220] assumes that binding affinity is uniform throughout all phases of sodium channel kinetics but that access to and from the receptor site is interdicted or facilitated by conformational changes in the protein macromolecules. The receptor is "guarded" by the conformation of pore proteins. Both hypotheses are robust, as frequency-dependent block can be explained by either hypothesis: repeated stimulation causes local anesthetic to be bound to an enhanced number of sodium channels (Fig. 58-9).

Through the aforementioned mechanisms, local anesthetics decrease the amplitude of the action potential, slow the rate of depolarization, increase firing threshold, slow impulse conduction, and prolong the refractory period. Neural blockade is achieved when these changes prevent the membrane potential from reaching the firing threshold (Fig. 58-5).[178]

Benzocaine

Benzocaine, a topical local anesthetic, does not fit the model of the cationic species being the "active" local anesthetic moiety, because it is uncharged and hydrophobic. Benzocaine should reach the receptor site by an alternate pathway that does not require passage through the sodium channel in-

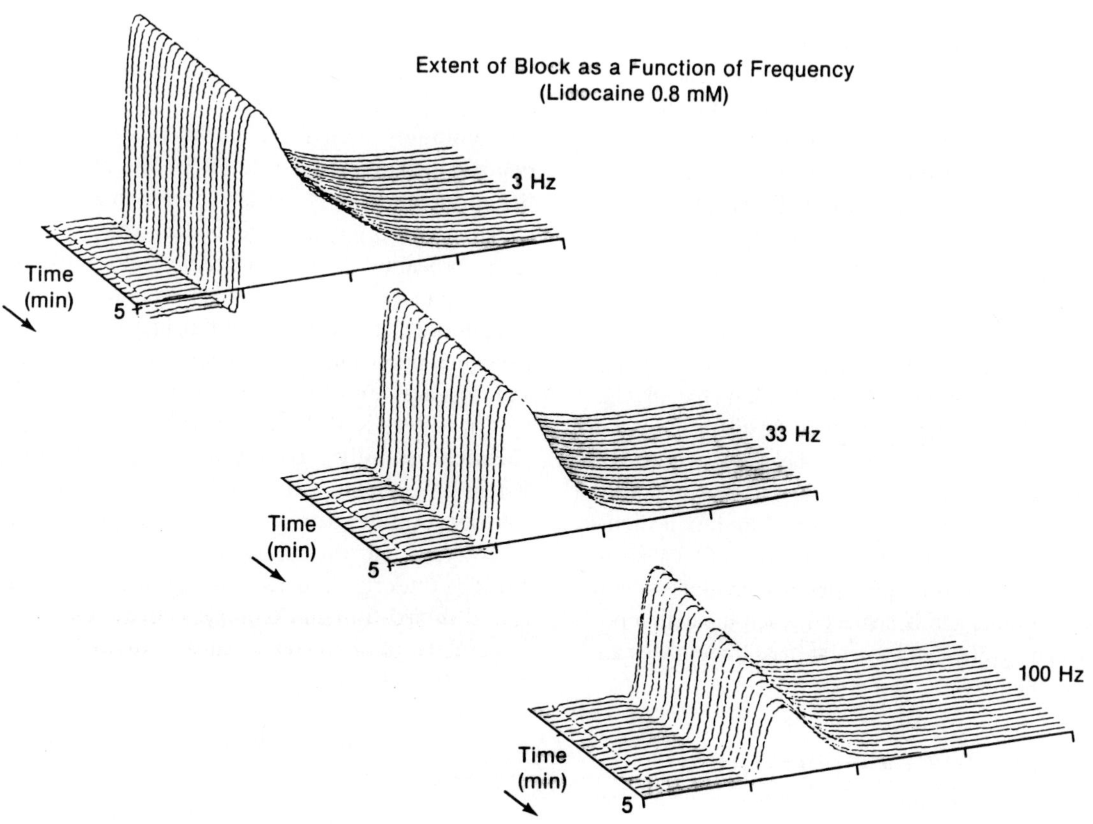

Fig. 58-9. Frequency-dependent block. With increasing frequency of nerve stimulation at a uniform concentration of local anesthetic, the amplitude of the action potential decreases over time. (From Covino BG, Scott DB: *Handbook of epidural anaesthesia and analgesia,* Orlando, 1985, Grune & Stratton.)

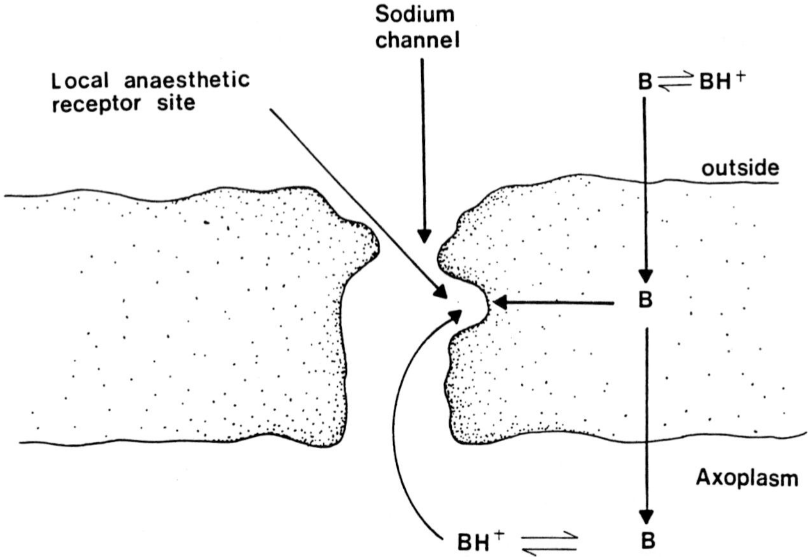

Fig. 58-10. Local anesthetic-receptor binding. Local anesthetic base (B) diffuses through the membrane to the axoplasm. Within the axoplasm, the cationic species (BH^+) is then formed, which diffuses back into the hydrophilic channel to bind to the receptor. Benzocaine is unique. As a hydrophobic local anesthetic base, benzocaine gains access to the receptor through the lipid membrane independent of channel gating kinetics. (From Covino BG: Local anesthetics. In Ferrante FM, VadeBoncouer TR, editors: *Postoperative pain management,* New York, 1993, Churchill-Livingstone.)

ternal aperture, which is corroborated by the fact that benzocaine does not produce frequency-dependent block. Benzocaine (as an uncharged local anesthetic base) can dissolve in the lipid membrane, diffuse toward the channel protein macromolecules and the receptor site, and bind to the receptor without forming a cationic moiety (Fig. 58-10). Thus, benzocaine gains access to the receptor site independent of the channel kinetic state, thereby explaining its inability to elicit frequency-dependent block.[112,205]

Myelinated axons

The myelin sheath increases the efficiency of impulse propagation via saltatory conduction. In addition, the myelin sheath acts as a diffusion barrier to local anesthetics[36] except at the nodes of Ranvier.[89] Sodium channel density is 100 or more times greater at the node than in the myelin-coated section of a nerve. Sodium transmembrane ion flux is therefore concentrated at the node. Thus, restriction of local anesthetic access to the nodal region does not preclude neural blockade. Neural blockade is achieved when the action potential is reduced by 50% and when at least three nodes are exposed to anesthetic.[7,237]

PHARMACOLOGIC CLASSIFICATION OF LOCAL ANESTHETICS

A variety of chemical structures are capable of blockade of nerve conduction in intact or isolated nerves: amino esters, amino carbamates, amino ketones, amino amides, alcohols, thioesters, thioethers, thioamides, ureas, phosphoric esters, polyethers, simple amines, and guanidine-type structures.[51] Traditionally, local anesthetics with clinical use have possessed the chemical arrangement: aromatic portion—intermediate chain–amino portion.

Commonly used local anesthetics are classified into two distinct groups (Table 58-2): the amino esters and the amino amides. The esters possess an ester link between the aromatic portion and intermediate chain of the molecule (e.g., procaine, 2-chloroprocaine, and tetracaine). The amides possess an amide link between the aromatic portion and intermediate chain of the local anesthetic molecule (e.g., lidocaine, prilocaine, mepivacaine, etidocaine, bupivacaine, and ropivacaine).

The esters and amides differ with respect to their chemical stability, biodegradation, and allergenicity. Esters have short shelf-lives, being somewhat unstable in solution. Amides are very stable compounds. Esters are hydrolyzed in the plasma by pseudocholinesterase. Amides undergo hepatic biodegradation via the microsomal mixed-function oxidase system. The potential allergenicity of the ester local anesthetics resides in the production of para-aminobenzoic acid (PABA) as one of the primary products of biotransformation. Because amides are not metabolized to PABA, allergic reactions are extremely rare.[55]

Physicochemical Properties and Structure-Activity Relationships

The physicochemical properties of the various esters and amides determine anesthetic potency, rapidity of onset of

Table 58-2 Structure and physicochemical properties of local anesthetics

Agent	Aromatic lipophilic	Intermediate chain	Amine hydrophilic	Molecular weight (base)	pKa (25°C)	Partition coefficient	Percent protein binding
Esters							
Procaine	H-N(H)-⟨ring⟩-	$COOCH_2CH_2$	$-N(C_2H_5)_2$	236	8.9	0.02	5.8
Tetracaine	H_9C_4N(H)-⟨ring⟩-	$COOCH_2CH_2$	$-N(CH_3)_2$	264	8.6	4.1	75.6
Chloroprocaine	H-N(H)-⟨ring, Cl⟩-	$COOCH_2CH_2$	$-N(C_2H_5)_2$	271	8.7	0.14	—
Amides							
Prilocaine	⟨ring⟩-, CH_3	NHCOCH(CH_3)	-N(H)(C_3H_7)	220	7.7	0.9	~ 55
Lidocaine	⟨ring⟩-, CH_3, CH_3	$NHCOCH_2$	$-N(C_2H_5)_2$	234	7.7	2.9	64.3
Mepivacaine	⟨ring⟩-, CH_3, CH_3	NHCO	piperidine N-CH_3	246	7.6	0.8	77.5
Bupivacaine	⟨ring⟩-, CH_3, CH_3	NHCO	piperidine N-C_4H_9	288	8.1	27.5	95.6
Etidocaine	⟨ring⟩-, CH_3, CH_3	NHCOCH(C_2H_5)	-N(C_2H_5)(C_3H_7)	276	7.7	141	94

(From Covino BG, Scott DB: *Handbook of epidural anaesthesia and analgesia,* Orlando, 1985, Grune & Stratton.)

amides determine anesthetic potency, rapidity of onset of neural blockade, and duration of activity. Minor alterations in the aromatic portion, the intermediate chain, or in the amine portion of the local anesthetic molecule have dramatic effects on lipid solubility, protein binding, and pK_a (Table 58-2).

Structure-activity relationships

The aromatic portion of the local anesthetic molecule is believed to be responsible for the lipophilic properties of a compound, whereas the amine portion is responsible for the innate hydrophilicity. Changes in the aromatic or amine portions of a local anesthetic will alter its partition coefficient and protein-binding capacity. For example, addition of a butyl group to the aromatic portion of procaine results in a hundredfold increase in lipid solubility (increasing the partition coefficient) and a tenfold increase in protein binding.[241] Increasing the molecular weight of an amide or ester by lengthening the intermediate chain or by addition of carbon atoms to the ends of a molecule will increase potency to a maximum. Any further increases in molecular weight will decrease potency.[234]

Stereochemistry and stereospecificity. Many local anesthetics (e.g., cocaine, bupivacaine, etidocaine, ropivacaine) possess a chiral carbon atom. Such local anesthetics can be configured around the chiral carbon atom as two three-dimensional mirror images. Each optical isomer possesses different physicochemical properties and sometimes different biologic properties.[55]

The observation that different enantiomers of local anesthetics could confer different biologic properties has been known for some time.[145,203] Cocaine was well known to be a purely levorotatory isomer.[145,203] This observation took on new clinical importance with the discovery of the cardiotoxic effects of bupivacaine. Sodium channel receptor affinity is threefold greater for R(+) than for S(−) bupiva-

dissociation time during diastole for the R(+) bupivacaine enantiomer.[134]

Lipid solubility

Lipid solubility is the physicochemical property primarily responsible for anesthetic potency (Fig. 58-11).[47,131,245] For example, bupivacaine (one of the most lipid soluble amines) is formed by addition of a butyl group to the amine portion of mepivacaine, which results in a four-fold increase in potency, a thirty-fivefold increase in the partition coefficient, and a major increase in protein binding.[245] In general, potency increases as a function of lipid solubility until reaching a partition coefficient of approximately four. As predicted from structure-activity relationships, any further increase in partition coefficient (lipid solubility) does not translate into any appreciable increase in anesthetic potency (Fig. 58-11).[46]

Lipid solubility also correlates with rapidity of onset of block and time to recovery from neural blockade,[44] although lipid solubility is not their primary determinant.

Protein binding

Neural blockade occurs after the binding of local anesthetic to a protein receptor within the sodium ion channel.[47] Because the receptor is proteinaceous in nature, substances with greater binding affinity for protein should remain within the channel for a longer time, thereby resulting in increased duration of neural blockade. Thus, duration of anesthesia is primarily related to the extent of protein binding of local anesthetics. It is assumed that the extent of binding of local anesthetics to plasma proteins represents the extent of binding to membrane proteins (Fig. 58-12).[47]

Rapidity of onset

The rapidity of onset of neural blockade of local anesthetics is primarily determined by the pK_a of the individual agents,[47,230] at least *in vitro* (Fig. 58-13). *In vivo,* onset of action may be affected by the ability of local anesthetic to diffuse through nonneural tissue. Because the unionized form of a local anesthetic is responsible for diffusion across the nerve membrane,[185] speed of onset of neural blockade will be determined by the amount of drug in the base (unionized) form at physiologic pH. At pH equals 7.4, the percentage of local anesthetic moiety found in the base form is inversely proportional to the pK_a of the local anesthetic. Thus, agents with low pK_as (e.g., lidocaine, prilocaine, mepivacaine, etidocaine; see Table 58-2) have relatively rapid onsets of action (Fig. 58-13). Agents with high pK_as have relatively slow onsets of action (e.g., procaine, tetracaine; see Table 58-2; Fig. 58-13). As predicted by pK_a, the onset of neural blockade with bupivacaine is intermediate.

Differential sensory/motor blockade

With the introduction of bupivacaine and ropivacaine into clinical practice, local anesthetics can be distinguished on the basis of their ability to produce a differential blockade of sensory and motor fibers. Bupivacaine[215] and ropivacaine[11,53] show relative differential selectivity for blockade of sensory fibers in lieu of motor fibers. All other local anesthetics ex-

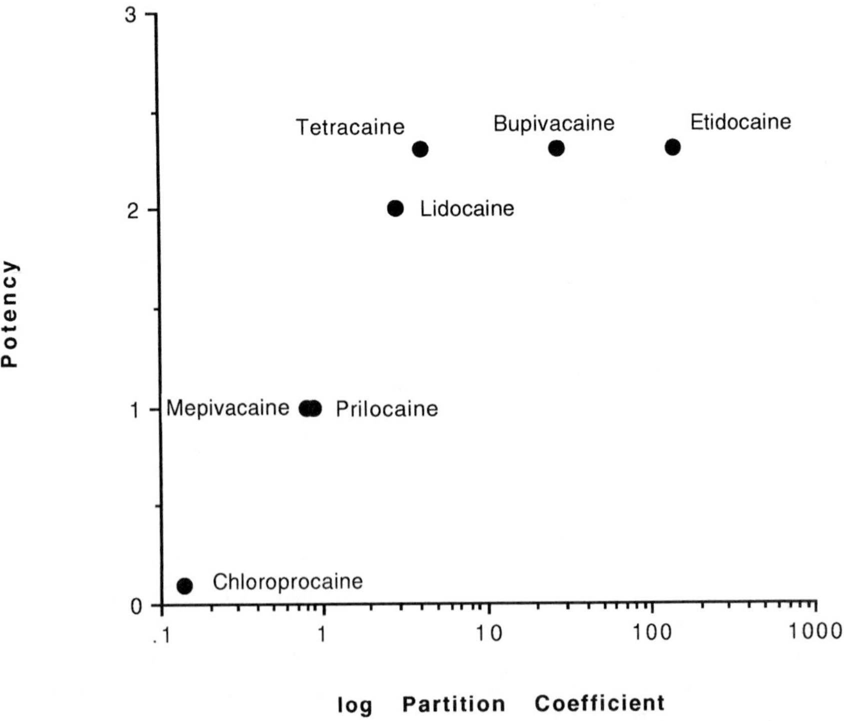

Fig. 58-11. Relationship between lipid solubility and anesthetic potency.

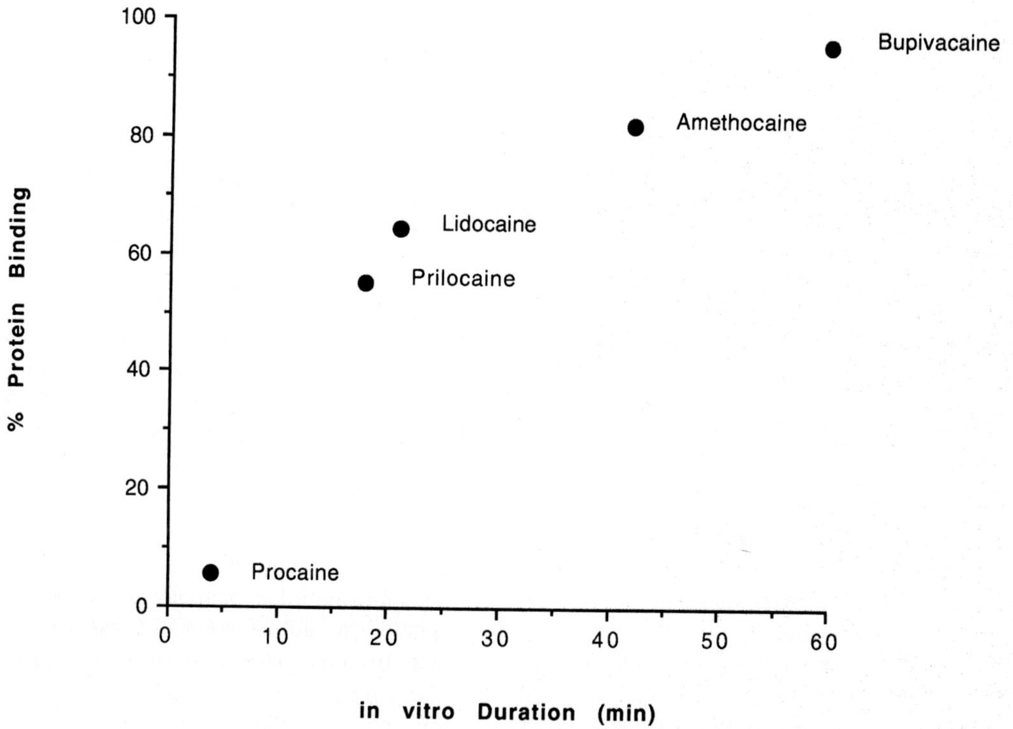

Fig. 58-12. Relationship between protein binding and the rate of recovery from block in an isolated nerve preparation.

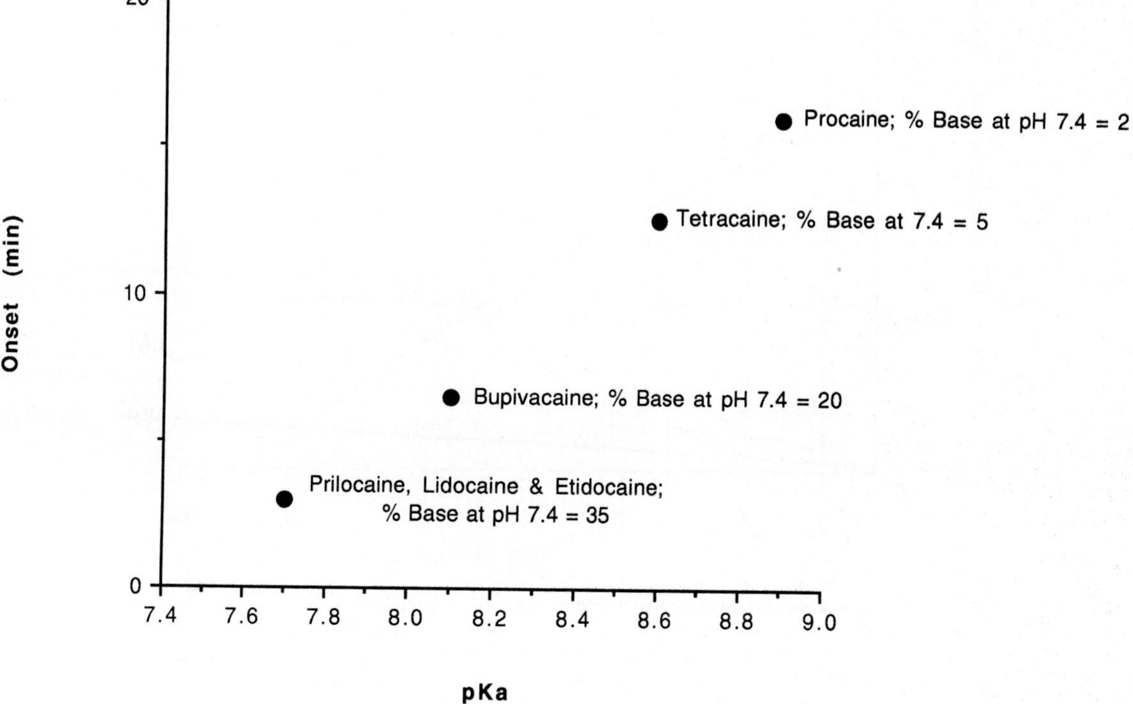

Fig. 58-13. Relationships between the *in vitro* rapidity of onset of neural blockade, pK_a, and the percentage of drug in the base (unionized) form.

hibit minimal discrimination between sensory versus motor neural blockade.

In addition to the structure-activity relationships and physicochemical properties of local anesthetics, other factors are responsible for clinical effects. Most of these factors involve the intentional clinical manipulation of uptake, but an understanding of the distribution and elimination of local anesthetics still is crucial to their effective use. Thus, a discussion of pharmacokinetics is pertinent to understanding nonpharmacodynamic factors influencing local anesthetic activity.

PHARMACOKINETICS

Kinetic Modeling

The uptake, distribution, and elimination of local anesthetics can be described by a two- or three-compartment model.[9,185,243] The term *disposition* represents the combined processes of distribution and clearance, excluding the process of absorption.[243,249]

Although local anesthetics are sometimes released directly into the bloodstream after intravenous (IV) regional anesthesia[190] or are used therapeutically as IV analgesics[80] and antiarrhythmics,[95] the magnitude of most initial blood concentrations will be determined by the amount absorbed from a tissue depot during traditional regional anesthesia (Fig. 58-14). Irrespective of whether local anesthetic is absorbed or administered intravenously, it is rapidly diluted in the blood and quickly taken up by highly perfused, rapidly equilibrating tissues (e.g., brain, lung, kidney, liver; Fig. 58-15). This α-phase is responsible for the rapid exponential disappearance of local anesthetic from the blood. Very quickly, disappearance from the blood slows. This β-phase or distribution phase represents access of local anesthetic to less perfused or slowly equilibrating tissues (e.g., skeletal muscle) that act as storage buffers. The capacity of this reservoir can be gauged by the volume of distribution (V_d). Local anesthetics with large volumes of distribution have lesser peak concentrations (e.g., etidocaine, which is highly protein bound and lipid soluble; Table 58-2). The converse is similarly true. The distribution phase is sometimes divided into a third or clearance phase (γ-phase), representing metabolism and excretion.[122] Disappearance of local anesthetic from the blood is linear in the γ-phase.

Absorption into the bloodstream occurs after oral ingestion, topical application, or depot injection of local anes-

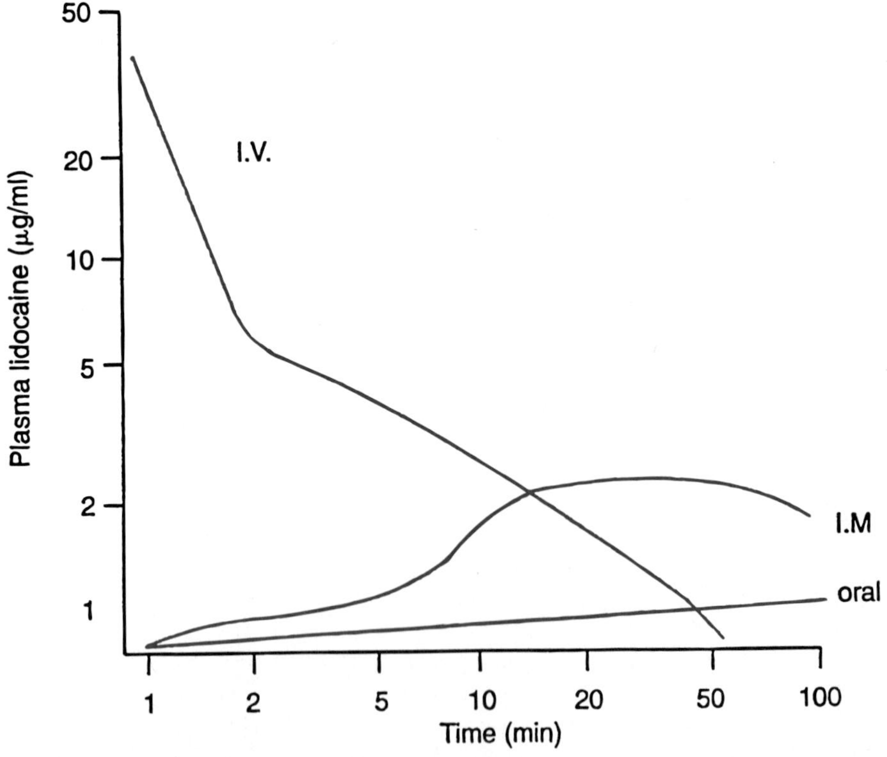

Fig. 58-14. Plasma concentration as a function of route of administration. After an intravenous injection of 100 mg of lidocaine, plasma levels decline exponentially as lidocaine is taken up by well-perfused tissues. During the distribution phase, plasma levels decrease linearly. Absorption after a 250-mg intramuscular injection resembles the absorption pattern associated with regional anesthesia. Peak plasma concentrations are seen in 10 to 30 minutes. After oral dosing (250 mg), absorption occurs slowly with peak plasma concentrations achieved in 1 to 2 hours. (From de Jong RH: *Local anesthetics,* St. Louis, 1994, Mosby.)

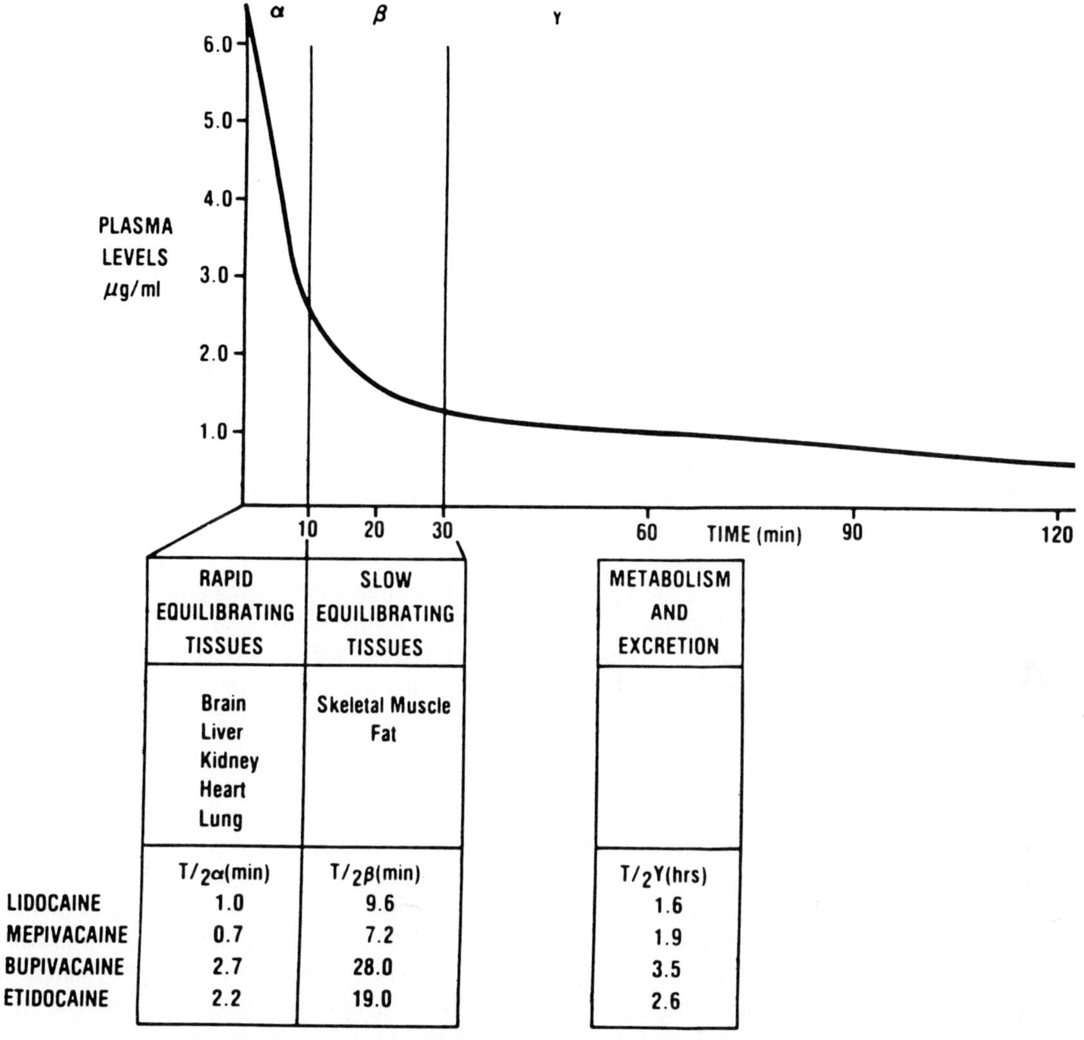

Fig. 58-15. Plasma concentration–decay curve after intravenous injection of local anesthetic. α-Phase represents redistribution into rapidly equilibrating, well-perfused tissues. β-Phase represents redistribution of local anesthetic into slowly equilibrating, poorly perfused tissues. The γ-phase represents metabolism and excretion. (From Covino BG: Local anesthetics. In Ferrante FM, VadeBoncouer TR, editors: *Postoperative pain management,* New York, 1993, Churchill-Livingstone.)

thetic (i.e., regional anesthesia). Resulting blood concentrations are distinct from those achieved after IV administration (Fig. 58-14) and are the result of multiple factors (to be discussed), although the physiology of transit through rapidly and slowly equilibrating tissues is essentially the same as outlined previously.

The final disposition phase (γ-phase) for local anesthetic represents clearance. Clearance is independent of the route of administration (unlike dilution or absorption). The physiologic determinants of clearance are blood flow, protein binding, and the intrinsic function of the biotransformation and elimination mechanisms.[122] Representative clearances for amide local anesthetics are listed in Table 58-3.

The concept of half-life gives a readily interpretable measure of clearance with respect to time. A half-life can be defined for each phase of disposition, although the $t_{1/2}\alpha$ is exceedingly short (e.g., lidocaine, 10 minutes; bupivacaine, 2.1 minutes; ropivacaine, 1.4 minutes)[10] and can be essentially ignored unless comparing rates of redistribution from blood to tissues. Thus, $t_{1/2}\beta$ is more useful for calculating when steady state is achieved (3.3 half-lives) during continuous drug administration or when clearance is complete (5 half-lives) after the final dose of drug. Representative half-lives are listed in Table 58-3.

Protein binding

Plasma proteins bind local anesthetics and affect uptake into and release from the vascular compartment. Once bound, these local anesthetic molecules are essentially removed from the processes of distribution, biotransformation, and

Table 58-3 Pharmacokinetic parameters for amino-amide local anesthetics

Local anesthetic	Vd_{ss} (l)	Clearance (l/min)	$t_{1/2}\beta$ (hr)
Prilocaine*	261	2.84	1.6
Lidocaine	91	0.95	1.6
Mepivacaine	84	0.78	1.9
Etidocaine	133	1.11	2.7
Bupivacaine	73	0.58	2.7

*Data for prilocaine are based on a two-compartment model. All other values are based on a three-compartment model.[41]

elimination. Protein binding is one determinant of how quickly a local anesthetic is distributed to tissue sites and eventually cleared. The free unbound fraction of local anesthetic more closely relates to pharmacologic and toxic effects than the total (bound plus free) concentration of local anesthetic.[60,146,169,243–245,259]

The major protein complex responsible for local anesthetic binding is α_1-acid glycoprotein.[146,168,194] Albumin makes up the greatest proportion of plasma protein, but local anesthetic binding is low,[245] although some bupivacaine is bound to albumin.[238] Various diseases, physiologic states, and medications can affect the plasma concentration of α_1-acid glycoprotein, thereby increasing or decreasing the free concentration of local anesthetic. Cancer,[116] trauma,[69] uremia,[69,100] and myocardial infarction[195] will increase the plasma concentration of α_1-acid glycoprotein and therefore decrease the free concentration of local anesthetic. Conversely, pregnancy[246] and oral contraceptives will reduce the concentration of α_1-acid glycoprotein, increasing the free concentration of local anesthetic.[260] Moreover, there may be differential binding of the enantiomers of racemic local anesthetics, and this may account for differences in pharmacologic activity of the optical isomers.[247]

There is a limited binding capacity to plasma proteins. As the concentration of local anesthetic increases, saturation of α_1-acid glycoprotein binding sites occurs, and proportionately more local anesthetic is found in the free unbound form (Fig. 58-16).[164,243]

Sampling: blood versus plasma; arterial versus venous

Pharmacokinetic analysis requires the ability to determine minute concentrations of local anesthetic in the blood and other body fluids. Gas–liquid chromatography is the standard assay technique,[242] but very different results will be obtained, depending on whether the sample is whole blood or plasma or arterial or venous in nature.

Besides being bound to plasma proteins, local anesthetics also may be adsorbed to the surface of erythrocytes, essentially sequestering local anesthetic from disposition. The concentration of local anesthetic in whole blood represents the total concentration (bound plus unbound fraction). Assay of plasma water would give a better measure of biologic activity of the local anesthetic, as the free (unbound) concentration is a more accurate reflection of the active concentration. Thus, whole blood concentrations always are greater than plasma levels (Fig. 58-17).[248]

Arterial blood (or plasma) contains local anesthetic before extraction by tissues. Peripheral venous blood (or plasma) contains local anesthetic after a certain fraction has been taken up by various organ groups. Thus, the concentration of local anesthetic in arterial blood (or plasma) is always higher than in venous blood (or plasma), especially before steady state distribution has been attained (Fig. 58-17).[32,153]

Other factors affecting pharmacokinetics

Uptake by lung. The lung rapidly extracts large quantities of local anesthetic because it is well perfused, part of the rapidly equilibrating tissue group, and has substantial tissue mass.[142,153] This has particular importance for those receiving IV regional anesthesia,[244] intercostal nerve blocks,[193] and interpleural regional analgesia,[231] wherein uptake in the lung may confer some protection against development of toxic concentrations.

Interestingly, the lung has been implicated as an extrahepatic site of prilocaine metabolism *in vitro.*[2] This has not been confirmed by *in vivo* studies.

Age and weight. Plasma concentrations of local anesthetics after regional anesthesia correlate poorly with age[160] and weight.[154,155,209,250] There is a trend toward more rapid absorption in the elderly population[83,90,160] and in children.[67,68]

Other drugs. Any drug that decreases hepatic blood flow or enzymatic activity could decrease the clearance of the amide local anesthetics. Such a phenomenon has been described for propanolol[163] or cimetidine,[78] when administered in conjunction with IV lidocaine.

Disease states. Any disease that reduces hepatic perfusion would likely reduce clearance of the amide local anesthetics. Reduced clearance of local anesthetics has been described in those with congestive heart failure,[14,240] hepatic cirrhosis,[240] and orthostatic hypotension.[77]

Absorption

Except for IV regional anesthesia[190] and the therapeutic infusion of lidocaine[141] or 2-chloroprocaine[166] in the management of neuropathic pain, local anesthetics enter the bloodstream by absorption. Intrinsically, local anesthetics differ from other drugs because they are deposited as a depot in proximity to target neural structures to attain a sufficient intraneural concentration to block conduction (i.e., regional anesthesia and analgesia). A notable exception is the administration of oral congeners of lidocaine, such as mexiletine, for the management of neuropathic pain.[38] When local anesthetic is injected into a tissue or body fluid, the processes of bulk movement, spread, and diffusion carry the local anesthetic away from the site of injection. Thus, factors that in-

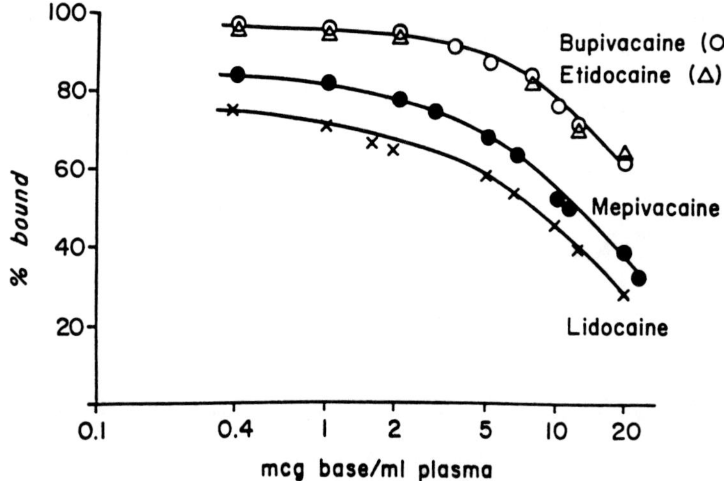

Fig. 58-16. Plasma binding of amide local anesthetics. As the total concentration of local anesthetic increases in the plasma, α_1-acid glycoprotein binding sites become saturated. Thus, more local anesthetic is found in the free (active) form at greater plasma concentrations. (From Tucker GT, Mather LE: Pharmacokinetics of local anaesthetic agents, *Br J Anaesth* 47:213, 1975.)

fluence movement of local anesthetic toward its neural target and factors that influence absorption and uptake of local anesthetic into the bloodstream may increase or decrease the quantity of local anesthetic available for neural blockade (Fig. 58-18). Such factors may have an appreciable effect on the onset, intensity, and duration of neural blockade.

Dose

The dose of administered local anesthetic is a prime factor responsible for rapidity of onset and the intensity and duration of neural blockade.[211,249] **Increasing the number of moieties available for diffusion will speed the onset, increase the intensity, and prolong the duration of neural blockade.** In clinical practice, the dose of local anesthetic is increased by administering a greater volume or concentration of drug, which has lead to certain misconceptions.

Volume

Increasing the volume of local anesthetic will increase its spread and may increase the dermatomal distribution of neural blockade, particularly in the epidural[74,211] and subarachnoid[98,99] spaces. Enhanced spread will increase the possibility of adsorption onto nerve but also the absorption into the vasculature, thereby somewhat dissipating the effect of enhanced volume. In situations such as postlaminectomy syndrome, wherein spread of local anesthetic is restricted because of fibrous tissue, hyaluronidase is sometimes used to enhance spread and to increase the rapidity of onset and intensity of block.[24] Volume is not a determinant of rapidity of onset, intensity, or duration of neural blockade. No clinically significant difference in onset, intensity, or duration of blockade is seen when the same dose of local anesthetic is administered in a large volume as a dilute solution or in a small volume as a concentrated solution.[52]

Concentration. It is a widely (and incorrectly) held belief that more concentrated solutions of local anesthetic will yield faster absorption, increased blood levels, and greater chance of toxicity irrespective of the volume of injectate if dosage is held constant. This belief is fallacious.[43,117,209] To achieve differing concentrations with uniform dosage, volume of injectate should be altered. The attendant differences in spread counterbalance the differences in concentration so that uniform blood levels, onset, intensity, and duration of block are achieved.

Thus, total dosage rather than volume or concentration of local anesthetic determines anesthetic activity.

pH

Commercially available local anesthetic is injected as a salt in aqueous solution. Once injected, the salt dissociates into cationic and basic forms, their ratio depending on the pK_a of the local anesthetic (see Table 58-2) and the pH of the milieu into which it is injected. The pH depends on the patient's acid–base status, the site of administration, and local buffer capacity (e.g., the epidural and subarachnoid spaces have limited buffering reserve[186]). As pK_a approaches pH, more local anesthetic is found in the basic form, and the base form has greatest ability to penetrate membranes. This explains the failure of local anesthesia in the presence of infection (acidosis), which results in a preponderance of cationic moieties that cannot penetrate nerve membranes.

Tachyphylaxis. The development of decreased effect with repetitive bolus injection or continuous infusion of local anesthetic is called *tachyphylaxis*. The theories surrounding the genesis of tachyphylaxis are multiple, and ex-

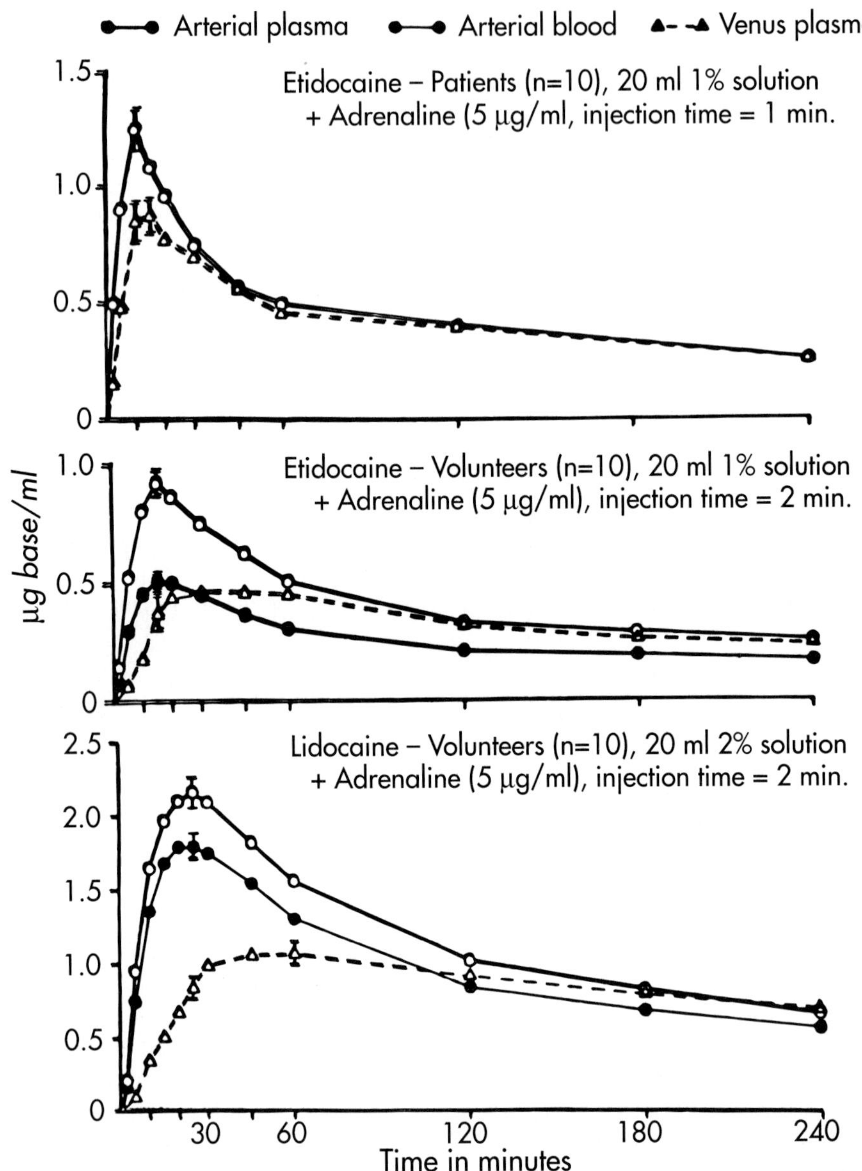

Fig. 58-17. Mean concentrations of etidocaine and lidocaine after epidural injection. Note that whole blood concentrations of local anesthetic are greater than plasma concentrations over the first 60 minutes. Similarly, arterial concentrations of local anesthetic are greater than venous concentrations over the same time period. (From Tucker GT, Mather LE: Pharmacokinetics of local anaesthetic agents, *Br J Anaesth* 47:213, 1975.)

cellent reviews are found elsewhere.[81] One possible mechanism involves the repeated administration of commercial local anesthetics (pH 4 to pH 6). If repeatedly administered to body spaces with limited buffering capacity (e.g., the subarachnoid space in continuous spinal anesthesia, the epidural space in postoperative epidural analgesia), buffering capacity may be overwhelmed.[42] Over time, the cationic moiety of the local anesthetic would predominate, as previously described, and neural blockade would be less efficacious.

The probability that tachyphylaxis will occur is directly proportional to the pK_a of the local anesthetic. Local anesthetics with pK_as close to physiologic pH (e.g., lidocaine, mepivacaine; Table 58-2) have the greatest incidence of tachyphylaxis.

pH adjustment. The pH of commercially available solutions of local anesthetics may be increased by the addition of sodium bicarbonate to increase the proportion of uncharged base form and speed onset of block. The pH adjustment of solutions of bupivacaine and lidocaine has been reported to speed the onset of neural blockade for brachial plexus[111] and epidural blockade.[61] One milliliter of sodium bicarbonate is added to every 9 ml of mepivacaine or lidocaine, whereas 0.1 ml of bicarbonate is added to every 9.9 ml of bupivacaine (greater concentrations of sodium bicar-

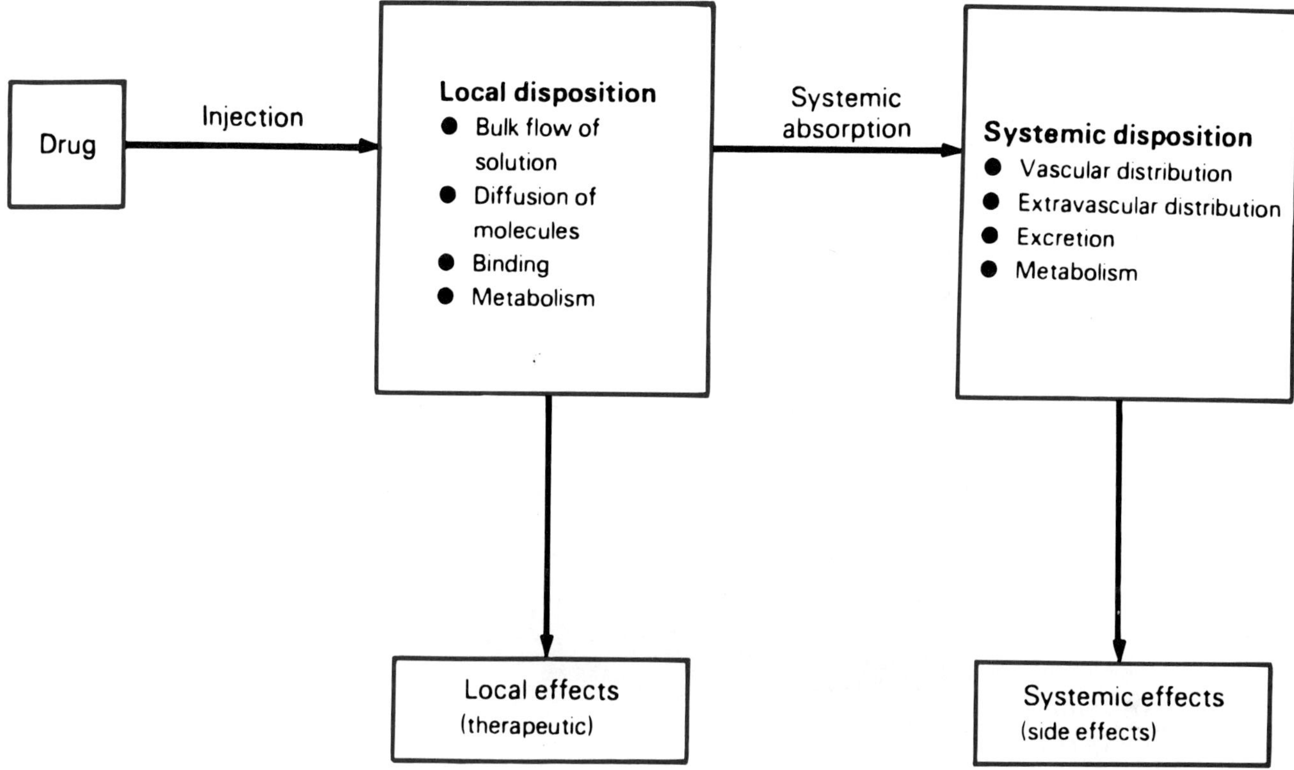

Fig. 58-18. Local and systemic disposition of local anesthetics. (From Mather LE, Cousins MJ: Local anaesthetics and their current clinical use, *Drugs* 18:185, 1979.)

bonate cause the local anesthetic to precipitate out of solution).

Site of injection

For a particular site of injection and a standardized uniform dose (so dose is no longer a contributing factor), partition coefficient of the local anesthetic, factors affecting diffusibility (degree of adiposity, presence of scar), pH of the local environment, tissue vascularity, total area for absorption, and regional blood flow determine the rate of absorption. Of these factors, regional blood flow appears to be rate-limiting.[196] Thus, different injection sites will yield different peak blood or plasma concentrations of local anesthetic after a uniform dose (Fig. 58-19). Independent of the local anesthetic used, absorption from varying sites of injection decrease in the following order: (interpleural?)[251] > intercostal > caudal > epidural > brachial plexus > sciatic and femoral nerve block > subarachnoid.[31]

Intercostal and interpleural. Intercostal neural blockade has been reported to produce the greatest systemic concentrations of local anesthetic after injection.[209,250] The intercostal space is well vascularized, and the dose is dispersed over a large absorptive surface.

Theoretically, the pleura would supply a greater absorptive surface, and interpleural injection could result in even greater systemic concentrations. Interpleural regional analgesia[180] was shown to be associated with a 50% greater plasma concentration of bupivacaine as compared with intercostal block after administration of approximately equianalgesic doses.[251] Blood concentrations after interpleural analgesia are highly variable,[149,232] and further research is necessary to resolve this issue.

Epidural space. Absorption from the epidural space has been well studied (e.g., Fig. 58-17). While the epidural space is filled with venous plexuses, these veins traverse the space to supply adjacent structures rather than actually drain the space. Moreover, the large quantities of fat within the epidural space sequester local anesthetic and delay absorption.[209] Vascular uptake from different regions of the epidural space (thoracic, cervical, lumbar) appears to be similar,[149] except for absorption from the caudal region,[62] which may be a result of the greater vascularity of bony tissue in the caudal canal.[62]

Brachial plexus. The slowest onset and the longest durations of neural blockade are associated with brachial plexus anesthesia.[49] The onset of anesthesia is prolonged because local anesthetic is not deposited in the immediate vicinity of its neural target and should diffuse some distance. The long duration of brachial plexus blockade is a result of the large dosages used and of the relatively decreased vascularity of the injection site, which slows removal of local anesthetic by absorption.[49] Peak plasma concentrations are similar after using the interscalene or axillary technique for brachial plexus blockade.[254]

Subarachnoid space. After injection into the cerebrospinal fluid (CSF), the concentration of local anesthetic decreases exponentially (Fig. 58-20). **Absorption from the subarachnoid space yields the least local anesthetic blood concentrations compared with other sites of injection.**[31] Systemic absorption is believed to occur via diffusion through the arachnoid granulations into the relatively more vascular epidural space[41] and through blood vessels of the cord and pia mater.[98]

After injection, local anesthetic is diluted and dispersed within the CSF and adsorbed onto spinal roots and the cord.[248] Onset of neural blockade is rapid because local anesthetic is placed in the immediate vicinity of its neural target: the spinal cord and nerve roots. Unlike in peripheral nerves, a nerve sheath does not surround these structures thus facilitating diffusion. The short duration of anesthesia is a result of the relatively small quantities of local anesthetic used to achieve spinal anesthesia.[49]

Infiltration anesthesia. Along with subarachnoid injection, subcutaneous infiltration of local anesthetic has the

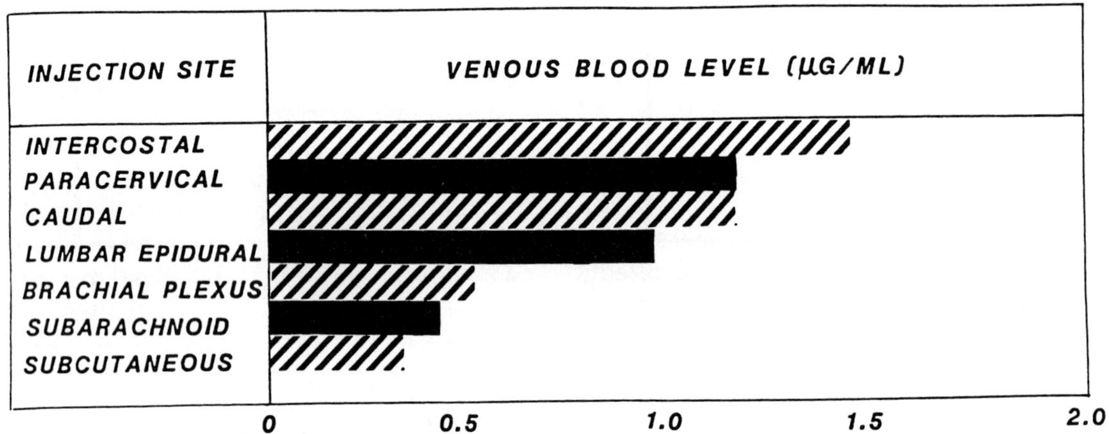

Fig. 58-19. Concentration of local anesthetic in the blood after injection of a uniform standardized dose (100 mg of lidocaine in this case) as a function of the site of injection. (From Covino BG: Local anesthetics. In Ferrante FM, VadeBoncouer TR, editors: *Postoperative pain management,* New York 1993, Churchill-Livingstone.)

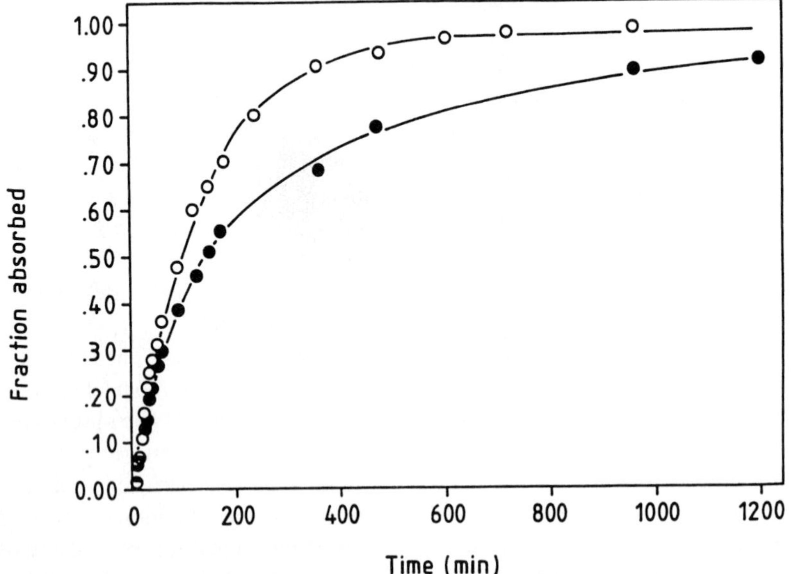

Fig. 58-20. Absorption of local anesthetic from the subarachnoid space. Absorption is expressed as a fraction of total dose on the y-axis. (From de Jong RH: *Local anesthetics,* St. Louis, 1994, Mosby.)

shortest latency of onset but also the shortest duration of action.[49] Alkalinization has been reported to reduce the pain associated with infiltration of lidocaine.[221]

Individual local anesthetics

The rate and amount of vascular absorption also may be affected by the pharmacologic characteristics of local anesthetics. When comparing local anesthetics of equivalent potency, lidocaine and mepivacaine are absorbed more rapidly after epidural injection than is prilocaine;[2] bupivacaine is absorbed more rapidly than etidocaine.[144] These rates of absorption reflect intrinsic differences in vasodilator activity (lidocaine, mepivacaine > prilocaine) and lipid solubility (etidocaine > bupivacaine). Although there is no innate difference in vasodilator activity between bupivacaine and etidocaine, etidocaine has greater sequestration in epidural fat because of its lipid solubility, which leads to decreased absorption and lower peak concentrations after epidural administration.[210]

Addition of vasoconstrictors

There are no mechanisms intrinsic to individual tissues by which local anesthetic can be inactivated. Clearance from the circulation occurs in distant organs. Absorption into the circulation is the first step in removal of the drug, and absorption is proportional to blood flow. By use of vasoconstrictors, more local anesthetic will remain at the site of injection over time, increasing the intensity and prolonging the duration of neural blockade. Epinephrine and phenylephrine have been used as vasoconstrictors. Epinephrine is used most commonly in a concentration of 1:200,000 (5 μg/ml) because it has been reported to produce effective vasoconstriction when used with lidocaine for epidural and intercostal block.[26]

The decrease in absorption caused by a vasoconstrictor varies directly by the extent of perfusion and the absorptive surface area at the injection site. For instance, the rate of absorption of local anesthetic would be decreased the most for infiltration anesthesia compared with epidural block and greatly decreased for epidural anesthesia compared with intercostal nerve block (Fig. 58-21).[209]

The effect of epinephrine on the duration of anesthesia also varies as a function of the specific local anesthetic. Epinephrine will increase the duration of epidural anesthesia when added to procaine, mepivacaine,[97] or lidocaine.[28,233] The reduced vasodilator activity of prilocaine compared with lidocaine or mepivacaine decreases the effectiveness of epinephrine in prolongation of neural blockade.[233] The effect of epinephrine on epidural administration of bupivacaine and etidocaine depends on the concentration of the local anesthetic. The intensity and duration of epidural anesthesia will be increased by use of epinephrine with dilute solutions (0.125% and 0.25%).[138] At higher concentrations, the greater lipid solubility and protein binding of etidocaine and bupivacaine make addition of epinephrine superfluous,[30,138,172]

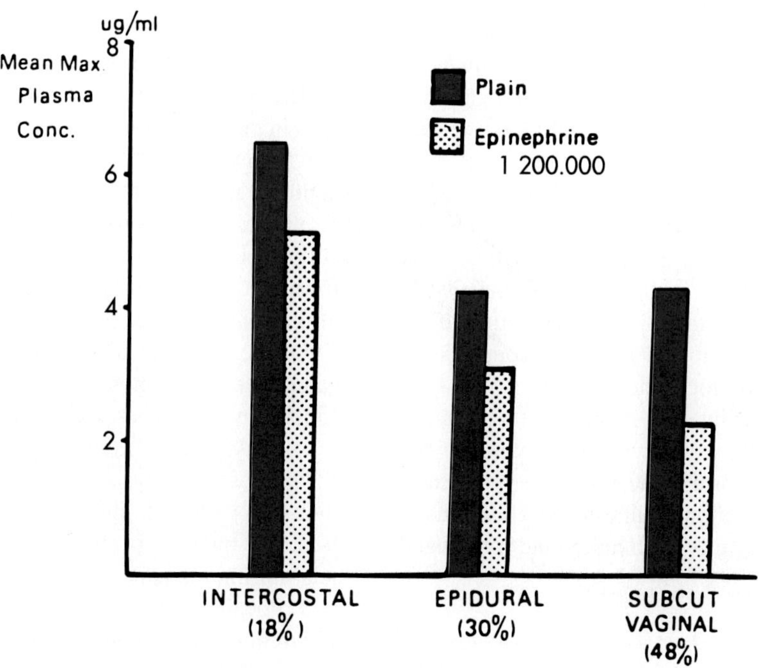

Fig. 58-21. Mean maximum concentrations of lidocaine with and without 1:200,000 epinephrine administered at three different sites. The most marked reduction in systemic plasma concentration occurs with subcutaneous injection (48%) as compared with 30% for epidural and 18% for intercostal injection. (From Covino BG: Clinical pharmacology of local anesthetic agents. In Cousins MJ, Bridenbaugh PO, editors: *Neural blockade in clinical anesthesia and management of pain,* ed 2, Philadelphia, 1988, JB Lippincott.)

although use of epinephrine with these agents may increase the intensity of motor blockade.[217]

Elimination

Amino-ester local anesthetics

The first step in elimination of the ester local anesthetics is cleavage of the ester linkage (Fig. 58-22). The individual esters differ in the rate (Table 58-4) and site of hydrolysis of the ester bond. Derivatives of PABA (Fig. 58-22; i.e., procaine, 2-chloroprocaine, and tetracaine) are hydrolyzed in the plasma by pseudocholinesterase. Cocaine is a double ester and is metabolized by plasma and liver cholinesterases.

Procaine is the parent compound of the PABA-derived group of ester-linked local anesthetics. On hydrolysis, it is broken down into PABA and diethylaminoethanol (DEAE).[27] Hydrolysis is exceedingly rapid ($t_{1/2}\beta$ = 43 seconds).[66] PABA has no intrinsic local anesthetic activity, and DEAE has anesthetic potency similar to procaine.[33,34] The longer than anticipated duration of local anesthetic activity associated with procaine may be caused by DEAE.[33]

Addition of a chloride to the 2-carbon position of the aromatic ring of procaine yields 2-chloroprocaine. The addition of chloride increases the rate of hydrolysis fourfold[86] (Table 58-4) and doubles the potency. This faster hydrolysis makes the drug much less toxic with IV injection. For this reason, 2-chloroprocaine has been touted by some authorities as a superior choice to lidocaine for IV administration in the management of neuropathic pain.[1]

Tetracaine is synthesized by substitution of a butylamino radical for the para-amino group on the procaine aromatic ring with shortening of the alkylamino tail (Table 58-2). These alterations yield a local anesthetic that is 10 times as potent and four times more slowly hydrolyzed than procaine, resulting in greater intensity of neural blockade and longer duration of action.[55]

The enzyme responsible for hydrolysis of the ester local anesthetics (pseudocholinesterase) is found almost completely in the blood,[121] with trace amounts found in nervous tissue.[161] Pseudocholinesterase is the same enzyme that is responsible for the metabolism of succinylcholine. True cholinesterase is widely distributed in the nervous system but does not hydrolyze ester local anesthetics.[86]

Low levels of pseudocholinesterase may be found in patients with advanced liver disease and in those who are homozygotic for the atypical form of the enzyme, a genetically determined trait. Administration of an ester local anesthetic to these patients may result in toxicity and prolonged apnea.[87]

Amino-amide local anesthetics

Unlike the amino-ester local anesthetics, metabolism of the amino-amide local anesthetics occurs in the endoplasmic reticulum of hepatocytes, catalyzed by NADPH-linked oxidative enzymes.[25] In general, tertiary amines are metabolized into secondary amines that are then hydrolyzed by amidases. Liver disease may reduce the metabolism of the amide local anesthetics, resulting in greater plasma levels and the possibility of systemic toxicity.[4,214]

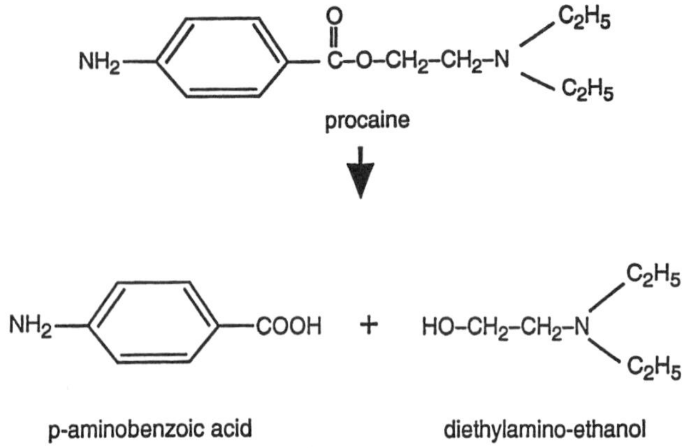

NH_2–C_6H_4–C(=O)–O–CH_2–CH_2–N(C_2H_5)$_2$
procaine
↓
NH_2–C_6H_4–COOH + HO–CH_2–CH_2–N(C_2H_5)$_2$
p-aminobenzoic acid diethylamino-ethanol

Fig. 58-22. The hydrolysis of procaine. (From de Jong RH: *Local anesthetics*, St. Louis, 1994, Mosby.)

Table 58-4 Rate of hydrolysis of amino-ester local anesthetics

	$t_{1/2}\beta$[66,162] (sec)	Rate of hydrolysis[86] µM/ml/hr
Procaine	43	1.2
2-Chloroprocaine	21	4.7
Tetracaine	—	0.3

The biotransformation of the amide local anesthetics results in the formation of a large variety of metabolites. There also is considerable variation in the rate of metabolism of individual amide local anesthetics. The following is an approximate rank order for rate of metabolism:[51] prilocaine > etidocaine > lidocaine > mepivacaine > bupivacaine. Excellent references are available for in-depth examination of the complex topic of amide biotransformation.[54]

Of the amide local anesthetics, the metabolism of lidocaine has been most extensively studied (Fig. 58-23). Lidocaine undergoes oxidative deethylation to form the secondary amine monoethylglycinexylidide (MEGX).[54] Subsequent hydrolysis causes the formation of glycine-xylidide (GX) and xylidine. MEGX and GX are less toxic than lidocaine but have been implicated in the occurrence of toxicity during lidocaine administration.[101,214]

Prilocaine is a lidocaine homologue with a potency similar to lidocaine but with markedly lower systemic toxic potential.[72,86] Prilocaine is a unique amide local anesthetic because it is a secondary amine. Unlike lidocaine, it requires no preparatory metabolic step before hydrolysis. Prilocaine is rapidly hydrolyzed to o-toluidine and N-propylalanine (Fig. 58-24). Orthotoluidine is subsequently oxidized to a pair of aminophenyls (toluene derivatives).[93]

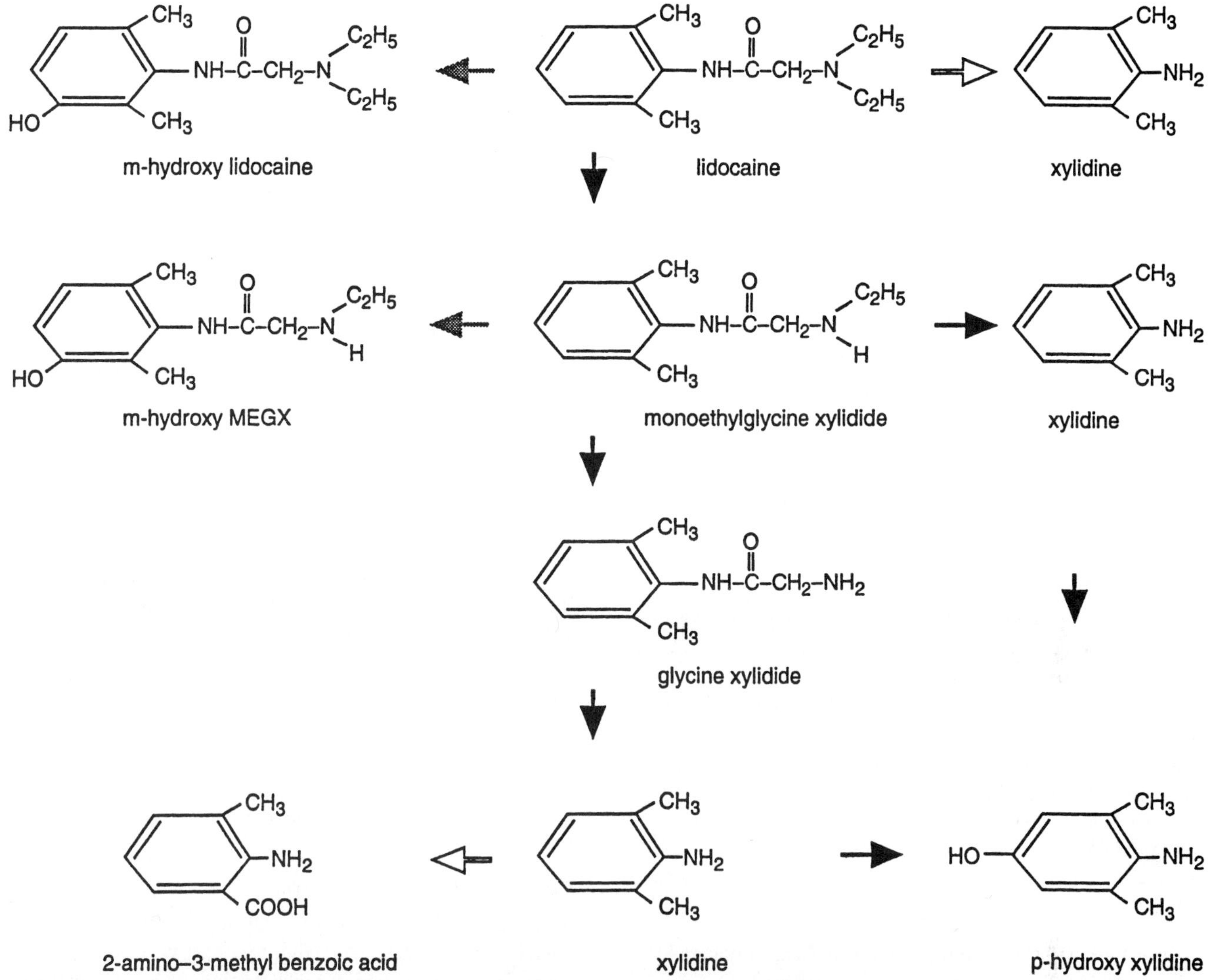

m-hydroxy lidocaine
lidocaine
xylidine
m-hydroxy MEGX
monoethylglycine xylidide
xylidine
glycine xylidide
2-amino–3-methyl benzoic acid
xylidine
p-hydroxy xylidine

Fig. 58-23. Lidocaine metabolism. Lidocaine undergoes initial metabolism to form the secondary amine monoethylglycinexylidide. Hydrolysis subsequently forms glycinexylidide and xylidine. Minor breakdown products include m-hydroxy derivatives. The unfilled arrow represents metabolic pathways present in nonhuman species. (From de Jong RH: *Local anesthetics,* St. Louis, 1994, Mosby.)

2-Amino-3-hydroxytoluene and 2-amino-5-hydroxytoluene oxidize hemoglobin to methemoglobin.[123] Doses of prilocaine greater than 600 mg may result in sufficient methemoglobinemia to cause cyanosis, although desaturation may be detected by pulse oximetry at lower doses.[113] The levels of methemoglobinemia that are achieved cause only slight impairment of oxygen transport in healthy subjects, although methemoglobinemia can be reversed with IV administration of reducing agents such as methylene blue (1 to 5 mg/kg).[113,173]

The lung has been suggested as a possible extrahepatic site for metabolism of prilocaine,[2] although initial *in vitro* studies have not been confirmed *in vivo.*[2]

Hepatic clearance and renal excretion

Perfusion not only affects absorption and distribution but also elimination. The amount of amide local anesthetic delivered to the liver for biotransformation and the amount of metabolites delivered to the kidney for excretion are related to cardiac output. Thus, blood levels of amide local anesthetics vary as a function of cardiac output.[222,239]

Hepatic clearance is determined by the hepatic extraction ratio, i.e., the proportion of molecules that are metabolized after entering the liver. Hepatic extraction of local anesthetics is considerable. Approximately 75% of lidocaine in the hepatic artery is cleared by a single pass through the liver.[9] The hepatic extraction ratio is determined largely by the extent of protein binding of the local anesthetic. Moderately protein-bound amide local anesthetics (e.g., lidocaine, mepivacaine) have high extraction ratios. Their hepatic clearance is flow-limited and varies with hepatic blood flow. Highly protein-bound local anesthetics (e.g., bupivacaine) have extraction ratios of less than 50%, and their clearance

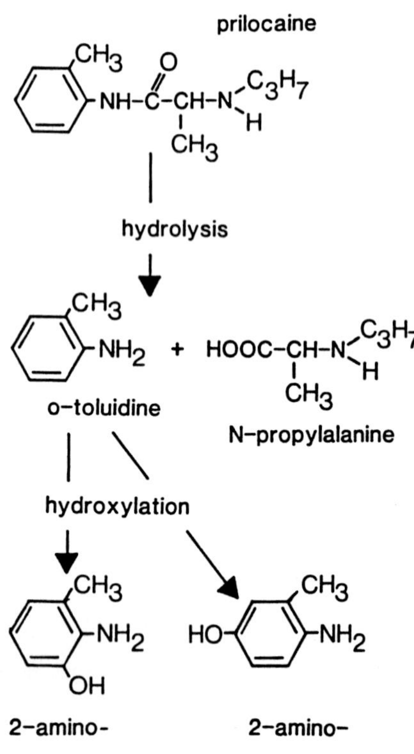

Fig. 58-24. Prilocaine metabolism and the genesis of methemoglobinemia. Orthotoluidine is formed by hydrolysis as prilocaine is a secondary amine. Subsequent oxidation of o-toluidine forms toluene derivatives, which oxidize hemoglobin to methemoglobin. (From de Jong RH: *Local anesthetics,* St. Louis, 1994, Mosby.)

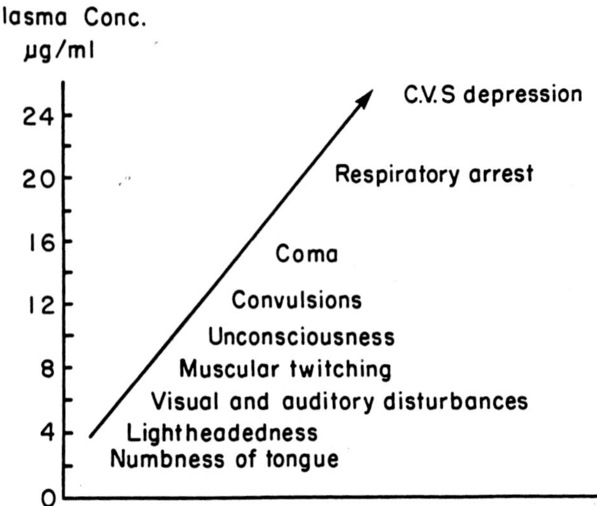

Fig. 58-25. Central nervous system toxicity. Increasing plasma concentrations of local anesthetic eventually result in seizures and then cardiovascular (CVS) depression. The notable exception to this phenomenon is bupivacaine, wherein cardiotoxicity is achieved at subconvulsant concentrations of local anesthetic. (From Covino BG: Clinical pharmacology of local anesthetic agents. In Cousins MJ, Bridenbaugh PO, editors: *Neural blockade in clinical anesthesia and management of pain,* Philadelphia, 1988, JB Lippincott.)

is rate-limited by the concentration of free, unbound local anesthetic.[55]

The liver has sufficient metabolic reserve, and clearance is little affected by alcoholic liver disease.[239] Advanced liver disease may reduce the metabolism of amide local anesthetics, and the resulting increased blood levels may increase the risk of systemic toxicity.[4,9,214] Alterations in hepatic perfusion (e.g., heart failure) have the greatest influence on hepatic extraction ratio, at least for the modestly bound local anesthetics.

Only a small percentage of local anesthetic is excreted unchanged in the urine; metabolic breakdown products and their conjugates are found in abundance. Thus, renal dysfunction affects local anesthetic blood levels less than alterations in hepatic clearance.[9]

Toxicity of Local Anesthetics

The toxicity associated with local anesthetics may be categorized as systemic toxicity, contact toxicity (neurotoxicity and local tissue reactions), and allergic phenomena.

Systemic toxicity

Systemic toxicity manifests as alterations in function of the central nervous system (CNS) and the cardiovascular system. CNS[86,207,208] and cardiovascular system toxicities[79,224] are related to intrinsic anesthetic potency and dosage.

Central nervous system toxicity

The signs and symptoms of local anesthetic-induced CNS toxicity are well described (Fig. 58-25).[51] With a progressive increase in the systemic concentration of local anesthetic, the patient will first experience dry mouth, dizziness, and lightheadedness, followed by visual (difficulty in focusing) and auditory (tinnitus) disturbance. Muscle twitching and tremors will then occur. As the blood concentration of local anesthetic increases, tonic–clonic seizures may occur. The preceding events are symptomatic of CNS excitation. This initial state of CNS excitation is caused by blockade of inhibitory pathways in the cerebral cortex.[56,235] Initial inhibition of inhibitory pathways would allow unopposed activity of facilitatory neurons, leading to the excitatory manifestations of CNS toxicity. With further increase in systemic local anesthetic concentration, CNS depression, respiratory arrest, and ultimately cardiovascular depression occur as inhibitory and excitatory CNS neurons cease to function.

Potency, rapidity of increase in systemic blood level, and acidosis influence CNS toxicity and, in particular, the convulsive threshold (blood level). Studies of IV local anesthetics in human volunteers have consistently shown a relationship between anesthetic potency and the dosage of local anesthetic required to induce CNS toxicity.[207,208] Moreover, a correlation exists between potency and seizure threshold. Venous blood levels of 2 to 4 µg/ml of etidocaine and bupivacaine can cause convulsions.[17,46,207] Lidocaine produces convulsions in venous concentrations in excess of 10 μg/ml.[46] Rapidity of injection and the consequent accelerated rate of increase in blood concentration will decrease the concentration necessary to elicit convulsions.[206] Acidosis will affect the CNS activity of local anesthetics and reduce the threshold for seizure activity also.[73]

Cardiovascular system toxicity

The cardiovascular toxicity associated with local anesthetics is attributable to their direct effects on cardiac muscle (contractility, automaticity, rhythmicity, and conductivity) and on peripheral vascular smooth muscle.

Cardiac effects of local anesthetics

Contractility. Local anesthetics have a negative ionotropic effect on cardiac muscle that is dose-related and intrinsic to local anesthetic potency.[21,102,182,198,236] Atrial and ventricular contractility are depressed,[182] although the atria are less susceptible.[198] Hypercapnia, acidosis, and hypoxia potentiate myocardial depression.[198] The mechanism underlying depression of myocardial contractility is poorly and incompletely understood but may result from: (1) differential release of local anesthetics from sodium channel binding sites,[45] and (2) in part, calcium channel binding.[8] At IV doses of 2 to 4 mg/kg in humans, the effect of lidocaine on cardiac contractility is minimal.[102] Larger IV doses (in animal models) produce a dose-related decrease in iontropy and an increase in left ventricular end-diastolic pressure.

Local anesthetic-induced depression of cardiac contractility is directly related to potency (Fig. 58-26).[21,224] Thus, tetracaine, bupivacaine, and etidocaine depress ionotropy more than lidocaine, mepivacaine, and procaine.[21,236]

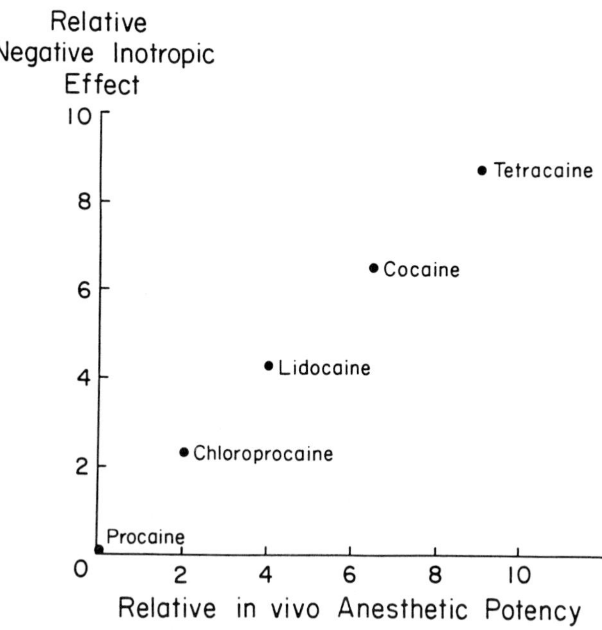

Fig. 58-26. Relationship between local anesthetic potency and depression of cardiac contractility. (From Covino BG: Clinical pharmacology of local anesthetic agents. In Cousins MJ, Bridenbaugh PO, editors: *Neural blockade in clinical anesthesia and management of pain,* Philadelphia, 1988, JB Lippincott.)

The greater negative iontropic effect of bupivacaine may be in part a result of its greater lipophilicity[45,58] and, in part, due to calcium channel binding.[8] More importantly, the greater negative iontropy of bupivacaine (and, in part, its greater cardiotoxic potential) results from intrinsic kinetics of association–dissociation from the local anesthetic receptor in cardiac sodium channels (to be discussed).[40]

Automaticity. With respect to chronotropy, the sinoatrial node is somewhat resistant to the effects of local anesthetics.[109] When well perfused and bathed in 50 μg/ml lidocaine or 5 μg/ml bupivacaine, guinea pig atria showed only modest depression of chronotropy.[198] Increasing dose[136] or the presence of hypercapnia, acidosis, or hypoxia[109,198] potentiate the negative chronotropic effects of local anesthetics.

Rhythmicity and conductivity. Ventricular arrhythmias are rarely seen with tetracaine, mepivacaine, and lidocaine. Bupivacaine (at subconvulsant doses) and, to a lesser extent, etidocaine (at supraconvulsant doses) can cause ventricular tachycardia and ventricular fibrillation.[57,70,197] Many of the cardiotoxic reactions associated with bupivacaine have occurred in pregnant women. It is uncertain whether the physiologic state of pregnancy enhances toxicity.[157] Hypercapnia, acidosis, and hypoxia potentiate the negative ionotropic and chronotropic effects of local anesthetics[198] and markedly increase the cardiotoxicity of bupivacaine.[127,189] Resuscitation after bupivacaine cardiotoxicity is difficult in patients and in animals.[189] Little information is available on the ease of resuscitation after cardiac depression with other local anesthetics.

The potential for ventricular dysrhythmias differs between bupivacaine and other local anesthetics and gives some insight into the mechanisms responsible for bupivacaine-induced arrhythmias. Mepivacaine and bupivacaine share the same piperidine ring structure (Table 58-2), yet ventricular arrhythmias are rarely seen with mepivacaine. Etidocaine, which is more lipid soluble but equally as protein bound (Table 58-2), has a lesser incidence of ventricular dysrhythmias than bupivacaine. Thus, structure-activity relationships and the physicochemical properties of the bupivacaine molecule are not responsible for ventricular dysrhythmogenesis.[46]

Unlike other anesthetics, cardiac dysrhythmias are seen at subconvulsant doses of bupivacaine.[97,128] This violates the usual relationship between signs and symptoms of toxicity and dosage (Fig. 58-25). Electrophysiologically, bupivacaine markedly depresses the rapid phase of depolarization of the cardiac action potential and can prolong recovery phase, resulting in conduction blockade and decreased electrical excitability. Thus, undirectional block of conduction pathways with bupivacaine may generate reentrant types of arrhythmias.[40,58]

Centrally-mediated neurogenic mechanisms may play a role in bupivacaine cardiotoxicity also. Injection of bupivacaine into the brain in experimental models results in arrhythmias,[18,108] which indicates that the cardiac effects of bupivacaine (and perhaps other local anesthetics) may be at least in part centrally mediated.

The differential cardiotoxicity of local anesthetics also may be attributable to kinetic differences in association–dissociation with local anesthetic receptors.[39,40,152] Lidocaine preferentially and rapidly binds to the receptor in the open activated state; bupivacaine rapidly binds in the inactivated state.[40] For both drugs, binding affinity is least in the resting, closed channel state, although the dissociation rate constants differ. The dissociation time constant for lidocaine is 0.15 seconds, whereas bupivacaine is tenfold slower at 1.5 seconds.[8] Lidocaine and bupivacaine are similar in that they rapidly bind to open or inactivated sodium channels during early systole. The difference lies in the speed with which they dissociate from the receptor during diastole. Thus, lidocaine kinetics can be described as "fast-in, fast-out," and bupivacaine kinetics can be described as "fast-in, slow-out."[40] The slower dissociation of bupivacaine from its receptor site may contribute to bupivacaine's greater cardiotoxicity.[40] Interestingly, there seems to be stereospecificity to bupivacaine cardiotoxicity. There is a fourfold prolongation of dissociation time for the R(+) enantiomer during diastole.[134]

Effects on peripheral vascular smooth muscle

Local anesthetics exhibit biphasic action on vascular smooth muscle as a function of dose.[20,140] *In vitro*[20] and *in vivo*[118] studies confirm the differential effect of dosage: at lesser doses, local anesthetics vasoconstrict by stimulating spontaneous myogenic contraction of smooth muscle; at greater doses local anesthetics produce vasodilation by inhibition of contraction.

Cocaine is unique because it is a vasoconstrictor at most doses. The vasoconstrictive properties of cocaine are not a direct but rather an indirect effect of the drug. By inhibition of the catecholamine reuptake pump, cocaine results in excess-free norepinephrine. Thus, a profound state of vasoconstriction is achieved.[46]

Contact Toxicity

The potential for toxic reactions caused by direct contact with local anesthetics is real. Toxic phenomena can be categorized into neurotoxic, myotoxic, and histotoxic reactions.

Neurotoxicity

The use of local anesthetics rarely produces nerve damage,[12,137,167,219] which has been shown clinically in large clinical studies[167,252,253] and in the laboratory.[12,137,219] Studies on isolated frog sciatic nerve preparations have shown that concentrations of local anesthetic required to cause irreversible conduction block are far in excess of those used clinically.[219] At clinically used concentrations, local anesthetic quickly washes out from isolated nerve preparations after suppressing the compound action potential, with return of the potential to preblock status.[219] *In vivo* bathing of neural structures such as the vagus nerve[12] or the aortic nerve[137] with clinically used concentrations of local anesthetic yields similar results. Neurotoxicity has occurred in the settings of: (1) posttraumatic neuropathy and intraneural injection, (2) continuous spinal anesthesia with hyperbaric solutions, and (3) subarachnoid administration of 2-chloroprocaine.

Posttraumatic neuropathy and intraneural injection. Usually, local anesthetic is administered in close proximity to nerves rather than into neural tissue, to avoid the possibility of direct nerve trauma. Inadvertently, local anesthetic is sometimes deposited into the nerve itself. Such occurrences cause exquisite pain on injection that should prompt cessation of injection. Injection of mepivacaine or lidocaine into the ulnar nerves of volunteers resulted in local tenderness, paresthesiae, and conduction abnormalities for several weeks postinjection.[139] Intraneural injection of saline caused the same changes, suggesting that subsequent alterations were more the result of posttraumatic neuropathy than toxicity of the local anesthetic *per se*.[139]

Continuous spinal anesthesia with hyperbaric solutions. Great consternation erupted in the early 1990s when cauda equina syndrome was elicited after repetitive injections of hyperbaric lidocaine during continuous spinal anesthesia through small-bore subarachnoid catheters.[184,201] Because of these events, the Food and Drug Administration (FDA) removed the sale of these catheters from the marketplace.[16] The FDA Safety Alert did not attempt to define the etiology of the cauda equina syndrome. The question arises as to whether the catheter itself, the local anesthetic, any additives (e.g., 7.5% glucose), a distribution pattern caused by use of the small bore catheter, or a combination of these events was responsible for the syndrome.

Several models implicated poor mixing of hyperbaric local anesthetic with spinal fluid and pooling of the local anesthetic at the sacral site of the lumbar lordosis.[129,183,191] Several factors affected maldistribution, including catheter size, tip configuration, tip position, injection rate, and velocity, resulting in pooling and stasis of local anesthetic around lumbosacral nerve roots.[183,191] Sacrally directed catheter tips increase the likelihood of sacral pooling of hyperbaric local anesthetic.[183] The resultant poor spread to higher lumbothoracic levels would result in poor anesthesia and would invite further dosing that would lead to still more pooling, and the cycle would repeat itself.[129,191]

Unfortunately, the hydromechanics of small-bore catheter injection may not be the entire story because neurologic toxicity (transient radiculopathy) has been reported after traditional single subarachnoid injections of 5% hyperbaric lidocaine.[202] Moreover, exposure of isolated myelinated amphibian nerves to concentrated solutions of lidocaine and tetracaine caused irreversible impulse blockade.[130] In this[130] and another study,[199] the addition of 7.5% glucose to local anesthetic did not affect neurotoxic potential.

A number of factors can be responsible for neurotoxicity

associated with spinal anesthesia. Despite the excellent safety history of subarachnoid administration of local anesthetics,[167,252,253] it is perhaps prudent to at least reexamine the question of their overall innate neurotoxicity.

Subarachnoid administration of 2-chloroprocaine. Cauda equina syndrome was reported after subarachnoid administration of 2-chloroprocaine also.[156,181] The commercial formulation of 2-chloroprocaine at that time contained an antioxidant (sodium bisulfite) that prolonged shelf-life. Also, pH was adjusted to approximately 3.0 in the commercial preparation. As can be seen from Table 58-5, the preponderance of evidence suggested the local anesthetic itself was innocuous, but the antioxidant was considered to be neurotoxic. Sodium bisulfite combined with low pH was believed to be responsible for production of sulfur dioxide.[96] Unfortunately, one study does not entirely absolve 2-chloroprocaine itself (Table 58-5),[120] although these findings were not evident in other investigations.

Because of concern regarding sodium bisulfite, the commercial preparation was reformulated substituting ethylenediamine tetra-acetate (EDTA), a calcium-chelating agent, for sodium bisulfite (Nesacaine MPF). The addition of EDTA is not without concern because of its calcium-chelating property. Subarachnoid administration of EDTA in dogs causes spinal nerve root degenerative and functional changes.[257] These changes can be prevented by previous administration of calcium chloride, suggesting the toxic effects are a result of leaching of calcium from nerve tissue.[257] Autopsies of humans receiving subarachnoid morphine (with EDTA) fail to show neurotoxicity.[218] This may perhaps be a result of the more generous volume of CSF in humans than in dogs.

Myotoxicity

All local anesthetics cause muscle necrosis to some extent. The effect is reversible, with muscle regeneration being essentially complete at 2 weeks after injection.[15] Extent of damage ranged from changes in muscle alone (bupivacaine, lidocaine, procaine, tetracaine) or those involving muscles, surrounding blood vessels, and nerves (chloroprocaine, lidocaine with epinephrine).[88] Regeneration also was slower with chloroprocaine and lidocaine with epinephrine.[88]

2-chloroprocaine and lumbar muscle spasm. The use of large volumes (> 40 ml) of 2-chloroprocaine (Nesacaine MPF, containing EDTA) has been associated with severe lumbar muscle spasm after otherwise uneventful epidural injections.[223] The calcium-chelating properties of EDTA may interfere with muscle excitation–contraction coupling.[223] EDTA-containing solutions and preservative-free solutions can cause lumbar muscle spasm when given in large volumes.[223]

Histotoxicity

Because of the widespread use of infiltration anesthesia, the potential toxicity of local anesthetics on the integument and their effects on wound healing are of special importance. Local anesthetics exhibited no histotoxicity when administered intradermally or subcutaneously.[15] Moreover, repeated exposures were devoid of irritant effects.[6] Local anesthetics had no deleterious effects on wound healing, and lidocaine may promote it.[75]

Allergenicity

Systemic toxic reactions[85] are often misdiagnosed as true allergic reactions to local anesthetics.[200] Because ester local anesthetics are metabolized to PABA, an allergen, all ester local anesthetics may exhibit true allergic or hypersensitivity reactions.[5] Moreover, cross-sensitivity exists among the ester local anesthetics and the other PABA esters (e.g., sunscreens and preservatives [e.g., methylparaben]).[165] In contrast, true allergic reactions to amide local anesthetics are exceedingly rare.[84,187]

Table 58-5 Neurotoxicity studies of 2-chloroprocaine

Reference #	Study model	Intensity of neurotoxicity		
		Commerical 2-chloroprocaine with sodium metabisulfite	2-chloroprocaine (without antioxidant)	$NaHSO_3$†
Barsa et al.[13]	Isolated rabbit vagus nerve	3+	—	—
Pizzalato et al.[170]	Intact rabbit sciatic nerve	0	—	—
Ravindran et al.[176]	Dog—total spinal	3+	—	—
Rosen et al.[188]	Sheep—total spinal	1+	—	—
Rosen et al.[188]	Monkey—total spinal	1+	—	—
Myers et al.[158]	Intact rat sciatic nerve	3+	—	—
Gissen et al.[96]	Isolated rabbit vagus nerve	3+	—	3+
Wang et al.[256]	Rabbit—spinal	3+	—	3+
Kalichman et al.[120]	Intact rat sciatic nerve	2+	3+	1+

0, no effect; —, not studied; $NaHSO_3$, sodium bisulfite.

*All preparations of 2-chloroprocaine in this column were commercial and contained the antioxidant sodium bisulfite.

†Only three studies specifically tested for the production of $NaHSO_3$ itself.

Commercial preparations of local anesthetics contain preservatives (methylparaben[5]) and antioxidants (metabisulfite in epinephrine-containing local anesthetic solutions[64,204]) that are truly allergenic. Often a reaction to the preservative or antioxidant is attributed to the local anesthetic. Intradermal testing of preservative-free local anesthetic and of the preservative or antioxidant in commercial preparations, can differentiate the source of the allergic phenomenon.[85]

NEW AGENTS AND DELIVERY SYSTEMS

New Agents

Ropivacaine

Ropivacaine (Fig. 58-27) is the N-propyl homologue of bupivacaine and mepivacaine. Unlike either bupivacaine or mepivacaine, the commercial preparation of ropivacaine contains only the S(-) enantiomer; the other compounds exist as racemic mixtures. The S(-) enantiomer of ropivacaine compared with the R(+) enantiomer produces a longer duration of sensory blockade and is severalfold less arrhythmogenic. Compared with bupivacaine, ropivacaine dissociates more rapidly from sodium channels, produces less accumulation of sodium channel blockade at physiologic heart rates, and overall, is less cardiotoxic than bupivacaine.[8,11,110,150]

With respect to physicochemical and pharmacokinetic characteristics, pK_a and protein binding of ropivacaine are similar to bupivacaine. Lipid solubility of ropivacaine is intermediate between lidocaine and bupivacaine (Table 58-6).

In contrast to bupivacaine, ropivacaine may enhance differential sensory and motor blockade.[3,11] The enhanced sensory and motor discrimination suggested by initial investigations in animal models[3,11] has been confirmed in some[29,53] but not all[151,225] human studies. Most studies in humans have shown similar potency and duration of sensory anesthesia between ropivacaine and bupivacaine.[29,110,261] Further clarification of differential sensory and motor blockade by ropivacaine should await further study and clinical use.

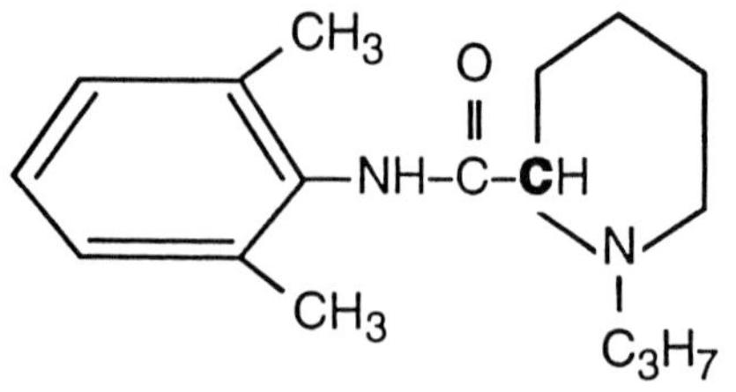

S-ropivacaine

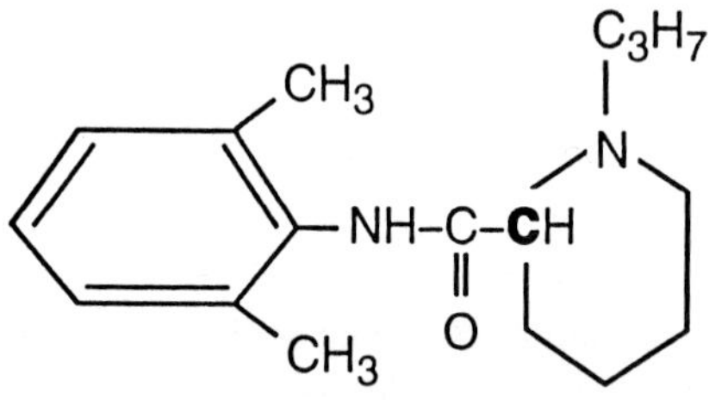

R-ropivacaine

Fig. 58-27. Optical isomers of ropivacaine. (From de Jong RH: *Local anesthetics,* St. Louis, 1994, Mosby.)

Table 58-6 Physiochemical and pharmacokinetic characteristics of ropivacaine, bupivacaine, and lidocaine

Characteristic	Ropivacaine	Bupivacaine	Lidocaine
Physicochemical			
pK_a	8.0	8.1	7.9
Protein binding (%)	94	95	65
Relative lipid solubility	2.9	10	1
Pharmacokinetic			
Vd_{ss} (l)	59	73	91
$t_{½}$ (hr)	1.8	2.7	1.6
Cl (l/min)	0.73	0.58	0.95

Ultralong duration local anesthetics

The development of a local anesthetic with a protracted duration of action has focused on investigation of compounds with nontraditional molecular structures and novel mechanisms of neural blockade (one-way dissociation, potassium channel blockade).

Cyclizing local anesthetics are uncharged tertiary amines that cross nerve membranes to form quaternary amines by cyclization in the axoplasm.[192] Via a polar phenomenon, the long amino-alkyl chain curls around on itself to form a charged cyclic piperidinium ring. The drug is thereby trapped within the axoplasm and produces anesthesia of several days duration. Unfortunately, the haloalkyl amine moiety that is necessary for cyclization is a carcinogen, and cyclization often occurs before nerve membrane penetration.[258]

A permanently charged quaternary ammonium derivative of lidocaine (N-β-phenylethyl lidocaine) has been synthesized.[258] The compound does not undergo cyclization. The local anesthetic gains access through the nerve membrane because its positive charge is shielded by surrounding hydrophobic arms. Within the axoplasm, the local anesthetic is trapped because it is a charged moiety. Using *in vitro* and *in vivo* models, N-β-phenylethyl lidocaine has produced protracted anesthesia.[258]

Tetraethylammonium and its derivatives have long been known to block potassium channels.[55] By blockade of the potassium channel, repolarization is impeded, and the resting membrane potential approaches neutrality. A series of N-alkyl-substituted tetraethylammonium derivatives were found to produce blockade of 17 to 20 days' duration.[213] Unfortunately, subsequent testing revealed the effects to be neurotoxic rather than from high binding affinity of a local anesthetic.[137]

Although development of local anesthetics with novel molecular structures and novel mechanisms of action continues, most current efforts are directed toward modification of formulations of existing local anesthetics to yield new delivery systems.

New Delivery Systems

Eutectic mixture of local anesthetics (EMLA)

A eutectic mixture is a mixture of crystalline substances with a melting point that is less than that of either its individual components.[91] One gram of EMLA contains lidocaine (25 mg), prilocaine (25 mg), an emulsifier, a thickener, and distilled water (adjusted to a pH of 9.4). EMLA is a liquid at room temperature that contains uncharged base in concentrations up to 80%. EMLA is more effective than other topical anesthetic preparations because the high concentrations of uncharged base aid dermal penetration and diffusion.[76]

One to two grams of EMLA cream are applied per 10 cm^2 of skin and covered with an occlusive dreassing.[91] Topical anesthesia is produced by diffusion of EMLA through the skin to block activation of nociceptors. Typically, onset of anesthesia occurs over 45 to 60 minutes. Depth of skin penetration is a function of time of application up to a maximum of 2 hours. Often, penetration continues over the first 30 minutes after removal of the cream from the skin.[19]

Maximum systemic concentrations of lidocaine and prilocaine are well below toxic levels if appropriate dosing guidelines are followed.[71,106,119] Peak blood concentrations occur 2 to 3 hours after application. Application to areas of broken or inflamed skin, mucous membranes, and other areas of high perfusion may result in excessive absorption.[119] Repetitive daily use in children increases the potential for development of methemoglobinemia[59] as does concomitant use of methemoglobin-producing agents (e.g., acetaminophen, benzocaine, nitrofurantoin, phenobarbital, phenytoin, quinine, and sulfonamides).[126]

EMLA has a number of clinical uses. EMLA provides good local anesthesia for IV catheter insertion and for a number of dermal procedures in children.[126] The delivery system has been found to be effective for provision of analgesia in those with chronic pain syndromes such as reflex sympathetic dystrophy[175] or postherpetic neuralgia.[226]

Nonimmediate release delivery systems

In an attempt to prolong the duration of neural blockade with existing local anesthetics, delayed release and sustained release delivery systems have been developed.

Delayed release delivery systems. Delayed release delivery systems involve repeated, intermittent dosing from immediate-release units incorporated into a single dosage form.[143] Delayed release systems for local anesthetics have included peanut oil vehicle,[48] substituted dextrans,[103–105,212] and lipid solutions (iophendylate).[132,133]

An early delayed release delivery system involved procaine in peanut oil. The formulation was locally irritating, highly allergenic, and neurotoxic (causing transverse myelitis).[48]

The addition of substituted dextrans to prilocaine, lidocaine, or bupivacaine has yielded variable results.[103–105,212] Substituted dextrans have been shown to be immunogenic and neurotoxic, and further research with this delivery system has been essentially abandoned.

Lipid carriers such as iophendylate (Pantopaque) have been examined experimentally in animals for the delivery of local anesthetics.[132,133] Longer but less intense motor block was achieved with iophendylate, although potential complications associated with its use include adhesive arachnoiditis[133] and embolic phenomena after inadvertent intravascular injection.

Sustained release delivery systems. By definition, sustained release drug delivery systems achieve slow release of a drug over a protracted interval.[143] A controlled release delivery system maintains constant blood or tissue levels of a drug. If duration of action is extended but continuous blood levels are not achieved, the system is termed a prolonged release system.[143] Essentially, all sustained release delivery systems under investigation for local anesthetics are prolonged release systems.

Lidocaine, etidocaine, tetracaine, and bupivacaine have been encapsulated into micelle-like structures called liposomes.[63,135,147] Local anesthetics are encapsulated in liposomes by addition to a lipid (e.g., lecithin) emulsifier in an aqueous vehicle, followed by sonification. The local anesthetic and aqueous carrier are trapped in the center of the resultant lipid bilayer. Similarly, volatile anesthetics have been encapsulated in lecithin.[107,124] In both systems, the drug is slowly and continuously released from the liposome.

Local anesthetics in crystalline form may be encapsulated also.[22,125] A lipid monolayer surrounds the crystal, which is in turn surrounded by a lipid bilayer. A secondary coating, composed of smaller lipid vesicles and unilamellar membranes, surrounds the entire preparation.

Initial efforts with liposome-encapsulated agents were directed at cutaneous anesthesia.[94,107,124,125] Subsequently, liposome-encapsulated lidocaine has been administered epidurally to dogs, with a resultant threefold increase in the duration of neural blockade.[147] Drug toxicity has been examined by IV infusion of bupivacaine-encapsulated liposomes. Interestingly, the arrhythmogenic and convulsant dose of bupivacaine more than doubled, probably because liposomes do not cross blood–organ barriers.[23]

A biodegradable polymer system of cylindrical pellets containing bupivacaine has been shown to provide prolonged sciatic nerve block after surgical implantation in rats.[148] Sustained release of local anesthetic is believed to be achieved by enzymatic degradation of the polymeric system.[174] Potentially, such biodegradable polymeric systems could be injected for production of regional anesthesia and analgesia.

Of all the aforementioned delivery systems, encapsulation of local anesthetics within lipid micellar preparations or biodegradable polymers holds the most promise for ultralong anesthesia or analgesia.

KEY POINTS

- Local anesthetic agents act by binding to a protein receptor in the sodium channel.
- The gating model of sodium channel kinetics states that sodium channels may be opened or closed, although protein macromolecules of the channel can exist in three separate conformations. Thus, there are three kinetic states of the sodium channel: resting, open, and inactivated. The inactivated state is a transitional state.
- Local anesthetics diffuse through the nerve membrane to the axoplasm, wherein they become charged species. The cationic species of local anesthetic is the active moiety that binds to the receptor. Benzocaine is the exception and gains entrance to the receptor from the membrane itself.
- Local anesthetic agents can be separated chemically into two groups: amino-ester and amino-amide agents. They differ in chemical stability, site of action, method of biodegradation, and allergic potential.
- Local anesthetic agents differ in anesthetic potency, onset and duration of action, and differential sensorimotor blockade. The profile of individual agents is determined by their structure-activity relationships and physiochemical characteristics.
- Lipid solubility is a primary determinant of intrinsic anesthetic potency because the site of action of local anesthetics is the nerve membrane, which consists primarily of lipids.
- The duration of action of local anesthetics is related primarily to the extent of protein binding. Greater protein binding of a specific agent is presumed to result in a longer period of sodium channel blockade and a longer duration of anesthesia.
- In isolated nerves, onset time is correlated with the pK_a of the various agents. Lipid solubility also influences onset of action.
- Bupivacaine shows the most dramatic separation between sensory anesthesia and motor blockade.
- Factors that influence the success rate of regional anesthetic procedures include dosage, site of administration, pH adjustment of local anesthetic solutions, addition of a vasoconstrictor to the local anesthetic solution, and confounding physiologic variables such as pregnancy, infection, or renal failure.
- Increasing the dosage of a local anesthetic usually results in a more dense block, longer duration of anesthesia, and a shorter latency interval.
- Epinephrine frequently is added to local anesthetic solutions to decrease the rate of vascular absorption, which improves the density and duration of anesthesia.
- The shortest duration of action occurs after subarachnoid or subcutaneous administration. The longest latencies and durations occur after major peripheral nerve blocks.
- Alkalinization of local anesthetic solutions by adding sodium bicarbonate also decreases onset of conduction blockade.
- The vascular absorption of local anesthetic agents is related to the injection site, dosage, addition of a vasoconstrictor agent, and the specific agent used.
- The vascular distribution of local anesthetic agents falls into two phases: a rapid disappearance (α) phase and a slower disappearance (β) phase from blood. The α-phase is related to uptake by tissues with high vascular perfusion. The β-phase is mainly a function of distribution to slowly equilibrating tissues. Sometimes the β-phase is subdivided into a γ-phase, which represents biotransformation and excretion of the compound.
- The esters of procaine-like drugs are hydrolyzed in plasma by pseudocholinesterase. The amide agents are metabolized primarily in the liver.
- The elimination of local anesthetics is influenced by the patient's hepatic and cardiac status.
- Local anesthetic-induced systemic toxicity primarily involves the CNS and the cardiovascular system.
- Initial symptoms of local anesthetic-induced CNS toxicity are lightheadedness and dizziness. These often are followed by visual and auditory disturbances.
- Anesthetic potency and CNS toxicity of various IV agents are positively correlated.
- Local anesthetics have direct effects on cardiac muscle and vascular smooth muscle.
- Bupivacaine may produce severe cardiac dysrhythmias. Ropivacaine may produce less severe dysrhythmias.
- Local anesthetics depress myocardial contractility. All local anesthetics exert a dose-dependent negative inotropic action on isolated cardiac tissue that is proportional to the conduction-blocking potency of the various agents in isolated nerves.

- Methemoglobinemia may follow large doses of prilocaine.
- Ester agents, such as procaine, produce allergic reactions. Amide local anesthetics rarely produce allergic reactions.
- Prolonged sensorimotor deficits may follow the subarachnoid injection of large doses of 2-chloroprocaine.
- Severe back spasms may follow the epidural administration of large volumes of 2-chloroprocaine solutions containing EDTA.

KEY REFERENCES

Covino BG: Pharmacology of local anesthetic agents, *Br J Anaesth* 58:701, 1986.

Covino BG: Clinical pharmacology of local anesthetic agents. In Cousins MJ, Bridenbaugh PO, editors: *Neural blockade in clinical anesthesia and management of pain,* ed 2, Philadelphia, 1988, JB Lippincott.

Covino BG, Scott DB: *Handbook of epidural anaesthesia and analgesia,* Orlando, 1985, Grune and Stratton.

Covino BG, Vassallo HG: *Local anesthetics: mechanisms of action and clinical use,* New York, 1976, Grune & Stratton.

de Jong RH: *Local anesthetics,* St. Louis, 1994, Mosby.

Strichartz GR: *Local anesthetics. Handbook of experimental pharmacology,* vol 81, Berlin-Heidelberg, 1987, Springer-Verlag.

Tucker GT: Pharmacokinetics of local anesthetics, *Br J Anaesth* 58:717, 1986.

Tucker GT, Mather LE: Properties, absorption and disposition of local anesthetic agents. In Cousins MJ, Bridenbaugh PO, editors: *Neural blockade in clinical anesthesia and management of pain,* ed 2, Philadelphia, 1988, JB Lippincott.

REFERENCES

1. Ackerman WE, Phoro JC, McDonald JS: Analgesia with intravenous local anesthetics. In Raj PP, editor: *Practical management of pain,* St. Louis, 1992, Mosby.
2. Akerman B, Astrom A, Ross S, et al: Studies on the absorption, distribution and metabolism of labeled prilocaine and lidocaine in some animal species, *Acta Pharmacol Toxicol* 24:389, 1966.
3. Akerman B, Hellberg IB, Trossvik C: Primary evaluation of the local anesthetic properties of the amino amide agent ropivacaine (LEA 103), *Acta Anesthesiol Scand* 32:571, 1988.
4. Aldrete JA, Homatas J, Boyes RN, et al: Effects of hepatectomy on the disappearance rate of lidocaine from blood in man and dog, *Anesth Analg* 49:687, 1970.
5. Aldrete JA, Johnson DA: Evaluation of intracutaneous testing for investigation of allergy to local anesthetic agents, *Anesth Analg* 49:173, 1970.
6. Aldrete JA, Klug DK: Alteration of skin reactivity to local anesthetic drugs in guinea pigs, *Int J Dermatol* 9:142, 1970.
7. Arbuthnott R, Boyd IA, Kalu KV: Ultrastructural dimensions of myelinated peripheral nerve fibers in the cat and their relation to conduction velocity, *J Physiol Lond* 308:125, 1980.
8. Arlock P: Actions of three local anesthetics: lidocaine, bupivacaine and ropivacaine on guinea pig papillary muscle sodium channels (V_{max}), *Pharmacol Toxicol* 63:96, 1988.
9. Arthur GR: Pharmacokinetics of local anesthetics. In Strichartz GR, editor: *Local anesthetics. Handbook of experimental pharmacology,* vol 81, Berlin-Heidelberg, 1987, Springer-Verlag.
10. Arthur GR, Feldman HS, Covino BG: Comparative pharmacokinetics of bupivacaine and ropivacaine, a new amide local anesthetic, *Anesth Analg* 67:1053, 1988.
11. Bader AM, Datta S, Flanagan H, et al: Comparison of bupivacaine- and ropivacaine-induced conduction blockade in the isolated rabbit vagus nerve, *Anesth Analg* 68:724, 1989.
12. Barsa J, Batra M, Fink BR, et al: A comparative in vivo study of local neurotoxicity of lidocaine, bupivacaine, 2-chloroprocaine, and a mixture of 2-chloroprocaine and bupivacaine, *Anesth Analg* 61:961, 1982.
13. Barsa JE, Batra M, Fink BR, et al: Prolonged neural blockade following regional analgesia with 2-chloroprocaine, *Anesth Analg* 61:961, 1982.
14. Bax ND, Tucker GT, Woods HF: Lignocaine and indocyanine green kinetics in patients following myocardial infarction, *Br J Clin Pharmacol* 10:353, 1980.
15. Benoit PW, Belt WD: Some effects of local anesthetic agents on skeletal muscle, *Exp Neurol* 34:264, 1972.
16. Benson JS: *FDA Safety Alert: Cauda equina syndrome associated with use of small-bore catheters in continuous spinal anesthesia,* May 29, 1992.
17. Berde CB: Convulsions associated with pediatric regional anesthesia, *Anesth Analg* 75:164, 1992.
18. Bernards CM, Artu AA: Hexamethonium and midazolam terminate dysrhythmias and hypertension caused in intracerebroventricular bupivacaine in rabbits, *Anesthesiology* 74:89, 1991.
19. Bjerring P, Andersen PH, Arendt-Nielsen L: Vascular response of human skin after analgesia with EMLA cream, *Br J Anaesth* 63:655, 1989.
20. Blair MR: Cardiovascular pharmacology of local anaesthetics, *Br J Anaesth* 47:247, 1975.
21. Block A, Covino BG: Effect of local anesthetic agents on cardiac conduction and contractility, *Reg Anesth* 6:55, 1981.
22. Boedeker BH, Lojeski EW, Haynes DH: Microencapsulated tetracaine demonstrated to be an ultralong-duration local anesthetic, *Anesthesiology* 77:A799, 1992.
23. Boogaerts J, Declercq A, Lafont N, et al: Toxicity of bupivacaine encapsulated into liposomes and injected intravenously: comparison with plain solution, *Anesth Analg* 76:353, 1993.
24. Borg PAJ, Krijnen HJ: Hyaluronidase in the management of pain due to post-laminectomy scar tissue, *Pain* 58:273, 1994.
25. Boyes RN: A review of the metabolism of amide local anaesthetic agents, *Br J Anaesth* 47:225, 1975.
26. Braid DP, Scott DB: The systemic absorption of local analgesic drugs, *Br J Anaesth* 37:394, 1965.
27. Brodie BB, Lief PA, Poet R: The fate of

procaine in man following its intravenous administration and methods for the estimation of procaine and diethylaminoethanol, *J Pharmacol Exp Ther* 94:359, 1948.
28. Bromage PR: A comparison of the hydrochloride and carbon dioxide salts of lidocaine and prilocaine in epidural analgesia, *Acta Anaesthesiol Scand Suppl* 16:55, 1965.
29. Brown DL, Carpenter RL, Thompson GE: Comparison of 0.5% ropivacaine and 0.5% bupivacaine for epidural anesthesia in patients undergoing lower extremity surgery, *Anesthesiology* 72:633, 1990.
30. Buckley FP, Littlewood DG, Covino BG, et al: Effects of adrenaline and the concentration of solution on extradural block with etidocaine, *Br J Anaesth* 50;171, 1978.
31. Burm AG, van Kleef JW, Gladines MP, et al: Plasma concentrations of lidocaine and bupivacaine after subarachnoid administration, *Anesthesiology* 59:191, 1983.
32. Burm AGL, van Kleef JW, Vermeulen NPE, et al: Pharmacokinetics of lidocaine and bupivacaine following subarachnoid administration in surgical patients: simultaneous investigation of absorption and disposition kinetics using stable isotopes, *Anesthesiology* 69:584, 1988.
33. Butterworth IV JF, Cole LR: Low concentrations of procaine and diethylaminoethanol reduce the excitability but not the action potential amplitude of hippocampal pyramidal cells, *Anesth Analg* 71:404, 1990.
34. Butterworth IV JF, Lief PA, Strichartz GR: The pH-dependent local anesthetic activity of diethylaminoethanol, a procaine metabolite, *Anesthesiology* 68:501, 1988.
35. Butterworth IV JF, Strichartz GR: Molecular mechanisms of local anesthesia: a review, *Anesthesiology* 72:711, 1990.
36. Catchlove RFH: The influence of CO_2 and pH on local anesthetic action, *J Pharmacol Exp Ther* 181:298, 1972.
37. Cerbón J: NMR evidence for hydrophobic interaction of local anesthetics. Possible relation to their potency, *Biochim Biophys Acta* 290:51, 1972.
38. Chabal C, Jacobson L, Mariano A, et al: The use of oral mexiletine for the treatment of pain after peripheral nerve injury, *Anesthesiology* 76:513, 1992.
39. Chernoff DM: Kinetic analysis of phasic inhibition of neuronal sodium currents by lidocaine and bupivacaine, *Biophys J* 58: 53, 1990.
40. Clarkson CW, Hondeghem LM: Mechanism of bupivacaine depression of cardiac conduction: fast block of sodium channels during the action potential with slow recovery from block during diastole, *Anesthesiology* 62:396, 1985.
41. Cohen EN: Distribution of local anesthetic agents in the neuraxis of the dog, *Anesthesiology* 29:1002, 1968.
42. Cohen EN, Levine DA, Colliss JE, et al: The role of pH in the development of tachyphylaxis to local anesthetic agents, *Anesthesiology* 29:994, 1968.
43. Cohen LS, Rosenthal JE, Horner DW, et al: Plasma levels of lidocaine after intramuscular injection, *Am J Cardiol* 29:520, 1972.
44. Courtney KR, Kendig JJ, Cohen EN: Frequency-dependent conduction block, *Anesthesiology* 48:111, 1978.
45. Courtney KR, Stirchartz GR: Structural elements which determine local anesthetic activity. In Strichartz GR, editor: *Local anesthetics. Handbook of experimental pharmacology,* vol 81, Berlin-Heidelberg, 1987, Springer-Verlag.
46. Covino BG: Clinical pharmacology of local anesthetic agents. In Cousins MJ, Bridenbaugh PO, editors: *Neural blockade in clinical anesthesia and management of pain,* ed 2, Philadelphia, 1988, JB Lippincott.
47. Covino BG: Pharmacology of local anaesthetic agents, *Br J Anaesth* 58:701, 1986.
48. Covino BG: Ultralong-acting local anesthetic agents, *Anesthesiology* 54:263, 1981.
49. Covino BG, Bush DF: Clinical evaluation of local anesthetic agents, *Br J Anaesth* 56: 147, 1984.
50. Covino BG, Scott DB: *Handbook of epidural anaesthesia and analgesia,* ed 1, Orlando, 1985, Grune & Stratton.
51. Covino BG, Vassallo HG: *Local anesthetics: mechanism of action and clinical use,* New York, 1976, Grune & Stratton.
52. Crawford OB: Comparative evaluation in peridural anesthesia of lidocaine, mepivacaine, and L-67, a new local anesthetic agent, *Anesthesiology* 25:321, 1964.
53. Datta S, Camann W, Bader A, et al: Clinical effects and maternal and fetal plasma concentrations of epidural ropivacaine versus bupivacaine for cesarean section, *Anesthesiology* 82:1346, 1995.
54. de Jong RH: Biotransformation. In de Jong RH, editor: *Local anesthetics,* St. Louis, 1994, Mosby–Year Book.
55. de Jong RH: *Local anesthetics,* St. Louis, 1994, Mosby–Year Book.
56. de Jong RH, Robles R, Corbin RW: Central actions of lidocaine-synaptic transmission, *Anesthesiology* 30:19, 1969.
57. de Jong RH, Ronfeld RA, DeRosa RA: Cardiovascular effects of convulsants and supra-convulsant doses of amide local anesthetics, *Anesth Analg* 61:3, 1982.
58. de la Coussaye JE, Bassoul B, Albat B, et al: Experimental evidence in favor of role of intracellular actions of bupivacaine in myocardial depression, *Anesth Analg* 74:698, 1992.
59. de Waard-van der Spek FB, van der Berg GM, Oranje AP: EMLA cream: an improved local anesthetic. Review of current literature, *Ped Dermatol* 9:126, 1992.
60. Denson DD, Myers JA, Hartrick CT, et al: The relationship between free bupivacaine concentration and central nervous system toxicity, *Anesthesiology* 63:A211, 1984.
61. DiFazio CA, Carron H, Grosslight KR, et al: Comparison of pH-adjusted lidocaine solutions for epidural anesthesia, *Anesth Analg* 65:760, 1986.
62. DiGiovanni AJ: Inadvertent intraosseous injection—a hazard of caudal anesthesia, *Anesthesiology* 34:92, 1971.
63. Djordjevich L, Ivankovich AD, Chigurupati R, et al: Efficacy of liposome-encapsulated bupivacaine, *Anesthesiology* 65:A 185, 1986.
64. Dooms-Goossens A, de Alam AG, Degreef H, et al: Local anesthetic intolerance due to metabisulfite, *Contact Dermatitis* 20:124, 1989.
65. Drachman D, Strichartz G: Potassium channel blockers potentiate impulse inhibition by local anesthetics, *Anesthesiology* 75:1051, 1991.
66. DuSouich P, Erill P: Altered metabolism of procainamide and procaine in patients with pulmonary and cardiac disease, *Clin Pharmacol Ther* 21:101, 1977.
67. Ecoffey C, Desparmet J, Berdeaux A, et al: Pharmacokinetics of lignocaine in children following caudal anesthesia, *Br J Anaesth* 56:1399, 1984.
68. Ecoffey C, Desparmet J, Macry M, et al: Bupivacaine in children: pharmacokinetics following caudal anesthesia, *Anesthesiology* 63:447, 1985.
69. Edwards DJ, Lalka D, Cerra F, et al: Alpha 1-acid glycoprotein concentration and protein binding in trauma, *Clin Pharmacol Ther* 31:62, 1982.
70. Eicholzer AW, Feldman HS: Acute toxicity of etidocaine following various routes of administration in the dog, *Toxicol Appl Pharmacol* 37:13, 1976.
71. Engberg G, Danielson K, Henneberg S, et al: Plasma concentrations of prilocaine and lidocaine and methaemoglobin formation in infants after epicutaneous application of a 5% lidocaine-prilocaine cream (EMLA), *Acta Anaesthesiol Scand* 31:624, 1987.
72. Englesson S, Eriksson E, Wahlqvist S, et al: Differences in tolerance to intravenous Xylocaine and Citanest (L67), a new local anesthetic. A double blind study in man. *Proc 1st Eur Congr Anesthesiol* 2:206, 1962.
73. Englesson S, Greusten S: The influence of acid-base changes on central nervous system toxicity of local anesthetic agents. II, *Acta Anaesthesiol Scand* 18:88, 1974.
74. Erdimir HA, Soper LE, Sweet RB: Studies of factors affecting epidural anesthesia, *Anesth Analg* 44:400, 1965.
75. Eriksson AS, Sinclair R, Cassuto J, et al: Influence of lidocaine on leukocyte function in the surgical wound, *Anesthesiology* 77:74, 1992.
76. Evers H, von Dardel O, Juhlin L, et al: Dermal effects of compositions based on the eutectic mixture of lignocaine and prilocaine (EMLA). Studies in volunteers, *Br J Anaesth* 57:997, 1985.
77. Feely J, Wade D, McAlliste CB, et al: Effect of hypotension on liver blood flow and lidocaine dispositions, *N Engl J Med* 307:866, 1982.
78. Feely J, Wilkinson GR, McAllister CR, et al: Increased toxicity and reduced clearance of lidocaine by cimetidine, *Ann Intern Med* 96:592, 1982.
79. Feldman HS, Covino BG, Sage DJ: Direct chronotropic and ionotropic effects of local anesthetic agents in isolated guinea pig atria, *Reg Anesth* 7:149, 1982.
80. Ferrante FM, Paggioli J, Cherukuri S, et al: The analgesic response to intravenous lidocaine in the treatment of neuropathic pain, *Anesth Analg* 82:91, 1996.
81. Ferrante FM, VadeBoncouer TR: Epidural analgesia with combinations of local anesthetics and opioids. In Ferrante FM, VadeBoncouer TR, editors: *Postoperative pain management,* New York, 1993, Churchill-Livingstone.

82. Fink BR, Cairns AM: Lack of size-related differential sensitivity to equilibrium conduction block among mammalian myelinated axons exposed to lidocaine, *Anesth Analg* 66:948, 1987.
83. Finucane BT, Hammonds WD: Influence of age on vascular absorption of lidocaine injected epidurally in man, *Reg Anesth* 9:36, 1984.
84. Fisher M: Intradermal testing after anaphylactoid reaction to anaesthetic drugs: practical aspects of performance and interpretation, *Anaesth Intensive Care* 12:115, 1984.
85. Fisher M, Graham R: Adverse responses to local anesthetics, *Anaesth Intensive Care* 12:325, 1984.
86. Foldes FF, Davidson GM, Duncalf D, et al: The intravenous toxicity of local anesthetic agents in man, *Clin Pharmacol Ther* 6:328, 1965.
87. Foldes FF, Foldes VM, Smith JC, et al: The relation between plasma cholinesterase and prolonged apnea caused by succinylcholine, *Anesthesiology* 24:208, 1963.
88. Foster AH, Carlson BM: Myotoxicity of local anesthetics and regeneration of the damaged muscle fibers, *Anesth Analg* 59:727, 1980.
89. Franz DN, Perry RS: Mechanisms for differential block among single myelinated and non-myelinated axons by procaine, *J Physiol Lond* 199:319, 1968.
90. Freund PR, Bowdle TA, Slattery JT, et al: Caudal anesthesia with lidocaine or bupivacaine: plasma local anesthetic concentration and extent of sensory spread in old and young patients, *Anesth Analg* 63:1017, 1984.
91. Gajraj NM, Pennant JH, Watcha MF: Eutectic mixture of local anesthetics (EMLA) cream, *Anesth Analg* 78:574, 1994.
92. Gasser HS, Erlanger J: The role of fiber size in the establishment of a nerve block by pressure or by cocaine, *Am J Physiol* 88:581, 1929.
93. Geddes IC: Studies on the metabolism of Citanest C[14], Acta Anaesthesiol *Scand Suppl* 26:37, 1965.
94. Gesztes A, Mezei M: Topical anesthesia of the skin by liposome-encapsulated tetracaine, *Anesth Analg* 67:1079, 1988.
95. Gintant GA, Hoffman BF: The role of local anesthetic effects in the actions of antiarrhythmic drugs. In Strichartz GR, editor: *Local anesthetics. Handbook of experimental pharmacology,* vol 81, Berlin-Heidelberg, 1987, Springer-Verlag.
96. Gissen AJ, Datta S, Lambert D: The chloroprocaine controversy II. Is chloroprocaine neurotoxic? *Reg Anesth* 9:135, 1984.
97. Grambling ZW, Ellis RG, Valpitto PP: Clinical experience with mepivacaine (Carbocaine), *J Med Assoc Ga* 53:16, 1964.
98. Greene NM: Distribution of local anesthetic solutions within the subarachnoid space, *Anesth Analg* 64:715, 1985.
99. Greene NM: *Physiology of spinal anesthesia,* ed 2, Baltimore, 1969, Williams and Wilkins.
100. Grossman SH, Davis D, Kitchell BB, et al: Diazepam and lidocaine plasma protein binding in renal disease, *Clin Pharmacol Ther* 31:350, 1982.
101. Halkin H, Meffin P, Melmon KL, et al: Influence of congestive heart failure on blood levels of lidocaine and its monodeethylated metabolite, *Clin Pharmacol Ther* 17:669, 1975.
102. Harrison DC, Sprouse JH, Morrow AG: The antiarrhythmic properties of lidocaine and procaine amide; clinical and physiologic studies of their cardiovascular effects in man, *Circulation* 28:486, 1963.
103. Hassan AG, Akerman B, Renck H, et al: Effects of adjuvants to local anesthetics on their duration. III, *Acta Anaesthesiol Scand* 29:385, 1985.
104. Hassan HG, Renck H, Lindberg B, et al: Effects of adjuvants to local anesthetics on their duration. I, *Acta Anaesthesiol Scand* 29:375, 1985.
105. Hassan HG, Renck H, Lindberg B, et al: Effects of adjuvants to local anesthetics on their duration. II, *Acta Anaesthesiol Scand* 29:380, 1985.
106. Haugstredt S, Friman AM, Danielson K: Plasma concentrations of lidocaine and prilocaine and analgesic effect after dermal application of EMLA cream 5% for surgical removal of mollusca in children, *Z Londercjor* 45:148, 1990.
107. Haynes DK, Kirkpatrick AF: Long duration local anesthesia with lecithin-coated microdroplets of methoxyflurane: studies with human skin, *Reg Anesth* 16:173, 1991.
108. Heavner JE: Cardiac dysrhythmias induced by infusion of local anesthetics into the lateral cerebral ventricle of cats, *Anesth Analg* 65:133, 1986.
109. Heavner JE, Dryden CF, Sanghani V, et al: Severe hypoxia enhances central nervous system and cardiovascular toxicity of bupivacaine in lightly anesthetized pigs, *Anesthesiology* 77:142, 1992.
110. Hickey R, Hoffman J, Ramamurthy S: A comparison of ropivacaine 0.5% and bupivacaine 0.5% for brachial plexus block, *Anesthesiology* 74:639, 1991.
111. Hilgier M: Alkalinization of bupivacaine for brachial plexus block, *Reg Anesth* 10:59, 1985.
112. Hille B: Local anesthetics: hydrophilic and hydrophobic pathways for the drug-receptor reaction, *J Gen Physiol* 69:497, 1977.
113. Hjelm M, Holmdahl HM: Methaemoglobinemia following lignocaine, *Lancet* 1:53, 1965.
114. Hondeghem LM, Katzung BG: Antiarrhythmic agents: the modulated receptor mechanism of action of sodium and calcium channel-blocking drugs, *Ann Rev Pharmacol Toxicol* 24:387, 1984.
115. Hondeghem LM, Katzung BG: Time- and voltage-dependent interactions of antiarrhythmic drugs with cardiac sodium channels, *Biochim Biophys Acta* 472:373, 1977.
116. Jackson PR, Tucker GT, Woods HF: Altered plasma drug binding in cancer: role of α_1-glycoprotein and albumin, *Clin Pharmacol Ther* 32:295, 1982.
117. Jebson P: Intramuscular lignocaine 2% and 10%, *BMJ* 3:566, 1971.
118. Jorfeldt L, Lfstrom JB, Pernow P, et al: The effect of mepivacaine and lidocaine on forearm resistance on capacitance vessels in man, *Acta Anaesthesiol Scand* 14:183, 1970.
119. Juhlin L, Hagglund G, Evers H: Absorption of lidocaine and prilocaine after application of a eutectic mixture of local anesthetics (EMLA) on normal and diseased skin, *Acta Derm Benereol Stockh* 69:18, 1989.
120. Kalichman MW, Powell HC, Reisner LS, et al: The role of 2-chloroprocaine and sodium bisulfite in rat sciatic nerve edema, *J Neuropathol Exp Neurol* 45:566, 1986.
121. Kalow W: Hydrolysis of local anesthetics by human serum cholinesterase, *J Pharmacol Exp Ther* 104:122, 1952.
122. Katz J: The distribution of ^{14}C-labeled lidocaine injected intravenously in the rat, *Anesthesiology* 29:249, 1968.
123. Kiese M: Relationship of drug metabolism to methemoglobin formation, *Ann N Y Acad Sci* 123:141, 1965.
124. Kirkpatrick AF, Lavallee-Grey M, Haynes DH: Long duration local anesthesia with lecithin-coated microdroplets of methoxyflurane: studies with rat skin, *Reg Anesth* 16:164, 1991.
125. Kline MD, Boedeker BH, Mattix ME, et al: Intradermal toxicity of lecithin-coated microcrystalline tetracaine, *Anesthesiology* 77:A800, 1992.
126. Koren G: Use of the eutectic mixture of local anesthetics in young children for procedure-related pain, *J Pediatrics* 122:S30, 1993.
127. Kotelko DM, Shnider SM, Dailey PA, et al: Bupivacaine-induced cardiac arrhythmias in sheep, *Anesthesiology* 60:10, 1984.
128. Kyttä J, Heavner JE, Badgwell JM, et al: Cardiovascular and central nervous system effects of coadministered lidocaine and bupivacaine in piglets, *Reg Anesth* 16:89, 1991.
129. Lambert DH, Hurley RJ: Cauda equina syndrome and continuous spinal anesthesia, *Anesth Analg* 72:817, 1991.
130. Lambert LA, Lambert DH, Strichartz GR: Irreversible conduction block in isolated nerve by high concentrations of local anesthetics, *Anesthesiology* 80:1082, 1994.
131. Langerman L, Bansinath M, Grant GJ: The partition coefficient as a predictor of local anesthetic potency for spinal anesthesia: evaluation of five local anesthetics in a mouse model, *Anesth Analg* 79:490, 1994.
132. Langerman L, Golomb B, Benita S: Spinal anesthesia: significant prolongation of the pharmacologic effect of tetracaine with lipid solution of the agent, *Anesthesiology* 74:105, 1991.
133. Langerman L, Grant GJ, Zakowski M, et al: Prolongation of spinal anesthesia using a lipid drug carrier with procaine, lidocaine and tetracaine, *Anesth Analg* 75:900, 1992.
134. Lee-Son S, Wang GK, Concus A, et al: Stereoselective inhibition of neuronal sodium channels by local anesthetics. Evidence for two sites of action? *Anesthesiology* 77;324, 1992.
135. Legros F, Luo H, Pourgeors P, et al: Influence of different liposomal formulations on pharmacokinetics of encapsulated bupivacaine, *Anesthesiology* 73:A851, 1990.
136. Lieberman NA, Harris RS, Katz RI, et al: The effects of lidocaine on the electrical and mechanical activity of the heart, *Am J Cardiol* 22:375, 1968.
137. Lipfert P, Seitz RJ, Arndt JO: Ultralong-

lasting nerve block: triethyldodecylammonium bromide is probably a neurotoxin rather than a local anesthetic, *Anesthesiology* 67:896, 1987.

138. Littlewood DG, Scott DB, Wilson J, et al: Comparative anaesthetic properties of various local anesthetic agents in extradural block in labor, *Br J Anaesth* 49:75, 1977.
139. Löfstrom JB: Clinical evaluation of local anesthetics, *Clin Anesth* 1969:20, 1971.
140. Löfstrom JB: The effect of local anesthetics on the peripheral vasculature, *Reg Anesth* 17:1, 1992.
141. Löfstrom JB: Tissue distribution of local anesthetics with special reference to the lung, *Int Anesthesiol Clin* 16:53, 1978.
142. Löfstrom JB, Alan BG, Bertler A, et al: Lung uptake of lidocaine, *Acta Anaesthesiol Scand* 70:80, 1978.
143. Longer MA, Robinson JR: Sustained-release drug delivery systems. In Gennaro AR, editor: *Remington's pharmaceutical sciences,* ed 18, Easton, PA, 1990, Mack Publishing.
144. Lund PC, Bush DF, Covino BG: Determinants of etidocaine concentration in the blood, *Anesthesiology* 42:497, 1975.
145. Maier HW: *Ker Kokainismus-Geschicte/ Pathalogie medizinische und behördliche Bekäpfung,* Leipzing, 1962, Verlag.
146. Marathe PH, Shen DD, Artru AA, et al: Effects of serum protein binding on the entry of lidocaine into brain and cerebrospinal fluid of dogs, *Anesthesiology* 75: 804, 1991.
147. Mashimo T, Uchida I, Pak M, et al: Prolongation of canine epidural anesthesia by liposome encapsulation of lidocaine, *Anesth Analg* 74:827, 1992.
148. Masters DB, Berde CB, Dutta SK, et al: Prolonged regional nerve blockade by controlled release of local anesthetic from a biodegradable polymer matrix, *Anesthesiology* 79:340, 1993.
149. Mayumi T, Dohi S, Takahashi T: Plasma concentrations of lidocaine associated with cervical, thoracic and lumbar epidural anesthesia, *Anesth Analg* 62:578, 1983.
150. McCloskey JJ, Haun SE, Deshpande JK: Bupivacaine toxicity secondary to continuous caudal epidural infusion in children, *Anesth Analg* 75:287, 1992.
151. McCrae AF, Jozwiak H, McClure JH: Comparison of ropivacaine and bupivacaine in extradural analgesia for the relief of pain in labour, *Br J Anaesth* 74:261, 1995.
152. Moller R, Covino BG: Cardiac electrophysiologic properties of bupivacaine and lidocaine compared with those of ropivacaine, a new amide local anesthetic, *Anesthesiology* 72:322, 1990.
153. Moore DC, Bridenbaugh LD, Bridenbaugh PO, et al: Caudal and epidural blocks with bupivacaine for childbirth. Report of 657 parturients, *Obstet Gynecol* 37:667, 1971.
154. Moore DC, Mather LE, Bridenbaugh PO, et al: Arterial and venous plasma levels of bupivacaine following peripheral nerve blocks, *Anesth Analg* 55:763, 1976.
155. Moore, DC, Mather LE, Bridenbaugh LD, et al: Arterial and venous plasma levels of bupivacaine (marcaine) following epidural and intercostal nerve blocks, *Anesthesiology* 45:39, 1976.
156. Moore DC, Spierdijk, Van Kleef JD, et al: Chloroprocaine neurotoxicity: four additional cases, *Anesth Analg* 61:155, 1982.
157. Morishima HO, Pederson H, Finster M, et al: Bupivacaine toxicity in pregnant and nonpregnant ewes, *Anesthesiology* 63:134, 1985.
158. Myers RR, Kalichman MW, Reisner LS, et al: Neurotoxicity of local anesthetics: altered perineurial permeability, edema, and nerve fiber injury, *Anesthesiology* 64:29, 1986.
159. Narahashi T, Frazier DT: Site of action and active form of procaine in squid giant axons, *J Pharmacol Exp Ther* 194:506, 1975.
160. Nation RL, Triggs EJ, Selig M: Lignocaine kinetics in cardiac patients and aged subjects, *Br J Clin Pharmacol* 4:439, 1977.
161. Nordqvist P: The occurrence of procaine esterase in peripheral nerve and its influence on procaine block, *Acta Pharmacol Toxicol* 8:217, 1952.
162. O'Brien JE, Abbey V, Hinsvark O, et al: Metabolism and measurement of chloroprocaine, an ester-type local anesthetic, *J Pharm Sci* 68:75, 1979.
163. Ochs, HR, Carstens G, Greenblatt DJ: Reduction in lidocaine clearance during continuous infusion and co-administration of propanolol, *N Engl J Med* 303:373, 1980.
164. Pardridge WM, Sakiyama R, Fierer G: Transport of propanolol and lidocaine through the rat blood-brain barrier. Primary role of globulin-bound drug, *J Clin Invest* 71:900, 1983.
165. Patterson RP, Anderson J: Allergic reactions to drugs and biologic agents, *JAMA* 248:2637, 1982.
166. Phero JC, McDonald JS, Raj PP, et al: Controlled intravenous administration of chloroprocaine for intractable pain management, *Reg Anesth* 9:51, 1984.
167. Phillips OC, Ebner H, Nelson AT: Neurologic complications following spinal anesthesia with lidocaine: a prospective review of 10,440 cases, *Anesthesiology* 30:284, 1969.
168. Piatsky MM, Knoppert D: Binding of local anesthetics to α_1-acid glycoprotein, *Clin Res* 26:836A, 1978.
169. Pieper JA, Wyman MG, Goldreyer BN, et al: Lidocaine toxicity: effects of total versus free lidocaine concentrations, *Circulation* 62:181, 1980.
170. Pizzalato D, Reneger OJ: Histopathologic effects of long exposure to local anesthetics on peripheral nerves, *Anesth Analg* 38:138, 1959.
171. Radsdale DS, McPhee JC, Schever T, Catterall WA: Molecular determinants of state-dependent block of Na^+ channels by local anesthetic, *Science* 265:1724, 1995
172. Raj PP, Knarr D, Vigdorth E, et al: Difference in analgesia following epidural blockade in patients with postoperative or chronic low back pain, *Pain* 34:21, 1988.
173. Ralston DH, Shnider SM: The fetal and neonatal effects of regional anesthesia in obstetrics, *Anesthesiology* 48:38, 1978.
174. Ranade VV: Drug delivery systems: 3B. role of polymers in drug delivery, *J Clin Pharmacol* 30:107, 1990.
175. Rashiq S, Knight B, Ellsworth J: Treatment of reflex sympathetic dystrophy with EMLA cream (letter), *Reg Anesth* 19:434, 1994.
176. Ravindran RS, Turner MS, Muller T: Neurological effects of subarachnoid administration of 2-chloroprocaine CE, bupivacaine and low pH normal saline in dogs, *Anesth Analg* 61:279, 1982.
177. Raymond SA, Gissen AJ: Mechanisms of differential nerve block. In Strichartz GR, editor: *Local anesthetics. Handbook of experimental pharmacology,* vol 81, Berlin-Heidelberg, 1987, Springer-Verlag.
178. Raymond SA, Strichartz GR: Further comments on the failure of impulse propagation in nerves marginally blocked by local anesthetics, *Anesth Analg* 70:121, 1990.
179. Raymond SA, Strichartz GR: The long and short of differential block, *Anesthesiology* 20:725, 1989.
180. Reiestad F, Strömskag KE: Interpleural catheter in the management of postoperative pain. A preliminary report, *Reg Anesth* 11:89, 1986.
181. Reisner LS, Hochman BN, Plumer MH: Persistent neuralgia deficit and adhesive arachnoiditis following intrathecal 2-chloroprocaine injection, *Anesth Analg* 58: 452, 1980.
182. Richards RK, Smith NT, Katz J: The effects of interaction between lidocaine and pentobarbital on toxicity in mice and guinea pig atria, *Anesthesiology* 29:493, 1968.
183. Rigler ML, Drasner K: Distribution of catheter-injected local anesthetics in a model of the subarachnoid space, *Anesthesiology* 75:684, 1991.
184. Rigler ML, Drasner K, Krejcie TC, et al: Cauda equina syndrome after continuous spinal anesthesia, *Anesth Analg* 72:275, 1991.
185. Ritchie JM, Ritchie B, Greengard P: The active structure of local anesthetics, *J Pharmacol Exp Ther* 150:152, 1965.
186. Robin ED, Whaley RD, Crump CH, et al: Acid-base relations between spinal fluid and arterial blood with special reference to control of ventilation, *J Appl Physiol* 13: 385, 1958.
187. Rood JP: A case of lignocaine hypersensitivity, *Br Dent J* 135:411, 1973.
188. Rosen MA, Baysinger CL, Shnider SM, et al: Evaluation of neurotoxicity of local anesthetics following subarachnoid injection, *Anesthesiology* 57:A196, 1982.
189. Rosen MA, Thigpen JW, Shnider SM, et al: Bupivacaine-induced cardiotoxicity in hypoxic and acidotic sheep, *Anesth Analg* 64:1089, 1985.
190. Rosenberg PH: Intravenous regional anesthesia: nerve block by multiple mechanisms, *Reg Anesth* 18:1, 1993.
191. Ross BK, Coda B, Heath CH: Local anesthetic distribution in a spinal model: a possible mechanism of neurologic injury after continuous spinal anesthesia, *Reg Anesth* 17:69, 1992.
192. Ross SB, Akerman BA: Cyclization of three N-W-Haloalkyl-N-Methylamino-aceto-2,6 Xylidide derivatives in relation to their local anesthetic effect in vitro and in vivo, *J Pharmacol Exp Ther* 182:351, 1972.

193. Rothstein P, Arthur GR, Feldman HS, et al: The lung modifies arterial concentrations of bupivacaine in humans, *Reg Anesth* 8:44, 1983.
194. Routledge PA, Barchowsky A, Bjornsson TD, et al: Lidocaine plasma protein binding, *Clin Pharmacol Ther* 27:347, 1980.
195. Routledge PA, Shand DG, Barchowsky A, et al: Relationship between alpha 1-acid glycoprotein and lidocaine disposition in myocardial infarction, *Clin Pharmacol Ther* 30:154, 1981.
196. Rowland M: Local anesthetic absorption, distribution and elimination. In Eger EI, editor: *Anesthesia uptake and action,* Baltimore, 1974, Williams and Wilkins.
197. Sage DJ, Feldman H, Arthur GR, et al: Cardiovascular effects of lidocaine and bupivacaine in the awake dog, *Anesthesiology* 59:A210, 1983.
198. Sage DJ, Feldman HS, Arthur GR, et al: Influence of lidocaine and bupivacaine on isolated guinea pig atria in the presence of acidosis and hypoxia, *Anesth Analg* 63:1, 1984.
199. Sakura S, Chan VWS, Ciriales R, et al: The addition of 7.5% glucose does not alter the neurotoxicity of 5% lidocaine administered intrathecally in the rat, *Anesthesiology* 82: 236, 1995.
200. Schatz M, Fung DL: Anaphylactic and anaphylactoid reactions due to anesthetic agents, *Clin Rev Allergy* 4:215, 1986.
201. Schell RM, Brauer FS, Code DJ, et al: Persistent sacral root deficits after continuous spinal anesthesia, *Can J Anaesth* 38: 908, 1991.
202. Schneider M, Ettlin T, Kaufmann M, et al: Transient neurologic toxicity after hyperbaric subarachnoid anesthesia with 5% lidocaine, *Anesth Analg* 76:1154, 1993.
203. Schönenberger H, Peter A, Zwez W: *Zum Wirkungmechanismus der Localanästhetica, Arch Pharmacol* 38:209, 1968.
204. Schwartz HJ, Gilbert IA, Lenner KA, et al: Metabisulfite sensitivity and local dental anesthesia, *Ann Allergy* 62:83, 1989.
205. Schwarz W, Palade PT, Hille B: Local anesthetics: effect of pH on use-dependent block of sodium channels in frog muscle, *Biophys J* 20:343, 1977.
206. Scott DB: Evaluation of clinical tolerance of local anaesthetic agents, *Br J Anaesth* 47:328, 1975.
207. Scott DB: Evaluation of the toxicity of local anaesthetic agents in man, *Br J Anaesth* 47:56, 1975.
208. Scott DB: Toxicity caused by local anaesthetic drugs, *Br J Anaesth* 53:533, 1981.
209. Scott DB, Jebsen PJ, Braid DP, et al: Factors affecting plasma levels of lignocaine and prilocaine, *Br J Anesth* 44:1040, 1972.
210. Scott DB, Jebson PJ, Boyes RN: Pharmacokinetic study of the local anesthetic bupivacaine (Marcaine) and etidocaine (Duranest) in man, *Br J Anaesth* 45:1010, 1973.
211. Scott DB, McClure JH, Giasi RM, et al: Effects of concentration of local anaesthetic drugs in extradural block, *Br J Anaesth* 52:1033, 1980.
212. Scurlock JE, Curtis BM: Dextran-local anesthetic interactions, *Anesth Analg* 59: 335, 1980.
213. Scurlock JE, Curtis BM: Tetraethylammonium derivatives: ultralong-acting local anesthetics, *Anesthesiology* 54:265, 1981.
214. Selden R, Sasahara AA: Central nervous system toxicity induced by lidocaine. Report of a case in a patient with liver disease, *JAMA* 202:908, 1967.
215. Sheskey MC, Rocco AG, Bizzari-Schmidt M, et al: A dose-response study of bupivacaine for spine anesthesia, *Anesth Analg* 62:931, 1983.
216. Sigelbaum SA, Koester J: Ion channels. In Kandel ER, editor: *Principles of neural science,* ed 3, Norwalk, CT, 1991, Appleton-Lange.
217. Sinclair CJ, Scott DB: Comparison of bupivacaine and etidocaine in extradural blockade, *Br J Anaesth* 56:147, 1984.
218. Sjöberg M, Karlson P-Å, Nordberg C, et al: Neuropathologic findings after long-term intrathecal infusion of morphine and bupivacaine for pain treatment in cancer patients, *Anesthesiology* 76:173, 1992.
219. Skou JC: Local anesthetics. II. The toxic potencies of some local anesthetics and butyl alcohol, determined on peripheral nerve, *Acta Pharmacol Toxicol* 10:292, 1954.
220. Starmer CF: Theoretical characterization of ion channel blockade. Competitive binding to periodically accessible receptors, *Biophys J* 52:405, 1987.
221. Steinbrook RA, Hughes N, Fanciullo G, et al: Effects of alkalinization of lidocaine on the pain of skin infiltration and intravenous catheterization, *J Clin Anesth* 5:456, 1993.
222. Stenson RE, Constantino RT, Harrison DC: Interrelationship of hepatic blood flow, cardiac output, and blood levels of lidocaine in man, *Circulation* 43:215, 1971.
223. Stevens RA, Urmey WF, Urquhart BL, et al: Back pain after epidural anesthesia with chloroprocaine, *Anesthesiology* 78:492, 1993.
224. Stewart DM, Rogers WP, Mahaffrey JE, et al: Effect of local anesthetics on the cardiovascular system in the dog, *Anesthesiology* 24:620, 1963.
225. Stienstra R, Jonker TA, Bourdrez P, et al: Ropivacaine 0.25% versus bupivacaine 0.25% for continuous epidural analgesia in labor: a double-blind comparison, *Anesth Analg* 80:285, 1995.
226. Stow PJ, Glynn CJ, Minor B: EMLA cream in the treatment of post-herpetic neuralgia. Efficacy and pharmacokinetic profile, *Pain* 39:301, 1989.
227. Strichartz GR: Molecular mechanisms of nerve block by local anesthetics, *Anesthesiology* 45:421, 1976.
228. Strichartz GR, Rando T, Wang GK: An integrated view of the molecular toxicology of sodium channel gating in excitable cells, *Ann Rev Neurosci* 10:237, 1987.
229. Strichartz GR, Ritchie JM: The action of local anesthetics on ion channels of excitable tissues. In Strichartz GR, editor: *Local anesthetics. Handbook of experimental pharmacology,* vol 81, Berlin-Heidelberg, 1987, Springer-Verlag.
230. Strichartz GR, Sanchez V, Arthur G, et al: Fundamental properties of local anesthetics. II. Measured octanol: buffer partition coefficients and pK_a values of clinically used drugs, *Anesthesiology* 71:158, 1990.
231. Strömskag KE, Minor BG, Post C: Distribution of bupivacaine after interpleural injection in rats, *Reg Anesth* 16:43, 1991.
232. Strömskag KE, Reiestad F, Holmquist ELO, et al: Intrapleural administration of 0.25%, .375% and 0.5% bupivacaine with epinephrine after cholecystectomy, *Anesth Analg* 67:430, 1988.
233. Swerdlow M, Jones R: The duration of action of bupivacaine, prilocaine and lignocaine, *Br J Anaesth* 42:335, 1970.
234. Takman BH, Boyes RN, Vassallo HG: *Local anesthetics medicinal chemistry,* ed 4, New York, 1974, John Wiley & Sons.
235. Tanaka K, Yamasaki M: Blocking of cortical inhibitory synapses by intravenous lidocaine, *Nature* 209:207, 1966.
236. Tanz RD Heskett T, Loehning RW, et al: Comparative cardiotoxicity of bupivacaine and lidocaine in the isolated perfused mammalian heart, *Anesth Analg* 63:549, 1984.
237. Tasaki I: *Nervous transmission.* Springfield, IL, 1953, Thomas.
238. Terasaki T, Pardridge WM, Denson DD: Differential effect of plasma protein binding of bupivacaine on its in vivo transfer into brain and salivary gland of rats, *J Pharmacol Exp Ther* 239:724, 1986.
239. Thompson PD, Melmon KL, Richardson JA, et al: Lidocaine pharmacokinetics in advanced heart failure, liver disease and renal failure in humans, *Ann Intern Med* 78:499, 1973.
240. Thompson PD, Rowland M, Melmon K: Influence of heart failure, liver disease and renal failure on the disposition of lidocaine in man, *Am Heart J* 82:417, 1971.
241. Truant AP, Takman B: Differential physical-chemical and neuropharmacologic properties of local anesthetic agents, *Anesth Analg* 38:478, 1959.
242. Tucker GT: Determination of bupivacaine (Marcaine) and other anilide-type local anesthetics in human blood and plasma by gas chromatography, *Anesthesiology* 32: 255, 1970.
243. Tucker GT: Pharmacokinetics of local anesthetics, *Br J Anaesth* 58:717, 1986.
244. Tucker GT, Boas RA: Pharmacokinetic aspects of intravenous regional anesthesia, *Anesthesiology* 34:538, 1971.
245. Tucker GT, Boyes RN, Bridenbaugh PO, et al: Binding of anilide-type local anesthetics in human plasma. I. Relationships between binding, physicochemical properties, and anesthetic activity, *Anesthesiology* 33:287, 1970.
246. Tucker GT, Boyes RN, Bridenbaugh PO, et al: Binding of anilide-type local anesthetics in human plasma. II: Implications in vivo with special reference to transplacental distribution, *Anesthesiology* 33:303, 1970.
247. Tucker GT, Lennard MS: Enantiomer specific pharmacokinetics, *Pharmacol Ther* 45:309, 1990.
248. Tucker GT, Mather LE: Pharmacokinetics of local anaesthetic agents, *Br J Anaesth* 47:213, 1975.

249. Tucker GT, Mather LE: Properties, absorption, and disposition of local anesthetic agents. In Cousins MJ, Bridenbaugh PO, editors: *Neural blockade in clinical anesthesia and management of pain,* ed 2, Philadelphia, 1988, JB Lippincott.
250. Tucker GT, Moore DC, Bridenbaugh PO, et al: Systemic absorption of mepivacaine in commonly used regional block procedures, *Anesthesiology* 37:277, 1972.
251. van Kleef JW, Burm AG, Vletter AA: Single-dose interpleural versus intercostal blockade: nerve block characteristics and plasma concentration profiles after administration of 0.5% bupivacaine with epinephrine, *Anesth Analg* 70:484, 1990.
252. Vandam LD, Dripps RD: A long-term follow-up of 10,098 spinal anesthetics. II. Incidence and analysis of minor sensory neurological defects, *N Engl J Med* 255:110, 1956.
253. Vandam LD, Dripps RD: Long-term follow-up of patients who received 10,098 spinal anesthetics. IV. Neurological disease incident to traumatic lumbar puncture during spinal anesthesia, *JAMA* 172:1483, 1960.
254. Vester-Andersen T, Christiansen C, Hansen A, et al: Interscalene brachial plexus blocks area of analgesia, complications and blood concentrations of local anesthetics, *Acta Anaesthesiol Scand* 25:81, 1981.
255. Wang AW, Jay ZY, Narahashi T: Interaction of spin-labeled local anesthetics with the sodium channel of squid axon membranes, *J Membr Biol* 66:227, 1982.
256. Wang BC, Hillman DE, Spiedholz NI, et al: Chronic neurological deficits and Nesacaine-CE—an effect of the anesthetic, 2-chloroprocaine, or the antioxidant, sodium bisulfite, *Anesth Analg* 63:445, 1984.
257. Wang BC, Li D, Hiller JM, et al: Lumbar subarachnoid ethylenediaminetetraacetate induces hind limb tetanic contractions in rats: prevention by $CaCl_2$ pretreatment, observation of spinal nerve root degeneration, *Anesth Analg* 75:895, 1992.
258. Wang GK, Quan C, Vladmirov M, et al: Quaternary ammonium derivative of lidocaine as a long-acting local anesthetic, *Anesthesiology* 83:1293, 1995.
259. Wood M: Plasma binding and limitation of drug access to site of action, *Anesthesiology* 75:721, 1991.
260. Wood M, Wood AJ: Changes in plasma drug binding and alpha 1 acid glycoprotein in mother and newborn infant, *Clin Pharmacol Ther* 29:522, 1981.
261. Wood MB, Rubin AP: A comparison of epidural 1% ropivacaine and 0.75% bupivacaine for lower abdominal gynecologic surgery, *Anesth Analg* 76:1274, 1993.

CHAPTER 59

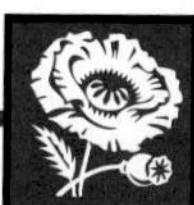

Spinal Anesthesia

FRANCIS X. RIEGLER

Spinal anesthesia results from the delivery of anesthetic agents into the cerebrospinal fluid (CSF). It is one of the simplest regional anesthetic techniques to perform, and was first described in humans by August Bier[9] in 1899. Despite its long history, spinal anesthesia remains an area of vibrant research in contemporary anesthesiology. It is chiefly distinguished from its cousin epidural anesthesia by the production of subarachnoid neural blockade covering wide areas of the body with minute quantities of anesthetic agents. Safe practice of spinal anesthesia includes properly selecting and preparing the patient, accessing the CSF, administering appropriate anesthetic drugs and adjuvants, managing physiologic side effects, and overseeing the patient throughout the procedure as well as in the early recovery process.

INDICATIONS AND CONTRAINDICATIONS

Indications

Spinal anesthesia is ideal for operations on the lower torso or the lower extremities. Box 59-1 lists surgical procedures that can be performed under spinal anesthesia. Operations in the upper abdomen may be performed under high spinal

BOX 59-1
OPERATIONS FOR WHICH SPINAL ANESTHESIA IS INDICATED

Lower abdominal surgery

Appendectomy

Gynecologic surgery

Dilation and curettage
Cone biopsy
Tubal ligation
Laparoscopy
Hysterectomy
Ovarian cystectomy

Obstetric surgery

Cesarean section
Vaginal delivery
Cerclage

Herniorrhaphies

Ventral
Inguinal

Lower limb surgery

Orthopedic
Vascular
Amputations
Skin grafts

Urologic surgery

Transurethral resections
Cystoscopy
Open prostatectomy
Penile implant
Orchiectomy

Perineal and rectal surgery

Bartholin's cyst
Rectal fissure
Hemorrhoids

From Covino BG, Lambert DH: Epidural and spinal anesthesia. In Barash PG, Cullen BF, Stoelting RK, editors: *Clinical anesthesia,* Philadelphia, 1989, JB Lippincott.

anesthesia; however, because of the difficulty of eliminating visceral traction stimuli it may be necessary to employ heavy sedation or light general anesthesia.

Contraindications

The only absolute contraindication to spinal anesthesia is patient refusal (Box 59-2). Other contraindications to spinal anesthesia are relative and for a given patient should be balanced against the expected benefits of the technique, as well as the comparative risks and benefits of alternative forms of

BOX 59-2
CONTRAINDICATIONS TO SPINAL ANESTHESIA

Patient refusal
Uncorrected hypovolemia
Uncorrected coagulopathy
Bacteremia
Infection at lumbar puncture site
Anatomic abnormalities that make lumbar puncture impossible
Elevated intracranial pressure
Certain neurologic disorders

anesthesia. Relative contraindications include: (1) infection, either local to the dural puncture site or systemic; (2) uncorrected hypovolemia; (3) uncorrected coagulation defects; (4) anatomic factors that make CSF access difficult or impossible; (5) certain chronic neurologic disorders such as multiple sclerosis, which may be exacerbated by the perioperative stresses of anesthesia and surgery (the concern here is usually more legal than medical); and (6) elevated intracranial pressure

Use of aspirin or nonsteroidal anti-inflammatory drugs (NSAIDs) per se does not appear to be a contraindication,[6, 55] nor does planned intraoperative anticoagulation following atraumatic dural puncture[86] which is performed at a time of normal coagulation function. The predictive value of Ivy bleeding times for hemorrhagic complications of regional anesthesia in patients taking aspirin and NSAIDs has not been established.[55]

PATIENT SELECTION AND PREPARATION

Patients may be offered spinal anesthesia when it is expected to be adequate for the planned procedure, and when in the judgment of the anesthesiologist the patient is an appropriate candidate for spinal anesthesia. The surgeon's willingness to operate with spinal anesthesia should also be considered. Patients should be told why spinal anesthesia is being offered to them, the potential advantages, and the possible side effects and complications. They should be informed of what they may see or hear in the operating room. Any concern about being awake during the operation can be assuaged, and the patient reassured that adequate sedation can be given to decrease anxiety and ensure comfort. An essential element of preparation by the anesthesiologist for spinal anesthesia is the formulation of a complete backup plan for general anesthesia including airway management if this is required for any reason during the procedure.

A common source of concern for patients in considering spinal anesthesia is the fear of "paralysis" or other permanent neurologic injury. Clusters of case reports of this phenomenon were published in the 1950s,[22, 60] and again in the early 1990s concerning continuous spinal anesthesia with microcatheters and/or 5% lidocaine in 7.5% dextrose.[90] Advances in pharmacology and technology have allowed the development of modern drugs and materials for spinal anesthesia that have a proven record of safety. (In 1992 spinal microcatheters were withdrawn from the market following a safety alert by the US Food and Drug Administration.[37]) A 1981 review of neurologic complications associated with spinal and epidural anesthesia identified 65,304 patients from various series who had undergone spinal anesthesia using currently accepted drugs and techniques, with only one permanent lesion possibly related to spinal anesthesia.[58] Transient neurologic sequelae following spinal anesthesia do occur, but these also appear to be rare.[58] For comparison purposes, numerous recent studies have indicated that the risk of death with modern anesthesia techniques is in the range of one in 10,000 to one in 200,000 (see Chapter 32). More often than not, patients accept spinal anesthesia when they feel they have a good rapport with the anesthesiologist and have made an informed decision to proceed.

The core preanesthesia history, physical examination, and laboratory assessment should be the same as for general anesthesia. A complete medication history is important because certain drugs can alter physiologic responses to spinal anesthesia. Any abnormalities in the neurologic history or examination should be documented on the chart. A coagulation profile may be indicated in patients who have received major anticoagulant drugs preoperatively, or in whom the review of systems suggests a bleeding diathesis. The planned skin puncture site and bony landmarks should be examined to confirm that spinal anesthesia is technically feasible. Operating room setup should be the same as for general anesthesia.

ANATOMY

Spinal anesthesia results from the distribution of anesthetic agents into the cerebrospinal fluid in the spinal subarachnoid space and their uptake by neuronal elements of the spinal cord. Knowledge of the functional anatomy of the region is essential to the safe conduct of anesthesia.

Spinal Canal

The spinal canal descends from the foramen magnum caudally to the sacral hiatus. The bony perimeter of the canal is formed by the posterior elements of the vertebral bodies. Normally, there are 7 cervical, 12 thoracic, and 5 lumbar vertebral bodies, along with the fused sacral and coccygeal vertebrae. The vertebrae along the spinal canal vary in size and shape. The lumbar vertebrae are the largest because of their weight bearing function. The articulation of the lumbar facet joints allows significant flexion and extension. This is in contrast to the thoracic facet joints, which allow predominately rotational movement. Lumbar spine flexion facilitates accessing the CSF with a needle. Vertebral discs space the bodies and cushion the spinal column.

Although anesthetic agents can be injected at any point along the spinal canal, this is routinely done only below the second lumbar vertebrae (L2-3 interspace and below) because the spinal cord proper usually terminates caudally at the level of the first lumbar vertebra. Therefore, lumbar puncture below this level is unlikely to cause spinal cord trauma. Fig. 59-1 is representative of a lumbar vertebra. It consists of a vertebral body anteriorly, two pedicles, two transverse processes, the laminae, facet joints for articulation with the vertebrae above and below, and a spinous process which forms the surface landmark. Lumbar puncture is performed by inserting a spinal needle in the skin between the spinous processes and directing it anteriorly so that the tip punc-

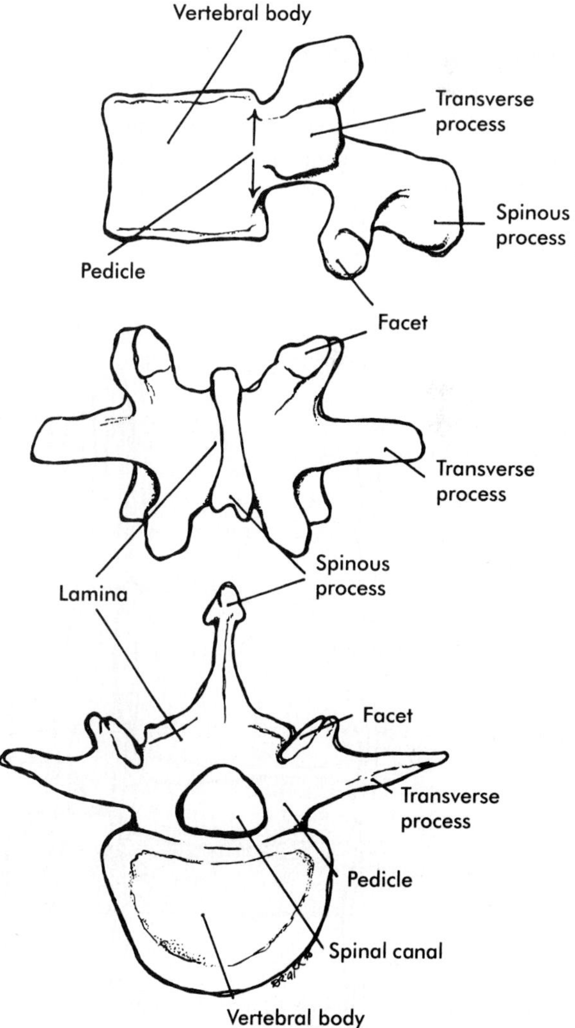

Fig. 59-1. Anatomy of a lumbar vertebra. (From Lee JA, Atkinson RS: *Sir Robert MacIntosh's lumbar puncture and spinal analgesia. Intradural and extradural,* ed 4, Edinburgh, 1978, Churchill-Livingstone.)

tures the dura in the space bounded by the lamina above and below and the facet joints laterally.

Ligaments

The spinal column is stabilized by numerous ligaments, several of which the needle tip traverses during lumbar puncture. Posteriorly, the supraspinous ligament connects the tips of the spinous processes, the interspinous ligaments run between the spinous processes, and the ligamentum flavum connects the laminae. Anterior to the spinal canal, the longitudinal ligaments connect the vertebral bodies to one another. The posterior longitudinal ligament runs along the posterior surface of the vertebral bodies, and the anterior longitudinal ligament runs from the base of the skull to the sacrum, attaching to the intervertebral discs and vertebral bodies. In the lumbar cistern of the spinal canal below L2, the segmental spinal nerves of the cauda equina exit the spinal canal laterally via the vertebral foramina formed between the bony pedicles. These relationships are shown in Figs. 59-2 and 59-3.

Spinal Cord and Meninges

Fig. 59-4 illustrates in transverse section the contents of the spinal canal. Progressing from dorsal to ventral lie the ligamentum flavum, the epidural space, the dura mater, the nerve roots of the cauda equina suspended in the CSF, the dorsal root ganglion and dorsal and ventral nerve roots of a spinal segmental nerve, and the vertebral body. Not shown are the arachnoid mater and the potential subdural space between the arachnoid mater and the dura mater.

Fig. 59-3 depicts views of the lower thoracic, lumbar, and sacral area of the spinal column. Lumbar puncture for spinal anesthesia is usually performed below the second lumbar vertebra down to the L5-S1 interspace. The only subarachnoid neural structure in this region is the cauda equina. The nerve roots extend for some distance within the spinal canal caudally before exiting, providing a large surface area for contact with injected anesthetic agents. The filum terminale is a band of connective tissue that runs from the termination of the spinal cord down to the region of the coccyx.

Cerebrospinal Fluid

The CSF occupies the potential space between the pia mater and the arachnoid mater and forms the volume of distribution for spinal anesthetic agents to the spinal cord structures. Ninety percent of the CSF is formed in the choroid plexus in the lateral and third and fourth cerebral ventricles.[96] The remaining 10% is derived from brain substance. The volume of CSF formed daily is believed to be equal to the volume present in the central nervous system (approximately 150 ml). When CSF is removed (as is believed to occur in post dural puncture headache), however, there is enough reserve capacity to produce several liters per day. CSF is removed via the arachnoid villi, a cluster

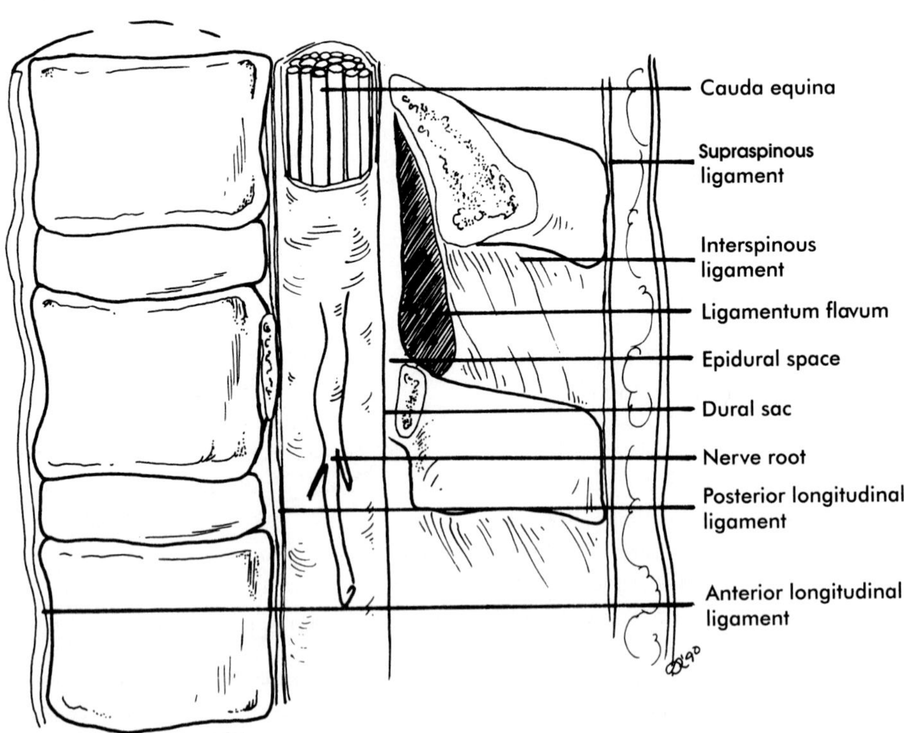

Fig. 59-2. Longitudinal section through the lumbar spine showing the ligaments and contents of the dural sac. (Modified from Lee JA, Atkinson RS: *Sir Robert MacIntosh's lumbar puncture and spinal analgesia. Intradural and extradural,* ed 4, Edinburgh, 1978, Churchill-Livingstone.)

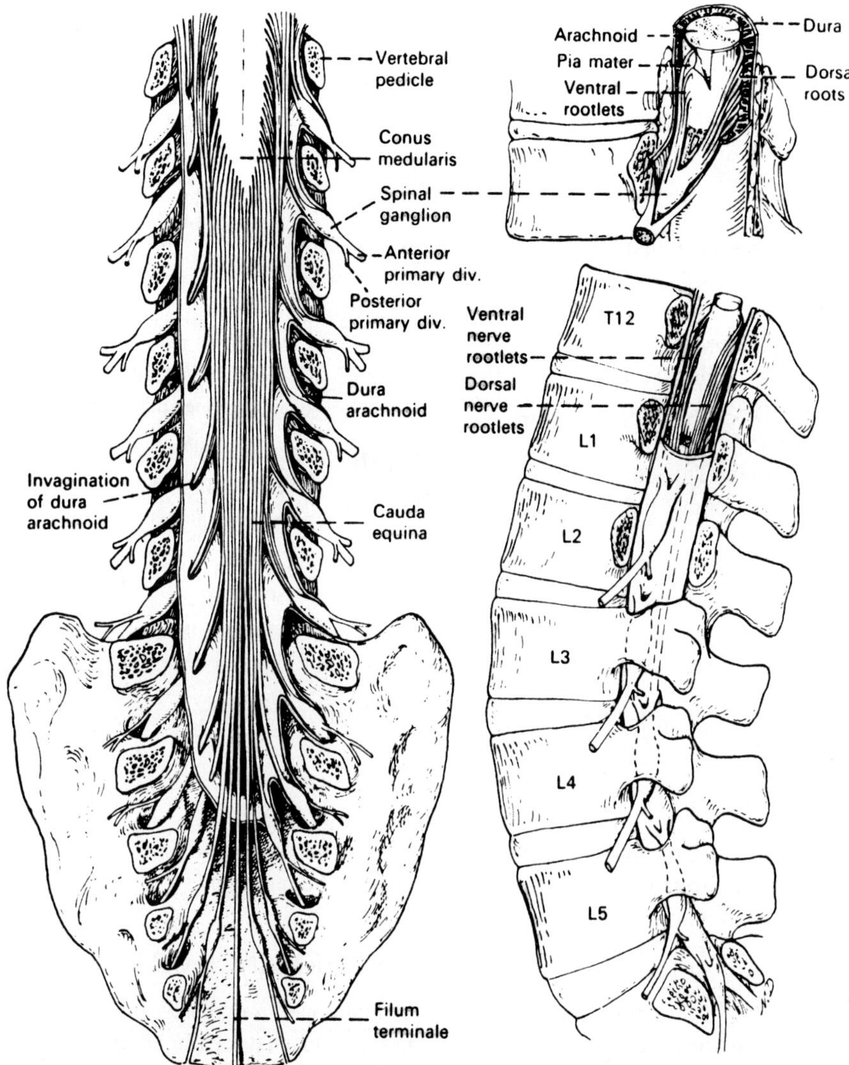

Fig. 59-3. Diagram of the cauda equina and the lumbosacral spine. (From Bonica JJ: *Management of pain,* ed 2, Philadelphia, 1990, Lea & Febiger.)

of cells that project into the subarachnoid space adjacent to the major dural venous sinuses. When CSF pressure exceeds pressure in the venous sinus, tiny tubules in the villi allow CSF to flow into the sinus. When venous sinus pressure is greater than CSF pressure, the tips of the villi close and reverse flow is prevented. The CSF cascades downward from the third ventricle through the cerebral aqueduct into the fourth ventricle and then through the foramina of Luschka and Magendie into the spinal subarachnoid space. It continues to flow inferiorly and then superiorly, bathing the spinal cord, cauda equina, and brain. The CSF maintains a physiologically stable environment and buffering capacity for the central nervous system (CNS), ensuring the regulation of biochemical functions,[45] as well as providing buoyancy and regulation of the contents of the skull.

The CSF is a hydrophilic environment. Ninety percent is water. It forms a clear colorless fluid with a specific gravity of 1.003 to 1.009, pH of 7.39 to 7.50, and it contains 40–80 mg/dl glucose, 15–45 mg/dl protein, 3–5 mononuclear cells/mm^3, 138 mEq/L sodium, 2–3 mEq/L potassium, 2–3 mEq/L calcium, 2–3 mEq/L magnesium, and 1–4 mEq/L chloride. In the lateral recumbent position, the normal pressure of CSF ranges between 60 and 150 mm H_2O.

MECHANISM OF SPINAL ANESTHESIA

Local anesthetics are the core agents of spinal anesthesia. Following injection the local anesthetic mixes with and is diluted by CSF. The extent of anesthesia is dependent on distribution within CSF and uptake by spinal nerve roots. Although local anesthetics also bathe the spinal cord itself, spinal anesthesia is believed to result from neural blockade

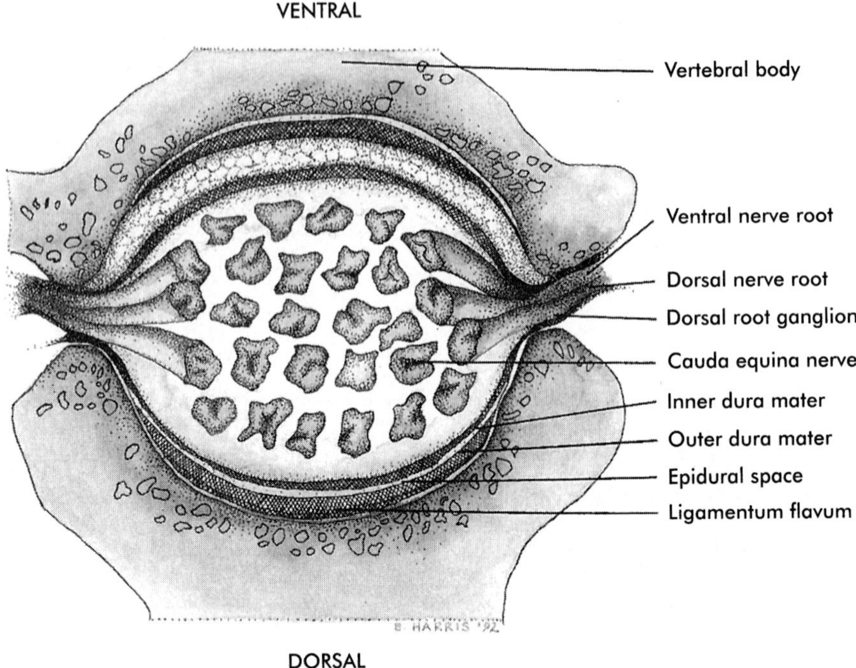

Fig. 59-4. Cross-section of the lumbar spine.

at the root level. The nerve roots leaving the spinal canal are not covered by epineurium, and are directly exposed to the local anesthetic within the CSF. Afferent impulses entering the CNS via the dorsal roots and efferent impulses leaving via the ventral roots are blocked during spinal anesthesia. Neural blockade in superficial areas of the spinal cord is not believed to play a meaningful role in the production of anesthesia.[46] **Spinal anesthesia is not therefore a "chemical transection" of the spinal cord, but rather a phenomenon mediated at the level of the nerve roots within the subarachnoid space. The result of this neural blockade includes anesthesia, analgesia, sympathetic blockade, and usually complete muscle relaxation.**

EQUIPMENT

A variety of self-contained disposable kits are available commercially to facilitate the performance of spinal anesthesia. The minimum equipment required to perform single shot spinal anesthesia includes swabs to apply antiseptic (usually betadine) to the skin, a sterile towel or gauze to remove excess antiseptic, a small gauge needle to raise a skin wheal, a spinal needle, and a syringe containing local anesthetic. When employing 24-gauge or smaller spinal needles it may be desirable to use a larger introducer needle through which the spinal needle can be inserted. These small gauge needles can be used by experienced operators to perform lumbar puncture without an introducer. Needle size, tip shape, and angle of dural puncture are important factors in determining the risk of postdural puncture headache (see below). If continuous spinal anesthesia is planned, a catheter will also be required.

PERFORMANCE OF LUMBAR PUNCTURE

As mentioned previously, lumbar puncture for spinal anesthesia is usually performed at an interspace somewhere between the second lumbar and the first sacral vertebrae because the spinal cord, in most adults, terminates at the L1/L2 interspace and this decreases the likelihood of spinal cord trauma. Positions for lumbar puncture include the sitting, lateral decubitus, and occasionally the prone jackknife position. The lateral decubitus position has advantages for the performance of lumbar puncture in patients who have been sedated, while the sitting position usually allows better identification of the bony midline, especially in obese patients. Selection of a position for lumbar puncture may also be influenced by the desired distribution of nonisobaric solutions following injection (see below).

During the process of lumbar puncture, a clear three-dimensional mental image of the structures of the posterior spine should be visualized. It is important to gain as much flexion of the lumbar spine as is practical throughout the procedure in order to spread the spinous processes and open the interlaminar spaces, through which the tip of the spinal needle must pass to reach the CSF. This is done by producing flexion of the hips, knees, head, and neck (Figs. 59-5 and 59-6). In the lateral decubitus position, the patient is placed on his or her side with the hips, back, and shoulders near the edge of the operating table. An imaginary line drawn be-

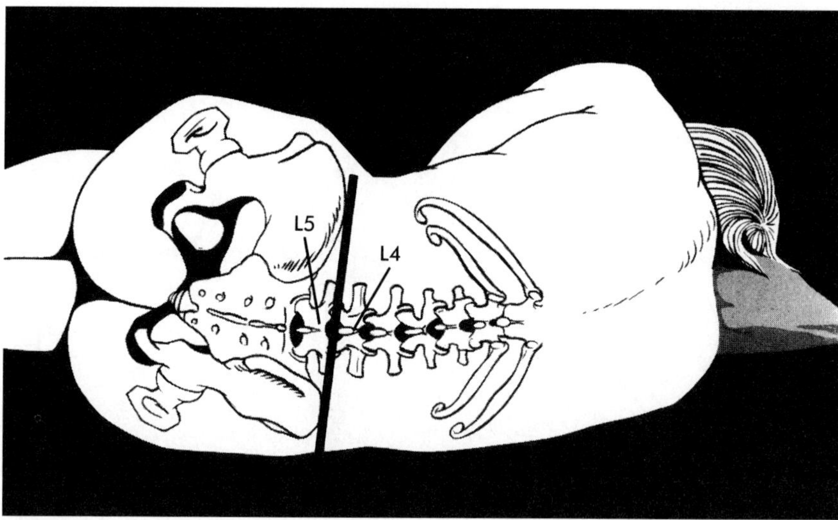

Fig. 59-5. Proper position for lumbar puncture. A line drawn between the iliac crests intersects the lumbar spine at the L4/L5 interspace. (From Covino BG, Lambert DH: Epidural and spinal anesthesia. In Barash PG, Cullen BF, Stoelting RK, editors: *Clinical anesthesia,* ed 2, Philadelphia, 1991, JB Lippincott.)

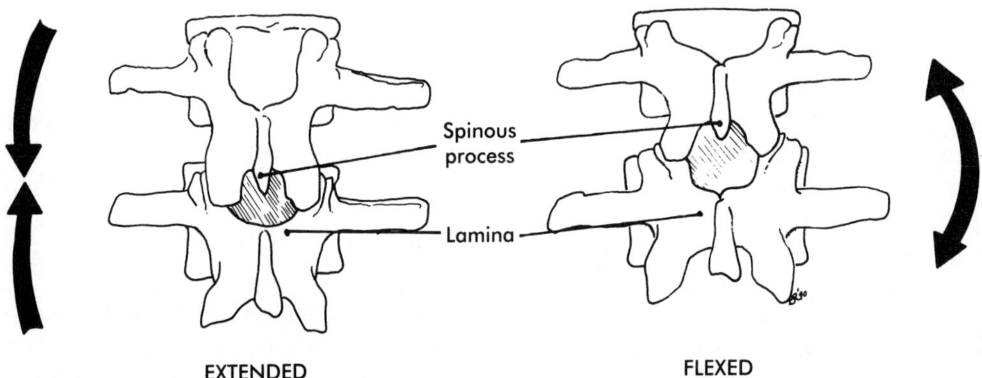

Fig. 59-6. The effects of flexion and extension of the lumbar spine. Flexion enlarges the opening between the spinous processes and the laminae, enhancing the chance for successful lumbar puncture. (Modified from Lee JA, Atkinson RS: *Sir Robert MacIntosh's lumbar puncture and spinal analgesia. Intradural and extradural,* ed 4, Edinburgh, 1978, Churchill-Livingstone.)

tween the superior portions of the iliac crests usually passes through the L4 vertebra or the L4/5 interspace.[53] This line can be used as a landmark from which to identify the lumbar interspaces. The widest interspace below L2 is identified, and antiseptic solution applied. Local anesthetic is injected intradermally in the bony midline of the selected interspace using a 25-gauge or smaller needle. Deeper infiltration of the ligamentous structures and surrounding tissues with a 22-gauge or smaller 1-inch needle may add to patient comfort and allows the operator to probe the interspace for bony landmarks. The needle (or introducer) should be inserted in the bony midline perpendicular to the plane of the back near the bottom of the interspace, and advanced in a slightly cephalad direction, while maintaining a mental image of the structures of the spine. As the tip of the spinal needle engages the ligamentum flavum, an increase in resistance to advancement can be felt. As the needle tip penetrates the ligamentum flavum and enters the epidural space, a decrease in resistance is often appreciated. As the needle is advanced further and penetrates the dura, a "click" or "pop" is usually felt. When the stylet of the needle is removed, the appearance of CSF in the hub indicates proper placement of the needle tip. In the majority of adult cases the distance from the skin to the CSF will be between 4 and 6 cm.

Occasionally, bony obstruction to passage of the needle tip will be encountered prior to dural puncture. In this case the operator should reverify that the needle is being advanced in the true bony midline and that the patient is properly positioned for optimal flexion of the lumbar spine. The most likely obstructions are the superior or inferior spinous processes or the supe-

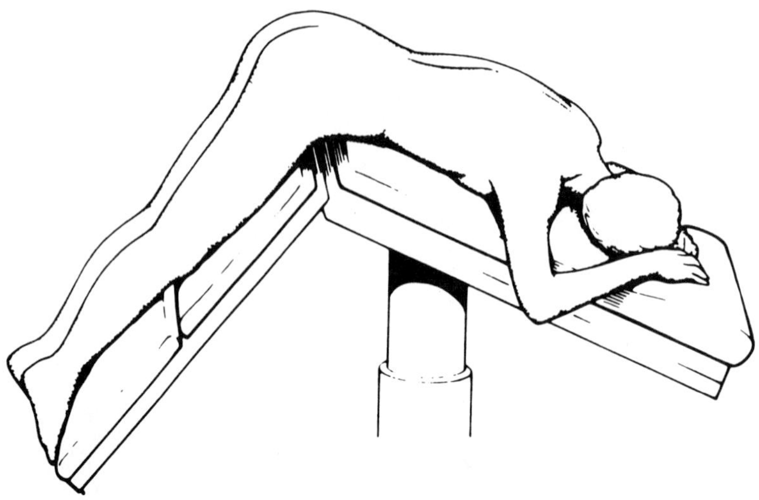

Fig. 59-7. Prone jackknife position. The lumbar spine is extended and lumbar puncture with the midline approach may be difficult. A lateral approach is often used with this position. (Modified from Lambert DH, Covino BG: Hyperbaric, hypobaric and isobaric spinal anesthesia, *Res Staff Phys* 33:79, 1987.)

rior or inferior laminae on either side. **When attempting to redirect the tip of a standard 3.5-inch spinal needle, it is important to withdraw the needle tip all the way to the subcutaneous tissue before reinserting. Experience with fluoroscopically guided nerve block procedures verifies that failure to do so does not redirect the needle tip and merely results in bending of the needle shaft.** Inexperienced operators usually fail to appreciate that small changes in hub position result in proportionately larger changes in needle tip position.[54] The direction of the needle bevel (if beveled) also produces a certain deviation of the needle tip over longer distances.[61]

In certain instances a midline approach to the CSF may prove difficult, such as in elderly patients with densely calcified ligaments. A paramedian or lateral approach may prove successful, because the needle tip need not traverse the supraspinous and interspinous ligaments. A local anesthetic skin wheal is raised 0.5 to 1 cm lateral to the bony midline at the upper border of the lower spinous process. The needle is directed at an angle which will allow the tip to penetrate the dura in the midline. If bone is encountered with this approach the needle should be withdrawn and redirected in either a cephalad or caudad direction so as to "walk off" the lamina and into CSF. If difficulty is encountered at a particular interspace and lumbar puncture is not successful after several attempts it is wisest to try another interspace or abandon the procedure.

For patients in the sitting or prone positions the procedure is similar. In the sitting position, flexion of the lumbar spine can be obtained by having the patient lean forward and rest the arms on a Mayo stand. In obese patients, it is easier to locate the bony midline in the sitting position. In the prone jackknife position the spine will not be maximally flexed, so a lateral approach for this position may prove easier (Fig. 59-7).

Another approach described in many textbooks is the Taylor approach. It is essentially a paramedian approach to the L5-S1 interspace, which is usually the largest interspace in the vertebral column.[100] A skin wheal is raised 1 cm medial and 1 cm caudad to the posterior superior iliac spine. The spinal needle is inserted through the skin wheal in a direction cephalad and medial to enter the CSF in the midline of the lumbosacral (L5/S1) interspace (Fig. 59-8).

INJECTION OF LOCAL ANESTHETIC

Prior to injection of the anesthetic solution, the clinician must be certain the tip of the needle is properly located within the CSF. When using a beveled spinal needle, confirming flow of CSF in four quadrants confirms ideal needle tip position. In most cases, it should be possible to aspirate CSF prior to injection. A "tripod" position of the nondominant hand, with the dorsum on the patient's back and the thumb and index fingers stabilizing needle tip position, will help to ensure that the entire dose of anesthetic is delivered to the CSF. Once CSF flow is demonstrated, the anesthetic should be injected at a rate of 1 ml every 5 to 10 seconds. Confirming the ability to aspirate CSF midway through the injection and again at the conclusion provides reassurance that the entire dose has been delivered to the CSF.

PHARMACOLOGIC CONSIDERATIONS

Selection of anesthetic agents is determined by the nature of the operative procedure and its anticipated duration.

Definition of Density, Specific Gravity, and Baricity

Density is the weight in grams of 1 ml of solution at a specific temperature. Specific gravity is the ratio of the density

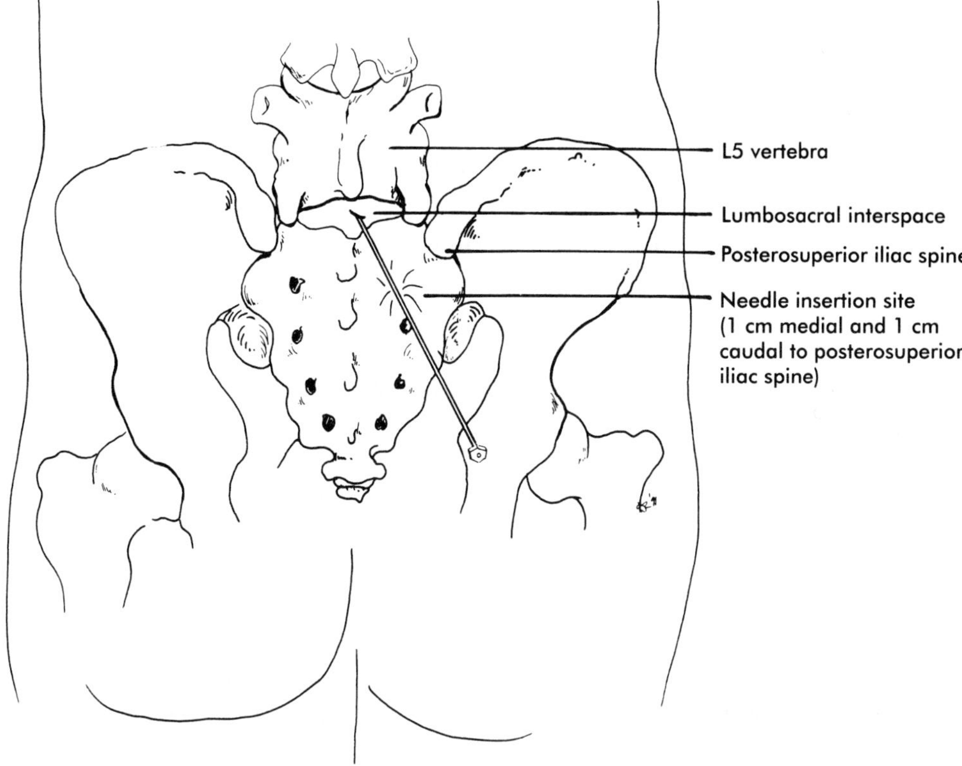

Fig. 59-8. Taylor or lumbosacral approach to lumbar puncture. The spinal needle is inserted 1 cm medial and 1 cm caudal to the posterosuperior iliac spine and directed toward the midline and the L5/S1 interspace. (Modified from Lee JA, Atkinson RS: *Sir Robert MacIntosh's lumbar puncture and spinal analgesia. Intradural and extradural,* ed 4, Edinburgh, 1978, Churchill-Livingstone.)

of a solution at a specific temperature to the density of water at the same temperature. Baricity is the ratio of the density of a local anesthetic at a specified temperature to the density of CSF at the same temperature. Baricity may also be defined in terms of specific gravity, i.e., the ratio of the specific gravity of a local anesthetic solution at a specified temperature to the specific gravity of CSF at the same temperature, but this is less accurate than using density.[46]

By definition, an isobaric solution has a baricity of one, a hyperbaric solution has a baricity greater than one, and a hypobaric solution has a baricity less than one.[49] Because density varies inversely with temperature, local anesthetics are denser when injected at room temperature than at 37° in the CSF. Clinically, the most important density of a local anesthetic solution is the one at body temperature, because the solution quickly reaches this after injection.[36]

Fig. 59-9 shows the effect of local anesthetic solution density on baricity when used at body temperature in CSF for spinal anesthesia. Local anesthetic solutions with baricity less than 0.9998 at 37° C are hypobaric in all patients; local anesthetic solutions with baricity greater than 1.008 are hyperbaric; and local anesthetic solutions with baricity between these values are considered isobaric.[68] Because of the normal range of CSF density, however, it is difficult to know that an isobaric solution is truly isobaric in all patients. For clinical purposes local anesthetic solutions with a density between 0.9998 and 1.0008 behave as if they have the same density as CSF (i.e., isobaric).

Clinical Use of Local Anesthetics for Spinal Anesthesia

Any local anesthetic will produce spinal anesthesia when injected into the CSF. Table 59-1 lists the local anesthetics commonly used for spinal anesthesia. Commonly, local anesthetics are formulated with normal saline to make them isosmotic. The specific gravity of such solutions usually renders them isobaric at body temperature, but 0.5% bupivacaine is slightly hypobaric and 2% lidocaine is slightly hyperbaric. Because of its low potency, procaine is formulated as a 10% solution for spinal anesthesia and, because of its high concentration, is hyperbaric. Commercially prepared hyperbaric solutions of lidocaine and bupivacaine are commonly available. The solutions are made by adding dextrose, which raises their density to greater than 1.008. Although dextrose is usually used to make local anesthetic solutions hyperbaric, 1% tetracaine can be made hyperbaric by adding 10% procaine.[17] Hypobaric solutions are prepared clinically by diluting the local anesthetic with distilled water to achieve a density of less than 0.9998.[91] Because the density of CSF is close to that of water it is necessary to add large

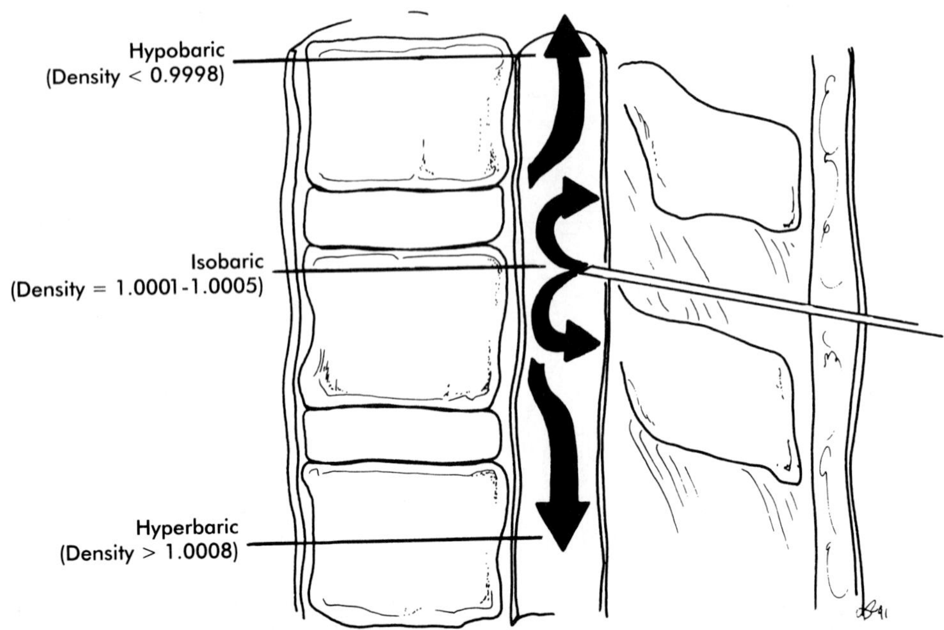

Fig. 59-9. Diagrammatic illustration of the effect of density on the distribution of local anesthetic in the subarachnoid space. Hypobaric solutions "float" to the least dependent areas, hyperbaric solutions seek the lowest point, while isobaric solutions remain in the vicinity of the injection site.

Table 59-1 Drugs used for spinal anesthesia

Agent	Concentration (percent)	Baricity	Dosage (mg)	Duration* (hrs)
Procaine†	2.5–10	Hyperbaric	50–200	< 1
Lidocaine	5 (7.5% dextrose)	Hyperbaric	50–100	< 2
Lidocaine	2	Hyperbaric	50–80	< 2
Lidocaine	1	Isobaric	50–80	< 2
Lidocaine‡	0.5	Hypobaric	50	< 2
Bupivacaine	0.75 (8.25% dextrose)	Hyperbaric	15	< 3
Bupivacaine	0.75	Isobaric	15	< 3
Bupivacaine	0.5	Isobaric	15	< 3
Bupivacaine‡	0.25	Hypobaric	15	< 3
Tetracaine	0.5 (5% dextrose)	Hyperbaric	15	< 4
Tetracaine	0.5	Isobaric	15	< 4
Tetracaine‡	< 0.33	Hypobaric	10	< 4

*Refer to *approximate* duration in the lumbosacral dermatomes. Duration will be less in the higher dermatones.
When a dose range is specified, duration will be longer with the larger dose.
†Procaine is available as a 10% solution. Dilutions with saline to as little as 2.5% are hyperbaric.
‡Diluted with sterile distilled water.

amounts of water to produce a truly hypobaric solution. Such dilution results in having to inject large volumes of local anesthetic to achieve adequate anesthesia. On the other hand, adding small volumes of 10% dextrose will reliably make a local anesthetic hyperbaric. Hence, higher concentrations of local anesthetic are achievable and smaller volumes need be injected for hyperbaric spinal anesthesia.

Tables 59-2, 59-3, and 59-4 summarize information on the density and baricity of local anesthetic solutions and their preparation for clinical use in spinal anesthesia.

The role of 5% lidocaine in 7.5% dextrose in spinal anesthesia

Recently, the safety of the 5% preparation of lidocaine in 7.5% dextrose for spinal anesthesia has been questioned.[29] Clusters of case reports, ranging from transient lumbosacral monoradiculopathy after single-dose

Table 59-2 Density and baricity of local anesthetics commonly used for spinal anesthesia

Agent	Usual concentration (%)	Glucose concentration (%)	Density (37° C)	Baricity (37° C)
Cerebrospinal fluid			1.0003	1.000
Procaine	2.5	DW	0.9986	0.9983 (HO)
Procaine	10.0		1.0107	1.0104 (H)
Lidocaine	2.0	S	1.0007	1.0004 (H)
Lidocaine	5.0	7.5	1.0265	1.0262 (H)
Bupivacaine	0.5	S	0.9993	0.9990 (HO*)
Bupivacaine	0.75	8.25	1.0230*	1.0227 (H)
Tetracaine	< 0.33	DW	< 0.9980	< 0.9977 (HO)
Tetracaine	0.5	S	1.0000	0.9997(HO*)
Tetracaine	0.5	5.0	1.0136	1.0133 (H)

*Approximate value calculated from specific gravity.
CSF density (37° C) 99.9% confidence limits = 0.9998–1.0008.
DW — distilled water; S — saline; HO — hypobaric; I — isobaric; H — hyperbaric; HO* — solution considered to be clinically isobaric.
From Lambert DH, Covino GB: Hyperbaric, hypobaric and isobaric spinal anesthesia, *Res Staff Phys* 33:79, 1987.

Table 59-3 Dilutions for hyperbaric, isobaric, and hypobaric solutions

	Hyperbaric* (ml local: ml dextrose (10%))	Isobaric (ml local: ml sterile distilled water)	Hypobaric (ml local: ml sterile distilled water)
2% Lidocaine	3:0 (2/20)†	3:5 (0.75/7.5)	3:9 (0.5/5)
1% Tetracaine	1:1 (0.5/5)	1:1 (0.5/5)	1.5:3 (0.33/3.3)
0.75% Bupivacaine	2:1 (0.5/5)	2:1 (0.5/5)	2:2.5 (0.33/3.3)

*Hyperbaric solutions of lidocaine (7.5% dextrose) and bupivacaine (8.25% dextrose) are commercially available.
†Number in parentheses — percent concentration of local anesthetic/mg local anesthetic per ml of solution.

Table 59-4 Percent solutions required for hyperbaricity, isobaricity, and hypobaricity

	Hyperbaric (SG > 1.007)	Isobaric (SG 1.004–1.007)	Hypobaric (SG < 1.004)
% Lidocaine	> 1	0.55–1.0	< 0.55
% Tetracaine	> 0.65	0.35–0.65	< 0.35
% Bupivacaine	> 0.65	0.35–0.65	< 0.45

All solutions prepared by diluting 2% lidocaine, 1% tetracaine, and 0.75% bupivacaine with sterile distilled water.
SG — specific gravity.

administration[94] to cauda equina syndrome following continuous spinal anesthesia[90] with this preparation have been published. A variety of factors, either alone or in combination, have been postulated to have contributed to the neurotoxicity in these and other cases: the high concentration of lidocaine (5%), high osmolarity with 7.5% dextrose, high density, pooling and related maldistribution of the solution on the sacral side of the lumbar lordotic hump with injection via small-bore needles or microcatheters, and stretching or ischemia of affected nerve roots with the lithotomy position. The role of 5% lidocaine in 7.5% dextrose in contemporary spinal anesthesia practice is the subject of vigorous controversy on both sides of the issue. The safety of dextrose-free solutions of lidocaine for spinal anesthesia has not been questioned.

Effect of Local Anesthetic on Duration of Spinal Anesthesia

In CSF the duration of action of plain local anesthetic in spinal nerve roots is determined by lipid solubility and protein binding. The local anesthetics used for spinal anesthesia can be rank ordered in regard to duration as follows: procaine < lidocaine < bupivacaine < tetracaine. Table 59-1 contains guidelines for the use of local anesthetic solutions for spinal anesthesia.[66] The durations listed in Table 59-1 are only approximate and may be shorter or longer in a given patient. Thus procaine is used for brief operations (dilation and curettage, cerclage); lidocaine for intermediate-duration operations (hernia, lower limb amputation); and bupivacaine and tetracaine for longer operations (knee and hip replacement).

Vasoconstrictors

Vasoconstrictors can be added to local anesthetics to prolong the duration of action.[23] It is believed that vasoconstriction decreases vascular uptake and egress of the local anesthetic, making more available for penetration into neural tissue. When a higher fraction of the local anesthetic penetrates the nerves, the duration of anesthesia is prolonged. Epinephrine, phenylephrine, and ephedrine have been used to prolong spinal anesthesia.[20] Ephedrine is least effective and not commonly used. Epinephrine (1:1000), 0.1 to 0.5 ml, or phenylephrine (1% solution), 2 to 5 mg (0.2 to 0.5 ml), have been added to prolong spinal anesthesia.

Vasoconstrictor prolongation of spinal anesthesia is not reported to be uniform and may depend on particular circumstances and the operational definition of prolongation. Chambers et al.[15,16] found no "useful" prolongation of lidocaine or bupivacaine spinal anesthesia by epinephrine. In contrast, Armstrong et al.[3] observed a prolongation of tetracaine spinal anesthesia by phenylephrine, whereas epinephrine increased the duration of tetracaine anesthesia in the lumbar and sacral dermatomes only. In these studies, "useful" prolongation meant that regression of two or four segments from the most cephalad extent of the block (thoracic dermatomes) was delayed. Although the authors felt that prolongation in the lumbar and sacral dermatomes was "not useful," it is certainly beneficial for operations confined to these areas. Further, contrary to the studies of Chambers et al. and Armstrong et al., recent results indicate that the duration of lidocaine and bupivacaine spinal anesthesia *is* prolonged by phenylephrine and/or epinephrine.[2,69,78,85,101]

It should be appreciated that the local anesthetics themselves have independent effects on vascular tone. Spinal cord and dural blood flow in the dog are increased by lidocaine and tetracaine, but decreased by bupivacaine.[62–64] Since increased duration of spinal anesthesia due to vasoconstrictors is believed to result from vasoconstriction, it seems logical that vasoconstrictors would be efficacious when added to lidocaine and tetracaine as these agents cause vasodilatation but less so with bupivacaine, which causes vasoconstriction.

Vasoconstrictors such as epinephrine and phenylephrine also have direct antinociceptive effects on the dorsal horn of the spinal cord. Adrenergic agonists interact with specific receptors in the spinal cord to produce analgesia. As a result, these agents may prolong duration of anesthesia via vasoconstriction or activation of spinal antinociceptors or both.[19]

In summary the available data and the weight of clinical experience suggest that epinephrine and phenylephrine prolong spinal anesthesia, particularly in the lumbar and sacral dermatomes, and addition of these agents for longer operations in these dermatomes is advantageous. Addition of adrenergic agonists to local anesthetics used for spinal anesthesia has not been associated with ischemia of the spinal cord and does not appear to be hazardous.

Other Additives

In addition to beta adrenergic agonists such as epinephrine and the alpha 1 adrenergic agonist phenylephrine, two other agents have been described as additives for spinal anesthesia: fentanyl and alpha 2 adrenergic agonists.

In animal models, spinally administered opioids and local anesthetics have been shown to be synergistic for somatic analgesia. Opioids act primarily in spinal cord grey matter (cell bodies), while local anesthetics act primarily in white matter (axons). Intrathecal opioids preferentially inhibit afferent synaptic transmission in nociceptive pathways with preservation of efferent conduction in sympathetic pathways. Addition of 20 μg fentanyl to 5% hyperbaric lidocaine in volunteers has been shown to prolong sensory block in both thoracic and lumbar dermatomes.[72] Duration of tolerance of tourniquet induced pain was increased on average by 48%. Neither motor block nor time to void was prolonged with fentanyl. It was hypothesized that synergistic blockade of A delta and C fiber conduction by intrathecal fentanyl allowed subtherapeutic concentrations of hyperbaric lidocaine to maintain nerve block during regression of spinal anesthesia. Enhancement of intraoperative spinal anesthesia in patients undergoing cesarean section with 0.5% bupivacaine plus fentanyl (0.25 μg/kg) has also been demonstrated.[5] Higher doses of intravenous fentanyl (50–150 μg) have also been shown to increase the sensory level of intraoperative spinal anesthesia, an effect which was reversed by naloxone.[92] Thus, it appears that low dose intrathecal fentanyl and higher dose systemic fentanyl enhance the distribution of spinal anesthesia and low dose intrathecal fentanyl enhances the quality of spinal anesthesia (see Chapter 64).

The alpha 2 adrenergic agonist clonidine has independent spinal analgesic effects, as well as local vasoconstrictive effects. Intrathecally administered clonidine prolongs bupivacaine spinal anesthesia, but is associated with bradycardia, hypotension, and sedation due to the peripheral hemodynamic effects of systemically absorbed drug.[80] Like intravenous fentanyl, orally administered clonidine also prolongs spinal anesthesia.[83] No data are available concerning the quality of spinal anesthesia with clonidine supplementation. In the United States, clonidine is only approved for oral administration as of 1995.

FACTORS INFLUENCING THE SENSORY DISTRIBUTION OF SPINAL ANESTHESIA

An advantage of spinal anesthesia is that profound neural blockade can be produced over large areas of the body with small quantities of drug. An attendant challenge in clinical practice is to limit the CSF distribution of drug so that it produces adequate anesthesia for the procedure, without excessively increasing the likelihood of morbid side effects. Because the lower lumbar and sacral spinal nerve roots travel some distance in the lumbar CSF as part of the cauda equina, these dermatomes are nearly always blocked with lumbar injection of spinal anesthetics. The ultimate extent of cephalad neural blockade is less predictable. A clinical reality of spinal anesthesia is that the same technique of spinal anesthesia may produce significantly variant sensory distributions and physiologic consequences across a population of patients. The dilemma for the individual practitioner is to select a technique which is likely to produce acceptable conditions in an individual patient. This same dilemma was even noted by Bier[9] in his landmark report of the first spinal anesthesia in humans.

Greene[49] reviewed numerous factors that are believed to influence the distribution of local anesthetics in the CSF (Box 59-3). In actual practice, any one of these factors may materially influence the ultimate sensory distribution of anesthesia in a particular patient under a specific set of circumstances. **The consensus view is that across patients the most consistently important factors in clinical practice are the density (baricity) of the local anesthetic solution, the conformation of the spinal canal, and the position of the spine during and immediately after the local anesthetic solution is injected.**[66]

BOX 59-3
FACTORS INFLUENCING DISTRIBUTION OF LOCAL ANESTHETICS IN CEREBROSPINAL FLUID*

Patient characteristics

- Age
- Height
- Weight
- Gender
- Intraabdominal pressure
- Anatomic configuration of spinal column
- Position

Technique of injection

- Site of injection
- Direction of injection
  - Direction of needle
  - Direction of bevel
- Turbulence
  - Rate of injection
  - Barbotage

Diffusion

- Characteristics of spinal fluid
  - Composition
  - Circulation
  - Volume
  - Pressure
  - Density

Characteristics of anesthetic solution

- Density
  - Hypobaric
  - Isobaric
  - Hyperbaric
- Amount of anesthetic
- Concentration of anesthetic
- Volume injected
- Addition of vasoconstrictors

*Hypothetical or demonstrable.
From Greene NM: Distribution of local anesthetic solutions within the subarachnoid space, *Anesth Analg* 64:715, 1985.

Effect of Baricity and Patient Position on the Level of Spinal Anesthesia

Baricity of the anesthetic solution and patient position are clearly major determinants of the distribution of local anesthetic in CSF. The effect of these factors is shown in Figs. 59-10, 59-11, and 59-12. The models in Fig. 59-10 graphically simulate the effect of injecting hyperbaric, isobaric, and hypobaric local anesthetic solutions into the CSF of a patient who is seated during the injection and immediately turned to the supine horizontal position. Injection of a hyperbaric solution in the sitting position results in the local anesthetic moving downward. When the patient is turned to the supine horizontal position, the majority of the local anesthetic remains caudal to the lumbar curve (lordosis), but a meaningful quantity enters the thoracic hollow. An isobaric solution remains in the vicinity of the injection both during and after the injection, regardless of position. A hypobaric solution rises in the CSF in the seated position. Therefore, the longer the patient remains seated following injection of a hypobaric solution, the higher the level of anesthesia will be once the patient is placed in the supine position. In fact, if the patient is not placed in the head down (Trendelenburg) position after injection, a hypobaric solution will continue to rise and may eventually produce total spinal anesthesia.

Fig. 59-11 shows the effect of injecting the local anesthetic in patients in the lateral decubitus position who are then turned to the supine horizontal position. A hyperbaric solution spreads out horizontally in the lateral position so that when the patient is turned supine, some of the solution enters the sacral region and some descends into the thoracic area because of the lumbar lordosis. An isobaric solution is not affected by patient position and remains in the area of injection. A hypobaric solution rises within the CSF so that when the patient assumes the supine horizontal position, the solution remains near the site of injection but displaced toward the apex of the lumbar lordosis.

Fig. 59-12 illustrates the effect of injecting the various solutions into a patient who is in the prone jackknife position. Hyperbaric solutions should not be used with this position because, as shown, the solutions will descend within the spinal canal (towards the head) and achieve excessively high levels likely to produce respiratory arrest. Isobaric and hypobaric solutions can be used with this position because iso-

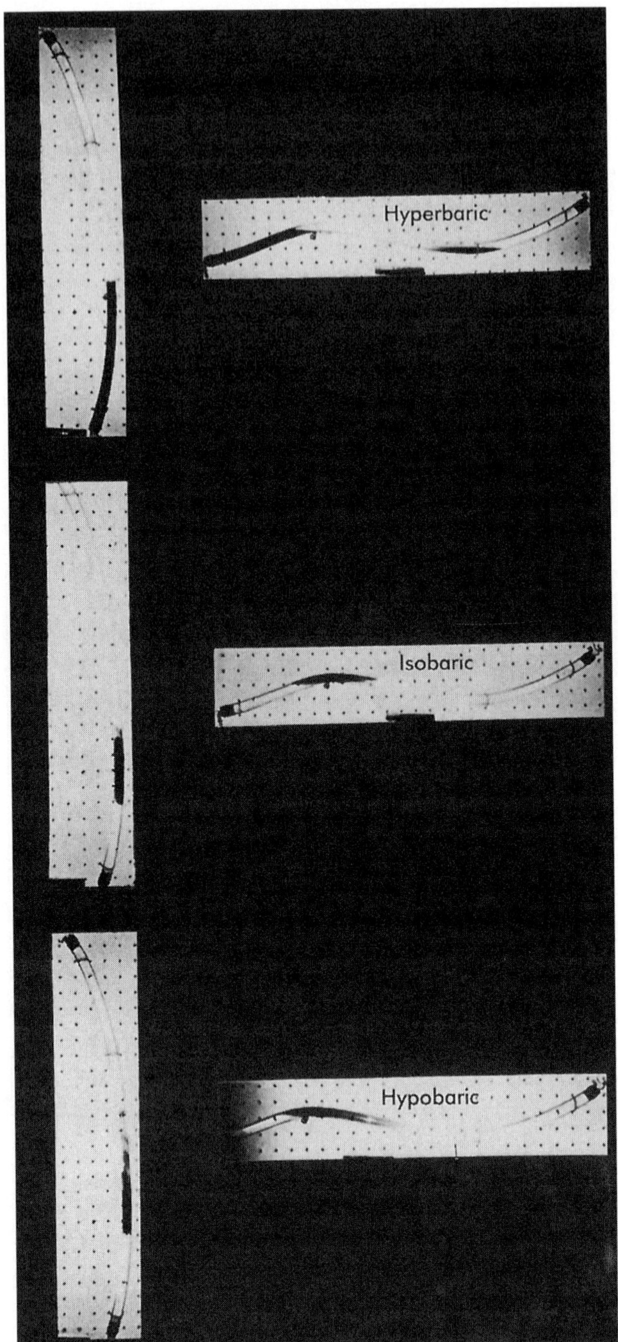

Fig. 59-10. Spinal canal model showing the effect of baricity and position on the distribution of local anesthetic in the seated position. The model is a plastic tube that contains saline (density similar to CSF) and bent to mimic the contour of the spinal canal during spinal anesthesia. The local anesthetic (15 mg bupivacaine) is colored with methylene blue. The injections were made with the model in the "seated" position (*left*) and immediately turned "supine" and horizontal (*right*). *Top* to *bottom,* solutions were hyperbaric, isobaric, and hypobaric.

baric solutions are unaffected by the patient's position and hypobaric solutions "ascend" within the spinal canal to produce lumbosacral levels of anesthesia.

These descriptions indicate the importance of understanding the effects of baricity and patient position during and after injection of local anesthetic solution for appropriate and safe

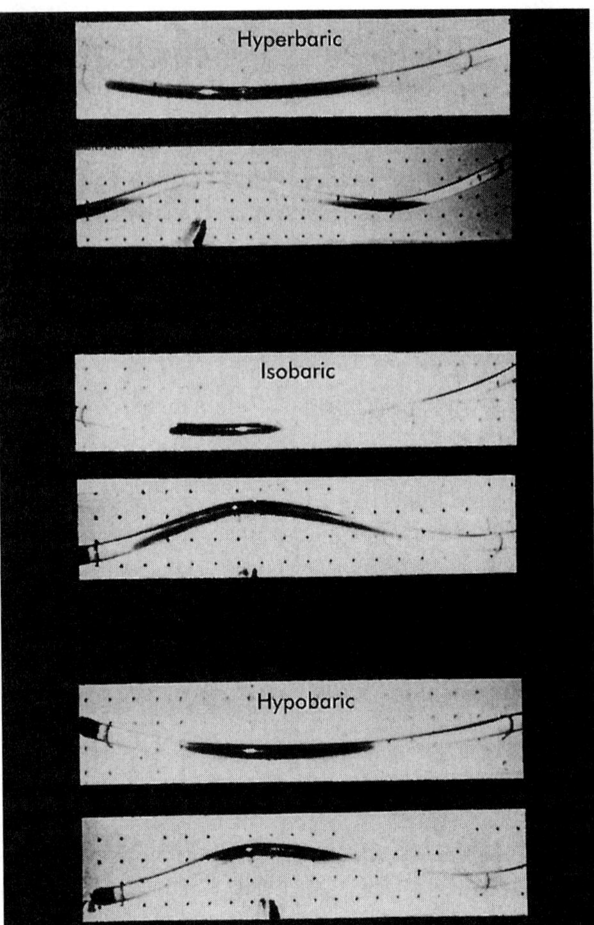

Fig. 59-11. Spinal canal model showing the effect of baricity and position on the distribution of local anesthetic in the lateral position. The model is a plastic tube that contains saline (density similar to CSF) and bent to mimic the contour of the spinal canal during spinal anesthesia. The local anesthetic (15 mg bupivacaine) is colored with methylene blue. The injections were made with the model in the "lateral" position (*top*—view of the model is from above) and immediately turned "supine" and horizontal. *Top* to *bottom,* solutions were hyperbaric, isobaric, and hypobaric.

distribution of local anesthetic within the CSF. As a clinical example, consider the patient with peripheral vascular disease undergoing a right lower extremity distal bypass procedure employing the lateral decubitus position for lumbar puncture and anesthetic injection. For a hyperbaric solution, the optimum patient position would be the right lateral decubitus, in a slight head up position. For an isobaric solution, either the right or left lateral decubitus position would be appropriate. With a hypobaric solution, the optimum position would be the left lateral decubitus position, but in a slight head down position. The head down position would also facilitate venous return and counteract arterial hypotension.

Effect of Dose on the Level of Spinal Anesthesia

Figs. 59-13 and 59-14 and Table 59-5 show the effect of density on the spread of local anesthetic and its clinical duration of action within the spinal canal. **Despite common assumptions and practices, a convincing relationship between dose**

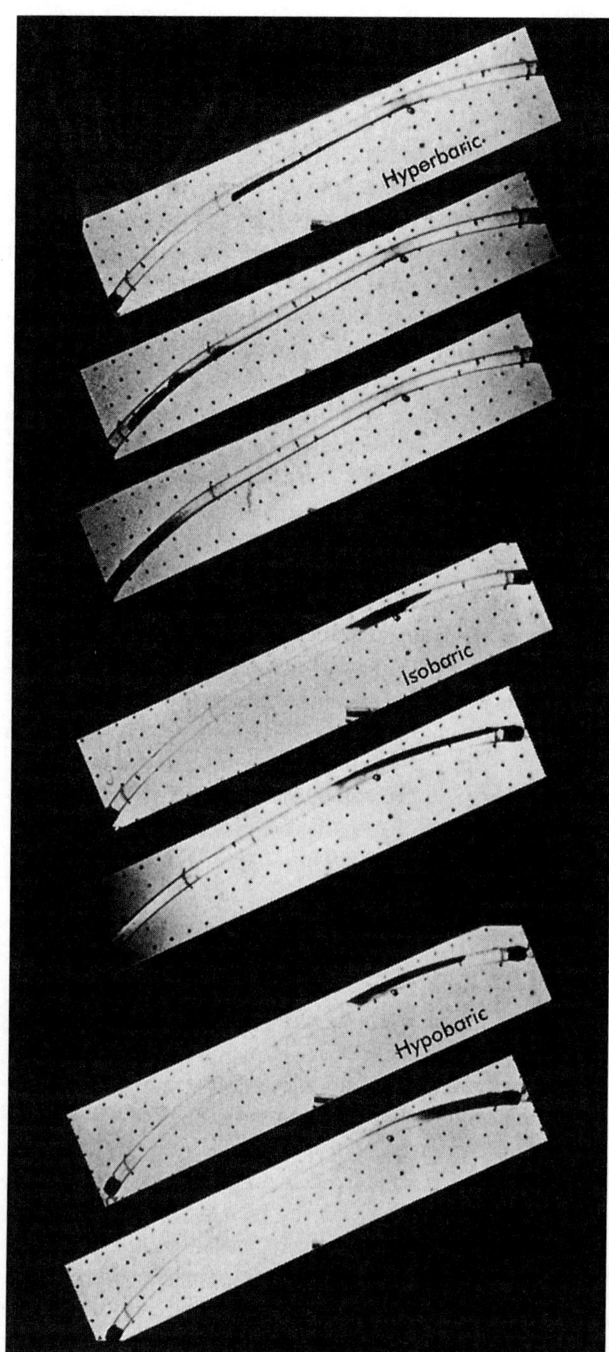

Fig. 59-12. Spinal canal model showing the effect of baricity and position on the distribution of local anesthetic in the prone jackknife position. The model is a plastic tube that contains saline (density similar to CSF) and bent to mimic the contour of the spinal canal during spinal anesthesia. The local anesthetic (15 mg bupivacaine) is colored with methylene blue. The injections were made with the model in the "prone jackknife" position. *Top* to *bottom,* solutions were hyperbaric, isobaric, and hypobaric. Clearly the hyperbaric solution must not be used with this position. The time between injection and final distribution of the dye is 5 minutes.

(mass) of drug injected and the ultimate height of the block has never been substantiated.[66] Fig. 59-13 shows that despite increasing doses, hyperbaric local anesthetic solutions tend to gravitate to the same point in the thoracic concavity with the patient supine and horizontal, resulting in a similar level of

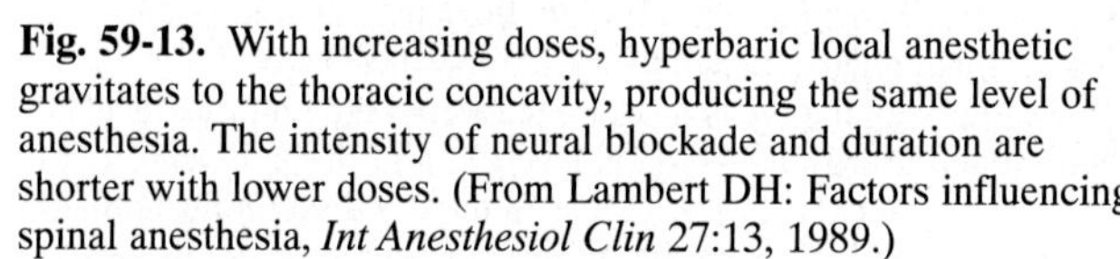

Fig. 59-13. With increasing doses, hyperbaric local anesthetic gravitates to the thoracic concavity, producing the same level of anesthesia. The intensity of neural blockade and duration are shorter with lower doses. (From Lambert DH: Factors influencing spinal anesthesia, *Int Anesthesiol Clin* 27:13, 1989.)

anesthesia. Lower doses simply provide less intense neural blockade of shorter duration, because less of the drug is spread over the same volume. A more reasoned approach would be to administer an empiric dose of local anesthetic (Table 59-6).[66]

Effect of Patient Height on the Level of Spinal Anesthesia

Many anesthesiologists believe there is a relationship between patient height and the sensory level of spinal anesthesia. This seems logical, and older textbooks depict guidelines relating dose to patient height.[33] **Nonetheless, newer data show that when a fixed dose of local anesthetic is given, regardless of height or spinal column length, no correlation is seen between these factors and the final level of anesthesia (Fig. 59-15).**[81] Therefore, an approach to spinal anesthesia based on density and patient position is better than an approach based on dose and height, and less emphasis should be placed on attempting to precisely control the segmental level of spinal anesthesia. Instead, an average empirically determined dose of local anesthetic, irrespective of the patient's height, should be injected (Table 59-6).

Estimating the Necessary Level of Spinal Anesthesia

It is necessary to achieve a segmental level of spinal anesthesia that will block the nerves innervating both the skin

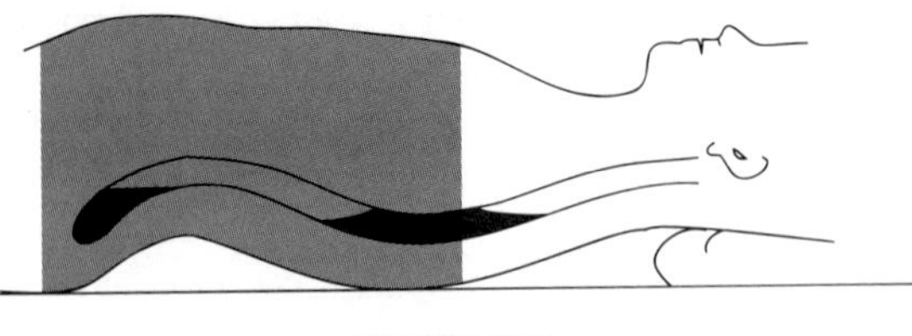

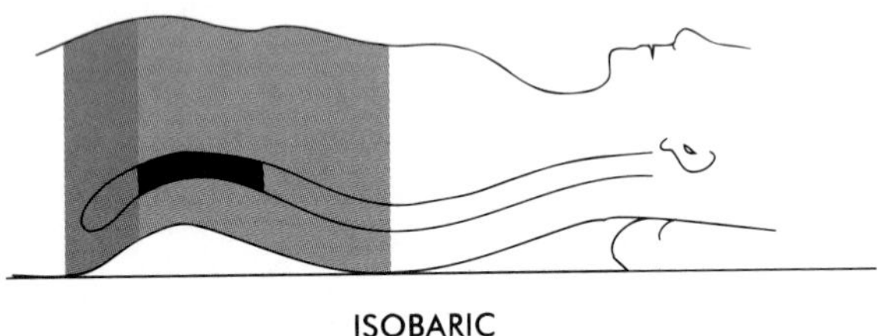

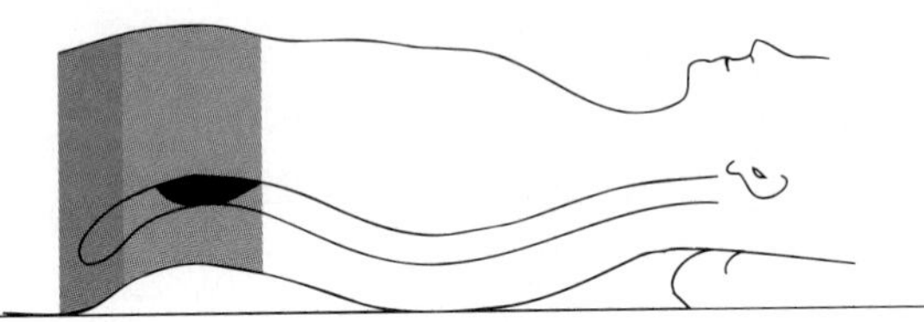

Fig. 59-14. Anticipated effects of injecting hyperbaric, isobaric, and hypobaric local anesthetics into the subarachnoid space. The dark stippled areas represent surgical anesthesia (see Table 59-5). The lighter stippled areas indicate that often the pinprick level (but not necessarily the surgical level) of anesthesia extends considerably cephalad. The dark areas in the dural sac indicate that hyperbaric solutions gravitate to dependent areas, isobaric solutions remain uniformly at the site of injection, and hypobaric solutions rise in the CSF. (From Lambert DH: Factors influencing spinal anesthesia, *Int Anesthesiol Clin* 27:13, 1989.)

Table 59-5 Effect of baricity on anesthetic level and duration of spinal anesthesia

Local anesthetic	Baricity	Average peak level	Average maximum duration (min)
Bupivacaine (15 mg)	Hyperbaric	T5	250
	Isobaric	T9	350
	Hypobaric	Data not available	
Tetracaine (15 mg)	Hyperbaric	T6	285
	Isobaric	T10	332
	Hypobaric	T11	360

Modified from Chambers WA, et al: Effect of baricity on spinal anaesthesia with bupivacaine, *Br J Anaesth* 53:279, 1981; and Brown DT, et al: Effect of baricity on spinal anaesthesia with amethocaine, *Br J Anaesth* 52:589, 1980.

and the visceral structures affected by the procedure. For example, consider total abdominal hysterectomy. Although it may be possible to make the low transverse abdominal incision at the twelfth thoracic dermatome, a spinal anesthetic level limited to this dermatome will not be adequate to complete the operation because the innervation of the uterus is via the tenth, eleventh, and twelfth thoracic nerves. Further, because the operation will result in traction on the uterus and peritoneum, a mid thoracic (T6) level of spinal anesthesia would be preferable. This will block the visceral "traction reflexes," which cause pain or vague discomfort. Therefore, an understanding of the somatic and visceral segmental levels of spinal anesthesia necessary for various types of surgery is required for the successful practice of spinal anesthesia. Fig. 59-16 shows the approximate segmental levels required for surgery involving particular viscera. The dermatomal distribution is illustrated in Fig. 60-3.

As a practical guide, it useful to define surgical procedures as involving nerves above or below the first lumbar (L1) dermatome. For procedures above L1, hyperbaric solutions should be used. In patients turned supine and horizontal after injection of the local anesthetic, hyperbaric solutions gravitate to the thoracic hollow (kyphosis), assuring an adequate level of spinal anesthesia. Because the thoracic kyphosis is located at T6 in the average patient, a T6 level of spinal anesthesia is usually achieved (Box 59-4). For procedures below L1, isobaric solutions are ideal because they linger in the lumbar cistern, providing anesthesia of the lumbar dermatomes for a prolonged duration. Depending on the nature of the procedure and the anticipated position of the patient it may also be appropriate to use hypobaric solutions (Box 59-5).

CARDIOVASCULAR EFFECTS OF SPINAL ANESTHESIA

Arterial hypotension commonly accompanies spinal anesthesia. The reduction in blood pressure usually signifies clinically successful anesthesia. The primary cause of hypotension during spinal anesthesia is preganglionic sympathetic neural blockade. The amount of hypotension is directly related to the extent of sympathetic blockade.[47] Fig. 59-17 shows the change in mean arterial blood pressure due to spinal anesthesia with 15 mg isobaric bupivacaine. The blood pressure decreases an average of 2.5% per spinal segment blocked. The figure also shows considerable variability in the hemodynamic response to spinal anesthesia. The variability is attributed to varying amounts of sympathetic blockade. Mark and Steele[75] reviewed the circulatory changes associated with spinal anesthesia. Their review indicates that arteriolar resistance is reduced 5% to 20%, stroke volume 5% to 20%, heart rate 5% to 25%, cardiac output 10% to 30% and arterial blood pressure 15% to 30%.

Bradycardia, when it occurs, results from block of the cardioaccelerator nerves and decreased venous return. Levels of spinal anesthesia that block the T1–T4 dermatomes not only inhibit the cardioaccelerator nerves but also result in total preganglionic sympathetic blockade that produces venodilatation and reduces venous return. Decreased venous return reflexly slows the heart rate by activating receptors in the right atrium and great veins.[46] **The fall in mean arterial blood pressure is due to a decrease in cardiac output, which results from venodilatation and decreased stroke volume. Any decline**

Table 59-6 Guidelines for the employment of hyperbaric and isobaric solutions in spinal anesthesia

Surgical site	Solution	Concentration (%)	Usual dose (mg)	Usual volume (ml)	Approximate duration with no EPI (hr)	Approximate duration with 0.2 mg EPI (hr)
Above L1	Bupivacaine	0.75	15	2	2	2
(hyperbaric)	Tetracaine	0.5	15	3	3	3
	Lidocaine	5.0	50–100	1–2	1	1
Below L1	Bupivacaine*	0.5	15	3	3–4	4–6
(isobaric)	Tetracaine	0.5	15	3	3–4	4–6
	Lidocaine*	2.0	60	3	1–2	2–4

EPI—epinephrine.
*Isobaric solutions of bupivacaine and lidocaine are not approved by the FDA for spinal anesthesia. However, this use has been reported to numerous publications. Solutions intended for spinal anesthesia should NOT contain any preservatives or antioxidants such as methylparaben, sodium bisulfite, or sodium metabisulfite.
From Lambert DH, Covino BG: Hyperbaric, hypobaric and isobaric spinal anesthesia, *Res Staff Phys* 33:79, 1987.

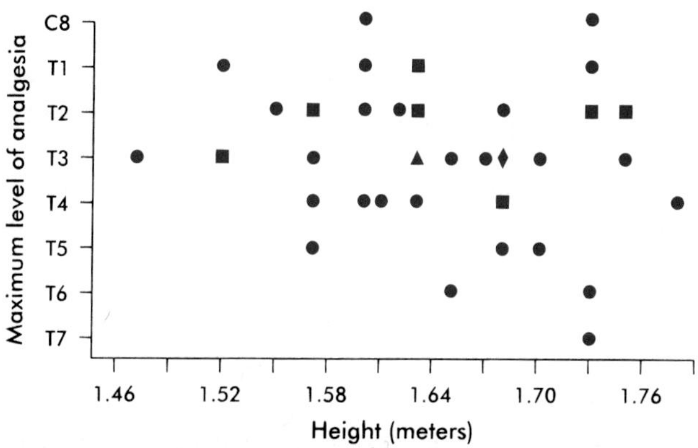

Fig. 59-15. Relationship between height and maximum cephalad spread of blockade after administration of 12 mg hyperbaric bupivacaine in 50 term parturients. *Circles,* 1 patient; *squares,* 2 patients; *triangle,* 3 patients; *diamond,* 4 patients. (From Norris MC: Height, weight, and the spread of subarachnoid hyperbaric bupivacaine in the term parturient, *Anesth Analg* 67:555, 1988.)

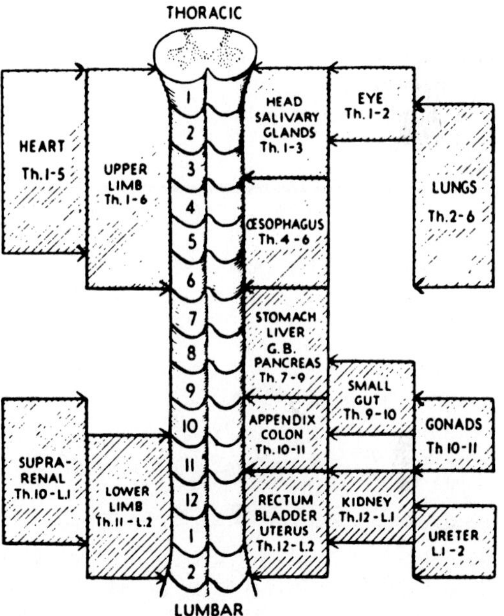

Fig. 59-16. Spinal levels of sympathetic connector cells and the level required for adequate spinal anesthesia. Although knowledge is limited about the specific levels, this diagram acts as a helpful guide in determining the appropriate levels of analgesia needed for surgery on particular viscera. (From Last RJ: *Anatomy: regional and applied,* ed 6, Edinburgh, 1978, Churchill-Livingstone.)

in peripheral vascular resistance (i.e., arteriolar dilatation) contributes little to the fall in mean arterial blood pressure. It should be appreciated that all of the cardiovascular effects seen with spinal anesthesia result from preganglionic sympathetic blockade by local anesthetic.

RESPIRATORY EFFECTS OF SPINAL ANESTHESIA

Spinal anesthesia has only modest effects on respiration.

Respiratory Mechanics

Even with high thoracic levels of spinal anesthesia, inspiratory muscle function is little affected.[4] This is not surprising because the principal muscle of inspiration is the diaphragm, which is innervated by the phrenic nerve (root origin C3–C5). Therefore, a high thoracic level of spinal anesthesia will not affect diaphragmatic function. In fact, spinal anesthesia may enhance contraction of the diaphragm by producing abdominal muscle paralysis, which decreases the force the diaphragm must generate to displace the abdominal viscera during inspiration.

Unlike inspiratory function, active expiratory efforts are reduced in proportion to the anesthetic level, and substantial reductions in maximal expiratory pressure and flow rates are seen with thoracic levels of anesthesia. The abdominal wall muscles are primarily responsible for expiration, and effective coughing requires active expiratory efforts. It is theoretically possible that patients with chronic obstructive pulmonary disease may be adversely affected by spinal anesthesia because

BOX 59-4
SURGERY ABOVE THE L1 DERMATOME

Hernias
Any intraabdominal operation
Radical orchiectomy (groin incision)
Gynecologic operation requiring T10 dermatomal level (dilation and curettage, cerclage, cone biopsy)
Cesarean section

BOX 59-5
SURGERY BELOW THE L1 DERMATOME

Lower limb orthopedic surgery, including hip surgery
Genitourinary surgery (transurethral resection of prostate, transurethral resection of bladder tumor, cystoscopy, penile implant, scrotal orchiectomy)
Perineal surgery (Bartholin's cyst)
Lower limb vascular surgery
Amputation of the lower limbs
Rectal surgery

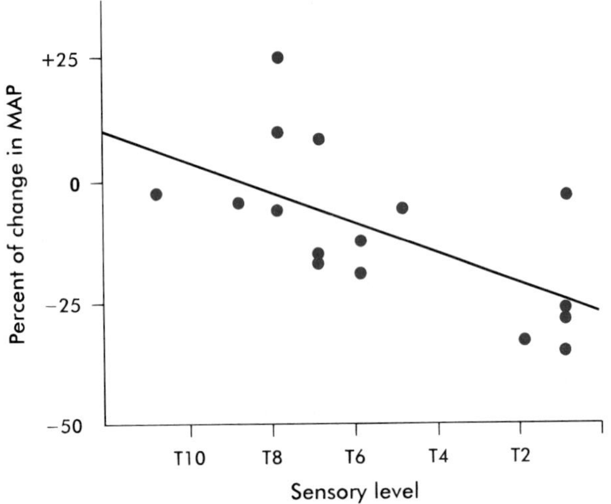

Fig. 59-17. Relationship between the percent change in mean arterial blood pressure (MAP) and the sensory level of spinal anesthesia produced by 15 mg of isobaric bupivacaine in 16 patients undergoing knee joint replacement. (From Mark JB, Steele SM: Cardiovascular effects of spinal anesthesia, *Int Anesthesiol Clin* 27:31, 1989.)

their ability to cough and clear secretions may be impaired.[35] Nonetheless, clinically, patients with chronic obstructive pulmonary disease do well with spinal anesthesia.

Pulmonary Gas Exchange

Spinal anesthesia has little effect on pulmonary gas exchange independent of the effect of sedating drugs. Numerous studies have confirmed the absence of a significant effect of spinal anesthesia on respiratory minute ventilation, dead space ventilation, alveolar-to-arterial differences for oxygen or carbon dioxide, intrapulmonary shunting, or arterial tension of oxygen or carbon dioxide.[28]

Control of Breathing

Respiratory arrest caused by high levels of spinal anesthesia is attributed to brainstem ischemia caused by hypotension, rather than any direct effect of spinal anesthesia on the respiratory control center.[46] However, spinal anesthesia sometimes produces dyspnea, which may be caused by decreased afferent input from the abdominal and chest walls. This proprioceptive information normally inhibits the drive to breathe and when this inhibition is prevented by high spinal anesthesia, the patient may experience dyspnea.[97]

Intrathecal administration of narcotics as an adjuvant for intraoperative anesthesia and to facilitate postoperative analgesia can be associated with delayed respiratory depression (see Chapter 64).

CONTINUOUS SPINAL ANESTHESIA

Continuous spinal anesthesia (CSA) has a history nearly as long as that of single injection spinal anesthesia, having first been reported in 1907.[30] Reports of paralysis with spinal anesthesia in the 1950s and the advent of continuous epidural anesthesia nearly made the literature on CSA extinct until a resurgence of interest occurred with the development and marketing of spinal microcatheters for CSA in the 1980s. When compared with continuous epidural anesthesia, CSA has two advantages: (1) visualization of CSF flow as an endpoint increases success, and (2) it requires 10 to 15 times less local anesthetic, eliminating the likelihood of systemic toxic reactions. When compared to the single injection method of spinal anesthesia, CSA has several advantages[95,98] related to safety and duration (Box 59-6).[56] CSA is potentially safer in elderly or debilitated patients who will not tolerate hemodynamic instability, which can be avoided by carefully titrating small amounts of local anesthetic until the desired level of anesthesia is achieved. Although the single injection method of spinal anesthesia will suffice for most operations, there are instances when duration will need to be prolonged and CSA can be prolonged indefinitely. In addition, subarachnoid catheters can be used effectively for postoperative analgesia with local anesthetics and/or opioids.[8]

All of the equipment and materials necessary for CSA can be found in currently available disposable kits for epidural anesthesia. The method of lumbar puncture is the same as described for single injection spinal anesthesia. Once lumbar puncture has been successfully completed, the catheter is passed 2 to 3 cm into the subarachnoid space. The needle is withdrawn over the catheter and the catheter taped up the patient's back so that injections can be made from the head of the operating table. Injection of the local anesthetic solution is made after the patient has been positioned for

BOX 59-6
ADVANTAGES AND DISADVANTAGES OF CONTINUOUS SPINAL ANESTHESIA

Advantages

Less local anesthetic required
  Less chance of systemic toxicity
Cardiovascular stability
  Injection of local anesthetic after positioning
  Allows incremental dosing
Facilitates surgical schedule
  Placement of catheter in induction area
Recovery period shorter
  Low doses of short-acting agents usable
Duration may be prolonged indefinitely
Possibility of postoperative analgesia

Disadvantages

Requires time for catheter insertion
  May be difficult or impossible
Spinal headache
Potential for infection, nerve injury, hemorrhage

surgery. Injecting small increments of isobaric local anesthetic (20 mg, 2% lidocaine, or 5 mg, 0.5% bupivacaine) while waiting for anesthesia to develop minimizes hemodynamic changes. Because the onset of spinal anesthesia is so rapid, it is not necessary to redose until vague discomfort is felt by the patient. At this point, additional small doses will quickly restore anesthesia, and help prevent accumulation of local anesthetic and a prolonged recovery room stay. Small doses of lidocaine (20 mg) and bupivacaine (5 mg) can be expected to last 30 and 60 minutes, respectively. **Based on recent reports,[29] hyperbaric lidocaine as the 5% solution in 7.5% dextrose should be used with caution for CSA and in limited doses because of its association with neurotoxicity.** If the expected cephalad distribution of spinal anesthesia does not develop following an initial dose of hyperbaric lidocaine, the catheter tip may have threaded to the sacral side of the lumbar lordotic hump with pooling of the anesthetic solution there. An isobaric solution of 0.5% bupivacaine should then be used to extend the cephalad distribution of anesthesia.

The greatest disadvantage of CSA is the potential for postdural puncture headache (PDPH). Currently used equipment from commercially available epidural kits includes 17- or 18-gauge thin-wall needles with a long bevel, and 19- or 20-gauge catheters. For patients over the age of 60 the risk of PDPH appears to be acceptably low and in the range of a few percentage points.[31,44] Retrospective studies suggest that dural edema and inflammation from catheter irritation seal the dural rent, decrease leakage of CSF, and help prevent PDPH even in younger patients.[31,74] This has been discredited by more recent, prospective work.[71] The risk of PDPH with CSA in younger patients is more substantial and consistent with the concept that the probability of PDPH is related primarily to the size of the needle used.[18,82]

Another disadvantage of CSA is the occasional difficulty of passing the catheter into the CSF. The exact cause for this difficulty is not clear. For 19- and 20-gauge catheters passing through a long beveled Tuohy needle, it is possible that the bevel does not completely enter the subarachnoid space. This may result in abundant CSF flow, but with obstruction of catheter passage by the dura (Fig. 59-18). Alternatively, inability to thread the catheter may result from the catheter striking the anterior wall of the subarachnoid space so that there is not enough room for the catheter to bend and thread easily (Fig. 59-19). Rotating or moving the needle in or out may overcome these problems (see Lambert[67] for more details). If the spinal needle tip is located centrally in the CSF and away from the walls of the dural sac, the catheter should thread easily. Repeating the lumbar puncture and trying to thread the catheter at another interspace may be the best solution. Theoretical disadvantages include potential for infection, nerve injury, and hemorrhage, but these have not been documented with the use of 19- and 20-gauge catheters.

It is occasionally difficult to remove spinal subarachnoid as well as epidural catheters, and there have been reports of some of the catheters breaking during removal. When resistance to removal is encountered, the patient should be positioned in the lateral decubitus with maximum flexion of the lumbar spine. This will usually release the pressure preventing removal, and the catheter can be extracted easily.[56] If this maneuver does not facilitate catheter withdrawal, other positions should be tried.[67]

In an effort to decrease the potential for headache with CSA and thus broaden its application, kits with microcatheters as small as 32 gauge were developed and marketed in the 1980s. Unfortunately, the microcatheters were plagued by technical problems, failed spinals, and published clusters of postoperative cauda equina syndrome. This culminated in the publication by the US Food and Drug Administration of a safety alert, and resulted in withdrawal of spinal microcatheters from the North American market.[1]

COMBINED SPINAL AND EPIDURAL ANESTHESIA

Combined single-injection spinal and continuous catheter epidural anesthesia is purported to have several advantages over either technique alone: rapid development of neural blockade and assurances of profound muscle relaxation with subarachnoid local anesthetics plus the ability to extend the block with additional epidural local anesthetic, the development of more profound sensory blockade with combined subarachnoid and epidural local anesthetics,[32] the ability to use smaller bore needles for dural puncture using the Tuohy needle as an "introducer," additional feedback as to whether the needle tip is in the epidural space (because the CSF should be within millimeters of the epidural needle tip), and

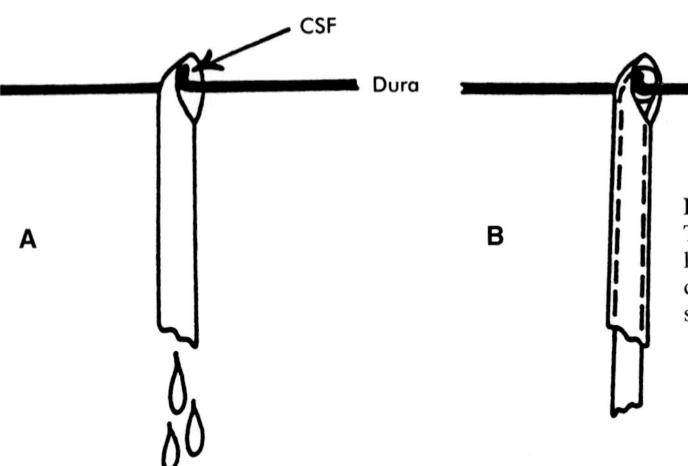

Fig. 59-18. Failure to thread with the long bevel 17- or 18-gauge Touhy needle. **A,** The bevel only partially penetrates the dura allowing abundant CSF return. **B,** Dura and arachnoid prevent the catheter from entering the CSF. (From Lambert DH: Continuous spinal anesthesia, *Anesthesiol Clin North Am* 10:87, 1992.)

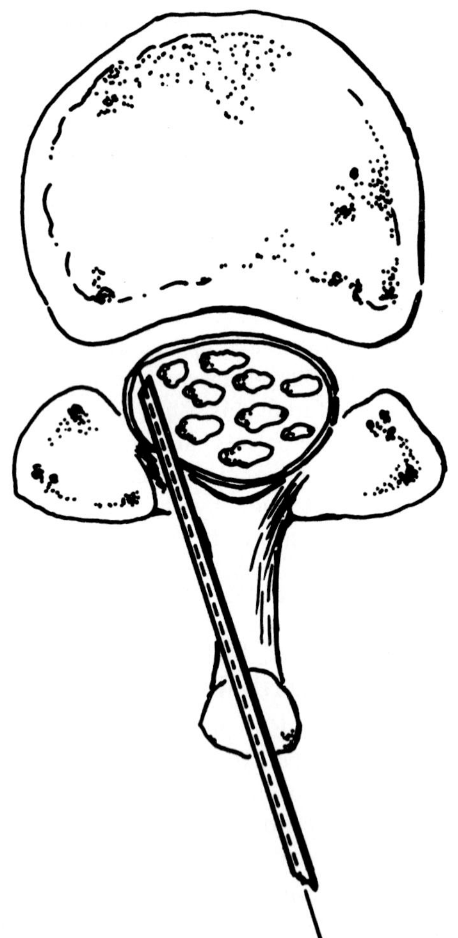

Fig. 59-19. Inability to thread the spinal catheter into the subarachnoid space. A possible cause is the catheter hitting the anterior wall of the dural sac. (From Lambert DH: Continuous spinal anesthesia, *Anesthesiol Clin North Am* 10:87, 1992.)

the ability to use the epidural catheter to extend postoperative analgesia. The technique was recently reviewed and is reported to be useful in anesthesia for obstetrics and orthopaedic surgery.[38] The eventual role of combined spinal and epidural anesthesia in contemporary practice is unknown.

COMPLICATIONS OF SPINAL ANESTHESIA

Clinically relevant complications of spinal anesthesia include arterial hypotension, extensive cephalad spread of local anesthetic resulting in respiratory impairment, spinal headache, and back pain. More serious complications consist of isolated nerve injuries, meningitis, cauda equina syndrome, subdural hemorrhage, brain damage, and death.[65]

Arterial Hypotension and Its Management

Arterial hypotension is the most common complication of spinal anesthesia and results from widespread sympathetic blockade. The cardiovascular effects of spinal anesthesia are discussed in an earlier section of this chapter. **Arterial hypotension is due to diminished venous return from venous pooling and secondarily to decreases in heart rate, resulting in decreased cardiac output. The decrease in venous return is proportional to the extent of sympathetic blockade and the patient's position.** Replenishment of vascular volume before induction of spinal anesthesia and proper positioning once spinal anesthesia is induced will improve venous return and raise cardiac output and arterial blood pressure. Administration of 500 to 1000 ml of crystalloid will lessen the effects of venodilatation during spinal anesthesia. Patients with congestive heart failure usually require less crystalloid because of their congested vascular volume. Restoration of vascular volume in dehydrated patients before induction of spinal anesthesia decreases arterial hypotension. After the spinal anesthetic has been injected, the patient is positioned to ensure adequate venous return. If blood pressure cannot be maintained in the desired range in a euvolemic patient in the supine horizontal position, slight head-down tilt should be employed to increase venous return and cardiac output.[47] Five to 10 degrees of head down tilt may improve venous return and blood pressure without greatly increasing the cephalad spread of anesthesia, though the uniform utility of this maneuver has been disputed.[77] An alternative strategy is to elevate the legs above the level of the heart to facilitate venous return. It is illogical to position the patient with head up when there is extensive cephalad spread of the anesthetic. The level of the anesthetic will not regress rapidly enough to be beneficial but venous pooling will worsen, decreasing cardiac output and lowering arterial blood pressure further.

When fluid therapy and patient positioning does not maintain the blood pressure in an acceptable range, a vasopressor drug should be given. Because the major vascular change contributing to arterial hypotension during spinal anesthesia is decreased venous return (arteriolar tone is only minimally decreased), a vasoconstrictor drug is the preferred treatment.[11,12] Ephedrine (5 to 10 mg) and mephentermine (5 to 15 mg) are commonly administered intravenously. These drugs have both alpha and beta receptor agonist activity whereas phenylephrine (50 to 100 μg), another often used vasopressor agent, is an alpha receptor agonist and potent arteriolar constrictor. In addition to raising blood pressure, ephedrine and mephentermine also increase heart rate. Phenylephrine, on the other hand, increases blood pressure by arteriolar constriction and, as a result, may reflexly slow the heart rate through the baroreceptor mechanism.[48]

Repeated administration or infusion of ephedrine or mephentermine results in decreased effectiveness (tachyphylaxis).[42] Persistent hypotension despite multiple injections of these vasoconstrictor drugs and slight head-down tilt suggests unrecognized hypovolemia. This may result from surgical blood loss or excessive preoperative dehydration and should be treated by volume infusion. When it is necessary to administer a vasoconstrictor for prolonged periods, phenylephrine (10 mg in 250 ml) may be infused. Alternatively, ephedrine may be given intramuscularly (25 to 50 mg) before or immediately after injection of the spinal local anesthetic to prevent hypotension. The amount of hypotension that can be safely tolerated depends on the patient's age and general health. Patients with cardiac or cerebrovascular disease are at risk for ischemia when blood pressure falls during spinal anesthesia. The limit of arterial hypotension that can safely be tolerated in these patients cannot be known *a priori*. The usual recommendation is that arterial blood pressure not be allowed to fall more than 30% in such patients. In healthy individuals, greater falls in blood pressure are better tolerated and may even help to decrease blood loss during surgery.

Postdural Puncture Headache

Postdural puncture headache is a common complication of spinal anesthesia that results from decreased CSF pressure consequent to loss of CSF through the dural puncture site. The most important diagnostic finding is that the headache and associated symptoms are made worse by the erect posture and lessened in the horizontal position. The headache is usually frontal or occipital and occasionally accompanied by other stigmata such as tinnitus, photophobia, or diplopia. The generally accepted pathophysiology is stretching of sensitive structures of the CNS (e.g., cranial nerves) as it "sags" on assumption of an erect posture. Symptoms may present immediately after dural puncture, but usually occur 24 to 72 hours later. Vandam and Dripps[103] identified gender, age, and needle diameter as affecting the incidence of PDPH (Table 59-7). Women develop PDPH more frequently than men, and the incidence is inversely related to age (Fig. 59-20) and directly related to the diameter of the spinal needle (Fig. 59-21). A previous history of PDPH has been identified as a significant predictor of another headache.[73] The diagnosis of PDPH is always one of exclusion, and during assessment other potential causes should be borne in mind.

Midline approaches to the subarachnoid space cause greater leakage of CSF than paramedian insertion. There-

Table 59-7 Relation of sex, age, and needle gauge used for lumbar puncture to incidence of postdural puncture headache

Factors	Number of spinal anesthetics	Number of headaches	Percent
Sex			
Male	4063	302	7
Female	5214	709	14
Vaginal delivery	938	300	22
Other procedures	4276	489	12
Totals	9277	1011	11
Age (years)			
10–19	537	51	10
20–29	1994	321	16
30–39	1833	261	14
40–49	1759	192	11
50–59	1736	133	8
60–69	1094	45	4
70–79	297	7	2
80–89	27	1	3
Totals	9277	1011	11
Needle gauge			
16	839	151	18
19	154	16	10
20	2698	377	14
22	4952	430	9
24	634	37	6

From Vandam LD, Dripps RD: Long term follow up of patients who received 10,098 spinal anesthetics, III. Syndrome of decreased intracranial pressure (headache and ocular and auditory difficulties), *JAMA* 161:586, 1956.

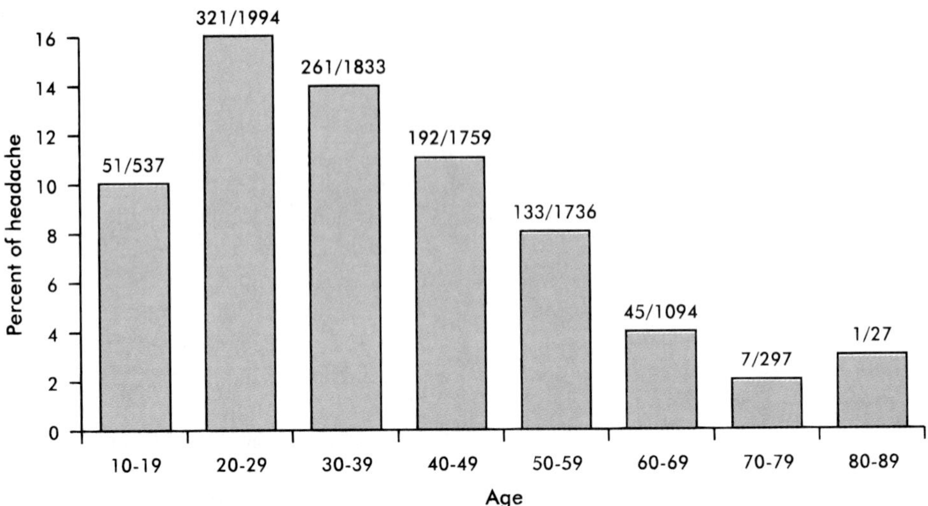

Fig. 59-20. The incidence of postdural puncture headache is inversely related to age. The ratio above each bar is the number of headaches to the total number of spinal anesthetics given to that age group. (From Vandam LD, Dripps RD: Long term follow up of patients who received 10,098 spinal anesthetics: III. Syndrome of decreased intracranial pressure (headache and ocular and auditory difficulties), *JAMA* 161:586, 1956.)

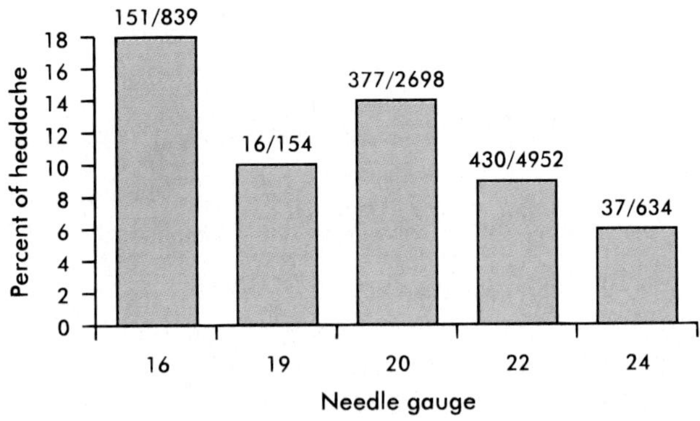

Fig. 59-21. The incidence of postdural puncture headache is inversely related to the gauge of the spinal needle used for lumbar puncture. The ratio above each bar is the number of headaches to the total number of spinal anesthetics given with that gauge needle. (From Vandam LD, Dripps RD: Long term follow up of patients who received 10,098 spinal anesthetics: III. Syndrome of decreased intracranial pressure (headache and ocular and auditory difficulties), *JAMA* 161:586, 1956.)

fore, the incidence of PDPH with the midline approach may be higher than with a paramedian approach.[51,88]

The direction of the spinal needle bevel in relation to the orientation of the longitudinal dural fibers is also believed to influence the incidence of PDPH (Fig. 59-22, Table 59-8).[76] Inserting the bevel parallel to the orientation of the dural fibers cuts fewer fibers than when the bevel is oriented perpendicular. Therefore, parallel insertion results in less fluid leak and a lower incidence of PDPH than perpendicular insertion.

An alternative explanation for the lower incidence of PDPH with the paramedian approach as well as with the bevel of the needle parallel to the longitudinal axis of the dura has been offered by Hatfalvi.[52] He demonstrated in a cadaver model that with the midline approach to lumbar puncture, a side-facing bevel (bevel parallel) will cause bending of the needle shaft as the tip traverses tissues, resulting in a tangential puncture of the dura (Fig. 59-23). This has the effect of creating a valvular "flap" opening in the dura that can be closed by CSF pressure from within.

Another independent factor influencing PDPH incidence is spinal needle tip design. Blunt, conical, or rounded-point needles such as the Green, Sprotte, and Whitacre are said to spread dural fibers less traumatically, allowing them to close more effectively following puncture.[26] A recent metaanalysis of several articles[50] concluded that noncutting needles for spinal anesthesia generally produce a lower incidence of PDPH than cutting needles. Additionally, smaller needles produce less headache than larger needles of the same type. Nonetheless, very-small-gauge cutting needles (< 26 gauge) may prove difficult to use and may have a higher failure rate than larger noncutting needles. This analysis also determined that size or design does not influence the incidence of postoperative low back pain.

The treatment of PDPH includes (1) analgetic therapy, bedrest, and hydration; (2) intravenous or oral caffeine; (3) epidural saline infusion; and (4) epidural blood patch. In rare cases, surgical closure of the dura will be required.[10] The majority (80% to 85%) of cases of PDPH will resolve within 5 days without any therapy. Bed rest, analgetic therapy, and hydration are usually satisfactory treatment for patients who have had extensive surgery and are not likely to be ambulatory immediately. Hydration will increase the production of CSF. When CSF production exceeds loss through the dural rent, normal CSF pressure will be maintained. The symptoms of PDPH are mild in 50% of patients and do not interfere with normal activity. Thirty-five percent are bothered enough to return to bed periodi-

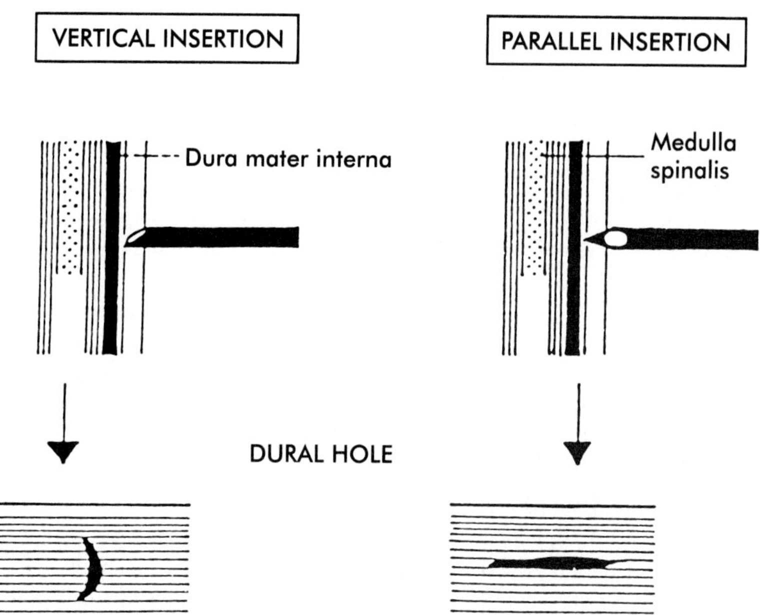

Fig. 59-22. The type of needle insertion for lumbar puncture may affect the incidence of spinal headache. The bevel of the spinal needle can be inserted through the dura perpendicular (vertically) or parallel to the longitudinal dural fibers. The number of severed dural fibers is greater with the vertical insertion. (From Mihic DN: Postspinal headache and relationship of needle bevel to longitudinal dural fibers, *Reg Anesth* 10:76, 1985.)

Table 59-8 Incidence of postdural puncture headache in relation to orientation of needle bevel during insertion through the longitudinal dural fibers

	Vertical insertion*		Parallel insertion	
Needle gauge	Number of patients	Number of headaches	Number of patients	Number of headaches
22	29	5 (17%)	140	1 (0.7%)
25	33	5 (15%)	280	0
Total	62	10 (16%)	420	1 (0.2%)

*Vertical insertion shows in all comparisons a higher incidence of spinal headache ($P < 0.001$).
From Mihic DN: Postspinal headache and relationship of needle bevel to longitudinal dural fibers, *Reg Anesth* 10:76, 1985.

cally to obtain relief, and in 15% the headache is so severe that they cannot sit up long enough to eat.[41] Several controlled studies have demonstrated no significant difference in the incidence of PDPH between patients placed at 4 to 24 hours of bed rest versus those who are allowed to ambulate immediately.[21] During PDPH there is a compensatory vasodilatation of intracranial blood vessels to restore intracranial volume. Thus, there may be a vascular (i.e., cerebral vasodilatation) component to PDPH. Because caffeine is a cerebral vasoconstrictor, it has been used for treatment. Eighty percent of patients experience significant improvement following infusion of 500 mg of caffeine sodium benzoate in 1000 ml of Ringer's lactate solution followed by another liter of Ringer's lactate.[57] Similar improvement has been found if the caffeine is given as a single 300 mg oral dose.[13]

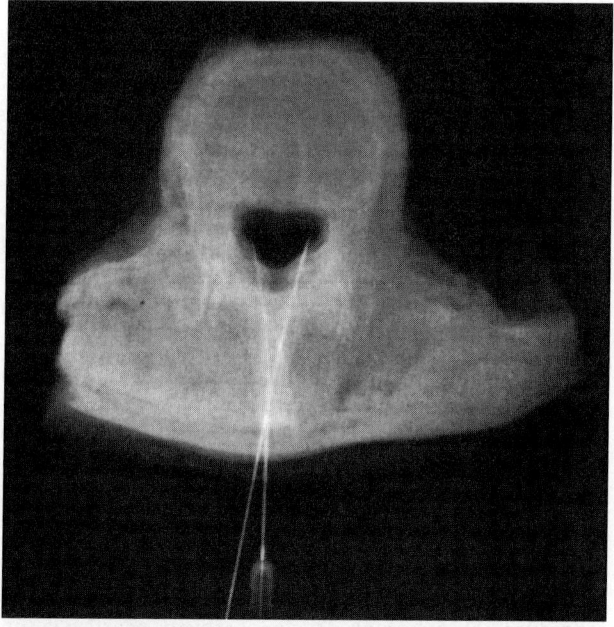

Fig. 59-23. The deviation of 22- and 25-gauge needles, with bevels facing each other. The 25-gauge needle is shown with introducer. (From Hatfalvi BI: The dynamics of post-spinal headache, *Headache* 17:64, 1977.)

Epidural infusion of saline has also been used to treat PDPH. Single injections do not maintain high enough epidural pressures to prevent CSF leaks. To be effective, large volumes of saline (15 to 25 ml/hr infused for at least 24 hours) are required.[24]

If the headache is incapacitating and persists for more than 24 hours following conservative therapy, an epidural blood patch is indicated. The patch simultaneously seals the hole in the dura and displaces CSF into the head and is usually immediately curative. An epidural blood patch is performed by placing a needle into the epidural space in the vicinity of the previous dural puncture and aseptically injecting 10 to 20 ml of autologous blood.[99] If the patient feels a fullness in the back prior to completion of the injection, the injection should then be terminated. The procedure is 90% to 95% effective but may be repeated if relief has not been obtained within 24 hours. Failure of two epidural blood patches is probably due to improper diagnosis. Serious complications associated with the epidural blood patch have not been reported, although low back pain and nuchal discomfort may occur. These usually resolve within 24 to 48 hours and may be treated with analgetics.

Prophylactic epidural blood patch has been evaluated in cases where there is an unintentional dural puncture followed by successful epidural catheterization on a subsequent attempt. Available data concerning the efficacy of this approach are mixed, and the role of prophylactic epidural blood patches remains unsettled.[79]

Extensive Spread of Spinal Anesthesia

Extensive spread of local anesthetic within the subarachnoid space leading to respiratory and cardiovascular compromise can occur in any patient undergoing spinal anesthesia. This usually happens shortly after the induction of spinal anesthesia, but may be delayed. **The signs and symptoms of extensive spread may include apprehension, agitation, nausea and vomiting, arterial hypotension, anxiety, respiratory insufficiency, apnea, and unconsciousness. Treatment consists of airway maintenance, oxygenation, assisted ventilation, and restoration of blood pressure.** Blood pressure should be maintained by fluid administration, repositioning the patient head down to increase venous return and cardiac output, and administration of vasopressor drugs. Often the phrenic nerves are spared and diaphragmatic breathing is sufficient. In the parturient, however, the enlarged uterus may interfere with diaphragmatic excursions. General anesthesia with endotracheal intubation should be considered if the patient is at risk for pulmonary aspiration. During high levels of spinal anesthesia, the amount of local anesthetic in the cervical region is small. Therefore the high level is usually brief in duration and respiratory function ordinarily returns to normal quickly.

Backache

Severe backache following spinal anesthesia is relatively uncommon. It may be caused by periosteal trauma, muscular hematoma, ligamentous injury, or reflex muscle spasm. The profound muscle relaxation that can accompany spinal anesthesia may cause lumbar ligamentous strain in patients in the lithotomy position. Although the overall incidence of backache in patients following spinal anesthesia is low, the incidence in younger healthy outpatients has been reported to be 32% to 55%.[39] Only 3% of these outpatients considered the backache severe, and 12% considered it moderate.[84] Therefore, it appears that spinal anesthesia should not be discouraged in outpatients for this reason. Treatment of backache following spinal anesthesia consists of ruling out neurologic damage, reassurance, rest, local application of heat, and oral analgesics. Backache following spinal anesthesia is usually transient, resolving in 48 hours with conservative therapy. When paraspinous muscle spasm is the cause, a trigger point injection with a local anesthetic or oral diazepam (acting as a mild muscle relaxant) may be helpful.

Nausea and Vomiting

Nausea and vomiting is believed to occur in 13% to 42% of patients undergoing spinal anesthesia. It may be a symptom of major hypotension producing cerebral hypoxia. **Therefore, when nausea and vomiting occur during spinal anesthesia, immediate attention should be turned to whether hypotension is present and blood pressure should be restored while providing oxygen therapy.** It has been shown that immediate treatment of arterial hypotension in parturients minimizes the incidence of nausea during cesarean section.[27] Nausea and vomiting may also be caused by traction-mediated parasympathetic reflexes provoked by surgical manipulation or by the vasovagal response.[25] Atropine (0.4 mg intravenously) may help. Nausea due to administration of narcotics can be treated with droperidol (0.625 mg intravenously). For a review of this topic see Crocker and Vandam.[25] Rarely, nausea and vomiting may be severe enough to warrant induction of general anesthesia.

The Failed Spinal

Occasionally, spinal anesthesia may prove inadequate for the planned surgical procedure. In some cases there is an adequate distribution of sensory anesthesia, but the patient is unable to tolerate the procedure. Often in such instances there is a simple failure to provide adequate sedation. The need for such sedation should not be misconstrued as a "failed block." In other cases, the spinal anesthetic agents fail to distribute themselves sufficiently for the procedure. Additionally, for single injection spinal anesthesia, failure to obtain free flow of CSF following needle placement has been associated with failure of spinal anesthesia.[70] In some of these cases the drug may be injected into the subdural space, which is the potential space between the dura and the arachnoid.

Rarely, seemingly correct placement of spinal anesthetic fails to provide spinal anesthesia. This phenomenon has long been recognized, occurs with single shot as well as continuous spinal anesthesia, and has been identified with numerous local anesthetics. There is a temptation to ascribe these failures to "bad drug," but Schmidt et al.[93] reported a series of "truly failed" spinal anesthetics. In five cases lidocaine administered via spinal catheter failed to produce sensory anesthesia. CSF from these patients was confirmed to have lidocaine present, and drug from the same lot produced anesthesia in other patients. In four of the five cases, bupivacaine produced successful anesthesia. It has been postulated that some patients may have a physiologic resistance to lidocaine spinal anesthesia.[7,93]

Major Neurologic Sequelae

Major neurologic sequelae are extremely rare following spinal anesthesia. This is due in part to the use of disposable spinal anesthesia equipment, the safety of local anesthetics currently in use, and the small quantity of local anesthetic required for spinal anesthesia. One review indicated 31 cases of neurologic sequelae in approximately 65,000 patients having spinal anesthesia; 12 of these events represented exacerbations of preexisting neurologic disease.[102] The causes of neurologic damage associated with spinal anesthesia include: (1) trauma from lumbar puncture; (2) chemical or bacterial contamination of the local anesthetic solution; (3) toxic reactions to the local anesthetic; (4) subarachnoid hemorrhage; and (5) spinal cord ischemia.

Trauma is an infrequent cause of injury and usually results when multiple attempts are made at lumbar puncture.[102] Contamination of local anesthetic solutions with bacteria, detergents, or other chemicals has caused neurologic sequelae. Aseptic meningitis has been attributed to cleaning reusable spinal anesthesia syringes with detergents and antiseptics.[40] Use of disposable equipment has virtually eliminated this complication, as well as bacterial meningitis.

Local anesthetics used for spinal anesthesia are free of neurolytic effects. Nevertheless, a number of cases of cauda equina syndrome occurred when large volumes of chloroprocaine, intended for epidural anesthesia, were accidentally injected into the subarachnoid space.[87,89] The neurotoxicity was due to the effect of sodium bisulfite, a preservative in the chloroprocaine solution.[43] Since then, chloroprocaine has been formulated without sodium bisulfite and additional cases of neurotoxicity have not been reported. As has been discussed, a number of cases of neurotoxicity following spinal anesthesia with the 5% preparation of lidocaine in 7.5% dextrose have been reported. They ranged from transient monoradiculopathy to cauda equina syndrome and occurred with single injection as well as continuous spinal anesthesia.[29]

An expanding epidural or subarachnoid hematoma can damage the spinal cord. Laceration of a blood vessel during lumbar puncture may rarely result in continued bleeding in patients given anticoagulants.[34] It should be remembered that spontaneous hemorrhages have been reported in patients receiving anticoagulants who did not undergo spinal or epidural anesthesia.

Spinal cord ischemia is exceedingly rare. In fact, in the review by Kane[58] involving 65,000 patients, there were no cases of spinal cord ischemia following spinal or epidural anesthesia. It is theoretically possible in certain patients with preexisting compromise of the anterior spinal artery, because spinal cord ischemia has occurred following arterial hypotension in patients having epidural or general anesthesia.

When a neurologic complication occurs after spinal anesthesia, a detailed neurologic examination, consultation by a neurologist, and documentation of relevant information should be completed. Whereas nerve injury can be caused by an errantly placed needle or injection of the wrong substance into the subarachnoid space, it can also result from causes other than spinal anesthesia itself. For example, preexisting neurologic lesions, pressure on nerves from surgical retractors, or faulty positioning and descent of the fetal head through the pelvis during parturition have presented as postoperative nerve damage in patients having spinal or epidural anesthesia.

Except for emergency drainage of a hematoma or abscess, treatment of neurologic complications following spinal anesthesia is symptomatic. The best approach is to prevent nerve injury. When lumbar puncture proves difficult, it is often best to abandon the procedure rather than risk injury from trauma.

A report on 900 closed insurance claims for the period 1978 to 1986 disclosed 14 cases (1.6%) of unexpected cardiac arrest resulting in brain damage or death following spinal anesthesia.[14] The patients were young and healthy and having relatively minor surgical procedures with a T4 level of spinal anesthesia. Some of the patients were sedated to the point of unconsciousness and by the time the anesthesiologist realized something was wrong, the patient had become cyanotic or asystolic. There was also a delay between recognition of the problem and institution of appropriate resuscitative measures.[59] **If profound sedation is necessary for patient comfort or surgical need, then control of the airway and respiration should be considered. Some form of apnea monitoring and continuous use of pulse oximetry is strongly recommended in all patients having spinal anesthesia.**

CONCLUSION

Spinal anesthesia is a core anesthetic technique that all anesthesiologists should be able to safely administer. It has many advantages, but like all anesthetic methods it also has disadvantages and complications. Fortunately, the complications are usually mild and self-limiting. Spinal anesthesia is potentially applicable in nearly all operations of the lower torso and lower extremities. This chapter has presented the principles for the safe and successful practice of spinal anesthesia.

Current research themes in spinal anesthesia include:

- The role of combined spinal and epidural anesthesia in contemporary practice
- The role of adjuvants such as opioids and alpha 2 agonists in spinal anesthesia

- Optimum use of hypnotic drugs such as propofol during spinal anesthesia
- Further definition of the role of spinal anesthesia in ambulatory surgery
- Factors contributing to potential neurotoxicity with 5% lidocaine in dextrose
- Factors contributing to cardiovascular morbidity with spinal anesthesia and their management
- The role of spinal anesthesia in pediatric surgery
- Factors influencing the incidence of postdural puncture headache in spinal anesthesia

KEY POINTS

- Spinal anesthesia results from subarachnoid neural blockade. It is characterized by the production of anesthesia over large areas of the body by small quantities of drug. Spinal anesthesia is potentially applicable for nearly all operations of the lower torso and lower extremities.
- Patients undergoing spinal anesthesia must receive the same preparation and care as patients undergoing general anesthesia. Patients should be informed of why spinal anesthesia was selected, the potential advantages, and potential complications. They should be informed of what they may see or hear in the operating room. Any concern about being awake in the operating room should be assuaged and the patient reassured that sedation will be available to treat anxiety and ensure comfort.
- Major neurologic injuries, including paraplegia, are rare events in spinal anesthesia. They appear to occur with approximately the same frequency as death attributable to general anesthesia.
- Preoperative use of aspirin or NSAIDs does not appear to be a contraindication to spinal anesthesia. The Ivy bleeding time is neither sensitive nor specific enough to reliably identify patients at risk of spinal hematoma following spinal anesthesia. Anticoagulation with heparin or warfarin-like drugs at the time of lumbar puncture remains a contraindication to spinal or epidural anesthesia.
- Baricity is a term related to the density of the local anesthetic solution used for spinal anesthesia. It is the ratio of the density of the anesthetic solution at a specified temperature to the density of CSF at the same temperature.
- Local anesthetic solutions with baricity less than 0.9998 at 37° C are hypobaric in all patients; local anesthetic solutions at 37° C with baricity greater than 1.008 are hyperbaric in all patients; and local anesthetic solutions with baricity between these values are considered isobaric. Because of the range of CSF density, however, it is difficult to know that a solution is truly isobaric in a given patient.
- The local anesthetics used for spinal anesthesia can be ranked in regard to duration as follows: procaine < lidocaine < bupivacaine < tetracaine.
- Recently, the safety of the 5% preparation of lidocaine in 7.5% dextrose for spinal anesthesia has been questioned. Clusters of case reports, ranging from transient lumbosacral monoradiculopathy after single dose administration to cauda equina syndrome following continuous spinal anesthesia with this preparation have been published. The safety of lidocaine in dextrose-free solution is not in question.
- Vasoconstrictors such as epinephrine and phenylephrine prolong the duration of spinal anesthesia. Small doses of opioids such as morphine and fentanyl increase the intensity and quality of subarachnoid neural blockade, as well as provide a longer duration of analgesia following the procedure. When opioids are added to spinal anesthesia, patients require monitoring for delayed respiratory depression.
- Many factors may influence the distribution of local anesthetics within the CSF and thus the ultimate sensory level of anesthesia obtained in a particular patient. The most important are the density of the local anesthetic solution, the conformation of the spine at the time of injection, and the position of the patient during and immediately following injection.
- The primary cause of hypotension during spinal anesthesia is preganglionic sympathetic neural blockade by local anesthetic, which results in decreased venous return and cardiac output. The degree of hypotension is proportional to the extent of sympathetic blockade. Bradycardia contributes to the decrease in cardiac output, and is accentuated by blockade of T1–T4, which comprise the cardioaccelerator nerves.
- Complications of spinal anesthesia include arterial hypotension, nausea and vomiting, extensive spread of the local anesthetic resulting in respiratory impairment, PDPH and back pain. More serious complications consist of isolated nerve injuries, meningitis, cauda equina syndrome, subdural hemorrhage, hypoxic brain injury, and death. Injury from cardiovascular or respiratory compromise is largely preventable through vigilant monitoring and prompt intervention.
- Spinal headache (PDPH) is a common complication of spinal anesthesia that results from decreased CSF pressure owing to a loss of CSF through the dural puncture site. Use of the smallest gauge needle possible, use of conical or blunt-tipped needles, advancement of beveled needles with the bevel parallel to the long axis of the dura,

and a paramedian approach decrease the likelihood of PDPH.

- The treatment of PDPH includes (1) analgesic therapy, bedrest, and hydration; (2) intravenous or oral caffeine; (3) epidural saline infusion; and (4) epidural blood patch. Epidural blood patch displaces CSF into the head and seals the dural rent simultaneously. Failure to respond to two epidural blood patches should call into question the diagnosis of PDPH.
- Continuous spinal anesthesia is appropriate for older or debilitated patients in whom it is especially important to minimize hemodynamic instability. Small doses of local anesthetic can be titrated until the desired level of anesthesia is achieved. Using isobaric or hypobaric local anesthetic solutions in CSA avoids pooling and maldistribution of hyperbaric solutions on the sacral side of the lumbar lordosis in the supine position. Currently available equipment for CSA, because of large needle size, may produce an unacceptably high incidence of PDPH in younger patients.
- Specialized kits for microcatheter CSA were developed and marketed in hopes of minimizing the risk of PDPH and allowing wider use of the technique. Nonetheless, the microcatheters were plagued by technical failures and cases of cauda equina syndrome associated with their use. Following a safety alert by the US Food and Drug Administration in 1992, the catheters were withdrawn from the North American market.

KEY REFERENCES

Covino BG, Scott DB, Lambert DH: *Handbook of spinal anaesthesia and analgesia,* Philadelphia, 1994, WB Saunders.

De Jong RJ: Last round for a "heavyweight"? *Anesth Analg* 78:3, 1994.

Greene NM: Distribution of local anesthetic solutions within the subarachnoid space, *Anesth Analg* 64:715, 1985.

Hatfalvi BI: Postulated mechanisms for postdural puncture headache and review of laboratory models, *Reg Anesth* 20:329, 1995.

Mark JB, Steele SM: Cardiovascular effects of spinal anesthesia, *Int Anesthesiol Clin* 27:31, 1989.

REFERENCES

1. Scientific Publications ASRA Continuous Spinal Anesthesia Symposium, *Reg Anesth* 18:387–484, 1993.
2. Abouleish EI: Epinephrine improves the quality of spinal hyperbaric bupivacaine for Cesarean section, *Anesth Analg* 66:395, 1987.
3. Armstrong IR, Littlewood DG, Chambers WA: Spinal anesthesia with tetracaine-effect of added vasoconstrictors, *Anesth Analg* 62:793, 1983.
4. Askrog VF, Smith TC, Eckenhoff JE: Changes in pulmonary ventilation during spinal anesthesia, *Surg Gynecol Obstet* 119:563, 1964.
5. Belzarena SD: Clinical effects of intrathecally administered fentanyl in patients undergoing cesarean section, *Anesth Analg* 74:653, 1992.
6. Benzon HT, Brunner EA, Vaisrub N: Bleeding time and nerve blocks after aspirin, *Reg Anesth* 86, 1984.
7. Bevacqua BK, Cleary WF: Relative resistance to intrathecal local anesthetics, *Anesth Analg* 78:1024, 1994.
8. Bevacqua BK, Stucky AV: Intrathecal lidocaine/fentanyl infusion for post-operative analgesia, *Anesth Analg* 72:520, 1991.
9. Bier A: Experiments regarding cocainization of the spinal cord, *Chir* 51:361, 1899.
10. Brown BA, Jones OW: Prolonged headache following spinal puncture: response to surgical treatment, *J Neurosurg* 19:349, 1962.
11. Butterworth IV JF, et al: Augmentation of venous return by adrenergic agonists during spinal anesthesia, *Anesth Analg* 65:612, 1986.
12. Butterworth IV JF, et al: Effect of total spinal anesthesia on arterial and venous responses to depamine and dobutamine, *Anesth Analg* 66:209, 1987.
13. Camman WR, et al: Effects of caffeine on postdural puncture headache: a double blind, placebo controlled trial, *Anesth Analg* 70:181, 1990.
14. Caplan RA, et al: Unexpected cardiac arrest during spinal anesthesia: a closed claims analysis of predisposing factors, *Anesthesiology* 68:5, 1988.
15. Chambers WA, Littlewood DG, Logan MR, et al: Effect of added epinephrine on spinal anesthesia with lidocaine, *Anesth Analg* 60:417, 1981.
16. Chambers WA, Littlewood DG, Scott DB: Spinal anesthesia with hyperbaric bupivacaine: effect of added vasoconstrictors, *Anesth Analg* 63:134, 1982.
17. Chantigian RC, et al: Anesthesia for cesarean delivery utilizing spinal anesthesia: tetracaine versus tetracaine and procaine, *Reg Anesth* 9:195, 1984.
18. Chen L, et al: Postdural puncture headache and continuous spinal anesthesia, *Reg Anesth* 15:268, 1990.
19. Collins JG, Kitahata LM, Matsumoto LM, et al: Spinally administered epinephrine suppresses noxiously evoked activity of WDR neurons in the dorsal horn of the spinal cord, *Anesthesiology* 60:269, 1984.
20. Concepcion M, Maddi R, Francis D, et al: Vasoconstrictors in spinal anesthesia with tetracaine-a comparison of epinephrine and phenylephrine, *Anesth Analg* 63:134, 1984.
21. Cook PT, Davies MJ, Beavis RE: Bedrest and postlumbar puncture headache: the effectiveness of 24 hours' recumbency in reducing the incidence of postlumbar puncture headache, *Anaesthesia* 44:389, 1989.
22. Cope RW: The Wooley and Roe case: Wooley and Rose versus the Ministry of Health and others, *Anesthesia* 9:247, 1954.
23. Covino BG, Vassallo HG: *Local anesthetics: mechanism of action and clinical use,* New York, 1976, Grune & Stratton.
24. Crawford JS: Prevention of headache consequent on dural puncture, *Br J Anaesth* 44:598, 1972.
25. Crocker JS, Vandam LD: Concerning nausea and vomiting during spinal anesthesia, *Anesthesiology* 20:587, 1959.
26. Cruickshank RH, Hopkinson JM: Flow through dural puncture sites: An in vitro

comparison of needle point types, *Anaesthesia* 44:415, 1989.
27. Datta S, et al: Method of ephedrine administration and nausea and hypotension during spinal anesthesia during cesarean section, *Anesthesiology* 56:68, 1982.
28. de Jong RH: Arterial carbon dioxide and oxygen tensions during spinal block, *JAMA* 191:608, 1965.
29. de Jong RH: Last round for a "heavyweight," *Anesth Analg* 78:3, 1994.
30. Dean HP: Discussion on the relative value of inhalation and injection methods of inducing anaesthesia, *Br Med J* 2:869, 1907.
31. Denny N, Masters R, Pearson D, et al: Postdural puncture headache after continuous spinal anesthesia, *Anesth Analg* 66: 791, 1987.
32. Dirkes WE, et al: The effect of subarachnoid lidocaine and combined subarachnoid lidocaine and epidural bupivacaine on electrical sensory thresholds, *Reg Anesth* 16:262, 1991.
33. Dripps RD, Eckenhoff JG, Vandam LD: *Introduction to anesthesia: the principles of safe practice,* ed 5, Philadelphia, 1977, WB Saunders.
34. Eddie L, et al: Spinal subarachnoid hematoma after lumbar puncture and heparinization: a case report, review of the literature, and discussion of anesthetic complications, *Anesth Analg* 65:1201, 1986.
35. Egbert LD, Tamersoy K, Deas TC: Pulmonary function during spinal anesthesia: the mechanism of cough depression, *Anesthesiology* 22:882, 1961.
36. Ernst EA: In vitro changes of osmolality and density of local anesthetic solutions, *Anesthesiology* 29:104, 1968.
37. FDA Safety Alert: Cauda equina syndrome associated with the use of small-bore catheters in continuous spinal anesthesia, Washington, DC, 1992, Food and Drug Administration.
38. Felsby S, Juelsgaard P: Combined spinal and epidural anesthesia, *Anesth Analg* 80:821, 1995.
39. Flatten H, Raeder J: Spinal anesthesia for outpatient surgery, *Anesthesiology* 40: 1108, 1985.
40. Garfield JM, et al: Prolonged diabetes insipidus subsequent to an episode of chemical meningitis, *Anesthesiology* 64:253, 1986.
41. Gielen M: Postdural puncture headache, *Reg Anesth* 14:101, 1989.
42. Gilman AG, Goodman AS, Gilman A: *The pharmacologic basis of therapeutics,* ed 6, New York, 1980, MacMillan Publishing.
43. Gissen AJ, Datta S, Lambert DH: The chloroprocaine controversy: II. Is chloroprocaine neurotoxic? *Reg Anesth* 9:135, 1984.
44. Gold BS, et al: Continuous spinal anesthesia for ambulatory surgery patients, *Anesthesiology* 71:A722, 1989.
45. Goldstein GW, Betz AL: The blood-brain barrier, *Sci Am* 255:74, 1986.
46. Greene NM: *Physiology of spinal anesthesia,* ed 3, Baltimore, 1981, Williams & Wilkins.
47. Greene NM: Preganglionic sympathetic blockade in man: a study of spinal anesthesia: The Torston Gordh Lecture 1980, *Acta Anaesth Scand* 25:463, 1981.
48. Greene NM: Perspectives in spinal anesthesia (Abbott lecture), *Reg Anesth* 7:55, 1982.
49. Greene NM: Distribution of local anesthetic solutions within the subarachnoid space, *Anesth Analg* 64:715, 1985.
50. Halpern S, Preston R: Postdural puncture headache and spinal needle design, metaanalyses, *Anesthesiology* 81:1376, 1994.
51. Hatfalvi BI: The dynamics of post spinal headache, *Headache* 17:64, 1995.
52. Hatfalvi BI: Postulated mechanisms for postdural puncture headache and review of laboratory models, *Reg Anesth* 20:329, 1995.
53. Hogan QH: Tuffier's line: the normal distribution of anatomic parameters, *Anesth Analg* 78:194, 1994.
54. Horlocker TT: A trigonometric analysis of needle redirection and needle position during neural block, *Reg Anesth* 21:30, 1996.
55. Horlocker TT, Wedel DJ, Schroder DR, et al: Preoperative antiplatelet therapy does not increase the risk of spinal hematome associated with regional anesthesia, *Anesth Analg* 80:303, 1995.
56. Hurley RJ: Continuous spinal anesthesia, *Int Anesthesiol Clin* 27:46, 1989.
57. Jarvis AP, Greenwalt JW, Fagraeus L: Intravenous caffeine for post-dural puncture headache, *Reg Anesth* 11:42, 1986.
58. Kane RE: Neurologic deficits following epidural or spinal anesthesia, *Anesth Analg* 60:150, 1981.
59. Keats AS: Anesthesia mortality-a new mechanism, *Anesthesiology* 68:2, 1988.
60. Kennedy F, Effron AS, Perry G: The grave spinal cord paralysis caused by spinal anesthesia, *Surg Gynecol Obstet* 91:385, 1950.
61. Kopacz DJ, Allen HW: Comparison of needle deviation during regional anesthesia techniques in a laboratory model, *Anesth Analg* 86:630, 1995.
62. Kozody R, Ong B, Palahniuk RJ, et al: Subarachnoid bupivacaine decreases spinal cord blood flow in dogs, *Can Anaesth Soc J* 32:216, 1985.
63. Kozody R, Palahniuk RJ, Biehl DR: Spinal cord blood flow following subarachnoid lidocaine, *Can Anaesth Soc J* 32:472, 1985.
64. Kozody R, Palahniuk RJ, Cumming MO: Spinal cord blood flow following subarachnoid tetracaine, *Can Anaesth Soc J* 32:23, 1985.
65. Lambert DH: Complications of spinal anesthesia, *Int Anesthsiol Clin* 27:51, 1989.
66. Lambert DH: Factors influencing spinal anesthesia, *Int Anesthesiol Clin* 27:13, 1989.
67. Lambert DH: Continuous spinal anesthesia, *Int Anesthesiol Clin* 27:46, 1992.
68. Lambert DH, Covino BG: Hyperbaric, hypobaric and isobaric spinal anesthesia, *Res Staff Phys* 33:79, 1987.
69. Lawrence VS, et al: Spinal anesthesia with isobaric lidocaine 2% and the effect of phenylephrine, *Reg Anesth* 9:17, 1984.
70. Levy JH, et al: A retrospective study of the incidence and causes of failed spinal anesthetics in a university hospital, *Anesth Analg* 64:705, 1985.
71. Liu N, Montefiore A, Kermarec N, et al: Prolonged placement of spinal catheters does not prevent postdural spinal headache, *Reg Anesth* 15:285, 1993.
72. Liu S, Chiu AA, Carpenter RL, et al: Fentanyl prolongs lidocaine spinal anesthesia without prolonging recovery, *Anesth Analg* 80:730, 1995.
73. Lybecker H, et al: Incidence and prediction of postdural puncture headache: A prospective study of 1021 spinal anesthesias, *Anesth Analg* 70:389, 1990.
74. Mahisekar UL, Winnie AP, Vasireddy AR, et al: Continuous spinal anesthesia and postdural puncture headache: A retrospective study, *Reg Anesth* 16:107, 1991.
75. Mark JB, Steele SM: Cardiovascular effects of spinal anesthesia, *Int Anesthesiol Clin* 27:31, 1989.
76. Mihic DN: Postspinal headache and relationship of needle bevel to longitudinal dural fibers, *Reg Anesth* 10:76, 1985.
77. Miyabe M, Namiki A: The effect of head-down tilt on arterial blood pressure after spinal anesthesia, *Anesth Analg* 76:549, 1993.
78. Moore DC, Chadwick HS, Ready LB: Epinephrine prolongs lidocaine spinal: pain in the operative site the most accurate method of determining local anesthetic duration, *Anesthesiology* 67:416, 1987.
79. Neal JM: Management of postdural puncture headache, *Anesthesiol Clin North Am* 10:163, 1992.
80. Niemi L: Effects of intrathecal clonidine on duration of bupivacaine spinal anesthesia, haemodynamics, and postoperative analgesia in patients undergoing knee arthroscopy, *Acta Anaesth Scand* 38:724, 1994.
81. Norris MC: Height, weight, and the spread of hyperbaric bupivacaine in the term parturient, *Anesth Analg* 67:555, 1988.
82. Norris MC, Leighton BL: Continuous spinal anesthesia after unintentional dural puncture in parturients, *Reg Anesth* 15:285, 1990.
83. Ota K, Namiki A, Iwasaki H, et al: Dose-related prolongation of tetracine spinal anesthesia by oral clonidine in humans, *Anesth Analg* 79:1121, 1994.
84. Perz RR, Johnson DL, Shinozaki T: Spinal anesthesia for outpatient surgery, *Anesth Analg* 67:S168, 1988.
85. Racle JP, Benkhadra A, Poy JY, et al: Effect of increasing amounts of epinephrine during isobaric bupivacaine spinal anesthesia in elderly patients, *Anesth Analg* 66:882, 1987.
86. Rao TLK, El-Etr AA: Anticoagulation following placement of epidural and subarachnoid catheters: an evaluation of neurologic sequelae, *Anesthesiology* 55:618, 1981.
87. Ravindran RS, et al: Prolonged neural blockade following regional anesthesia with 2-chloroprocaine, *Anesth Analg* 58: 447, 1980.
88. Ready LB, et al: Spinal needle determinants of rate of transdural fluid leak, *Anesth Analg* 69:457, 1989.
89. Reisner LS, Hochman BN, Plumer MH: Persistent neurologic deficit and adhesive arachnoiditis following intrathecal 2-chloroprocaine injection, *Anesth Analg* 59: 452, 1980.
90. Rigler ML, Drasner K, Krejcie TC, et al: Cauda equina syndrome after continuous spinal anesthesia, *Anesth Analg* 72:275, 1991.

91. Rosenberg H: Density of tetracaine-water mixtures and the effectiveness of 0.33% tetracaine in hypobaric spinal anesthesia, *Anesthesiology* 45:682, 1976.
92. Sarantopoulos C, Fassoulaki A: Systemic opiods enhance the spread of sensory analgesia produced by intrathecal lidocaine, *Anesth Analg* 79:94, 1994.
93. Schmidt SI, et al: A series of truly failed spinal anesthetics, *J Clin Anesth* 2:336, 1990.
94. Schneider M, Ettlin T, Kauffmann M, et al: Transient neurologic toxicity after hyperbaric subarachnoid anesthesia with 5% lidocaine, *Anesth Analg* 76:1154, 1993.
95. Shroff PK, Skerman JH, Blass NH: Continuous spinal blockade: an old technique revisited, *South Med J* 81:178, 1988.
96. Spector R, Johanson CE: The mammalian choroid plexus, *Sci Am* p 68, 1989.
97. Steinbrook RA: Respiratory effects of spinal anesthesia, *Int Anesthesiol Clin* 27: 40, 1989.
98. Stutter PA, Gamulin Z, Forster A: Comparison of continuous spinal and continuous epidural anesthesia for lower limb surgery in elderly patients: a retrospective study, *Anaesthesia* 44:47, 1989.
99. Szeinfeld M, et al: Epidural blood patch: evaluation of the volume and spread of blood injected into the epidural space, *Anesthesiology* 64:820, 1986.
100. Taylor JA: Lumbosacral subarachnoid tap, *J Urol* 43:561, 1940.
101. Vaida GT, Moss P, Capan LM, et al: Prolongation of lidocaine spinal anesthesia with phenylephrine, *Anesth Analg* 65:781, 1986.
102. Vandam LD, Dripps RD: Exacerbation of pre-existing neurologic disease after spinal anesthesia, *N Engl J Med* 255:843, 1956.
103. Vandam LD, Dripps RD: Long term follow-up of patients who received 10,098 spinal anesthetics: III. Syndrome of decreased intracranial pressure (headache and ocular and auditory difficulties), *JAMA* 161:586, 1956.

CHAPTER 60

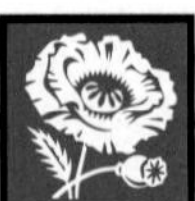

Epidural Anesthesia

ROBERT R. GAISER

Corning is credited with being the first to use epidural anesthesia in 1885 when he postulated that medications injected within the spinal canal might be taken up by the rich plexuses of blood vessels in the neighboring region.[16] The first approach to the epidural space was demonstrated by Cathelin in 1901. He found that fluids injected into the epidural space through the sacral hiatus rose to a height proportional to the amount injected. His objective was to develop a method of anesthesia equally effective to spinal anesthesia but less dangerous.[12] Although these caudal injections were far from ideal for surgical operations, they were successfully used for labor analgesia. Pages, in 1921, described the midline lumbar approach to the epidural space and segmental epidural anesthesia. Since these early pioneers, epidural anesthesia has increased in popularity for the anesthesiologist and the public. This popularity is largely attributed to its acceptance and use for analgesia. With current epidural infusion mixtures, it is possible to manage postoperative and chronic pain with minimal side effects. Like many other forms of regional anesthesia, epidural anesthesia offers the ability to perform major surgery in conscious patients. Unlike spinal anesthesia, it may be extended postoperatively. Epidural anesthesia also may be combined with general anesthesia. This combination offers the advantage of excellent relaxation of the abdominal musculature without the use of muscle relaxants. Patients can awaken from the general anesthetic relatively quickly because their pain will be controlled without requiring medications that have sedative side effects. Successful epidural anesthesia requires good training and a thorough understanding of the anatomy and technique.

ANATOMY

Spinal Canal

A thorough knowledge of the anatomy of the spinal canal and the bones and ligaments that form it is essential for the performance of epidural blockade.

The spinal column consists of seven cervical, twelve thoracic, five lumbar, and five fused sacral vertebrae (Fig. 60-1). A vertebra consists of a vertebral body with an arch posteriorly. It is through this arch that the spinal cord travels. The arch consists of two pedicles anteriorly and two laminae posteriorly. At the junction of the pedicle and the lamina is the transverse process; where the laminae meet is the spinous process. Whereas the laminae and the spinous processes are joined by ligaments, the pedicles are not. The gaps between the pedicles form the foramina, through which the spinal nerves leave the canal.

The spinal canal contains the spinal cord with its three coverings: the pia mater, the arachnoid mater, and the dura mater. The pia mater is closely attached to the spinal cord, and the arachnoid mater is a thin membrane lying close to the dura mater, from which it is easily separated. Three spaces are created. The epidural space is located outside the dura mater. The subdural space is located between the dura and arachnoid mater. Subdural injection of local anesthetic is a rare complication (1:10,000; see Complications). The last space is the subarachnoid space, which is discussed in the chapter on spinal anesthesia.

Ligaments

The anterior and posterior longitudinal ligaments run between the anterior and posterior aspects of the vertebral bodies. The supraspinous ligament stretches from C7 to the sacrum, acquiring maximum thickness in the lumbar area. The interspinous ligament runs between spinous processes. The ligamentum flavum, which consists of yellow elastic fibers, runs from the anterior and inferior aspects of the vertebral laminae to the posterior and superior aspects of the laminae below. The ligamentum flavum is most dense in the lumbar area, 3.0 to 3.5 mm, and is the final barrier to a needle before it enters the spinal canal. Because it is tougher than the other ligaments but does not offer the total resistance of bone, it usually can be readily identified with an epidural needle.

Epidural Space

The epidural space is located outside the dural canal, extending from the base of the skull to the sacral hiatus. The epidural space lies between two layers of dura mater. The outer periosteal layer blends with the periosteum of the vertebra, whereas the inner layer encloses the spinal cord (Fig. 60-2). The two layers of the spinal dura are firmly adherent to the base of the skull at the foramen magnum. Thus, the superior boundary to the epidural space is the foramen magnum. Although it is possible to achieve high sensory levels of anesthesia, it is impossible to achieve "total" spinal (blockade of the cranial nerves) anesthesia because the foramen magnum limits the cephlad spread. The inferior boundary is the sacrococcygeal membrane. The lateral boundaries are the pedicles of the vertebrae and the intervertebral foraminae. Although the epidural space often is considered to be an open space because injected fluid could escape into

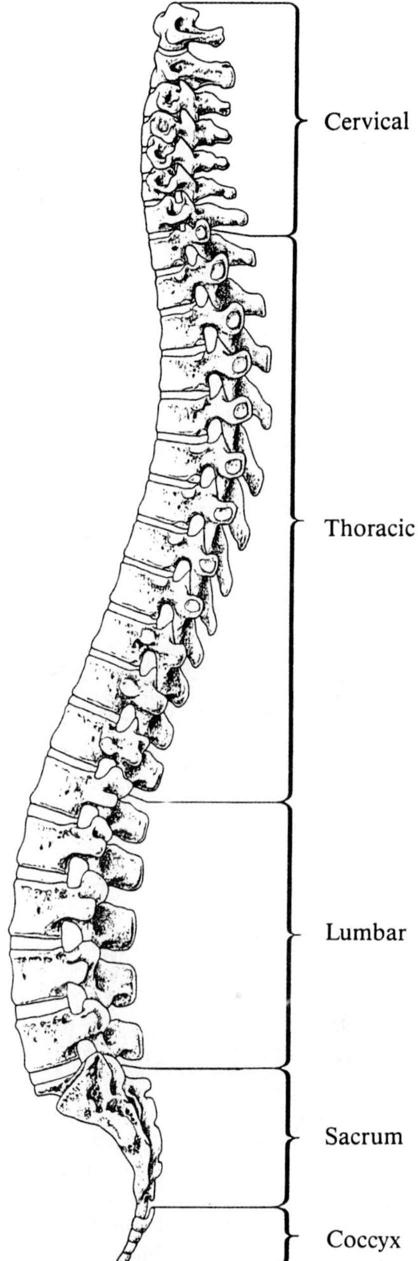

Fig. 60-1. The spinal column contains the spinal canal. The thoracic kyphosis and lumbar lordosis are important considerations when performing major conduction anesthesia. (Reprinted by permission from Scott DB: *Techniques of regional anaesthesia,* Norwalk, 1989, Appleton & Lange.)

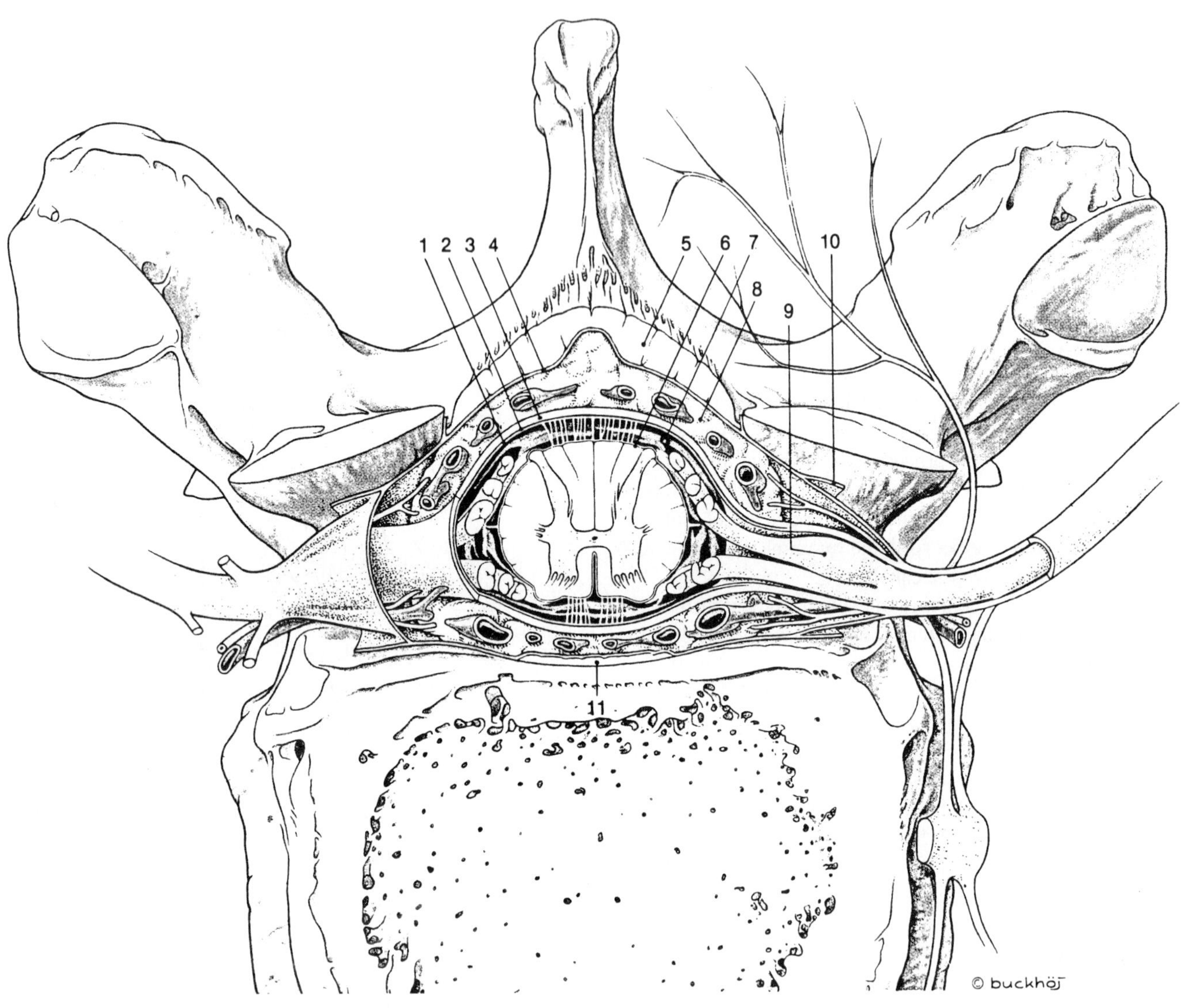

Fig. 60-2. The epidural space extends from the foramen magnum to the coccyx. The spinal dura actually is a two-layered structure. The outer layer is closely applied to the wall of the spinal canal covering bones, discs, and ligaments, which make up the canal. 1, Arachnoid mater; 2, subdural space; 3, dura mater; 4, dura mater; 5, ligamentum flavum; 6, pia mater; 7, subarachnoid space; 8, epidural space; 9, dorsal root ganglion; 10, periosteum; 11, posterior longitudinal ligament. (Reprinted by permission from Scott DB: *Techniques of regional anaesthesia,* Norwalk, 1989, Appleton & Lange.)

the paravertebral space through the intervertebral foramina, there is little evidence that this occurs. For practical purposes, the epidural space should be considered to be closed.

The epidural space contains nerve roots, fibrous tissue, fat, blood vessels, and lymphatics. The epidural fat constitutes an important depot for injected local anesthetics. Lymphatic networks surrounding and draining the dura run anteriorly from each intervertebral foramen and empty into longitudinal channels in front of the vertebral column.

Epidural veins are numerous. They are easily distensible because they have thin walls. These veins run vertically and are primarily arranged into two main systems found on the sides of the epidural space. There are interconnections between the two sides completing a vascular ring at each level. The veins are valveless and help establish communication between the pelvic and the intracranial venous sinuses, connecting with the vertebral, azygous, and lumbar veins. **Unintentional venous cannulation while performing epidural blockade always is a possibility, thus requiring appropriate test dosing (see test dose).**

The anterior and posterior spinal roots join to form the spinal nerve, which contains motor, sensory, and, in most nerves, autonomic fibers. Spinal nerves leave the spinal canal through the intervertebral foraminae and quickly divide into anterior and posterior primary rami. The latter supply the skin and muscles of the back. The anterior rami supply the rest of the trunk and the limbs. Their dermatomal distribution is shown in Fig. 60-3.

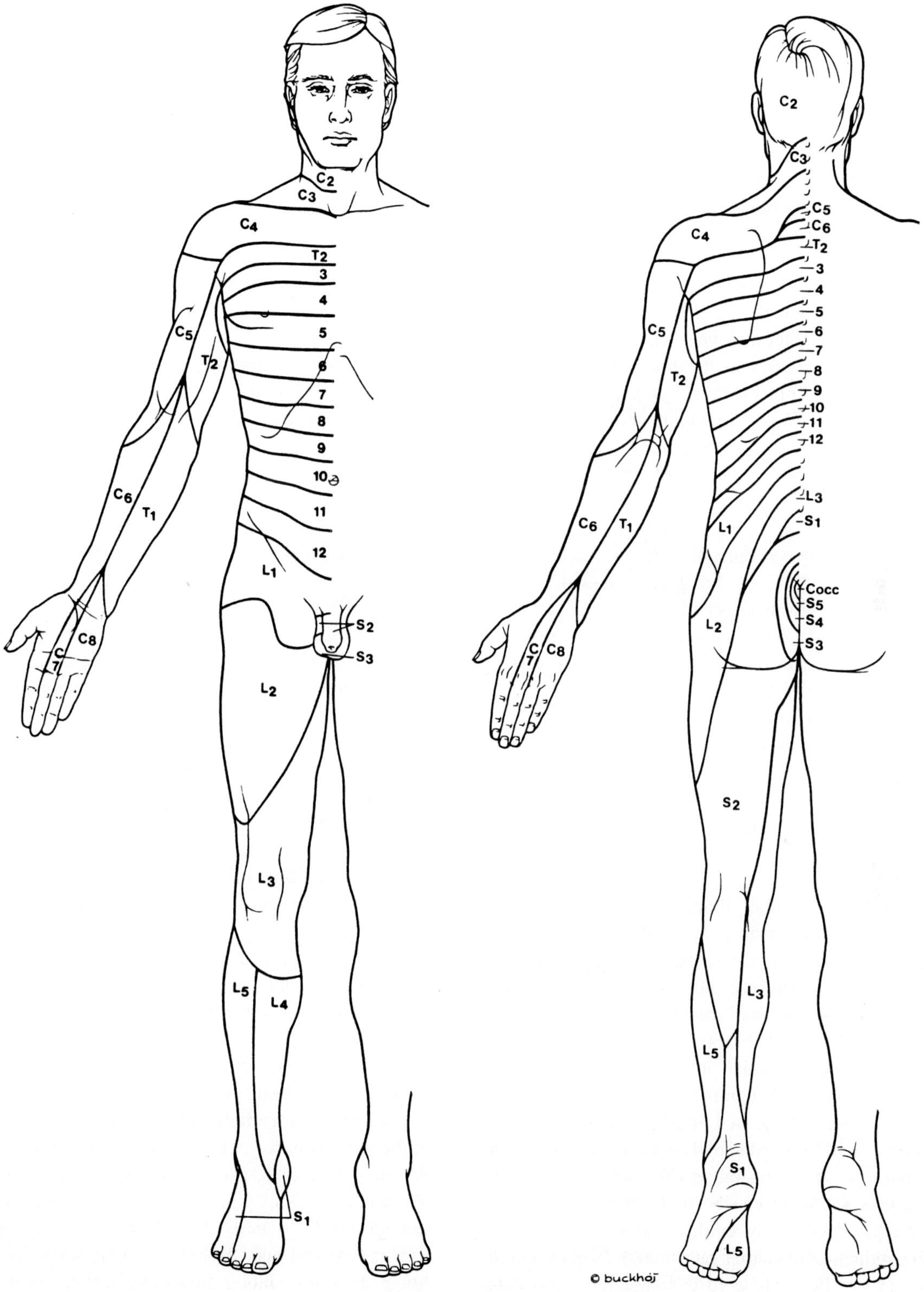

Fig. 60-3. Dermatomal distribution. (Reprinted by permission from Scott DB: *Techniques of regional anaesthesia,* Norwalk, 1989, Appleton & Lange.)

Each spinal nerve is covered for a short distance by a dural cuff as the nerve leaves the canal through its intervertebral foramen. Efferent sympathetic nerve fibers exit the spinal cord in the ventral nerve roots from spinal segments T1 to L2. Some of the parasympathetic nerve fibers leave the spinal cord at the S2- to S4-spinal segments (the sacral parasympathetic outflow). Additionally, parasympathetic fibers join the vagus, oculomotor, facial, glossopharyngeal, and accessory nerves (the cranial parasympathetic outflow). Cranial parasympathetic outflow is unaffected by epidural blockade. Autonomic nervous system anatomy is more fully discussed in Chapter 37.

PHYSIOLOGY

Mechanism of Epidural Blockade

Local anesthetics produce reversible neural blockade by preventing the passage of sodium ions through the nerve membrane.[10] When injected into the epidural space, most of the drug is absorbed into the venous blood system.[6] Some is retained in the fatty tissue, whereas the rest reaches target nerve fibers within the spinal nerves and nerve roots.[9]

Although the dura mater and the connective tissue of the spinal nerves offer a barrier to the local anesthetic from reaching the nerve membranes, they do not completely prevent the drugs from directly blocking nerve conduction. Another mechanism for neural blockade assumes that local anesthetic passes through the dura and arachnoid maters to reach the spinal cord itself. Epidural anesthesia tends to resemble spinal blockade as it progresses.[60]

All modalities of nerve function—motor, sensory, and autonomic—can be effectively blocked, provided a sufficient concentration of local anesthetic is used. Unlike with use of spinal anesthesia, it is relatively easy to obtain a differential block by administering a dilute solution of certain local anesthetics, e.g., 0.25% bupivacaine.[56] Moreover, because the epidural space may be entered at any spinal level and because spread of local anesthetic is governed by the amount administered, the blockade can be confined to a smaller number of spinal nerves than usually is possible with a subarachnoid injection.

Cardiovascular

The major circulatory effect of epidural anesthesia is related to its accompanying sympathetic blockade. Blockade to the midthoracic region causes a considerable decrease in sympathetic activity, resulting in vasodilation in the lower part of the body. Venodilation decreases venous return to the heart and decreases cardiac output. The decrease in cardiac output is more pronounced with high (mid-thoracic) compared with low (lumbar) epidural anesthesia.[47] Decreased arteriolar tone appears to play a lesser role in hypotension. The addition of epinephrine attenuates the hypotension as the epinephrine is absorbed, and its systemic effects become evident.[33]

Although the decrease in cardiac output is largely attributed to a reduction in venous return, high thoracic epidural anesthesia has been show to decrease left ventricular contractility. Even patients without myocardial disease have altered left ventricular contractility as evidenced by echocardiography.[28] The etiology may be from a reduction in sympathetic tone to the heart. Further, with blockade to the upper five thoracic segments, the cardiac accelerator fibers are blocked, and the heart may slow. Both factors contribute to a decrease in cardiac output.

Some prefer epidural anesthesia to general anesthesia in high-risk patients with myocardial disease. In one study, patients undergoing peripheral vascular surgery were randomized to receive either epidural or general anesthesia. Both groups received epidural analgesia postoperatively. There was a reduction in the overall postoperative complication rate and in the incidence of cardiovascular failure in the epidural group.[61] Although this study stimulated an interest in epidural anesthesia, subsequent studies have failed to detect any difference between epidural anesthesia and a well-conducted general anesthetic in patients with myocardial disease.[21]

Pulmonary

Epidural blockade rarely causes respiratory complication, even in patients with serious respiratory disease.[20] The advantage to epidural anesthesia is that it avoids airway manipulation and controlled ventilation. To affect respiration, a high block would be required because the diaphragm is innervated by the spinal segments C3 to C5, although intercostal muscle function is affected if the blockade extends to the thoracic levels.

Endocrine

Epidural anesthesia has been shown to modify the "stress response" to surgery. **As compared with general anesthesia, epidural anesthesia inhibits the increase in cortisol, catecholamines, and blood glucose associated with the stress of surgery.**[51] This altered response is a result of blocking the afferent neurogenic impulses from the area of surgery.

Gastrointestinal

Reduction of sympathetic activity in the gut leaves the vagus unopposed, and an increase in gastrointestinal motility is common.[2] This effect leads to better gastric emptying and tends to oppose the effect of opioids. The incidence of colonic anastomotic dehiscence has been reported to be reduced with epidural blockade, particularly when epidural analgesia was continued postoperatively.[37]

Hematologic

Epidural anesthesia can potentially decrease the risks of venous thromboembolism and postoperative pulmonary embolism. This reduction has been shown for patients undergoing hip, knee, and major abdominal operations.[36,40,42] The mechanisms by which epidural anesthesia accomplishes this are not fully understood. Blockade of the sympathetic nervous system may decrease venous stasis by increasing lower extremity blood flow. Further, epidural anesthesia lessens the metabolic response to stress, which has been shown to promote platelet aggregation during trauma. Finally, a higher circulating level of plasminogen-activator has been observed in patients undergoing hip surgery during epidural anesthesia.[43]

Epidural anesthesia reduces intraoperative blood loss during hip surgery, prostatectomy, or cesarean section.[50,58] The decrease in blood pressure caused by epidural anesthesia does not completely explain why less bleeding occurs as blood loss does not always correlate with intraoperative blood pressure.

Uterine Blood Flow

Lumbar epidural analgesia is commonly used for pain relief during labor. Provided hypotension is avoided or promptly managed, intervillous and uterine blood flow are improved as a result of a decrease in uteroplacental vascular resistance.[49]

TECHNIQUE

Identification of the Epidural Space

Locating the epidural space depends on identifying the moment the needle penetrates the ligamentum flavum to prevent further advancement through the dura and arachnoid maters into the subarachnoid space.

Distance between the ligamentum flavum and the dura mater

The greatest distance between the ligamentum flavum and the dura is found in the midline at the second lumbar interspace, where the distance is about 5 or 6 mm in men. In the midthoracic region, the distance is somewhat less, in the range of 3 to 5 mm at the midline. In the lower cervical region, the distance narrows to 1.5 to 2.0 mm; below C7, it widens again, especially during flexion and at the first thoracic interspace.

Epidural pressure

Inspiration causes an insignificant negative pressure in the lumbar epidural space unless the inspiratory effort is great, the needle is in the upper lumbar region, and the patient is lying in the lateral decubitus position. **Most negative pressure effects seen in the lower lumbar region are a result of coning of the dura by the advancing needle point.** As described by Bromage,[8] the needle tents the dura as it advances, resulting in negative pressure. In the thoracic region, respiratory negative pressures are transmitted effectively to the epidural space. Pregnancy, abdominal masses, ascites, or obesity increases the pressure in the lumbar epidural space, which may even become positive.[41]

Loss of resistance

The most popular method to locate the epidural space is the *loss of resistance technique.* An epidural needle is inserted through a skin wheal and advanced in the midline sagittal plane slightly cephalad until the spinal ligaments are entered. The stylet is removed, and an air- or normal saline-filled syringe is attached. The syringe should have a freely mobile plunger. If the needle tip is in a spinal ligament (engaged), it is difficult to inject the syringe. The needle is advanced in small increments, and the plunger of the syringe is depressed. As soon as the needle traverses the ligamentum flavum and enters the spinal canal, there is no further resistance to the plunger, and it is now easy to inject. If bone is contacted, it probably is the lamina of the lower vertebra. The needle should be withdrawn and redirected cephalad to walk off the lamina of the inferior spinous process.

Hanging drop

The *hanging drop technique* uses the negative pressure within the epidural space to ensure correct placement. A drop of fluid is placed at the hub of the needle after engaging the interspinous ligament. When the ligamentum flavum is penetrated, the drop of fluid is sucked into the epidural space, and correct identification of the space can be confirmed by injection of fluid or air without resistance.

Single Shot Versus Continuous Technique

For brief procedures, a single dose of local anesthetic solution may be sufficient. A catheter is required for procedures of long or uncertain duration and to provide postoperative analgesia. The catheter is advanced through the needle, and the point at which it reaches the bevel is identified by the markings on the catheter. A slight resistance is felt as the catheter emerges from the bevel. The catheter is passed 2 to 5 cm into the epidural space. Advancing beyond 5 cm in adults increases the likelihood of epidural vein puncture or migration of the catheter out of the spinal canal, resulting in a patchy or unilateral block. Advancing less than 2 cm increases the possibility the catheter may become dislodged from the space.[4] The catheter should be held in place during removal of the needle to prevent unintentional removal of the catheter. Once the needle leaves the skin, the catheter is grasped at the exit hole, and the needle totally removed. When finished using the catheter, the entry site is dressed, and a note is made recording that the tip of the catheter was removed intact.

Epidural Needles

The loss of resistance is most easily detected with large bore needles (i.e., 16-, 17-, and 18-gauges). These needles allow the catheter to pass easily through them. Most epidural needles have a Huber point, which causes the catheter to leave the needle at an angle, reducing the possibility of directly impinging on the dura or the spinal canal wall. The Huber point may be sharp or blunt, according to personal preference. Some needles have a wing at the hub end of the needle to allow for a two-handed insertion. Many have 1-cm graduations marked on the shaft to measure the depth of the epidural space from the skin. All have a removable stylet, which protects the orifice while the needle advances through the skin from occlusion with a tissue plug (Fig. 60-4).

Equipment

The epidural kit, which should be sterile, typically contains (1) an epidural needle; (2) a loss-of-resistance syringe, which is either glass or plastic; (3) a syringe with a small gauge needle for skin infiltration; (4) swabs, solution receptacles, and sterile drapes. It is important to prevent contamination of the epidural needle or catheter with the iodine preparation solution, which is neurotoxic.

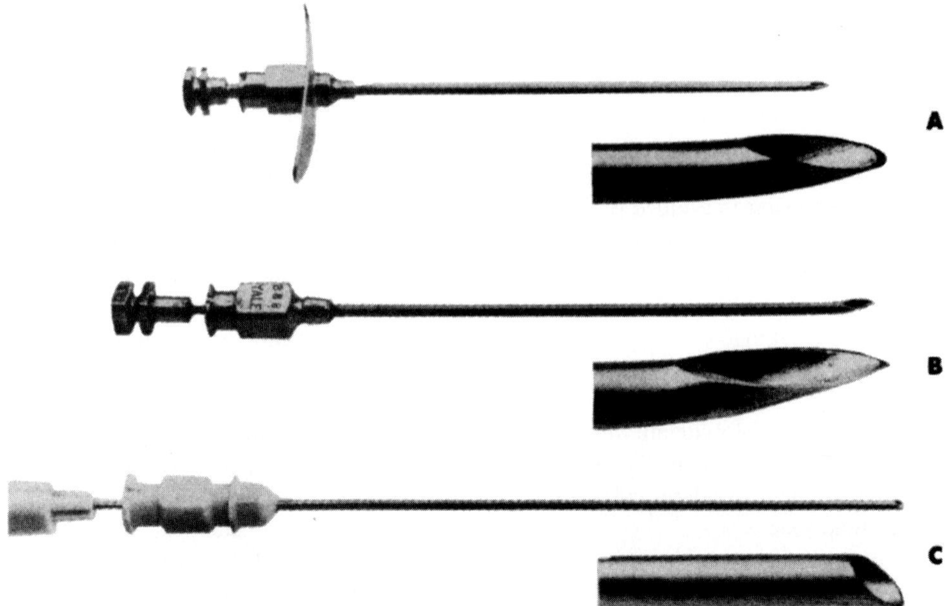

Fig. 60-4. Needles commonly used for epidural anesthesia: Weiss needle with wings **(A),** standard Tuohy needle **(B),** Crawford needle **(C).** (Reprinted by permission from Covino BG, Scott DB: *Handbook of epidural anaesthesia,* Orlando, 1985, Grune & Stratton.)

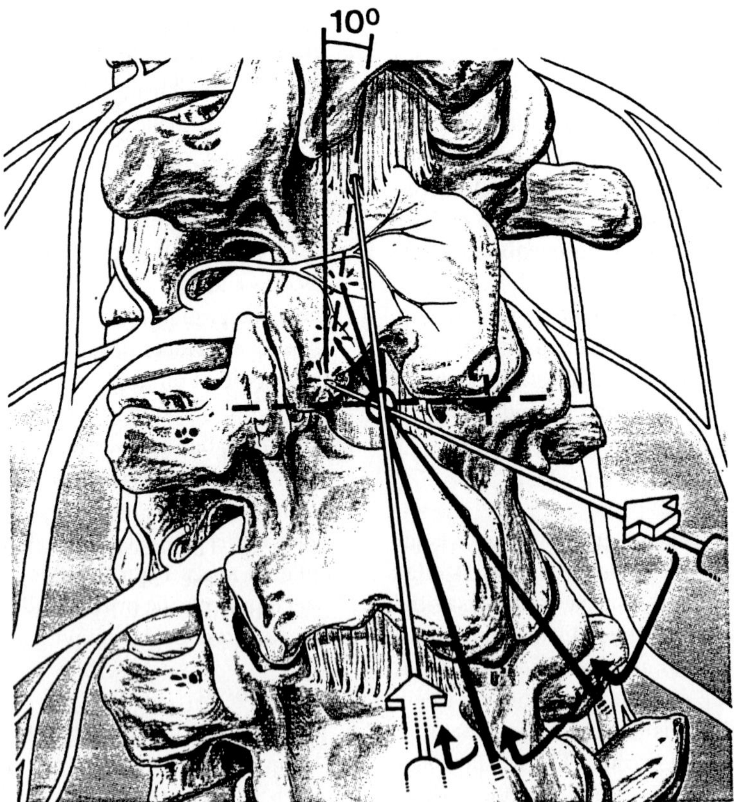

Fig. 60-5. The paramedian approach is used when the midline approach is not possible. The needle is inserted 1.0 to 1.5 cm from the upper border of the spinous process below the chosen interspace, but the needle tip should ultimately enter the epidural space at the midline. (Reprinted by permission from Scott DB: *Techniques of regional anaesthesia,* Norwalk, 1989, Appleton & Lange.)

An epidural catheter, if required, may be in its own sterile package. There are two types of catheters: single and multiport. The single port has one opening at the tip, whereas the multiport has several openings at the tip. One has not been shown to be superior over the other. The catheter may contain a stylet for easier insertion. Although the stylet has been associated with a higher incidence of dural puncture, it may be required in patients with a poorly compliant epidural space. The catheter has a darkened tip for confirmation of complete, intact removal when finished. A bacterial filter may be attached to the injection port to ensure all injections through the catheter are bacteria-free. The technique is performed in a sterile manner.

Patient Position

One of two positions may be chosen: (1) lateral decubitus—the spine and hips are maximally flexed with the knees drawn up to the abdomen and the patient's head bent toward the knees; or (2) sitting—sitting on the operating table with the feet resting on a stool, elbows resting on the knees, and the spine maximally flexed. The sitting position is preferred in obese patients because the midline may be more easily identified.

Paramedian Approach

If the spinal ligaments are calcified, as may occur with aging, or if the patient is difficult to position with the spine flexed, the midline approach may not be possible. A paramedian approach is an alternative in these patients. The skin is punctured 1.5 to 2.0 cm from the midline adjacent to the inferior spinous process to the chosen interspace. The needle is advanced slightly medial and cephalad through paraspinous muscles. Ultimately, the epidural needle should enter the space in the midline. Any bone the needle encounters is likely to be ipsilateral lamina, and the needle is walked off superiorly (Fig. 60-5). Disadvantages to the paramedian approach include an increased likelihood of encountering an epidural vein and a less definite loss of resistance.

Thoracic

The thoracic spinous processes, especially between T3 and T7, have greater caudad angulation than the lumbar spinous processes. This greater angulation requires steeper angles of needle insertion than in the lumbar area (Fig. 60-6). It may be easier to use a paramedian approach. The advantage of thoracic epidural anesthesia over the lumbar route is it can provide a more localized effect, sparing the lower extremities and permitting less drug usage with superior analgesia of the thorax.

Caudal

The sacral portion of the spinal canal can only be reached through the sacral hiatus or, less commonly, the posterior sacral foraminae, as the five sacral vertebrae are fused. The sacral hiatus is formed by the absence of the laminae of S5. The hiatus is covered by part of the sacrococcygeal ligament

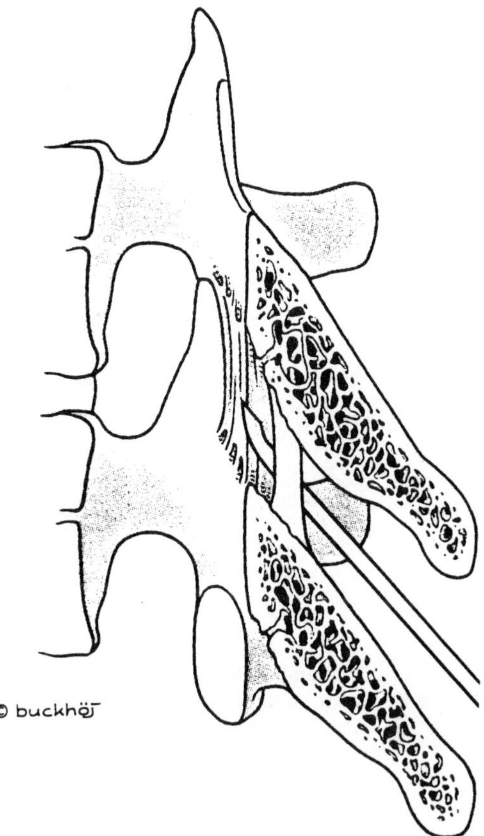

Fig. 60-6. The spinous processes of the vertebral bodies in the thoracic region are not horizontal, rather they are angulated downward, requiring a cephalad direction of the epidural needle to enter the epidural space. (Reprinted by permission from Scott DB: *Techniques of regional anaesthesia,* Norwalk, 1989, Appleton & Lange.)

and has two cornuae, one on each side, which are palpable through the skin in most patients.

The caudal approach to the epidural space is performed either in the lateral or prone position. The sacral cornuae on each side of the hiatus are palpated; the depression between them is the sacral hiatus. After appropriate local anesthetic infiltration at the chosen entry site, the needle (for a single shot technique, a short 21- to 23-gauge needle may be used) is advanced toward the hiatus at 45° to the skin and pointing cephalad. The sacrococcygeal ligament is pierced, and the bony resistance of the anterior wall of the sacral canal encountered. The needle is redirected more cephalad until it can be advanced 1.0 to 1.5 cm into the canal. After examining the needle hub for the absence of fluid or blood, local anesthetic is given, or a catheter is advanced. During injection, the skin over the sacrum is observed for subcutaneous swelling, which indicates a wrongly placed needle tip or catheter (Fig. 60-7).

Epidural Medications

Local anesthetics

Most local anesthetic drugs may be used for epidural blockade. The thickness of the spinal nerves and their coverings

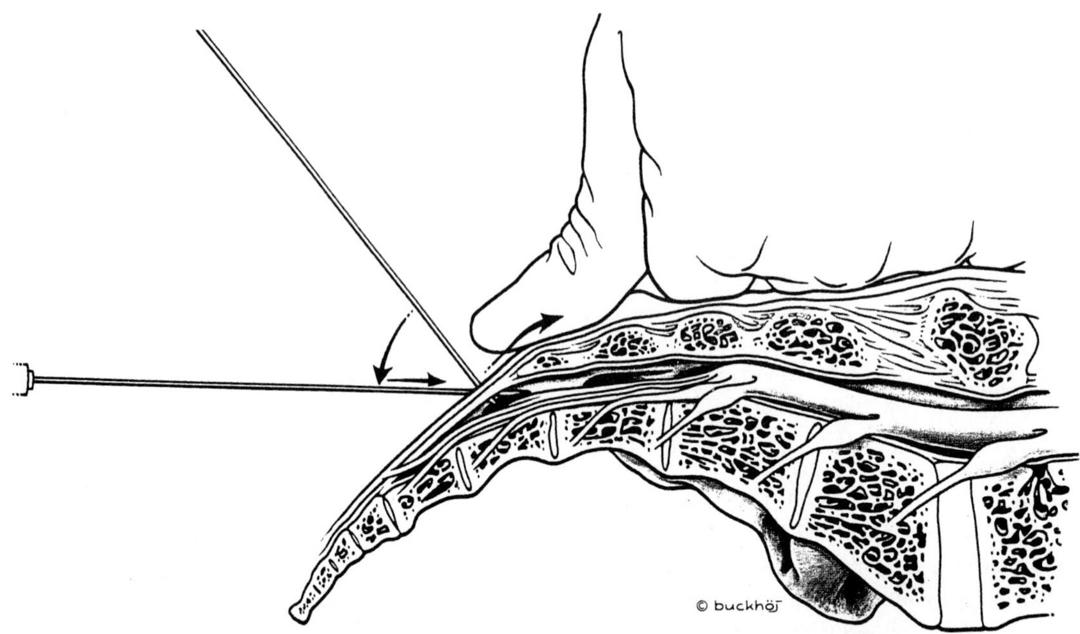

Fig. 60-7. Caudal anesthesia is widely used in pediatrics. It is relatively easy to perform because there are less anatomic variations than in adults. (Reprinted by permission from Scott DB: *Techniques of regional anaesthesia,* Norwalk, 1989, Appleton & Lange.)

dictate that high concentrations are required if somatosensory and motor blockade is desired.[27] Pain mediated through autonomic sensory nerves (e.g., labor pains) can be relieved by lower concentrations. For a single shot technique, the drug is chosen with regard to its duration. If a catheter is used, the choice of drug is not as important.

The volume of injectate is important in regard to spread, although it should be emphasized that the relationship between spread and volume is not linear.[25] The first few milliliters of solution can spread a considerable distance from the injection site, but it may be unilateral. Further quantities fill the epidural space, ensuring biltateral spread. As drug travels cephalad and caudad, a given quantity may not increase the sensory level as cephalad as expected. Larger quantities of local anesthetic create a denser and longer-lasting nerve block. Predicting the spread of solution within the epidural space is not an exact science. Using a catheter reduces the problem considerably as the level of blockade may be increased progressively by injecting 5-ml aliquots until the desired height is reached. With conscious patients undergoing surgery, anesthesia several segments above the surgical site is recommended.

Epinephrine

Local anesthetics exhibit a biphasic effect on the vascular smooth muscle of the epidural veins. Low concentrations enhance muscle activity, causing vasoconstriction. In the more commonly used higher concentrations, vasodilation occurs, resulting in faster removal of drug from the epidural space.[5] The addition of epinephrine decreases the rate of vascular absorption, allowing more anesthetic molecules to reach the nerve membrane and to improve the depth and duration of anesthesia. Epinephrine also decreases systemic blood concentrations of all local anesthetics after epidural administration.[26] Small amounts of epinephrine absorbed from the epidural space produce predominantly beta-adrenergic effects, decreasing systemic vascular resistance and increasing heart rate.[33]

Epidural opioids

The use of epidural opioids solely or combined with local anesthetics has gained increasing popularity for intraoperative management and for postoperative analgesia (see Chapter 64). By combining opioids to the local anesthetic, less local anesthetic is required to produce equal or improved analgesia. The principal advantage of epidural opioids is that they do not cause sympathetic blockade like epidural local anesthetics. A single dose of epidural opioid can provide prolonged analgesia. The exact site of action of epidural opioids is debatable, although the preponderance of evidence supports a direct spinal action, with proportionately more drug reaching the cerebrospinal fluid through the epidural route compared with IV narcotics. Opioids block pain-related transmission by binding at presynaptic and postsynaptic receptor sites in the spinal cord.[14] **Side effects include respiratory depression, urinary retention, nausea, and pruritus.** It is possible to relieve the side effects without reversing the analgesia by titrating small amounts (40 μg) of IV naloxone.[53]

The most commonly used epidural opioids include

preservative-free morphine, fentanyl, and sufentanil. Meperidine and alfentanil also have been used, but they are not as popular.[44,54] Lipid solubility is a major determinant of opioid action. The greater the lipid solubility, the faster the onset.[30] Fentanyl and sufentanil are more lipid-soluble than morphine, and both have a more rapid onset of action. The disadvantage of this high lipid solubility is that these agents have a shorter duration of action. Compared with intrathecal administration, dosages are greater when administered epidurally (Table 60-1).

Alpha-2 agonists

Alpha-2 agonists, when administered epidurally, result in analgesia. The antinociceptive effect is assumed to result from activation of alpha-2 adrenergic receptors in the dorsal horn of the spinal cord.[24] Clonidine at a dose of 300 μg has been used for postoperative analgesia and in the management of cancer pain.[22,52] Side effects include sedation, bradycardia, and hypotension.

Test Doses

Because the dose required to achieve adequate epidural anesthesia can cause serious problems if the injection is made unintentionally into the subarachnoid space or into a blood vessel, a test dose should be administered before injection. An adequate test dose will rule out intravascular or subarachnoid injection.

The most commonly used test dose is a small amount of local anesthetic containing at least 15 μg of epinephrine. If administered intravenously, the patient's heart rate increases by 20% within 60 seconds.[46] If the patient is taking beta-blocking medication, the heart rate may be unaffected, but the blood pressure still increases because of unopposed alpha stimulation. The amount of local anesthetic for a test dose should be adequate to produce sensory blockade only if it is administered subarachnoid, and no discernible sensory level if it is administered epidurally (e.g., 60 mg of lidocaine).

Other test doses have been devised because many question the reliability of the local anesthetic and epinephrine test dose. Higher doses of local anesthetic (e.g., 100 mg of lidocaine or chloroprocaine) produce systemic symptoms of local anesthetic toxicity if the catheter or needle is intravascular. These symptoms include circumoral numbness, tinnitus, and a metallic taste in the mouth. This dose results in an obvious spinal blockade, if intrathecal, and a patchy sensory level of a couple of dermatomes, if epidural.[15]

An air test dose also has been used.[35] To successfully use the air test dose, a Doppler probe should be placed over the precordium. One milliliter of air is rapidly injected through the epidermal catheter. If the catheter is IV, the mill-wheel murmur typical of air embolism is heard. This test dose does not detect intrathecal injection and poses the risk of paradoxical air embolus if the patient has a patent foramen ovale.

No matter which test is used, a negative test dose does not guarantee correct placement. The main injection always should be given slowly or in increments, and the patient should be constantly monitored for symptoms of toxicity.

INDICATIONS FOR EPIDURAL BLOCKADE

Epidural blockade can be used for surgical and obstetrical operations and for the relief of acute and chronic pain.

Surgical Operations

The most common approach to the epidural space is the lower lumbar region. Local anesthetic drug injected into the lumbar epidural space can provide excellent thoracic and sacral anesthesia (Table 60-2). If a more discrete band of anesthesia is required, then the local anesthetic is injected at or near the center point of that band, which may involve entering the epidural space in the thoracic or cervical region. The benefit of using smaller volumes of local anesthetic is weighed against the inherent danger of spinal cord trauma when using these higher locations.

Relief of Acute Pain

Obstetrics

Epidural blockade has its widest application in the relief of labor pain, and it is by far the most effective method for this purpose.[17] The pain of uterine contractions is transmitted through sympathetic sensory fibers entering the spinal nerves at T10 to L1. During the second stage of labor as the fetus descends through the birth canal, somatic sensory nerve blockade of S2 to S4 is necessary.

Postoperative pain

With appropriate catheter placement, a band of neural blockade produces excellent analgesia with minimal side ef-

Table 60-1 Epidural opioid dosages

Epidural opioid	Dose	Duration of analgesia (hr)
Morphine	1–5 mg	5–24
Fentanyl	25–100 μg	1–2
Sufentanil	10–50 μg	2–3

Table 60-2 Suggested minimum cutaneous level for major conduction anesthesia

Lower extremity	T12
Hip	T10
Prostate or bladder	T10
Testes	T6
Herniorraphy	T4
Intraabdominal	T4

fects. As a result, epidural blocks have become popular for postoperative pain relief.[38] Although local anesthetics or opioids can be used, a combination of the two produces the best results and the fewest complications.[6] Because these agents have a different site and mode of action, they have additive effects in regard to the analgesia produced, but their side effects tend to be dose related and are not additive. Thus, the dosage of each can be reduced while still retaining highly effective analgesia. Likewise, the lower doses required when used in combination reduce the incidence of serious complications, such as hypotension or respiratory depression.

Relief of Chronic Pain

The introduction of epidural opioids has had a dramatic effect, particularly for the management of cancer pain. Implantable systems that require small volumes of injectate are now available. The judicious addition of local anesthetic drugs improves otherwise incomplete analgesia without resorting to large doses of opioids. Epidural injection of local anesthetic together with steroids is popular in the management of chronic back pain, but its long-term effectiveness has been challenged. Finally, many painful conditions (e.g., phantom limb pain) are thought to benefit from nerve blockade for several days. The epidural route has many advantages for such a strategy, with either intermittent bolus injections or continuous infusions.

CONTRAINDICATIONS FOR EPIDURAL BLOCKADE

The few absolute contraindications to epidural anesthesia are listed in Box 60-1. Disc herniation or back pain does not preclude epidural anesthesia, although the level of disc herniation usually is avoided. The presence of neurologic disease, such as multiple sclerosis, is not a contraindication because there is no evidence that such conditions are worsened by epidural blockade, although many anesthesiologists avoid epidural anesthesia in these patients because postoperative exacerbation of an existing neurologic problem is possible.

BOX 60-1
CONTRAINDICATIONS TO EPIDURAL ANESTHESIA

Absolute

Patient refusal
Coagulopathy
Infection at site

Relative

Hypovolemia
Sepsis
Preexisting neurologic disease

COMPARISON OF EPIDURAL AND SPINAL BLOCKADE

Although there are obvious similarities between epidural and spinal blockade, there are several clinically important differences.

Spinal blockade is achieved by the diffusion of local anesthetic in the cerebrospinal fluid (CSF) after injection. Epidural blockade is achieved by the local anesthetic drug bathing the spinal nerves. With spinal anesthesia, the dose of drug and its baricity are more important than the volume of injectate, whereas with epidural anesthesia, the volume injected is the main determinant of spread.

In the subarachnoid space, multiple rootlets unite into roots that join to form a mixed spinal nerve as they pierce the dura and enter the epidural space. Thus, a single spinal nerve is derived from 10 or more small rootlets. These rootlets together with the spinal cord itself have only a thin covering of connective tissue (the pia mater), which provides little barrier to the entry of local anesthetic drug. In the epidural space, the spinal nerves, which are much larger than the rootlets, have a much thicker covering derived from the arachnoid and dura maters; this covering offers a considerable impediment to penetration by local anesthetic drugs.

The exact site of action of local anesthetic drugs injected into the epidural space is disputed, although the mixed spinal nerves (or the anterior and posterior roots if they have not joined before leaving the subarachnoid space) appear to be the prime targets. Drug can penetrate into the CSF and be available for diffusion into the rootlets and into the spinal cord, or it can travel in the epidural space and diffuse across the dura to reach the spinal cord.[8] At the upper limit of its spread, there is little gradation between the blocked and the unblocked nerves because there is little dilution of the drug as it spreads during injection. With spinal blockade, there is a decrease of local anesthetic concentration as the drug diffuses through the CSF. As a result, it is relatively easy to show a difference between pinprick and touch over the upper two or three segments of a spinal block.

Because of the different sensitivities of nerve fibers (autonomic, sensory, and motor) to local anesthetics, it is possible to produce a differential block by choosing an appropriate concentration of drug. For example, the pain of labor can be reduced with minimal or no motor blockade. This is relatively easy to achieve with epidural anesthesia, but more difficult with spinal blockade. Conversely, total neural blockade of the spinal nerves is much easier to achieve with spinal than with epidural blockade (Box 60-2).

PERIOPERATIVE MANAGEMENT

As with any anesthetic, patients considered for epidural blockade are seen preoperatively to assess their physical sta-

BOX 60-2
EPIDURAL VERSUS SPINAL ANESTHESIA

Advantages to spinal anesthesia

- Quick onset
- Technically easier to perform
- Excellent sacral anesthesia

Advantages to epidural anesthesia

- Lower incidence of hypotension
- Unlimited duration
- Able to use for postoperative analgesia
- Less risk of headache

tus and the appropriateness of the procedure. The procedure and possible complications are explained to obtain informed consent. The patient's spine is inspected for evidence of infection, previous surgery, or scoliosis (which may make the procedure technically more difficult). Premedication is administered at the discretion of the anesthesiologist.

Epidural anesthesia is administered with appropriate resuscitation equipment immediately available. This equipment includes a means for positive pressure ventilation, a source of oxygen, and suction. An IV catheter is placed before starting (except for epidural steriod injection), and monitoring is similar to general anesthesia.

If a patient is to remain conscious, the whole surgical team is made aware and conducts themselves accordingly. Sedation, consisting of a benzodiazepine or opioid or both, is used at the discretion of the anesthesiologist. Benzodiazepines are popular, especially if the patient appears nervous. Because these drugs have no analgesic properties, they are not useful by themselves if a patient complains of pain. Opioids are analgesic and sedative. Opioids and benzodiazepines in combination possess synergistic respiratory depressant effects.[3]

Combined general anesthesia with epidural anesthesia is appropriate for many patients. This technique offers advantages for patients who prefer to be asleep, and it speeds the preparation for surgery because it is not necessary to await complete blockade. Positioning, skin cleaning, and draping can all be done on the unconscious patient during the development of the block. Before induction of general anesthesia, the level of blockade can be checked to confirm that the epidural catheter is positioned correctly and that the block is bilateral. By using epidural blockade, intraoperative narcotic requirements are decreased because the epidural block provides excellent analgesia. Epidural blockade is an effective technique for producing induced hypotension. Combining epidural block with general anesthesia avoids the nausea and vomiting that conscious patients sometimes experience with hypotension. Finally, if the procedure is prolonged, the patient remains comfortable without risking oversedation.

Hypotension is not uncommon and usually is easily managed. The etiology for the hypotension is sympathetic blockade with vasodilation in the lower extremities. Although somewhat controversial, most clinicians believe that the severity of hypotension can be lessened by the previous administration of IV fluids to increase the intravascular volume,[39] although large volumes of fluid may not be desirable in certain patients who may have trouble mobilizing this fluid once the block recedes. In these patients, IV vasopressors may be a better choice. The vasopressors most commonly used are ephedrine, an indirect alpha and beta receptor agonist, and phenlyephrine, an alpha-agonist.

Like all patients after major surgery, the blood pressure can be labile for 1 or 2 hours postoperatively, and special care is necessary when moving the patient from the operating table. The patient should remain in the postanesthesia care unit until the block begins to recede with evidence of returning motor function and a decreasing sensory level. If desired, the epidural block can be continued for postoperative analgesia.

COMPLICATIONS

Complications occur not only intraoperatively, but also postoperatively. Very infrequently, the adverse effects can be permanent. The majority of serious complications can be avoided. If diagnosed promptly and managed quickly, the possibility of permanent sequelae is lessened.

Local Anesthetic Toxicity

The large doses of local anesthetic used in epidural anesthesia impose the risk of systemic toxicity. Immediate toxicity results from direct intravascular administration of local anesthetic, whereas delayed toxicity follows systemic uptake of local anesthetics.

The epidural space contains a large venous plexus made up of thin walled veins. Although these veins may be entered by the epidural needle, it is more common for the plastic epidural catheter to do so. **The fact that blood does not appear in the catheter during aspiration does not guarantee that the catheter is not intravascular, because the vein may collapse with aspiration. The appropriate use of test doses before every injection lessens the risk of intravascular injection.**

In regard to delayed toxicity, drugs are readily absorbed from the epidural space, achieving a peak plasma concentration in 20 to 30 minutes.[1,59] This is much slower than in patients receiving an intravascular injection, and very few toxic reactions have been reported as a result of absorption. The addition of epinephrine to the local anesthetic reduces the uptake of local anesthetic from the epidural space.[19]

Signs and symptoms

Because the brain is more sensitive to local anesthetic drugs than the heart, the early signs of toxicity are related to the central nervous system. Symptoms consist of

lightheadedness, dizziness, a metallic taste in the mouth, numbness of the tongue or lips, slurred speech, or tinnitus. These symptoms occur with doses lower than those required to cause unconsciousness and seizures. Seizures are typical grand mal epileptiform convulsions. Management consists of halting the injection and hyperventilation with 100% oxygen. If the seizure does not terminate with ventilation, IV diazepam or thiopental is indicated.

Usually central nervous system toxicity is exhibited before cardiovascular toxicity. Cardiovascular effects occur at high plasma concentrations. Toxic doses inhibit phase 0 depolarization of the cardiac conduction cycle.[13] Conduction and contractility are affected. Hypotension, bradycardia, or ventricular tachycardia may occur. Management consists of supporting the circulation until the concentration of the local anesthetic decreases.

The lipid-soluble and highly protein bound local anesthetics, such as bupivacaine, tend to cause serious arrythmias, particularly ventricular tachycardia,[18] which is thought to result from their pharmacokinetic behavior in the myocardium. Like other local anesthetics such as lidocaine, they rapidly gain access to the myocardial calls ("fast in"). Unlike lidocaine, they leave the myocardium slowly ("slow out") because of protein binding.

Cardiovascular toxicity is likely only if a large dose of drug is given by rapid IV injection. The appearance and diagnosis of central nervous system toxicity during a slow injection allows the administration to be stopped before dangerous cardiovascular effects develop.

Unintentional Subarachnoid Injection

Given the relatively large doses of local anesthetic drug required for epidural block compared with spinal anesthesia, an accidental subarachnoid injection resulting in a high or total spinal block always is a potential risk. If the subarachnoid space is entered with a large-bore epidural needle, the escape of CSF usually becomes obvious. An incompletely inserted needle bevel may be confusing. It also is possible to insert a multiorifice catheter, with the distal hole subarachnoid and the proximal holes epidural. Catheters properly positioned in the epidural space have been reported to rarely migrate intrathecally. **The steps used to avoid a massive intrathecal injection are identical to those used to avoid an IV injection: aspiration, the use of an adequate test dose, and careful titration of the epidural dose of local anesthetic.** A sufficient intrathecal test method consists of administering local anesthetic, lidocaine, 40 to 60 mg, or bupivacaine, 8 to 10 mg, and waiting 3 to 5 minutes before administering more local anesthetic.

Signs and symptoms

Sensory levels higher than T2 are frequently associated with dyspnea. Absence of proprioceptive input from the afferent fibers from the abdomen and intercostals contributes to the sensation of dyspnea. If the C3, C4, and C5 segments are affected, paralysis of the diaphragm may occur and, combined with intercostal paralysis, leads to respiratory arrest. If the local anesthetic enters the cranium intrathecally through the foramen magnum, blockade of the cranial nerves—a "total spinal"—occurs. With such a high level and the absence of sympathetics, profound hypotension is typical.

Management of a high or total spinal consists of positive pressure ventilation. A vasopressor is required to maintain arterial pressure. Endotracheal intubation may be needed if the patient is at risk of aspiration or if the patient requires prolonged assisted ventilation. The duration of a high spinal blockade depends on the local anesthetic used.

Unintentional Subdural Injection

The subdural space is located between the dura and arachnoid mater. Although uncommon (0.1%), unintentional injection into the subdural space is possible.[48] Characteristics of a subdural block include a weak patchy block spread mainly in a cephalad direction, severe hypotension, and a high level of blockade from a small amount of local anesthetic. Management is directed to the maintenance of adequate respiratory and circulatory function.

Postdural Puncture Headache

One of the most common complications of epidural blockade is accidental dural puncture. It occurs in approximately 1% of all attempted epidural blockades. If the dura and arachnoid maters are punctured with the epidural needle, three courses of action are possible: (1) A subarachnoid catheter may be placed, and the patient treated as if given a continuous spinal anesthetic. All involved caregivers should be made aware the catheter is not epidural but subarachnoid. (2) A single dose of local anesthetic is administered to produce spinal anesthesia. (3) The needle is removed, and epidural anesthesia is attempted at another interspace. If this last route is chosen, higher levels of anesthesia should be expected because local anesthetic may gain access to the spinal cord through the dural puncture.[31] In these patients, it is especially important to fractionate the dose of local anesthetic, frequently checking the sensory level to prevent higher levels than desired.

The risk of headache after unintentional dural puncture with an epidural needle is great, approximately 80% in parturients with a 17-gauge needle. Headache caused by a dural puncture, postdural puncture headache (PDPH), was described by Bier in 1898. The postulated etiology is the leakage of CSF through the dural puncture hole into the epidural space (see Chapter 59). This leakage of fluid allows the brain and its supporting structures to sag, placing traction on the pain-sensitive vascular structures. The headache is strongly related to posture, being exacerbated in the upright position and relieved in the supine position. The pain may be frontal, occipital, or both, and it may be accompanied by visual or auditory symptoms. Although it may present immediately after dural puncture, it usually occurs 24 to 72 hours later.[34]

Management begins with conservative measures. IV or

oral hydration is believed to encourage CSF production and replace lost CSF. Because bedrest does not prevent the occurrence of headache, there is no routinely recommended time period for which a patient should remain supine after dural puncture. Oral or IV caffeine may be helpful.[11] Caffeine increases cerebral arteriolar resistance, decreases cerebral blood flow and volume, and decreases CSF pressure.

The most effective management for PDPH is the epidural blood patch. In 1960, Gormley noted that patients with "bloody" lumbar punctures had a decreased incidence of headache. He postulated that clotted blood covers the dural hole and prevents the leakage of CSF. He successfully showed that blood placed in the epidural space relieves the headache.[29] It is more likely that it works by increasing the CSF pressure by acting as a space filler in the epidural space. Its effect almost always is immediate in relieving the headache. Blood is a nonirritant substance that is slowly absorbed from the epidural space.[23] Indications for a blood patch include a postural headache that does not improve within 48 hours, a severe headache with associated nausea and vomiting, and diplopia (related to stretching of the sixth cranial nerve, which supplies the lateral rectus muscle of the eye). The incidence of success from the first blood patch has been observed to be as high as 96%; in a few patients, a second or third patch may be necessary. Main causes of failure of the blood patch are wrong diagnosis or improper placement of the patch. Some advocate the use of a prophylactic epidural blood patch if a dural puncture occurs and if an epidural catheter has been placed, whereas other investigators question its effectiveness. To perform an epidural blood patch, 10 to 20 ml of autologous blood is obtained aseptically and slowly injected into the epidural space. The most common complication is transient back pain and lower extremity pain.

Neurologic Damage

Prolonged or permanent nerve damage rarely occurs after epidural blockade. Neurologic damage can be divided into three types: mechanical, caused by needle trauma or hematoma formation; chemical, caused by the toxic effects of the injectate; or vascular.[32]

Trauma usually is confined to a nerve root, resulting in a radiculopathy for which the patient presents with a sensory deficit in a dermatomal distribution. The patient usually complains of a pain or a "shock" shooting to the lower extremity at the time of needle insertion or injection. Disruption of nerve fibers may lead to a prolonged neuropathy, but in the majority of patients, the pain and numbness resolve within a few weeks.

Spinal cord compression may result from an epidural hematoma or abscess. An epidural hematoma causes back pain with a progressive weakness and sensory deficit. Management involves immediate diagnosis by computed tomography or magnetic resonance imaging, followed by emergency decompressive laminectomy. A hematoma develops faster than an abscess, which can take several days to cause symptoms.

An epidural hematoma may be associated with anticoagulation perioperatively, but most cases have been reported as spontaneous occurrences in the absence of anticoagulation. Opinions differ, but there is support for proceeding with epidural blockade if the catheter is inserted before an anticoagulant is administered, assuming a normal coagulation screen.

Adhesive arachnoiditis results in sensory and motor deficits with chronic pain. The most important cause is the injection of an irritant solution, usually by mistake. Many substances have been injected accidentally into the epidural space with varying degrees of damage. The initial injection is painful, with a progressive loss of nerve function occurring over a period of hours or days.

A feared vascular injury is the anterior spinal artery syndrome, which causes a rapid, painless paraplegia. The exact cause is not well understood, although the tenuous arterial blood supply of the lower spinal cord is an important factor. Severe hypotension and clamping or retraction of the aorta during surgery have been implicated. Arteriovenous anomalies also may be important but can seldom be diagnosed before the block is performed.

KEY POINTS

- A proper knowledge of the spinal anatomy is essential to the successful use of epidural blockade.
- The epidural space can be entered at any part of the spine, but the risk to spinal cord trauma is the least at the lumbar level.
- The epidural space, that part of the spinal canal outside the dura mater, contains fat, the spinal nerves, and blood vessels that supply the spinal cord, spinal nerves, and vertebrae. Numerous veins have thin walls and are easily distended; therefore, unintentional cannulation is a distinct possibility.
- Local anesthetics injected into the epidural space not only reach the spinal nerves, but they also pass through the dura and arachnoid maters into the subarachnoid space to reach the roots and the spinal cord itself.
- The major circulatory effects of epidural anesthesia are related to sympathetic blockade.
- Epidural blockade can reduce cardiac output by three main mechanisms: (1) reducing venous return by removing sympathetic vasoconstriction to the lower extremities; (2) slowing the heart, requiring blockade of the upper five thoracic segments; and (3) reducing sympa-

thetic tone of the heart, thereby reducing myocardial contraction.

- Locating the epidural space with a needle allows the physician to identify the moment that the ligamentum flavum has been penetrated and to prevent further advancement through the dura and arachnoid maters. The most common method used is the "loss of resistance" technique.
- Although the relationship between spread and dosage is not linear, the volume of the injectate is an important determinate of the height of an epidural block.
- Drugs are readily absorbed from the epidural space, achieving a peak plasma concentration in 20 to 30 minutes, which is much slower than with intravascular injection, and few toxic reactions are related to absorption itself.
- Epidural opioids allows the amount of local anesthetic required and their associated complications to be decreased without decreasing the amount of analgesia. Side effects of epidural opioids include respiratory depression, pruritus, and sedation.
- Because of the relatively large doses of local anesthetic drugs required for epidural blockade, a test dose should be administered before injection. An appropriate test dose would detect an IV or subarachnoid catheter. Lidocaine with epinephrine is the most common test dose. With this test dose, an IV catheter would cause tachycardia and hypertension, and a subarachnoid catheter would result in a sensory and motor deficit of the lower extremities.
- One of the most common complications of epidural blockade is accidental dural puncture. It occurs in about 1% of all attempted epidural injections, and it may result in a headache, especially if the patient is young.
- Although rare, prolonged or permanent nerve damage can occur after epidural blockade.

KEY REFERENCES

Beilin Y, Bernstein HH, Zucker-Pinchoff B: The optimal distance that a multiorifice epidural catheter should be threaded into the epidural space, *Anesth Analg* 81:301, 1995.

Bromage PR: Mechanism of action of extradural analgesia, *Br J Anaesth* 47:199, 1975.

Butterworth JR, Strichartz GR: Molecular mechanisms of local anesthesia: a review, *Anesthesiology* 72:711, 1990.

Cushieri RJ, Morran CG, Howie JC, et al: Postoperative pain and pulmonary complications: comparison of three analgesic regimens, *Br J Surg* 72:495, 1985.

Kane RE: Neurologic deficits following epidural or spinal anesthesia, *Anesth Analg* 60:150, 1981.

McCrae AF, Wildsmith JAW: Prevention and treatment of hypotension during central neural block, *Br J Anaesth* 70:672, 1993.

Moore DC, Batra MS: The components of an effective test dose prior to epidural block, *Anesthesiology* 55:693, 1981.

Nishimura N, Kajimoto Y, Kabe T, et al: The effects of volume loading during epidural analgesia, *Resuscitation* 13: 31, 1985.

Yeager MP, Glass DD, Neff RK, et al: Epidural anesthesia and analgesia in high-risk surgical patients, *Anesthesiology* 66:729, 1987.

REFERENCES

1. Abdel-Salan AR, Vonwiller JB, Scott DB: Evaluation of etidocaine in extradural block, *Br J Anaesth* 47:1081, 1975.
2. Ahn H, Bronge H, Johansson K, et al: Effect of continuous postoperative epidural analgesia on intestinal motility, *Br J Surg* 75:1176, 1988.
3. Bailey PL, Pace NK, Ashburn MA, et al: Frequent hypoxemia and apnea after sedation with midazolam and fentanyl, *Anesthesiology* 73:826, 1990.
4. Beilin Y, Bernstein HH, Zucker-Pinchoff B: The optimal distance that a multiorifice epidural catheter should be threaded into the epidural space, *Anesth Analg* 81:301, 1995.
5. Blair MR: Cardiovascular pharmacology of local anesthetics, *Br J Anaesth* 47S:247, 1975.
6. Braid DP, Scott DB: The systemic absorption of local analgesic drugs, *Br J Anaesth* 37:394, 1965.
7. Bromage PR, Naquib M, El-Fagih S, et al: Epinephrine and fentanyl as adjuvants to 0.5% bupivacaine for epidural analgesia, *Reg Anesth* 14:189, 1989.
8. Bromage PR: Mechanism of action of extradural analgesia, *Br J Anaesth* 47:199–211, 1975.
9. Bromage PR: Spread of analgesic solutions in the epidural space and their site of action: a statistical study, *Br J Anaesth* 34:161, 1962.
10. Butterworth JR, Strichartz GR: Molecular mechanisms of local anesthesia: a review. *Anesthesiology* 72:711, 1990.
11. Carbaat PAT, van Grevel H: Lumbar puncture headache: controlled study on the preventive effect of 24 hour's bed rest, *Lancet* 2:1133–1135, 1981.
12. Cathelin MF: Une Novelle vige d'injection rachidienne. Methode des injections epidurales par le procede du canal sacre. Applications a l'homme, *C R Soc Biol (Paris)* 53:452, 1901.
13. Clarkson CW, Hohdieshen LM: Mechanism for bupivacaine depression of cardiac conduction: fast block of sodium channels during the action potential with slow recovery from block during diastole, *Anesthesiology* 62:396, 1985.
14. Coda BA, Brown MC, Schaffer R, et al: Pharmacology of epidural fentanyl, alfentanil, and sufentanil in volunteers, *Anesthesiology* 81:1149–1161, 1994.

15. Colonna-Romano P, Lingaraju N, et al: Epidural test dose: lidocaine 100 mg, not chloroprocaine is a symptomatic marker of IV injection in labouring parturients, *Can J Anaesth* 40:714, 1993.
16. Corning JL: Spinal anesthesia and local medication of the cord, *N Y J Med* 42:483, 1885.
17. Covino BG, Scott DB: *Handbook of epidural anaesthesia and analgesia,* Orlando, 1985, Grune & Stratton.
18. Covino BG: Toxicity of local anesthetics, *Adv Anesth* 3:37–65, 1986.
19. Craft JB, Epstein BS, Coakley CS: Effect of lidocaine with epinephrine versus lidocaine (plain) on induced labor, *Anesth Analg* 51: 243, 1972.
20. Cushieri RJ, Morran CG, Howie JC, et al: Postoperative pain and pulmonary complications: comparison of three analgesic regimens, *Br J Surg* 72:495, 1985.
21. Davies MJ, Bilbert BS, Mooney PJ, et al: Combined epidural and general anaesthesia versus general anaesthesia for abdominal aortic surgery: a prospective randomised trial, *Anesth Intensive Care* 21:790, 1993.
22. DeKock M, Crochet B, Morimont C, et al: Intravenous or epidural clonidine for intra- and post-operative analgesia, *Anesthesiology* 79:525, 1993.
23. DiGiovanni AJ, Dunbar BS: Epidural injections of autologous blood for postlumbar-puncture headache, *Anesth Analg* 49:268, 1970.
24. Eisenach J, Detweiler D, Hood D: Hemodynamic and analgesic actions of epidurally administered clonidine, *Anesthesiology* 78: 277, 1993.
25. Erdermir HA, Sopier LE, Sweet RB: Studies of the factors affecting peridural anesthesia, *Anesth Analg* 44:400, 1965.
26. Fink BR, Ansheim GM, Levy BA: Neural pharmacokinetics of epinephrine, *Anesthesiology* 48:263, 1978.
27. Galindo A, Hernandez J, Benauides O, et al: Quality of spinal extradural anaesthesia: the influence of spinal nerve root diameter, *Br J Anaesth* 47:41, 1955.
28. Goertz AW, Seeling W, Heinrich H, et al: Influence of high thoracic epidural anesthesia on left ventricular contractility assessed using end-systolic pressure-length relationship, *Acta Anaesth Scand* 37:38, 1993.
29. Gormley JB: Treatment of postspinal headache, *Anesthesiology* 21:565, 1960.
30. Grass JA: Sufentanil: clinical use as postoperative analgesia—epidural/intrathecal route, *J Pain Sympt Management* 7:271, 1992.
31. Hodgkinson R: Total spinal block after epidural injection into an interspace adjacent to an inadvertant dural perforation, *Anesthesiology* 55:593, 1981.
32. Kane RE: Neurologic deficits following epidural or spinal anesthesia, *Anesth Analg* 60:150, 1981.
33. Kerkkamp HE, Gielen MJ: Hemodynamic monitoring in epidural blockade: cardiovascular effects of 20 ml of 0.5% bupivacaine with and without epinephrine, *Reg Anesth* 15:137, 1990.
34. Lee JJ, Roberts RB: Paresis of the fifth cranial nerve following spinal anesthesia, *Anesthesiology* 49:217, 1978.
35. Leighton BL, Gross JB: Air: an effective indicator of intravenously located epidural catheters, *Anesthesiology* 71:648, 1989.
36. Lieberman JR, Huo MM, Hanway J, et al: The prevalence of deep venous thrombosis after total hip arthroplasty with hypotensive epidural anesthesia, *J Bone Joint Surg* 76: 341, 1994.
37. Liu SS, Carpenter RC, Mackey DC, et al: Effects of perioperative analgesia technique on rate of recovery after colon surgery, *Anesthesiology* 83:757, 1995.
38. Loper KA, Ready LB, Ness M: Epidural morphine provides greater pain relief than patient controlled intravenous morphine following cholecystectomy, *Anesth Analg* 69: 826, 1989.
39. McCrae AF, Wildsmith JAW: Prevention and treatment of hypotension during central neural block, *Br J Anaesth* 70:672, 1993.
40. Mellbring G, Dahlgren S, Reiz S: Thromboembolic complications after major abdominal surgery: effect of thoracic epidural analgesia, *Acta Chir Scand* 149:263, 1983.
41. Messih H: Epidural space pressures during pregnancy, *Anaesthesia* 36:775, 1981.
42. Mitchell D, Friedman RJ, Baker JD, et al: Prevention of thromboembolic disease following total knee arthroplasty. Epidural versus general anesthesia, *Clin Orthop* 269: 109, 1991.
43. Modig J, Borg J, Bagg I, et al: Role of extradural and of general anaesthesia in fibrinolysis and coagulation after total hip replacement, *Br J Anaesth* 55:625, 1983.
44. Mohan VK, Batra YK, Vaidyanathan S, et al: Analgesic and urodynamic effects of epidural meperidine and pentazocine—a comparative study, *Int J Clin Pharm Therapeut* 33: 34, 1993.
45. Moller RA, Covino BG: Cardiac electrophysiologic effects of lidocaine and bupivacaine, *Anesth Analg* 67:107, 1988.
46. Moore DC, Batra MS: The components of an effective test dose prior to epidural block, *Anesthesiology* 55:693, 1981.
47. Nishimura N, Kajimoto Y, Kabe T, et al: The effects of volume loading during epidural analgesia, *Resuscitation* 13:31, 1985.
48. Pavlin DJ, McDonald JS, Child B, et al: Acute subdural hematoma—an unusual sequela to lumbar puncture, *Anesthesiology* 52:166, 1980.
49. Petrikovsky BM, Cohen M, Tancer ML: Uterine and umbilical blood flow during cesarean section under epidural anesthesia, *Acta Obstet Gynecol Scand* 67:737, 1988.
50. Ploeckinger B, Ulm MR, Chalubinski K, et al: Epidural anaesthesia in labour: influence of surgical delivery rates, intrapartum fever and blood loss, *Gynecol Obstet Invest* 39:24, 1995.
51. Rao MV, Chari P, Malhotra SK, et al: Role of epidural analgesia on endocrine and metabolic responses to surgery, *Indian J Med Res* 92:13, 1990.
52. Rockeman MG, Seeling W, Brinkmann A: Analgesic and hemodynamic effects of epidural clonidine, clonidine/morphine, and morphine after pancreatic surgery—a double blinded study, *Anesth Analg* 80:869, 1995.
53. Saiah M, Borgeat A, Wilder-Smith OH, et al: Epidural-morphine-induced pruritus: propofol versus naloxone, *Anesth Analg* 78:110, 1994.
54. Salomaki TE, Leppaluoto J, Laitnen JO, et al: Epidural versus intravenous fentanyl for reducing hormonal, metabolic, and physiologic responses after thoracotomy, *Anesthesiology* 79:672, 1993.
55. Sechzer P, Abel L: Post-spinal analgesia headache treated with caffeine: evaluation with the demand method, *Curr Therap Res* 24:307, 1978.
56. Scott DB, McClure JH, Gias RM, et al: Effects of concentration of local anaesthetic drugs in extradural block, *Br J Anaesth* 52: 1033, 1980.
57. Sharrock NE, Mineo R, Urguhart B, et al: The effect of two levels of hypotension on intraoperative blood loss during total hip arthroplasty performed under lumbar epidural anesthesia, *Anesth Analg* 76:580, 1993.
58. Shir Y, Raja SN, Frank SM, et al: Intraoperative blood loss during radical retropubic prostatectomy: epidural versus general anesthesia, *Urology* 45:993, 1995.
59. Tucker GT, Mather LE: Clinical pharmacokinetics of local anaesthetics, *Clin Pharmacokinet* 4:241, 1979.
60. Urban BJ: Clinical observations suggesting a changing site of action during induction and recession of spinal and epidural anesthesia, *Anesthesiology* 39:496–503, 1973.
61. Yeager MP, Glass DD, Neff RK, et al: Epidural anesthesia and analgesia in high-risk surgical patients, *Anesthesiology* 66: 729–736, 1987.

CHAPTER 61

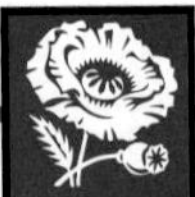

Plexus Anesthesia

ALON P. WINNIE
CARLOS D. FRANCO

Although regional blocks, when properly administered, may provide a safe and reliable form of anesthesia for many surgical procedures, they are frequently not used, even when indicated. Why? The most important reason is that, in the vast majority of cases, anesthesiologists select general anesthesia over regional because during their residency training they had insufficient experience with the techniques of regional anesthesia to develop the same confidence and expertise which they had acquired for the various general anesthetic techniques. Recent evidence indicates that the use of regional anesthesia in residency training programs has increased over the past decade (from 21.3% to 29.8%), but there is still wide variability among residency programs with respect to its use (as little as 2.8% in some programs and as much as 58.5% in others).[6] Furthermore, much of the overall increase is accounted for by more than double the use of epidural anesthesia, which increased from 7% to 16%, most likely because of the increasing involvement of residents in obstetrics and pain management. Unfortunately, during this same time, the use of nerve block anesthesia increased only from 5% to 7%, and this is still insufficient to develop the confidence and competence that will allow the choice of this form of anesthesia even when indicated. It has been clearly demonstrated that anesthesiologists trained in regional anesthesia continue to use regional techniques in practice.[3] Hopefully, the new "Minimum Clinical Experience Requirements" of the Residency Review Commitee for Anesthesiology, which includes a minimum of 40 peripheral blocks for surgery and 25 for pain, will improve the proficiency and confidence of graduating residents and will cause them to choose regional anesthesia more frequently in their practice. Such proficiency should be all the more important to anesthesiologists, because the majority of anesthesiologists prefer a block over general anesthesia for their own surgery.[2,5]

The second most important reason for the underuse of regional anesthesia is that surgeons have always felt that regional anesthesia is undesirable because the time required to perform blocks and the delay until the anesthesia is complete is excessive. Indeed, the traditional multiple-injection techniques *were* time consuming to perform, and these techniques *did* frequently result in a fairly high incidence of unsatisfactory anesethesia. As a result, supplemental general anesthesia was required, and the surgical schedule was delayed. The more recently developed single-injection techniques have simplified nerve block procedures, reduced the time necessary to carry them out, and enhanced the success rate. Because paresthesias are not *mandatory* with *many of these* techniques, the neurological complications have been reduced markedly.[16,26] Apparently, these developments *have* had a positive impact on the attitude of surgeons; in a recent survey, the vast majority of surgeons expressed a preference for regional anesthesia over general for themselves, if feasible.[11]

Of course, the greatest deterrent to the use of regional anesthesia is usually the patient. In a recent survey, only 31% of 800 patients preferred a local or regional over a general anesthetic.[15] Although 22% of the patients expressed a preference for a technique that allowed them to remain awake and aware throughout the procedure, many more patients preferred to be asleep. Interestingly, a very small percentage of the patients surveyed were concerned about the dangers of regional anesthesia. Patients with previous exposure to regional anesthesia continued to prefer regional anesthesia for subsequent surgery, implying that increased patient education about the benefits and desirability of regional anesthesia is extremely important. Obviously, all of the objections to regional anesthesia can be overcome if anesthesiologists are better trained in the various techniques of regional anesthesia, as the resultant increase in successful blocks will convince surgeons of the value of regional anesthesia (when indicated), and ultimately the surgeons, anesthesiologists, and patients will agree that, when indicated, regional anesthesia *is* a highly desirable form of anesthesia. However, there must be no apparent disagreement between the surgeon and the anesthesiologist if the patient is going to accept this form of anesthesia. If a patient fears possible pain or awareness during the administration of a block and during the operation, this apprehension may be alleviated: (1) by appropriate counseling by the surgeon; (2) by the reinforcement of this information by the anesthesiologist on the preoperative visit, when the details of a particular technique can be explained; (3) by the judicious choice of adjunctive preoperative and intraoperative medications to provide tranquility, amnesia, and sleep; and (4) by explaining that one of the advantages of regional anesthesia is the extension of analgesia postoperatively to control postoperative pain. If all of these measures are observed, it is the rare patient who will not "prefer" regional anesthesia, and as alluded to above, once a patient has experienced a "successful" regional anesthetic, patients often request regional anesthesia, when appropriate, in the future.[15] Appropriate technical expertise begins with a complete understanding of the anatomy, followed by adequate clinical experience during the residency training.

THE CONCEPT OF PLEXUS ANESTHESIA

If all regional techniques could be carried out by a single injection, as is done with spinal and epidural anesthesia, then most, if not all, of the objections to regional anesthesia by surgeons, anesthesiologists, and patients would be overcome. By its very simplicity, a single-injection technique minimizes the degree of skill and experience required to perform a successful block, markedly reduces the time required to perform a successful block, and enhances its safety because the incidence of complications such as intravascular injection and postinjection neuropathy is known to be related to the number of injections. Obviously, it is also preferable to the patient if one "needle stick" can replace many.

The concept of "plexus anesthesia" was introduced nearly 30 years ago to provide a system of single-injection techniques for blocking all of the major plexuses, cervical, brachial, lumbar, and sacral. The concept is based on the fact that all of the plexuses, at some point in their formation and/or distribution, pass between two muscles and hence may be considered to be invested by the fascia of these muscles.[20,22,24,25] Thus, at this point, each plexus lies in a potential "interfascial compartment," so if this compartment can be identified and entered by a needle, the plexus can be blocked by a single injection of an appropriate volume of local anesthetic. With these techniques, just as with spinal and epidural techniques, the local anesthetic solution, rather than the needle, "seeks out the nerves of the plexus," obviating the multiple injections required by earlier techniques.

PLEXUS ANESTHESIA FOR UPPER EXTREMITY SURGERY

Anatomic Considerations

The brachial plexus is derived from the anterior primary divisions of the fifth, sixth, seventh, and eighth cervical spinal nerves and the first thoracic nerve, with frequent contributions from the fourth cervical and second thoracic nerves (Fig. 61-1). After leaving their respective intervertebral foramina, the roots of the plexus travel laterally in the "gutters" atop the cervical transverse processes, pass between the anterior and posterior tubercles at the tips of the transverse processes, and then descend toward the first rib, above which the roots of C5 and C6 fuse to form the superior trunk of the plexus, the roots of C8 and T1 fuse to form the infe-

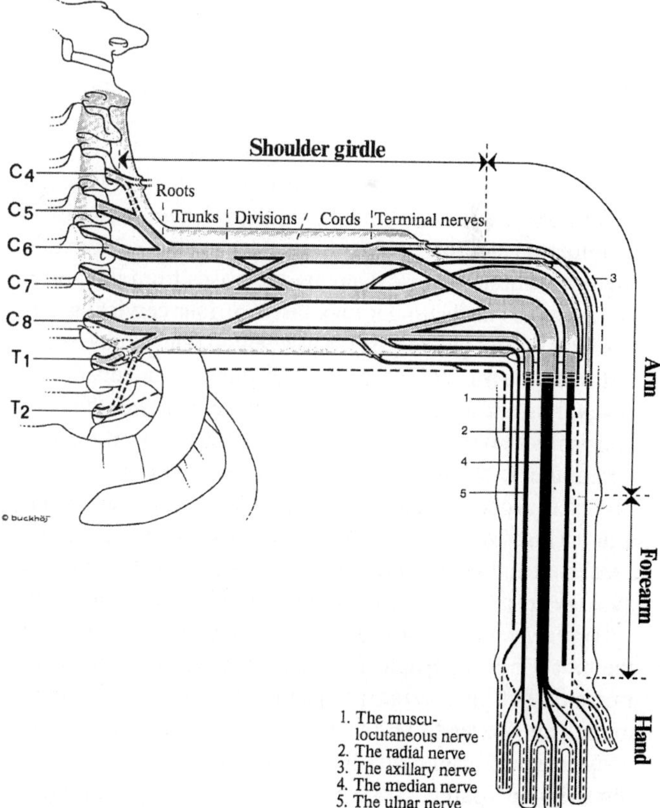

Fig. 61-1. Schematic representation of the formation and distribution of the brachial plexus and the level at which the various components leave the sheath. (From Winnie AP: *Plexus anesthesia,* vol 1, Philadelphia, 1990, WB Saunders and Mediglobe SA, Fribourg, Switzerland. Used with permission.)

rior trunk, and the root of C7 continues between these two trunks as the middle trunk of the plexus. It is important clinically to appreciate that these three trunks are "stacked" on top of one another as they cross the first rib, not one behind the other as depicted in so many textbooks of anesthesia.[12] Then, under cover of the clavicle, the fibers within the trunks regroup to form the six divisions of the plexus—three anterior and three posterior.

The divisions are important because the destination of all the fibers contained therein is determined at this level; the fibers within the three anterior divisions (after regrouping one last time) provide the nerves that innervate the anterior surface of the upper extremity and shoulder girdle and the fibers in the posterior divisions innervate the posterior surface. Then, as the plexus emerges from under the clavicle, the divisions have regrouped to form the three cords of the plexus; the anterior divisions provide the fibers that form the medial and lateral cords, and the posterior divisions provide the fibers that form the posterior cord. Finally, it is from the cords that the terminal nerves of the brachial plexus are derived. This is accomplished in a very "schematic" fashion in that each cord, before terminating as or contributing to a major nerve, gives off another major branch. Thus, the posterior cord gives off the axillary nerve before continuing into the arm as the radial nerve; the lateral cord gives off the musculocutaneous nerve before providing the lateral head of the median nerve; and the medial cord gives rise to the ulnar nerve before providing the medial head of the median nerve. In addition, just proximal to the point where the ulnar nerve leaves the medial cord, this cord gives rise to the medial brachial cutaneous nerve and the medial antibrachial cutaneous nerve, in that order.

To apply the concept of "plexus anesthesia" to brachial plexus block, an understanding of the perineural anatomy is as important as (or even more important than) the neural anatomy. The middle scalene muscle arises from the posterior tubercles of the upper two, three, or four cervical vertebrae and inserts on the first rib just behind (and in close contact with) the trunks (Fig. 61-2). The anterior scalene muscle arises from the anterior tubercles of the upper two, three, or four cervical transverse processes, descends toward the first rib parallel to the middle scalene muscle, and inserts on the rib just in front of (and in close contact with) the subclavian artery (Fig. 61-3). Thus, the two scalene muscles form a "scalene sandwich" that contains the brachial plexus. The analogy to a sandwich is an appropriate one, because the space between the scalene muscles, like the space between the bread in a sandwich, is very narrow in the anteroposterior axis but very extensive in the vertical and horizontal axes. This proves to be of great clinical significance to the anesthesiologist who wishes to carry out a brachial plexus block above the clavicle (see later discussion of techniques).

Because the roots and trunks of the brachial plexus are "sandwiched" between the anterior and middle scalene muscles, they are invested by the fascia surrounding these muscles (i.e., the scalene fascia derived from the prevertebral fascia). Furthermore, when the neurovascular bundle passes over the first rib and under the clavicle, it invaginates the scalene (or prevertebral) fascia, taking it along as a tubular investment of the neurovascular bundle in the axilla and forming the axillary perivascular space, a lateral extension of the subclavian perivascular space. The axillary perivascular space and the

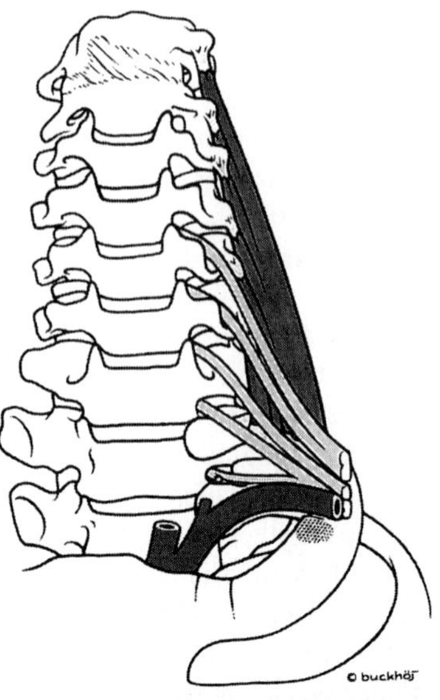

Fig. 61-2. Middle scalene muscle, in front of which the five roots of the plexus combine to form the three trunks, functions as the posterior wall of the interscalene compartment. (From Winnie AP: *Plexus anesthesia,* vol 1, Philadelphia, 1990, WB Saunders and Mediglobe SA, Fribourg, Switzerland. Used with permission.)

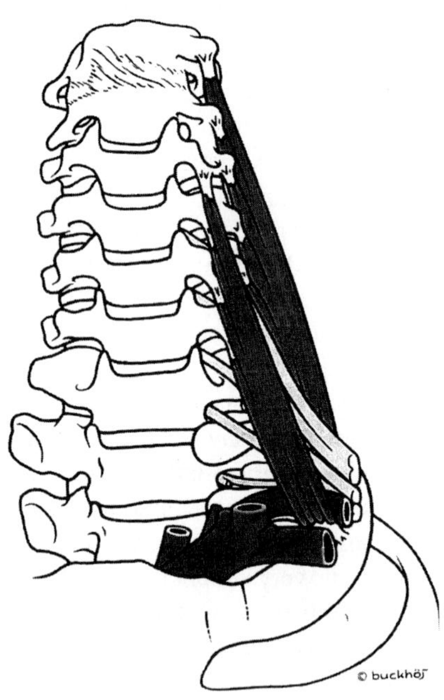

Fig. 61-3. Anterior scalene muscle functions as the anterior wall of the interscalene compartment. The fascia of the middle and anterior scalene muscles form a "sheath" around the plexus above the level of the first rib and clavicle. (From Winnie AP: *Plexus anesthesia,* vol 1, Philadelphia, 1990, WB Saunders and Mediglobe SA, Fribourg, Switzerland. Used with permission.)

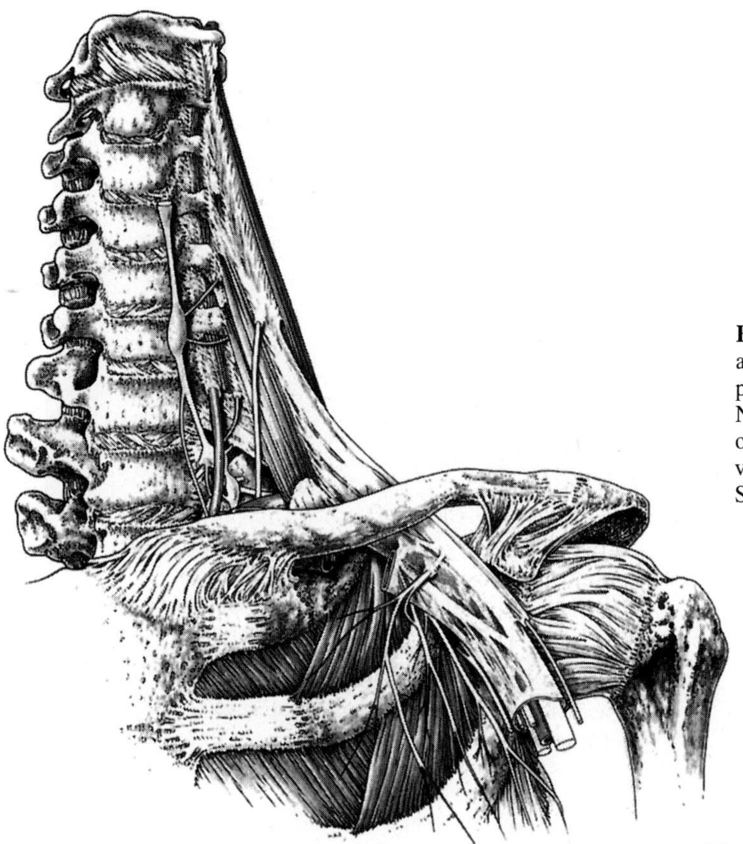

Fig. 61-4. Fascial investment of the brachial plexus forms a continuous perineural and perivascular space around the plexus from the intervertebral foramina to the distal axilla. Note that the axillary sheath is a lateral, tubular extension of the scalene fascia. (From Winnie AP: *Plexus anesthesia,* vol 1, Philadelphia, 1990, WB Saunders and Mediglobe SA, Fribourg, Switzerland. Used with permission.)

plexus contained therein terminate in the distal axilla, ending as they began, namely, sandwiched between two muscles, the coracobrachialis muscle superiorly and the long head of the triceps muscle inferiorly. In the axilla, the neurovascular bundle runs in a protective "valley," the walls of which are formed by the two muscles mentioned previously—the floor being formed by the shaft, neck, and head of the humerus.

The entire brachial plexus does not stay within the axillary perivascular space as the neurovascular bundle traverses the axilla toward the upper arm. The musculocutaneous nerve leaves the axillary perivascular space high in the axilla and immediately enters the coracobrachialis muscle, within which it travels throughout its entire length, giving off its motor branches to the powerful flexors of the forearm. Just above the elbow, it leaves the coracobrachialis muscle and travels in the subcutaneous tissue just lateral to the biceps tendon to become the lateral antibrachial cutaneous nerve. This is important because the local anesthetic injected into the axillary sheath must be injected in a volume sufficient to reach the level where the musculocutaneous nerve lies within the sheath, or the flexors of the forearm will not be blocked and the entire lateral aspect of the forearm will not be anesthetized. In addition, the axillary nerve leaves the sheath at a similar level, as do the intercostobrachial and medial brachial cutaneous nerves. These nerves must be blocked if a tourniquet is to be used, or the patient simply will not tolerate the tourniquet. The axillary nerve is blocked by a volume sufficient to reach the musculocutaneous nerve, and the intercostobrachial and medial brachial cutaneous nerves can be blocked by simply depositing a small amount of local anesthetic just superficial to the axillary arterial pulse (see later discussion of techniques).

In summary, the brachial plexus is surrounded by a fascia, which forms a perineural and perivascular space that extends from the intervertebral foramina to the distal axilla (Fig. 61-4). Therefore, just as with peridural techniques, a single injection of a local anesthetic can provide anesthesia of the entire brachial plexus, the extent of which depends upon the level of injection and the volume of local anesthetic injected at that level. Extending the analogy of perivascular techniques of brachial plexus block to peridural techniques, an axillary perivascular brachial block is the "caudal anesthetic of the upper extremity," the subclavian perivascular technique of brachial plexus block is the "lumbar epidural of the upper extremity," and the interscalene technique is the "thoracic epidural of the upper extremity."

Technical Considerations

The three techniques most frequently used to provide anesthesia in the distribution of the brachial plexus are the interscalene, the subclavian perivascular, and the axillary perivascular techniques of brachial plexus block.

Interscalene technique

This technique of brachial plexus block[20] is carried out as follows. The patient is placed in the dorsal recumbent position with the head turned somewhat to the side opposite that to be blocked. The block is carried out at the C6 level, which is determined by simply extending a line laterally from the cricoid cartilage (Fig. 61-5). After careful explanation of the procedure, the patient is asked to elevate the head slightly to bring the clavicular head of the sternocleidomastoid muscle into prominence. The anesthesiologist then places his or her index finger and middle finger immediately behind the lateral edge of the muscle and instructs the patient to relax. As the sternocleidomastoid muscle relaxes, the palpating fingers will actually move medially behind this muscle. The palpating fingers are now rolled laterally across the belly of the anterior scalene muscle until the interscalene groove—the groove between the anterior and middle scalene muscles—is encountered. With both the index finger and middle fingers in the interscalene groove, a 22-gauge, $1\frac{1}{2}$-inch, short-bevel needle is inserted between the fingers at the level of C6 in a direction that is perpendicular to the skin in every plane (i.e., mostly mesiad but slightly dorsad and slightly caudad) (Figs. 61-6 and 61-7). The needle is advanced slowly until a paresthesia is

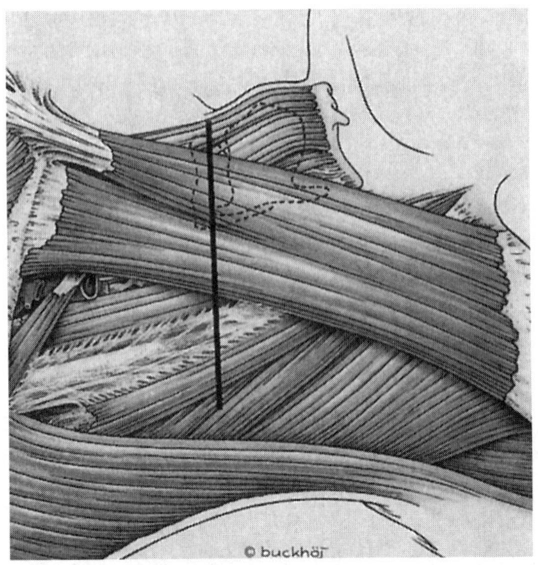

Fig. 61-5. The first step in carrying out the interscalene technique of brachial plexus block is to determine the level of C6 by extending a line laterally from the cricoid cartilage. (From Winnie AP: *Plexus anesthesia,* vol 1, Philadelphia, 1990, WB Saunders and Mediglobe SA, Fribourg, Switzerland. Used with permission.)

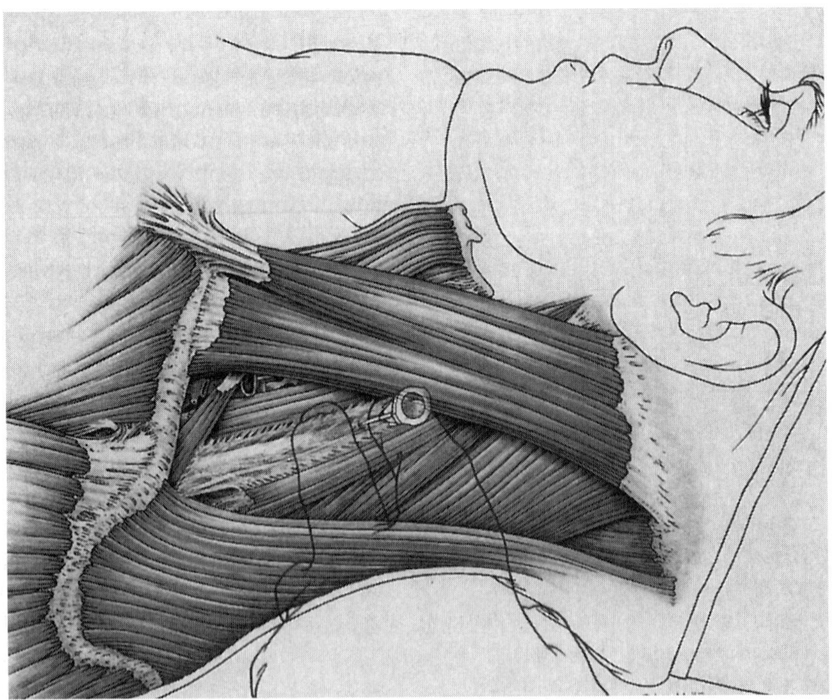

Fig. 61-6. After rolling the index and middle fingers laterally across the belly of the anterior scalene muscle to the interscalene groove, the needle is inserted between the fingers in a direction that is perpendicular to the skin in every plane. (From Winnie AP: *Plexus anesthesia,* vol 1, Philadelphia, 1990, WB Saunders and Mediglobe SA, Fribourg, Switzerland. Used with permission.)

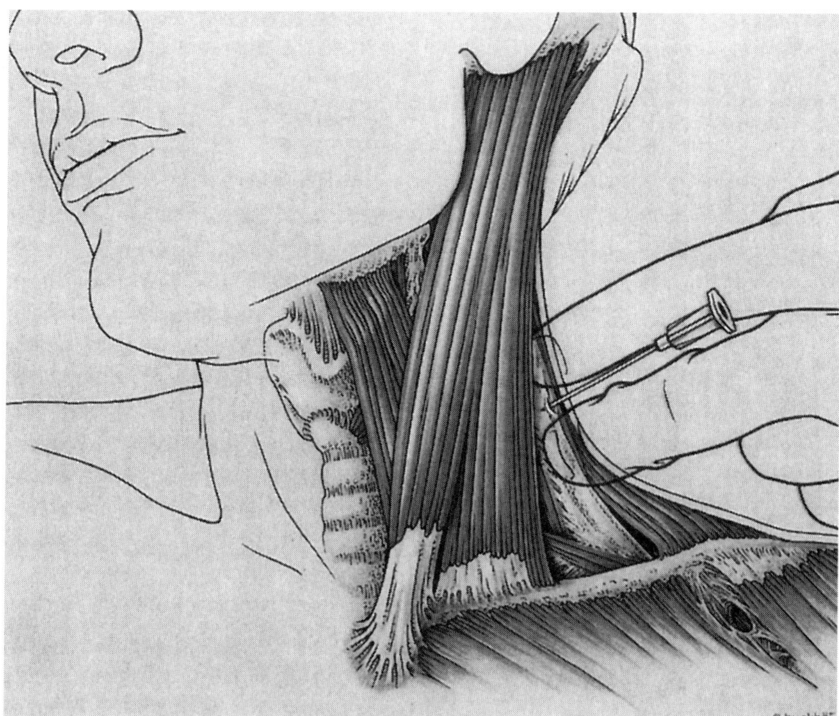

Fig. 61-7. View from the front shows that the properly directed needle has a slightly caudad direction, which is essential for safety. (From Winnie AP: *Plexus anesthesia,* vol 1, Philadelphia, 1990, WB Saunders and Mediglobe SA, Fribourg, Switzerland. Used with permission.)

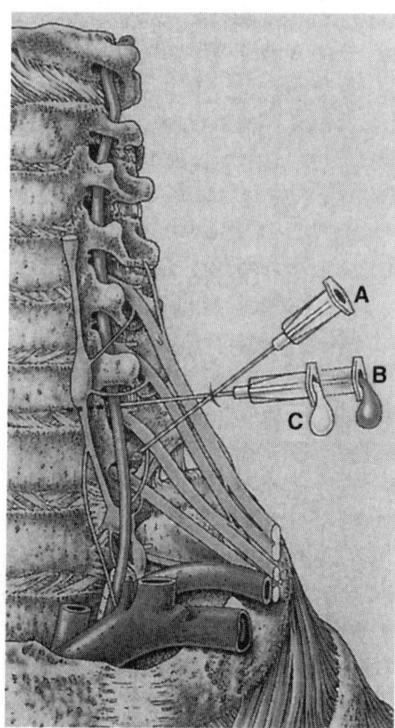

Fig. 61-8. Slight caudad direction (A) will cause the needle to encounter bone if it misses the roots of the plexus. A more horizontally directed needle is free to advance past the tip of the transverse process and enter the vertebral vessels (B) or even the subarachnoid space (C). (From Winnie AP: *Plexus anesthesia,* vol 1, Philadelphia, 1990, WB Saunders and Mediglobe SA, Fribourg, Switzerland. Used with permission.)

elicited or until a transverse process is encountered. The patient must be instructed to say "stop" when he or she feels an electric shock to the arm and to tell the anesthesiologist where the paresthesia is experienced. Only a paresthesia below the shoulder is acceptable. The reason is that the only sensory branch from the plexus above the clavicle is the suprascapular nerve. Thus, a paresthesia to the shoulder could result from stimulation of the suprascapular nerve outside the sheath. If bone is contacted without producing a paresthesia, the U-shaped end of the transverse process is walked millimeter by millimeter until a paresthesia is evoked. A slightly caudad direction of the needle is absolutely essential to the safety of the interscalene technique (Fig. 61-8). It assures the anesthesiologist that, if the needle misses the roots of the plexus, it will be stopped by bone (Fig. 61-8*A*). If the needle is inserted horizontally in a directly mesiad direction, it may penetrate the vertebral vessels or enter the epidural space or spinal canal (Fig. 61-8*B* and *C*). The likelihood of eliciting paresthesias on the first insertion of the needle is increased with this technique if one remembers that the roots of the brachial plexus lie slightly closer to the middle than to the anterior scalene muscle, so when the needle is inserted between the palpating fingers into the interscalene groove, it should be inserted and advanced slightly closer to the middle than to the anterior scalene muscle. After a paresthesia has been obtained distal to the shoulder and verifying that the needle is

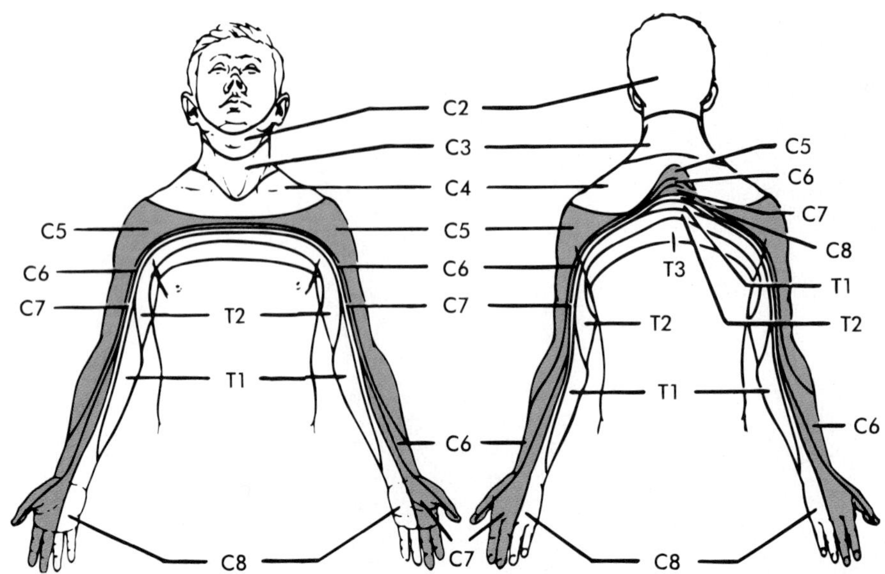

Fig. 61-9. Injection of 20 ml into the interscalene space may be insufficient to diffuse down to C8 and T1, so the skin in the distribution of these roots may not be anesthetized with this volume.

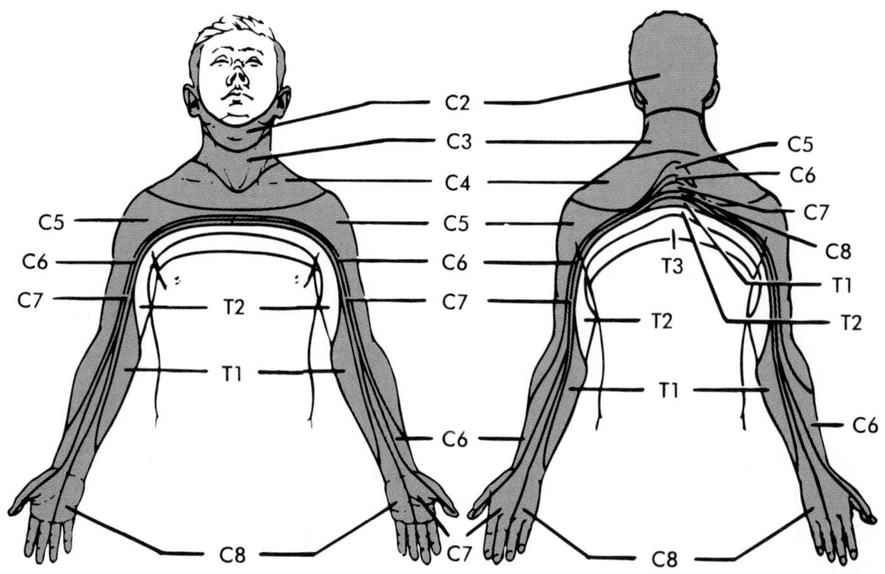

Fig. 61-10. Injection of 40 ml into the interscalene space is usually sufficient to anesthetize all of the roots of the brachial plexus and, in addition, all of the cervical plexus.

not intravascular (by aspirating for blood in several quadrants), an appropriate volume of local anesthetic is injected with repeated aspiration throughout the injection. Because the injection is being made at such a high level, 20 ml is frequently inadequate to diffuse far enough inferiorly to reach the lower roots of the plexus and, as a result, anesthesia in the distribution of C8 and T1 is not infrequently delayed and occasionally absent with this volume (Fig. 61-9). In most patients, an injection of 40 ml of local anesthetic will fill the entire interscalene space from the transverse processes of the upper cervical vertebrae down to the cupola of the lung. Therefore, although anesthesia in the distribution of C8 and T1 may be somewhat delayed as compared with other techniques, a 40-ml injection into the interscalene space will usually provide anesthesia not only of the entire brachial plexus but of the cervical plexus as well (Fig. 61-10). If anesthesia in the distribution of the cervical plexus is not necessary for the surgical procedure, firm digital pressure applied superiorly throughout the interscalene injection will inhibit cephalad flow and promote caudad flow of the local anesthetic, thus reducing the volume of anesthetic necessary to provide complete anesthesia of the entire brachial plexus. With this technique of brachial plexus block, as with any other, the intercostobrachial and

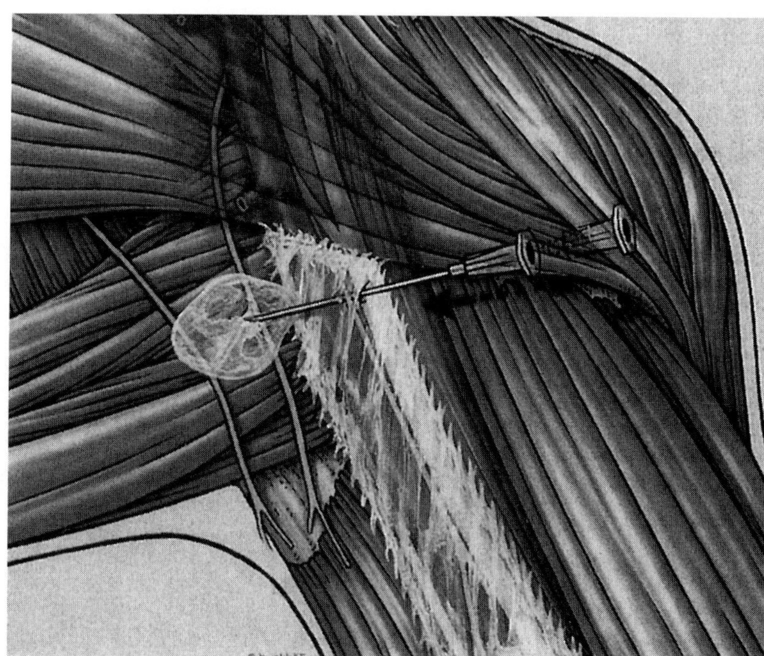

Fig. 61-11. When performing any of the perivascular techniques of brachial plexus block, a few milliliters of local anesthetic must be injected subcutaneously superficial to the arterial pulse to block the intercostobrachial and medial brachial cutaneous nerves to allow the use of a pneumatic tourniquet. (From Winnie AP: *Plexus anesthesia,* vol 1, Philadelphia, 1990, WB Saunders and Mediglobe SA, Fribourg, Switzerland. Used with permission.)

medial brachial cutaneous nerves must be blocked separately by the subcutaneous injection of a few milliliters of local anesthetic over the axillary artery pulse if a tourniquet is to be used during the surgical procedure (Fig. 61-11). Because the local anesthetic is injected into the upper part of the brachial plexus with the interscalene technique of brachial plexus block, obviously it becomes the technique of choice for operation on the upper arm and shoulder. However, if the clinical situation indicates, interscalene brachial plexus block can be used with large volumes of local anesthetic and firm digital pressure for operation on all parts of the upper extremity.

Subclavian perivascular technique

This technique[22] is carried out as follows: the patient is placed in the dorsal recumbent position with the head turned somewhat to the side opposite that to be injected. The patient is asked to lift the head off the table slightly to bring the clavicular head of the sternocleidomastoid muscle into prominence; then the index finger is placed immediately behind or posterior to the lateral border of the sternocleidomastoid muscle at the level of C6, which is lateral from the cricoid cartilage (see Fig. 61-5). The patient is now told to put his or her head back on the table. As the taut sternocleidomastoid muscle relaxes, the palpating finger actually moves medially and the fingernail on the palpating finger almost disappears behind the sternocleidomastoid muscle. The palpating finger is now rolled laterally across the belly of the anterior scalene muscle until it encounters the interscalene groove (Fig. 61-12). When the interscalene groove has been identified, the palpating finger is moved inferiorly along the groove as far as it can be palpated; with the finger still in the groove and possibly on the artery, a $1^1/_2$-inch, 22-gauge, short-bevel needle is inserted just above the palpating finger in a direction that is directly caudad but not mesiad or dorsad (Figs. 61-13 and 61-14). During the insertion and advancement of the needle, it is important that the hub of the properly directed needle actually lie against the skin of the neck. With this technique, the needle must be held between the thumb and forefinger or forefingers, because there is no room between the hub of the needle and the neck for the anesthesiologist to use the traditional pencil grip. The needle is advanced slowly and directly caudad until a paresthesia below the shoulder confirms that the needle lies within the subclavian perivascular space. The trunks of the brachial plexus lie slightly closer to the middle scalene muscle than to the anterior, so the needle should be inserted slightly closer to the middle scalene muscle than to the anterior scalene muscle. The patient should be instructed to say "stop" when he or she feels an electric shock to the arm, at which point the anesthesiologist must be certain that the paresthesia was felt below the shoulder. Again, a paresthesia to the shoulder is unacceptable because it may indicate that the needle has simply contacted the suprascapular nerve, and it is impossible then to tell whether this nerve has been contacted inside or outside the sheath of the brachial plexus. Only a paresthesia that radiates to a point below the shoulder is acceptable.

Because of the caudad direction of the needle, the anesthesiologist actually has three chances to produce a paresthesia as the needle is advanced (Fig. 61-15*A* through *D*). If the needle fails to touch the superior trunk (*A*), it may contact the middle trunk (*B*); if it fails to contact the middle trunk, it may touch the inferior trunk (*C*); should it miss all three, it will encounter the first rib on which scalene muscles

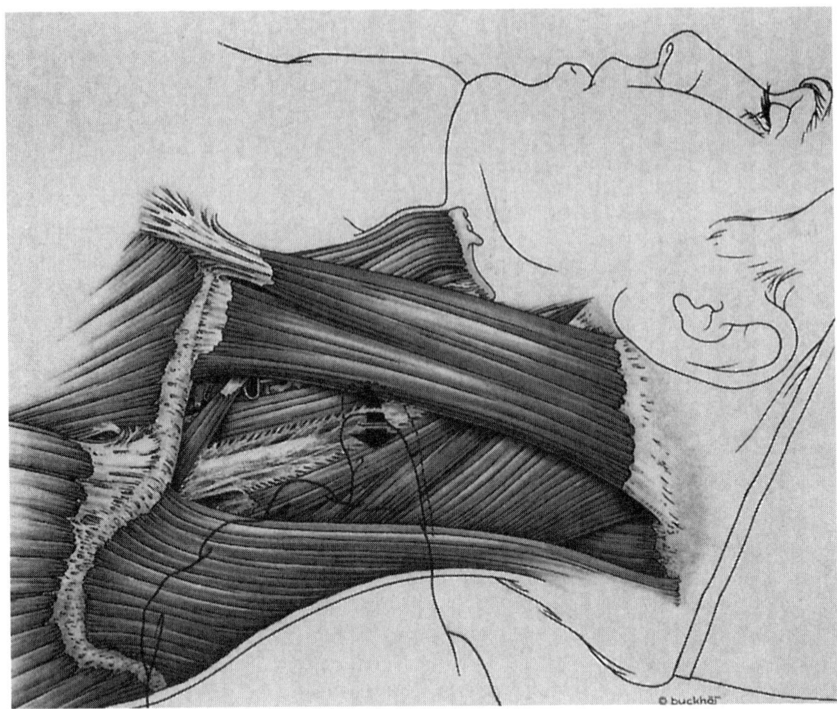

Fig. 61-12. In carrying out a subclavian perivascular block, the index finger is rolled laterally across the belly of the anterior scalene muscle at the level of C6 until the interscalene groove is encountered. (From Winnie AP: *Plexus anesthesia,* vol 1, Philadelphia, 1990, WB Saunders and Mediglobe SA, Fribourg, Switzerland. Used with permission.)

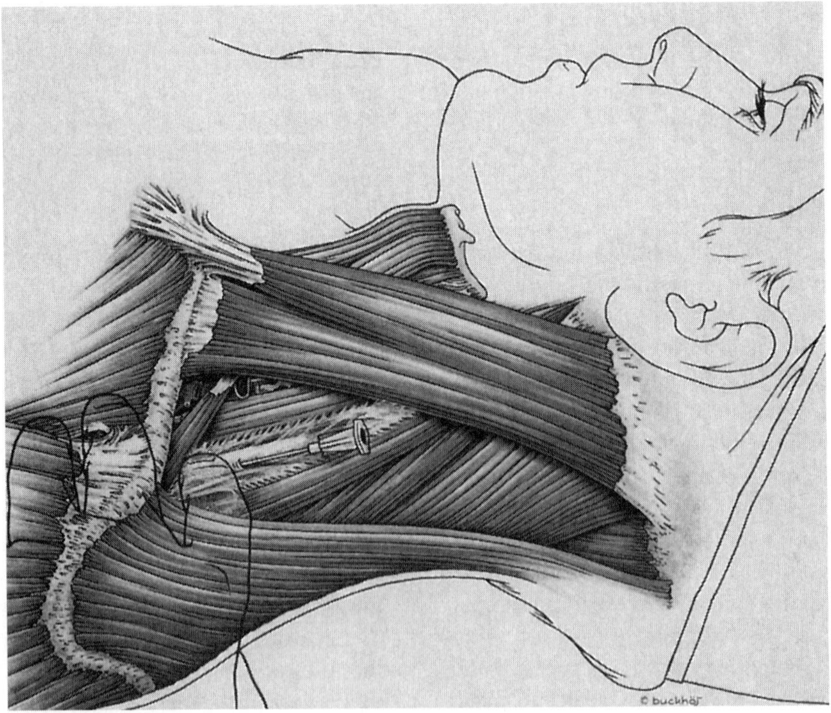

Fig. 61-13. When the index finger has been moved inferiorly in the groove as far as it can be palpated, a needle is inserted just above the finger and advanced in a direction that is directly caudad but not mesiad or dorsad. (From Winnie AP: *Plexus anesthesia,* vol 1, Philadelphia, 1990, WB Saunders and Mediglobe SA, Fribourg, Switzerland. Used with permission.)

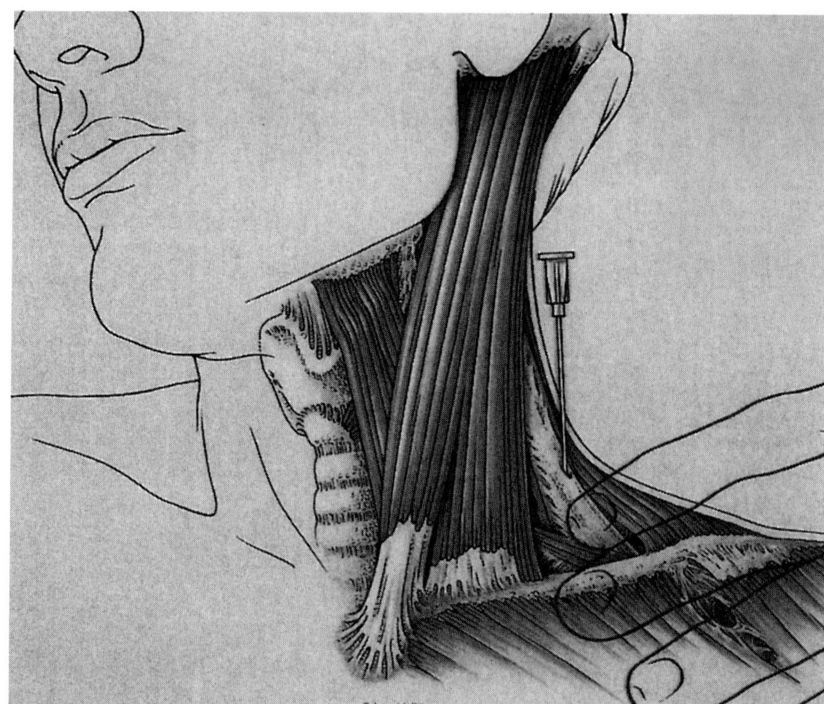

Fig. 61-14. View from the front shows that the properly directed needle is advanced directly caudad with the hub of the needle in contact with the neck. (From Winnie AP: *Plexus anesthesia,* vol 1, Philadelphia, 1990, WB Saunders and Mediglobe SA, Fribourg, Switzerland. Used with permission.)

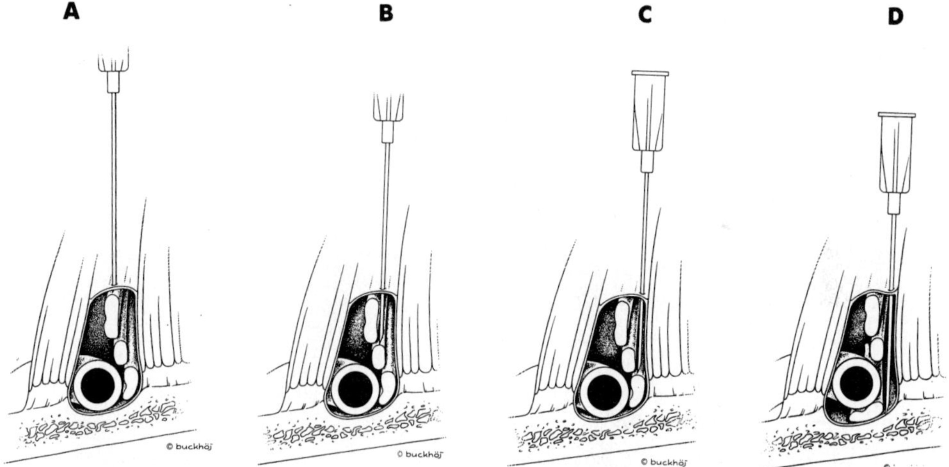

Fig. 61-15. Because the three trunks cross the first rib "stacked" one atop the other and because the needle is advanced in a directly caudad direction, if the advancing needle misses the superior (*A*) trunk, it will hit the middle (*B*) or inferior (*C*) trunk. If it misses all three trunks, the needle will encounter the first rib (*D*), preventing further advancement. (From Winnie AP: *Plexus anesthesia,* vol 1, Philadelphia, 1990, WB Saunders and Mediglobe SA, Fribourg, Switzerland. Used with permission.)

always insert (*D*). So, although contact with the first rib is not sought with this technique, the rib does provide a backstop that prevents further advancement of the properly directed needle. After the desired paresthesia has been obtained and aspiration in several quadrants confirms that the needle is not intravascular, an appropriate volume of local anesthetic is injected with frequent aspirations throughout the injection. Because the subclavian perivascular technique is carried out at a level where the entire plexus is contained in the fewest component parts, a smaller volume of local anesthetic is required with this technique than with any other. Thus, 20 ml is usually sufficient to block the entire brachial plexus (Fig. 61-16). However, if the injection is made fairly high in the subclavian perivascular space, the onset of anesthesia may be delayed or even absent in the distribution of the inferior trunk. Unless it is contraindicated, a

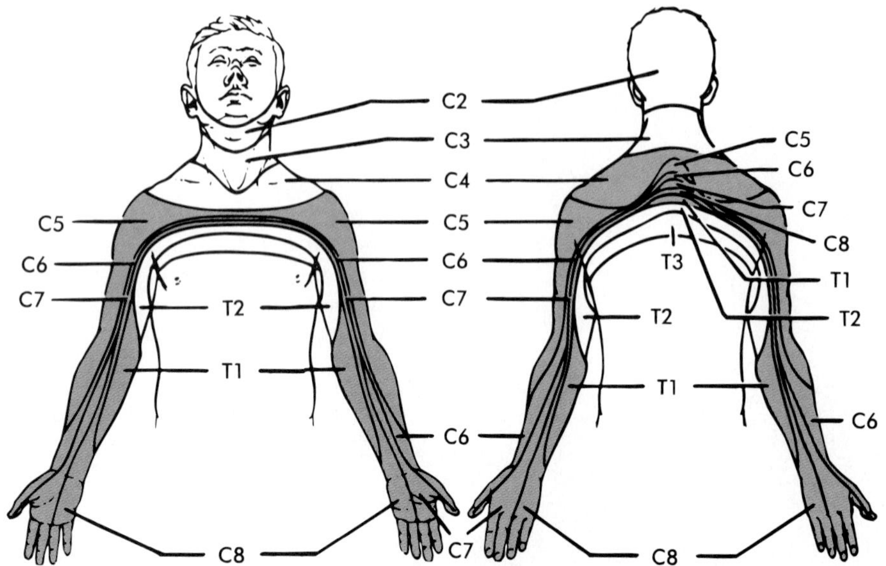

Fig. 61-16. With the subclavian perivascular technique, injection of 20 ml of local anesthetic is usually sufficient to anesthetize the skin in the distribution of all three trunks of the plexus.

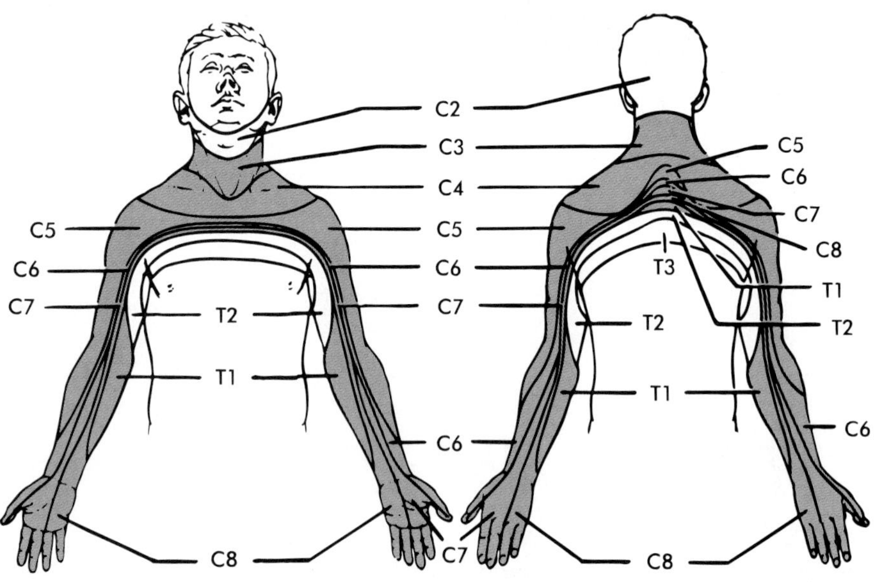

Fig. 61-17. Injection of 20 ml will usually anesthetize not only the trunks of the brachial plexus but also the lower roots of the cervical plexus.

larger volume is probably preferable. An injection of 40 ml of local anesthetic not only fills the subclavian perivascular space but also spreads proximally into the upper interscalene space and distally into the axialry perivascular space to give anesthesia not only of the brachial plexus but also of the lower cervical plexus (Fig. 61-17). Finally, with this technique as with any other, the intercostobrachial and middle brachial cutaneous nerves must be blocked separately by the subcutaneous injection of a few milliliters of local anesthetic over the axillary artery pulse if a tourniquet is to be used during the surgical procedure (see Fig. 61-11). Although each of the brachial plexus block techniques have specific advantages and disadvantages depending upon the clinical situation, the subclavian perivascular block is probably the one technique that provides the greatest extent of anesthesia with the least volume of local anesthetic, so it has greater clinical use in more surgical situations than any of the other techniques.

Axillary perivascular technique

The axillary perivascular technique of brachial plexus block[21] is carried out as follows: the patient is placed in the supine position with the arm abducted to 90° and the forearm flexed and externally rotated so that the dorsum of the hand lies on the table next to the patient's head. The axillary artery pulse is palpated and followed proximally as far as possible, which is usually the point where it disappears under the pectoralis major muscle. At this point (Fig. 61-18), with the index finger directly over the pulse, an immobile needle,[19] a $1^{1}/_{2}$-inch, 22-gauge, short-bevel needle connected to a filled syringe by a length of extension tubing, is inserted just above the fingertip toward the apex of the axilla such

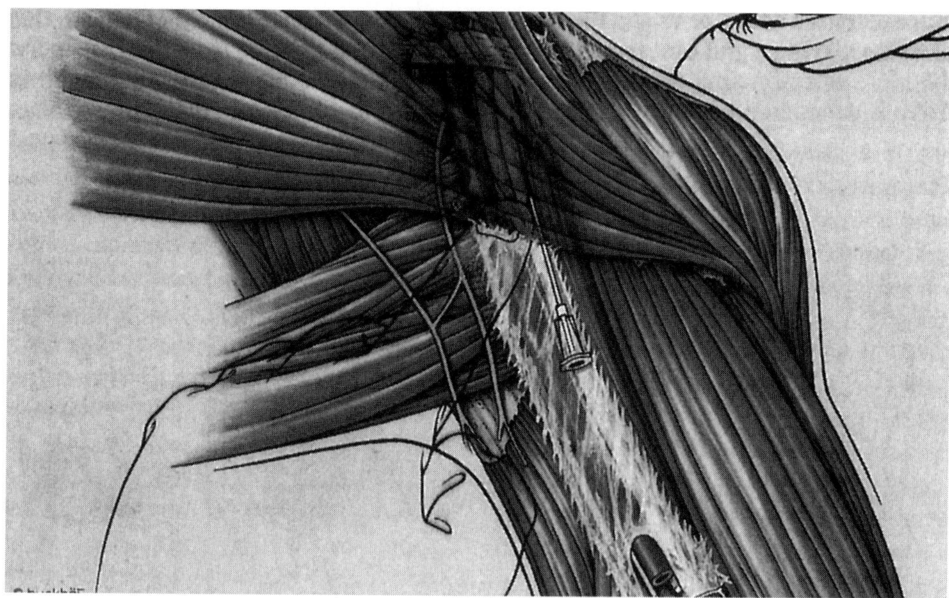

Fig. 61-18. In carrying out the axillary perivascular block, the index finger follows the arterial pulse as far proximally as possible, at which point a needle is inserted just above the fingertip toward the apex of the axilla, such that it forms an approximately 10° angle with the artery. The needle is advanced until one of the four endpoints indicates penetration of the sheath. (From Winnie AP: *Plexus anesthesia,* vol 1, Philadelphia, 1990, WB Saunders and Mediglobe SA, Fribourg, Switzerland. Used with permission.)

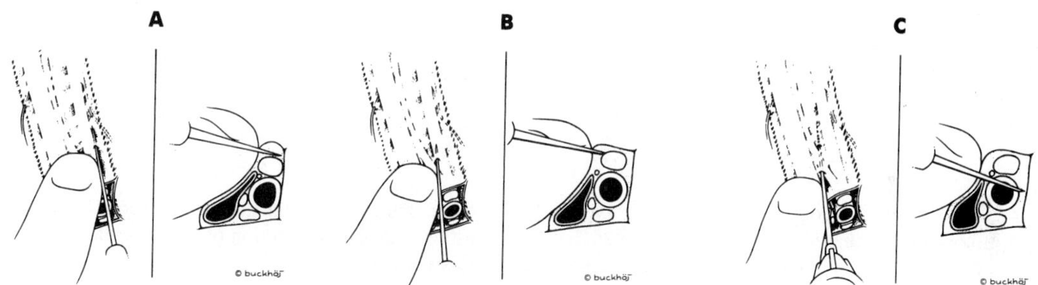

Fig. 61-19. Endpoints that indicate penetration of the sheath by the needle include a fascial "click" (*A*), a paresthesia (*B*), and arterial blood (*C*). In addition, an appropriate motor response to a nerve stimulus may be presumed to indicate placement within the sheath. (From Winnie AP: *Plexus anesthesia,* vol 1, Philadelphia, 1990, WB Saunders and Mediglobe SA, Fribourg, Switzerland. Used with permission.)

that it will form a 10° to 20° angle with the artery as it is advanced. The artery is thus approached gradually until one of four endpoints is achieved (Fig. 61-19):

(1) The anesthesiologist perceives a definite "click" as the needle penetrates the axillary sheath (*A*). If the needle is appropriately placed within the sheath, it should clearly pulsate, although pulsation of the needle in the absence of a perceptible "click" is not a satisfactory endpoint.

(2) A paresthesia is elicited during the introduction of the needle (*B*) (with or without a perceptible "click"), which means the needle is obviously within the axillary sheath. Even if one attempts to avoid paresthesias, they will be evoked in 40% of axillary blocks.[14]

(3) Arterial blood appears in the hub of the needle, which means the angle of the needle should be changed quickly and the needle advanced rapidly until the inability to aspirate blood indicates penetration of the posterior arterial wall. Recent studies indicate that such a "transarterial technique," when deliberately used, may provide the highest success rate of all four endpoints.[4]

(4) An appropriate muscle group in the hand and/or forearm responds at a current of 0.5 milliamps or less when a nerve stimulator is used, indicating proper placement within the sheath.[10]

Whichever endpoint is used, after placement of the needle tip within the sheath and aspiration in several quadrants for blood, 20 ml (Fig. 61-20) to 40 ml (Fig. 61-21) of local anesthetic is injected slowly in 4- to 5-ml increments with repeated aspiration for blood between increments. The volume of local anesthetic used will depend on the patient's size, and the choice of agent will depend on the anticipated duration of surgery. Obviously, after the appropriate agent and volume have been determined, the anesthesiologist must ascertain that the total dose of local anesthetic required is less than accepted limits to avoid systemic toxicity. If the surgical procedure requires blockade of the musculocutaneous nerve, the needle must be placed as high in the axilla as possible, the maximal acceptable volume should be used, and digital pressure should be applied just behind the needle to force the solution as high as possible within the sheath.[23] If the increased volume of anesthetic required to reach the musculocutaneous and axillary nerves cannot be used because of coexisting disease, a low-volume technique may be used, whereby 10 ml of local anesthetic is injected into the axillary perivascular compartment and the musculocutaneous nerve is blocked separately by reinserting the needle superior to the entire neurovascular bundle and injecting 5 to 8 ml into the body of the coracobrachialis muscle. It is not necessary to obtain a paresthesia of the musculocutaneous nerve, because the fascia of this muscle will confine the injected solution and render blockade almost cer-

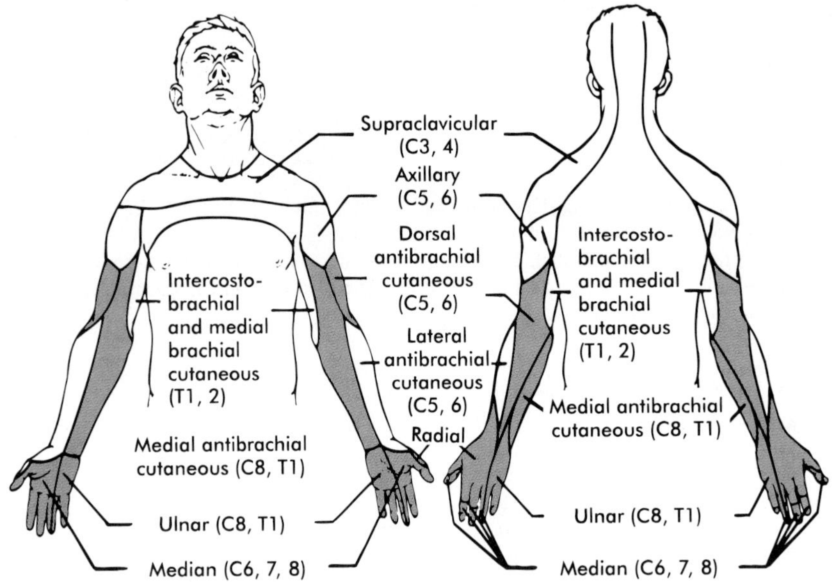

Fig. 61-20. Injection of 20 ml into the axillary perivascular space may be insufficient to reach those nerves that leave the sheath at a high level, so anesthesia in the distribution of the musculocutaneous and axillary nerves may not be provided by this volume.

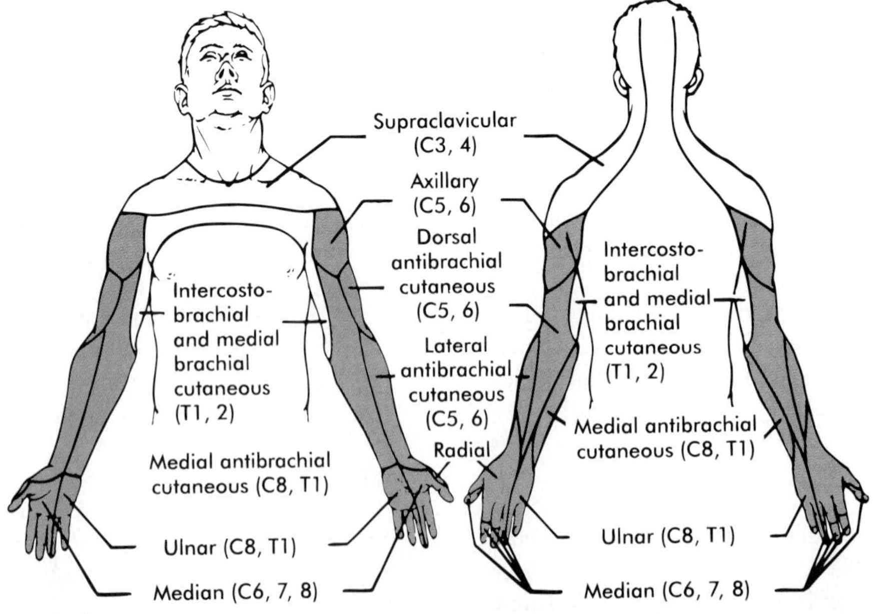

Fig. 61-21. Injection of 40 ml into the axillary perivascular space is usually sufficient to block the entire plexus.

tain. After the completion of the injection within the sheath and the subcutaneous injection of local anesthetic to block the intercostobrachial nerve (see Fig. 61-11), the patient's arm should be brought to the side and digital pressure and massage in the axilla continued to prevent the possible obstruction to the central flow of local anesthetic by the humeral head.

Multiple Compartment Concept

Approximately 25 years ago Rorie described "septa" extending inward from the sheath surrounding the neurovascular bundle,[12] and approximately 15 years ago Thompson and Rorie demonstrated what they interpreted to represent "compartmentalization of dye" injected into the axillary sheath on computed tomography (CT) scans.[17] As a result of these studies, those authors felt that the perivascular space surrounding the brachial plexus was subdivided into multiple compartments by these connective tissue septa, that these septa interfered with circumferential spread of injected local anesthetics, and that these septa explained the occasional occurrence (termed "not uncommon" by Thompson) of a profound block of rapid onset in one nerve and a partial or absent block in others after any of the perivascular techniques of brachial plexus block were used. More recently, Partridge, Katz, and Benirschke carried out 36 axillary dissections that clearly demonstrated that these "septa" do indeed exist, but that they are thin and incomplete and that a single injection (of latex and methylene blue) into the sheath reaches all of the nerves contained therein.[9] Further evidence of the lack of clinical significance of these "septa" is provided by the fact that in most published series of brachial plexus blocks using single-injection techniques, the incidence of partial block is the exception rather than the rule.[13] So, these septa appear to be of little clinical significance.

PLEXUS ANESTHESIA FOR LOWER EXTREMITY SURGERY

Anatomic Considerations

As with the roots of the brachial plexus, the roots of the lumbar plexus are sandwiched between two muscles, the quadratus lumborum muscle posteriorly and the psoas major muscle anteriorly (Fig. 61-22).[24] Therefore, at the level of its formation, the lumbar plexus is invested by the fascia of these two muscles. Once formed, the three nerves to the leg derived from the lumbar plexus take widely divergent courses through the pelvis and into the leg, but of the three, only the femoral nerve remains in close proximity to the psoas major muscle throughout its descent. This nerve, which is the largest derivative of the lumbar plexus, forms behind the psoas major muscle from the posterior divisions of the second, third, and fourth lumbar nerves, and in its descent toward the leg, it appears at the lateral margin of the psoas major muscle at approximately the junction of the middle and lower thirds of that muscle. However, as it continues on its course to the thigh, the femoral nerve remains in the "gutter" between the psoas major and iliacus muscles, so that above the inguinal ligament (Fig. 61-23,

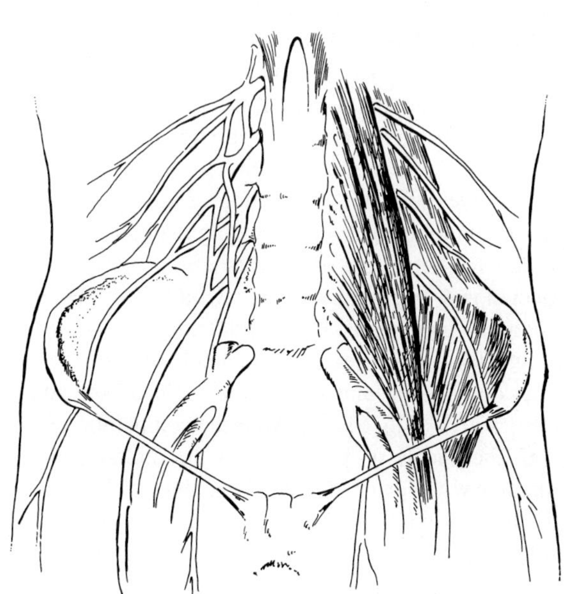

Fig. 61-22. The lumbar plexus is formed between the quadratus lumborum and psoas major muscles and is, therefore, sandwiched between the two layers of fascia investing them. (From Winnie AP: The inguinal paravascular technic of lumbar plexus anesthesia: The 3-in-1 block. *Anesth Anal* 52:989–996, 1973. Copyright © International Anesthesia Research Society.)

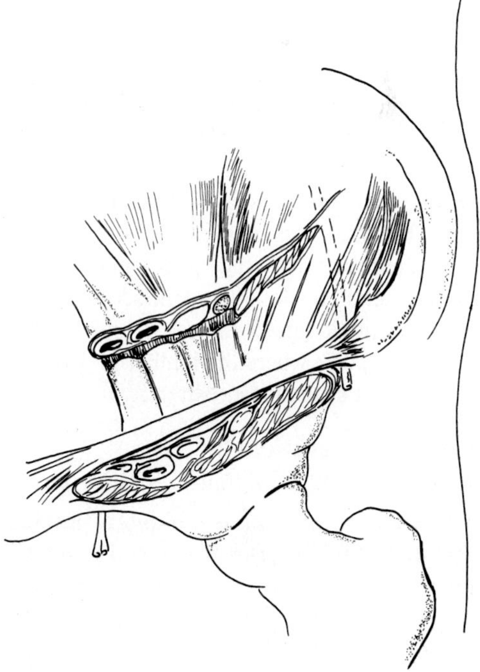

Fig. 61-23. Cross sections just above and below the inguinal ligament show the contributions to the fascial envelope surrounding the femoral nerve on its passage through the pelvis and into the leg. (From Winnie AP: Regional anesthesia of the extremities. In *ASA Refresher Courses* [19:233], Philadelphia, 1991, JB Lippincott.)

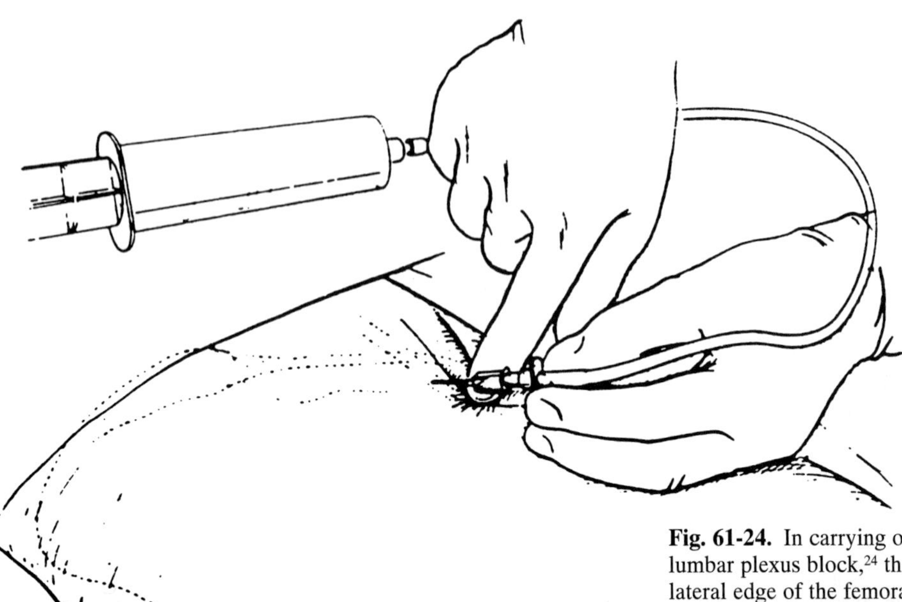

Fig. 61-24. In carrying out the inguinal paravascular technique of lumbar plexus block,[24] the index finger palpates and identifies the lateral edge of the femoral artery and a needle is inserted at this point in a cephalad direction and advanced until a paresthesia indicates penetration of the sheath. (From Winnie AP: Regional anesthesia of the extremities. In *ASA Refresher Courses* [19:233], Philadelphia, 1991, JB Lippincott.)

upper section) the nerve is bounded posterolaterally by the fascia of the iliacus muscle, medially by the fascia of the psoas major muscle, and anteriorly by the transversalis fascia. In its pelvic descent toward the thigh, the nerve is enveloped in a fascial extension of the compartment in which it formed above the pelvic brim. As the nerve passes under the inguinal ligament into the thigh (Fig. 61-23, *lower section*), the fused iliopsoas fascia continues to provide a posterolateral boundary of this compartment, the fascia lata (a continuation into the thigh of the transversalis fascia) continues to provide an anterior boundary, and the thick iliopectoneal fascia provides a continuation of the medial boundary. Throughout its course from the point of its formation to its termination in the upper leg, the femoral nerve travels in a fascial envelope that can serve as a conduit to carry local anesthetic injected into it below the inguinal ligament up to the point where the lumbar plexus gives origin to its three nerves to the lower extremity.

Technical Considerations

Inguinal paravascular technique of lumbar plexus block

The inguinal paravascular technique of lumbar plexus block ("3-in-1 block")[24] uses the fascial envelope around the femoral nerve described previously **to serve as a conduit to allow local anesthetic injected below the inguinal ligament to reach the level where the lumbar plexus forms. Thus a single injection into this envelope can provide anesthesia not only of the femoral nerve, but also of the obturator and lateral femoral cutaneous nerves.**

The technique is carried out as follows (Fig. 61-24): the patient is placed in the supine position with the anesthesiologist standing on the side opposite the site of the anticipated operation. After the usual preparation of the skin, the anesthesiologist palpates the lateral edge of the femoral artery pulse, and an immobile needle[19] is inserted in a cephalad direction just lateral to the tip of the palpating finger. The technique is actually very similar to the technique for an axillary perivascular block, with the needle advanced just distal to the fingertip in a cephalad direction. However, with the inguinal paravascular technique, a paresthesia of the femoral nerve must be obtained, not only because a paresthesia is necessary to obtain anesthesia of the femoral nerve, but because a paresthesia indicates that the tip of the needle is actually within the perineural envelope surrounding the femoral nerve. After the production of the paresthesia, the needle is immobilized, and following aspiration in several quadrants for blood, the desired volume of local anesthetic is injected in 4- to 5-ml increments with intermittent aspiration between increments. Firm digital pressure should be applied just distal to the needle throughout the injection to prevent retrograde flow and to promote cephalad spread of the local anesthetic (Fig. 61-25). After the completion of the injection, the needle is removed, but the digital pressure is maintained with cephalad-caudad massage of the area. In an adult, the approximate volume is 20 to 30 ml of local anesthesic, the actual volume depending upon the height of the patient. Nonetheless, even in short patients the volume should not be less than 20 ml, and in very tall patients a volume of 30 ml need not be exceeded. The clinical significance of this technique in terms of safety, simplicity, and success should be apparent. Moore has emphasized that "open operations on or above the knee cannot be carried out

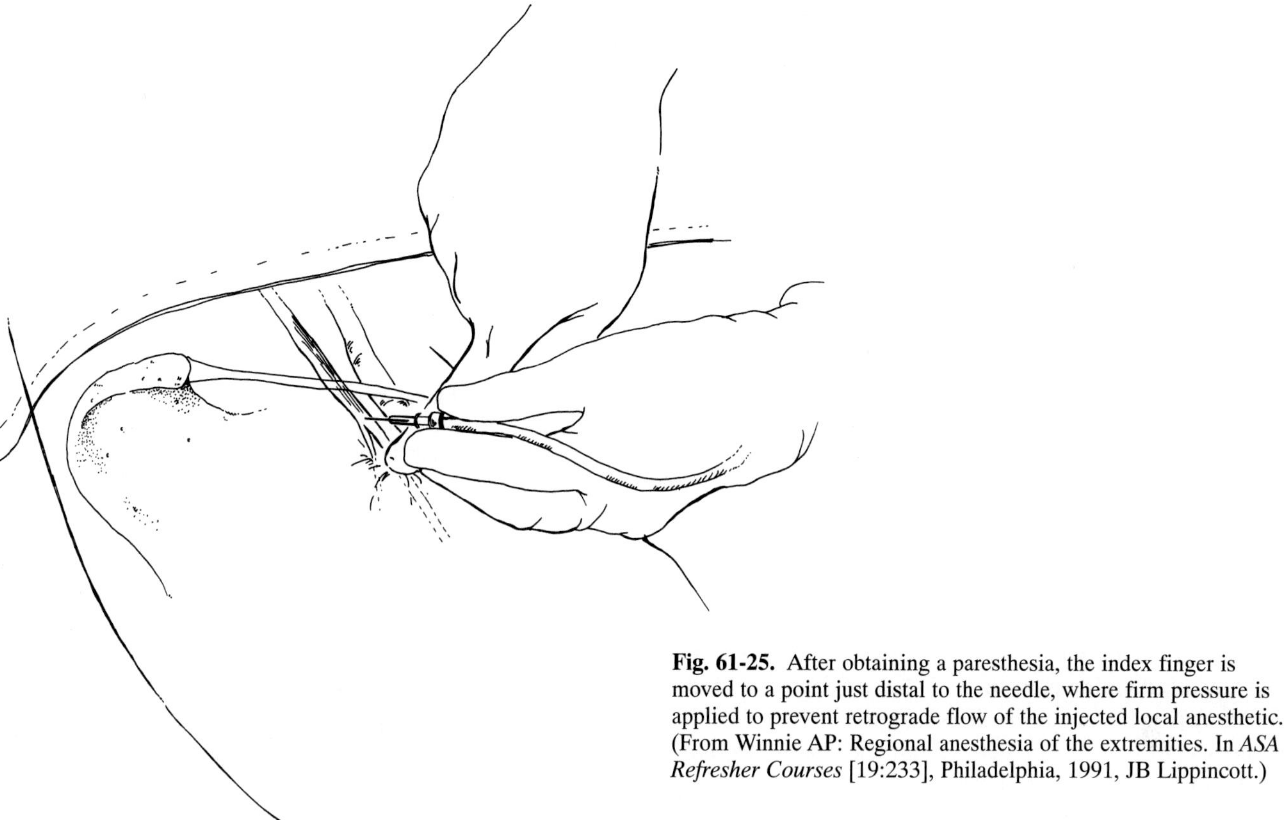

Fig. 61-25. After obtaining a paresthesia, the index finger is moved to a point just distal to the needle, where firm pressure is applied to prevent retrograde flow of the injected local anesthetic. (From Winnie AP: Regional anesthesia of the extremities. In *ASA Refresher Courses* [19:233], Philadelphia, 1991, JB Lippincott.)

under the combination of sciatic and femoral nerve blocks *unless* the lateral femoral cutaneous and obturator nerves are also blocked."[7] He has also stated that "even in the most experienced hands, blocking of the obturator nerve is often unsatisfactory. Therefore, if the patient's physical status dictates that regional anesthesia should be employed in these cases, it seems best to resort to a more certain method, e.g., spinal block."[8] However, if an anesthesiologist is able to provide anesthesia for operations on the lower leg and foot with a combination of a sciatic and femoral block, anesthesia of the *entire* leg can be achieved with the same combination of blocks by modifying the technique of femoral block, by eliciting a paresthesia, and by increasing the volume of the local anesthetic injected. In other words, open operations on or above the knee *can* be carried out under the combination of inguinal paravascular lumbar plexus block and sciatic block.

Further, the use of the inguinal paravascular technique of lumbar plexus block enhances the simplicity and increases the extent of anesthesia; it also reduces the possibility of side effects. In attempting to provide block anesthesia of all four nerves by conventional techniques, as many as 10 to 15 needle insertions and as much as 65 to 95 ml of local anesthetic may be required. Therefore, the chance of complications is decreased by the inguinal paravascular technique in three ways: (1) the possibility of postanesthetic neuropathy is decreased because the incidence of this complication increases with the number of times a needle penetrates a nerve; (2) the possibility of intravascular injection is decreased because this possibility also increases as the number of injections increases; and (3) the potential for overdosage and systemic toxicity is decreased because the possibility of a toxic reaction decreases as the total volume and the total dose of the local anesthetic injected decrease. Thus, by reducing the number of injections and the volume of local anesthetic required, the inguinal paravascular technique markedly reduces the chances of complications, either neural or systemic.

Of course, if the inguinal paravascular technique of lumbar plexus block is selected, unless the operation is confined to the areas innervated by the femoral, lateral femorocutaneous, and obturator nerves (such as a skin graft donor site), a sciatic nerve block must also be carried out.

If the patient can be turned to the lateral position, a modification of Labat's technique can be used to achieve sciatic block, which is carried out as follows.[25] With the patient in Sims' position, lying on the side opposite the one to be injected, a primary line is drawn from the superior border of the greater trochanter to the posterior iliac spine (Fig. 61-26). This line is then bisected and a second line is drawn perpendicular to the first, passing inferiorly beginning at its midpoint. A third line is drawn between the superior border of the greater trochanter and the sacral hiatus, and the point where this third line crosses the perpen-

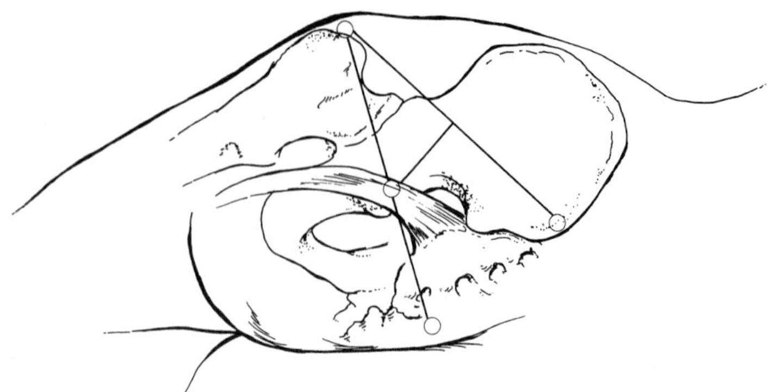

Fig. 61-26. The author's modification of Labat's technique of sciatic block[25] is carried out by extending two lines from the top of the greater trochanter—one to the posterosuperior iliac spine and the other to the sacral hiatus. A line perpendicular to the first line is dropped from its midpoint, and at the point where that line intersects the second line, a needle is inserted until contact with the sciatic nerve produces a paresthesia. (From Winnie AP: Regional anesthesia of the extremities. In *ASA Refresher Courses* [19:233], Philadelphia, 1991, JB Lippincott.)

dicular line determines a point that is usually directly over the sciatic nerve. A $3^1/_2$, 22-gauge needle is inserted here and advanced until a paresthesia indicates contact with the sciatic nerve. Local anesthetic is injected in 4- to 5-ml increments (with aspiration between incremental doses) until a total of 20 ml has been administered. This technique locates the position of the sciatic nerve more accurately than any other method. This is because the angle inscribed by the two lines originating at the superior border of the greater trochanter will depend upon the length of the sacrum; the length of the sacrum will, in turn, depend upon the height of the patient. Thus, the distance along the perpendicular line at which the needle is inserted will vary with the height of the patient. Other more traditional techniques insert the needle a fixed distance down the perpendicular line, and obviously this distance will vary with the patient's size. As a result, this modification allows a reduction in the number of needle insertions required to find the nerve, and this contributes significantly both to patient acceptance and, more importantly, to a lower incidence of postanesthetic neuropathy.

If the patient cannot be turned to the lateral position, after the completion of the lumbar plexus block, the "supine sciatic technique"[25] can be used (Fig. 61-27). The patient remains in the supine position, and the hip is slightly adducted and flexed to 90° or greater by an assistant, with the knee similarly flexed and supported in a position that may be altered to minimize discomfort. At this level, the sciatic nerve lies in the readily palpable hollow between the greater trochanter and the ischial tuberosity. These landmarks are palpated and a needle is inserted at the midpoint of a line connecting these two points. A 3-inch, 22-gauge needle is inserted parallel to the table (horizontally) in a direction that is cephalad and slightly mesiad until it encounters the sciatic nerve. After a paresthesia is produced in the distribution of the sciatic nerve, 15 to 20 ml of local anesthetic is injected in 4- to 5-ml increments with aspiration between increments and with firm digital pressure distal to the needle throughout the entire injection.

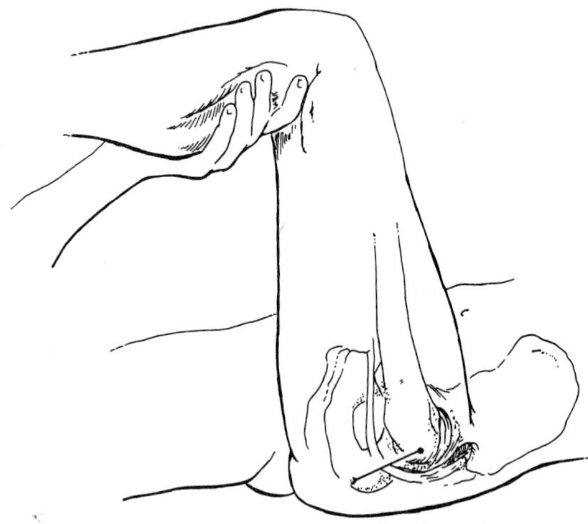

Fig. 61-27. The author's technique of supine sciatic block[25] is carried out by inserting a needle at the midpoint of a line drawn between the greater trochanter and the ischial tuberosity with the patient's hip and knee flexed 90°. The needle is advanced until paresthesia indicates contact with the nerve. (From Winnie AP: Regional anesthesia of the extremities. In *ASA Refresher Courses* [19:233], Philadelphia, 1991, JB Lippincott.)

Combined lumbrosacral plexus block

If the inguinal paravascular and/or sciatic block techniques are contraindicated (as by infection with enlarged inguinal lymph nodes, etc.), if the patient can be turned to the lateral position, and if spinal and/or epidural anesthesia are undesirable or contraindicated (by patient refusal, anticoagulants, etc.), it is possible to block both the lumbar and sacral plexuses by a lumbar paravertebral approach.[25] The technique of lumbrosacral plexus block is carried out as follows (Fig. 61-28): the patient is placed in the lateral recumbent position, lying on the side opposite that to be blocked. A line is drawn

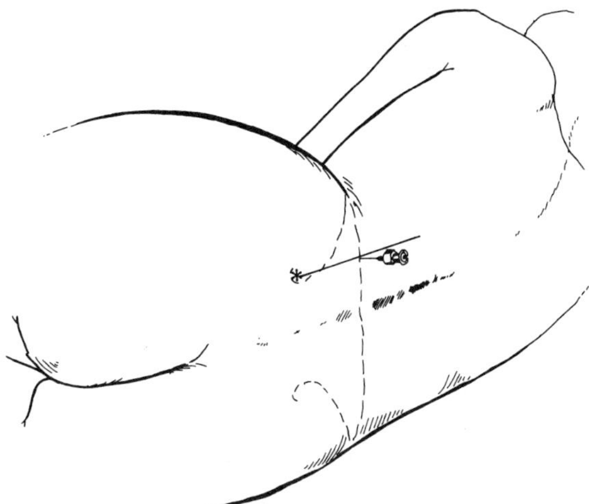

Fig. 61-28. Lumbosacral plexus block[25] is carried out with the patient in the lateral recumbent position. A spinal needle is inserted at the intersection of the intercristal line and a line is drawn through the posterosuperior iliac spine parallel to the vertebral column. As the needle is advanced, if the transverse process of L4 is contracted, the needle is redirected slightly more caudad and advanced until a paresthesia is produced, at which point the local anesthetic is injected. (From Winnie AP: Regional anesthesia of the extremities. In *ASA Refresher Courses* [19:233], Philadelphia, 1991, JB Lippincott.)

connecting the superior borders of both iliac crests, indicating the L4 to L5 interspace, and a second line is drawn parallel to the spine passing through the posterosuperior iliac spine. At the point where the intercristal line crosses the paraspinous line, a $3^1/_2$-inch, 22-gauge needle is inserted perpendicular to the skin in every plane. As the needle is advanced, if the transverse process of the fourth lumbar vertebra is encountered, the needle is redirected slightly more caudad and advanced until a paresthesia is produced. If a paresthesia cannot be elicited (which occurs in 20% to 25% of the cases), a nerve stimulator may be useful to elicit a response of the quadratus femoris muscles. If and when a paresthesia is elicited (or an appropriate response to nerve stimulation is evoked), the tip of the needle must lie between the quadratus lumborum and the psoas major muscles. At that point the needle is immobilized, and the injection of 40 ml of local anesthetic will usually block the roots of both the lumbar and sacral plexuses.

CHOICE OF LOCAL ANESTHETICS FOR PLEXUS ANESTHESIA

Single-injection techniques have overcome most of the objections of surgeons, anesthesiologists, and patients to peripheral block anesthesia for extremity surgery. In addition, the development of numerous local anesthetics with different pharmacologic profiles has helped to make plexus anesthesia the anesthetic of choice in many clinical situations. The advantages provided by the relatively new, long-acting local anesthetics are greatest when these agents are used for peripheral nerve blocks because their prolonged duration of action compared with the older local anesthetic agents increases as one moves away from the central nervous system. For example, as one moves from spinal to epidural block, the duration of anesthesia provided by bupivacaine doubles, and, as one goes from epidural to plexus block, duration increases two- to threefold.

The wide spectrum of activity of local anesthetic agents, particularly in duration of action, has expanded the usefulness of regional anesthesia to include situations in which this type of anesthesia was previously unacceptable. Until recently, the need to provide an appropriate duration limited the use of a regional anesthetic procedure. Today, anesthetic agents are available that are capable of providing excellent plexus anesthesia for a duration that ranges from approximately 30 minutes to 14 hours, depending upon the concentration and volume of the local anesthetic and the presence or absence of vasoconstrictors. For example, if one wishes to provide anesthesia for a short procedure of 20 minutes duration, one may choose 2-chloroprocaine or procaine; for a 1- to 2-hour procedure, one may choose lidocaine; for procedures lasting 3 to 4 hours, one may choose lidocaine with epinephrine, or if one wishes to avoid epinephrine, one may choose mepivacaine; for procedures lasting 5 to 7 hours, one may choose a mixture containing 1% mepivacaine, 0.2% tetracaine, and epinephrine 1:200,000; for even longer procedures, or more frequently, when anesthesia and/or analgesia are desirable well into the postoperative period, the anesthesiologist may choose to use bupivacaine. If profound motor block and long duration of anesthesia are desirable, etidocaine may be a useful choice.

With such a wide variety of agents available, regional anesthesia is appropriate for most clinical situations. For example, in outpatient surgery, where one wishes the anesthesia to be terminated rapidly upon completion of the surgical procedure, a short- or moderate-duration agent, such as chloroprocaine or lidocaine, may be used. Where it is advantageous to provide analgesia well into the postoperative period, to maintain the sympathetic block to enhance blood flow, or to prolong the motor block to maintain immobilization, agents such as bupivacaine or etidocaine may be useful. For inpatients a continuous (catheter) technique can be used for postoperative pain control, a procedure that has been shown to provide significantly better pain relief than patient-controlled analgesia (PCA).[1] In outpatients, the addition of buprenorphine to the local anesthetic can provide up to 2 full days of complete analgesia, something that cannot be accomplished by any of the other opioid agents.[18]

An additional advantage offered by the long-acting local anesthetics used to provide a plexus anesthesia, especially for inpatients, is a logistic one. Frequently, it is stated that if a particular anesthesiologist's surgical schedule includes a mixture of cases requiring general and regional anesthesia, the regional anesthetic might delay the surgical schedule inordinately. In this situation, the use of a plexus block can expedite the surgical schedule *if* the blocks can be carried out well before the beginning of the surgical schedule. After regional anesthesia is established, the anesthesiologist can leave the patients in the care of nursing personnel until the patient to be operated under plexus anesthesia can be brought into the operating room fully anesthetized, thus abolishing any "turnover time" between cases resulting from anesthesia.

In summary, the usefulness of regional anesthesia has been extended tremendously by the current availability of local anesthetics that range from ultra-short to ultra-long durations of activity. When these agents are used to provide plexus anesthesia, the anesthesiologist is able to provide the patient undergoing operation on the extremities a safe and effective form of anesthesia.

KEY POINTS

- If regional anesthesia is to be satisfactory to the patient, surgeon, and anesthesiologist, they must agree that regional anesthesia is the best form of anesthesia in this case.
- If all regional techniques could be carried out by a single injection, as with spinal and epidural anesthesia, then most, if not all, of the objections to regional anesthesia by surgeons, anesthesiologists, and patients would be overcome.
- The concept of "plexus anesthesia" was introduced nearly 30 years ago to provide a system of single-injection techniques for blocking all of the major plexuses—cervical, brachial, lumbar, and sacral. The concept is based on the fact that all of the plexuses, at some point in their formation and/or distribution, pass between two muscles and hence may be considered invested by the fascia of these muscles. Thus, each plexus lies in a potential "interfascial compartment," so if this compartment can be identified and entered by a needle, the plexus can be blocked by a single injection of an appropriate volume of local anesthetic.
- The brachial plexus is invested by a fascial envelope, which forms a perineural and perivascular space that extends from the intervertebral foramina to the distal axilla. Therefore, just as with peridural techniques, a single injection of local anesthetic can provide anesthesia of the entire brachial plexus, the extent of which depends upon the level of injection and the volume of local anesthetic injected at that level.
- As with the roots of the brachial plexus, the roots of the lumbar plexus are sandwiched between two muscles—the quadratus lumborum muscle posteriorly and the psoas major muscle anteriorly. Therefore, at the level of its formation, the lumbar plexus is invested by the fascia of these two muscles.
- The inguinal paravascular technique of lumbar plexus block ("3-in-1 block") uses the fascial envelope around the femoral nerve to serve as a conduit to allow local anesthetic injected below the inguinal ligament to reach the level where the lumbar plexus forms. Thus, a single injection into this envelope can provide anesthesia not only of the femoral nerve but also of the obturator and lateral femoral cutaneous nerves.

KEY REFERENCES

Raj PP, Rosenblatt R, Montgomery SJ: Use of the nerve stimulator for peripheral blocks, *Reg Anesth* 5:14, 1980.

Winnie AP: *Plexus anesthesia. I. The perivascular techniques of brachial plexus block,* Philadelphia, 1983, WB Saunders.

Winnie AP, Ramamurthy S, Durrani Z, et al: Plexus blocks for lower extremity surgery, *Anesthesiol Rev* 1:11–16, 1974.

REFERENCES

1. Ali MJ, Dobkowski W, Hawkins R, et al: Continuous interscalene analgesia versus patient controlled analgesia for shoulder surgery, *Anesthesiology* 73:A827, 1990.
2. Broadman LM, Mesrobian R, Ruttimann U, McGill WA: Do anesthesiologists prefer a regional or a general anesthetic for themselves? *Reg Anesth* 11:57, 1986.
3. Buffington CW, Ready LB, Horton WG: Training and practice factors influence the use of regional anesthesia: Implications for resident evaluation, *Reg Anesth* 11:2, 1986.
4. Cockings E, Moore PL, Lewis RC: Transarterial brachial plexus blockade using high doses of 1.5% mepivacaine, *Reg Anesth* 12:159, 1987.
5. Katz J: A survey of anesthetic choice among anesthesiologists, *Anesth Analg* 52(3):373, 1973.
6. Kopacz DJ, Bridenbaugh LD: Are anesthesia residency programs failing regional anesthesia? The past, present and future, *Reg Anesth* 18:84, 1993.
7. Moore DC: Sciatic and femoral nerve block, *JAMA* 150:550, 1952.
8. Moore DC: Block of the sciatic and femoral

nerves. In Moore DC, editor: *Regional block,* Springfield, 1973, Charles C Thomas.
9. Partridge BL, Katz J, Benirschke K: Functional anatomy of the brachial plexus sheath: Implications for anesthesia, *Anesthesiology* 66:743, 1987.
10. Raj PP, Rosenblatt R, Montgomery SJ: Use of the nerve stimulator for peripheral blocks, *Reg Anesth* 5:14, 1980.
11. Rice LJ, Trescot AM, Guzzetta P, Ruttimann U: Regional vs. general anesthesia: What would surgeons choose for themselves? *Reg Anesth* 13:82, 1988.
12. Rorie DK: The brachial plexus sheath, *Anatomic Rec* 187:451, 1974.
13. Selander D: Axillary plexus block: Paresthetic or perivascular? (editorial) *Anesthesiology* 66:726, 1987.
14. Selander D, Edshage S, Wolff T: Paresthesiae or no paresthesiae? Nerve lesions after axillary blocks, *Acta Anaesthesiol Scand* 23:27, 1979.
15. Shevde K, Panagopoulos G: A survey of 800 patients' knowledge, attitudes, and concerns regarding anesthesia, *Anesth Analg* 73:190, 1991.
16. Stan TC, Krantz MA, Solomon DL, Poulos JG: The incidence of neurovascular complications following axillary brachial plexus block using a transarterial approach: A prospective study of 1,000 consecutive patients, *Reg Anesth* 20:484, 1995.
17. Thompson GE, Rorie DK: Functional anatomy of the brachial plexus sheaths, *Anesthesiology* 59:117, 1983.
18. Viel EJ, Bledjam JJ, de la Coussage JE, et al: Brachial plexus block unit opioids for postoperative pain relief: Comparison between buprenorphine and morphine, *Reg Anesth* 14:274–278, 1989.
19. Winnie AP: An immobile needle for nerve blocks, *Anesthesiology* 31:577, 1969.
20. Winnie AP: Interscalene brachial block, *Anesth Analg* 49:455, 1970.
21. Winnie AP: *Plexus anesthesia. I. The perivascular techniques of brachial plexus block,* Philadelphia, 1983, WB Saunders.
22. Winnie AP, Collins VJ: The subclavian perivascular technique of brachial plexus anesthesia, *Anesthesiology* 25:353, 1964.
23. Winnie AP, Radonjic R, Akkineni SR, et al: Factors influencing distribution of local anesthetic injected into the brachial plexus sheath, *Anesth Analg* 58:225, 1979.
24. Winnie AP, Ramamurthy S, Durrani Z: The inguinal paravascular technic of lumbar plexus anesthesia, *Anesth Analg* 52:989–996, 1973.
25. Winnie AP, Ramamurthy S, Durrani Z, et al: Plexus blocks for lower extremity surgery, *Anesthesiol Rev* 1:11–16, 1974.
26. Winnie AP: Does transarterial technique of axillary block provide a higher success rate and a lower complication rate than a paresthesia technique? New evidence and old. *Reg Anesth* 20(6):482, 1995.

CHAPTER 62

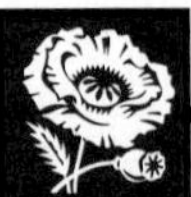

Peripheral Nerve Blocks

MICHAEL F. MULROY

Trunk
- Intercostal nerve block
- Paravertebral block
- Ilioinguinal block

Upper Extremity
- Peripheral nerve blocks of the arm
- Digital nerve block
- Intravenous regional block

Lower Extremity
- Popliteal fossa blockade
- Ankle block

Head and Neck
- Trigeminal nerve block
- Cervical plexus block
- Occipital nerve block
- Airway anesthesia

The major nerve blocks have been described in other chapters, including blockade of the brachial plexus, sacral plexus, and the neuraxis itself with epidural and subarachnoid approaches. Alternative approaches to the peripheral nerves of the trunk, arm, leg, and head are described in this chapter.

TRUNK

Intercostal Nerve Block

In some situations, a narrower band of thoracic or abdominal anesthesia is preferred to spinal or epidural blockade, or the latter are more hazardous because of infection or coagulopathy. Anesthesia of the intercostal nerves of the lower six ribs can provide both motor and sensory anesthesia of the abdominal wall from the xiphoid to the pubis (Table 62-1).[1,9]

Anatomy

The somatic nerves of the chest emerge from their respective intervertebral foramina and pass into the intercostal groove along the ventral caudad surface of each rib. An artery and vein travel along with each of these nerves in the groove under the protection of the overhanging external edge of the rib. The fascia of the internal and external intercostal muscles are the internal and external borders of this intercostal groove. As the nerves travel beyond the midaxillary line, they form a lateral sensory branch. The intercostal groove becomes less well defined anterior to the midaxillary line, and the nerve begins to move away from its protected position. The lowest intercostal nerve (the twelfth) is less closely applied to its accompanying rib.

Technique of blockade

The sixth through the eleventh ribs are identified, and their accompanying nerves are blocked by injections along the easily palpated, sharp posterior angulation of the ribs that occurs 5 to 7 cm from the midline in the back. Ribs above the fifth are difficult to palpate because of the overlying scapula and paraspinous muscles and are thus most easily blocked using the paravertebral technique (described later in this chapter).

The patient should be placed in the lateral, sitting, or prone position. The prone position is most practical. A pillow can be placed under the patient's abdomen to provide slight flexion of the thoracic spine. The patient's arms should be draped over the edge of the stretcher or operating table so that each scapula falls away laterally from the midline. The physician should stand at the side of the patient, so that his or her dominant hand is toward the patient's feet.

The spinous processes should be marked in the midline from T6 through T12, and the ribs identified along the line of their most extreme posterior angulation. For the twelfth rib, this is usually 7 cm from the midline. At the level of the sixth rib, this posterior angulation is best appreciated somewhat more medially, usually 5 cm from the midline. These two ribs can be marked at their inferior borders and a line drawn between these two points. The rest of the ribs can be identified and marked between them on their inferior bor-

Table 62-1 Intercostal blocks

Indications	Comments
Upper abdominal surgery—cholecystectomy, gastrectomy	Usually requires supplemental general anesthesia and intubation; can be used with supplemental celiac plexus block
Rib fractures	Requires anesthesia of one or two ribs on either side
Chest tubes, percutaneous biliary drainage procedures	—
Postoperative analgesia[1]	Long-acting amide local anesthetics provide postoperative analgesia for 8 to 12 hours
Diagnosis of neuralgia	—

ders, along the angled line between the sixth and the twelfth ribs (Fig. 62-1).

After aseptic preparation, light sedation should be provided for the patient and a skin wheal raised at each mark. The nerves should be blocked starting with the lowest rib and moving upward.

The physician should place an index finger of his or her cephalad hand on the skin above the identifying mark for the lowest rib; this finger should lie immediately over the midpoint of the rib. The skin can be retracted in a cephalad direction so that the previous mark now lies over the rib itself. A 22-gauge, 1-inch needle (attached to a 10-ml syringe) should be inserted directly but gently onto the rib with the other hand, holding the syringe and needle so that they maintain a constant 10° cephalad angulation (Fig. 62-2).

Once the needle is safely "parked" on the dorsal surface of the rib, tension can be released on the skin and the needle and syringe controlled with the cephalad hand. This is done by placing the ulnar border of the hand against the skin and grasping the hub of the needle firmly between the thumb and index finger. The middle finger of this hand should rest along the shaft of the needle to provide guidance. Once the syringe is firmly gripped by the cephalad hand, the fingers of the caudad hand should be placed in an "injection" position—either in the rings of a three-ring syringe or on the plunger of a straight syringe.

The needle and syringe are raised slightly off the bone and repositioned in a caudad direction until they pass below the inferior border of the rib. The entire needle and syringe unit should be kept at a 10-degree cephalad angle to the rib at all times. As it passes the inferior border, the needle should be advanced 4 to 6 mm under the rib, with the needle pointing slightly cephalad into the intercostal groove (Fig. 63-3).

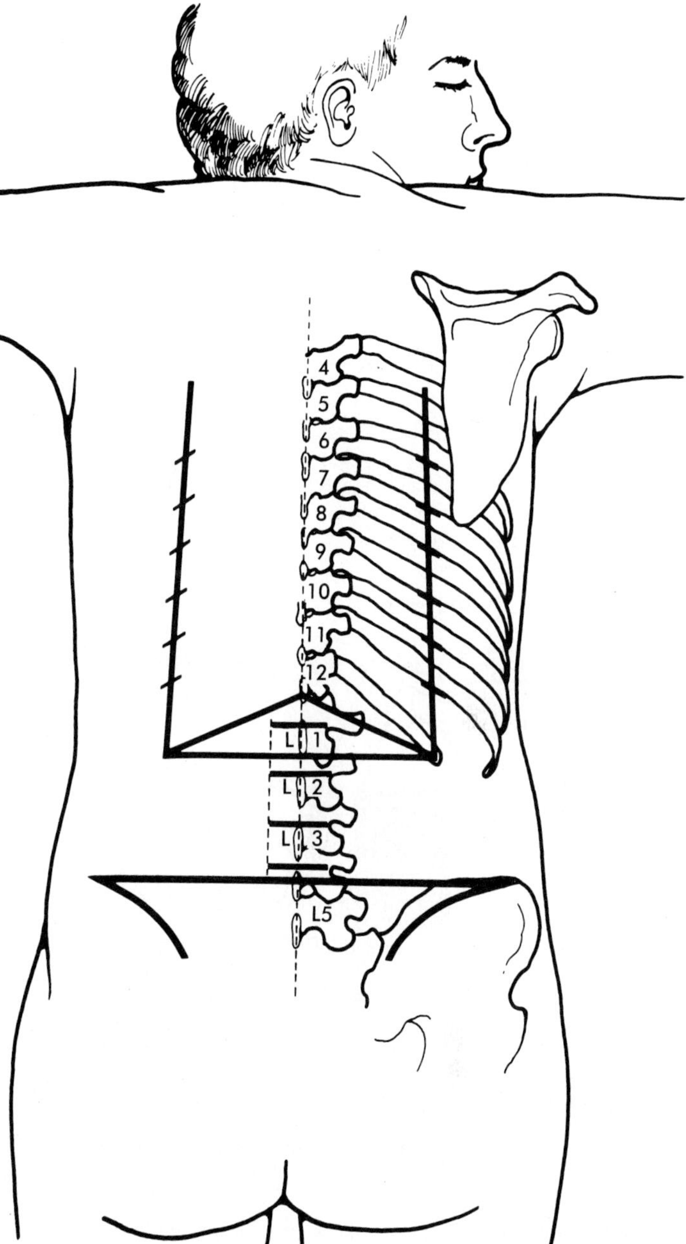

Fig. 62-1. Superficial skin markings for intercostal blocks. (From Mulroy MF: *Regional anesthesia: an illustrated procedural guide,* Philadelphia, 1996, Lippincott-Raven.)

Once in the groove, and after a negative aspiration of blood, 3 to 5 ml of local anesthetic solution is injected. Generally, 0.25% bupivacaine produces good sensory anesthesia, whereas 0.5% bupivacaine is required for prolonged anesthesia with motor blockade. Aspiration is not reliable in preventing intravascular injection of the anesthetic; a slight "jiggling" motion of the needle during the injection reduces this occurrence by allowing the needle to remain in a vessel only transiently.

As soon as the injection is complete, the needle is withdrawn from the groove and moved cephalad and parked again

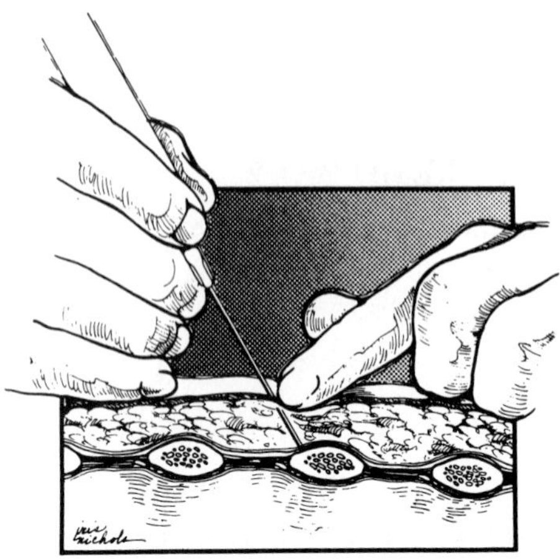

Fig. 62-2. Hand and needle position for intercostal blocks, identifying the rib. (From Mulroy MF: *Regional anesthesia: an illustrated procedural guide*, Philadelphia, 1996, Lippincott-Raven.)

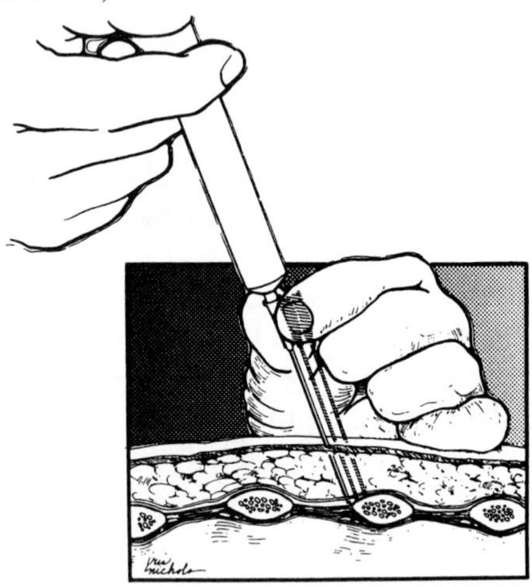

Fig. 62-3. Hand and needle position for intercostal blocks, during injection. (From Mulroy MF: *Regional anesthesia: an illustrated procedural guide,* Philadelphia, 1996, Lippincott-Raven.)

on the safe dorsal surface of the rib. The fingers of the caudad hand are removed from the injection position and control resumed of the syringe. The cephalad hand now relinquishes control and is moved up to the next rib to repeat this process.

The six or seven designated ribs are blocked on each side by progressively moving up the back, with control of the syringe alternating between the cephalad and caudad hands at the time of injection. The ribs on the opposite side are blocked in a similar manner. This can be performed by standing on the same side and reaching across the back, or by moving to the opposite side of the patient. If the contralateral blocks are performed from the opposite side of the bed, hands can be switched so that the functions of cephalad and caudad hand remain the same even though the right and left hands have changed roles. It is sometimes more difficult for operators to control the syringe with their nondominant hand, but it is worth the effort, because attempting to hold the syringe with the cephalad hand makes maintenance of the proper cephalad angulation difficult. The syringe often is rotated along its long axis as it is moved to the caudad edge of the rib, so that by the time the needle moves off the rib it is pointed in a caudad rather than cephalad direction. This injects solution away from the nerve rather than into the groove.

If the intercostal blocks are to be supplemented with somatic paravertebral blocks or sympathetic blockade of the celiac plexus, perform these blocks at the end of intercostal anesthesia. The total dosage of drug is adjusted in such combination techniques so that the maximum recommended amounts are not exceeded.

Complications

Pneumothorax is the greatest concern but is rare when performed by experienced clinicians; the occurrence of pneumothorax was less than 1% in one series.[8] The incidence can be reduced by the "safe" habit of identifying the rib first and parking the needle on the rib before and after each injection. If there is any suspicion (such as coughing or pain during performance of the block), a radiograph should be taken and a chest tube placed, if indicated.

Respiratory insufficiency can occur in patients with chronic obstructive lung disease dependent on intercostal muscles for tidal ventilation.[2] Respiratory depression can also occur when these blocks are used for postoperative analgesia if excessive narcotics are given before the block. Respiratory depression most commonly occurs when excessive sedation is administered during performance of the block with the patient in the prone position. This is hazardous not only because of potential airway obstruction, but also because of the risk of regurgitation and aspiration. A second person providing monitoring and sedation during performance of the block reduces the likelihood of this complication.

Spinal or epidural anesthesia can be produced if the injection is made too close to midline.[14] This may result in unexpected hypotension, but is rare if the standard injection positions described are used.

Paravertebral Block

In the upper thoracic region, the upper five ribs are more difficult to palpate, and blockade of their associated intercostal nerves is best performed with a paravertebral injection. This approach is technically more difficult, and has slightly greater potential for complications,[3] because of the proximity of the lung and of the intervertebral foramina. In the lumbar region, the paravertebral approach is the only alternative for individual somatic nerve block, and is performed with greater ease. This approach is used almost exclusively for diagnostic and therapeutic blocks and is rarely needed for surgery, and thus is described in Chapter 63.

Ilioinguinal Block

For the lower abdominal wall, the upper lumbar nerve roots form the ilioinguinal nerves, which provide innervation of the groin region (Table 62-2).

Table 62-2 Ilioinguinal block

Indications	Comments
Hernia repair	Needs local supplement, especially in children
Postoperative analgesia	—

Anatomy

The L1 nerve root (occasionally joined by a branch of the T12 root) provides sensory anesthesia to the lowest portion of the abdominal wall and the groin by means of its superior iliohypogastric branch and inferior ilioinguinal branch. These nerves travel in a path similar to that of the intercostal nerves but without the convenient bony landmark of a rib to identify them. Nevertheless, they can be anesthetized relatively easily in the groin because of their relationship to the anterior superior iliac spine.

Technique of blockade

The block is performed with the patient in the supine position and can be administered with the patient awake or anesthetized. The patient should be placed in a supine position. The anterior superior iliac spine is identified and an "x" is placed on the skin 2.5 cm medial to it and slightly cephalad. After aseptic preparation, a skin wheal is raised at the "x."

A 1-inch, 22-gauge needle is introduced through the "x" and directed perpendicular to the skin until it reaches the fascia of the external oblique muscle. A "wall" of local anesthetic solution is injected between this point and the iliac spine, and along an imaginary line extending toward the umbilicus on the opposite side of the mark. The solution is injected at and below the level of the external oblique with some solution injected at the level of the internal oblique. A total of 10 to 15 ml of anesthetic is usually required. A solution of 1% lidocaine, 0.25% bupivacaine, or an equivalent is adequate.

If field anesthesia for hernia repair is required, further subcutaneous infiltration of anesthetic should be performed along the skin crease of the groin and along the imaginary line extending to the umbilicus. For hernia operations, further anesthesia of the spermatic cord is required, in the form of local injections in the area of the cord and the internal ring. Although epinephrine is useful in the subcutaneous and ilioinguinal block, it should be avoided in solutions used to anesthetize the base of the penis or the spermatic cord.

Further anesthesia of the groin area and below can be obtained by block of the femoral and lateral femoral cutaneous nerves.

Complications

Hematoma of the injection area is the most common problem, but is insignificant in normal patients. Motor block of the leg can occur if the femoral nerve is anesthetized and can delay ambulation of outpatients.

UPPER EXTREMITY

Brachial plexus block techniques have been described elsewhere (Chapter 61). The terminal branches can also be anesthetized by a local anesthetic injection along their peripheral courses as they cross the joint spaces, or by the injection of a dilute local anesthetic solution intravenously (IV) distal to a pneumatic tourniquet on the upper arm (IV regional block).

Peripheral Nerve Blocks of the Arm

Peripheral block is usually not quite as dense as a central block, but may be useful in anesthetizing one branch that was missed with a central block[7] or in providing very localized anesthesia on the hand.

Anatomy

The nerves to the forearm are most closely approximated in the brachial plexus. The terminal branches are separated below the level of the axilla, but the individual nerves can be identified with relative ease as they traverse the two joints of the arm, where they lie superficially, usually close to a bony landmark. **The sensory branches to the forearm from the musculocutaneous nerve and the internal cutaneous nerve branch extensively before they cross the elbow joint, so that injection of other nerves (which basically supply the hand) at this level does not improve forearm anesthesia. Thus, block at the elbow produces no greater anesthesia than block at the wrist.**

Technique of blockade

Block at the elbow. Two nerves to the hand cross this joint on its inner aspect, whereas the ulnar travels posteriorly in its well-known superficial groove.

The ulnar nerve can be blocked by injecting 3 to 5 ml of local anesthetic just proximal to the groove formed by the medial condyle of the humerus and the olecranon. This is easily done with the joint flexed at approximately 30°. Further flexion may cause the nerve to roll medially and anterior to the condyle. Paresthesias can usually be obtained, but direct injection on a paresthesia or directly into the groove is not advised because of the risk of damage to the nerve.

The median nerve crosses the joint in the company of the brachial artery. A line can be drawn between the two condyles on the inner aspect of the joint, and a skin wheal raised at the point where this line crosses the pulsation of the brachial artery—usually 1 cm to the ulnar side of the biceps tendon. A needle is introduced perpendicularly at this point and paresthesias immediately sought adjacent to the artery. Five milliliters of solution is sufficient to produce anesthesia; intraneural injection should be carefully avoided.

The radial nerve lies along the same intracondylar line,

approximately 2 cm lateral to the biceps tendon. Another skin wheal is raised here, and a needle inserted to search for paresthesias in a fan-shaped pattern. If paresthesias are not obtained, a wall of anesthetic solution is deposited here, but there will be less chance of reliable anesthesia.

Block at the wrist. The nerves lie more superficially at this joint and are closely associated with easily identified landmarks (Fig. 62-4). For this reason, this level of block is usually preferred over the elbow.

The ulnar nerve lies between the ulnar artery and the flexor carpi ulnaris. A skin wheal is raised at the level of the styloid process on the palmar side of the forearm between these two landmarks. A small-gauge needle is inserted and 3 ml of solution injected in the area, with or without paresthesias.

At the same level on the forearm, the median nerve lies between the tendons of the palmaris longus and the flexor carpi radialis. If only the palmaris longus can be felt, the nerve should rest just to the radial side of this tendon. A skin wheal can be raised and a needle inserted until it pierces the deep fascia. Three milliliters of solution is injected to produce anesthesia.

The radial nerve requires a broader injection because it has already started to ramify as it crosses the wrist. The anatomic "snuff box" formed by the tendons of the extensor pollicis longus and extensor pollicis brevis tendons is located and 3 ml of solution injected here. A subcutaneous wheal is raised extending from this point over the dorsum of the wrist and onto the back of the hand.

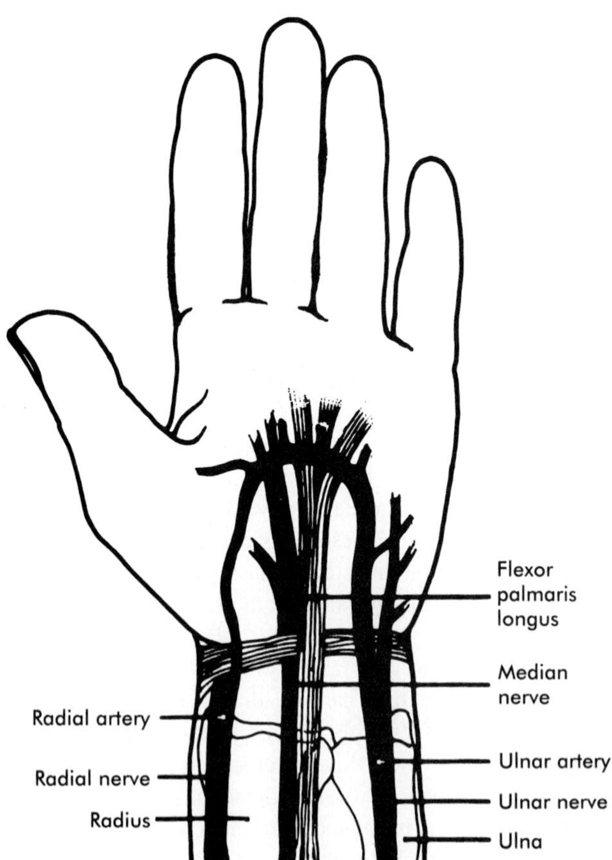

Fig. 62-4. Terminal nerves to the hand, as identified at the wrist. (From Mulroy MF: *Regional anesthesia: an illustrated procedural guide,* Philadelphia, 1996, Lippincott-Raven.)

Complications

Neuropathy is the most common complication of peripheral nerve injections, and is often associated with intraneural injection. Hematoma can also occur but is a minor complication.

Digital Nerve Block

The terminal nerves of the fingers can be blocked by injections on each side of the base of each digit. The most common problem with this form of anesthesia is that insufficient time is allowed for anesthesia to develop before a procedure is undertaken. Ten to 15 minutes may be required for adequate analgesia.

Technique of blockade

Some sedation is usually necessary for injections in this tender area.

The patient's hand can be rested on a flat surface with the palm down and the fingers extended. For each finger, an "x" is placed on the skin of the web space between the metacarpal heads. This is usually at the point where the skin texture changes from the rough character of the dorsal hand to the smooth texture of the palm. A 25-gauge needle is introduced here and directed down toward the metacarpal head of the digit to be blocked (Fig. 62-5). One to 2 ml of solution is injected along the ventral head and 1 ml along the dorsal head to anesthetize both the dorsal and ventral branches.

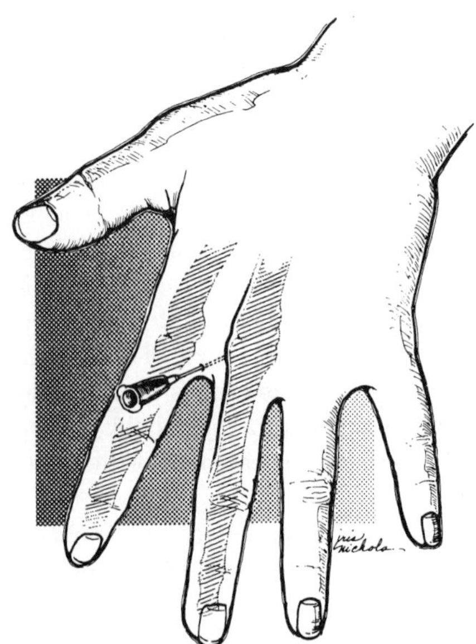

Fig. 62-5. Needle position for digital nerve block. (From Mulroy MF: *Regional anesthesia: an illustrated procedural guide,* Philadelphia, 1996, Lippincott-Raven.)

Both sides of each digit must be blocked. For the outside aspects of the index and little fingers, the solution is injected along the appropriate borders of the hand at the level of the metacarpal heads. For the thumb, similar injections are made on each side of the metacarpal head.

No epinephrine is used in these terminal digit blocks.

Intravenous Regional Block

The simplest technique of arm anesthesia is the injection of local anesthetic into the venous system distal to an occluding tourniquet. This appears to produce anesthesia by direct diffusion of the anesthetic from the vessels into the nearby nerves. The technique is often referred to as a Bier block and is named after August Bier, who first described anesthesia produced in this manner. His technique required a cutdown and ligation of a vein; the modern adaptation is elegant in its simplicity (Table 62-3).

Technique of blockade

This block is best performed with the patient in the supine position.

A small-gauge (20- or 22-gauge) IV plastic catheter is introduced in the dorsum of the patient's hand on the arm to be blocked. It should be taped firmly in place and a heparin port or small syringe attached and saline solution injected to maintain patency. A pneumatic tourniquet is applied over the upper arm.

The arm is elevated to promote venous drainage. An elastic or rubber bandage may be applied to produce further exsanguination (Fig. 62-6). After exsanguination, the tourniquet is inflated to 300 mm Hg or two times the systolic blood pressure and carefully tested for adequate occlusion of the radial pulse.

The patient's arm is returned to the horizontal position. A 50-ml syringe with 0.5% lidocaine or prilocaine (or 0.25% bupivacaine) is attached to the previously inserted cannula and the contents injected. The forearm will discolor and the patient will perceive a transient "pins and needles" sensation as anesthesia ensues over the following 5 minutes.

For short procedures, the cannula can be removed at this point. If surgery may extend beyond 1 hour, the cannula can be left in place and reinjected after 90 minutes.

Beyond 45 minutes of surgery, many patients experience discomfort at the level of the tourniquet. Special double-cuff tourniquets are available for this block to alleviate this problem. The proximal cuff should be inflated first, allowing anesthesia to be induced in the area under the distal cuff. If discomfort ensues, the distal cuff can be inflated over the anesthetized area of skin and the uncomfortable proximal cuff released. This step is critical, because the major risk of this procedure is premature release of anesthetic into the circulation. If a double cuff is used, both cuffs should be tested before starting, and the proper sequence for inflation and deflation meticulously followed. Because of this risk, and the greater risk of leakage under the narrower width cuffs of the double tourniquet, a single standard-width surgical tourniquet is probably better for short procedures.

If surgery is completed in less than 20 minutes, the tourniquet should remain inflated for at least that period of time (Fig. 62-7).[15] If 40 minutes have elapsed, the tourniquet can be deflated as a single maneuver. Between 20 and 40 minutes, deflate the cuff, reinflate immediately, and finally deflate after a minute.

The duration of anesthesia is minimal beyond the time of tourniquet release. Although bupivacaine may provide a slight prolongation of analgesia, any advantage is short-lived.

Table 62-3 Intravenous regional block

Indications	Comments
Surgery	Superficial hand surgery
Orthopedics: closed reduction of simple fractures (e.g., Colles)	———
Pain therapy (e.g., bretyllium)	For sympathetically mediated pain

Complications

Systemic toxicity is the greatest risk because a potentially toxic quantity of local anesthetic is injected directly into the vascular system. This problem is related to ei-

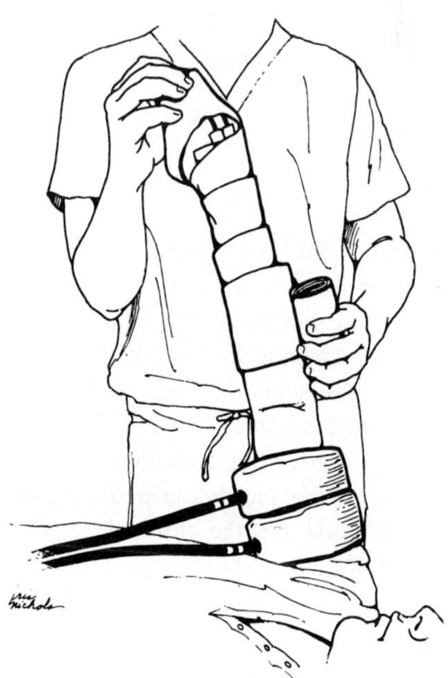

Fig. 62-6. Intravenous regional anesthesia with a double cuff and exsanguinating bandage. (From Mulroy MF: *Regional anesthesia: an illustrated procedural guide,* Philadelphia, 1996, Lippincott-Raven.)

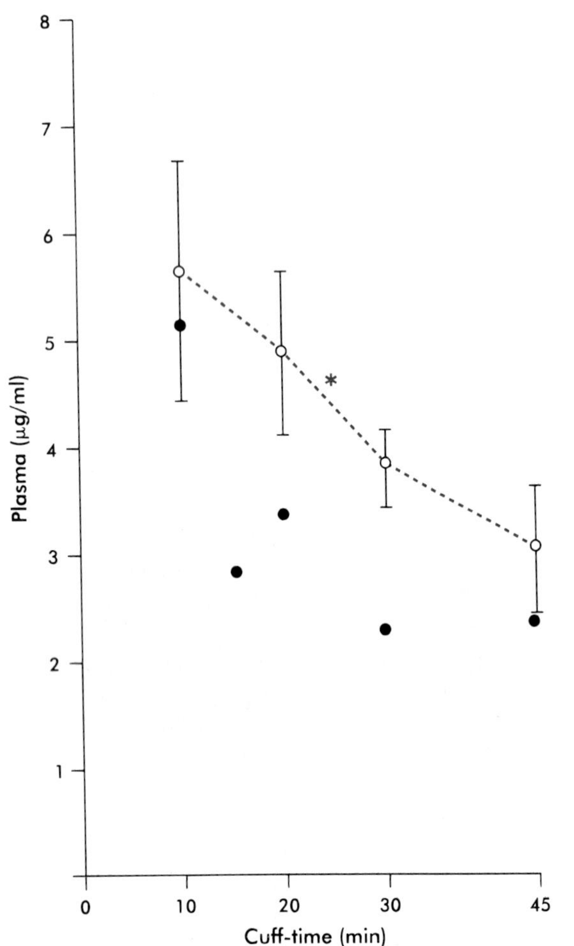

Fig. 62-7. Plasma levels of lidocaine after varying periods of cuff release. Open circles represent mean +/− SD after 50 ml 1% solution; closed circles represent individual blood levels following 50 ml 0.5% solution; * = $p < 0.05$. (From Tucker GT, Boas RA: Pharmacokinetic aspects of intravenous regional anesthesia, *Anesthesiology,* 34:538, 1971.)

ther a leak under the tourniquet or premature release.[5] Factors that reduce the potential for leakage include use of a distal IV site, slow injection, and adequate pressure in a wide cuff. A supplemental IV line should be placed in the opposite arm for resuscitation drugs, and the mental status of the patient must be monitored constantly.

Phlebitis is rare after this technique. Use of chloroprocaine was avoided in the past because of one report of a 10% incidence of phlebitis, but the current formulation of drug has been used in dilute concentrations, such as 0.5 to 0.75%.[10]

LOWER EXTREMITY

The nerves to the lower extremity are most easily blocked by the spinal, caudal, or epidural techniques. However, there are occasions when anesthesia by these routes is contraindicated because of systemic sepsis or coagulopathy. For outpatient surgery, many prefer to avoid the possible risks of postspinal headache, urinary retention, or prolonged immobilization sometimes associated with axial blocks. Thus, peripheral blockade still has a role in lower-extremity anesthesia. Proximal anesthesia of the lumbosacral trunks is described elsewhere, but there are (as in the arm) opportunities to block the peripheral nerves more distally as they cross the joints of the leg.

Popliteal Fossa Blockade

Blockade at the level of the knee (unlike the blockade of the arm at the elbow) produces excellent anesthesia of the lower leg and foot. It is simpler to perform than the five injections required for blockade at the ankle, and it may provide anesthesia for the discomfort of a calf tourniquet.[11] It is particularly useful in outpatients because motor function of the proximal muscles is preserved, and ambulation with crutches is easier than with sciatic-femoral blockade.

Anatomy

The sciatic nerve bifurcates high in the popliteal fossa into the peroneal nerve and the tibial nerve. The former courses laterally around the tibial head and provides the motor and sensory fibers to the anterior calf and dorsum of the foot. The latter remains posterior and provides sensation to the calf and sole of the foot. Thus, there are three major branches that cross the knee—the femoral, the tibial, and the peroneal.

Technique of blockade

Anesthesia at the level of the knee depends on locating the sciatic nerve near its bifurcation into the tibial and peroneal branches high in the popliteal fossa (Fig. 62-8). Supplemental anesthesia of the femoral nerve is needed to block its terminal saphenous branch, which serves the medial anterior calf and the dorsum of the foot.

The patient should be placed in a prone position. The triangular borders of the popliteal fossa can be outlined by drawing the central borders of the biceps femoris and of the semitendinosus muscles. The base of the triangle is the skin crease behind the knee. The patient can help to identify the muscles by slightly flexing the lower leg.

After the triangle is drawn, a perpendicular line is dropped from the midpoint of the base to the apex of the triangle. An "x" is drawn 6 cm from the base and 1 cm lateral to this bisecting line. After aseptic skin preparation, a skin wheal is raised at the "x."

A 3- or 4-inch needle is introduced through the "x" and directed 45° cephalad along the middle of the triangle. The nerves pass down the back of the leg parallel to the bisecting line of the triangle. A fanwise search is conducted perpendicular to this line until the nerve is contacted. If the femur is contacted by the needle, the depth should be noted. The nerve should be midway between the skin and the femur.

Once a paresthesia is obtained, the needle is fixed in position and 30 to 40 ml of local anesthetic solution is injected. The femoral branches can be injected in the same position

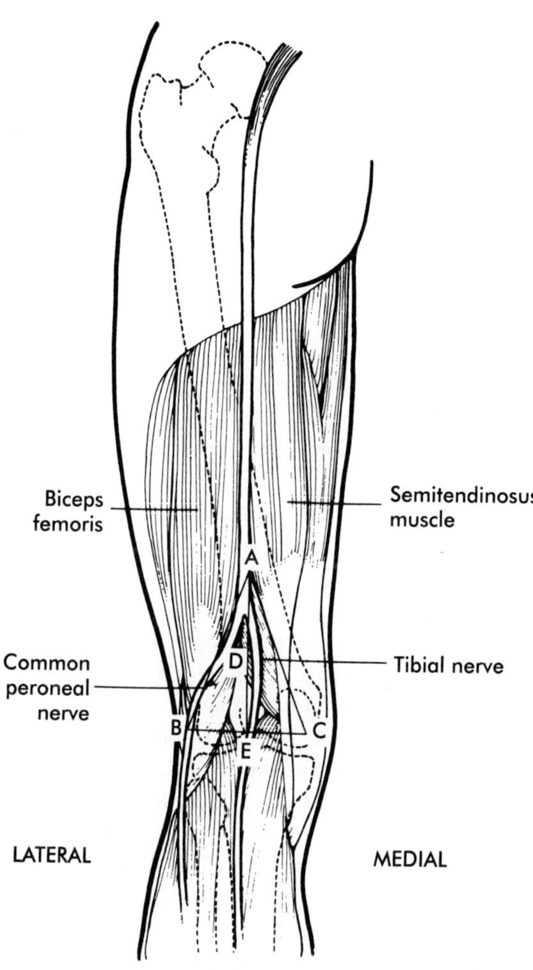

Fig. 62-8. Anatomy of the sciatic nerve at the knee. A, B, and C define the triangle formed by the borders of the popliteal fossa. The perpendicular is dropped from the apex to the midpoint of the base [E], and the point of injection [D] is 6 cm above the baseline and 1 cm lateral to this line. (From Mulroy MF: *Regional anesthesia: an illustrated procedural guide,* Philadelphia, 1996, Lippincott-Raven.)

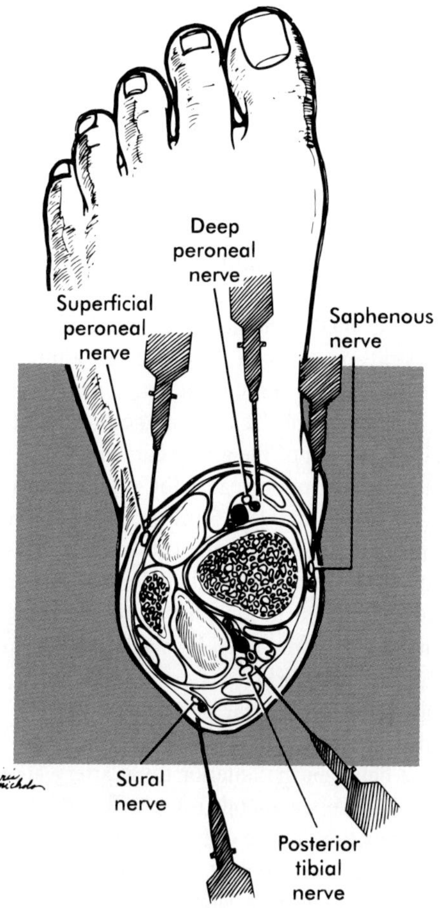

Fig. 62-9. Positions for injection of local anesthetics at the ankle. (From Mulroy MF: *Regional anesthesia: an illustrated procedural guide,* Philadelphia, 1996, Lippincott-Raven.)

by raising a subcutaneous wheal of 5 to 10 ml of local anesthetic along the medial tibial head just below the knee.

Ankle Block

The nerves of the foot can all be blocked at the level of the ankle.[12] Although this approach is ideal in producing the least amount of immobility of the lower extremity, it is technically more difficult because at least five nerves must be anesthetized. It is useful for superficial operations of the foot when a tourniquet is not required.

Anatomy

As described, two main branches of the sciatic nerve provide sensation for the foot, whereas terminal branches of the femoral nerve (as the saphenous nerve) innervate a small portion of the dorsum of the foot. The two main trunks have divided before the level of the ankle (Fig. 62-9). The posterior tibial nerve is the main branch of the tibial, but the sural nerve has separated from it to provide innervation to the lateral sole of the foot. Anteriorly, the deep peroneal nerve similarly continues as the main terminal branch to the dorsum of the foot, but it has formed multiple superficial branches before crossing the ankle joint.

Technique of blockade

Several of these nerves can be blocked by simple infiltration of a "wall" of anesthesia, but increased reliability can be produced by seeking paresthesias of the major branches. If paresthesias are not sought, this block may actually be less time consuming than other techniques, although five separate injections are required.

The posterior tibial nerve is the major nerve to the sole of the foot. It should be approached with the patient either in the prone position or supine with the hip and knee flexed so that the foot rests on the bed. The medial malleolus is identified and the pulsation of the posterior tibial artery behind it. A needle is introduced through the skin just behind the posterior artery and directed 45° anteriorly, seeking a paresthesia in the sole of the foot; 5 ml of a local anesthetic produces anesthesia if a paresthesia is identified. If not, a fan-shaped injection of 10 ml is performed in the triangle formed by the artery, the Achilles tendon, and the tibia itself.

The sural nerve (the other posterior nerve of the ankle) is blocked with the foot in the same position, by injection on the lateral side. A subcutaneous ridge of anesthesia is injected behind the lateral malleolus, filling the groove between it and the calcaneus to produce anesthesia of the sural nerve; this requires another 5 ml of local anesthetic.

The rest of the nerves are anterior, and one must either turn the patient supine or extend the leg. The saphenous nerve is anesthetized by infiltrating 5 ml of local anesthetic around the saphenous vein at the level where this vein passes anterior to the medial malleolus. A wall of anesthesia between the skin and the bone itself suffices to block the nerve.

The deep peroneal nerve is the major nerve to the dorsum of the foot and lies in the deep plane of the anterior tibial artery. The pulsation of the artery can be located at the level of the skin crease on the anterior midline surface of the ankle. If it can be palpated, 5 ml of local anesthetic can be injected just lateral to this point. If the artery is not palpable, the tendon of the extensor hallucis longus can be identified by asking the patient to extend the big toe. The anesthetic can be injected into the deep planes below the fascia using either of these landmarks.

To block the superficial peroneal branches, a subcutaneous ridge of anesthetic solution can be injected along the skin crease between the anterior tibial artery and the lateral malleolus. This subcutaneous ridge will overlie the previous subfascial injection for the deep peroneal nerve. Another 5 to 10 ml of local anesthetic may be required to cover this area.

Anesthesia of the foot should ensue within 10 minutes after performance of these five injections.

Complications

As in peripheral nerve block of the arm, neuropathy is the most serious complication. Intraneural injection, or "pinning" any of the nerves against bone during injection, must be avoided. Hematoma also occurs but is usually inconsequential.

HEAD AND NECK

Regional anesthesia of the head and neck has limited surgical application. Concern about control and maintenance of the airway makes many anesthesiologists uncomfortable with regional techniques when intraoperative airway intervention is awkward. Nevertheless, there are occasional patients who may benefit from regional techniques on the head or neck. More commonly, the techniques of trigeminal nerve block and occipital nerve block are used for diagnostic or neurolytic blocks for chronic pain syndromes. Cervical plexus block is useful for some surgical procedures on the neck, and topical/regional airway anesthesia is effective in reducing the subjective discomfort and hemodynamic responses to intubation.

Trigeminal Nerve Block

Anatomy

Sensory and motor nerve function of the face are provided by the branches of the fifth cranial (trigeminal) nerve. The roots of this nerve arise from the base of the pons and send sensory branches to the large gasserian (or semilunar) ganglion, which lies on the superior margin of the petrous bone just inside the skull above the foramen ovale. A smaller motor fiber nucleus lies behind it, and sends motor branches to one terminal nerve, the mandibular nerve. The three major branches of the trigeminal nerve have separate exits from the skull. The uppermost ophthalmic branch passes through the sphenoidal fissure into the orbit. The main terminal fibers of this nerve—the frontal nerve—bifurcate into the supratrochlear and supraorbital nerves. These two branches traverse the orbit along the superior border and exit on the front of the face in the easily palpated supraorbital notch for the former, and along the medial border of the orbit for the latter.

The two major branches of the trigeminal nerve are the middle (maxillary) and lower (mandibular). The maxillary nerve contains only sensory fibers and exits the skull through the foramen rotundum. It passes beneath the skull anteriorly through the sphenomaxillary fossa. At this point, it lies medial to the lateral pterygoid plate on each side. At the anterior end of this channel, it again moves superiorly to reenter the skull in the infraorbital canal in the floor of the orbit. Within the sphenomaxillary fossa, it branches to form the sphenopalatine nerves and into the posterior dental branches. The anterior dental nerves arise from the main trunk as it passes through the infraorbital canal. The terminal infraorbital nerve emerges from the infraorbital foramen just below the eye and lateral to the nose, and it branches into the terminal palpebral, nasal, and labial nerves.

The mandibular nerve is the third and largest branch of the trigeminal, and the only one that contains motor fibers. It exits the skull through the foramen ovale. At this point, it is just posterior to the lateral pterygoid plate of the sphenoid bone. The motor nerves separate into an anterior branch immediately below the foramen ovale. The main branch continues as the inferior alveolar nerve medial to the ramus of the mandible. This nerve curves anteriorly to follow the mandible and exits as a terminal branch through the mental foramen. The mental nerve provides sensation to the lower lip and jaw.

Technique of blockade

Gasserian ganglion block. Ideally, the simplest block of the trigeminal nerve is performed in the central ganglion, which includes all three branches, and is frequently recommended for treatment of disabling trigeminal neuralgia. **This block is technically the most difficult and has the most potential for the complications of subarachnoid injection of anesthetic during neurolytic block.** It is described in the chapter on pain management (see Chapter 63) and is mentioned here only to advise against its use for surgical anesthesia.

Superficial trigeminal nerve branch blocks. Fortunately, most anesthetic applications of trigeminal block can be more easily performed by injection of the individual terminal superficial branches. This is relatively simple because the three superficial branches and their associated foramina all lie in the same sagittal plane on each side of the face (Fig. 62-10). Each foramen is readily palpable, and these nerves can be easily blocked with superficial injections of small quantities of local anesthetic. The bony landmarks are usually sufficient. Each of these blocks can be performed with the patient in the supine position.

The supraorbital notch can be palpated along the medial superior rim of the orbit, usually 2.5 cm from the midline. Two to 3 ml of local anesthetic is injected immediately in the vicinity of the notch to produce anesthesia of the ipsilateral forehead. The supratrochlear nerve is anesthetized by superficial infiltration of the medial aspect of the orbital rim if the desired band of anesthesia crosses the midline.

The infraorbital foramen lies below the inferior orbital rim in the same plane at approximately the same distance from the midline as the supraorbital notch (usually 2.5 cm). If the foramen cannot be palpated directly, it can be found by gently probing with a small-gauge needle. This needle is introduced through a skin wheal approximately 0.5 cm below the expected opening, because the canal angles cephalad from this point toward the orbital floor. Injection of a small quantity of local anesthetic immediately in the vicinity of the foramen produces anesthesia of the middle third of the ipsilateral face.

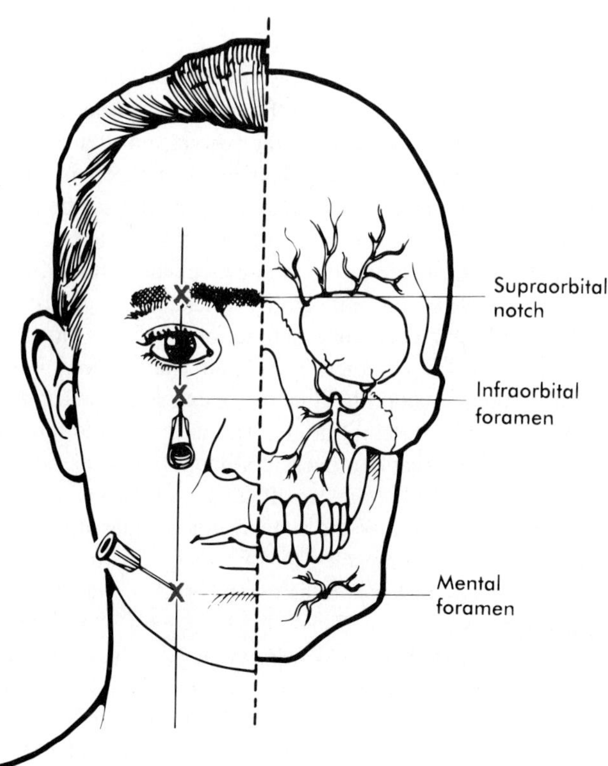

Fig. 62-10. Terminal branches of the trigeminal nerve on the face and their foramina. (From Mulroy MF: *Regional anesthesia: an illustrated procedural guide,* Philadelphia, 1996, Lippincott-Raven.)

The mental nerve also emerges approximately 2.5 cm from the midline, usually midway between the upper and lower border of the mandible. The mental canal angles medially and inferiorly; therefore, in this case needle insertion should start approximately 0.5 cm above and 0.5 cm lateral to the anticipated location of the orifice, if it cannot be palpated directly. In older patients, resorption of the superior margin of the mandibular bone makes the foramen appear to lie more superiorly along the ramus. Again, 2 ml of local anesthesia injected into the canal produces anesthesia of the mandibular area.

Maxillary nerve block. If anesthesia of the superior dental nerves is required, or if a superficial infraorbital nerve block does not produce adequate anesthesia, proximal block of the maxillary nerve is required. This can be performed by a lateral approach to the sphenopalatine fossa.

The patient should be positioned supine with a small towel placed under the occiput and the head turned slightly away from the side to be blocked. The zygomatic arch is marked along its course and the patient is asked to open and close the mouth slowly so that the curved upper border of the mandible can be identified. The lowest point of the mandibular notch is palpated and an "x" is marked at this spot, which is usually at the midpoint of the zygoma. A skin wheal is raised at the "x" after the appropriate skin preparations.

With the patient's jaw in the open position, a 3-inch needle is introduced through the "x" and directed 45° cephalad and slightly anterior. This direction should be toward the imagined posterior border of the globe of the eye (Fig. 62-11).

The needle should contact the pterygoid plate. It is withdrawn slightly and redirected slightly anterior until it passes beyond the pterygoid plate. At this point, the nerve should lie approximately 1 cm deeper. A paresthesia in the nose or the upper teeth confirms the nerve localization.

Five milliliters of solution is injected into the fossa, either on obtaining the paresthesia or blindly by advancing 1 cm beyond the plate.

Mandibular nerve block. This nerve can also be blocked for inferior dental pain. It is the only branch with which anesthesia carries the risk of loss of motor (mastication) function.

Head position and landmarks are the same as described for the maxillary nerve block. A 2-inch needle is introduced through the skin wheal and directed medially but slightly posterior and without the cephalad angulation required for maxillary nerve anesthesia; this leaves the needle approximately perpendicular to the skin in all planes.

When the pterygoid plate is contacted, the needle is redirected posteriorly until it passes beyond the plate. It should contact the nerve 0.5 to 1 cm deep to this point (Fig. 62-12).

Paresthesia of the jaw or cheek confirms identification of the nerve. Five to 10 ml of solution is injected incrementally at this point, to produce anesthesia of the terminal branches. If paresthesias are essential, the fossa can be explored gently cephalad and caudad from the initial point where the needle passes posterior to the plate. As with maxillary block,

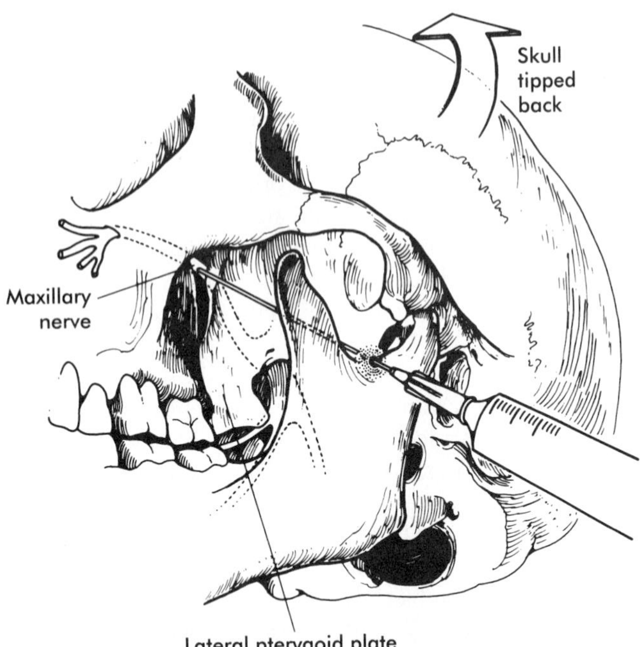

Fig. 62-11. Lateral approach to the maxillary nerve. (From Mulroy MF: *Regional anesthesia: an illustrated procedural guide,* Philadelphia, 1996, Lippincott-Raven.)

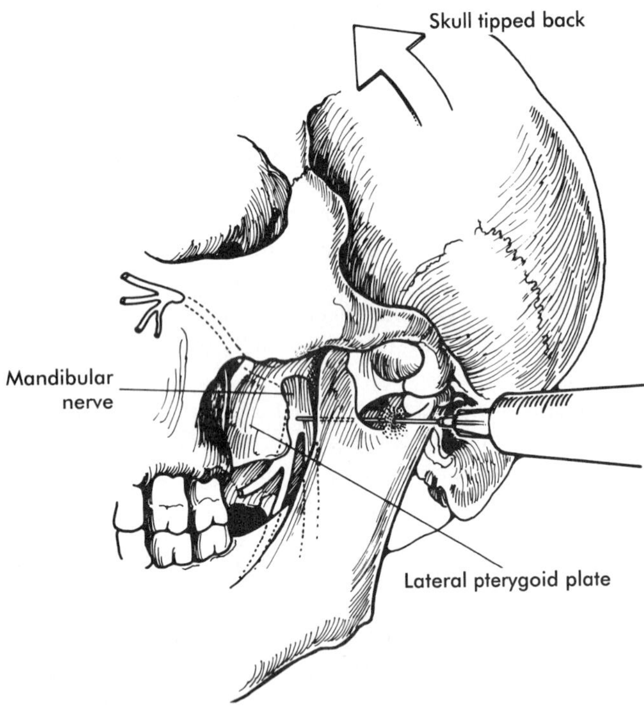

Fig. 62-12. Lateral approach to the mandibular nerve. (From Mulroy MF: *Regional anesthesia: an illustrated procedural guide,* Philadelphia, 1996, Lippincott-Raven.)

paresthesias can be painful to the patient, and the use of an assistant to secure the head is occasionally needed.

Complications

Spread of anesthetic to adjacent nerves and tissues is common, as in the orbit or the facial nerve. This is not serious unless neurolytic drugs are used. Intravascular injection is another possibility in the highly vascular head and neck region, and incremental injection of small quantities of anesthetic is warranted.

Table 62-4 Cervical plexus block

Indications	Comments
Thyroid surgery	—
Carotid endarterectomy	May need local infiltration of carotid bifurcation
Shoulder surgery	Rarely adequate alone; need brachial plexus anesthesia

Cervical Plexus Block

Anesthesia of the neck by blockade of the cervical nerve roots can be used to facilitate thyroid surgery, carotid endarterectomy, and shoulder surgery. For these procedures, many anesthesiologists are insecure about control of the airway during surgery and may elect to proceed with a supplemental intubation and light general anesthesia. Shoulder surgery can be performed with nerve block alone, but usually requires full brachial plexus blockade (Table 62-4).

Anatomy

Sensory and motor fibers of the neck and posterior scalp arise from the nerve roots of the second, third, and fourth cervical nerves (Fig. 62-13). This cervical plexus is unique in that the sensory fibers separate from the motor fibers early in their course and can be blocked separately. Classic plexus anesthesia along the tubercles of the vertebral body produces both motor and sensory blockade. The transverse processes of the cervical vertebrae form peculiar elongated troughs for the emergence of their nerve roots. These troughs lie just lateral to a medial opening for the cephalad passage of the vertebral artery. The trough at the terminal end of the transverse process divides into an anterior and posterior tubercle, which can often be easily palpated. These tubercles also serve as the attachments for the anterior and the middle scalene muscles, thus forming a compartment for the cervical plexus as well as for the brachial plexus immediately below.

The compartment at the cervical level is less developed than the one formed around the brachial plexus. The motor branches (including the phrenic nerve) curl anteriorly around the lateral border of the anterior scalene and proceed caudad and medially toward the muscles of the neck. They branch anteriorly to the sternocleidomastoid muscle as they pass behind it. The sensory fibers also emerge behind the anterior scalene muscle but separate from the motor branches and continue laterally to emerge superficially under the posterior border of the sternocleidomastoid. They provide sen-

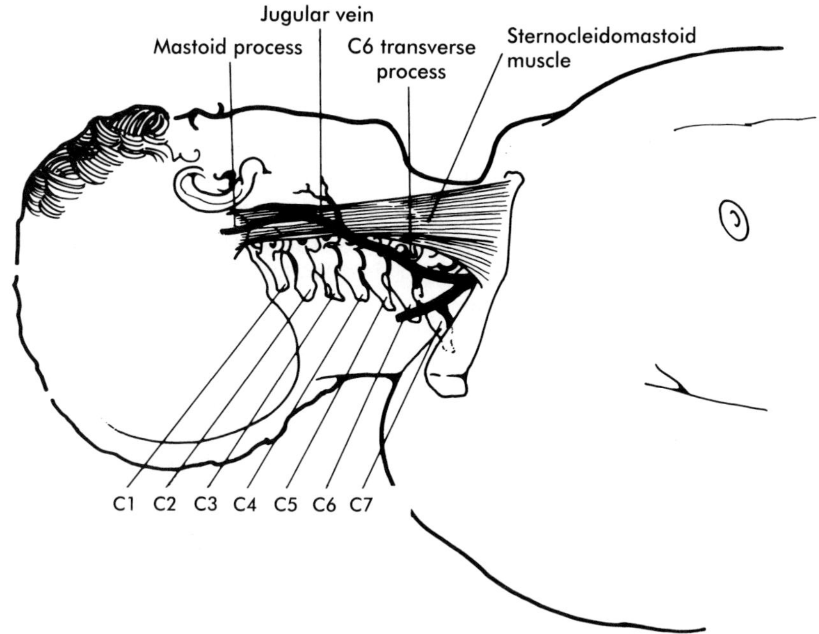

Fig. 62-13. Anatomy of the deep cervical plexus. (From Mulroy MF: *Regional anesthesia: an illustrated procedural guide,* Philadelphia, 1996, Lippincott-Raven.)

sory anesthesia to the anterior and posterior skin of the neck and shoulder.

Technique of blockade

Deep cervical plexus block. These fibers can be blocked by either the classic "deep" plexus block or a superficial sensory block.

The patient should be placed in the supine position with a small towel under the head and the head turned slightly to the side opposite the one to be blocked.

The mastoid process should be identified and marked. The transverse processes can often be palpated; if not, the most prominent tubercle—that of the sixth cervical vertebra—should be marked and a line drawn between it and the mastoid process.

The cervical processes are palpated approximately 0.5 cm posterior to the line drawn between the mastoid and the sixth cervical tubercle. The second vertebral process should lie approximately 1.5 cm below the mastoid itself. (There is no process for the first vertebra.)

The third and fourth processes lie approximately 1.5 cm below their respective superior neighbors. An "x" is placed over each transverse process.

Skin wheals are raised at the three "x" marks that have been placed over the transverse processes.

A 1.5-inch needle is introduced perpendicular to the skin and directed posterior and slightly caudad at each "x" until it rests on the transverse process. It is important to maintain a caudad direction to avoid entry directly into the intervertebral foramina. The needle is walked caudad; it should slip off the bone if it is truly on the process rather than continuing to contact bone if it is on the vertebral body. It is important to contact the transverse process as far laterally as possible to avoid any contact of the needle with the vertebral artery.

Paresthesias are usually not necessary. A syringe is connected directly to the needle and 5 ml of local anesthetic solution is injected along the transverse process itself. Anesthesia in the distribution of the nerve should follow within 5 minutes.

Superficial cervical plexus block. This method is useful if only sensory anesthesia is desired.

An "x" is marked along the posterior border of the sternocleidomastoid muscle at the level of the fourth cervical vertebra. This usually corresponds with the junction of the external jugular vein as it crosses the posterior border of the muscle.

A skin wheal is raised at this mark and superficial local anesthetic infiltration performed along the posterior border of the sternocleidomastroid muscle 4 cm above and below the level of the "x." Ten to 12 ml of local anesthetic solution usually provide sensory anesthesia of the anterior neck and shoulder.

Complications

Intravascular injection into the vertebral artery with deep cervical plexus blockade is the greatest risk. Careful aspirations and incremental injection are critical. Phrenic nerve block also occurs and is a relative contraindication to performing these blocks bilaterally. Hematoma can also occur, usually with the superficial technique. Unlike peripheral nerve blocks, this can be a significant problem in the neck if associated with airway compression or interference with the proposed surgery.

Occipital Nerve Block

Injection of the terminal branches of the cervical nerves can be used for minor surgical procedures of the posterior scalp but is more commonly applied in the evaluation and treatment of headaches.

Anatomy

Whereas the ophthalmic branch of the trigeminal nerve provides sensory innervation of the forehead and anterior scalp, the remainder of the scalp is innervated by fibers of the greater and lesser occipital nerves. These terminal branches of the cervical plexus can be blocked by superficial injection at the point on the posterior skull where they emerge from below the muscles of the neck (Fig. 62-14).

Technique of blockade

It is not necessary to shave the scalp for this block. The block is performed with the patient in the sitting position, leaning the head forward to expose the prominent nuchal ridge of bone at the posterior base of the skull.

The external occipital protuberance is identified in the midline, and a mark is made lateral to this prominence along the nuchal line at the lateral border of the insertion of the erector muscles of the neck, usually 2.5 cm from the midline. The branches of the greater occipital nerve usually pass laterally from behind the muscle to cross the nuchal line at this point.

After skin preparation, a small needle is introduced through the mark to the depth of the skull itself. A ridge of 3 to 5 ml of local anesthetic (1% lidocaine or equivalent) is deposited across the path of the emerging nerves just above the level of the bone. Paresthesias are occasionally encountered but are not essential to obtaining simple skin anesthesia.

If more anterior anesthesia of the scalp is required, the lesser occipital nerve branches are blocked by advancing the needle subcutaneously from this point in an anterior direction toward the mastoid process. A band of anesthetic solution is deposited along the line between the skin entry and the mastoid. A larger volume (6 to 8 ml) will be required.

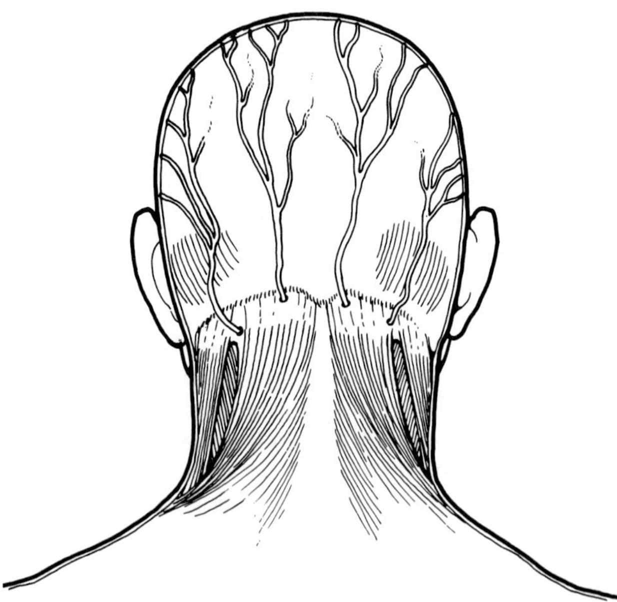

Fig. 62-14. Occipital nerves. (From Mulroy MF: *Regional anesthesia: an illustrated procedural guide,* Philadelphia, 1996, Lippincott-Raven.)

Complications

Local hematoma is a common and minor complication. The only serious complication is injection of local anesthetic into the foramen magnum if the needle is advanced below the nuchal ridge.

Airway Anesthesia

Manipulation of the airway during either laryngoscopy or intubation can be associated with laryngospasm, coughing, and cardiovascular reflexes that are undesirable. Similarly, long-term intubation is uncomfortable and stimulating to patients in the intensive care unit.[4] The anesthesiologist can abolish or blunt these responses by anesthetizing one or all of the sensory pathways involved.

Anatomy

The nasal mucosa is innervated by fibers of the sphenopalatine ganglion, a branch of the middle division of the fifth cranial nerve. These branches lie on the lateral wall of the nasal passages on each side, under the mucosa just posterior to the middle turbinate. The branches of these fibers continue caudad to provide sensory innervation to the superior portion of the pharynx, the uvula, and the tonsils. Anesthetizing the maxillary branch of the trigeminal is possible but is not a practical solution for airway anesthesia. Transmucosal topical application of local anesthetic is more appropriate. Below the sphenopalatine fiber distribution, sensory innervation of the oral pharynx and supraglottic regions is provided by branches of the glossopharyngeal nerve. These nerves lie laterally on each side of the pharynx submucosally in the region of the posterior tonsillar pillar. Direct submucosal injection can be performed, but carries a hazard of unintentional intravascular injection into several blood vessels in this area. Topical anesthesia of the terminal branches in the mouth and throat provides an easier approach. The larynx itself is innervated by the superior laryngeal branch of the vagus nerve in the area above the vocal cords. This branch leaves the main vagal trunk in the carotid sheath and passes anteriorly. Its internal branch penetrates the thyrohyoid membrane and divides to provide the sensory fibers to the cords, epiglottis, and arytenoids.

The recurrent laryngeal nerve provides innervation to the areas below the vocal cords, including motor innervation for all but one of the intrinsic laryngeal muscles. The trachea itself is also innervated by the recurrent laryngeal nerve. Topical anesthesia is the simplest approach to this nerve.

Technique of blockade

The airway can be anesthetized with the patient in the supine position, although many patients find it more comfortable to be semiupright or sitting when topical anesthesia is sprayed into the posterior pharynx. These positions allow them greater ease in swallowing excess solution and may reduce gagging. Regardless of the position chosen, there should be a firm support behind the head to reduce the possibility of involuntary withdrawal motions by the patient, which may dislocate needles used for injections.

For nasal mucosal anesthesia, cotton pledgets soaked with anesthetic solution are introduced through the nares and along the turbinates all the way to the posterior end of the nasal passage (Fig. 62-15). A second set of pledgets is placed with a cephalad angulation to follow the middle turbinate back to the mucosa overlying the sphenoid bone. This set of pledgets is the more critical one, because anesthesia in this mucosal area is most likely to anesthetize the branches of the sphenopalatine ganglia as they pass along the lateral wall of the airway. Bilateral anesthesia is preferable even if a nasal tube is to be inserted only on one side; bilateral blockade of the sphenopalatine fibers also produces posterior pharyngeal anesthesia caudad to this level. The pledgets should be allowed to remain in contact with the nasal mucosa for at least 2 to 3 minutes to allow adequate diffusion. Cocaine in a 4% solution has been the traditional topical anesthetic for this application, because of the unique vasoconstrictive properties of cocaine that produce shrinkage of the mucosa and reduce the chance of bleeding. Because of the toxicity of cocaine and the significant abuse problem in this country, alternate solutions have been recommended, primarily a mixture of 3% to 4% lidocaine and 0.25% to 0.5% phenylephrine.[6,13]

Topical anesthesia of the posterior pharynx can be performed while the nasal applicators are in place. A commercial spray or an atomizer filled with a 4% solution of lidocaine (a higher concentration of local anesthetics is required to penetrate mucosal membranes) can be used. For effective anesthesia in the posterior pharyngeal wall, topical application is performed in two stages. First, the tongue itself is sprayed with a local anesthetic and the patient is encouraged to gargle and swallow the residual liquid in the mouth. The numb tongue can be grasped with a gauze pad with one hand while the spray device is inserted in the mouth with the other. The patient should be encouraged to take rapid deep breaths ("pant like a puppy"), then the posterior pharynx is sprayed on inspiration. The inspiratory flow of gases should be enough to draw the lidocaine solution into the posterior pharynx and even to the vocal cords. If the superior laryngeal nerve block has been performed before this, there is a good likelihood that the aerosol will be carried into the trachea. A few minutes are needed for adequate onset of topical anesthesia in the pharynx.

Superior laryngeal nerve block can also be performed while the nasal pledgets are in place. This nerve is blocked bilaterally by identifying the superior ala of the thyroid cartilage, which usually lies just inferior to the posterior position of the hyoid bone on each side (Fig. 62-16). A 5-ml syringe with a 1% lidocaine solution should be used with a 23-gauge 5/8-inch needle. The skin of the neck is retracted caudad down over the thyroid cartilage with the index finger of one hand. Then the needle is inserted until it rests on the superior margin of the cartilage. Tension on the skin is released and the needle withdrawn slightly and allowed to walk superiorly off the cartilage. The needle is reinserted and passed through the thyrohyoid membrane, which is felt as a discernible resistance. After careful aspiration, 2.5 ml of solution is injected into the space below the membrane, and the procedure is repeated on the opposite side. This block can be performed as part of total airway anesthesia, or can be used independently to provide increased acceptance of indwelling endotracheal tubes in patients in the intensive care unit.

Tracheal anesthesia is performed with a direct transcricoid injection. A small skin wheal is raised over the cricothyroid membrane. A 20-gauge IV catheter is inserted gently through the skin wheal and through the membrane it-

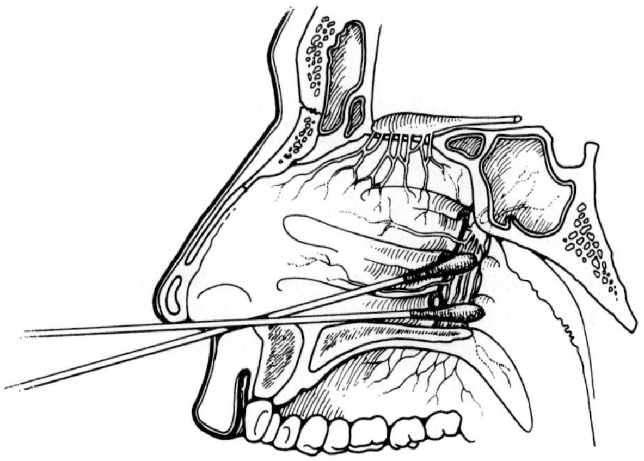

Fig. 62-15. Topical anesthesia of the nasal mucosa and sphenopalatine ganglion. (From Mulroy MF: *Regional anesthesia: an illustrated procedural guide,* Philadelphia, 1996, Lippincott-Raven.)

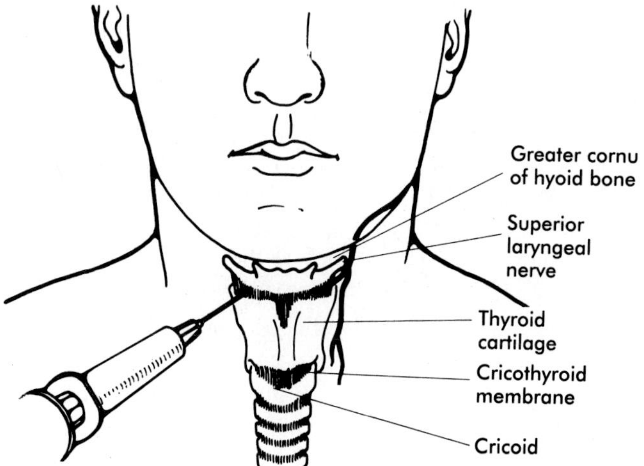

Fig. 62-16. Superior laryngeal nerve block. (From Mulroy MF: *Regional anesthesia: an illustrated procedural guide,* Philadelphia, 1996, Lippincott-Raven.)

self. Entry into the trachea is confirmed by the ability to aspirate air through the catheter. The steel stylet is removed and the plastic catheter left in the trachea. A syringe with 4 ml of 4% lidocaine is attached to the catheter and the local anesthetic sprayed into the trachea during inspiration (Fig. 62-17). The inflow of air usually carries the local anesthetic caudad; the resultant cough will spread the anesthetic up to the underside of the vocal cords and the larynx.

After these steps have been completed, the pledgets are removed from the nasal passages and nasal intubation performed. If tracheal or laryngeal anesthesia has been omitted because of concern of aspiration, there can be some pharmacologic intervention to reduce the cardiovascular response to the passage of the tube into the trachea. This may be facilitated by the IV use of beta blockers or by the administration of sedation beforehand or rapid-acting thiobarbiturates immediately after the airway is secured.

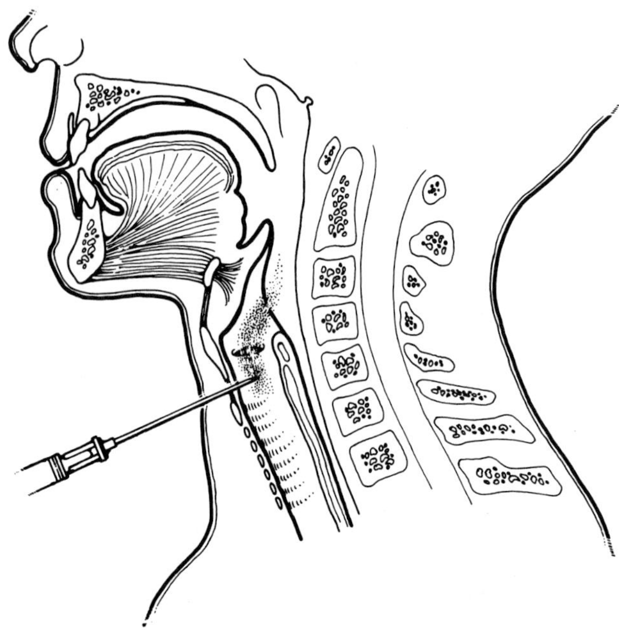

Fig. 62-17. Transtracheal injection. (From Mulroy MF: *Regional anesthesia: an illustrated procedural guide,* Philadelphia, 1996, Lippincott-Raven.)

Complications

Systemic toxic reaction to the local anesthetic is easily produced with the large volumes of multiple drugs commonly used and with the total quantities often exceeding recommended doses. Fortunately, transmucosal absorption is less than with direct injection. Careful attention to total dosage is necessary, with constant monitoring of the patient's mental status. Cocaine is the most toxic agent, and the dosage can be reduced by substituting other vasoconstrictors.[6,13]

Aspiration of gastric contents can occur if airway protective reflexes are blocked in presence of a full stomach. In this situation, limited anesthesia and sedation are more appropriate.

KEY POINTS

- Anesthesia of the intercostal nerves of the lower six ribs can provide both motor and sensory anesthesia of the abdominal wall from the xiphoid to the pubis. Pneumothorax, although rare when anesthesia is provided by experienced clinicians, remains the greatest concern with this technique.
- Because the sensory branches to the forearm from the musculocutaneous nerve and the internal cutaneous nerve branch extensively before they cross the elbow joint, injection of other nerves at this level does not improve forearm anesthesia. Thus, block at the elbow produces no greater anesthesia than block at the wrist.
- The terminal nerves of the fingers can be blocked by injections on each side of the base of each digit.
- The simplest technique of anesthesia for the arm is the injection of local anesthetic into the venous system distal to an occluding tourniquet. This technique appears to produce anesthesia by direct diffusion of the anesthetic from the vessels into the nearby nerves. Because a Bier block involves injection of a potentially toxic quantity of local anesthetic directly into the vascular system, systemic toxicity is a serious risk.
- The nerves to the lower extremities are most easily blocked by the spinal, caudal, or epidural techniques. These techniques are contraindicated in cases of systemic sepsis or coagulopathy. In outpatient surgery, peripheral blockade may be preferred for lower extremity anesthesia because it avoids the risks of postdural-puncture headache, urinary retention, or prolonged immobolization sometimes associated with axial blocks.
- Regional anesthesia of the head and neck has limited surgical application, particularly because of concern about control and maintenance of the airway when intraoperative airway intervention is awkward.
- Anesthesia of the neck and shoulder by blockade of the cervical nerve roots can be used to facilitate thyroid surgery, carotid endarterectomy, and shoulder surgery. With deep cervical plexus blockade, intravascular injection into the vertebral artery poses the greatest risk. Careful aspirations and incremental injection are critical.

Phrenic nerve block can occur also, and is a relative contraindication to performing these blocks bilaterally.

- Manipulation of the airway, either during laryngoscopy or intubation, can be associated with laryngospasm, coughing, and undesirable cardiovascular reflexes. These responses can be abolished or blunted by anesthetizing one or all of the sensory pathways involved. This is accomplished by topical anesthesia of the mucosa of the trachea, nose and/or oropharynx, plus blockade of the superior laryngeal nerves.

KEY REFERENCES

Bridenbaugh PO, DuPen SL, Moore DC, et al: Postoperative intercostal nerve block analgesia versus narcotic analgesia, *Anesth Analg* 52:81, 1973.

Cory P, Mulroy MF: Postoperative respiratory failure following intercostal block, *Anesthesiology* 54:418, 1981.

Grice SC, Morell RC, Balestrieri FJ, et al: Intravenous regional anesthesia; evaluation of leakage under the tourniquet, *Anesthesiology* 65:316, 1986.

Lanz E, Theiss D, Jankovic D: The extent of blockade following various techniques of brachial plexus block, *Anesth Analg* 62:55, 1983.

Schurman DJ: Ankle block anesthesia for foot surgery, *Anesthesiology* 44:342, 1976.

Tucker GT, Boas RA: Pharmacokinetic aspects of intravenous regional anesthesia, *Anesthesiology* 34:538, 1971.

REFERENCES

1. Bridenbaugh PO, DuPen SL, Moore DC, et al: Postoperative intercostal nerve block analgesia versus narcotic analgesia, *Anesth Analg* 52:81, 1973.
2. Cory P, Mulroy MF: Postoperative respiratory failure following intercostal block, *Anesthesiology* 54:418, 1981.
3. Eason MJ, Wyatt R: Paravertebral thoracic block—a reappraisal, *Anaesthesia* 34:638, 1979.
4. Gotta AW, Sullivan CA: Anesthesia of the upper airway using topical anesthesia and superior laryngeal nerve block, *Br J Anaesth* 53:1055, 1981.
5. Grice SC, Morell RC, Balestrieri FJ, et al: Intravenous regional anesthesia; evaluation and prevention of leakage under the tourniquet, *Anesthesiology* 65:316, 1986.
6. Gross JB, Hartigan ML, Schaffer DW: A suitable substitute for 4% cocaine before blind nasotracheal intubation:3% lidocaine-0.25% phenylephrine nasal spray, *Anesth Analg* 63:915, 1984.
7. Lanz E, Theiss D, Jankovic D: The extent of blockade following various techniques of brachial plexus block, *Anesth Analg* 62:55, 1983.
8. Moore DC, Bridenbaugh LD: Pneumothorax: its incidence following intercostal nerve block, *JAMA* 182:1005, 1962.
9. Moore DC, Bush WH, Scurlock JE: Intercostal nerve block: a roentgenographic anatomic study of technique and absorption in humans, *Anesth Analg* 59:815, 1980.
10. Palas TAR: Don't forget chloroprocaine for IVRA, *Reg Anesth* 15:271, 1990.
11. Rorie DK, Byer DE, Nelson DO, et al: Assessment of block of the sciatic nerve in the popliteal fossa, *Anesth Analg* 59:371, 1980.
12. Schurman DJ: Ankle block anesthesia for foot surgery, *Anesthesiology* 44:342, 1976.
13. Sessler CN, Vitaliti JC, Cooper KR, et al: Comparison of 4% lidocaine/0.5% phenylephrine with 5% cocaine: which dilates the nasal passages better? *Anesthesiology* 64: 274, 1986.
14. Sury MRJ, Bingham RM: Accidental spinal anaesthesia following intrathoracic intercostal nerve blockade, *Anaesthesia* 41:401, 1986.
15. Tucker GT, Boas RA: Pharmacokinetic aspects of intravenous regional anesthesia, *Anesthesiology* 34:538, 1971.

CHAPTER 63

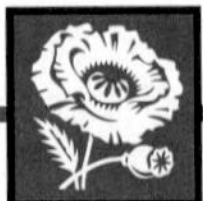

Nerve Blocks and Other Procedures for Pain Therapy

FRANCIS X. RIEGLER
RAY H. d'AMOURS

AN OVERVIEW OF PAIN MANAGEMENT

Pain Management and Anesthesiology

Pain remains the most common reason patients seek health care services. Unrelieved pain and related disabilities comprise an enormous, worldwide ongoing social and economic problem. Low back pain and related symptoms—the most commonly presenting pain syndrome in pain clinics—is the second leading reason for physician office visits in the United States alone.[127] Anesthesiology initially developed out of a practical need to control intraoperative pain. As early as 1922, the world's oldest organization of anesthesiologists, the International Anesthesia Research Society, adopted as its slogan "We strive always for world conquest of pain." Expertise with techniques of regional anesthesia, familiarity with the pharmacology of local anesthetics and systemic analgesics, and a generally expanding role outside the operating room in locations such as the pain clinic and the intensive care unit have uniquely positioned anesthesiologists to lead in the development and clinical application of pain management strategies.

Greater understanding of pain and the pain experience as an integrated, multidimensional phenomenon has led to the development of modern pain management regimens which are based on a comprehensive, multidisciplinary approach to the patient. In almost all cases, anesthesiologists seeking to gain expertise in the management of pain need to develop clinical skills and understanding beyond the realm of the operating room. The American Board of Anesthesiology (ABA) has supported the development of anesthesiologists as pain management specialists by developing and initiating the issuance of Certificates of Added Qualifications in Pain Management. Certification requires demonstration of additional training and experience in pain management as well as successful completion of a written examination. This is currently the only pain management certification that is recognized by the American Board of Medical Specialties, and it is only available to diplomates of the ABA.[4] Anesthesia-based fellowships in pain management are ideally designed to engender a broader understanding of the discipline through exposure to the relevant aspects of related fields such as psychology, neurology, and physical therapy. Anesthesiologists engaged in the field of pain management should have sufficient knowledge of these areas to coordinate appropriate consultation when indicated (Fig. 63-1).

The Human Pain Experience

The International Association for the Study of Pain has defined the human pain experience as "an unpleasant sensory and emotional experience associated with actual or potential tissue damage or described in terms of such damage."[144] In some circumstances, it may be a valuable phenomenon which signals disease or prevents further injury. In other circumstances, it serves no useful purpose and is maladaptive. Implicit in the term "*pain management*" is an acknowledgment that complete relief of pain and related symptomatology cannot always be obtained for all patients. In many cases, optimal management is ongoing and entails minimizing the degree of symptoms experienced, maximizing functional capacity, and initiating therapy to reduce associated psychologic distress.

Because of its ultimately subjective nature, the human pain experience is not a phenomenon which can be reliably quantified by parameters external to the patient such as laboratory tests or vital signs. Figure 63-2 schematizes an integrated model of the pain experience, which can be likened to an onion. At the core of the model is nociceptive input, which results from actual or potential tissue damage. The emotional and sensory perception of nociceptive input results in "pain." In turn, these are integrated with cognitive and affective factors

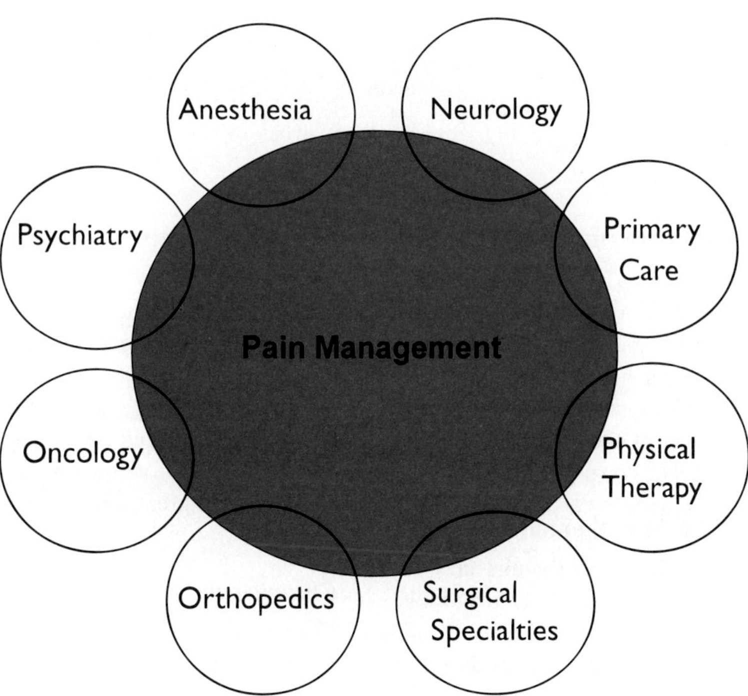

Fig. 63-1. Modern pain management incorporates aspects of numerous medical specialties. The pain management expert must have sufficient awareness of each specialty to arrange appropriate consultation.

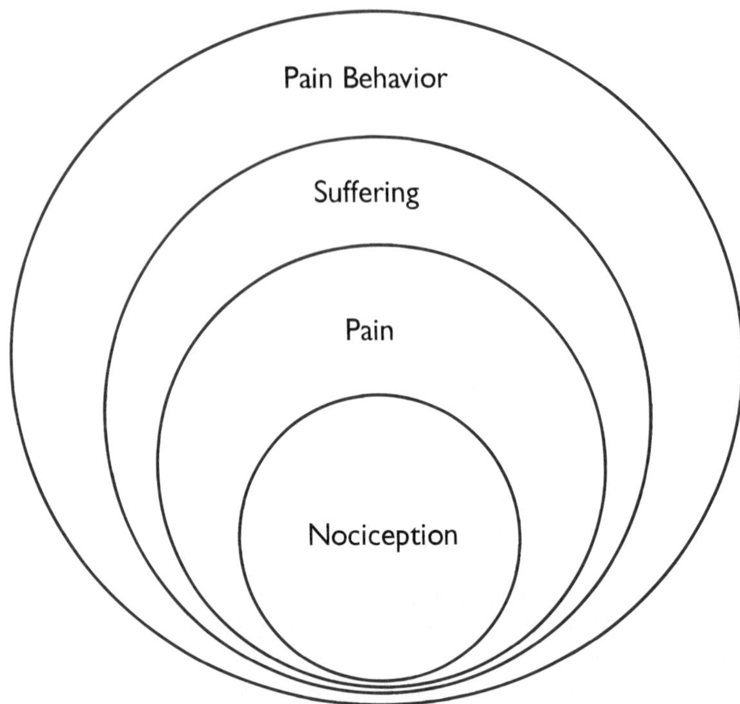

Fig. 63-2. A conceptual model of the pain experience. In the assessment of pain, only pain behavior can be directly observed. (From Loeser JD: Concepts of pain. In Stanton-Hicks M, Boas R, editors: *Chronic low back pain,* New York, 1982, Raven.)

Table 63-1 Clinical dimensions of pain syndromes and their management

	Acute pain	Cancer pain	Chronic pain
Care setting	Inpatient	Inpatient/Outpatient	Outpatient
Emotional component of pain	+	+ +	+ + +
Duration of therapeutic relationship	Short	Intermediate	Long
Extent of relief commonly achieved	+ + +	+ +	+
Utility of nerve blocks as a single mode of treatment	+ + +	+ +	+
Role of opioid therapy	Primary	Primary	Limited

unique to the patient, which may result in "suffering." None of the foregoing components is directly measurable. The integration of them results in observable pain behaviors on the part of the patient. To some extent, these are quantifiable by measures such as verbal pain rating between 0 and 10, but ultimately such measures depend on the patient's own self report.

Clinical Approaches to Pain Management

Clinically, pain syndromes in children and adults may be broadly classified as acute, chronic, or cancer related (Table 63-1). Each involves distinctive features of pathogenesis and ultimately requires an individualized approach for optimal management.

Acute pain

Examples of acute pain syndromes include postoperative pain and trauma pain. Symptoms typically have a clear causal relationship to tissue injury. Healing of the injured area is expected to occur quickly and is accompanied by resolution of symptoms. Treatment of acute pain is primarily directed at inhibiting nociception until healing occurs, with less emphasis placed on the psychologic and emotional aspects of pain. Nerve blocks and opioid analgesics can both be used with great effectiveness in the treatment of acute pain.

Chronic pain

Chronic pain syndromes are defined as those with a duration of greater than six months or which greatly outlast the expected period of healing for demonstrable causative pathology. Common examples include chronic low back pain and postherpetic neuralgia ("shingles"). Chronic pain may also exist in the absence of nociceptive input from the periphery (e.g., phantom limb pain). Many treatments which are dramatically successful in the management of acute pain are only partially effective for chronic pain.[178] Prolonged neural blockade is difficult to achieve in practice, and the long-term use of opioid analgesics may be complicated by the development of tolerance and psychological dependence. **Chronic pain is commonly associated with significant psychological and emotional components. Treatment may need to be directed largely at these aspects and may frequently be much less successful than treatment of acute pain.** The lack of success can be frustrating for both the patient and the physician.

Cancer pain

Cancer-related pain syndromes may result from solid or liquid tumors, as well as their treatment, which may include surgery, chemotherapy, and radiotherapy. An example would be recurrent head and neck cancer with localized pain related to tumor progression and oral mucositis pain secondary to radiation therapy. Cancer-related pain frequently manifests elements of both acute and chronic pain. Symptoms generally have a clear relationship to tissue injury, but may persist for months or years. Healing of damaged tissue may never occur. Psychological and emotional factors may be prominent. Opioid analgesics can be used with great effectiveness and the problem of tolerance is often obviated by limited life expectancy. Nerve blocks with local anesthetics or neurolytic agents can be invaluable in selected patients. When death is imminent, patients may be willing to tolerate side effects such as sensory or motor deficits which would otherwise be unacceptable. Effective management of cancer pain can be challenging but is almost always achievable. It can dramatically improve the quality of life for patients and their loved ones.

Nerve blocks have been used in the diagnosis and treatment of pain for over a century. Skillfully administered, they are among the most effective currently available methods of relieving acute and chronic pain. Despite long-standing use of this technique, there are still misconceptions about its proper role in the management of chronic pain.

The basis of efficacy for nerve blocks in chronic pain management is the interruption of sensory and nociceptive pathways. Sensory nerve blocks relieve pain and interrupt the afferent limbs of an abnormal reflex mechanism. Low concentrations of local anesthetic agents block unmyelinated C fibers and small A delta fibers without significantly impairing motor function. In many instances, blocks with short-acting local anesthetic agents produce pain relief that greatly outlasts the pharmacologic action of the drug. The exact mechanism of this long-lasting effect is not yet known. Neurodestructive agents such as alcohol and phenol produce prolonged pain relief by chemical destruction of nociceptive pathways.

Nerve blocks are used diagnostically to distinguish specific pain pathways. Prognostic blocks are useful in predicting the effects of prolonged interruption. They also afford the patient an opportunity to experience the numbness and/or other side effects that follow prolonged or permanent blocks. Therapeutic blocks can be achieved with either a local anesthetic agent or a neurolytic agent.

Local anesthetic blocks are useful for relieving severe pain in the head and neck, chest, abdomen, pelvis, and extremities. Continuous pain relief for prolonged periods in terminally ill cancer patients can be achieved by continuous segmental epidural or peripheral nerve block with local anesthetics or narcotics. To obtain optimal results, it is essential to adhere to certain basic principles, as outlined by Bonica[29]: "a willingness to devote the necessary time to evaluate the patient thoroughly; proper diagnosis of the etiology, mechanism, and distribution of pain; adequate skill in the procedure; and ensuring that the patient and the patient's family have been informed about the procedure and its consequences."

TYPES OF NERVE BLOCKS USEFUL FOR PAIN RELIEF

Nerve blocks used in chronic pain management include somatic peripheral nerve blocks, intravertebral central neural blocks, and visceral sympathetic blocks. These same nerve blocks can be spectacularly effective in acute postoperative and dental pain management, where they interrupt transmission of nociceptive stimuli from the peripheral to the central nervous system (CNS). However, because the mechanisms operant in maintenance of chronic pain are frequently different from those of acute pain, nerve blocks may be less effective in chronic pain states. Nevertheless, they still have an important part to play in the diagnosis and management of chronic pain.

INDICATIONS FOR NERVE BLOCKS

Acute Pain

Nerve blocks effectively control acute pain by temporarily uncoupling the nociceptive pain source from conscious levels, as may occur, for example, with an intercostal block for broken ribs. In acute pain, the diagnosis is usually not problematic, and nerve blocks are used as therapy. Analgesia can be maintained in certain cases by continuous catheter techniques. There remains a great need for an agent that will produce a reversible sensory nerve block that will last for days rather than hours.

Chronic and Cancer Pain

Nerve blocks can be used to ascertain whether interruptible ongoing nociception is contributing to the patient's pain complaint, and if so, diagnostic blocks can help distinguish the afferent nerve pathway of such nociception. Although the information can be useful diagnostically, nerve blocks alone may be less useful in long-term management. This is because the maintenance of chronic pain states often results from a complex interplay of psychosocial and neurologic phenomena.

If neurosurgical ablative procedures (e.g., rhizotomy, sympathectomy) are being considered, nerve blocks can be used prognostically to allow the patient to experience the effects of such denervation and to aid in deciding whether to proceed with surgery. It is critically important that all parties concerned appreciate that although the immediate numbness experienced after a prognostic block may provide pain relief, over time the numbness itself can become distressing. In fact, denervation dysesthetic sensations that follow chronic deafferentation can become as distressing as the original nociception. Therefore, although prognostic blocks are useful in helping patients and surgeons make decisions, they do not guarantee long-term satisfaction with neurodestructive procedures.

PATIENT PREPARATION

Facilities

For invasive procedures such as nerve blocks, the facilities of a pain control center should promote an atmosphere of comfort and relaxation for the patient. Adequate space and equipment are imperative to ensure proper preparation and care of the patient.

Large treatment rooms are necessary to perform the more invasive procedures, such as epidural blocks, celiac plexus blocks, lumbar sympathetic blocks, and stellate ganglion blocks. The rooms should be equipped to accommodate possible emergencies. Following is a list of equipment that is essential for such invasive procedures:

- Locking stretcher or surgical table that can be easily and quickly placed into many different positions
- Oxygen tank with Ambu-bag, oxygen mask, and nasal cannula
- Suction machine and catheter
- Cardiac monitor with defibrillator
- Emergency crash cart with medication and equipment for airway management and intravenous (IV) access
- Radiograph view box

Role of the Nurse

Nurses (or other assistants) can play an important role in preparing and educating the patient before a procedure. The nurse may help the physician inform the patient of the purpose of the procedure, how the procedure is performed, the expected outcome, and the side effects and risks. An information sheet given to the patient will reinforce the verbal explanation. Written, informed consent is obtained.

Commonly, the chronic pain patient, when first seen at the pain-control center, has already seen many professionals in various hospitals and has endured numerous tests and procedures. This experience may leave the patient fearful of seeing a new set of medical professionals. Futher, nerve blocks are often foreign to patients and can engender apprehension. The nurse should help to reassure the patient that nerve blocks are a standard form of therapy and are performed by experts at the pain-control center.

During the procedure, the nurse sets up equipment, positions the patient, monitors vital signs, and assists as required. The nurse can help the patient relax by employing relaxation, distraction, or other techniques. The patient should be informed at each step of the procedure. Sudden, unexpected movement can be avoided if the patient has an idea of what is to happen. The nurse should have a thorough knowledge of the procedure and anticipate any complications, side effects, and emergencies.

After the procedure, patients are closely monitored as long as necessary, usually 30 minutes to 1 hour. The patient is given verbal and written instructions before discharge and must be accompanied home by a responsible adult escort. A list and description of side effects that commonly occur with the block should be included. Patients are also informed of how and when to contact personnel in the pain-control center.

ADJUVANT TECHNIQUES FOR SUCCESSFUL NERVE BLOCK

Fluoroscopy

Many procedures that involve catheter placement, visceral nerve block, or neurolytic block can be performed under fluoroscopy. An IV line is started in all patients. The invasive nature of these blocks and the presence of large pieces of radiograph apparatus increase the patient's apprehension. After the procedure, the patient is monitored as necessary. A postblock pain assessment is completed to evaluate the success of the block, and arrangements are made for the safe transfer of the patient either to a hospital bed or to the pain-control center before discharge.

Radiologic localization is also indicated when difficulty is anticipated because of poor landmarks or anatomic anomalies, or when deep nerves or plexuses are to be blocked. It is absolutely necessary for most neurolytic procedures.

Contrast materials

Contrast materials in conjunction with fluoroscopy can be useful in ruling out intravascular needle tip location or in defining tissue planes in the area of injection.[201] They should not be employed in patients with a history of allergy to iodine-containing solutions. **For injections in and around the spinal canal, or where there is a possibility of subarachnoid injection, only nonionic contrast materials, such as Isovue™ or Omnipaque™, may be used. Unintentional intrathecal administration of ionic contrast media can be catastrophic.**[25] Otherwise, an ionic contrast material, such as Conray™, may be used. There is as much as a tenfold increase in cost for the newer nonionic compared with ionic materials. In general, the smallest possible volumes should be injected. Although the newer agents, and especially the nonionic agents, are relatively free of adverse reactions, complications remain a possibility.[39] Ionic contrast can be irritating to nerves if injected without local anesthetic.

Peripheral Nerve Stimulation

Nerve stimulation with appropriately low amperage may be used to localize any peripheral nerve with a motor component.[170,179] As the tip of a needle connected to a nerve stimulator approaches a nerve, twitches are observed in the distribution of the corresponding motor unit. Many of the stimulators in use for monitoring neuromuscular blockade may be used for nerve localization if they generate variable, low-output currents (6.0 mAmps or less) with digital readouts.

An electrical field at the tip of a stimulating needle induces depolarization of myelinated motor efferents as the needle tip approaches a peripheral nerve. The current required to produce a twitch decreases as the needle tip nears the nerve in three dimensions. Empirically, current requirements of 1.0 mAmp or less appear to indicate sufficient proximity of the needle tip to produce a successful block. Advantages of the technique include an objective endpoint for neural localization and the ability to systematically guide the needle tip closer to the nerve by observing the changes in required current. Properly conducted neurostimulation at low current levels is usually painless for the conscious patient because the depolarization threshold for myelinated motor efferents is lower than for unmyelinated sensory afferents. It has been suggested that the chances for neural injury are less than with paresthesia techniques because the needle tip can be directed close to the nerve but need not contact it to produce a motor response at less than 1.0 mamp. Disadvantages include an inability to use the technique for purely sensory nerves and the potential for equipment failure.

Standard unsheathed needles are adequate for peripheral nerve stimulation. Nonetheless, sheathed and coated needles are more efficacious and require less current to stimulate the nerve. Various kits are available with sheathed needles of different lengths and sizes connected to an extension set and an alligator clip.

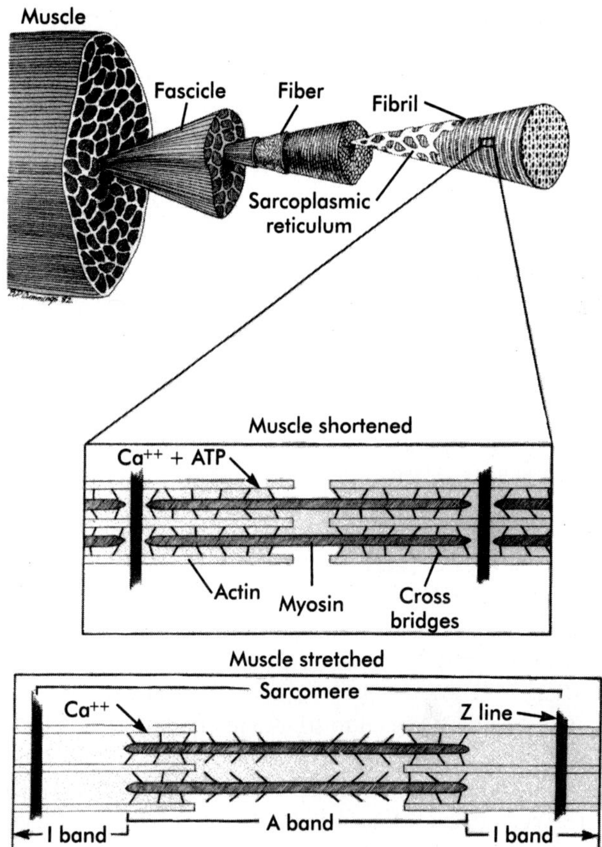

Fig. 63-3. Subunits of a skeletal muscle with the microanatomy of the myofibril, showing the relationship between Ca^{++} and ATP during muscle contraction and relaxation. (From Travell J, Simons DG: Myofascial pain and dysfunction. In *The trigger point manual,* Baltimore, 1983, Williams & Wilkins.)

MANAGEMENT OF MYOFASCIAL PAIN

Skeletal muscle accounts for 40% of body weight. Muscle tissue is subject to the wear and tear of daily activities. Any muscle can develop myofascial trigger points that can cause pain and muscle spasms.

Pathophysiology of a Trigger Point

Many researchers believe myofascial trigger points begin as neuromuscular dysfunction[174] and evolve into a histologically distinct lesion.[146] Miehlke et al.[146] reported biopsy findings supporting the existence of an initial dysfunction phase, followed by a dystrophic phase.

Acute muscle strain may overload fibrils in one region of the muscle, causing tissue damage that involves the sarcoplasmic reticulum with release of stored calcium. The presence of normal adenosine triphosphate (ATP) and excess calcium initiates and maintains a sustained contracture (Fig. 63-3). The body may respond with local vasoconstriction to this region of uncontrolled metabolism within the muscle. This may be a local or a reflex response. The taut fibers are palpable as a band in the muscle (Boxes 63-1 and 63-2).

BOX 63-1
PATHOPHYSIOLOGY OF A TRIGGER POINT
First Mechanism

Acute muscle strain
Damages sarcoplasmic reticulum
↓
Ca^{++} ion release and accumulation
Presence of ATP and excess Ca^{++}
↓
Initiates and maintains sustained contracture
Produces a region of uncontrolled metabolism
↓
Body responses with local vasoconstriction
There is now a region of increased metabolism, decreased circulation, and shortened muscle fiber
↓
Taut and palpable band in the muscle
↓
Trigger point

BOX 63-2
PATHOPHYSIOLOGY OF A TRIGGER POINT
Second Mechanism

Tissue injury
↓
Releases histamine
Serotonin
Kinins
Prostaglandins
↓
Further ischemia
Increased metabolism with reduced circulation
↓
Accumulates metabolic products
↓
Increases further sensitizing products
↓
Active trigger point

Table 63-2 Common myofascial nerve entrapments

Muscle	Nerve entrapped
Frontalis	Supraorbital
Semispinalis capitis	Greater occipital
Scaleni	Brachial plexus
Brachialis	Radial (sensory)
Triceps	Radial
Supinator	Deep radial
Flexor carpi ulnaris	Ulnar
Interossei (hand)	Digital (palmar)
Pectoralis minor	Brachial plexus
Paraspinal muscle	Posterior primary rami
Piriformis	Sciatic
Peroneous longus	Common peroneal
Tarsal tunnel	Tibial
Interossei (foot)	Digital (plantar)

Other factors related to trigger injury may contribute to the pathophysiology of trigger points.[9] Inflammatory mediators such as histamine, serotonin, kinins, and prostaglandins may be released locally,[146,198] and mast cells also proliferate at sites of muscle injury.

Clinical Presentation

Myofascial pain may begin acutely with muscle strain or may develop insidiously because of chronic muscular fatigue. Pain may continue for months or years.[107] Regardless of the mode of onset, the pain associated with a myofascial trigger point is steady, deep, and aching. It is exacerbated by strenuous use of the involved muscle, passive stretching, pressure on the trigger point, cold or damp weather, viral infections, stress, and fatigue.

A limited range of motion, stiffness, and weakness usually accompany the pain. These symptoms are worse in the morning and recur after periods of overactivity or immobilization during the day. Patients may report symptoms of autonomic dysfunction (e.g., excessive lacrimation, pilomotor activity, and changes in sweat patterns). The involved extremity may feel cold because of reflex vasoconstriction. Concurrent depression and sleep disturbances may lower the pain threshold.

A myofascial trigger point is a hyperirritable locus, located in a tight band of skeletal muscle or its associated fascia.[206] The trigger point is painful on compression and can evoke a characteristic referred pain and an autonomic response. Myofascial trigger points must be distinguished from tender spots in skin, ligaments, and periosteum (Table 63-2).

Trigger points can be either active or latent. An active trigger point causes pain, while a latent trigger point may restrict movement and weaken the affected muscle. The latent trigger point persists for years after recovering from injury and predisposes to acute exacerbations of pain. Precipitating factors include jerky motion, fatigue, cold and damp surroundings, and emotional upset.

Objective Data

Routine laboratory tests show no significant abnormalities in patients with a myofascial pain syndrome. The erythrocyte sedimentation rate, SMA, blood count, and serum muscle enzymes are all normal. Radiographs and computed tomography (CT) scans are normal. Electromyography (EMG) may show insertion potential, an increased number of polyphasic potentials in muscles with trigger points. Thermograms of skin overlying active trigger points may show areas of increased skin temperature.[71] Conversely, some investigators have found decreased skin temperature in the same areas.[120,188] Sola and Williams[196] observed low skin resistance over trigger points.

Management

The goals of treatment are to decrease pain to tolerable levels, improve function, and prevent permanent disability. These goals can be achieved by muscle relaxation through either spray-and-stretch techniques, trigger-point injections, an exercise program, or stimulation analgesia.

Stretch-and-spray technique

The stretch-and-spray procedure is the workhorse of myofascial therapy. It inactivates myofascial trigger points quickly with less patient discomfort than local myoneural injection. A recent onset of muscle spasm responds with full return of pain-free function if the vapocoolant spray is applied when the muscle is passively stretched.[208] When more than one muscle is involved, a stretch-and-spray procedure is a practical means of covering a large area to make

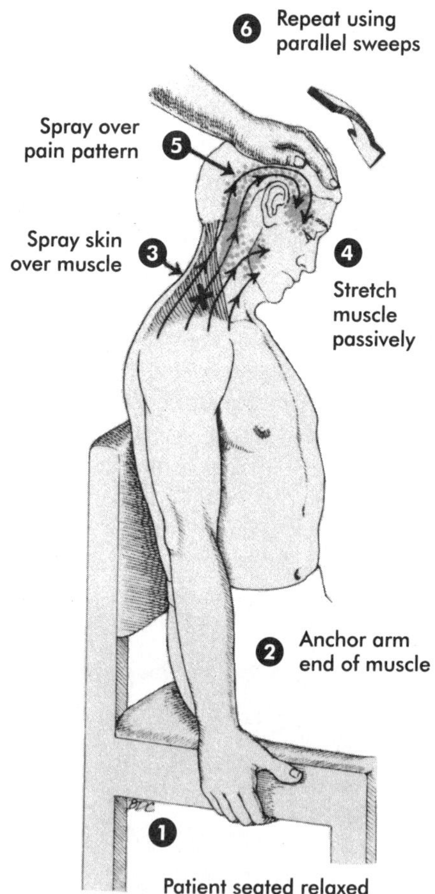

Fig. 63-4. The stretch-and-spray technique. (From Travell J, Simons DG: Myofascial pain and dysfunction. In *The trigger point manual,* Baltimore, 1983, Williams & Wilkins.)

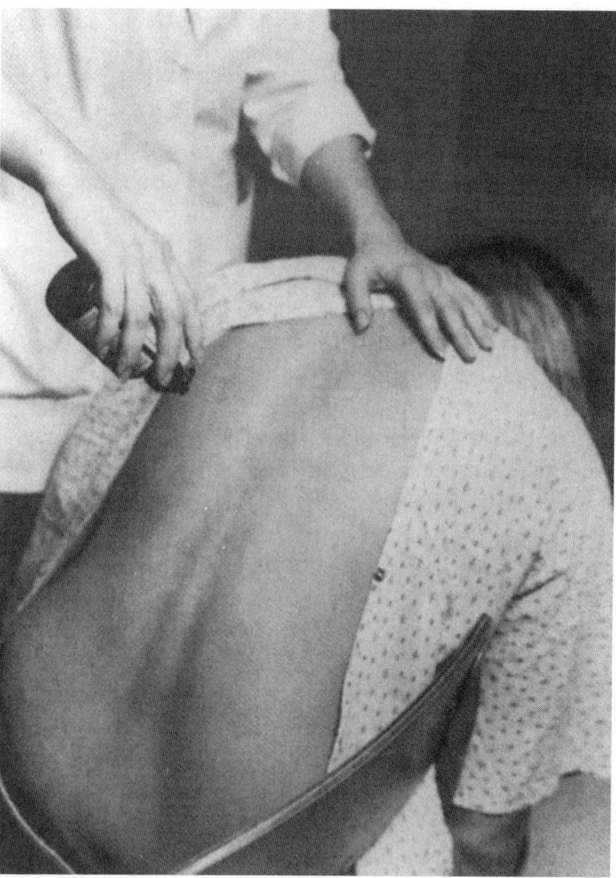

Fig. 63-5. Fluori-Methane Stretch-n-Spray being used on the thoracic and lumbar paraspinals while the muscles are stretched to increase the length of the muscle fibers and deactivate trigger points. The bottle is held 12 to 18 inches from the surface to be treated, and the fluid is sprayed at a 30- to 45-degree angle to the skin in unidirectional sweeps.

significant progress toward pain relief. The technique does not require precise localization of the trigger point. However, considerable skill is required to coordinate the course of spray so that it covers fibers that are being maximally stretched.

The patient must be positioned comfortably to permit voluntary relaxation (Fig. 63-4). One end of the muscle must be anchored so that pressure can be applied to the other end to passively stretch it. With the patient properly positioned, the first sweep of spray is applied before any stretching. The vapocoolant spray is applied in one direction only. The spray is swept over the entire length of the affected muscle and then over the referred pain pattern. The stretch-and-spray steps are repeated until full muscle length is achieved. Time must be allowed after a series of two or three sprays to rewarm the skin. After the skin is rewarmed, the stretch-and-spray procedure can be repeated with several cycles of full active range of motion.

Detailed descriptions of the vapocoolant stretch-and-spray technique have been published.[77,142,207,209,222] Both ethylchloride and fluoromethane can be used and are commercially available. However, ethylchloride, a local anesthetic, is flammable, explosive, and very cold when applied. If inhaled it can cause unconsciousness.

Fluoromethane is nonflammable, nonexplosive, and a good alternative. It is made up of a mixture of 85% trichloromonofluoromethane and 15% dichlorodifluoromethane. The fluorocarbon (Freon) has been tested for toxicity.[75] It has no effect on pulmonary function and does not change tracheal mucociliary transport.

The fluoromethane spring cap, which seals the nozzle of the bottle, permits on-off application. The bottle must be inverted so that the fluid will flow from it (Fig. 63-5). After adequate instruction, patients may be given fluoromethane spray for home use.

The jet stream of vapocoolant is directed at an acute angle (30°) to the skin and is swept parallel over the affected muscle in one direction only. The bottle is held approximately 18 inches from the skin. Slow, even sweeps over the skin at approximately 4 inches/sec are spaced to slightly overlap. Two or three sweeps are usually maximum before the skin must be rewarmed. Frosting of the skin can cause ulceration.[149] When the spray is applied for the first time over very irritable trigger points, the skin may be hypersensitive to the cold. However, after several passes of the spray, the hypersensitivity usually abates (Fig. 63-6).

The patient further benefits by soaking in a hot bath after stretch-and-spray treatments. Activities such as strenuous swimming should be avoided, but unstrained stretch and painless range-of-motion exercises are desirable.

The precise mechanism by which the vapocoolant spray exerts its effect has not been determined. It may act indirectly via skin afferent nerves rather than by direct cooling of the muscle. The stimulation of skin afferent nerves may produce trigger point inhibition, spinal inhibition, or supraspinal inhibition.

The patient is seen again several days after treatment. If pain relief is adequate on follow-up, the patient is encouraged to pay more attention to the muscle strain and to avoid reactivating the trigger points. If within a few hours the patient experiences severe cramping pain in the general region of the treatment, the stretch-and-spray procedure has produced shortening activation of an antagonist muscle. This phenomenon can be avoided by systematically treating both the agonist and antagonist groups of muscles. When active trigger points do not subside after stretch-and-spray treatments, the physician should look for perpetuating factors. These may be inadequate spraying of all trigger points, a nervous patient, inadequate technique, or chronicity of trigger points.[143,207]

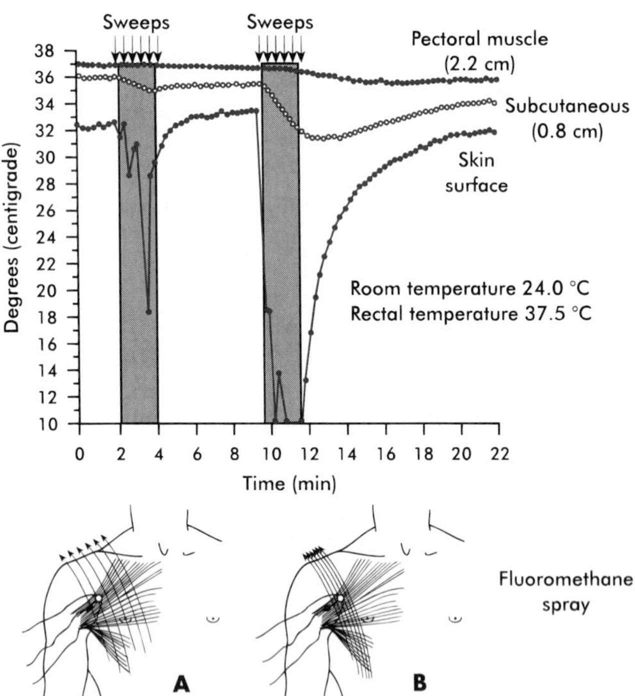

Fig. 63-6. Temperature changes that occur in skin, subcutaneous structures, or muscle with the stretch-and-spray technique, **A,** Results of first sweep of the spray. **B,** Results of second sweep (2 minutes sweep each time). (From Travell J, Simons DG: Myofascial pain and dysfunction. In *The trigger point manual,* Baltimore, 1983, Williams & Wilkins.)

Trigger-point injection

Trigger-point injection is helpful when a few discrete trigger points are present and the muscle cannot stretch because of excessive pain.

An aseptic technique is required for injection of the trigger points. The solutions, needles, and syringes should be properly sterilized before use. Localization of a trigger point is done mainly by feel. The trigger point is the most sensitive spot in the palpable band. The muscle is placed on sufficient stretch so that one can palpate the tight band and hold the trigger point in position.

With flat palpation, the trigger point can be localized by feeling the band roll back and forth between the fingers

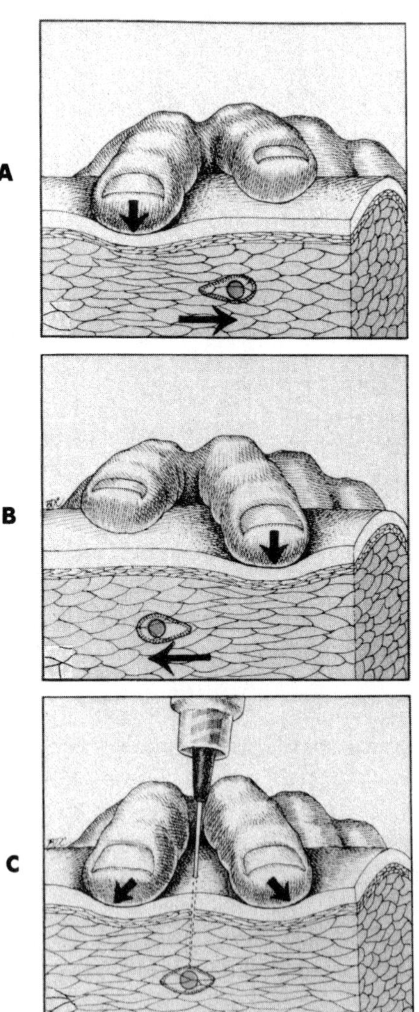

Fig. 63-7. Method of palpating and fixing the trigger point in the muscle with two fingers before inserting the needle tip in the trigger point for injection. **A,** Fixation of trigger point by the proximal finger. **B,** Fixation of trigger point by the distal finger. **C,** Needle on the trigger point. (From Travell J, Simons DG: Myofascial pain and dysfunction. In *The trigger point manual,* Baltimore, 1983, Williams & Wilkins.)

(Figs. 63-7 and 63-8). The trigger point is then fixed by keeping it between the fingers. The needle is inserted perpendicular to the skin and slowly advanced to the depth of the trigger point. The patient is asked to indicate when the pain is worse. At that site, the needle will usually impale the trigger point.

Dry needling of trigger points without injecting any solution may be effective but does not equal the therapeutic effectiveness of injecting a local anesthetic. Kraus[122] noted that postinjection pain follows dry needling. Sola and Kuitert[195] treated a series of 100 patients with isotonic saline injected in the trigger points.[195] They found saline to be effective in relieving the pain. Hameroff et al., on the other hand, found long-acting local anesthetics—bupivacaine and etidocaine—to provide better and longer pain relief for up to 70 days after injection. Travell and Simons[210] advocate use of procaine for trigger-point injections. They argue that procaine has less systemic and local toxicity, in addition to its vasodilator effect and curarelike action at the myoneural junction. We have used a mixture of 0.5% etidocaine and 0.375% bupivacaine and achieved a long-lasting effect without systemic toxicities or myotoxicity. In our experience, this mixture has produced better relief than dry needling, saline, or lidocaine.

Role of corticosteroids

Travell and Simons[210] advocate mixing corticosteroid with a local anesthetic for trigger-point injection for only two groups of patients: those with soft-tissue inflammation (adhesive capsulitis) and those with postinjection muscle soreness. They prefer oral steroids and believe that long-acting steroids are contraindicated because of their myotoxic properties[171] and delayed sequelae (Cushing's syndrome). We have used dexamethasone (4 mg/10 ml of local anesthetic solution), mixed with bupivacaine and etidocaine, in more than 10,000 patients, without sequelae from its use. It is true that a steroid may cause a burning sensation in the area of injection 24 to 48 hours after injection. This subsides, however, and patients continue to have prolonged pain relief 7 to 10 days later. If patients are informed at the outset about the burning and its duration, they tolerate it better.

Postinjection maneuvers

Stretch after trigger-point injections is important.[122,222] Vapocoolant spray or heat may also be applied after injection during stretching of the muscle to full length.

Alternative techniques to stretch-and-spray and trigger-point injections have also been practiced for myofascial pain. They include ischemic compression techniques, massage, deep heat, transcutaneous electrical nerve stimulation (TENS), biofeedback, acupuncture, and central modulation.[148,175,215] A combination of some or all may be required in patients with chronic intractable trigger-point pain. Commonly, however, the techniques employed are stretch-and-spray, trigger-point injection, and TENS therapy, in conjunction with muscle relaxants, nonsteroidal anti-inflammatory drugs (NSAIDS), and exercises. The earlier the patient is treated, the more effective and long-lasting the treatment. Generally, for chronic trigger-point pain (6 to 12 months) a series of six injections at weekly intervals must be completed in conjunction with other therapy before any appreciable improvement in pain relief. The management plan

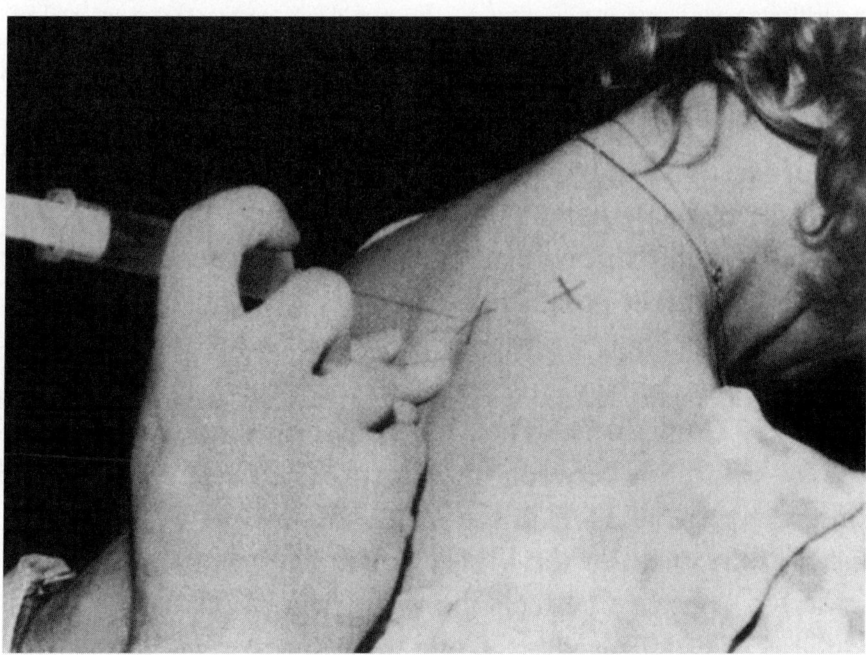

Fig. 63-8. Method of fixing the trigger point in a flat shoulder muscle for injection of a local anesthetic-steroid mixture. *X's* denote the position of the trigger points.

should be evaluated periodically, and alternative treatments employed if the current one is not effective.

CRANIAL NERVES

Block of the trigeminal ganglion and the branches of the trigeminal nerve is discussed in Chapter 62 ("Peripheral Nerve Blocks").

Glossopharyngeal Nerve Block

Anatomy

The glossopharyngeal nerve (CN IX) is the sensory nerve that supplies the posterior third of the tongue and the pharynx from the level of the soft palate down to the laryngeal opening. A block of the glossopharyngeal nerve can produce analgesia in this distribution.

The nerve leaves the cranium through the middle compartment of the jugular foramen along with the accessory nerve (CN XI) and diverges to follow the course of the styloid process before curving forward into the pharynx. The styloid process is the bony landmark for this nerve.

Indications

Intraoral glossopharyngeal nerve block is most commonly performed for the control of acute pain in perioral endoscopy procedures. In the control of chronic pain, it is most commonly performed in patients with invading carcinomas of the posterior third of the tongue or pharynx that are unresponsive to other therapies. Because extraoral blocks of the glossopharyngeal nerve can readily spread to the vagus and accessory nerves, neurolytic blocks often produce analgesia of the hemilarynx and/or trapezius muscle, and sternomastoid paralysis on the ipsilateral side. These complications are often acceptable to patients with terminal cancer pain. Glossopharyngeal nerve block is occasionally used in the exceedingly rare condition of idiopathic glossopharyngeal neuralgia.

Technique

The needle is inserted at the midpoint of the line joining the tip of the mastoid process with the angle of the mandible. The needle passes through the substance of the sternomastoid muscle, and, at a depth of approximately 3 cm, contact is sought with the bony styloid process. The needle is walked off the posterior border of the styloid process. A small bolus of 1 to 2 ml of local anesthetic injected at this point will produce anesthesia of the glossopharyngeal nerve. Because of the proximity of the accessory and the vagus nerves, these are frequently blocked as well.

The terminal distribution of the glossopharyngeal nerve can also be blocked at the midpoint of the posterior pillar of the fauces via an intraoral approach. An injection of 1 to 2 ml of a local anesthetic at this site will produce rapid analgesia of the posterior third of the tongue and the adjacent pharynx (Fig. 63-9).

Often patients with pharyngeal cancer will have undergone a radical neck dissection, and the sternomastoid muscle will have been removed. This makes identification of the styloid process and performance of the block much easier because this particular bony landmark is now almost subcutaneous.

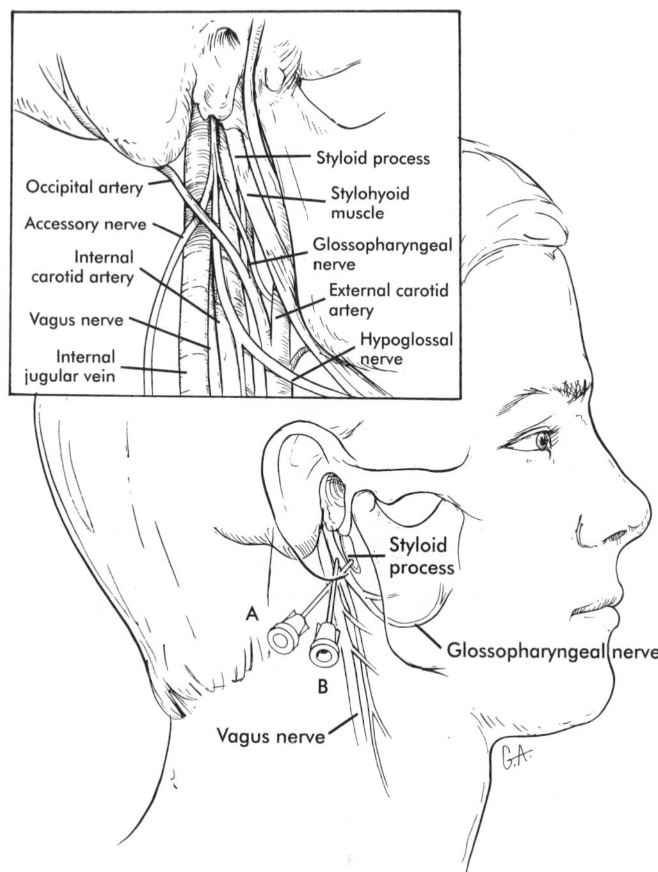

Fig. 63-9. Glossopharyngeal nerve block. *A,* The 5-cm, 22-gauge needle is inserted halfway between the mastoid process and the angle of the mandible, seeking the styloid process. When the bony endpoint has been located, the needle is "walked" off the anterior aspect of the styloid process at the same depth (usually about 3 cm). A glossopharyngeal paresthesia should be obtained. A small bolus of 1 to 2 ml of either a local anesthetic or a neurolytic agent is sufficient for block at this site. Note the proximity of the underlying internal carotid artery and internal jugular vein, necessitating meticulous attention to aspiration testing. *B,* Point of entry of needle for glossopharyngeal and vagal nerve block: (1) the needle is inserted at the point of entry perpendicularly to the skin until it touches the styloid process; (2) the needle tip is slipped anteriorly and seeks paresthesia of the glossopharyngeal nerve; (3) for vagal nerve block the needle tip is slipped posteriorly to the same depth (approximately 3 cm).

Complications

Because of the proximity of the internal carotid artery and the internal jugular vein, the risks of intravascular injection are always significant, demanding meticulous aspiration tests. With the temporary and perhaps permanent analgesia that comes with these blocks, a degree of swallowing dysfunction and a potential risk of aspiration must be

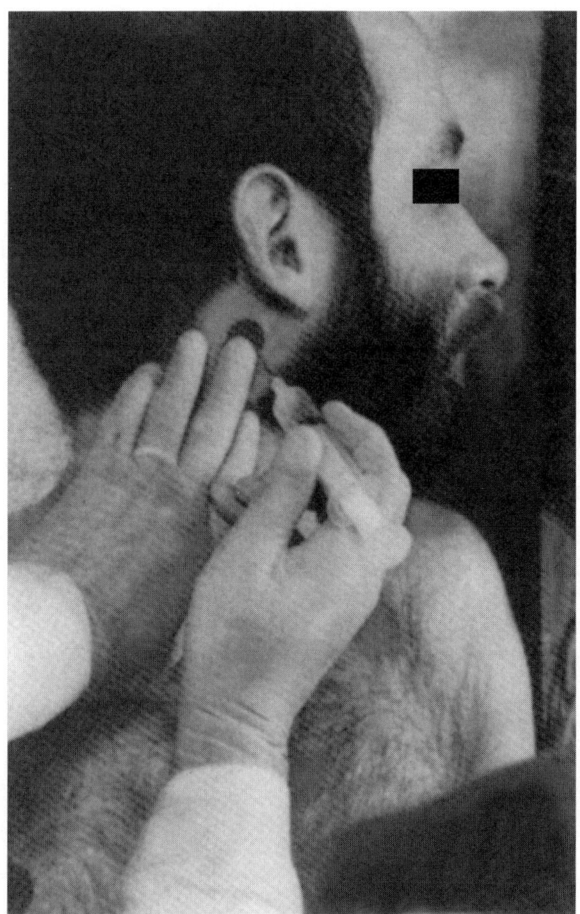

Fig. 63-10. Spinal accessory nerve block. Illustration shows injection of 5 ml of local anesthetic in the substance of the sternocleidomastoid muscle.

appreciated. Numbness of the pharynx and larynx can severely compromize ingestion and swallowing.

Spinal Accessory Nerve Block

Anatomy

The accessory nerve is the eleventh cranial nerve. After it exits the jugular foramen, the cranial portion separates and joins the vagus. The spinal accessory portion continues into the upper part of the sternocleidomastoid muscle and emerges from its posterior border at the junction of the lower and middle thirds. There, it crosses the neck to supply the trapezius muscle. The nerve can be blocked in the substance of the sternocleidomastoid muscle.

Indications

The spinal accessory nerve block has been useful as an adjunct to cervical plexus block for carotid surgery, and as an adjunct to brachial plexus block with or without cervical plexus block for proximal shoulder surgery. It also may be helpful for acute and chronic torticollis.

Technique

A 23-gauge, 2.5-cm needle is inserted into the sternocleidomastoid muscle 2 cm below the tip of the mastoid process. The patient's head should be turned to the opposite side to make the muscle prominent. An injection of 5 ml of the local anesthetic will block the branches to the sternocleidomastoid and the trapezius muscles (Fig. 63-10). A neurolytic block can be performed using 3 ml of 50% alcohol or 3% to 6% phenol. Using a nerve stimulator and looking for trapezius contractions will increase the accuracy of the injection.

Complications

A spinal accessory nerve block results in weakness of the sternocleidomastoid and trapezius muscles. A successful block is recognized by the absence of contraction of the sternocleidomastoid muscle when the patient turns the head to the opposite side, and weakness of the trapezius muscle when the patient attempts to shrug the shoulders. The patient has difficulty lifting the head off the bed, turning the head, or raising an arm above the head. No serious complications should be encountered if the local anesthetic is placed in the substance of the muscle. A lesser occipital nerve block may result in numbness behind the ear.

SPINAL NERVE ROOTS

Thoracic

Anatomy

The 12 pairs of thoracic nerve roots can be blocked as they emerge from the thoracic intervertebral foramina. The spinous processes of the thoracic vertebrae extend downward, especially in the midthoracic area; therefore the tip of the spinous process in the thoracic region may be opposite the intervertebral foramen as far as two levels caudad. However, from T1 to T3 and from T9 to T12 this overlap does not exceed one level.

Indications

A thoracic nerve root block is useful for diagnostic, prognostic, and therapeutic purposes, and for pain secondary to nerve root irritation or compression at the foramina level or distally. It can be used for treatment of intercostal neuralgia secondary to herpes zoster, fractured ribs, tumors, or metastasis.

Technique

A thoracic nerve root block can be performed with the patient prone or in the lateral position with the affected side facing up. Vertebrae can be counted down from C7 and checked again by counting up from L4. Fluoroscopy is essential.

A 22-gauge, 8-cm needle is advanced perpendicularly through a skin wheal 3 cm lateral to the level of the cephalad edge of the vertebrae to contact the transverse process. The needle is then withdrawn and advanced slightly medially (25°) and caudally (20°). If paresthesias are obtained, 5 ml of a local anesthetic are injected. If paresthesias are not obtained, the needle is advanced 2.5 cm deeper than the transverse process or until it contacts the posterolateral aspect of the vertebra, where the local anesthetic is injected.

The development of cutaneous analgesia in the appropriate dermatome indicates a successful block. It is hard to confirm analgesia of one dermatome because of the overlap of dermatomes. Three roots may have to be blocked to provide good analgesia in one dermatome.

Complications

Pneumothorax is possible but unlikely. **If the patient has a coughing spasm or if air is aspirated, the pleura has been punctured. The patient should then be observed for development of a pneumothorax.**

Epidural or subarachnoid spread of the injected solution can occur, especially if there is a long dural sleeve. Segmental sympathetic block can result from the block of the sympathetic fibers that accompany the root.

If the volume is increased, solution can spread paravertebrally or epidurally up and down, and more roots may be anesthetized. It is particularly important to use small volumes (1 to 3 ml) of local anesthetic when performing a neurolytic block. In addition, use of a small volume will define the contribution of the individual nerve root to the patient's pain.

Lumbar

Anatomy

The spine of the lumbar vertebra is straight and has a rectangular surface under the skin. The upper edge of the spine corresponds to the transverse process of the same vertebra. The line joining the highest part of the iliac crest corresponds to the L4 vertebra or the L4–L5 interspace.

Indications

A lumbar nerve root block is indicated for relief of acute or chronic radiculopathy pain secondary to disc prolapse or tumor.

Technique

A lumbar nerve root block is similar to a thoracic nerve root block. A 22-gauge, 8-cm needle is advanced perpendicularly

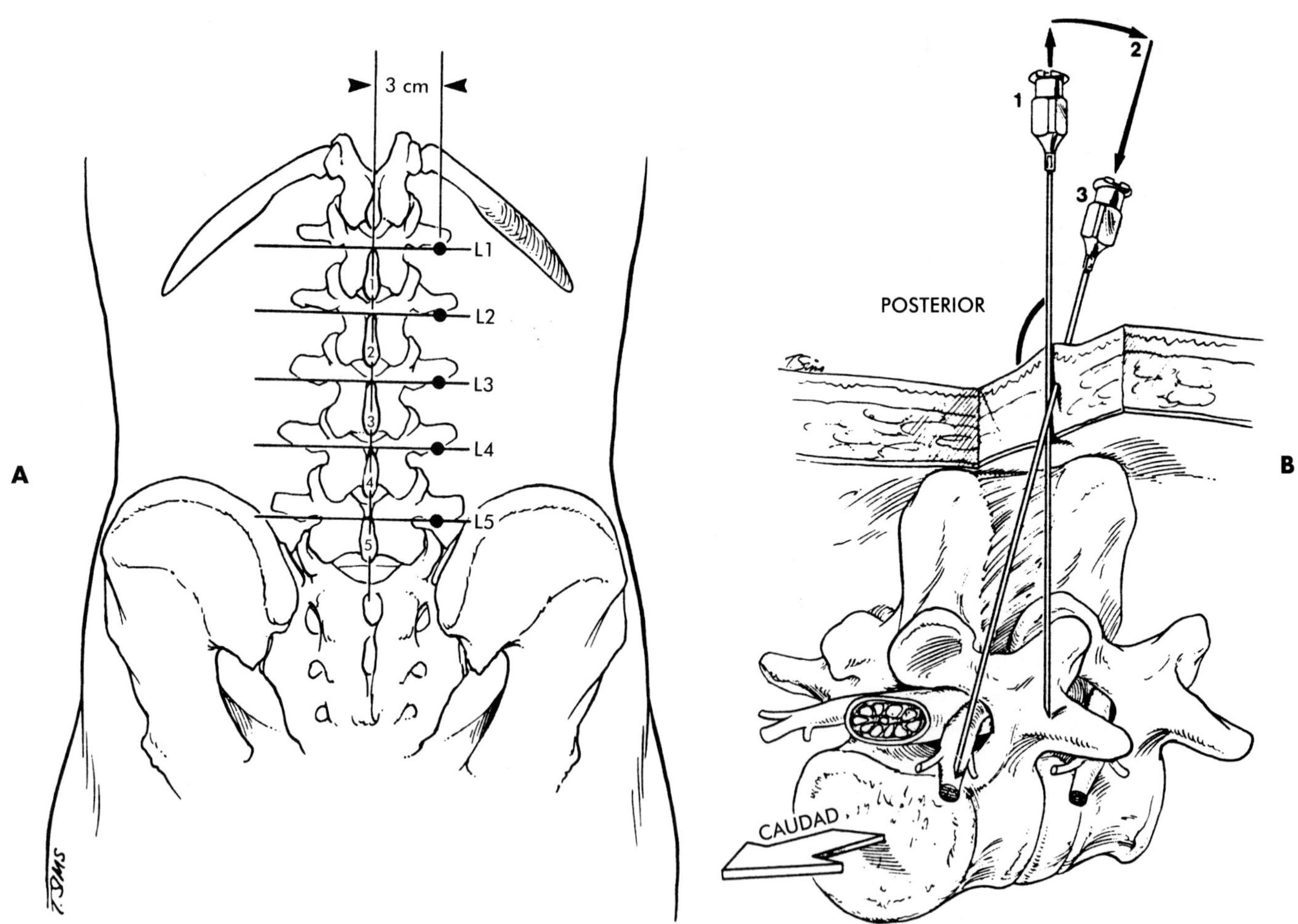

Fig. 63-11. Lumbar nerve root block. **A,** Needle is inserted 3 cm lateral to the tip of the spinous processes of the lumbar vertebrae perpendicularly until it touches the transverse process. **B,** An 8-cm, 22-gauge needle touching the transverse process (position *1*). Positions *2* and *3* show the needle directed caudally to touch the nerve root at a deeper level. (From Raj PP: Chronic pain. In Raj PP, ed: *Handbook of regional anesthesia,* New York, 1985, Churchill-Livingstone.)

through a skin wheal 4 cm lateral to the cephalad edge of the lumbar spine (Fig. 63-11). The needle is advanced until it impinges on the transverse process. It is then withdrawn and reinserted caudally and medially. If paresthesia is obtained, 5 ml of a local anesthetic solution are injected. If no paresthesia is obtained and if the posterolateral aspect of the vertebra is encountered, the needle is withdrawn 1 cm and the solution is injected.

Complications

A successful block is recognized by hypesthesia in the appropriate dermatome. Because all lumbar nerves innervate postural muscles, a lumbar root block may result in weakness and inability to stand or walk. Epidural or subarachnoid injection can result if the anesthetic solution is injected through the intervertebral foramen or into a long dural sleeve.

SUPRASCAPULAR NERVE BLOCK

Anatomy

The suprascapular nerve is a branch of the superior trunk of the brachial plexus which originates from the fifth and sixth cervical nerves. After leaving the brachial plexus it enters the scapular region through the suprascapular notch on the cephalad border of the scapula and then innervates the supraspinatus and infraspinatus muscles. It supplies a large sensory component to the shoulder joint, with a variable cutaneous branch to the cephalad and lateral aspects of the upper extremity just below the deltoid insertion.

Indications

The suprascapular nerve is blocked diagnostically for pain around the shoulder in an attempt to see if the pain is arising from within the shoulder joint. Therapeutically, repeated blocks can be performed for arthritic shoulder pain, although this is usually not a satisfactory long-term solution.

Technique

The operator identifies the spine of the scapula and then draws a line vertically through the midpoint of the spine and parallel to the vertebral column. The upper and outer quadrant so formed is bisected, and a needle is inserted at a distance of 2 cm along this line (Fig. 63-12). The needle is inserted at a right angle to the skin and advanced until the dorsal surface of the scapula is located. The needle is then walked along this dorsal surface until the suprascapular notch is identified. If a nerve stimulator is used, contractions of the supraspinatus and infraspinatus muscles will confirm placement. At this location, 5 ml of local anesthetic are injected. It is not always possible to verify any dermal analgesia as a result of this block. If motor blocking concentrations of drug are used, a successful block will compromize arm abduction for the first 15° before the deltoid muscle takes over (Fig. 63-13).

Complications

The main concern with this block is the risk of pneumothorax if the needle, during its initial advancement, passes over the superior border of the scapula and enters the thoracic cavity between the ribs. Also, if and when the needle is walked over the suprascapular notch, it should not be advanced, because pleural puncture with subsequent pneumothorax could occur. The nerve is accompanied by the cor-

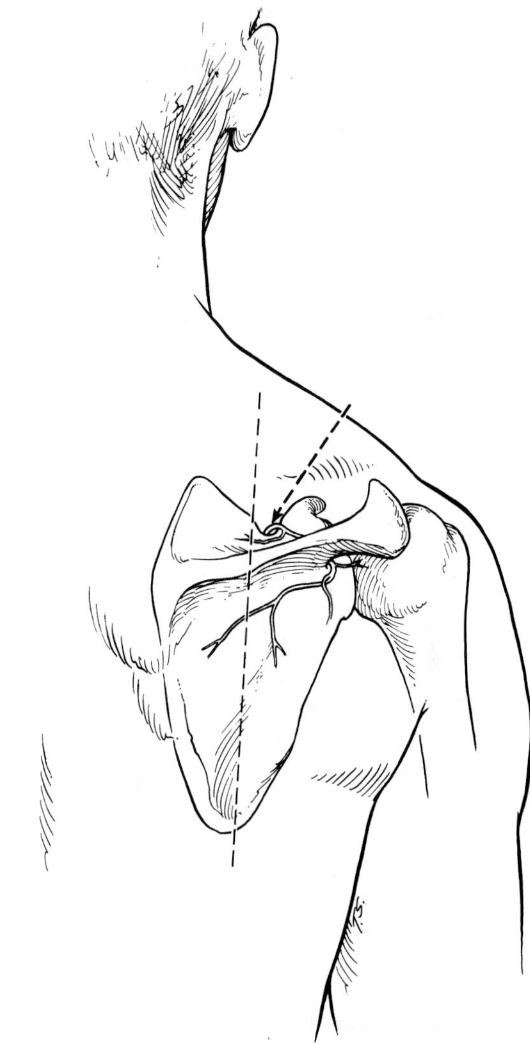

Fig. 63-12. Suprascapular nerve block. The nerve is blocked in the suprascapular fossa. The spine of the scapula is divided by a vertical line, the upper and outer quadrant so formed is bisected, and a needle is introduced 2 cm along this line and advanced to a depth of approximately 5 to 6 cm, at which point the dorsal surface of the scapula should be located. If this endpoint is not reached at this depth, the needle should be withdrawn and repositioned. When osseous contact is achieved, the needle is "walked" until the suprascapular notch is located, or, if an electrical stimulator is used, needle placement is confirmed by movements of the suprascapular and infrascapular muscles. At this point 5 ml of local anesthetic is injected.

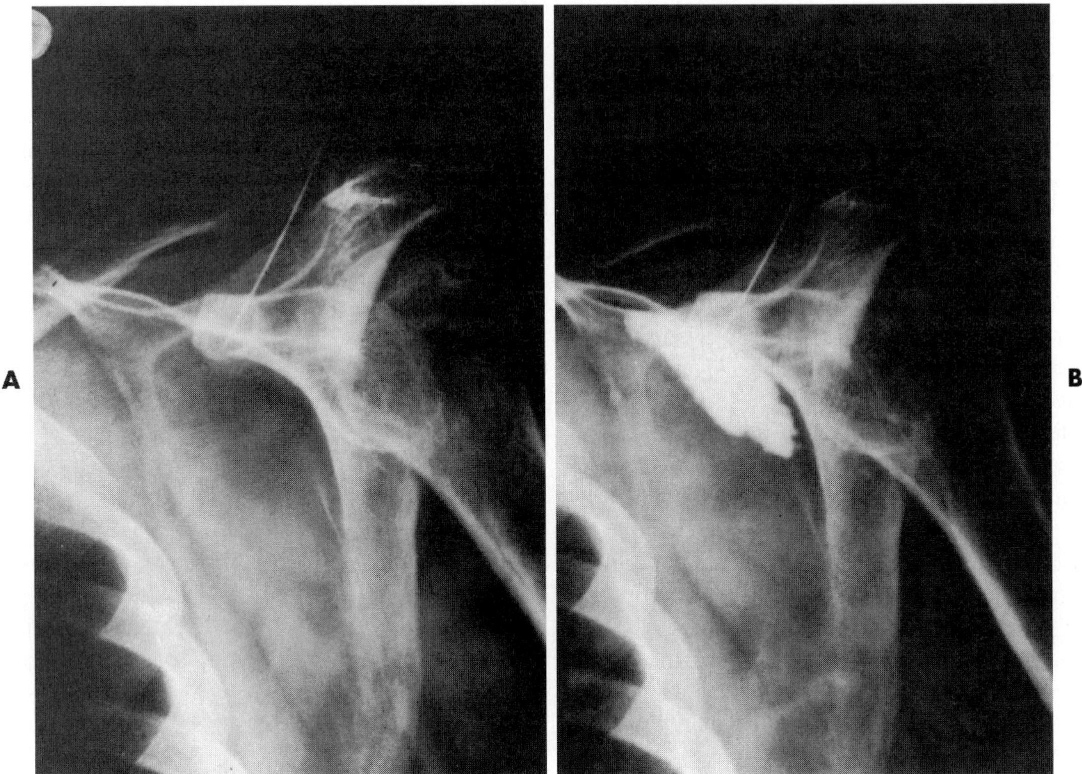

Fig. 63-13. Needle placement on the suprascapular nerve (**A**) and the radiographic spread (**B**).

responding suprascapular vessels, and intravascular injection is possible.

PUDENDAL NERVE BLOCK

Anatomy

The pudendal nerve (S2, S3, S4) arises from the sacral plexus. After crossing the ischial spine and the sacrospinous ligament, it enters the lesser sciatic foramen and runs on the medial side of the ischium with the pudendal vessels in the pudendal canal (Alcock canal). At the anterior end of the canal, it sends branches to the perineal region. The inferior hemorrhoidal nerve innervates the anal region, whereas the other branches innervate the urogenital region.

Indications

A pudendal nerve block is indicated for obstetric vaginal procedures (e.g., vaginal delivery and forceps delivery) and for somatic perineal pain.

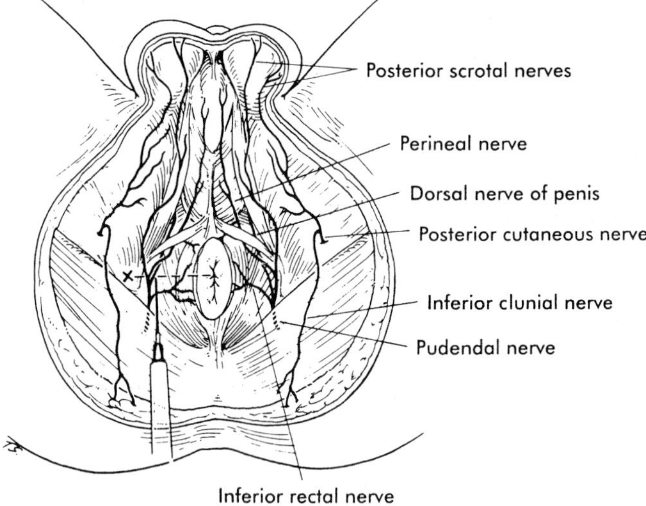

Fig. 63-14. Anatomy and technique of pudendal block (perineal route). (From Raj PP: Chronic pain. In Raj PP, ed: *Handbook of regional anesthesia,* New York, 1985, Churchill-Livingstone.)

Technique

Equipment needed for a pudendal nerve block are an Iowa trumpet and a 12- to 14-cm, 20-gauge needle. The patient is placed in the lithotomy position. Landmarks are the ischial spine, sacrospinous ligament, and ischial tuberosity.

In the transvaginal approach, the needle is guided within the Iowa trumpet along the operator's index and middle finger; the needle progresses transvaginally toward the ischial spine after piercing the sacrospinous ligament. Local anesthetic is injected into the pudendal canal.

In the perineal approach, a skin wheal is raised 2 to 3 cm posteromedially to the ischial tuberosity. A 12- to 15-cm, 22-gauge needle is introduced through the skin wheal in a posterior and lateral direction (Fig. 63-14); it is guided by the operators' finger in the rectum or vagina toward the ischial spine. After the needle pierces the sacrospinous ligament, 10 to 15 ml of local anesthetic is injected around the ligament.

SYMPATHETIC NERVE BLOCKS

Anatomy

The autonomic nervous system is comprised of the sympathetic and parasympathetic nervous systems, each consisting of preganglionic and postganglionic nerves (Fig. 63-15). Preganglionic nerves of the sympathetic system arise from the thoracic and lumbar segments of the spinal cord, and parasympathetic nerves arise from the brain stem and sacral cord. These divisions are termed *thoracolumbar* and *craniosacral,* respectively. Most visceral structures are innervated by both the sympathetic and parasympathetic systems, although some structures, such as blood vessels and sweat glands, have only single innervation.

Axons of preganglionic sympathetic nerves exit from the intermediolateral and intermedial columns of the spinal cord and join ventral nerve roots from T2 to L2. Anatomic variations exist, with some preganglionic sympathetic nerves exiting at C7 and others from L3 and L4.[6,99,151,180] More important for the anesthesiologist performing sympathetic blocks are the variations that occur intraspinally. Preganglionic sympathetic nerves have been shown to travel up to 12 segments intraspinally before exiting the spinal cord.[6] Similarly, axons to thoracic ganglia remain ipsilateral, but those to lumbar ganglia take both ipsilateral and contralateral pathways.[66] Finally, preganglionic nerves will often travel several segments within the sympathetic chain before synapsing, or synapse in ganglia closer to their respective visceral structures.[123,124] Variations in neuroanatomy account for some of the disappointing results obtained in seemingly well-performed sympathetic blocks.

Paravertebral sympathetic ganglia lie on both sides of the vertebral column. In the cervical and thoracic regions, the chain is in close proximity to somatic nerves. Cervically, the ganglia can be found just anterior to the transverse processes; in particular, the superior cervical ganglion is associated with the upper four cervical levels; the middle ganglion, when present, is related to C5 and C6; and the inferior ganglion comprises C6 and C7 output. In as many as 82% of cases, the inferior ganglion is fused with the first thoracic ganglion to form the stellate ganglion.[6,10,86,111,124] If not connected, the first thoracic ganglion is termed the stellate ganglion.[104]

In the thoracic region up to 11 ganglia will be present lying near the necks of the ribs. Four ganglia exist in the lumbar and sacral regions although variations commonly occur. The position of the sympathetic chain and ganglia in the lumbar region differs and is found at the anterior lateral border of the vertebral bodies, separated from somatic nerves by both the psoas muscle and psoas fascia (Fig. 63-16 on page 1463).

Sympathetic innervation of the abdominal viscera differs from innervation above the diaphragm, with preganglionic nerves passing through the sympathetic chain. These become the splanchnic nerves and synapse at collateral ganglia around the abdominal aorta, following branches of the aorta to each respective visceral structure. These collateral ganglia are diffuse and more appropriately represent a plexus of nerves, termed the *celiac plexus.*

Preganglionic sympathetic nerves exit the spinal cord with ventral nerve roots and connect to the sympathetic chain by the white communicating rami. These fibers are myelinated, thus giving a whitish appearance to the nerve bundle. Postganglionic nerves form a sympathetic chain and communicate with the spinal nerve en route to the periphery. These are unmyelinated and grayish in appearance and are known as the *gray communicating rami.* Each presynaptic fiber may synapse with as many as 30 postsynaptic nerves; this diffuseness allows amplification of the stress response seen when the sympathetic system is activated.[6,147]

Sympathetic fibers traverse deep fascial planes and are more inaccessible than somatic nerves. Blockade can be accomplished at numerous locations: at the sympathetic chain; as an interruption of the somatic nerve that blocks the corresponding sympathetic fibers; as perivascular infiltration; as IV regional anesthesia; or as an intraspinal block. Although any of these techniques theoretically will result in a sympathetic block, a successful block must always be monitored and documented, because alternative sympathetic pathways may exist.

The site most appropriate for blockade depends on each patient's clinical status. A patient can present with signs and symptoms suggestive of sympathetically mediated pain, but the diagnosis may be inconclusive. In these cases, a diagnostic sympathetic block should be performed. The best location for a diagnostic block is the sympathetic chain. A block at this level affects only sympathetic nerves, and, if pain relief is achieved, one can be satisfied that the sympathetic system contributes to the pain experienced. An alternative is the differential intraspinal (epidural or intrathecal) block. The drawback to this block is the relative inability to administer a local anesthetic that can selectively block only sympathetic nerves. Thus, the epidural or intrathecal route is not recommended for definitive diagnosis of sympathetically mediated pain.

Evaluation of sympathetic blockade completeness

Whenever possible, the effectiveness of a sympathetic block should be monitored. With the exception of blocks involving visceral structures (e.g., thoracic sympathetic chain block, splanchnic nerve block, and celiac plexus block), all sympathetic blocks can be evaluated for completeness.

Many tests have been reported that monitor sympathetic activity. Unfortunately, many lack applicability for the practicing clinician because of the intricate apparatus involved, cost and time for set up. The tests described below can be

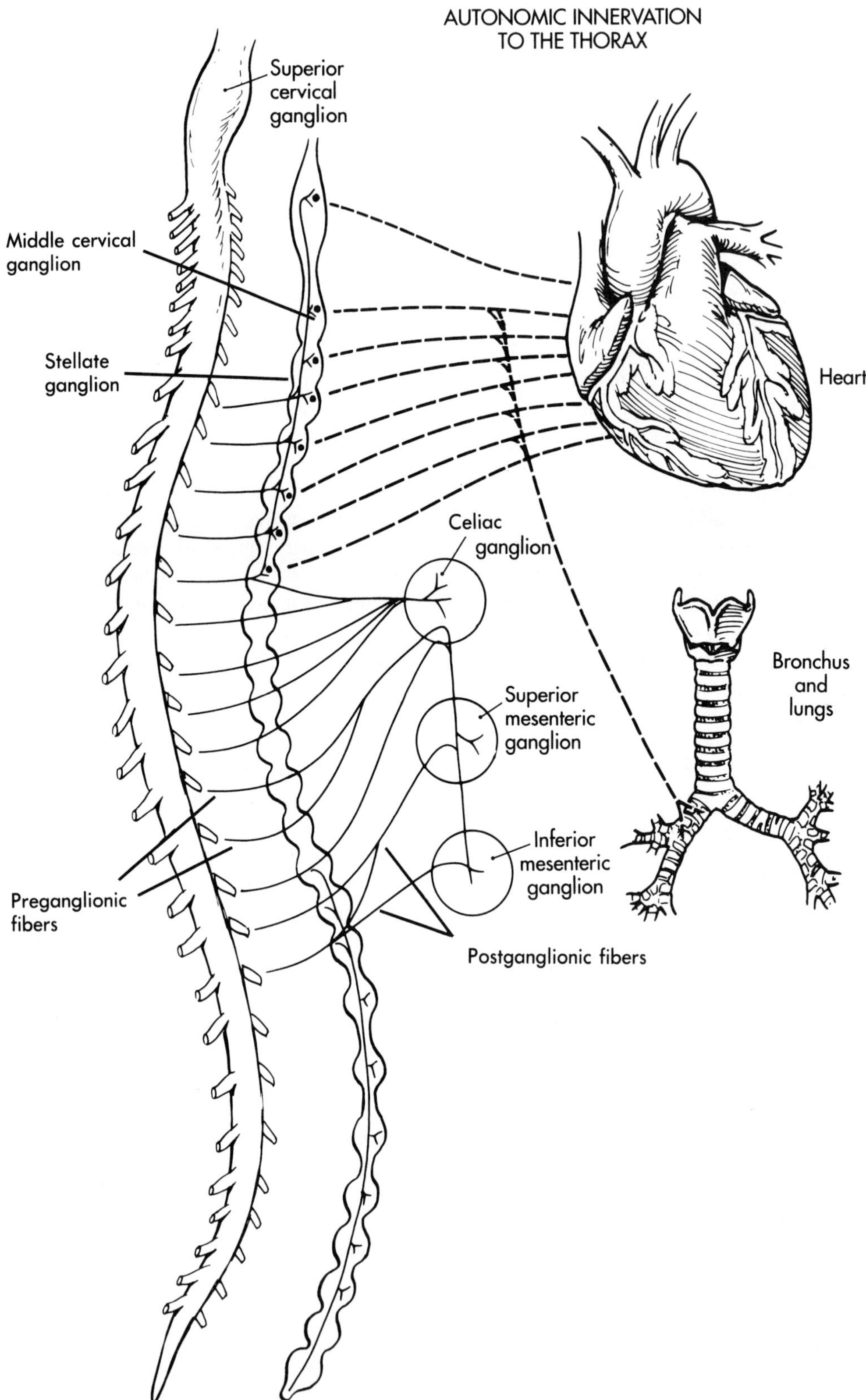

Fig. 63-15. Innervation of the sympathetic nervous system. Preganglion and postganglion fibers are distinguished. (From Raj PP: *Practical management of pain*, ed 2, St Louis, 1992, Mosby–Year Book.)

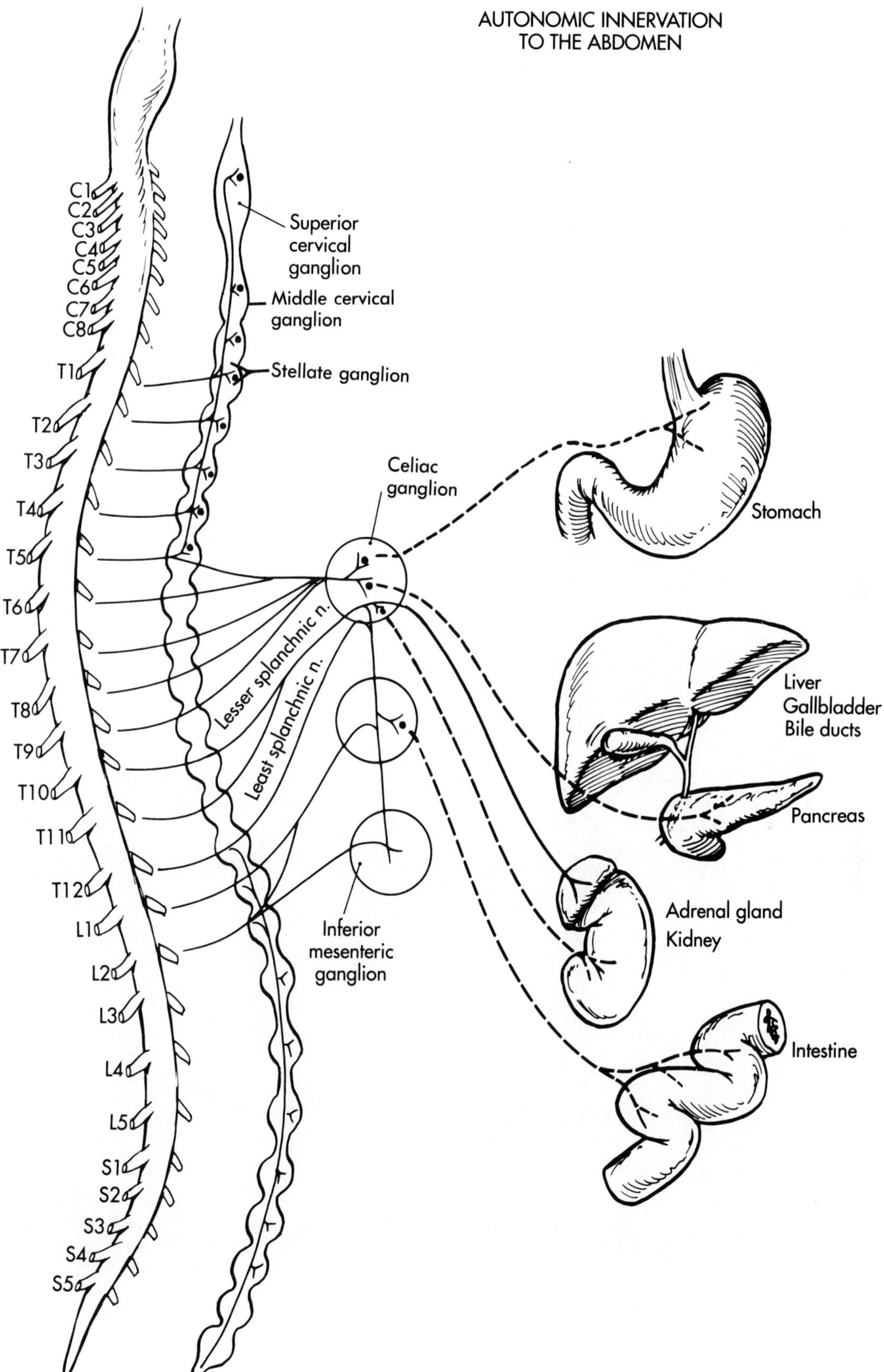

Fig. 63-15, cont'd. For legend see opposite page. *(Continued)*

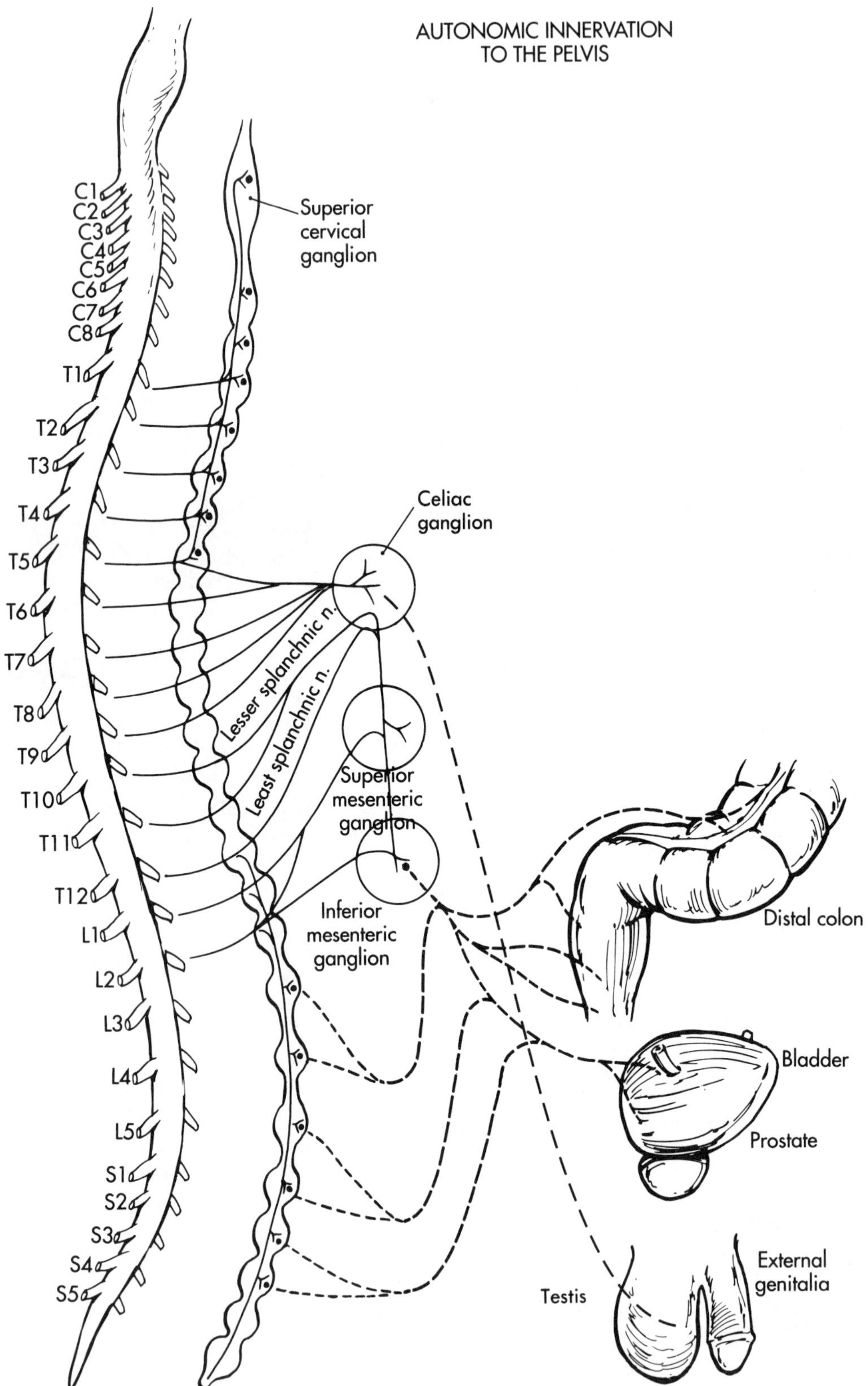

Fig. 63-15, cont'd. Innervation of the sympathetic nervous system.

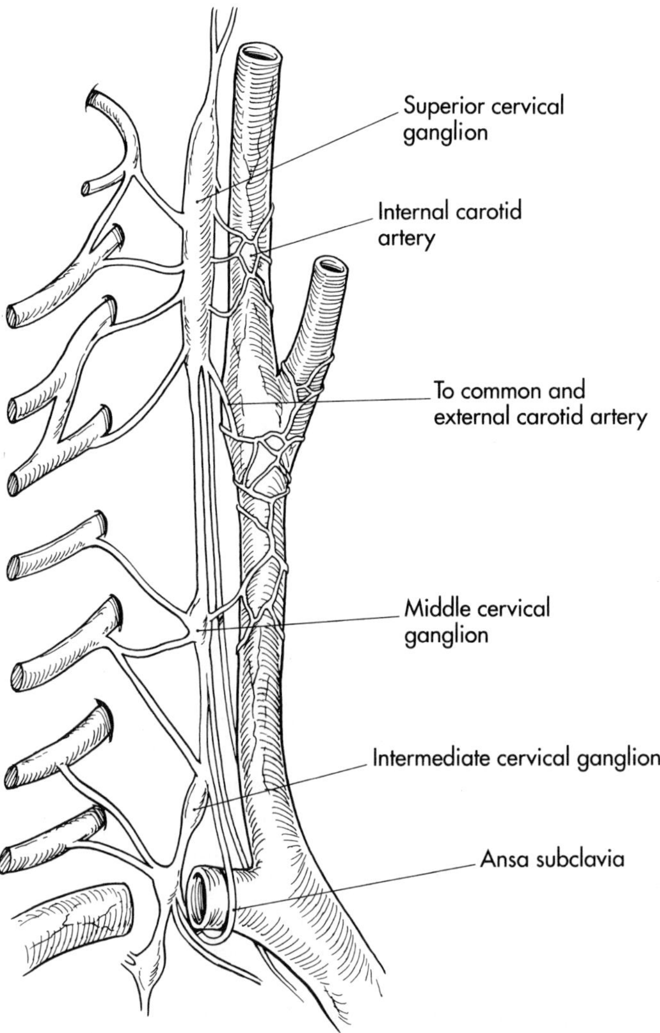

Fig. 63-16. Schematic of the upper thoracic and cervical sympathetic chain. (From Raj PP: *Practical management of pain,* ed 2, St Louis, 1992, Mosby–Year Book.)

performed at the patient's bedside, and one or two of these should be used to monitor all blocks.

Surface temperature monitoring

Skin temperature recording represents the easiest and fastest way to test sympathetic blockade. Modern temperature monitors have two or three channels combined with very sensitive sensors and digital displays. For upper-extremity blocks, the shoulder, flexor surface of the forearm, dorsum of the hand, and one of the digits, preferably the thumb, can be monitored. Lower extremity temperature is best measured on the anterior thigh, medial aspect of the leg, dorsum of the foot, and the great toe.

Skin temperature should be measured 15 to 20 minutes before block to allow for equilibration with the ambient surroundings. Wrapping of the extremities reduces any environmental effects. Both affected and unaffected (i.e., control) sides should be monitored.

Thermography has been advocated for documentation of sympathetic blockade. It records skin temperature by either an infrared technique or liquid crystals. Both methods effectively demonstrate changes in skin temperatures.

A minimum positive change of 2° C should be found after sympathetic block. At times, this may not occur despite appropriate blockade. Some reflex sympathetic dystrophy patients present with a very warm extremity that will not further warm with sympathetic blockade.

Sympathogalvanic reflex

If a skin temperature change cannot be evoked or further documentation is deemed necessary, the sympathogalvanic reflex (SGR) can be recorded. Initially described by Lewis in 1955, this reflex is also called *skin conductance response, galvanic skin reaction, electrodermal reaction,* and *psychogalvanic reflex.*

This reflex arc tests efferent sympathetic nerves, spinal and supraspinal nerves, and primary afferent neurons. The measured response involves electrical activity in the skin, specifically special cells surrounding the sweat glands. The reflex cannot be elicited if the sympathetic efferents are blocked.

To measure the SGR, standard electrocardiograph (ECG) electrodes are placed on the dorsal and plantar surfaces of the distal extremity (i.e., foot or hand) with a third grounding electrode remotely located. The skin should be made free of epithelial cells before electrode placement.

The patient is allowed to rest in silence for several minutes to permit the tracing to return to baseline. A short deep breath, loud noise, or pinch of the skin usually suffices to elicit the response, which is recorded as a deflection on the ECG paper. The deflection lasts for 4 to 5 seconds, and changes of 1 to 3 mV are normal. Both blocked and unblocked extremities should be measured. At 20 to 30 minutes postprocedure, the blocked side should have an absent SGR.

The presence of the SGR varies between patients, with younger patients having much greater deflections and unstable baseline patterns. All patients do not have an elicitable SGR, particularly the elderly, diabetic, or significantly depressed individuals. Drugs such as opiates, barbiturates, atropine, and other centrally-acting agents can blunt or abolish the SGR. Habituation can also occur, with smaller deflections occuring after repeated stimuli.

Sweat test

Three methods of sweat testing have been used clinically to test sympathetic blockade. The ninhydrin test relies on a protein in sweat to change its color to yellow.[58] A blocked extremity will not sweat and will show no color change. The test is considered very accurate but requires a lot of time and cannot produce immediate results for clinical use. The cobalt blue test uses filter papers that are saturated with cobalt blue, then dried and stored in a desiccator. The presence of sweat changes the paper from blue to pink. An extremity that has been sympathetically denervated shows no color change when pressed onto the paper. The starch-iodine test also relies on color change. Its principal drawback is the long cleanup required after the starch-iodine application.

Blood flow measurements

The most common blood flow measurement has been the indirect Doppler measurement. Blood pressures using a Doppler probe are calculated in the brachial and dorsalis pedis (or anterior tibial) arteries after standard blood pressure cuffs have been applied. An index is then determined. After a sympathetic block a decrease in pressure is expected in the blocked extremity.

Direct measurement techniques have been devised using a flowmeter, either electromagnetic or ultrasonic, applied directly to the blood vessel during surgery. Muscle blood flow can also relate to sympathetic block, and techniques available include venous occlusion, plethysmography, xenon clearance, and mass spectrometery to measure muscle Po_2.

Pain assessment

The assessment of pain pre- and postblock also provides some indication of sympathetic blockade. Pain relief can be almost immediate after a block or can be delayed for several hours in some patients. Narcotics or sedative drugs can render pain assessment scores meaningless in the immediate postblock period. Patients should be instructed to keep pain diaries to aid assessment of each block's effectiveness.

Stellate Ganglion Block

Anatomy

Cell bodies of preganglionic axons lie in the anterolateral horn (ALH) of the spinal cord. Fibers destined for the head and neck originate in the first and second thoracic spinal cord segments, whereas preganglionic nerves to the upper extremity originate in segments T2 to T8 and occasionally T9.

Head and neck. Preganglionic fibers to the head and neck exit with the ventral roots of T1 and T2, then travel as white communicating rami before joining the sympathetic chain and passing cephalad to synapse at the inferior (stellate), middle, or superior cervical ganglion. Postganglionic nerves either follow the carotid arteries (external or internal) to the head or integrate as the gray communicating rami before joining the cervical plexus or upper cervical nerves to innervate structures of the neck (Fig. 63-17). To achieve successful sympathetic denervation of the head and neck, one should block the stellate ganglion because all preganglionic nerves either synapse here or pass through on their way to more cephalad ganglia. Blockade of the middle or superior ganglia will miss the contribution of sympathetic fibers traveling from the stellate ganglion to the vertebral plexus and ultimately to the corresponding areas of the cranial vault supplied by the vertebral artery.

Upper extremity. Sympathetic nerves to the upper extremity exit the spinal cord from T2 to T8 with ventral spinal roots, travel as white communicating rami to the sympathetic chain, then pass cephalad to synapse at the second thoracic ganglion, first thoracic or inferior cervical ganglion (stellate), and occasionally middle cervical ganglion. Most postganglionic nerves leave the chain as gray communicating rami and join the anterior divisions of C5 to T1 which form the brachial plexus. Some postganglionic nerves pass directly from the chain to form the subclavian perivascular plexus, and innervate the subclavian, axillary, and upper part of the brachial arteries.[154]

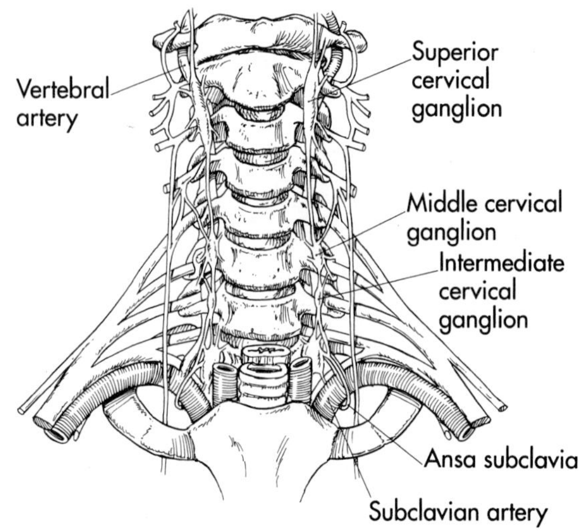

Fig. 63-17. Cervical sympathetic ganglia and stellate ganglion. Note the relationship of structures to the respective ganglia. (From Raj PP: *Practical management of pain,* ed 2, St Louis, 1992, Mosby–Year Book.)

Most individuals will have the inferior cervical ganglion fused to the first thoracic ganglion, thus forming the stellate ganglion. This ganglion commonly measures 2.5 cm long, 1.0 cm wide, and 0.5 cm thick. It usually lies in front of the neck of the first rib and extends to the interspace between C7 and T1. When elongated, it may lie over the anterior tubercle of C7, and in individuals with unfused ganglia the inferior cervical ganglion rests over C7 and the first thoracic ganglion over the neck of the first rib. From a three-dimensional perspective, the stellate ganglion is limited medially by the longus colli muscle, laterally by the scalene muscles, anteriorly by the subclavian artery, posteriorly by the transverse processes and prevertebral fascia, and inferiorly by the posterior aspect of the pleura (Fig. 63-18). At the level of the stellate ganglion, the vertebral artery lies anterior, having originated from the subclavian artery. After passing over the ganglion, the artery enters the vertebral foramen and is located posterior to the anterior tubercle of C6 (Fig. 63-19). Because the classic approach to blockade of the stellate ganglion is at the level of C6 (Chassaignac's tubercle), the needle is positioned anterior to the artery. Other structures posterior to the stellate ganglion include the anterior divisions of the C8 and T1 nerves (inferior aspects of the brachial plexus).

The stellate ganglion supplies sympathetic innervation to the upper extremity through gray communicating rami travelling with C7, C8, T1, and occasionally C5 and C6. Other

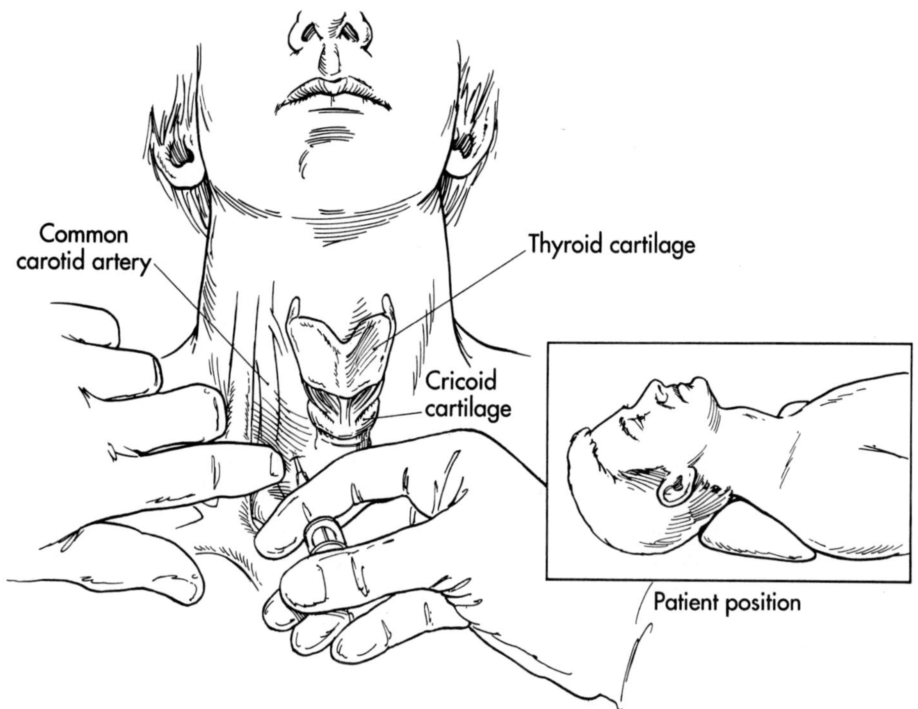

Fig. 63-18. Stellate ganglion block. C6 anterior tubercle is directly beneath the operator's index finger. The carotid artery is retracted laterally when necessary. The needle is perpendicular to all skin planes and is inserted directly posterior. *Inset*, Patient positioned for stellate ganglion block. A pillow or roll should be between the shoulders to extend the neck, to bring the esophagus midline, and to facilitate palpation of Chassaignac's tubercle. (From Raj PP: *Practical management of pain,* ed 2, St Louis, 1992, Mosby–Year Book.)

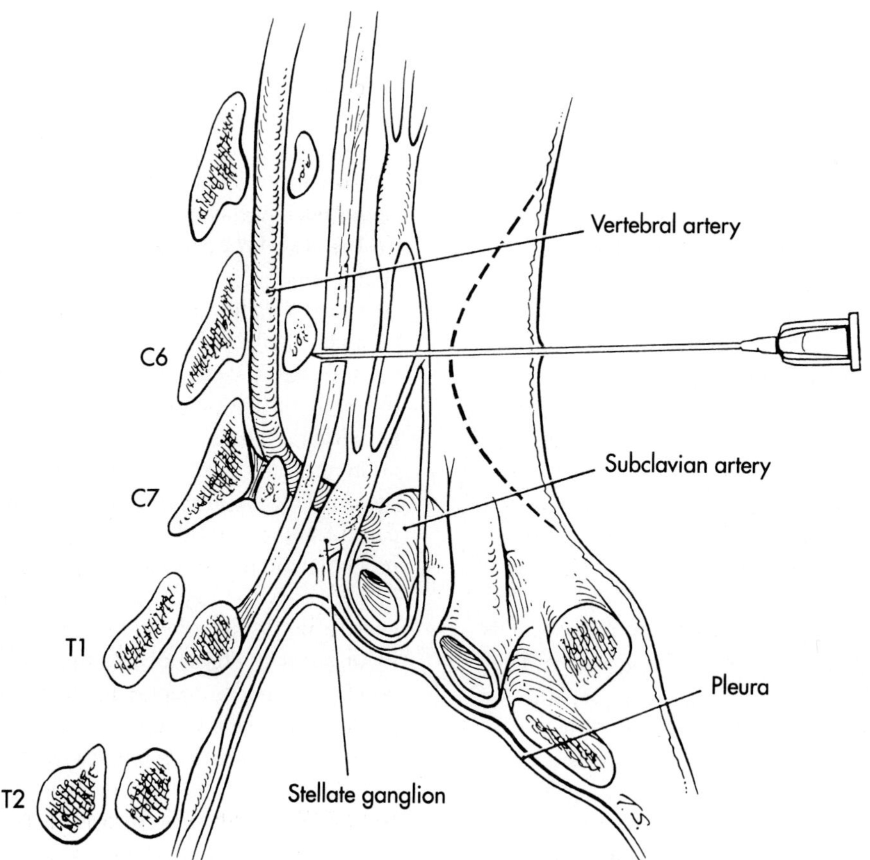

Fig. 63-19. Saggital view of the sympathetic chain. Note that the stellate ganglion is positioned directly posterior to the vertebral artery. The longus colli muscle separates the ganglia from the bone at C6 level. The needle is superior to the stellate ganglion. (From Raj PP: *Practical management of pain,* ed 2, St Louis, 1992, Mosby–Year Book.)

inconstant contributions to the upper extremity come from the T2 and T3 gray communicating rami. The latter fibers do not pass through the stellate ganglion, but rather join the brachial plexus and ultimately innervate distal structures of the upper extremity. These fibers have sometimes been implicated in inadequate relief of sympathetically mediated pain, despite evidence of a satisfactory stellate block. The anomalous pathways have been termed *Kuntz's nerves* and can be reliably blocked only by a posterior approach. Although technically more difficult than the classically taught anterior approach, the use of nerve-imaging techniques (e.g., CT) can help prevent the principal risk of pneumothorax. If a local anesthetic block is successful using this approach, neurolysis can be performed using low volumes of either aqueous phenol or alcohol. Because most, if not all, sympathetic fibers to the upper extremity pass through these upper thoracic ganglia, the results of this neurolytic block can be quite successful.

Other efferent fibers from the stellate ganglion follow the major vascular structures, including the subclavian and common carotid arteries. The subclavian arterial plexus also receives contributions from the ansa cervicalis (originating from the stellate ganglion) and the intermediate cervical ganglion.

Indications

The following clinical conditions have been treated with sympathetic block of the cervicothoracic chain.

- **Pain**
  - Reflex sympathetic dystrophy
  - Causalgia
  - Herpes zoster (shingles)
  - Postherpetic neuralgia, early
  - Phantom limb pain
  - Paget's disease
  - Neoplasm
  - Postradiation neuritis
  - Pain from CNS lesions
  - Intractable angina pectoris
- **Vascular insufficiency**
  - Raynaud's disease
  - Frostbite
  - Vasospasm
  - Occlusive vascular disease
  - Embolic vascular disease
  - Scleroderma
- **Other**
  - Hyperhidrosis
  - Meniere's disease
  - Shoulder/hand syndrome
  - Stroke
  - Sudden blindness
  - Vascular headaches

Many of these indications remain controversial, and reports of efficacy are based largely on case reports and not large, well-designed studies. In particular, treatment with stellate ganglion block for phantom limb pain, postherpetic neuralgia, vascular occlusion of large vessels, stroke, and Meniere's disease has yielded questionable results. Others, such as angina pectoris, require blockade of the upper five thoracic sympathetic ganglia in addition to the stellate ganglion to provide relief.

Technique

Patient preparation. Preparation of the patient for the initial block ideally begins at a visit before the procedure. Patients are much more likely to remember discharge instructions and expected side effects if these are explained during a prior visit when they are not apprehensive about an impending procedure. Conversations about the realistic expectations of sympathetic blockade should be held before any procedures. Patients are much less likely to experience frustration or despair if they understand beforehand what can be expected. If the pain etiology is unclear and the intended block is considered diagnostic, a complete explanation to the patient will enable him or her to record valuable information concerning the effectiveness of the procedure.

An IV line placed before the block is not considered mandatory at all pain clinics. Its placement will facilitate the use of IV sedation, when indicated, and provide access for the administration of resuscitative drugs should a complication occur. In skilled hands, a stellate ganglion block can be performed quickly and relatively painlessly. In these situations, an IV may not be necessary although all standard resuscitative drugs, suction, O_2, cardiac defibrillators, and instruments for tracheal intubation need to be readily accessible.

Anterior approach. The patient lies supine with the head resting flat on the table, without the use of a pillow. A folded sheet or thin pillow should be placed under the shoulders of most patients to further facilitate extension of the neck and make palpation of bony landmarks easier (Fig. 63-18). The head should be kept midline with the mouth slightly open to relax the anterior cervical musculature.

The site of needle entry is the C6 level—Chassaignac's tubercle—and can be most readily identified by first locating the cricoid cartilage (Fig. 63-19). For most individuals, this will be approximately 3.0 cm cephalad to the sternoclavicular joint. Palpation of the tubercle can be expected at the medial border of the sternocleidomastoid muscle, approximately 1.5 cm lateral to the midline. Location of the carotid artery should be noted; its position is most commonly lateral to the C6 tubercle. In some individuals, it will be necessary to retract the common carotid artery laterally, away from the site of entry.

In either a left-handed or right-handed stellate ganglion block, the nondominant hand should be used for palpating landmarks. A jabbing motion is not well tolerated by the patient; gentle but firm probing can easily define the borders of the tubercle. A single finger—the index finger—relays the most specific tactile information. An alternative approach traps the tubercle between the index and middle fingers.[34]

The skin is antiseptically prepared and the needle inserted, penetrating the skin at the tip of the operator's index finger. A prior skin wheal with local anesthetic is rarely necessary except in some teaching situations or in the case of patients with obese necks, in which repeated punctures may be anticipated. A 23-gauge needle, 4 to 5 cm long, is used and should puncture the skin directly downward (posteriorly), perpendicular to the table in all planes. Although a smaller gauge (e.g., 25-gauge) needle can be used, its added flexibility and smaller caliber can make it more difficult to reliably ascertain when bone is encountered and then maintain the proper location for injection.

The needle passes through the underlying tissue until it contacts either Chassaignac's tubercle or the junction of the C6 vertebral body and the tubercle. The depth of these structures differs, with the tubercle itself being more anterior than the junction of body and tubercle. Regardless, if the skin is properly displaced posteriorly by the nondominant index finger, the depth is rarely beyond 2.0 to 2.5 cm.

An important difference between medial and lateral location of bone at C6 relates to the presence of the longus colli. It is located over the lateral aspect of the vertebral body and medial aspect of the transverse process. It does not cover the C6 tubercle; only the prevertebral fascia that invests the longus colli covers the C6 tubercle. Therefore, if the needle contacts the medial aspect of the transverse process at a depth somewhat greater than expected, the physician should be prepared to withdraw the needle 0.5 cm to avoid injection into the longus colli muscle. Injection into the muscle belly can prevent caudad diffusion of local anesthetic to the stellate ganglion. Location of the needle on the superficial tip of the C6 anterior tubercle requires only withdrawal of the needle from periosteum before injection.

The procedure is most easily performed if the syringe is attached before needle placement. This prevents accidental dislodgement of the needle from the bone, which is possible if attachment is attempted after needle placement. After bone is encountered, the palpating finger maintains its pressure, the needle is withdrawn 2 to 5 mm, and the medication is injected. Alternatively, after bone is met, the palpating hand can release and fix the needle by grasping its hub. The dominant hand is now free to aspirate and inject.

Injection of medication must be performed in a routine and systematic fashion. An initial test dose must be injected in all cases. **Less than 1 ml of solution injected intravascularly into the vertebral artery has resulted in loss of consciousness and seizure activity. Before any injections, careful aspiration must be performed, for either blood or cerebrospinal fluid (CSF).** If the aspiration is negative, 0.5 to 1.0 ml of solution is administered and the patient is asked to raise the thumb to indicate he or she is having no adverse symptoms. The patient should be reminded that talking will move the neck musculature and can dislodge the needle from its proper location. To maintain verbal contact, the patient can be asked to point a thumb or finger upward during the procedure. After the initial test dose, the remainder of the solution can be injected, carefully aspirating after each 3 to 4 ml.

During injection or needle placement, a paresthesia of the arm or hand may be elicited. This signifies that placement of the needle is deep to the anterior tubercle, adjacent to the C6 or C7 nerve root. Repositioning the needle will be necessary. Any aspiration of blood or CSF also necessitates repositioning of the needle.

The total volume of solution necessary depends on the block desired. If placed properly, 5 ml of solution will block the stellate ganglion. This will not reliably block all sympathetic fibers to the upper extremities because contributions from T2 and T3 may be present. Injection of 10 ml of solution will more reliably block all innervation to the upper extremity, even in patients with anomalous Kuntz nerves. If blockade is being performed for sympathetically mediated pain of the thoracic viscera including the heart, 15 to 20 ml of solution should be administered.

Evidence of block. Sympathetic interruption to the head, supplied by the stellate ganglion, can be easily documented by the presence of Horner's syndrome: myosis (pinpoint pupil); ptosis (drooping of the upper eyelid); and enophthalmos (sinking of the eyeball). Associated findings include conjunctival injection, nasal congestion, and facial anhidrosis. However, these signs can be present without complete interruption of the sympathetic nerves to the upper extremity.

Evidence of sympathetic blockade to the upper extremity includes visible engorgement of the veins on the back of the hand and forearm, psychogalvanic reflex (PGR), plethysmography, thermography, and sweat test. A rise in skin temperature also occurs provided the preblock temperature does not exceed 33° C to 34° C.

Complications

Common complications of a stellate ganglion block occur from the diffusion of local anesthetic into nearby nervous structures. These include the recurrent laryngeal nerve with complaints of hoarseness, feeling of a lump in the throat, and sometimes a subjective shortness of breath. **Bilateral stellate blocks are rarely advised because bilateral blocking of the recurrent laryngeal nerve can result in respiratory compromise and loss of laryngeal reflexes. Block of the phrenic nerve results in temporary paralysis of the diaphragm and can result in respiratory embarrassment in patients whose respiratory reserve is already severely compromised.**

Partial brachial plexus block can also result secondary to spread along the prevertebral fascia[44] or if the needle location is too posterior. The patient should be discharged with a sling and careful instructions on how to care for a partially blocked arm, should this occur. The specificity of a diagnostic stellate ganglion block for sympathetically maintained pain is compromised when somatic sensory fibers of the brachial plexus are also blocked. In this circumstance, the block should be repeated at another time when the results of a solely sympathetic block can be observed.

The two most feared complications from a stellate ganglion block include an intraspinal injection and seizures from an intravascular injection. Respiratory embarrassment and the need for mechanical ventilation can result from injection into either the epidural space (if high concentrations of local anesthetic are used) or intrathecal space. Should this occur, patients need continual reassurance that everything is being appropriately managed and that they will recover without sequelae. Some sedation is required while the local anesthetic wears off. No muscle relaxants are necessary for tracheal intubation because profound anesthesia of the larynx can be expected.

Intravascular injection most commonly occurs in the vertebral artery. Small amounts of local anesthetic result in unconsciousness, respiratory paralysis, seizures, and sometimes severe arterial hypotension. IV fluid resuscitation, vasopressors, O_2, and endotracheal (ET) intubation may be necessary. If the quantity of drug injected into the artery is small (< 2 ml), the preceding sequelae are self-limited, with O_2 and fluid administration often being the only needed therapy. One must be careful when performing a stellate ganglion block that no air is injected from the syringe. Preventable cerebral air embolisms have been reported.[3,153,154]

Side effects of a stellate ganglion block should be distinguished from complications. Most unpleasant side effects result from development of a Horner's syndrome as outlined previously.

Alternative approaches

C7 anterior approach. The anterior approach to the stellate ganglion at C7 is similar to the approach described at C6. However, unlike the C6 tubercle, C7 has only a vestigial tubercle that is very difficult to palpate. To identify C7, one must usually first find Chassaignac's tubercle (C6), then move one finger-breadth caudad from the inferior tip. The patient must be positioned with a pillow under the shoulders to extend the cervical spine and help make the tubercle more superficial.

The advantage to blockade at C7 is the lower volume of local anesthetic necessary to provide complete interruption of the upper-extremity sympathetic innervation. Six to 9 ml of solution will suffice. Recurrent laryngeal nerve block is less frequent with this approach. The technique carries two important disadvantages. Less-pronounced landmarks cause needle positioning to be less reliable, and the risk of pneumothorax increases because the dome of the lung is in close proximity. The latter occurs more easily in thin, tall individuals whose pleural cupulae extend more cephalad.

Posterior approach. The ease of performing a stellate ganglion block by the anterior approach has rendered the posterior approach unnecessary except for specific indications.[60] The posterior approach is useful for patients who develop Horner's syndrome with an anterior approach but fail

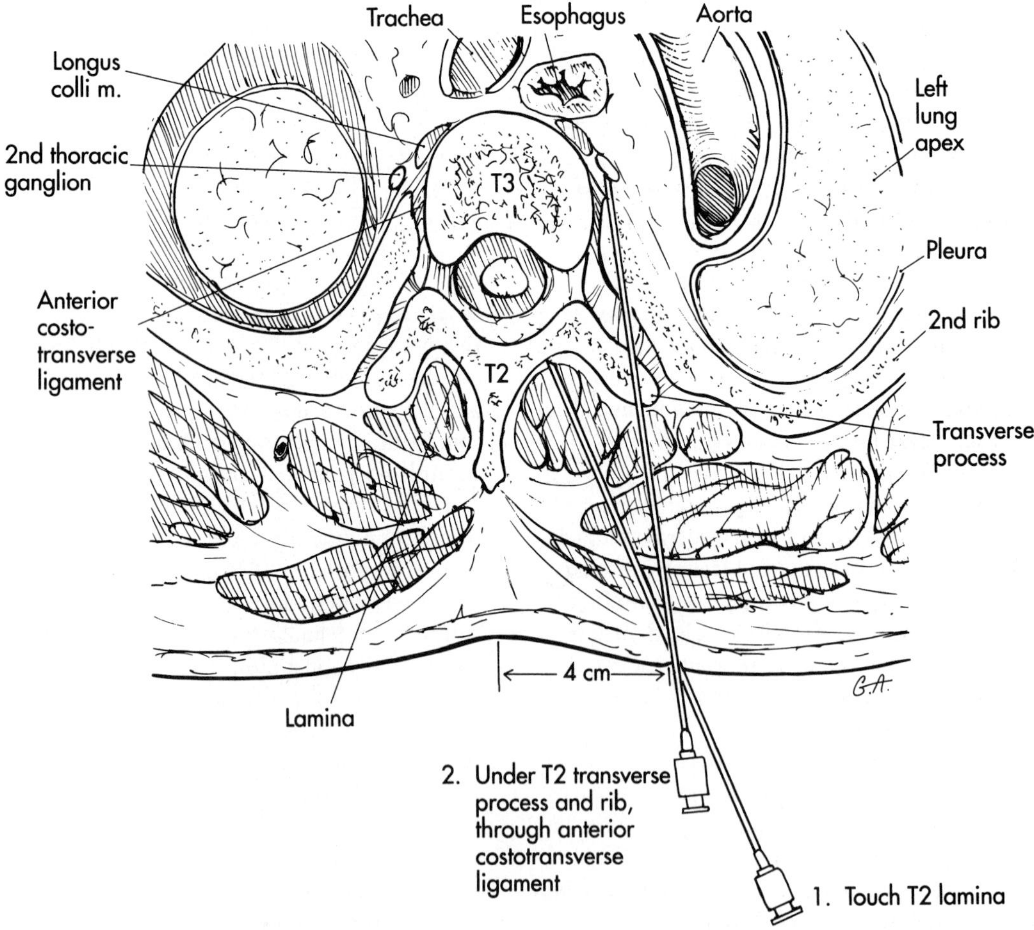

Fig. 63-20. Posterior approach to upper thoracic sympathetic chain block. Needle is introduced 4 cm from midline, then walked off the T2 lamina. The needle should always be directed medially. (From Raj PP: *Practical management of pain,* ed 2, St Louis, 1992, Mosby–Year Book.)

to show other signs of sympathetic denervation to the upper extremity. Should this occur despite repetitive, well-placed blocks, the patient may have a fascial tissue barrier preventing caudad diffusion of the drug. The posterior approach at the T2 or T3 level provides sympathetic interruption to the upper extremity.

Patients chosen for chemical neurolytic sympathectomy of the upper extremity should be blocked with the posterior approach. Although dilute solutions of phenol have been injected by the anterior approach at C6, the smaller volume used may prevent reliable diffusion to the stellate ganglion.[176] If one increases the volume, the risk of spread to the recurrent laryngeal nerve, phrenic nerve, or brachial plexus is unacceptably high. Also, Horner's syndrome invariably develops if complete neurolytic destruction occurs by the anterior approach. Although the posterior approach usually avoids Horner's syndrome, the patient must understand and accept this potentially permanent complication before neurolysis.

A major disadvantage of sympathetic block by the posterior approach is the high risk of pneumothorax (Fig. 63-20). The apex of the lung lies in close proximity to the sympathetic chain at T2 and can be difficult to avoid by even the most experienced of operators. With the use of CT, precise needle location can be more readily achieved.[60] Whenever neurolysis is anticipated, placement should be guided by CT scan.

Celiac Plexus and Splanchnic Nerve Block

Anatomy

Sympathetic innervation of the abdominal viscera originates in the ALH of the spinal cord. Preganglionic axons from T5 to T12 leave the spinal cord with the ventral spinal nerve roots to join the white communicating rami en route to the sympathetic chain. In contrast to other preganglionic sympathetic nerves, these axons do not synapse in the sympathetic chain; rather they pass through the chain to synapse at distal sites, including the celiac, aorticorenal, and superior mesenteric ganglia. Postganglionic nerves accompany blood vessels to their respective visceral structures (Fig. 63-21).

The celiac plexus receives innervation from the greater splanchnic (T5 to T10), lesser splanchnic (T10 to T11), and

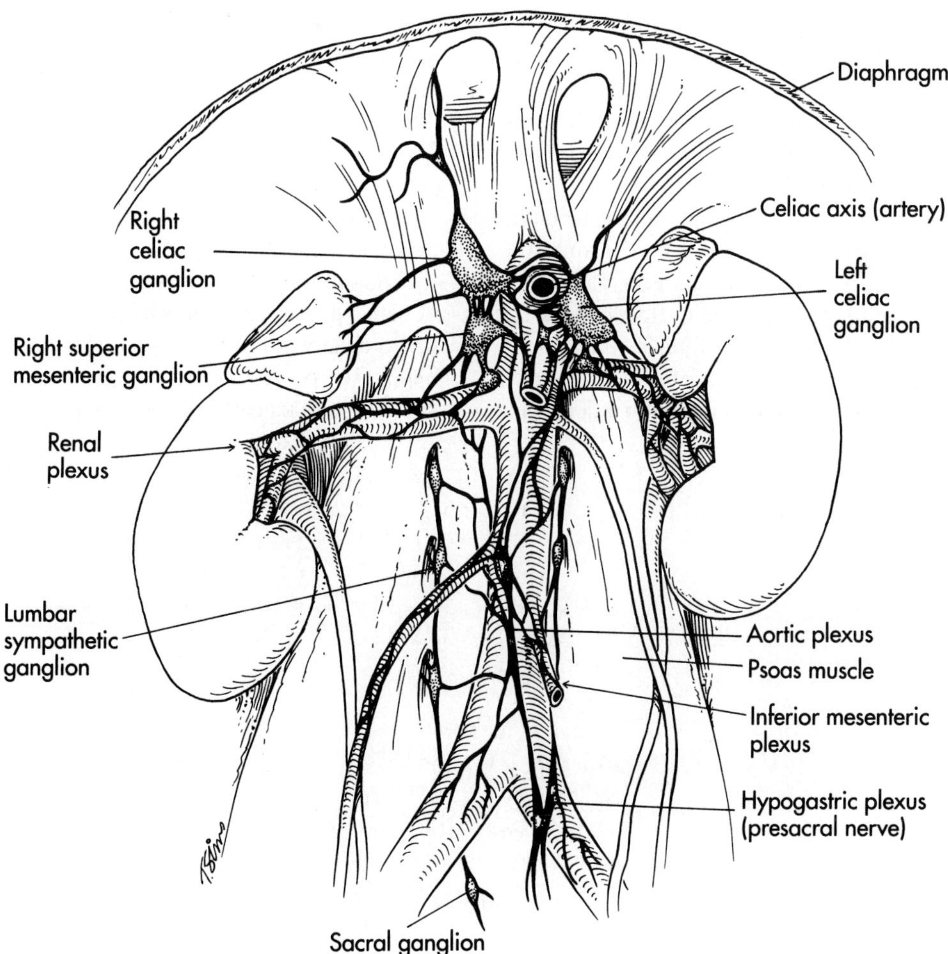

Fig. 63-21. Anterior view of the celiac plexus. The relationship to nearby structures is shown. Note the dense, diffuse intertwining network of nerves that form the plexus. (From Raj PP: *Practical management of pain,* ed 2, St Louis, 1992, Mosby–Year Book.)

least splanchnic (T12) nerves. This innervation indicates an alternative approach of interrupting visceral pain if celiac plexus block has failed or is inappropriate because of tumor invasion: a segmental epidural neurolysis from T5 to T12 can produce visceral pain interruption.

Preganglionic nerves from T5 to T9, and occasionally T4 and T10, travel caudally after joining and separating from the sympathetic chain along the lateral and anterolateral aspects of the vertebral bodies. At the level of T9 and T10, the axons coalesce to form the greater splanchnic nerve, pierce the diaphragm, and end as numerous terminal endings in the celiac plexus. Most travel ipsilaterally, but a few will cross and synapse with contralateral postganglionic cell bodies.

Sympathetic nerves from T10 to T11, and occasionally T12, combine to form the lesser splanchnic nerve. Their course parallels the greater splanchnic nerve in a posterolateral position and ends in either the celiac plexus or aorticorenal ganglion. The least splanchnic nerves arise from T12, parallel the lesser splanchnic nerve, and synapse in the aorticorenal ganglion.

The previously mentioned sympathetic nerves are efferent nerves that maintain important characteristics in reflexive sympathetically mediated pain. Afferent, nociceptive information from abdominal viscera travels in afferent nerves which accompany the efferent sympathetic nerves.

The celiac plexus lies anterior to the aorta and epigastrium (Fig. 63-21). It is also located just anterior to the crus of the diaphragm. The plexus extends for several centimeters in front of and laterally to the aorta (Fig. 63-22). Fibers within the plexus arise from preganglionic splanchnic nerves, parasympathetic preganglionic nerves from the vagus, some sensory nerves from the phrenic and vagus nerves, and sympathetic postganglionic fibers. Afferent fibers concerned with nociception pass diffusely through the celiac plexus and represent the main target of celiac plexus blockade. These afferent fibers coalesce to form a dense, intertwining network of autonomic nerves. Three pairs of ganglia exist within the plexus: (1) the celiac ganglia; (2) the superior mesenteric ganglia; and (3) the aortic renal ganglia. Postganglionic nerves from these ganglia innervate all the abdominal viscera with the exception of part of the transverse colon, the left colon, the rectum, and pelvic viscera. The latter, including the uterus and cervix, ultimately have nociceptive synapses from T10 to L1 spinal levels.

Indications

Any pain originating from visceral structures innervated by the celiac plexus can be effectively alleviated by blockade of the plexus. This includes the pancreas, liver, gallbladder, omentum, mesentery, and alimentary tract from the stomach to the transverse portion of the large colon (see Fig. 63-15). The particular disease state determines the effectiveness of a celiac plexus block in producing sustained pain relief beyond the duration of the local anesthetic solution. The pain syndrome involved dictates whether a local anesthetic block, neurolytic injection, catheter placement, or steroid injection should be employed.

The best indication for neurolytic celiac plexus block is upper-abdominal malignancy, pancreatic cancer, in particular. This was initially described by Kapis[112] in 1914. The pain is described as severe and unremitting, and narcotics often poorly alleviate the pain. The rapid progression of the disease makes the time from diagnosis to death very short, often less than 6 months. These factors, together with the excellent analgesia achieved with neurolytic blockade, make celiac plexus block an excellent choice for pancreatic cancer pain when more conservative measures have failed.

An additional benefit in these patients may be the effect of celiac plexus block on gastric motility. Complete sympathetic denervation of the gastrointestinal (GI) tract allows unopposed parasympathetic activity and increased peristalsis. Although diarrhea has been reported in a few patients, a

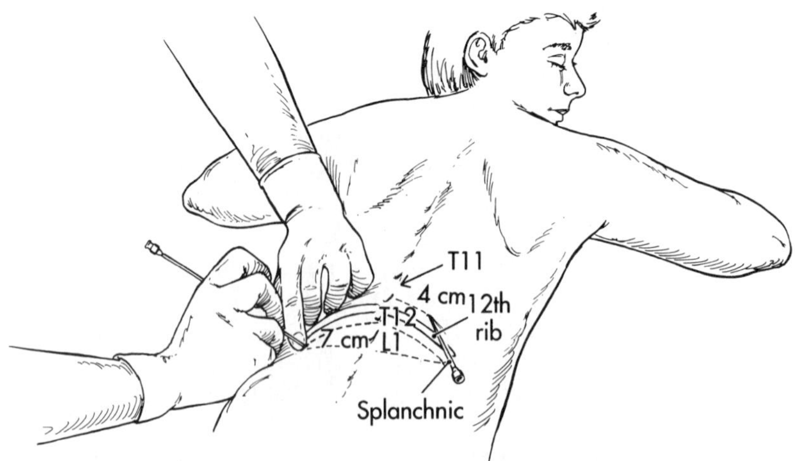

Fig. 63-22. Surface landmarks for splanchnic nerve block or celiac plexus blocks. The diagram drawn resembles a flat isoceles triangle. (From Raj PP: *Practical management of pain,* ed 2, St Louis, 1992, Mosby–Year Book.)

concomitant decrease in the incidence of nausea and vomiting has also been reported. The presence of severe nausea and vomiting has been cited as a primary problem with pancreatic cancer in patients whose pain might otherwise be reasonably managed with oral narcotics.[35]

An alternative to neurolysis for patients who have had multiple abdominal surgeries and continue to complain of pain is the addition of a corticosteroid preparation to the local anesthetic solution. Best results can be expected in patients who have an inflammatory component involving the celiac plexus. Betamethasone (Celestone) has dual properties of excellent tissue dispersion, which are essential for the diffuse celiac plexus, and depot characteristics that would help to prolong the effect from blockade. However, good controlled studies are lacking.

The etiology of abdominal pain cannot always be clearly elucidated at initial evaluation, especially in patients who have undergone multiple abdominal surgeries. In these patients, it can be difficult to differentiate abdominal wall pain from underlying visceral pain. Either a local-anesthetic celiac plexus block or an intercostal nerve block should be considered a pain-specific block which will identify visceral and somatic pain, respectively.

The long-term effectiveness of a neurolytic celiac plexus block in patients with nonmalignant abdominal pain has been variable.[13,83,102,129,165] Often, regeneration of new pathways or development of a deafferent pain syndrome has occurred in these patients by 6 to 12 months. Although long-term success with neurolytic celiac blocks has not been high, short-term relief may allow some patients with intractable, intolerable abdominal pain to gain coping skills and learn to manage their pain. This alternative may prove superior to unmerited surgical reexploration. Neurolytic celiac plexus block may be indicated in patients whose pain is uncontrolled, who have required repeated pain-related hospital admissions, who have had multiple surgical procedures for pain without benefit, and who are debating further surgical explorations. If temporary pain relief is achieved with a local anesthetic celiac plexus block and the addition of steroids is ineffective, a neurolytic celiac plexus block should be considered.

Image intensification

Image intensification techniques can aid the performance of celiac plexus blocks and include radiographs, fluoroscopy, and CT.[109,110,156] Because many pain clinics do not have these facilities on site, these blocks may have to be performed in the radiology suite. This is rarely necessary for diagnostic blocks or when local anesthetics are the sole agents used. The potential seriousness and permanency of complications with neurolytic solutions, however, make image intensification preferable.

Fluoroscopy and CT-guided placement each have advantages.[40,102,193] Fluoroscopy yields a real-time display during the injection of solutions. Verification of needle placement can be performed before injection. Intravascular, intraspinal, or lateral spread of solution into the psoas muscle or along the diaphragm can easily be seen. Proper, diffuse spread can be monitored as the total volume is injected[102] (Fig. 63-23).

The advantage of CT-guided placement rests with the precision of needle location (Fig. 63-24). If anatomic variations are expected secondary to extensive disease, CT can easily identify these before placement and aid technically difficult placements. After they are positioned, needle tips can be discretely seen in relation to all nearby structures. Instillation of small volumes of air through the needles clearly shows where the solution can be expected to spread.

Computed tomography also is a good teaching instrument, demonstrating the close proximity of previously mentioned structures, including the kidneys, great vessels, and diaphragmatic crus. The high cost of CT precludes its use in routine cases, especially if fluoroscopy is available.

Lateral technique

After insertion of an IV catheter, the patient is positioned prone with a pillow under the lower abdomen to remove the lumbar lordosis and to allow easier palpation of the spinous processes. In patients whose pain will not allow them to lie prone or in highly anxious patients, premedication is given through the IV. In situations when the block is performed for diagnostic purposes, one may wish to avoid premedication. Although the block can be performed in the lateral position, technical considerations make needle placement more difficult.

Landmarks drawn with an indelible skin marker greatly facilitate needle placement, even for those experienced with the procedure (Fig. 63-25). This may be performed before preparing and draping the patient, or with a sterile marker after preparation. Landmarks to be drawn include the spinous processes T12 and L1, and the inferior border of the twelfth rib. The T12 spinous process should be correctly identified and marked by following the twelfth rib medially and counting cephalad from the L5 spinous process.

The site for needle entry is marked 7- to 8-cm lateral from the spinous process. Either 20- or 22-gauge needles, 12 to 18 cm long, are used. The exact length depends on body habitus. The insertion point should be immediately inferior to the border of the twelfth rib and should not exceed 8 cm from midline (7 cm in thin individuals) to avoid the risk of placing the needle through renal parenchymal tissue. Likewise, it is extremely important that the needles not be placed immediately beneath the T11 rib, because a pneumothorax can result.

The ultimate directional positioning of the needle toward the midline will depend on whether the splanchnic nerves or celiac plexus are to be blocked (Fig. 63-26 on page 1474). Classically, needles have been directed to the L1 spinous process for block of the celiac plexus. Splanchnic nerves are blocked by positioning the needles more cephalad toward the eleventh or twelfth thoracic spinous process. If the L2 spinous process is mistaken for the L1 process, inadequate cephalad spread of solution may result.

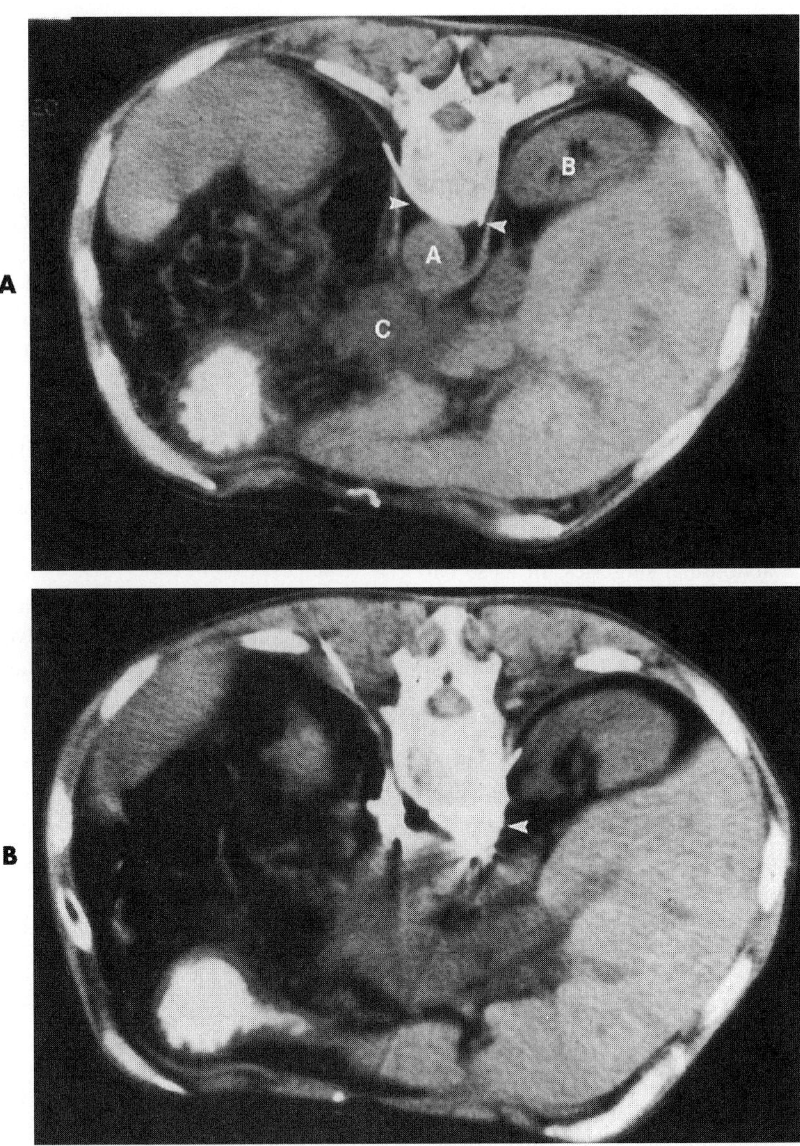

Fig. 63-23. A, CT radiograph of the celiac plexus block. Precise needle location (*arrow*) is observed with respect to surrounding structures. *A,* Aorta; *B,* kidney; *C,* pancreas. **B,** Contrast material fills the periaortic space (*arrow*). (From Raj PP: *Practical management of pain,* ed 2, St Louis, 1992, Mosby–Year Book.)

Anatomically, the crus of the diaphragm determines whether the block performed represents a true celiac plexus block or a splanchnic nerve block. If the tip of the needle lies posterior to the crus, the nerves blocked will belong to the splanchnic nerves. When the needles are advanced anteriorly, they pass transcrurally and solution injected blocks nerves to the celiac plexus. Needles placed at the T11 vertebral body always are located posteriorly to the crus. Below this level, the crus migrates posteriorly to attach to the T12 vertebral bodies.[147] At the T12 or L1 level, the needles can be placed either anterior or posterior to the crus. The classically taught needle placement at the anterior border of the vertebral body most often results in placement posterior to the crus. For reliable placement anterior to the crus, the needle needs to be placed transcrurally, often through the abdominal aorta.

Infiltration of deep-muscular structures and periosteum with local anesthetics lessens the need for sedation. Heavy sedation should especially be avoided whenever a diagnostic block is being performed. With advancement of the needle, two bony landmarks—the twelfth rib and the transverse process of L1—can be mistaken for the vertebral body. Both are superficial to the vertebral body; the twelfth rib is quite superficial, but the transverse process can sometimes be misleading. If any question remains after bone is encountered, the needle should be removed and redirected cephalad. Caudad redirection can create a final placement at L2 which is less than optimal.

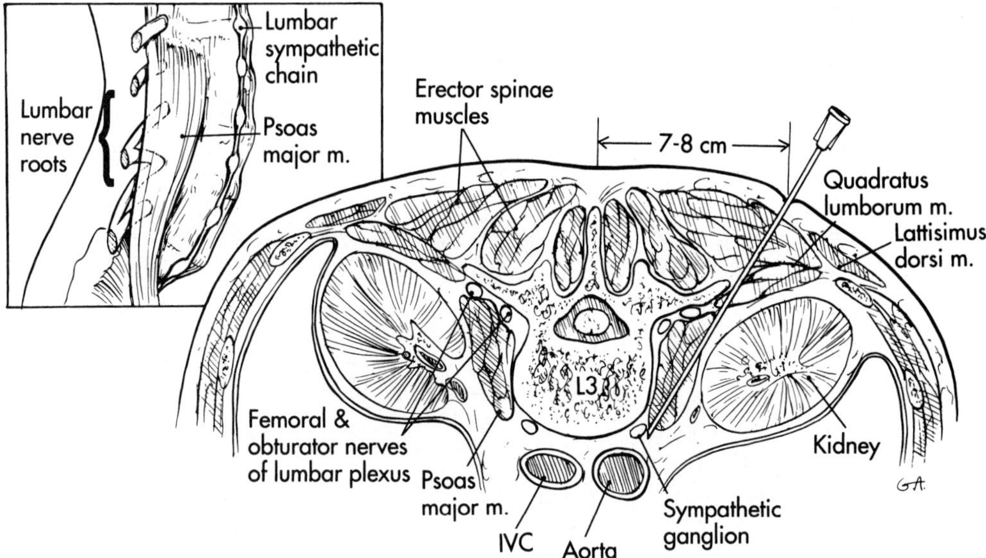

Fig. 63-24. Anatomy of the lumbar sympathetic chain. The sympathetic chain has migrated to the anterolateral border of the vertebral bodies. The chain is separated from the somatic nerve roots by the large psoas muscle. (From Raj PP: *Practical management of pain,* ed 2, St Louis, 1992, Mosby–Year Book.)

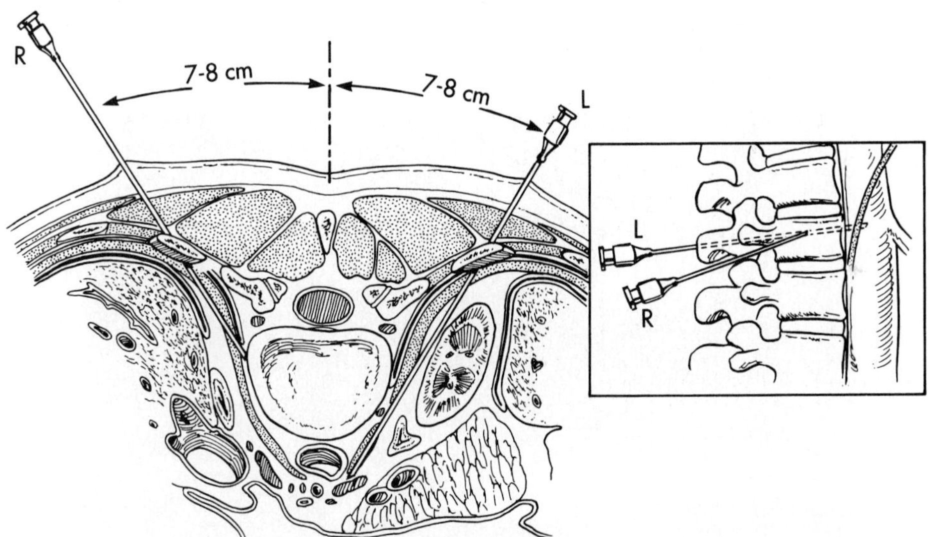

Fig. 63-25. Retrocrural and transcrural needle placement for celiac plexus block. *L,* Needle is retrocrural and will result in solution spreading and blocking the splanchnic nerves. *R,* Needle is transcrural, and solution will block the celiac plexus directly. (From Raj PP: *Practical management of pain,* ed 2, St Louis, 1992, Mosby–Year Book.)

After the vertebral body has been reached, a marker is placed on the needle 2 to 3 cm from the skin. The needle tip is then walked laterally until it just slips off the lateral surface of the vertebral body (Fig. 63-27). To make accurate small adjustments, the needle must first be withdrawn to superficial, subcutaneous structures. If adjustments with the smaller 22-gauge needle are attempted when the needle is deep, either it will be unsuccessful or the degree of change will be unpredictable. The needle should be first withdrawn to the skin and then a small change in the angle made before reinsertion. The skin may be considered a fulcrum with the celiac plexus being quite far from this point. Anything greater than small changes in the needle angle at the skin will result in a much larger change in position at the ultimate destination of the needle tip.

After the lateral aspect of the vertebral body has passed, a "pop" is often felt when the needle passes through the psoas fascia. At this point, the needles approach the great vessels and should be advanced slowly. The aorta is encountered from the left and the interior vena cava (IVC)

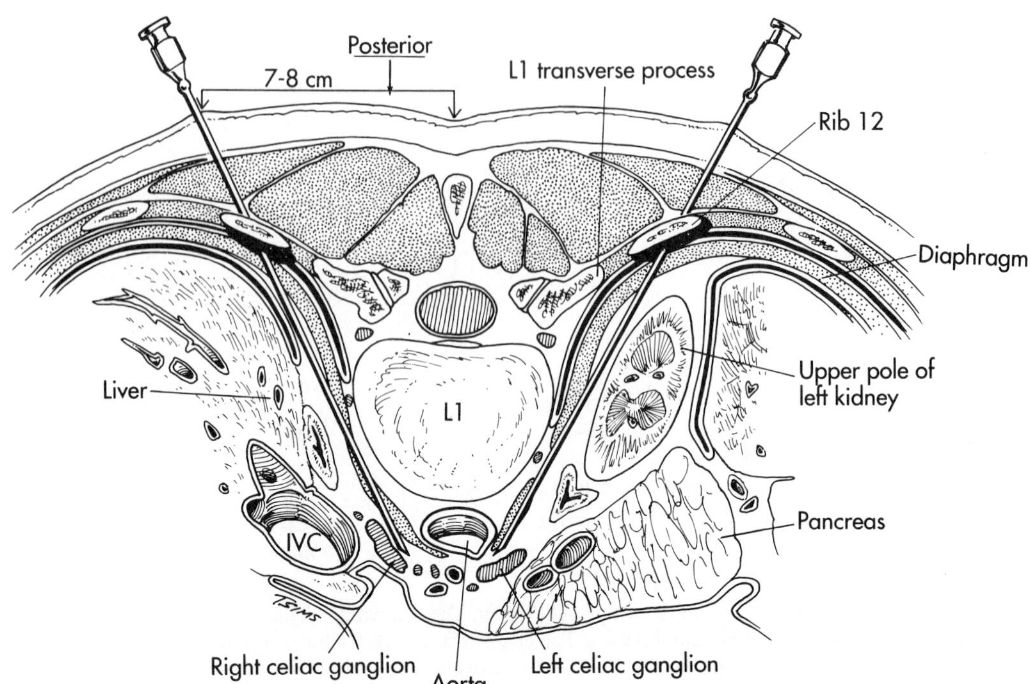

Fig. 63-26. Cross-section of celiac plexus block. Note the proximity of renal parenchymal tissue, necessitating needles placed no farther than 7 to 8 cm from midline. (From Raj PP: *Practical management of pain,* ed 2, St Louis, 1992, Mosby–Year Book.)

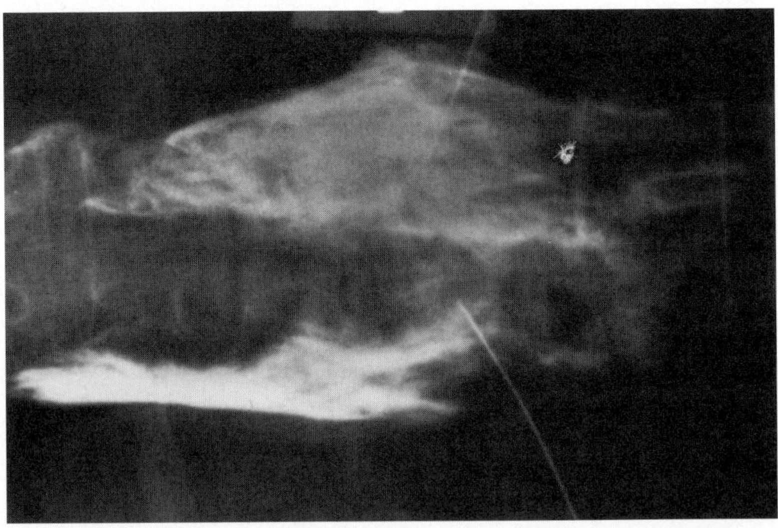

Fig. 63-27. Radiograph taken under direct fluoroscopic control. Spread of solution is monitored. No lateral diffusion is seen, and good confluence of contrast is seen anterior to the vertebral body. This is further confirmed by lateral cross-table radiograph. (From Raj PP: *Practical management of pain,* ed 2, St Louis, 1992, Mosby–Year Book.)

from the right. Pancreatic or other intra-abdominal masses often distort the structures laterally and posteriorly along the vertebral column. One can easily check for optimal location of the needle by feeling for arterial pulsation. These pulsations can also be observed visually if the needle approximates the aorta. These checks should be performed as the needle passes its final 2 to 3 cm past the lateral part of the vertebral body.

After proper placement of the needles, a careful aspiration of both needles is performed before injection. If blood is encountered, the needle is slowly withdrawn until negative aspiration is achieved. Alternatively, on the aortic side, the needle can be advanced through the aorta until no blood is returned and injection made at this location.

Initially, 2 to 3 ml of a local anesthetic solution containing epinephrine is injected to further test for either intravascular or intraspinal placement. If this test is negative, 15 ml of bupivacaine 0.5% with epinephrine 1:200,000 is injected through each needle.

Alternative approaches

Single-needle approach. A single-needle approach using the left side has been reported with good results.[70,93] The technique for needle placement is similar to that previously described for bilateral placement. Final location of the needle has been reported both posterior to the aorta and anterior by a transaortic approach. An adequate volume (20 to 30 mL) must be used because only one needle is used and the celiac plexus is a diffuse network.

Anterior approach. An anterior approach to the celiac plexus has been employed with the needle inserted through the abdominal wall at the T12 level. A thin, 22-gauge needle should be used because bowel will often be perforated, unlike other abdominal percutaneous radiographic procedures.[113] The needle tip will locate anterior to the aorta at the exact position of the celiac plexus. For patients who cannot lie prone, this approach may have applicability. However, many patients undergoing this procedure have either a large pancreatic mass or other intra-abdominal tumor anterior to the plexus, and a needle through these often vascular masses should be avoided.

Catheter placement

Patients with nonmalignant abdominal pain often fare poorly after neurolytic blockade of the celiac plexus, despite deriving temporary benefit from local anesthetic blockade. Because this pain is sympathetically mediated and reflexively perpetuated, continuous denervation of the plexus by local anesthetic infusion may provide prolonged analgesia.

The technique for placement is similar to that described previously.[83] Instead of 22-gauge needles, a 6-inch or 8-inch catheter system (Becton and Dickinson, Longdwel Catheter) is placed bilaterally. After placement, the catheters are secured at the skin with either a 2.0-cm silk skin suture or benzoin and steristrips, and covered with a sterile, clear dressing. Local anesthetic solution (bupivacaine 0.1%) is infused at 6 to 8 ml per hour. These catheters can be maintained for 4 to 7 days if placed sterilely and the sites checked daily.

Neurolytic block

Patients with pancreatic cancer or other isolated upper-abdominal malignancies are the most commonly chosen for a neurolytic celiac plexus block. The technique is similar to that previously described, with image intensification employed whenever possible.

In choosing patients for a neurolytic celiac plexus block, one must try to differentiate somatic pain from visceral pain. Retroperitoneal extension into somatic structures or distant metastases is not effectively blocked with a celiac plexus block. If both visceral and somatic etiologies are present, the celiac plexus block may serve only to unmask the somatic component of pain. Although this may be sufficient to bring the patient's pain to a state manageable with oral narcotics, it is always best to determine these factors before neurolytic blockade with a diagnostic local anesthetic block.

Reports of success with this procedure average 85%, with a range of 70% to 100%, giving this procedure the highest success rate compared with other neurolytic blocks. The duration of pain relief is perhaps more difficult to ascertain because most patients died within 1 month. One report cited a patient having pain relief for 1.5 years.[91]

The preferred agent to be employed continues to be debated. No comparative studies have been performed examining the effectiveness of the two most commonly used compounds—phenol and alcohol.[205] Concentrations of alcohol used have ranged from 50% to 100%. The greatest disadvantage with absolute alcohol is the immediate and severe pain experienced on injection.[48] Patients describe this sensation as a "forceful kick to the abdomen." Although this sensation provides good confirmation of proper needle location, some patients do not easily forget it and have occasionally refused subsequent blocks. An alternative to absolute alcohol is a mixture of bupivacaine 0.5% with alcohol in a 1:1 mixture. The bupivacaine decreases or eliminates the immediate discomfort from the alcohol injection. Although no good comparative studies are available, long-term results from the two preparations appear similar. Regardless of the strength of alcohol used, the volume injected is important to ensure adequate block. A total of 50 ml—25 ml through each bilaterally placed needle—has been the standard volume injected. This ensures adequate diffusion throughout the celiac plexus.

Phenol was initially prepared for celiac plexus blocks in a 6% solution. Studies of smaller groups of patients using 6% phenol reported pain relief similar to the previously mentioned alcohol studies.[76] The 6% solutions were classically used because of the inability of phenol to remain in solution at higher concentrations. This has been overcome as solutions of 12% are now easily prepared in contrast media. At higher concentrations, no accurate data exist concerning the pharmacokinetics of phenol; toxicity limits have not been determined.

Complications

The main side effect of celiac plexus block is backache, which usually results from passage of needles through the musculature of the back. This can be minimized by gentle advancement of the needles, minimal repositioning, and adequate local infiltration. The back pain is self-limiting but can be a significant complaint requiring a nonsteroidal anti-inflammatory drug (NSAID), muscle relaxant, or heating pad.

Hypotension, secondary to vasodilation of the large splanchnic bed, can be expected from a well-placed celiac plexus block. In otherwise healthy patients, this can be avoided or minimized with a 500- to 1000-ml IV bolus of lactated Ringer's solution before the block. In sicker patients, when volume preloading may not be desirable, neosynephrine directly counters the peripheral vasodilatory effects of the block. The magnitude of the initial hypotensive response does not depend on the agent used (a local anesthetic or neurolytic).

The orthostatic hypotensive response caused by a neurolytic block can persist after compensatory mechanisms have adjusted for splanchnic vasodilation. In most cases, this is self-limiting and becomes insignificant within 1 or 2 weeks. The efficacy of a local anesthetic block performed before the neurolytic injection in identifying those patients who might have long-term problems is questionable.

Other complications of celiac plexus block can be subdivided into those resulting from needle placement and those caused by the agent injected. Needles can inadvertently pass through a dural cuff, resulting in a spinal headache. Repeated puncture of an intervertebral disc produces back pain that can be slow to resolve. Puncture of the great vessels, most commonly the aorta, can result in a retroperitoneal hemorrhage. Placement of a needle through the L1 somatic nerve root can produce a paresthesia and possibly a painful neuropathy. Injection into the artery of Adamkiewicz was postulated to be the cause of paraplegia after an attempted celiac plexus block with phenol.[184] Injection into this artery results in paraplegia because it is the main blood supply to portions of the spinal cord.

Measured laterally from the spinous process, the point of entry for needles should never exceed 7 cm in thin individuals or 8 cm in obese patients.[156] If placed more laterally, the risk of piercing renal parenchymal tissue is greatly enhanced, leading to renal hemorrhage or nephrocutaneous fistula. The close proximity of the kidneys to the advancing needle can be easily checked with CT imagery.

A potentially serious complication from needle placement occurs if the twelfth rib is not correctly identified and the needles are inadvertently inserted under the eleventh rib. Although pulmonary parenchymal tissue does not extend to this level, the pleural reflection and subpleural space are present and a pneumothorax can result. If an imaging technique is used, the site of entry and its relation to the twelfth rib should be noted before needle advancement.

Complications can also result from the local anesthetic or neurolytic agent employed. Local anesthetic complications secondary to intravascular injection can easily occur if careful, repeated aspirations with concurrent monitoring are not performed. The aorta and IVC are not infrequently punctured and this may not be recognized with the longer needles necessary to perform these blocks. The use of epinephrine-containing solutions and incremental dosing may help avoid this problem. Unintentional injection of a local anesthetic solution into a dural cuff or the intraspinal canal can result in a total spinal block. Resuscitative equipment must always be readily available to handle such emergencies. Accidental injection of either alcohol or phenol into the intraspinal space can be catastrophic.

A more common complication of neurolytic blockade occurs when the drug diffuses laterally and posteriorly into the psoas muscle. Image intensifiers can greatly reduce this likelihood. When it does happen, the effect is most often limited to the L1 nerve root. This is predominantly a sensory root, and its block will cause numbness over the anterior groin region. Involvement of the lumbar plexus, beginning at L2 and passing through the psoas muscle, is less likely but can result in significant loss of motor function, particularly in the quadriceps.

Lumbar Sympathetic Block

Anatomy

The lumbar sympathetic chain lies at the anterolateral border of the vertebral bodies. Compared with the more cephalad portion, the lumbar chain has more variable anatomy. The chain rarely appears as the same size or shape, or in the same location among individuals. The number of ganglia is also quite variable, with four sets being more common than five—a result of fusion of the T12 and L1 ganglia. They can be segmentally located or closely grouped between the second and fourth lumbar vertebrae. The size of the ganglion varies from 3 to 5 mm in width to 10 to 15 mm in length.

The lumbar sympathetic chain consists of preganglionic axons and postganglionic neurons. The cell bodies of the preganglionic nerves arise from T11, T12, L1, L2, and occasionally T10 and L3. Their axons leave the spinal canal with the corresponding anterior spinal nerves, join the chain as white communicating rami and then synapse in the appropriate ganglia.

Postganglionic axons depart the chain either directly to form a diffuse plexus around the iliac and femoral arteries, or, more commonly, as gray communicating rami to combine with spinal nerves of the lumbar and sacral plexuses. They join the major nerves of the lower extremity and ultimately end with the corresponding vessels. Most fibers traveling this network pass through the second and third lumbar sympathetic ganglia; blockade of these ganglia results in near-complete sympathetic denervation of the lower limb.

Preganglionic efferent axons for visceral structures synapse most commonly in the inferior three thoracic and first lumbar ganglia. They join hypogastric and aortic plexuses en route to the pelvic viscera. Afferent, nociceptive fibers in this region accompany the sympathetic fibers and relay pain sensations from kidney, ureter, bladder, distal portion of transverse colon, left (descending) colon, rectum, prostate, testicle, cervix, and uterus.

The anatomic positioning of the lumbar sympathetic chain at the anterolateral border of the vertebral body differs from more cephalad portions of the chain and allows it to be removed from somatic nerves (Fig. 63-28). The aorta is positioned anteriorly and slightly medial to the chain on the left side. The IVC is closer to the chain on the right in an anterior plane. Many other small lumbar arteries and veins are positioned near the sympathetic chain. The psoas

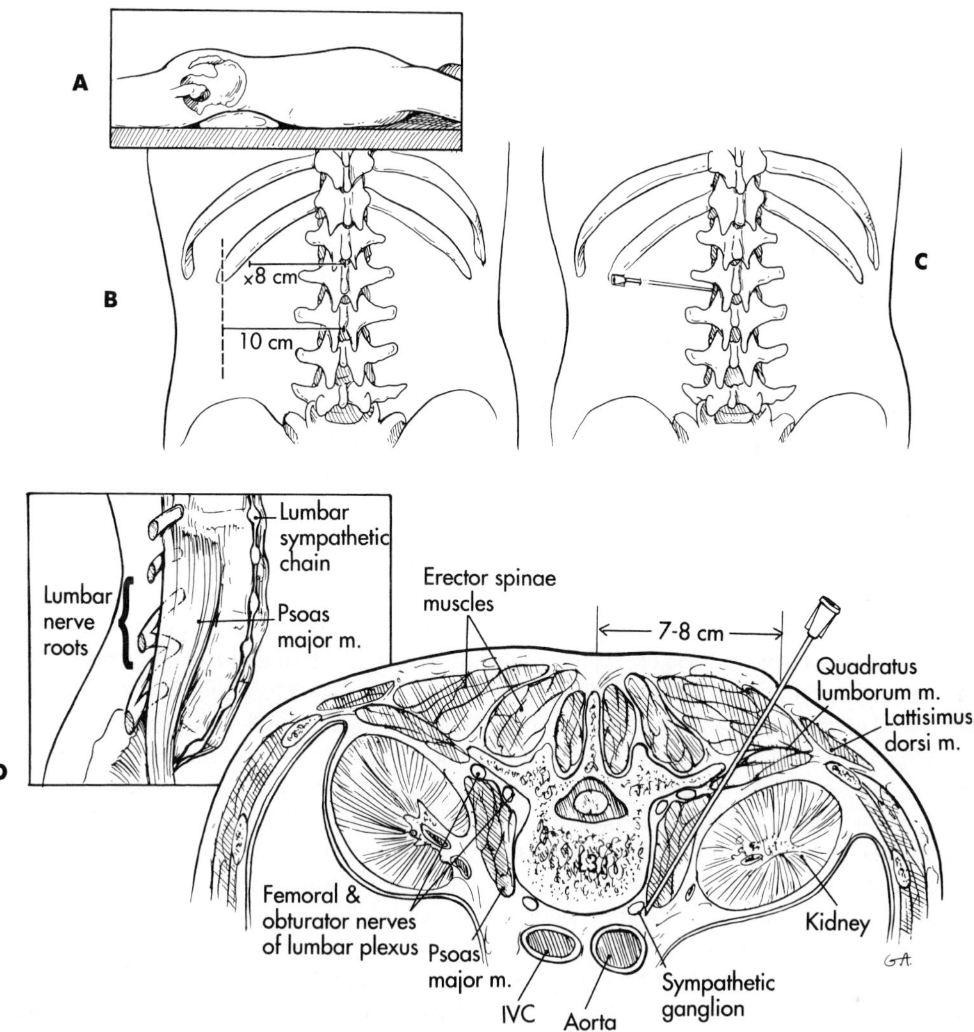

Fig. 63-28. Lateral approach to lumbar sympathetic nerve block. **A,** Patient is positioned prone with a pillow beneath the anterior iliac spines. **B,** Skin landmarks include the twelfth rib, the posterior iliac crest, and the cephalad tip of the L2 spinous process. **C,** The needle is inserted 7 to 8 cm from midline, perpendicular to the spinal canal at L2. **D,** Cross-sectional view of the final needle placement. (From Raj PP: *Practical management of pain,* ed 2, St Louis, 1992, Mosby–Year Book.)

muscle is situated posteriorly and lateral to the sympathetic chain.

Indications

Lumbar sympathetic blocks have been used extensively in the treatment of reflex sympathetic dystrophy and causalgia. Blockade of the sympathetic nerves can also be performed with a spinal, epidural, or peripheral nerve block, but pain relief after a lumbar sympathetic block most specifically delineates the painful etiology as sympathetically mediated. Most fibers headed for the lower extremity pass through the second and third lumbar ganglia, such that a sympathetic block placed at this level provides almost complete sympathetic denervation to the lower extremity. The pain relief obtained is usually immediate and can be long-lasting, although a delay of several hours can be seen in some patients.

Peripheral vascular insufficiency represented the initial indication for lumbar sympathetic block, performed in 1926 by Mandl,[136] and continues to be a major reason for sympathetic block. Although proximal, fixed lesions are more amenable to surgical correction, diffuse distal disease often responds better to sympathectomy. If pain relief or signs of vascular improvement are observed, most patients require a chemical or surgical sympathectomy for a prolonged effect.

Patients with acute herpes zoster and possibly postherpetic neuralgia can benefit from lumbar sympathetic blockade. Improved circulation to the vasa nervosum and peripheral structures can decrease inflammation and prevent further neuronal damage caused by the virus. Sympathetic blockade alone should not be viewed as sufficient treatment in most cases of acute herpes zoster; epidural placement of local anesthetics and corticosteroids in combination with intralesion injections peripherally is necessary for effective early resolution of symptoms.

Deafferent pain syndromes, in particular phantom limb pain, respond variably to sympathetic blocks. Truly deafferented pain would not be expected to benefit from sympathetic block, yet it is known that many deafferent pain syndromes do have a component of sympathetically mediated pain. A recent study involving patients with symptoms of sympathetic pain after traumatic myelopathy demonstrated good relief of pain with lumbar sympathetic blocks.[50] Pain from cancer of the lower extremity, of the GI tract distal to the transverse colon, or of visceral structures confined to the pelvis can be relieved by lumbar sympathetic block. The pain often has a neurogenic etiology, involving the lumbar or lumbosacral plexuses in particular, with a resulting sympathetic component. Other space-occupying lesions of the pelvis may produce pain relieved in part by sympathetic block. Acute radiation neuritis and some chronic postradiation neuralgias can be partially relieved with sympathetic blocks.

Many of the previously mentioned cancer pain syndromes have a mixed somatic and visceral etiology. Narcotics, whether oral, parenteral, or intraspinal, often inadequately relieve visceral pain. Thus, although sympathetic denervation may not provide complete pain relief it can make management with narcotics acceptable to patients. A local anesthetic sympathetic block should be initially performed to demonstrate therapeutic efficacy. If it is initially effective but symptoms recur, serious consideration should be given to permanent neurolysis.

Technique

Two techniques will be described: (1) a lateral approach first described by Reid[183] and (2) a classic prone position initially reported by Mandl.[136] Informed consent is obtained before the block, and an IV line is placed. Sedation is not essential and can be avoided in diagnostic cases if sufficient local anesthetic is infiltrated along the proposed needle course and ongoing rapport is maintained with the patient.

Lateral approach. The patient is positioned prone with one or two pillows placed under the lower abdomen across the anterior iliac crest (Fig. 63-16). This allows flexion of the lower lumbar spines, making skin landmarks easier to palpate and opening the spaces between transverse processes. The spinous processes of L2, L3, and L4 are marked and outlined. These can be confirmed by marking the inferior border of T12 and the posterior iliac crest. The midpoint between these two lines, 7.0 cm from the midline, places the mark at the L2 to L3 region. This mark should be perpendicular to the caudad aspect of the L2 vertebra. This corresponds to the interspace between the transverse processes of L2 to L3.

The optimal distance from midline for needle insertion is reported to be from 4 to 10 cm.[28,34] Distances beyond 8 cm may subject the kidney to puncture. Distances of 4 to 5 cm do not allow much cross-sectional area of the vertebral body for contact by the advancing needle tip. For inexperienced operators, this can make identification of the vertebral body more difficult. Reid described 7 cm from midline as the optimal distance to provide easy identification of the vertebral body and to avoid puncture of renal parenchymal tissue.

Traditionally, two or three needles have been placed at the L2, L3, and L4 levels. Injection of contrast material with subsequent radiograph or image-intensification has demonstrated good longitudinal spread of solution along the anterolateral border of the vertebral bodies with a single-needle technique. Likewise, temperature rises of the distal extremity have provided clinical verification of a sympathetic block. The use of multiple-needle techniques can be reserved for situations when a temperature increase does not occur despite adequate placement, or pain relief is not achieved in patients with known sympathetic pain.

After a skin wheal is raised, local anesthetic solution can be injected for deeper infiltration along the anticipated tract for subsequent needle placement. Injection of too much solution should be avoided because spillover onto the lumbar plexus can occur and result in a false distal temperature rise of the measured extremity.

A 22-gauge, 12- to 18-cm needle is inserted slowly toward the vertebral column until it comes in contact with the vertebral body. The angle of the needle in relation to the skin can be as shallow as 45° in thin individuals and somewhat steeper in more obese patients. The transverse process can be located on insertion of the needle, which is then redirected either cephalad or caudad to find the intertransverse space and vertebral body.[34] This step, however, is not essential because if the transverse process is not encountered during the initial pass, further insertion of the needle will locate the vertebral body. If one bypasses the transverse process, it is important to recognize that the first bone encountered is the vertebral body. The distinction between the transverse process and the vertebral body may seem intuitive considering the difference in depths of these two structures, but in obese patients the long distance between skin and the transverse process may be misleading.

After the vertebral body has been appropriately identified, a rubber marker should be placed on the needle 2 to 3 cm from the skin. The needle is partially removed and then redirected at a slightly steeper angle. The length of the needles necessitates small-angle changes at the skin to prevent large changes at the distal end. With correct repositioning, the needle will pass just lateral to the vertebral body and rest at the anterolateral border. When the needle tip is in the proper location, it lies anterior to the vertebral insertion of the psoas fascia.

Before injection, careful aspiration should be carried out with the needle bevel in two planes. The aorta on the left and the IVC on the right both lie close to the sympathetic chain. Test injections of an epinephrine-containing local anesthetic solution protects against both unintentional intraspinal placement and intravascular injection.

Most preservative-free local anesthetics at commercially

prepared concentrations will block the sympathetic chain. If a single-needle technique is used, 15 ml of volume should be injected to ensure proper cephalad and caudad spread of solution.

Initial injection with 2-chloroprocaine yields a faster onset of block as manifested by a recorded temperature rise of the distal extremity. This short-lasting agent will prevent 18 to 24 hours of quadriceps weakness, should the needle be in the psoas muscle and the lumbar plexus unintentionally blocked. If a temperature rise is noted (which can take 15 to 20 minutes in some individuals) and no weakness is found, 15 ml of bupivacaine 0.5% with epinephrine 1:200,000 can be instilled.

Classic "paramedian" approach. The patient is placed prone and the spinous processes of L2, L3, and L4 are outlined. Skin wheals are raised 4 to 5 cm lateral to the midline. Shorter 8- to 12-cm, 20-gauge needles are used and inserted at a 70° to 80° angle toward the midline. A needle is advanced until it makes contact with the transverse process; at a depth of 4 to 6 cm, a marker should be placed 3 to 5 cm from the skin. The needle is then repositioned inferiorly and medially to slip off the transverse process and pass to the vertebral body, approximately 2.0 cm deep to the transverse process. The needle is further repositioned to slip off the vertebral body and is advanced to the previously positioned skin marker. The needle tip should now lie anterior to the psoas fascia at the anterolateral border of the vertebral body. The process is repeated with the other two needles, and anesthetic solution is injected as previously described.

Neurolytic block. Neurolysis of the lumbar sympathetic chain is easily performed and is one of the most useful neurolytic procedures.[24] It may be indicated for recalcitrant reflex sympathetic dystrophy, causalgia, peripheral vascular disease, pelvic malignancies, and deafferentation pain syndromes. **Neurolysis should be considered only after local anesthetic blocks of the lumbar sympathetic chain have documented efficacy, but have failed to produce long-lasting relief.**

Needle placement for neurolysis does not differ from local anesthetic lumbar sympathetic block. Image-intensification, in particular fluoroscopy, greatly facilitates placement, allows real-time visualization of drug diffusion, and helps prevent complications caused by ill-placed needles or neurolytic solution. When a single-needle technique is used, fluoroscopy documents adequate cephalad spread to the upper limits of L2 and caudad diffusion of drug to L4. Needle placement should be checked before the injection of contrast material. This can be done in both anteroposterior and lateral planes. C-arm fluoroscopy is ideal and allows real-time visualization of both planes. Myelography suites commonly image in only one plane but allow spot films to be taken in the lateral position.

Distal skin temperatures should be monitored during neurolysis for further documentation of block. If any questions remain after the placement of needles, a local anesthetic solution can be injected before neurolysis and its efficacy evaluated by a temperature rise and relief of symptoms.

The spread of contrast material is characteristic and reproducible. The dye confines itself to the anterolateral border of the vertebral body in a tight, linear fashion. Movement of contrast is cephalad and caudad with no lateral diffusion of drug to the vertebral bodies. Contrast that diffuses laterally most often is being deposited either in the psoas muscle or on the fascia. This may appear as a roundish, poorly circumscribed density or a bandlike area with muscular striations visibly present. In either situation, neurolytic agents should not be injected.

Phenol is the agent of choice for neurolysis. It has been shown to cause a lower incidence of neuralgias than equivalent injections with alcohol.[49] Although volumes as small as 2 ml through each of three needles have been used, larger volumes (15 ml) through a single needle have been equally efficacious. Concentrations of 6% phenol may be replaced with a 10% or 12% solution. Evidence in cat sciatic nerves suggests that higher concentrations provide more permanent neurologic destruction.[90] After the neurolytic agent has been administered, 1 ml of saline should be injected to prevent any neurolytic agent from spilling onto somatic nerves during withdrawal.

Catheter placement

Six- or 8-inch, 16-gauge, extracatheters with stylet (Longdwel catheters, Becton & Dickinson) are easily placed on the lumbar sympathetic chain for short-term infusions of local anesthetics. If effective and indicated, a neurolytic solution can be injected.

Catheter placement is best performed with the lateral approach as described previously. Image intensification, although not mandatory, should be used whenever possible because precise location allows infusion of lower volumes of solution. If neurolysis is planned after a period of local anesthetic infusion, image intensification can verify that the catheter has not been dislodged since initial placement.

The length of infusion necessary varies with each clinical situation. Infusions lasting 7 days or longer have been managed with a single catheter. Strict sterile technique must be used during placement, and the exit site should be kept sterile and visible for daily checks.

The most common long-term management problem with a catheter system is posterior dislodgment into the psoas muscle, manifested by decreased sensation and weakness of the quadriceps muscles. Nurses must be adequately educated and patients warned to prevent falls. Dislodgment occurs most often in obese or active patients and results from excessive movements of the underlying tissues.

Bupivacaine has been the most common agent used for infusions. Initial doses and infusion settings are 0.1% at 6 ml/hr. Both the concentration and rate can be increased if an adequate block cannot be maintained. Rates of 20 ml/hr have been necessary in refractory cases. Concentrations of

0.25% have been used if tachyphylaxis develops near the end of the infusion period.

A catheter system and infusion of local anesthetics can provide continuous denervation of the sympathetic nervous system. Patients with recalcitrant reflex sympathetic dystrophy, who derive only temporary benefit from a routine lumbar sympathetic block, may receive long-term benefit from catheter placement. Concomitant, aggressive physical therapy should be prescribed and will be better tolerated when the catheter is in place.

Complications

The most common side effect of a lumbar sympathetic block is backache, which results from needle placement through the paravertebral muscles of the back. This side effect should be carefully explained to patients before blockade. A heating pad, ice packs, rest, and muscle relaxants may be necessary.

Intravascular injections of large volumes of local anesthetics can produce serious, systemic toxic reactions. This reaction is best avoided using test doses, repeated aspiration, and epinephrine-containing solutions in combination with appropriate monitoring.

Unintentional subarachnoid injections can rarely occur if the needle is mistakenly positioned in a dural cuff. The length of the needle and its small diameter hinder free back-flow of CSF. The high pressure generated during aspiration of the small 22-gauge needle can suck the arachnoid mater against the bevel, resulting in no flow of CSF. Initially, injecting a small amount of local anesthetic and waiting for a spinal effect avoids a subsequent total spinal block.

Not uncommonly, the needle passes through the intervertebral disc. The sensation of "passing through swiss cheese" is easily appreciated, necessitating removal of the needle and repositioning. Medication cannot be easily injected into a disc. No sequelae have been reported from this occurrence, and any extrusion of disc material would be lateral, away from the spinal canal, and not of any clinical significance.

Renal trauma or puncture of a ureter can occur if proper technique is not followed. Most importantly, the needle should not be inserted more than 7 to 8 cm from the midline. Sequelae are minimal unless a neurolytic agent is injected, resulting in possible ureteral stricture or extravasation of urine.

Blockade of the genitofemoral nerve, or the lumbar plexus within the psoas muscle, can occur if the needle is placed too far laterally or posteriorly. If a local anesthetic solution is used, a resulting numbness or weakness can occur in the groin, anterior thigh, or quadriceps. To avoid the 18- to 24-hour weakness experienced with bupivacaine, a short-duration agent (e.g., 2-chloroprocaine) can be injected initially and the strength of the quadriceps tested.

Lateral spread of neurolytic solution from the lumbar sympathetic chain can result in genitofemoral neuralgia and, less often, lumbar plexus involvement (Fig. 63-29).[29,49,52,181] Neuralgia can result despite appropriate technique and the appearance of adequate spread within the proper fascial plane.

Boas et al.[23] report a 6% incidence of genitofemoral neuralgia in their patients. Cousins et al.[49] reported on 35 patients receiving 100% alcohol using a technique without image intensification. Mild neuralgia (< 1 week) occurred in 14%, and severe neuralgia (> 1 week) occurred in 26%. Use of a similar technique with phenol resulted in respective incidence of 6% and 16%. Sensory loss was reported in 5% of patients and motor weakness in 6%.[49]

The genitofemoral nerve is most susceptible at the L4 to L5 vertebral level after it has emerged from the psoas major muscle and lies anterior to the fascia in close proximity to the sympathetic chain. Most mild neuralgias can be treated with nonnarcotic analgetics and reassurance that this complication is transient. For severe cases, Boas et al.[23] have reported success using 1 to 2 mg/kg IV lidocaine over 2 to 3 minutes, which is sufficient to produce light toxicity symptoms. The pain typically disappears and normal cutaneous sensation returns. In refractory cases, TENS, tricyclic antidepressants, or antiepileptic agents may be necessary.

Hypogastric Plexus Block

Anatomy

The superior hypogastric plexus is a retroperitoneal structure located bilaterally at the level of the fifth lumbar and first sacral vertebral bodies, in proximity to the bifurcation of the common iliac vessels. The plexus innervates pelvic viscera via the hypogastric nerves. Neurolytic nerve block or surgical interruption of the hypogastric plexus (presacral neurectomy) have effectively relieved a variety of painful pelvic conditions.

Indications

Chronic pelvic pain is a notoriously difficult problem with numerous causes. Possible cancerous etiologies include the cervix, uterus, bladder, rectum, prostate, testis, vulva, and colon. In addition, pelvic autonomic nerves may generate pain referred to the pelvis that is not a result of the previously listed causes (i.e., postlaminectomy pelvic pain, posttraumatic, postparaplegic, and nonspecific pelvic, rectal, and/or vaginal pains). Previous therapeutic interventions were limited to presacral neurectomy with a 50% success rate and limited duration of pain relief.[184] Because pain fibers that travel through the hypogastric plexus bypass the lower spinal cord, selective spinal and epidural nerve blocks may be ineffective.

Hypogastric plexus block offers a new technique for relieving pelvic pain, especially in patients suffering from cancer-caused autonomic pain originating in the pelvis. In addition, noncancer-origin intractable pain also responds to local anesthetic and neurolytic injection of 6% phenol into the superior hypogastric plexus and into the presacral nerves. Patients for neurolytic block must be highly

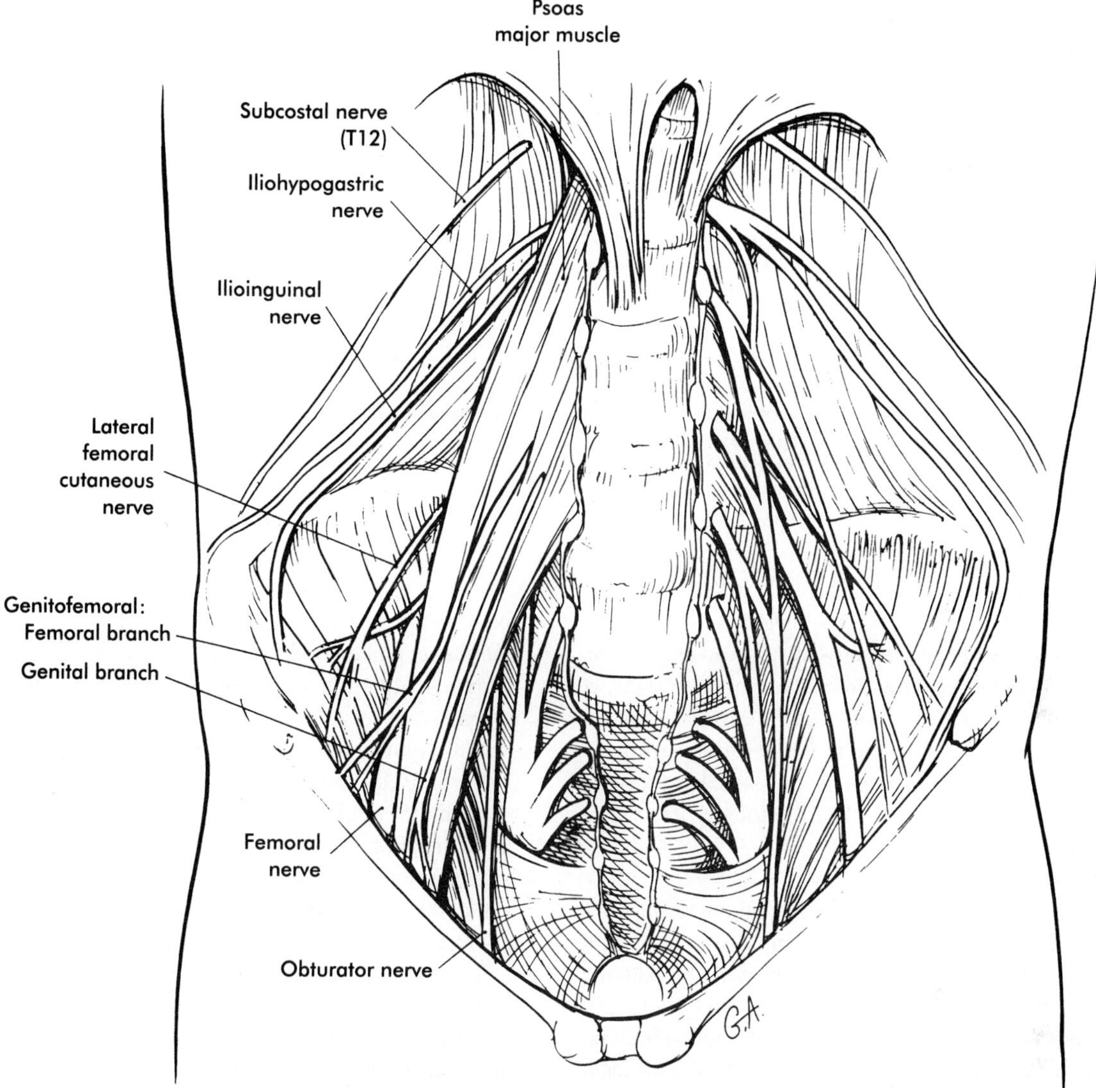

Fig. 63-29. Anterior view of the nerves from the lumbar plexus as they exit the musculature of the back. Note the genitofemoral nerve on the psoas major muscle. (From Raj PP: *Practical management of pain,* ed 2, St. Louis, 1992, Mosby–Year Book.)

selected, but diagnostic hypogastric plexus block is safe using the technique described (Tables 63-3 and 63-4).

Racz[177] has employed hypogastric plexus blocks for intractable pelvic pain syndromes where multiple diagnostic blocks confirm the pain to be mediated through the hypogastric plexus. The neurolytic injections are usually unilateral. Because of the proximity of the ureter to the hypogastric plexus, only 6% phenol may be used to prevent serious sequelae. Many patients have been treated safely with 6% phenol for noncancerous, sympathetically mediated pain in the vicinity of the ureter (lumbar sympathetic and celiac plexus blocks).[177]

Table 63-3 Patient profile for hypogastric plexus block

	Number of patients	Average age	Age range
Male	18	50.2	32–75
Female	16	54.2	30–82
Total	34	52.4	30–82

Technique

The needle is placed under fluoroscopic control (Fig. 63-29) with the patient in the prone position. Alternatively, guidance with CT can be employed.[213] Padding is placed beneath the pelvis to flatten the lumbar lordosis, and the posterior lumbosacral region is prepped and draped. Skin wheals are raised 5 to 7 cm from the midline at the level of the iliac crests (L4 to L5). Seven-inch, 22-gauge spinal needles are inserted through the skin wheals perpendicular in all planes to the skin with their tips directed toward the anterolateral aspect of the L5 vertebral body. When the needle tip is prop-

Table 63-4 Pain relief by hypogastric plexus block according to diagnosis*

	Significant relief on discharge		Duration of relief (in months)			
Type of pain	Yes	No	<1	1–3	3–6	Unspecified
Pelvic pain	15 (83%)	3 (16%)	5 (33%)	7 (46%)		3 (20%)
Vaginal pain or dyspareunia	3 (60%)	2 (40%)	1 (33%)	2 (66%)		
Scrotal/perineal pain	2 (40%)	3 (60%)	2 (100%)			
Coccydynia	4 (100%)		2 (50%)	2 (50%)		
Buttock/ischial pain	19 (63%)	11 (36%)	6 (31%)	2 (10%)	3 (15%)	8 (42%)
Iliac/inguinal pain	5 (33%)	10 (66%)	1 (20%)		1 (20%)	3 (60%)
Thigh pain		6 (100%)				

* Many patients had two or more complaints or areas of pain for which hypogastric block was performed. The total, therefore, exceeds the actual number of blocks performed.
From Raj PP: *Practical management of pain,* ed 2, St. Louis, 1992, Mosby–Year Book.

erly positioned, fluoroscopy or CT will show it to be just off the midline and anterior to the body of L5 near its junction with S1. After injection, contrast spreads from the midline at L5 to S1 to the lateral pelvic wall and inferiorly to the S1 nerve root. The injection must be in the posterior retroperitoneal space (Fig. 63-30), which is outlined by thin-line spread of contrast material in the lateral radiographic view.

Complications

Recent reports by Plancarte et al.[172] of 20 patients using 10% phenol, 8-ml volume, resulted in 70% improvement of pain for 3 to 12 months. They also supplemented the somatic component of the pain with epidural steroids and dilute (2% to 3%) phenol. These patients all had advanced carcinoma: cervical, prostatic, testicular, and rectal. The only significant complication was vascular puncture. Bilateral injections were performed to alleviate midline pelvic pain.

Surgical presacral neurectomy has been shown to be remarkably free of serious bladder and sexual dysfunction complications. Although unilateral neurolytic hypogastric nerve blocks appear safe, it may be advisable not to attempt bilateral blocks in men because of the risk of sexual dysfunction.

Intravenous Regional Sympathetic Block

Indications

When local anesthetic blocks of the sympathetic chain fail to improve sympathetically maintained pain in an extremity, IV regional block with sympatholytic drugs may be an appropriate alternative.

Mechanism of action

Guanethidine monosulfate selectively inhibits the sympathetic nervous system while leaving the parasympathetic system intact. The site of action is the postganglionic neuron at the neuroeffector junction. Guanethidine is actively transported into the postganglionic neuron by the norepinephrine (NE) pump. It displaces NE from presynaptic vesicles and inhibits reuptake of NE. A brief release of NE is followed by depletion, although the relative degree of each varies among patients.

With sympathetic stimulation, guanethidine and NE are both released from storage vesicles. It is believed that guanethidine does not act as a false neurotransmitter because the sympatholytic effect does not depend on the degree of NE depletion. Rather, the mode of action is hypothesized to result from inhibition of neuronal transmission at the outer membranes of the postganglionic sympathetic axon.

Reserpine has also been administered IV and may have a mechanism of action similar to that of guanethidine. The main difference with reserpine is that it crosses the blood–brain barrier and causes significant CNS effects. Bretylium blocks the coupling of the action potential to NE release and also blocks NE reuptake.

Technique

The extremity is prepared for a Bier block as described in Chapter 62. After inflation of the tourniquet, 20 mg of guanethidine with lidocaine 0.5% (total volume, 25 to 30 ml) is injected for the upper extremity, and 40 mg of guanethidine (total volume, 40 to 50 ml) is injected for the lower extremity. Lidocaine is used to decrease the burning otherwise experienced with the injection of guanethidine. Five hundred to 1000 units of heparin has been advocated by some experts to prevent stasis. The tourniquet is kept inflated for 20 to 30 minutes to "fix" the guanethidine and prevent its release into the systemic circulation.

Reserpine is administered in the same fashion as guanethidine, except that 1 or 1.5 mg of reserpine is substituted for upper and lower extremities, respectively.[17] The extremity is likewise prepared for bretylium injection (5 mg/kg). Intra-arterial injection of reserpine has been reported, using 1.0 to 1.5 mg diluted with 5 ml normal saline and injected into the axillary, brachial, or femoral artery.[2] A

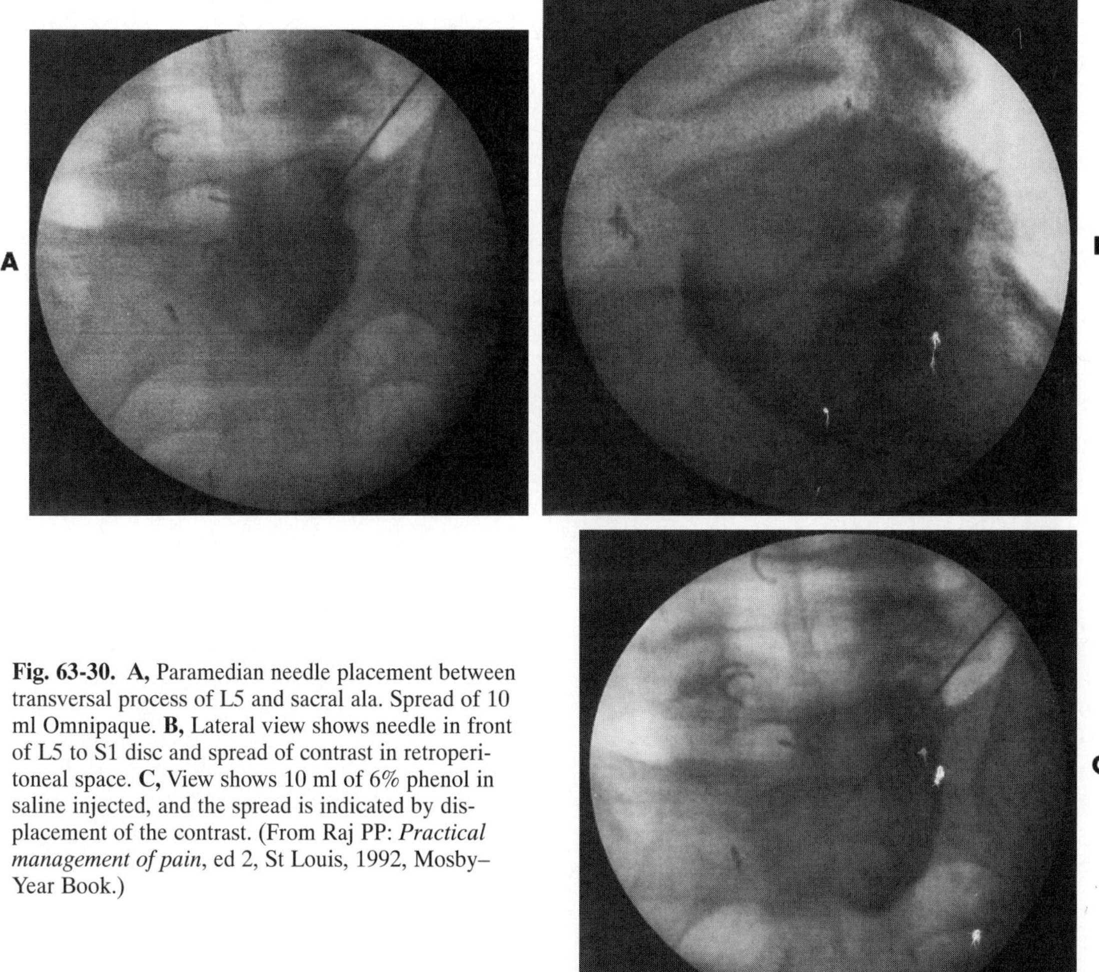

Fig. 63-30. **A,** Paramedian needle placement between transversal process of L5 and sacral ala. Spread of 10 ml Omnipaque. **B,** Lateral view shows needle in front of L5 to S1 disc and spread of contrast in retroperitoneal space. **C,** View shows 10 ml of 6% phenol in saline injected, and the spread is indicated by displacement of the contrast. (From Raj PP: *Practical management of pain*, ed 2, St Louis, 1992, Mosby–Year Book.)

tourniquet placed on the extremity is inflated to just below diastolic blood pressure for 5 minutes.

Effectiveness

The most widely studied drug for IV regional sympathetic (IVRS) block has been guanethidine. The best series[63,81,94,96,105,132] included over 180 patients. In a study of 31 patients by Glynn et al.[81] patients with RSD (N = 28) or Raynaud's disease (N = 3) were treated with two injections: 10 ml of NaCl and 20 mg of guanethidine in 10 ml NaCl. Pain was significantly reduced ($p < 0.001$) with guanethidine but returned to baseline after 7 days. No change in palmar sweating was noted, which was expected because this effect is mediated by acetylcholine at the postganglionic junction. Blood flow was significantly increased ($p < 0.001$) and remained elevated at 7 days follow-up ($p < 0.001$). Significant changes (percentage decrease) were also recorded for the ice response ($p < 0.001$) and were still present at 7 days after the block ($p < 0.001$).

A comparison of guanethidine and reserpine documented that only guanethidine increased temperature after a cold stress test, an effect that persisted for 3 days.[141] Administration of guanethidine every 4 days (maximum of four blocks) showed effects similar to stellate ganglion blocks performed every other day (maximum of eight blocks) in follow-up at 1 and 3 months.[26]

Complications

Reported complications of IVRS guanethidine include orthostatic hypotension, local piloerection, pain on injection, and edema of the extremity. With release of guanethidine into the systemic circulation, potential complications, including bradycardia, diarrhea, edema, nausea, and bleeding (if heparin was administered with the guanethidine), can occur. Guanethidine should not be administered to patients taking monoamine oxidase (MAO) inhibitors or those with known or suspected pheochromocytoma.

FACET BLOCK

Facet Syndrome

The degenerative changes and associated muscle spasm developing when a facet joint is involved in a sprain from a forceful or violent twisting motion were termed the *facet*

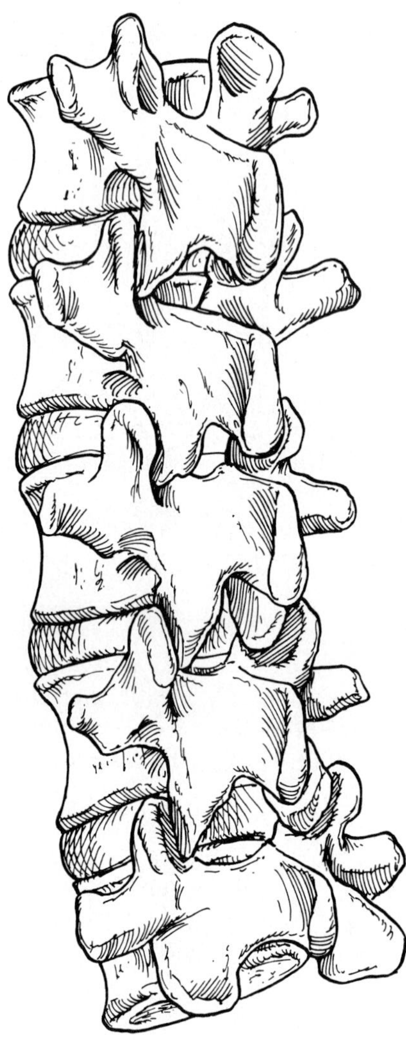

Fig. 63-31. Lumbar facet joints are best visualized with 30-degree to 45-degree obliquity. The inferior articular facet from the vertebra above and the superior articular facet from the vertebra below articulate to form the facet joint. (From Raj PP: *Practical management of pain,* ed 2, St Louis, 1992, Mosby–Year Book.)

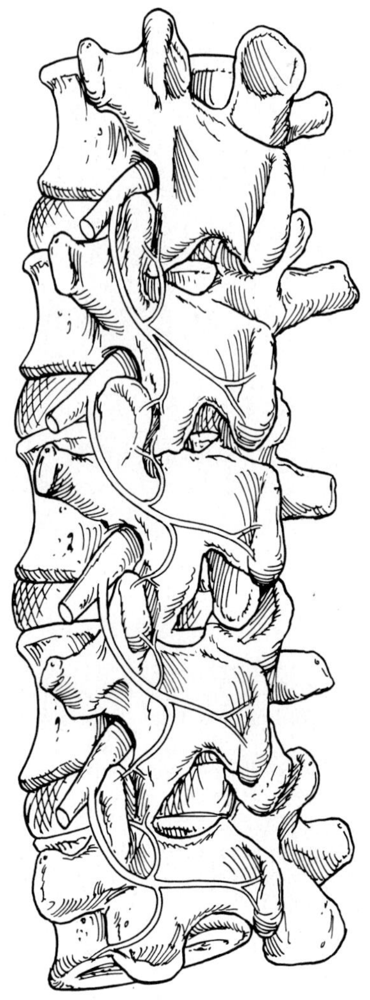

Fig. 63-32. Each articular facet is innervated by branches from the posterior ramus at the same level and the level above, resulting in a dual nerve supply. (From Raj PP: *Practical management of pain,* ed 2, St Louis, 1992, Mosby–Year Book.)

syndrome in 1933. The intra-articular facet joints are subject to trauma at all levels of the spinal column.

Anatomy

The apophyseal articulations are formed by the superior articular facet of one vertebra and the inferior articular facet of the adjacent vertebra (Fig. 63-31). The articular surfaces of the facets are covered by hyaline cartilage. The joints are lined by synovium and—where the surfaces of the facets are not in contact—tabs of synovial tissue project into the joint from the joint margins.[92] The fibrous joint capsule forms superior and inferior joint recesses that may contain small synovial villi.[130] The inferior and posterior portions of the recesses are larger, allowing a wide range of motion. Medially and anteriorly, the capsule blends with the ligamentum flavum and is adjacent to the neural foramen and the nerve root.

The joint capsule is richly innervated.[92,158,169] Each dorsal ramus sends branches to the facet joint at its own level and to the level caudad (Fig. 63-32). Consequently, each posterior ramus innervates two facet joints, and each facet joint has innervation from two levels.

The articular facets in the cervical spine extend laterally from the junction of the lamina and pedicles and are oriented in the coronal plane to permit flexion, extension, and lateral bending (Fig. 63-33). In the thoracic spine, the facets extend superiorly and inferiorly from the junctions of the laminae and pedicles. The apophyseal joints are oriented approximately 20° off the coronal plane (Fig. 63-34). The superior facets in the lumbar spine are concave posteriorly, and the inferior facets are convex anteriorly. The lumbar facet joints are oriented approximately 45° off the sagittal plane, but, because of the curvature of the joints, the posterior portion of the joint is much closer to the sagittal plane (Fig. 63-35).

Cervical Facet Syndrome

A cervical facet syndrome may result from athletic or occupational injuries, sleeping with a twisted neck, or a sudden jerk of the neck resulting in overriding of the superior facet

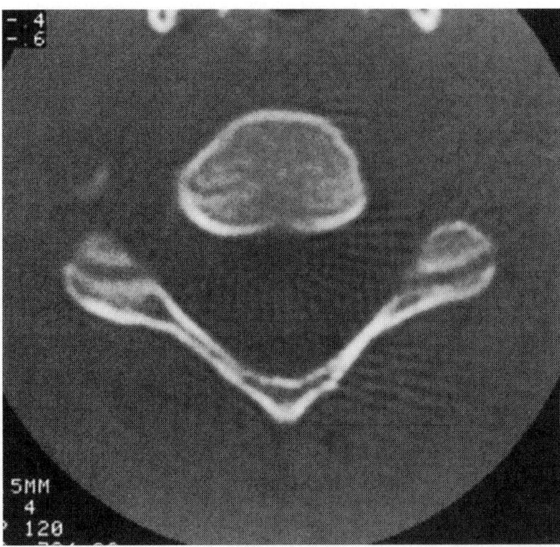

Fig. 63-33. CT scan through the midcervical region showing the facet joints oriented in the coronal plane. (From Raj PP: *Practical management of pain,* ed 2, St Louis, 1992, Mosby–Year Book.)

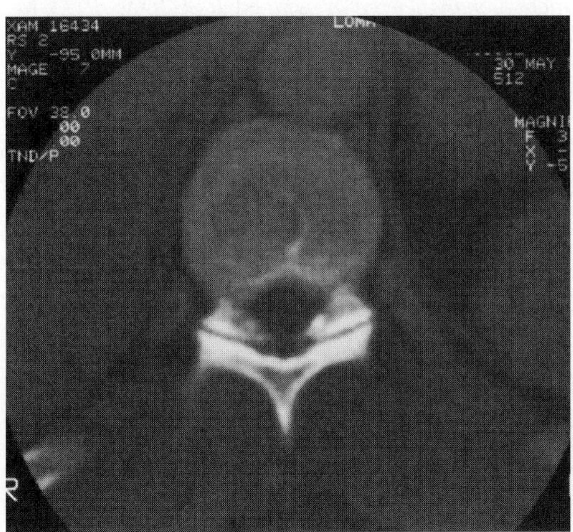

Fig. 63-34. CT scan through the midthoracic region showing the facet joints oriented just off the coronal plane. (From Raj PP: *Practical management of pain,* ed 2, St Louis, 1992, Mosby–Year Book.)

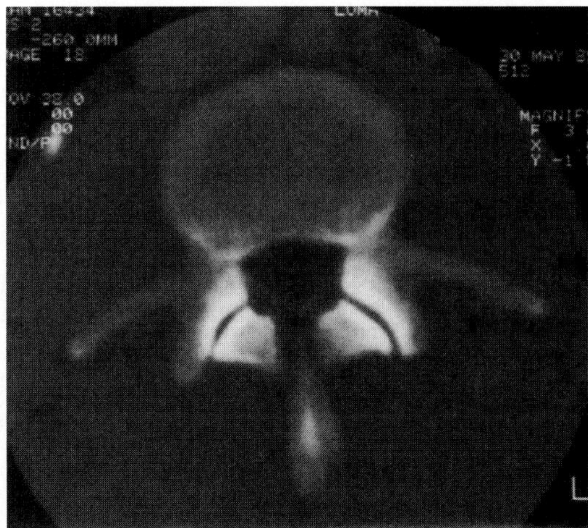

Fig. 63-35. CT scan through the lower lumbar region showing the curved facet joints oriented approximately 45 degrees off the sagittal plane. (From Raj PP: *Practical management of pain,* ed 2, St Louis, 1992, Mosby–Year Book.)

on the inferior articular facet (e.g., automobile accident). Degenerative changes, including joint capsular hypertrophy, osteophyte formation, and increased fibrous layer formation, may cause intense muscle spasm on the ipsilateral side.

In cervical facet syndrome, there is pain on palpation of the transverse process and decreased range of motion at the involved level. Rotating motion and hyperextension may particularly aggravate the pain, which is described as dull and aching, most frequently radiating to the occipital region, shoulder, arm, and cervicoscapular area. The head may be held to one side, and the patient is unable to touch the ear to the shoulder of the affected side.[28]

Diagnosis

The diagnosis of a cervical facet syndrome is made by history, physical examination, and radiographic evaluation. Carrera[41] suggests that CT may have an important role in diagnosing lumbar facet syndrome. Cervical facet arthrography may or may not indicate joint pathology, which appears to have no correlation with the degree of symptoms the patient experiences.

Treatment

Treatment of the cervical facet syndrome includes conservative measures such as local heat, traction, NSAIDs, local myofascial trigger-point injections, and local injection in the paravertebral muscles. Manual manipulation may be required to reduce the subluxation. Arthrography with local anesthetic and steroid injection under fluoroscopy may prove beneficial, with up to 12 months of pain relief.[61] Because of the possibility of subarachnoid and epidural injection, it is recommended that the cervical facet joint injections be undertaken with fluoroscopic control.

Thoracic Facet Syndrome

The thoracic facet joint syndrome results from a sudden twisting motion, twisting while lifting overhead, or unguarded rotating motion of the thoracic spine. The resultant pain may be mild, dull, and aching with radiation encircling the chest, or it may be sharp, pleuritic-type pain that can affect functional vital capacity and become debilitating to the patient. There is usually decreased motion in the portion of the spine involved, and examination of the patient may reveal a loss of the thoracic curve or muscle spasm causing localized scoliosis.

Diagnosis

Diagnosis is made by history, physical examination, and plain radiographs. CT scan may provide a more precise diagnosis of the area of involvement, but radiographic findings may not correlate with the clinical picture.

Treatment

Treatment consists of local heat, NSAIDs, or local muscle (myofascial) injections. Intercostal nerve blocks may help with splinting and guarding, especially if vital capacity is decreased.[28] Hydrotherapy, consisting of swimming in warm water (95° F), may significantly improve thoracic facet syndrome. If the articular facet involved is identified, the joint may be indirectly blocked with a paravertebral somatic nerve block using an adequate volume of local anesthetic and steroid solution. However, because of the anatomic location of the joint and the proximity of the joint to the rib and the epidural space, individual facet joint blocks in the thoracic spine are not described. Fluoroscopic control is recommended when performing any thoracic nerve block procedure.

Lumbar Facet Syndrome

The lumbar facet joints present the most frequently encountered problems involving any of the facet joints of the spine. Low-back pain with or without radiation is the primary presenting complaint. The lumbar facet syndrome should be one of the differential diagnoses of low-back pain after other etiologies such as degenerative disc disease, disc herniation, or trauma have been evaluated. The pain of an aggravated lumbar facet is described as a dull ache that radiates into the low back, buttocks, hip, and posterior or lateral thigh down to the knee. Hamstring pain and muscle spasm, decreased straight-leg raising, and depressed deep tendon reflexes may be present.[152] The pain only occasionally radiates below the knee, and when it does it is usually associated with pronounced pathologic changes of the involved facet. The pain may then present as sciatica. On examination, the patient complains of tenderness to deep palpation over the facet joint, sharp aching pain on extension of the lumbar spine, and pain with simultaneous rotation and flexion of the lumbar spine. Frequently, there is muscle spasm of the ipsilateral paraspinous muscles.

Diagnosis

The diagnosis is based on history, physical examination, and possibly changes noted on plain radiography or CT scan examination.

Treatment

Treatment consists of local heat, NSAIDs, electroacupuncture therapy, local myofascial trigger-point injections to the paraspinous muscles, and, most precisely, by injection of a single-level or multiple-level lumbar articular facet joint.

Facet Arthrography

The normal facet joint has an S-shaped contour in the oblique projection. There are small superior and larger inferior recesses. The articular cartilage is seen as a thin lucency between the contrast and cortex of the adjacent facets (Fig. 63-36). The capacity of the joint is 1 to 2 ml.[80] The joint usually ruptures along the medial or lateral aspect of the inferior recess with injection of the local anesthetic and steroid (Fig. 63-37).[56,61]

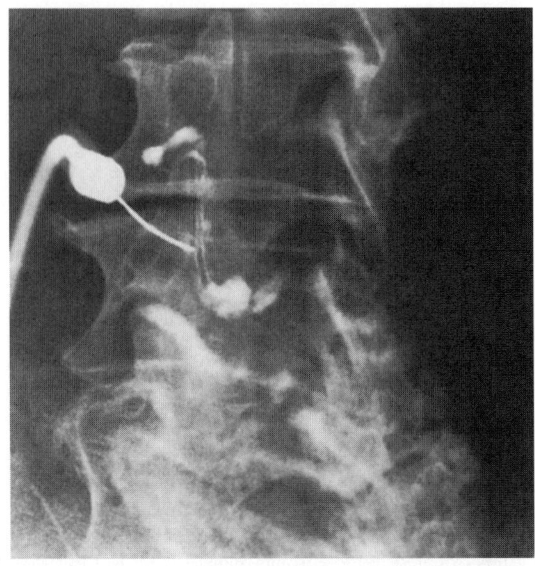

Fig. 63-36. Facet arthrogram showing the S-shaped contour with filling of the smaller recess and larger inferior recess. (From Raj PP: *Practical management of pain,* ed 2, St Louis, 1992, Mosby–Year Book.)

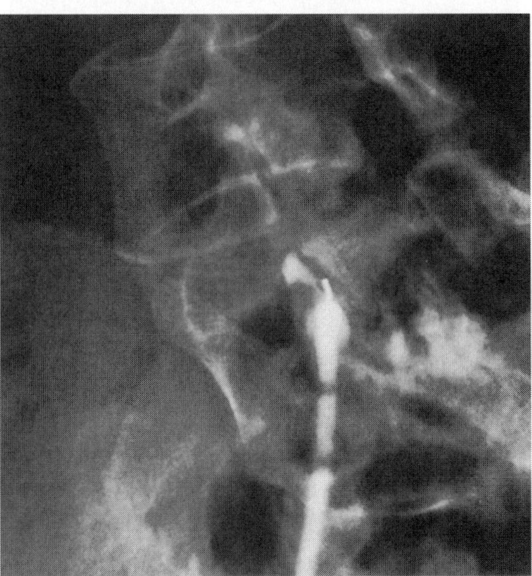

Fig. 63-37. L5 to S1 facet arthrogram showing rupture of the inferior recess with contrast injection. (From Raj PP: *Practical management of pain,* ed 2, St Louis, 1992, Mosby–Year Book.)

With degenerative arthritis, there is thinning of the articular cartilage and hypertrophy of the facets. With inflammation, filling defects from synovial proliferation have been observed (Fig. 63-38).[56,61] Contraction of the joint capsule may occur and probably has a pathogenesis similar to that described in other joints with adhesive capsulitis.[56]

The defect in the pars interarticularis in patients with spondylolysis may fill with contrast when a facet arthrogram is conducted (Fig. 63-39). Mooney and Robertson[152] first noticed a relationship between the "facet syndrome" and spondylolysis. Ghelman and Doherty[78] first reported com-

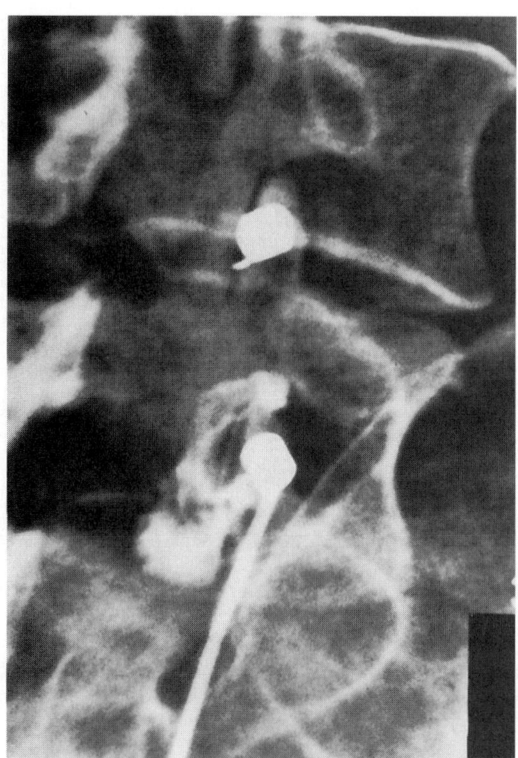

Fig. 63-38. L5 to S1 facet arthrogram with filling defects in the inferior recess secondary to synovial proliferation. A needle is also in place in the L4 to L5 facet joint. (From Raj PP: *Practical management of pain,* ed 2, St Louis, 1992, Mosby–Year Book.)

munication of a facet joint with an adjacent defect in the pars interarticularis. Maldague et al.[135] and Park et al.[167] further documented that a high percentage of patients with spondylolysis have communication of the facet joint with the defect and have relief of pain with injection of the facet joint.

Indications

The findings on conventional radiographs correlate poorly with the clinical symptoms.[41,56] There may be better correlation between symptoms and findings on CT.[42,185] Facet arthrography with injection of local anesthetic and an antiinflammatory agent is a diagnostic procedure that is in many cases therapeutic, with relief of symptoms lasting much longer than expected from the pharmacologic effects of the injected agents.[36,56,61,152]

The major indications for facet injection include focal tenderness over a facet joint, chronic low-back pain with or without radiation but with a normal radiographic work-up, back pain with evidence of disc disease and facet arthritis, and postlaminectomy syndrome without arachnoiditis or recurrent disc disease.[56,79]

Local anesthetic injection to determine the cause of back pain may also be useful in patients with spondylolysis to demonstrate an abnormal communication between the facet joint and the defect in the pars interarticularis. In patients with a transitional vertebra at the lumbosacral junction, anesthetic injection is helpful to determine if there is a

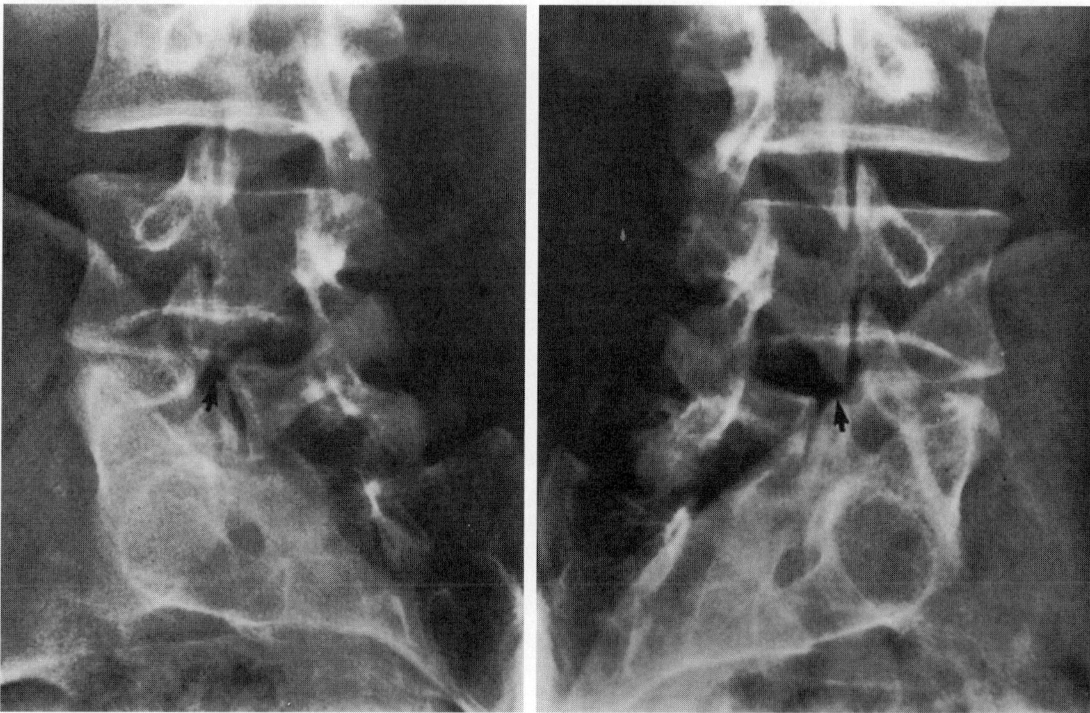

Fig. 63-39. Oblique radiographs of the lower lumbar spine showing spondylolysis with bilateral defects in the pars interarticularis at L5 (arrows). (From Raj PP: *Practical management of pain,* ed 2, St Louis, 1992, Mosby–Year Book.)

painful pseudoarthrosis between the transverse process and the sacrum (Fig. 63-40). In patients with posterolateral spine fusion in whom there is a question of painful pseudoarthrosis, anesthetic injection may delineate the cause of the pain.

Technique

Blind technique. The lumbar facet joint injection may be attempted by a "blind" technique. The patient is placed prone and rotated obliquely 30° with a pillow placed under the iliac crest of the side to be injected. This helps position the posterior facet joints on a vertical plane and allows the needle to advance perpendicular to the table at an approximate 60° angle to the skin. The needle is placed about 6 to 8 cm lateral to the midportion of the spinous process. The L5-S1 facet joint is difficult to reach because of the overriding effect of the posterosuperior iliac crest. After sterile preparation and drape, a 22-gauge, 3-inch spinal needle is advanced until bone is encountered. Aspiration for CSF or blood is performed before injection of any local anesthetic or steroid solution. If injection of 1 to 3 ml of hypertonic saline reproduces the pain, then 2 to 5 ml of local anesthetic and steroid solution may be injected.

Radiographic technique. Radiographic documentation of the intra-articular position of the tip of the needle during arthrography eliminates any question about a technique-related response to the injection. Although arthrography and injection of the cervical facets using fluoroscopy have been described,[61] virtually all referrals for facet injection are for low-back pain. This discussion of radiographic technique, therefore, deals only with the lumbar facets.

Patients with facet syndrome usually have pain localized to one side. The localization of the level for injection is made difficult, however, because of the frequency of multiple-level disease, the dual nerve supply of each facet joint, and the fact that similar symptoms can result from disease at different levels.[128,135,137] Thus, it may be necessary to inject two or three levels to determine the etiology of the symptoms.

Facet joints can be entered only from a posterior approach. The patient is placed in the prone position on the radiographic table, and the symptomatic side is rotated up while the facet joint is visualized under fluoroscopy to determine the optimal obliquity (Fig. 63-41). Because of the curvature of the facet joints in the lumbar spine, the 45° obliquity that best shows the facet joints on plain radiographs demonstrates the anterior portion of the joint and not the posterior portion that is necessary for facet injection. The minimum obliquity that allows visualization of the facet joint is usually best for facet injection. This may be close to the sagittal plane. At the L5-S1 level, care must be taken not to place the patient in too steep an obliquity or the posterior ileum will be positioned over the facet joint. A wedge sponge is placed beneath the patient's abdomen, and the hip and knee on the symptomatic side are flexed to maintain position and decrease the lumbar lordosis. The skin is marked where the needles are to be inserted (Fig. 63-42, A and B).

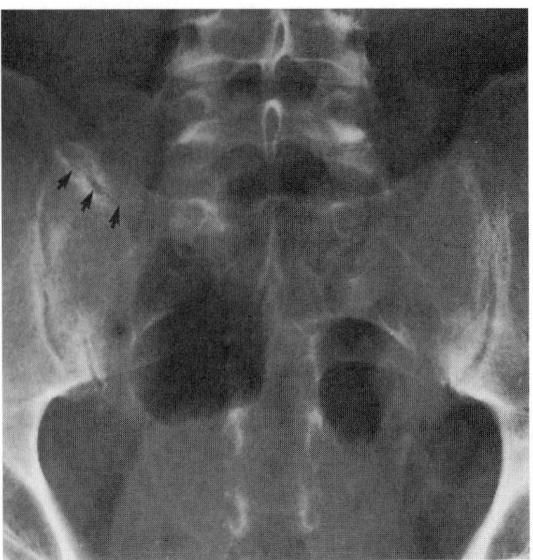

Fig. 63-40. Anteroposterior radiograph of the sacrum and lower lumbar spine showing partial sacralization of L5 on the right, with pseudoarthrosis between the enlarged transverse process of L5 and the superior margin of the sacrum (*arrows*). (From Raj PP: *Practical management of pain,* ed 2, St Louis, 1992, Mosby–Year Book.)

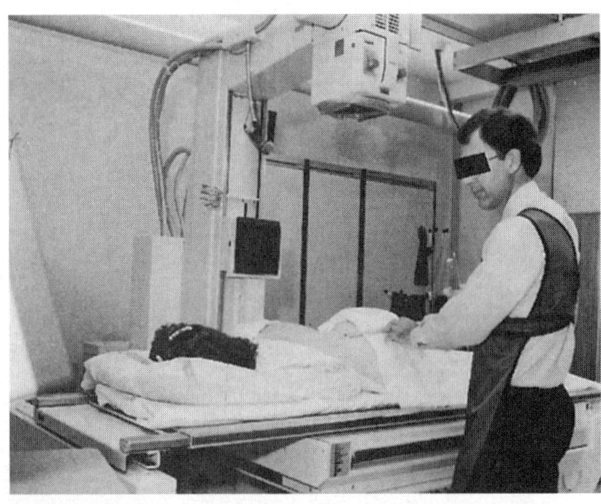

Fig. 63-41. With the patient placed in the prone position and the facet joint observed fluoroscopically, the patient is positioned to determine the optimal obliquity for entering the posterior aspect of the joint. (From Raj PP: *Practical management of pain,* ed 2, St Louis, 1992, Mosby–Year Book.)

The tray for facet injection includes a 3-ml syringe and a 22-gauge, 3-inch spinal needle for each facet to be injected. A syringe filled with contrast material and attached to an extension tube is used for arthrography. A 10-ml syringe filled with 1% lidocaine is used for local anesthesia. Each 3-ml syringe is filled with 1.5 ml of 0.5% bupivacaine and 20 mg of methylprednisolone acetate (Depo-Medrol) (Fig. 63-43).

The skin is sterilely prepared and draped. After the skin is anesthetized, the 22-gauge spinal needle is directed vertically toward the facet joint. Local anesthesia is achieved in the soft tissues overlying the facet joint by injection of lidocaine through the spinal needle when it is advanced. Care

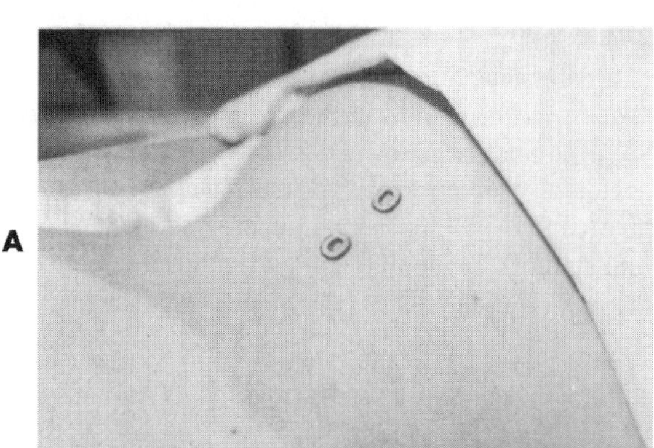
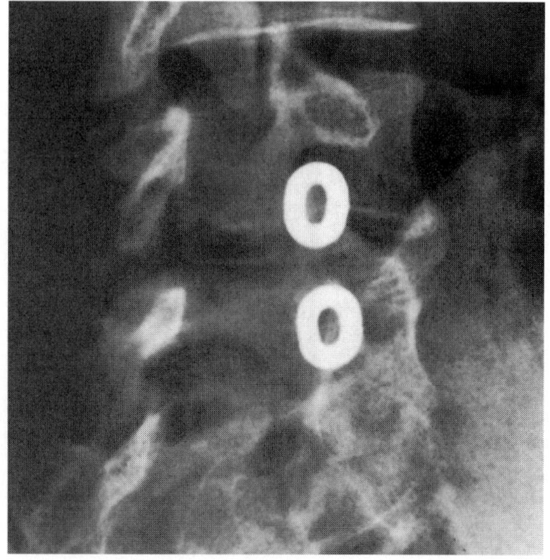

Fig. 63-42. A, Injection sites for L4 to L5 and L5 to S1 facet blocks localized on overlying skin. **B,** Spot film shows the lead markers overlying the L4 to L5 and L5 to S1 facet joints. (From Raj PP: *Practical management of pain,* ed 2, St Louis, 1992, Mosby–Year Book.)

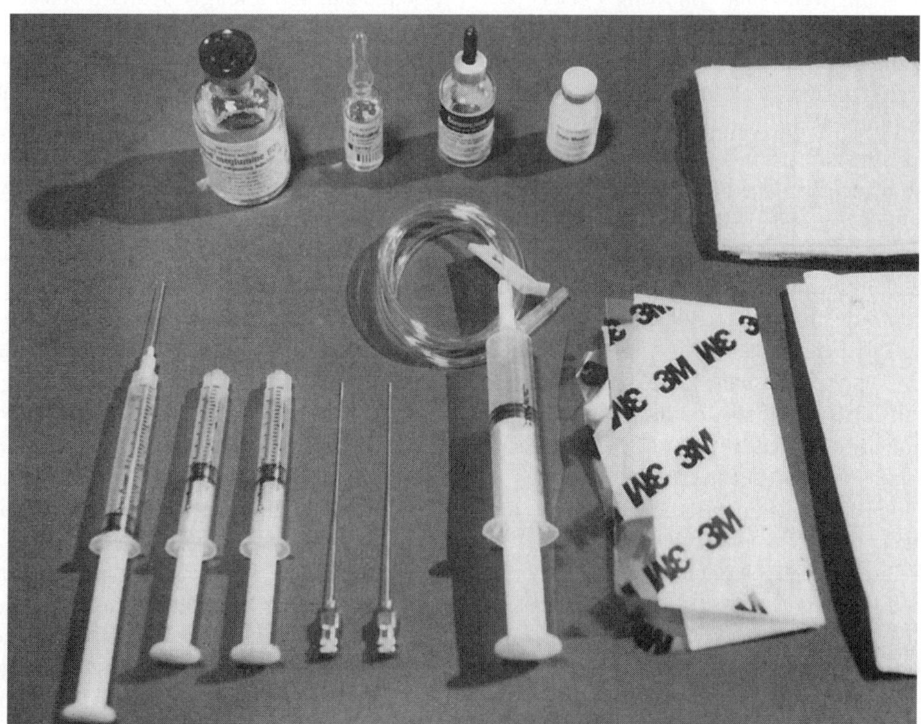

Fig. 63-43. Supplies used for facet block include a syringe for lidocaine with 25-gauge needle for skin anesthesia, a 3-ml syringe and 3.5-inch 22-gauge spinal needle for each facet to be injected, a 10-ml syringe with extension tubing for arthrography, drapes, radiographic contrast medium, 1% lidocaine, 0.5% bupivacaine, and methylprednisolone acetate. (From Raj PP: *Practical management of pain,* ed 2, St Louis, 1992, Mosby–Year Book.)

should be taken to pass the tip of the needle directly toward the facet joint by observing it frequently with fluoroscopy. Sometimes puncture of the joint capsule can be felt. More often, however, joint entry is signaled by the prevention of further needle advancement by bone. When the tip of the needle is superimposed on the facet joint and the needle cannot be advanced further, the needle tip should be in or very near the facet joint. Small adjustments can be made in needle position by retracting the needle 1 to 2 cm and readvancing. To prevent working around already positioned needles, it is most convenient to start with the most cephalad joint and work caudally when injecting multiple joints.

When the needle tip is positioned within the joint, aspiration is attempted to be certain the needle has not entered the subarachnoid space. If there is no return of CSF, the extension tubing with contrast material is attached, and 1 ml of iodinated contrast material is injected. A spot film is exposed with each facet injection to document the intra-articular position of the needle tip. After the needle position has been documented, 1.5 ml of 0.5% bupivacaine and 20 mg of methylprednisolone acetate are injected into each joint, and the needles are removed.

Results

Most patients experience little or no pain during injection of facet joints. If the injected facet is the cause of the pain, there is frequently dramatic relief of pain immediately after the injection. The patient is asked to sit, climb off the table, and walk while still in the radiographic procedure room. He or she is questioned concerning any immediate change in symptoms and instructed to keep track of any change in pain over the next 24 hours, as well as the following weeks.

The immediate response to the injection and long-term relief of pain is significant. The test is considered positive if there is complete relief of low-back pain and sciatica after intra-articular facet block, if the pain continues to be absent during the 24 hours after the study, and if the patient's normal activities do not exacerbate the pain.[41,61,79]

Initial pain relief has been reported in 54% to 65% of patients undergoing facet block. Between 20% and 30% of these patients had continued pain relief for more than 6 months.[41,56,152] Patient selection and technique are important factors in achieving satisfactory results.

Raymond et al.[182] reported that when maximum volumes of contrast material, local anesthetic, and steroid injection were strictly controlled to prevent rupture of the joint capsule, the overall response rate in 25 patients dropped to 16%, and there was no long-term therapeutic benefit. These authors' findings suggest that many patients responding favorably to facet blocks are affected by an extra-articular disorder, and the diffusion of the injected material into the tissues surrounding the facet joint after rupture of the joint capsule is the reason for the therapeutic effect of the injection.

Complications

The only absolute contraindications to facet block is infection in the overlying soft tissues. A relative contraindication is allergy to contrast agents. Facet injection can be accomplished, however, without injection of contrast material, and the newer nonionic contrast agents also decrease the risk in allergic individuals.

Complications from facet blocks are rare and include infection, allergic reaction, and transient radicular pain. Theoretically, the subarachnoid space could be entered during a facet block. It is important to aspirate before any injection to be certain there is no return of CSF. Placement of the needle under fluoroscopic visualization and proper technique ensure against this possibility.

EPIDURAL STEROIDS

Epidural injection of local anesthetics, steroids, and other agents has been used in the treatment of lumbosacral nerve root compression since the early 1900s. The first use of epidural hydrocortisone for the relief of back pain was reported in the 1950s. Numerous reports on the use of epidural steroids for lumbosacral radiculopathy, both controlled and uncontrolled, have been published since then.

Drug Choice

The steroid used is either methylprednisolone acetate (Depo-Medrol), or triamcinolone diacetate (Aristocort intralesional). The dose of methylprednisolone ranges from 80 to 120 mg;[36] most anesthesiologists choose 80 mg. Kepes and Duncalf,[117] after a review of the literature, stated that methylprednisolone was found to be less irritating, more beneficial, and a longer acting medication. The dose of triamcinolone ranges from 2 (50 mg)[7] to 3 ml (75 mg).[221] Delaney et al.[55] prefer triamcinolone because of its excellent anti-inflammatory effect, its low potential for sodium retention, and the fact that it remains in suspension in the local anesthetic for a longer time. Although no study has compared the relative effectiveness of methylprednisolone and triamcinolone, they appear to be equally effective. Most anesthesiologists dilute the steroid with a local anesthetic or saline. The results are apparently comparable with either diluent.[204] The addition of a local anesthetic is advisable in the presence of muscle spasm,[115,212] and the induction of sensory blockade also indicates correct epidural placement. However, inclusion of local anesthetic adds some risks, including hypotension and convulsion from intravascular injection. Because the results are the same with either diluent,[204] the use of saline is probably sufficient, especially in a busy outpatient practice.

The volume of the diluent depends on the injection site, whether lumbar or caudal. Although large volumes (average of 72 ml) have been used in the past,[53] they do not offer any advantage over smaller volumes of injectate.[103] The injection of a 6 to 10 ml volume has been recommended in lumbar epidural injections because this amount has been found adequate to bathe the areas involved in most lumbar disc derangements.[98] Smaller (2 to 3 ml) volumes are not recommended for two reasons. Several nerve roots, other than those immediately adjacent to a herniated or bulging disc, may also be inflamed.[15,157] In addition, the polyethylene glycol vehicle in the steroid preparation needs to be diluted because this vehicle has been found to cause degenerative lesions in rat sciatic nerves,[218] and, in higher concentrations, it has been shown to impair nerve transmission in rabbit vagus nerves.[18]

If the caudal route is chosen, a larger volume (20 to 25

ml) is necessary to reach the desired level.[103,204] The caudal route is quite effective[84] and is probably indicated in postlaminectomy patients. However, the lumbar approach should be used whenever possible because there is less anatomic variation, needle placement is easier, and it allows injection of the agent closer to the lesion.[212]

Indications

The primary indication for epidural steroid injection is nerve root irritation[14,87] and accompanying inflammation. Inflammation of the nerve in the presence of a herniated disc has been confirmed during surgery,[157] on myelography,[19] and on histologic examinations.[131,139] Improvement in clinical signs and symptoms has been shown to coincide with resolution or decrease of nerve root edema in the presence of persistent disc herniation.[19]

Steroids decrease inflammation by inducing the biosynthesis of a phospholipase A2 inhibitor which prevents prostaglandin generation.[73,85] Phospholipase A2 liberates the fatty acid substrates required for prostaglandin synthesis[85]; prostaglandins of the E series have been shown to cause hyperalgesia.[68] The mechanism of the antiprostaglandin effect of steroids differs from that of aspirin, which prevents prostaglandin generation by inhibiting the cyclo-oxygenase enzyme.

White et al.[214] observed the response of 304 consecutive patients with low-back pain to an epidural steroid injection. When they tabulated their results according to the etiology of the back pain, they found that the common denominator of success was the presence of nerve root irritation (Table 63-5). They also found a longer duration of pain relief in patients with acute pain (signs and symptoms < 2 weeks), and in those without psychologic overlay. Whereas short-term success rates were the same, 24% of the patients without psychologic overlay were still relieved of their pain at 6 months, compared with only 1.5% of the patients with large psychologic overlay.[214] The short-term success rates of the acute- and chronic-pain groups were also found to be the same. However, pain relief at 6 months was 34% in the acute-pain group, compared with 12% in the chronic-pain group.[214]

The effectiveness of epidural steroids for back pain secondary to a herniated disc has been documented. Sustained response of over 1 year has been documented in 41% of patients with herniated lumbar disc.[88] They have also been used in back pain secondary to degenerative spine with disc space narrowing,[103,166] with spondylolysis or spondylolisthesis,[88,98,103] after trauma,[82] and after laminectomy.[82,216]

Epidural steroid injections have probably been overused by "block-oriented" anesthesiologists because of anecdotal reports of their effectiveness. The use of epidural steroids in patients with bony abnormalities such as spinal stenosis, scoliosis, spondylolysis, or spondylolisthesis is questionable. If a patient known to have a bony abnormality for years complains of an acute radiculopathy, a trial of epidural steroid injection may be conducted. We have rarely seen

Table 63-5 Effectiveness of epidural steroid injections on the different causes of back pain*

Causes of back pain	Effect of steroid injections
Annulus tear ("back sprain")	Hastens recovery
Chronic lumbar degenerative disc disease	Transient relief
Herniated nucleus pulposus without neurologic deficit	Transient relief
Herniated nucleus pulposus with nerve root compression	Therapeutic
Spondylolysis	Therapeutic if nerve root irritation is present
Facet arthropathy	Steroid injection into the apophyseal joint may be successful
Scoliosis	May be effective if nerve root entrapment is present
Ankylosis spondylitis	Ineffective
Spinal stenosis	Transient relief
Functional low-back pain	Ineffective

*Derived from the results of White et al.[214]
From Benzon HT: Epidural steroid injections for low back pain and lumbosacral radiculopathy, *Pain* 24:277, 1986.

prolonged (2-year) relief in patients with years of documented spinal stenosis who developed an acute radiculopathy. If these patients initially respond, but the pain recurs within 6 to 9 months, repeat injection is probably not indicated. Rather, the patient may need surgical decompression because the pressure on the nerve by the bony abnormality results in recurrent nerve inflammation and can eventually lead to nerve fibrosis.[157]

Results with epidural steroids in postlaminectomy patients are generally poor. Although one study showed a 76% success rate after three injections of 125-mg hydrocortisone acetate and 30-ml 1% procaine,[82] others have reported very low success rates.[36,45] The lack of improvement may be caused by chronicity of the problem, the occurrence of accompanying arachnoiditis, and scarring around the nerve roots.[53,87] Brown[36] noted relief in postlaminectomy patients who experienced a recurrence of pain after a significant duration of pain relief, and in the patients whose radiculopathies were different from the one originally treated surgically.

Efficacy

Kepes and Duncalf[116] concluded that the rational use of epidural steroids in back pain has not been scientifically demonstrated (Table 63-6). Benzon, on the other hand,

Table 63-6 Effect of epidural injections on relief of chronic back pain in controlled studies

Patients		Methods			
Experimental	Control	Experimental	Control	Statistical significance	Remarks
20	20	Epidural local	Bed rest	Not determined	Experimental ambulation in 11 days vs. control in 31 days
24	24	Epidural steroid + local	Epidural local	None	Followed for 3 months
51	49	Epidural steroid	Epidural local	Yes	Followed for 3 months
27	24	Epidural steroid	Saline	None	Two-year follow-up
35	35	Epidural and subarachnoid	Nothing	None	Intraoperative injections
Crossover 16	19	Epidural local + steroid	Epidural local + saline	Yes	Improvement: experimental 63%; control 25%
Crossover 20		Saline/local	Saline + steroid Local + steroid	None	Four groups

From Kepes ER, Duncalf D: Treatment of backache with spinal injections of local anesthetics, spinal and systemic steroids. A review, *Pain* 22:33, 1985.

Table 63-7 Success rate of epidural steroid injections in relation to duration of back pain*

Cause of back pain	Drug injected	Concurrent treatment	Duration of symptoms (mo)	Number of patients	Success rate
Degenerated disc†	MP, 80 mg	None	3	12	10 (83%)
			6	12	8 (67%)
			≥ 12	26	15 (58%)
Herniated disc; 20 patients had laminectomy	MP, 120 mg in 3 ml 1% lidocaine‡	None	< 3	14	14 (100%)
			> 3	22	5 (23%)
			> 3	42§	8 (19%)
Disc disease, degenerated spine	MP, 80 mg in 20 ml 1% lidocaine	SM and SS in 38 patients	< 6	31	(81%)
			> 6	65	(44%)
Herniated disc	MP, 80 mg in 4 to 6 ml saline	None	≤ 3	34	(88%)
			> 3	26	(44%)
Disc disease, spondylosis, spondylolisthesis, s/p laminectomy	MP, 80 mg; hydrocortisone acetate, 25 mg	SM, SS	< 12	370	(69%)
			> 12	130	(46%)

MP — methylprednisolone; SM — spine manipulation; SS — sciatic stretch.
*All studies were anecdotal series. Their improvement criteria were symptomatic improvement. Heyse-Moore also looked at the improvement in straight leg raising and spinal mobility.
†Additional findings in nine patients; spondylolisthesis, sacralization, apophyseal joint change, osteitis condensans ilii, metastatic prostate cancer.
‡An intrathecal injection of 80-mg methylprednisolone was given in some patients (number of patients was not stated).
§Includes the 20 postlaminectomy patients.
From Benzon HT: Epidural steroid injections for low back pain and lumbosacral radiculopathy, *Pain* 24:275, 1986.

noted that three of five prospective, controlled studies showed better results with epidural steroids.[14] Carron[43] recently questioned the use of epidural steroids in back pain. He believed that, because of the natural course of the disease, any therapy completed within 4 to 6 weeks of an acute episode of low-back pain produces improvement in more than 90% of patients. He raised the possibility that epidural steroids may shorten the period of recovery. There has been no study addressing this issue. Coomes[47] has shown shortened recovery after caudal injection of procaine (11 days) compared with bed rest alone (31 days) in patients with sciatica. However, this study compared bed rest with caudal local anesthetic injection, not epidural steroid injection. Although several studies[12,32,204] showed better results with local anesthetic combined with steroid compared with local anesthetic alone, a study is needed comparing the period of recovery with epidural steroid with the period of recovery with bed rest. It should also be noted that not all patients

Table 63-8 Results of well-controlled studies on epidural steroid injections

Type of study	Cause of back pain	Duration of symptoms	Treatments studied, route	Number of injections	Success rate (%) steroid vs. control
P, R	Disc lesion	Not specified	MP, 80 mg in 42 ml 0.5% procaine vs. 42 ml 0.5% procaine, caudal	1 to 2	18/24 (75%); 75% vs. 67%
P, R, DB	Herniated disc, spinal stenosis S/P laminectomy	13 weeks to 36 months	MP, 80 mg (in 2 ml sterile water) in 5 ml 1% procaine vs. 2 ml NS + 5 ml 1% procaine, lumbar	1	25/42 (61%); 61% vs. 62.5%
P, R, DB	Degenerated disc	≤ 1 year	MP, 80 mg in 10 ml NS vs. 1 ml NS lumbar	1 to 2	21/35 (60%); 60% vs. 31%
P, R, DB	Herniated disc	1 to 3 weeks	MP, 80 mg vs. 2 ml NS, lumbar	1	Same results (25% to 70%)

P — prospective; R — randomized; DB — double-blind; MP — methylprednisolone; NS — normal saline.

with an acute episode of back pain require prolonged bed rest. Deyo et al.[57] showed that patients with mechanical low-back pain, without marked neurologic deficits, required only 2 days of bed rest for recovery.

Patients with acute radiculopathies respond better to epidural steroid injections than patients with chronic pain. Several studies (Table 63-7) show that the success rate ranges from 83% to 100% when the back pain is 3 months old or less[36,88,98] and 57% to 81% when the back pain is 6 months old or less.[98,103] Patients with pain for more than 1 year had an improvement rate of only 46%.[212] Sustained relief was also found to be more likely in patients whose symptoms were acute. The success rate at 6 months after an epidural steroid injection was found to be 34% in patients with acute pain (< 2 weeks duration), compared with only 12% for patients who had chronic pain.[214]

None of the preceding studies were controlled. **Even so, they suggest that epidural steroid injections for chronic back pain and radiculopathy are not effective and are therefore not advisable. Patients with chronic back pain may respond if they had a symptom-free interval and if the new symptoms were of recent onset at the time of injection.**[36] **Patients with new onset of a different radiculopathy may also respond.**[36] These patients may therefore have a trial epidural steroid injection. If they don't respond to one steroid injection, there is no reason to repeat it.

If epidural steroid injections are generally not recommended for chronic back pain, are they recommended in acute lumbosacral radiculopathies? A reevaluation of the results of prospective, controlled studies is shown in Table 63-8.

Beliveau[12] studied 48 patients; 24 patients were given caudal injections of 42-ml 0.5% procaine in normal saline with 80-mg methylprednisolone, the rest had caudal injection of procaine and saline. Although the study was randomized (assignment to a group was done in an alternate fashion), it was not a blinded study. There was also no distinction as to whether the patients had acute or chronic unilateral sciatica. Despite these shortcomings, this study demonstrated no difference between the two treatment groups; improvement was 67% to 75% in both groups.

A frequently quoted study, especially among orthopedic surgeons, is that of Cuckler et al.[51] They evaluated 73 patients with lumbar radicular pain syndromes. Of these, 42 patients were given an epidural injection of 2-ml sterile water containing 80 mg of methylprednisolone combined with 5 ml of 1% procaine, whereas the control patients were given 2-ml saline and 5 ml of 1% procaine. Patients were evaluated 24 hours after the injection. No statistical difference was found between the two groups. Of the patients given the epidural steroid, 61% (25 of 42) reported some degree of improvement, compared with 62% (20 of 31) in the control group. Long-term follow-up also did not reveal any sustained relief. This study can be criticized on several grounds. The patients studied were not homogeneous. Some patients had acute herniated disc, and others had spinal stenosis. Although the authors reported the number of patients who had a disc problem or spinal stenosis, they did not report the number of patients who had had laminectomy. The inclusion of postlaminectomy patients adds a degree of uncertainty as to whether the patients had acute or chronic pain. The control group was not really a placebo because procaine was injected. We know, from Coomes'[47] study, that epidural local anesthetic injections result in a significantly greater probability of improvement. The patients were evaluated at 24 hours after the injection; this time was not adequate to observe the steroid effect. Green et al.[88] found that, although 37% of patients (who responded to the injection) noted relief within 2 days or less, 59% experienced relief between 4 and 6 days. Cuckler et al.[51] also gave a second injection of steroid in patients who had less than 50% improvement; these injections were given in an unblinded fashion. The lack of long-term effectiveness of the steroid injection is bothersome. Cuckler et al.[51] contacted their patients for a final assessment by telephone rather than by face-to-face subjective and objective evaluation.

Two prospective, randomized, double-blind reports[59,194] come closer to being ideal studies. In both, the cause and duration of the back pain and radiculopathy are comparable; the route (epidural) and the type, but not volume, of steroid injected were the same. In addition, patients studied did not have any previous treatment, and concurrent treatments (bed rest, physical therapy, and analgetics) were the same.

The study of Dilke et al.[59] found significantly better results in the steroid group; 21 of 35 patients (60%) reported relief of pain compared with 11 of 36 patients (31%) in the placebo group. At 3 months' follow-up, a smaller number of patients in the steroid group had severe residual pain (1 of 44 versus 6 of 38 patients) or were taking analgetics daily (7 of 44 versus 14 of 38 patients) than in the placebo group. In addition, a greater number of patients who were given the placebo injection (14 versus 3 patients in the steroid group) were still not working.

Although Dilke et al.[59] showed significantly better results with the epidural steroid injection, Snoek et al.[194] did not. Snoek et al.[194] did not find any difference between the epidural steroid and placebo injections although both groups exhibited generalized improvement. Although the percentages of subjective and objective improvements were generally better in the steroid group, these results did not attain statistical significance. The percentage of improvement after the epidural steroid injection ranged from 25% with relief of impulse pain to 70% when judged by a physiotherapist.[194]

The difference in the results between the two studies may be the result of several factors. Dilke[59] used a 10-ml volume of saline and steroid, but Snoek[194] used only 2-ml of undiluted steroid. Snoek et al.[194] may also have missed the improvement in some of their patients. They evaluated the result of their steroid injection at 24 to 48 hours compared with up to 6 days by Dilke.[59] As previously noted, 59% of patients who respond to a steroid injection do so after 4 to 6 days.[88]

The follow-up period after epidural steroid injections has varied greatly between studies. Evaluation intervals include 3 months,[59] 6 months,[214] 8 to 20 (14 + or − 6) months[16,94] to 30 (average: 20.85) months,[51] and 1 to 2 years[7] after the injections (Table 63-9). At 3 months, Dilke et al.[59] noted that 16 of the 44 patients (36%) who were given an epidural steroid injection had no pain at all, compared with 8 of 38 (21%) patients given a placebo. Of the 44 patients, 40 (91%) had either no pain or no "severe pain," compared with 28 of 38 patients (74%) in the placebo group.

White et al.[214] followed their patients initially for 6 months, then up to 2 years for the patients that responded to the steroid injection. At 6 months' follow-up, 34% of the patients with acute (< 2 weeks) pain were still improved. However, only 1.3% of the patients were still without recurrence at their 2-year follow-up.[214]

Green et al.[88] observed 49 patients with protruded disc for an average of 1.5 years. Of those who responded, less than 11 patients (22%) had sustained relief for 6 months, and 20 patients (41%) had sustained relief for 1 year or more.

Snoek et al.[194] followed 51 patients. At 14 plus or minus 6 months after the injection, 52% of patients given the steroid had laminectomy, compared with 58% of those who had the placebo.

Cuckler et al.[51] followed 73 patients; 46 had the epidural steroid injection. At 13 to 30 months' follow-up, 6 of 23 patients (26%) who had herniated disc were considered improved (75% improvement). This contrasted with 2 of 13 (15%) control patients. In their patients with spinal stenosis, 22% (5 of 73) of patients given epidural steroid and 14% (2 of 14) of control patients were still improved.[51]

Arnhoff et al.[7] retrospectively followed 151 patients who were given either epidural or subarachnoid steroid injections. The majority (89 patients, 59%) of their patients had chronic pain, and some had laminectomy. Their initial success rate was 58.3%. At 1 to 2 years' follow-up, 21 patients (14%) reported complete pain relief. The number of patients whose pain was always present decreased from 97 (64%) to 40 (26.5%). In addition, the number of patients who "spent less time in bed" increased from 26 (17%) to 87 (72%).[7]

One can see from Table 63-9 that the studies[59,88,214] that followed patients who had pain for less than a year reported a 1.3% to 41% success rate. The low success rate of White et al.[214] is probably the result of the heterogeneity of the causes of the low-back pain in his patients. The patients of Dilke[59] and Green[88] had sustained response; these patients had disc problems. As White et al.[214] noted, epidural steroids were therapeutic in the patients with herniated disc with nerve root irritation.

These results should be compared with three studies that noted the long-term natural history of nonsurgically treated herniated disc. From these studies[74,87,168] (Table 63-10), we can see that 68% to 82% of the patients had no pain or only mild pain during the follow-up period. The investigators concluded that a large majority of patients have only mild residual pain or no further recurrence after an acute attack of pain subsides.

The overuse of epidural steroid injections involves not only questionable indications but also the number of injections. Some authors advise against repeat injections if there is no response to the first one. On the other hand, several investigators recommend repeat injections[59,98,204,212] because they have noted some patients who improved after subsequent injections despite initial failure. There is no need to repeat the injection after obtaining complete relief. If relief is partial, up to three injections may be given. More than three injections do not confer additional relief.[89] We rarely give three injections because in our experience one or two

Table 63-9 Follow-up results of epidural steroid injections

Treatment, route	Duration of pain	Duration of follow-up	Follow-up success rate
MP, 80 mg in 10 ml saline, lumbar	≤ 1 year	3 months	36%, 91%*
MP, 120 mg in 20 ml 0.25% bupivacaine, caudal; MP + 10 ml bupivacaine, lumbar	1 day to 6 months	6 months 24 months	34% (acute); 12% (chronic) 1.3
MP, 80 mg in 4 to 6 ml saline, lumbar	≤ 6 months	1.5 years (6 months to 5 years)	41%
MP, 80 mg in 2 ml water + 5 ml 1% procaine, lumbar	13 weeks to 36 months	20.85 months (13 to 30 months)	26% (HNP); 22% (SS)
TA, 50 mg in 6 ml 1% lidocaine, lumbar*	3 months to ≥ 60 months	1 to 2 years	14%

MP — methylprednisolone; TA — triamcinolone; HNP — herniated nucleus pulposus; SS — spinal stenosis.
*See text.

Table 63-10 Long-term natural history of nonsurgically treated herniated discs

	Group I	Group II	Group III
Number of patients	80	36	68
Treatment	IM dexamethasone	Bed rest and back support	Bed rest
Follow-up			
Range (months)	3 to 34	18 to 120	0 to 156
Average (months)	15.4	60	96
No pain	12 (15%)	17 (47%)	18 (26.5%)
Mild pain	54 (67.5%)	11 (31%)	28 (41%)
Severe pain	14 (17.5%)	8 (22%)	22 (32.4%)
Number of patients who had surgery	11 (12%)		5 (7%)

*Ninety-one patients were originally followed. Eleven (12%) of the 91 patients had surgery. The remaining 80 patients had conservative treatment.
From Benzon HT: Epidural steroid injections for low back pain and lumbosacral radiculopathy, *Pain* 24:277, 1986.

injections are usually adequate. How soon can the epidural steroid injection be repeated if the pain recurs after a good response to a prior injection? Preferably, there should be a 1-year interval.

It should be realized that epidural steroid injection only reduces nerve root inflammation and that there are other nonoperative treatments, including bed rest, muscle relaxants, anti-inflammatory agents and analgetics, that are important during the acute stage. The patient should receive physical therapy and be trained in proper body mechanics. Identification and treatment of any work-related, financial, psychologic, or marital problems should be undertaken.[5,37,199]

Complications

Epidural steroid injections are relatively safe; no major complication was reported after 500 injections.[36] Unintentional dural puncture has been reported in 1% of attempted epidurals.[212] It should be noted that the incidence of dural puncture headache in chronic pain patients is the same as in the general surgical population.[16] Rare cases of Cushing's syndrome have been reported; the authors recommended upper dosages of 3 mg/kg for methylprednisolone to prevent salt and water retention.[118] A case of congestive heart failure (CHF) from salt and water retention has been reported.[82] Other possible complications include exacerbation of diabetes mellitus, epidural abscess,[191] and spinal meningitis.[62] Intraocular hemorrhage had been ascribed to a marked and sudden increase in CSF pressure from rapid injection of large volumes into the epidural space.

In contrast to the epidural route, intrathecal steroid injections are fraught with complications. Cases of adhesive arachnoiditis[163]; aseptic,[163] cryptococcal,[191] and tuberculous meningitis[187]; transient inability to micturate[211]; sclerosing spinal pachymeningitis[21]; and conus medullaris syndrome[46] have been reported. Adhesive arachnoiditis is probably caused by the polyethylene glycol vehicle which has been shown to cause axonal and myelin degeneration. Because of these complications and overall ineffectiveness,[1] some have advised against intrathecal steroid injections.[14,20]

NEUROLYTIC AGENTS

Injection of neurolytic agents to interrupt pain pathways for a prolonged period of time has been practiced for many years. Such injections destroy the nerve fibers and thus pro-

Table 63-11 Concentration, nerve fiber effect, and efficacy of commonly used neurolytic agents

Agent	Concentration (%)	Nerve fiber affected	% success (approximate)
Alcohol	100	All fibers	58
	75	Sensory and C fibers	
	50	C fibers	
Phenol in glycerin or	6–12	Motor, sensory, and C fibers	60
Renografin or metrizamide	3	C fibers	
Ammonium sulfate	10	C fibers	40
Cold saline	Hypertonic	C fibers	30

From Raj PP: *Practical management of pain,* ed 1, Chicago, 1986, Year Book Medical Publishers.

duce a prolonged and sometimes permanent nerve block which resembles a nerve section. Neurodestruction with these agents may benefit patients with severe intractable pain and in whom neurosurgical procedures are contraindicated (e.g., those in poor physical condition).

Over the years, a variety of agents and combinations of agents have undergone clinical trials, with varying results. Ethyl alcohol and phenol have received considerable attention and, based on reasonable long-term results, have remained the neurolytic agents of choice. Despite a few pharmacologic and pathologic studies, there remains a paucity of scientific information for physicians managing intractable pain to make rational choices.

Alcohol

The effect of alcohol on somatic nerves was studied by Schlosser,[190] who found that alcoholization was followed by degeneration and absorption of all the components of the nerve except the neurolemma. There is general agreement that with 95% and absolute alcohol, the destruction includes sympathetic, sensory, and motor components of a mixed somatic nerve. Thus, it is undesirable to block a mixed nerve with such a concentration of alcohol. However, there is a great discrepancy in the conclusions concerning the effect of alcohol in concentrations below 80% on motor fibers (Table 63-11 and Fig. 63-44). Labat and Greene[125] reported quite satisfactory clinical results in the management of painful disorders by employing 33% alcohol without any resulting muscular paralysis or even paresis.

Ethyl alcohol is a potent neurolytic agent that can nonselectively destroy spinal and peripheral nerves. The neuronal action of ethanol involves the extraction of phospholipid, cholesterol, and cerebroside. Precipitation of mucoproteins and lipoproteins is also noted. In peripheral nerves, these actions result in a separation of the myelin sheath and edematous Schwann cell and axon. After subarachnoid injection, alcohol disappears from the CSF extremely rapidly,[140] declining from an initial concentration of 25.6% to 3.1% after only 109 minutes. Unfortunately, plasma concentrations were not measured, and the absolute neural uptake could not be accurately assessed.

The minimum concentration of alcohol required for neurolysis has not been definitely established. It has been stated that 30% ethanol in the subarachnoid space temporarily destroys sensory but not motor fibers, and that 80% ethanol causes only a reversible sensory block. *In vitro* studies on rabbit sciatic nerves showed equivalent suppression of large-diameter and small-diameter nerve fibers when exposed to 35% ethanol.[72] Fisher et al.[72] concluded there was no evidence that either fiber diameter or conduction velocity affected susceptability to neurolysis.

For subarachnoid block, alcohol concentrations between 50% and 100% are generally selected (Fig. 63-45). The reported volumes required for neurolysis have ranged from 0.3 ml/segment to a maximum of 0.7 ml/segment of absolute alcohol[61] or 0.5 to 1 ml/segment to a maximum of 1.5 ml/segment.[65] For celiac plexus block, volumes of 10 to 20 ml of absolute alcohol bilaterally may be used.[65] Similar volumes have been reported for lumbar sympathetic block. Often, 100% alcohol is diluted 1:1 with a local anesthetic agent before injection.

Alcoholic neuritis

The use of alcohol to effect prolonged nerve block presents one great disadvantage—the possible occurrence of alcoholic neuritis. This complication is so serious that many clinicians have rejected this method of nerve blocking.

It has been postulated that alcoholic neuritis is caused by incomplete destruction of somatic nerves. This is probably so, because neuritis has not been observed when the intraneural injection of a cranial or somatic nerve produces a complete block. Alcoholic neuritis occurs frequently after paravertebral block of the thoracic sympathetics because the sympathetic ganglia lie so close to the intercostal nerves that the alcohol, intended for the ganglion, also bathes and partially destroys the somatic nerve. During the period of regeneration, hyperesthesia and intense burning pain with occasional sharp shooting pain occur. These pains are sometimes so severe that they are worse than the original pain. Fortunately, in most instances these symptoms subside within a few weeks or a month. Occasionally, however, this complication persists for many months, requiring sedation, and in some instances it is necessary to perform a rhizotomy or sympathectomy.

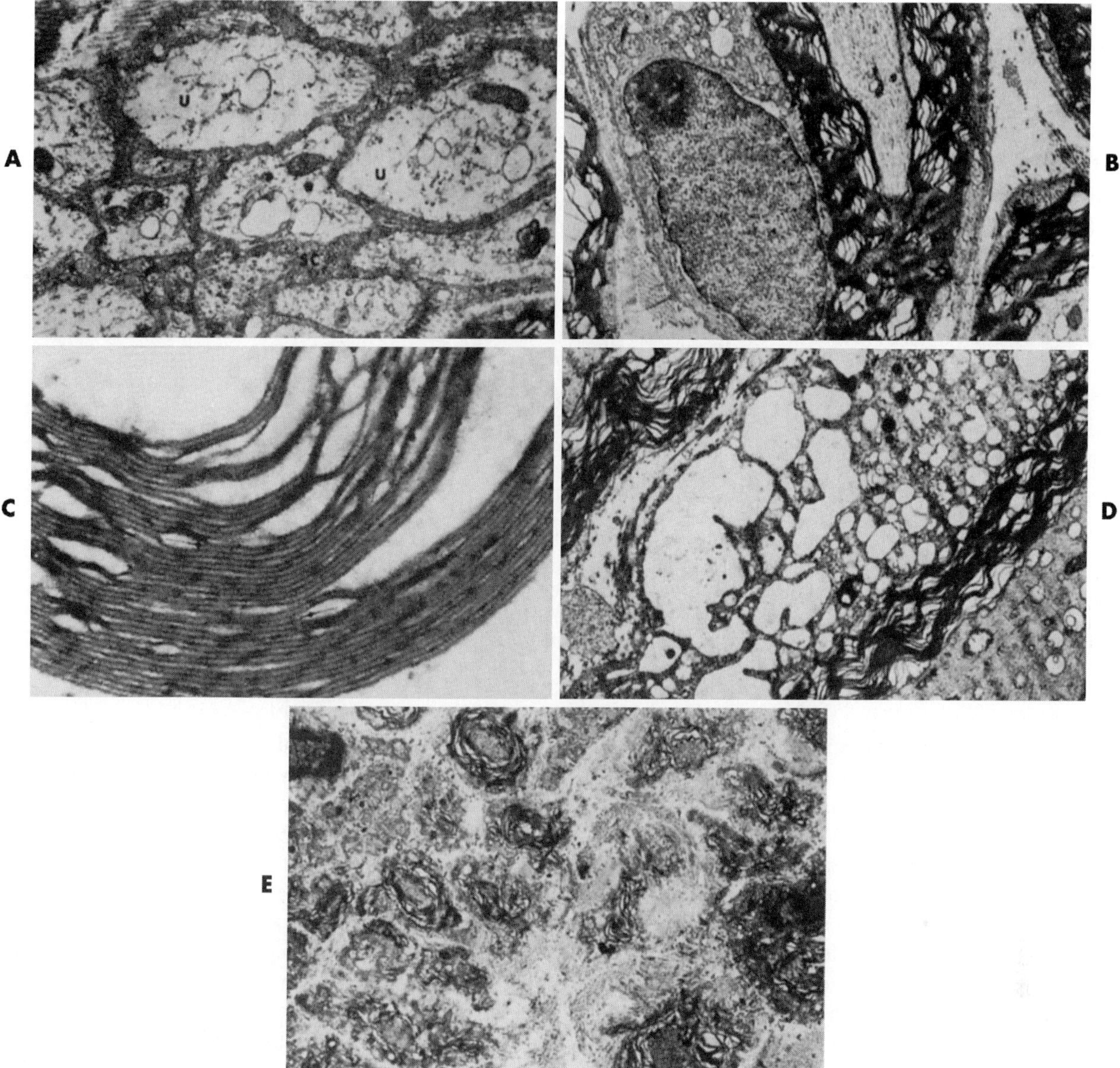

Fig. 63-44. A, Effect of alcohol on the peripheral nerve, 15 seconds after application. Electron micrograph shows the sciatic nerve of a mouse after topical application of 100% alcohol. *u,* Swelling of unmyelinated nerve fibers; *sc,* Schwann cell cytoplasm that is clumped and granular Schwann cell destruction (× 5000). **B,** Effect of alcohol on the peripheral nerve, 15 seconds after application. Electron micrograph shows the Schwann cell after exposure to 100% alcohol. Note spilling of the myelin sheath and dilated endoplasmic reticulum, indicating acute injury to the Schwann cell and myelin sheath (× 4300). **C,** Effect of alcohol on the peripheral nerve, 1 minute after application. Electron micrograph shows spilling of the myelin sheath after exposure to 100% alcohol (× 9600). **D,** Effect of alcohol on the peripheral nerve, 24 hours after a 15-second exposure to 100% alcohol. Note degenerating axons, spilling myelin lamelae, and beginning of connective tissue reaction (× 2200). **E,** Effect of alcohol on the peripheral nerve, 4 hours after a 15-second exposure. Electron micrograph shows vacuolization in the Schwann cell after exposure to 100% alcohol. (From Woolsey RM, Taylor JJ, and Nagel JH: Acute effects of topical ethyl alcohol on the sciatic nerve of the mouse, *Arch Phys Med Rehab* 53:410, 1972.)

Prevention of alcoholic neuritis. Mandl[138] recommends, as a prophylactic measure against this complication, the injection of a local anesthetic during the insertion of the needle, at the site of injection before the alcohol is injected, and on withdrawing the needle. With this technique he has observed only two instances of alcoholic neuritis.

Treatment. Mild cases of alcoholic neuritis are treated conservatively with mild analgetics such as aspirin or with small doses of codeine. Moderate cases of alcoholic neuritis

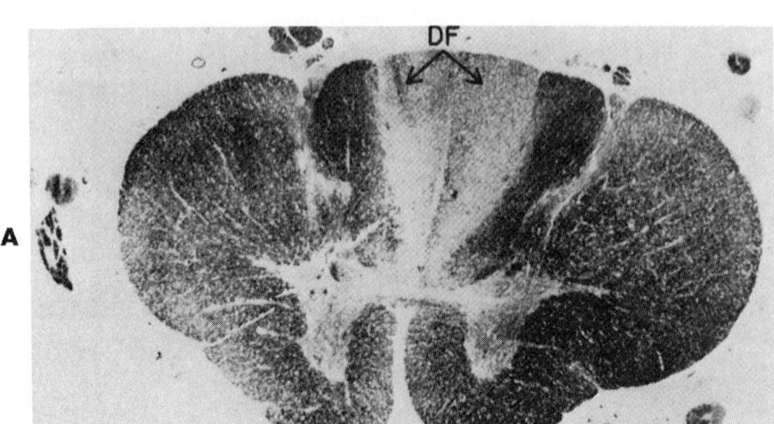

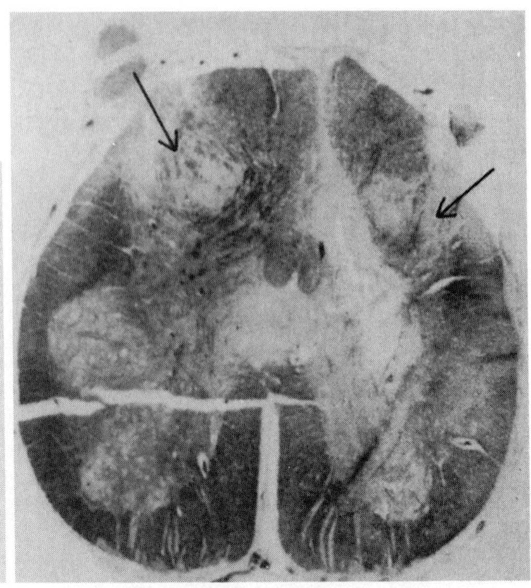

Fig. 63-45. **A,** Effect of alcohol on the spinal cord, 4 days after neurolytic block. Cross-section through the spinal cord at T4 shows degeneration of the dorsal fasciculus (*DF*) after injection of 100% alcohol several interspaces lower. **B,** Effect of alcohol on the spinal cord, 50 days after direct cord injection. Note necrosis and degeneration (*arrows*) after accidental injection of 100% alcohol into the spinal cord. (From Gallagher HS, Yonezawa T, Hay RC et al: Subarachnoid alcohol block II. Histologic changes in the central nervous system, *Am J Pathol* 35:679, 1961.)

may require more aggressive therapy. IV histamine (2.75 mg dissolved in 500 ml of 5% glucose in distilled water) administered twice daily has provided some relief. Several patients have been helped by the IV administration of local anesthetics. Bonica[27] has found tetracaine (250 mg dissolved in 500 ml of fluid) superior to procaine. In one patient, IV procaine had been administered several times with only transient relief of pain, yet one infusion of tetracaine effected prolonged relief. In some cases, daily sympathetic blocks have been employed, with excellent results. Serial caudal blocks performed at regular intervals can effect complete relief of pain caused by neuritis after lumbar sympathetic blocks.

Severe cases of alcoholic neuritis that do not respond to these conservative methods may require sympathectomy or rhizotomy. De Takats[54] reported three cases in which sympathectomy was required.

Phenol

The ability of phenol to destroy tissue has been known since its discovery. Apparently its first deliberate use to destroy nervous tissue was by Doppler[22] in Germany in 1925. After trying it in rabbits, he applied it on ovarian vessels and noted downstream vasodilation and flush. Later, Doppler reported treating peripheral vascular disease in the lower extremity by exposing and painting the femoral arteries with a 7% aqueous solution. He reported improvement in 12 patients but did not give a failure or complication rate. In France in 1933, Binet[22] reported painting ovarian vessels with 7% phenol. Both researchers attributed their good results to destruction of perivascular sympathetic fibers.

The first use of phenol by injection for the purpose of neurolysis was reported by Putnam and Hampton[176] in 1936 for neurolysis of the gasserian ganglion. The use of phenol as a local anesthetic had already been reported by Nechaev in the Russian literature in 1933.[162]

Mandl[137] in 1947 suggested the injection of phenol to obtain permanent sympathectomy. In 1950, he reported its use in 15 patients without complications, suggesting that it was preferable to alcohol.[138] In 1949 Haxton[100] and Boyd et al.[30] also reported on the paravertebral injection of phenol for peripheral vascular disease. In 1955, Maher[134] introduced it as a hyperbaric solution for intrathecal use in intractable cancer pain, with the famous remark that "it is easier to lay a carpet than to paper a ceiling." Thereafter, he reported its epidural use as well.

By 1959, phenol was established as a neurolytic agent for the relief of chronic pain. Kelly and Gautier-Smith[114] and Nathan[159] simultaneously reported on the intrathecal injection of phenol in hyperbaric solution with positioning to fix it on anterior nerve roots, thus relieving spasticity caused by upper motor neuron lesions. Since then, phenol has been widely used for neurolysis in the treatment of both pain and spasticity (Fig. 63-46).

Phenol is not available as a ready-to-use pharmaceutical preparation. It must be prepared from sterile ampules of analytic grade phenol by a hospital pharmacist. When it is to be mixed with glycerin, great care must be taken that both phenol and glycerin are free of water, or the necrotizing effect of the mixture will be much greater than anticipated. Phenol is highly soluble in glycerin and diffuses from it slowly, an advantage in intrathecal injection that allows for

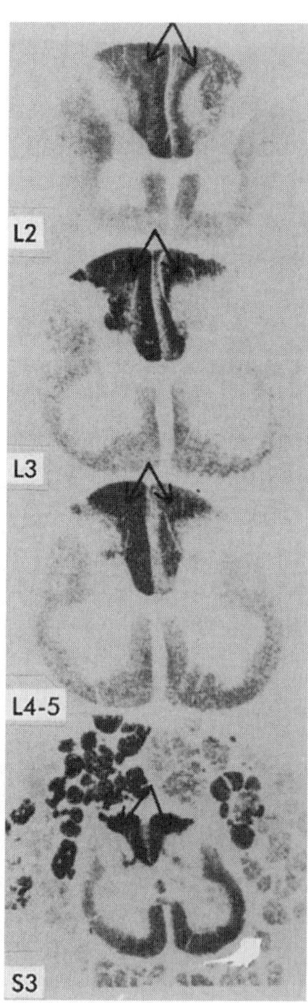

Fig. 63-46. Effect of phenol on the spinal cord. Micrographs of transverse sections at levels L2, L3, L4 to L5, and S3. They show degeneration of the posterior column after subarachnoid injection of phenol at L3 to L4. (From Smith MC: Histological findings following intrathecal injections of phenol solutions for relief of pain, *Br J Anaesth* 36:387, 1964.)

limited spread and highly localized tissue fixation. Phenol has also been prepared in sterile water, normal saline, and contrast material. We prefer 6% to 12% phenol in ionic contrast for extraspinal injections and phenol in nonionic contrast for epidural or intrathecal use.

Its mode of action as a neurolytic agent has been extensively studied and was reviewed by Felsenthal in 1974.[67] Maher,[134] seeking the ideal strength solution, tried concentrations of phenol in glycerin varying from 3.3% to 10% in the subarachnoid space. The stronger concentration produced motor damage, and there was gradation of block according to the concentration, with pain sensation being blocked at lower concentrations (5%) than were touch and proprioception. The 3.3% concentration was ineffective. Iggo and Walsh[106] followed with a study of action potentials in cat spinal rootlets and concluded that 5% phenol in either Ringer's solution or oil contrast medium produced selective block of smaller nerve fibers. Simultaneously, Nathan and Sears,[160] using the same preparation, arrived at the same conclusion. For a long time thereafter, the idea prevailed that phenol caused selective destruction of smaller nerve fibers with slower conduction rates, the C afferents carrying slow pain, the A delta afferents carrying fast pain, and the A gamma efferents controlling muscle tone.

These observations led to histopathologic studies. Stewart and Lourie[200] in 1963 saw nonselective degeneration in cat rootlets, the severity paralleling the concentration. Nathan et al.[161] repeated their action potential studies and looked at the histopathology. This time, they found evidence of A alpha and A beta damage in the electrophysiologic experiments and confirmed the nonselectivity of damage by histologic examination. They pointed out that phenol in low concentrations is a local anesthetic and when acting as such has a selective effect, as do other local anesthetics. However, when time of exposure and concentration are adequate, protein denaturing results, and this effect is nonselective.

Since this report, various researchers have confirmed the overall destructive effect of phenol. Knott et al.[119] noted damage from phenol in saline or in dimethylsulfoxide; Moller et al.,[150] after comparing low concentrations of phenol with low concentrations of alcohol, concluded that 3% phenol was similar to 40% alcohol. Schaumberg et al.[189] performed a meticulous combined electrophysiologic and histologic study, and Burkel et al.[38] included electron microscopic observations and noted severe damage to the perineural vascular elements, maximum degeneration in 2 weeks, maximum recovery at 14 weeks, and no identifiable binding site for tritium-labeled phenol.

The block produced by phenol tends to be less profound and of shorter duration than that produced by alcohol. Axons of all sizes are affected by therapeutic concentrations and, as with ethyl alcohol, appear edematous. The posterior root ganglia are unaffected by phenol. Similar pathologic changes occur in peripheral nerves when exposed to phenol. The composition of phenol solutions determines the neurolytic potency, that is, aqueous solutions of phenol are far more potent than those prepared in glycerin. Solutions of phenol are subject to oxidative degradation on prolonged storage. Concentrations of 3% to 10% have been evaluated, but the most commonly selected concentrations are between 6% and 8%. Recent studies of 6%, 9%, and 12% phenol in calsaphenous nerves show 12% phenol to be the most effective neurolytic concentration.[90]

No pharmacokinetic data are available to describe the systemic absorption after neurolytic administration. Phenol is efficiently metabolized by liver enzymes. The principal pathways are conjugation to the glucuronides and oxidation to equinol compounds or to CO_2 and water, and excretion as a variety of conjugates via the kidneys.

Clinical Usage of Neurolytic Agents

Patient selection criteria for chemical neurolysis

Proper patient selection is perhaps the most important criterion for success with neurolytic blockade. Unfortunately, most published studies on the use of neurolytic blocks have not been uniform in their selection criteria. The most common application of neurolytic blockade is in the management of cancer pain. The following criteria need to be seriously considered according to Brechner:[31]

A. Medical criteria
   1. Pain is localized to a few dermatomes.
   2. Performance of the procedure will not compromise the patient's existing medical condition or hasten the patient's demise.
   3. Performance of the procedure will not compromise bodily functions important to the patient and/or family.
   4. Medical conditions such as coagulopathy do not contraindicate insertion of needles.
   5. Expert pharmacologic tailoring has not succeeded in significantly decreasing the patient's pain without increasing intolerable side effects.
   6. Other nondestructive procedures, such as use of intrathecal morphine pump, are not appropriate or are not cost effective.
   7. The nature of the specific cancer indicates a progressive disease even with oncologic treatment and pain is the most predominant symptom.

B. Behavioral criteria
   1. Diagnostic block results in at least 50% pain relief
   2. Patient and family understand the procedure and potential side effects.
   3. Behavioral observation indicates positive indices of comfort with diagnostic block, such as decreased medication intake, increased alertness, more relaxed posture.

C. Psychosocial criteria
   1. Patient's and family's expectations are realistic in terms of the intended results and possible side effects.
   2. Family support exists for providing help to the patient if motor and/or sensory deficits limit the patient's functionality.

The decision to proceed with the neurolytic block depends on exploring these various criteria with the patient. If the patient does not wish to proceed, this should be respected and alternative treatments suggested.

Common Neurolytic Procedures

The use of neurolysis in stellate ganglion block, celiac plexus block, lumbar sympathetic block, and hypogastric plexus block is described above.

Intrathecal neurolysis

Intrathecal neurolysis with phenol or alcohol can be useful in patients with unilateral pain localized to three or four dermatomes, especially in the chest/thoracic wall or extremities. The positioning of the patient is of paramount importance. If absolute alcohol (a hypobaric solution) is used, the patient is positioned so that the alcohol can "layer" on top of the cerebrospinal fluid close to the neural roots to be interrupted.[101] If phenol in glycerol (a hyperbaric solution) is used, the positioning is such that the area of pain is in the most dependent part of the spinal canal to allow the solution to layer at the bottom of the cerebrospinal fluid (Figs. 63-47 and 63-48).[203]

For example, for intrathecal neurolysis to block the pain associated with unilateral thoracic wall pain secondary to multiple rib metastases on the right side, the patient is placed in two different positions depending on whether alcohol or phenol is used. If hyperbaric phenol is chosen, the patient is positioned with the painful side down on an operating table. The table is flexed so that the neural roots to be blocked are the most dependent part of the body, and the whole table is rotated back 45°. This allows the phenol to gravitate toward the neural components at the paravertebral foramina. The 45° tilt directs the hyperbaric solution primarily toward the dorsal sensory root and away from the ventral motor root.

With 100% alcohol, the patient is positioned so that the alcohol floats up toward the intended neural roots. Therefore, the patient is positioned with the painful side up and the body tilted forward to preferentially affect the dorsal roots.

There are important differences between alcohol and phenol that need to be pointed out. First, alcohol can be painful on injection, and phenol is painless. Therefore, patient movement should be anticipated with alcohol injection and the needle anchored carefully to prevent injection to the spinal cord with resultant catastrophic neurologic damage. Second, alcohol acts immediately on contact with the dorsal root, but phenol may take 10 to 15 minutes to fully penetrate the dorsal root. Phenol injection produces a sentinel "warm sensation" along the dermatologic distribution of the nerve roots that initially come in contact with it. If the warm sensation does not occur on the intended dermatomes, then one has up to 10 minutes to adjust the operating table to allow migration of the solution toward the intended dermatomes. Finally, 4% to 6% phenol in absolute glycerol cannot be injected through a spinal needle smaller than 20 gauge because of its high density, but alcohol can be injected through a 25- or 27-gauge spinal needle. After injection with either alcohol or phenol, the patient's position is maintained for 45 minutes.

Pathologic and postmortem examinations indicate variable effects of alcohol and phenol injection. For example, 95% alcohol injected into a peripheral nerve blocks the sympathetic, sensory, and motor fibers, whereas 80% alcohol affects the motor component unpredictably. In animal models, recovery from motor nerve block did not relate to the evidence of nerve degeneration or regeneration.[219] In human studies, recovery of motor function did not consistently correlate with the alcohol concentration.[97]

Despite 60 years of use, the success rate of intrathecal neurolysis has been consistently 45% to 60%.[202] The technique has not changed much despite decades of use. Criteria for success vary from one study to another, making comparison difficult. In addition, prospective comparisons of this technique with newer methods of pain control (i.e., intrathecal morphine pump, deep brain stimulation, dorsal root entry

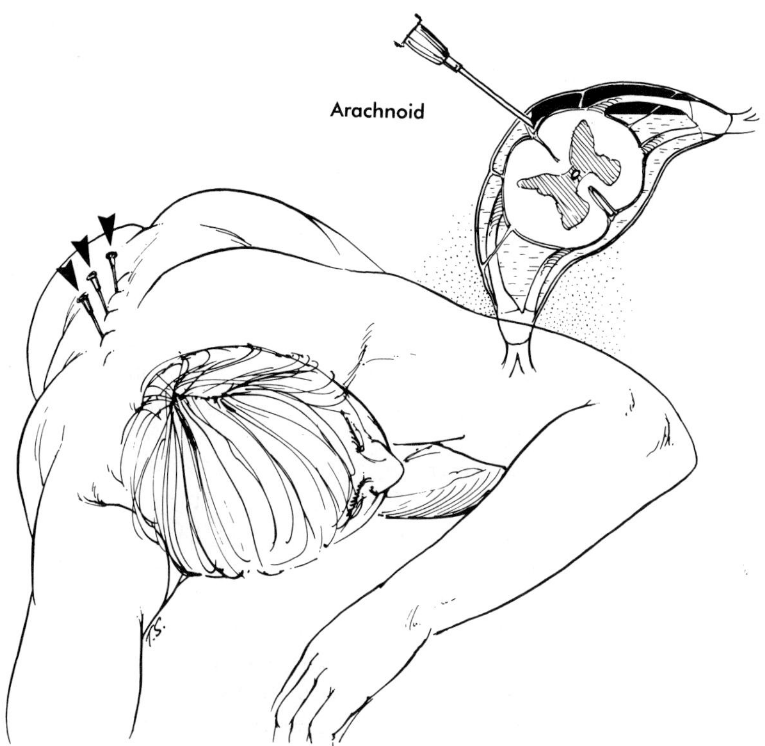

Fig. 63-47. Technique of alcohol neurolysis in the subarachnoid space. The painful part is uppermost, and the angle is 45 degrees to position the posterior nerve roots uppermost. (From Raj PP: *Practical management of pain,* ed 2, St Louis, 1992, Mosby–Year Book.)

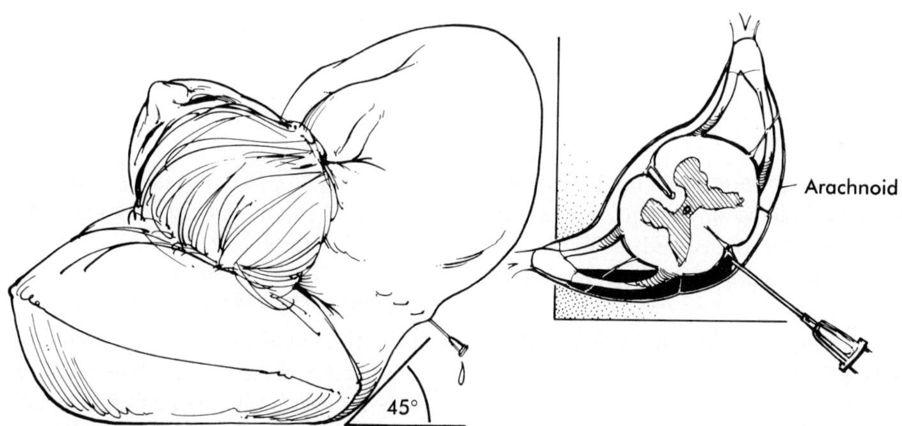

Fig. 63-48. Phenol neurolysis in the subarachnoid space. The painful part is lowermost, and the angle is 45 degrees to position the posterior nerve roots lowermost. (From Raj PP: *Practical management of pain,* ed 2, St Louis, 1992, Mosby–Year Book.)

zone lesions) have not been performed, making it difficult to assess its real value in the modern world of pain control.

Complications. Complications of intrathecal neurolysis include bladder, bowel, and motor paresis.[217] In patients with pelvic pain and intact bladder sphincter control, intrathecal/epidural morphine pump may be better for long-term pain control to allow preservation of this important function.

Epidural neurolysis

Indications for epidural neurolysis include pain in the shoulder or upper extremities, thoracic wall, and pleural upper-abdominal wall pain. Advantages of epidural neurolysis over intrathecal phenol are that the positioning is less critical and that neurolysis can be carried out over a period of 2 to 3 days by intermittent injection of phenol or alcohol through the epidural catheter. Epidural neurolysis is indicated over intrathecal when a wide segmental block is indicated.

Fluoroscopy with employment of radiopaque catheters is recommended. With the patient in a lateral position and painful side down, the tip of an epidural catheter is placed as close to the intended neural roots as possible. For the shoulder and arm area, a Tuohy needle is inserted at C7-T1 and a

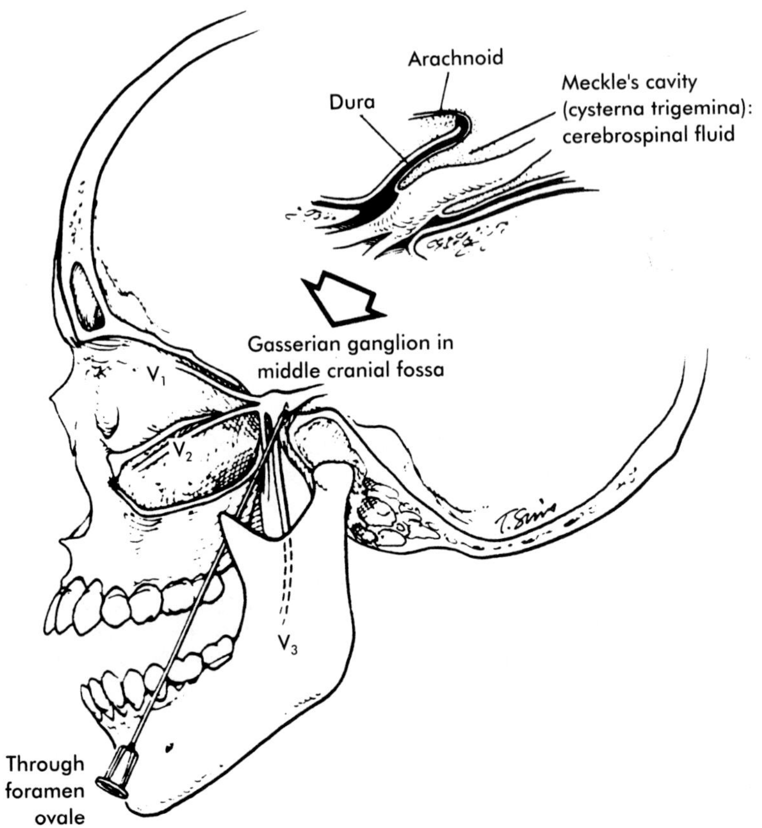

Fig. 63-49. Technique of gasserian ganglion block. Lateral skeletal view showing the needle traversing the foramen ovale. Inset shows relationships of the gasserian ganglia in Meckle's cavity.

catheter directed slightly upward; for upper-thoracic wall pain, the catheter is directed downward. For lower-thoracic wall pain, the catheter is inserted at T7-T8 and directed upward; for the upper-abdominal wall, it is directed downward.

After negative aspiration, 1% lidocaine is injected, in 5-ml increments every 15 minutes until there is evidence of decreased pinprick sensation over the area of pain. If pain (clinical pain estimate or visual analog scale) is decreased more than 75% and is satisfactory to the patient, the lidocaine block is allowed to wear off totally. Then 15% phenol in glycerol (75% of the lidocaine volume necessary to block the painful dermatomes) is injected through the epidural catheter. After 15 minutes, the presence of pinprick sensation over the area of pain is examined and, if absent, no further injection is necessary. If not, phenol in 1- to 2-ml increments is injected every 30 minutes until sensory block is demonstrated over the painful area. The catheter is left in place, and the patient is observed for the next 12 hours for narcotic need and pain levels, recorded hourly in a diary form. If the pain relief is not complete, the injection is repeated the next day. Alcohol can be used in concentrations of 30% to 100%, phenol in concentrations of 6% to 15%. Success rates with this procedure have not been adequately studied, although anecdotal reports of success have been reported ranging from 33% to 90%.[69,121]

Cranial nerve neurolysis

The trigeminal nerve is the major somatic nerve of the head and neck area (see Chapter 62). It is primarily a sensory nerve, and its major branches anatomically separate, thereby lending themselves to regional nerve blocking techniques (Figs. 63-49 through 63-51). In head and neck cancer, the branches can be separately anesthetized with local anesthetics to determine which major or peripheral branches contribute to the pain. For the ophthalmic area, the frontal and supraorbital nerve can be blocked to relieve pain, first with local anesthetic, then with 0.5 to 1 ml of 95% alcohol. The maxillary nerve can be blocked through the extraoral approach (Fig. 63-51). Alcohol block with 0.5 to 2 ml can produce immediate pain relief. The mandibular nerve can be approached laterally or extraorally through the mandibular notch or intraorally through the buccal fold (Fig. 63-52). One problem with this method is that the motor fibers to masticatory muscles can be blocked, resulting in impaired chewing. For carcinoma of the tongue, a separate lingual nerve block may be

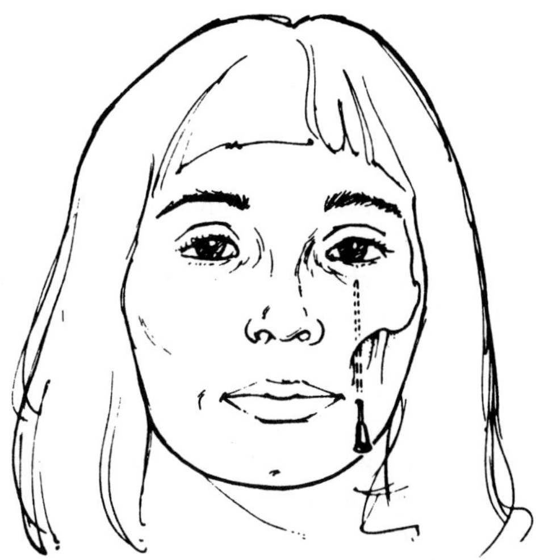

Fig. 63-50. Technique of gasserian block. Anteroposterior direction of the needle.

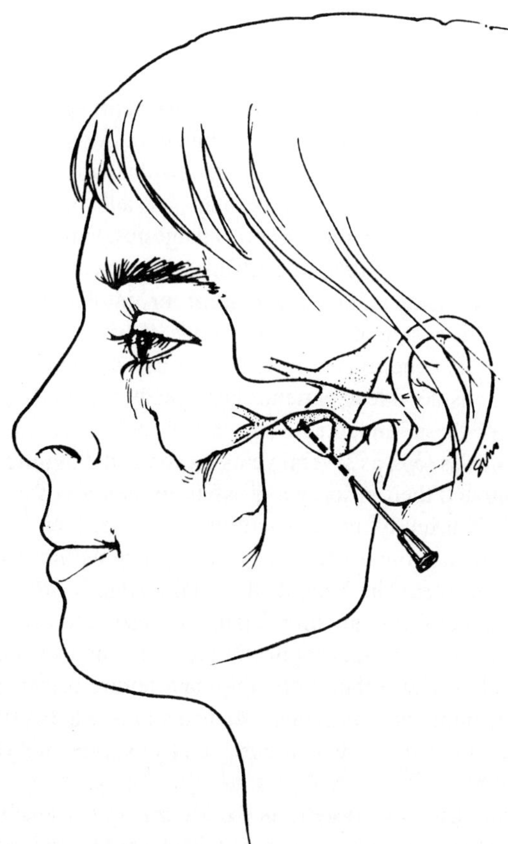

Fig. 63-51. Technique of gasserian block. Lateral direction of the needle.

indicated and performed with minute amounts of alcohol (0.25 to 0.5 ml).

SPINAL CORD STIMULATORS

Electrical stimulation of the spinal cord is a nondestructive technique which can be an effective means of providing

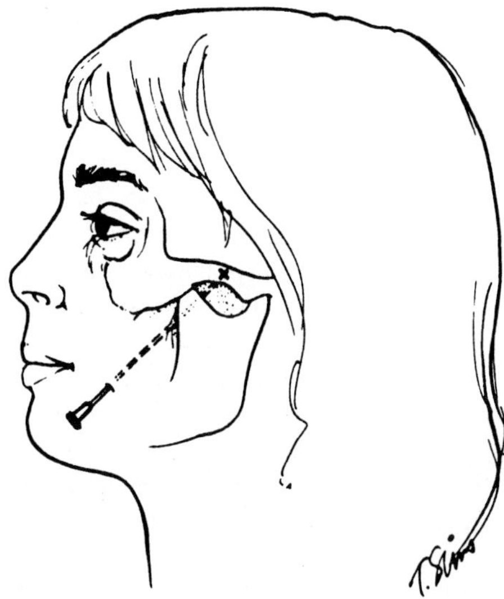

Fig. 63-52. Technique for the external block of the mandibular nerve is essentially the same as that for the maxillary block, except that the needle is directed upward and posteriorly, so that the mandibular nerve is contacted as it exits the foramen ovale.

analgesia for patients with certain chronic pain syndromes. The concept was first applied by Shealy[192] in 1967, and was original termed *Dorsal Column Stimulation.* Although the exact mechanism of action remains poorly understood, several possibilities have been proposed. **The original explanation, and the one most widely accepted, is that electrical stimulation of the dorsal columns activates large sensory neurons with resultant inhibition of afferent input from small nociceptive fibers.** Other experts have suggested that the antinociceptive effects of electrical stimulation may result from release of neuromodulatory chemicals in the spinal cord or activation of supraspinal centers.[8,145] Stimulation of the ventral aspects of the spinal cord also has been shown to provide analgesia.[126] Because the exact site of effect remains uncertain, the technique is now more commonly termed *spinal cord stimulation* (SCS). Clinical application of this concept involves implantation of stimulating electrodes near the spinal cord which are connected to small portable or completely implantable electrical pulse generators. When used in conjunction with strict patient selection criteria, success rates of greater than 50% for certain pain syndromes have been reported with a minimal incidence of serious complications.[164]

Indications

In current practice, SCS is an appropriate method for management of certain pain syndromes when alternative treatments have failed. The primary indication is for patients with chronic pain in the lower back which radiates down the leg, in whom surgical treatment has failed (Failed Back Syndrome). Isolated low-back pain without a radicular component is much less likely to be treated successfully. Other indications include phantom limb pain, lesions of the brachial, lumbar or cervical plexi, reflex sympathetic dystrophy, peripheral nerve injury or pain from peripheral vascular disease. The quality that unifies all of these indications is the presence of some form of neuropathic pain.

Patients should not be considered for SCS until an extensive search for reversible pathology has been conducted. All other conventional alternative therapies should be tried first. Formal psychologic evaluation of candidates is required to identify those with significant psychological overlay or secondary gain issues, because these patients are much less likely to achieve satisfactory results.[133] Patients who have passed psychological screening should then undergo a trial of spinal cord stimulation with temporary devices before proceeding to permanent implantation. The effect of TENS is not useful in predicting benefit from SCS.[197]

Implantation technique

Whereas early SCS electrodes required laminectomy for placement, modern electrodes are small enough that they are typically inserted into the epidural space percutaneously, through modified Touhy needles. The procedure is performed under local anesthesia with patients in either the prone or lateral position. Sterile technique must be scrupulously maintained to avoid infection. Under fluoroscopic guidance, the electrodes are guided from their point of insertion cephalad toward an area posterior to the spinal cord, at or above the spinal cord segmental level which corresponds to the distribution of symptoms. Middle- to lower-thoracic placement is common for patients with lower-extremity pain. For treatment of pain in the upper extremities, the electrodes are placed in the upper-cervical or lower-thoracic levels of the spine. The final location for the electrode is determined empirically with the help of electrical stimulation. The electrode position is adjusted until the patient reports a tingling sensation exactly in the painful area. Modern electrodes contain multiple discrete stimulating segments which can be independently selected with controls on the generator. These can be used to finely adjust the point of stimulation during placement, or to regain proper stimulating distribution should the electrode move from its original position. If paresthesias in the appropriate area cannot be achieved, successful treatment of pain is unlikely. Implanted electrodes can be attached to a portable external generator for a temporary trial of SCS, or to a permanent generator which is surgically placed in a subcutaneous pocket. Implantable pulse generators can be powered by self-contained batteries (which require periodic replacement) or through external power sources which transmit energy by radio frequency. The most common complications are minor wound infections and dislodgment of electrodes with resultant loss of effectiveness. Continuous refinement of SCS technology has made equipment failures much less common that in the past.

Implantable Spinal Catheters

The discovery of opioid receptors in the spinal cord in 1976[220] has led to the clinical use of spinally administered opioids and other agents for the treatment of a variety of pain syndromes, including postoperative pain and pain resulting from malignancy. *Spinal analgesia* is the term used to describe the administration of analgesic agents into either the epidural or subarachnoid spaces. The desire to administer spinal analgesics safely and reliably for prolonged periods in the treatment of chronic pain has resulted in development of new types of implantable catheter systems designed for long-term use. These systems span the technological spectrum from the very simple (ordinary epidural catheters taped securely, or sutured in place) to totally implantable, programmable, microprocessor controlled infusion pumps. The minor operative procedure needed to implant these systems can be performed either by a surgeon or a properly trained and clinically credentialed anesthesiologist. Prerequisite to the proper use of the systems is an understanding of the pharmacology of spinal analgesics and this has become the domain primarily of anesthesiologists.

Indications

The primary indication for initiating long-term spinal analgesia is pain associated with malignancy. Most patients with cancer-related pain do not require spinal analgesia because such pain can usually be managed adequately with systemic opioids and non-narcotic analgesics. However, approximately 5% to 10% of patients with cancer pain will experience inadequate pain control or intolerable side effects with systemic analgesics alone. A subset of these patients can benefit greatly from the use of spinal analgesics. Considerable experience has already accumulated in the use of these implantable systems in individual patients for periods as long as several years. Several studies have not demonstrated their efficacy and safety for control of cancer pain.[64,173] Currently, most practitioners restrict their use to patients with limited life expectancies, such as those with terminal cancer. The benefit of spinal analgesia for treatment of other forms of chronic pain not related to cancer is much less clear and this application remains somewhat controversial. The likelihood of equipment failure or development of significant drug tolerance make implanted systems less useful in patients who are expected to survive for years or decades.

In contrast to neurolytic nerve blocks, spinal analgesia has the advantage of being completely reversible, and can be used to treat pain experienced over a wide area, usually without associated sensory or motor blockade. A preimplantation trial of spinal analgesia is easily accomplished at low cost using standard epidural or subarachnoid catheters. One disadvantage of implanted systems is the high cost of equipment and follow-up patient care.

Types of implantable systems

Implantable systems for spinal analgesia can be categorized into two main types: externalized catheters and totally implantable systems. The simplest systems available for long-term administration of spinal analgesics are externalized catheters originally designed for intraoperative use. These plastic catheters can be inserted into the epidural or subarachnoid space in the usual fashion and sutured in place at the skin. With careful maintenance, these catheters may remain functional for several weeks. Their use can be extended if the catheter is tunneled subcutaneously for a distance away from the insertion site. Tunneling helps anchor the catheters in place and serves as a barrier to prevent infection from reaching the CNS. Catheters specifically designed for implantation and tunneling, such as the DuPen™ catheter, are available and are more flexible and durable than traditional catheters. The DuPen™ catheter features a silver impregnated antibacterial cuff intended to prevent superficial infections from reaching the meninges. Experience with this device has demonstrated a significant but low incidence of serious CNS infection.[64] Externalized catheters can be injected manually by visiting nurses, or by reliable patients or family members. More often they are attached to pumps to provide continuous infusions with or without a patient-controlled analgesia (PCA) feature. These catheters can be inserted into either the epidural or subarachnoid space, although many practitioners remain concerned about the risk of CNS infection when externalized catheters are placed intrathecally.

Several systems are available which can be implanted entirely beneath the skin. These may be preferable in patients with longer life expectancies because of a decreased risk of infection, as well as for cosmetic considerations. The simplest completely implantable systems involve catheters which are tunneled under the skin to a subcutaneous injection port. Injection of drugs into the catheter requires piercing the skin and port membrane with a specially designed noncoring needle.

The most sophisticated spinal analgesia system available is the Medtronics Synchromed™ infusion pump. This totally implantable device incorporates a battery, drug reservior, and micrprocessor-controlled infusion pump in a single small unit which can be placed in a subcutaneous pocket. The implanted device is connected to a catheter leading to the subarachnoid space. The pump can be "programmed" much like a pacemaker, by placing a programming wand over the unit. Drug delivery rate is thus easily adjusted. The unit can also be instructed to deliver preprogrammed boluses or to have different infusion rates for day and night. Periodic replenishment of the drug reservoir is accomplished by injection through a subcutaneous port. Battery changes require a minor surgical procedure to move the device. The high initial cost for purchase of these pumps may be offset by the reduced cost of follow-up home care in patients with longer life expectancies.[11]

Choice of Spinal Analgesics

Opioids are by far the most commonly used agents in implantable spinal catheter systems. These drugs are notable for their ability to provide profound analgesia without affecting other sensory modalities. Morphine is frequently chosen because of its high degree of water solubility, which affords a prolonged duration of action, extensive spread throughout the CSF, and relatively low systemic drug concentrations. Local anesthetics may be used in dilute concentrations to augment opioid analgesia and can enhance the relief of pain associated with movement. They are most effectively used with catheters placed in the epidural space. Clonidine and other alpha$_2$-adrenergic agonists will soon be available for spinal administration and are typically used in combination with opioids. They may be particularly effective in the treatment of neuropathic pain.

Complications

The most common complications associated with use of implantable spinal catheters are equipment failure and infection. When used with appropriate care, most infections are limited to the superficial tissues. Most deeper infections have been successfully treated with antibiotics and catheter removal. Equipment failures include catheter dislodgment, kinking, or fracture. Catheters placed in the epidural space may become occluded by accumulation of fibrous tissue. Tumors that compress the spinal cord or prevent the flow of drugs in the epidural space can limit the effectiveness of spinally administered agents. Massive overdose from drug administration errors have occurred.

KEY POINTS

- Anesthesiology initially developed out of a practical need to control intraoperative pain. Greater understanding of pain and the pain experience as an integrated, multidimensional phenomenon has led to the development of modern pain management regimens which are based on a comprehensive, multidisciplinary approach to the patient. In almost all cases, anesthesiologists seeking to gain expertise in the management of pain need to develop clinical skills and understanding beyond the realm of the operating room.
- Implicit in the term "*pain management*" is an acknowledgment that complete relief of pain and related symptomatology cannot always be obtained for all patients. In many cases, optimal management is ongoing and entails

minimizing the degree of symptoms experienced, maximizing functional capacity, and initiating therapy to reduce associated psychologic distress.

- Clinically, pain syndromes in children and adults may be broadly classified as acute, chronic, or cancer related. Each involves distinctive features of pathogenesis and ultimately requires an individualized approach for optimal management.
- Nerve blocks used in chronic pain management include somatic peripheral nerve blocks, intravertebral central neural blocks, and sympathetic blocks.
- A myofascial trigger is a hyperirritable locus in a taut band of skeletal muscle. The trigger point is painful when compressed and can evoke referred pain and an autonomic response.
- The stretch-and-spray procedure is the workhorse of myofascial therapy. It inactivates myofascial trigger points quickly with less patient discomfort than local myoneural injection. Although precise localization of the trigger point is not needed, considerable skill is required to coordinate the course of spray so that it covers fibers that are being placed on maximum tension by passive stretch.
- Glossopharyngeal nerve block is used for control of acute pain in perioral endoscopy procedures, for chronic pain in patients with invading carcinoma of the posterior third of the tongue or pharynx unresponsive to other therapies, and in the rare condition of idiopathic glossopharyngeal neuralgia.
- Thoracic nerve block is used for pain secondary to nerve root irritation or compression at the foramina level or distally and to treat intercostal neuralgia secondary to herpes zoster, fractured ribs, tumors, or metastasis.
- The site of needle entry for a stellate ganglion block is Chassaignac's tubercle, which can be most readily identified by first locating the cricoid cartilage at the C6 level. Palpation of the tubercle can be expected at the medial border of the sternocleidomastoid muscle, approximately 1.5 cm lateral to the midline.
- Sympathetic interruption to the head following stellate ganglion block can be documented by the presence of any of the signs of Horner's syndrome: myosis, ptosis, or enophthalmos. Associated findings include conjunctival infection, nasal congestion, and facial anhidrosis. These signs can be present without complete interruption of the sympathetic nerves to the upper extremity.
- Pain originating from visceral structures innervated by the celiac plexus can be alleviated by celiac plexus blockade. The particular disease state determines the effectiveness of a celiac plexus block in producing sustained pain relief and the use of a local anesthetic block, neurolytic injection, catheter placement, or steroid injection.
- Guanethidine monosulfate selectively inhibits the sympathetic nervous system, acts at the postganglionic neuron of the neuroeffector junction, and is actively transported into the postganglionic neuron by the NE pump where it displaces NE from presynaptic vesicles and inhibits reuptake of NE.
- The cervical facet syndrome is initially treated conservatively: local heat, traction, NSAIDs, local myofascial trigger-point injections, and local injection in the paravertebral muscles. Arthrography with local anesthetic and steroid injection may give up to 12 months pain relief. Because of the possibility of subarachnoid and epidural injection, cervical facet joint injections should be performed with fluoroscopic control.
- Facet injection is used for focal tenderness over a facet joint, chronic low-back pain with a normal radiographic work-up, back pain with evidence of disc disease and facet arthritis, or postlaminectomy syndrome without arachnoiditis or recurrent disc disease.
- Patients with "facet syndrome" usually have pain localized to one side. Determining the level for injection is difficult because multiple-level disease is common; each facet joint has a dual nerve supply, and similar symptoms can result from disease at different levels. Injection at two or three levels may be needed.
- Epidural steroid injection is used for acute nerve root irritation and inflammation. Other indications—especially in chronic pain states—are questionable.
- Injection of neurolytic agents interrupts pain pathways for a prolonged duration, acting by destroying the nerve fibers. These agents are reserved for severe, intractable pain when neurosurgical procedures are contraindicated.
- Intrathecal neurolysis with phenol or alcohol can be used for unilateral pain localized to three or four dermatomes, especially in the chest wall or extremities. The positioning of the patient is of paramount importance. With absolute alcohol, a hypobaric solution, the patient is positioned so that the alcohol can layer on top of the CSF close to the neural roots to be interrupted. With phenol in glycerol, a hyperbaric solution, the patient is positioned so that the area of pain is in the most dependent part of the spinal curve to allow the solution to layer at the bottom of the CSF close to the targeted nerve roots.
- Phenol block is less profound and of shorter duration than alcohol. It affects axons of all sizes, but does not affect posterior root ganglia. The usual concentrations are between 6% and 8%. Phenol block can be achieved with a painless injection and may take 10 to 15 minutes to fully penetrate the dorsal root, so the clinician has time to adjust the table to allow migration to intended dermatomes.
- Alcohol can cause alcoholic neuritis which is so objectionable that many clinicians have rejected its use. It can also be painful on injection, so patient movement should be anticipated and the needle anchored to prevent injection to the spinal cord and resultant neurologic damage. Alcohol acts immediately on contact with the dorsal root so patient positioning must be precise.

- After injection with either alcohol or phenol the patient's position should be maintained for 45 minutes.
- In current practice, SCS is an appropriate method for management of certain pain syndromes when alternative treatments have failed. The primary indication is for patients with chronic pain in the lower back which radiates down the leg, in whom surgical treatment has failed (Failed Back Syndrome).
- The desire to administer spinal analgesics safely and reliably for prolonged periods in the treatment of chronic pain has resulted in development of new types of implantable catheter sysems designed for long-term use. These systems span the technological spectrum from the very simple (ordinary epidural catheters taped securely, or sutured in place) to totally implantable, programmable, microprocessor-controlled infusion pumps.

KEY REFERENCES

Bonica JJ, editor: *The management of pain,* ed 2, Philadelphia, 1990, Lea & Febiger.

Cousins MJ, Bridenbaugh PO, editors: *Neural blockade in clinical anesthesia and pain management,* ed 2, Philadelphia, 1988, JB Lippincott.

Patt RB, editor: *Cancer pain,* Philadelphia, 1993, JB Lippincott.

Raj PP: *Practical management of pain,* ed 2, St. Louis, 1992, Mosby–Year Book.

Travell J, Simons DG: Myofascial pain and dysfunction. In: *The trigger point manual,* Baltimore, 1983, Williams & Wilkins.

REFERENCES

1. Abram SE: Subarachnoid corticosteroid injection following inadequate response to epidural steroids for sciatica, *Anesth Analg* 57:313, 1978.
2. Abram SE: Intraarterial reserpine, *Anesth Analg* 59:889, 1980.
3. Adelman MH: Cerebral air embolism complicating stellate ganglion block, *J Mt Sinai Hosp* 15:28, 1948.
4. Booklet of Information, November, 1995, *The American Board of Anesthesiology.*
5. Anderson TP, Cole TM, Gullickson G, et al: Behavior modification of chronic pain; a treatment program by a multidisciplinary team, *Clin Orthop* 129:96, 1977.
6. Appenzeller O: *The autonomic nervous system,* New York, 1982, Elsevier Biomedical Press.
7. Arnhoff FN, Triplett HB, Pokorney B: Followup status of patients treated with nerve blocks for low back pain, *Anesthesiology* 46:170, 1977.
8. Atweh SF, Dajani BM, Saade NE, et al: Supraspinal inhibition of trigeminal input into subnucleus caudalis by dorsal column stimulation, *Brain Res* 348:401, 1985.
9. Awad EA: Interstitial myofibrositis: hypothesis of the mechanism, *Arch Phys Med Rehab* 54:440, 1973.
10. Becket RF, Grunt JA: The cervical sympathetic ganglia, *Anat Rec* 127:1, 1956.
11. Bedder MD, Burchiel K, Larson A: Cost analysis of two implantable narcotic delivery systems, *J Pain Symp Man* 6:368, 1991.
12. Beliveau PA: A comparison between epidural anesthesia with and without corticosteroid in the treatment of sciatica, *Rheum Phys Med* 11:40, 1971.
13. Bell S, Cole R, Robert Thomason IC: Coeliac plexus block for control of pain in chronic pancreatitis, *Br Med J* 281:1604, 1980.
14. Benzon HT: Epidural steroid injections for low back pain and lumbosacral radiculopathy, *Pain* 24:277, 1986.
15. Benzon HT, Braunschweig R, Molloy RE: Delayed onset of epidural anesthesia in patients with back pain, *Anesth Analg* 60: 874, 1981.
16. Benzon HT, Braunschweig R, Molloy RE, et al: Postdural puncture headache in patients with chronic pain, *Anesthe Analg* 60:874, 1980.
17. Benzon HT, Chomka CM, Brenner EA: Treatment of reflex sympathetic dystrophy with regional intravenous reserpine, *Anesth Analg* 59:500, 1980.
18. Benzon HT, Gissen AJ, Strichartz GR, et al: The effect of polyethelene glycol on mammalian nerve impulses, *Anesth Analg* 65:553, 1987.
19. Berg A: A clinical and myelographic studies of conservatively treated cases of lumbar intervertebral disc protrusion, *Acta Chir Scand* 104:124, 1953.
20. Bernat JL: Intraspinal steroid therapy, *Neurology* 39:1124, 1981.
21. Bernat JL, Sadowsky CH, Vincent FM, et al: Sclerosing spinal pachymeningitis; a complication of intrathecal steroid administration of depomedrol for multiple sclerosis, *J Neurol Neurosurg Psych* 39:1124, 1976.
22. Binet A: Valeur de la sympathectomie chimique en gynecologie, *Cynecol Obstet* 27:393, 1933.
23. Boas RA: Sympathetic blocks in clinical practice, *Int Anesth Clin,* vol 16(4), Boston, 1978, Little Brown.
24. Boas RA, Covino BG, Shahnarian A: Lumbar sympathectomy; a percutaneous chemical technique, *Adv Pain Res Ther* 54: 501, 1976.
25. Bohn HP, Reich L, SuljagaPetchel K: Inadvertent intrathecal use of ionic contrast media for myelography, *Amer J Neuro* 13:1515, 1992.
26. Bonelli S, Conoscente F, Movilia PG, et al: Regional intravenous guanethidine vs. stellate ganglion block in reflex sympathetic dystrophies; a randomized trial, *Pain* 16: 297, 1983.
27. Bonica JJ: Regional anesthesia with tetracaine, *Anesthesiology* 11:606, 1950.
28. Bonica JJ: *The management of pain,* Philadelphia, 1953, Lea & Febiger.
29. Bonica JJ, Buckley FP: Regional anesthesia with local anesthetics. In Bonica JJ, editor: *The management of pain,* ed 2, Philadelphia, 1990, Lea & Febiger.
30. Boyd AM, Ratcliff AH, Jepson RP, et al: Intermittent claudication, *J Bone Joint Surg* 3:325, 1949.
31. Brechner T: Regional analgesia: local anesthetics and neurolytic agents. In Raj PP, editor: *Practical management of pain,* ed 2, St. Louis, 1992, Mosby–Year Book.
32. Breivick H, Hesla PE, Molnar I, et al: Treatment of chronic low back pain and sciatica: comparison of caudal epidural steroid injections of bupivacaine and methylprednisolone with bupivacaine followed by saline. In Bonica JJ, AlbeFessard

D, editors: *Advances in pain research and therapy,* New York, 1976, Raven Press.

33. Bridenbaugh LD, Moore OC, Campbell DD: Management of upper abdominal cancer pain, *JAMA* 190:99, 1964.
34. Bridenbaugh PO, Cousins MJ: *Neural blockade in clinical anesthesia and management of pain,* Philadelphia, JB Lippincott.
35. Brown D: Personal communication.
36. Brown FW: Management of discogenic pain using epidural and intrathecal steroids, *Clin Orthop* 129:72, 1977.
37. Brown FW: Protocol for management of acute low back pain with or without radiculopathy, including the use of epidural and intrathecal steroids. In Brown FW, editor: *American Academy of Orthopedic Surgeons Symposium on the Lumbar Spine,* St. Louis, 1981, CV Mosby.
38. Burkel WE, McPhee M: Effect of phenol injection into peripheral nerve of rat; electron microscope studies, *Arch Phys Med Rehab* 51:391, 1970.
39. Bush WH, Swanson DP: Acute reactions to intravascular contrast media: Types, risk factors, recognition, and specific treatment, *Amer J Roentgenol* 157:1153, 1991.
40. Buy JN, Muss AA, Singler RC: CT guided celiac plexus and splanchnic nerve neurolysis, *J Com Assist Tomogr* 6:315, 1982.
41. Carrera GF: Lumbar facet joint injection in low back pain and sciatica; preliminary results, *Radiology* 137:665, 1980.
42. Carrera GF, Williams AL, Haughton VM: Computed tomography in sciatica, *Radiology* 137:433, 1980.
43. Carron H: The changing role of the anesthesiologist in pain management, *Reg Anesth* 14:4, 1989.
44. Carron H, Litwiller R: Stellate ganglion, *Anesthe Analg* 54:567, 1975.
45. Carron H, Toomey TC: Epidural steroid therapy for low back pain. In Stanton-Hicks ME, Boas RA, editors: *Chronic low back pain,* New York, 1982, Raven Press.
46. Cohen FL: Conus medullaris syndrome following intrathecal corticosteroid injections, *Arch Neurol* 36:228, 1979.
47. Coomes EN: A comparison between epidural anaesthesia and bed rest in sciatica, *Brit Med J* 1:20, 1961.
48. Copping J, Willix R, Kraft R: Palliative chemical splanchnicectomy, *Arch Surg* 98:418, 1969.
49. Cousins MJ, Reeves TS, Glynn CJ, et al: Neurolytic lumbar sympathetic blockade; duration of denervation and relief of rest pain, *Anaesth Intens Care* 7:121, 1979.
50. Cremer SA, Maynard F, Davidoff G: The reflex sympathetic dystrophy syndrome associated with traumatic myelopathy; report of 5 cases, *Pain* 37:187, 1989.
51. Cuckler JM, Bernini PA, Wiesel SM, et al: The use of epidural steroids in the treatment of lumbar radicular pain, *J Bone Joint Surg* 67:63, 1985.
52. Dam WH: Therapeutic blockade, *Acta Chair Scand* 343:89, 1965.
53. Davidson JT, Robin CG: Epidural injections in the lumbosciatic syndrome, *Brit J Anaesth* 33:595, 1961.
54. De Takats G: Discussion of paper by HS Ruth: diagnostic, prognostic and therapeutic nerve blocks, *JAMA* 102:419, 1934.
55. Delaney TJ, Rawlingson JC, Carron H, et al: Epidural steroid effects on nerves and meninges, *Anesth Analg* 59:610, 1980.
56. Destouet JM, Gilula LA, Murphy WA, et al: Lumbar facet joint injection: indication, technique, clinical correlation, and preliminary results, *Radiology* 145:321, 1982.
57. Deyo RA, Diehl AK, Rosenthal M: How many days of bed rest for acute low back pain? A randomized clinical trial, *N Engl J Med* 315:1064, 1986.
58. Dhuner KG, Edshage S, Wilhelm A: Ninhydrin test: objective method for testing local anesthetic drugs, *Acta Anaesth Scand* 4:189, 1960.
59. Dilke TFW, Burry HC, Grahame R: Extradural corticosteroid injection in management of lumbar nerve root compression, *Brit Med J* 2:635, 1973.
60. Dondelinger TF, Kurdziel JC: Percutaneous phenol block of the upper thoracic sympathetic chain with computer tomography guidance, *Acta Radiologica* 28:511, 1987.
61. Dory MA: Arthrography of the lumbar facet joints, *Radiology* 140:23, 1981.
62. Doughtery JH, Fraser RH: Complications following intraspinal injections of steroids, *J Neurosurg* 48:1023, 1978.
63. Driessen JJ, et al: Clinical effects of regional intravenous guanetidine (Ismelin) in reflex sympathetic dystrophy, *Acta Anaesth Scand* 27:505, 1983.
64. DuPen SL, Peterson DG, Bogosian AC, et al: A new permanent exteriorized epidural catheter for narcotic self-administration to control cancer pain, *Cancer* 59:986, 1987.
65. Dwyer B, Gibb D: Chronic pain and neurolytic neural blockade. In Cousins MJ, Bridenbaugh PO, editors: *Neural blockade clinical anesthesia and management of pain,* Philadelphia, 1980, JB Lippincott.
66. Faden AL, Petras JM: An interspinal sympathetic preganglionic pathway: anatomic evidence in the dog, *Brain Res* 144:358, 1978.
67. Felsenthal G: Pharmacology of phenol in peripheral nerve blocks: a review, *Arch Phys Med Rehab* 55:13, 1974.
68. Ferreira SH: Prostaglandin: peripheral and central analgesia. In Bonica JJ, editor: *Advances in pain research and therapy,* vol 5, New York, 1983, Raven Press.
69. Ferrer-Brechner T: Epidural and intrathecal phenol neurolysis for cancer pain: review of rationale and techniques, *Anesth Rev* 8:14, 1981.
70. Filshier J, Golding S, Robbie DS, et al: Unilateral computerized tomography guided celiac plexus block: a technique for pain relief, *Anaesthesia* 38:498, 1983.
71. Fischer AA: Thermography and pain, *Arch Phys Med Rehab* 62:542, 1981.
72. Fisher E, Cress RH, Haines G, et al: Evoked nerve conduction after nerve block by chemical means, *Am J Phys Med* 49: 333, 1970.
73. Fowler RJ, Blackwell GJ: Antiinflammatory steroids induce biosynthesis of an phospholipase A, inhibitor which prevents prostaglandin generation, *Nature* 28:456, 1979.
74. Friedenberg ZB, Shoemaker RC: The results of nonoperative treatment of ruptured lumbar discs, *Am J Surg* 88:933, 1954.
75. Friedman M, Dougherty R, Nelson SR, et al: Acute effects of an aerosol hair spray on tracheal mucociliary transport, *Am Rev Respir Dis* 116:281, 1977.
76. Galizia EJ, Lahiri SK: Paraplegia following coeliac plexus bloc with phenol, *Br J Anaesth* 46:539, 1974.
77. Gardner DA: The use of ethyl chloride spray to relieve somatic pain, *J Am Osteopath Assoc* 49:525, 1950.
78. Ghelman B, Doherty FH: Demonstration of spondylolysis by arthrography of the apophyseal joint, *AJR* 130:986, 1978.
79. Ghelman B, Goldman AB: Lumbar facet injection. In Goldman AB, editor: *Procedures in skeletal radiology,* ed 1, Orlando, 1984, Grune & Stratton.
80. Glover JR, Chir B: Arthrography of the joint of the lumbar vertebral arches, *Orthop Clin North Am* 8:37, 1977.
81. Glynn CJ, Basedow RW, Walsh JA: Pain relief following postganglionic sympathetic blockade with IV guanetidine, *J Anesth* 1297, 1981.
82. Goebert HW, Jallo ST, Gardner WS, et al: Painful radiculopathy treated with epidual injections of procaine and hydrocortisone acetate: result in 113 patients, *Anesth Curr Res* 40:130, 1961.
83. Gorbitz C, Leavens ME: Alcohol block of the celiac plexus for control of upper abdominal pain caused by cancer and pancreatitis, *J Neurosurg* 34:575, 1971.
84. Gordon J: Caudal extradural injection for the treatment of low back pain, *Anaesthesia* 35:553, 1987.
85. Granstrom E: Biochemistry of the prostaglandins, thromboxanes, and leukotrienes. In Bonica JJ, Lindblom U, Iggo A, editors: *Advances in pain research and therapy,* vol 5, New York, 1983, Raven Press.
86. Grant RT, Holing HE: Further observations on vascular responses of human limb to body warming; evidence for sympathetic vasodilator nerves in human subjects, *Clin Sci* 3:273, 1938.
87. Green LN: Dexamethasone in the management of symptoms due to herniated lumbar disc, *J Neurol Neurosurg Psychiatr* 38: 1211, 1975.
88. Green PWB, Burke AJ, Weiss CA, et al: The role of epidural cortison injection of treatment of discogenic low back pain, *Clin Orthop* 153:121, 1980.
89. Greenwood JJ, McGuire TH, Kimbell F: A study of the causes of failure in the herniated intervertebral disc operation, *J Neurosurg* 9:15, 1952.
90. Gregg RV, Constantini CH, Ford DJ, et al: Electrophysiologic and histopathologic investigation of phenol in renografin as a neurolytic agent, *Anesthesiology* 63:A239, 1985.
91. Greiner L, Vlatowsk L, Prohm P: Sonographically guided and intraoperative alcohol block of the celiac ganglia in conservatively uncontrolled cancer induced epigastric pain, *Ultrashall Med* 4:57, 1983.
92. Hadley LA: Anatomicoroentgenographic

studies of the posterior spinal articulations, *AJR* 86:270, 1961.

93. Hankemeier V: Neurolytic celiac plexus block for cancer related upper abdominal pain using the unilateral puncture technique and lateral position, *Pain* 4:S135, 1987.
94. Hannington-Kiff JG: Intravenous regional sympathetic block with guanethidine, *Lancet* 1019, 1974.
95. Hannington-Kiff JG: Relief of Sudeck's atrophy by regional intravenous guanethidine, *Lancet* 1:1132, 1977.
96. Hannington-Kiff JG: Relief of causalgia in limbs by regional intravenous guanethidine, *Br Med J* 367, 1979.
97. Hansebout RR, Cosgrove JBR: Effects of intrathecal phenol in man: a histological study, *Neurology* 16:277, 1966.
98. Harley C: Extradural corticosteroid infiltration. A followup study of 50 cases, *Ann Phys Med* 9:22, 1967.
99. Harriman DGF, Summer DF, Ellis FR: Malignant hyperpyrexia myopathy, *Quart J Med* 42:639, 1973.
100. Haxton HA: Chemical sympathectomy, *Br Med J* 1:1026, 1949.
101. Hay RC: Subarachnoid alcohol blocks in the control of intractable pain: report of results in 252 patients, *Anaesth Analg* 41:12, 1962.
102. Hegedus V: Relief of pancreatic pain by radiography guided block, *AJR* 133:1101, 1979.
103. Heyse-Moore G: A rational approach to the use of epidural medication in the treatment of sciatic pain, *Acta Orthop Scand* 49:36, 1978.
104. Hoffman HH: An analysis of the sympathetic trunk and rami in the cervial and upper thoracic regions in man, *Ann Surg* 145:94, 1957.
105. Holland JR: The causalgia syndrome treated with regional intravenous guanethidine, *Clin Exp Neurol* 15:166, 1978.
106. Iggo A, Walsh EG: Selective block of small fibres in the spinal roots by phenol, *Brain* 83:701, 1960.
107. Ingle JI, Beveridge EE: *Endodontics,* ed 2, Philadelphia, 1976, Lea & Febiger.
108. Ischia S, Luzzani A, Ischia A, et al: A new approach to the neurolytic block of the celiac plexus: the transaortic technique, *Pain* 16(333):1983.
109. Jackson SH, Jacobs JB, Epstein RA: A radiographic approach to celiac plexus block, *Anesthesiology* 31:373, 1969.
110. Jacobs JB, Jackson SH, Doppman JL: A radiography approach to celiac ganglion block, *Radiology* 92:1372, 1969.
111. Jamieson RW, Smith DB, Anson BJ: The cervical sympathetic ganglia. An anatomical study of 100 cervicothoracic dissections, *Quart Bull NW Univ Med Sch* 26:219, 1952.
112. Kappis M: *Ertahrungen mit Local-anasthesiadej Bauchuperationen,* Verhandl der Deutsch Gesellsch 1 Chir 43:87, 1914.
113. Karsteadt N: Personal communication.
114. Kelly RE, Gautheir-Smith PC: Intrathecal phenol in the treatment of reflex spasms and spasticity, *Lancet* 2:1102, 1959.
115. Kelman H: Epidural injection therapy for sciatic pain, *Am J Surg* 64:183, 1944.
116. Kepes ER, Duncalf D: Treatment of backache with spinal injections of local anesthetics, spinal and systemic steroids. A review, *Pain* 22:33, 1985.
117. Kepes ER, Duncalf D: Treatment of backache with spinal injections of local anesthetics, spinal and systemic steroids. A review, *Pain* 22:33, 1985.
118. Knight CL, Burnell JC: Systemic side-effects of extradural steroids, *Anaesthesia* 35:593, 1980.
119. Knott LW, Katz J, Rubenstein LJ: Separate and combined effects of phenol, hyaluronidase, and dimethyl sulfoxide on the sciatic nerve of the rat, *Arch Phys Med Rehab* 49:100, 1968.
120. Kohlrausch W: Die sportbehindernden Wirkungen muskularer Erkankungen, *Med Klin* 32:1420, 1936.
121. Korevaar WC, Kline MT, Donnelly CC: Thoracic epidural neurolysis using alcohol, *Pain Suppl* 4:S133, 1987.
122. Kraus H: *Clinical treatment of back and neck pain,* New York, 1970, McGrawHill.
123. Kuntz A: *The autonomic nervous system,* Philadelphia, 1953, Lea & Febiger.
124. Kuntz A: Components of splanchnic and intermesenteric nerves, *J Comp Neurol* 105:251, 1956.
125. Labat G, Greene MB: Contributions to the modern method of diagnosis and treatment of socalled sciatic neuralgias, *Am J Surg* 11:435, 1931.
126. Larson SJ, Sances A, Cusick JF, et al: A comparison between anterior and posterior spinal implant systems, *Surg Neurol* 4:180, 1975.
127. Lemrow N, Adams D, Coffey R, et al: *The 50 most frequent diagnosis-related groups (DRG's), diagnoses and procedures: statistics by hospital size and location,* DHHS Publication no. (PHS) 90-3465, Hospital Studies Program Research Note 13, Agency for Health Care Policy and Research, Public Health Service, Rockville, 1990.
128. Leriche R: Simple methods in easing pain in the extremities in arterial diseases and in certain vasomotor disorders, *Pres Med* 49:799, 1941.
129. Leung JW, BowenWright M, Aveling W, et al: Coeliac plexus block for pain in pancreatic cancer and chronic pancreatitis, *Br J Surg* 70:730, 1983.
130. Lewin T, Moffett B, Viidik A: The morphology of the lumbar synovial intervertebral joints, *Acta Morphol Neerl Scand* 4:299, 1961.
131. Lindahl O, Rexed B: Histolic changes in spinal nerve roots of operated cases of sciatica, *Acta Orthop Scand* 20:215, 1950.
132. Loh L, et al: Effects of regional guanethidine infusion in certain painful states, *J Neurol Neurosurg Psych* 43:446, 1980.
133. Long DN, Erickson DE, Campbell J, et al: Electrical stimulation of the spinal cord and peripheral nerves for pain control—10 years experience, *Appl Neurophysiol* 44:207, 1981.
134. Maher RM: *Phenol for pain and spasticity,* Pain: Henry Ford Hospital International Symposium, Boston, 1966, Little Brown.
135. Maldague B, Maturin P, Malghen J: Facet arthrography in lumbar spondylolysis, *Radiology* 140:29, 1981.
136. Mandl F: *Die paravertebral injection,* Vienna, 1926, SpringerVerlag.
137. Mandl F: *Paravertebral block,* New York, 1947, Grune & Stratton.
138. Mandl F: Aqueous solution of phenol as a substitute for alcohol insympathetic block, *J Int Coll Surg* 13:566, 1950.
139. Marshall LL, Trethwie ER: Chemical irritation of nerve root in disc prolapse, *Lancet* 2:230, 1973.
140. Matsuki M, Kato Y, Ichiyangi L: Progressive changes in the concentrations of ethyl alcohol in the human and canine subarachnoid space, *Anesthesiology* 36: 617, 1972.
141. McKain CW, Bruno JU, Goldner JL: The effects of intravenous regional guanethidine and reserpine, *J Bone Joint Surg* 6: 808, 1983.
142. Mennell J: Spraystretch for relief of pain from muscle spasm and myofascial trigger points, *J Am Podiatr Assoc* 6:873, 1976.
143. Mennell JM: The therapeutic use of cold, *J Am Osteopath Assoc* 74:1146, 1975.
144. Merskey H, Boduk N: *Classification of chronic pain syndomes and definition of pain terms,* Seattle, 1994, IASP Press: p. 210.
145. Meyerson BA, Broden E, Linderoth B: Possible neurohumoral mechanisms in CNS stimulation for pain suppression, *Appl Neurophysiol* 48(175):1985.
146. Miehlke K, Schulze G, Eger W: Klinische und experimentelle untersuchungen zum fibrositissyndrome, Z Rheumaforsch 1: 310, 1960.
147. Mitchell GAG: *Anatomy of the autonomic nervous system,* Edinburgh, 1953, E & S Livingstone.
148. Modell W, Travell J, et al: Treatment of painful disorders of skeletal muscle, NY *State J Med* 48:2050, 1948.
149. Modell W, Travell J, Kraus H, et al: Relief of pain by ethyl chloride spray, *NY State J Med* 52:1550, 1952.
150. Moller JE, Helweg-Larson J, Jacobsen E: Histopathological lesions in the sciatic nerve of the rat following perineural application of phenol and alcohol solutions, *Dan Med Bull* 16:116, 1969.
151. Monro PAG: *Sympathectomy,* London, 1959, Oxford University Press.
152. Mooney V, Robertson JU: The facet syndrome, *Clin Orthop* 115:149, 1976.
153. Moore DC: *Stellate ganglion block,* Springfield, 1954, Charles C Thomas.
154. Moore DC: *Regional block,* ed 4, Springfield, 1975, Charles C Thomas.
155. Moore DC: Celiac (splachnic) plexus block with alcohol for cancer pain of the upper intraabdominal viscera. In Bonica JJ, Ventafridda V, editors: *Pain research and therapy,* vol 2, New York, 1979, Raven Press.
156. Moore DC, Bush WH, Burnett LL: Celiac plexus block: a roentgenographic, anatomic study of technique and spread of solution in patients and corpses, *Anesth Analg* 60:369, 1981.
157. Murphy RW: Nerve roots and spinal nerves in degenerated disc disease, *Clin Orthop* 129:46, 1977.

158. Nade S, Bell E, Wyke BD: The innervation of the lumbar spinal joints and its significance, *J Bone Joint Surg* 62:255, 1980.
159. Nathan PW: Intrathecal phenol to relieve spasticity in paraplegia, *Lancet* 2:1099, 1959.
160. Nathan PW, Sears TA: Effects of phenol on nervous conduction, *J Physiol* (London) 150:565, 1960.
161. Nathan PW, Sears TA, Smith MC: Effects of phenol solutions on the nerve roots of the cat: an electrophysiologic and histological study, *J Neurol Sci* 2:7, 1965.
162. Nechaev VA: *Solutions of phenol in local anesthesia,* Soviet Khir 5:203, 1933.
163. Nelson DA, Vates TS, Thomas RB: Complications from intrathecal steroid therapy in patients with multiple sclerosis, *Acta Neurol Scand* 49:176, 1973.
164. North RB, Ewend MG, Lawton MT, et al: Failed back surgery syndrome: five year follow up after spinal cord stimulator implantation, *Neurosurgery* 28:692, 1991.
165. Owitz S, Koppolu S: Celiac plexus block: an overview, *Mt Sinai J Med* 50:486, 1983.
166. Parisien V: Conservative treatment of low back pain with epidural steroids, *J Med Assoc* 71:83, 1980.
167. Park WM, McCall JW, Benson D, et al: Spondylarthrography: the demonstration of spondylolysis by apophyseal joint arthrography, *Clin Radiol* 36:247, 1980.
168. Pearce J, Moll JMH: Conservative treatment and natural history of acute lumbar disc lesions, *J Neurol Neurosurg Psychiatr* 30:13, 1967.
169. Pederson HE, Blunck CFJ, Gardiner E: The anatomy of lumbosacral posterior rami and meningeal branches of spinal nerves (sinuvertebral nerves), *J Bone Joint Surg* 38(A):377, 1956.
170. Pither CE, Raj PP: The use of peripheral nerve stimulators for regional anesthesia: a review of experimental characteristics, techniques, and clinical applications, *Reg Anaesth* 10:2, 1985.
171. Pizzolato P, Mannheimer W: *Histopathologic effects of local anesthetic drugs and related substances,* Springfield, 1961, Charles C Thomas.
172. Plancarte R, et al: Hypogastric plexus block: retroperitoneal approach, *Anesthesiology* 71:A739, 1989.
173. Plummer JL, Cherry DA, Cousins MJ, et al: Long term spinal administration of morphine in cancer and non-cancer pain: a retrospective study, *Pain* 44:215, 1991.
174. Popelianskii II, Zaslavskii ES, Veselovskii VP: Medicosocial significance, etiology, pathogenesis, and diagnosis of nonarticular disease of soft tissues of the limbs and back (Russian), *Vopr Revm* 3:38, 1976.
175. Prudden B: Pain erasure: *the Bonnie Prudden way,* New York, 1980, M Evans.
176. Putnam TJ, Hampton AO: A technique of injection into the gasserian ganglion under roentegenographic control, *Arch Neurol Psychiatr* 35:92, 1936.
177. Racz G: *Techniques of neurolysis,* Boston, 1989, Kluwer Academie Publishing.
178. Raj PP, Knarr D, Vigdorth E, et al: Difference in analgesia following epidural blockade in patients with postoperative or chronic low back pain, *Pain* 34:21, 1988.
179. Raj PP, Rosenblatt R, Montgomery SJ: Use of the nerve stimulator for peripheral blocks, *Reg Anaesth* 5:19, 1980.
180. Randall WC, Cox JW, Alexander WF: Direct examination of the sympathetic outflows in man, *J Appl Physiol* 7:688, 1955.
181. Raskin NH, Levinson SA, Hoffman PM, et al: Postsympathectomy neuralgia amelioration with diphenylhydantoin and carbamazepine, *Am J Surg* 128:75, 1974.
182. Raymond J, Dumas J: Intraarticular facet block: diagnostic test or therapeutic procedure? *Radiology* 151:333, 1984.
183. Reid W, Watt JK, Gray TG: Phenol injection of the sympathetic chain, *Fr J Surg* 57:45, 1970.
184. Renaer M: *Chronic pelvic pain in women,* New York, 1981, SpringerVerlag.
185. Risius B, Mordic MT, Hardy RW, et al: Sector computed tomographic spine scanning in the diagnosis of lumbar root entrapment, *Radiology* 143:109, 1982.
186. Rizzi R, Biscvola G, Visentin M: Celiac plexus block: how anatomical alterations due to cancer growth can modify diffusion of contract medium, *Pain Suppl* 4:S135, 1987.
187. Roberts M, Shepard GL, McCormick RL: Tuberculosis meningitis after intrathecally administered methylprednisolone acetate, *JAMA* 200:894, 1967.
188. Ruhmann W: Muskelrheuma and tastmassage 2. Muskelrheumatische disposition, *Med Klin* 27:1242, 1931.
189. Schaumberg HN, Byck R, Weller RO: The effect of phenol on peripheral nerves: A histological and electrophysiological study, *J Neuropathol Exp Neurol* 29:615, 1970.
190. Schlosser H: Erfahrungen in der neuralgiebehandlung mit alkoholeinspritzungen, *Verh Dtsch Ges Inn Med* 24:49, 1907.
191. Shealy CN: Dangers of spinal injections without proger diagnosis, *JAMA* 197:1104, 1966.
192. Shealy CN, Mortimer JT, Reswick J: Electrical inhibition of pain by stimulation of the dorsal column: preliminary reports, *Anesth Analg* 46:489, 1967.
193. Singler RC: An improved technique for alcohol neurolysis of the celiac plexus, *Anesthesiology* 56:137, 1982.
194. Snoek W, Weber H, Jorgensen B: Double blind evaluation of extradural methylprednisolone for herniated lumbar discs, *Acta Orthop Scand* 48:635, 1977.
195. Sola AE, Kuitert JH: Myofascial trigger point pain in the neck and shoulder girdle, *Northwest Med* 54:980, 1955.
196. Sola AE, Williams RL: Myofascial pain syndromes, *Neurology* 6:91, 1956.
197. Spiegelmann R, Friedman W: Spinal cord stimulation: a contemporary series, *Neurosurgery* 28:65, 1991.
198. Stenger RJ, Spiro D, Scully RE, et al: Ultrastructural and physiologic alterations in ischemic skeletal muscle, *Am J Pathol* 40:1, 1962.
199. Sternbach RA: Physiological aspects of chronic pain, *Clin Orthop* 129:150, 1977.
200. Stewart WA, Lourie H: An experimental evaluation of the effects of subarachnoid injection of phenolpantopaque in cats, *J Neurosurg* 20:64, 1963.
201. Stolberg HO, Mc Clennan BL: Ionic versus nonionic contrast, *Curr Prob Diagn Radiol* 20:47, 1991.
202. Swerdlow M: Subarachnoid and extradural neurolytic block. In Bonica JJ, Ventafridda V, editors: *Advances in pain research and therapy,* vol 2, New York, 1979, Raven Press.
203. Swerdlow M: Intrathecal and extradural block in pain relief. In Swerdlow M, editor: *Relief of intractable pain,* ed 3, Amsterdam, 1984, Elsevier Scientific.
204. Swerdlow M, SayleCreer W: A study of extradural medication in the relief of lumbosciatic syndrome, *Anaesthesia* 25:341, 1970.
205. Thompson GE, Moore DC, Bridenbaugh LD, et al: Abdominal pain and alcohol celiac plexus nerve block, *Anesth Analg* 56:1, 1977.
206. Travell J: Basis for the multiple uses of local block of somatic trigger areas (procaine infiltration and ethyl chloride spray), *Miss Valley Med J* 71:13, 1949.
207. Travell J: Ethyl chloride spray for painful muscle spasm, *Arc Phys Med Rehab* 33: 291, 1952.
208. Travell J: Rapid relief of acute "stiff neck" by ethyl chloride spray, *J Am Med Wom Assoc* 4:89, 1959.
209. Travell J: Identification of myofascial trigger point syndromes: a case of atypical facial neuralgia, *Arch Phys Med Rehab* 62: 100, 1981.
210. Travell J, Simmons DG: *Myofascial pain and dysfunction. The trigger point manual,* Baltimore, 1983, Williams & Wilkins.
211. Van Buskirk, Poffenbarger AL, Capriles LF, et al: Treatment of multiple sclerosis with intrathecal steroids, *Neurology* (Minneapolis) 14:595, 1964.
212. Warr AC, Wilkinson JA, Burn JMB, et al: Chronic lumbosciatic syndrome treated by epidural injection and manipulation, *Practitioner* 209:53, 1972.
213. Wechsler RJ, Maurer PM, Halpern EJ, et al: Superior hypogastric plexus block for chronic pelvic pain in endometriosis: CT techniques and results, *Radiology* 196:103, 1995.
214. White AH, Derby R, Wynne G: Epidural injections for the diagnosis and treatment of low back pain, *Spine* 5:78, 1980.
215. Williams HL, Elkins EC: Myalgia of the head, *Arch Phys Ther* 23:14, 1942.
216. Winnie AP, Hartman JT, Meyers HL, et al: Pain Clinic II: intradural and extradural corticosteroids for sciatica, *Anesth Analg* 54:370, 1972.
217. Wood K: The use of phenol as a neurolytic agent: a review, *Pain* 5:205, 1978.
218. Wood KM, Arguelles J, Norenberg MD: Degenerative lesions in rat sciatic nerves after local injections of methylprednisolone in aqueous solution, *Reg Anesth* 5:13, 1980.
219. Woolsley RM, Taylor JJ, Nagel JH: Acute effects of topical ethyl alcohol on the sciatic nerve of the mouse, *Arch Phys Med Rehab* 53:410, 1972.
220. Yaksh TL, Rudy TA: Analgesia mediated by a direct spinal action of narcotics, *Science* 192:1357, 1976.
221. Yates DW: A comparison of the types of epidural injection commonly used in the treatment of low back pain and sciatica, *Rheumatol Rehab* 17:181, 1978.
222. Zohn DA, Mennell JM: *Musculoskeletal pain: diagnosis and treatment,* Boston, 1976, Little Brown.

CHAPTER 64

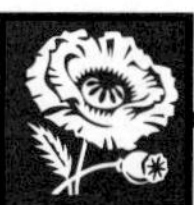

Spinal and Epidural Opioids

RAYMOND S. SINATRA
CEPHAS P. SWAMIDOSS

The remarkable increase in analgesic efficacy provided by intrathecal and epidurally administered opioids has clearly advanced the management of postsurgical, obstetric, and chronic pain. Rarely has a concept so rapidly progressed from preliminary laboratory observations to successful applications in clinical medicine.[237] Acceptance of such therapy was facilitated by two factors. First, a number of anesthesiologists experienced with spinal/epidural techniques became familiar with department-sponsored basic research and appreciated the clinical applications of this relatively novel concept. Second, the gains in analgesic intensity and duration were far superior to those achieved with parenterally administered opioids. This ability to provide nearly complete relief of severe malignancy-associated and postsurgical pain impressed both patients and clinicians and mandated follow-up evaluation in a variety of clinical settings.[228] During the past 15 years, thousands of literature citations have confirmed the efficacy of spinally acting (neuraxial) opioids.

EXPERIMENTAL PHARMACOLOGY AND INITIAL CLINICAL STUDIES

Although systemically administered opioids have been known to influence spinal function,[114] definitive neurophysiologic studies performed in the early 1970s[41,119,120] demonstrated that morphine selectively suppressed dorsal horn lamina I and V neurons, which mediate noxious information, yet had no effect on lamina IV neurons, which process light touch and proprioceptive input. The fact that enkephalin-containing neurons and opioid receptors were almost exclusively localized to the substantia gelatinosa provided evidence of an intrinsic spinal modulatory system whose activation could attenuate release of substance-P and other nociceptive transmitters.[10,119,127,171,243, 244,245] This concept was substantiated by Duggan et al.[78] who noted selective inhibition of nociceptive transmission following iontophoretic administration of opiates directly into substantia gelantinosa.

A number of behavioral investigations added to the understanding of spinal opioid analgesia. In a combined behavioral-autoradiographic study,[162] peak suppression of noxious stimulation in rats correlated with the time that highest concentrations of intrathecally administered 3H-morphine had penetrated into substantia gelatinosa. In primates, intrathecal morphine significantly elevated response thresholds to noxious stimuli.[241,242] Analgesic benefits were dose dependent, antagonized by naloxone and exhibited tolerance that could be reversed by alpha-2 and serotonin agonists. This effect was quite selective, because non-nociceptive sensation was unaffected.[242]

Based on different behavioral responses observed in animal models, three major opioid receptor subtypes appear to modulate nociceptive input in the substantia gelatinosa.[144,145,197,198] Activation of mu and delta receptors produced dose-dependent inhibition of cutaneous thermal responses (hot plate, tail flick), whereas activation of kappa receptors resulted in suppression of visceral chemical responses (writhing) while having no effect on somatic nociception. A recent investigation employing a different opioid agonist, stimulus and animal model,[104] provided conflicting data suggesting that spinal mu and delta receptors may play the major role in modulating visceral nociception. Other behavioral evaluations provided reassuring evidence that spinally administered opioids had little neurotoxic potential. Yaksh reported that macaque monkeys given epidural morphine for up to 16 months developed no abnormal neurohistologic changes or neurologic dysfunction.[241]

Wang et al.,[231,232] familiar with ongoing behavioral research in primates, took the requisite first step and employed spinal opioids to treat eight patients with intractable pain related to genitourinary tract malignancy. In this double-blind study, patients receiving intrathecal morphine (0.5 mg and 1 mg) experienced complete relief of pain lasting 12 to 24 hours, whereas others treated with parenteral morphine reported less effective analgesia. Although excessive sedation, pruritus, and respiratory depression were not reported, the patients enrolled in the study were most likely tolerant to these effects, having received parenteral opioids for prolonged periods of time. Despite the small size of this preliminary evaluation, its findings were soon recognized as among the most important recent advances in anesthesiology.[237] The term "selective" spinal analgesia[61,200] was coined to underscore the therapeutic advantage of neuraxial opioids over local anesthetics in blocking pain. Although it was recognized that selective spinal analgesia involved suppression of synaptic transmission and neuronal excitation rather than nonselective blockade of axonal conduction, little was known regarding opioid kinetics in cerebrospinal fluid (CSF) or the extent and importance of vascular uptake. Although spinal opioid analgesia avoided the hypotension, convulsions, and risk of cardiovascular collapse associated with the use of local anesthetics, the technique was soon associated with a number of its own unique and occasionally serious side effects. It became evident that controlled studies concerning pharmacokinetics and pharmacodynamics of neuraxial opioids were required to ensure safe clinical application.

NEURAXIAL OPIOIDS: PHARMACOKINETICS AND PHARMACODYNAMICS

The complex pharmacokinetics that follow intrathecal and epidural deposition of opioid analgesics have been outlined[59,60,98,208] and must be appreciated to understand the benefits and possible complications of spinal analgesia. Opioids deposited at either site provide effective dose-dependent neuraxial analgesia; however, epidural administration is complicated by factors related to dural penetration, absorption in fat, higher dose requirements and the consequences of systemic uptake.

Spinal Opioid Receptors

Activation of spinal opioid receptors is associated with decreased presynaptic release of nociceptive neurotransmitters as well as inhibition of postsynaptic responses. Opioid receptors are coupled to guanosine (G)—effector proteins, which mediate the changes in calcium and potassium ion flux and membrane polarity necessary to modulate nociceptive input.[239,241] Activation of kappa receptors directly inhibits substance P release at primary afferent terminals by blocking calcium influx required for transmitter release.[241,243] Mu and delta receptors appear to be coupled to voltage-dependent potassium channels.[239] In this regard, stimulation of mu and delta receptors leads to increased potassium conductance and neuronal hyperpolarization. This effect is mediated by G-protein inhibition of cyclic adenosine monophosphate synthesis and directly counters the pronounced decrease in potassium permeability caused by the nociceptive transmitter substance P (Fig. 64-1).[243] Antinociception induced by morphine is mediated by stimulation of mu, delta, and kappa receptors, whereas fentanyl analgesia is mediated by mu receptors only.[74] This ability to interact with a variety of receptor subtypes may underlie morphine's neuraxial specificity and high analgesic efficacy.

The term "affinity" describes the attraction and successful attachment of opioid ligands to the binding site, whereas "efficacy" characterizes the ability to activate the effector mechanisms.[114] In this regard, both naloxone and sufentanil have high receptor affinity; however, the antagonist has zero efficacy, whereas the agonist is a powerful activator of G-proteins. Opioid agonists that have high receptor efficacy require occupancy of fewer receptors to achieve a desired analgesic effect. The term "potency" correlates analgesic response versus dose requirement and is influenced by several factors, including receptor binding affinity and intrinsic efficacy.[108] At the spinal level, potency is also related to gains in analgesic effectiveness as compared with systemic administration of an equivalent dose.[225] Because spinal administration bypasses the blood–brain barrier, hydrophilic opi-

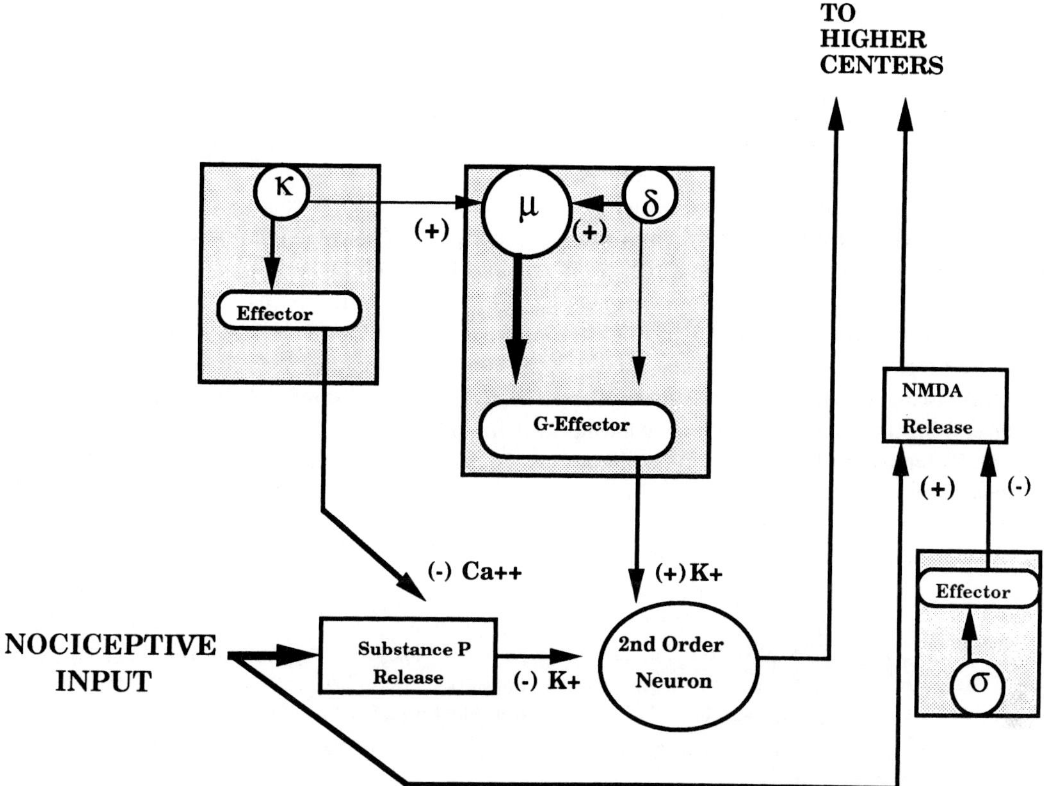

Fig. 64-1. Generalized overview of opioid receptor subtypes mediating spinal analgesia. Ligand specific binding at mu (μ) and delta (δ) subtypes result in receptor conformational changes and activation (coupling) of guanosine nucleotide effector proteins. Guanosine-protein activation inhibits adenylate cyclase resulting in decreased cyclic adenosine monophosphate (cAMP) synthesis, increased K^+ conductance, and neuronal hyperpolarization. Kappa (κ) receptors activate an uncharacterized effector protein, which decreases Ca^{++} ion flux required for substance P release. Sigma (σ) receptor subtypes modulate pain at supraspinal sites by inhibiting N-methyl-D-aspartate (NMDA) release. Mu and delta receptors may exist as a complex within the same neuron. Activation of delta and kappa subtypes may enhance mu receptor–mediated analgesia. (From Sinatra RS: Pharmacokinetics and pharmacodynamics of spinal opioids. In Sinatra RS, Hord AH, Ginsberg B, Preble LM, editors: *Acute pain: Mechanisms and management,* St Louis, 1992, Mosby–Year Book.)

oids such as morphine have increased receptor accessibility and gains in analgesic potency relative to systemic administration.[79,105,114,225] Analgesic efficacy is further increased when neuraxial opioids are administered prior to surgical injury.[29,238] When compared with intraoperative or postoperative dosing, preincisional "preemptive" administration of epidural morphine[161] and fentanyl[117] is associated with reductions in postsurgical pain scores and analgesic consumption.

Analgesic Onset

After intrathecal administration, the amount of drug that leaves the CSF and enters spinal tissues is inversely proportional to both its lipid solubility and pKa and directly influences time to analgesic onset.[59,60] **Lipophilic and weakly ionized opioids rapidly exit the aqueous CSF compartment and penetrate into lipid-rich spinal tissue to activate opiate receptors.**[60,75,121,175,210,211] In contrast, hydrophilic opioids such as morphine have difficulty traversing neural and vascular membranes and tend to remain in CSF. Morphine's delay in reaching spinal sites of activity underlies its observed latency to clinical onset and peak analgesic effect.[60,175,211] Additional delay has also been related to morphine's low intrinsic efficacy because a greater number of opioid receptors must be occupied to provide a similar intensity of spinal analgesia as that observed with potent agonists such as sufentanil.[73,216]

Differences in onset are further magnified following epidural administration. Lipophilic opioids traverse dural membranes easily and provide a rapid onset of analgesia.[175] Morphine penetrates the dura slowly and in proportion to the concentration gradient associated with epidural deposition. Factors other than lipid solubility may also delay analgesic onset. In a study evaluating drug transfer across cadaveric dura mater, morphine's globular chemical structure was associated with less efficient transport than that observed with the more spindle-shaped phenylpiperidine-based opioids.[150]

Duration and Analgesic Efficacy

Lipid solubility, polarity, and the amount of un-ionized drug remaining in CSF play key roles in determining duration of spinal analgesia.[60,175] **Unlike systemically administered opioids, drug metabolism does not influence the duration of spinal activity to a clinically significant degree.**[114] **In contrast, clearance from epidural and intrathecal sites of deposition plays a major role in determining duration of action. Principle routes of clearance include both rapid vascular absorption and slow rostral diffusion in CSF with elimination at the arachnoid granulations (Fig. 64-2).**[59,60,210] Increasing lipid solubility facilitates vascular uptake; therefore, this route of clearance has greater importance with lipophilic opioids such as fentanyl and sufentanil. As significant amounts of lipophilic drug are taken up by the epidural venous plexus and spinal blood vessels or become trapped in fatty tissues,[59,60] concentrations at sites of activity rapidly decline. Pregnancy, portal hypertension, and other conditions associated with epidural venous engorgement may further increase vascular uptake.[60,208]

Morphine's hydrophilic properties and polarity allow significant amounts of drug to remain sequestered in CSF for relatively long periods.[92,163,164] In this regard, morphine CSF concentrations approach 1000 ng/ml, or 1/200 of the injected epidural dose, 1 hour after administration.[164] A 0.5-mg bolus of intrathecal morphine results in CSF concentrations greater than 10,000 ng/ml, with barely detectable

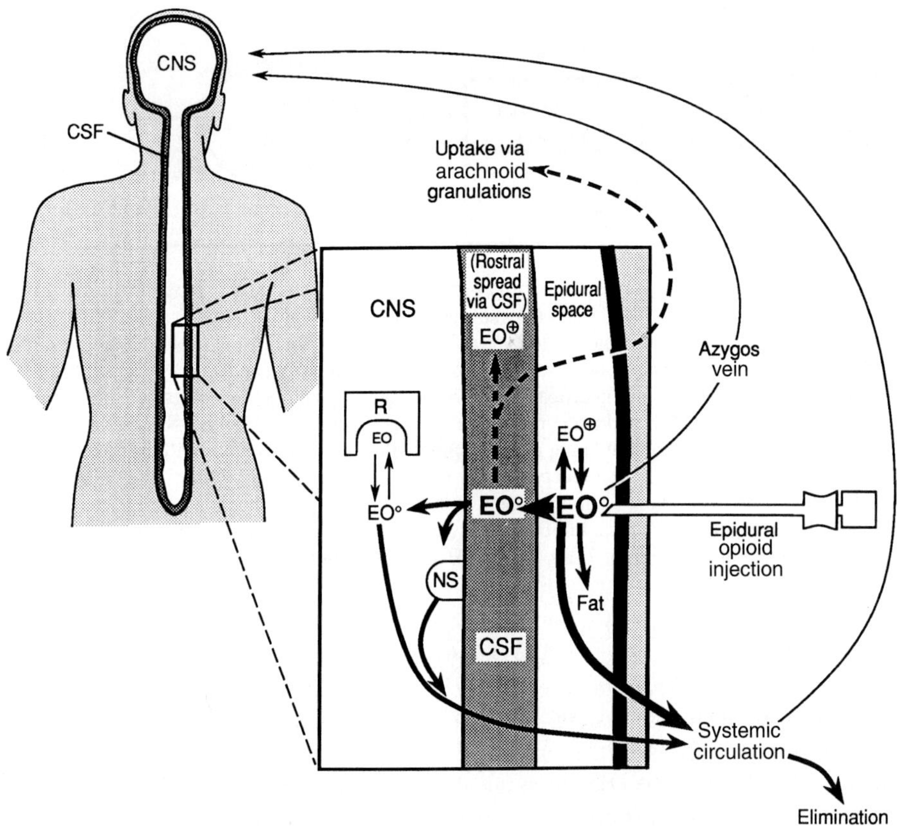

Fig. 64-2. Factors that influence dural penetration, cerebrospinal fluid (CSF) sequestration, and vascular clearance of epidurally administered opioids. The major portion of epidurally-administered opioids (EO) is taken up by the epidural and spinal blood vessels or absorbed into epidural fat. Molecules taken up by the epidural plexus and azygos system may be delivered to supraspinal centers and mediate central opioid effects. A smaller percentage of uncharged molecules (EO°) traverse the dura and enter CSF. Lipophilic opioids rapidly exit the CSF and penetrate spinal tissue. As with intrathecal dosing, the majority of these molecules are either trapped within lipid membranes (nonspecific binding sites [NS]) or are removed by spinal vascular uptake. A small fraction of molecules bind to and activate spinal opioid receptors (R). Hydrophilic opioids penetrate pia and arachnoid membranes and spinal tissue slowly. A larger proportion of these molecules remain sequestered in CSF and are slowly transported rostrally. This CSF depot permits more continuous spinal uptake, greater dermatomal spread, and a prolonged duration of activity. (From Sinatra RS: Pharmacokinetics and pharmacodynamics of spinal opioids. In Sinatra RS, Hord AH, Ginsberg B, Preble LM, editors: *Acute pain: Mechanisms and management,* St Louis, 1992, Mosby–Year Book.)

plasma levels.[163] Similar CSF pharmacokinetics have been observed with epidural and intrathecal bolus doses of hydromorphone.[36,175] Molecules trapped in CSF ensure continued receptor binding by replenishing those that have dissociated from spinal sites of activity. Lipid-soluble opioids that lack a CSF depot must be continually infused to extend their limited duration of activity.[220,253] Zakowski and colleagues[253] reported that a 25 μg bolus of fentanyl produced analgesic CSF levels of 200 ng/ml; however, concentrations declined to less than 50 ng/ml at 30 minutes and a nonanalgesic level of 15 ng/ml at 90 minutes. Receptor dissociation kinetics also influence analgesic duration, as agents associated with greater drug-receptor complex stability provide prolonged activity. Of the opioids used clinically, alfentanil has the shortest receptor dissociation kinetics, followed by fentanyl, sufentanil, methadone, morphine, and lofentanil.[108,112,114] Relationships between lipid physiochemistry and both onset and duration of epidural analgesia are presented in Table 64-1.

Total dose of opioid administered and volume of injectate represent two additional variables which may influence duration of activity and dermatomal spread of analgesia. With highly lipophilic agents, little or no change in analgesic duration was noted by increasing the epidural dose above a critical amount (fentanyl 75 to 100 μg, sufentanil 50 μg)[93,154,156,158]; however, dose-dependent prolongation of effect was observed with morphine.[129,164] Nordberg et al.[164] reported significant dose-related increases in epidural morphine analgesia, with 2, 4, and 6 mg providing 8.6, 13, and 15.6 hours of pain relief, respectively. Lanz et al.[129] evaluated the optimal dose of epidural morphine, noting that although 2 mg was the lowest dose capable of providing analgesia, 5 mg offered the longest duration of pain relief. Sjostrom et al.[213] observed no difference in CSF morphine levels when similar doses were administered in volumes of 1 or 10 ml. Nevertheless, we have found that larger volumes of injectate (10 to 15 ml) reduce the time required for lumbar epidural doses of morphine to control pain originating at higher dermatomal sites.[207] As described earlier, a significant proportion of lumbar epidural morphine gains access to CSF and is slowly transported rostrally.[33,59,210] This concept is important, for unlike local anesthetics which block nerve fibers at spinal segments immediately adjacent to their site of administration, opioids must migrate to higher levels (T6 to T12) in order to bind spinal receptors and block pain originating at higher dermatomes (Fig. 64-3). Gourlay et al.,[92] using similar size injectate volumes, noted that fentanyl, in contrast to morphine and meperidine, did not migrate to higher interspaces after lumbar epidural administration. This lack of rostral spread underlies fentanyl's "segmental" spinal analgesic profile that results from its rapid incorporation into epidural fat and vascular clearance from epidural and intrathecal sites of deposition. Dermatomal spread of lipophilic opioids appears to be directly related to the dural surface area in contact with the drug and may be increased following administration in larger volumes of solution.[20,155]

Table 64-1 Spinal opioid physiochemistry and pharmacodynamics

Opioid	Molecular weight	Lipid solubility*	Parenteral potency	pKa	Mu-receptor affinity	Dissociation kinetics	Potency gain (epidural vs. IV or SC)	Onset of analgesia	Duration of analgesia
Morphine	285	1.4	1	7.9	Moderate	Slow	10	Delayed	Prolonged
Meperidine	247	39	0.1	8.5	Moderate	Moderate	2–3	Rapid	Intermediate
Methadone	309	116	2	9.3	High	Slow	2	Rapid	Intermediate
Hydromorphone	285	1.9	8	—	High	Slow	4	Rapid	Intermediate
Alfentanil	417	129	25	6.5	High	Very rapid	1	Very rapid	Short
Fentanyl	336	816	80	8.4	High	Rapid	1	Very rapid	Short
Sufentanil	386	1727	800	8.0	Very high	Moderate	1	Very rapid	Short

IV — intravenous; SC — subcutaneous.
*Octanol-water partition coefficient (at pH of 7.4).
Data compiled from references 19, 108, 112, 114, 210.

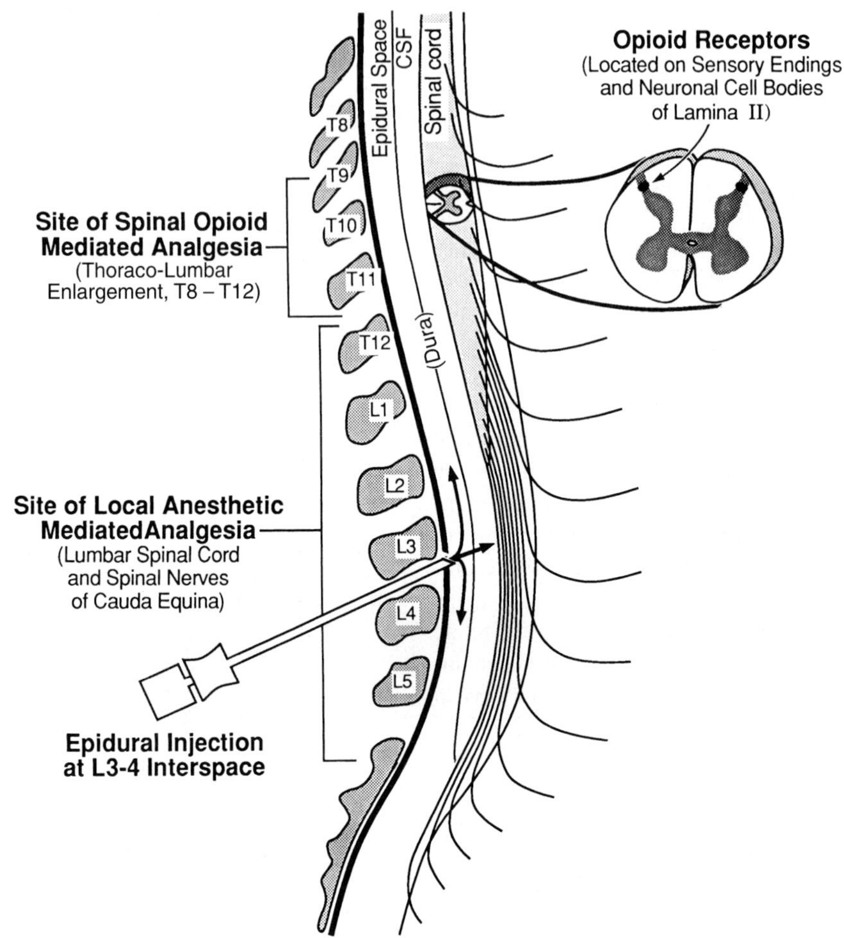

Fig. 64-3. Age versus 24-hour epidural morphine dose. Relationships between epidural deposition of opioid analgesics and local anesthetics in regard to sites of activity. (From Sinatra RS: Pharmacokinetics and pharmacodynamics of spinal opioids. In Sinatra RS, Hord AH, Ginsberg B, Preble LM, editors: *Acute pain: Mechanisms and management,* St Louis, 1992, Mosby–Year Book.)

In this regard, Birnbach et al.[20] reported improved postoperative analgesia, presumably related to greater dermatomal spread when epidural fentanyl was administered with increased volumes of diluent. Similar benefits were appreciated when epidural sufentanil (50 μg) was administered in larger injectate volumes.[155]

Although epidural opioids offer gains in analgesic effect, the total dose administered may result in clinically significant plasma levels. This is particularly so with the more lipophilic opioids. Spinal analgesia provided by epidural morphine and hydromorphone is perceived and maintained, despite serum levels that are significantly lower than the minimal effective analgesic concentration (MEAC) attained with parenteral administration.[36,225,229,230] In contrast, vascular uptake of meperidine results in higher plasma levels and a significant "central" analgesic effect during the first 1 to 2 hours following epidural administration.[91] Plasma concentrations of highly lipophilic opioids rise rapidly following epidural deposition, and during continuous infusion, approach or exceed intravenous (IV) MEAC.[39,87,89,139,209] **The observation that both IV and epidural infusions of either fentanyl or sufentanil[87,89,139] provide similar plasma concentrations and identical levels of pain relief has raised questions regarding the neuraxial selectivity of analgesia provided by lipophilic opioids.** The decline in analgesic specificity observed with opioids of increasing lipophilicity was clearly illustrated by Van den Hoogen et al.,[225] who compared the potency of subcutaneous and epidural dosing. Linear inverse relationships between potency gain and increasing lipid-to-water partition coefficients were apparent as morphine (apparent partition coefficient [APC = 1.4]) achieved a greater than tenfold increase in analgesic specificity, whereas analgesia associated with epidural sufentanil (APC = 1600) was equivalent to that observed with subcutaneous doses. Despite its high lipophilicity, the potent opioid agonist remifentanil offers high neuraxial specificity as molecules absorbed from the epidural space are rapidly deactivated by plasma esterases. Preliminary laboratory investigations of epidural remifentanil have reported rapid onset of analgesia, and extremely low plasma concentrations with supraspinal activity.[40]

INTRATHECAL AND EPIDURAL OPIOIDS: POSTSURGICAL APPLICATIONS

Intrathecal Opioids

Morphine, the most widely investigated and extensively used spinal opioid, was first to receive FDA approval for epidural and intrathecal use. The quantity of intrathecal morphine required to provide a given level of analgesia is typically much smaller than the amount that must be given IV or intramuscular (IM). One may realize as much as a hundredfold decrease in 24-hour dose requirements (where 0.5 mg of intrathecal morphine = 5 mg of epidural morphine = 50 to 70 mg of parenteral morphine). **Despite this reduction in dosage, peak CSF morphine concentrations are many times higher than that attained when equivalent doses are injected parenterally.**[59,163]

Intrathecal morphine in doses of 0.2 to 0.6 mg provides highly effective analgesia and improved postoperative pulmonary function in patients recovering from orthopedic, prostatic, major vascular and gynecologic surgery.[13,14,101,102,111,246,247] Intrathecal morphine appears to be particularly useful in gallbladder surgery as doses of 0.2 mg provided up to 24 hours of complete analgesia with minimal risk of associated Sphincter of Oddi spasm.[247] Gwirtz et al.[101] recently presented a series of 4135 patients treated with intrathecal morphine over a period of 5 years. Doses ranged from 0.2 to 0.8 mg and were generally administered upon completion of surgery. Eighty-five percent of patients experienced effective analgesia (good to excellent pain control on postoperative day 1). There were no serious or life-threatening side effects; however 2.3% of patients experienced slowed respiration (defined as a respiratory rate of 8 breaths or less per minute). The major disadvantage of intrathecal morphine is the limited duration of analgesia such therapy provides, which is generally 12 to 24 hours. Benefits including the relative absence of pain during the immediate postoperative period and a smooth transition to parenteral opioid analgesia may compensate for the added costs associated with intrathecal delivery. Intrathecal morphine doses for patients recovering from a variety of surgical procedures are presented in Table 64-2.

Since the withdrawal of subarachnoid microcatheters, lipophilic opioids are by themselves rarely administered intrathecally as the limited duration of analgesia provided by single doses does not warrant the time, cost, and risk of postdural puncture headache. In a recent dose response study,[186] elderly patients treated with either 10 or 20 μg of intrathecal fentanyl experienced only 66 and 119 minutes duration of analgesia. Patients given 40 μg experienced 300 minutes of satisfactory analgesia with minimal side effects. Lipophilic opioids are commonly employed as analgesic adjuncts to spinal anesthesia. The combination of 0.75% bupivacaine plus small doses of fentanyl (12.5 to 20 μg) was found to be more effective than bupivacaine alone in decreasing pain associated with peritoneal traction and lower extremity tourniquet pain.[5,109] Sufentanil offers additional advantages in this setting, because the smaller dose (5 μg) and volume of injectate is less likely to influence the baricity and volume of the local anesthetic solution.[76,110] Fentanyl and sufentanil may also be combined with intrathecal morphine.[133,156] Intrathecal combinations of lipophilic opioids with morphine have been advocated to avoid morphine's latency in onset and peak analgesic effect while providing useful duration of analgesia.[55,101,102]

Table 64-2 Recommended doses of intrathecal morphine for postsurgical analgesia

Procedure	Dose (mg)
Vaginal hysterectomy	0.1–0.2
Cesarean section	0.1–0.2
Hip procedures	0.2–0.25
Knee surgery	0.25–0.3
Lower abdominal surgery	0.2–0.4
Upper abdominal surgery	0.4–0.5
Nephrectomy	0.4–0.6
Cholecystectomy	0.4–0.5
Abdominal aortic aneurysm	0.4–0.6
Whipple procedure	0.4–0.6
Retroperitoneal dissection	0.4–0.6
Thoracotomy	0.5–0.7

Use lowest recommended dose in patients greater than 60 years of age. (Modified from Gwirtz KH: Single-dose opioids in the management of acute postoperative pain. In RS Sinatra, AH Hord, B Ginsberg, LM Preble, editors: *Acute Pain Mechanisms and Management,* St. Louis, 1992, Mosby–Year Book.)

Single and Intermittent Boluses of Epidural Opioids

Intermittent boluses of epidural opioids are commonly used for control of postsurgical pain. Although this method of administration provides effective analgesia and does not require sophisticated delivery systems, CSF concentrations of opioid rise abruptly following each epidural bolus and may be responsible for a high incidence of annoying and potentially serious side effects.[33,34,79,105,177,185,192] The technique provides limited analgesic duration and generally excludes the postsurgical use of local anesthetics. Despite these deficiencies, single-bolus and intermittent dosing may be safely employed providing that dose and dosing interval are carefully adjusted in older or high-risk patient populations.[183,184] Contraindications for epidural opioid administration include infection at the insertion site, septicemia, epidural mass or metastases, history of herpes simplex labialis (refer to section on obstetrical use), and coagulopathy.

Three different classes of opioid analgesics have been advocated for epidural administration; these medications include the hydrophilic opioid morphine, less hydrophilic opioids, such as hydromorphone and meperidine, and highly lipophilic agents including fentanyl and sufentanil.

Morphine

Epidural boluses of morphine effectively relieve both the visceral pain associated with abdominal or pelvic surgery and somatic pain following thoracotomy and orthopedic procedures.[16,25,59,60,70,140,179,206] Doses ranging from 2 to 10 mg are usually administered via lumbar catheters; however, thoracic administration may provide more effective control of upper-abdominal or thoracic pain.[130,206] Analgesic onset and duration of effect following single-dose administration vary according to the surgical stimulus, dose, and site of administration. In general onset is appreciated after 30 to 60 minutes, peak effect occurs at 90 to 120 minutes, and duration extends from 12 to 24 hours.[35,59,60,189,211] Ready and coworkers[184] studied age as a predictor of epidural morphine bolus–dose requirements in postsurgical patients. The therapeutic goal of their evaluation was to produce a pain-free or nearly pain-free state with minimal adverse effects. Despite considerable interpatient variability, a correlation between patient age and effective 24-hour epidural morphine dose was noted (dose requirement in milligrams = 18 − (age × 0.15)) (Fig. 64-4). On the other hand, analgesic quality and frequency of side effects did not change in relation to increasing patient age. In a larger follow-up investigation employing careful dose adjustment and frequent assessment, intermittent boluses of morphine provided safe and effective analgesia for patients recovering on routine postsurgical wards.[182] Of importance was the fact that morphine boluses were administered by the ward nurses under the supervision of the anesthesiology-based acute pain service.

The superiority of epidural morphine analgesia (as determined by descriptive and visual analog scores) over pain relief offered by parenteral opioids has been demonstrated following a wide variety of postsurgical settings.[79,105,140,179,181] Following gallbladder surgery, epidural morphine provided a more uniform level of analgesia and more effective respiratory effort than that noted with IM narcotic or intercostal nerve block.[181] In three comparison studies, the quality and uniformity of postoperative analgesia provided by epidural morphine was significantly better than that offered by IM morphine or morphine patient-controlled analgesia (PCA), while requiring only 1/15 the parenteral dose over the 24-hour study period.[79,105,140] In addition to providing optimal pain relief, single doses of epidural morphine significantly reduce supplemental IV narcotic requirements and associated dose-dependent side effects throughout the postsurgical period (Fig. 64-5).[161]

Hydromorphone

Hydromorphone is a semisynthetic opioid agonist which displays intermediate lipophilicity and high analgesic potency.[19,135,175,191] Although it has not received FDA approval

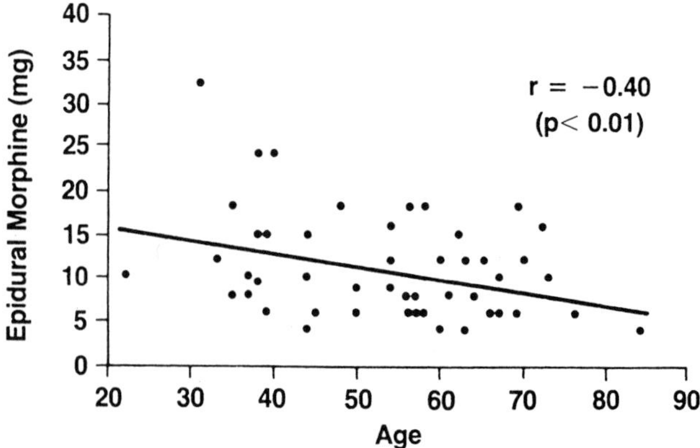

Fig. 64-4. Age versus 24-hour epidural morphine dose requirements in patients recovering from intra-abdominal gynecologic surgery. (From Ready LB, Chadwick, Ross B: Age predicts effective epidural morphine dose after abdominal hysterectomy, *Anesth Analg* 66:1215, 1987.)

for epidural administration, its safety and efficacy have been demonstrated in a number of clinical evaluations.[36,46,53,77,135,167,168,205,223] The clinical behavior of epidural hydromorphone including onset, duration, and dermatomal spread appears optimally positioned between that observed with morphine and the more lipophilic opioids. Despite similar CSF kinetics,[36] the greater potency and high receptor affinity of hydromorphone provide a more rapid onset of analgesia than morphine.[32,53] Significant reductions in pain scores are noted at 15 minutes and peak effect is noted at 30 minutes following epidural administration.[32,36,46] Hydromorphone's removal from the epidural space is slower than that of highly lipophilic opioids, although its ability to remain in CSF and spread rostrally is greater.[32,135,167] These properties provide important clinical advantages. First, doses administered via lumbar catheters can control pain at higher dermatomal segments. When lumbar doses of hydromorphone are used to control pain associated with upper-abdominal and thoracic surgery, the volume of epidural infusate should be increased from 10 to 15 ml[107]; second, epidural administration is associated with superior analgesia and greater potency than that observed when similar doses are given parenterally. Equianalgesic doses of epidural hydromorphone are 55% to 75% lower than IV requirements.[135,167,168,223] Intermittent epidural doses range from 0.5 to 1.5 mg and provide 5 to 12 hours of pain relief.[36,53] The safety and side effect profile of epidural hydromorphone is superior to morphine as equivalent doses are associated with less respiratory depression, pruritus, and sedation.[32,36,46]

Meperidine

The physiochemical properties of meperidine, including its moderate lipid solubility, mu receptor specificity, and dilute local anesthetic properties, suggested a useful role as an epidural analgesic. In an initial evaluation, Glynn et al.[91] reported a rapid onset of postsurgical analgesia after 100 mg

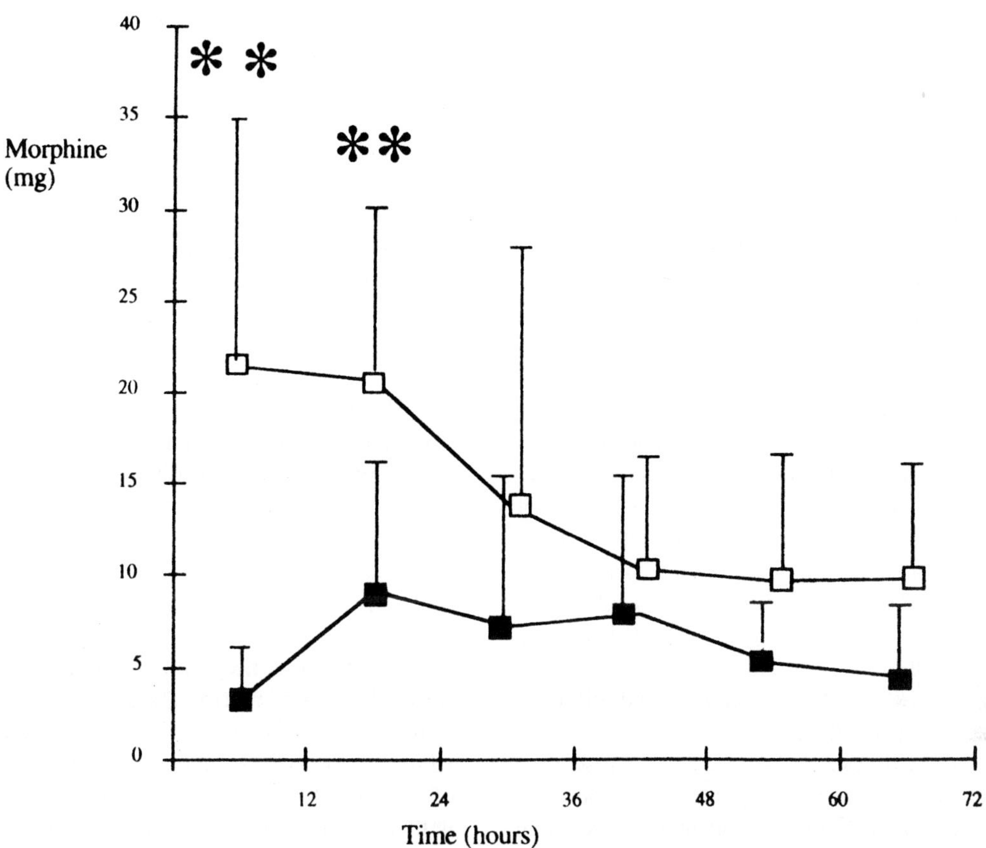

Fig. 64-5. Intravenous patient-controlled analgesia (IV-PCA) morphine requirement per 12-hour period following surgery (mean ± SD), white box = control group; black box = group given 5 mg epidural morphine prior to surgery, $^{**}p < 0.01$ between groups. (From Negre I, Gueneron JP, Jamali SJ, et al: Preoperative analgesia with epidural morphine, *Anesth Analg* 79:298, 1994.)

epidural meperidine. Pain relief was noted at 5 minutes, peaked at 30 minutes, and lasted 8 hours. Onset of analgesia paralleled an equally rapid rise in CSF meperidine levels. In this regard, peak levels were noted between 15 and 45 minutes and occurred significantly sooner than the 60- to 120-minute latency in the CSF peak reported with morphine.[214] These investigators noted few side effects and no evidence of delayed respiratory depression, findings that larger controlled trials[12,169,214] have since confirmed. Early-onset respiratory depression has been reported after epidural meperidine, most commonly associated with doses exceeding 75 mg.[91,169] Meperidine has gained popularity for use as a continuous epidural infusion analgesic. Its lipophilic characteristics are intermediate between morphine and fentanyl and match those of bupivacaine.[19,92] Epidural infusions of 0.1% meperidine and 0.1% bupivacaine appear to spread equally and provide greater than additive analgesic benefit.[207]

Lipophilic opioids

Highly lipophilic opioids, such as fentanyl and sufentanil, are frequently employed as epidural analgesics because they provide rapid and effective pain relief with minimal adverse effects.[89,93,99,154,157] Epidural boluses of fentanyl and sufentanil are associated with less pruritus and nausea/vomiting than morphine and a reduced incidence of delayed respiratory depression.[93,154] Drawbacks associated with single boluses or intermittent doses include:

(1) Bolus dose requirements are high (fentanyl 50 to 100 μg, sufentanil 30 to 40 μg).
(2) Significant early onset ventilatory depression can occur.
(3) The duration of action of single boluses is quite limited.[89,93,154,187,190]

The analgesic efficacy and safety profile of fentanyl have have made it the lipophilic opioid of choice for postsurgical analgesia. Although not FDA approved for epidural administration, fentanyl is marketed in a preservative-free solution. Naulty et al.[154] reported that single doses of epidural fentanyl (50 to 100 μg) provided 4 to 5 hours of excellent postoperative analgesia. This preliminary report evaluated patients who had received epidural bupivacaine (0.75%). However, subsequent studies in patients treated with short-duration local anesthetics found that similar doses of fentanyl provided only 90 to 120 minutes of postoperative analgesia.[187,202] Single doses of epidural fentanyl administered prior to surgical incision provide superior analgesia with reduced parenteral opioid requirements than that observed when similar doses are administered following surgical manipulation.[117]

The high lipid solubility and potency of sufentanil suggested optimal characteristics for use as an epidural analgesic.[75,134,190,226] **Although approved by the FDA for obstetrical epidural analgesia, sufentanil's risk of clinically significant immediate-onset respiratory depression have limited its use in the general surgical patient population.** In a controlled comparison study,[190] the onset of postoperative analgesia was more rapid with epidural sufentanil (50 μg) than with morphine (5 mg). Sufentanil alleviated pain with movement within 10 minutes, three to five times faster than morphine. On the other hand, morphine analgesia lasted twice as long as that with sufentanil. In patients recovering from major abdominal surgery epidural sufentanil in doses between 25 and 70 μg provided extremely effective analgesia; however, the duration of pain relief (in which patients were totally pain free) was limited to just 140 and 224 minutes.[93] Duration of analgesia may be extended with the addition of epinephrine.[132]

Intermittent boluses of highly lipophilic opioids offer advantages in the following settings:

(1) Augmentation of intraoperative epidural anesthesia: fentanyl may be combined with subtherapeutic doses of bupivacaine to achieve "additive" analgesia which may effectively blunt intraoperative and postoperative pain while having minimal effect on sympathetic tone or motor strength.[109] This technique is useful in patients who require effective anesthesia, but because of pulmonary or cardiac disease, cannot tolerate intercostal muscle weakness or the extensive sympathectomy that follows high dermatomal blockade with more concentrated solutions of local anesthetic.

(2) Rapid control of postoperative discomfort in patients experiencing severe breakthrough pain.

(3) Facilitating the transition between regression of epidural anesthesia and the initiation of IV PCA in settings where postsurgical epidural analgesia cannot be provided.[202,211]

(4) As the rapid-acting component of combination epidural analgesic therapy: in this regard, fentanyl or sufentanil may be combined with low-to-moderate doses of epidural morphine in order to minimize delay in analgesic onset.[55,211]

Other lipophilic opioids, including heroin, methadone, butorphanol, and buprenorphine have been reported to provide effective analgesia following epidural administration; however, none have offered a therapeutic advantage over the more commonly used agents.[3,43,151,233] Epidural methadone (5 mg) offers a more rapid onset than morphine (5 mg); however, duration is only of intermediate length (7 hours).[233] Epidural heroin has a similar onset yet a longer analgesic duration than fentanyl.[151] These characteristics reflect rapid spinal uptake of lipophilic heroin molecules with subsequent hydrolysis to its long duration hydrophilic metabolites, monoacetyl morphine, and morphine.[114] The lipophilic mixed-agonist butorphanol has been advocated as a spinal analgesic; however, significant central effects resulting from absorption and recirculation to the CNS have limited its overall usefulness.[3,42] In this regard, epidural butorphanol dosage is equivalent to parenteral requirements and dose-dependent improvements in analgesic duration parallel significant increases in sedation.[42] Caution must be exercised when administering epidural butorphanol to patients with opioid dependency, because this mixed agonist/antagonist may precipitate symptoms of acute withdrawal.

Continuous Infusion of Epidural Opioids

Continuous "low-dose" infusion of epidural opioids has been advocated as a method to control severe pain following surgery and trauma with fewer adverse effects than intermittent bolus techniques.[81,138,222,251] **Continuous infusions permit analgesia to be more precisely titrated to the level of pain stimulus and rapidly terminated if problems should occur. The technique avoids the peak CSF concentrations that follow intermittent epidural boluses and reduces the risk of rostral spread and delayed respiratory depression.**[59,81] Other benefits include decreased time spent administering agents and assessing effect and a reduced risk of contamination and medication errors when compared with intermittent dosing techniques. Continuous infusion techniques also provide greater therapeutic versatility, because shorter-acting opioids and dilute local anesthetic solutions may be administered.

Epidural infusions of morphine, meperidine, and hydromorphone provide greater pain relief and lower dose requirements than IV administration.[32,81,84] El-Baz et al.[81] evaluated the effectiveness of a continuous epidural morphine (0.5 mg/hr) infusion versus intermittent doses of morphine or bupivacaine for post-thoracotomy analgesia. They noted that morphine infusions provided effective analgesia yet avoided most of the troublesome side effects observed with intermittent boluses. Patients in the continuous infusion group experienced less urinary retention, pruritus, and oversedation than patients treated with morphine boluses and less urinary retention and hypotension than individuals receiving intermittent doses of bupivacaine.

Both animal and human studies have documented additive, and possibly synergistic, analgesic effects when intrathecal or epidural morphine is combined with bupivacaine.[69,70,219] Dahl et al.[68,69] reported that patients recovering from major abdominal surgery and treated with epidural infusions of morphine with 0.1% bupivacaine benefited from improved dynamic or movement-associated pain following cough and ambulation as compared with individuals receiving morphine alone. Patients recovering from abdominal aortic surgery and treated with epidural infusions of morphine with bupivacaine 0.125% experienced a more rapid time to extubation and lower visual analog scale (VAS) pain scores than others treated with intravenous patient-controlled analgesia (IV-PCA) morphine.[25] In a recent retrospective analysis of more than 4000 patients, de Leon Casasola et al.[70] reported that epidural morphine-bupivacaine infusions provided excellent analgesia, were associated with an extremely low incidence of serious adverse events (3 episodes of severe respiratory depression and 126 cases of hypotension), and could be safely administered to patients recovering on postsurgical wards.

Continuous infusions of epidural hydromorphone provide effective analgesia for patients recovering from a variety of surgical procedures. Such therapy is associated with rapid onset to peak effect, less sedation, and significantly less pruritus than equianalgesic doses of morphine.[32,37,46] Brodsky et al.[32] reported a series of 44 patients receiving continuous lumbar epidural infusions of hydromorphone (0.5%) for post-thoracotomy analgesia. Postsurgical analgesia was excellent with greater than 90% of patients reporting no pain or mild discomfort during the 48-hour study interval. The incidence of hypoventilation, pruritus, and nausea was lower than that observed with equipotent doses of epidural morphine. Chaplan et al.[46] compared a 3:1 dose ratio of morphine:hydromorphone for continuous epidural infusions, with patients in the hydromorphone group receiving between 0.15 and 0.3 mg/hr. They reported that each opioid provided effective epidural analgesia; however, patients treated with hydromorphone infusions experienced fewer adverse effects. The incidence of moderate-to-severe pruritis and the need for treatment were significantly higher in the morphine group.

Highly lipophilic opioids such as fentanyl, are commonly employed as continuous epidural infusions.[11,60,87,194,195,235] Welchew and Thornton[235] were among the first to evaluate continuous fentanyl infusions, reporting that such therapy offered rapid and effective analgesia and improved respiratory volume and flow rates in patients recovering from thoracotomy. In subsequent evaluations, patients receiving continuous infusions of fentanyl (60 to 70 μg/hr) following upper-abdominal surgery or cesarean section experienced superior pain relief with less-troubling side effects such as pruritus and nausea, than individuals treated with parenteral opioids.[11,84,199,251]

Continuous epidural infusions of sufentanil have also been used for the control of postoperative pain.[47,87] Cheng et al.[47] reported that continuous infusions of sufentanil 0.3 μg/kg/hr provided rapid and sustained analgesia with few side effects in patients recovering from intra-abdominal surgery.

Significant amounts of fentanyl and sufentanil are absorbed by epidural and spinal vasculature resulting in progressive increases in plasma concentration.[23,56,87,89] **Comparisons of patients receiving IV and epidurally administered fentanyl revealed no differences in postoperative pain scores and dose requirements (Fig. 64-6).**[87,89,139] These results questioned the specificity of epidural dosing because plasma levels after 18 hours exceeded the minimum effective analgesic concentration (MEAC) of fentanyl. In a randomized, double-blind study, Geller et al.[87] compared

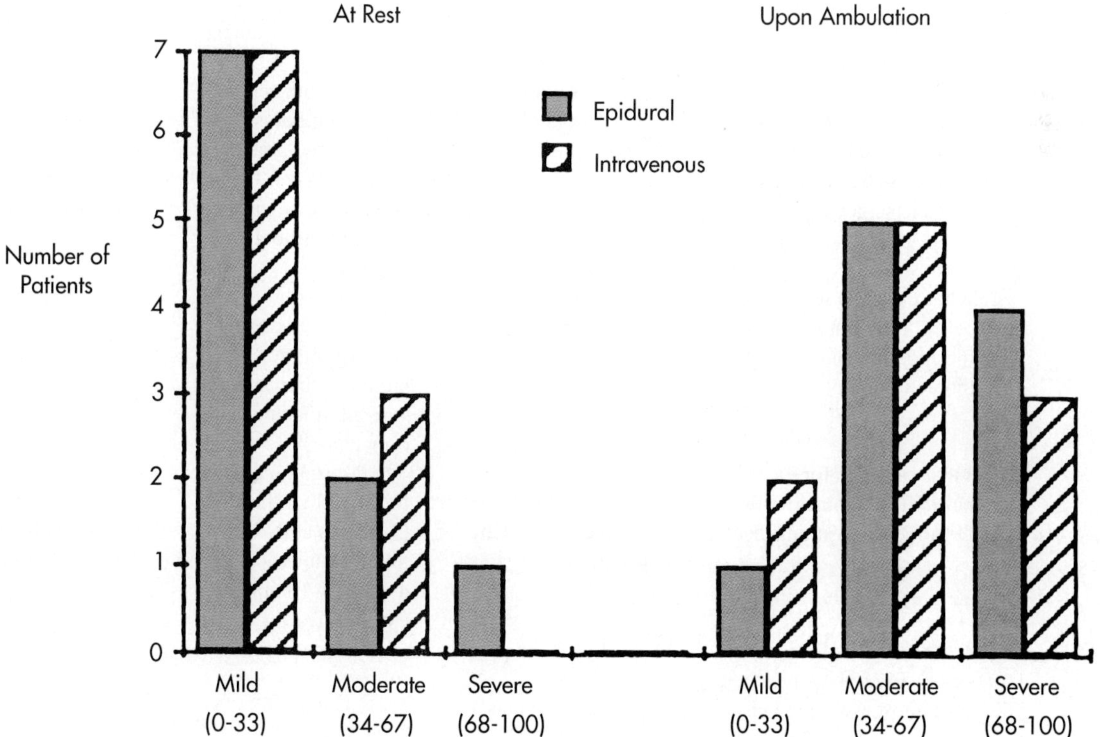

Fig. 64-6. Pain scores at rest and upon ambulation in patients receiving epidural (gray bars) or intravenous (hatched bars) fentanyl infusions following lower extremity orthopedic surgery. (From Loper KA, Ready LB, Downey M, et al: Epidural and intravenous fentanyl infusions are clinically equivalent after knee surgery, *Anesth Analg* 70:72, 1990.)

epidural infusions of either sufentanil (5 μg/hr) or fentanyl (20 μg/hr) with IV infusions of sufentanil. They noted equivalent intragroup pain scores and dose requirements; however, patients treated with IV sufentanil experienced greater sedation and a higher incidence of respiratory depression.

Continuous infusion with large volumes of diluent may help promote rostral spread and control surgical pain at higher dermatomal sites.[20,155] Snijdelaar et al.[215] observed improvements in post-thoracotomy pain scores when thoracic epidural doses of sufentanil were administered as high-volume infusions (0.7 μg/ml at 7 ml/hr) rather than an equivalent-dose low-volume (4 μg/ml at 1.3 ml/hr) infusion. Administration of lipophillic opioids via catheters placed at interspaces adjacent to the site of surgery and in combination with dilute concentrations of bupivacaine may also improve epidural analgesia.[84,137,199] Guinard et al.[99] reported that thoracic epidural infusions were superior to lumbar epidural and IV sites of administration in reducing fentanyl dose requirements and total hospital stay in patients recovering from thoracotomy. Scott et al.[199] found that the combination fentanyl/bupivacaine infusions offered effective postsurgical analgesia with minimal risk of side effects in the non–intensive care unit setting. Their conclusions were based on a prospective analysis in which the incidence of complications and adequacy of analgesia were evaluated in 1014 patients. Lui and coworkers[137] suggest that 0.05% bupivacaine is the optimal concentration for use with epidural fentanyl for post-thoracotomy analgesia. This concentration was associated with significant fentanyl dose sparing while avoiding hypotension and motor weakness observed with 0.1% bupivacaine. Dosing guidelines for intermittent opioid bolus doses and continuous epidural infusions are presented in Table 64-3.

Patient-Controlled Epidural Analgesia

Epidural patient-controlled analgesia (Epi-PCA) is a pain management technique that offers greater reduction in pain intensity with lower opioid dose requirement than IV PCA, while providing increased control and

Table 64-3 Dosing guidelines for epidural opioid analgesia

Opioid	Site of administration	Intermittent bolus technique	Continuous infusion technique*	Adjunctive therapy
Morphine	Lumbar catheters for incisions below T8, thoracic catheters for upper-abdominal and thoracic surgery	Administer 3 to 8 mg bolus in 10 ml preservative free saline every 8–24 hours as clinically indicated	2 to 4 mg bolus followed by infusion (5 μg/ml) at 8–15 ml/hr (lumbar catheters); 4–8 ml/hr (thoracic catheters)	IV Ketorolac 15–30 mg q6hr Epidural bupivacaine 0.1%–0.03%
Hydromorphone	Lumbar catheters for incisions below T8, thoracic catheters for upper-abdominal and thoracic surgery	0.5 to 1.5 mg bolus every 5–10 hours	0.5 to 1.5 mg bolus followed by infusion (10 μg/ml) at 8–15 ml/hr (lumbar catheters) 4–8 ml/hr (thoracic catheters)	IC Kerorolac 15–30 mg q6hr Epidural bupivacaine 0.1%–0.03%
Meperidine	Lumbar catheters for incisions below T10, thoracic catheters for upper-abdominal and thoracic surgery	50 to 75 mg bolus every 3–5 hours	50 to 75 mg bolus followed by infusion (100 μg/ml) at 8–15 ml/hr (lumbar catheters) 4–8 ml/hr (thoracic catheters)	IV Ketorolac 15–30 mg q6hr Epidural bipivacaine 0.1%–0.03%
Fentanyl	Lumbar catheters for incisions below T12, thoracic catheters for almost everything else	50 to 100 μg bolus every 2–3 hr (not recommended)	50 to 100 μg bolus followed by infusion (5 μg/ml) at 8–15 ml/hr (lumbar catheters) 4–8 ml/hr (thoracic catheters)	IV Ketorolac 15–30 mg q6hr Epidural bupivacaine 0.05%–0.1% or less
Sufentanil	Lumbar catheters for incisions below T12, thoracic catheters for almost everything else	20 to 30 μg bolus every 2–3 hr (not recommended)	20 to 30 μg/ml bolus followed by infusion (1–2 μg/ml) at 8–15 ml/hr (lumbar catheters); 4–8 ml/hr (thoracic catheters)	IV Ketorolac 15–30 mg q6hr Epidural bupivacaine 0.05%–0.1% or less

*Dependent on age, physical status, height, extent of surgical dissection, and so on.

higher patient satisfaction than either single doses or continuous infusions of epidural opioids. Epi-PCA combines the best aspects of self-administration dosing regimens, including increased analgesic titratability, as well as the superior pain relief associated with neuraxial sites of activity.[141,167,230] The technique involves standard placement of an epidural catheter (ideally at interspaces immediately adjacent to the site of surgery), administration of an analgesic loading dose (opioids, local anesthetic, or both), and initiation of a continuous epidural infusion with superimposed patient-activated epidural boluses. Development of specialized infusion devices that offer precise epidural PCA dosing and 250 to 500 ml analgesic solution capacity have increased the safety, reliability, and overall acceptance of the technique. The potential advantages of Epi-PCA versus IV-PCA and single-bolus or continuous epidural opioid analgesia are presented in Box 64-1.

Most of the early works describing the concept of Epi-PCA were performed in Europe.[64,213] Chrubasik et al.[64,65] compared the efficacy of three different opioids administered epidurally on demand. They noted that the dose of self-administered epidural morphine required to provide effective analgesia was significantly less than amounts used with either continuous Epi- or IV-PCA techniques. Sjostrom et al.[213] evaluated Epi-PCA with morphine (1 mg intermittent bolus with a 30-minute lockout interval) in 30 patients. These investigators noted that the average consumption was 0.5 mg/hour and that serum morphine levels were well below minimum effective plasma concentrations associated with parenteral administration. In a subsequent clinical evaluation performed at the University of Kentucky, Epi-PCA morphine provided high clinical efficacy and safety in over 4000 patients recovering from a variety of surgical procedures.[229,230] Walmsley et al.[230] reported that total self-administered dose and plasma morphine concentrations required to provide effective analgesia were significantly less than amounts observed with IV-PCA (Fig. 64-7). According to their protocol, patients are "loaded" with 2 to 3 mg of epidural morphine. Thereafter, a basal infusion of 0.4 mg/hr is started and patients are allowed to self-administer 0.2 mg morphine every 10 to 15 min with a maximum dose of 1.2 mg/hr.

BOX 64-1
POTENTIAL ADVANTAGES OF EPIDURAL PATIENT-CONTROLLED ANALGESIA VERSUS TRADITIONAL EPIDURAL OPIOID TECHNIQUES

Epidural PCA versus epidural opioid boluses or infusions
- Improved patient control and autonomy
- Increased patient satisfaction
- Decreased anxiety
- Reduced opioid requirement
- Reduced movement pain scores

Epidural PCA versus IV-PCA
- Increased analgesic efficacy
- Reduced opioid requirement
- Decreased opioid side effects
- Improved postsurgical outcome

PCA—patient-controlled analgesia; IV-PAC—intravenous patient-controlled analgesia.

Lipophilic opioids have also been evaluated for use in this setting.[89,94,95,97,209] In a well-designed evaluation of Epi-PCA versus IV-PCA fentanyl, Glass et al.[89] noted no intragroup differences in pain scores or total fentanyl dose requirement in patients recovering from major surgery. Nevertheless, Grant et al.[94] observed dose-sparing advantages when Epi-PCA fentanyl was compared with IV-PCA in patients recovering from thoracotomy. Patients using Epi-PCA self-administered significantly less fentanyl while achieving equivalent levels of pain relief. Unfortunately, serum opioid concentrations were not measured. The combination of Epi-PCA fentanyl plus IV ketorolac provided superior control of movement-associated pain, reduced fentanyl dose requirements, and a more rapid return of gastrointestinal function than Epi-PCA fentanyl alone (Fig. 64-8).[96]

Sufentanil has also been advocated for use with Epi-PCA. Grass et al.[96] noted that onset to peak analgesic effect occurred more rapidly and pain associated with movement was better controlled with Epi-PCA sufentanil than with IV-PCA morphine. A major criticism of this and other evaluations of Epi-PCA sufentanil was the omission of an IV-PCA control group[95,97]; thus, it remained unclear whether epidural administration, the opioid selected, or both factors are responsible for improvements in outcome. In a recent double-blind evaluation, Sinatra and coworkers[209] were unable to detect differences between Epi-PCA and IV-PCA sufentanil in patients recovering from abdominal hysterectomy. Patients treated with either IV or epidural sufentanil 0.1 μg/kg/hr infusion and 2 μg bolus every 6 minutes benefitted from a more rapid analgesic onset, improved resting and dynamic pain scores, and less reduction in postoperative forced vital capacity than patients treated with IV-PCA morphine. However, when epidural and IV sufentanil groups were compared, no differences in pain scores, total PCA attempts, dose requirements, or plasma sufentanil concentrations were observed (Fig. 64-9). In agreement with a previous report by Geller et al., who compared IV versus epidural infusions,[87] patients receiving IV sufentanil experienced greater sedation and respiratory depression.

Thoracic epidural administration may take advantage of sufentanil's highly segmental analgesic properties and improve the effectiveness of Epi-PCA. However, Swenson and coworkers[218] found no clinical advantage between thoracic versus lumbar Epi-PCA sufentanil with respect to quality of analgesia, self-administered dose, and pulmonary function in patients recovering from thoracotomy.

Hydromorphone offers neuraxial selectivity and a high margin of safety when employed for Epi-PCA.[135,167,168,223]

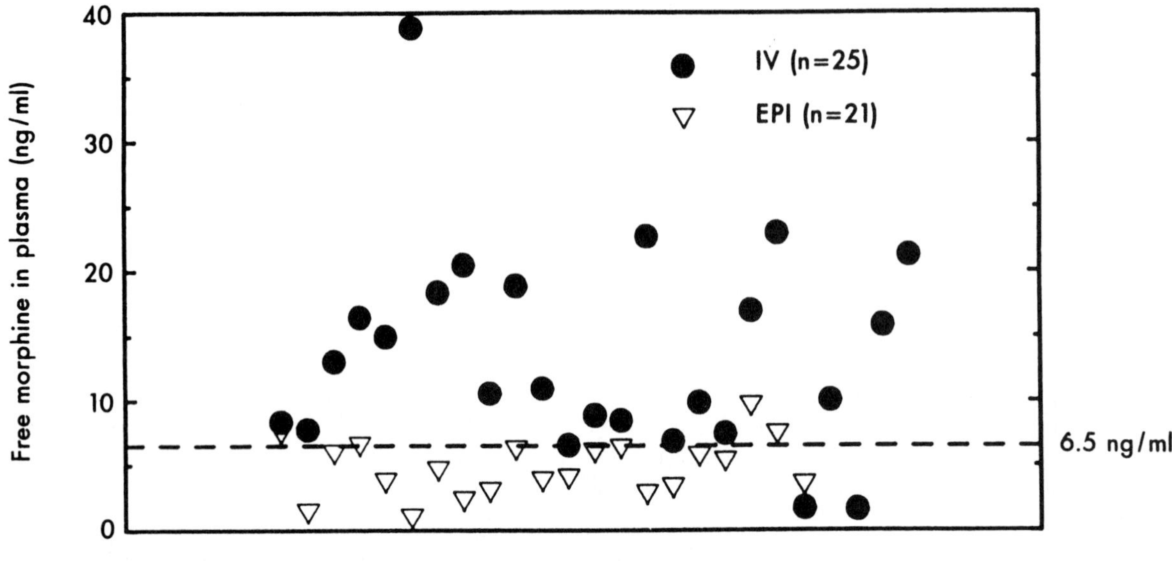

Fig. 64-7. Free, unconjugated morphine serum levels after 24 hours of patient-controlled epidural analgesia and intravenous patient-controlled analgesia using morphine in 46 patients. Samples were drawn at least 30 minutes after the last PCA bolus. EPI—epidural; IV—intravenous; GC/MS—gas chromatography-mass spectrometry; MS—morphine sulfate. (From Walmsley PNH: Patient-controlled epidural analgesia. In Sinatra RS, Hord AH, Ginsberg B, Preble LM, editors: *Acute pain: Mechanisms and management,* St Louis, 1992, Mosby–Year Book.)

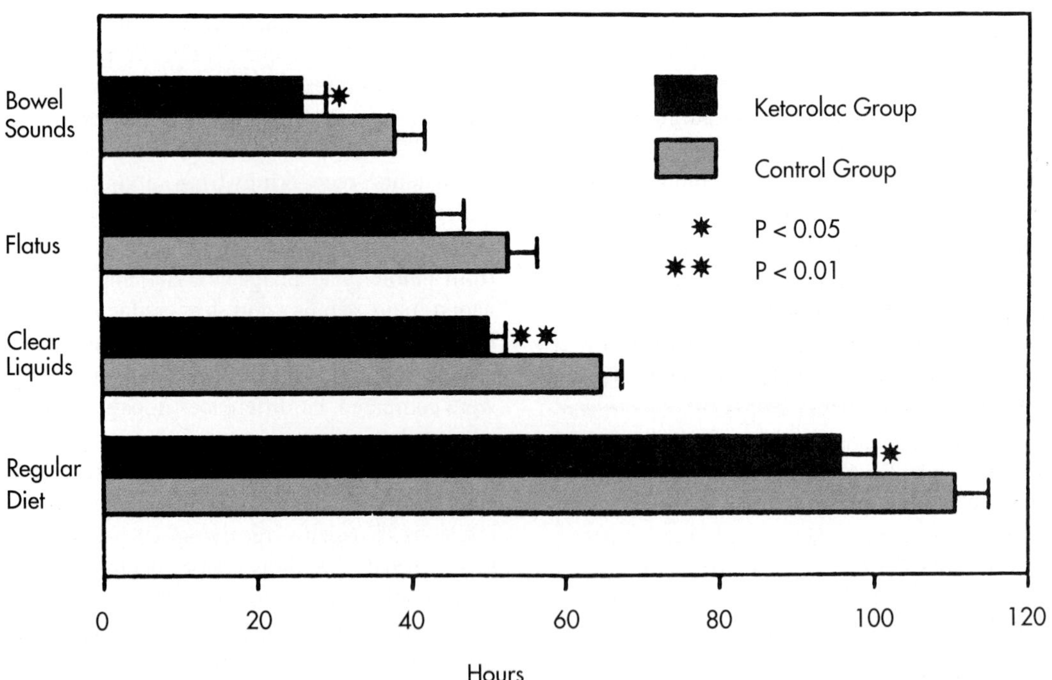

Fig. 64-8. Recovery of gastrointestinal function. Times (in hours) to return of several measures of gastrointestinal function for patients receiving epidural patient-controlled analgesia (Epi-PCA) fentanyl (control) and Epi-PCA fentanyl plus intravenous ketorolac following radical prostatectomy. (From Grass JA, Sakima NT, Valley M, et al: Assessment of ketorolac as an adjuvant to fentanyl patient-controlled epidural analgesia after radical retropubic prostatectomy, *Anesthesiology* 78:642,1993.)

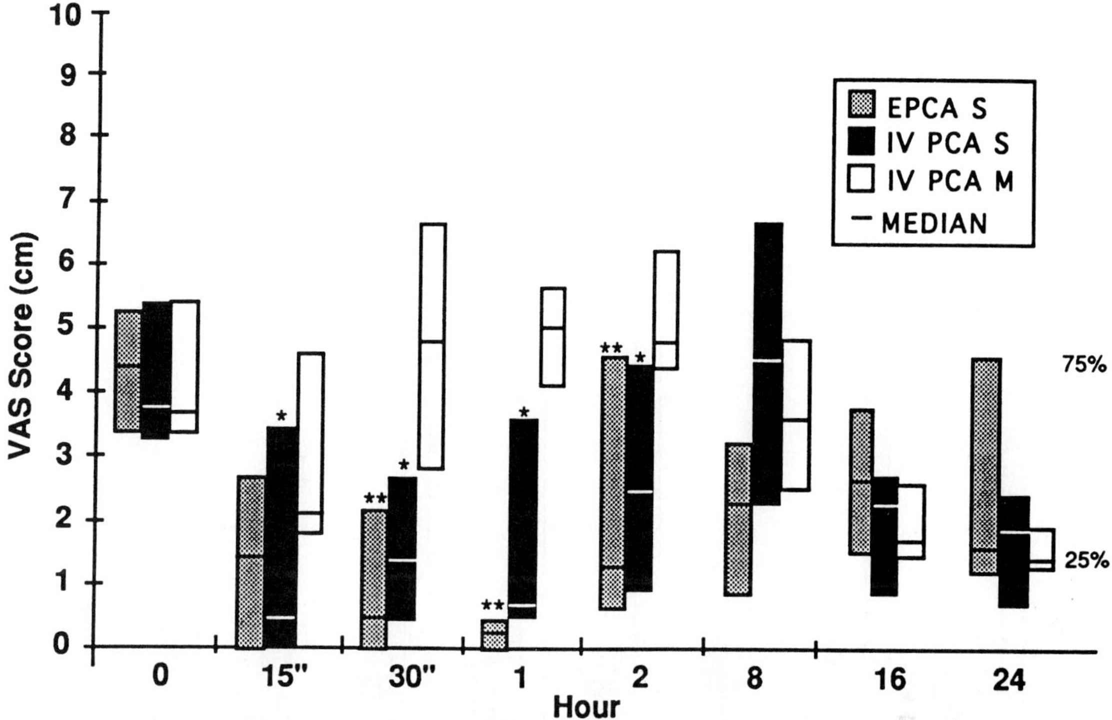

Fig. 64-9. Visual analog scale pain scores at rest taken at various intervals following initiation of patient-controlled analgesia (PCA); median scores (line) and 25% and 75% range (bars) are presented for each group. * $p \leq 0.05$ for differences between Group 3 (IV-PCA morphine) and Group 2 (IV-PCA sufentanil). ** $p \leq 0.05$ for differences between Group 3 and Group 1 (Epi-PCA sufentanil). (From Sinatra RS, Sevarino FB, Paige D: Patient-controlled analgesia with sufentanil: a comparison of two different methods of administration, *J Clin Anesth* 8:123–129, 1996.)

Parker and White[167,168] reported Epi-PCA with hydromorphone was a safe and more effective alternative to IV-PCA hydromorphone, offering the advantage of reduced opioid dose requirement and more rapid recovery, that is shorter time to return of bowel sounds, resumption of solid diet, discontinuation of analgesic therapy and hospital discharge (Fig. 64-10). These authors speculated that the neuraxial specificity and dose-sparing effect of Epi-PCA hydromorphone was partly responsible for significant improvements in gastrointestinal function. In a more recent comparison of IV versus Epi-PCA hydromorphone for patients recovering from radical prostatectomy, Liu et al.[135] reported similar reductions in dose requirement (50% reduction in self-administered hydromorphone) and a higher incidence of pruritus in the Epi-PCA group. Despite reductions in opioid dose, this relatively small 16-patient study was unable to detect intergroup differences in times to return of gastrointestinal function or hospital discharge. IV ketorolac may be employed to augment Epi-PCA hydromorphone. Singh et al.[212] reported that Epi-PCA hydromorphone plus IV ketorolac provided superior analgesia and improved pulmonary function in patients recovering from thoracotomy when compared with Epi-PCA hydromorphone alone. In two different investigations, the addition of bupivacaine to the epidural infusate did not improve the quality of pain relief provided by Epi-PCA hydromorphone.[168,212] At Yale New Haven hospital, both IV ketorolac (15 mg every 6 hr) and epidural bupivacaine are combined with Epi-PCA hydromorphone unless medical or surgical contraindications exist. In reviewing records of more than 2800 patients recovering from major surgical procedures who were treated with Epi-PCA hydromorphone with 0.03% bupivacaine, greater than 90% reported good to excellent analgesia. Thirty-five percent reported no pain at rest. Side effects, especially pruritus, nausea, and sedation were significantly less common than that previously observed with epidural morphine or hydromorphone.[135,168,207] Epi-PCA is initiated with a 0.5 to 1.5 mg hydromorphone loading dose. A basal infusion (10 μg/ml) at a rate of 8 to 12 ml/hr plus a PCA dose of 3 to 4 ml with a 6 to 8 min lockout is initiated in the postanesthesia care unit. Continuous epidural infusion rates are decreased by one third when administered via thoracic catheters. Alternatively, the loading dose may be reduced by 50% (0.25 to 0.75 mg) and the basal infusion started in the operating room. Epi-PCA dosing is added as required when the patient is awake and alert in the postanesthesia care unit. Bupivacaine 0.031% is added to Epi-PCA solutions except in situations where postsurgical hypovolemia is present. In agreement with previous findings,[70,135] we have found that epidural combinations of opioids with extremely dilute local

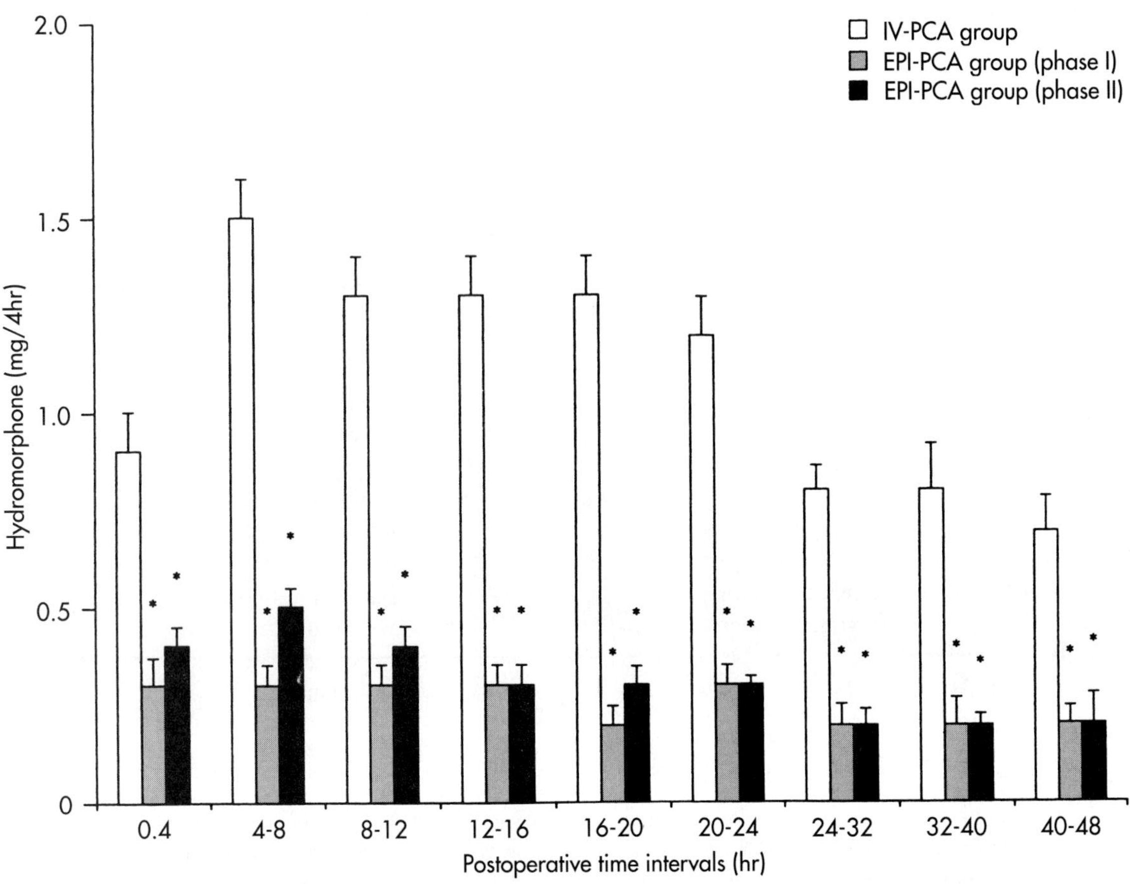

Fig. 64-10. Postoperative hydromorphone use (mg/4-hr interval) when administered via intravenous patient-controlled analgesia (IV-PCA) (white bars) or epidural patient-controlled analgesia (Epi-PCA) in patients recovering from cesarean section delivery. Results are expressed as mean ± standard error of mean. $*p < 0.05$, significantly different from IV-PCA group. (From Parker RK, White PF: Epidural patient-controlled analgesia: An alternative to intravenous patient-controlled analgesia for pain relief after cesarean delivery, *Anesth Analg* 75:245, 1992.)

anesthetics improve postsurgical analgesia, especially dynamic pain, without increasing the incidence of orthostatic hypotension or interfering with safe assisted ambulation. Dosing guidelines for Epi-PCA are presented in Table 64-4.

OTHER CLINICAL APPLICATIONS OF INTRATHECAL AND EPIDURAL OPIOIDS

Obstetrics

Laboring parturients face the dilemma of either continued suffering or neonatal exposure to large parenteral doses of narcotic. These concerns, coupled with the fact that they represent a healthy, homogeneous study population, make this group an ideal choice for evaluating the benefits of spinal opioid analgesia.

Labor and delivery

Relatively high doses of intrathecal morphine (1 to 2 mg) may provide adequate pain relief in the first stage of labor[4]; however, a high percentage of patients experience distressing side effects, incomplete analgesia in the second stage, and require local anesthetic supplementation. Leighton et al.[133] noted improvements in analgesic efficacy following intrathecal administration of morphine (0.25 mg) and fentanyl (25 μg) to patients in labor. Onset of analgesia was appreciated within 15 minutes of administration and lasted through the second stage. Pain relief was not associated with delayed respiratory depression or the significant incidence of pruritus and nausea previously observed with higher doses of morphine alone. Intrathecal fentanyl in doses of 20 to 25 μg offers effective labor analgesia of limited duration (90 to 100 minutes) and is not associated with maternal hypotension in prehydrated parturients.[106,152] In recent years, sufentanil has become the intrathecal opioid of choice for labor analgesia.[42,110,224] Intrathecal sufentanil may be employed as primary therapy or in combined spinal-epidural techniques. Duration of intrathecal sufentanil analgesia is dose dependent with doses of 7.5 to 10 μg providing optimal pain relief, the longest duration of analgesia (80 to 90 minutes) and lowest incidence of pruritus.[109,224] Unlike epidural administration, increases in the volume of intrathecal injectate from 1 to 10 mL did not in-

Table 64-4 Epidural PCA dosing guidelines

Opioid	Concentration	Loading dose*	EPI-PCA dose*	Lockout (min)	Continuous rate*	4 hour limit
Morphine	50 μg/ml	2–4 mg	2–4 ml	10–15	6–12 ml/hr	40–70 ml
Hydromorphone	10 μg/ml	500–1500 μg	2–4 ml	6–10	6–12 ml/hr	40–70 ml
Fentanyl	5 μg/ml	75–100 μg	2–4 ml	6	6–15 ml/hr	40–70 ml
Sufentanil	2 μg/ml	0.5 μg/kg	2–4 ml	6	0.1 μg/kg/hr	40–70 ml

*Dependent upon site of epidural catheter, extent of surgery, and patient physical status.

fluence the quality or duration of intrathecal sufentanil analgesia.[110] More recently, Campbell et al.[42] reported that the intrathecal combination of bupivicaine (2.5 mg) plus sufentanil (10 μg) offered rapid and effective labor analgesia during the first stage without maternal hypotension or fetal compromise. **Intrathecal opioid analgesia is most beneficial for parturients who desire to ambulate as well as those with significant cardiac disease because it offers effective pain relief without sympathetic blockade and cardiovascular compromise.**

Epidurally administered opioids have found even wider application in the obstetric setting and are often employed as adjuncts for epidural analgesia during labor and delivery. Epidural opioids usually provide insufficient analgesia for labor, especially second stage, unless supplemented with local anesthetic.[12,159,160] **In this regard, the combination of fentanyl or sufentanil and low concentrations of bupivacaine offers the benefit of additive analgesia with reduced risk of motor and autonomic blockade or potential cardiotoxicity associated with more concentrated solutions of local anesthetic.**[159,160,172,173] Some anesthesiologists allow patients in early labor to ambulate following administration of epidural opioids alone or in combination with mini doses of local anesthetic (4 to 6 mL of 0.25% of bupivacaine). As contractions become stronger during late first and early second stage, the parturient is returned to her bed and additional analgesia may be provided.

When compared with epidural local anesthetic techniques, analgesia provided by solutions of opioids plus dilute bupivacaine may improve delivery outcome by reducing the incidence of cesarean section and forceps delivery.[50,51,52] Continuous infusion of 0.125% bupivacaine and either fentanyl (2 to 3 μg/ml) or sufentanil (0.3 μg/ml) provide effective and uniform levels of analgesia without delaying onset or prolonging the duration of the second stage.[50,159,160] Sufentanil (0.3 μg/ml) and 0.125% bupivacaine[172,173] have also been advocated for labor and delivery analgesia; however, high dose requirements have raised concerns about potential maternal-fetal depression following accidental IV injection. Combinations of lipophilic opioid plus bupivacaine may also be administered via Epi-PCA. This method of administration provides labor analgesia equivalent to that observed with continuous epidural infusions, but with significant reductions in total anesthetic dose.[86] At Yale-New Haven hospital, patients, obstetricians, and anesthesiologists have been pleased with the safety, efficacy, and reliability of epidural hydromorphone for labor analgesia.[207] A loading dose of hydromorphone (150 to 200 μg with 10 ml 0.25% bupivicaine) followed by an infusion (hydromorphone 5 μg/ml with bupivacaine 0.03%) provides rapid and highly effective analgesia with minimal sensory and motor blockade, hypotension, or urinary retention. This solution is employed as a walking epidural and allows patients to sit or ambulate with assistance within the labor room.

Postcesarean section analgesia

Because the majority of cesarean deliveries are performed during spinal anesthesia,[51,88] intrathecally administered opioids provide an attractive option for postoperative analgesia. Small doses of intrathecal morphine (0.3 to 0.5 mg) offer similar duration of postcesarean section analgesia and a comparable incidence of adverse side effects as that observed with epidural morphine. Abboud et al.[2] reported that patients treated with smaller doses of intrathecal morphine (0.1 to 0.25 mg) experienced superior and more prolonged analgesia than patients receiving intrathecal placebo with "rescue" doses of subcutaneous morphine. Patients in the placebo group had the most profound changes in minute ventilation response to CO_2. Because of the high safety and efficacy of minidose intrathecal morphine, some clinicians routinely add 0.1 to 0.15 mg to hyperbaric bupivacaine for spinal anesthesia.[51,166] We have found the combination of intrathecal meperidine (10 mg) plus "minidose" morphine (0.15 mg) offers a number of clinical advantages including augmentation of intraoperative anesthesia, effective (albeit not complete) postoperative analgesia, a significant reduction in the need for supplemental parenteral opioids, and a very low incidence of side effects. Supplemental analgesia, when required, is best provided with reduced doses of IV-PCA opioids.[55,207]

Epidurally administered opioids also provide superior postcesarean analgesia with no appreciable increase in risk over that noted with IM narcotics. This is especially important considering that the rate of cesarean-section delivery exceeds 20% in many hospitals.[88] Leicht et al.[131] studied 1000 patients who received 5 mg of epidural morphine during cesarean section. Duration of pain relief averaged 23 hours, with 16% of patients not requiring additional analgesics for the remainder of their hospital stay. Similar findings were noted in a study of 3000 patients.[85] In both studies, the incidence of respiratory depression (respiratory rate less than 10 breaths/min) averaged 2.5 to 4 patients/1000 studied.

An unusual side effect noted with epidural morphine in this patient population is reactivation of herpes simplex virus infection. Crone et al.[63] reported recurrent lesions in 9.3% of patients treated with epidural morphine during cesarean delivery versus a 1% recurrence rate in untreated individuals. What remains unclear is whether this represents a direct morphine effect or viral reactivation secondary to spinal opioid analgesia.

In a prospective, randomized, double-blind study, Chestnut and colleagues[53] evaluated the safety and analgesic efficacy of epidural hydromorphone (1 mg) versus epidural bupivacaine (0.25%, 10-ml bolus) following cesarean delivery. Patients treated with epidural hydromorphone benefited from superior analgesia, prolonged time to first analgesic intervention, and reduced total dose of IV hydromorphone rescue during the first 24 hours. Respiratory depression was not observed; however, vomiting and pruritus were more common in the hydromorphone group. Parker et al.[168] compared four groups of patients treated with Epi-PCA hydromorphone for postcesarean-section analgesia. The results showed that pain relief provided by self-administered hydromorphone was not improved by adding 0.08% bupivacaine or a basal hydromorphone infusion (0.0375 mg/hr) after cesarean section. There were no significant differences between treatment groups when compared for pain, sedation, fatigue, anxiety, pruritus, times to recovery of bowel function, ambulation, resumption of a solid diet, discontinuation of PCA therapy, and hospital discharge.

Epidural fentanyl is frequently employed for intraoperative augmentation of epidural anesthesia although single-bolus doses provide only limited analgesia after cesarean section.[187,202] Epidural fentanyl infusions are widely used in this setting as they offer effective analgesia with minimal adverse effects. Youngstrom et al.[250] evaluated a continuous epidural infusion of fentanyl (4 μg/ml) and epinephrine (1.6 μg/ml) for postcesarean analgesia. Patients who received continuous infusion at a rate of 15 ml/hr obtained excellent pain relief and required minimal amounts of IV opioid supplementation.[250] In a prospective evaluation of 3823 patients who had received epidural opioids after cesarean section, those treated with epidural fentanyl-epinephrine infusions reported fewer side effects than patients who had received 4 to 5 mg of morphine.[251]

Sufentanil has also been used for analgesia after cesarean surgery and offers advantages in settings where rapid onset of analgesia is desired. Sufentanil's dose-dependent duration of analgesia appears to be slightly longer than that noted with fentanyl when administered with 2% lidocaine or 0.5% bupivacaine epidural anesthesia, and it ranged between 200 and 400 minutes with doses of 30 to 75 μg.[190] The duration of sufentanil analgesia after cesarean delivery may be extended by the addition of epinephrine (300 μg/ml) or when administered in larger volumes of epidural injectate.[132,155]

BOX 64-2
SPINAL OPIOID ANALGESIA AFTER CESAREAN SECTION CURRENT CLINICAL PRACTICE AT YALE–NEW HAVEN HOSPITAL

Most patients receive a single dose of preservative-free morphine (0.25 mg), which is mixed with hyperbaric bupivacaine (12 mg). Alternatively, we add two opioids to the local anesthetic solution: preservative-free **meperidine** (10 mg) and **morphine** (0.15 mg). This combination provides better analgesia than morphine alone during the first several hours after cesarean section.

All patients receive IV **metoclopramine** (10 mg) before administration of spinal anesthesia. This dose of antiemetic is readministered every 6 hours for 24 hours after surgery. Patients who complain of moderate-to-severe pruritus receive IV **diphenhydramine** (12.5 to 25 mg), **naloxone** (0.04 to 0.08 mg), or **nalbuphine** (5 mg).

Patients are also provided low-dose IV-PCA **meperidine** (5 to 8 mg every 6 to 10 min as needed) for supplemental analgesia. Patients who receive the smaller dose (0.15 mg) of intrathecal morphine are provided PCA immediately after arrival to the postanesthesia care unit, whereas patients who receive the larger dose (0.25 mg) do not begin PCA until 8 to 12 hours after adminstration of spinal anesthesia. IV PCA is continued for 24 to 30 hours, and then switched to oral analgesics. All patients are followed by the Acute Pain Service. Standard orders include an hourly assessment of respiratory rate and level of sedation and intermittent use of pulse oximetry.

Cohen et al.[57] compared Epi-PCA fentanyl and sufentanil in the postcesarean section setting and found that both groups achieved adequate analgesia and patient satisfaction. Patients in the sufentanil group required fewer PCA attempts and self-administered less drug; nevertheless, they also experienced a higher rate of nausea and vomiting. Recommendations for intrathecal and epidural opioid analgesia following cesarean section are outlined in Boxes 64-2 and 64-3.

Pediatrics

For a variety of reasons, including physician fears of cardiorespiratory depression and development of drug dependence, as well as the child's limited ability to articulate complaints of pain and fear of shots, the pediatric population commonly experiences undermedication of pain.[146,196] Because children have the same right to effective pain relief (and its associated benefits) as do adults, spinal opioid therapy has been modified and made available for control of pediatric pain. Indications for spinal opioid analgesia include postoperative pain of moderate-to-severe intensity following

BOX 64-3
EPIDURAL OPIOID ANALGESIA AFTER CESAREAN SECTION CURRENT CLINICAL PRACTICE AT YALE–NEW HAVEN HOSPITAL

We give most patients a small dose of epidural fentanyl (50 to 75 μg) to augment intraoperative anesthesia. We delay epidural fentanyl administration until after the umbilical cord is clamped in cases of: (1) severe fetal distress; (2) thick meconium-stained amniotic fluid; (3) preterm delivery; and (4) other conditions associated with an increased risk of neonatal respiratory depression. After delivery, we give a combination of either preservative-free **morphine** (2 to 3 mg) plus **meperidine** (40 mg) or **hydromorphone** (0.5 to 0.6 mg) epidurally. We add saline so that the total volume is 10 mL. These doses of hydromorphone or morphine-meperidine may be readministered every 6 hours or 12 hours respectively for 24 hours. Alternatively, the catheter may be removed, and IV-PCA initiated 6 to 12 hours after epidural administration of opioid. Some patients receive a 24-hour continuous epidural infusion of **hydromorphone** (10 μg/ml) at a dose of 0.1 mg/hr or a continuous epidural infusion of **fentanyl** (5 μg/ml) at a dose of 40 to 60 μg/hr. Patient-controlled bolus doses (5–15 μg of fentanyl or 5 to 10 μg of hydromorphone every 8 minutes) may be combined with a lower background epidural infusion rate.

We administer metoclopramide for treatment of nausea and vomiting and give small doses of **diphenhydramine, naloxone,** or **nalbuphine** for treatment of pruritus. We give a small dose of **ketorolac** (15 mg slow IV bolus every 6 hours) for breakthrough pain (unless contraindicated).

thoracotomy, upper abdominal, urogenital, and lower extremity orthopedic surgery. Selective spinal analgesia may be gained from single doses or continuous infusions of opioid analgesics administered at epidural, caudal, and intrathecal sites.[9,17,116,124,125] The caudal space is used frequently in children because it is simple to locate and offers reliable results with minimal complications.[124,248] On the other hand, lumbar epidural catheters are somewhat more difficult to insert, especially in smaller children. Experience with caudal, lumbar, and thoracic epidural routes of morphine administration has been reported with dosages ranging between 0.05 and 0.12 mg/kg.[9,103,124,125] As in adults, the dose and total volume of diluent may be varied depending on sites of injection and surgical incision.

Caudal analgesia with morphine offers considerable versatility and when administered in appropriate volumes of solution, can blunt pain from sacral sites to high thoracic dermatomal regions. In this regard, fairly high volumes of diluent are required to blunt pain at higher thoracic dermatomes such as sternotomy or thoracotomy.[31,45,103,188] Krane et al.[124,125] compared caudal morphine (0.1 mg/kg), caudal bupivacaine, and intravenous morphine in 46 children after orthopedic or genitourinary surgery, noting analgesia of 8 to 24 hours, 5 hours, and 45 minutes, respectively. Although no episodes of delayed respiratory depression were observed, a follow-up investigation by the same group reported an adverse event occurring 3.5 hours following caudal injection of morphine.[123] **Caudal morphine doses of 0.05 mg/kg (in 5 ml of preservative-free saline) appear to be associated with a lower risk of respiratory depression.[31,103,125] Nevertheless, most authors recommend appropriate monitoring in a high visibility setting by experienced personnel for 24 hours after injection. This is particularly important in premature infants due to the high risk of postoperative apnea.**

Epidurally administered opioids also provide effective postoperative analgesia.[9,17,203] Attia et al.[9] reported pharmacokinetic and CO_2 responses in children receiving epidural morphine (0.05 mg/kg) for relief of upper abdominal surgical pain. All patients noted excellent analgesia; however, CO_2 sensitivity was impaired for 22 hours following administration. Some investigators suggest that more lipophilic opioids (hydromorphone, fentanyl, sufentanil) would offer advantages over morphine, including rapid analgesic onset and less tendency to spread rostrally in CSF following epidural administration.[17,18,103] In this regard, Benlabed et al.[17] noted that epidurally administered sufentanil (0.75 μg/kg) provided analgesia for 200 minutes following urologic surgery; however, respiratory depression lasted more than 240 minutes. The short duration of pain relief and associated respiratory compromise led these authors to conclude that bolus doses of sufentanil offer limited clinical advantage in this setting.

Intrathecal opioids are also used in pediatric patients and offer effective relief following more extensive and painful procedures. Jones et al.[116] reported that intrathecal morphine offered effective postoperative analgesia in 59 children recovering from open heart surgery. Sixty percent of patients noted excellent pain relief for up to 22 hours; however, 9 children experienced significant respiratory depression. Broadman et al.[30] reported that intrathecal morphine (0.01 mg/kg) provided excellent postoperative pain relief lasting up to 18 hours in 10 children following Harrington rod instrumentation for scoliosis surgery. Dalens and Tanguy[67] who used larger doses (0.025 mg/kg) of intrathecal morphine, noted excellent pain relief and no evidence of respiratory depression in patients recovering from spinal fusion surgery. Intrathecal, epidural, and caudal doses of opioid analgesics for pediatric patients are presented in Table 64-5.

Respiratory depression is the most feared adverse effect associated with spinal opioid analgesia. As in adults, clinically significant respiratory depression occurs most commonly with morphine, is most often observed during the first 6 to 12 hours following administration, and is exacerbated by concomitant administration of par-

Table 64-5 Recommended agents and rates of infusion for pediatric epidural, caudal, and intrathecal analgesia

	Surgical site		
	Lower extremity lower abdomen	Upper abdomen	Thoracic
Thoracic catheter		(1) 0.1–0.5 ml/kg/hr (3) 0.1–0.5 ml/kg/hr	(1) 0.1–0.5 ml/kg/hr (3) 0.1–0.5 ml/kg/hr (4) 0.1 – 0.5 ml/kg/hr (5) 0.05–0.25 ml/kg/hr
Lumbar or caudal catheters	(1) 0.1–0.5 ml/kg/hr (3) 0.1–0.5 ml/kg/hr	(1) 0.1–0.5 ml/kg/hr (3) 0.1–0.5 ml/kg/hr (4) 0.1–0.5 ml/kg/hr (6) 0.1–0.5 ml/kg/hr	(1) 0.1–0.5 ml/kg/hr (3) 0.1–0.5 ml/kg/hr (5) 0.1–0.25 ml/kg/hr (7) 0.1–0.25 ml/kg/hr
Caudal (single dose)	(2) 0.05 ml/kg/segment	(8) 0.05–0.10 mg/kg in 3 ml preservative-free normal saline	(8) 0.05–0.10 mg/kg in preservative-free normal saline
Intrathecal		(8) 0.01–0.02 mg/kg	(8) 0.01–0.02 mg/kg

(1) — bupivacaine 0.1%; (2) — bupivacaine 0.25%; (3) — bupivacaine 0.1% and fentanyl 2 μg/ml; (4) — bupivacaine 0.1% and hydromorphone 10 μg/ml; (5) — bupivacaine 0.1% and hydromorphone 20 μg/ml; (6) — hydromorphone 10 μg/ml; (7) — hydromorphone 20 μg/ml; (8) — morphine, preservative free. (From: Haber DW, Berde CB: Spinal opioids for pediatric pain management, In RS Sinatra, AH Hord, B Ginsberg, LM Preble, editors: *Acute pain mechanisms and management*, St Louis, 1992, Mosby–Year Book.)

enteral narcotics.[18,103,248] In addition to respiratory depression, pediatric patients experience a similar incidence and severity of pruritus, nausea or vomiting, and urinary retention as noted in adults. Itching is more an annoyance than a major problem and responds to diphenhydramine and low-dose naloxone (0.005 mg/kg). Urinary retention is also observed following genital surgery and can be a problem if a urinary catheter is not left in place. Pediatric patients may occasionally become agitated despite excellent postoperative analgesia when placed in unfamiliar intensive care surroundings or following prolonged separation from their parents. Such changes in behavior may require judicious administration of anxiolytic agents (midazolam 0.05 to 0.1 mg/kg every 2 hours), as well as increased vigilance in assessing ventilatory status following initiation of such therapy.[18,103]

Chronic Pain

Although the chronic pain patient population was first offered and potentially has most to gain from spinal opioid analgesia, a relatively small number of patients suffering from pain of terminal cancer or chronic pain syndromes have benefited from the technique. Many patients suffering intractable malignancy pain do not achieve satisfactory analgesia with systemic opioids until the dosage is increased to the point of marked sedation or confusion. The gain in analgesic potency achieved with spinal opioids can offer these patients superior pain relief, minimal sedation, and an improved quality of life. As an added benefit, the troublesome spinal opioid side effects noted in postsurgical patients are uncommon in this population because chronic exposure to systemic opioids often results in significant tolerance to these problems.

Prolonged periods of effective spinal analgesia have been reported in terminal malignancy patients treated with intrathecal and epidurally administered opioids. Both methods involve permanent percutaneous placement of a catheter and bolus dosing with a syringe, continuous infusion using an external pump, or continuous infusion using a totally implanted pump.[58,59,176,231,232]

Intrathecal dosing has the advantage of lower dose requirements and more selective analgesic effect, but it can be complicated by dural puncture headache, meningitis, and arachnoiditis.[60,231] Epidural catheter placement and prolonged administration of drug often lead to epidural fibrosis, a condition which impedes dural penetration and may increase analgesic dose requirements. The efficacy of epidurally administered opioids may also be compromised by an unrecognized epidural tumor mass in patients with widespread metastatic disease.[49]

Bolus doses of intrathecal morphine (0.5 to 2 mg) were noted to provide effective analgesia in 46 to 72 patients suffering from intractable pain secondary to cancer of the pelvic organs.[231,232] Complications including CSF leakage, infection, and progressive tolerance development were noted; however, patients did not experience significant respiratory depression and most were able to remain at home and participate in their usual everyday activities. **Caution must be applied when initiating intrathecal morphine analgesia in patients previously managed with oral or parenteral narcotics because acute withdrawal may be precipitated by sharp reductions in total analgesic requirements.**

Continuous infusion of epidural and intrathecal opioids at constant, slow rates may lower the risk of tolerance development by avoiding high peak CSF levels and cephalad migration of drug.[23,56] Infusion techniques also lower the incidence of catheter occlusion commonly observed with bolus injection. Continuous administration of intrathecal morphine offers the advantage of potent, highly selective analgesia (hundredfold reduction in parenteral morphine dose requirement over 24 hours) and improved versatility in dosing. Postmortem studies after long-term continuous intrathecal infusions of morphine or morphine-bupivacaine were not associated with neuronal or myelin damage of the spinal cord.[228]

Continuous infusion devices are commercially available and following subcutaneous implantation, slowly release low doses of opioid for periods of 2 to 4 weeks, after which time the patient returns to the hospital to have the reservoir recharged.[176] Coombs et al.[58] reported effective relief of malignancy pain in a group of patients receiving continuous morphine doses of 2 mg/day initially and 6.6 mg/day at the end of 12 weeks. Unfortunately, some patients required rapid escalation in infusion rate and total dose requirements. Efforts to overcome tolerance development with trials of delta opioid receptor agonists (DADL),[240] the alpha-agonist clonidine[80] and potent opioids, such as sufentanil,[73] have provided some degree of success. Best results have been noted with "holiday" protocols in which intraspinal local anesthetics are substituted for opioids to provide several days of analgesia while improving spinal opioid-receptor sensitivity.

Spinal opioids offer effective relief of a variety of chronic pain syndromes, including low back pain and phantom limb pain. Penn and Paice[170] reported that patients suffering from chronic low back pain of benign origin experienced excellent analgesia with epidural or intrathecal morphine for periods of 6 months or longer. These investigators emphasize that patients were carefully selected, hospitalized, and screened for a 3- to 5-day course of epidural morphine delivery before being sent home with an indwelling catheter and programmable administration device. Although many practitioners are reluctant to institute long-term narcotic therapy in patients with pain of benign origin, the increased analgesic efficacy noted with intrathecal opioids offers a useful alternative that, in difficult cases, should not be dismissed out of hand. Lumbar intrathecal administration of fentanyl and morphine[113] in patients with severe postamputation phantom limb pain has been reported to provide complete relief of discomfort. This dramatic response in a setting where parenteral opioids were completely ineffective suggests that the spinal cord plays an important role in the genesis of phantom pain. Further investigations testing the applicability of spinal opioids for treatment of other nerve injury syndromes are warranted.

SIDE EFFECTS OF SPINAL OPIOIDS

Morphine's ability to remain sequestered in CSF offers the advantages of prolonged duration, higher analgesic potency, and an extended dermatomal level of activity; however, progressive rostral spread leads to major therapeutic liabilities, which, in selected settings may limit the overall utility of this agent. Polar, hydrophilic morphine molecules are slowly transported cephalad via bulk CSF flow, eventually reaching higher spinal segments and brainstem nuclei.[33] This concept was substantiated by the finding that morphine CSF concentrations sampled at the C7 interspace peaked within 3 hours following lumbar epidural administration.[92] **This cephalad progression of epidural morphine analgesia parallels a predictable onset of pruritus at 3 hours, nausea and vomiting at 4 to 6 hours, and "delayed" respiratory depression at 6 to 10 hours.**[33,34,82]

Respiratory Depression

Respiratory depression associated with morphine occurs at two distinct intervals.[59,82,100] An early phase occurring soon after administration reflects absorption and circulatory redistribution to the brain and is of similar magnitude to that noted when equally sized doses are administered parenterally. A later, more insidious, delayed-onset depression results from morphine's migration in CSF to brainstem respiratory centers.[33,59,82,118]

Kafer et al.[118] were first to describe morphine's biphasic respiratory depressive effect, documenting maximal depression of minute ventilation response to CO_2 at 2 and 8 hours following epidural administration. In a multicenter study of 14,000 patients treated with epidural morphine, the incidence of significant respiratory depression ranged between 0.25% and 0.40%, with all episodes occurring within 12 hours of administration.[177] **Risk factors underlying delayed respiratory depression include high doses of morphine, patients over 65 years of age, presence of pulmonary disease, and most importantly, concomitant parenteral administration of narcotics and sedative hypnotics (Box 64-4).** Intrathecal administration was originally associated with higher risk, although greater clinical experience has shown that careful dose adjustment is associated with rates of respiratory depression comparable with that observed with epidural dosing. Even in the absence of the above mentioned factors, the incidence of clinically significant respiratory compromise with both epidural and intrathecal morphine ranges between 0.1% and 0.4%,[59,82,177] while less troublesome depression of CO_2 response occurs more frequently, especially in postsurgical settings. In two comparisons of postoperative analgesic techniques, declines in O_2 saturation were less common but of greater magnitude with epidural morphine than with IV morphine (Fig. 64-11).[2,37]

Although delayed respiratory depression is usually gradual in onset and reversible with small doses of naloxone, its risk mandates frequent respiratory checks, and increased nursing supervision.[90,182,183] Some authors advocate respiratory depression "prophylaxis" with low dose naloxone infusions,[115,118B] nalbuphine infusions,[118B] or intermittent doses of long acting opioids such as oral naltrexone.[66] Older patients treated with long-acting CNS depressants appear to be highly sensitive to epidural morphine. Pro-

BOX 64-4
FACTORS PREDISPOSING TO THE DEVELOPMENT OF RESPIRATORY DEPRESSION FOLLOWING THE ADMINISTRATION OF EPIDURAL OPIOIDS

Drug-related factors

Hydrophillic opioids
Excessive dose
Large injectate volume
Excessive dose frequency
Concomitant administration of IM narcotics

Patient-related factors

Age greater than 60 years
Debilitated individuals
Morbid obesity
Sleep apnea syndrome
Coexisting respiratory disease
Unintentional intrathecal administration
Raised intrathoracic pressure
Shock wave lithotripsy
Trendelenberg position

found sedation, confusion, and airway obstruction may be observed in patients treated with large preoperative or intraoperative doses of midazolam, lorazepam, and scopolamine. The activity of these CNS depressants appears to be magnified and more prolonged if postsurgical pain has been virtually eliminated. Increased postsurgical sedation may be reversed safely with small doses of flumazenil and physostigmine.[207]

Epidural hydromorphone has a lower tendency to migrate rostrally in CSF and a lower risk of delayed respiratory depression than morphine.[32,207] Its safety in this setting was revealed in a letter to the editor which described a patient who inadvertently received a 5-mg rather than 0.5-mg epidural dose without significant sequelae.[149]

Compared with morphine, the rostral spread of more lipophilic opioids is of smaller magnitude and usually of little clinical significance.[6,126] Wells and Davies[236] observed CNS depression and severe bradypnea following extracorporeal shock wave lithotripsy in a patient who had received 100 μg of epidural fentanyl. These symptoms took 4 hours to resolve. Whether the shock waves used with this procedure were associated with cephalad spread of fentanyl is not clear; however, the patient's morbid obesity and intraoperative administration of midazolam (4.5 mg) and nalbuphine

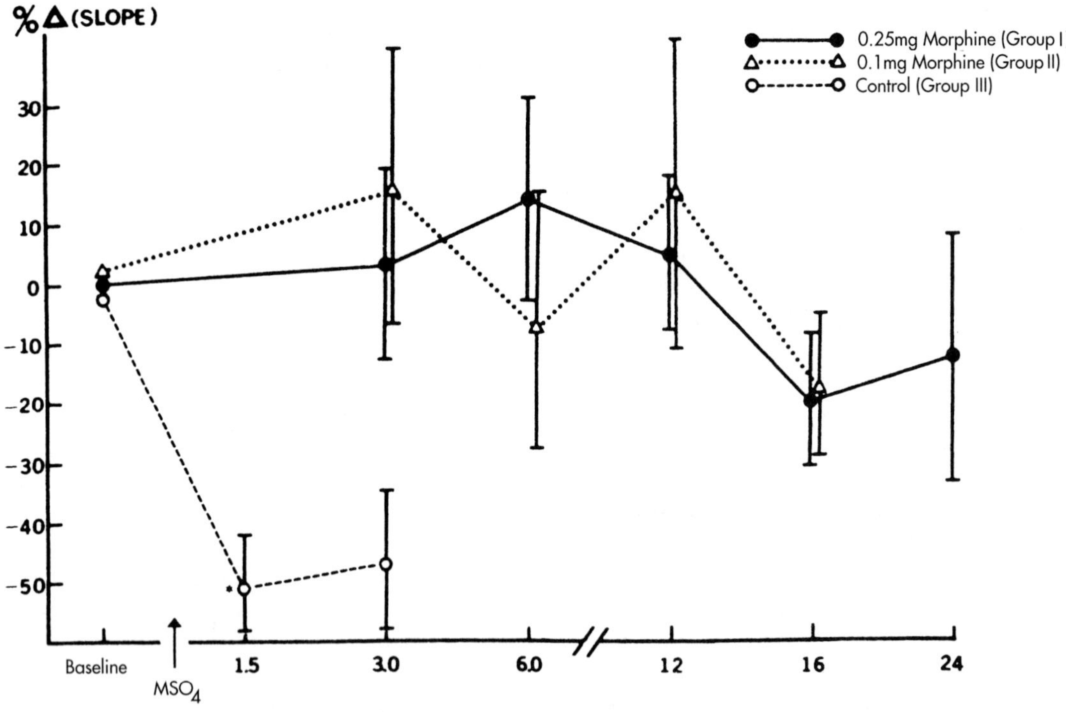

Fig. 64-11. Percent change in CO_2 response slopes ($l \cdot min^{-1} \cdot mm\ Hg^{-1}$) from baseline values after patients received intrathecal (solid circle, triangle) or subcutaneous morphine control (open circle). (From Abboud TK, Dror A, Mosaad P, et al: Mini-dose intrathecal morphine for the relief of post-cesarean section pain: Ventilatory responses to carbon dioxide, *Anesth Analg* 67:137, 1988.)

(2.5 mg) were believed to have contributed to the CNS depression. It is unclear whether the risk of delayed-onset respiratory depression increases in the setting of continuous infusions where prolonged elimination kinetics may lead to significant systemic accumulation.[47,56]

Early-onset respiratory depression is more common with potent lipophilic opioids and reflects vascular uptake and rapid circulation to brainstem respiratory centers.[6,82,93,121,217] Although measurable and occasionally serious,[6,21,93,121] such depression is usually of less significance than delayed respiratory compromise, as it is more likely to occur in highly visible, controlled settings (operating room, recovery room, intensive care unit) in which the anesthesiologist is present or immediately available. Graf et al.[93] cautioned against using large single-bolus doses to extend duration, inasmuch as respiratory arrest occurred in one patient within seconds of administering 70 μg sufentanil. Other episodes of immediate-onset respiratory depression have been reported after large or repeat boluses.[6,21,82,91,217] Immediate respiratory depression may be related to inadvertent puncture of an epidural vein with intravascular administration or may simply reflect sufentanil's rapid vascular uptake. In this regard, sufentanil plasma levels peak within 2 minutes and approach 0.31 ng/ml.[44,47] When administering sufentanil, precautions similar to those used when administering any local anesthetic should be used; that is, a test dose (5 μg) is followed by small and slowly administered increments.[93]

Nausea and Vomiting

The high incidence of nausea and vomiting noted with intrathecal and epidurally administered morphine is also related to rostral CSF flow with transport of molecules to the chemoreceptor trigger zone (area postrema) in the brainstem.[33,34,59] In a series of 1200 postsurgical patients treated with bolus doses of epidural morphine, 17% suffered severe nausea and vomiting,[185] a figure comparable to that observed with parenterally administered opioids. Nausea is a more frequent side effect in young adults recovering from abdominal surgery and in obstetric patients, occurring in 20% to 30% of postcesarean patients treated with epidural morphine.[79,105] Lussos et al.[143] found that metoclopramide administered before induction of spinal anesthesia for cesarean section decreased symptomology without adverse effects. Significant reductions in the incidence and severity of nausea associated with epidural fentanyl may be achieved when small amounts of droperidol (0.05 mg) are added to the infusate.[7] Ondansetron (2 to 4 mg) also provides effective antiemetic benefit; however, prohibitive cost often restricts its routine use as primary therapy.[207] In the presence of intractable nausea and vomiting, a small bolus of naloxone followed by a continuous infusion will usually attenuate the symptoms without significant loss of analgesia. Abboud et al.[1] found that naltrexone (6 mg) is an effective oral prophylactic against both pruritis and vomiting but at the cost of a shortened duration of intrathecal morphine analgesia. Transdermal scopolamine patch preparations have also proven effective in this setting but require 2 to 4 hours before significant antiemetic benefits are appreciated.[122] The incidence of nausea and vomiting is reduced when opioids are administered via continuous infusion and is rarely observed in patients receiving long-term therapy for malignancy pain.

Pruritus

Pruritus is frequently observed with epidural opioids and represents the most common side effect noted in obstetric patients. In some individuals, pruritus may be so severe and distressful that it interferes with sleep and compromises the benefits of superior analgesia. In young adults and parturients treated with epidural morphine, mild pruritus, usually of the face and chest, occurs in 70% to 90% of patients,[79,105,201] whereas more severe symptoms, often associated with rash and requiring treatment are noted in 40%.[34,60,79,105] Although the etiology of pruritus is unclear its occurrence appears unrelated to direct opioid-induced histamine release as the peak onset occurs 3 to 6 hours after administration.[201,252] Furthermore, mild pruritus, usually isolated to the abdomen, is also observed with intrathecal and epidurally administered hydromorphone, fentanyl and sufentanil, opioids that are not associated with systemic release of histamine.[60] Pruritus may reflect alterations in spinal and trigeminal processing of afferent information, whereby spinal modulation of nociceptive input is reinterpreted as itch at higher centers.[201] A recent report suggests that changes in spinal efferent outflow may indirectly release histamine at peripheral sites.[252] This finding may explain why antihistamine may provide effective therapy. Other effective forms of treatment include cold compresses, naloxone infusion, and single doses of naltrexone.[1,66] Rawal and coworkers[178] reported that a naloxone infusion of 2.5 to 5 μg/kg/min reduced both the incidence and severity of pruritis in patients treated with epidural morphine. Small doses of IV propofol also provide effective relief of pruritus; however, multiple doses may be required, because its duration of antipruritic activity is limited to 60 to 90 minutes.[26,193] Our current regimen of treating moderate-to-severe pruritis is to administer 40-μg naloxone bolus followed by 0.4 mg/1000 ml of maintenance fluid to run at 100 ml/hr. Such dosing effectively counteracts pruritic side effects and maintains excellent analgesia.

Urinary Retention

A final serious adverse effect which adds to the morbidity of spinal opioid analgesia is urinary retention. This complication occurs most often, but not exclusively, in young men and has been related to relaxation of the bladder detrusor muscle.[60,180] Urinary retention is rarely observed in obstetric patients or in individuals receiving long-term epidural opioid therapy. Urinary retention is disturbing to both patient

YALE-NEW HAVEN HOSPITAL

DOCTOR'S ORDERS

PLEASE USE BALL POINT PEN – BEAR DOWN

INSTRUCTIONS

1. EACH TIME A PHYSICIAN WRITES A MEDICATION ORDER, DETACH TOP COPY AND SEND TO PHARMACY
2. RULE OFF UNUSED LINES AFTER LAST COPY (PINK) HAS BEEN SENT TO PHARMACY. IMPRINT NEW SET AND PLACE IN CHART

DO NOT USE THIS SHEET UNLESS A NUMBER SHOWS ▶ 3

HOLD HERE WHILE REMOVING YELLOW COPIES

DATE	TIME	ORDERS	DOCTOR'S SIGNATURE	NURSE'S SIGNATURE

ACUTE PAIN SERVICE/DEPARTMENT OF ANESTHESIOLOGY

CONTINUOUS EPIDURAL/INTRATHECAL INFUSION ORDERS

1. INFUSION: Drug(s) and concentration(s) ____________
   rate: ________ cc/hr
2. HEAD OF BED greater than ____ degrees. ACTIVITY: per surgeon.
   VITAL SIGNS per routine, except respiratory rate q __ h x ___ hours,
   then q __ h x __ hours, then q4h. MAINTAIN IV access while
   epidural catheter is in place.
3. PULSE OXIMETRY Yes __; No __. Continuous ___ for ___ hours;
   Intermittent ___ q ___ hours for ___ hours.
4. Naloxone (Narcan) two (2) ampules in patient's unit dose cassette
5. NO SYSTEMIC NARCOTICS/SEDATIVES TO BE GIVEN EXCEPT AS ORDERED BY APS.
6. Treatment of nausea/vomiting:
   Yes __; No __ droperidol (Inapsine) 0.2ml (0.5mg) IV q2h prn x 2 doses
   Yes __; No __ metoclopramide (Reglan) __mg IV q4h prn x 2 doses
   Yes __; No __ transderm scopolamine patch (mastoid area) for 72 hours
   Yes __; No __ other: ____________
7. Treatment of pruritus (itching):
   Benadryl 12.5mg IV q30 minutes prn x 2 doses
8. Prophylactic infusion for itching: Yes __; No __.
   Naloxone __; or Nalbuphine __. Add ___ ampule(s) per liter of
   maintenance IV fluid x ___ liter(s)
9. Adjuvant therapy: Yes __; No __.
   Ketorolac, loading dose of __mg __(route); then __mg __(route)
   q __h PRN; or __mg __(route) q __ hours for ___ doses.
10. Notify APS, beeper 128-2154, for:
    a) somnolence or confusion
    b) respiratory rate of 10 or less
    c) inadequate analgesia
    d) pruritus or nausea/vomiting unresponsive to treatment
    e) oxygen saturation less than 90%
    f) leakage or redness around insertion site

Date: ____________ ____________ MD

F-854 (Rev. 7/87)

Fig. 64-12. Standardized orders for continuous epidural analgesia used at Yale-New Haven Hospital.

and surgeon, especially when its severity requires frequent catheterization. Although mechanisms underlying urinary retention remain unclear, IV naloxone and urocholine represent effective therapy in selected cases.

Monitoring Requirements

What is the most appropriate method of respiratory monitoring for patients treated with epidural/intrathecal morphine or continuous opioid infusions? This question is difficult, and no single solution appears applicable to every institution. In the absence of any generally accepted standards for monitoring patients treated with such therapy, the decision of whether to use long-acting opioids such as morphine or hydromorphone and how best to monitor patients must be left to the judgment of each individual practitioner in conjunction with the nursing staff on postsurgical wards.

Various noninvasive monitors have been advocated including pulse oximetry, and end-tidal PCO_2 monitoring; however, none of these methods has become universally accepted. In most published studies, hourly monitoring of respiratory rate has been the most common method used to detect respiratory compromise. Apnea monitors may be prone to annoying false alarms, do not detect hypoventilation, and require cooperation from patients and nurses for turning them off while caring for the newborn and prior to ambulation. Pulse oximeters share the drawbacks of patient inconvenience, frequent motion artifact alarms and an inability to detect hypercapnia. The speed with which epidural

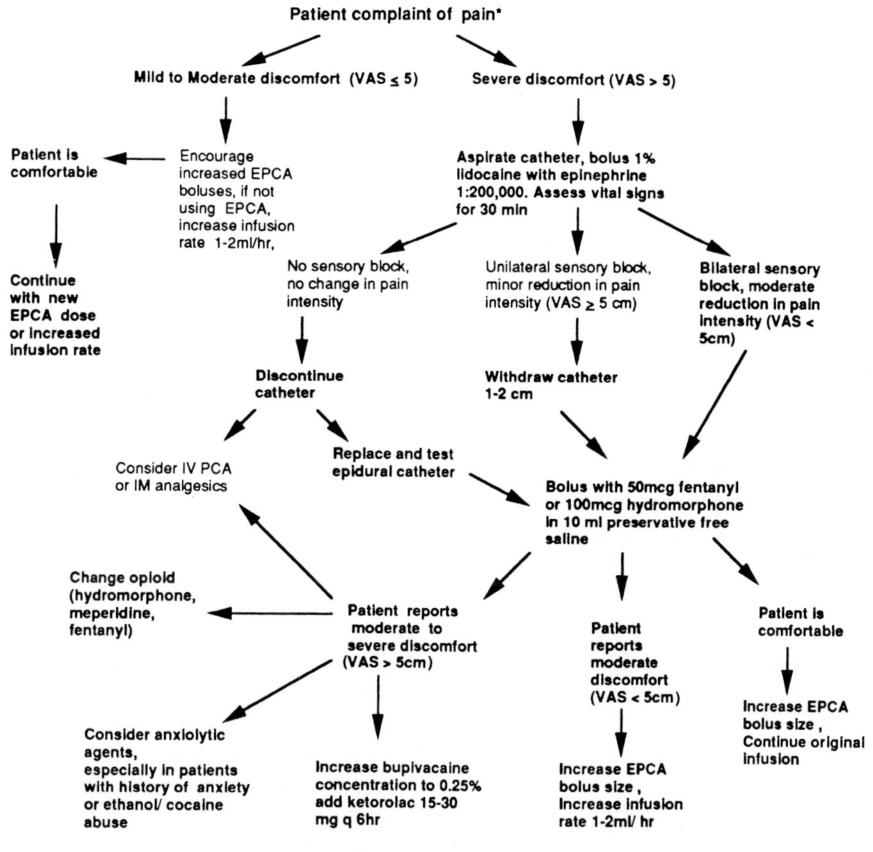

Fig. 64-13. Algorithim used for assessing and treating inadequate epidural analgesia.

morphine-induced respiratory depression develops is not sudden, but slowly progressive. **Respiratory rate is often a poor indicator of ventilatory depression; increasing somnolence offers a more reliable warning of respiratory compromise and should be continuously monitored.**[182,183] **Vigilant nursing education, standardized orders, frequent patient assessment and level-of-consciousness checks provide the best insurance in avoiding serious respiratory depression.**[183] With appropriate nursing staff education and standardized orders, neuraxial opioids may be safely administered to a majority of patients recovering from surgery or trauma. In this regard, two recent large-scale evaluations noted that intermittent doses and continuous infusions of morphine were safely provided on postsurgical wards where nurses were well trained with respect to dose, patient assessment, and treatment of side effects.[70,182] Standardized orders for epidural opioid analgesia at Yale-New Haven hospital are presented in Figure 64-12. We agree with the recommendation that an acute pain service or 24-hour in-house anesthesia personnel be immediately available to back up the nursing staff in settings of spinal opioid overdose or inadequate analgesia.[183] Inadequate analgesia may be the result of catheter-related problems, undermedication, and patient-related variability. An algorithim used to assess patients' level of comfort and treat inadequate analgesia is presented in Figure 64-13.

ANESTHETIC OUTCOME AND NEURAXIAL OPIOIDS

The current practice of medicine dictates that both quality and cost of medical care be examined and improved. In an increasingly competitive marketplace, anesthesiologists are being asked with increasing frequency to provide proof of outcomes from services rendered. Costs associated with epidural placement and infusion devices, drug preparation, and supervision are considerably higher than traditional forms of analgesia. To justify this increased expenditure, studies have been undertaken to determine whether optimal postsurgical analgesia can decrease morbidity and duration of hospital stay.[54,71,72,96,97,136,221] Improvements in outcome and length of hospital stay are difficult variables to measure, because a variety of factors other than pain management may influence time to discharge from the surgical ward. These include hospital census, individual surgeon's criteria for discharge, and differences in nursing, physical therapy, and nutritional support.

In addition to providing superior postsurgical analgesia, epidural administration of opioid analgesics alone or in combination with dilute bupivacaine is more effective than IV-PCA and IM administered opioids in suppressing release of catecholamines and stress hormones and maintaining hemodynamic stability.[15,27,28,38,148,165,234] Patients who benefit most from epidural analgesia are those recovering from extensive surgical procedures where parenteral opioid dose requirements are high and pulmonary compromise secondary to inadequate analgesia is common.[15,38,71,72] Therapeutic gains are dramatic in patients with underlying cardiovascular and pulmonary disease,[28,48,54,72] and less obvious in healthy individuals recovering from minimally invasive procedures. **Optimally administered epidural analgesia and Epi-PCA can reduce myocardial oxygen requirements, improve respiratory function, and decrease the incidence of DVT.[22,204] Such therapy has also been shown to reduce mortality, hospital stay, and overall costs.[54,71,72,96,97,136]** These desirable attributes outweigh the greater invasiveness and potential side effects associated with epidural placement and indwelling catheters.

Improvements in physiologic parameters observed with epidural opioids may be more important than reductions in pain scores. Using improvements in respiratory effort as an index of pain relief, Bromage et al.[35] noted significant benefit in patients receiving epidural morphine (forced expiratory volume [FEV_1] = 67% of baseline versus 45% noted with IV morphine). Morbidly obese patients recovering from major abdominal surgery and treated with epidural morphine benefited from a more rapid return of peak expiratory flow and fewer pulmonary complications than others treated with parenteral opioids.[179] Shulman et al.[205] evaluated post-thoracotomy pain and pulmonary function following epidural and systemic morphine administration in 30 patients undergoing thoracotomy for lung resection. The patients were randomized to receive either epidural or IV morphine for management of analgesia. Patients receiving epidural morphine had less pain at 2 and 8 hours and, although both groups showed a decrease in FEV_1, functional residual capacity (FRC), and peak expiratory flow rate (PEFR), the epidural group consistently showed less of a decrease in all three categories during the first 24 hours. Salomaki et al.[194,195] compared epidural and IV fentanyl infusions for post-thoracotomy analgesia in a randomized, double-blind fashion and found that respiratory function was better preserved, and the incidence of nausea, oversedation, and excessive neuroendocrine response was reduced in the epidural group. In 1987, Yeager et al.[249] compared two groups in a randomized, controlled clinical trial to evaluate the effects of epidural anesthesia and postoperative analgesia on postoperative morbidity in a group of high-risk surgical patients. Patients randomized to the epidural anesthesia and postoperative analgesia group had a reduction in both overall postoperative complications and in the incidence of cardiovascular failure. Using urinary cortisol as a marker of the stress response, they found a significantly diminished level in the epidural group when compared with the control group. Tuman and colleagues[221] evaluated the interaction of epidural anesthesia, coagulation status, and outcome after lower extremity revascularization in 80 patients prospectively randomized to receive either general anesthesia and postoperative epidural analgesia or general anesthesia plus IV-PCA. They found that the duration of postoperative intensive care unit stay as well as the incidence of cardiovascular and infectious postoperative complications to be significantly reduced in the general-epidural group. Additionally, they noted that their study population of vascular patients were hypercoagulable compared with controls. In a study of 100 patients randomized to receive either epidural anesthesia or general anesthesia with IV-PCA for elective lower extremity revascularization procedures, Christopherson et al.[54] found comparable rates of cardiac morbidity, however the incidence of reoperation for inadequate tissue perfusion was significantly lower in the epidural anesthesia group. Liu et al.[136] found that in patients recovering from colectomy, epidural analgesia with the combination of bupivacaine and morphine provided the best balance of analgesia and side effects while accelerating postoperative recovery of gastrointestinal function (Fig. 64-14). de Leon-Casasola et al.[72] studied the incidence of postsurgical myocardial ischemia and myocardial infarction in patients at high risk for coronary artery disease. Patients received either epidural bupivacaine and morphine or general anesthesia followed by IV-PCA morphine. They noted that patients receiving epidural anesthesia/analgesia benefited from a reduction in postoperative tachycardia, ischemia, and myocardial infarction. In a second study, de Leon-Casasola et al.[71] found that, although satisfactory analgesia was achieved by patients receiving either epidural or IV-PCA after oncologic surgery, patients receiving epidural anesthesia and analgesia experienced faster recovery as judged by shorter mechanical ventilation time and decreased surgical intensive care unit and hospital stays, and lower overall hospitalization costs. Reductions in surgical morbidity and shortened time to hospital discharge represent clinical value-added advantages that outweigh the greater cost and invasiveness of epidural analgesic techniques.

In summary, epidural administered opioids offer an excellent analgesic alternative to parenteral narcotics or epidural local anesthetics. This application is a new one for an old family of drugs,[8,237] yet these agents appear ideally suited to selectively block pain as it first enters the CNS. Potential advantages of spinal/epidural analgesia must be carefully balanced on a case-by-case basis against dose-associated side effects and the greater invasiveness of the technique. Nevertheless, the higher intensity of pain relief noted with continuous epidural opioid infusions is capable of providing "pain prevention" or lack of pain perception.[8,69,227] Pain prevention is an important goal in high risk and debilitated individuals, as it is associated with reduced catecholamine re-

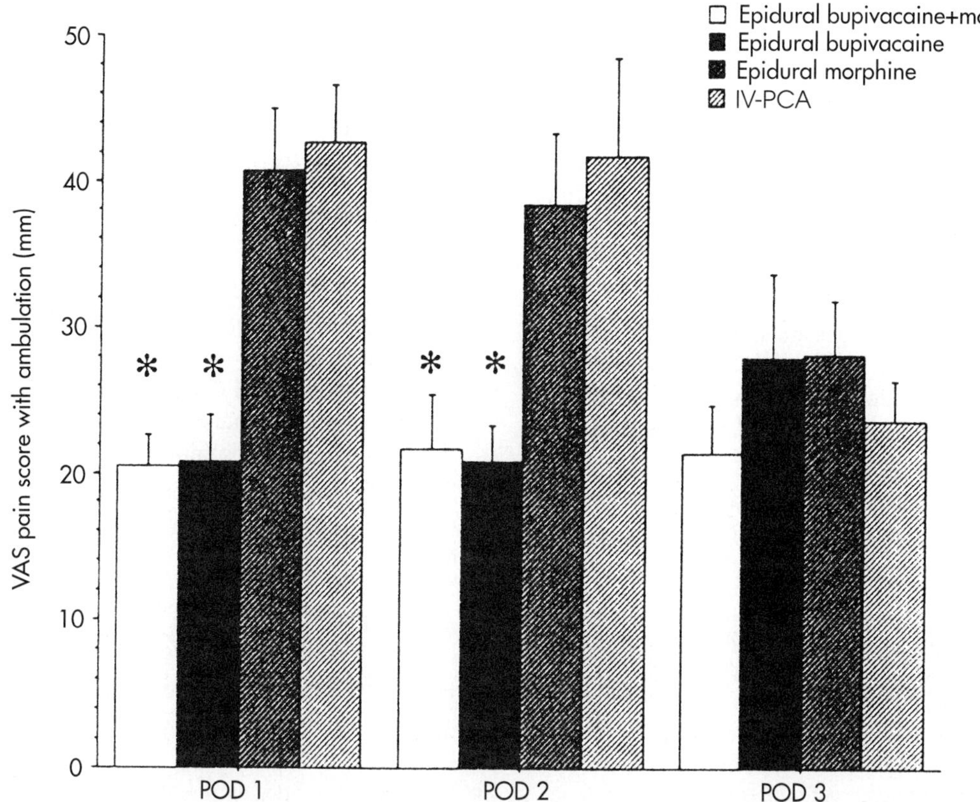

Fig. 64-14. Pain scores with morning ambulation. Mean and standard error displayed. *Significant difference from intravenous patient-controlled analgesia (IV-PCA) and epidural morphine groups ($p < 0.01$). (From Liu S, Carpenter RL, Mackey DC, et al: Effects of perioperative analgesic technique on rate of recovery after colon surgery, *Anesthesiology* 83:757–765, 1995.)

sponse, better cardiovascular stability, and improved pulmonary function in the immediate postsurgical period.[15,27,48,69,72]

FUTURE DEVELOPMENTS

Spinal opioid analgesia remains among the most promising of techniques available for the effective and safe relief of severe pain. Further understanding of pharmacokinetics and pharmacodynamics will increase the usefulness and clinical application of the technique. In their 1984 review, Cousins and Mather[60] outlined a number of questions regarding spinal opioid analgesia, and although many answers have been provided, important concepts require continued investigation. These include: (1) optimal opioid agents and dosage in geriatric and pediatric and chronic pain populations; (2) improvements in neuraxial analgesic efficacy and postsurgical outcome associated with continuous infusion and Epi-PCA techniques; (3) methods to decrease tolerance in chronic pain settings; (4) nonopioid "multimodal" supplementation of neuraxial analgesia; (5) improved prophylaxis and treatment of neuraxial opioid side effects.

Future areas of investigation will include the following:

- Enhancement of spinal opioid analgesia with concomitant administration of nonopioid adjuncts, including alpha-adrenergic agonists, N-methyl-D-aspartate–receptor agonists, nonsteroidal inflamatory drugs, neostigmine, and serotonergic agonists.[2,24,83,147,153,174]
- New kappa agonists and mu_1-selective agonists may be employed for effective spinal analgesia with reduced potential for respiratory depression.[62]
- In preliminary animal studies, intrathecal administration of tramadol, a mu receptor agonist which also inhibits monoamine reuptake, provided intense analgesia of prolonged duration.[142] The finding that tramadol analgesia was not associated with hemodynamic instability or respiratory depression suggests important clinical application.
- Epidural preparations of lipophilic opioids encapsulated in liposomes permiting slow sustained analgesic effects that may be safer than continuous infusions or large doses of morphine.[128]
- Remifentanil has been shown to provide powerful spinal and highly specific opioid activity in animals and it is being evaluated in clinical studies.[40] Its neuraxial specificity is related to the fact that systemically absorbed agent is rapidly inactivated by plasma esterases.

KEY POINTS

- Spinally administered opioids provide powerful regional analgesia without associated motor blockade or excessive CNS depression.
- Morphine selectively suppresses neurons of dorsal horn laminae I and V, mediating noxious information, while having no effect on lamina IV neurons, known to process light touch and proprioceptive input.
- Enkephalin-containing neurons are almost exclusively localized to the substantia gelatinosa, offering evidence that there is an intrinsic modulatory system whose activation could attenuate release of substance P and other nociceptive transmitters.
- Three major opioid receptor subtypes are involved in nociceptive input modulation: mu and delta receptors produce dose-dependent inhibition of cutaneous-thermal responses, whereas activation of kappa receptors results in powerful suppression of visceral-chemical responses while having no effect on somatic nociception.
- Following intrathecal administration, the amount of drug remaining in cerebrospinal fluid at any given time is inversely proportional to the lipid solubility and pKa of the agent employed and directly influences the onset of spinal analgesia. Spinal analgesia after the administration of highly lipophilic opioids is more rapid in onset than that noted with highly ionized lipid-insoluble opioids such as morphine.
- In addition to lipid solubility, total dose administered and volume of injectate represent two variables that can influence duration of activity and dermatomal spread.
- The amount of intrathecally administered opioid required to provide a given level of analgesia is typically much smaller than the amount that must be given IV or IM.
- Morphine is: (1) widely employed for postoperative analgesia and relief of various chronic pain syndromes; (2) usually given epidurally at lumbar sites in doses from 3 to 10 mg; and (3) has an onset and duration in epidural form after single-dose administration that varies according to surgical stimulus and dose and site of administration, with onset in 30 to 60 minutes, peak effect at 90 to 120 minutes, and duration of 12 to 24 hours.
- The clinical behavior of epidural hydromorphone, including onset, duration, and dermatomal spread, appears optimally positioned between that observed with morphine and the more lipophilic opioids. The greater potency and high receptor affinity of hydromorphone provides a more rapid onset of analgesia than morphine, with significant reductions in pain scores noted at 15 minutes and peak effect at 30 minutes following epidural administration.
- Highly lipophilic opioids, such as fentanyl and sufentanil, are frequently employed as epidural analgesics because they provide rapid and effective pain relief with minimal adverse effects.
- Drawbacks associated with single boluses or intermittent doses include: (1) bolus dose requirements are high (fentanyl 50 to 100 μg, sufentanil 30 to 40 μg) (2) significant early onset ventilatory depression can occur; and (3) duration of action (although dose dependent) is quite limited.
- Continuous epidural infusions permit analgesia to be more precisely titrated to the level of pain stimulus and rapidly terminated if problems should occur. The technique avoids the peak CSF concentrations that follow intermittent epidural boluses and reduces the risk of rostral spread and delayed respiratory depression.
- Epidural infusions of morphine, meperidine, and hydromorphone provide superior pain relief with decreased dose requirement compared with IV administration. Morphine infusions (0.5 mg/hr) provided effective analgesia following thoracotomy yet avoided most of the troublesome side effects observed with intermittent boluses.
- Fentanyl's reliability, rapid onset, and short duration make it ideally suited for continuous epidural infusion techniques.
- Sufentanil provides extremely rapid and effective analgesia with no evidence of delayed respiratory depression, but dose requirements are surprisingly high, early-onset ventilatory depression is observed, and the duration of pain relief appears to be no greater than that provided by fentanyl.
- Significant amounts of fentanyl and sufentanil are absorbed by epidural and spinal vasculature resulting in progressive increases in plasma concentration.[23,56,87,89] Comparisons of patients receiving IV and epidurally administered fentanyl revealed no differences in postoperative pain scores and dose requirements.
- Epidural patient-controlled analgesia (Epi-PCA) is a pain management technique that offers greater reduction in pain intensity with lower opioid dose requirement than IV-PCA, while providing increased control and higher patient satisfaction than either single doses or continuous infusions of epidural opioids.
- Epi-PCA with hydromorphone is a safe and more effective alternative to IV-PCA hydromorphone, offering the advantage of reduced opioid dose requirement and more rapid recovery, that is shorter times to return of bowel sounds, resumption of solid diet, discontinuation of analgesic therapy, and hospital discharge.
- In recent years, sufentanil has become the intrathecal opioid of choice for labor analgesia.[42,109,224] Intrathecal sufentanil may be employed as primary therapy or in combined spinal-epidural techniques.
- Epidurally administered opioids provide insufficient analgesia for labor, especially second stage, unless supple-

mented by local anesthetic. The combination of bupivacaine and fentanyl is especially efficacious.

- The caudal space is used frequently in children, because it is simple to locate and offers reliable results with minimal complications. Caudal analgesia with morphine offers considerable versatility and when administered in appropriate volumes of solution can blunt pain from sacral sites to high thoracic dermatomal regions.
- Prolonged periods of effective spinal analgesia have been reported in terminal malignancy patients treated with intrathecally and epidurally administered opioids. Both methods involve permanent percutaneous placement of a catheter and either bolus dosing with a syringe, continuous infusion using an external pump, or continuous infusion using a totally implanted pump.
- Spinal opioids offer effective relief of a variety of chronic pain syndromes, including low back pain and phantom limb pain.
- Respiratory depression associated with morphine occurs at two different intervals: (1) an early phase occurring soon after administration reflects absorption and circulatory redistribution to the brain and is similar in magnitude to that noted when equal-sized doses are administered parenterally; and (2) a later, more insidious, delayed-onset depression reflects morphine's transport via CSF to brainstem respiratory centers.
- Risk factors underlying delayed respiratory depression include high doses of morphine, thoracic epidural administration, patients over 65 years of age, presence of pulmonary disease, and most importantly, concomitant parenteral administration of narcotics and sedative-hypnotics.
- The incidence of clinically significant respiratory compromise ranges from 0.1% to 0.4%, while the less troublesome depression of CO_2 response occurs more frequently, especially in postsurgical settings. IV naloxone may eliminate or reduce the severity of side effects associated with intraspinal opioids without affecting the quality or duration of analgesia.
- The high incidence of nausea and vomiting noted with intrathecal and epidurally administered morphine is also related to rostral CSF flow with the transport of molecules to the chemoreceptor trigger zone (area postrema) in the brainstem.
- Pruritus is frequently observed with epidural opioids and represents the most common side effect noted in obstetric patients.
- Urinary retention occurs most often in young men and has been related to relaxation of the bladder detrusor muscle.
- With appropriate nursing staff education standardized orders, spinal opioids may be safely administered to a majority of patients recovering from surgery or trauma.
- Patients who benefit most from epidural analgesia are those recovering from extensive surgical procedures where parenteral opioid dose requirements are high, and those with pulmonary compromise secondary to inadequate analgesia.
- Therapeutic gains are dramatic in patients with underlying cardiovascular and pulmonary disease and less obvious in healthy individuals recovering from minimally invasive procedures. Optimally administered epidural analgesia and Epi-PCA can reduce myocardial oxygen requirements, improve respiratory function, and decrease the incidence of deep vein thrombosis.

KEY REFERENCES

Beattie WS, Buckley DN, Forrest JB: Epidural morphine reduces the risk of postoperative myocardial ishemia in patients with cardiac risk factors, *Can J Anesth* 40:532–541, 1993.

Berde CB: Pediatric postoperative pain management, *Pediatr Clin North Am* 36:921–940, 1989.

Breslow MJ, Jordan DA, Christopherson R, et al: Epidural morphine decreases postoperative hypertension by attenuating sympathetic nervous system hyperactivity, *JAMA* 261:3577–3581, 1989.

Bromage PR, Camporesi EM, Durant PAC, et al: Rostral spread of epidural morphine, *Anesthesiology* 56:431, 1982.

Chaplan SR, Duncan SR, Brodsky JB, Brose WG: Morphine and hydromorphone epidural analgesia: a prospective, randomized comparison, *Anesthesiology* 77:1090–1094, 1992.

Chestnut DH: Effect on the progress of labor and method of delivery. In Chestnut DH, editor: *Obstetric Anesthesia: Principles and Practice.* St. Louis, 1994, Mosby–Year Book, pp 403–417.

Cousins MJ, Cherry DA, Gourlay GK: Acute and chronic pain: use of spinal opioids. In Counsins MJ, Bridenbaugh PO, editors: *Neural Blockade in Clinical Anesthesia and Management,* ed 2, Philadelphia, 1987, JB Lippincott, pp 993-996.

Cousins MJ, Mather LE: Intrathecal and epidural administration of opioids, *Anesthesiology* 61:276, 1984.

Dahl JB, Rosenberg J, Hansen BL, et al: Differential analgesic effects of low-dose epidural morphine and morphine-bupivacaine at rest and during mobilization after major abdominal surgery, *Anesth Analg* 74:362–365, 1992.

de Leon-Casasola OA, Parker B, Lema MJ, et al:

Postoperative epidural-bupivacaine-morphine therapy: experience with 4,227 surgical cancer patients, *Anesthesiology* 81:368–375, 1994.

Etches RC, Sandler A, Daley MD: Respiratory depression and spinal opioids, *Can J Anaesth* 36:165, 1989.

Glass PSA, Estok P, Ginsberg B, et al: Use of patient-controlled analgesia to compare the efficacy of epidural to intravenous fentanyl administration, *Anesth Analg,* 74: 345–51, 1992.

Gwirtz KH, Young JV, Walker SG, et al: Intrathecal opioid analgesia for acute postoperative pain: experience with 4,134 surgical patients, *Anesthesiology* 83:A780, 1995.

Harrison DM, Sinatra R, Morgese L: Epidural narcotic and patient controlled analgesia for post-cesarean section pain relief, *Anesthesiology* 68:454, 1988.

Kafer ER, Brown JT, Scott DD, et al: Biphasic depression of ventilatory responses to CO_2 following epidural morphine, *Anesthesiology* 58:418–427, 1983.

Kitahata LM, Collins JG: Spinal action of narcotic analgesics, *Anesthesiology* 54:153–163, 1981.

Negre I, Gueneron JP, Jamali SJ, et al: Preoperative analgesia with epidural morphine, *Anesth Analg* 79: 298–302, 1994.

Parker RK, White PF: Epidural patient-controlled analgesia: an alternative to intravenous patient-controlled analgesia for pain relief after cesarean delivery, *Anesth Analg* 75: 245–251, 1992.

Rawal N, Sjostrand UH, Dahlstrom B, et al: Epidural morphine for postoperative pain relief: a comparative study with intramuscular narcotic and intercostal block, *Anesth Analg* 61:93, 1982.

Ready LB, Loper KA, Nessly M, Wild L: Postoperative morphine is safe on surgical wards, *Anesthesiology* 75: 452–456, 1991.

Van den Hoogen RH, Colpaert FC: Epidural and subcutaneous morphine, meperidine, fentanyl, and sufentanil in the rat, *Anesthesiology* 66:186–194, 1987.

Wamsley PNH: Patient-controlled epidural analgesia. In: Sinatra RS, Hord AH, Ginsberg B, Preble LM: *Acute Pain Mechanisms and Management,* St Louis, 1992, Mosby–Year Book.

Yaster M, Maxwell LG: Pediatric regional anesthesia, *Anesthesiology* 70:324, 1989.

Yeager MP, Glass DG, Neff RK: Epidural anesthesia and analgesia in high-risk surgical patients, *Anesthesiology* 66:729–636, 1987.

REFERENCES

1. Abboud TK, Lee K, Zhu J, et al: Prophylactic oral naltrexone with intrathecal morphine for cesarean section, *Anesth Analg* 71:367–370, 1990.
2. Abboud TK, Dror A, Mosaad P, et al: Mini-dose intrathecal morphine for the relief of post-cesarean section pain: ventilatory responses to carbon dioxide, *Anesth Analg* 67:137, 1988.
3. Abboud TK, Moore M, Zhu J, et al: Epidural butorphanol and morphine for relief of post-cesarean section pain, *Anesth Analg* 66:887, 1987.
4. Abboud TK, Shnider SM, Dailey PA: Intrathecal administration of hyperbaric morphine for the relief of pain in labor, *Br J Anaesth* 56:1351, 1984.
5. Ackerman WE, Colclough GW, Juneja MM: Epidural fentanyl significantly decreases nausea and vomiting during uterine manipulation in awake patients, *Anesthesiology* 69:A679, 1988.
6. Ahuja BR, Strunin L: Respiratory effects of epidural fentanyl, *Anaesthesia* 40:949, 1985.
7. Aldrete AJ, Vascello LA: Reduction of nausea and vomiting from epidural opiates by adding droperidol, *Anesthesiology* 81:A967, 1994.
8. Armitage EN: Postoperative pain prevention or relief, *Br J Anaesth* 63:136–137, 1989.
9. Attia J, Ecoffey C, Sanddouk P, et al: Epidural morphine in children: pharmacokinetics and CO2 sensitivity, *Anesthesiology* 65:590, 1986.
10. Atweh SA, Kuhar MJ: Autoradiographic localization of opiate receptors in rat brain. I. Spinal cord and lower medulla, *Brain Res* 124:53, 1977.
11. Bailey PW, Smith BE: Continued epidural infusion of fentanyl for postoperative analgesia, *Anesthesia* 35:1002, 1980.
12. Baraka A, Matkabi M, Noueihid R: Epidural meperidine-bupivacaine for obstetric analgesia, *Anesth Analg* 61:652, 1982.
13. Baraka A, Noueihid R, Hajj S: Intrathecal injection of morphine for obstetric analgesia, *Anesthesiology* 54:136, 1981.
14. Barron DW, Strong JE: Postoperative analgesia in major orthopedic surgery, *Anaesthesia* 36:937, 1981.
15. Beattie WS, Buckley DN, Forrest JB: Epidural morphine reduces the risk of postoperative myocardial ishemia in patients with cardiac risk factors, *Can J Anesth* 40:532–541, 1993.
16. Behar M, Magora F Olshwang D, et al: Epidural morphine in the treatment of pain, *Lancet* 1:527–528, 1979.
17. Benlabed M, Ecoffey C, Levron JC, et al: Analgesia and ventilatory response to CO_2 following epidural sufentanil in children, *Anesthesiology* 67:948, 1987.
18. Berde CB: Pediatric postoperative pain management, *Pediatr Clin North Am* 36:921–940, 1989.
19. Bernards CM, Hill HF: Physical and chemical properties of drug molecules governing their diffusion through the spinal meninges, *Anesthesiology* 77:750–756, 1992.
20. Birnbach DJ, Arcurio T, Johnson MD, et al: Effect of diluent volume on analgesia produced by epidural fentanyl, *Reg Anesth* 60:13, 1988.
21. Blackburn C: Respiratory arrest after epidural sufentanil, *Anaesthesia* 42:665, 1987.
22. Blomberg S, Emanuelsson H, Kvist H, et al: Effects of thoracic epidural anesthesia on coronary arteries and arterioles in patients with coronary artery disease, *Anesthesiology* 73:840–847, 1990.
23. Boersma FP, Noorduin H, Pieters W, et al: Sufentanil concentrations in the spinal cord after long-term epidural infusion, *Anesthesiology* 71:A706, 1989.
24. Bouaziz H, Tong C, Eisenach JC: Postoperative analgesia from intrathecal neostigmine in sheep, *Anesth Analg* 80: 1140–1144, 1995.
25. Boylan J, Vosu H, Klinck J, et al: A comparison of patient controlled analgesia and epidural analgesia in aortic surgery, *Anesthesiology* 81:A1052, 1994.
26. Borgeat A, Saiah M, Wildersmith O, et al: Subhypnotic doses of propofol relieves pruritus induced by epidural and intrathecal morphine, *Anesthesiology* 76:510–512, 1992.
27. Breslow MJ, Jordan DA, Christopherson R, et al: Epidural morphine decreases postoperative hypertension by attenuating sympathetic nervous system hyperactivity, *JAMA* 261:3577–3581, 1989.
28. Breslow MJ: Neuroendocrine responses to surgery. In Breslow MJ, Miller CF,

Rogers MC, editors: *Perioperative management,* St Louis, 1990, Mosby–Year Book.

29. Bridenbaugh PO: Preemptive analgesia-is it clinically relevant? (editorial) *Anesth Analg* 78:203–204, 1994.
30. Broadman LM, Higgins TT, Hannallah RS, et al: Intraoperative subarachnoid morphine for postoperative pain control following Harrington rod instrumentation in children, *Can J Anaesth* 34:S96, 1987.
31. Broadman LM, Hannallah RS, Norden JM, et al: "Kiddie caudals," experience with 1154 consecutive cases without complications, *Anesth Analg* 66:S18, 1987.
32. Brodsky JB, Chaplan SR, Brose WG, Mark JBD: Continuous epidural hydromorphone for postthoracotomy pain relief, *Ann Thorac Surg* 50:888–893, 1990.
33. Bromage PR, Camporesi EM, Durant PAC, et al: Rostral spread of epidural morphine, *Anesthesiology* 56:431, 1982.
34. Bromage PR, Camporesi EM, Durant PAC et al: Non-respiratory side effects of epidural morphine, *Anesth Analg* 61:490–495, 1982.
35. Bromage PR, Camporesi E, Chestnut D: Epidural narcotics for postoperative analgesia, *Anesth Analg* 59:473–480, 1980.
36. Brose WG, Tanelian DL, Brodsky JB, Mark JBD, et al: CSF and blood pharmacokinetics of hydromorphone and morphine following lumbar epidural administration, *Pain* 45:11–15, 1991.
37. Brose WF, Cohen SE: Oxygen desaturation following cesarean section: comparison of three analgesic regimens, *Proc Soc Obstet Anesth Perinatol* 21:45, 1989.
38. Brown DL, Carpenter RL: Perioperative analgesia: a review of risks and benefits, *J Cardiothoracic Anesth* 4:368–383, 1990.
39. Bullingham RES, McQuay JH, Moore RA: Unexpectedly high plasma fentanyl levels after epidural use, *Lancet* 1:1361, 1980.
40. Buerkle H, Yaksh TL: Comparison of the spinal actions of the Mu-Opioid remifentanil with alfentanil and morphine in the rat, *Anesthesiology* 84:94–102, 1996.
41. Calvillo O, Henry JL, Neuman RS: Effects of morphine and naloxone on dorsal horn neurons in the cat, *Can J Physiol Pharmacol* 52:1207, 1974.
42. Cambell DC, Cammann WR, Datta S: The addition of bupivacaine to intrathecal sufentanil for labor analgesia, *Anesth Analg* 81:305–309, 1995.
43. Camman WR, Loferski BL, Franciullo GI, et al: Does epidural butorphanol offer any clinical advantage over the intravenous route? *Anesthesiology* 76:216–220, 1992.
44. Camu F, Verborgh C, Van der Auwern A, et al: Pharmacokinetics and analgesic effect of epidural sufentanil, *Acta Anaesthesiol Scand* 80(suppl):82, 1985.
45. Carr AS, Markakis MA, Holtby HM, et al: Caudal morphine for thoracotomy in infants undergoing extracardiac vascular surgery, *Anesthesiology* 81:A1001, 1994.
46. Chaplan SR, Duncan SR, Brodsky JB, Brose WG: Morphine and hydromorphone epidural analgesia: a prospective, randomized comparison, *Anesthesiology* 77:1090–1094, 1992.
47. Cheng EY, Koebert RF, Hopwood MA, et al: Continuous epidural sufentanil infusion for postoperative analgesia, *Anesthesiology* 67:A233, 1987.
48. Chernow B: Hormonal responses to a graded surgical stress, *Arch Intern Med* 147:1273–1278, 1987.
49. Cherry DA, Gourlay GK, Cousins MJ: Epidural mass associated with lack of efficacy of epidural morphine and undetectable CSF morphine concentrations, *Pain* 25:69, 1986.
50. Chestnut DH: Effect on the progress of labor and method of delivery. In Chestnut DH editor: *Obstetric anesthesia: Principles and practice.* St Louis, 1994, Mosby–Year Book, pp. 403-417.
51. Chestnut DH: What is new in obstetric anesthesia? Review course lecture: International Anesthesia Research Society, *Anesth Analg* 68(suppl):1, 1989.
52. Chestnut DH, Vandewalker GE, Owen CL, et al: The influence of continuous epidural bupivacaine analgesia on the second stage of labor and method of delivery in nulliparous women, *Anesthesiology* 66: 774, 1987.
53. Chestnut DH, Choi WW, Isbell TJ: Epidural hydromorphone for postcesarean analgesia, *Obstet Gynecol* 68:65–69, 1986.
54. Christopherson R, Beattie C, Meinert CL, et al: Perioperative morbidity in patients randomized to epidural or general anesthesia for lower extremity vascular surgery, *Anesthesiology* 79: 1–12, 1993.
55. Chung JH, Sinatra RS, Fermo L, et al: Efficacy of intrathecal meperidine-morphine combination for postoperative analgesia in cesarean section patients, *Anesthesiology* 81:A931, 1994.
56. Coda BA, Kawata J, Ross BK: Plasma sufentanil concentration during prolonged epidural infusion for postoperative analgesia, *Anesth Analg* 76:S49, 1993.
57. Cohen S, Amur D, Pantuck CB et al: Postcesarean delivery epidural patient-controlled analgesia: fentanyl or sufentanil, *Anesthesiology* 78:486–491, 1993.
58. Coombs DW, Saunders RL, Gaylor MS: Relief of continuous chronic pain by interspinal narcotic, *JAMA* 250:2336, 1983.
59. Cousins MJ, Cherry DA, Gourlay GK: Acute and chronic pain: use of spinal opioids. In Cousins MJ, Bridenbaugh PO, editors: *Neural blockade in clinical anesthesia and management of pain,* ed 2, Philadelphia, 1987, JB Lippincott, pp 993-996.
60. Cousins MJ, Mather LE: Intrathecal and epidural administration of opioids, *Anesthesiology* 61:276, 1984.
61. Cousins MJ, Mather LE, Glynn CJ, et al: Selective spinal analgesia, *Lancet* 1:1141, 1979.
62. Cowan A, Vasthare U, Tuma RF, et al: Pharmacological profile of ICI 204448, a peripherally acting kappa-selective opioid agonist, *Anesthesiology* 83:A875, 1995.
63. Crone LAL, Conly JM, Clark KM, et al: Recurrent herpes simplex virus labialis and the use of epidural morphine on obstetric patients, *Anesth Analg* 66:887, 1987.
64. Chrubasik J, Wiemers K: Continuous-plus-on demand epidural infusions of morphine for postoperative pain relief, *Anesthesiology* 62:263–268, 1985.
65. Chrubasik J, Wust H, Schulte-Monting J, et al: Relative analgesic potency of epidural fentanyl, alfentanil, and morphine in the treatment of postoperative pain, *Anesthesiology* 68:929, 1988.
66. Cullen M, Altstatt AH, Kwon NJ, et al: Naltrexone reversal of the side effects of epidural morphine, *Anesthesiology* 69: A336, 1988.
67. Dalens B, Tanguy A: Intrathecal morphine for spinal fusion in children, *Spine* 13:494, 1988.
68. Dahl JB, Rosenberg J, Hansen BL, et al: Differential analgesic effects of low-dose epidural morphine and morphine-bupivacaine at rest and during mobilization after major abdominal surgery, *Anesth Analg* 74:362–365, 1992.
69. Dahl JB, Rosenberg J, Dirkes WE, et al: Prevention of postoperative pain by balanced analgesia, *Br J Anaesth* 64:518–520, 1990.
70. de Leon-Casasola OA, Parker B, Lema MJ, et al: Postoperative epidural-bupivacaine-morphine therapy: experience with 4, 227 surgical cancer patients, *Anesthesiology* 81:368–375, 1994.
71. de Leon-Casasola OA, Parker BM, Lema MJ, et al: Epidural analgesia versus intravenous PCA, *Reg Anesth* 19:307–315, 1994.
72. de Leon-Casasola OA, Karabella D, Harrison P, Lema MJ: A decrease in postoperative myocardial ishemia and infarction by epidural bupivacaine-morphine after upper abdominal surgery, *Reg Anesth* 18:66–71, 1993.
73. de Leon-Casasola OA, Lema MJ: Epidural sufentanil provides superior analgesia for opioid tolerant patients unresponsive to epidural morphine (abstract), *Anesthesiology* 77:A855, 1992.
74. Dervisogullari A, Kampine JP, Abram S, Tseng LF: Delta, kappa, and mu receptors involvement in spinal opioid analgesia in rats: comparison between fentanyl and morphine, *Anesthesiology* 83:A870, 1995.
75. Donadoni R, Rolly G, Noordvin H: Epidural sufentanil for postoperative pain relief, *Anaesthesia* 40:634, 1985.
76. Donadoni R, Vermeulen H, Noordwin H, et al: Intrathecal sufentanil as a supplement to subarachnoid anesthesia with lignocaine, *Br J Anaesth* 59:1523, 1987.
77. Dougherty RTB, Baysinger CL, Henenberger D, et al: Epidural hydromorphone for postoperative analgesia, *Anesth Analg* 68:318, 1989.
78. Duggan AW, Hall JG, Headley PM: Suppression of transmission of nociceptive impulses by morphine: selective effects of morphine administered in the region of the substantia gelatinosa, *Br J Pharmacol* 61:65, 1977.
79. Eisenach JC, Grice SC, Dewan DM, et al: Patient controlled analgesia following cesarean section: a comparison with intramuscular and epidural narcotics, *Anesthesiology* 70:585, 1989.

80. Eisenach JC, Rauck RL, Buzzanelli C, et al: Epidural clonidine analgesia for intractable cancer pain: phase I, *Anesthesiology* 71:647, 1989.
81. El-Baz NMI, Faber LP, Jensik RJ: Continuous epidural infusion of morphine for treatment of pain after thoracic surgery: a new technique, *Anesth Analg* 63:757–764, 1984.
82. Etches RC, Sandler A, Daley MD: Respiratory depression and spinal opioids, *Can J Anaesth* 36:165, 1989.
83. Fisher BC, Zornow MH, Yaksh TL: Antinociceptive effects of intrathecal dexmedetomidine in rats, *Anesth Analg* 70:5450, 1990.
84. Fisher RL, Lubenow TR, Liceaga A, et al: Comparison of continuous epidural infusion of fentanyl-bupivacaine and morphine-bupivacaine in management of postoperative pain, *Anesth Analg* 67:559–563, 1988.
85. Fuller JG, McMorland GH, Douglas J, et al: Epidural morphine for postoperative pain after cesarean section: a review, *Proc Soc Obstet Anesth Perinatol* 20:94, 1988.
86. Gambling DR, Yu P, Cole C, et al: A comparative study of PCEA and continuous infusion epidural analgesia during labor, *Can J Anaesth* 35:249, 1988.
87. Geller E, Chrubasik J, Graf R, et al: A randomized double-blind comparison of epidural sufentanil versus intravenous sufentanil or epidural fentanyl analgesia after major abdominal surgery, *Anesth Analg* 76:1243–1250, 1993.
88. Gibbs CP, Krischer J, Peckham BM, et al: Obstetric anesthesia: a national survey, *Anesthesiology* 65:298, 1985.
89. Glass PSA, Estok P, Ginsberg B, et al: Use of patient-controlled analgesia to compare the efficacy of epidural to intravenous fentanyl administration, *Anesth Analg* 74:345–351, 1992.
90. Glass PS: Respiratory depression following only 0.4 ng of intrathecal morphine, *Anesthesiology* 60:256, 1984.
91. Glynn CJ, Mather LE, Cousins MJ: Peridural meperidine in humans, *Anesthesiology* 55:520–526, 1981.
92. Gourlay GK, Cherry DA, Plummer JL, et al: The influence of drug polarity on the absorption of opioid drugs into CSF, *Pain* 31:297, 1987.
93. Graf G, Frasca A, Sinatra RS, et al.: Epidural sufentanil: for postoperative analgesia: a dose-response study, *Anesth Analg* 73:405–409,1991.
94. Grant R, Dolman J, Harper J, et al: Patient controlled lumbar epidural fentanyl compared with patient controlled intravenous fentanyl for post-thoracotomy pain, *Can J Anaesth* 39:214–219, 1992.
95. Grass JA, Zuckerman RL, Sakima NT, Harris AP: Patient controlled analgesia after cesarean delivery—epidural sufentanil versus intravenous morphine, *Reg Anesth* 19:90–97, 1994.
96. Grass JA, Sakima NT, Valley M, et al: Assessment of ketorolac as an adjuvant to fentanyl patient-controlled epidural analgesia after radical retropubic prostatectomy, *Anesthesiology* 78:642–648, 1993.
97. Grass JA, Zuckerman RL, Tsao H, et al: Patient controlled epidural analgesia results in shorter hospital stay after cesarean section, *Reg Anesth* 16:26, 1991.
98. Gregg R: Spinal analgesia, *Anesthesiol Clin North Am* 7(1):79, 1989.
99. Guinard JP, Mavrocordatos P, Cuttat JF, Carpenter R: A randomized comparison of intravenous versus lumbar and thoracic epidural fentanyl for analgesia after thoracotomy, *Anesthesiology* 77:1108–1115, 1992.
100. Gustafsson LL, Schildt B, Jacobsen K: Adverse effects of extradural and intrathecal opiates, *Br J Anaesth* 54:479, 1982.
101. Gwirtz KH, Young JV, Walker SG, et al: Intrathecal opioid analgesia for acute postoperative pain: experience with 4,134 surgical patients, *Anesthesiology* 83: A780, 1995.
102. Gwirtz KH: Single-dose opioids in the management of acute postoperative pain. In Sinatra RS, Hord AH, Ginsberg B, Preble LM, editors: *Acute pain mechanisms and management,* St Louis, 1992, Mosby–Year Book.
103. Haber DW, Berde CB: Spinal opioids for pediatric pain management, In: Sinatra RS, Hord AH, Ginsberg B, Preble LM, editors: *Acute pain mechanisms and management,* St Louis, 1992, Mosby–Year Book.
104. Harada Y, Nishioka K, Kitahata LM, et al: Contrasting actions of intrathecal U50, 488H, Morphine or (D-Pen2, D-Pen5) enkephalin on the visceromotor response to colorectal distension in the rat, *Anesthesiology* 83:336–343, 1995.
105. Harrison DM, Sinatra R, Morgese L: Epidural narcotic and patient controlled analgesia for post-cesarean section pain relief, *Anesthesiology* 68:454, 1988.
106. Hays R, Palmer CM, Van Maren G, et al: Intrathecal fentanyl for labor analgesia, *Anesthesiology* 81:A1149, 1994.
107. Horan CT, Beeby DG, Brodsky JB et al: Segmental effect of lumbar epidural hydromorphone: a case report, *Anesthesiology* 62:84–85, 1985.
108. Hug CC: Pharmacokinetics of new synthetic narcotic analgesics. In Estafanous FG, editor: *Opioids in anesthesia,* Boston, 1984, Butterworth, pp. 50–60.
109. Hunt CO, Datta SJ, Hauch M, et al: Perioperative analgesia with subarachnoid fentanyl-bupivacaine, *Anesthesiology* 67:A621, 1987.
110. Isaacson W, Arkoosh VA, Kinsella SM, et al: Intrathecal sufentanil labor analgesia: the effect of diluent volume, *Anesthesiology* 81:A1154, 1994.
111. Isaacson IJ, Weitz FI, Berry AJ, et al: Intrathecal morphine's effect on the postoperative course of patients undergoing abdominal aortic surgery, *Anesth Analg* 66:S86, 1987.
112. Janssen PAJ: The development of new synthetic narcotics. In Estafanous FG, editor: *Opioids in anesthesia,* Boston, 1984, Butterworth, pp. 37-44.
113. Jacobson L, Chabal C, Brody MC: Relief of persistent post-amputation stump and phantom limb pain with intrathecal fentanyl, *Pain* 37:317, 1989.
114. Jaffe JH: Narcotic analgesics. In Goodman LS, Gilman A, editors: *The pharmacological basis of theraputics,* London 1970, Macmillan, pp. 237-275.
115. Johnson A: Influence of intrathecal morphine and naloxone intervention on postoperative ventilatory regulation in elderly patients, *Acta Anaesthesiol Scand* 36: 436–444, 1992.
116. Jones SEF, Beasley JM, McFarlane D, et al: Intrathecal morphine for postoperative pain relief in children, *Br J Anaesth* 56: 137, 1984.
117. Katz J, Kavanagh BP, Sandler AN, et al: Preemptive analgesia:clinical evidence of neuroplasticity contributing to postoperative pain, *Anesthesiology* 77:439–446, 1992.
118. Kafer ER, Brown JT, Scott DD, et al: Biphasic depression of ventilatory responses to CO_2 following epidural morphine, *Anesthesiology* 58:418–427, 1983.
118b. Kendrick WD, Woods AM, Daly MY, et al: Naloxone versus nalbuphine infusion for propylaxis of epidural morphine-induced pruritus, *Anesth Analg* 82:641–647, 1996.
119. Kitahata LM, Collins JG: Spinal action of narcotic analgesics, *Anesthesiology* 54: 153–163, 1981.
120. Kitahata LM, Kosaka Y, Taub A, et al: Lamina-specific suppression of dorsal horn activity by morphine sulfate, *Anesthesiology* 41:39, 1974.
121. Klepper ID, Sherrill DL, Bromage PR: Analgesic and respiratory effects of sufentanil in volunteers, *Br J Anaesth* 59:1147, 1987.
122. Kotelko DM, Rottman RL, Wright WC, et al: Transdermal scopolamine decreases nausea and vomiting following cesarean section in patients receiving epidural morphine, *Anesthesiology* 71:675–679, 1989.
123. Krane EJ: Delayed respiratory depression in a child after caudal epidural morphine, *Anesth Analg* 67:79, 1988.
124. Krane EJ, Jacobson LE, Lynn AM, et al: Caudal morphine for postoperative analgesia in children: a comparison with caudal bupivacaine and intravenous morphine, *Anesth Analg* 67:79, 1988.
125. Krane EJ, Tyler DC, Jacobson LE, et al: The dose response of caudal morphine in children, *Anesthesiology* 71:48, 1989.
126. Lam AM, Knill RL, Thompson WR, et al: Epidural fentanyl does not cause delayed respiratory depression, *Can Anaesth Soc J* 30:578–579, 1983.
127. LaMotte C, Pert CB, Snyder SH: Opiate receptor binding in primate spinal cord: distribution and changes after dorsal root section, *Brain Res* 112:407, 1976.
128. Langerman L, Golomb E, Benita S, Tverskoy M: Intrathecal opiates: a new way for prolongation of pharmacological effect, *Anesthesiology* 71:A697, 1989
129. Lanz E, Kehrberger E, Theiss D: Epidural morphine: a clinical double-blind study of dosage, *Anesth Analg* 64:786, 1988.
130. Larsen VH, Iversen AD, Christensen A, et al: Postoperative pain treatment after upper abdominal surgery with epidural morphine at thoracic or lumbar level, *Acta Anaesthesiol Scand* 29:566, 1985.
131. Leicht CH, Hughes SC, Dailey PA, et al: Epidural morphine sulfate: a prospective

report of 1000 patients, *Anesthesiology* 65:A366, 1986.

132. Leicht CH, Kelleher AJ, Robinson DE, et al: Prolongation of postoperative epidural sufentanil analgesia with epinephrine, *Anesth Analg* 70:323, 1990.
133. Leighton BL, DeSimone C, Norris MC, et al: Intrathecal narcotics for labor revisited: the combination of fentanyl and morphine, *Anesth Analg* 69:122, 1989.
134. Leysen JE, Neiemegeers CJE: 3H-sufentanil: a superior ligand for mu-opiate receptors, *Eur J Pharmacol* 87:209, 1983.
135. Liu S, Carpenter RL, Mulroy MF, et al: Intravenous versus epidural administration of Hydromorphone, *Anesthesiology* 82:682–688, 1995.
136. Liu S, Carpenter RL, Mackey DC, et al: Effects of perioperative analgesic technique on rate of recovery after colon surgery, *Anesthesiology* 83:757–765, 1995.
137. Liu S, Angel J, Owens BD, Carpenter RL: .05% bupivacaine is an optimal concentration for use with fentanyl for post-thoracotomy analgesia, *Anesthesiology* 81:A975, 1994.
138. Logas WG, El-Baz N, El-Ganzouri A, et al: Continuous thoracic epidural analgesia for postoperative pain relief following thoracotomy: a randomized prospective study, *Anesthesiology* 67:787–791, 1987.
139. Loper KA, Ready LB, Downey M, et al.: Epidural and intravenous fentanyl infusions are clinically equivalent after knee surgery, *Anesth Analg* 70:72–75, 1990.
140. Loper KA, Ready LB: Epidural morphine after anterior cruciate ligament repair: a comparison with PCA morphine, *Anesth Analg* 68:350–352, 1989.
141. Lubenow TR, Tanck EN, Hopkins EM, McCarthy RJ, et al: Comparison of patient assisted epidural analgesia with continuous-infusion epidural analgesia for postoperative patients, *Reg Analg* 19:206–211, 1994.
142. Lubenow TR, McCarthy RJ, Kroin JS, Ivankovich AD: Analgesic, hemodynamic and respiratory responses to intrathecal tramadol in dogs, *Anesthesiology* 83: A822, 1995.
143. Lussos SA, Bader AM, Thornhill ML, Datta S: The antiemetic efficacy and safety of prophylactic metoclopramide for elective cesarean delivery during spinal anesthesia, *Reg Anesth* 17:126–130, 1992.
144. Malmberg AB, Yaksh TL: Pharmacology of the spinal action of ketorolac, morphine, ST-91, U50488H, and L-PIA on the formalin test, *Anesthesiology* 79:270–281, 1993.
145. Martin WF, Eades CG, Fraser HF, et al: Use of hindlimb reflexes of the chronic spinal dog for comparing analgesics, *J Pharmacol Exp Ther* 144:8, 1964.
146. Mather L, Mackie J: The incidence of postoperative pain in children, *Pain* 15: 271–277, 1983.
147. Mogensen T, Eliasen K, Ejlersen E, et al: Epidural clonidine enhances postoperative analgesia from a combined low dose epidural bupivacaine morphine regimen, *Anesth Analg* 75:607–610, 1992.
148. Moller IW, Dinesen K, Sondergard S, et al: Effect of patient controlled analgesia on plasma catecholamine, cortisol and glucose concentrations after cholecystectomy, *Br J Anaesth* 61:160–164, 1988.
149. Moon RE, Clements FM: Accidental epidural overdose of hydromorphone, *Anesthesiology* 63:238–239, 1985.
150. Moore RA, Bullingham RES, McQuay JH, et al: Dural permeability to narcotics: in vitro determination and application to extradural administration, *Br J Anaesth* 54:1117–1128, 1982.
151. Moore A, Bullingham R, MacQuay H, et al: Spinal fluid kinetics of morphine and heroin, *Clin Pharmacol Ther* 35:40, 1984.
152. Moses M. Cascio M, Zakowski MI, et al: Hemodynamic effect of intrathecal fentanyl in term parturients, *Anesthesiology* 81:A1150, 1994.
153. Motsch J, Graber E, Ludwig K: Addition of clonidine enhances postoperative analgesia from epidural morphine, *Anesthesiology* 73:1067–1073, 1990.
154. Naulty JS, Datta S, Ostheimer GW: Epidural fentanyl for post cesarean delivery pain management, *Anesthesiology* 63:694, 1985.
155. Naulty JS, Ross R: The effect of diluent volume on analgesia produced by epidural sufentanil, *Proc Soc Obstet Anesth Perinatol* 20:124, 1988.
156. Naulty JS, Ross R: Epidural fentanyl and morphine for post-cesarean delivery analgesia, *Proc Soc Obstet Anesth Perinatol* 20:18, 1988.
157. Naulty JS, Hertwig L, Hunt CO, et al: Duration of analgesia of epidural fentanyl following cesarean delivery: effects of local anesthetic drug, *Anesthesiology* 65:A180, 1986.
158. Naulty JS, Sevarino FB, Lema J, et al: Epidural sufentanil for post-cesarean delivery pain management, *Anesthesiology* 65:A396, 1986.
159. Naulty JS, Smith R, Ross R, Epstein BS: Effect of changes in labor analgesic practice on labor outcome, *Proc Soc Obstet Anesth Perinatol* 20:129, 1988.
160. Naulty JS: Continuous infusions of local anesthetics and narcotics for epidural analgesia in the management of labor, *Anesthesiol Clin* 28:17–24, 1990.
161. Negre I, Gueneron JP, Jamali SJ, et al: Preoperative analgesia with epidural morphine, *Anesth Analg* 79:298–302, 1994.
162. Nishio Y, Sinatra RS, Kitahata LM, et al: Spinal cord distribution of 3H-morphine after intrathecal administration: Relationship to analgesia, *Anesth Analg* 69: 323, 1989.
163. Nordberg G, Hedner T, Mellstrand T: Pharmacokinetic aspects of intrathecal morphine analgesia, *Anesthesiology* 60: 448–454, 1984.
164. Nordberg G, Hedner T, Mellstrand T, Dahlstrom B: Pharmacokinetic aspects of epidural morphine analgesia, *Anesthesiology* 58:545–551, 1983.
165. Norris E, Parker S, Breslow M, et al: The endocrine response to surgical stress: a comparison of epidural anesthesia/analgesia vs general anesthesia/PCA, *Anesthesiology* 75:A696, 1991.
166. Palmer CM, Voulgaropoulos D, Van Maren G, et al: What is the optimal dose of subarachnoid morphine for post cesarean analgesia? *Anesthesiology* 81: A1151, 1994.
167. Parker RK, White PF: Epidural patient-controlled analgesia: an alternative to intravenous patient-controlled analgesia for pain relief after cesarean delivery, *Anesth Analg* 75:245–251, 1992.
168. Parker RK, White PF: Epidural patient-controlled analgesia: influence of bupivacaine and hydromorphone basal infusion on pain control after cesarean section, *Anesth Analg* 75:740–746, 1992.
169. Paech MJ: Post caesarean section pain relief with epidural pethidine or fentanyl, *Anaesth Inten Care* 17:157–165,1989.
170. Penn RD, Paice JA: Chronic intrathecal morphine for intractable pain, *J Neurosurg* 67:182, 1987.
171. Pert CB, Kuhar MJ, Snyder SH: Autoradiographic localization of the opiate receptor in rat brain, *Life Sci* 16: 1849–1854, 1975.
172. Phillips GH: Epidural sufentanil/bupivacaine combinations for analgesia during labor: effect of varying sufentanil doses, *Anesthesiology* 67:835, 1987.
173. Phillips GH: Combined epidural sufentanil and bupivacaine for labor analgesia, *Reg Anesth* 12:165, 1989.
174. Plummer JL, Cmielewski PL, Gourlay GK, Owen H, Cousins MJ: Antinociceptive and motor effects of intrathecal morphine combined with intrathecal clonidine, noradrenaline, carbachol and midazolam in rats, *Pain* 49:145–152, 1992.
175. Plummer JL, Cmielewski GD, Reynolds GK, Gourlay GK: Influence of polarity on dose response relationships of intrathecal opioids in rats, *Pain* 40:339–347, 1987.
176. Poletti CE, Cohen AM, Todd DP, et al: Cancer pain relieved by long-term epidural morphine with permanent indwelling systems for self-administration, *J Neurosurg* 55:581, 1981.
177. Rawal N, Arner S, Gustafsson LL, et al: Present state of extradural and intrathecal opioid analgesia in Sweden, *Br J Anaesth* 59:791, 1987.
178. Rawal N, Schott U, Dahlstrom B, et al: Influence of naloxone infusion on analgesia and respiratory depression following epidural morphine, *Anesthesiology* 64: 194–201, 1986.
179. Rawal N, Sjostrand UH, Christofferson E: Comparisons of intramuscular and epidural morphine for postoperative analgesia in the grossly obese: influence on postoperative ambulation and pulmonary function, *Anesth Analg* 63:584–592, 1984.
180. Rawal N, Mollefors K, Axelsson K, et al: An experimental study of the urodynamic effects of epidural morphine and of naloxone reversal, *Anesth Analg* 62:641–647, 1983.
181. Rawal N, Sjostrand UH, Dahlstrom B, et al: Epidural morphine for postoperative pain relief: a comparative study with intramuscular narcotic and intercostal block, *Anesth Analg* 61:93, 1982.
182. Ready LB, Loper KA, Nessly M, Wild L:

Postoperative morphine is safe on surgical wards, *Anesthesiology* 75:452–456, 1991.
183. Ready LB, Oden R, Chadwick HS, et al: Development of an anesthesiology-based postoperative pain management service, *Anesthesiology* 68:100, 1988.
184. Ready LB, Chadwick HS, Ross B: Age predicts effective epidural morphine dose after abdominal hysterectomy, *Anesth Analg* 66:1215–1218, 1987.
185. Reiz S, Westberg M: Side effects of epidural morphine, *Lancet* 2:203, 1980.
186. Reuben SS, Dunn SM, Duprat KM, O'Sullivan P: An intrathecal fentanyl dose-response study in lower extremity revascularization procedures, *Anesthesiology* 81:1371–1375, 1994.
187. Robertson K, Douglas MJ, McMorland GH: Epidural fentanyl with and without epinephrine for post-cesarean section analgesia, *Can Anaesth Soc J* 32:502, 1985.
188. Rosen KR, Rosen DA: Caudal epidural morphine for control of pain following open heart surgery in children, *Anesthesiology* 70:418, 1989.
189. Rosen MA, Hughes SC, Shnider SM, et al: Epidural morphine for the relief of postoperative pain after cesarean delivery, *Anesth Analg* 62:666, 1983.
190. Rosen MA, Dailey PA, Hughes SC, et al: Epidural sufentanil for postoperative analgesia after cesarean section, *Anesthesiology* 68:448, 1988.
191. Roy SD, Flynn GL: Solubility and related physiochemical properties of narcotic analgesics, *Pharm Res* 5:580–586, 1988.
192. Rutter DV, Skewes DG, Morgan M: Extradural opioids for postoperative pain, *Br J Anaesth* 53:915, 1981.
193. Saiah M, Borgeat A, Wilder-Smith OHG, et al: Epidural-morphine induced pruritus: Propofol versus naloxone, *Anesth Analg* 78:1110–1113, 1994.
194. Salomaki TE, Leppaluoto J, Laitinen JO, et al: Epidural versus intravenous fentanyl for reducing hormonal, metabolic, and physiologic responses after thoracotomy, *Anesthesiology* 79:672–679, 1993.
195. Salomaki TE, Laitinen JO, Nuutinen LS: A randomized double-blind comparison of epidural versus intravenous fentanyl infusion for analgesia after thoracotomy, *Anesthesiology* 75:790–795, 1991.
196. Schecter NL, Allen DA, Hanson K: Status of pediatric pain control: a comparison of hospital analgesic usage in children and adults, *Pediatrics* 77:11, 1986.
197. Schmauss C, Doherty C, Yaksh TL: The analgesic effects of an intrathecally administered partial opiate agonist, nalbuphine hydrochloride, *Eur J Pharmacol* 86:1, 1983.
198. Schmauss C, Yaksh TL: In vivo studies on spinal opiate receptor systems mediating antinociception. II. Pharmacological profiles suggesting a differential association of mu, delta and kappa receptors, *J Pharmacol Exp Ther* 228:1, 1984.
199. Scott DA, Beilby DS, McClymont C: Postoperative analgesia using epidural infusions of fentanyl with bupivacaine, *Anesthesiology* 83:727–737, 1995.
200. Scott DB, McClure J: Selective epidural analgesia, *Lancet* 1:1410–1411, 1979.
201. Scott PU, Fischer HBJ: Intraspinal opiates and itching: a new reflex? *Br Med J* 284:1015, 1982.
202. Sevarino FB, Sinatra RS, et al: Epidural fentanyl effect on IV PCA requirements, *Can J Anesth* 38:450–453, 1991.
203. Shapiro LA, Jedeikin RJ, Shalev D, et al: Epidural morphine analgesia in children, *Anesthesiology* 61:210, 1984.
204. Sharrock NE, Haggett MJ, Urquhart B, et al: Does postoperative epidural analgesia reduce deep vein thrombosis? *Anesthesiology* 73:A69, 1990.
205. Shulman MS, Wakerlin G, Yamaguchi L, Brodsky JB: Experience with epidural hydromorphone for post-thoracotomy pain relief, *Anesth Analg* 66:1331–1335, 1987.
206. Shulman M, Sandler An, Bradley JW, et al: Post-thoracotomy pain and pulmonary function following epidural and systemic morphine, *Anesthesiology* 61:569–575, 1984.
207. Sinatra RS: Unpublished observations, 1994–1996.
208. Sinatra RS: Postoperative analgesia: epidural and spinal techniques. In Chestnut DH, editor: *Obstetric anesthesia: Principles and practice,* St Louis, 1994, Mosby–Year Book, pp. 513–547.
209. Sinatra RS, Sevarino FB, Paige D: Patient-controlled analgesia with sufentanil: a comparison of two different methods of administration, *J Clin Anesth* 8: 123–129, 1996.
210. Sinatra RS: Pharmacokinetics and pharmacodynamics of spinal opioids. In Sinatra RS, Hord AH, Ginsberg B, Preble LM, editors: *Acute pain: Mechanisms and management,* St Louis, 1992, Mosby–Year Book.
211. Sinatra RS, Sevarino FB, Chung JH, et al: Comparison of epidurally administered sufentanil, morphine and sufentanil-morphine combination for postoperative analgesia, *Anesth Analg* 72:522–527, 1991.
212. Singh H, Bossard RF, White PF: Epidural PCA: effect of ketorolac vs bupivacaine supplementation on pulmonary functions after thoracotomy, *Anesthesiology* 83: A874, 1995.
213. Sjostrom S, Hartvig P, Persson P, et al: Pharmacokinetics of epidural morphine and meperidine in humans, *Anesthesiology* 67:877, 1987.
214. Skjoldebrand A, Garle M, Gustafsson LL, et al: Extradural pethidine with and without adrenaline during labor, *Br J Anaesth* 54:415, 1982.
215. Snijdelaar DG, Hasenbos MA, van Egmond J, Wolff AP, et al: High thoracic epidural sufentanil with bupivacaine: continuous infusion of high volume versus low volume, *Anesth Analg* 78:490–494, 1994.
216. Sosnowski M, Yaksh TL: Differential cross-tolerance between intrathecal morphine and sufentanil, *Anesthesiology* 73: 1141–1147, 1990.
217. Steinstra R, Van Poorten F: Immediate respiratory arrest after caudal sufentanil, *Anesthesiology* 71:993, 1989.
218. Swenson JD, Hullander M, Bready RJ, Leivers D: A comparison of patient controlled epidural analgesia with sufentanil by the lumbar versus thoracic route after thoracotomy, *Anesth Analg* 78:215–218, 1994.
219. Tejwani GA, Rattan AK, McDonald JS: Role of spinal opioid receptors in the antinociceptive interactions between intrathecal morphine and bupivacaine, *Anesth Analg* 74:726–734, 1992.
220. Torda TA, Pybus DA: A comparison of four opiates for epidural analgesia, *Br J Anaesth* 54:291, 1982.
221. Tuman KJ, McCarthy RJ, March RJ, et al: Effects of epidural anesthesia and analgesia on coagulation and outcome after major vascular surgery, *Anesth Analg* 73:696–704, 1991.
222. Ullman D, Fortune SB, Greenhouse BB, et al: The treatment of patients with multiple rib fractures using continuous thoracic epidural narcotic infusion, *Reg Anesth* 14:43–47, 1989.
223. Urquhart ML, Klapp K, White PF: Patient controlled analgesia: a comparison of intravenous vs subcutaneous hydromorphone, *Anesthesiology* 69:428–432, 1988.
224. Van Decar T, Callicot R, Jones R, Herman N: Determination of a dose response curve for intrathecal sufentanil in labor, *Anesthesiology* 81:A1148, 1994.
225. Van den Hoogen RH, Colpaert FC: Epidural and subcutaneous morphine, meperidine, fentanyl, and sufentanil in the rat, *Anesthesiology* 66:186–194, 1987.
226. Van der Auwern A, Verborgh C, Camu F: Analgesic and cardiorespiratory effects of epidural sufentanil and morphine, *Anesth Analg* 66:999–1003, 1987.
227. Wall PD: The prevention of postoperative pain (editorial), *Pain* 33:289–290, 1988.
228. Wagemans MFM, van de Valk, Zuurmond WW, de Lange JJ: Safety of long-term intrathecal administration of morphine or morphine bupivacaine mixture in cancer pain patients, *Anesthesiology* 83:A818, 1995.
229. Wamsley PNH: Patient-controlled epidural analgesia. In Sinatra RS, Hord AH, Ginsberg B, Preble LM, editors: *Acute pain mechanisms and management,* St Louis, 1992, Mosby–Year Book.
230. Wamsley PNH, McDonnell FJ, Colclough GW, et al: A comparison of epidural and intravenous PCA after gynecological surgery, *Anesthesiology* 73:A1268, 1990.
231. Wang JK: Intrathecal morphine for intractable pain secondary to cancer of the pelvic organs, *Pain* 21:99, 1985.
232. Wang JK, Nauss LA, Thomas JE: Pain relief by intrathecally applied morphine in man, *Anesthesiology* 50:149–150, 1979.
233. Wang J, Denson D, Knarr D, et al: Continuous epidural methadone in the management of postoperative pain following lower abdominal surgery, *Reg Anesth* 13:58, 1988.
234. Wayslak TJ, English MJM, Jeans ME: Reduction of postoperative morbidity following patient-controlled morphine, *Can J Anesth* 37:726–731, 1990.
235. Welchew EA, Thornton JA: Continuous thoracic epidural fentanyl, *Anaesthesia* 37:309–316, 1982.

236. Wells DG, Davies G: Profound CNS depression from epidural fentanyl for extracorporeal shock wave lithotripsy, *Anesthesiology* 67:991–992, 1987.
237. Winnie AP: New uses for old drugs, *Anesthesiol Rev* 7:8–10, 1980.
238. Woolf CJ, Wall PD: Morphine-sensitive and morphine-insensitive actions of C-fiber input on the rat spinal cord, *Neurosci Lett* 64:221–225, 1986.
239. Worth AR, Williams JT, Surprenant A: Mu and delta receptors belong to a family of receptors that are coupled to potassium channels, *Proc Natl Acad Sci* US 84: 5487–5491, 1987.
240. Yaksh TL, Harty GJ: Effects of etorphan on the antinociceptive actions of intrathecal (DADL) enkephalin, *Eur J Pharmacol* 79:293, 1982.
241. Yaksh TL: Spinal opiate analgesia: characteristics and principles of action, *Pain* 11:293, 1981.
242. Yaksh TL, Reddy SVR: Studies in the primate on the analgesic effects associated with intrathecal actions of opiates, alpha adrenergic agonists and baclofen, *Anesthesiology* 54:451, 1981.
243. Yaksh TL, Jessell TM, Gamse R, et al: Intrathecal morphine inhibits substance P release in vivo from mammalian spinal cord, *Nature* 286:155, 1980.
244. Yaksh TL, Rudy TA: Studies on the direct spinal action of narcotics in the production of analgesia in the rat, *J Pharmacol Exp Ther* 202:411, 1977.
245. Yaksh TL, Rudy TA: Analgesia mediated by a direct spinal action of narcotics, *Science* 192:1357–1358, 1976.
246. Yamaguchi H, Watanabe S, Fukuda T, et al: Minimal effective intrathecal morphine dose for pain relief after abdominal hysterectomy, *Anesth Analg* 70:537, 1989.
247. Yamaguchi H, Watanabe S, Motokawa K, et al: Intrathecal morphine dose response data for pain relief after cholecystectomy, *Anesth Analg* 70:168–171, 1990.
248. Yaster M, Maxwell LG: Pediatric regional anesthesia, *Anesthesiology* 70:324, 1989.
249. Yeager MP, Glass DG, Neff RK: Epidural anesthesia and analgesia in high-risk surgical patients, *Anesthesiology* 66:729–636, 1987.
250. Youngstrom P, Hoyt P, Herman M, et al: Dose response study of continuous infusion epidural fentanyl-epinephrine for post-cesarean analgesia, *Anesthesiology* 73:A984, 1990.
251. Youngstrom P, Boyd B, Rhoton F: Complaints of side effects from post-cesarean epidural opioid analgesia: fewer with fentanyl-epinephrine infusion than with morphine bolus, *Anesthesiology* 77:A859, 1992.
252. Zakowski M, Ramanathan S, Khoo P, et al: Plasma histamine with intraspinal morphine in cesarean section, *Anesth Analg* 70:S40, 1990.
253. Zakowski M, Minn M, Hoskins I, et al: Pharmacokinetics and effects of intrathecal fentanyl for labor analgesia, *Anesthesiology* 83:A942, 1995.

CHAPTER 65

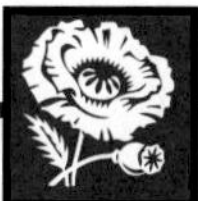

Cardiovascular Drugs

DAVID BRONHEIM
MARK ABEL
DANIEL M. THYS

People over 65 years of age represent the fastest growing segment of the American population, and the percentage of people over 75 years of age is increasing even faster. Advanced age and concurrent chronic diseases are no longer viewed as presenting major restrictions to complex surgical interventions. Cardiovascular diseases such as hypertension, congestive heart failure (CHF), and coronary artery disease have become increasingly prevalent in patients undergoing anesthesia and surgery.

These patients are frequently treated with one or several chronic medications. To provide optimal anesthetic care, one must clearly understand the implications of concurrent medical therapy. This chapter reviews frequently used cardiovascular medications and provides information about anesthetic considerations associated with their use.

ANTIHYPERTENSIVE MEDICATIONS

Many antihypertensive agents are currently available for treatment of essential hypertension. Selection of one or several medications often depends on degree of hypertension, effectiveness of certain drugs within a given population, side effects, and concurrent diseases. **Patients with hypertension and angina are frequently treated with regimens that include beta-adrenergic blocking agents and calcium channel blockers.** Hypertensive individuals with chronic obstructive pulmonary disease are managed with drugs that do not increase bronchial tone or interact with bronchodilators. Certain medications are most useful in combination with a diuretic, whereas diuretics are contraindicated in patients with certain diseases (e.g., gout). Also, combinations of drugs in low doses may be better tolerated than single medications at higher dosages.

In the 1950s, after several episodes of cardiovascular collapse were described in anesthetized patients treated with reserpine for hypertension, it became common practice to withdraw antihypertensive therapy before anesthesia and surgery to "preserve normal autonomic function." Subsequently, it was noted that hypertensive patients in whom therapy had been withheld often had difficult intraoperative courses and exacerbated postoperative hypertension. With the recognition that patients who continued taking antihypertensive medications had no greater decreases in blood pressure during anesthesia than normal patients,[196] came today's usual recommendation *not* to discontinue these drugs prior to anesthesia and surgery. Growing awareness indicated that discontinuation of certain antihypertensive agents, such as clonidine or beta-adrenergic blocking agents, could even precipitate withdrawal syndromes with catastrophic consequences.[92,129]

Today is it recommended, except occasionally for diuretics, that oral antihypertensive therapy be continued up until surgery and be reinstituted as soon as possible postoperatively. If oral intake is precluded, intravenous (IV), transdermal, or sublingual therapy can be substituted.

Diuretics

Patients with evidence of cardiovascular disease frequently are treated with a regimen that includes a diuretic for control of hypertension, treatment of CHF, or for related diseases. Dosage schedules and side effects for more commonly prescribed diuretics are listed in Table 65-1.

Thiazides

The thiazides and related agents are the most frequently prescribed antihypertensive medications. They act directly on distal kidney tubules to increase sodium, chloride, and water excretion (Fig. 65-1).[15] This is not the direct mechanism by which thiazides treat hypertension. Chronically, these drugs have little effect on cardiac output and decrease plasma volume by only 5%.[53] Blood pressure is lowered by the arte-

Table 65-1 Diuretics

Agent	Usual daily dose (mg)	Precautions and special considerations	Side effects
Thiazides and related sulfonamide diuretics			
Bendroflumethiazide (Naturetin)	2.5–5	May be ineffective in renal failure except for indapamide and metolazone; hypokalemia increases digitalis toxicity; may cause an increase in blood levels of lithium. Decrease in urinary calcium excretion. May precipitate acute gout.	Hypokalemia, hypomagnesemia, hyperuricemia, glucose intolerance, insulin resistance, hypercholesterolemia, increased low-density lipoprotein cholesterol, hypertriglyceridemia, hypercalcemia, sexual dysfunction, weakness, photosensitivity (except for ethacrynic acid), leukopenia, allergic skin rash.
Benzthiazide (Exna)	12.5–50		
Chlorothiazide (Diuril)	125–500		
Chlorthalidone (Hygroton)	12.5–50		
Hydrochlorothiazide (Hydrodiuril, Esidrex)	12.5–100		
Hydroflumethiazide (Saluron, Diucardin)	12.5–50		
Indapamide (Lozol)	2.5–5		
Methylchlothiazide (Enduron)	2.5–5		
Metolazone (Zaroxolyn)	2.5–5		
Polythiazide (Renese)	1–4		
Quinethazone (Hydromox)	25–100		
Trichlormethiazide	1–4		
Loop diuretics			
Bumetanide (Bumex)	0.5–5	Effective in chronic renal failure. Increase urinary calcium excretion.	As above, except for hypercalcemia
Ethacrynic acid (Edecrin)	25–100		
Furosemide (Lasix)	20–320		
Potassium-sparing agents			
Amiloride (Midamor)	5–10	Danger of hyperkalemia in patients receiving a potassium supplement, a potassium-containing salt substitute or an angiotensin-converting enzyme inhibitor, and in patients with renal failure; can cause renal failure in patients treated with a nonsteroidal anti-inflammatory drug (indomethacin and triamterene). May increase blood levels of lithium. Spironolactone interferes with digoxin immunoassay. Danger of renal calculi (triamterene).	Hyperkalemia for all three agents. For spironolactone only: gynecomastia, mastodynia, gastrointestinal irritation, drowsiness, lethargy, irregular menses or postmenopausal bleeding, hirsutism.
Spironolactone (Aldactone)	25–100		
Triamterene (Dyrenium)	50–200		

Modified from Gifford RW: Treatment of patients with systemic arterial hypertension. In Schlant RG, Alexander FW, editors: *Hurst's The Heart,* New York, 1994, McGraw Hill, pg. 1430.

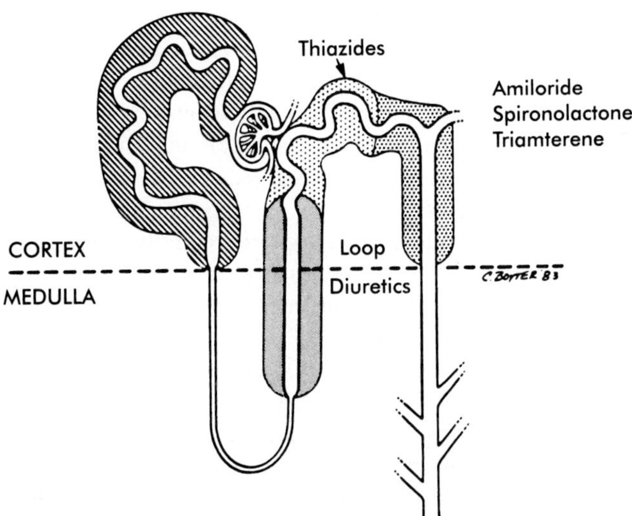

Fig. 65-1. Approximate sites of action of diuretics within the nephron. (Modified from Delaney VB, Bourke E: Diuretics. In Hurst JW, editor: *The heart,* New York, 1990, McGraw-Hill.)

riolar dilation that accompanies diuretic-induced sodium excretion.[246] These drugs are also used in treatment of CHF, edema secondary to liver disease, diabetes insipidus, and urinary calculi in patients with hypercalciuria. Side effects may include hypokalemia, hypomagnesemia, hypercalcemia, hyperglycemia, metabolic alkalosis, hyponatremia, orthostatic hypotension, dysrhythmias, hyperuricemia and gout.[178]

Loop diuretics

Furosemide, bumetanide, and ethacrynic acid are unrelated chemically but act on the kidney at the level of the thick ascending limb of Henle's loop to prevent reabsorption of sodium, chloride, and water (Fig. 65-1). Again, this may not be the "loop diuretics'" sole effect. When given parenterally, furosemide causes systemic vasodilation and reduction of left ventricular filling pressure before a diuretic effect is apparent.[24,41,58] Loop diuretics are substantially more effective diuretics than thiazides with respect to removal of excess fluid and are indicated in treatment of acute and chronic CHF, as well as edema of hepatic or renal origin. Loop diuretics are less effective than thiazides in treatment of hypertension, except when the hypertension is associated with chronic renal insufficiency.[119,204,205] Side effects include ototoxicity, hypokalemia, hypomagnesemia, hyperuricemia, metabolic alkalosis, dehydration, and hyponatremia. Treatment with loop diuretics may lower serum calcium levels; in combination with hydration, these medications are used for the acute therapy of hypercalcemia. Finally, loop diuretics have been used for management of high intracranial pressure and to convert acute oliguric renal failure to nonoliguric renal failure.

Potassium-sparing agents

Spironolactone is a competitive aldosterone antagonist. By inhibiting the effects of aldosterone on the nephron's distal convoluted tubule and collecting system (Fig. 65-1), spironolactone decreases renal sodium absorption and potassium excretion. A mild diuretic, its most common use is with thiazides or loop diuretics to attenuate their substantial potassium depletion. Spironolactone may be used to treat patients with primary hyperaldosteronism or for gentle diuresis in patients with hepatic cirrhosis.[127]

Triamterene and amiloride are also potassium-sparing diuretics. They are not aldosterone inhibitors but work directly on distal convoluted tubules to prevent sodium-potassium exchange. As with spironolactone, triamterene and amiloride are used in combination with thiazides to treat hypertension and to reverse or prevent hypokalemia.[54] All three drugs occasionally may cause hyperkalemia.

Anesthetic considerations

Major anesthetic considerations with diuretics relate to their effects on fluid balance and electrolytes. Because intravascular volume may be decreased after diuretic administration current recommendations for patients taking diuretics call for withholding diuretics on the day of surgery unless evidence suggests volume overload or signs and symptoms of CHF. Physical examination should include careful evaluation of vital signs, with particular attention to orthostatic blood pressure changes and other signs or symptoms of dehydration. If hypovolemia goes unrecognized, anesthetic induction may result in hypotension and tachycardia.

Diuretics can also cause profound electrolyte imbalances; serum electrolyte levels must be verified preoperatively. Patients receiving chronic therapy with loop diuretics or thiazides may have decreased total body potassium, evidence for which is found in low serum potassium levels. Chronic diuretic use, especially in patients with hypokalemia, has been associated with increased incidence of preoperative dysrhythmias.[114] Rapid correction of mild-to-moderate hypokalemia before surgery in asymptomatic patients is not considered indicated for the following reasons:

(1) Acute replacement may itself be dangerous and cause life-threatening hyperkalemia.[136]
(2) Little can be done to rapidly correct total body potassium. The difference between a serum potassium level of 2.5 and 3.5 mEq/L may be as much as 200 to 400 mEq in a 70 kg individual.
(3) Recent studies suggest that chronic hypokalemia does not increase incidence of intraoperative dysrhythmias.[251]
(4) In stable patients with chronic mild-to-moderate hypokalemia without signs or symptoms of hypokalemia (e.g., muscle weakness, ileus, nephropathy) and in the absence of dysrhythmias or digitalis use, anesthesia and surgery can proceed.

Accordingly, there is no absolute serum potassium value below which elective surgery is contraindicated. This does *not* mean, in a given patient who is hypokalemic and symptomatic (i.e., with arrythmias already), that elective surgery can proceed.

Diuretics enhance the effects of neuromuscular-blocking agents.[180]

Centrally Acting Alpha$_2$ Adrenoreceptor Agonists

Sympatholytics act centrally to decrease sympathetic outflow. Within this group, four drugs are commercially available: clonidine, guanabenz, guanfacine, and alpha-methyldopa. Usual dosages and related information are listed in Table 65-2.

The mode of action of clonidine is complex, but its major effect as an antihypertensive is as a centrally acting alpha$_2$ agonist. (Note that clonidine is an agonist, not an antagonist, despite its role as an antihypertensive.) This agonism somehow reduces sympathetic and increases parasympathetic tone.[122] Clonidine decreases heart rate, systemic vascular resistance, plasma renin activity, and epinephrine and norepinephrine levels. Side effects include hypotension, sedation, dry mouth, and dizziness. Because clonidine may cause fluid retention, it is most effective with a diuretic. Important anesthetic considerations pertain to clonidine. Sudden discontinuation may result in a withdrawal syndrome including rebound hypertension or even hypertensive crisis, plus restlessness, insomnia, agitation, nausea, and sweating. These disturbances usually occur 18 to 36 hours after the last dose.[92] Withdrawal may be treated by reinstitution of clonidine therapy or by administration of alpha- and beta-adrenergic blocking agents.

Clonidine now can be given as a transdermal patch, allowing continued application in most patients, even those unable to take oral medications. The clonidine patch is available in 3.5, 7.0, and 10.5 cm^2 sizes, equivalent to oral doses of 0.1, 0.2, and 0.3 mg per day, respectively. Patients receiving clonidine therapy who require surgery should be given clonidine transdermally to prevent withdrawal if unable to take it orally. Clonidine is effective in prevention of narcotic withdrawal and has been studied for a possible role in reducing hemodynamic variability during anesthesia.[93,165] Clonidine has been shown to lower the minimum alveolar concentration (MAC) of anesthetics in animals[18] and to decrease intraoperative requirements for isoflurane[165] and narcotics.[70,93,94] Oral clonidine premedication 2 to 4 ug/kg has been shown to improve postoperative analgesia in children. Similarly, intravenous (IV) infusion of clonidine after spinal fusion in adults has been shown to decrease pain and morphine requirements.[179] Suffice it to say that clonidine is a very complex and widely acting drug. Interactions with various anesthetics are complex and imperfectly understood.

Table 65-2 Centrally acting alpha$_2$ adrenoceptor agents

Agent	Dosage (mg)	Duration of action (hr)	Mode of elimination
Clonidine	0.1–1.0 bid	6–12	Hepatic/renal
Clonidine TTS (patch)	3.5, 7.0, 0, 10.5 cm^2 weekly	7 days	Hepatic/renal
Guanabenz	4–64 bid	6–12	Hepatic
Guanfacine	1 – 3 daily	12–24	Renal
Alpha-methyldopa	250–1000 bid	6–12	Renal/hepatic

Guanabenz and guanfacine are centrally acting agonists with modes of action and anesthetic considerations similar to those of clonidine, including similar withdrawal syndromes.[104,256]

Alpha-methyldopa is a widely used antihypertensive agent. Its major pharmacologically active metabolite, alpha-methylnorepinephrine, is a potent alpha$_2$ agonist that stimulates brainstem postsynaptic alpha$_2$ receptors. This decreases sympathetic tone and systemic vascular resistance.[149] As with clonidine, alpha-methyldopa must be used with diuretics to prevent tolerance secondary to volume expansion. Common side effects include orthostatic hypotension, dizziness, sedation, dry mouth, nasal congestion, headache, and impotence. Less common but more serious side effects include leukopenia, hepatitis, thrombocytopenia, and a lupuslike syndrome. Approximately 20% of patients develop a positive direct Coombs' test, and hemolytic anemia occurs in a few (5% of the 20%) of these patients.[48,263] Rebound syndromes may occur following discontinuation of alpha-methyldopa, but these are infrequent compared with clonidine. Patients unable to take oral medications postoperatively may receive the IV form.

Peripherally Acting Sympatholytic Agents

Alpha-adrenergic blocking agents (Table 65-3)

Prazosin, terazosin, and doxazosin. These drugs competitively block postsynaptic alpha$_1$-adrenergic receptors in vascular smooth muscle. They reduce blood pressure with little effect on cerebral and renal vascular blood flow or heart rate. Prazosin, terazosin, and doxazosin may be used for treatment of hypertension and for afterload reduction in patients with CHF. More recently, these drugs have been widely used for treatment of benign prostatic hypertrophy.[31] Side effects include orthostatic hypotension, dizziness, and even frank syncope after the initial dose, especially in patients already receiving other antihypertensive medications. Side effects may be reduced by administration of small ini-

Table 65-3 Alpha-adrenergic blocking agents

Agent	Dosage (mg)	Duration of action
Prazosin	1–10 bid	4–8 hr
Terazosin	1–20 daily	12–24 hr
Doxazosin	1–16 daily	24 hr
Phenozybenzamine	10–40 bid or tid	3–4 days

tial doses. Subsequent dosages are generally well tolerated.[37] Less common side effects include palpitations, headaches, sedation, dry mouth, gastrointestinal symptoms, tachycardia, and edema. As with clonidine, a diuretic must be added to prevent fluid retention when these drugs are used as antihypertensive agents.[100]

Phenoxybenzamine and phentolamine. Phenoxybenzamine is a noncompetitive, nonselective alpha antagonist with a half-life of 24 hours. It is predominantly used for long-term control of hypertension associated with pheochromocytomas. Phentolamine is also a nonselective alpha antagonist. Because of its short half-life, it is used IV for perioperative management of hypertension associated with pheochromocytomas. Common side effects of these drugs include hypotension and tachycardia, which are manifestations of its blocking properties.

Anesthetic implications. With alpha-adrenergic blocking agents, normal responses to catecholamine stimulation may be inhibited, and anesthetic agents that decrease preload may have more marked effects on blood pressure.

Adrenergic neuronal blocking agents

Guanethidine and guanadrel. Guanethidine and guanadrel are antihypertensive agents which have limited current use because of the availability of drugs with fewer side effects. They are selective inhibitors of postganglionic adrenergic neurons; their exact mechanisms of action are not completely understood. Guanethidine must be actively transported into the neuron, where it accumulates in neuronal storage vesicles and causes norepinephrine storage depletion. Although norepinephrine stores are depleted, the antihypertensive effect of guanethidine may not actually depend on this depletion. Its major mode of action may be to inhibit nerve pulse transmission at the outer neuronal or vesicular membrane. With chronic administration, peripheral vascular resistance decreases.

Side effects include expansion of intravascular volume, necessitating guanethidine's use with a diuretic as well as orthostatic and exercise-induced hypotension, diarrhea, and sexual dysfunction. Tricyclic antidepressants, amphetamines, chlorpromazine, and ephedrine may interfere with its effectiveness by their effect on the uptake mechanism of guanethidine. Guanethidine is contraindicated in patients with pheochromocytomas and should not be given to those receiving monoamine oxidase (MAO) inhibitors.

The anesthetic implications of guanethidine involve the decrease in norepinephrine concentration, which may cause the pharmacologic equivalent of denervation hypersensitivity. Therefore direct-acting sympathomimetics may cause exaggerated hemodynamic responses. Decreased norepinephrine neuronal tissue stores render indirect-acting agents (e.g., ephedrine) less effective.[261]

Reserpine. This Rauwolfia alkaloid was the first really effective oral antihypertensive agent. It exerts its effect at the postganglionic neuron; its action is believed to be related to inhibition of norepinephrine and dopamine uptake into terminal vesicles, resulting in increased norepinephrine degradation and decreased conversion of dopamine to norepinephrine. Reserpine crosses the blood–brain barrier and decreases central nervous system (CNS) serotonin and dopamine. Although this effect is believed to be unrelated to its antihypertensive effect, it may be the mechanism by which reserpine causes depression, nightmares, and sedation. Because of vasodilation, reserpine may increase intravascular volume; therefore concurrent diuretic use is important. With reserpine and guanethidine, depletion of norepinephrine stores renders ephedrine and indirect-acting agents less effective, whereas effects of direct-acting agonists may be accentuated.[261]

Vasodilators (Table 65-4)

Hydralazine

Hydralazine is a vasodilator used in treatment of hypertension and CHF.[46] Its pharmacologic effect is a direct action on arteriolar smooth muscle.[242] In response to arteriolar vasodilation, a baroreceptor-mediated increase in plasma volume, heart rate, cardiac output, and stroke volume often occurs.[2] As a result, hydralazine must be used with a diuretic and/or a beta-adrenergic blocking agent to remain effective. Additional side effects include palpitations, headaches, flushing, nasal congestion, and worsening angina in patients with coronary artery disease. Especially in higher dosages, it may cause a lupuslike syndrome, which is reversible on discontinuation.[196] Hydralazine may be given by oral, IV, and intramuscular (IM) routes. Perioperatively, hydralazine is useful when titrated intravenously for control of hypertension, particularly for patients in whom beta-blockade is contraindicated (e.g., presence of CHF).

Minoxidil

Minoxidil is a direct-acting arteriolar vasodilator. As with hydralazine, it must be used with a beta-adrenergic blocking agent to prevent tachycardia and with a diuretic to prevent fluid retention. Minoxidil is effective when used for hypertension, especially in patients with renal failure. Side effects, such as facial hirsutism, pulmonary hypertension, and fluid retention, have limited its use to patients with severe hypertension.[198] Minoxidil is currently widely applied topi-

Table 65-4 Direct acting vasodilators

Agent	Dosage (mg)	Duration of action (hr)
Minoxidil	2.5–30 mg daily or bid	8–12
Hydralazine	Oral: 10–200 bid or tid	6–12
	Intravenous: 5–40 tid or qid	4–8

cally to grow hair. How this use interacts with anesthesia administration is unknown.

Angiotensin-Converting Enzyme (ACE) Inhibitors (Table 65-5)

Angiotensin-converting enzyme (ACE) inhibitors are antihypertensive agents that have also found use in treatment of CHF. They are increasingly replacing older agents in treatment of hypertension because they are better tolerated. They have been shown to reduce symptoms and improve survival in patients with CHF. The number of ACE inhibitors in use has dramatically increased over the past several years. Commercially available ACE inhibitors include captopril, enalapril, lisinopril, ramipril, quinapril, fosinopril and benzapril, with more drugs under investigation.[30] Their primary mode of action is to competitively inhibit the enzyme that converts angiotensin I to the potent vasoconstrictor angiotensin II (Fig. 65-2). They also may decrease aldosterone levels, potentiate the vasodilating kallikrein-kinin system,[11] and may affect prostaglandin levels. ACE inhibitors dilate both venous capacitance and arteriolar resistance vessels. Precipitous reductions in blood pressure may occur following initiation of therapy, particularly in hypovolemic patients. Reversible renal insufficiency and hyperkalemia may occur with ACE inhibitors. A dry cough may occur in as many as 10% of patients taking these drugs.[11] Other side effects include proteinuria and rash.

Table 65-5 Angiotensin-converting enzyme (ACE) inhibitors

Agent	Dosage	Duration of action	Elimination
Captopril	12.5–50 mg bid-tid	4–8 H	Renal
Enalapril	5–20 mg bid	12–24 H	Renal
Enalaprot	1.25 mg IV qid	6	Renal
Lisinopril	10–40 mg daily	24 H	Renal
Benazepril	10–40 mg daily-bid	24 H	Renal/hepatic
Fosinapril	10–40 mg daily-bid	24 H	Renal/hepatic
Quinapril	5–80 mg daily-bid	24 H	Renal/hepatic
Ramipril	1.25–20 mg daily-bid	24 H	Renal/hepatic

Enalaprilat, the active metabolite of enalapril, is available in IV form. Early administration of IV enalaprilat has been shown to limit myocardial infarct extension and to improve subsequent left ventricular function in acute myocardial infarctions (MI).[221] Recent studies show that IV enalaprilat is effective in reducing blood pressure and left ventricular afterload in hypertensive patients undergoing coronary artery bypass graft.[19,20]

Angiotensin Receptor Antagonists

Losartan is the prototype of this new class of cardiovascular drugs and several more are in development. Angiotensin II is the end product of the renin-angiotensin system which medicates the vasoconstriction and aldosterone secretion responses to the system. Type I (AT_1) receptors are responsible for these effects. Losartan and several investigational agents exert their effects by blocking this receptor. Oral doses of losartan are well absorbed, but undergo extensive (14%) first-pass hepatic metabolism; it is converted to a more active metabolite. The usual oral dose for the management of hypertension is 50 to 100 mg/day and has been shown to reduce blood pressure in hypertensive patients as well as normal subjects.[126] Early results in patients with CHF suggest that the new drugs effectively reduce afterload

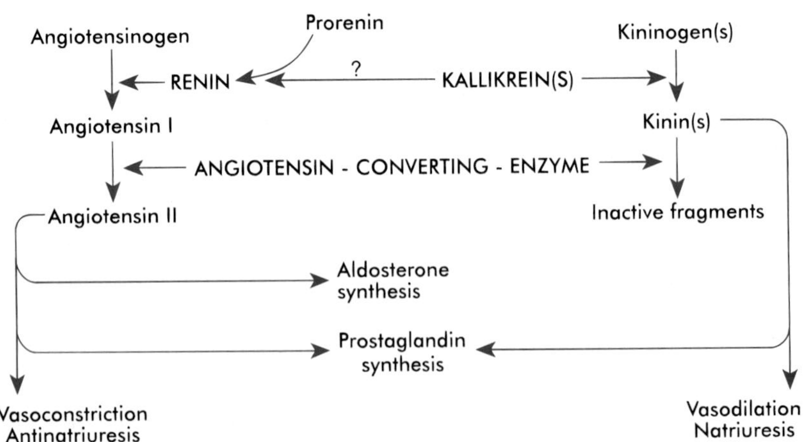

Fig. 65-2. Schematization of the renin-angiotensin-aldosterone system and the kallikrein-kinin system and their interaction with the angiotensin-converting enzyme. (From Borek M, Charlap S, Frishman WH: Enalapril, *Pharmacotherapy* 7:135, 1987.)

and increase cardiac output.[50,97] Data regarding long-term use of losartan in CHF are not yet available. Side effects are uncommon and related to the hypotensive effect of losartan. Dizziness occurs with an incidence of 4% to 5%. Hyperkalemia occurs occasionally. Side effects of ACE inhibitors which are usually attributed to their nonspecific actions on bradykinin or neurokinin pathways, such as dry cough, are not seen with losartan, because losartan is specific for the renin-angiotensin system.[126] Therefore, losartan may be useful in patients who could benefit from ACE inhibitors but who are unable to tolerate the side effects attributable to nonspecific actions of the latter drugs.

Beta-adrenergic blocking agents, calcium channel blockers, and nitrates may also be used as antihypertensive agents. They are discussed in the following section.

ANTIANGINAL AGENTS

Three groups of drugs, namely nitrates, beta-adrenergic blocking agents, and calcium channel blockers, alone or in combination, are effective in managing angina. Choosing a class of drugs or a particular drug within each class depends primarily on patient tolerance of side effects, ventricular function, presence or absence of conduction disease, and relative indications or contraindications caused by additional illnesses.

Nitrates

Nitrates in many forms have been used in treatment and prevention of angina for more than 100 years. **Nitrates are arterial and venous smooth muscle dilators that affect venous capacitance more than arterial resistance at lower doses (Fig. 65-3).**[91,121]

Other hemodynamic effects include decreases in left ventricular end-diastolic pressure, pulmonary artery pressure, pulmonary vascular resistance, and right ventricular end-diastolic pressure. Decreases in mean arterial pressure are usually slight and smaller than in the other hemodynamic parameters.[69] Low doses have little effect on cardiac output and heart rate in patients with normal or increased intravascular volume. Rapid administration or high doses of nitrates, especially in patients with volume-contracted states, may decrease left ventricular end-diastolic pressure, stroke volume, cardiac output, and mean arterial pressure and cause reflexive increases in heart rate and sympathetic tone.[101,249]

The antianginal use of nitroglycerin stems from its effect on the relationship between myocardial oxygen (O_2) supply and demand. By increasing venous capacitance and thus decreasing left ventricular end-diastolic pressure and volume, nitroglycerin decreases systolic ventricular wall tension, which is the major determinant of myocardial energy consumption.

An additional benefit of nitrates is improved flow to areas of ischemia.[12,117,159] This effect is related to higher myocardial perfusion pressure, resulting from lower left ventricular diastolic pressure, and/or to redistribution of coronary blood flow to subendocardial tissue.

Nitroglycerin is a direct coronary arterial vasodilator, especially of large epicardial vessels.[29,67,91] Dilation of large coronary arteries explains nitrates' beneficial effects when angina is caused by coronary spasm. In patients with classic angina due to coronary insufficiency, coronary blood flow does not increase following administration of nitroglycerin.[98] It has been postulated that dilation of large epicardial vessels or improvement of cardiac perfusion pressures causes an autoregulated increase in coronary vascular resistance in well-perfused arteriolar resistance vessels distal to large coronary arteries. This increased resistance shunts coronary flow to areas of ischemia where the arterioles are dilated. Effects of nitrates on coronary blood flow distribution are much different (indeed opposite) from those of sodium nitroprusside and dipyridamole. The latter drugs dilate arteriolar resistance vessels and can lead to myocardial steal syndromes. There seems also to be relationship between nitroglycerin, prostacyclin synthesis, and arterial dilation.[247]

Clinical studies have shown that nitroglycerin's effects on both systemic and coronary circulations are important. Intracoronary injections of nitroglycerin are considered by some investigators to be not as effective as IV nitroglycerin in treatment of pacer-induced ischemia.[84] Beneficial systemic effect is suggested by the observation that intracoronary injection is less effective, despite increased coronary blood flow. Conversely, other studies have shown that intracoronary nitroglycerin in doses without systemic effect de-

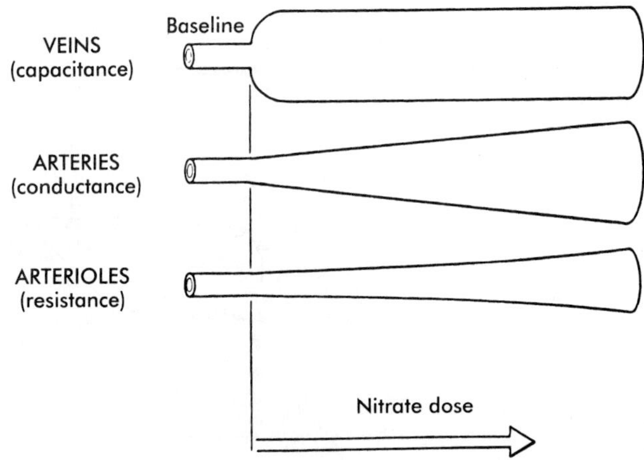

Fig. 65-3. Hemodynamic effects of nitrates on major vascular beds. At low doses, the venous capacitance vessels are nearly maximally dilated. The systemic arteries begin to dilate at low doses. This effect increases in a dose-dependent fashion. Arteriolar vasodilation occurs only with very high doses, which are probably not clinically achievable. (From Abrams J: Hemodynamic effects of nitroglycerin and long-acting nitrates, *Am Heart J* 110:216, 1985.)

creases ST segment elevations, improves systolic and diastolic function, and enhances flow to ischemic tissue.[163]

Nitroglycerin's relaxation of vascular smooth muscles stems from the intracellular reaction of organic nitrates with a sulfydryl moiety on the nitrate receptor to form inorganic nitrite. Nitrite is then oxidized to form nitric oxide. Nitric oxide in combination with tissue thiols forms *s*-nitroso-thiol, an activator of guanylate cyclase, the enzyme that catalyzes the formation of cyclic guanylic acid (cGMP) (Fig. 65-4).[120] The exact mechanism of action of cGMP is unclear, but elevated cGMP levels may inhibit use of intracellular calcium. Dephosphorylation of light-chain myosin occurs through a cGMP-mediated protein kinase, causing smooth-muscle relaxation. Higher intracellular levels of cGMP also mediate bronchial, biliary, gastrointestinal, ureteral, and uterine smooth-muscle relaxation.

Clinically, nitrates may be used transdermally or orally for chronic therapy, on an intermittent basis via the sublingual route, or intravenously for acute therapy (Table 65-6). Clinical indications include classic exertional, Prinzmetal's variant and unstable angina, acute MI, and coronary artery spasm. Patients taking nitrates who are to have surgery should continue to receive therapy until and possibly throughout surgery. If a substantial perioperative or postoperative lapse is expected, nitrate ointments or IV nitroglycerin may be used. All nitrates cause rapid development of tolerance, but a drug-free interval will reverse this condition.

Perioperatively, IV nitroglycerin may be used for treatment of myocardial ischemia, CHF, acute volume overload, systemic and pulmonary hypertension, and coronary artery spasm. Patients receiving acute nitroglycerin therapy can exhibit exaggerated hemodynamic responses to anesthetics. Nitroglycerin may prolong the neuromuscular blockade of pancuronium.[95]

Beta-Adrenergic Blocking Agents

The many beta-adrenergic blocking agents have a wide spectrum of therapeutic uses beyond treatment of hypertension and angina (Box 65-1). They are among the most widely prescribed cardiac medications. Variations among beta-adrenergic blocking agents result from their differing pharmacologic properties in regard to $beta_1$ selectivity, alpha-adrenergic blocking activity, presence of intrinsic sympathomimetic activity (ISA) or membrane-stabilizing activity (MSA), potency, lipid solubility, first-pass effect, half-life, and mode of metabolism and excretion. All beta-adrenergic blocking agents competitively block effects of catecholamines on receptors in the heart, lung, vasculature, kidney, and brain, and the therapeutic value stems from these effects.

As a group, these drugs have significant cardiovascular effects. Beta-adrenergic blocking agents decrease blood pressure, but the mechanism is debated (Box 65-2). Beta blockers decrease myocardial contractility and heart rate and thus cardiac output, but even at dosages lower than necessary to cause substantial decreases in cardiac output, propranolol can be an effective antihypertensive. Beta blockers with ISA, such as pindolol, decrease cardiac output less, yet are similarly effective antihypertensives. Hypertensive patients with high plasma renin activity (PRA) respond well to propranolol, which decreases PRA, yet beta blockers which do not decrease PRA (e.g., pindolol) are also effective.

Evidence suggests that beta blockers cross the blood–brain barrier, and a CNS mechanism involving reduction of receptor-mediated sympathetic outflow has been pro-

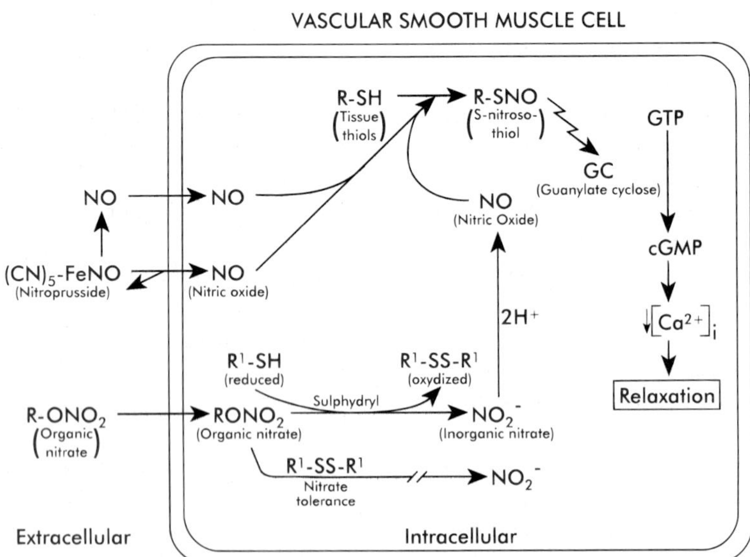

Fig. 65-4 Cellular mechanism of action of nitroglycerin and nitroprusside. (From Ignarro LJ, Lippton H, Edwards JC, et al: Mechanism of vascular smooth muscle relaxation by nitrates, nitroprusside and nitric oxide, *J Pharmacol Exp Ther* 218:739, 1981.)

Table 65-6 Nitrate preparations and dosages

Nitroglycerin	
Sublingual tablets—Nitrostate	0.3–0.6 mg PRN (up to 3 tablets)
Translingual spray—Nitrolingual	0.4 mg/spray (up to three sprays)
Transmucosal tablets—Nitrograd (Forest)	1–3 mg q5 h three times a day
Oral extended-release	2.5–6.5 bid to quid
Ointment—2%	1″–2″ q4 h for 12–14 hr day
Transdermal patches	one patch 12–14 hr/day
Isosorbide dinitrate	
Sublingual tablets—immediate release	2.5–10 mg q2–3 h
Oral tablets	30 mg bid or 20 mg tid in morning and afternoon
Extended-release tablets and capsules	40–80 mg once daily to tid
Isosorbide-5-mononitrate	
Immediate release	20 mg in morning and afternoon, 7 hours apart
Extended-release	60–120 mg once daily

posed. On the other hand, lipophilic drugs, such as propranolol and metoprolol, are not more effective than hydrophilic compounds such as atenolol. Other proposed mechanisms of action include resetting of baroreceptors, attenuation of pressor responses to stress and exercise and blockade of prejunctional receptors that normally facilitate norepinephrine release.[76,83,170,171,197] Despite unclear exact mechanism(s) of action, beta blockers are among the most frequently prescribed antihypertensive medications.

In angina pectoris, beta-adrenergic blocking agents decrease heart rate, blood pressure, and contractility, and therefore reduce myocardial O_2 consumption. They may improve perfusion by increasing diastolic coronary filling time.[83,235,236] Other mechanisms have been suggested (Box 65-3). In patients with poor ventricular function, increased wall tension, secondary to elevated left ventricular end-diastolic pressure, may negate other gains. Treatment of angina pectoris with beta blockers, in combination with nitrates and/or calcium channel blockers, represents the current standard of care, if no contraindications exist.

Competitive beta-receptor inhibition has useful antidysrhythmic effects (Table 65-7). Beta blockers decrease the action potential's phase-4 depolarization slope and decrease automaticity. This explains their therapeutic efficacy in patients with dysrhythmias associated with enhanced automaticity, such as that seen with thyrotoxicosis, digitalis toxicity, pheochromocytoma, and MI. By decreasing atrioventricular (AV) node conduction, beta blockers have proved useful in heart rate control in patients with atrial fibrillation, atrial flutter, and paroxysmal atrial tachycardia.[75] More recently, they have been shown to be useful in treatment of ventricular dysrhythmias associated with ischemia and mitral valve prolapse after papillary muscle dysfunction or infarction.[158,200] Patients who survive an MI have decreased morbidity, less sudden death, and fewer recurrent infarctions when treated with beta blockers.[82] Whether this represents an antidysrhythmic or anti-ischemic effect is unclear.[87]

Other cardiovascular syndromes in which beta-blocker therapy has proved useful include mitral valve prolapse, preexcitation syndromes, hypertrophic cardiomyopathy, tetralogy of Fallot, aortic aneurysm, prolonged QT-interval syndromes, and even advanced cardiomyopathies. Noncardiac

BOX 65-1
REPORTED USES FOR BETA-ADRENORECEPTOR BLOCKING DRUGS

Cardiovascular

- Hypertension*
- Angina pectoris*
- Supraventricular dysthythmias*
- Ventricular dysthythmias*
- Reducing the risk of mortality and reinfarction in survivors of acute myocardial infarction*
- Hyperacute phase of myocardial infarction*
- Dissection of the aorta
- Hypertrophic cardiomyopathy*
- Digitalis intoxication
- Mitral valve prolapse
- "QT interval" prolongation syndrome
- Tetralogy of Fallot
- Mitral stenosis
- Congestive cardiomyopathy
- Fetal tachycardia
- Neurocirculatory asthenia

Noncardiovascular

- Neuropsychiatric
  - Migraine prophylaxis*
  - Essential tremor*
  - Anxiety
  - Alcohol withdrawal (delirium tremens)
- Endocrine
  - Thyrotoxicosis
  - Hyperparathyroidism
  - Pheochromocytoma (to be used with alpha-blockers)*
- Other
  - Glaucoma*
  - Portal hypertension and gastrointestinal bleeding

*Approved indications by the Food and Drug Administration.
From Frishman WH: Beta-Adrenergic Blockers, *Med Clin North Am* 72:50 1988. With permission.

BOX 65-2
PROPOSED MECHANISMS TO EXPLAIN THE ANTIHYPERTENSIVE ACTIONS OF BETA BLOCKERS

Reduction in cardiac output
Inhibition of renin
Reduction in plasma volume
Central nervous system effects
Reduction in peripheral vascular resistance
Resetting of baroreceptor levels
Reduction in venomotor tone
Effects on prejunctional beta receptors—reductions in norepinephrine release
Most important effect of beta blockers—prevents the pressor response to catecholamines with exercise and stress

From Frishman WH: *Clinical Pharmacology of the B-Adrenoceptor Blocking Drugs,* ed 2, Norwalk, 1984, Appleton-Century-Crofts, p 28. Adapted and reproduced with permission.

BOX 65-3
POSSIBLE MECHANISMS BY WHICH BETA-BLOCKERS PROTECT THE ISCHEMIC MYOCARDIUM

Reduction in myocardial oxygen consumption, heart rate, blood pressure, and myocardial contractility
Augmentation of coronary blood flow
- Increase in diastolic perfusion time by reducing heart rate
- Augmentation of collateral blood flow
- Redistribution of blood flow to ischemic areas

Alterations in myocardial substrate use
Decrease in microvascular damage
Stabilization of cell and lysosomal membranes
Shift to oxyhemoglobin dissociation curve to the right
Inhibition of platelet aggregation

From Frishman WH: *Clinical Pharmacology of the B-Adrenoceptor Blocking Drugs,* ed 2, Norwalk, 1984, Appleton-Century-Crofts, p 306. With permission.

uses have included prevention of bleeding in patients with portal hypertension and treatment of glaucoma, thyrotoxicosis, migraines, essential tremors, delirium tremens, and situational anxiety.

These important drugs are not without significant side effects. Beta blockers may precipitate overt CHF in patients with impaired ventricular function. Patients with sinus node dysfunction or AV block may develop symptomatic bradycardias following administration. Stimulation of $beta_2$ receptors in lungs causes bronchodilation; conversely, treatment with beta blockers may cause bronchospasm. Their use is problematic in bronchospastic disease. Even beta blockers with relative $beta_1$ selectivity (e.g., metoprolol, atenolol, betaxolol, esmolol) occasionally cause bronchoconstriction when used in doses within usual therapeutic range.[74,142,228] Beta blockade may decrease cardiac output and block $beta_2$-mediated coronary or peripheral arterial dilation, allowing unopposed constriction (e.g., spasm). Symptoms of peripheral and coronary vascular disease may worsen after beta-blocker therapy.[109] Additional concerns include impotence, decreased sympathetic manifestations of hypoglycemia in patients taking insulin or hypoglycemic agents.[164] The problem of impotence, the mechanism of which is unclear, seems often to lead physicians to prescribe the calcium blockers instead of beta adrenergic blockers for men. The calcium blockers are likely less effective in therapy. CNS effects such as depression, psychosis, and obtundation may occur. Multiple interactions between beta-adrenergic blocking agents and other drugs have been described. Abrupt withdrawal of beta blockers may result in hypertension, tachycardia, exacerbation of anginal syndromes, and even MI or death.[181]

The beta-adrenergic blocking agents most frequently used in the United States today are described in the following sections (Table 65-7).

Propranolol

Propranolol is the standard against which all other beta-adrenergic blocking agents are measured. It is not cardioselective and has no ISA. Although propranolol has MSA, this occurs only at doses far beyond therapeutic and is not clinically relevant except following massive overdoses. After oral absorption, propranolol undergoes major first-pass hepatic metabolism. Thus the usual oral dosage of propranolol is 40 to 320 mg/day, whereas reasonable IV dosage is only 0.025 to 0.15 mg/kg. Cimetidine decreases hepatic metabolism and blood flow and may decrease propranolol's therapeutic dose. Propranolol is highly lipophilic and crosses the blood–brain barrier, which may explain its many CNS effects. Its usual oral half-life is about 4 hours. Propranolol is also available as a long-acting preparation, a marked advantage for treatment of patients with angina pectoris.[75]

Metoprolol, atenolol, bisoprolol, and betaxolol

Metoprolol is a cardioselective beta blocker with no ISA or MSA. It primarily undergoes hepatic metabolism, with a half-life of 3 to 7 hours. When used in low doses, metoprolol may be preferable to propranolol for smokers and other patients who may have bronchospastic components, who nonetheless could benefit from beta blocker therapy. Although relatively cardioselective, metoprolol still may precipitate bronchospasm.[142] It is less likely than propranolol to mask symptoms of hypoglycemia.[51] Its usual dosage is 50 to 200 mg twice daily. As with propranolol, metoprolol is available in IV form, with usual dosage of 0.025 to 0.15 mg/kg. It is now available as an extended release preparation.

Atenolol is a long-acting cardioselective beta blocker

Table 65-7 Pharmacologic properties of beta-blockers

Agent	Relative $beta_1$ selectivity	ISA	MSA	Alpha activity	Elimination half-life charts	Predominant mode of elimination	Oral dosage (mg)	IV dosage
Acebutolol	+	+	+	–	3–4 hr	Renal/hepatic	200–600 bid	
Atenolol	+ +	–	–	–	6–7 hr	Renal	50–200 daily	5–10 titrated at 1 mg/min
Betaxolol	+ +	–	+	–	16–22 hr	Hepatic/renal	10–40 mg daily	
Bisoprolol	+ +	–	–	–	9–13	Renal/hepatic	10–20 mg daily	
Carteolol	–	+	–	–	5–6 hr	Renal	2.5–10 daily	
Esmolol	+ +	–			9 min	Erythrocyte esterases		0.5–1 mg/kg bolus, then 100 – 300 μg/kg/min
Labetalol	–	–	–	+	6–8 hr	Hepatic	200–1200 bid	5–20 mg initially, then 40 mg q 10 min up to 300 mg as boluses or 2 mg/min as infusion
Metoprolol	+	–	–	–	3–7 hr	Hepatic	50–200 bid	0.1–0.15 mg/kg titrated slowly to effect
Metoprolol extended-release	+ +	–	–	–	?	Hepatic	50–400 daily	
Nadolol	–	–	–	–	20–24 hr	Renal	40–240 daily	
Penbutolol	–	+	–	–	5 hr	Renal	20 daily	
Pindolol	–	+ +	+	–	3–4 hr	Renal/hepatic	5–30 bid	
Propranolol	–	–	+ +	–	4 hr	Hepatic	40–320 daily, bid or qid	0.1–0.15 mg/kg titrated slowly to effect
Propanolol extended-release	–	–	+ +	–	10 hr	Hepatic	80–320 daily, bid	
Timolol	–	–	–	–	4–5 hr	Renal	10–30 bid	

with no ISA or MSA. It is eliminated by renal excretion, with a half-life of 6 to 7 hours. Its usual dosage is 50 to 200 mg daily. It is available in an IV form, with a recommended dosage of 5 to 10 mg given slowly. Besides being cardioselective and requiring only a single daily intake, other possible advantages include relative lipophobia and minimal blood–brain barrier crossing. Unfortunately, in clinical trials with atenolol, this has not been reflected by a lower incidence of CNS side effects.[36,74] Atenolol is sufficiently long-acting that, if given on the day of cardiovascular surgery, substantial drug presence can be a problem during attempted emergence from bypass.

Bisoprolol, a long-acting cardioselective beta blocker with no ISA or MSA,[125] is renally eliminated with 50% unchanged in the urine with the remaining 50% appearing in the urine as inactive metabolites.[155] Its half-life of 9 to 13 hours makes it suitable for once a day administration.[125,155]

Betaxolol is an oral, long-acting cardioselective beta blocker with some MSA but no ISA. Undergoing predominantly hepatic metabolism, its half-life of 16 to 22 hours makes it suitable for once-a-day administration.[42] As with timolol, betaxolol is also available in a topical form for treatment of glaucoma.

Nadolol

Nadolol is a noncardioselective beta blocker with no ISA or MSA. Unlike propranolol, it is renally excreted, with a half-life of 20 to 24 hours, allowing once-a-day administration. This is nadolol's major therapeutic advantage when compared with propranolol. The usual dosage is 40 to 240 mg/day.[77]

Timolol

Timolol is a noncardioselective beta blocker with no MSA or ISA. Its usual dosage is 10 to 30 mg twice a day, with a half-life of 4 to 5 hours. It undergoes both hepatic and renal excretion. Otherwise, it is similar to propranolol. Timolol is frequently used as an eye drop for therapy of glaucoma. In this form, it may be systemically absorbed and produce effects similar to those after oral ingestion.[74]

Acebutolol, carteolol, penbutolol, and pindolol

These four beta blockers exhibit ISA and partial agonist effects. With the patient at rest, these drugs may decrease heart rate to a lesser extent than other beta blockers. They are efficacious in blunting exercise-induced hemodynamic response. These drugs are believed to produce fewer lipid abnormalities and peripheral vascular complications with less myocardial depression and bronchospasm. Specifically, pindolol produces less depression of heart rate and fewer nocturnal pauses in patients with sick sinus syndrome compared with agents lacking agonist effects.[40,241] Another possible advantage may be absence of rebound after discontinuation, but no large-scale trials are available to support these claims. No data are available to support the use of these drugs after MI. Dosages and other properties of acebutolol, carteolol, penbutolol, and pindolol are listed in Table 65-7.[38,73,78]

Labetalol

Labetalol is unique among presently available beta-adrenergic blockers in that it also possesses alpha-adrenergic antagonism in a ratio of about 5:1 (beta/alpha). This alpha-blocking activity can be used to decrease arterial pressure with somewhat better maintenance of cardiac output. Labetalol is available in both IV and oral forms (Table 65-7). Its use is well established in acute therapy of severe hypertension in the emergency room, operating room, and recovery suite, but it is seldom employed as a long-term medication.

Esmolol

Esmolol, is a highly cardioselective $beta_1$-adrenergic blocker with no intrinsic ISA or MSA. It has a distribution half-life of 2 minutes and an elimination half-life of 9 minutes, due to rapid hydrolysis by erythrocytes esterases. Its short duration of action makes it particularly valuable in management of perioperative patients. Esmolol is typically used as a bolus with or without an infusion. Steady-state plasma levels are obtained within 5 minutes. Usual bolus dosages are 0.5 to 1 mg/kg. Infusion rates of 50 to 300 ug/kg/minute are titrated to clinical effect. On discontinuation of an esmolol infusion, significant recovery occurs within 10 to 20 minutes, and blood concentrations are undetectable within 30 minutes. Because esmolol is metabolized by erythrocyte esterase, metabolism and elimination are not affected by *plasma* cholinesterase inhibitors. Esmolol allows beta-blocker use in acute situations when quick withdrawal may be necessary because of the patient's changing clinical status. Esmolol has been used intraoperatively to attenuate response to intubation, prevent and/or treat tachycardia and ischemia, and to produce deliberate hypotension. The time course for attainment of heart rate decreases is faster than for changes in blood pressure.[191] More recently, it has been used to attenuate the increased heart rate and mean arterial pressure associated with rapidly increased inspired desflurane concentrations.[255] Postoperatively, it has been useful in treatment of hypertension, myocardial ischemia, and supraventricular dysrhythmias.[130]

Celiprolol

Celiprolol is a third-generation, cardioselective beta blocker currently being evaluated for FDA approval. It is unique among beta blockers in that it is a $beta_1$ blocker and a partial $beta_2$ *agonist*.[140] It may have bronchosparing properties in asthmatic patients compared with other beta blockers.[201]

Anesthetic considerations

Anesthetic considerations about beta-adrenergic blocking therapy are numerous. When they were first introduced, beta blockers and antihypertensives were discontinued before anesthesia and surgery because of concern that their effects might be additive to those of general anesthetic agents. Unfortunately, this sudden withdrawal tended to result in rebound effects with worsening of both angina and hypertension.[181,194] **Present recommendations are to continue the patient's usual beta-adrenergic blocking regimen until surgery and to restart the drugs as soon as possible postoperatively.**

Because of their pharmacologic effects, beta blockers may attenuate the sympathomimetic effects of cyclopropane or ether anesthesia[49] and of intraoperative stresses such as hypercarbia.[72] Beta blockers have additive negative inotropic effects with potent inhalation agents. In dogs at 1.0 MAC of enflurane, propranolol causes mild decreases in myocardial contractility, heart rate, and cardiac output. These changes are more pronounced at deeper anesthetic concentrations. Circulatory depression, although present, is less when halothane or isoflurane are combined with propranolol compared with enflurane. In dogs anesthetized with halothane, isoflurane, or enflurane, propranolol produces additive slowing of heart rate and AV node conduction.[107,116,206]

Patients maintained on beta blockers, particularly when these medications are combined with calcium channel blockers, are at risk for severe bradyarrhythmias when anesthesia is induced with high-dose fentanyl or sufentanyl. These bradyarrhythmias also occur with muscle relaxants which lack vagolytic effects. When high-dose narcotics are given to patients who take beta blockers, with or without calcium channel blockers, vagolytic muscle relaxants such as pancuronium can be used to offset the bradycardic affects of the narcotics combined with the adrenergic blockade.[1]

Several currently available IV beta blockers—propranolol, metoprolol, atenolol, labetalol, and esmolol—may be administered perioperatively to attenuate hemodynamic responses to intubation or surgical stress, tre and ischemia, slow heart rates, or treat dysrhy

Calcium Channel Blockers

The calcium channel blockers represent a dive of compounds with dissimilar structures and pha logic effects. *In vitro,* they inhibit slow channel–me cell membrane transport of calcium and thus modulate cium's intracellular effects (Fig. 65-5).[5,139,188] They all ha vasodilatory properties and depress both contractility an cardiac conduction.[25,26,71,182] Unlike beta blockers, which all depend on receptor blockade for their activity, the sites and mechanisms of action of individual calcium channel blockers vary, as do their individual actions on different tissues. **These medications are not nearly as interchangeable as beta blockers.**[25]

Used predominantly in antianginal and antihypertensive therapy (Fig. 65-6), calcium channel blockers are also used in treatment of syndromes as diverse as paroxysmal supraventricular tachycardia (PSVT) and migraine headaches.[225,234]

Until recently, three calcium channel blockers—verapamil, diltiazem and nifedipine—were available in the United States. These comprise three different molecular classes. Recently, several dihydropyridine derivative calcium channel blockers—nisoldipine, nicardipine, nimodipine, amlodipine, isradipine, and felodipine—have become available. Bepridil, which is structurally distinct, is available as well (Table 65-8).

Verapamil

Verapamil, which is structurally similar to papaverine, has a complex mode of action. It is a racemic mixture, with each isomer having different cellular actions.[139] The net effect is to depress both slow channel activation and recovery from inactivation. Via its effects on calcium channels, verapamil substantially decreases myocardial contractility[229] and di-

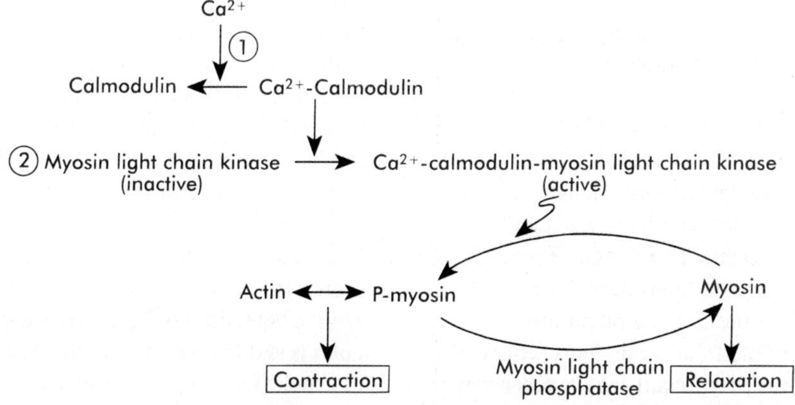

Fig. 65-5. Activation sequence of mechanical contraction in vascular smooth muscle. The calcium (Ca^{2+}) calmodulin complex (1) activates myosin light-chain kinase (2), which catalyzes the phosphorylation of myosin (P-myosin). Cross-bridge formation between P-myosin and actin produces mechanical contraction. (From Anderson KE, et al: On the mechanism of action of calcium antagonists, *Acta Med Scand* 681(suppl):11, 1984.)

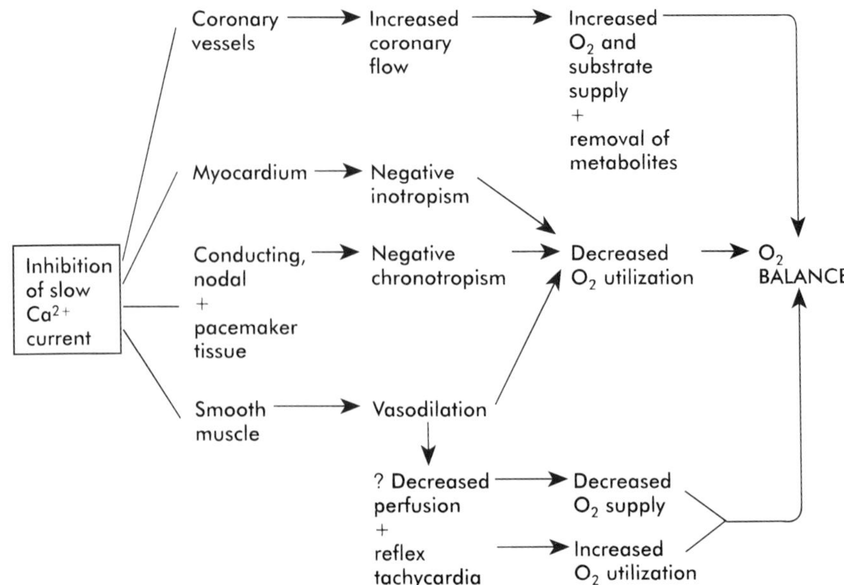

Fig. 65-6. Consequences of calcium channel blockers on myocardial O_2 balance. Because of reflex responses, negative chronotropism and inotropism may not be important. (From Nayler WG, Dillon JS, Daly MF: Cellular sites of action of calcium antagonists and β-adrenoceptor blockers. In Opie LH, editor: *Perspectives in cardiovascular research,* vol 9, Calcium antagonists and cardiovascular disease, New York, 1984, Raven Press.)

lates coronary and peripheral vascular beds.[25,26] It therefore increases coronary blood flow and and systemic vascular resistance. In contrast to nitrates, verapamil and all calcium channel blockers have little effect on venous capacitance.[267] By blocking calcium channels in the SA node, verapamil slows heart rate. By decreasing heart rate, contractility, and peripheral resistance, verapamil decreases myocardial O_2 consumption. By increasing diastolic filling time and coronary blood flow while decreasing coronary vascular resistance, verapamil increases myocardial O_2 delivery. By directly antagonizing coronary vascular spasm, verapamil is useful in treatment of classic and Prinzmetal's variant angina.[229]

The electrophysiologic effects of verapamil are substantial. It slows spontaneous rates of firing and increases sinoatrial (SA) node recovery time, thereby decreasing heart rate. In the AV node, it directly decreases conduction and increases effective refractory period. Because verapamil substantially prolongs AV node conduction, it is effective in slowing ventricular response in atrial fibrillation and flutter. It can successfully convert PSVTs to sinus rhythm,[147,254] with an effectiveness of greater than 90%. Verapamil has also been shown useful in the control of multifocal atrial tachycardia. It should be noted that in patients with Wolff-Parkinson-White syndrome, verapamil may worsen tachycardia by preferential AV slowing, which may increase conduction through accessory pathways.[106]

The net effect of verapamil in lowering both systolic and diastolic blood pressures with few side effects makes it efficacious for treatment of hypertension.[80,239] Possibly as a result of improvement in diastolic function, verapamil improves exercise tolerance and decreases symptoms in patients with hypertrophic cardiomyopathy.[216]

In acute IV therapy, the recommended dose of verapamil is 0.075 to 0.15 mg/kg over 1 minute. Peak vasodilatory effect occurs at approximately 5 minutes and may persist for 30 minutes, although the antidysrhythmic effect may persist substantially longer. IV distribution half-life is 3.5 minutes, and elimination half-life is 110 minutes. A second dose may be given at 30 minutes. Anesthetics or other drugs that decrease liver blood flow will increase the half-life of verapamil.

The side effects of verapamil are related to its pharmacologic and therapeutic actions. Verapamil may exacerbate sinus node and AV node dysfunction, especially in patients with underlying disease or those treated with digitalis or beta blockers.[139] Verapamil may worsen symptoms of CHF, especially if used in combination with beta blockers.[193] Digitalis levels increase by an average of 70% after initiation of therapy with verapamil.[141]

Diltiazem

Diltiazem, a benzothiazepine, is a calcium channel blocker with a spectrum of pharmacologic effects between verapamil and the dihydropyridines. Diltiazem like all calcium channel blockers is an effective coronary artery dilator, but has relatively mild effects on peripheral vessels. It is a mild negative inotrope, but less so than verapamil. Diltiazem has little effect on cardiac output.[25,26,108,139] Reflex tachycardia is not a problem because it slows conduction through the SA and AV nodes, but less so than verapamil.[182] Although diltiazem may be used in combination with beta blockers, the ef-

Table 65-8 Pharmacologic effects of the calcium channel blockers

	HR acute	Conduction: SA node	Conduction: AV node	Myocardial contractility	PVR	CO	CBF	MVO_2	Oral	Intravenous dose (mg)	T½ (hrs)
Diltiazem	↓	↓	↓	↓	↓	V	↑	↓	30–90 q 6–8 hr	0.25 mg/kg (bolus then 0.15 ng/kg/hr	2–6
Bepridil	↓	↓	↓	V	—	V	↑	↓	200–400 OD	—	24–48
Verapamil	↓	↓	↓	↓↓	↓	↓	↑	↓	80–120 q 6–2 hr	0.75–0.15 mg/kg (bolus) then 0.075–0.15 mg/kg	3–7
Amlodipine	↑	—	—	↓ —	↓↓	↑	↑	V	2.5–10 OD	—	36–45
Felodipine	↑	—	—	—	↓↓	↑	↑	V	2.5–10 OD	—	triexponential 4.8 min 1.5 hr; 9.1 hr
Isradipine	↑	—	—	—	↓↓	↑	↑	V	2.5–10 OD	—	6–11
Nicardipine	↑	—	—	—	↓↓	↑	↑	V	10–20 8 hr	5–15/hr	2
Nifedipine	↑	—	—	↓ —	↓↓	↑	↑	V	10–40 q 8 hr	—	1.5–5
Nimodipine	↑	—	—	—	↓↓	↑	↑	V			
Nisoldipine	↑	—	—	—	↓↓	↑	↑	V	20–40 OD hr	—	10

↑, increase; ↓, decrease; —, no change; V — variable; SA — sinoatrial; AV — atrioventricular; HR — heart rate; MVO_2 — myocardial oxygen comsumption; PVR — peripheral vescular resistance; CO — cardiac output; CBF — coronary blood flow.

fects may be additive, causing SA and AV node dysfunction in patients with underlying conduction disease. Verapamil, with its potent conduction depression, should not be used in combination with beta blockers, except perhaps in patients with idiopathic hypertrophic subaortic stenosis.

Because of its depressant effect on the AV node, diltiazem may be used for control of heart rate in atrial fibrillation. Recently, an IV preparation of diltiazem has become available for rate control in rapid atrial fibrillation and flutter as well as conversion of PSVT to sinus rythm. The usual dose of IV diltiazem is 0.25 mg/kg as a slow bolus, followed by an infusion of 0.15 mg/kg. An additional bolus of 0.35 mg/kg may be administered if needed. Oral diltiazem may be used for the chronic management of these problems.[217] Preliminary results indicate that IV diltiazem may be useful in managment of acute hypertension.[3]

The dihydropyridines

Nifedipine. *In vitro,* nifedipine has significant effects on both smooth muscle and myocardium.[108] *In vivo,* however, it is an effective coronary and systemic arterial dilator at doses that have little effect on myocardial contractility or conduction tissue.[108] As a result of its afterload reduction, nifedipine may cause reflex sympathetic-mediated increases in heart rate and cardiac output.[63] As an antianginal, it is more effective than verapamil in decreasing coronary vascular resistance and coronary spasm and improving coronary blood flow.[25,26] Because it is an effective peripheral vasodilator, nifedipine may decrease both afterload and myocardial O_2 demand. Because it has little inotropic or conduction effects, nifedipine may be used in combination with beta blockers. Indeed, beta blockers eliminate nifedipine's potentially detrimental reflex increases in heart rate.[52,79]

Clinically, nifedipine effectively improves exercise tolerance and decreases the frequency of anginal attacks in patients with exercise-induced angina. Because it decreases afterload and increases cardiac output, nifedipine may be safely used for treatment of angina and hypertension in patients with CHF.[166] Nifedipine is an effective antihypertensive both chronically[80,239] and in acute hypertensive emergencies.[63,81] Because it is light sensitive, IV nifedipine is not commercially available in the United States. The side effects of nifedipine include headaches, pedal edema, hypotension, and exacerbation of angina. As with verapamil, nifedipine increases serum digitalis levels.[14] A recent highly publicized study concluded that in patients with coronary disease, moderate-to-high doses of the short-acting form of nifedipine were associated with an increase in mortality. The study was a retrospective, meta-analysis of 16 prior studies.[88] Although the conclusions are controversial, an FDA advisory panel has recommended that physicians no longer prescribe short-acting nifedipine preparations to patients with angina.

Nicardipine. Nicardipine has structural and pharmacologic properties similar to those of nifedipine. Like nifedipine, nicardipine is a potent coronary and systemic vasodilator with little effect on contractility.[22,66,199,39] It is available as an IV agent for treatment of hypertension in acute care settings, including the perioperative period. Its elimination is triexponential with an alpha redistribution half life of 2.7 minutes. An initial IV bolus of 2 mg is followed by an initial infusion rate of 5 mg/hr, which may be increased in 2.5 mg increments every 15 minutes up to a maximum infusion rate of 15 mg/hr.[3]

Nimodipine. Nimodipine, a nifedipine analog, is a calcium channel blocker with some degree of specificity for cerebrovascular smooth muscle.[138] It has been reported to be useful in prevention of cerebral vasospasm and neurologic deficits after the occurrence of subarachnoid hemorrhage. This finding is controversial. In addition, nimodipine is used for therapy of migraine headache and for preservation of neurologic function after ischemic stroke.[90,177]

Amlodipine, isradipine, felodipine, and nisoldipine. These drugs are structurally and pharmacologically similar to the dihydropyridine prototype, nifedipine. They dilate coronary and peripheral arteries with minimal effects on cardiac conduction and contractility. Clinically, these drugs are effective for the treatment of hypertension and angina and may be safely used in patients with CHF.[28,145,266]

The individual agents are distinct from each other in some ways. For example, amlodipine does not alter serum digitalis levels.[224] Some studies show that isradipine generally is not associated with reflex tachycardia.[28,167]

Bepridil

Bepridil is structurally unrelated to other calcium channel blockers. It blocks slow calcium channels in both cardiac and vascular smooth muscle as well as fast sodium channels in cardiac muscle. Unlike the dihydropyridines, bepridil has negative chronotropic and dromotropic effects, and is a mild negative inotrope.[115] It is effective in reducing the frequency of exercise-induced angina.[268] It is well tolerated in patients with left ventricular impairment without overt heart failure.[55] Besides slowing conduction through the SA and AV nodes, bepridil has electrophysiologic effects similar to class Ia antidysrhythmics. It prolongs the QT interval on ECG and may be proarrythmic. It may precipitate *torsades de pointes*.[115] Bepridil also has been associated with agranulocytosis and pancytopenia.[258]

Because of its serious side-effects profile, bepridil only should be used in patients with angina that has not responded to other agents.

Anesthetic considerations

When used in combination with high-dose narcotics in patients with normal conduction systems and ventricular function, IV verapamil decreases systemic vascular resistance and mean arterial pressure with no change in cardiac output or pulmonary capillary wedge pressure. Although lengthening of the PR interval has been observed, neither first-degree nor more advanced AV node block occurred.[137]

In combination with inhalation agents in isolated guinea pig hearts, verapamil decreases spontaneous heart rate and peak left ventricular pressure in dose-dependent manner. It decreases AV conduction with halothane, isoflurane, and to a greater extent with enflurane anesthesia.[172] AV dissociation occurred in a small number of patients receiving enflurane.

In dogs, verapamil in combination with inhalation anesthetics lengthened AV conduction time; the combination of verapamil and enflurane sometimes even resulted in complete heart block.[6] In another canine model, verapamil plus enflurane or isoflurane produced additive decreases in contractility and cardiac output compared with inhalation agents alone. In this study, enflurane again appeared less well tolerated than halothane or isoflurane when combined with verapamil.[131] One human case report describes a cardiac arrest following administration of IV verapamil during halothane anesthesia.[184]

In a study of patients chronically taking beta blockers and who were undergoing coronary artery bypass surgery under halothane anesthesia, IV verapamil caused decreased mean arterial pressure, contractility, and cardiac index and a 3-mm Hg increase in left ventricular end-diastolic pressure with little effect on heart rate.[222]

To prevent possible increases in ischemia or worsening hypertension, current recommendations are to continue verapamil perioperatively. Verapamil has many perioperative uses. It has been used for intraoperative control of PSVT. (Verapamil is not indicated in WPW syndrome.) It has also been shown to protect the heart against epinephrine- and aminophylline-induced dysrhythmias in dogs anesthetized with halothane.[132,162] During cardiopulmonary bypass, verapamil has been shown to terminate refractory ventricular fibrillation following aortic cross-clamp removal.[118] Intraoperative myocardial ischemia refractory to IV nitroglycerin has been successfully treated with verapamil (7.5 mg IV).[190] Verapamil also may play a role in myocardial preservation.

Diltiazem, in combination with potent inhalation agents, has been shown to lengthen AV conduction time[8] and to additively depress contractility similar to verapamil.[27,134] Combined with enflurane, diltiazem is particularly depressive to conduction. Together, they may cause first-degree AV block, Mobitz I AV block, or sinus node dysfunction.[215] Diltiazem also may protect against halothane-associated dysrhythmias[128] and may have some use in myocardial preservation.[10]

Nifedipine and nicardipine, when given with fentanyl, decrease systemic vascular resistance with little effect on cardiac output or heart rate.[102,248] *In vitro,* nifedipine and halothane produce additive decreases in contractility. *In vivo,* when nifedipine was combined with inhalation anesthesia, cardiac output was largely unchanged, although mean arterial pressure and systemic vascular resistance decreased.[226,238]

Perioperatively, nifedipine and nicardipine have been used for control of hypertension,[248] myocardial preservation,[44,143] and treatment of ischemia.[143,154,156]

Calcium channel blockers may potentiate effects of depolarizing and nondepolarizing neuromuscular blocking agents.[61] In contrast with beta-adrenergic blocking agents, calcium channel blockers have not been shown to be effective in prevention of intraoperative ischemia.[43]

DIGITALIS

More than 200 years have passed since William Withering published "An account of the Foxglove and some of its Medical Uses."[260] Now, two centuries and a myriad of new drugs later, digitalis remains a mainstay of cardiac therapeutics.[230]

The mechanism of action of the cardiac glycosides is unique. They bind to and directly inhibit the membrane-bound, sodium-potassium adenosine-triphosphatase (ATPase) pump of the myocardial cell, causing increased intracellular sodium and decreased intracellular potassium. The increase in intracellular sodium changes the sodium concentration gradient and produces decreased exchange of extracellular sodium for intracellular calcium. This leads to a net increased inward calcium current and intracellular calcium concentration. As the intracellular concentration of calcium increases, it becomes more readily available to contractile proteins and enhances myocardial contractility. Digitalis remains the most prominent inotrope available for chronic use and has been shown clinically to decrease symptoms of CHF.[6,32,153,174] Most inotropes increase myocardial O_2 consumption. However, by decreasing ventricular radius and heart rate, digitalis may actually improve angina symptoms in patients who have angina pectoris with CHF. Cardiac glycosides have substantial electrophysiologic effects. Digitalis substantially enhances parasympathetic tone while causing some decrease in cardiac sympathetic activity.[192] These effects are the reason digitalis is efficacious in treatment of supraventricular dysrhythmias.[253] By inhibiting the sodium-potassium ATPase pump, digitalis may have effects on conduction independent of vagal tone.[214] In normal subjects, digoxin has only a small SA node effect. In one study, it decreased average heart rates from 75 to 68 beats. Digoxin may be safely used in patients with sinus bradycardias without decreasing heart rates, with the exception that patients with evidence of sick sinus syndrome who are given digitalis may have lengthened SA node conduction and recovery times.[21]

The major effects of digitalis on atrial and AV node tissue are also vagally mediated. In humans, therapeutic dosages decrease conduction velocity and either have no effect or increase effective atrial refractory period.[96] Digitalis causes prolongation of both conduction time and effective refractory period of the AV node. In the accessory pathway of patients with Wolff-Parkinson-White syndrome, digitalis may shorten the refractory period of the antegrade pathway[124] without affecting the retrograde pathway.[57,226] Therefore, it should not be used in patients with Wolff-Parkinson-White syndrome. In the ventricle, digitalis shortens the effective refractory period[96] while having little indirect effect.[213]

At toxic levels, in addition to causing anorexia, nausea, fatigue, visual disturbances, and confusion, digitalis also may cause severe conduction disturbances. The ECG manifestations may include sinus bradycardia or SA node exit block, AV block, premature atrial contractions, junctional tachycardias, premature ventricular contractions, and ventricular tachycardia and fibrillation.

Treatment of digitalis toxicity may include several measures, from simply stopping further dosages, to monitoring, to treating hypokalemia in patients without symptoms, to initiating oral therapy with activated charcoal and placement of a transvenous pacemaker (for patients with symptomatic bradycardia or AV dissociation). Atrial, junctional, and ventricular ectopy are amenable to therapy with phenytoin or procainamide. Ventricular ectopy is usually successfully treated with lidocaine. Anecdotal data suggest that magnesium, bretylium, and amiodarone may suppress severe life-threatening dysrhythmias. Amiodarone itself may increase digoxin levels by 100%. In general, drugs that increase serum digitalis levels (e.g., quinidine, propafenone, verapamil) should be avoided.

Availability of IV digoxin-specific Fab fragments has dramatically changed therapy for severe toxicity. (These are fragments of antibodies which are thought to contain the specific antigen binding site.) These fragments bind to digoxin and pharmacologically inactivate it.[231,257]

Therapeutic indications for digitalis use include management of CHF, termination of PSVT and prevention of its recurrence, and control of heart rate in atrial fibrillation or flutter.

The usual dosage of digoxin is approximately 0.25 mg/day, with half of that dose prescribed for elderly patients or for patients with renal insufficiency. When acute therapy is necessary, a loading dose of 1 to 1.5 mg is given over 24 hours. Digitoxin, because of its very long half-life, is now infrequently used. Its loading dose is 0.8 to 1.2 mg over 24 hours, with a maintenance dose of 0.1 to 0.15 mg daily. Ouabain is no longer commercially available.

Some authors have suggested prophylactic administration of digitalis in patients undergoing cardiovascular or intrathoracic surgery if atrial fibrillation or flutter, previous heart failure, cardiomegaly, valvular lesion, or ischemia on ECG is present.[176] Possible advantages of digitalization must be weighed against the consequences of administering such a long-acting medication with a very narrow therapeutic/toxic ratio. Perioperatively, potassium levels and renal function may fluctuate substantially, which may increase the likelihood of digitalis toxicity.

Dysrhythmias occur often during the perioperative period. In patients receiving digitalis therapy, digitalis toxicity must be considered as the dysrhythmia source. This could delay introduction of drugs (e.g., verapamil) that substantially increase serum digitalis levels or delay use of cardioversion, which may precipitate ventricular fibrillation in the presence of digitalis toxicity. These considerations become even more important when one realizes that powerful inotropes and antidysrhythmics with shorter half-lives than digitalis are available for acute administration if necessary.[150]

Some data suggest that halothane, enflurane, ether, methoxyflurane, ketamine, droperidol, and curare may reduce the likelihood of digitalis-induced ventricular dysrhythmias. Thiopental and fentanyl have no effect, whereas succinylcholine, neostigmine, and diazepam may induce dysrhythmias in patients taking digitalis. More important to any discussion of digitalis-associated dysrhythmias and toxicity is prevention of hypokalemia, acid-base imbalance, hypoxia, hypercalcemia, and catecholamine excess states and avoidance of medications that acutely increase digitalis serum levels.[7]

ANTIDYSRHYTHMIC AGENTS

Antidysrhythmic agents are indicated for prevention and treatment of symptomatic dysrhythmias or for therapy of asymptomatic dysrhythmias of malignant potential. Reasons for selecting one drug over another are frequently complex; the choice may depend on type of dysrhythmia, a particular drug's therapeutic index, a medication's effectiveness during electrophysiologic studies, or a patient's tolerance of side effects.

Antidysrhythmic drugs are classified on the basis of their major pharmacologic effects on myocardial electrophysiology, as originally proposed by Vaughan Williams[250] and now modified to include newer agents (Box 65-4). Although now loosely used to group drugs, this classification was originally proposed to rigorously classify patterns of pharmacologic action. This is a subtle but important difference. Many antidysrhythmics, although classified into one group or another, have (1) multiple actions in a given tissue; (2) different actions in different heart tissues; and (3) active metabolites with different actions than the parent compound.

Agents with class I actions include drugs that affect the fast inward sodium current of phase 0, the period of rapid depolarization of the action potential (Fig. 65-7). They have been further divided into three groups: Ia, Ib, and Ic. Antidysrhythmics with class Ia action include quinidine, procainamide, disopyramide, and moricizine. They all decrease the maximal velocity (V_{max}) and amplitude of phase 0 depolarization of the action potential. Effective refractory period (ERP), action potential duration (APD), and ratio of ERP/APD are increased. Automaticity, represented by the decreased slope of phase 4 of the action potential (Fig. 65-6), also is decreased with these drugs. These agents produce measurable increases in refractoriness of cardiac tissue and lengthening of the QTc interval on the ECG.

Drugs with class Ib actions, such as lidocaine, mexiletine, tocainide, and phenytoin, have more moderate effects on phase 0 of the action potential. They shorten APD and ERP and increase the ERP/APD ratio. They show little ECG effect.

Antidysrhythmics with class Ic actions, such as encainide, flecainide, and propafenone, have the greatest effect on phase O of the action potential with little effect on repo-

BOX 65-4
CLASSIFICATION OF ANTIDYSRHYTHMIC AGENTS

Class Ia	Class Ib	Class Ic
Quinidine	Lidocaine	Encainide
Procainamide	Mexiletine	Flecainide
Disopyramide	Tocainide	Propafenone
Moricizine	Phenytoin	

Class II beta blockers

Propranolol
Atenolol
Timolol
Metoprolol
Acebutolol
Esmolol

Class III

Bretylium
Amiodarone
(N-acetyl-procainamide)

Class IV calcium channel blockers

Verapamil
Diltiazem

Other agents not formally classified

Digoxin
Adenosine
Ibutilide

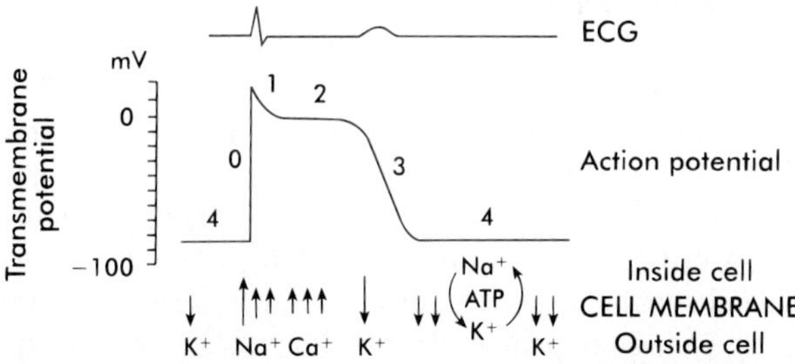

Fig. 65-7. Schematic representation of the action potential in a ventricular myocardial cell as it correlates with the electrocardiogram (ECG). Arrows indicate times of major ionic movement across the cell membrane. (From Lewis AJ: Monitoring and dysrhythmia recognition in advanced cardiac life support. In McIntyre KM, Lewis AJ, editors: *Textbook of advanced cardiac life support,* Dallas, 1994, American Heart Association.)

larization. On the ECG, PR and QRS intervals are lengthened, but QTc intervals are largely unchanged.

Class II actions refer to antidysrhythmic effects associated with beta-adrenergic antagonism. Therefore class II agents include all beta-adrenergic blocking agents.

Approved class III agents include amiodarone, bretylium and sotalol. Their predominant effect is to prolong APD and increase ERP via action on potassium channels. The ERP to APD ratio is increased.

Class IV action refers to antidysrhythmic effects of calcium channel antagonism and therefore includes all calcium channel blockers.

Some newer drugs, such as adenosine and ibutilide, do not fit into any of these categories and are as such unclassified.

Class Ia Agents (Table 65-9)

Quinidine

Quinidine, the *d*-isomer of quinine, has been used effectively alone or in combination with other agents[59] for conversion of atrial fibrillation, atrial flutter,[232] and PSVT[264] and for maintenance of sinus rhythm after conversion. Also, quinidine has proved useful in suppression of ventricular ectopy, tachycardia, and fibrillation.[34,259] As previously mentioned, quinidine decreases V_{max}, increases the APD, and to an even greater extent, increases ERP. It decreases automaticity in atrial and ventricular tissue and in the His-Purkinje and pacemaker fibers.[111] ECG changes occur with quinidine; most noticeably, the QTc interval lengthens.

In the normal dosage range, the mild negative inotropic effects of quinidine are outweighed by its blockade-mediated vasodilation, and it is thus well tolerated by patients with CHF. Quinidine's direct effects on SA node automaticity are balanced by its anticholinergic effects, which speed conduction through the SA and AV nodes. Quinidine thus causes little change in heart rate.[219] Quinidine sulfate is typically initiated at 200 mg every 6 hours and increased to 800 to 2400 mg/day, titrated to drug levels and therapeutic effect. It undergoes hepatic metabolism (60% to 80%) and renal excretion (20% to 40%), with a variable half-life of 4 to 10 hours.[233] The metabolites of quinidine also possess antidysrhythmic activity.[244] Quinidine may be administered cautiously intramuscularly when oral intake is not possible. Although available in an IV form, this route is almost always avoided if alternatives are available because of profound hypotensive effects.

As with all antidysrhythmics, quinidine may be prodysrhythmic in some patients. Patients with CHF are at greater risk. With congenital prolongation of the QT interval or bradycardia associated with hypokalemia, quinidine, by further lengthening the QT interval, may initiate *torsades de pointes,* a serious, potentially lethal dysrhythmia.[210] If *torsades de pointes* occurs, therapy should include increasing heart rate with isoproterenol or pacing, correction of hypokalemia and hypomagnesemia, and discontinuation of quinidine. Lidocaine may prove helpful.

Because of its anticholinergic effects on the AV node, quinidine may increase ventricular response in atrial fibrillation and flutter.[219] Therefore, if quinidine is used for conversion of atrial dysrhythmias, digoxin, verapamil, or a beta blocker should be administered concurrently. If quinidine therapy is initiated in a patient receiving digitalis, one must be aware that quinidine may double the digitalis plasma concentration and possibly lead to digitalis toxicity. Digitalis dosages should therefore be decreased by half.[152] Evidence of quinidine-induced cardiac toxicity may be manifested by

Table 65-9 Class Ia antidysrhythmic agents

Drug	Usual dosage and interval	Effect on ECG	Adverse Effects
Quinidine	PO: 200–400 q4–6 h	Prolongs QRS, QT interval and PR (±)	Diarrhea and other GI symptoms, cinchonism, hepatic granulomas and necrosis, thrombocytopenia, rashes, hypotension, heart blocks, tachyarrhymias, torsades de pointes, fever, lupuslike syndrome
Procainamide	PO: 50 mg/kg/day in divided doses q3–4 h or q6 h (long-acting) IV loading; no more than 100 mg q5min to 1 g (12 mg/kg) IV maintenance; 2–4 mg/min	Prolongs QRS, QT interval and PR (±)	Lupuslike syndrome, confusion, disorientation, GI symptoms, rash, hypotension, arrhythmias, torsades de pointes, blood dyscrasias, fever
Disopyramide	PO: 100–200 mg q6 h	Prolongs QRS, QT interval and PR (±)	Anticholinergic effects, hypotension, heart failure, tachyarrhythmias, torsades de pointes, heart block, nausea, vomiting, diarrhea, hepatic toxicity, acute psychosis, agranulocytosis, constipation, hypoglycemia
Moricizine	200–300 mg tid	Prolongs QRS interval	May be prodysrhythmic; CHF, interventricular conduction delays

Modified from Abramowicz M, editor: Drugs for cardiac arrhythmias, *Med Lett Drugs Ther* 33:59, 1991.

greater than 50% increase in QT interval, widening of QRS complex, and SA or AV node disturbances. Noncardiac adverse effects typically occur with quinidine. In 30% to 40% of patients, therapy must be withdrawn because of gastrointestinal (GI) intolerance. Quinidine may cause CNS toxicity, as manifested by tinnitus and delirium. Other adverse effects include fever, rash, anaphylaxis, thrombocytopenia, hemolytic anemia, and agranulocytosis.

In surgical patients, quinidine should be continued preoperatively and resumed as soon as possible. If oral intake is impossible, IV procainamide or lidocaine may be substituted, depending on the original reason for initiating quinidine therapy. Quinidine increases the neuromuscular blockade of decamethonium, curare, and succinylcholine[103] and may worsen neuromuscular blockade in myasthenia gravis.[144]

Procainamide

Procainamide, a congener of procaine, has a pharmacologic effect and a set of clinical indications similar but not identical to those of quinidine.[111] Although both are class Ia agents, each may be effective in suppression of dysrhythmias that are unresponsive to the other drug. This is not surprising, because procainamide's major metabolite, *N*-acetylprocainamide (NAPA), actually has class III actions.[207] In addition, because procainamide is readily available in stable IV form, it is useful for acute management of atrial fibrillation and flutter, PSVT, and dysrhythmias associated with Wolff-Parkinson-White syndrome. It may also be used for acute suppression of ventricular dysrhythmias following acute MI, and in treatment of ventricular tachycardia.

Procainamide is available orally, but its short half-life, even in its sustained-release form, requires three or four daily administrations. Usual dosages are about 50 mg/kg/day. When given intravenously, it may produce vasodilation by a ganglionic blocking action and should therefore be administered slowly over approximately 20 minutes. A loading dose up to 1 g may be given, followed by an infusion at 1 to 4 mg/min.[161] Procainamide undergoes acetylation to NAPA, with half the population being fast acetylators. Subsequently, both substances are renally excreted. Therefore, dosage should be adjusted in patients with renal dysfunction. Procainamide and NAPA levels may prove useful to facilitate dosage adjustment.[135]

As with quinidine, procainamide may be prodysrhythmic and may cause *torsades de pointes*.[23] It may also cause sinus node and conduction system dysfunction.[265] It should therefore not be used in patients with prolonged QT interval, hypokalemia, or history of *torsades de pointes*. A significant noncardiac adverse effect that develops in 15% to 20% of patients is a lupuslike syndrome. It usually resolves with drug discontinuation. Interestingly, all patients will develop positive antinuclear antibody titers, but therapy should only be discontinued if symptoms develop.[145] Preoperatively, procainamide should be continued until surgery. In the perioperative period, procainamide may be given as an IV infusion and used as a substitute for quinidine or disopyramide in treatment of atrial and ventricular dysrhythmias.

Disopyramide

Disopyramide is a class Ia agent similar to quinidine and procainamide and effective over a broad range of dysrhythmias. Its modes of action in decreasing automaticity and V_{max} and

Usually effective plasma concentrations	Metabolism	Indications	Half-life
2–7 μg/ml	Hepatic (60%–80%); renal (20%–40%)	Ventricular and superventricular arrhythmias, including PAT, AF, atrial flutter, WPW, junctional tachycardias	4–10 h increased in elderly
4–10 μg/ml NAPA 10–20 μg/nl	Hepatic; excreted in urine by filtration and active secretion	As above	2–5 h increased in renal failure
2–8 μg/ml	Hepatic; 50% excreted unchanged in urine	As above	4–10 h 8–18 h with renal dysfunction
0.2–1.5 μg/ml	Hepatic; with biliary and urinary excretion	Ventricular dysrhythmias	9.2 hr

increasing ERP and APD are similar to those of the other class Ia agents.[13] Unlike quinidine and procainamide, disopyramide has significant negative inotropic effects.[110] Even more than quinidine, it has substantial anticholinergic effects. These two properties limit the usefulness of disopyramide. If it is tolerated, little additional chronic toxicity occurs.

The usual dosage of disopyramide is 100 to 400 mg, three to four times daily, up to 800 mg total. Its half-life elimination is 4 to 10 hours[99] and is usually increased in patients with cardiac or renal disease. Fifty percent is excreted unchanged by the kidney and the remainder as an active metabolite.

As with all Ia agents, disopyramide should not be used in patients with congenital prolongation of the QT interval, hypokalemia, or history of *torsades de pointes*. It may cause severe bradycardia in patients with sinus node dysfunction or conduction system disease. Because of negative inotropic effects, disopyramide is contraindicated in patients with CHF. In combination with a beta blocker or verapamil, this drug will precipitate CHF. Disopyramide is the drug of choice in management of dysrhythmias in patients with idiopathic hypertrophic subaortic stenosis, for which its negative inotropic effect is an advantage. Because of its anticholinergic effects, it is contraindicated in patients with glaucoma and obstructive uropathy. In addition, disopyramide may cause dry mouth, constipation, urinary retention, and esophageal reflux.[183] These symptoms may be alleviated by concomitant use of physostigmine or neostigmine.[243]

Moricizine

Moricizine, a phenothiazine derivative, is an unusual class IA antidysrhythmic in that it also has some characteristics of class Ib and Ic agents. Moricizine decreases V_{max} to an extent similar to class Ia agents. As with Ib agents, it shortens APD and increases the ERP/APD ratio. On the ECG, moricizine prolongs the QRS complex with little effect on the QT interval, a characteristic of IC agents.

In clinical studies, moricizine has been effectively used for treatment of chronic complex ventricular dysrhythmias and prevention of ventricular tachycardia and fibrillation. In its IV form (which remains clinically unavailable) moricizine terminates supraventricular tachycardias, including those with accessory pathways.

Moricizine is well absorbed orally and undergoes hepatic metabolism to many different metabolites, which as yet are unstudied for therapeutic effect. Moricizine then undergoes biliary and urinary excretion, with a half-life of 9.2 hours. Recommended dosages are 600 to 900 mg three times daily. Adverse reactions include dizziness, nausea, and headaches. Intraventricular conduction delays may occur in up to 9% of patients. Moricizine may be prodysrhythmic or worsen CHF in 2% to 5% of patients. Few data are available regarding interactions with anesthetic agents.[34]

Class Ib Agents (Table 65-10)

Lidocaine

Although lidocaine, the prototypical class IB agent, was first introduced as a local anesthetic, it is now the most widely used IV antidysrhythmic agent. Lidocaine is the drug of choice in acute treatment and suppression of all ventricular dysrhythmias, except those associated with prolonged QT intervals and *torsades de pointes*. After acute MI, it is effective in prevention of ventricular fibrillation.[160]

Table 65-10 Class Ib antidysrhythmic agents

Drug Ib	Usual dosage and interval	Effect on ECG	Adverse Effects
Lidocaine (Xylocaine; and others)	IV loading: 1 mg/kg given over 2 min, then 2 mg/kg over 20 min or 50 mg given over 1 min and repeated every 5 min × 3 or 20 mg/min infused over 10 min IV maintenance: 30 μg/kg each min for 24–30 hr	No significant change	Drowsiness or agitation, slurred speech, tinnitus, disorientation, coma, seizures, paresthesias, cardiac depression, especially with excessive accumulation in heart failure or liver failure or infusions for more than 24 hours
Phenytoin (Dilantin; and others)	PO: loading 14 mg/kg PO: maintenance: 200–400 mg/day IV loading: 50 mg q6 min to total dose of 1000 mg (± 12 mg/kg) IV maintenance: 200–400 mg/day	No significant change	Ataxia, nystagmus, drowsiness, coma, blood dyscrasias, cardiac toxicity with rapid IV injection, fever, rash, hepatic granulomas, and necrosis
Mexiletine (Mexitil)	PO initial dose: 100–200 mg q8 h taken with food PO maintenance: 100–300 mg q6–12h, maximum 1200 mg/day	No significant change	GI upset, fatigue, nervousness, dizziness, tremor, sleep upset, convulsions, infrequent aggravation of arrhythmias, visual disturbances, psychosis, fever, hepatic toxicity, blood dyscrasias
Tocainide (Tonocard)	PO initial dose: 200–400 mg q8 h PO maintenance: 200–600 mg q8 h, maximum 2400 mg/day	No significant change	GI upset, paresthesias, dizziness, tremor, confusion, nightmares, psychotic reactions, coma, seizures, rash, fever, arthralgia, infrequent cytosis, aplastic anemia, thrombocytopenia, hepatic granulomas interstitial pneumonitis

Modified from Abramowicz M, editor: Drugs for cardiac arrhythmias, *Med Lett Drugs Ther* 33:59, 1991.

As with all class I agents, lidocaine decreases V_{max} to some extent. Unlike class Ia agents, it shortens APD and ERP of Purkinje fibers.[17] In addition, lidocaine decreases the slope of phase 4 of the action potential and thus reduces automaticity. Lidocaine has little effect on atrial tissue and thus is ineffective against supraventricular tachycardias.[169]

Because lidocaine undergoes rapid first-pass elimination, with clearance approximately equal to liver blood flow,[240] it is unavailable as an oral agent. IV lidocaine is usually given as a 1 mg/kg bolus, followed by repeat small boluses of an additional 2 mg/kg over 15 minutes and an infusion of 1 to 4 mg/min. An infusion is necessary because of lidocaine's rapid distribution out of the central compartment with termination of the antidysrhythmic activity. Elimination is significantly longer than central compartment redistribution. Therefore, a steady-state lidocaine infusion may be discontinued without "tapering." The blood levels will gradually decrease over 8 to 10 hours.

Modifications of infusion rates are required in the elderly and in patients with liver disease or CHF with decreased liver blood flow.[245] Normal individuals show great variability is plasma levels. Thus, the patient's ECG, blood pressure, and mental status should be carefully monitored so that infusions or boluses may be discontinued if toxicity develops. If dysrhythmias persist at usual doses and no toxic symptoms are present, lidocaine administration may be increased after a drug level has been obtained. If dysrhythmias persist with plasma lidocaine concentrations greater than 9 μg/ml, another agent should be used, even without symptoms of toxicity. Lidocaine provides little antidysrhythmic effect at levels less than 1.5 μg/ml, and toxicity often occurs at levels greater than 5 μg/ml.

Potential adverse reactions to lidocaine include drowsiness, dizziness, confusion, delirium, dysarthria, dyesthesias (especially periorally), and even coma and seizures. Seizures may occur with nontoxic doses if they are given too rapidly. Lidocaine may occasionally cause sinus and AV nodal dysfunction in patients with underlying conduction disease. In patients with atrial fibrillation, lidocaine may increase ventricular response rates. Animal model studies have evaluated cardiac toxicity associated with lidocaine. Lidocaine clearly has cardiac toxicity, but this occurs at levels approximately four times higher than those associated with CNS toxicity. Characteristic ECG findings in these studies were sinus arrest, increased PR intervals, AV block, widening QRS complexes, ectopy, and tachydysrhythmias.[9,56] In dogs, lidocaine in combination with

Usually effective plasma concentrations	Indications	Half-life	Metabolism
1.5–6 μg/mg	Ventricular dysrhythmias	1.5–2.0 h	Hepatic, < 10% excreted in urine
5–20 μg/ml	Dyrhythmias associated with digitalis toxicity	22 h	Hydroxylated in liver, excreted in urine
0.5–2 μg/ml	Ventricular dysrhythmias	10–12 h	Hepatic
3–10 μg/ml	Ventricular dysrhythmias	15 h	Hepatic biotransformation 55%; excreted unchanged in urine 45%

isoflurane and calcium channel blockers caused hypotension and AV block, which was reversed with calcium chloride.[133]

Tocainide and mexiletine

Tocainide is a lidocaine analog available as an oral medication. As such, it is indicated for chronic treatment of complex ventricular dysrhythmias. Tocainide has proved useful alone and in combination with class Ia, class II, and class III drugs in treatment of ventricular dysrhythmias unresponsive to other agents.[112,168,209] Response to lidocaine is often, but not always, predictive of response to tocainide and mexiletine. Also, tocainide and mexiletine are not necessarily interchangeable.

Like lidocaine, tocainide is not effective against supraventricular dysrhythmias. At therapeutic levels, it has little effect on sinus or AV nodes. As a class Ib agent, tocainide decreases V_{max}, APD, ERP, and automaticity of Purkinje and ventricular fibers. Following oral administration, peak blood levels occur at 1 to 2 hours. Tocainide undergoes both hepatic metabolism and renal elimination, with a 15-hour half-life.[148] Adverse reactions following oral administration occur in approximately 40% of patients. These reactions include nausea, vomiting, tremor, paresthesias, rash, and less often, agranulocytosis and pulmonary fibrosis.[195,252] Tocainide worsens symptoms of CHF in approximately 5% of patients and may be prodysrhythmic in 1% to 8%.

Mexiletine is an orally active congener of lidocaine with similar indications and modes of action as tocainide. As with tocainide, mexiletine has been used effectively in combination with class Ia and even class II and III agents against ventricular dysrhythmias.[60,151,218] It undergoes predominantly hepatic elimination, with a half-life of 10 to 12 hours and, unlike tocainide, may be safely administered to patients with renal failure.[262]

Mexiletine has little hemodynamic effect and is well tolerated in patients with CHF. Adverse reactions, such as dizziness, tremor, visual blurring, and nausea, are usually dose related. Rash occurs less often with mexiletine than with tocainide, but thrombocytopenia and positive antinuclear antibody testing occur occasionally. Mexiletine may be prodysrhythmic in 10% of patients. Both these drugs should be continued perioperatively and restarted postoperatively as soon as possible. If oral intake is not possible, a lidocaine infusion may be substituted.

Phenytoin

Although mainly used as an anticonvulsant, phenytoin has been used in patients with atrial and ventricular dys-

Table 65-11 Class Ic antidysrhythmic agents

Drug	Usual dosage and interval	Effect on ECG	Adverse effects
Flecainide (Tambocor)	PO initial dose: 100 mg q12 h, increase q4–6 days if required, by 50 mg q12 h PO maintenance: up to 400 mg/day	Prolongs PR and QRS intervals	Bradycardia, heart block, new ventricular fibrillation, sustained ventricular tachycardia, heart failure, dizziness, blurred vision, nervousness, headache, GI upset, neutropenia
Encainide (Enkaid)	PO initial dose: 25 mg q8 h, increase q4–6 days if required to 35 mg q8 h, and then to 50 mg q8 h PO maintenance: up to 200 mg/day	Prolongs PR and QRS intervals	Bradycardia, heart block, new ventricular fibrillation, sustained ventricular tachycardia, heart failure, dizziness, headache, visual disturbances, diarrhea, GI upset, glucose intolerance
Propafenone (Rythmol)	PO initial dose: 150 mg q8 h, increase (q3–4 days if required PO maintenance: 150–300 mg q8 h	Prolongs PR and QRS intervals	Bradycardia, heart block, new ventricular fibrillation, sustained ventricular tachycardia, heart failure, dizziness, light-headedness, metallic taste, dysgeusia, GI upset, bronchospasm

Modified from Abramowicz M, editor: Drugs for cardiac arrythmias, *Med Lett Drugs Ther* 33:60, 1991.

rhythmias, digitalis toxicity, and chronic ventricular dysrhythmias. It can be used alone or in combinations. Its action is similar to the other class Ib agents. Phenytoin has only a slight effect on V_{max}, but decreases APD. In addition, possibly via centrally mediated sympatholysis, phenytoin may decrease sympathetic flow to myocardium and thus has additional antidysrhythmic effects. It is well tolerated orally in doses of 300 mg/day, titrated to serum blood levels and side effects. A usual loading dose is 1000 mg given at a rate that does not exceed 50 mg/min, and the ECG and blood pressure are monitored to prevent hypotension and cardiovascular collapse.

Phenytoin undergoes hepatic metabolism with excretion in the bile, enterohepatic reabsorption, and subsequent urinary excretion. It has a 22-hour half-life. Common adverse effects include nystagmus, ataxia, slurred speech, confusion, and dizziness. Rarer but serious reactions include severe dermatitis and even Stevens-Johnson syndrome, which is a lupuslike syndrome. Whether it causes rare hematologic malignancy is controversial. In patients with liver disease or any altered metabolic state, or when given with a wide range of other medications, phenytoin levels should be reassessed.[16]

Class Ic Agents (Table 65-11)

Flecainide

Flecainide, as a class Ic agent, substantially depresses V_{max} of the action potential in Purkinje and ventricular fibers. PR and QRS intervals are increased, even at therapeutic doses. Flecainide is effective in suppressing both ventricular and supraventricular tachycardias, including Wolff-Parkinson-White syndrome.[208] Data from the Cardiac Arrhythmia Suppression Trials that suggested increased mortality with class Ic agents after MI have limited their use.[33] Usual doses are 200 to 400 mg daily given in divided doses. Although it undergoes hepatic metabolism, approximately 30% of flecainide is renally excreted, with a usual half-life of 12 to 27 hours.[47]

As with all antidysrhythmics, flecainide may be prodysrhythmic in a subset of patients. In addition, it aggravates CHF in approximately 15% of patients and can cause sinus arrest, AV block, and intraventricular conduction disturbances.[128,186] Flecainide may even increase pacemaker thresholds up to 200% and therefore should be used with caution in patients with conduction disease.[105] Other adverse effects include dizziness, blurred vision, GI upset, and neutropenia. Flecainide dosages may need to be reduced when administered with cimetidine or amiodarone. Digoxin and propranolol doses must be reduced when flecainide is introduced. Finally, beta-adrenergic blocking agents and flecainide may have additive negative effects on myocardial contractility. Few data are available regarding interaction with anesthetics.

Encainide

Encainide has a mode of action similar to flecainide. It is effective in treatment of both ventricular and supraventricular dysrhythmias, including Wolff-Parkinson-White syndrome.[185] The pharmokinetics of encainide are complicated by its biphenotypic metabolism. In 93% of the population, encainide undergoes first-pass hepatic metabolism, with a 0.5- to 4-hour half-life. The remaining 7% undergo metabolism at a slower rate, with an elimination half-life of 8 to 20 hours.[202] Usual dosages are 25 to 50 mg every 8

Usually effective plasma concentration	Indications	Half-life	Metabolism
0.2–1 μg/ml	Ventricular dysrhythmias	12–27 h	Hepatic; 10%–50% excreted unchanged renally
Active metabolites preclude establishment	Ventricular dysrhythmias	12 h	Hepatic metabolism; renal excretion
Active metabolites preclude establishment	Ventricular dysrhythmias	6–7 h	Hepatic metabolism; renal excretion

hours. As with flecainide, encainide may aggravate CHF and worsen underlying dysrhythmias. It may cause sinus arrest, AV block, and intraventricular conduction defects. Few data are available regarding interaction with anesthetics.

Propafenone

Propafenone, an antidysrhythmic agent approved for management of ventricular dysrhymias, is a sodium channel blocker with mode of action similar to the other approved class Ic agents, flecainide, and encainide.[85] Because data from the Cardiac Arrhythmia Suppression Trial Investigators[33] suggested increased mortality in patients taking encainide and flecainide, these drugs were relabeled. Currently, they are only approved in patients with life-threatening dysrhythmias. Because propafenone has a mode of action similar to these two agents, it also was approved for the same indications.

Propafenone has shown evidence *in vitro* and *in vivo* of beta-adrenergic blocking properties. Oral propafenone increases human lymphocyte B adrenoreceptor density, a phenomenon observed with other beta blockers. In healthy patients and asthmatic persons, propafenone decreases heart rate during exercise, increases airway reactivity to methacholine, and decreases hemodynamic response to isoproterenol.[85] As with other class Ic agents, propafenone increases the QRS interval, even at normal heart rates. QTc intervals are increased only to the extent that QRS intervals increase. The PR, AH, and HV intervals may also increase. Propafenone depresses sinus node automaticity and increases refractoriness in atrium, AV node, ventricle, and accessory pathways.[227] It has a negative inotropic effect, which may reduce ejection fraction in normal subjects and produce symptoms of CHF in approximately 0.8% to 2.5% of patients. As with other class Ic agents, propafenone may worsen conduction system disease.[227]

After oral administration and absorption, propafenone undergoes a cytochrome P-450 metabolism that varies genetically. In 93% of the population, the half-life is 6 to 7 hours; the remaining 7% have an elimination half-life of 12 to 32 hours.[85] Usual starting doses are 150 mg every 8 hours, which may be increased up to 1200 mg/day. Propafenone increases plasma concentrations of digoxin, warfarin, and metoprolol; therefore, dosages of these drugs may need adjustment.

In clinical studies, propfenone has been effective in suppression of frequent ventricular ectopy, nonsustained ventricular tachycardia, and exercise-induced ventricular ectopy. Propafenone has proved useful in prevention of atrial fibrillation and suppression of AV node and accessory pathway supraventricular dysrhythmias. Even when propafenone is not able to suppress these dysrhythmias, it is effective at slowing the heart rate.

Other adverse effects include worsening of asthma and bronchoconstriction, dizziness, and CNS and GI disturbances. Rare cases of cholestatic jaundice have been reported.[85]

Class III Agents (Table 65-12)

Amiodarone

Amiodarone is perhaps the most efficacious antidysrhythmic agent, but unfortunately, it is also the most toxic. Amiodarone is effective in prevention of ventricular tachycardia and fibrillation, in treatment of supraventricular

Table 65-12 Class III antidysrhythmic agents

Drug	Usual dosage and interval	Effect on ECG	Adverse Effects
Amiodarone (Cordarone)	PO loading: 800–1600 mg/day 1–3 weeks then 600–800 mg/day for 4 weeks PO maintenance: 100–400 mg/day IV/150 mg over 10 minutes then 1 mg/minute × 6 hr then 0.5 mg/min. May be rebolused for breakthrough arrhythmias	Prolongs PR, QRS, and QT intervals; sinus bradycardia	Bradycardia, heart block, new ventricular fibrillation, sustained ventricular tachycardia, torsades de pointes, GI upset, alcoholiclike hepatitis, phospholipidosis, ataxis, tremor, dizziness, acute pulmonary toxicity, pulmonary fibrosis, photosensitivity, blue-gray skin, corneal microdeposits, hyper- or hypothyroidism, increased serum cholesterol
Bretylium (Bretylol, and others; Bretylate in Canada)	IV loading: 5 mg/kg with additional doses of 10 mg/kg to maximum of 30 mg/kg (effect may be delayed) IV maintenance: 5–10 mg/kg q6 h or continuous infusion 1–2 mg/min	No change; sinus bradycardia	Orthostatic hypotension, nausea and vomiting, increased sensitivity to catecholamines, initial increase in dysrhythmias
Sotalol	PO 40–80 mg q12 h increased to 320 q12 h as necessary IV 0.2 mg/kg initially, increasing to 1.5 mg/kg over 5 minutes	Prolongs PR and QT interval	Bradycardia, heart block, torsades de pointes, CHF, bronchospasm, worsening arrhythmics

Modified from Abramowicz M, editor: Drugs for cardiac arrhythmias, *Med Lett Drugs Ther* 33:60, 1991.

tachycardias with and without preexcitation syndromes and in conversion and control of paroxysmal atrial fibrillation and flutter and dysrhythmias associated with hypertrophic cardiomyopathies.[173] Because of toxicity, the use of amiodarone is limited to treatment of dysrhythmia syndromes found unresponsive to other therapies.

Amiodarone is an iodinated benzofuran with a structural similarity to procainamide and thyroxine. It prolongs APD and ERP. It also decreases phase 4 automaticity in all cardiac tissues. On the ECG, the PR, QT, and QRS intervals are all lengthened.[173] Amiodarone is usually fairly well tolerated in patients with CHF but may cause symptomatic heart block requiring permanent pacemaker insertion in approximately 4% of patients. Its incidence of prodysrhythmic effects in 1% to 2% of patients is less than that associated with other antidysrhythmics.[146]

Noncardiac effects of amiodarone are dose related and occur often. These include photosensitivity dermatitis (which sometimes results in a striking iridescent blue-gray skin discoloration), corneal microdeposition, hyperthyroidism and hypothyroidism, pulmonary infiltration and fibrosis, tremor, ataxia, neuropathies, myopathies, hepatitis, and GI symptoms.[203] Drug interactions are numerous. Usual loading doses of amiodarone vary widely, ranging from 600 to 1400 mg/day for 2 to 21 days; maintenance doses are usually about 200 to 600 mg/day. Although efficacy may improve with higher dosages, toxicity is clearly dose related, and therefore the lowest effective dose during therapy is maintained.

Amiodarone is poorly and highly variably absorbed. After GI absorption, it undergoes extensive liver metabolism and is rapidly concentrated in myocardium. With time, it undergoes redistribution to adipose and muscle tissue until a steady state is reached. This leads to an extremely slow, extraordinarily variable elimination half-life of 26 to 107 days.[146] The very long half-life makes preoperative discontinuation impossible, and serious adverse effects have been reported for patients anesthetized when receiving amiodarone. In one series of 16 patients, 10 patients developed nodal rhythms or complete heart block. Six of 12 patients required intra-aortic balloon counterpulsation following cardiopulmonary bypass, and two patients developed hypotension secondary to decreased systemic vascular resistance. Three patients died.[157] As a result, invasive monitoring and AV pacing should be considered preoperatively, and inotropes and vasoconstrictors should be available and administered as necessary. In an isolated animal heart model amiodarone in conjunction with potent inhalation agents caused an additive decrease in heart rate and inotropy along with prolongation of AV conduction time. This animal data may be related to the reports of increased risks of amiodarone and anesthesia.[212] Amiodarone is now available for IV use in treatment of hemodynamically unstable ventricular tachycardia and fibrillation. The drug has received recent attention as a "last ditch" agent for treating these life-threatening arrythmias during emergence from cardiopulmonary bypass in critically ill patients. Initially, 150 mg is administered over 10 minutes followed by 1 mg/min for 6 hours.

Usually effective plasma concentration	Indication	Half-life	Metabolism
Not established	Ventricular and supraventricular dysrhythmias	26–107 days	Hepatic
Not established	Ventricular dysrhythmias	8 hr; increased in renal failure	Renal
0.8–2.6 mg/ml	Ventricular dysrhythmias (used for supraventricular arrhythmics in Europe)	12 hr	Renal

Subsequently, an infusion of 0.5 mg/min is administered. Rapid IV injection can cause hypotension, bradycardia, and AV nodal block.

Bretylium

Bretylium was first evaluated in the 1950s as an oral preparation for hypertension. Because of sympatholytic-mediated orthostatic hypotension and variable oral absorption, bretylium was abandoned. Subsequently, after its antidysrhythmic activity was noted, bretylium was approved as IV therapy for life-threatening dysrhythmias. Because of its indirect autonomic effects, its use is reserved for acute management of patients with ventricular dysrhythmias unresponsive to lidocaine.

Bretylium has a direct class III action, with increased APD and ERP. In addition, bretylium initially causes release of norepinephrine from postganglionic neurons. Following uptake into these neurons, it blocks further release of norepinephrine.[189] When given intravenously to patients without cardiac arrest, bretylium is administered as a 5-mg/kg loading dose over 10 to 20 minutes, which may be repeated up to a total dose of 20 mg/kg if no response occurs. Subsequently, one may use a maintenance infusion of 1 to 4 mg/min. Because bretylium is eliminated unchanged in the urine, maintenance infusions must be decreased if creatinine clearance is reduced.

In cardiac emergencies, bretylium is given as a rapid bolus in doses of 5 to 10 mg/kg. In awake patients, a rapid infusion may cause nausea, vomiting, and hypotension in volume-depleted patients. Orthostatic hypotension occurs in almost all patients and may persist for days after discontinuation of the drug. Otherwise, bretylium has little effect on contractility.

The anesthetic implications for patients receiving bretylium are worth noting. By blocking catecholamine release, bretylium causes the equivalent of a denervated state. Direct-acting catecholamines may cause exaggerated responses, and indirect agents may be less effective. Recently, IV bretylium has been used for regional blockade in reflex sympathetic dystrophy.[62] Bretylium may also be used to treat bupivicaine-induced ventricular arrhythmias.[68]

Sotalol

Sotalol is another class III antiarrhythmic agent that has mixed properties. Sotalol is a racemic mixture of d- and l-sotalol isomers. It provides significant noncardioselective beta-adrenergic antagonist effects without any intrinsic sympathomimetic activity or membrane-stabilizing effects. The d-sotalol isomer contributes nearly pure class III activity by blocking outward K^+ channels. The beta-blocking effects of sotalol occur with considerably lower doses than the class III effects.[187]

The electrophysiologic effects of sotalol include an increase in APD and prolongation of ERP. Automaticity is decreased and, in a manner similar to other beta-blockers, sotalol decreases heart rate and slows conduction through the AV node. Unlike all other beta-blockers, sotalol provides additional antiarrhythmic and antifibrillatory effects be-

Table 65-13 Unclassified antiarrhythmic agents

	Usual dosages	Effects on ECG	Adverse reactions
Adenosine	6–12 mg IV (may repeat 12 mg × 2)	Increased PR interval; AV block	High-grade block, asystole, hypotension, dizziness, nausea, headaches
Ibutilide	1–2 mg IV	Prolongs QT interval	May be proarrhythmic; CHF, conduction delays

Modified from Abramowicz M, editor: Drugs for cardiac arrhythmias, *Med Lett Drugs Ther* 33:59, 1991.

cause of its effects on APD and refractoriness. On ECG, the PR and QT intervals may increase.

The hemodynamic effects of sotalol are secondary to a combination of beta-adrenergic antagonist–mediated negative inotropic effects, and a propensity to increase contractility secondary to increased APD.[113]

The heart rate decreases and cardiac output is also decreased slightly. Contractility is actually increased despite the beta-blocking action of the drug. Care should still be taken, however, in prescribing sotalol to patients with compromised ventricular function because of its beta-blocking activity. Sotalol also demonstrates a property called "reverse-use dependence," which describes the fact that as heart rate increases, the prolongation of APD caused by sotalol is less. Therefore, sotalol may have less of an effect on refractoriness during tachycardia.[220]

Sotalol is FDA approved for treatment of life-threatening ventricular arrhythmias. It is also effective for treating supraventricular arrhythmias, as it slows sinus tachycardia, slows the ventricular response rate to atrial fibrillation, and has been shown to convert atrial flutter and fibrillation to normal sinus rhythm. In Europe, sotalol is available intravenously and used for conversion of supraventricular arrhythmias.

Table 65-12 summarizes the usual dosage, effective plasma concentration, half-life metabolism and side effects of sotalol. Notably, many of the adverse effects of sotalol are secondary to its beta-blocking activity. These effects include fatigue, dizziness, dyspnea, aggravation of bronchospasm, hypotension, and bradycardia which can be seen with other beta-blockers as well. Exacerbation of CHF occurs less often with sotalol.[86]

Any drug that can cause an increase in QT interval can induce *torsades de pointes,* which can occur in up to 4% of patients.[237] This is a consequence of the class III actions of sotalol. The occurrence of *torsades de pointes* may be more likely if there is concomitant hypokalemia, bradycardia, or if the patient is taking other drugs that prolong repolarization.[65,175] Sotalol also has drug interactions with other antiarrhythmics (e.g., amiodarone, disopyramide, and flecainide).

Halothane has been shown to interact in an additive fashion to prolong the QT interval with other antiarrhythmics (see section on quinidine). On this basis, caution should probably be taken when using halothane in patients taking sotalol, although there are no studies to support this theory. No data exist on the interactions between sotalol and anesthetics.

Other Nonclassified Agents

Adenosine and ibutilide (Table 65-13)

Adenosine is an endogenous nucleotide natural to all cells of the body. In pharmacologic doses, it slows conduction through the AV node and has proved highly efficacious as acute IV therapy for patients with paroxysmal supraventricular tachycardia in both reentry and accessory pathway (Wolff-Parkinson-White) dysrhythmias. After IV administration, adenosine undergoes rapid redistribution to erythrocytes and cells of the vascular endothelium, with a half-life estimated at less than 10 seconds. Subsequently, it is metabolized to inosine or adenosine monophosphate. After a bolus of 6 mg, approximately 60% of patients with PSVT will convert to sinus rhythm within 1 minute. If the initial bolus is unsuccessful, 12 mg given intravenously will convert most of the remaining patients, for a cumulative effectiveness of 92%. Transient high-grade blocks and even asystole may be seen following adenosine administration. These usually resolve rapidly and without therapy.

Adenosine is contraindicated in patients with sick sinus syndrome and second- or third-degree AV block. Hypotension may develop, especially when higher dosages are used. Other adverse side effects include facial flushing, headache, chest pain, dyspnea, dizziness, and nausea. Little data are yet available on the intraoperative use of adenosine, but its very short half-life may make it especially useful in the perioperative period for supraventricular tachydysrhythmias. One should remember that adenosine is also used to cause ischemia in both laboratory models of coronary steal with flow-limiting stenosis and clinically to elicit ischemia in adenosine-thallium scanning. Those considering the use of adenosine as a vasodilator must take this into account. The drug is *not* FDA approved for use as a vasodilator, or for deliberate intraoperative hypotension.

Ibutilide has recently been approved for IV use for termination of atrial fibrillation or flutter of recent onset. It acts by prolonging action potential in cardiac tissue but the

Usually effective plasma concentration	Indications	Half-life	Metabolism
?	Paroxysmal supraventricular tachycardias including Wolff-Parkinson-White syndrome	10 sec	Metabolized to inosine and adenosine monophosphate; adenosine monophosphate
?	Atrial fibrillation Atrial flutter	2–12 hr	Hepatic/renal

mechanism remains unknown. Half-life varies between 2 and 12 hours. The drug is extensively metabolized in liver and renally excreted. Clinical trials suggest conversion rates of 22% to 43% for atrial fibrillation and 48% to 70% in atrial flutter. Dosage is usually 1 mg over 10 minutes which may be repeated a second time. Adverse reactions include *torsades de pointes,* heart block and CHF.[4]

KEY POINTS

- Cardiovascular medications, with the exception of diuretics, should be continued and restarted as soon as possible through the perioperative period in order to control the underlying conditions and in the case of medications such as beta blockers and centrally acting $beta_2$ agonists to prevent dangerous rebound states with withdrawal.
- Preoperative diuretic use should lead to a more careful evaluation for evidence of intravascular depletion and electrolyte abnormalities.
- Centrally acting $alpha_2$ agonists reduce overall sympathetic tone and may reduce MAC and perioperative analgesic use.
- ACE inhibitors, which increase venous capacitance and decrease afterload, are now more frequently used for management of CHF in addition to hypertension. Side effects such as relative hypovolemia and hyperkalemia should be expected. They should be restarted orally or given intravenously as soon as possible.
- Nitrates work as antianginals by both decreasing preload and left ventricular end-diastolic pressure and volume enhancing blood flow to the subendocardium and areas of ischemia.
- Although the beta blockers may vary by half-life, relative beta selectivity, ISA, and MSA, they largely have similar effects, contraindications, and rebound syndromes.
- Esmolol, because of its short 9-minute half-life, may be titrated to effect through a rapidly changing perioperative period. Its uses include treatment of arrhythmias, hypertension, and coronary ischemia.
- Calcium channel blockers have markedly varied effects and must be understood individually rather than as a group. Verapamil, diltiazem, bepridil, and the dihydropyridine derivations may not be used interchangeably.
- During the perioperative period, verapamil and diltiazem are frequently used intravenously for control of supraventricular arrhythmias. Nicardipine is frequently used intravenously for control of hypertension.
- Antiarrhythmic drugs are classified on the basis of their major pharmacologic electrophysiologic effects, even though many drugs have effects which overlap more than one category. As the underlying problems necessitating their use are usually severe, they should be restarted as soon as possible.
- Lidocaine is the first-line drug for treatment of all ventricular arrhythmias except those associated with prolonged QT intervals and *torsades de pointes.*
- Amiodarone has a half-life of up to 107 days. The availability of blood levels has decreased its relative toxicity with chronic usage. For intractable ventricular fibrillation and tachycardia, patients may be loaded intravenously.
- Adenosine, with a half-life measured in seconds, is especially useful for evaluating and treating supraventricular arrhythmias, but should not be used for vasodilation or deliberate intraoperative hypotension.

KEY REFERENCES

Atlee JL, Hammann BR, Brownlee SW, et al: Comparison of the effects of inhalation anesthetics and diltiazem, nifedipine or verapamil on specialized atrioventricular conduction times in spontaneously beating dog hearts, *Anesthesiology* 68:519, 1988.

Bauer JH: Angiotensin converting enzyme inhibitors, *Am J Hyperten* 3:331, 1990.

Chung F, Houston PL, Cheng DCH, et al: Calcium channel blockade does not offer adequate protection from perioperative ischemia, *Anesthesiology* 69:343, 1988.

Flacke JW, Bloor BC, Flacke WE, et al: Reduced narcotic requirements by clonidine with improved hemodynamic and adrenergic stability in patients undergoing coronary artery bypass, *Anesthesiology* 67:11, 1987.

Frishman WH: Beta-adrenergic blockers, *Med Clin North Am* 50, 1988.

Frishman WLT: Multifactorial action of beta-adrenergic blocking drugs in ischemic heart disease, *Circulation* 67(suppl 1):11, 1983.

Gerson H, Allen FB, Seitzer JL, et al: Arterial and venous dilation by nitroprusside and nitroglycerin, *Anesth Analg* 61:256, 1982.

Greenberg H, Dwyer EM, Jameson AG, et al: Effects of nitroglycerin on the major determinants of myocardial oxygen consumption, *Am J Cardiol* 36:426, 1975.

Hohnloser SH, Woosley RL: Sotalol, *N Eng J Med* 331: 31–39, 1994.

Kaplan J: Role of ultrashort-acting beta blockers in the perioperative period, *J Cardiovasc Anesthiol* 2:683, 1988.

Kapur PA, Bloor BC, Flacke WE, et al: Comparison of cardiovascular responses to verapamil during enflurane, isoflurane, or halothane anesthesia in the dog, *Anesthesiology* 61:156, 1984.

Prasad T, Kaplan JA: Nicardipine, a new intravenous antagonist, *J Cardiothor Anesth* 3:344, 1989.

Smith TW: Digitalis, Mechanism of action and clinical use, *N Engl J Med* 318:358, 1988.

Vitez IS: Chronic hypokalemia and intraoperative dysrhythmias, *Anesthesiology* 63:130, 1985.

REFERENCES

1. Abel M, Book WJ, Eisenkraft JB: Adverse effects of nondepolarising neuromuscular blocking agents. Incidence, prevention and management, *Drug Safety* 10:420–438, 1994.
2. Ablad B: A study of the mechanism of the hemodynamic effects of hydralazine in man, *Acta Pharmacol Toxicol* 20(suppl 1):1, 1963.
3. Abdelwahab W, Frishman W, Landau A: Management of hypertensive urgencies and emergencies, *Clin Pharmacol* 35:747, 1995.
4. Abramowicz M: Ibutilide, *Med Lett Drugs Ther* 38:38, 1996.
5. Anderson KE, Högestätt ED: On the mechanism of action of calcium antagonists, *Acta Med Scand* 681(suppl):11, 1984.
6. Arnold SB, Byrd RC, Meister W, et al: Long-term digitalis therapy improves left ventricular function in heart failure, *N Engl J Med* 303:1443, 1980.
7. Atlee J: *Perioperative cardiac dysrhythmias,* ed 2, Chicago, 1990, Mosby–Year Book.
8. Atlee JL, Hammann BR, Brownlee SW, et al: Comparison of the effects of inhalation anesthetics and diltiazem, nifedipine or verapamil on specialized atrioventricular conduction times in spontaneously beating dog hearts, *Anesthesiology* 68:519, 1988.
9. Avery P, Reden D, Sahaenzer G, et al: The influence of serum potassium on the cerebral and cardiac toxicity of bupivacaine and lidocaine, *Anesthesiology* 61:134, 1984.
10. Barner HB, Jellinek M, Standeven JW, et al: Cold blood diltiazem cardioplegia, *Ann Thorac Surg* 33(1):55, 1982.
11. Bauer JH: Angiotensin converting enzyme inhibitors, *Am J Hypertens* 3:337,1990
12. Becker LC, Fortuin NS, Pitt B: Effect of ischemia and antianginal drugs on the distribution of radioactive microspheres in the canine left ventricle, *Circ Res* 28:263, 1971.
13. Befeler B, Castellanos A, Wells DE, et al: Electrophysiologic effects of the antiarrhythmic agent disopyramide phosphate, *Am J Cardiol* 35:282, 1975.
14. Belz GG, Aust PE, and Munkes R: Digoxin plasma concentrations and nifedipine, *Lancet* 1:844, 1981.
15. Beyer KH, Baer JE: The site and mode of action of some sulfonide-derived diuretics, *Med Clin North Am* 59:735, 1975.
16. Bigger JT, Hoffman BF: Antiarrhythmic drugs. In Goodman LS, Gillman AG, editors: *The pharmacological basis of therapeutics,* New York, 1985, Macmillan.
17. Bigger JT Jr, Mandel WJ: Effect of lidocaine on the electrophysiological properties of ventricular muscle and Purkinje fibers, *J Clin Invest* 49:63, 1970.
18. Bloor BC, Flacke WE: Reduction in halothane anesthetic requirements by clonidine, an alpha adrenergic agent, *Anesth Analg* 61:741, 1982.
19. Boldt J, Schidler E, Harter K, et al: Influence of intravenous administration of angiotensin-converting enzyme inhibitor enalaprilat on cardiovascular mediators in cardiac surgery patients, *Anesth Analg* 80: 480, 1995.
20. Boldt J, Schindler E, Wollbruck M, et al: Cardiorespiratory response of intravenous angiotensin converting enzyme inhibitor enalaprilat in hypertensive cardiac surgery patients, *Cardiothorac Vasc Anesth* 9:44, 1995.
21. Bolognesi R, Benedini G, Ferrari R, et al: Inhibitory effect of acute and chronic administration of digitalis on the sick sinus node, *Eur Heart J* 7:334, 1986.
22. Bongranis S, Razzetti R, Schianetta P: Cardiovascular effects of nicardipine in anesthetized open chest dogs in the absence and presence of beta-adrenergic receptor blockade, *J Cardiovasc Pharmacol* 7:899, 1985.
23. Brachmann J, Scherlag BJ, Rosenshtraukh LV, et al: Bradycardia-dependent triggered activity: Relative to drug-induced multiform ventricular tachycardia, *Circulation* 68:846, 1983.
24. Brater DC: Pharmacodynamic considerations in the use of diuretics, *Ann Rev Pharmacol Toxicol* 23:45, 1983.
25. Braunwald E: Calcium-channel blockers: Pharmacologic considerations, *Am Heart J* 104:665, 1982.
26. Braunwald E: Mechanism of action of calcium-channel blocking agents, *N Engl J Med* 307:1618, 1983.
27. Broadbent MP, Swan PC, Jones RM: Interactions between diltiazem and isoflurane: An in vitro investigation in isolated guinea pig atria, *Br J Anesth* 57:1018, 1985.
28. Brogden RN, Sorkin EM: Isradipine, an update of its pharmakodynamic and phar-

makokinetic properties and therapeutic efficacy in the treatment of mild to moderate hypertension, *Drugs* 49:618, 1995.

29. Brown BG: Response of normal and diseases epicardial coronary arteries to vasoactive drugs: Quantitative arteriographic studies, *Am J Cardiol* 56:283, 1985.
30. Burris JF: The expanding role of angiotensin converting enzyme inhibitors in the management of hypertension. *Clin Pharmacol* 35:337, 1995.
31. Caine M: Alpha adrenergic blockers for treatment of benign prostatic hyperplasia. *Urol Clin North Am* 17:641, 1990.
32. Captopril-Digoxin Multicenter Research Group: Comparative effects of therapy with captopril in patients with mild to moderate heart failure, *JAMA* 259:539, 1988.
33. Cardiac Arrhythmia Suppression Trial Investigators: Preliminary report: effect of encainide and flecainide on mortalityin a randomized trial of arrhythmia suppression after myocardial infarction, *N Engl J Med* 321:406, 1989.
34. Carliner NH, Crouthamel WG, Fisher ML et al: Quinidine therapy in hospitalized patients with ventricular arrhythmias, *Am Heart J* 98:708, 1979.
35. Carnes CA, Loyle JD: Moricizine: a novel antiarryhythmic agent, *Ann Pharmacother* 24:745, 1990.
36. Carney RM: Prevalence of major depressive disorders in patients while receiving beta blocker therapy versus other medications, *Am J Med* 83:223, 1987.
37. Carruthers SG: Adverse effects of alpha-1 adrenergic blocking drugs, *Drug Safety* 11:12, 1994.
38. Abramowicz M, editor: Carteolol and penbutolol for hypertension, *Med Lett Drugs Ther* 31:35, 1989.
39. Charlap S, Kimmel B, Laifer L, et al: Twice daily nicardipine in the treatment of patients with mild to moderate hypertension, *J Clin Hypertens* 2:271, 1986.
40. Channer KS, James MA, MacConnell J, et al: β-adrenoreceptor blockers in atrial fibrillation: The importance of partial agonist activity, *Clin Pharmacol* 37:53, 1994.
41. Chennavesin A: Pharmacodynamic analysis of the furosemide-probenecid interaction in man, *Kidney Intern* 16:187, 1979.
42. Chrysant SG, Bittar N: Betaxolol in the treatment of stable angina pectoris, *Cardiology* 84:316, 1994
43. Chung F, Houston PL, Cheng DCH, et al: Calcium channel blockade does not offer adequate protection from perioperative ischemia, *Anesthesiology* 69:343, 1988.
44. Clark RD, Magovern GJ, Christlief IY, et al: Nifedipine cardioplegia experience: Results of a 3-year cooperative clinical study, *Ann Thorac Surg* 36:654, 1983.
45. Clavijo GA, Clavijo IV, Weart CW: Amlodipine: A new calcium antagonist, *Am J Hosp Pharm* 51:59, 1994.
46. Cohn JN, Franciosa JA: Vasodilator therapy of cardiac failure, *N Engl J Med* 297:27, 1977.
47. Conrad GJ, Ober RE: Metabolism of flecainide, *Am J Cardiol* 53:41B, 1984.
48. Corstairs KD, Breckenridge A, Dollery CT, et al: Incidence of a positive direct Coombs' test in patients on alpha-methyldopa, *Lancet* 2:133, 1966.
49. Craythorne NWB, Huffington PE: Effect of propanolol in the cardiovascular response to cyclopropane and halothane, *Anesthesiology* 27:580, 1966.
50. Crozier I, Ikram H, Awan N, et al: Losartan in heart failure: Hemodynamic effects and tolerability, *Circulation* 91:691, 1995.
51. Daacon SP, Barnett D: Comparison of atenolol and propanolol during insulin induced hypoglycemia, *Br Med J* 2:7, 1976.
52. Dargie HJ, Lynch PG, Krikler DM, et al: Nifedipine and propranolol: A beneficial drug interaction, *Am J Med* 71:676, 1981.
53. DeCarvalho JGR: Hemodynamic correlates of prolonged thiazide therapy: Comparison of responders and nonresponders, *Clin Pharmacol Ther* 22:875, 1977.
54. DeCarvalho JGR: Spironolactone and triamterene in volume dependent essential hypertension, *Clin Pharmacol Ther* 27:53, 1980.
55. DeMarco T, Deedwania P, Chatterjee K: Systemic and coronary hemodynamic effects of bepridil in patients with depressed left ventricular function, *Am J Cardiol* (suppl) 69:31D–36D, 1992.
56. De Jong RH, Ronfeld RA, De Rosa RA: Cardiovascular effects of convulsant and superconvulsant doses of amide local anesthetics, *Anesth Analg* 610:3, 1982.
57. Dhingra RC, Palileo EV, Strasberg B, et al: Electrophysiologic effects of ouabain in patients with preexcitation and circus movement tachycardia, *Am J Cardiol* 47: 139, 1981.
58. Dikshitik A: Renal and extra renal hemodynamic effects of furosemide in congestive heart failure after acute myocardial infection, *N Engl J Med* 288:1087, 1973.
59. Duff HG, Roden DM, Primm RK, et al: Mexiletine for resistant ventricular tachycardia: Comparison with lidocaine and enhancement of efficacy by combination with quinidine, *Am J Cardiol* 47:438, 1981.
60. Duff HJ, Roden D, Primm RK, et al: Mexiletine in the treatment of resistant ventricular arrhythmias: Enhancement of efficacy and reduction of dose-related side effects by combination with quinidine, *Circulation* 67:1124, 1983.
61. Durant NN, Nguyen K, Katz RL: Potentiation of neuromuscular blockade by verapamil, *Anesthesiology* 60:298, 1984.
62. Dzwierzynski WW, Sanger JR: Reflex sympathetic dystrophy, *Hand Clin* 10:29 1994.
63. Ellrodt AG, Ault M, Riedinger MS, et al: Efficacy of sublingual nifedipine in hypertensive emergencies, *Am J Med* 79:19, 1985.
64. Ellrodt G, Chew CYC, Singh BN: Therapeutic implication of slow-channel blockade in cardiocirculatory disorders, *Circulation* 62:669, 1980.
65. Elonen E, Neuvonen PJ, Tarssanen L, et al: Sotalol intoxication with prolonged Q-T interval and severe tachyarrhythmias. *B Med J* 1: 1184, 1979.
66. Famamura T, Ronishi T, Matsuda H, et al: Electrophysiological effects of nicardipine hydrochloride on the isolated: Sinoatrial and atrioventricular nodes of the rabbit, *Jpn Circ J* 47:817, 1983.
67. Feldman RL, Pepine CJ, Curry RC, et al: Coronary arterial responses to graded doses of nitroglycerin, *Am J Cardiol* 43:91, 1979.
68. Feldman HS, Arthur CR, Pitkanen M, et al: Treatment of acute systemic toxicity after rapid intravenous injection of ropivicaine and bupivicaine in the conscious dog, *Anesth Analg* 73: 373, 1991.
69. Ferrer MI, Bradley SE, Wheeler HD, et al: Some effects of nitroglycerin upon the splanchnic, pulmonary and systemic circulations, *Circulation* 33:357, 1966.
70. Flacke JW, Bloor BC, Flacke WE, et al: Reduced narcotic requirements by clonidine with improved hemodynamic and adrenergic stability in patients undergoing coronary artery bypass, *Anesthesiology* 67:11,1987.
71. Fleckenstein A: Specific pharmacology of calcium in myocardium, cardiac pacemakers, and vascular smooth muscle, *Ann Rev Pharmacol Toxicol* 17:149, 1977.
72. Foex P, Prys-Roberts C: Interaction of beta-receptor blockade and PCO_2 levels in the anesthetized dog, *Br J Anaesth* 48:315, 1976.
73. Frishman WH: Acebutolol, *Cardiol Rev Rep* 6:979, 1985.
74. Frishman WH: Atenolol and timolol: Two new systemic adrenoreceptor antagonists, *N Engl J Med* 306:1456, 1984.
75. Frishman WH: Beta adrenergic blockers, *Med Clin North Am* 72:37, 1988.
76. Frishman WH: *Clinical pharmacology of β-adrenoceptor blocking drugs,* ed 2, Norwalk, 1984, Appleton-Century-Crofts.
77. Frishman WH: Nadolol: A new beta adrenoreceptor antagonist, *N Engl J Med* 305:678, 1981.
78. Frishman WH: Pindolol: A new beta-adrenoreceptor antagonist with partial agonist activity, *N Engl J Med* 308:940, 1983.
79. Frishman WH, Charlap S, Kimmel B, et al: Diltiazem compared to nifedipine and combination treatment in patients with stable angina: Effects on angina, exercise tolerance and the ambulatory ECG, *Circulation* 77:774, 1988.
80. Frishman WH, Stroh JA, Greenberg SM, et al: Calcium-channel blockers in systemic hypertension, *Med Clin North Am* 72:454, 1988.
81. Frishman WH, Weinberg P, Peled H, et al: Calcium-entry blockers for the treatment of severe hypertension and hypertensive emergencies, *Am J Med* 77(2B):35, 1984.
82. Frishman WLT: Beta-adrenergic blockade for survivors of acute myocardial infarction, *N Engl J Med* 310:830, 1984.
83. Frishman WLT: Multifactorial action of beta-adrenergic blocking drugs in ischemic heart disease, *Circulation* 67(suppl 1):11, 1983.
84. Fuchs Rm, Brinker JA, Gusman PA, et al: Regional coronary blood flow during relief of pacing induced angina by nitroglycerin, *Am J Cardiol* 51:19, 1983.
85. Funck-Brentano C, Kroemer HK, Lee JT, et al: Propafenone, *N Engl J Med* 322:518, 1990.
86. Funck-Brentano C, Kibleur Y, Le Coz F, et al: Rate dependence of sotalol-induced prolongation of ventricular repolarization during exercise in humans. *Circulation* 82:2235, 1990.
87. Furberg CD: Effects of propanolol in post

infarction patients with mechanical or electrical complications, *Circulation* 69:761, 1984.

88. Furberg CD, Psaty BM, Meyers JV: Dose related increase in mortality in patients with coronary heart disease, *Circulation* 92:1326, 1995.
89. Gallagher JD, Gessman LJ, Moura P, et al: Electrophysiologic effects of halothane and quinidine on canine purkinje fibers: Evidence for a synergistic interaction, *Anesthesiology* 65:278, 1986.
90. Gelmers HJ, Gorter K, De Weerdt CJ, et al: A controlled trial of nimodipine in acute ischemic stroke, *N Engl J Med* 318:203, 1988.
91. Gerson H, Allen FB, Seitzer JL, et al: Arterial and venous dilation by nitroprusside and nitroglycerin, *Anesth Analg* 61:256, 1982.
92. Geykes GE, Boer P, Raferty EJ: Clonidine withdrawal, mechanism and frequency of rebound hypertension, *Br J Clin Pharmacol* 7:55, 1976.
93. Ghignone M, Calvillo O, Quintin L: Anesthesia and hypertension: The effect of clonidine on perioperative hemodynamics and isoflurane requirements, *Anesthesiology* 67:3, 1987.
94. Ghignone M, Quinton L, Duke PC, et al: Effects of clonidine on narcotic requirements and hemodynamic response during induction of fentanyl anesthesia and endotracheal intubation, *Anesthesiology,* 64: 361, 1986.
95. Glisson SN, Sanchez MM, El-Etr AA, et al: Nitroglycerin and neuromuscular blockade produced by gallamine, succinylocholine, d-turbocurare and pancuronium, *Anesth Analg* 59:117, 1980.
96. Gomes JAD, Dhatt MS, Akhtar M, et al: Effects of digitalis on ventricular myocardial and His-Purkinje refractoriness and reentry in man, *Am J Cardiol* 42:931, 1978.
97. Goodfriend TL, Elliott ME, Catt, KJ: Angiotensin Receptors and their antagonists, *N Engl J Med,* 344:1649, 1996.
98. Gorlin R, Brachfield N, MacLeod C, et al: Effects of nitroglycerin on coronary circulation in patients with coronary artery disease or increased left ventricular work, *Circulation* 19:705, 1959.
99. Gottdiener JS, DiBianco R, Bates R, et al: Effects of disopyramide on left ventricular function: Assessment by radionuclide cineangiography, *Am J Cardiol* 51:1554, 1983.
100. Graham RM, Pettinger WA: Drug therapy: Prazosin, *N Engl J Med* 300:232, 1979.
101. Greenberg H, Dwyer EM, Jameson AG, et al: Effects of nitroglycerin on the major determinants of myocardial oxygen consumption, *Am J Cardiol* 36:426, 1975.
102. Griffin RM, Dimich I, Jurado R, et al: Cardiovascular effects of nifedipine infusions during fentanyl anesthesia, *Anesthesiology* 61:A10, 1984.
103. Grogono AW: Anesthesia for atrial fibrillation: Effect of quinidine on muscle relaxation, *Lancet* 2:1039, 1963.
104. Harris AL: Aspects of clonidine therapy, *N Engl J Med* 294:845, 1976.
105. Hellestrand KJ, Burnett PJ, Milne JR, et al: The effect of the antiarrhythmic agent flecainide on acute and chronic pacing thresholds, *PACE* 6:892, 1983.
106. Heng MK, Singh BN, Roche AHG, et al: Effects of intravenous verapamil on cardiac arrhythmias and on the electrocardiogram, *Am Heart J* 90:487, 1975.
107. Henriksson BA, Biber B, Haggendal J, et al: Cardiovascular effects of enflurane and asphyxia during long term beta-adrenoceptor blockade, *Acta Anaesthesiol Scand* 29:363, 1985.
108. Henry PD: Comparative pharmacology of calcium antagonists: Nifedipine, verapamil and diltiazem, *Am J Cardiol* 46:1047, 1980.
109. Hiatt WR: Effects of beta-adrenergic blockers on the peripheral circulation in patients with peripheral vascular disease, *Circulation* 72:1226, 1985.
110. Hinderling PH, Garrett ER: Pharmacodynamics of the anti-arrhythmic disopyramide in healthy humans, *J Pharamco Biopharm* 4:231, 1976.
111. Hoffman BF, Rosen MR, Wit AL: Electrophysiology and pharmacology of cardiac arrhythmias. VII. Cardiac effects of quinidine and procainamide, *Am Heart* J 90:117, 1975.
112. Hohnloser SH, Lange HW, Raeder EA, et al: Short- and long-term therapy with tocainide for malignant ventricular tachyarrhythmias, *Circulation* 73:143, 1986.
113. Hohnloser SH, Woosley RL: Sotalol, *N Engl J Med* 331: 31, 1994.
114. Holland OB: Diuretic induced ventricular ectopic activity, *Am J Med* 70:762, 1981.
115. Hollingshead LM, Faulds D, Fitton A: Bepridil: A review of its pharmacological properties and therapeutic use in stable angina pectoris, *Drugs* 44:835–857, 1992.
116. Horan BF, Prys-Roberts C, Roberts JG, et al: Haemodynamic responses to isoflurane anaesthesia and hypovolemia in the dog and their modification by propanolol, *Br J Anaesth* 49:179, 1979.
117. Horowitz LD, Gorlin R, Taylor WJ, et al: Effects of nitroglycerin on regional myocardial blood flow in coronary artery disease, *J Clin Invest* 50:1578, 1971.
118. Humphrey LS, Blanck TJJ: Intraoperative use of verapamil for nitroglycerin-refractory myocardial ischemia, *Anesth Analg* 64:88, 1985.
119. Humphreys MH, Rector FC Jr: Pathophysiology of edema formation. In Seldin DW, Giebisch G, editors: *The Kidney: physiology and pathophysiology,* New York, 1985, Raven Press, p 1163.
120. Ignarro LJ, Lippton H, Edwards JC, et al: Mechanism of vascular smooth muscle relaxation by nitrates, nitroprusside and nitric oxide, *J Pharmacol Exp Ther* 218:739, 1981.
121. Imhof PR, Ott B, Frankhauser P, et al: Differences in nitroglycerin dose-response in venous and arterial beds, *Eur J Clin Pharmacol* 31:193, 1981.
122. Isaac L: Clonidine in the central nervous system: Site of mechanism of hypotensive action, *J Cardiovasc Pharmacol* 2(suppl 1):S5, 1980.
123. Iwatsuki N, Katoh M, Ono K, et al: Antiarrhythmic effect of diltiazem during halothane anesthesia in dogs and in humans, *Anesth Analg* 64:964, 1985.
124. Jedeikin R, Gillette P, Zinner A: Effect of ouabain on the antegrade effective refractory period of accessory atrioventricular connections in children, *Circulation* 66(abstact):171, 1982.
125. Johns TE, Lopez LM: Bisoprolol: Is this just another beta-blocker for hypertension angina? *Ann Pharmacother* 29:403, 1995.
126. Johnson CI: Angiotensin receptor antagonists: focus on losartan, *Lancet* 346:1403, 1995.
127. Johnson LC, Greible HG: Treatment of hypertensive disease with diuretics. V. Spironolactone, an aldosterone antagonist, *Arch Intern Med* 119:225, 1967.
128. Josephson MA, Ikeda N, Singh BN: Effects of flecainide on ventricular function: Clinical and experimental correlations, *Am J Cardiol* 53:95B, 1984.
129. Kadish A, Oka Y, Becker R, et al: Propanolol withdrawal: Cause of postcoronary bypass arrhythmias and hypertension, *Circulation* 60:104, 1979.
130. Kaplan J: Role of ultrashort acting beta-blockers in the perioperative period, *J Cardiovasc Anesth* 2:683, 1988.
131. Kapur PA, Bloor BC, Flacke WE, et al: Comparison of cardiovascular responses to verapamil during enflurane, isoflurane, or halothane anesthesia in the dog, *Anesthesiology* 61:156, 1984.
132. Kapur PA, Flacke WE: Epinephrine-induced arrhythmias and cardiovascular function after verapamil during halothane anesthesia in the dog, *Anesthesiology* 55: 218, 1981.
133. Kapur PA, Grogan DL, Fournier DJ: Cardiovascular interactions of lidocaine with verapamil or diltiazem in dogs, *Anesthesiology* 68:79, 1988.
134. Kapur PA, Tippit SE: Correlation of cardiovascular effects with plasma levels of diltiazem during isoflurane anesthesia, *Anesthesiology* 61:A12, 1984.
135. Karlsson E: Clinical pharmacokinetics of procainamide, *Clin Pharmaco* 3:97, 1978.
136. Kassiner JP, Harrington JJ: Diuretics and potassium metabolism: a reassessment of the need, effectiveness and safety of potassium therapy, *Kidney Intern* 11:505, 1967.
137. Kates RA, Kaplan JA: Cardiovascular responses to verapamil during coronary artery bypass graft surgery, *Anesth Analg* 62:821, 1983.
138. Kazda S, Towart R: Nimodipine: A new calcium antagonistic drug with a preferential cerebrovascular action, *Acta Neurochi (Wien)* 63:259, 1982.
139. Keefe D, Frishman WH: Clinical pharmacology of the calcium-channel blocking drugs. In Packer M, Frishman WH, editors: *Calcium-channel antagonists in cardiovascular disease,* Norwalk, 1984, Appleton-Century-Crofts.
140. Kendall MJ, Rajman I: A risk-benefit assessment of celiprolol in the treatment of cardiovascular disease, *Drug Safety* 10:220, 1994.
141. Klein HO, Lang R, Weiss E, et al: The influence of verapamil on serum digoxin concentrations, *Circulation* 65:998, 1982.
142. Koch-Weser J: Metoprolol, *N Engl J Med* 301:698, 1979.
143. Koolen JJ, Van Wezel HB, Vissen CA: Nicardipine for preservation of myocardial metabolism and function in patients under-

going coronary artery surgery, *Anesthesiology* 71:508, 1989.

144. Kornfeld P, Horowitz SH, Genkins G, et al: Myasthenia gravis unmasked by antiarrhythmic agents, *Mt Sinai J Med* 43:10, 1976.
145. Kosowsky BD, Taylor J, Lown B, et al: Long-term use of procainamide following acute myocardial infarction, *Circulation* 47:1204, 1973.
146. Kreeger RW, Hammill SC: New antiarrhythmic drugs, *Mayo Clinic Proc* 62: 1033, 1987.
147. Krikler DM, Spurrell RAJ: Verapamil in the treatment of paroxysmal supraventricular tachycardia, *Postgrad Med J* 50:447, 1974.
148. Lalka D, Meyer MB, Duce BR, et al: Kinetics of the oral antiarrhythmic lidocaine congener, tocainide, *Clin Pharmacol Ther* 19:757, 1976.
149. Langan SZ, Cauero I, Massiyhamr I: Recent developments in noradrenergic neurotransmission and its relevance to the mechanism of action of certain anti-hypertensive agents, *Hypertension* 2:372, 1980.
150. Lawson NW, Wallfisch HK: Cardiovascular pharmacology: A new look at the pressors. In Stoelting RK, editor: *Advances in anesthesia,* Chicago, 1986, Mosby–Year Book.
151. Leahey EB Jr, Heissenbuttel RH, Giardina EGV, et al: Combined mexiletine and propranolol treatment of refractory ventricular arrhythmia, *Br Med J* 281:357, 1980.
152. Leahey EB Jr, Reiff JA, Giardina EGV, et al: The effect of quinidine and other oral antiarrhythmic drugs on serum digoxin: A prospective study, *Ann Intern Med* 92:605, 1980.
153. Lee DC, Johnson RA, Bingham JB, et al: Heart failure in outpatients: A randomized trial of digoxin vs placebo, *N Engl J Med* 306:699, 1982.
154. Lee TH, DiSesa VJ, Cohn LH, et al: Correction of intraoperative diastolic myocardial dysfunction with nifedipine, *Clin Cardiol* 6:549, 1983.
155. Leopold G, Pabst J, Ungethum W, et al: Basic pharmacokinetics of bisoprolol, a new highly selective beta 1 adrenoreptor antagonist, *J Clin Pharm* 26:616, 1986.
156. Lewis BH, Muller JE, Rutherford J, et al: Nifedipine for coronary artery spasm after revascularization, *N Engl J Med* 306:992, 1982.
157. Liberman BA, Teasdale SJ: Anaesthesia and amiodarone, *Can Anaesth Soc J* 32(6): 629, 1985.
158. Lichstein E: Effects of propanolol on ventricular arrhythmias, *Circulation* 67:15, 1983.
159. Lichtlen P, Halter J, Gattiker K: The effects of isosorbide dinitrate on coronary blood flow, coronary resistance and left ventricular dynamics under exercise in patients with coronary artery disease, *Basic Res Cardiol* 69:402, 1974.
160. Lie KI, Wellens HJJ, van Capelle FJ, et al: Lidocaine in the prevention of primary ventricular fibrillation: A double-blind, randomized study of 212 consecutive patients, *N Engl J Med* 291:1324, 1974.
161. Lima JJ, Goldfarb AL, Conti DR, et al: Safety and efficacy of procainamide infusions, *Am J Cardiol* 43:98, 1979.
162. Lina AA, Leon-Ruiz EN, Fouts KE, et al: Influence of verapamil and aminophylline on epinephrine dysrhythmias under halothane anesthesia, *Anesthesiology* 63: A84, 1985.
163. Liu P, Houle S, Burns RJ, et al: Effect of intracoronary nitroglycerin on myocardial blood flow and distribution in pacing induced angina pectoris, *Am J Cardiol* 55: 1270, 1985.
164. Lloyd-Mostyn RH, Oram S: Modification by propanolol of cardiovascular effects of induced hyperglycemia, *Lancet* 2:1213, 1975.
165. Longnecker DE: Alpine anesthesia: can pretreatment with clonidine decrease the peaks and valley? *Anesthesiology* 67:1, 1987.
166. Losardo AA, Klein NA, Beer N, et al: Beneficial effects of sublingual nifedipine in patients with ischemic heart disease and depressed left ventricular function, *Angiology* 33:811, 1982.
167. Lund-Johansen P: Cardiac effects of isradipine in patients with hypertension, *Am J Hypertens* 6:294S, 1993.
168. Maloney JD, Nissen RG, McColgan JM: Open clinical studies at a referral center: Chronic maintenance tocainide therapy in patients with recurrent sustained ventricular tachycardia refractory to conventional antiarrhythmic agents, *Am Heart J* 100: 1023, 1980.
169. Mandel WJ, Bigger JT Jr: Electrophysiologic effects of lidocaine on isolated canine and rabbit atrial tissue, *J Pharmacol Exp Ther* 178:81, 1971.
170. Manin`t Veld: Effect of 10 different beta adrenoreceptor antagonists on hemodynamics, plasma renin activity and plasma norepinephrine in hypertension, *J Cardiovasc Pharmacol* 5:530, 1983.
171. Manin`t Veld: Mechanism of action of beta blockers in hypertension. In Kostis JB, DeFelice EA, editors: *Beta blockers in treatment of cardiovascular disease,* New York, 1984, Raven Press.
172. Marijic J, Bosnjak ZJ, Stowe DF, Kampine JP: Effects and interaction of verapamil and volatile anesthetics on the isolated perfused guinea pig heart, *Anesthesiology* 69:914, 1988.
173. Mason JW: Amiodarone, *N Engl J Med* 316:455, 1987.
174. Mathur PN, Powles P, Pugsley SO, et al: Effect of digoxin on right ventricular function in severe chronic airflow obstruction, *Ann Intern Med* 95:283, 1981.
175. McKibbin JK, Pocock WA, Barlow JB, et al: Sotalol, hypokalemia, syncope, and torsades de pointes. *Br Heart J* 51:157, 1984.
176. Meyer J: Concerning the question of pre-, intra-, and postoperative digitalis adminsitration, *Surg Anesthesiol* 16:9, 1972.
177. Meyer JS, Hardenberg J: Clinical effectiveness of calcium entry blockers in prophylactic treatment of migraine and cluster headaches, *Headache* 23:266, 1983.
178. Michael R: Older and newer diuretics. In Drayer JIM, Lowenthal M, Weber A, editors: *Drug therapy in hypertension,* New York, 1988, Marcel Dekker.
179. Mikawa K, Nishina K, Maekawa N, et al: Oral clonidine premedication reduces postoperative pain in children, *Anesth Analg* 82:225, 1996.
180. Miller RD: Enhancements of d tubocurarine neuromuscular blockade in man, *Anesthesiology* 45:422, 1967.
181. Miller RR: Propanolol withdrawal rebound phenomenon: exacerbation of coronary events after abrupt withdrawal of antianginal therapy, *N Engl J Med* 293:416, 1975.
182. Mitchell LB, Schroeder JS, Mason JW: Comparative clinical electrophysiologic effect of diltiazem, verapamil and nifedipine—a review, *Am J Cardiol* 49:629, 1982.
183. Mokler CM, Hillman RA: Nature of the anticholinergic action of some drugs, *Pharmacol Res Com* 4:171, 1972.
184. Moller IW: Cardiac arrest following IV verapamil combined with halothane anaesthesia, *Br J Anaesth* 59: 522, 1987.
185. Morganroth J: Encainide for ventricular arrhythmias: Placebo-controlled and standard comparison trials, *Am J Cardiol* 58: 74C, 1986.
186. Morganroth J, Anderson JL, Gentzkow GD: Classification by type of ventricular arrhythmia predicts frequency of adverse cardiac events from flecainide, *J Am Coll Cardiol* 8:607, 1986.
187. Nattel S, Feder-Elituv R, Matthews C, et al: Concentration dependence of class III and beta-adrenergic blocking effects of sotalol in anesthetized dogs, *J Am Coll Cardiol* 13: 1190, 1989.
188. Nayler WG, Dillon JS, Daly MF: Cellular sites of action of calcium antagonists and β-adrenoceptor blockers. In Opie LH, editor: *Perspectives in cardiovascular research,* vol 9, Calcium antagonists and cardiovascular disease, New York, 1984, Raven Press.
189. Nishimura M, Watanabe Y: Membrane action and catecholamine release action of bretylium tosylate in normoxic and hypoxic canine Purkinje fibers, *J Am Coll Cardiol* 2:287, 1983.
190. Nussmeier NA, Slogoff S: Verapamil treatment of intraoperative coronary artery spasm, *Anesthesiology* 62:539, 1985.
191. Ornstein E, Young WL, Ostapkovich N, et al: Are all effects of esmolol equally rapid in onset? *Anesth and Analg,* 81:297, 1995.
192. Pace DG, Gillis RA: Neuroexcitatory effects of digoxin in the cat, *J Pharmacol Exp Ther* 199:583, 1976.
193. Packer M, Leon MB, Bonow RO, et al: Hemodynamic and clinical effects of combined therapy with verapamil and propranolol in ischemic heart disease, *Am J Cardiol* 50:903, 1982.
194. Panten J, Haggendal J, Milocco I, et al: Long term metoprolol therapy and neuroleptanesthesia in coronary artery surgery: Withdrawal versus maintenance of β_1-adrenoreceptor blockade, *Anesth Analg* 62: 380, 1983.
195. Perlow GM, Jain BP, Pauker SG, et al: Tocainide-associated interstitial pneumonitis, *Ann Intern Med* 94:489, 1981.
196. Perry HM: Late toxicity to hydralazine resembling systemic lupus erythematous or rheumatoid arthritis, *Am J Med* 54:58, 1973.
197. Pickering TS: Effects of autonomic blockade on the baroreflex in man at rest and during exercise, *Circ Res* 30:177, 1972.
198. Pottinger WA: Minoxidil and the treatment of severe hypertension, *N Engl J Med* 303: 922, 1980.

199. Prasad T, Kaplan JA: Nicardipine, a new intravenous antagonist, *J Cardiothorac Anesth* 3:344, 1989.
200. Pratt C: Ventricular antiarrhythmic effects of beta adrenergic blocking drugs, *J Clin Pharmacol* 22:335, 1982.
201. Pujet JC, Dubreuil C, Fleury B, et al: Effects of celiprolol, a cardioselective beta blocker on respiratory function in asthmatic patients, *Eur Resp J* 5:196, 1992.
202. Quart B: Polymorphic encainide oxidation: What is the clinical significance (abstract), *Acta Pharmacol Toxicol* 59(suppl V, pt 1):116, 1986.
203. Raedor EA, Podrid PJ, Lawn B: Side effects and complications of amiodarone therapy, *Am Heart J* 109:975, 1985.
204. Reubi FC: Clinical use of furosemide, *Ann NY Acad Sci* 139:433, 1966.
205. Reubi FC, Cottier PT: Effects of reduced glomerular filtration rate on responsiveness to chlorothiazide, *Circulation* 23:200, 1961.
206. Roberts JE, Foex P, Clarke TNS, et al: Hemodynamic interactions of high dose propanolol pretreatment and anaesthesia in the dog. I. Halothane dose reponse studies, *Br J Anaesth* 48:315, 1976.
207. Roden DM, Reele SB, Higgins SB, et al: Antiarrhythmic efficacy, pharmacokinetics and safety of N-acetyl procainamide in human subjects: Comparison with procainamide, *Am J Cardiol* 46:463, 1980.
208. Roden DM, Woosley RL: Flecainide, *N Engl J Med* 315:36, 1986.
209. Roden DM, Woosley RL: Tocainide, *N Engl J Med* 315:41, 1986.
210. Roden DM, Woosley RL, Primm RK: Quinidine-induced long QT syndrome: Incidence and presenting features, *Am Heart J* 111:1088, 1986.
211. Rogers A, Curling PE, Cooper S, et al: Intravenous nifedipine for treatment of intraoperative hypertension, *Anesthesiology* 63:A24, 1985.
212. Rooney RF, Marij CJ, Stommel KA, et al: Additive cardiac depression by volatile anesthetics in isolated hearts after chronic amiodarone treatment, *Anesth Analg* 80: 917, 1995.
213. Rosen MR, Gelband H, Hoffman BF: Correlation between effects of ouabain in the canine electrocardiogram and transmembrane potentials of isolated Purkinje fibers, *Circulation* 47:65, 1973.
214. Rosen MR, Wit AL, Hoffman BF: Electrophysiology and pharmacology of cardiac arrhythmias. IV. Cardiac antiarrhythmic and toxic effects of digitalis, *Am Heart J* 89:391, 1975.
215. Rosenthal T, Ezra D: Calcium antagonists. Drug interactions of clinical significance, *Drug Safety* 13:157, 1995.
216. Rosing DR, Bonow RO, Packer M, et al: Verapamil therapy for the management of hypertrophic cardiomyopathy. In Packer M, Frishman WH, editors: *Calcium channel antagonists in cardiovascular disease,* Norwalk, 1984, Appleton-Century-Crofts.
217. Roy D: Efficacy of diltiazem in recurrent supraventricular tachyarrhythmias, *Can J Cardiol* 11:538, 1995.
218. Ruskin JN, DiMarco JP, Garan H: Out-of-hospital cardiac arrest: electrophysiologic observations and selection of long-term antiarrhythmic therapy, *N Engl J Med* 303:607, 1980.
219. Schmid PG, Nelson LD, Mark AL, et al: Inhibition of adrenergic vasoconstriction by quinidine, *J Pharmacol Exp Ther* 188:124, 1974.
220. Schmitt C, Brachmann J, Karch M, et al: Reverse use-dependent effects of sotalol demonstrated by recording monophasic action potentials of the right ventricle, *Am J Cardiol* 68:1183, 1991.
221. Schulman SP, Weiss JL, Becker LC: Effect of early enalapril therapy on left ventricular function and structure in acute myocardial infarction, *Am J Cardiol* 76:764, 1995.
222. Schulte-Sasse V, Hess W, Markschies-Hornung A, et al: Combined effects of halothane anesthesia and verapamil on systemic hemodynamics and LV myocardial contractility in patients with ischemic heart disease, *Anesth Analg* 63:791, 1984.
223. Schulte-Sasse V, Hess W, Markschies-Hornung A, et al: Cardiovascular interactions of halothane anesthesia and nifedipine in patients subjected to elective coronary artery bypass surgery, *Thorac Cardiovasc Surg* 31:261, 1983.
224. Schwartz JB: Effects of amlodipine on steady state digoxin concentrations and renal digoxin clearance, *J Cardiovasc Pharm* 12:1, 1988.
225. Schwartz ML, Rotmensch HH, Frishman WH, et al: Potential applications of calcium channel antagonists in the management of noncardiac disorders. In Packer M, Frishman WH, editors: *Calcium channel antagonists in cardiovascular disease,* Norwalk, 1984, Appleton-Century-Crofts.
226. Sellers TD Jr, Bashore TM, Gallagher JJ: Digitalis in the pre-excitation syndrome: Analysis during atrial fibrillation, *Circulation* 56:260, 1977.
227. Shan EN, Sung RJ, Morady F, et al: Electrophysiologic and hemodynamic effects of intravenous propaferone in patients with recurrent ventricular tachycardia, *J Am Coll Cardiol* 3:1291, 1984.
228. Sheppard D: Effects of esmolol on airway function in patients with asthma, *J Clin Pharmacol* 26:169, 1986.
229. Singh BN, Chew CYC, Josephson MA, et al: Hemodynamic mechanisms underlying the antianginal actions of verapamil, *Am J Cardiol* 50:886, 1982.
230. Smith TW: Digitalis: Mechanism of action and clinical use, *N Engl J Med* 318:358, 1988.
231. Smith TW, Butler VP Jr, Haber E, et al: Treatment of life-threatening digitalis intoxication with digoxin-specific Fab antibody fragments, *N Engl J Med* 307:1357, 1982.
232. Sodermark T, Edhag O, Sjogren A, et al: Effect of quinidine on maintaining sinus rhythm after conversion of atrial fibrillation or flutter: A multicenter study from Stockholm, *Br Heart J* 37:486, 1975.
233. Sokolow M, Edgar AL: Blood quinidine concentrations as a guide in the treatment of cardiac arrhythmias, *Circulation* 1:576, 1950.
234. Solomon GD, Steele JG, Spaccavento LJ: Verapamil prophylaxis of migraine: A double-blind placebo-controlled study, *JAMA* 250:2500, 1988.
235. Sonnenblick EH: Myocardial energetics, *N Engl J Med* 25:688, 1971.
236. Sonnenblick EH: Oxygen consumption of the heart, *Am J Cardiol* 22:328, 1968.
237. Soyka LF, Wirtz C, Spangenberg RB: Clinical safety profile of sotalol in patients with arrhythmias, *Am J Cardiol* 65:74, 1990.
238. Spiss CK, Zadrobilck E, Weinlmayr-Goettel M, et al: Nifedipine induced hypotension in man: Hemodynamic response during isoflurane and halothane anesthesia, *Anesthesiology* 63:A93, 1985.
239. Spivak C, Ocken S, Frishman WH: Calcium antagonists: Clinical use in treatment of systemic hypertension, *Drugs* 25:154, 1983.
240. Stenson RE, Constantino RT, Harrison DC: Interrelationships of hepatic blood flow, cardiac output, and blood levels of lignocaine in man, *Circulation* 43:205, 1971.
241. Strickberger SA, Fish RD, Lamas GA, et al: Comparison of effects of propanolol versus pindolol on sinus rate and pacing frequency in sick sinus syndrome, *Am J Cardiol* 71:53, 1993.
242. Stunkard A, Werthheimer L, Redisch W: Studies on hydralazine: Evidence for a peripheral site of action, *J Clin Invest* 3:1047, 1954.
243. Teichman SL, Ferrick A, Kim SG, et al: Disopyramide-pyridostigmine interaction: Selective reversal of anticholinergic symptoms with preservation of antiarrhythmic effect, *J Am Coll Cardiol* 10:633, 1987.
244. Thompson KA, Blair IA, Woosley RI, et al: Comparative in vitro electrophysiology of quinidine, its major metabolites and dihydroxyquinidine, *J Pharmacol Exp Ther* 241:84, 1987.
245. Thompson PD, Melmon KL, Richardson JA, et al: Lidocaine pharmacokinetics in advanced heart failure, liver disease and renal failure in humans, *Ann Intern Med* 78:499, 1973.
246. Tobian L: Why do thiazide diuretics lower blood pressure in pressure essential hypertension? *Annu Rev Pharmacol* 7:399, 1967.
247. Trimarco B, Cuocolo A, Van Dorne D, et al: Late phase of nitroglycerin-induced coronary vasodilation blunted inhibition of prostaglandin synthesis, *Circulation* 71:840, 1985.
248. Van Wezel HB, Kooken JJ, Visser CA, et al: The efficacy of nicardipine and nitroprusside in preventing poststernotomy hypertension, *J Cardiol Anesth* 3:707, 1989.
249. Vatner SF, Pagani M, Rutherford JD, et al: Effects of nitroglycerin on cardiac function and regional blood flow in conscious dogs, *Am J Physiol* 234:244, 1978.
250. Vaughan Williams EM: A classification of antiarrhythmic actions reassessed after a decade of new drugs, *J Clin Pharmacol* 24:129, 1984.
251. Vitez IS: Chronic hypokalemia and intraoperative dysrhythmias, *Anesthesiology* 63:130, 1985.
252. Volosin K, Greenberg RM, Greenspon AJ: Tocainide associated agranulocytosis, *Am Heart J* 109:1392, 1985.
253. Watanabe AK: Digitalis and the autonomic nervous system, *J Am Coll Cardiol* 5:35A, 1985.
254. Weiner I: Verapamil therapy for atrial flut-

ter and fibrillation. In Packer M, Frishman WH, editors: *Calcium channel antagonists in cardiovascular disease,* Norwalk, 1984, Appleton-Century-Crofts.

255. Weiskopf RB: Cardiovascular effects of desflurane in experimental animals and volunteers, *Anaesthesia* 50:(suppl)14, 1995.
256. Wendt RL: Guanebenz. In Suriabine A, editor: *Pharmacology of antihypertensive drugs,* New York, 1980, Raven Press.
257. Wenger TL, Butler VP, Haber E, et al: Treatment of 63 severely digitalis-toxic patients with digoxin-specific antibody fragments, *J Am Coll Cardiol* 5:118A, 1985.
258. Weiss RJ: Bepridil and agranulocytosis, *Am Heart J* 125: 1819, 1993.
259. Winkle RA, Gradman AH, Fitzgerald JW: Antiarrhythmic drug effect assessed from ventricular arrhythmia reduction in the ambulatory electrocardiogram and treadmill test: Comparison of propranolol, procainamide and quinidine, *Am J Cardiol* 42: 473, 1978.
260. Withering W: An account of the foxglove and some of its medical uses: With practical remarks on dropsy, and other diseases, Birmingham, London, 1785, GGJ and J Robinson.
261. Wollem GL, Gifford RW, Tarazi RC: Clinical pharmacology of antihypertensive drugs. In Gross F, Naegli SR, Kirkwood AH, editors: *Antihypertensive therapy, principles and practice; proceedings of an international symposium,* New York, 1966, Springer.
262. Woosley RL, Wang T, Stone W, et al: Pharmacology, electrophysiology, and pharmacokinetics of mexiletine, *Am Heart J* 107:1058, 1984.
263. Worlberdge SM, Lanstairs KC, Decie JV: Autoimmune hemolytic anemia associated with alpha-methyldopa therapy, *Lancet* 2: 135, 1966.
264. Wu D, Hung JS, Kuo CT, et al: Effects of quinidine on atrioventricular nodal reentrant paroxysmal tachycardia, *Circulation* 64:823, 1981.
265. Wyse DG, McAnulty JH, Rahimtoola SH: Influence of plasma drug level and the presence of conduction disease on the electrophysiologic effects of procainamide, *Am J Cardiol* 43:619, 1979.
266. Zannad F: Clinical pharmacology of nisoldipine coat core, *Am J Cardiol* 75:41E, 1995.
267. Zsoter TT, Church JG: Calcium antagonist–pharmacodynamic effects and mechanism of action, *Drugs* 25:93, 1983.
268. Zusman RM, Higgins J: Bepridil improves left ventricular performance in patients with angina pectoris, *J Cardiovasc Pharm* 22:474, 1993.

CHAPTER 66

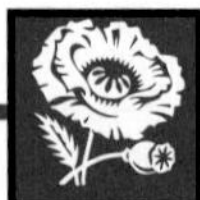

Anesthetic Considerations in the Use of Corticosteroids and Antibiotics

CLIFFORD S. DEUTSCHMAN

CORTICOSTEROIDS

The Perioperative Use of Glucocorticoids

Synthetic analogs of hormones secreted by the adrenal cortex are used in the treatment of a number of disorders. The use of exogenous glucocorticoids, however, alters the responsiveness of the endogenous system. This system is of central importance in the maintenance of metabolic homeostasis, fluid and electrolyte balance, and normal cardiodynamic responsiveness, especially in response to surgical or traumatic stress. It has long been believed that adrenal insufficiency in the presence of stress or injury is associated with a increased mortality and morbidity. Therefore, most physicians go to great lengths to provide patients who have been administered exogenous steroids with "stress" steroid coverage, by administering large doses of steroids throughout the perioperative period. Nonetheless, there are concerns that overadministration of adrenocorticoids is associated with impaired wound healing and immune function. This chapter will review glucocorticoid physiology, pharmacology, and toxicity with regard to these concerns, in order to arrive at an evidence-based strategy for steroid administration in the perioperative period. Specifically, the following questions will be addressed:

(1) Does the administration of exogenous steroids really surpress the endogenous system?
(2) Are steroids an essential component of the response to perioperative stress, do exogenous steroids alter this response and, if so, why?
(3) Is there evidence that exogenous steroids increase perioperative complications?
(4) What is the basis for the administration of the large doses of exogenous steroids often given in the perioperative period?
(5) Is there a more rational approach?

Physiology, pharmacology and secretory control of glucocorticoids

The adrenal cortex is responsible for the secretion of three classes of hormones: (1) glucocorticoids, which primarily affect substrate metabolism; (2) mineralocorticoids, which are involved in the regulation of sodium, potassium, and acid/base homeostasis; and (3) sex hormones, primarily androgens. Anatomically, the gland is divided into three zones.[230] Each of the three major classes of adrenocorticosteroids was once believed to originate from a unique anatomic location. It is now known that each zone has a preferential, but not exclusive, synthetic pattern. Aldosterone, the primary mineralocorticoid, is manufactured in the outermost layer, the zona glomerulosa.[144] Most cortisol—the major glucocorticoid in humans—is produced in the central zona fasciculata, although some is produced in the innermost zona reticularis.[144,230] This inner zone is the major producer of sex steroids, although some are produced in the zona fasciculata. The functions of these hormones overlap to some extent; cortisol has mineralocorticoid properties as well as exerting effects on metabolism.

Biosynthesis. All adrenal corticoids arise from cholesterol, which in turn is either synthesized by the gland from acetate or absorbed from low-density lipoproteins (Fig. 66-1).[88,162] The zona fasciculata is rich in cholesterol and comprises a pool that can be rapidly mobilized in response acute synthetic demand.[11,88,230] Cholesterol is converted to ΔE^4-pregnenolone in adrenal mitochondria by a complex series of reactions culminating in side chain cleavage.[11,162] This reaction is the rate-limiting step in steroid synthesis and is closely regulated. ΔE^4-pregnenolone is then synthesized into one of two compounds.[11,162] The major pathway in the fasciculata involves the conversion of the parent compound by 17-α-hydroxylase to 17-hydroxypregnenolone, a precursor of cortisol, androgens, and estrogens. A minor pathway in the fasciculata is synthesis of progesterone, which in turn can be converted to 11-deoxycorticosterone, corticosterone, and aldosterone.[11,162] This is the preferred pathway in the zona glomerulosa.

Pharmacokinetics and pharmacodynamics. From 10

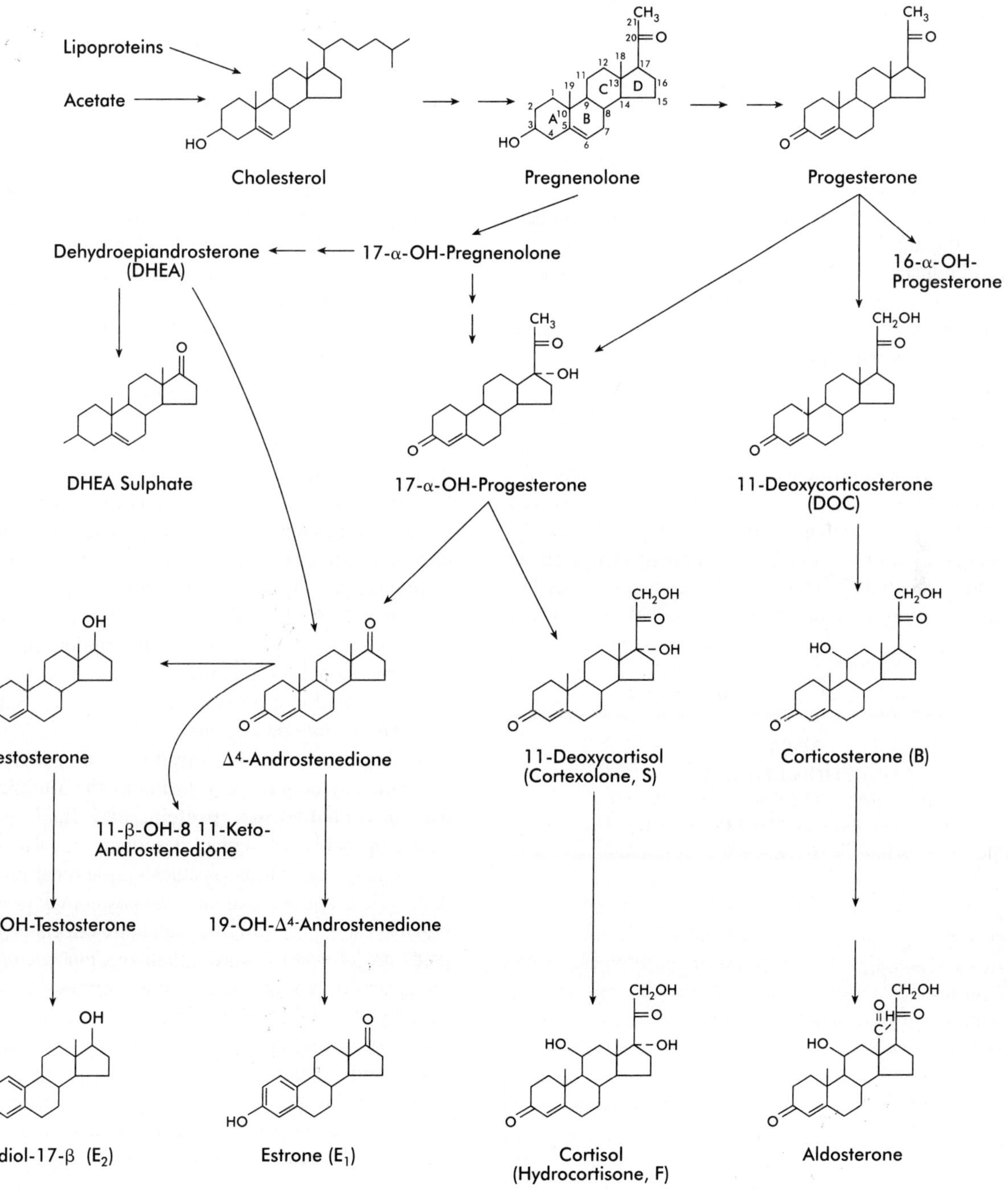

Lipoproteins
Acetate
Cholesterol
Pregnenolone
Progesterone
Dehydroepiandrosterone (DHEA)
17-α-OH-Pregnenolone
16-α-OH-Progesterone
DHEA Sulphate
17-α-OH-Progesterone
11-Deoxycorticosterone (DOC)
Testosterone
Δ^4-Androstenedione
11-Deoxycortisol (Cortexolone, S)
Corticosterone (B)
11-β-OH-8 11-Keto-Androstenedione
19-OH-Testosterone
19-OH-Δ^4-Androstenedione
Estradiol-17-β (E_2)
Estrone (E_1)
Cortisol (Hydrocortisone, F)
Aldosterone

Fig. 66-1. Synthesis of adrenocorticosteroids.

to 20 mg of cortisol are secreted daily by the zona fasciculata and zona reticularis of the adrenal cortex. The serum half-life of free cortisol is 80 to 110 minutes, but this is probably a very poor indicator of activity. **Biologic effects persist for 12 to 24 hours after the administration of cortisol.** In all probability, this discrepancy is due to the fact that 97% of secreted hormone is rapidly bound to carrier molecules that render it inactive.[11,187] Of circulating cortisol, 90% is bound to cortisol binding globulin (CBG or transcortin).[7] The remaining 7% is carried by albumin.[7] Binding to other plasma proteins occurs but is negligible.

CBG is synthesized in the liver[187] and is subject to regulation by a number of hormones including estrogen and thyroxine.[11] Therefore, conditions that affect circulating levels of binding globulins, such as malnutrition, inflammation, diabetes, pregnancy or oral contraceptive use, and altered thyroid function, will alter cortisol effects (Box 66-1). Binding of cortisol to CBG is linear up to cortisol concentrations of about 25 μmg/dl.[7] Above this value, CBG becomes saturated and cortisol concentrations become less predictable.[7] CBG also binds other substances, most notably progesterone in the third trimester of pregnancy.[7] Most exogenously administered synthetic corticoids have negligible CBG binding (an exception is prednisone).

Cortisol release is subject to diurnal variation. The mechanism is unknown but appears to involve intracranial events associated with similar episodic release of adrenocorticotropic hormone (ACTH) as well as other, non–ACTH related causes.[11] Peak serum levels occur in the morning with a second, lower peak occurring in the evening. Chronic diseases (liver failure, congestive heart failure [CHF]) as well as general anesthesia and operation can interrupt the spontaneous pattern.[215] Cortisol is released in bursts characterized by a rapid concentration increase and a gradual decline. The interval separating these bursts varies from 40 minutes to 1 hour.[11]

BOX 66-1
CONDITIONS THAT ALTER CIRCULATING CORTICOSTEROID BINDING GLOBULIN (CBG)

Increased CBG
- Pregnancy
- Oral contraceptive use
- Hyperthyroidism
- Diabetes
- Hematologic disorders

Decreased CBG
- Liver disease
- Multiple myeloma
- Hypothyroidism
- Obesity
- Nephrosis

As stated, the half-life of cortisol in blood is 80 to 120 minutes,[158] but this does not appear to correlate well with duration of biologic effect. Urinary-free cortisol, however, shows a better correlation, with approximately 70% of a radiolabeled dose being excreted in 24 hours.[158] Almost none of the dose is recovered as unmetabolized cortisol; the hydrophobic nature of cortisol is such that renal resorption is extensive.[11,158] **Thus hepatic metabolism is necessary to transform cortisol into inactive, water-soluble products,[26] which are ultimately excreted as 17-hydroxycorticosteroids in the urine. Chronic hepatic insufficiency or hypothyroidism may decrease metabolism.[158] In contrast, renal failure has little effect.[11,158]**

Mechanism of action. Glucocorticoids exert their effects on specific intracellular protein receptors.[169] The hormones probably enter the cell via passive diffusion[11] or perhaps through a specific membrane "pore." Most evidence indicates that glucocorticoid receptors are in the cytoplasm,[111] but some authors argue that they are intranuclear.[221] Binding of the hormone to the receptor is followed by a second event termed "activation" or "transformation,"[111,169] which appears to involve dissociation of an inhibitory factor, likely a major heat-shock protein, HSP-90.[176] The activated hormone-receptor complex then binds to DNA at nuclear sites known as glucocorticoid regulatory elements.[229] These sites serve as promoters, enhancers, or repressors for numerous gene sequences.[11,169] Thus the effects of glucocorticoids, as with all steroid receptors, involve changes at the transcriptional level. The mRNA transcripts created may code for enzymes or proteins that exert their effects directly or, alternatively, may bind to another portion of the genome and act in turn as promoters, enhancers, or repressors.[11] In unusual cases, glucocorticoids may act via nontranscriptional mechanisms, as in the feedback mechanism on ACTH release (discussed following), which appears to occur too rapidly to involve transcription. In humans, the predominant action is permissive, that is, activated glucocorticoids bind to a promoter and enhance or potentiate effects exerted by other agents.

Biologic activity. The predominant effects of glucocorticoids involve the regulation of the mobilization and use of carbohydrate, protein, and lipid as fuel.[11,127] Glucocorticoids also enhance sodium and water retention and control epinephrine synthesis in adrenal medulla. The metabolic properties can alter the physiology of most major organ systems. Overall, the metabolic effects of glucocorticoids are directed toward enhancing gluconeogenesis and are generally thought of as being "permissive," that is, potentiating the effects of other metabolically active hormones. This may be reflected in a shift of the dose response curve of these other compounds or by increasing the magnitude of the maximal response obtainable to other hormones.

Carbohydrate metabolism. **A primary effect of glucocorticoids is to increase hepatic gluconeogenesis. This occurs both directly and via enhancement of the effects of glucagon and epinephrine.** In particular, control of the actions of alanine aminotransferase,[42] which converts alanine to pyruvate, and phosphoenolpyruvate carboxykinase, the rate-limiting step in the conversion of pyruvate to glucose, is regulated by cortisol.[42,183] In addition, glucose-6-phosphatase is stimulated by cortisol, enhancing the conversion of glucose-6-phosphate to glucose.[127] Glucocorticoids directly inhibit glucose uptake by adipose tissue, fibroblasts,[31] and lymphoid cells.[137] Direct inhibition of uptake by skeletal muscle has not been demonstrated,[136] although glucocorticoids decrease overall uptake of glucose as a function of blood level independent of insulin levels.[11]

Glycogen deposition in the liver is increased by glucocorticoid administration, but the net effect represents a balance between glycogen synthesis and mobilization and may be a function of the age of the organism studied.[11,94,95,127] Glucocorticoid administration increases net glycogen deposition in liver[195] and increases activation (or decreases inactivation) of hepatic glycogen synthetase.[109] Glucose-6-phosphatase, which catalyzes the conversion of glucose-6-phosphate to glucose and allows glucose release, is also enhanced.[220] In the periphery, glucocorticoids appear to be required for the epinephrine-stimulated activation of glycogen phosphorylase.[180] This results in the release of glucose-1-phosphate, which can enter the glycolytic pathway. Glycogenolysis in muscle is catecholamine driven, enhanced by steroids, and often associated with increased lactate production.[11,127] Lactate can also serve as a gluconeogenic precursor.[63]

Glucocorticoids, as a result of their effects on protein and lipid metabolism, increase the availability of gluconeogenic precursors (see following paragraphs).[11,127]

Lipid metabolism. Alterations in lipid metabolism are an important function of glucocorticoids. Glycerol from lipolysis is a gluconeogenic precursor and can enhance hepatic gluconeogenesis, whereas fatty acids serve as a source of energy substrate for hepatic cells. Glucocorticoids directly inhibit glucose uptake by adipose cells,[31,127] impairing the availability of glycerol and acetyl coenzyme A as substrates for triglyceride synthesis. The mechanism for this inhibition appears to involve decreased synthesis of enzymes or proteins needed to transport glucose into the cells.[46,65,119]

Glucocorticoids directly and indirectly increase lypolysis in adipose tissue and cause an increase in plasma free fatty acids.[11,64,127] This effect is in part driven by the decrease in glucose uptake, which limits the amount of glycerol available for fatty acid esterification. Hormone-sensitive lipase, which breaks down intracellular triglycerides, may be stimulated, or lipoprotein lipase, which catalyzes the esterification of free fatty acids from the plasma, may be inhibited.[11,56,127,192] The lipolytic effects of catecholamines[11,64,65,127] and glucagon[11,64,56] are enhanced by glucocorticoids. A tendency to stimulation of ketosis[64,185] is overridden by gluconeogenesis and the resultant rise in serum insulin levels.[11]

Protein metabolism. Glucocorticoids stimulate hepatic protein synthesis and block protein synthesis in muscle, skin, fibroblasts, and adipose and lymphoid tissues.[12,127] In addition, breakdown of these peripheral tissues is enhanced and uptake of amino acids is inhibited.[125] The resulting release of amino acids provides precursors for gluconeogenesis.[11,127] Plasma amino acids, especially valine, leucine, isoleucine, tyrosine, phenylalanine, and histidine are increased.[225] Plasma pyruvate and alanine increase also, reflecting conversion of other amino acids into these transport molecules.[11,127] The excretion of nitrogenous by-products in the urine varies. In fasting, nitrogen excretion does not increase but excretion of 3-methyl-histidine, a muscle breakdown product, is found.[120]

Other effects. Glucocorticoids have effects on immune function and inflammation, bone and mineral metabolism, fibroblast activity, and fluid and electrolyte balance. It is believed that endogenous glucocorticoids are important mediators of these actions, but most studies and clinical observations have been made in the presence of glucocorticoid deficiency or excess.

Cortisol deficiency. In adrenalectromized animals, hepatic gluconeogenesis and glycogen content fall and the gluconeogenic response to catecholamines or glucagon is impaired.[11,127] Both uptake and release of amino acids by perfused muscle also decrease.[105] Hepatic glycogen synthesis is decreased.[196] Peripheral hypoglycemia and hypolipidemia are noted.[11,127] **Cardiovascular responses to corticoid deficiency include electrocardiogram (ECG) changes,[54,114,127] hypotension, and decreased cardiac output that cannot be explained by fluid and electrolyte abnormalities alone and which cannot be corrected by salt and water repletion.[13,127] Circulatory collapse during stress in Addisonian patients may reflect loss of the enhanced response to catecholamines that steroids impart.[11,23,127]** Increased calcium uptake[23] by vascular smooth muscle, altered receptor affinity,[18,49] increased catechol metabolism,[98] and altered protein synthesis in cardiac[149] and vascular[146,147] tissue have all been implicated. A loss of cardiac glycogen,[11,127] decreased ATPase activity,[167] or altered electrolyte milieu[11,127] may also be involved. Renal function is altered, with an elevation in blood urea nitrogen (BUN) level despite decreased proteolysis. The inability of the kidney to excrete potassium,[11,197] acid,[11] and water[25] reflects a decreased glomerular filtration rate, impaired resorption, and an exaggerated response to vasopressin.[11,25,182] In addition, adrenelectomized animals are unresponsive to infused angiotensin, implying that the response to the renin-angiotensin axis may require glucocorticoids.[127] Hypercalcemia results from both renal dysfunction and complex interactions between cortisol, bone, and gastrointestinal and nonadrenal endocrine effects on calcium homeostasis.[11,57,127,142] Patients with Addison's disease are anorexic, lose weight, lack vigor, and are subject to severe bouts of depression[57]; frank psychosis may occur. In children and growing animals, growth may be impaired.

Conditions associated with adrenocorticoid insufficiency that are of importance to the anesthesiologist include tuberculosis, fungal infections, AIDS, metastatic cancer, lymphoma, pituitary disease, enzyme-inhibiting drugs such as metyrapone, some cytotoxic agents, and inborn errors of metabolism. Most of these are rare; **the most common causes of glucocorticoid deficiency are idiopathic (autoimmune) or arise secondary to cessation of chronic steroid administration.**

Cortisol excess. In response to excess cortisol, there are increases in basal energy expenditure, oxygen consumption, and carbon dioxide production.[19] Hepatic glucose and glycogen production are increased, and there is a tendency to hyperglycemia.[11,127] Glucose loads are poorly tolerated. This effect is magnified in diabetics, who may require increased insulin.[11] Glucose uptake is impaired in adipose and other tissues.[11,31,127] Glycosuria can occur. Glycogen is deposited in the liver and muscle.[11,127,195] Circulating levels of alanine are increased,[225] reflecting mobilization of peripheral muscle as substrate and the conversion of other amino acids, as well as pyruvate to alanine for transport.[11,127,188,212] Loss of muscle mass, especially of white glycolytic fibers, results.[11,125,127] Some authors believe that heart and diaphragmatic muscle may be spared,[127] but incorporation of labeled histidine into both these tissues is impaired after steroid administration in a manner identical to skeletal muscle.[228] Inhibition of hepatic and skeletal muscle DNA synthesis and RNA breakdown occur.[11,127]

Lipolysis and impaired reesterification increase glycerol and free fatty acid release, which is reflected in circulating levels.[11,65,127,188] Patients with Cushing's disease have increased circulating lipoproteins of all densities.[209] It is not clear why fat is deposited in some areas (e.g., the trunk) and lost in others (e.g., the extremities), resulting in the classic Cushingoid appearance.

In response to increased circulating glucocorticoids, the blood pressure is increased.[11] This may reflect enhanced vascular reactivity to catecholamines[24] and other vasoconstrictors,[11,18,127] or an increased cardiac output[174] from either a direct inotropic effect involving increased coupling of beta receptors and adenyl cyclase[49] or enhanced responsiveness to catecholamines.[11,127] Ultrastructural damage to cardiac muscle has been reported.[38] Levels of prorenin,[106] renin,[184] angiotensin converting enzyme,[76] and angiotensin II[11,127] increase after glucocorticoid administration and may play a role in the development of hypertension. Further, responsiveness to angiotensin II and norepinephrine is increased in glucocorticoid excess states.[11,127]

Glucocorticoids can increase the glomerular filtration rate (GFR) either via increased cardiac output or direct renal influences.[12] Atrial natriuretic factor is increased[11]; when a hormone such as dexamethasone, which has little mineralocorticoid effect, is administered, salt loss may occur.[11,12,89] In most cases of exogenous administration and in Cushing's syndrome, kaliuresis is the rule[11] with relative sodium retention. Acid loss results in a tendency toward alkalosis.[75,123,197]

Calcium and phosphate homeostasis and the dynamics of bone metabolism are significantly affected by steroid excess.[11,127] Serum phosphate and both urinary calcium and phosphate are increased in steroid excess states.[69] Urine values reflect a decrease in renal resorption of calcium and phosphate, and renal calculi may result.[166] There is a tendency toward hypocalcemia, reflecting the interplay of steroids, parathyroid hormone (PTH), 1,25-dihydroxycholecalciferol (1,25-$[OH]_2D_3$), and bone resorption.[11,127] Intestinal calcium absorption is somewhat impaired.[90] Bone formation is decreased by prolonged steroid use,[85] and bone resorption is enhanced.[10] This is the result of enhanced amounts and activity of PTH,[35,145] increased sensitivity to 1,25-$(OH)_2D_3$,[34,227] and blocking of the inhibitory effects of calcitonin.[21] Thus, osteoblasts are inhibited and osteoclasts stimulated. **Significant thinning of bone matrix, osteoporosis, and pathologic fractures may result. These problems represent some of the main limitations to long-term steroid use.[11,127]**

Steroids are often used therapeutically to suppress inflammation or pathologic inflammatory responses.[11,127,156] Glucocorticoids inhibit synthesis of prostanoids and phospholipase A2, block the actions of bradykinin, decrease accumulation of inflammatory cells at inflammatory sites, and block synthesis or release of numerous mediators, including tumor necrosis factor (TNF), interleukin (IL)-1, and IL-6.[11,127] Steroids cause lymphopenia, monocytopenia, and eosinopenia, which is an effect that peaks 4 to 6 hours after administration and is gone within 24 to 48 hours.[164] Release of polymorphonuclear cells by the bone marrow is enhanced.[127] Other changes associated with cortisol excess include euphoria, frank psychosis, peripheral neuropathy, polycythemia,[11,166] thrombocytopenia with a tendency to bleeding and bruising,[11] and eye changes, including intraocular hypertension[11] and the development of cataracts.[121]

Adrenocorticoid excess can result from exogenous administration or cortisol- or ACTH–secreting tumors. Most of these tumors are adrenal or pituitary adenomas, but other neoplasms that may secrete ACTH include oat cell carcinoma of the lung; thymoma; pancreatic islet cell tumors; carcinoids of the lung, GI tract, pancreas, or ovary; medullary cancer of the thyroid; and pheochromocytoma.[12]

Control of secretion. In order to address the first question raised in the introduction, regarding the ability of exogenous steroids to surpress the endogenous system, the control of the endogenous system must be examined. Multiple factors are involved in stimulating the release of cortisol but ultimately, control lies in the hypothalamic-pituitary-adrenal axis, a complex series of interrelated neural and endocrine structures (Fig. 66-2). The central focus lies in the ability to modulate levels of ACTH, the primary inducer of cortisol release. Initiation of ACTH release may come from exogenous or endogenous factors affecting descending neural pathways which begin in the supratentorial central nervous system. Under physiologic conditions, these pathways, which lead to the release of cortisol and the release of the factors that control cortisol levels, may involve

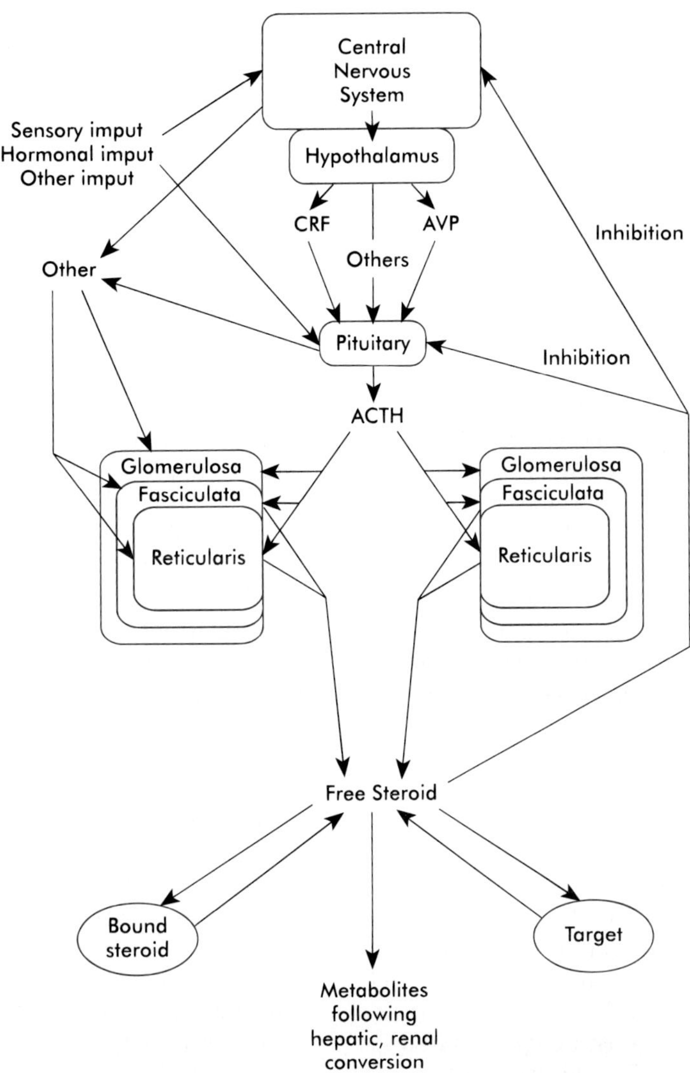

Fig. 66-2. Hypothalamic-pituitary-adrenal axis.

endogenous rhythms in the brain, physical or emotional "stress" or excitatory events, and the level of cortisol itself.[170]

Adrenocorticotropic hormone–releasing substances. Initiation of cortisol release begins in the paraventricular nucleus of the hypothalamus, where corticotropin releasing factor (CRF) and arginine vasopressin (AVP) are synthesized.[222] CRF is the primary and most potent stimulant of ACTH secretion.[82,211] This peptide contains 41 amino acids[194] and is ordinarily not detectable outside the hypophyseal circulation. Although its central function is in stimulating ACTH release (via a mechanism that may involve adenylyl cyclase[3]), receptors for CRF have also been found in the brain[52] (where they act to stimulate sympathetic outflow) and the GI tract.[152] CRF is carried to the anterior pituitary via a specific portal circulation.[81] AVP is also carried to the pituitary via this route. The role of AVP in the normal control of ACTH release is not as well understood as that of CRF.[11] It is clearly not essential for ACTH release[211] but can stimulate ACTH release itself and exerts a synergistic effect with CRF.[110]

Other factors that may contribute to ACTH release include catecholamines,[3,51,211] angiotensin II,[3] opiates,[5,51] somatostatin,[5,51] lymphocytic derived factors,[92] and cytokines. Finally, fever, hypoglycemia, stress, and falling cortisol levels also stimulate ACTH release.

Adrenocorticotropic hormone structure and synthesis. ACTH is produced by basophilic corticotropic cells in the anterior lobe of the pituitary.[165,169] It is one of a series of molecules derived from a common precursor, pro-opiomalanocortin (POMC).[108] A single mRNA directs the synthesis of all POMC derived molecules, with control exerted on the post-transcriptional level.[140] The precursor molecule is approximately 290 amino acids long. Cleavage of the c-terminus of POMC yields a protein that is subsequently cleaved to give ACTH and beta-lipotropin (β-LPH). β-LPH, in turn, can be split to yield beta-endorphin. Beta-endorphin and ACTH tend to be released stoichiometrically.[87] In different anatomic locations—such as the central nervous system—POMC can be cleaved to primarily yield alpha-melanocyte stimulating hormone (alpha-MSH), beta-endorphin, or corticotropinlike intermediate lobe protein (CLIP).[169]

ACTH consists of 39 amino acids arranged in a linear chain.[117,163] While the 10 residues on the amino terminal end of the peptide are required for biologic activity, the addition of the rest of the protein serves to lengthen the period of adrenal stimulation by the hormone. ACTH is rapidly cleared from the serum and may be inactivated even more quickly; thus immunoreactivity is present long after biologic activity has terminated.[11,151]

ACTH is secreted in bursts that occur 7 to 10 times per day.[11] Control is subject, under normal conditions, to diurnal variability, and the greatest amount of ACTH is secreted in the morning.[11] The stimulus for this variability appears to lie intracranially,[48] but its exact nature is unknown. Wake-sleep cycles have been implicated.[11]

Effects of ACTH on the adrenal gland. **Secretion of cortisol by the adrenal gland is regulated almost exclusively by ACTH, which initiates its effects via binding to a specific peptide receptor on the surface of cell membranes.**[33] Stimulation activates adenyl cyclase,[91,189] which in turn yields increased cyclic AMP, activation of Protein Kinase A and phosphorylation.[11] Calmodulin and calcium ions are involved,[69,91] and in all probability, the process involves membrane phospholipids. The major effect of this pathway is to stimulate conversion of cholesterol to ΔE^4-pregnenolone, the rate-limiting step in cortisol synthesis.[69,91] It has been postulated that this conversion involves an adrenal steroid carrier protein that moves with cholesterol into the inner mitochondria and from there to a P450 enzyme.[40] Inhibition of protein synthesis blocks the effects of ACTH on adrenal cortisol secretion.[91] ACTH stimulation of the adrenal gland results in secretion within 2 to 3 minutes implying the existence of a mobile pool. Long-term stimulation can yield hypertrophy of the gland.

ACTH increases cholesterol esterase activity via phosphorylation and decreases the activity of cholesterol ester synthetase.[189] These effects increase the supply of free cholesterol. Finally, ACTH stimulates lipoprotein uptake by the adrenal gland and also increases adrenal blood flow.[11]

Other factors involved in glucocorticoid release. Glucocorticoids themselves may inhibit steroidogenesis.[171] This will be further discussed with other aspects of negative feedback. Direct innervation of the adrenal gland has been implicated in the circadian rhythms associated with glucocorticoid release,[11] and there may be a role for beta-adrenergic receptors in the adrenal cortex.[186] All the factors previously cited as exerting affects on ACTH release may also be directly involved in the release of cortisol. In particular, opiates can decrease responsiveness to ACTH,[53] and prostanoids and growth hormone increase the effects of ACTH.[32,155]

Feedback inhibition. The dominant factor in decreasing both CFR and ACTH secretion is an increase in serum cortisol.[11,101,170] Studies in adrenelectomized animals and in patients with adrenal insufficiency have demonstrated three components to feedback inhibition.[101] A rapid component occurs within seconds to minutes of elevation of the serum cortisol levels and is proportional not to the absolute cortisol value, but rather to the rate of rise in cortisol.[68] This effect is exerted on both the hypothalamus and the pituitary gland and is more effective in blunting the response to histamine than to major surgery.[223] It is brief, leaving the hypothalamus-pituitary-adrenal (HPA) axis unresponsive to certain stimuli for several hours.[101] Clearly, this response is too fast to represent an effect mediated by altered gene expression and may well involve direct actions on the cell membrane.[11] Both the intermediate and delayed feedback loops are direct responses to serum cortisol levels that are dose dependent.[11] The intermediate feedback response involves inhibition of CRF and ACTH release but does not alter synthesis. Intermediate inhibition leaves the axis unresponsive to some, but not all, stimuli 1 to 2 hours after the initial stimulus and can last 10 to 24 hours.[11] The delayed loop is associated with a reduction in POMC mRNA production. Activation of this component of feedback inhibition requires several days of exogenous steroid administration and can leave the axis totally unresponsive to even massive stimuli for as long as several months.[11,86]

Thus, even a single dose of steroids can activate the rapid and intermediate components of feedback inhibition and may leave the HPA unresponse to normal physiologic stimuli for as long as 24 hours. Prolonged suppression, which involves the long-term feedback inhibition loop, requires exogenous steroid administration to occur over a significant period of time—at least several days. Studies defining classical feedback inhibition patterns have not been performed in the presence of surgical or inflammatory stress. This leads to a second question.

Importance of glucocorticoids in the response to surgical stress/inflammation

Normal response. In response to "stress" caused by operation, inflammatory disease, or trauma, a characteristic metabolic and physiologic state develops.[45,131,200] This condition involves increased resting energy expenditure,[102] oxygen consumption and carbon dioxide production, with substrate mobilization and altered hepatic protein synthesis. To facilitate repair of damaged tissue, increased delivery of oxygen and nutrients to numerous tissues is required and is met by increases in cardiac output, peripheral vasodilitation, and capillary leak. The magnitude of this response is proportional to the magnitude of the stress[36] and it persists for 5 to 7 days following the initiating stimulus. An interplay of numerous endogenous mediators, as well as a predictable alteration in neurohumoral activity, is involved; these include increased cortisol secretion.

Clearly, glucocorticoids are involved in the modulation of the stress response. Cortisol is important in the mobilization and synthesis of substrate and contributes, through its mineralocorticoid effects, to intravascular volume expansion. Infusion of cortisol into normal volunteers causes minor increases in metabolic rate, oxygen consumption, and carbon dioxide production.[19] In concert with other mediators, most notably epinephrine and glucagon, the "permissive" effects of cortisol become manifest. The combination of the three produces a synergistic pattern that mimics the metabolic changes seen in the perioperative or posttraumatic state.[19,185] Metabolic markers of the stress response, especially the increases in ACTH, cortisol, and epinephrine, can be blocked by deep general or neural axis anesthesia, but they return when the anesthetic is terminated.[41,116,141,196]

Evidence that normal function of the hypothalamic-pituitary-adrenal axis is essential in the perioperative period. Two types of studies have been cited to demonstrate that an intact, functional HPA axis is essential to recovery from surgical stress. In the first type, the HPA axis is anatomically disrupted, usually by adrenalectomy. In these investigations, conducted in animals, the adrenal gland is removed and the animal is subjected to surgery or trauma. In a series of classic studies, Swingle and coworkers showed that adrenalectomized dogs became hypovolemic and died after laparotomy or trauma, and they further demonstrated that the circulatory collapse could be prevented by administration of adrenaocortical extract.[202,203,204,205,206] It is unclear, however, whether the essential agent was a glucocorticoid, an adrenomedullary contaminant (i.e., catecholamines), or a mineralocorticoid. More recently, Udelsman et al.[216] demonstrated that primates subjected to operation without adequate exogenous steroid supplements had a substantial, although not universal, mortality. In a well-designed study of surgical stress in primates, these investigators found that adrenalectomized animals receiving subphysiologic steroid coverage before, during, and after a cholecystectomy had a 38% mortality rate as compared with a 14% rate in animals treated with physiologic or supraphysiologic doses of corticosteroids. This study clearly documents the potential occurrence of Addisonian crisis in the presence of inadequate levels of corticosteroids after even relatively low levels of surgical stress.

The second type of study involves investigations of patients who had been taking exogenous steroids prior to operation, did not receive glucocorticoids during the perioperative period and suffered an adverse occurrence. The first such report was by Fraser, Preuss, and Bigford in 1952.[73] This single case involved a cortisol dependent patient who died of cardiovascular collapse following hip surgery for rheumatoid arthritis. The patient did not respond to exogenously administered corticosteroids or epinephrine. Autopsy showed adrenal atrophy; therefore, the death was attributed to glucocorticoid-induced HPA suppression. Subsequent reports by Lewis et al.,[118] Salassa et al.,[172] and Marks[122] are similar. In 1961, Sampson, Brooke, and Winstone reported the case of a man on long-term glucocorticoid therapy for Crohn's disease. The steroids were discontinued on admission to the hospital, and he became hypotensive during operation but responded to administration of cortisone.[175] This pattern repeated itself during a second operation. Cortisol levels, estimated from urinary excretion, were decreased during the operation but increased appropriately when exogenous steroids were given. In a subsequent retrospective review, Winstone and Brooke reported on a group of steroid-dependent patients with ulcerative colitis who underwent colectomy.[224] In 17 patients who did not receive steroid coverage, there were four deaths, two of which were attributed to "pituitary-adrenal collapse." In a second group of 18 patients who received perioperative glucocorticoids, there were two deaths, neither attributed to "pituitary-adrenal collapse." In a third group, consisting of 22 patients who had never received steroids, there were three deaths. These studies illustrate that most of the data implicating glucocorticoid deficiency as a cause of perioperative vascular collapse is anecdotal. It appears that only some patients with adrenal suppression have problems if unsupplemented.

Evidence that normal function of the hypothalamic-pituitary-adrenal axis may not be essential in the perioperative period. In contrast to the studies previously presented, a number of investigators have reported data which suggest that the function of the HPA axis is not essential for recovery from surgical stress. Plumpton, Besser, and Cole[161] measured plasma cortisol in three groups of patients undergoing different types of surgical procedures. One group was receiving steroids which were discontinued prior to operation, a second group continued to receive steroids through the perioperative period and a third group served as a steroid-naive control. There were no differences in plasma cortisol or in outcome. Kehlet and Binder[100] studied 74 steroid-dependent patients undergoing major operation without steroid coverage. Thirty-nine patients had abnormal plasma glucocorticoid values 1 hour after incision, and 24 patients had abnormalities at 4 hours. Hypotensive episodes occurred in 18 patients; 11 were directly attributed to bleeding. Of the remaining seven, four had normal plasma cortisol and three were mildly decreased. Nonetheless, 33 patients with mildly decreased plasma cortisol values did not develop hypotension. Engquist, Backer, and Jarnum[59] studied two matched groups of 100 steroid-dependent patients each. One group received glucocorticoids in excess of their normal dose, the other group did not. Forty-four percent of the steroid-treated patients and 22% of the untreated patients had complications. Knudsen, Christiansen, and Lorentzen[103] reported on 250 patients who received steroids for inflammatory bowel disease. Fifty patients received high doses of glucocorticoids during the perioperative period, and 200 did not; 11 (22%) of those in the first group became hypotensive compared to 18 (9%) in the second. Finally, Bromberg et al.[28] reported that there was no evidence of adrenal insufficiency in 40 steroid-dependent (5 to 10 mg of prednisone/day) renal transplant patients admitted for a variety of surgical procedures and treated with only maintenance doses of prednisone.

Much as was the case with the earlier reports, there are a

number of difficulties with these studies. The combination is a confusing picture. It is therefore not clear whether or not HPA axis integrity is important to the response to surgical stress. Recent investigations into an additional aspect of the inflammatory response appears to clarify the issue.

Altered secretory control during inflammation

Attempts to stimulate the axis following suppression again involved either pain or hypoglycemia. Recent studies indicate that inflammation, as opposed to other forms of stress, may alter HPA behavior and modulate feedback inhibition. A study by Naito et al.[138] in 1991 examined the response of the HPA axis in a series of patients undergoing elective upper-abdominal surgery. First, values of CRF, ACTH, and cortisol were measured over time after operation. A biphasic response was apparent; on the day of surgery, all three were increased relative to the preoperative period, whereas on postoperative day two, CRF and ACTH were decreased compared with preoperative values. Cortisol was increased at both times. To explain these unusual findings, the response to administration of ACTH was examined. After the same dose of ACTH, plasma cortisol in the preoperative period increased from 400 to 800 nM, whereas the increase on postoperative day two was from 600 to 1400 nM. Suppression of the HPA with dexamethasone preoperatively and on postoperative day two revealed that exogenous steroids suppressed ACTH secretion to the same extent, but cortisol values were greater in the postoperative period. The data demonstrate that the secretion of cortisol is responding to something other than ACTH.

Other data indicate that the HPA axis may be responsive to inflammatory cytokines such as TNF, IL-1, and IL-6. Wolosky et al.[226] first reported in 1985 that IL-1 and IL-6 caused the release of ACTH from cultured pituitary cells. Since that report, studies in cultured cells,[78,213] experimental animals,[17,201,143,157,58,217] and humans[153,124,193] have demonstrated that TNF, IL-1, and IL-6 modulate the HPA axis. These cytokines increase release of CRF from the hypothalamus, ACTH from the pituitary, and also directly stimulate the adrenal cortex to release cortisol. In a follow-up study to examine the disparity between ACTH and cortisol levels, Naito et al.[139] studied the effects of neural axis blockade on ACTH, cortisol, and the cytokines TNF and IL-6 in two groups of patients. The first group underwent total hip replacement, the second pancreaticoduodenectomy. Patients in each group were randomly assigned to receive either general anesthesia alone or general plus epidural anesthesia throughout the operation. The epidural was used to block afferent neural impulse and thus eliminate activation of the HPA axis. In the patients undergoing total hip replacement, the addition of epidural anesthesia significantly attenuated plasma increases in ACTH and cortisol for 7 days postoperatively, whereas in patients receiving general anesthesia alone, cortisol and ACTH were increased for 8 hours postoperatively. No plasma TNF or IL-6 was detected in these patients. In contrast, patients who underwent pancreatic resection had significant levels of endotoxin, TNF, and IL-6 at least up to the third postoperative day. Most importantly, in this second group, the epidural had no effect on plasma levels of ACTH or cortisol, and cortisol remained increased through the third postoperative day.

These findings, taken in concert with the known effects of cytokines on the HPA axis, indicate that factors other than simple feedback inhibition are involved during major inflammatory stress such as surgery or trauma. Thus, the unpredictable and variable effects of exogenous steroid administration on HPA axis function in the perioperative period may be due to variable degrees of stimulation of CRF or ACTH and/or cortisol release by cytokines.

In summary, the effects of exogenous steroids on the behavior of the HPA axis in the presence of surgical stress is capricious, owing to the numerous factors likely to be involved in the modulation of adrenal function.

Adverse effects of exogenous steroids during inflammation

The data regarding the suppression of HPA axis function by exogneous steroids during perioperative stress indicate that the response is unpredictable. Thus, it would seem appropriate to administer steroids to these patients if therapy did not harm the patient in any significant way. This reasoning leads us to examine the evidence that perioperative use of high-dose steroid coverage is associated with an increased rate of complications. Both outcome-based and experimental approaches have been used to address this concern. Several studies which are pertinent have already been cited. Engquist, Backer, and Jarnum[60] examined two matched groups of 100 steroid-dependent patients; they found the overall complication rate was significantly greater (44% versus 22%) in patients who received perioperative stress-dose steroids. Winstone and Brooke, in their report on steroid-dependent patients undergoing colectomy for ulcerative colitis, reported that the patients who did not receive steroids had fewer complications (four perineal infections) compared with patients receiving steroids (four patients with bacterial septicemia, three with intra-abdominal sepsis, one lung abcess, one perineal infection, one wound infection/dehiscence).[224] Additionally, a number of randomized trials have investigated the use of high doses of glucocorticoids in the treatment of the systemic inflammatory response syndrome (SIRS, formerly called sepsis). In two recent meta-analyses of these trials, Cronin et al.[44] and Lefering and Neugebauer[115] independently demonstrated that patients who received steroids had worse outcomes and more complications than patients who did not receive steroids. Bohnen, Mustard, and Schouten prospectively examined APACHE II scores and mortality in patients admitted for treatment of intra-abdominal infection.[22] Mortality in steroid-dependent patients (who were treated with "stress doses") was double that of patients not receiving steroids and, more importantly, steroid-dependent patients had a probability of dying similar to that of patients with an

APACHE II score four points higher. The conclusion was that two to four "extra APACHE points" needed to be added to account for the effects of steroid treatment. **Thus, outcome based studies, although limited by design, indicate that there is an increased risk of death and major infectious complications in patients receiving high doses of glucocorticoids in the perioperative period.**

Animal and *in vitro* data indicate that glucocorticoids may have adverse effects on immune function and wound healing. Macrophage activation and cytokine production,[179] neutrophil adhesion and priming,[8] T-cell proliferation, gene expression, and immunoglobulin synthesis[84] are all inhibited after glucocorticoid treatment. A series of studies documented impaired wound and GI anastomotic healing in rats treated with corticosteroids.[61,178] Neither the immune nor the wound-healing effects have been directly demonstrated in patients, although numerous anecdotal reports exist.[6]

In patients with preexisting hypertension, diabetes, fluid retention, or altered mental status, perioperative administration of glucocorticoids would be expected to make these conditions worse. Steroids exacerbate abnormalities of gastric acid secretion and can induce the formation of stress ulcers. The actual effects of steroids on these conditions remains anecdotal.

In summary, **administration of high doses of glucocorticoids in the perioperative period is associated with altered outcome in clinical reports and a higher mortality for a given levels of risk as well as impaired wound healing and immune function in experimental animals and cell culture.**

The use of pharmacologic doses of corticosteroids and data regarding actual corticosteroid secretion in stress

The original recommendation for the use of pharmacologic doses of corticosteroids in the perioperative period appears to arise from a report by Lewis et al.[118] in 1953. These authors recommended a fourfold increase in glucocorticoid administration in the perioperative period—a practice that has been generalized and extended to cover a number of postoperative days. The rationale for these recommendations is unclear. Early studies in patients undergoing resuscitation, which used single measures of urinary metabolites to approximate 24 hour secretion, indicated that as much as 300 mg of cortisol/day may be generated in these moribund individuals.[70,177] In nine symptomatic asthmatics in whom maximal cortisol secretion was studied, Thomas and El-Shaboury found a mean value of 222 mg/24 hours with a range from 135 to 310 mg/24 hours.[210] Few other data are available.

A recent study indicates that normal volunteers secrete approximately 10 mg of cortisol/day and that five patients with Cushing's disease secondary to pituitary adenomas secreted 30 ± 9 mg/day.[62] A number of studies, summarized by Salem et al.,[173] indicate that cortisol secretion after major operation ranged from 60 to 300 mg/24 hours but rarely exceeded 200 mg/day. Kehlet and Binder[100] estimated that patients undergoing major surgery secreted 75 to 150 mg the day of operation with return to basal levels by postoperative day two or three. There are no data to justify the standard postoperative "slow taper" in the absence of documented HPA axis suppression.

A more rational approach

To arrive at a reasonable approach to perioperative glucocorticoid replacement, we must take into account a number of issues. The risk of suppression of the HPA axis is significant, if unpredictable, and must be accounted for because absence of any cortisol is associated with potential mortality. Nonetheless, assessment of the clinical literature indicates that replacement above the physiologic level is unnecessary. Indeed, this literature would seem to indicate that the endogenous response is sufficient in most cases. It may be useful to demonstrate that the endogenous system is capable of response; this can be accomplished with an ACTH stimulation test, in which 250 μg of ACTH is administered. An increase in plasma cortisol to greater than 18 to 20 μg/dl is defined as normal. A number of investigators have used this approach, supplementing only the nonresponders, with good results.[19,128] It has been noted that the response of the HPA axis is altered by inflammatory stress, and therefore the ACTH stimulation test may be abnormal in patients still capable of an adequate response. The adverse events in adrenal insufficiency are primarily cardiovascular and these can be monitored routinely in the perioperative period. It is therefore reasonable to administer the usual maintenance dose of glucocorticoids on the day of operation and then treat the patient symptomatically. An alternative approach would involve the routine use of moderate doses of supplemental exogenous steroids; recommendations from Salem et al.[173] are detailed in Table 66-1.

Mineralocorticoids

True mineralocorticoid abnormalities are rarely encountered by the anesthesiologist. **Exogenously administered glucocorticoids, however, have varying amounts of mineralocorticoid activity. Thus the anesthesiologist caring for the patient taking a glucocorticoid preparation may be faced with either excessive mineralocorticoid activity or in the patient taking a glucocorticoid with weak mineralocorticoid effects, relative mineralocorticoid deficiency.**

Biologic activity

The major mineralocorticoid is aldosterone. Both cortisol and 11-dehydroxycorticosterone also have mineralocorticoid properties.[11] These compounds are responsible for ionic balance; they act on epithelial cells[132] in the kidney,[37,123] gut,[20] salivary and sweat glands,[11] vascular tissues,[133,148] brain, and possibly the pituitary gland.[11] **The primary action of mineralocorticoids is to conserve sodium,[214] with the most important physiologic effects being exerted on the renal connecting segment and collecting tubules.[123,134,135,159,214]** Potassium secretion in the collecting

Table 66-1 Recommendations for supplementation of exogenous steroids in the perioperative period

Perioperative stress	Recommendation
Minor surgical stress	25 mg hydrocortisone equivalent on day of (e.g., inguinal hernia repair) operation only
Moderate surgical stress (e.g., open cholecystectomy, lower extremity vascular procedure, total joint replacement, segmental colon resection, hysterectomy)	50–75 mg hydrocortisone equivalent for 1–2 days, then preoperative dose
Major surgical stress (e.g., Whipple procedure, esophagogastrectomy, total colectomy, cardiopulmonary bypass)	100–150 mg hydrocortisone equivalent for 2–3 days, then preoperative dose

Adapted from Salem M, et al: A reassessment 42 years after emergence of a problem, *Ann Surg* 219:416–425, 1994.

segment and cortical collecting tubules and hydrogen ion secretion in the medullary collecting tubule[168] are also mediated via the actions of aldosterone. Magnesium and calcium ion excretion may be affected indirectly by aldosterone-induced sodium retention.[11] Aldosterone also exerts a permissive effect on the response of water to vasopressin, enhancing the resorption of water in the cortical collecting tubule.[123]

Mechanism of action

Mineralocorticoids show behavior typical of steroids.[27] Aldosterone binds to one of several cytosolic receptors (distinguishable from glucocorticoid receptors by their differing affinity for mineralocorticoids and glucocorticoids[123]); the resultant complex binds to a nuclear receptor, and the entire compound binds to chromatin.[11,123] Aldosterone exerts its effects, which occur within 30 minutes to 2 hours, via stimulation of transcription and protein synthesis.[11,27] This sequence results in the synthesis of several proteins,[80] which may exert a number of effects. Sodium resorption involves diffusion through membranous channels from tubular lumen into the tubular cell. Na^+ is then actively pumped, via a Na^+/K^+ ATPase, across the basolateral membrane into the blood.[27] Aldosterone-stimulated proteins may mediate the effects on sodium resorption via alteration of the permeability of the luminal membrane (apparently converting nonspecific channels into sodium-specific channels),[123,154] by increasing energy supply to the ATPase[123] or by increasing the activity of the pump.[43,123,132,134,135,159,214] All three effects are independent of potassium concentration.[123] It is less clear how aldosterone works with regard to secretion of potassium and acid.[27] Potassium excretion appears to be dependent on sodium intake; when sufficient Na^+ is delivered to the distal nephron, kaliuresis can occur, but sodium restriction leads to a failure of K^+ excretion in response to aldosterone.[123] Nonetheless, the relationship between sodium and potassium concentration is not stoichiometric.[123] Acid secretion occurs primarily in the medullary tubule and can be independent of effects on other cations.[123] Acid loss depends partially on sodium delivery to the distal nephron.[123] Mineralocorticoids may also exert some effects on calcium and magnesium homeostasis. These also appear to be secondary responses to sodium effects.[11]

Control of secretion

Renin-angiotensin system. The primary control of aldosterone release in humans is the renin-angiotensin system (Fig. 66-3).[11,207] Renin, synthesized in the kidney, acts on hepatic angiotensinogen to form angiotensin I, a decapeptide converted in the lung to angiotensin II by cleavage of two amino acids. Angiotensin II is responsible for the stimulation of aldosterone synthesis and release and is a potent vasoconstrictor also. This compound may be further modified to desaspartyl angiotensin II, also called angiotensin III, a seven–amino acid compound with potent aldosterone-stimulating properties but fewer vasopressor effects.[83] Angiotensinogenases, which are present in many tissues, inactivate these compounds.[207]

Renin is synthesized primarily in the juxtaglomerular cells located in the media of renal afferent arterioles just proximal to the glomeruli.[207] All renal tubules, after forming a loop, return to the area of the glomerulus from which they arise and by traversing near the arterioles. At this point, tubular epithelial cells, characterized by tall columnar cells with large nuclei, come in close contact with the juxtaglomerular cells. This region of the distal tubule is termed the *macula densa;* together with the juxtaglomerular cells, it forms the juxtaglomerular apparatus. These cells sense changes in the gradient of mean intra-arterial to interstitial pressure and respond by secreting renin. When the pressure gradient is large, renin is inhibited; narrowing of the gradient causes release. Thus a decrease in afferent blood pressure will increase renin release and subsequent vasoconstriction and conservation of salt and water. The sodium concentration of the fluid in the distal tubule also affects renin release.[218] Secondary influences include beta-adrenergic pathways to the kidney,[79] potassium levels in blood,[1] and prostaglandins.[207]

Angiotensin II and perhaps III are the most potent stimulators of aldosterone release.[207] Although angiotensin II and perhaps III exert some effect (like ACTH) on the conversion of cholesterol to ΔE^4-pregnenolone,[11,107,207] the primary mechanism of control over aldosterone formation exerted by these compounds appears to be via increasing the conversion of corticosterone to aldosterone.[11,107,207] This effect seems to be independent of adenyl cyclase or cyclic AMP formation.[77]

Angiotensin II binds to a specific receptor on the surface

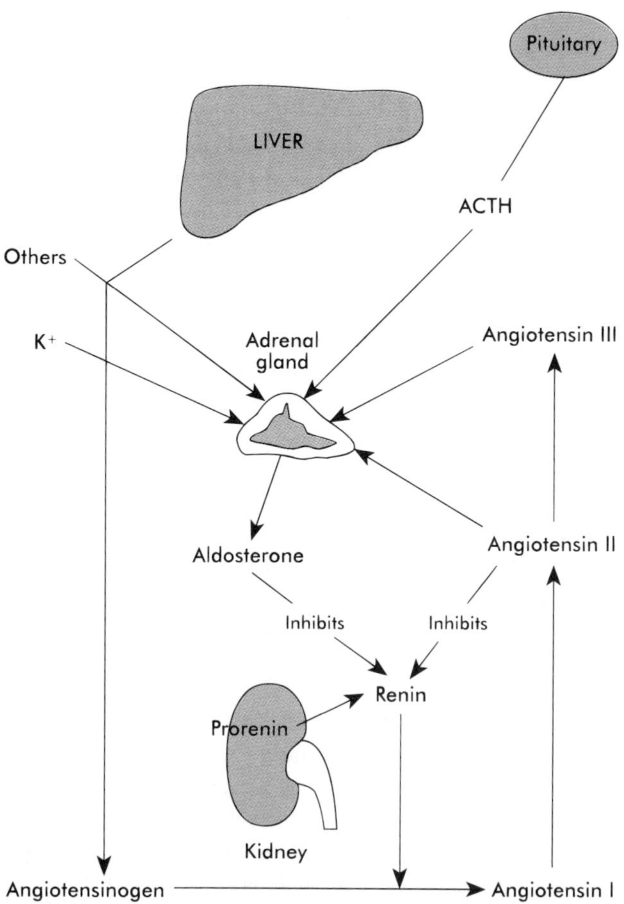

Fig. 66-3. Control of aldosterone secretion.

of cells in the zona glomerulosa and stimulates phosphatidylinositol hydrolysis, with resultant calcium mobilization, increased levels of phosphatidylinositol and phosphatidic acid, and activation of protein kinase C.[66] These steps then lead to enhanced cleavage of cholesterol side chains, as well as the previously mentioned changes in steroidogenesis.

Potassium. Increased potassium stimulates aldosterone secretion, whereas decreased potassium inhibits secretion.[67,74,126] These actions are exerted directly on the adrenal gland[207] and these are independent of sodium or renin-angiotensin effects.[66,67,74,126] In anephric patients, K^+ levels probably represent the major control mechanism for aldosterone release. Altered potassium results in changes both in the synthesis of ΔE^4-pregnenolone and corticosterone, as well as aldosterone itself.[126] Changes as small as 0.1 mEq/l can result in significant alterations in aldosterone production.[207] A direct effect on membrane depolarization with increased uptake of calcium, synthesis of phospholipids, and altered levels of cyclic AMP have been postulated.[66,67,104]

ACTH. Aldosterone secretion in response to sodium depletion may be under the control of ACTH (see Fig. 66-3). ACTH injection in humans increases aldosterone in the blood, presumably via a mass-action effect caused by increased conversion of cholesterol to γD^4-pregnenolone.[11,207]

Serum sodium. In isolated perfused adrenal glands, decreased sodium increases aldosterone secretion, *whereas increased sodium* has the opposite effect.[207] These effects appear to be mediated via renin but may also occur independently.[181]

Dopamine. Aldosterone release may be inhibited by dopaminergic mechanisms. The response of bovine adrenal cells to angiotensin II infusion is blunted by dopamine, although basal production of aldosterone is unaffected.[11]

Others. Growth hormone, prolactin, and pituitary factors other than ACTH (e.g., endorphins) modify aldosterone secretion. Acidosis stimulates aldosterone release.[11,207]

Pharmacokinetics and pharmacodynamics

Most aldosterone circulates unbound, and the free fraction of total aldosterone remains relatively constant. Some binding to albumin, erythrocytes, or CBG has been reported, but dissociation occurs so quickly that essentially all aldosterone is biologically available.[11] Circadian rhythms of spontaneous aldosterone release occur, and episodic release has been reported.[99] These alterations tend to be much less substantial than those noted in serum cortisol. The hormone is degraded by the liver, with the metabolic pathway being exclusively dependent on hepatic blood flow. Half-life is less than 15 minutes. Urinary metabolites tend to be conjugated to glucuronide, whereas some represents a modification to 21-deoxytetrahydroaldosterone, which appears to arise from eneterohepatic recirculation of tetrahydroaldosterone.[11]

Hormone deficiency

Mineralocorticoid deficiency induces hypovolemia, hyperkalemia, hyponatremia, hypochloremic acidosis, and hemoconcentration.[11,27] In general, the process is well-tolerated in the unstressed individual with normal sodium intake. Distal tubular sodium resorption and secretion of potassium and hydrogen ions are decreased and account for the clinical findings. The latter two are exacerbated by the decreased glomerular filtration, which serves to conserve sodium and water but results in decreased delivery of sodium to the distal tubule with impaired exchange of K^+ and H^+. Ultimately, this can lead to hypotension, vascular collapse, dysrhythmias, and cardiac arrest.[11,27,208]

Medications of importance to the anesthesiologist that are associated with mineralocorticoid deficiency include prolonged heparin administration and nonsteroidal anti-inflammatory drugs. Other conditions associated with this disorder include diabetes, renal insufficiency, hypokalemia, nephrectomy, inborn errors of metabolism, tumors of the sella turcica, and administration of steroid replacements with inadequate mineralocorticoid activity.[11,27]

Hormone excess

Primary hyperaldosteronism, or Conn's syndrome, is characterized by hypokalemia, sodium retention, and hypertension.[39] Because there are renal mechanisms to compensate for sodium retention, most of the manifestations of the hormonal excess will be mild, especially if sodium is restricted. Alkalosis may occur as acid is lost. In severe cases, polyuria, polydypsia, nocturia, weakness, and paresthesias or tetany may occur.[27] Primary hyperaldosteronism is most often due to adrenal tumors or hyperplasia. Secondary hyperaldosteronism occurs with congestive heart failure, nephrosis, cirrhosis, dehydration, as with chronic diuretic use, pregnancy (perhaps with exacerbation in toxemia), oral contraceptive use, and Bartter's syndrome; these often represent conditions in which effective blood volume is reduced. Other than in dehydration, edema is common and potassium wasting unusual, because little sodium is delivered distally and little exchange of K^+ or H^+ is necessary.[27,208]

Exogenous Steroids

The various steroid preparations have different relative potencies and different mineralocorticoid potency. A compendium of commonly available glucocorticoid preparations and their relative potencies and mineralocorticoid activity is presented in Table 66-2.

Adrenocorticoids and Anesthesia: Interactions Between Corticosteroids and Anesthetics

Opioids

When ACTH is cleaved from pro-opiomalonocortin, the residual molecules can be converted to a number of compounds with endogenous opioid properties. This has led several individuals to postulate potential interactions between steroids and opioids. To date, no such connection has been demonstrated, although bilateral adrenalectomy increases morphine potency and decreases its metabolism.

Etomidate and adrenal suppression

A number of studies have focused on the effects of etomidate on adrenal secretion; these studies demonstrate that **even a single dose of etomidate can suppress adrenal function.** Etomidate inhibits both cholesterol side-chain cleavage, as well as 11-β-hydroxylase (see Fig. 66-1) in both rats and humans.[50,219] **Use of etomidate in single-bolus form and both short and prolonged continuous infusions resulted in decreased circulating cortisol and increased ACTH for up to approximately 24 hours after the bolus or cessation of infusion.** Response to ACTH administration is blunted by etomidate. The only major adverse clinical effects associated with etomidate use are those associated with use in intensive care units,[72,112,113] where increased mortality and hypotension were observed in patients receiving etomidate as part of overall intensive care unit management.

Table 66-2 Exogenous glucocorticoid preparations

Compound	Trade name	Relative glucocorticoid potency	Relative glucocorticoid potency
Cortisone		1.0	1.0
Hydro-cortisone/cortisol	Solu-cortef, A-hydroCort	0.8	0.8
Prednisone	Deltasone	3.5–4.5	—
Prednisolone	Hydeltrasol	4.0	0.8
Methylpred-nisolone	Solu-Medrol	5.0	0.5
Triamcinolone	Aristocort, Aristospan, Cinelone, Kenalog	5.0	0.0
Dexametha-sone	Decadron, Hexadrol	30.0	0.0

ANTIBIOTICS

A full discussion of antibiotics is beyond the scope of this text. We will address two major issues: (1) the use of antibiotics as prophylaxis for wound infection or endocarditis; and (2) the interactions between antibiotics and drugs commonly administered by anesthesiologists.

Prophylactic Antibiotics

Prophylaxis for wound infection

Incidence of infection. The prevention of infection has become an increasingly important component of perioperative care. SIRS and the associated Multiple Organ Dysfunction Syndrome (MODS) account for an increasing percentage of perioperative mortality and morbidity. Although several of the basic methods prevent infection, such as meticulous surgical technique and the maintenance of appropriate host local and systemic physiology, are well documented,[30] it is increasingly clear that the major determinant for containing infection is the host resistance.[59] In turn, compromise of endogenous resistance can occur in the presence of a minute foreign body,[4,59] shock,[130] ischemia,[129] and immune impairment.[71] Even with uncomplicated procedures in "normal" patients, decreased immune function has been observed.[190] The contributions of anesthetics to this altered immunologic response are reviewed by Finlayson,[71] as well as Stevenson et al.[198] Studies have been performed to document the rate of infection and assess the use of antibiotics to compensate for acute immune deficiencies associated with the stress of surgery and anesthesia.[29] To prevent the potential hazards associated with misuse of antibiotics,[93] the Ad Hoc Committee of the American College of Surgeons Committee on Trauma established guidelines to classify surgical wounds in hope of defining appropriate candidates for prophylaxis.[2] This led to the commonly used scheme of classifying wounds as "clean," "clean-contaminated," "contaminated," and "dirty."

Use of antibiotics in clean-contaminated, contaminated, and dirty wounds has been demonstrated to be valuable in a number of clinical trials.[96,150] **In addition, data indicate a role for antibiotic prophylaxis in extensive procedures such as cardiac surgery**[97] **or procedures involving the placement of prosthetic devices despite their "clean" nature.** Further, several recent reports indicate a significant infection rate in "clean" procedures such as breast surgery or herniorrhaphy. Platt et al.[160] conducted a randomized, prospective double-blind trial of a single dose of cefonicid in breast surgery or inguinal herniorrhaphy and demonstrated a substantial reduction in the incidence and risk of infection. Although it is not clear that these results can be extended to other "clean" procedures, a reappraisal of antibiotic use and wound classification may well be appropriate. Anesthesiologists can expect to see the great majority of their patients receiving antibiotics before and during the operative procedure.

Overuse of antibiotics in the absence of documented infection is an important contributor to resistant strains of bacteria and resultant hospital-acquired infection. Thus, although the prophylactic use of antibiotics in the perioperative period may be warranted, their use should be limited to a short (24-hour) interval.

Timing and duration of prophylaxis. Antibiotic therapy is ineffective if delayed until the postoperative period.[199] As emphasized by Burke,[30] there appears to be a short period during which host mechanisms may be rendered inoperative and during which bacterial innoclulation occurs. Burke's early work has demonstrated that antibiotic coverage instituted before wound contamination renders susceptible bacteria inactive.[29] **Antibiotic prophylaxis should be instituted sufficiently before the incision (usually 30 to 120 min) to ensure that adequate tissue levels have been obtained and continued at least until the wound is closed.** Bergamini and Polk[14] recommended that parenteral antibiotics be given 30 minutes before an operation and indicate that tissue levels should remain adequate for several hours. Extending coverage beyond 24 hours is unnecessary, needlessly expensive, and may actually increase the risk of infection. Appropriate drugs, doses, and regimens are detailed in a number of reviews.[30,128,130,231]

Endocarditis prophylaxis

Prophylaxis for endocarditis is generally recommended for patients considered at risk who are undergoing procedures associated with bacteremia.[47] Conditions believed to be associated with a risk of endocarditis and some conditions in which prophylaxis is not recommended are noted in Box 66-2. Procedures associated with significant risk for bacteremia and endocarditis and some not believed to pose a risk are detailed in Box 66-3. Specific drug recommenda-

BOX 66-2
PATIENT CONDITIONS ASSOCIATED WITH ENDOCARDITIS RISK

Prophylaxis recommended in presence of:
- Prosthetic heart valve or other prosthetic material
- Previous infective endocarditis
- Most congenital heart defects
- Rheumatic and other acquired valvular heart diseases, even after surgical correction
- Hypertrophic cardiomyopathy
- Mitral valve prolapse with regurgitation

Prophylaxis not recommended in:
- Isolated secundum atrial septal defects
- Operations more than 6 months after repair of secundum atrial septal defects, ventricular septal defects, or patent ductus arteriosus
- Previous coronary bypass surgery
- Mitral valve prolapse without regurgitation
- Physiologic, functional, or innocent heart murmurs
- Previous Kawasaki's disease without valvular dysfunction
- Previous rheumatic fever without valvular disease
- Cardiac pacemakers or implantable defibrillators

BOX 66-3
PROCEDURES ASSOCIATED WITH ENDOCARDITIS RISK

Prophylaxis recommended for:
- Dental procedures causing bleeding, including cleaning
- Tonsillectomy or adenoidectomy
- Surgical operations involving intestinal or respiratory mucosa
- Rigid bronchoscopy
- Esophageal or gastric sclerotherapy
- Esophageal dilitation
- Gall bladder surgery
- Cystoscopy
- Urethral dilation
- Urethral catheterization in presence of urinary tract infection
- Urinary tract surgery in presence of infection
- Prostate surgery
- Incision and drainage of infected tissue
- Vaginal hysterctomy
- Vaginal bleeding in presence of infection

Prophylaxis not recommended in:
- Dental procedures not likely to cause mucosal or gingival bleeding
- Injection of intraoral local anesthetics
- Shedding of primary teeth
- Typanostomy tube insertion
- Endotracheal intubation
- Flexible bronchoscopy, even with biopsy
- Cardiac catheterization
- Gastrointestinal endoscopy even with biopsy
- Cesarean section
- In the absence of infection:
  - Urethral catheterization
  - Dilation and curettage
  - Uncomplicated vaginal delivery
  - Therapeutic abortion
  - Elective sterilization procedures
  - Insertion or removal of intrauterine devices

Table 66-3 Recommended regimens for endocarditis prophylaxis

Drug	Pediatric dose	Adult dose	Regimen
For dental, oral, and upper-respiratory procedures in patients at risk			
Amoxicillin	50 mg/kg	3 g	Orally 1 hr before
	25 mg/kg	1.5 g	Orally 6 hr later
If penicillin allergic:			
Erythromycin ethylsuccinate	20 mg/kg	800 mg	Orally 2 hr before, 6 hr later
or			
Erythromycin stearate	10 mg/kg	400 mg	Orally 2 hr before, 6 hr later
or			
Clindamycin	10 mg/kg	300 mg	Orally 1 hr before
	5 mg/kg	150 mg	Orally 6 hr later
For dental, oral, and upper-respiratory procedures in patients at high risk (prosthetic valves, history of endocarditis, surgically constructed pulmonary/systemic shunts or conduits)			
Ampicillin	50 mg/kg	2 g	Intravenous 30 min before
and Gentamycin	2 mg/kg	80–120 mg	Intravenous or intramuscular 30 min before
Follow-up with			
Amoxicillin	25 mg/kg	1.5 g	Orally 6 hr later
or			
Repeat initial regimen 8 hr later			
If penicillin/ampicillin allergic:			
Vancomycin	20 mg/kg	1 g	Intravenous 1 hr infusion started 1 hr before procedure
With or without gentamycin	2 mg/kg	80–120 mg	Intravenous or intramuscular 15 min before
Recommendations for gastrointestinal or genitourinary procedures:			
Ampicillin	50 mg/kg	2 g	Intravenous 30 min before
and Gentamycin	2 mg/kg	80–120 mg	Intravenous or intramuscular 30 min before
Follow-up with			
Amoxicillin	25 mg/kg	1.5 g	Orally 6 hr later
or			
Repeat initial regimen 8 hr later			
If penicillin/ampicillin allergic:			
Vancomycin	20 mg/kg	1 g	Intravenous 1 hr infusion started 1 hr before procedure
With or without Gentamycin	2 mg/kg	80–120 mg	Intravenous or intramuscular 15 min before
Repeat initial regimen 8 hr later			

tions are listed in Table 66-3. Of particular importance to the anesthesiologist is the risk of endocarditis associated with airway manipulation. Berry et al.[15] found a significant incidence of bacteremia after both orotracheal and nasotracheal intubation. Baltch et al.[9] found that 33% of patients intubated nasally for dental surgery had bacteremia, whereas Berry et al.[16] found a 12% incidence in children undergoing dental procedures. Berber et al.[13] dispute these findings, noting that they found no incidence with orotracheal or nasotracheal intubation for general anesthesia. More recently, Dinner et al.[55] have addressed the issue from the standpoint of trauma to the nasal mucosa and the effects of topical vasoconstrictors. Of 54 nasally intubated patients, all having intubations designated as atraumatic, 3 patients had positive blood cultures.

Table 66-4 Antibiotics known to interact with neuromuscular blocking agents

Antibiotic	Potentiation of D-tubocurarine	Potentiation of succinylcholine	Reversal of blockade by neostigmine	Reversal of blockade by calcium
Neomycin	Yes	Yes	Effective	Effective
Streptomycin	Yes	Yes	Effective	Effective
Gentamycin	Yes	Not studied	May be effective	Effective
Kanamycin	Yes	Yes	May be effective	May be effective
Neomycin	Yes	Yes	Effective	Effective
Polymixin A	Yes	Not studied	Not effective	Not effective
Polymixin B	Yes	Yes	Effective	Not effective
Colistin	Yes	Yes	Not effective	May be effective
Tetracycline	Yes	No	Partially effective	Partially effective
Clindamycin	Yes	Not studied	Partially effective	Partially effective

None of the 21 patients who had traumatic intubation had evidence of bacteremia, and 2 of the 3 patients with positive cultures had been treated with topical vasoconstrictors. The authors concluded that nasotracheal intubation poses a risk for bacteremia, but this is not related to mucosal damage and is not aided by vasoconstrictor application. Current guidelines by the American Heart Association do not recommend the use of antibiotics for simple endotracheal intubation. These guidelines stress that in high-risk patients (i.e., those with a prosthetic heart valve, a history of endocarditis, or a surgically constructed pulmonary/systemic shunt or conduit), prophylaxis may beappropriate.

Interactions Between Antibiotics and Muscle Relaxants

Potentiation of neuromuscular blockage by antibiotics represents the classic example of agents administered by anesthesiologists interacting with antibiotics. Although other potential interactions have been postulated, none has proven to be clinically relevant. Antibiotic-induced muscle relaxation is capricious. In some instances, blockade can be antagonized with cholinomimetics and in others with calcium. Therefore, despite extensive work at elucidating the mechanism of blockade, the nature of this potential complication remains uncertain. Antibiotics known to affect the neuromuscular junction and the effects of neostigmine or calcium on reversal are noted in Table 66-4.

KEY POINTS

- The adrenal cortex is responsible for the secretion of three classes of hormones: (1) glucocorticoids, which primarily affect substrate metabolism; (2) mineralocorticoids, which are involved in the regulation of sodium, potassium, and acid/base homeostasis; and (3) sex hormones, primarily androgens.
- Biologic effects persist for 12 to 24 hours after the administration of cortisol.
- Hepatic metabolism is necessary to transform cortisol into inactive, water-soluble products, which are ultimately excreted as 17-hydroxycorticosteroids in the urine. Chronic hepatic insufficiency or hypothyroidism may decrease metabolism. In contrast, renal failure has little effect.
- Glucocorticoids exert their effects on specific intracellular protein receptors.
- The predominant effects of glucocorticoids involve the regulation of the mobilization and use of carbohydrate, protein, and lipids as fuel.
- A primary effect of glucocorticoids is to increase hepatic gluconeogenesis. This occurs both directly and via enhancement of the effects of glucagon and epinephrine.
- Cardiovascular responses to corticoid deficiency include ECG changes, hypotension, and decreased cardiac output that cannot be explained by fluid and electrolyte abnormalities alone and which cannot be corrected by salt and water repletion. Circulatory collapse during stress in Addisonian patients may reflect loss of the enhanced response to catecholamines that is imparted by steroids.
- The most common causes of glucocorticoid deficiency are idiopathic (autoimmune) or arise secondary to cessation of chronic steroid administration.

- In response to increased circulating glucocorticoids, the blood pressure is increased. This may reflect enhanced vascular reactivity to catecholamines and other vasoconstrictors or an increased cardiac output from either a direct inotropic effect involving increased coupling of beta receptors and adenyl cyclase or enhanced responsiveness to catecholamines.
- Significant thinning of bone matrix, osteoporosis, and pathologic fractures may result. These problems represent some of the main limitations to long-term steroid use.
- Secretion of cortisol by the adrenal gland is regulated almost exclusively by ACTH, which initiates its effects via binding to a specific peptide receptor on the surface of cell membranes.
- Outcome-based studies, although limited by design, indicate that there is an increased risk of death and major infectious complications in patients receiving high doses of glucocorticoids in the perioperative period.
- Administration of high doses of glucocorticoids in the perioperative period is associated with altered outcome in clinical reports and a higher mortality for a given level of risk as well as impaired wound healing and immune function in experimental animals and cell cultures.
- Exogenously administered glucocorticoids have varying amounts of mineralocorticoid activity. Thus the anesthesiologist caring for the patient taking a glucocorticoid preparation may be faced with either excessive mineralocorticoid activity or, in the patient taking a glucocorticoid with weak mineralocorticoid effects, relative mineralocorticoid deficiency.
- The primary action of mineralocorticoids is to conserve sodium, with the most important physiologic effects being exerted on the renal connecting segment and collecting tubules.
- Mineralocorticoid deficiency induces hypovolemia, hyperkalemia, hyponatremia, hypochloremic acidosis, and hemoconcentration.
- Primary hyperaldosteronism, or Conn's syndrome, is characterized by hypokalemia, sodium retention, and hypertension.
- Use of etomidate in single-bolus form and both short and prolonged continuous infusions resulted in decreased circulating cortisol and increased ACTH for up to approximately 24 hours after the bolus or cessation of infusion.
- Use of antibiotics in "clean-contaminated," "contaminated," and "dirty" wounds has been demonstrated to be valuable in a number of clinical trials. In addition, data indicate a role for antibiotic prophylaxis in extensive procedures such as cardiac surgery or procedures involving the placement of prosthetic devices, despite their "clean" nature.
- Antibiotic prophylaxis should be instituted sufficiently before the incision (usually 30 to 120 min) to ensure that adequate tissue levels have been obtained and continued at least until the wound is closed.

KEY REFERENCES

Baxter JD, Tyrrell JB: The adrenal cortex. In Felig P, Baxter JD, Broadus AE, et al, editors: *Endocrinology and metabolism,* New York, 1987, McGraw-Hill.

Besdovsky HO, Del Rey A, Klusman I, et al: Cytokines as modulators of the hypothalamic-pituitary-adrenal axis, *J Ster Biochem Molec Biol* 40:613–618, 1991.

Bromberg JS, Alfrey EJ, Barker CF, et al: Adrenal suppression and steroid supplementation in renal transplant recipients, *Transplantation* 51:385–390, 1991.

Dajani AS, Bisno AL, Chung KJ, et al: Prevention of bacterial endocarditis. Recommendations by the American Heart Association, *JAMA* 264:2919–2922, 1990.

Dinner M, Tjeuw M, Artusio JF Jr: Bacteremia as a complication of nasotracheal intubation, *Anesth Analg* 66:460, 1987.

Naito Y, Fukata J, Tamai S, et al: Biphasic changes in hypothalamic-pituitary-adrenal function during the early recovery period after major abdominal surgery, *J Clin Endocrinol Metab* 73:111–117, 1991.

Naito Y, Tamai S, Shingu K, et al: Responses of plasma adrenocorticotropic hormone, cortisol and cytokines during and after upper abdominal surgery, *Anesthesiology* 77:426–431, 1992.

Platt R, Zaleznik CDF, Hopkins CC, et al: Perioperative antibiotic prophylaxis for herniorrhaphy and breast surgery, *N Engl J Med* 322:153, 1990.

Salem M, Tainsh RE Jr, Bromberg J, Loriaux DL, Chernow B: Perioperative glucocorticoid coverage: A reassessment 42 years after emergence of a problem, *Ann Surg* 219: 416–425, 1994.

Swingle WW, DaVanzo JP, Crossfield HC, et al: Glucocorticoids and maintenance of blood pressure and plasma volume of adrenalectomized dogs subjected to stress, *Proc Soc Exp Biol Med* 100:610–617, 1959.

Udelsman R, Ramp J, Gallucci WT, et al: Adaptation during surgical stress. A re-evaluation of the role of glucocorticoids, *J Clin Invest* 77:1377, 1986.

Woloski BM, Smith EM, Meyer WJ III, et al: Corticotropin-releasing activity of monokines, *Science* 230:1035–1037, 1985.

REFERENCES

1. Abbrecht PH, Vander AJ: Effects of chronic potassium deficiency on plasma renin activity, *J Clin Invest* 49:1510, 1970.
2. Ad Hoc Committee of the American College of Surgeons Committee on Trauma, National Research Council Division of Medical Sciences: factors influencing the incidence of wound infection, *Ann Surg* 160:S32, 1964.
3. Aguilera G, Harwood JP, Wilson JX, et al: Mechanisms of action of corticotropin releasing factor and other regulators of corticotropin release in rat pituitary cells, *J Biol Chem* 258:8039, 1983.
4. Anderson JR, Bucharth F, Larsen HW, et al: Polyglycolic acid, silk and topical ampicillin: their use in hernia repair and cholecytectomy, *Arch Surg* 115:293, 1980.
5. Axelrod J, Reisine TD: Stress hormones: Their interaction and regulation, *Science* 224:452, 1984.
6. Baker BL, Whitaker WL: Interference with wound healing by local action of adrenocortical steroids, *Endocrinology* 46:544, 1950.
7. Ballard PL: Delivery and transport of glucocorticoids to target cells. In Baxter JD, Rousseau GG, editors: *Glucocorticoid hormone action,* New York, 1979, Springer-Verlag.
8. Baltch AL, Hammer MC, Smith RP, et al: Comparison of the effects of three adrenal corticosteroids on human granulocyte function against Pseudomonas aeruginosa, *J Trauma* 26:525–533, 1986.
9. Baltch AL, Pressman HL, Hammer MC, et al: Bacteremia following dental extractions in patients with and without penicillin prophylaxis, *Am J Med Sci* 283:129, 1982.
10. Bar-Shavit Z, Kahn AJ, Pegg LE, et al: Glucocorticoids modulate macrophage surface oligosaccharides and their bone binding activity, *J Clin Invest* 73:754, 1984.
11. Baxter JD, Tyrrell JB: The adrenal cortex. In Felig P, Baxter JD, Broadus AE, et al, editors: *Endocrinology and metabolism,* New York, 1987, McGraw-Hill.
12. Bengele HH, McNamara ER, Alexander ER: Natriuresis after adrenal enucleation: effect of spironolactone and dexamethasone, *Am J Physiol* 233F:8, 1977.
13. Berber MA, Gastanaduy AS, Buckley JJ, et al: Risk of bacteremia after endotracheal intubation for general anesthesia, *South Med J* 7:1478, 1980.
14. Bergamini TG, Polk HC: *J Antimicrobial Chemother* 23:301, 1989.
15. Berry FA Jr, Blankenbaker WL, Ball CG: Comparison of bacteremia occurring with naostracheal and orotracheal intubation, *Anesth Analg* 52:873, 1973.
16. Berry FAS, Yarbrough S, Yarbrough N, et al: Transient bacteremia during dental manipulation in children, *Pediatrics* 51:476, 1973.
17. Besdovsky HO, Del Rey A, Klusman I, et al: Cytokines as modulators of the hypothalamic-pituitary-adrenal axis, *J Steroid Biochem Molec Biol* 40:613–618, 1991.
18. Besse JC, Bass AD: Potentiation by hydrocortisone of responses to catecholamines in vascular smooth muscle, *J Pharmacol Exp Ther* 154:224, 1966.
19. Bessey PQ, Watters JM, Aoki TT, et al: Combined hormonal infusion simulates the metabolic response to injury, *Ann Surg* 200:264, 1984.
20. Binder HJ: Effects of dexamethasone on electrolyte transport in the large intestine of the rat, *Gastroenterology* 75:212, 1978.
21. Binstock ML, Mundy GR: Effects of calcitonin and glucocorticoids in the hypercalcemia of malignancy, *Ann Intern Med* 93:269, 1980.
22. Bohnen JMA, Mustard RA, Schouten BD: Steroids, APACHE II score and the outcome of abdominal infection, *Arch Surg* 129:33–38, 1994.
23. Bohr DH: Contraction of vascular smooth muscle, *Can Med Assoc J* 90:174, 1964.
24. Bohr DH, Cummings G: Comparative potentiating action of various steroids on the contraction of vascular smooth muscle, *Fed Proc* 17:17, 1958.
25. Boykin J, deTorrente A, Erickson A, et al: Role of plasma vasopressin in impaired water excretion of glucocorticoid deficiency, *J Clin Invest* 62:738, 1978.
26. Bradlow HL, Mondor C, Zumoff B: Metabolism of cortoic acids in man, *J Clin Endocrinol Metab* 54:296, 1982.
27. Brand PH, Higgins JT Jr: Effects of adrenal hormones on water and electrolyte metabolism, In Mulrow PK, editor: *The adrenal gland.* New York, 1986, Elsevier.
28. Bromberg JS, Alfrey EJ, Barker CF, et al: Adrenal suppression and steroid supplementation in renal transplant recipients, *Transplantation* 51:385–390, 1991.
29. Burke JF: Effective period of preventive antibiotic action in experimental incisions and dermal lesions, *Surgery* 50:161, 1961.
30. Burke JF: The physiology of preventing infection: preventive antibiotics. In Burke JF, editor: *Surgical physiology,* 1983, WB Saunders.
31. Carter-Su C, Okomoto K: Effect of glucocorticoids on hexose transport in rat adipocytes, *J Biol Chem* 260:11091, 1985.
32. Castro-Magana M, Maddaiah VT, Collipp PJ, et al: Synergistic effects of growth hormone therapy on plasma levels of 11-deoxycortisol and cortisol in growth hormone deficient children, *J Clin Endocrinol Metab* 56:662, 1983.
33. Catalano RD, Stuve L, Ramachandran J: Characterization of corticotropin receptors in human adrenal cells, *J Clin Endocrinol* 62:300, 1986.
34. Chen TL, Cone CM, Morey-Holton E, et al: Glucocorticoid regulation of 1,25(OH)-2-vitamin D receptors in cultured mouse bone cells, *J Biol Chem* 257:13564, 1982.
35. Chen TL, Feldman D: Glucocorticoid potentiation of the adenosine 3′5′-monophosphate response to parathyroid hormone in cultured rat bone cells, *Endocrinology* 102:589, 1978.
36. Chernow B, Alexander R, Smallridge RC, et al: Hormonal responses to graded surgical stress, *Arch Intern Med* 147:1273, 1987.
37. Claire M, Oblin M-E, Steimer J-L, et al: Effect of adrenalectomy and aldosterone on modulation of mineralocorticoid receptors in rat kidney, *J Biol Chem* 256:142, 1981.
38. Clark AF, Tandler B, Vignos PJ: Glucocorticoid induced alterations in the rabbit heart, *Lab Invest* 47:603, 1982.
39. Conn JW: Primary hyperaldosteronism: new clinical syndrome, *J Lab Clin Med* 45: 3, 1955.
40. Connerly OM, Headon DR, Olson CD, et al: Intramitochondrial movement of adrenal sterol carrier protein with cholesterol in response to corticotropin, *Proc Natl Acad Sci U S A* 81:2970, 1984.
41. Cooper GM, Paterson JL, Ward ID, et al: Fentanyl and the metabolic response to gastric surgery, *Anaesthesia* 36:667, 1981.
42. Coufalik AH, Monder C: Stimulation of gluconeogenesis by cortisol in fetal rat liver in organ culture, *Endocrinology* 108:1132, 1981.
43. Cox M, Stevens RH, Singer I: The defense against hyperkalemia: the roles of insulin and aldosterone, *N Engl J Med* 299:525, 1978.
44. Cronin L, Cook D, Carlet J, et al: Corticosteroid treatment for sepsis: a critical appraisal and meta-analysis of the literature, *Crit Care Med* 23:1430–1439, 1995.
45. Cuthberson DP: Post-shock metabolic response, *Lancet* 1:433, 1942.
46. Czech MP, Fain JN: Dactinomycin inhibition of dexamethasone action on glucose metabolism in white fat cells, *Biochem Biophys Acta* 230:185, 1971.
47. Dajani AS, Bisno AL, Chung KJ, et al: Prevention of bacterial endocarditis. Recommendations by the American Heart Association, *JAMA* 264:2919–2922. 1990.
48. Dallman MF: Viewing the ventromedial hypothalamus from the adrenal gland, *Am J Physiol* 246R:1, 1984.
49. Davies AO, De Lean A, Lefkowitz RJ: Myocardial beta-adrenergic receptors from adrenalectomized rats: Impaired formation of high-affinity agonist-receptor complexes, *Endocrinology* 108:720, 1981.
50. De Coster R, Helmers JH, Noordiun H: Effect of etomidate on cortisol biosynthesis: site of action after induction of anesthesia, *Acta Endocrinologica* 110:526, 1985.
51. Degli Uberti EC, Patraglia F, Trasforini G, et al: Derorphin reduces the metapyrone-evoked release of adrenocorticotropin, beta-endorphin and beta lipotropin in man, *J Clin Endocrinol Metab* 61:1018, 1984.
52. De Sousa EB, Perrin MH, Insel TR, et al: Corticotropin-releasing factor receptors in rat forebrain: autoradiographic identification, *Science* 2234:1449, 1984.
53. De Sousa EB, Van Loon GR: D-ala2-met enkephalinamide, a potent opioid peptide, alters pituitary-adrenocortical secretion in rats, *Endocrinology* 111:1483, 1982.
54. De Vanzo JP, Crossfield HC, Swingle WW: Effect of various adrenal steroids on plasma magnesium and the electrocardiogram of adrenalectomized dogs, *Endocrinology* 68:825, 1958.

55. Dinner M, Tjeuw M, Artusio JF Jr: Bacteremia as a complication of nasotracheal intubation, *Anesth Analg* 66:460, 1987.
56. Divakaran P, Friedman N: A fast *in vitro* effect of glucocorticoids on hepatic lipolysis, *Endocrinology* 98:1550, 1976.
57. Downic WW, Gunn A, Paterson CR, et al: Hypercalcaemic crisis as a presentation of Addison disease, *Br Med J* 1:145, 1977.
58. Ebisui O, Fukata J, Murakami N, et al: Effects of IL-1 receptor antagonist and antiserum to TNF-a on LPS-induced plasma ACTH and corticosterone rise in rats, *Am J Physiol* 266:E986–E992, 1994.
59. Elek SD: Experimental staphylococcal infections in the skin of man, *Ann N Y Acad Sci* 65:85, 1956.
60. Engquist A, Backer OG, Jarnum S: Incidence of postoperative complications in patients subjected to surgery under steroid cover, *Acta Chir Scand* 140:343, 1974.
61. Erlich HP, Hunt TK: Effects of cortisone and vitamin A on wound healing, *Ann Surg* 167:324, 1968.
62. Estaban N, Loughlin T, Yergey A, et al: Daily cortisol production rate in man determined by stable isotope dilution, mass spectrometry, *J Clin Endocrinol Metab* 71:39–45, 1991.
63. Exton JH: Regulation of gluconeogenesis by glucocorticoids. In Baxter JD, Rousseau GG, editors: *Glucocorticoid hormone action,* New York, 1979, Springer-Verlag.
64. Fain JN: Inhibition of glucose transport in fat cells and activation of lipolysis by glucocorticoids. In Baxter JD, Rousseau GC, editors: *Glucocorticoid hormone action,* New York, 1979, Springer-Verlag.
65. Fain JN, Czech MP: Glucocorticoid effects on lipid mobilization and adipose tissue metabolism. In Blachko H, Sayers G, Smith AD, editors: *Handbook of physiology,* vol 6, Adrenal gland, Washington DC, 1975, American Physiologic Society.
66. Farese RV: Phospholipids as intermediates in hormone action, *Mol Cell Endocrinol* 35:1, 1984.
67. Farese RV, Larson RE, Sabir MA, et al: Effects of angiotensin II, K^+, adrenocorticotropin, serotonin, adenosine 3′5′-monophosphate, A23187, and EGTA on aldosterone synthesis and phospholipid metabolism in the rat adrenal zona glomerulosa, *Endocrinology* 113:1377, 1983.
68. Fehm HL, Voigt KH, Kummer G, et al: Differential and integral corticosteroid feedback effects on ACTH secretion in hypoadrenocorticism, *J Clin Invest* 63:247, 1979.
69. Findling JW, Adams ND, Lemann J Jr, et al: Vitamin D metabolites and parathyroid hormone in Cushing's syndrome: relationship to calcium and phosphorus homeostasis, *J Clin Endocrinol Metab* 54:1039, 1982.
70. Finlay WEI, McKee JI: Serum cortisol levels in severely stressed patients, *Lancet* 1:1414, 1982.
71. Finlayson DC: Immunologic changes in critically ill patients after anesthesia and surgery, *Anesthesiol Clin North Am* 7:883, 1989.
72. Fragen RJ, Shanks CA, Molteni A, et al: Effects of etomidate on hormonal response to surgical stress, *Anesthesiology* 61:652, 1984.
73. Fraser CG, Preuss FS, Bigford WD: Adrenal atrophy and irreversible shock associated with cortisone therapy, *JAMA* 149:1542–1543, 1952.
74. Fraser R, Mason PA, Buckingham JC, et al: The interaction of sodium and potassium states and ACTH and of angiotensin II in the control of corticosteroid secretion, *J Steroid Biochem Mol Biol* 11:1039, 1979.
75. Frieberg JM, Kinsella J, Sactor B: Glucocorticoids increase the Na^+/H^+ exchange and decrease Na^+ gradient dependent phosphate uptake in renal brush border membrane vesicles, *Proc Natl Acad Sci U S A* 79:4932, 1982.
76. Friedland J, Setton C, Silverstein E: Angiotensin converting enzyme induction by steroids in alveolar macrophages in culture, *Science* 197:64, 1977.
77. Fujita K, Aguilera G, Catt KJ: The role of cyclic AMP in aldosterone production by isolated glomerulosa cells, *J Biol Chem* 254:8567, 1979.
78. Fukata J, Usai T, Naitoh Y, et al: Effects of recombinant human interleukin-1α, -1β, 2 and 6 on ACTH synthesis and release in the mouse pituitary cell line AtT-20, *J Endocrinol* 122:33–39, 1989.
79. Ganong WF: Sympathetic effects on renin secretion: mechanisms and physiologic role, *Adv Exp Med Biol* 17:17, 1972.
80. Geheb M, Hercker E, Singer I, et al: Subcellular localization of aldosterone-induced proteins in toad urinary bladders, *Biochem Biophys Acta* 641:422, 1981.
81. Gibbs DM: Measurement of hypothalamic corticotropin factor in hypophyseal portal blood, *Fed Proc* 44:203, 1985.
82. Gilles GE, Linton EA, Lowry PJ: Corticotropin releasing activity of new CRF is potentiated several times by vasopressin, *Nature* 299:355, 1982.
83. Goodfriend TL, Peach MJ: Angiotensin III (des-aspartic acid)-angiotensin II: evidence and speculation for its role as an important agonist in the renin-angiotensin system, *Circ Res* 36(suppl I):38, 1975.
84. Goodwin JS, Atluru D, Dierakowdski S, et al: Mechanism of action of glucocorticoids-inhibition of T-cell proliferation and interleukin-2 production by hydrocortisone is reversed by leukotriene B4, *J Clin Invest* 77:1244–1250, 1986.
85. Gordon GS: Drug treatment of osteoporoses, *Annu Rev Pharmacol Toxicol* 18:253, 1978.
86. Graber AL, Ney RL, Nicholson WE, et al: Natural history of pituitary-adrenal recovery following long term suppression with corticosteroids, *J Clin Endocrinol Metab* 25:11, 1965.
87. Guillemin R, Vargo R, Rossier J, et al: Beta-endorphin and adrenocorticotropin are secreted concomitantly by the pituitary gland, *Science* 197:1367, 1977.
88. Gwynne JT, Strauss JF III: The role of lipoproteins in steroidogenesis and cholesterol metabolism in steroidogenic glands, *Endocr Rev* 3:299, 1982.
89. Haack D, Mohring J, Mohring B, et al: Comparative study on development of corticosterone and DOCA hypertension in rats, *Am J Physiol* 233F:403, 1977.
90. Hahn TJ, Halstead LR, Baran DT: Effects of short-term glucocorticoid administration on intestinal calcium absorption and circulating vitamin D metabolite concentrations in man, *J Clin Endocrinol Metab* 52:111, 1982.
91. Hall PF: Trophic stimulation of steroidogenesis: in search of the elusive trigger, *Recent Prog Horm Res* 41:1, 1985.
92. Healy DL, Hodgen GD, Schulte HM, et al: The thymus-adrenal connection: thymosin has corticotropin releasing activity in primate, *Science* 222:1353, 1983.
93. Hirschmann JV, Inui TS: Antimicrobial prophylaxis; a critique of recent trials, *Rev Infect Dis* 2:1, 1980.
94. Jost A: Problems of fetal endocrinology: the adrenal gland, *Recent Prog Horm Res* 22:541, 1966.
95. Jost A, Picon L: Hormonal control of fetal development and metabolism, *Adv Metab Disord* 4:123, 1970.
96. Kaiser AB: Antimicrobial prophylaxis in surgery, *N Engl J Med* 315:1129, 1986.
97. Kaiser AB, Petracek MR, Lea JW, et al: Efficacy of cefazolin, cefamandol and gentamycin as prophylactic agents in cardiac surgery; results of a prospective, randomized double-blinded trial in 1030 patients, *Ann Surg* 206:791, 1987.
98. Kalsner S: Mechanism of hydrocortisone potentiation of responses to epinephrine and norepinephrine in rabbit aorta, *Circ Res* 24:383, 1969.
99. Katz FH, Romfh P, and Smith JA: Diurnal variation of plasma aldosterone, cortisol and renin activity in supine man, *J Clin Endocrinol Metab* 40:125, 1975.
100. Kehlet H, Binder C: Adrenocortical function and clinical course during and after surgery in unsupplemented glucocorticoid treated patients, *Brit J Anaesth* 45:1043, 1973.
101. Keller-Woods ME, Dallman MF: Corticosteroid inhibition of ACTH secretion, *Endocr Rev* 5:1, 1984.
102. Kinney JM, Duke JH, Long CL, et al: Tissue fuel and weight loss after injury, *J Clin Pathol* 23(14):65, 1970.
103. Knudsen L, Christiansen LA, Lorentzen JE: Hypotension during and after operation in glucocorticoid treated patients, *Br J Anaesth* 53:295.
104. Kojima I, Kojima K, Rasmussen H: Role of calcium and cAMP in the actions of adrenocorticotropin on aldosterone secretion, *J Biol Chem* 260:4248, 1985.
105. Kostyo JL, Redmond AF: Role of protein synthesis in the inhibitory action of adrenal steroid hormones on amino acid transport by muscle, *Endocrinology* 79:531, 1966.
106. Krakoff LR, Elijovich F: Cushing's syndrome and exogenous glucocorticoid hypertension, *Clin Endocrinol Metab* 10:479, 1981.
107. Kramer RE, Gallant S, Brownie AC: Actions of angiotensin II on aldosterone biosynthesis in the rat adrenal cortex, *J Biol Chem* 255:3442, 1980.
108. Krieger DT: The multiple faces of pro-opiomelanocortin, a prototype precursor molecule, *Clin Res* 31:342, 1983.
109. Kreutner W, Goldberg ND: Dependence on

insulin of the apparent hydrocortisone activation of hepatic glycogen synthetase, *Proc Natl Acad Sci USA* 58:1515, 1967.
110. Lambertys SWJ, Verleun T, Oosterom R, et al: Corticotropin releasing factor (ovine) and vasopressin exert a synergistic effect on adrenocorticotropin release in man, *J Clin Endocrin Metab* 58:298, 1984.
111. Lan NC, Karin M, Nguyen T, et al: Mechanism of glucocorticoid hormone action, *J Steroid Biochem Mol Biol* 20:77, 1984.
112. Ledingham IM, Finlay WEI, Watt I, et al: Etomidate and adrenocortical function, *Lancet* 1:1434, 1983.
113. Ledingham IM, Watt I: Influence of sedation on mortality in critically ill multiple trauma patients, *Lancet* 1:1270, 1983.
114. Lefer AM: Corticosteroids and circulatory function. In Blashko H, Sayers G, Smith AD, editors: *Handbook of physiology,* vol 6, Adrenal gland, Washington DC, 1975, American Physiology Society.
115. Lefering R, Neugebauer EAM: Steroid controversy in sepsis and septic shock: a meta-analysis, *Crit Care Med* 23:1294–1303, 1995.
116. Lehtinen AM, Fyhrquist F, Kivalo I: The effect of fentanyl on arginine vasopressin and cortisol secretion during anesthesia, *Anesth Analg* 63:25, 1984.
117. Lerner AB, Buettner-Janusch J: The structure of human corticotropin (adrenocorticotrophic hormone), *J Biol Chem* 236: 2970, 1961.
118. Lewis L, Robinson RF, Yee J, et al: Fatal adrenal cortical insufficiency precipitated by surgery during prolonged continuous cortisone infusion, *Ann Intern Med* 39:116–125, 1953.
119. Livingston JN, Lockwood DH: Effect of glucocorticoids on the glucose transport system of isolated fat cells, *J Biol Chem* 250:8353, 1975.
120. Long CL, Birkhahn RH, Geiger JW, et al: Urinary excretion of 3-methylhistidine: an assessment of muscle protein catabolism in adult normal subjects and during malnutrition, sepsis and skeletal trauma, *Metabolism* 30:765, 1981.
121. Manabe S, Bucala R, Cerami A: Nonenzymatic addition of glucocorticoids to lens proteins in steroid induced cataracts, *J Clin Invest* 74:1803, 1984.
122. Marks LJ, Donovan MJ, Duncan FJ, et al: Adrenocortical response to surgical operation in patients treated with corticosteroids or corticotropin prior to surgery, *J Clin Endocrinol Metab* 19:1458–1470, 1959.
123. Marver D, Kokko JP: Renal target sites and the mechanism of action of aldosterone, *Min Elect Metab* 9:1, 1983.
124. Mastorakos G, Chrousos GP, Weber JS: Recombinant interleukin-6 activates the hypothalamic-pituitary-adrenal axis in humans, *J Clin Endocrinol Metab* 77:1690–1694, 1993.
125. Mayer M, Rosen F: Interaction of glucocorticoids and androgens with skeletal muscle, *Metabolism* 26:937, 1977.
126. McKena TJ, Island DP, Nicholson WE, et al: The effects of potassium on early and late steps in aldosterone biosynthesis in cells of the zona glomerulosa, *Endocrinology* 103:1411, 1978.
127. McPartland RP: Metabolic and pharmacologic actions of glucocorticoids. In Mulrow PK, editor: *The adrenal gland,* New York, 1986, Elsevier.
128. *Med Let* 31:105, 1989.
129. Miles AA: Natural resistance to infection, *Ann N Y Acad Sci* 66:356, 1956.
130. Miles AA, Mile BM, Burke JF: The value and duration of defense reactions of the skin to primary lodgement of bacteria, *Br J Exp Path* 38:79, 1957.
131. Moore FD: Bodily changes in surgical convalescence. I. The normal sequence–observations and interpretations, *Ann Surg* 137:289, 1953.
132. Morris DJ: The metabolism and action of mineralocorticoids, *Endocr Rev* 2:234, 1981.
133. Moura AM, Worcel M: Direct action of aldosterone on transmembrane 22Na efflux from arterial smooth muscle: rapid and delayed effects, *Hypertension* 6:425, 1984.
134. Mujais SK, Checkal MA, Jones WJ, et al: Regulation of renal Na-K-ATPase in the rat, *J Clin Invest* 73:13, 1984.
135. Mujais SK, Chekal MA, Jones WJ, et al: Modulation of renal sodium-potassium-adenosine triphosphatase activity by aldosterone, *J Clin Invest* 76:170, 1985.
136. Munck A: Steroid concentration and tissue integrity as factors determining the physiologic significance of effects of adrenal steroids *in vitro, Endocrinology* 77:356, 1965.
137. Munck A, Crabtree GR, Smith KA: Glucocortoid receptors and actions in rat thymocytes and immunologically-stimulated human peripheral lymphocytes. In Baxter JD, Rousseau GG, editors: *Glucocorticoid hormone action,* New York, 1979, Springer-Verlag.
138. Naito Y, Fukata J, Tamai S, et al: Biphasic changes in hypothalamic-pituitary-adrenal function during the early recovery period after major abdominal surgery, *J Clin Endocrinol Metab* 73: 111–117, 1991.
139. Naito Y, Tamai S, Shingu K, et al: Responses of plasma adrenocorticotropic hormone, cortisol and cytokines during and after upper abdominal surgery, *Anesthesiology* 77:426–431, 1992.
140. Nakanishi S, Kita T, Nakamura M, et al: Nucleotide sequence of cloned cDNA for bovine corticotropin-beta-lipoprotein precursor, *Nature* 278:423, 1979.
141. Namba Y, Smith JB, Fox GS, et al: Plasma cortisol concentrations during caesarian section, *Br J Anaesth* 52:1027, 1980.
142. Nerup J: Addison's disease–clinical studies: a report of 108 cases, *Acta Endocrinol* 76:127, 1974.
143. Neta R, Perlstein R, Vogel S, et al: Role of interleukin 6 (IL-6) in protection from lethal irradiation and in endocrine responses to IL-1 and tumor necrosis factor, *J Exper Med* 175:689–694, 1992.
144. Neville AM, Mackay AM: The structure of the human adrenal cortex in health and disease, *Clin Endocrin Metab* 1:361, 1972.
145. Ng B, Hekkelman JW, Heersche JMN: The effect of cortisol on the adenosine 3′5′-monophosphate response to parathyroid hormone on bone *in vitro, Endocrinology* 104:1130, 1979.
146. Nichols NR, Llpyd CJ, Mendelsohn FAO, et al: Glucocorticoid induced proteins in bovine endothelial cells, *Mol Cell Endocrinol* 32:245, 1983.
147. Nichols NR, McNally M, Campbell JH, et al: Overlapping but not identical protein synthetic domains in cardiovascular cells in response to glucocorticoid hormones, *Hypertension* 2:663, 1984.
148. Nichols NR, Nguyen HH, Meyer WJ III: Physical separation of aortic corticoid receptors with type I and type II specificities, *J Steroid Biochem Mol Biol* 22:577, 1985.
149. Nichols NR, Tracy KE, Funder JW: Glucocorticoid effects on newly synthesized proteins in muscle and non-muscle cells cultured from neonatal rat hearts, *J Steroid Biochem Mol Biol* 21:487, 1984.
150. Nichols RL: Postoperative wound infection, *N Engl J Med* 307:1701, 1982.
151. Nicholson WE, Liddle RA, Puett D, et al: Adrenocorticotrophic hormone biotransformation, clearance and catabolism, *Endocrinology* 103:1344, 1978.
152. Nieuwenhuijzen-Kruseman AC, Linton EA, Lowry PJ, et al: Corticotropin releasing factor immunoreactivity in human gastrointestinal tract, *Lancet* 2:1245, 1982.
153. Nolten WE, Goldstein D, Lindstrom M, et al: Effects of cytokines on the pituitary-adrenal axis in cancer patients, *J Interferon Res* 13:349–357, 1993.
154. Park SC, Edelman IS: Dual action of aldosterone on toad bladder: Na^+ permeability and Na^+ pump modulation, *Am J Physiol* 246F:517, 1984.
155. Parker LN, Odell WD: Control of adrenal androgen secretion, *Endocr Rev* 1:392, 1980.
156. Parrillo JE, Fauci AS: Mechanisms of glucocorticoid action on immune processes, *Ann Rev Pharmacol Toxicol* 19:219, 1979.
157. Perlstein RS, Whitnall MH, Abrams JS, et al: Synergistic roles of interleukin-6, interleukin-1 and tumor necrosis factor in the adrenocorticotropin response to bacterial lipopolysaccharide *in vivo, Endocrinol* 132:946–952, 1993.
158. Peterson RE: Metabolism of adrenal corticosteroids. In Christy NP, editor: *The human adrenal cortex,* New York, 1971, Harper & Row.
159. Petty KJ, Kokko JP, Marver D: Secondary effect of aldosterone on Na-K-ATPase activity in the rabbit cortical collecting tubule, *J Clin Invest* 68:1514, 1981.
160. Platt R, Zaleznik CDF, Hopkins CC, et al: Perioperative antibiotic prophylaxis for herniorrhaphy and breast surgery, *N Engl J Med* 322:153, 1990.
161. Plumpton FS, Besser GM, Cole PV: Corticosteroid treatment and surgery. An investigation of the indications for steroid cover, *Anaesthesia* 24:3, 1969.
162. Rapp JP: Adrenal steroid biosynthesis and metabolism. In Mulrow PK, editor: *The adrenal gland,* New York, 1986, Elsevier.
163. Rinkler B, Sieber P, Rittel W, et al: Revised amino-acid sequences for porcine and human adrenocorticotrophic hormone, *Nature* 235:114, 1972.
164. Roberts BV, Jessop JD, Dore J: Effects of gold salts and prednisolone on inflammatory cells. II. Suppression of inflammation and phagocytosis in the rat, *Ann Rheum Dis* 32:301, 1973.

165. Rochefort GJ, Saffran M: Distribution of adrenocorticotrophic hormone in the pituitary gland, *Can J Biochem Physiol* 35:471, 1957.
166. Ross EJ, Marshall-Jones P, Friedman M: Cushing's syndrome: diagnostic criteria, *Q J Med* 35:149, 1966.
167. Rovetto MJ, Murphy RA, Lefer AM: Cardiac impairment in adrenal insufficiency: reduced ATPase activity of myocardial contractile proteins, *Circ Res* 26:419, 1970.
168. Sabastian A, Sutton JM, Hutler HM, et al: Effects of mineralocorticoid replacement therapy on renal acid-base homeostasis in adrenalectomized patients, *Kidney Intern* 18:762, 1980.
169. Saffran J: Receptors for hormones of the adrenal cortex. In Mulrow PK, editor: *The adrenal gland,* New York, 1986, Elsevier.
170. Saffran M: Control mechanisms in the pituitary-adrenal system. In Mulrow PK, editor: *The adrenal gland,* New York, 1986, Elsevier.
171. Saito E, Ichikawa Y, Homma M: Direct inhibitory effect of dexamethasone on steroidogenesis on human adrenal *in vivo, J Clin Endocrinol Metab* 48:861, 1979.
172. Salassa RM, Bennett WA, Keating FR, et al: Post-operative adrenal cortical insufficiency; occurrence in patients previously treated with cortisone, *JAMA* 152:1509, 1953.
173. Salem M, Tainsh RE Jr, Bromberg J, Loriaux DL, Chernow B: Perioperative glucocorticoid coverage: a reassessment 42 years after emergence of a problem, *Ann Surg* 219:416–425, 1994.
174. Sambhi MP, Weil MH, Udhoji VN: Acute pharmacologic effects of glucocorticoids: cardiac output and related hemodynamic changes in normal subjects and patients with shock, *Circ Res* 31:523, 1965.
175. Sampson PA, Brooke BN, Winstone NE: Biochemical confirmation of collapse due to adrenal failure, *Lancet* 1:1377, 1961.
176. Sanchez ER, Housley PR, Pratt WB: The molybdate-stabilized glucocorticoid binding complex of L-cells contains a 98-100k dalton steroid binding phosphoprotein and a 90 kdalton nonsteroid binding phosphoprotein that is part of the murine heat-shock complex, *J Steroid Biochem* 24:9–18, 1986.
177. Sandberg AA, Eik-nes K, Migeon C, et al: The metabolism of adrenal steroids in dying patients, *J Clin Endocrinol Metab* 16:1001–1016, 1956.
178. Sandberg N: Time relationship between administration of cortisone and wound healing in rats, *Acta Chir Scand* 127:446, 1964.
179. Schaffner A: Therapeutic concentrations of glucocorticoids suppress the antimicrobial activity of human macrophages without impairing their responsiveness to gamma interferon, *J Clin Invest* 76:1755–1764, 1985.
180. Schaeffer LD, Chenoweth M, Dunn A: Adrenal corticosteroid involvement in the control of phosphorylase in muscle, *Biochem Biophys Acta* 192:304, 1969.
181. Scheider EG, Radke KJ, Ulderich DA, et al: Effect of osmolality on aldosterone secretion, *Endocrinology* 116:1621, 1985.
182. Schwartz J, Keil LC, Maselli J, et al: Role of vasopressin in blood pressure regulation during adrenal insufficiency, *Endocrinology* 112:234, 1983.
183. Seitz HJ, Kaiser M, Krone W, et al: Physiological significance of glucocorticoids and insulin in the regeneration of hepatic gluconeogenesis during starvation in rats, *Metabolism* 25:1545, 1976.
184. Seruta T, Suzuki H, Handa M, et al: Multiple factors contribute to the pathogenesis of hypertension in Cushing's syndrome, *J Clin Endocrinol Metab* 62:275, 1986.
185. Shamoon H, Soman V, Sherwin RS: The influence of acute physiologic increments of cortisol on fuel metabolism and insulin binding to monocytes in normal humans, *J Clin Endocrinol Metab* 50:495, 1980.
186. Shima S, Komoriyama K, Hirai M, et al: Studies on cyclic nucleotides in the adrenal gland. XI. Adrenergic regulation of adenylate cyclase activity in the adrenal cortex, *Endocrinology* 114:325, 1984.
187. Siiteri PK, Murai JT, Hammond GL, et al: The serum transport of steroid hormones, *Recent Prog Horm Res* 38:457, 1984.
188. Simmons PS, Miles JM, Gerich JE, et al: Increased proteolysis. An effect of increased plasma cortisol within the physiologic range, *J Clin Invest* 73:412, 1984.
189. Simpson ER, Waterman MR: Regulation by ACTH of steroid hormone biosynthesis in the adrenal cortex, *Can J Biochem Cell Biol* 61:692, 1983.
190. Slade MS, Simmons RL, Yunis E: Immunodepression after major surgery in normal patients. *Surgery* 78:363, 1975.
191. Smyreng T, Karlberg BE, Kagedal B, et al: Physiologic cortisol substitution of long term steroid treated patients undergoing major surgery, *Br J Anaesth* 53:949, 1981.
192. Soderlin TR, Corbin JD, Park CR: Regulation of adenosine 3,5-monophosphate-dependent protein kinase. II. Hormonal regulation of the adipose tissue enzyme, *J Biol Chem* 248:1822, 1973.
193. Spath-Schwalbe E, Born J, Schrenzenmeier H, et al: Interleukin-6 stimulates the hypothalic-pituitary-adrenocortical axis in man, *J Clin Endocrinol Metab* 79:1212–1214, 1994.
194. Spiess J, Rivier J, Rivier CC, et al: Primary structure of corticotropin releasing factor from ovine hypothalamus, *Proc Natl Acad Sci USA* 78:6517, 1981.
195. Stalmans W, Laloux M: Glucocorticoids and hepatic glycogen metabolism. In Baxter JD, Rousseau GC, editors: *Glucocorticoid hormone action,* New York, 1979, Springer-Verlag.
196. Stanley TH, Berman L, Green O, et al: Plasma catecholamine and cortisol responses to fentanyl-oxygen anesthesia for coronary-artery operations, *Anesthesiology* 53:250, 1980.
197. Stanton B, Giebisch G, Klein-Robbenhaar G, et al: Effects of adrenalectomy and chronic adrenal corticosteroid replacement on potassium transport in rat kidney, *J Clin Invest* 75:1317, 1985.
198. Stevenson GW, Hall SC, Rudnick S, et al: The effects of anesthetic agents on the human immune response, *Anesthesiology* 72:542, 1990.
199. Stone HH, Haney BB, Kolb LD, et al: Prophylactic and preventing antibiotic therapy: timing, duration, and economics, *Ann Surg* 189:691, 1979.
200. Stoner HB, Heath DF: The effect of trauma on carbohydrate metabolism, *Br J Anaesthes* 45:244, 1970.
201. Sweep F, Rijnkels C, Hermus A: Activation of the hypothalamic-pituitary-adrenal axis by cytokines, *Acta Endocrinol* 125:84–91, 1991.
202. Swingle WW, DaVanzo JP, Crossfield HC, et al: Glucocorticoids and maintenance of blood pressure and plasma volume of adrenalectomized dogs subjected to stress, *Proc Soc Exp Biol Med* 100:610–617, 1959.
203. Swingle WW, Hays HW, Remington JW, et al: The effect of primary doses of deoxycorticosterone acetate in preventing circulatory failure and shock in the adrenalectomized dog, *Am J Physiol* 132:249–258, 1949.
204. Swingle WW, Parkins WM, Taylar AR, Hays HW: A study of circulatory failure and shock following trauma to the healthy, vigorous adrenalectomized dog, *Am J Physiol* 124:22–29, 1938.
205. Swingle WW, Pfiffner JJ, Vars HM, et al: The function of the adrenal cortex hormone and the cause of death from adrenal insufficiency, *Science* 77:58–64, 1933.
206. Swingle WW, Remington JW, Drill VS, et al: Differences among adrenal steroids with respect to their efficacy in protecting the adrenalectomized dog against circulatory failure, *Am J Physiol* 136:567–576, 1942.
207. Tan SY: Control of adrenal secretion of mineralocorticoids. In Mulrow PK, editor: *The adrenal gland,* New York, 1986, Elsevier.
208. Tan SY: Diseases of hyper- and hypomineralocorticoid production. In Mulrow PK, editor: *The adrenal gland,* New York, 1986, Elsevier.
209. Taskinen M-R, Nikkila EA, Pelkonen R, et al: Plasma lipoproteins, lipolytic enzymes, and very low density lipoprotein triglyceride turnover in Cushing's syndrome, *J Clin Endocrinol Metab* 57:619, 1983.
210. Thomas JP, El-Shaboury AH: Aldosterone secretion in steroid-treated patients with adrenal suppression, *Lancet* 1:623–625, 1971.
211. Tilders FJH, Berkenbosh F, Vermes I, et al: Role of epinephrine and vasopressin in control of the pituitary adrenal response to stress, *Fed Proc* 44:1985.
212. Tomas FM, Munro HN, Young VR: Effect of glucocorticoid administration on the rate of muscle protein breakdown *in vivo* in rats as measured by urinary excretion of N-methylhistidine, *Biochem J* 178:139, 1979.
213. Tominaga T, Fukata J, Naito Y, et al: Prostaglandin-dependent *in vitro* stimulation of adrenocortical steroidogenesis by interleukins, *Endocrinology* 128:526–531, 1991.
214. Tomita K, Pisano JJ, Knepper MA: Control of sodium and potassium transport in the cortical collecting duct of the rat, *J Clin Invest* 76:132, 1985.
215. Udelsman R, Norton JA, Jelenich SE, et al:

Responses of the hypothalamic-pituitary-adrenal and renin-angiotensin axes and the sympathetic system during controlled surgical and anesthetic stress, *J Clin Endocrinol Metab* 64:986, 1987.

216. Udelsman R, Ramp J, Gallucci WT, et al: Adaptation during surgical stress. A reevaluation of the role of glucocorticoids, *J Clin Invest* 77:1377, 1986.
217. Van Der Meer MJM, Sweep CGJF, Pesman GJ, et al: Synergism between IL-1β and TNF-α on the activity of the pituitary-adrenal axis and on food intake of rats, *Am J Physiol* 268:E551–E557, 1995.
218. Vander AJ, Miller R: Control of renin secretion in the anesthetized dog, *Am J Physiol* 207:537, 1964.
219. Wagner RL, White PF, Kan PB, et al: Inhibition of adrenal steroidogenesis by the anesthetic etomidate, *N Engl J Med* 310:1415, 1984.
220. Weber G: Hormonal regulation and liver enzymes, *Gastroenterology* 53:984, 1967.
221. Welshons WV, Krummel BM, Gorski J: Nuclear localization of uncopied receptors for glucocorticoids, estrogens and progesterone in GH3 cells, *Endocrinology* 117:2140, 1985.
222. Whitnall MH, Mezey E, Gainer H: Co-localization of corticotropin releasing factor in median eminance neurosecretory vesicles, *Nature* 317:248, 1985.
223. Widmaier EP, Dallman MF: The effects of corticotropin releasing factor on adrenocorticotropin secretion from perfused pituitaries *in vitro:* Rapid inhibition by glucocorticoids, *Endocrinology* 115:2368, 1984.
224. Winstone NE, Brooke BN: Effects of steroid treatment on patients undergoing operation, *Lancet* 1:973, 1961.
225. Wise JK, Hendler R, Felig P: Influences of glucocorticoids on glucagon secretion and plasma amino acid concentrations in man, *J Clin Invest* 52:2774, 1973.
226. Woloski BM, Smith EM, Meyer WJ III, et al: Corticotropin-releasing activity of monokines, *Science* 230:1035–1037, 1985.
227. Wong GL, Kukert BP, Adams JS: Glucocorticoids increase osteoblast like bone cell response to 1,25$(OH)_2$ and D3, *Nature* 285:254, 1980.
228. Wool IG, Weinshelbaum EI: Incorporation of 14C-amino acids into protein of isolated diaphragms. Role of adrenal steroids, *Am J Physiol* 197:1089, 1959.
229. Yamamoto KR: Steroid receptor regulated transcription of specific genes and gene networks, *Ann Rev Genet* 19:209, 1985.
230. Yeasting RA: Selected morphological aspects of human suprarenal glands. In Mulrow PK, editor: *The adrenal gland,* New York, 1986, Elsevier.
231. Zintel HA, Nay HR: Postoperative complications of radical mastectomy, *Surg Clin North Am* 44:313–323, 1964.

PART III

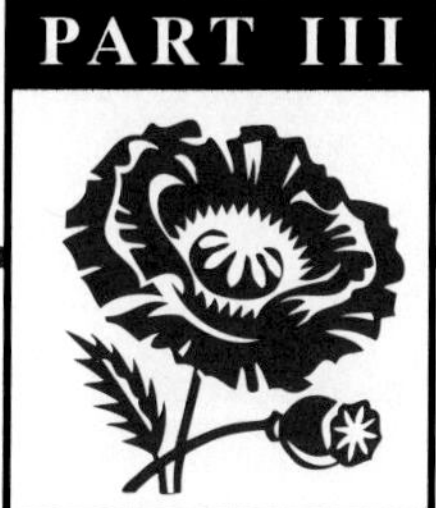

Specialty Areas of Anesthetic Practice

CHAPTER 67

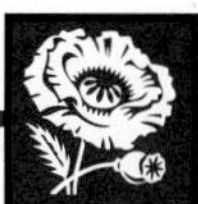

Neuroanesthesia: A Critical Review

MICHAEL M. TODD
DAVID S. WARNER
MAZEN A. MAKTABI

The idea that there is something different about anesthesia for neurosurgery is relatively new, despite occasional observations as early as the mid-1800s about effects of anesthetics on the condition of the brain; the subspecialty of neuroanesthesia arose only in the late 1960s and early 1970s. It developed because of newfound ability to measure variables such as intracranial pressure (ICP), cerebral blood flow (CBF), and cerebral metabolic rate (CMR). The relevance of such measurements was supported by the finding that volatile anesthetics could alter ICP in patients, a change apparently related to increased CBF. This was reinforced by the discovery that the barbiturates might be therapeutic in some patients. The result was a rapid growth in research and a simultaneous effort to use this information to guide clinical practice. The discipline has since grown to encompass many areas of neurophysiology as they apply to anesthesia, and to areas of the basic neurosciences that have no immediate application to clinical care.

Despite scientific expertise, neuroanesthesia is plagued by the fact that most physiologic parameters we regard as important (and which we enjoy measuring under experimental conditions) are difficult to record in patients; e.g., it is impossible to routinely "monitor" the effects of drugs on CBF, CMR, or ICP. There is no neuroanesthetic equivalent of the pulmonary artery (PA) catheter or the transesophageal echocardiograph (TEE) that permits a wide range of cerebral physiologic and pharmacologic effects to be followed easily in large numbers of patients. We can monitor the electroencephalogram (EEG), but we are unable to quantitatively link EEG patterns with changes in the other variables. We can insonate the cerebral vasculature with transcranial Doppler—but we do not know what the numbers really mean. We can do wonderful science with magnetic resonance imaging (MRI) or positron emission tomography—but we cannot bring these into the operating room. We are forced to extrapolate from findings made in the animal or clinical laboratory. This approach is fraught with potential error. It is unclear whether findings made in the laboratory can be easily extrapolated to the clinical setting. Because relatively few neurosurgical patients do poorly after routine surgery, regardless of anesthetic management methods, large numbers of patients would be needed to carry out valid studies relating drug-mediated changes in difficult-to-measure physiologic variables to outcome. Such studies have not been done and may never be. We can, for example, show that halothane increases cortical CBF to a greater degree than isoflurane, but the relationships between CBF and ICP are complex and it is not clear whether this means that halothane will produce a greater increase in ICP than will isoflurane. Because the relationship between drug-induced change in ICP and outcome is unknown, it is even less clear whether the CBF and ICP effects of halothane, isoflurane, N_2O, barbiturates, narcotics, and so forth have real effects on our patients.

These comments are not meant to deprecate the efforts of researchers dedicated to understanding the cerebrovascular, metabolic, or electrophysiologic effects of anesthetics nor are they meant to criticize those who have attempted to use such data to improve clinical care. We believe that an understanding of cerebrovascular physiology and pharmacology is important to anesthetists. As our knowledge grows, the connections between physiology and clinical management will become stronger, although some cherished beliefs will be discarded. We ask that the reader realize these limitations, refrain from making (or totally believing) dogmatic statements (including ours), and avoid carelessly translating physiologic and pharmacologic observations into clinical practice. Finally, we ask the reader to critically examine the clinical realities of anesthetic practice before deciding that some agent or technique is appropriate or inappropriate.

It is impossible to review the entire discipline of "neuroanesthesia." Several books have been written in an attempt to do that.[76,79,264] We have chosen not to deal with cerebral ischemia and protection nor will we discuss EEGs, evoked potentials and other forms of clinical monitoring except briefly. We will not deal with management of carotid endarterectomies (CEA) or neurosurgical intensive care. We will begin with an overview of the physiology and pharmacology of the cerebral circulation, with an emphasis on CBF, cerebral blood volume (CBV) and ICP. We will then describe what we believe to be rational approaches to management of certain clinical situations. We will focus on widely performed intracranial operations, with some remarks on cervical spine disease. Throughout, we will endeavor to exercise the skepticism we have asked of the reader and to distinguish between matters of academic/scientific interest and the realities of the neurosurgical operating room.

BASIC PHYSIOLOGY

Cerebral Blood Flow, Cerebral Blood Volume, and Cerebral Metabolic Rate

Measurement of CBF

Normal whole-brain and gray/white CBF values are shown in Table 67-1. These values are abstract and can be misinterpreted unless one knows how they are obtained. This might be untrue if CBF could be measured "mechanically" (i.e., with a flowmeter around the carotid arteries, or with a technique as simple as thermodilution cardiac outputs). Unfortunately, with few exceptions, such methods do not work. Venous outflow from the dog brain can be diverted through a flowmeter to allow continuous "mechanical" measurements, but this technique is not applicable to humans. Retrograde thermodilution catheters[430] or intravascular Doppler's[306] have been placed in the jugular vein of patients and research subjects, but none of these methods has been widely accepted (although they can be useful in selected circumstances). Therefore, we will begin with a review of those methods that have been widely used in either the operating room (OR) or intensive care unit (ICU), with some later comments on laboratory techniques or more complex clinical methods.

CBF and CMR methods for the OR

There are basically five methods that have been employed for CBF studies in the OR/ICU setting: (1) The Kety-

Table 67-1 "Normal" human values

Parameter	Whole brain	"Gray"	"White"
CBF (ml/100 g/min)	50	80	20
CBV (ml/100 g)	4	4–6	1.5–2.5
$CMRO_2$			
ml/100 g/min	2.7–3.6	3.4–4.3	0.7–1.1
μmole/g/min	1.2–1.6	1.5–1.9	0.3–0.5
CMRGlu			
mg/100 g/min	4.9	6.5–8.5	1.2–2.2
μmole/g/min	0.3–0.4	0.36–0.47	0.07–0.12
CMRLactate			
mg/100 g/min	−0.32	—	—
μmole/g/min	−0.035	—	—

All values represent the authors' best estimates based on many sources.
In PET measurements (which are used to derive regional data), an exact separation of gray and pure white matter is not possible. As a result, most of the gray matter values above might more accurately be described as "cortical" while white matter values are typically obtained from areas such as the internal capsule. Note that CMRlactate is a negative number, which reflects the fact that lactate is usually produced by brain rather than consumed (and hence the venous concentration is greater than arterial).

Schmidt method; (2) intracarotid ^{133}Xe injection; (3) intravenous (IV)/inhaled ^{133}Xe; (4) intra-aortic ^{133}Xe; and (5) transcranial Doppler sonography. Resultant CBF values can, with major limitations (Table 67-2), be used to calculated cerebral metabolic rates (CMR). We will also briefly discuss use of jugular venous O_2 sampling as a measure of flow-metabolism balance.

Kety-Schmidt method. Human CBF was first measured in 1945 by Kety and Schmidt, using a variation of the Fick principal.[194] Catheters were inserted into a peripheral artery and the jugular bulb (the internal jugular vein just as it exits the skull). A diffusible tracer (10% to 15% N_2O) was given by inhalation, and paired samples of blood entering and leaving the brain were obtained over the next 15 to 20 minutes. The arterial concentration of N_2O increases quickly, but because the tracer is being taken up by brain tissue, the cerebral*venous* concentration increases more slowly (Fig. 67-1). The rate at which tissue saturation is reached (i.e., when arterial and venous concentrations equilibrate) is a reflection of the rate of tracer delivery. If CBF is high, equilibrium will occur quickly; if flow is low, equilibration will be slow.

Even after 50 years, many investigators consider this method to be the gold-standard for whole-brain CBF measurements, and it has been widely used in the study of anesthetics. It is invasive, it provides only whole-brain CBF information and is "blind" to areas of near-zero flow (because areas that do not take up tracer don't contribute to the venous saturation curve). It is also time consuming, requiring 10 to 20 minutes to complete a single measurement. For these reasons, a number of other techniques have been developed.

Table 67-2 Limitations of various flow measurement methods

Method	Limitations
Human and laboratory methods	
Kety-Schmidt	Invasive No regional data Slow (10–20 min data acquisition) Blind to very low flow regions
Intracarotid ^{133}Xe	Invasive One hemisphere only Looks primarily at superficial cortex
Inhaled/IV ^{133}Xe	Looks primarily at superficial cortex Extracranial tracer delivery Computationally complex Tracer recirculation
Intra-aortic ^{133}Xe (CPB)	Looks primarily at superficial cortex Extracranial tracer delivery Underestimates CBF?
Transcranial Doppler sonography	Measures velocity only Accurately measures CBF changes—but not absolute CBF "Distorted" values if vessel diameter changes
Single photon emission computed tomography	Typically single measurement Not usable in the operating room or intensive care unit
Positron emission tomography	Extremely expensive and technically complex Not usable in the operating room or intensive care unit
Magnetic resonance imaging	Under development Not usable in the operating room or intensive care unit
Laboratory methods	
H_2 clearance	Very regional? (1–2 mm^3) Tissue injury? Requires craniectomy
Venous outflow	No regional information Forebrain only Deterioration with time Requires craniectomy
Radioactive microspheres	Limited number of flows (6–8) Requires complex surgery
Autoradiography	One measurement only Complex processing needed

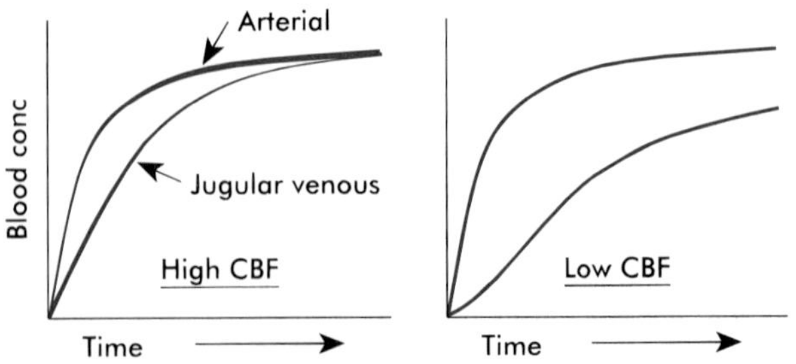

Fig. 67-1. Cerebral blood flow (CBF) as measured by the Kety-Schmidt (KS) method. Catheters are placed into an artery and into the jugular bulb. A diffusible tracer (e.g., N_2O) is then given by inhalation, and pair arterial and jugular venous samples are drawn over time (usually 15 to 20 min). Note that in both of the two sets of curves, the shape of the blood concentration versus time for the arterial curve is essentially the same. However, the time to arteriovenous equilibration is much longer in the low CBF curve (right) than on the left (in fact, equilibrium is never achieved on the left). Actual CBF is proportional to the area between the arterial and venous curves.

The Kety-Schmidt (KS) technique lends itself almost ideally to calculation of CMR, the rate at which the brain consumes or produces metabolic substrates or byproducts (e.g., oxygen [$CMRo_2$], glucose [CMRGlu], or lactate [CMRLact]). CMR plays a major role in the control of CBF and is dramatically altered by anesthetics. The standard method for its determination is based on the Fick principle—CBF is multiplied by the arteriovenous concentration difference of the compound of interest. Since the KS method requires both arterial and jugular venous sampling, obtaining the needed samples for CMR determinations is a trivial addition. For example, if CBF is 50 ml/100 g/min, arterial O_2 content is 20 ml/100 ml (0.20 ml O_2/ml blood), and cerebral venous O_2 content is 12 ml/100 ml (0.12 ml O_2/ml blood), then:

$$CMRo_2 = CBF\ (A - VO_2) = 50\ (0.20 - 0.12) = 4\ \text{ml}\ O_2/100\ \text{g/min (or 1.54}\ \mu\text{mol/g/min)}$$

Similar calculations yield the other CMR values shown in the first column of Table 67-1. Note that these have also been expressed as μmol/g/min, which is useful when attempting to examine the stoichiometry of energy metabolism. For example, if you wish to calculate the relative amount of glucose being converted in the brain to CO_2 and H_2O via oxidative metabolism:

$$CMRo_2/CMRGlu = (1.54\ \mu\text{mol/g/min})/(0.27\ \mu\text{mol/g/min}) = 5.7$$

This indicates that for every 5.7 mol of oxygen consumed, 1 mol of glucose is used. Because complete glucose oxidation uses 6 mole of oxygen/mole of glucose, this indicates that all of the glucose being consumed is not being oxidized but is being used in other processes. One can similarly calculate a respiratory quotient, lactate/glucose ratios, and so forth.

Radioactive tracer washout methods: intra-arterial ^{133}Xe. To obtain regional data, a diffusible radioactive tracer (e.g., ^{133}Xe in saline) can be injected as a bolus into the internal carotid artery. The rate at which radioactivity disappears from the head can then be monitored using extracranial radiation detectors.[304] If CBF is high, the slope of the washout curve will be steep; if slow, the rate of washout will be slow (Fig. 67-2, A). If multiple collimated detectors are used, separate washout curves can be recorded from different regions of the hemisphere ipsilateral to the injection. The individual washout curves can be mathematically separated into two components, one representing ^{133}Xe clearance from a high-flow compartment (gray matter), and one representing a slow flow compartment (white matter) (Fig. 67-2, B). The calculations needed to separate the fast and slow components of the washout curve are identical to those used when distinguishing the early redistribution phase of a drug from its terminal clearance (i.e., $t_{1/2}$-alpha versus $t_{1/2}$-beta).

Unlike the KS method, this techique can provide very high resolution regional CBF (rCBF) data from the hemisphere ipsilateral to the injection. Several mathematical processes have been developed to make it possible to compute flow indices in as little as 2 minutes after isotope injection (although a second flow can't be measured until more isotope is cleared). Unfortunately, it requires direct carotid puncture (or transfemoral cannulation of the internal carotid). Nevertheless, its technical simplicity has resulted in its widespread use for flow measurements during carotid surgery, and essentially everything known about the effects of anesthetics during carotid endarterectomies and the cerebral hemodynamic effects of carotid occlusion has been obtained with this method.

Radioactive tracer washout methods: Inhaled/IV ^{133}Xe methods. Intra-arterial ^{133}Xe injection is invasive and provides data from only one hemisphere. These limitations could be eliminated if an externally detectable tracer could be given IV or by inhalation (which would then be delivered to both hemispheres). Although this may seem simple, it is much more complex because of two problems.[304] First, an inhaled/IV tracer is delivered to *both* the brain and scalp (unlike tracer injected into the internal carotid artery). Hence the brain washout curve is "contaminated" by another curve representing flow in extracranial tissues. Second, the shapes of the arterial washin and washout curves are much more complex, depending on tracer redistribution throughout the body and its clearance from the lungs. These problems have been solved but require extensive computations. Although these calculations require some assumptions, the advantages of relative noninvasiveness and bilateral distribution appear to outweigh them, and hence this method is used by some centers for anesthesia-related studies,[7,310] but not during routine clinical anesthesia.

Radioactive tracer washout methods: Intra-aortic ^{133}Xe injection. One variation on the intra-arterial and intravenous ^{133}Xe method has been used during cardiac surgery.[369] A bolus of ^{133}Xe in saline is injected into the aortic root or into the aortic cannula. As with the intracarotid method, radioactivity is delivered to the brain as a bolus, and

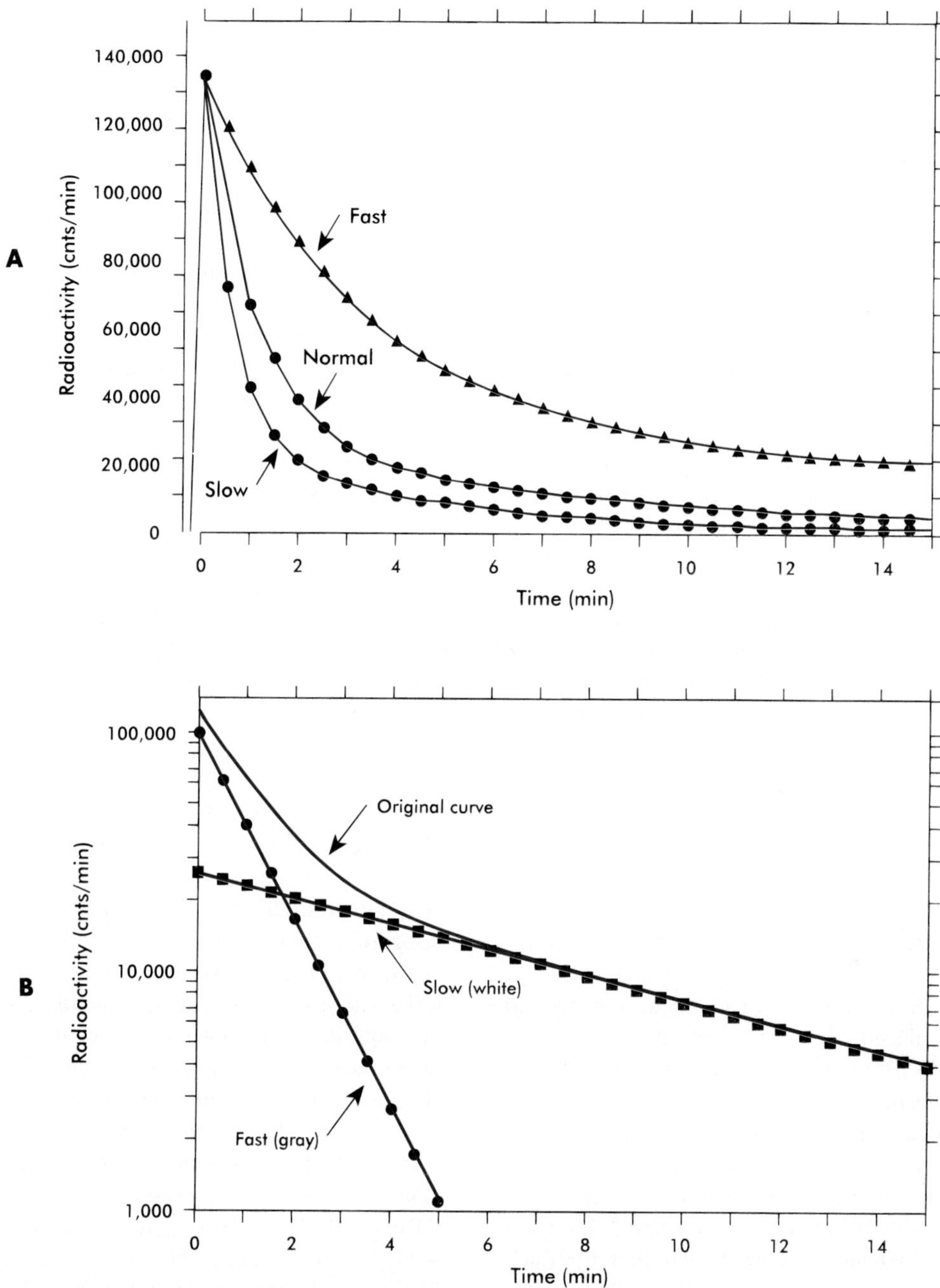

Fig. 67-2. Single channel curves showing the washout of radioactivity from the brain after the bolus injection of radioactive ^{133}Xenon into the internal carotid artery. The curves in **A** represent "raw data" plotted on a linear scale (counts vs. time). Injection was made just slightly before time zero. There are three curves, each with different slopes: the top representing a slow flow (low CBF), the middle a normal flow, and the bottom typical of a high flow state. In **B,** the middle (normal curve has been replotted on a log scale and is separated into monoexponential "fast" and "slow" components. Note that although these compartments are labeled as "gray" and "white," their exact anatomical nature is not defined. In **B,** the fast compartment has a flow of 80 ml/100 g/min, while that for the slow compartment is 20 ml/100 g/min. (From Hoedt-Rasmussen K: Regional cerebral blood flow, *Acta Neurol Scand* (Suppl 27) 43:13, 1967.)

the washout mathematics are relatively simple. Tracer is again delivered to extracranial tissues, and "contamination" remains a problem. During normothermia, CBF is much greater than scalp flow, making contamination a minor nuisance; during alpha-star hypothermia, CBF decreases and the contaminating influence of extracranial flow may become more of a problem. A recent study by Cook et al. comparing this method with the traditional KS technique suggests that serious underestimates of actual CBF may occur.

All three of the ^{133}Xe-based techniques have been combined with Fick-type measurements of arterial and venous blood samples to permit calculation of cerebral metabolic rate (CMR). CBF and the venous samples should represent the same tissue compartments. Blood from the jugular bulb is representative of blood draining the whole brain (with some hemispheric predominance, particularly in the presence of severe unilateral injury).[399] None of the ^{133}Xe-washout methods, strictly speaking, measure whole brain or hemispheric CBF; typically they yield a CBF value that is dominated by the cortical mantle. Hence calculation of CMR involves multiplying a whole brain arteriovenous difference value by a regional CBF value. As long as regional and global CBF change in parallel (e.g., during anesthetic administration), calculations of CMR should be reasonable (although the absolute values may differ from those based on KS flows). If the intervention or disease process being studied results in major flow redistribution or regional heterogenieity, calculated CMR may be misleading.

Transcranial doppler (TCD) sonography. Doppler-based methods for assessing blood flow in many vessels have been used. These formerly involved use of "continuous wave" Doppler methods, with the probe placed very close to the vessel of interest. In the early 1980s, "pulsed-wave" methods were developed; packets (brief bursts) of sound are emitted, with an interim period of silence during which reflected signal is used to measure time needed for the "round trip," which can be used to measure the distance from the probe to the target—and by adjusting the time interval during which the instrument will accept a returning signal ("range-gating"), the Doppler signal can effectively be *focused* on a target a given distance away. This is the basis for transcranial doppler (TCD).[31,298] In practice, a hand-held Doppler probe is placed over a relatively thin area of the skull (a "window"). By adjusting the insonation angle and depth it is possible to identify flow signals from multiple cerebral vessels. For example, from the temporal window, it is relatively easy to record signals from the internal carotid, middle cerebral, and anterior cerebral arteries. Other vessels can be found via other windows (e.g., transorbital, occipital). This method has been used extensively to aid in diagnosis of cerebral occlusive disease.

Physiologic and pharmacologically-induced changes in CBF can be assessed by following changes in TCD signal from a single vessel during some intervention. This is typically done using the middle cerebral artery (MCA). The probe is placed over the temporal window, and the MCA is identified as it moves toward the probe (which means a high-insensity signal can be recorded as the focal depth is adjusted over a range sometimes as great as 10 mm (e.g., from 45 to 55 mm from the skin). Because erythrocytes are moving almost directly toward the probe, the insonation angle is essentially zero, and flow-velocity is proportional to absolute flow (although absolute flow cannot be known without knowing vessel diameter). If probe position is fixed, changes in flow-velocity (denoted as Vmca) can be measured during various interventions (drug administration, CO_2 changes, etc.). As long as depth and insonation angle remains constant and the number of interventions are kept to a minimum, multiple studies have shown that changes in Vmca parallel changes in absolute CBF as measured with more traditional methods.

Transcranial doppler has now become the preferred method for examining the acute impact of anesthetic agents and adjuncts on CBF.[114,209,250,425] It is also increasingly used as a monitor during carotid surgery,[239] to aid in diagnosis of vasospasm in patients with subarachnoid hemorrhage (where a decrease in vessel diameter results in an increase in flow velocity),[274] and to measure flow and detect emboli during cardiac surgery.[56,331,429] This method does not yield absolute flow values—only flow velocities. Primary advantages are its noninvasive, nonradioactive nature, and its ability to monitor at least an index of CBF continuously, something that cannot be done with any other widely used method.

Although it is possible to multiply a Vmca value by an arteriovenous content difference, the resultant number cannot be called "CMR." Vmca is a velocity measurement (in cm/sec), not absolute flow (in ml/100 g/min). We have little or no information on the tissue compartment being perfused by the insonated vessel.

Jugular Venous Oximetry. It is often impractical to quantitate CBF (or CMR) in clinical practice. In an effort to obtain such information, many centers have begun monitoring cerebral venous oxygenation, particularly in the intensive care unit. This is performed either via intermittent sampling of jugular venous blood or continuously using an "oximetric" catheter. When combined with a measure of arterial saturation, this technique provides a measure of cerebral arteriovenous-oxygen content difference; if Sao_2 remains near $\approx$ 100%, one need not calculate $AVDo_2$, but simply follow the jugular venous saturation ($Sjvo_2$). This value is a measure of "the balance" between cerebral blood flow and $CMRo_2$, even though neither value can be directly calculated. If $Sjvo_2$ decreases, then one can conclude that CBF should be decreasing relative to demand (or, alternatively, $CMRo_2$ should be increasing disproportionately). This method has been advocated as an adjunct to ICP monitoring; an increase in ICP associated with an increase in $Sjvo_2$ is probably due to an increase in CBF and CBV, while an identical ICP change associated with a decrease in $Sjvo_2$ represents a different physiology (e.g., more edema). If venous lactates are also monitored, it may be possible to determine when a CBF reduction is "critical."[127,348,382] The obvious goal is to provide therapy "tailored" to physiology (e.g., to avoid treating "low-flow" intracranial hypertension with hypocapnia). Whether this will prove efficacious remains unclear. A similar approach has been proposed for the operating room[249] but has not been adequately evaluated.

Imaging techniques for physiologic studies

The methods noted above are those which can be used in the operating room or intensive care unit. The quest for greater information has lead to development of measurement methods that depend on complex imaging hardware. These include (1) stable xenon-enhanced computed tomography (CT); (2) single photon emission computed tomography (SPECT); (3) positron emission tomography (PET); and (4) functional magnetic resonance imaging (MRI).

Stable xenon CT. One of the first "functional imaging" methods was stable xenon computed tomography (CT). Xenon in high concentrations (40% to 60%) is radiopaque, and its regional concentration can be quantitated in a standard CT scanner. Rapid serial scans after discontinuation of xenon administration can be used to construct a large number of washout curves, one from each pixel of imaged tissue.[148] The limitations of this technique are the anesthetic and cerebrovascular effects of the high concentrations of xenon, and the radiation dose associated with the multiple scans. The method has been used to examine rCBF changes during anesthesia.[343] There are no methods for determining CMR related to this technique.

Single photon emission computed tomography (SPECT). Standard CT methods involve measuring attenuation of x-rays passed through the head. Similar analytical methods can also be used to examine the two-dimensional distribution of radioactivity emitted from tissue following the administration of a tracer (although this obviously requires a special scanning device).[454] In the earliest approaches, the concentration and distribution of ^{99m}Tc-labeled erythrocytes or plasma was used to calculate regional CBV,[356] with ^{133}Xe used as a flow tracer. More recently other tracers were employed including ^{99m}Tc-labeled compounds (e.g., ^{99m}Tc-hexamethylpropyleneamineoxime or HMPAO) that are tightly bound to brain tissue after injection, behaving similar to radioactive microspheres (see following paragraphs).[9] The tracer can be injected at some moment of interest (e.g., after equilibrium at a given anesthetic concentration), but the scan itself does not need to be obtained until hours later (e.g., after discharge from the recovery area). The regional concentration of tracer at the time of the scan reflects the distribution of flow at the time of injection. The major disadvantage is that only one measurement of flow can be obtained. Like xenon CT, this has had limited use in anesthetic studies.[344] There are also no related methods for determining CMR.

Positron emission tomography. Isotopes that decay by emitting positrons (positively charged electrons) have a uniquely useful place in cerebrovascular research. When a positron collides with an electron, two 511-Kev photons are emitted 180° apart (i.e., they fly off the parent atom in precisely opposite directions). If two detectors located at opposite diameters of circle record an event simultaneously (coincidence detection), then the source of the photons should lie on a line between the detectors. Using this physical property and a circular array of linked detectors, it is possible to determine the location of a positron-emitting isotope in two dimensions. The third dimension is added by scanning in multiple parallel planes. Using computational techniques similar to CT scanning, it is possible to generate three-dimensional images of the distribution of isotopes within the brain.[32,171]

The importance of PET scanning rests not with the scanning technology, but with the chemistry. Using a cyclotron, it is possible to generate positron-emitting isotopes of carbon (^{11}C), oxygen (^{15}C), fluoride (^{18}F), nitrogen (^{13}N) and many others.[359] A radiochemist can use these to label a wide variety of potentially valuable tracer compounds. For example, $^{15}O_2$ can be used to assess regional oxygen consumption ($CMRo_2$), whereas ^{18}F-fluorodeoxyglucose can be used to assess CMRGlu (just as ^{14}C-deoxyglucose is used in the animal lab). Labeled carbon monoxide ($C^{15}O$ or ^{11}CO) can be used to measure CBV, and oxygen-labeled water is a common CBF tracer. Many of these isotopes are extremely short-lived (e.g., 2 minutes for ^{15}O), and it is hence possible to rapidly measure several physiologic parameters in the same subject. A more recent development has been the positron-isotope labeling of various neurotransmitter receptor ligands, which allow sophisticated studies of regional receptor distribution and their binding kinetics.[134] A similar method has been used to determine binding kinetics and receptor distribution, using SPECT.[454]

PET methods have found only limited use in anesthesia-related research, at least until recently. It was first used to assess changes in cerebral blood volume.[11,12] It has now been used to examine the neuroanatomic substrates of pain and analgesia,[4,149] and the regional effects of anesthetics.[8,433]

Magnetic resonance imaging and resonance spectroscopy. Clinicians are familiar with MRI as an anatomic imaging method, but there has been a recent rapid growth in use of this method for physiologic imaging.[328,387] By appropriate tuning of pulses and magnets, it is now possible to "image" blood and hence to quantitate regional CBF and CBV. The "apparent diffusion coefficient (ADC)" of water can be determined as an index of ischemic brain injury and edema. Because oxyhemoglobin is paramagnetic, it is possible to follow changes in brain tissue oxygenation during normal and pathologic conditions.

Nuclear magnetic resonance spectroscopy has also been widely used.[387] Using surface coils in an MRI unit, it is possible to obtain a spectrum which reflects tissue concentrations of high-energy phosphate compounds (ATP, ADP, AMP, PCr, Pi) and also to assess changes in intracellular pH.[448] These methods have been extensively used in studies of cerebral ischemia. Recent technical developments hold the promise of permitting the actual imaging of high-energy phosphates in the brain as well.

Related laboratory methods

All of the aforementioned methods are used in clinical medicine or human research. All have also been used in the animal laboratory, but there are a variety of other techniques that are uniquely applicable to animals. The list is quite long, but the most common methods are: (1) H_2 clearance; (2) ^{14}C or ^{3}H based autoradiography (to measure both CBF and CMRGlucose); (3) radioactive microspheres; and (4) laser Doppler flowmetry.

H_2 clearance. H_2 is an excellent flow tracer. It is rapidly diffusible, it can be given by inhalation, and its washin/washout from brain can be monitored by small (10 to 250 μm diameter) platinum electrodes implanted in the brain or placed in the venous outflow from the brain.[457] The electrodes can be chronically implanted, allowing repeated rCBF measurements over long periods of time in awake animals. Difficulty involves unresolved concerns about tissue injury, particularly when measurements are made shortly after electrode implantation. It is also difficult to insert more than about five to 10 electrodes into a brain, and the smaller the brain, the greater the difficulty.

Autoradiography. H_2 clearance has limited resolution, although it allows multiple repeated flow measurements. If very high resolution is needed, ^{14}C- or ^{3}H-labeled tracers such as ^{14}C-iodoantipyrine, ^{14}C-butanol, ^{14}C-iodoamphetamine, or ^{3}H nicotine can be given as a brief (30 to 45 sec) intravenous infusion. The animal is then killed, the brain removed and either solubilized and counted, or cut into thin (20 μm) sections which are placed on film. When the film is developed, the regional concentrations of tracer can be determined (i.e., greater flow allows more tracer which produces greater film exposure by the radioactivity).[362] With careful processing, it is possible to determine CBF in tissue regions as small as 25 to 50 μm^2. Unfortunately, because the available tracers are not permanently trapped in tissue and because the brain should be removed, only one flow measurement can be made in each animal. Innumerable anesthesia-related studies have been done with such methods.[87,159,230,439] In addition, by using labeled glucose or glucose analogues (e.g., ^{14}-C-2-deoxyglucose), it is possible to determine local CMRGlu using analagous methods.[391]

Radioactive microspheres. If repetitive laboratory regional CBF measurements are needed, the most popular method involves the injection of 15-μm diameter radioactive microspheres into the arterial circulation (usually into the left atrium or ventricle).[169,236] These are trapped in the capillary bed, and the number of spheres reaching a given area is proportional to blood flow. Simultaneously, arterial blood is withdrawn at a known rate into a syringe; the ratio between the number of spheres in the syringe and those in the tissue permits absolute CBF calculations (after the tissue is weighed). Because these spheres are trapped, it is possible to make multiple flow measurements over time by injecting microspheres with different radiolabels. When the tissue is harvested, the number of each different sphere (and hence each different flow) can be determined using a gamma spectrophotometer. The total number of flows is limited (usually to six or eight). The regional resolution is much poorer than with autoradiographic techniques. Nevertheless, this method is very popular among researchers. If whole brain CBF is calculated, it is possible to determine CMR using arteriovenous blood sampling.

Laser Doppler flowmetry. Given the expense of isotope techniques (and isotope disposal) and the limited time resolution, a newer method is gaining popularity, at least in small animals. This is the so-called "laser-Doppler flowmeter (LDF)."[135,150,303] The cortical surface is exposed, and laser light (delivered via a fiber optic bundle) is beamed into the tissue. This light is reflected and scattered by the tissue—but light reflected from moving erythrocytes undergoes a Doppler frequency shift. The magnitude of this shift—which is proportional to CBF—is recorded. Although this method does not yield flow in traditional ml/100 g/min (but is typically expressed as LDF units), it has been well validated, and has the advantage of yielding continuous information relatively inexpensively. LDF has been used in humans, although with only limited enthusiasm.[52,151]

Significance of CBF and CMR: Control of Intracranial Pressure

Studies of regional CBF and CMR have provided invaluable information concerning the roles played by different anatomic structures in normal and pathologic brain function. Studies with anesthetics have provided some insights into the anatomic substrate of drug action, and other observations have improved our understanding of changes occurring during cerebral ischemia or after trauma. Such studies have not yet made much impact on clinical neuroanesthetic practice. Why should we be so interested in these variables? There seem to be two reasons: (1) CBF bears an important relationship to ICP; and (2) CBF and CMR are clearly important in the etiology of cerebral ischemia. Because this chapter will not deal directly with ischemia, we will direct our attention to the issue of ICP.

Physiology of intracranial pressure

The bulk of investigative efforts in neuroanesthesia have dealt with ICP. Why such intense interest? First, pressure within the intracranial space is defined by unique conditions. The brain is enclosed in a rigid container. Because neither water nor solids are compressible, any increase in total intracranial volume will result in a rapid increase in pressure. Second, large increases in ICP may have profound effects on the well-being of the brain. Intracranial hypertension can reduce global cerebral perfusion pressure (CPP = mean arterial pressure − ICP) or lead to physical shifts in the intracranial contents, with resultant focal compression of tissue against the falx, the tentorium, or the foramen magnum (Fig. 67-3); patients dying from intracranial mass lesions or trauma often have very high ICPs, and autopsy studies show clear evidence of compression-related ischemia.[178] If the skull is open, compression problems do not occur as readily, but the brain can swell out of the craniotomy site and impede the surgeon's ability to carry out the required procedures (or make closing the wound impossible). It may also be necessary to use excessive retraction pressure to obtain the necessary exposure, which can itself lead to tissue injury.[10] In extreme cases, the surgeon may be forced to am-

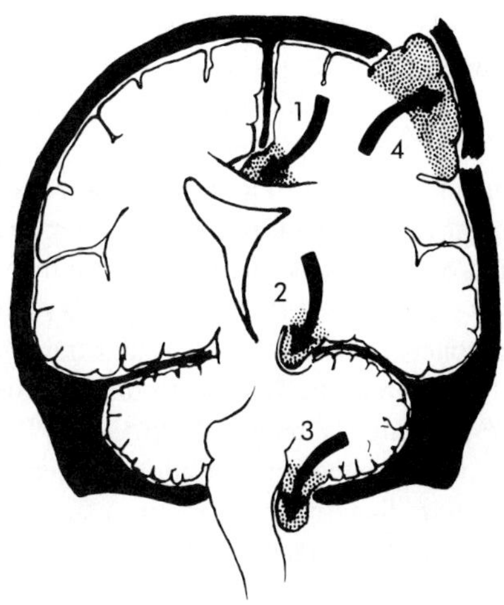

Fig. 67-3. Brain herniation patterns: (1) herniation of the cingulate gyrus under the falx; (2) transtentorial herniation of the temporal lobe; (3) herniation of the cerebellar tonsils through the foramen magnum; and (4) transcalvarial herniation (via a fracture site of craniectomy). In each case, an increase in brain volume combined with a physical shift of the intracranial contents results in intense compression of brain against some rigid structure. (From Fishman RA: Brain edema, *N Engl J Med* 293:706, 1975.)

putate portions of brain to achieve access (e.g., to an aneurysm) or to allow the dura/skull to be closed.

Any increase in total intracranial volume will increase ICP (or brain bulk). This phenomenon is shown as the "real" compliance curve in Fig. 67-4, which would be expected if we rapidly injected a noncompressible liquid into a rigid container. This real curve differs from the "typical" compliance curve presented in many reviews. The confusion arises because the x axis on the "typical curve" is often mislabeled as representing "intracranial volume." In fact, it does not represent total intracranial volume but rather "the volume of the growing mass." The initial portion of this typical curve is flattened because total volume does not change much during the early period of tumor growth (or hematoma expansion, etc.). This occurs because of "spatial compensation," a phenomenon shown schematically in Fig. 67-5.*

This diagram, the physiology of ICP, and its control are easier to understand if we conceptually divide the intracranial contents (weights/volumes given are relative to a "normal" brain) into four compartments:

- Solid material (≈ 12% or 168 g)
- Tissue water (≈ 78% or 1092 g)
- Cerebrospinal fluid (CSF) (75 ml)
- Blood (50 ml)

Increased mass of solid material occurs only during the growth of new cellular material (a tumor). In contrast, edema (an increase in either intra- or extracellular water) can occur without any alteration in tissue solids. CSF volume increases when: (1) its reabsorption is inhibited (e.g., hydrocephalus); or (2) the mass of solid material/tissue decreases (e.g., cerebral atrophy). Increases in CSF production are rare (but see following paragraphs). In many pathologic states, changes occur in all compartments: A growing tumor may increase interstitial fluid volume (edema) and either increase or decrease CBV. If the tumor obstructs CSF pathways, hydrocephalus can also occur.

The compartment that plays the greatest role in spatial compensation is CSF.* As a mass lesion expands, the CSF

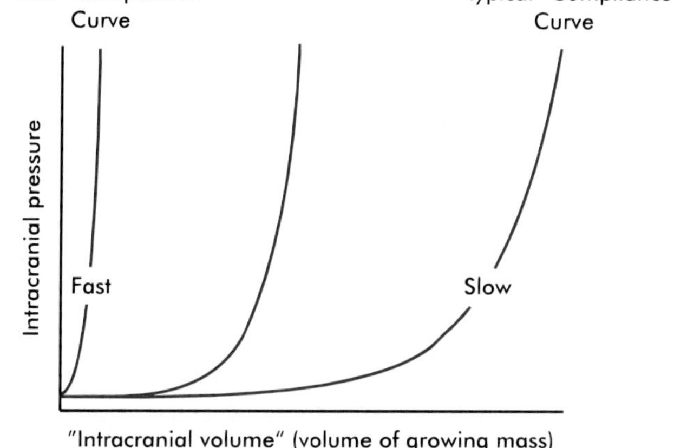

Fig. 67-4. Intracranial pressure "compliance curves." If intracranial contents are noncompressible and the skull were truly rigid, then the injection of any "extra" volume into the system would produce a very rapid increase in pressure (left curve, labeled *real*). However, this is not the pattern typically seen with a slowly growing mass lesion, which is shown on the right curve (labeled *typical*). Note however, that the x axis is often mislabeled. This should not read "intracranial volume" but rather "volume of growing mass." As a mass grows, total volume remains almost constant because of compensatory mechanisms (see Fig. 67-5). Only when these are exhausted does pressure rise precipitously. Note also that the faster volume is added, the more quickly are compensatory mechanisms exhausted.

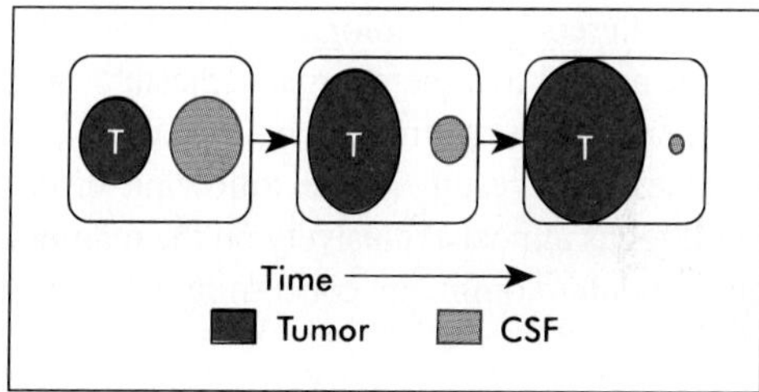

Fig. 67-5. Schematic depiction of spatial compensation. As a mass slowly increases in size (*solid ellipse, T*), the volume of some other compartment should get smaller. In most cases, this is CSF volume (*dotted ellipse*). Compensation can be said to be exhausted when this second compartment can no longer decrease in size, and hence total intracranial volume begins to rise.

*Contrary to popular belief, the major anatomic structure that determines "compliance" is the dura, not the skull.[380] Simply removing the bone has little impact on ICP or compliance.

*We do not discuss CSF physiology and pharmacology in detail in this chapter, because our emphasis is on blood flow and volume. There are two excellent and comprehensive reviews of this subject in the recent anesthesia literature.[19,20]

space will decrease by an ≈ equal volume. This is seen on a CT/MRI scan as a progressive reduction in cerebral ventricles and/or of the basal cisterns, etc. ICP will increase rapidly only when the CSF space can no longer be "squeezed" (see Fig. 67-6) or when intracranial compartmentalization results in some obstruction to CSF flow/absorption. Spatial compensation takes time, and rapidly increasing masses (e.g., hematomas) "exhaust" compensatory mechanisms quickly and can lead to severe increase in ICP much sooner than slowly growing lesions.

Control of intracranial hypertension can also be discussed in terms of these tissue compartments. ICP will increase when the volume of one or more of the compartments increases enough to exhaust compensatory mechanisms. To *decrease* ICP, we need only decrease the volume of one compartment. We can drain CSF via a ventriculostomy, alter its production rate with acetazolamide or furosemide, decrease peritumoral edema using steroids, or decrease interstitial (or even cell) volume using mannitol or furosemide. The surgeon can remove the tumor mass. Except for CSF drainage, most of these interventions are relatively slow, requiring hours or days.

Blood is the smallest of the four compartments. Its importance is related not to its size but to the fact that CBV can change very rapidly. For example, witness the rapid increase in ICP seen with jugular compression in Figure 67-6. Other than CSF drainage, the volume of no other compartment can be so rapidly altered by physiologic or pharmacologic methods. It can be argued that the neuroanesthesia provider is, in fact, an expert in the controlled manipulation of cerebral blood volume. As a result, in the following discussion of ICP, we will focus almost exclusively on the manipulation of CBV. We will defer comments concerning tissue water content to a later section dealing with the clinical management of the swollen brain.

Measurement of CBV

To determine the volume of blood in the intravascular space at any point in time (CBV), one should examine the brain concentration of a tracer that remains within the vasculature (which is not true of most flow tracers). CBV is calculated as the brain concentration of intravascular tracer divided by the arterial concentration. The most common method is to inject radio-iodinated albumin (RISA) or ^{99m}Tc-labeled erythrocytes, measure the concentration in arterial blood and determine the radioactivity in brain using an external counter.[145] This is complicated by the fact that counts seen by an external detector are emitted from both brain and scalp, and the resultant values are contaminated by extracranial blood (although this can be eliminated by SPECT). This does not invalidate the technique but does make it more suitable for examining *changes* in CBV rather than absolute volume. This problem can be resolved by using PET (see below) or other tomographic techniques to determine only the intracranial (and regional) concentration of an appropriate isotope.[32,327] A simpler semiquantitative approach is to use the subject's own erythrocytes as a volume tracer, with transcranial near-infrared absorbtion spectroscopy (NIRA) used to examine the changing concentrations of hemoglobin. To date, this method has proven useful only in infants in which transcranial illumination is feasible,[53] all intense developmental efforts are being made to extend it to adults. (NIRA technology may someday also be useful for the measurement of hemoglobin oxygenation in the brain,[207] and to monitor changes in CBF.)[113] In the animal laboratory, the accuracy of extracranial detector methods can be im-

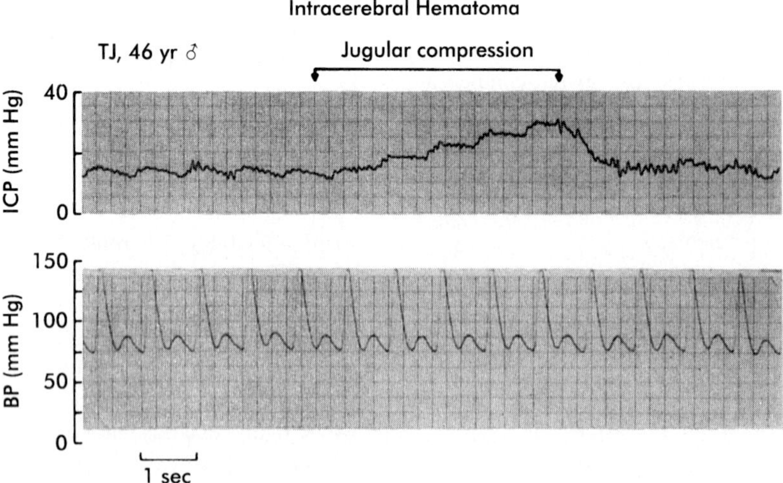

Fig. 67-6. Simultaneous intracranial pressure (ICP) and arterial pressure tracings before and during bilateral jugular vein compression. Note the "arterial" pulsation of both traces, and the "stairstep" rise in ICP when venous outflow is prevented. Each "step" represents the injection of a small increment of blood into the intracranial space.

proved by surgically removing extracranial material (e.g., muscle, skin, bone).[15] For more accurate measurements, it is necessary to sample brain tissue. Typically both an erythrocyte tracer (e.g., ^{99m}Tc- or ^{51}Cr-labeled erythrocytes) and a plasma tracer (e.g., RISA, ^{14}C dextran) are injected together. The animal is killed, preferably with a technique that does not allow the escape of blood from tissue, and the ratio of brain-to-blood concentrations is used to calculate "cerebral erythrocyte volume" and "cerebral plasma volume."[421] Total CBV is the sum of these.

CBV control

To increase CBV blood should go into the head faster than it leaves, at least until a new steady state is reached. This can be done in two ways: (1) impede the egress of blood; or (2) increase the rate at which it enters.

Impede the egress of blood. There are many ways to slow exit of cerebral venous blood. The most important are occlusion of the jugular veins or an increase in venous pressure. Of the many ways to occlude the jugular veins, the easiest is to rotate the head to one side, or to fully extend the neck (e.g., during a tracheostomy). Direct pressure is applied with circumferential neck ties (e.g., to secure an ET tube) or tight cervical collars. It may be possible to obstruct venous drainage by the placement of large catheters into the internal jugular vein (IJV); some clinicians avoid using the IJV in neurosurgical patients. The IJV is very large, and catheters occupy only a small portion of the lumen. At least one study has measured the diameter of the IJV by echo before and after IJ cannulation and showed no changes.[306] The real problems with IJV cannulation are the positions used during cannulation (head down/rotated). As a result, many experienced neuroanesthesia providers will first attempt to obtain central access via antecubital or subclavian routes, but may need to use the IJV as an alternative.

Venous distension can also occur by elevating right heart pressures (major volume overload, right heart failure), increasing intrathoracic pressure (PEEP, short expiratory phase, endotracheal tube obstruction, etc.), or placing the patient in a head-down posture. Positioning is a crucial factor in the control of CBV, and several studies have demonstrated the advantages of a modest head-up posture in minimizing ICP.[107,350,352] An angle greater than 30° above horizontal tends to reduce arterial pressure at the head more than it alters ICP and can reduce CPP (Fig. 67-7).[352] We believe that concerns about PEEP are overrated, and that the use of small amounts of PEEP to improve oxygenation intraoperatively is generally benign.[174] If a patient has lung disease serious enough to warrant high levels of PEEP, only a small fraction of the intrapulmonary pressure is transmitted to the intrathoracic space[222] and the ICP changes produced by PEEP are often minimal or can be offset by head-up posture.[70,219] A more likely problem is the unintentional or unwarranted application of PEEP in patients with normal lungs. PEEP can also increase respiratory dead-space volume and increase Pa_{CO_2}.

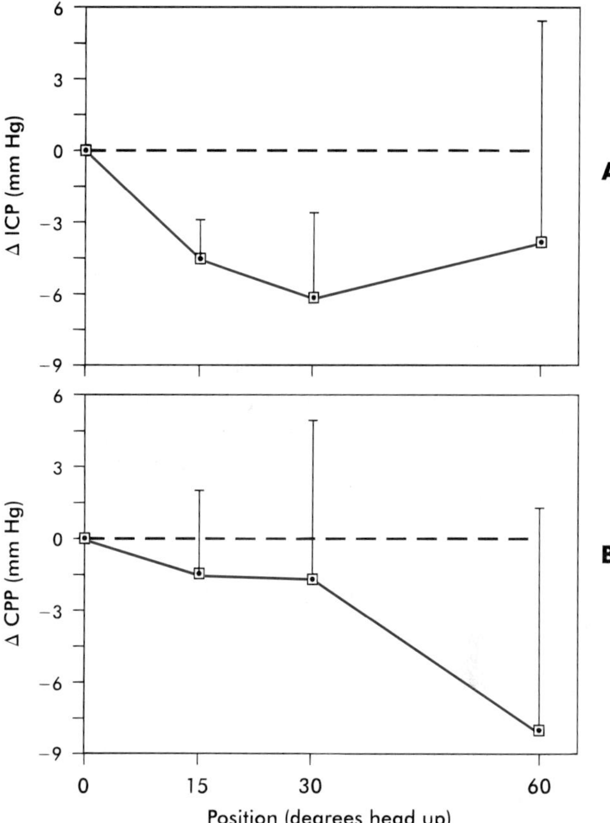

Fig. 67-7. Although a head-up posture can reduce intracranial pressure (ICP), it can also reduce perfusion pressure at the head. Changes in both ICP (**A**) and in calculated cerebral perfusion pressure (CPP) (**B**) at the head are shown (values are mean ± SD). Note that at 30° head up, ICP has been reduced to the lowest possible level without compromising CPP. (Data from Durward QJ, Amadner AL, Del Maestro RF, et al: Cerebral and vascular responses to changes in head elevation in patients with intracranial hypertension, *J Neurosurg* 59:938, 1983.)

A third (theoretical) way of increasing CBV is to pharmacologically increase intracranial venous capacitance. Because perhaps 90% of the blood in the brain is postcapillary, this could be important.[375] Venodilation is clearly produced by both volatile anesthetics and by drugs like sodium nitroprusside,[201] but the relevance of this to the ICP effects of these agents remains unknown.

Increase inflow. "Increase inflow" is just another way of saying "increase CBF," which will be the focus of the next section of this chapter. It is not quite correct to say that an increase in CBF will produce an increase in ICP. ICP changes in response to changes in *volume* not flow. When someone says that hypercapnia increases ICP because it increases CBF, what is really meant is that hypercapnia increases CBF, which is, in turn, accompanied by an increase in CBV.

Normal control of CBF and CBV

Before we can discuss the influence of drugs on CBF, CBV, and ICP, it is necessary to understand the "nor-

mal" factors that control them: $Paco_2$, Pao_2, arterial O_2 content, hydrostatic pressure (autoregulation), metabolism (flow-metabolism coupling), and the autonomic nervous system.

$Paco_2$. CBF varies with $Paco_2$ (Fig. 67-8).[225] This response is typically shown as a sigmoid curve, with lower and upper plateaus. The upper portion of the curve is of little interest in anesthesia, because it does not occur until $Paco_2$ is ≈ 80 to 100 mm Hg. In normal primates and humans, the lowest CBF that can be achieved by hyperventilation is ≈ 18 to 20 ml/100 g/min at 10 mm Hg.[147,151] In the midportion of the curve, CBF changes by 1.5 to 2.0 ml/100 g/min for each mm Hg change in $Paco_2$. The slope of the CBF–$Paco_2$ response curve depends on the baseline normocapnic flow values; as regional CBF increases, the slope of the response curve for that region also increases. As a result, CO_2 responsiveness in gray matter is greater than in white matter.

CO_2 responsiveness is driven by changing *extravascular/interstitial* H^+ concentration. As pH around the extraluminal surface of the vessel decreases, the vessel dilates. By contrast, the intravascular administration of a "fixed" acid or base has little effect. Because CO_2 readily diffuses across the blood–brain barrier into the interstitial space where it is converted to H^+ and HCO_3^-, an increase in intravascular CO_2 is accompanied by extravascular acidosis and hence vasodilation. The CBF response to changing $Paco_2$ is very fast. Severinghaus et al.[378] demonstrated that CBF reached a new steady state within less than 1 minute after a step-change in $Paco_2$. Transcranial doppler studies suggest that response may be even faster. This indirectly indicates that the site of action should be very close to the vessels themselves (because CO_2 can diffuse only a short distance in the time noted).

How does a change in pH change vascular diameter? Several mediators have been studied. Blockade of cyclooxygenase activity (with indomethacin) can blunt CO_2 response, suggesting some role for prostaglandins.[116] CO_2 responsiveness can be transiently abolished (for 12 to 24 hr) by events such as spreading depression that release of glutamate into tissue.[214] Given the well-known link between glutamate, the NMDA receptor, and nitric oxide (NO) release, this suggested that NO may play some role in CO_2 responsiveness. There is now substantial support for this. Treatment of rats with nitric oxide synthase inhibitors (e.g., L-nitroarginine methyl ester [L-NAME]) attenuate the response to hypercapnia.[119,177] Similar chemicals block the response to extravascular H^+. This hypothesis is incomplete, and NOS inhibition in primates does not dramatically alter hypercapnic CO_2 response.[257]

CBV and intracranial pressure. CBV also changes with CO_2, but the CBF and CBV response curves are not parallel. Grubb et al.[147] demonstrated a CBF/$Paco_2$ response curve in primates with a midrange slope of ≈1.8 ml/100 g/mm Hg change in $Paco_2$ (Fig. 67-8). A simultaneously determined CBV/$Paco_2$ curve was much flatter (0.041 ml/100 g/mm Hg) (Fig. 67-9). Hence decreasing $Paco_2$ from 40 to 20 mm Hg will decrease CBF by 36 ml/100 g/min (a 65% decrease), whereas CBV will decrease to 2.8 ml/100 g (a 28% change). This translates into a 10- to 14-ml decrease in whole brain volume. This seems to be small, but a brief explanation of intracranial compliance will demonstrate the contrary. Shapiro et al.[381] have shown that the amount of fluid that should be rapidly injected into or withdrawn from the intracranial space to change ICP tenfold (e.g., from 10 to

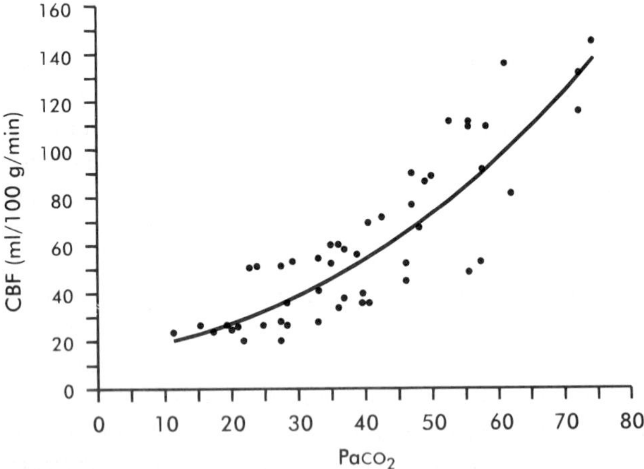

Fig. 67-8. The "bottom half" of a normal cerebral blood flow (CBF)/$Paco_2$ response curve. Each point represents one measurement. (From Grubb RL Jr, Raichle ME, Eichling JO, et al: The effects of changes in $Paco_2$ on cerebral blood volume, blood flow and vascular mean transit time, *Stroke* 5:630, 1974; Wollman H, Smith TC, Stephen GW, et al: Effects of extremes of respiratory and metabolic alkalosis on cerebral blood flow in man, *J Appl Physiol* 24:60, 1968.)

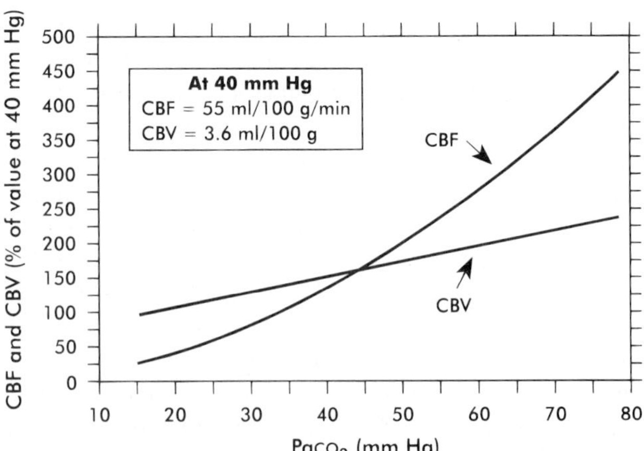

Fig 67-9. Cerebral blood flow (CBF) and cerebral blood volume (CBV) responses to $Paco_2$, with each value expressed as a percentage of that observed at a $Paco_2$ of 40 mm Hg. Note that the slope of the CBV/$Paco_2$ response curve is much flatter than for CBF. (Data from Grubb RL Jr, Raichle ME, Eichling JO: The effects of changes in $Paco_2$ on cerebral blood volume, blood flow, and vascular mean transit time, *Stroke* 5:630, 1974.)

100 mm Hg) is normally ≈ 26 ml. This is called the *pressure-volume index* (PVI). PVI values in patients with mass lesions or closed head injuries may be as low as 5 ml.[204] In such situations, a change in CBV of 10 to 15 ml would be enormous, and it is not surprising that hyperventilation has come to occupy such an important position in acute ICP/brain volume control.

The clinical utility of hypocapnia. **The ability of rapid reductions in $PaCO_2$ to acutely reduce ICP is indisputable.** Although cardiac arrest, stroke, subarachnoid hemorrhage, head trauma, and brain tumors can decrease the slope of the CBF/$PaCO_2$ curve, CO_2 responsiveness is almost never completely lost in a viable patient. It is hence unnecessary to worry whether responsiveness is present or absent in a given patient. If there is no CO_2 response, the patient will probably die or survive in only a severely debilitated state.

The more important questions are: (1) is profound hypocapnia detrimental? and (2) is there benefit to prolonged hypocapnia? In anesthetized animals, hypercapnia has little influence on $CMRO_2$ except at values greater than 200 mm Hg.[42] Moderate hyperventilation also does not alter $CMRO_2$. Nonetheless, during profound alkalosis ($PaCO_2$ ≈ 10 mm Hg) glucose consumption (GMRGlu) increases, as does lactate production. This has been interpreted as indicating excessive cerebral vasoconstriction and tissue ischemia. This may not be true, because alkalosis alone will stimulate glycolysis. Other studies indicate that excess lactate production and some depletion of high-energy phosphates may occur at $PaCO_2$ values of 10 to 15 mm Hg.[403] The electroencephalogram (EEG) slowing seen with extreme hypocapnia can also be reversed by increasing PaO_2, suggesting ischemia. This probably *does not* have any relevance in elective surgery. In a study of the most extreme conditions likely to be encountered clinically, Artru[18] examined cerebral metabolism and tissue high-energy phosphate concentrations during induced hypotension (mean arterial pressure = 40 mm Hg) in dogs with a $PaCO_2$ of 20 mm Hg. Although hypotensive/hypocapnic conditions resulted in increased tissue lactate, $CMRO_2$ and high-energy phosphate values were unchanged compared with normocapnic hypotension. What about hypocapnia in the presence of disease? It has long been argued that hypocapnia might constrict normal vessels, and redistribute blood into ischemic areas ("inverse steal"). Unfortunately, although theoretically attractive, such an event does not appear to occur; hypocapnia seems to increase the total amount of tissue "at risk" during focal ischemia, and primate outcome studies show no benefit.[265,355] Hypocapnia is commonly used to control ICP in head trauma. Available data do not provide much support for anything other than transient value. Robertson et al.[348] used CBF, arteriovenous O_2, and lactate measurements (via jugular venous catheters) to define different subgroups of head-injured patients. They have shown that a modest *increase* in $PaCO_2$ (from previously severe hypocapnia) in *some* patients with very low CBF values can reduce lactate production. Others have shown that reductions in $PaCO_2$, although reducing CBF and ICP, may result in evidence of tissue ischemia.[382] A small but important clinical trial compared chronic hypocapnia ($PaCO_2$ ≈ 25 mm Hg) with "normocapnia" ($PaCO_2$ ≈ 35 mm Hg) and with hypocapnia combined with infusions of THAM (an alkalinizing agent that crosses the blood–brain barrier and hence maintains CSF alkalosis).[290] ICP management was not improved in the hypocapnic patients, and there was a small suggestion of a worsened outcome.

In summary, although reducing $PaCO_2$ is of value in the acute control of ICP or brain bulk in an OR setting (and does not seem to be accompanied by any adverse consequences), essentially no data exist to demonstrate the value of prolonged hypocapnia. In patients with both stroke and head trauma, there is some reason to consider it detrimental.

PaO_2, arterial O_2 content, and hemodilution. Cerebral blood flow does not change much until PaO_2 is <50 mm Hg. It then increases progressively. Under normoxic condition, tissue PO_2 is ≈ 25 mm Hg (or less). Shinozuka[384] has shown that regional pH begins to decrease (and CBF to increase) when tissue PO_2 values decrease below this. This does not imply that H^+ is the direct mediator; it is likely that multiple "sensors" are involved, including endothelium, vascular smooth muscle, and neurons. Vasodilation may be the direct result of O_2-sensitive ion channels in smooth muscle or be produced by vasoactive substances released from multiple sites. Recent work suggests that adenosine, NO, prostacyclin (and other cyclo-oxygenase products) and angiotensin are involved, with vasopressin and opioids (met-enkephalin and leu-enkephalin) playing roles in the fetus and newborn.[120,177,316,322,326,431,437] This multiplicity of involved pathways strongly suggests that there is no single chemical or receptor responsible, but instead indicates the likelihood of substantial redundancy.

While the cerebral vasculature can directly "sense" changes in PaO_2, evidence also suggests that arterial O_2 *content* is an important determinant. This is teleologically sensible, because vasodilation occurring in response to a decreasing O_2 content should act to maintain O_2 delivery constant. It is hence not surprising that CBF will increase in a similar degree regardless of whether O_2 content is reduced by hypoxia, by reducing the O_2 content of erythrocytes, or by reducing the number of erythrocytes. It is commonly believed that hemodilution is "beneficial" because a decrease in viscosity increases CBF.[452] The argument regarding O_2 content suggests this is not entirely true. If so, hemodilution would lead to an *increase* in tissue PO_2, which does not occur.[61] Hemodilution therapy in patients with cerebral ischemia has also been unsuccessful. There is a clinically important corollary to this: if anything prevents the compensatory increase in CBF (e.g., carotid stenosis, trauma), any decrease in O_2 content may lead to tissue injury sooner than would occur in normal individuals.[217,339]

As might be expected from the changes in CBF, increases

in CBV and ICP have been noted during hypoxia in animals.[217,386] Work in our own laboratory has shown that isovolemic hemodilution results in increased CBV,[420] but it is not clear whether anemia can increase ICP in a clinically significant manner.

Autoregulation: CBF and CBV. Autoregulation refers to the maintenance of a constant CBF in the face of changes in *perfusion pressure.*[314] This should not be confused with the other factors that control flow. Most texts describe autoregulation with a curve similar to that in Fig. 67-10, A; in reality it is much less "distinct" (see Fig. 67-10, B). We typically say that CBF is "constant" as long as perfusion pressure is within the range of 50 to 120 to 150 mm Hg. The shape of the curve is similar whether perfusion pressure is altered by changing arterial pressure or changing ICP.[259] Artru et al.[24] have also shown that the lower knee of the autoregulatory curve occurs at the same arterial pressure in normocapnic and hypocapnic dogs, even though lesser flows are present during normotension in the hypocapnic animals. These studies suggest that *transmural* vessel tension is the controlling factor rather than flow or intraluminal pressure *per se* (but see[259]). This is supported by work in isolated ves-

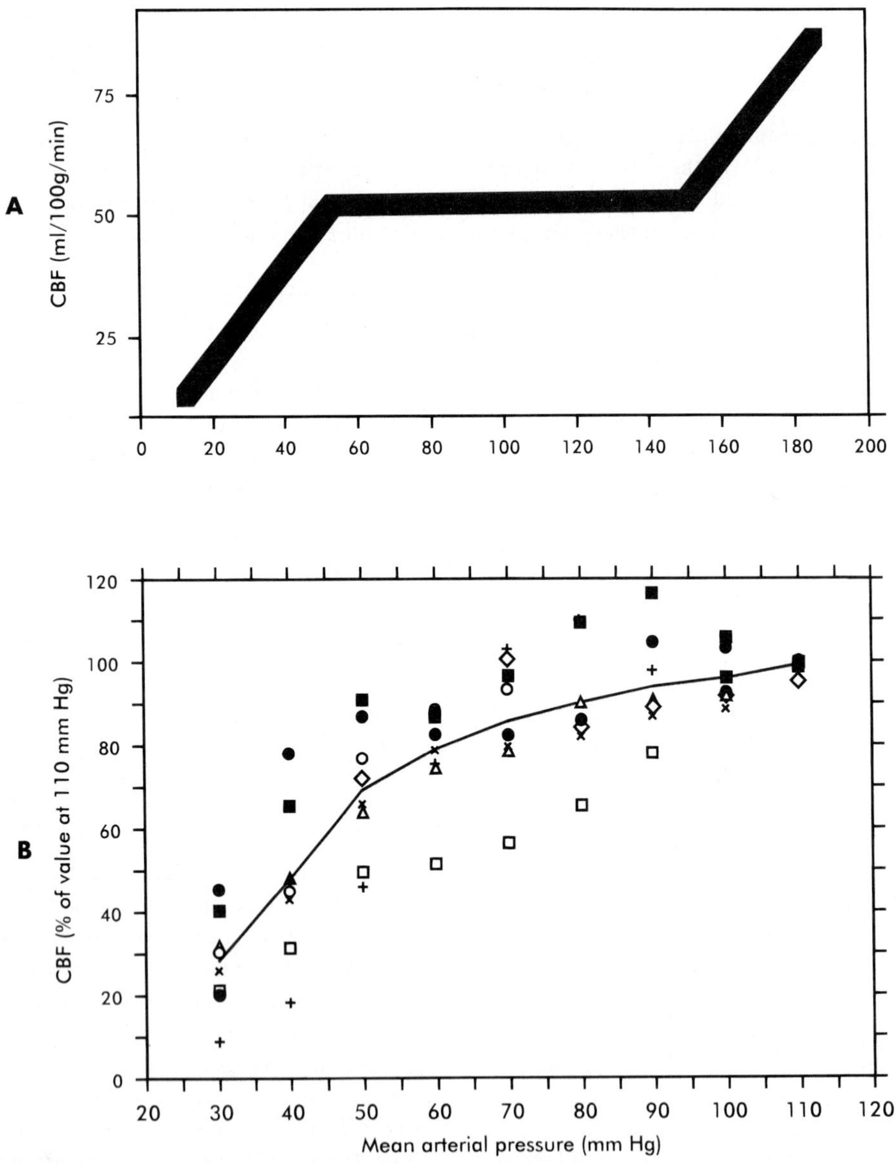

Fig. 67-10. Typical autoregulatory curve is shown in **A.** Flow is generally shown as being stable between mean arterial pressures (or more strictly, perfusion pressure) of 50 and 150 mm Hg. However, although this expresses the concept of autoregulation well, it does not depict reality. **B,** Data collected from eight rats during progressive hemorrhagic hypotension, with a fitted average line. Flow was measured continuously with a lasser Doppler but summarized in 10 mm Hg steps. Because the laser Doppler does not yield flow in typical units, cerebral blood flow (CBF) is expressed as percentage of flow at 110 mm Hg. Note the lack of a sharp "knee" and the wide scatter around the line.

sels, where several workers have shown that increasing transmural pressures result in depolarization of vascular smooth muscle with subsequent constriction.[198,299]

The sympathetic nervous system can modulate autoregulation. Both alpha blockade and cervical sympathectomy can change the lower limit of the autoregulatory curve (shifting it to the left), even though they do not change baseline flow.[110,156,192,357] Conversely, intense sympathetic stimulation and chronic hypertension can shift the curve to the right. Angiotensin also plays a possibly important role.[315,438]

There are several misconceptions regarding autoregulation. First, autoregulation is readily abolished. Changes in the shape of curve, shifts in the knees, or complete loss of autoregulation (i.e., parallel changes in CBF as BP changes) are commonly present in patients with tumors, arteriovenous malformations, ruptured aneurysms, strokes, and so forth. In fact, dysautoregulation is described in neurologically normal individuals and it is thus not clear that alterations in the curve *per se* have serious clinical implications. This, along with the typical scatter seen in Fig. 67-10, B, indicates that we cannot rely on the published "normal" limits for autoregulation, at least not in individual patients. Arguments supporting the safety of some hemodynamic intervention based on the idea, for example, that "the normal lower limit of autoregulation is not exceeded" are suspect. This is particularly true if tissue perfusion pressure is not known (e.g., with proximal carotid stenosis). Second, autoregulation is not instantaneous. Early studies suggested that the autoregulatory responses required 20 to 60 seconds. Recent studies using TCD indicate that the response is faster at least in normal subjects (i.e., 1 to 10 sec).[1] Abrupt blood pressure changes will lead to transient changes in CBF even when autoregulation is normal. In a patient with disrupted autoregulation, similar changes can lead to large and sustained alterations in CBF and presumably CBV and ICP. This is perhaps most relevant during the abrupt changes in BP produced by laryngoscopy and tracheal intubation, pin insertion, skin incision, tracheal suctioning, and so forth. Because volatile anesthetics appear to slow (and in high enough doses abolish) autoregulation, CBF responses to such stimuli may be exaggerated,[400,414] but these agents also decrease the BP pressure to the stimuli.

The lower end of the curve is of greatest concern during hypotension. CBF is adequately maintained down to perfusion pressures of 30 to 40 mm Hg during hypotension produced with nitroprusside, halothane, or isoflurane, but signs of cellular dysfunction (e.g., EEG and evoked response changes, acidosis, K^+ escape) appear at notably greater pressures with hemorrhage and with ganglionic blockers, indicating that direct vasodilators shift the knee to the right.[270,285] It is not clear that there are important differences between hypotensive agents at *clinically employed blood pressures* (e.g., MAP = 50 to 60 mm Hg), and no pharmacologic hypotensive technique has been clearly shown preferable. When autoregulation is altered (e.g., in a patient with vasospasm), hypotension, induced even with "good" drugs can exacerbate tissue injury.

Flow-metabolism coupling. There should be a constant matching of O_2/glucose delivery to metabolic demand. This is commonly referred to as "flow-metabolism coupling" and is reflected by parallel changes in CBF as CMR changes; tissue regions with high metabolic rates (e.g., gray matter) will have greater flows than regions with low CMR (Fig. 67-11).[208,221] This is reflected by a constant ratio between CBF and CMR (and by the straight line in Fig. 67-12). Under dynamic conditions, any change in CMR is rapidly matched by an appropriate change in CBF. A relationship between *functional* cerebral activity, CMR, and CBF is clearly present in humans.[215] For example, a light flashed into one visual field results in increases in both CBF and CMRGlu in the contralateral occipital visual cortex, and repeated clenching of one hand is accompanied by changes in contralateral sensorimotor cortex. Many studies indicate that coupling is probably the major mechanism by which the delivery of O_2 and nutrients is regionally modulated.

Although coupling "makes sense," its mechanism(s) are unknown and the subject of intense investigation. It was once assumed that if metabolism increased, regional acidosis would develop, leading to vasodilation, but this cannot explain the rapid responses seen to rapid increases in CMR or to neuronal activation, because flow increases before any acidosis develops. Other control mechanisms have been proposed. Cerebral vessels are well innervated by adrenergic,

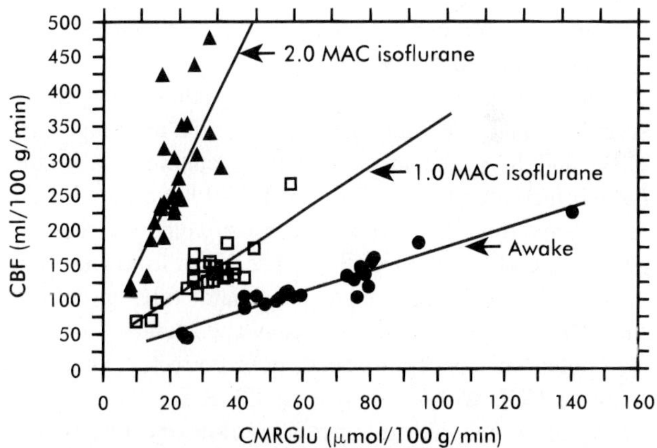

Fig. 67-11. Regression plots of regional cerebral metabolic rate for glucose (CMRGlu) versus regional cerebral blood flow (rCBF) in the rat. Each point on the curve represents the average CBF and CMRGlu value for one anatomic region (e.g., auditory cortex, caudate), determined by ^{14}C-iodoantipyrine and ^{14}C-deoxyglucose autoradiography, respectively. Animals were studied awake and at stable isoflurane doses of 1 and 2 MAC. For each situation, a significant straight-line relationship between CMRGlu and CBF is seen, indicating the persistence of a coupled relationship between these variables. As the concentration of isoflurane is increased, however, the slope of the regression line increases (i.e., higher CBF for a given CMRGlu value). This indicates that isoflurane is a cerebrovasodilator in the rat brain but that it does not uncouple flow and metabolism, even at 2 MAC. (Data from Maekawa T, Tommasino C, Shapiro HM, et al: Local cerebral blood flow and glucose utilization during isoflurane anesthesia in the rat, *Anesthesiology* 65:144, 1986.)

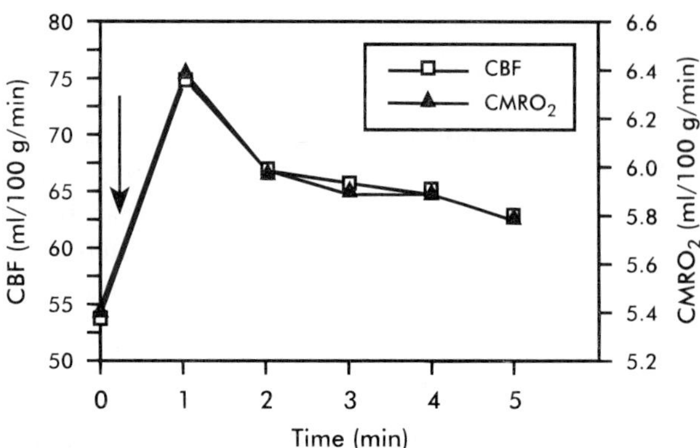

Fig. 67-12. Flow-metabolism coupling as a dynamic event. Dogs were prepared for the near-continuous measurement of both cerebral blood flow (CBF) and cerebral metabolic rate for oxygen ($CMRO_2$) using a venous outflow method. At the arrow, the femoral nerve was electrically stimulated. This is immediately followed by a matched increase in both $CMRO_2$ and CBF, demonstrating the presence of coupling. (Data from Kuramoto T, Oshita S, Takeshita H, et al: Modification of the relationship between cerebral metabolism, blood flow, and the EEG by stimulation during anesthesia in the dog, *Anesthesiology* 51:211, 1979.)

cholinergic, serotonergic, and GABAminergic nerve fibers.[404,437] It is probable that flow is under tight neurogenic control. Vasoactive compounds may be elaborated locally in response to metabolic activity. These might include acetylcholine, bradykinin, adenosine, and serotonin, NO, prostanoids, K^+, and so forth. Additional evidence shows that flow is more closely related to changing glucose consumption, not $CMRO_2$.[128]

Many situations encountered in anesthesia and neurosurgery change CMR and have the potential to change CBF, CBV, and ICP. The most dramatic example is a seizure (which increases CBF, CBV, and ICP-8)[106]; others include fever, shivering, and pain. The most common cause of changing CMR is the anesthetic itself (see following paragraphs). These CMR changes play major roles in defining the CBF changes produced by many anesthetics.

Another misconception needs to be corrected. Drugs that increase CBF without increasing CMR (or that decrease CMR) are often said to "uncouple" flow and metabolism. This divergence of CBF and CMR is seen with volatile anesthetics. These drugs do not *uncouple* CBF and CMR because the previously mentioned linear relationships (Fig. 67-11) persist during anesthesia with these drugs, except at very high concentrations.[159,230] True uncoupling can be demonstrated only by showing that increased either neuronal activity or CMR occurs without any accompanying increase in CBF.

Autonomic control. Many early reviews of anesthesia and cerebrovascular physiology ignored the effect of the autonomic nervous system. This stemmed largely from the observation that clinically relevant doses of most adrenergic and cholinergic agents have little effect on resting CBF. Brain vessels are well innervated by postganglionic sympathetic nerves that originate from the superior cervical sympathetic ganglia and by fibers that appear to modulate parasympathetic activity.[43,296,404,437] Under physiological conditions (normotension, normoxia and normocapnia), sympathetic nerves exert very little effect on cerebral blood flow. In contrast, high levels of sympathetic activity (such as that encountered during hemorrhagic shock) shifts the autoregulatory curve to right and blunts both hypoxic and hypercapnic vasodilation.[57,85,317] Conversely, adrenergic antagonists (e.g., phentolamine) or sympathetic ganglionectomy shift the curve to the left.[156,192,357] During acute hypertension, sympathetic nerves are activated and vasoconstrict cerebral vessels thus providing some protection against cerebral hyperemia and disruption of the blood–brain barrier. This phenomenon appears more effective in the brain stem than in the supratentorial part of the brain. Stimulation of parasympathetic pathways may play some role in cerebral vasodilation—particularly during anesthesia.[401] Atropine has relatively little influence of CBF except in huge doses.

Alpha-1 receptor agonists, such as phenylephrine and norepinephrine, exert little effect on cerebral vessels except in very high doses and then often only by shifting autoregulatory limits. This may be altered somewhat depending on the preexisiting state of the cerebral vasculature (e.g., in the presence of vasodilators),[313] but we believe that there is little reason for the oft-expressed concern that the clinical use of these drugs will somehow result in cerebral ischemia. In contrast, alpha-2 agonists such as clonidine and dexmetetomidine produce peripheral vasodilation and cerebral vasoconstriction.

Beta agonists (isoproterenol) exert important influences on CBF only if the blood–brain barrier is disrupted. Beta-receptors are present on neurons. When the barrier is open—or in very high doses—beta agonists may increase CMR with a resultant coupled increase in CBF. Whether this is of clinical relevance remains unclear.

CEREBROVASCULAR PHARMACOLOGY OF ANESTHETICS AND ADJUVANTS

As stated earlier, neuroanesthesia is the practice of applied cerebrovascular physiology and pharmacology, particularly the manipulation of CBV. Anesthetics affect all the parameters discussed in the previous sections, as does natural sleep.[229,367] The oft-noted attempt in the experimental laboratory to design a combination of anesthetic agents that have no such effects can only be viewed with disdain. Differing drug-induced changes do have some bearing on clinical practice, and it is important to understand them.

Intravenous Anesthetics

Barbiturates

Barbiturates were the first anesthetics whose cerebrovascular effects were examined. Thiopental is the prototype, and all other clinically used barbiturates are similar (although their pharmacokinetics differ). Increasing doses of thiopental progressively decrease CMR and CBF (assuming that

$Paco_2$ does not change).[187,262] The changes in CBF appear to occur as the result of metabolic suppression and coupled decreases in flow. If coupling is disrupted, if CMR is already maximally depressed *vasodilation* in response to barbiturates can be demonstrated.[261] This can also be seen in isolated vessels.[164,218,237,305] The relationship between dose and CBF/CMR is not linear, with large decreases seen with small doses and progressively less effect as blood concentrations increase further. The maximal decrease in both CBF and $CMRo_2$ occurs coincident with the appearance of isoelectricity on the EEG, and is ≈ 50% of awake normal (although the metabolic/CBF difference between burst-suppression and isoelectricity is small).[187,262] Thiopental even in very high doses does not appear to abolish autoregulation, Co_2 response, or flow-metabolism coupling. Barbiturates have also been shown to result in lesser CBV values than volatile agents.[419]

Propofol

Like thiopental, propofol produces dose-related EEG suppression (including isoelectricity) and progressive reductions in both CBF and CMR, with minimum CMR values of 40% to 60% of control values.[26,324,333,432] The relationship between these CBF changes and reductions in ICP was initially clouded by the decreases in BP sometimes seen with the recommended induction doses, but subsequent data indicate that propofol does reduce CBF independent of any systemic hemodynamic changes.[333] The only available CBV data again suggests similarities with the barbiturates.[419] The drug has been used successfully in many neurosurgical procedures and in neurosurgical intensive care units in both Europe and the United States.[54,168,390]

In recent years, case reports have appeared suggesting that propofol can induce seizures, but propofol has been given uneventfully to epileptic patients.[109,363]

Etomidate

Etomidate is remarkably barbituratelike, producing similar CBF and CMR changes. In dogs, etomidate reduces CBF more rapidly than $CMRo_2$, suggesting that it may have some direct cerebral vasoconstricting properties.[273,345] No CBV data are available, but the drug does reduce ICP.[84,92,273] It is possible to produce an isoelectric EEG, but this may be preceded by intermittent spiking, which may be associated with myoclonus.[341] True seizure activity (distinguished from myoclonus) is not typically seen in normal patients. In patients with convulsive disorders, small doses (8 to 12 mg) of etomidate can elicit true seizures. Etomidate has even been used to unmask seizure foci during operative EEG mapping.[108,341]

Recently, toxicity related to the propylene glycol solvent used for etomidate has been reported in patients given etomidate infusions for long periods of time.[216]

Ketamine

Ketamine can produce increases in CBF[175,409] and in ICP, particularly in spontaneously breathing patients.[78,379] It has also been reported to increase ICP when used for anesthetic induction.[41] For many years, ketamine was one of the few anesthetic agents for which use was deemed absolutely contraindicated in neuroanesthesia. The subsequent literature on this drug is quite contradictory. In 1982, Schwedler et al.[376] reported no important CBF changes in chronically-instrumented goats (as long as ventilation was supported). Others have reported significant increases in both rabbits and dogs.[23,342] In 1990, Werner et al.,[445] using TCD to assess CBF, demonstrated a clear dose-related CBF increase, whereas Mayberg et al.[251] saw no changes in either Vmca or ICP when the drug was given to anesthetized and ventilated individuals. Friesen et al.[131,132] found that ketamine could block the ICP response to intubation and infants, and had no direct ICP effects when ventilation was supported. It is difficult to draw firm conclusions from such data. We concur with suggestions that ketamine is probably inappropriate as a sole agent for neurodiagnositic procedures.

Eltanolone

Eltanolone is a new steroid hypnotic with a rapid onset of action and short duration of action.[59] Only one study of its cerebrovascular effects has appeared, and this demonstrates an action very similar to other intravenous agents.[449] The drug was withdrawn from the U.S.-approval clinical trial process recently.

Opiates

It was once believed that opiates had no effect on CMR or CBF because even 1 to 3 mg/kg doses of morphine have little effect on CBF and CMR in ventilated patients also receiving N_2O.[180] Drugs such as fentanyl have changed this picture. Low doses of fentanyl (e.g., 5 to 15 μg/kg) probably have little effect, but much larger doses of fentanyl (e.g., ≈ 50 to 100 μg/kg), sufentanil, alfentanil, and the newest agent, remifentanil, do progressively decrease CMR and CBF in many species including humans.[60,172,195,280,291,458] The maximum reduction is ≈ 40% to 50%, with $CMRo_2$ values of ≈ 2 ml/100 g/min and CBF values of 20 to 25 ml/100 g/min being observed in patients given "cardiac" doses of fentanyl (typically) combined with small doses of diazepam).[291,292] The CMR/CBF changes occur in parallel with progressive EEG slowing[377,442] although isoelectricity is not achievable. High doses of most opiates may produce rare seizures in humans[335,358] and seizure-associated histopathologic injury in some animals[203]; efforts to consistently demonstrate seizures in normal humans have been generally unsuccessful.[293] Low-voltage spikes, similar to discharges seen during sleep, have been recently reported in cardiac surgical patients[193] and seizures have been reported following high-dose fentanyl in patients with complex partial epilepsy.[412] Meperidine is a well-known convulsant, due to its metabolite, normeperidine.

Although opioids produce dose-related reductions in CBF and CMR, they have never found a major role in the control of ICP. One reason may relate to a unique property of these drugs. In 1990, Milde et al.[277] reported that bolus administration of 2 to 200 μg/kg doses of sufentanil produced transient but often pronounced increases in ICP in lightly anesthetized dogs.[272] This report was the subject of great debate, but several subsequent human studies have shown that the synthetic narcotics can increase ICP under some (poorly defined) conditions.[6,246,394] Fentanyl and sufentanil can also increase CBF (as measured by TCD) in normocarbic human volunteers.[425] The mechanism for such changes remains unclear—perhaps activation of mu (μ) receptors on cerebral vessels plays some role. Available clinical trials continue to suggest that opioid/N_2O anesthesia is acceptable for elective neurosurgery,[418] and show no clear advantages of any particular opioid.[133] This latter conclusion may change as experience is gained with the ultrashort-acting opioid remifentanil.[143,172]

The central nervous system (CNS) effects of naloxone have also been the subject of numerous studies. Naloxone alone probably has no important CBF/ICP effects.[27] When carefully titrated, it normalizes CBF and $CMRo_2$ in narcotized subjects.[248] Abrupt opioid reversal with excessive doses of naloxone has resulted in hypertension, pulmonary edema, dysrhythmias, and intracranial hemorrhage.[117,329]

Sedative Agents

Benzodiazepines and antagonists

Diazepam, midazolam, and lorazepam typically produce small decreases in CBF or $CMRo_2$, in both sedative and anesthetic doses.[124,126,199,347,433] A distinct ceiling effect is present, and an isoelectric EEG is not produced.[124] No data on CBV are available. The ICP effects of these drugs are consistently small.[141,411]

Recently, flumazenil has been introduced as a receptor-specific benzodiazepine antagonist. Like naloxone, it has little or no CNS effect when given alone.[125] It also appears to have no unique properties when used to reverse a benzodiazepine.[199,346] Fleischer et al.[124] have noted a dramatic rebound increase in canine CBF (and ICP) to values greater than baseline when a high-dose midazolam anesthetic is reversed by the bolus administration of a large dose of flumazenil. Similar changes in humans have been recorded by Chiolero et al.[62] This phenomenon is akin to the withdrawal phenomena seen when naloxone is given in large doses after narcotic anesthesia. Flumazenil is also known to precipitate seizures when given in large doses for abrupt diazepine reversal.

Butyrophenones (Droperidol)

Most data on droperidol were obtained when it was used in combination with opioids. Large doses (0.35 mg/kg) in dogs can reduce CBF by 40% but not change $CMRo_2$. This change occurred very gradually, and the pattern of decreasing CBF without changing $CMRo_2$ or BP is unique among anesthetics. In humans, the combination of droperidol (5 mg) and fentanyl (100 μg) uniformly reduced CBF and ICP, but droperidol alone (in relatively large doses) seems to produce a small increase.[64,275,278] In view of these data, it is unlikely that small antiemetic (0.0625 to 1.25 mg) or sedative (2.5 to 5 mg) doses of droperidol have any important CBF/ICP effects.

Dexmedetomidine

For roughly 10 years, there has been intense interest in the sedative/anesthetic properties of drugs that act as agonists at central alpha-2 adrenegeric receptors.[50,252,253] The best characterized (and most potent) of these agents is dexmedetomidine.[99] Although there is little clinical experience with this drug in neurosurgery, experimental studies demonstrate its ability to markedly reduce CBF in animals and humans[184,461] and to reduce ICP in animals.[462] It remains uncertain whether or not this vasoconstriction (which is at least partially independent of changes in CMR) is beneficial. The drug also may reduce seizure thresholds (and hence may be a "proconvulsant").[277]

Volatile Agents

When halothane was introduced in the 1950s, it was hailed as the neuroanesthetic of choice. It was nonflammable; induction and emergence were rapid and smooth (compared with ether); anesthetic depth and arterial pressure could be easily and quickly controlled; greater than 95% O_2 could be given; and ventilation was usually adequate or easily controlled to prevent severe brain swelling. In the late 1960s, it was discovered that halothane could increase ICP. Despite its decade-long record of success, the use of halothane in neurosurgery declined. This was accelerated by the enthusiasm for barbiturates that appeared in the early 1970s and by the development of short-acting opioids. A resurgence in the use of volatile anesthetics for neurosurgery was prompted by the introduction of insoluble ethers—first enflurane and then isoflurane. Both drugs were initially reported to have advantages over halothane in terms of CNS effects. Unfortunately, despite widespread beliefs, these "advantages" remain generally unproved.

Halothane, enflurane, and isoflurane

The effects of *halothane* on CBF were first examined in humans in 1964.[450] During normocapnic administration of ≈ 1.2% halothane (inspired), global CBF was 51 ml/100 g/min, as compared with awake normal values of 44 ml/100 g/min in the same group of subjects. The authors concluded that "halothane in the concentration studied was . . . a mild cerebral vasodilator." (Note: The magnitude of these CBF changes is similar to that produced by a 5 mm Hg change in $Paco_2$—see previous paragraph.) The first "clinical" correlate was reported by Jennett et al.[179] in 1969, who demonstrated ICP increases in neurosurgical patients (Fig. 67-13). This was confirmed by Adams et al.[3] in 1972. Neither group found any evidence of clinical deterioration in the patients given halothane, although Adams demonstrated that ICP changes were not seen in the presence of hypocapnia.

In 1973, *enflurane* was introduced into clinical practice,

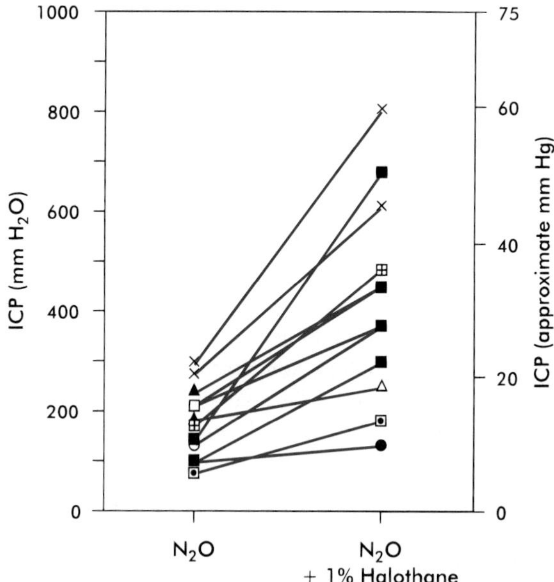

Fig. 67-13. Intracranial pressure (ICP) responses to the addition of ≈ 1% halothane in a series of patients with space-occupying intracranial lesions. ICP was measured with a ventriculostomy. (Modified from Jennett WB, Barker J, Fitch W, et al: Effects of anesthesia on intracranial pressure in patients with space-occupying lesions, *Lancet* I:61, 1969.)

followed in 1981 by *isoflurane.* Numerous human and animal studies have compared the CBF/CMR effects of these agents with those of halothane.[51,111,158,226-228,268,372,416,458] Because some of the earlier studies (particularly Eientrei et al.[111]) reported that halothane (at least in doses >1 MAC) resulted in the largest CBF changes, many clinicians concluded that isoflurane and enflurane were "better" than halothane. Because the capacity of enflurane to induce electroencephalographic seizures, particularly during hypocapnia, is viewed as "bad," the result was growth in the popularity of isoflurane as a neurosurgical anesthetic.

Unfortunately, this scenario may be problematic. Reported CBF differences among these drugs may be "artifacts" of specific measurement methods used. Recent work disputes the idea that volatile agents "uncouple" flow and metabolism and also supports the idea that changing CMR plays a major role in defining the CBF changes produced by the drugs. Finally, data exist concerning the relationships between the CBF, CBV, and ICP effects of these drugs, and lastly, it may be incorrect to conclude that differences in CBF can be translated into differences in clinical utility/safety.

Cerebral blood flow: flow distribution and method-related "artifacts." In an earlier section of this chapter, we cautioned against interpreting CBF measurements without understanding the limitations inherent in the specific measurement method used. This caveat applies to volatile anesthetics. In 1988, Hansen et al.[158] demonstrated that 1 MAC halothane and isoflurane produced identical hemispheric CBF values in rats; ^{14}C-iodoantipyrine autoradiography revealed that the two drugs produced remarkably different flow *patterns.* More recently, SPECT studies by Reinstrup et al.[344] confirm different flow distribution pictures. Halothane selectively increased flow to the cortex while reducing subcortical flow. Isoflurane resulted in more uniform flow patterns. This implied that if one were to compare the CBF effects of these volatile agents using a technique that selectively looked at the cortical mantle (e.g., most ^{133}Xe washout methods), halothane would appear to have the greater effect. By contrast, if whole brain flow were examined (e.g., using a KS technique), flows would be very similar.

There is animal and human evidence to support this hypothesis (Table 67-3). At least 13 studies compare halothane and isoflurane in some manner. These were all carried out at roughly 1 MAC doses but with variable background anesthetics (e.g., N_2O, morphine, subarachnoid tetracaine, etc.). Within each study, the CBF effects of the volatile agents were determined under similar conditions, and hence the differing background conditions do not confuse the comparison. When the method used to measure CBF provides cortically weighted data, flow values average 1.6 times greater with halothane than with isoflurane. However, when global measurements are compared, there are no differences between these agents.

This is circumstantial but compelling evidence. All volatile agents are mild cerebral vasodilators. There appear to be no major differences in the effects on *global* CBF. If the CBF/CBV relationships are similar for these different drugs, we predict that isoflurane and halothane would have similar CBV effects. Taking the argument one step further, we would also predict that these agents should have identical effects on ICP. This will be explored below.

It is tempting to dismiss regional differences in the CBF effects of these drugs as academic curiosities. In fact, such observations have important implications relative to the *mechanisms* by which volatile agents influence CBF. If these drugs acted by directly relaxing vascular smooth muscle, we would expect to see either more uniform flow distribution patterns or at least *similar* distribution patterns with different agents. The markedly different regional effect observed indicate that some factor should be acting as an intermediary. Additional support for this hypothesis comes from experiments in our laboratory, in which a focal cryogenic injury dramatically attenuated the CBF increase seen with isoflurane.[332] This altered flow response was seen in brain regions far removed from the site of injury, regions in which the response to CO_2 was unaltered. The nature of this hypothetical mediator is unknown at present but could be biochemical, metabolic, or neurogenic. This many reports suggest that either NO, a prostaglandin or acetylcholine, may play intermediary roles in the effects of volatile agents.[201,202,258,281,401,422]

CBV and ICP. Based on the apparent similarity of the CBF effects of halothane and isoflurane, we predicted that the two drugs should produce similar changes in CBV and ICP. In 1982, Artru[15,17] measured the acute changes in CBV

Table 67-3 The relative cerebral blood flow effects of volatile agents and the influence of measurement method

Authors	Reference	Year	Species	Method	Cortical/global	Halothane	Isoflurane	Halothane/isoflurane ratio
Todd et al.	416	1984	Cat	IC ^{133}Xe	Cortical	61 ± 15	48 ± 24	1.3
Eintrei et al.	111	1985	Human	Topical ^{133}Xe	Cortical	177 ± 39	67 ± 27	1.8
Scheller et al.	372	1986	Rabbit	H_2 clearance	Cortical	138 ± 94	62 ± 27	2.2
Michenfelder et al.	268	1987	Human	IC ^{133}Xe	Cortical	62 ± 24	37 ± 14	1.7
Hansen et al.	158	1988	Rat	Autoradiography	Cortical	185 ± 18	154 ± 19	1.2
Young et al.	458	1989	Human	IH/IV ^{133}Xe	Cortical	34	24	1.4
Madsen et al.	226–228	1986–87	Human	Kety-Schmidt	Global	36 ± 8	33 ± 11	1.1
Hansen et al.	158	1988	Rat	Autoradiography	Global	150 ± 16	147 ± 19	1.0

*Where available, all values are presented as mean ± SD (with SD calculated when SEM is reported in the original article). The designation of cortical vs. global refers to the primary area studied using the CBF method listed in the fourth column. For example, cortical measurements obtained with microspheres indicates that cortical tissue was specifically separated from underlying regions, whereas cortical measurements using H_2 clearance indicates electrode placement in the cortex. "Global" indicates that flow values reflect both cortical and deep structures combined (e.g., H_2 electrode placed in the confluence of venous sinuses).
In all cases, CBF values within a row are reported either in the same manuscript, or represent work from the same laboratory using the same methodology. Background anesthetics do differ from study to study, but are consistent within a row, except for the values listed in parenthesis. All measurements were made at approximately 1 MAC concentrations of volatile agent, except for Boarini et al. (1.3 MAC). The data from Michenfelder et al. represents values obtained prior to carotid cross-clamping in grade 1 patients undergoing carotid endarterectomies.

produced by 1 MAC concentrations of halothane, enflurane, and isoflurane in dogs ventilated with 70% N_2O. All three drugs produced 8% to 11% increases in volume with no statistical differences. More recently, Weeks et al.[443] quantitated cerebral plasma volume in rats anesthetized with 1 MAC halothane and isoflurane. There were no differences between these agents during normocapnia.

There is less information available regarding ICP. All three volatile agents are capable of increasing ICP.[2,3,146,179,287] The only human comparative data came from two studies by Adams et al.[2,3] with halothane and isoflurane. The two agents were not studied concurrently nor in equipotent doses, but both studies indicated that: (1) the two drugs could increase ICP when given during normocapnia; (2) neither drug had any ICP effect when given to hypocapnic patients; and (3) none of the ICP increases seen with either agent were associated with any adverse clinical outcome. Animal work by Scheller et al.[373] showed that in rabbits with severe brain injuries and preexistent intracranial hypertension, the ICP effects of the drugs were essentially identical (Fig. 67-14).

There are two possible exceptions to this "halothane = enflurane = isoflurane" hypothesis. Artru et al.[14,16,25] have

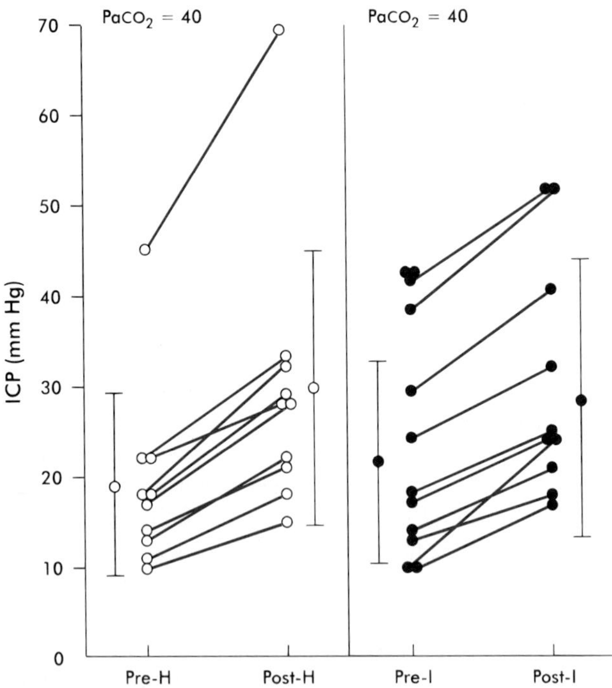

Fig. 67-14. Maximum intracranial pressure (ICP) responses to the addition of 1 MAC halothane (*on the left*) or isoflurane (*on the right*) to normocarbic rabbits after a focal cortical brain injury. The background anesthetic was morphine/N_2O. Baseline ICP in both groups was elevated by the injury (to ≈ 18–20 mm Hg), but the increases produced by the volatile agents were statistically identical. (From Scheller MS, Todd MM, Drummond JC, et al: The intracranial pressure effects of isoflurane and halothane administered following cryogenic brain injury in rabbits, *Anesthesiology* 64:598, 1986.)

shown that volatile agents have quite different effects on CSF production and reabsorption. Enflurane increases CSF production, and prolonged exposure can lead to slightly greater ICPs. Halothane decreases CSF production, a change that Maktabi et al.[232] suggest is mediated by vasopressin. Drummond et al.[104] and Scheller et al.[372] provided evidence of some unique interaction between CO_2 and isoflurane. Drummond et al.[104] reported that the slope of the CBF/$Paco_2$ response curve between 20 and 40 mm Hg was steeper for isoflurane than halothane, whereas Scheller et al.[372] noted that when isoflurane was given to hypocapnic rabbits, CBF actually decreased (but increased with halothane). Weeks et al.[443] found that although CBV was identical during normocapnic anesthesia with halothane and isoflurane, CBV fell more readily during hypocapnic isoflurane anesthesia than with halothane. Thus, it is possible that there may be agent-specific ICP differences during hypocapnia although this was not observed by Scheller et al.[373] in injured animals.

CMR

Volatile agents increase CBF at the same time CMR is decreasing. This was interpreted by many as indicating that these drugs "uncoupled" flow and metabolism. We now know that this is not true uncoupling. Kuramoto et al.[206] reported parallel increases in CBF and CMR during stimulation of the femoral nerve in dogs anesthetized with halothane. Further, Maekawa et al.[230] and Hansen et al.[159] indicated that coupled relationships between CBF and CMRGlu are maintained during halothane and isoflurane anesthesia, at least with concentrations of $\approx$ 1 MAC (and possibly greater) (see Fig. 67-11). These experiments demonstrate that coupling is present during these relatively modest doses of volatile agent, although Kuramoto et al.[206] did provide some evidence for true uncoupling at greater concentrations of halothane ($>$ 2 MAC).

The persistence of coupling has two implications. First, since the different volatile agents have different effects on CMR, observed variations in cortical flow may be the result of differing effects on metabolism, rather than different direct effects on the cerebral vasculature. With intact coupling, direct vasodilating effects of a drug may be offset by the indirect, metabolically linked vasoconstriction. Two agents with identical direct vasodilating properties, but with differing metabolic effects, may have very different effects on CBF. Persistence of coupling also suggests that CBF effects of a volatile agent may depend on metabolic brain conditions at the time of agent administration. This latter possibility was best demonstrated by Drummond et al.[105] who exposed rabbits to equi-MAC concentrations of halothane and isoflurane and noted that halothane appeared to produce a greater increase in cortical CBF (as expected). When baseline $CMRo_2$ was reduced by the administration of barbiturates, the flow effects of the two drugs were identical. Essentially the same experiment was carried out in humans by Matta et al.[250] using TCD with near-identical results. Such experiments suggest that the influence of a volatile agent may depend highly on the other drugs that have been given to the patient during that anesthetic.

Precautions. The previous comments indicate that the older wildely-held concepts concerning the different effects of volatile agents on the brain are not correct. Although it would be incorrect to state that there are no differences between volatile agents, these three agents are certainly more similar than heretofore believed. All three can increase CBF, CBV, and ICP. These drug-induced ICP increases have never been demonstrated to be detrimental and are easily counteracted by other ICP control measures (e.g., hyperventilation). To conclude that such agents are contraindicated in all but a tiny fraction of neurosurgical patients is a serious misinterpretation of available data. To conclude that "halothane is bad, but isoflurane is good (or better)" is incorrect with respect to cerebrovascular physiology.

Desflurane and sevoflurane

These newer agents may have some advantages over the current drugs because their low blood-gas solubility characteristics (0.6 for sevoflurane, 0.4 for desflurane) should allow more rapid titration of anesthetic depth and faster emergence. Several studies of the cerebrovascular effects of sevoflurane have appeared.[67,197,235,370,371] Essentially all of these showed modest decreases in flow, even under conditions where isoflurane resulted in small increases. It is tempting to conclude that this suggests some "advantage" to sevoflurane, but the reported differences were small. One potential problem with sevoflurane is that it is metabolized actively, releasing inorganic fluoride.[385] Prolonged use can lead to elevated fluoride concentrations[200]; this process can be accelerated in animals given enzyme-inducing drugs, such as phenobarbital and phenytoin.[170] Because many neurosurgical patients are taking such drugs, the potential for renal toxicity, particularly with long operations, needs to be addressed in future research studies.

In the early 1990s, the Mayo group reported dose-related increases in CBF with desflurane (as long as MAP was supported), and reductions in $CMRo_2$. When BP fell, CBF declined.[271] The most direct comparison of desflurane with isoflurane was performed in humans by Ornstein et al.[310] These measurements were made in hypocapnic patients undergoing craniotomy and indicated essentially identical reductions in CBF with both drugs after induction, with no subsequent increases as dose was raised. The one unique finding with desflurane is that it appears to produce a small but steady increase in ICP.[295] Artru[21] has demonstrated a decrease in intracranial compliance with desflurane, which may be the result of altered CSF dynamics.

None of these physiology studies have addressed the crucial issue of the clinical acceptability/advantages of these agents. Given the relatively minor differences seen between the cerebrovascular behavior of these drugs and isoflurane, it is unlikely that their use will pose important problems—

although it is equally uncertain that they offer practical advantages.

Nitrous Oxide

Many clinicians consider N_2O to have few cerebrovascular effects. This is not true. N_2O can increase CBF in animals and humans by more than 60% to 100%,[36,94,319] and can produce large ICP increases in patients with mass lesions.[166,288] Similar increases in CBF and ICP can be seen when N_2O is added to a volatile agent or narcotic background,[7,103,160,182,209,361] whereas Archer et al.[12] have shown that N_2O can increase CBV. The CBF changes are not altered by hypocapnia[415] although the ICP response can be blunted if compliance is improved. Similar alteration of the ICP response to N_2O can be achieved by administration of any agent that will decrease CBV (e.g., thiopental).[323]

Comparisons of CBF effects of N_2O with those produced by volatile agents suggest that N_2O may be a *more potent* vasodilator than either halothane or isoflurane. Hansen et al.[160] compared in rats the CBF effects of a 1 MAC anesthetic provided either with a volatile agent alone, or by a combination of 0.5 MAC volatile agent and 0.5 MAC N_2O. In all experiments, CBF was greater in the presence of N_2O. Similar results have now been obtained in two studies of humans.[7,209] Adding N_2O to a volatile agent background did not have any CMR effects, suggesting that one reason for the dramatic CBF effects of N_2O is that vasodilation is unopposed by indirect, CMR–mediated vasoconstriction.[338]

One unique property of N_2O is its propensity to diffuse rapidly into closed, airfilled spaces such as a pneumocephalus.[360] Because pneumocephalus is an almost uniform consequence of intracranial surgery,[311,340] some have argued against use of N_2O. As long as N_2O is used throughout the procedure and can equilibrate with any air bubble before the dura is closed, its use poses no problem. Indeed, discontinuation of N_2O can actually reduce ICP at the end of surgery.[97,389]

Adjuvant Drugs

Nondepolarizing muscle relaxants

Intracranial pressure effects. After many studies, one is struck by the extraordinarily benign nature of these agents in terms of CBF and ICP. The only suggestion of a detrimental effect follows the bolus administration of large doses of *d*-tubocurarine, where histamine release can increase both CBV and ICP.[410]

Interactions with phenytoin and other anticonvulsants. There is one practical concern regarding nondepolarizing relaxants and neurosurgery. Case reports and clinical studies have demonstrated that treatment of patients with phenytoin (and possibly carbamazepine) increases dose requirements for all nondepolarizers except perhaps atracurium and markedly reduces the duration of action.[308,309] The mechanism involves changes in both protein binding and in the number of acetylcholine receptors.[196,245]

Also occasionally complicating use of nondepolarizing relaxants in neurosurgery is presence of local neurologic deficits, particularly hemiplegia. Paretic/plegic extremities are relatively resistant to nondepolarizing relaxants.[282] Titration of relaxants in response to twitch monitoring *of this extremity* can lead to relative overdosage and difficulties with reversal. This can pose certain unique problems during intracranial surgery because the operating table is often positioned such that the paretic extemity is the most readily available (i.e., contralateral to the surgical hemisphere).

Succinylcholine

There is little question that succinylcholine increases ICP in humans.[241,276,289] In early work, these ICP changes could not be separated from those caused by laryngoscopy or changes in ventilation, but more recent studies indicate the drug has ICP effects clearly independent of other events.[276,398] Animal studies indicate that these changes are associated with increased CBF and may be related to increases in muscle spindle afferent activity.[210,211] These ICP effects can be completely blocked by prior paralysis or "precurarization" with pancuronium or metocurine,[161,210,276] indicating that the peripheral neuromuscular junctions play some role.

Does this mean that succinylcholine is contraindicated in neurosurgery? Probably not. The changes in ICP are modest and transient. There seems little reason to avoid the drug in situations where very rapid paralysis is needed. This does not apply to most elective situations, but under emergency conditions, the consequences of an unsecured airway and hypoxia/hypercapnia are far worse than any changes that might occur with succinylcholine. When succinylcholine is given to severely head-injured patients in intensive care unit situations (or to animals with intracranial hypertension), it does not have detrimental effects.[118,152,205]

Antihypertensives

Smooth muscle relaxants: nitroprusside, nitroglycerin and hydralazine. All antihypertensive drugs with direct smooth muscle relaxant properties are capable of increasing ICP in humans.[73,74,139,242,427] The idea that these drugs (at least nitroprusside and nitroglycerin) increase CBF as well as ICP has little support.[266] **Essentially all studies (human and animal) have reported either no change or a decrease in CBF.**[28,66,167,213,325] These drugs are capable of increasing CBV independently of their effects on flow. This possibility has been directly investigated in two studies. Michenfelder and Milde[266] gave dogs nitroprusside under conditions where BP was maintained constant and observed an increase in ICP without an increase in CBF. Dahl et al.[86] measured flow velocity in the basilar cerebral vessels using TCD methods and also measured CBF using SPECT during nitroglycerin infusion. They found that middle cerebral artery (MCA) flow velocity decreased while CBF was unchanged. These changes can be explained only by an increase in MCA diameter, *which did not translate into a flow change.* In both cases, the results are compatible with drug effects on CBV independent of CBF. This may be a manifestation of completely normal physiology. If autoregulation is intact, a reduction in arterial pressure should be accompanied by cerebral vasodilation, which acts to maintain CBF constant. This vasodilation is manifested by an increase in CBV (i.e., some of the ICP increases seen with antihypertensives or hypotensive agents may reflect normal rather than pathologic processes).

One can argue that increased ICP combined with decreased CBF may be detrimental. These changes have lead some to conclude that these drugs are contraindicated in patients with mass lesions. Nitroprusside can produce ICP-related neurologic deterioration in animals with mass lesions,[286] and there is one report of a decrease in the level of consciousness in a human given modest doses of the drug.[242] No similar observations have been made with nitroglycerin, but because most work suggests its ICP effects are identical, it is reasonable to accept the possibility. The difficulty with this caveat is that it limits the neuroanesthesia provider to a group of clearly less useful/reliable drugs (e.g., trimethaphan) ICP changes not studied. Nitrates (and hydralazine) have been successfully used for many years in patients with neurologic disorders. Part of this success probably relates to the techniques with which the drugs are used. Marsh et al.[240] documented that the magnitude of the ICP change is related to the speed of onset of drug effect. When the dose of nitroprusside was gradually increased over many minutes, no ICP changes were seen. Presumably this allowed time for spatial compensation. This is also probably the reason that hydralazine, which has a very slow onset, has been used so widely with such safety in neurosurgical practice. These drugs are most often used in combination with other drugs (e.g., beta-blockers, captopril, etc.) that act to reduce the total dose of vasodilator given and hence their ICP effects.

Antiadrenergic agents: alpha and beta blockers and trimethaphan. We stated previously that nonanesthetic adrenergic agonists and antagonists appear to have little effect on resting CBF. These drugs also have little effect on ICP. Labetalol has been studied extensively in animals and humans. Orlowski et al.[307] administered labetalol to 15 postoperative neurosurgical patients who previously had required nitroprusside for the control of hypertension. Mean ICP decreased from 11.3 mm Hg with nitroprusside to 8.6 mm Hg after conversion to labetalol. Esmolol has also been used for BP control in neurosurgical patients.[294] Its ICP effects have not been well evaluated but would be expected to be minor.

There is relatively little information available concerning the CBF/ICP effects of pure alpha-blocking drugs (e.g., phenoxybenzamine, prazocin) in neuroanesthesia, and much of this information is quite old. These agents probably have little direct CBF/ICP effects, but may shift the autoregulatory curve to the left, at least when hypotension is produced by hemorrhage.[156,192] Presumably, this results from blocking the effects of high circulating catecholamine concentrations.

For many years, the ganglionic blocker trimethaphan has been touted as an antihypertensive with little or no cerebral vascular effects. This information is probably untrue—or at least the drug is not considered remarkably "better" than nitroprusside.[266] This agent is now effectively obsolete and we will not discuss it further.

Calcium channel antagonists. Most work with calcium channel blockers has focused on their potential as cerebral protectants, but they are often used for acute control of hypertension. All available agents (e.g., verapamil, diltiazem, nifedipine, nimodipine, and nicardipine) increase ICP in animal models and humans.[35,38,137,138,301] They have no apparent cerebrovascular advantages over smooth muscle relaxants, except perhaps in patients with concomitant ischemic heart disease. They are relatively long acting; nifedipine can be given sublinqually. Nicardipine now has supplanted verapamil and diltiazem as an intravenous antihypertensive.

Adenosine. Adenosine has recently been released for treatment of supraventricular dysrhythmias.[58] This availability should ensure its trial for other purposes. It (or its analogue, ATP) can be given intravenously, and its effects are rapid in onset and of generally short duration. Unlike nitroprusside, the drug appears to have few toxic side effects, and tachyphylaxis is rare.[392] Modest degrees of BP reduction have been associated with increases in ICP.[428] It has not been well evaluated as an antihypertensive (as opposed to use for induced hypotension). It should be remembered that adenosine was the prototype drug used for the original annual production of coronary steal. Many neurology patients have concomitant coronary disease.

PRACTICAL CLINICAL MANAGEMENT

The challenge is to translate physiology and pharmacology into a rational approach to clinical management. This is not an easy task because few clinical management schemes have been subjected to objective trials. Most published material, including this chapter, is contaminated by personal opinion and by experiences that may be unique to a particular practice setting. We have chosen to concentrate on three major areas: (1) craniotomy for supratentorial tumor; (2) craniectomy for infratentorial tumor; and (3) craniotomy for intracranial vascular lesion. We also will comment briefly about the care of patients with cervical spine disease and those undergoing transsphenoidal surgeries.

Anesthesia for Supratentorial Craniotomy

Preoperative assessment

Neurosurgical patients require comprehensive preoperative medical evaluation as does any other individual scheduled for major surgery. Three specific neuro-related questions need to be asked: (1) Where is the mass lesion? (2) Is ICP already elevated? and (3) What is the patient's current neurologic status? The answer to the first question defines the surgical position and hence placement of monitoring. It also indicates the likely deficits that can arise. If retraction on the lateral sensorimotor cortex is needed to obtain exposure, the patient's contralateral upper extremity may be weak in the early postoperative period. If cranial nerve (CN) III should be manipulated by the surgeon, one pupil may be widely dilated postoperatively. Not all patients with mass lesions have intracranial hypertension (most do not). Conversely, clinically normal patients do not necessarily have normal ICPs. Determining the likelihood of intracranial hypertension requires examination of the patient and a preoperative CT or MRI scan. The clinical diagnosis of intracranial hypertension is obvious in some patients (e.g., diminished level of consciousness, nausea, vomiting, anisocoria, papilledema, etc.) Most patients do not have these "classic" signs and symptoms of intracranial hypertension and instead present with headaches, seizures, or focal neurologic deficits. The changes associated with intracranial hypertension include extensive edema surrounding the tumor and evidence for activation of compensatory mechanisms, including ventricular effacement, shifted midline structures, and compression of the basal cisterns. Alternatively, certain lesions, particularly those in the midline, may obstruct normal CSF flow and produce hydrocephalus. A brief neurologic examination provides the anesthesia provider with some basis for later comparison; the anesthesia provider may be the last person to see the patient before the induction of anesthesia and the first to see the patient awaken. This examination need not be complex. A simple, quick "move your arms, move your legs, open your eyes, where are you, what's your name. . . ." is sufficient.

Premedication and transportation

After evaluation, it is possible to make an intelligent decision regarding premedication. All sedatives (including benzodiazepines) can produce hypercapnia. Fortunately, a few mm Hg increase in $Paco_2$ is probably not important in the great majority of patients, and most experienced neuroanesthesia providers are comfortable with premedicant doses of midazolam. Narcotics are almost universally avoided. A 5-mg dose of midazolam may be appropriate for a neurologically intact patient with a small mass lesion, no midline shift, normal ventricular size, and so forth, but might be fatally inappropriate in an individual such as the one shown in Fig. 67-15. Most patients are not closely observed after premedicant drugs are given; they may deteriorate alone. Today, **sedatives are often given intravenously when patients arrive in the operating room area where they can be more closely observed.**

Given the value of a head-up posture for controlling ICP, we recommend that patients with mass lesions be transported with the head of the bed elevated 15° to 30°.

Monitoring

Monitoring decisions have become simpler in recent years because of the availability of capnography, pulse oximetry, and automated oscillometric BP monitors, as well as the routine acceptance of arterial catheters. Arterial catheters serve two roles. First, they assist in the management of arterial blood gases and blood chemistry. Second, they provide a beat-by-beat view of BP, which may be useful in conditions where autoregulation is disturbed. If a patient is cooperative, it is reasonable to place the catheter before the induction of anesthesia, but it is rarely mandatory. It may be entirely acceptable to induce anesthesia guided by expired CO_2, Spo_2, and a rapidly cycled automated cuff; the arterial

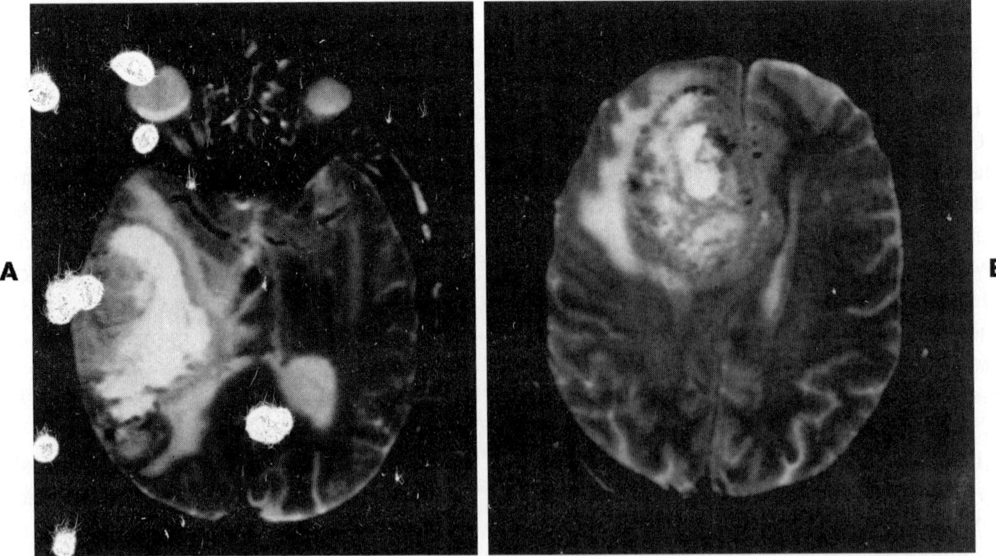

Fig. 67-15. MRI scans from two patients with very large intracranial lesions. In both cases there was significant edema, ventricular effacement, and some degree of midline shift (most noticable in **B**). In spite of similar apparent mass effects, however, intraoperative intracranial pressure (ICP) measured under identical anesthetic conditions ($Paco_2 \approx 30$ mm Hg, isoflurane/N_2O anesthesia, 10° head up, no mannitol until after measurements) was 12 mm Hg in **A,** and 55 mm Hg in **B.** The only difference between patients was that the family of B has noted the patient to be a bit more sleepy than usual.

catheter can be placed later. Some cases can be handled without an arterial catheter, particularly in healthy individuals with small and easily accessible tumors.

Central venous pressure (CVP) catheters are used less commonly. They provide information about intravascular volume when major blood loss is anticipated (e.g., during the resection of a large and highly vascular meningioma or hemangioblastoma). They also can monitor intrathoracic pressure, and can be invaluable in fluid management of patients at risk for development of diabetes insipidus, such as those undergoing resections of large suprasellar tumors such as craniopharyngiomas. There are very few "neurosurgical indications" for pulmonary artery catheterization. These include patients with significant cardiac disease or elderly patients for whom massive blood loss or a very long anesthetic is anticipated, or in whom profound induced hypotension is planned. (Use of PA catheters as a monitor for venous air embolism will be discussed later in this chapter.)

A recurrent question concerns the "indications" for the preanesthetic placement of ICP monitors. Approximately 10 to 15 years ago, some experts would have said that any patient with a large mass lesion, particularly a patient with an altered level of consciousness, should have a preoperative ICP monitor placed.[40] This is no longer reasonable. Our current understanding of ICP physiology and the effects of our agents has made it unnecessary to directly measure ICP for purely anesthetic reasons. The intraoperative measurement of ICP before opening the dura (e.g., with an epidural device) may prove useful in determining the need for mannitol, and there is some interest in postoperative monitoring, particularly in patients having posterior fossa procedures.[312,351] It is not possible at present to make firm recommendations in favor of such use.

Anesthetic induction and maintenance

There is no evidence that any one approach to anesthetizing these patients is better than any other. The fact that one drug increases CBF more than another or has a 10% small effect on ICP is not sufficient to conclude that it is a "bad" neuroanesthetic. Agents as halothane and N_2O have been used successfully in tens of thousands of patients. Most commonly "accepted" methods have goals in common. The first is a smooth induction without sudden hypertension or hypotension. The second is rapid achievement of hypocapnia before the administration of volatile agents and/or N_2O, and the third is that the technique be compatible with a rapid postoperative emergence. There are obviously many ways to accomplish such goals, and the following points represent only the most general guidelines.

Despite many years of effort and many alternative drugs (e.g., methohexital, althesin, etomidate, diazepam, midazolam, ketamine, alfentanil, propofol, eltanolone, etc.), no induction agent is clearly superior to thiopental. Hypotension during induction can usually be avoided by preinduction volume loading (e.g., 10 ml/kg of lactated Ringer's solution) and by adjusting the dose according to patient age and physical status. The patient should be in a modest head-up posture at the time of induction (i.e., 10°). When consciousness is lost, manual hyperventilation is begun with oxygen. When a patent airway is assured (using oral or nasal airways if needed), a paralyzing dose of a nondepolarizing relaxant is given, and administration of the primary agent is started gradually. The most common alternatives involve incremental loading with one of the synthetic opioids (e.g., fentanyl, sufentanil, alfentanil, or perhaps remifentanyl) combined with N_2O, or the administration of a volatile agent in progressively increasing concentrations (with or without N_2O). A propofol infusion can be used. Data now available do not indicate that any of these approaches offers major advantages[418] With respect to the three narcotics, fentanyl is equivalent to sufentanil and alfentanil and is much cheaper.[133] Remifentanil has recently been compared with fentanyl and again, offers no striking advantages other than somewhat more rapid emergence (Warner D, Hindman B, Young W, personal communication). The trachea is intubated when paralysis is complete. The hemodynamic response to intubation can be blunted in many ways. These include additional narcotics (e.g., fentanyl to a total loading dose of 10 to 12 μg/kg), supplementary thiopental, intravenous lidocaine (1 to 1.5 mg/kg) or short-acting antihypertensives (labetalol, esmolol, etc.). Topical anesthesia of the trachea is also widely used, although this does not alter the response to laryngoscopy per se.[157] Mechanical ventilation is begun, the endotracheal tube is secured, additional monitors are inserted (e.g., esophageal stethoscope, temperature probes, etc.), the patient's eyes are securely closed, and surgical positioning is begun. The patient is covered with blankets (or a forced air warmer) to maintain body temperature.

As with induction and maintenance, there are many ways of conducting wakeup. We believe BP should be restored to normal before the dura is closed, to verify adequacy of hemostasis. Normocapnia should be present before dural closure is complete; if the brain is so badly swollen that the dura cannot be closed, the patient should be taken to the ICU on controlled ventilation. Because uncontrolled hypertension is associated with an increased incidence of postoperative intracranial hemorrhage,[183] aggressive treatment is necessary. As with other aspects of management, the choice of antihypertensive drug is a matter of personal preference (see previous discussion). Some added BP control can be obtained by reducing the dose of atropine or glycopyrollate given at the time neuromuscular blockade is reversed, thereby avoiding any tachycardia. A brief period of coughing/gagging at the time of extubation is probably acceptable if BP is controlled, although this can be blunted with lidocaine if desired. We also believe that such patients should be transported to the postanesthesia care unit or surgical intensive care unit with at least some form of BP monitoring, particularly if the resection was bloody.

Management of severe intraoperative brain swelling. The preceding protocols will serve the majority of cases. The most serious deviation from routine involves management of the severely swollen brain. Some specific recommendations are appropriate. The course taken is defined by the answers to some simple questions:

- *Is this a major ventilatory disaster?*

  Is the brain swollen because of a disconnect, severe hypoxia, hypercapnia, or other cause? Is the chest moving appropriately? Does the patient have a reasonable expired CO_2 waveform, and what is the $ETCO_2$? What is the SpO_2? An arterial blood gas sample should be drawn immediately.
- *Is the swelling related to impaired cerebral venous drainage?*

  As noted earlier, the problems of venous drainage are often overlooked. We believe that the majority of swelling problems encountered in the neurosurgical operating room are related to poor venous drainage. The most common are: (1) excessive rotation of the neck; (2) inadequate head-up posture; and (3) some form of expiratory obstruction in the patient circuit. There is little reason for employing pharmacologic ICP control methods unless these mechanical problems have been corrected. Simply increasing the degree of head-up tilt is often sufficient.
- *Is the swelling hemodynamic?*

  Is the patient hypertensive and/or tachycardic? Is the anesthesia too light? In some cases, light anesthesia and/or inadequate paralysis can be manifested by chest tightness and increasing intrathoracic pressures, without other movement.

After the above causes have been ruled out, it is best to assume that the swelling is related to patient disease, not some iatrogenic factor. The next therapeutic step is to reduce $PaCO_2$ to between 20 and 25 mm Hg and verify that PaO_2 is greater than 100 mm Hg. Ideally, this should be achieved without increase in mean intrathoracic pressure, something accomplished by keeping an I:E ratio greater than 1:2. The limitations of greater degress of hypocapnia have been described.

Next, diuretic therapy is begun, typically with osmotic agents. Such compounds (e.g., mannitol, urea, glycerol, sorbitol, and hypertonic saline) all act in the same fashion: They produce an osmotic gradient across the intact blood–brain barrier which acts to "draw" water down its concentration gradient from brain to blood.[122] Their efficacy depends on the relative permeability of the BBB to the compound. If the BBB is disrupted, no osmotic gradient can be achieved (i.e., the compound equilibrates between blood and interstitium); all of these compounds act by removing water from areas with an intact barrier. Mannitol is the best characterized compound and remains the agent of choice when the patient's baseline osmolality is less than 290 mOsm/kg. A reasonable starting dose is 0.25 g/kg, a value derived from experience with ICP control after head trauma. There is a major difference between controlling ICP (where small volume changes can have huge ICP effects when compliance is poor) and controlling brain bulk (where much larger reductions in volume may be needed to facilitate surgical exposure). For this reason, there should be little hesitation to increase the dose to greater than 1 g/kg if swelling does not resolve. The upper dosage limit is defined only by osmolality, which should remain less than 310 to 320 mOsm/kg.[397] The pharmacokinetic half-life of mannitol is 2 to 3 hours.[63,165] There has been concern that mannitol might exacerbate brain swelling, particularly when administered rapidly.[75] Mannitol (and other hypertonic compounds) is a vasodilator[408] and can increase CBV and ICP when administered rapidly in large doses.[337] Ravussin et al.[336] have shown that in patients with intracranial hypertension, mannitol uniformly reduces ICP (and brain bulk) without any intervening increase (Fig. 67-16). Hence, the major "complications" of mannitol therapy are volume expansion,[354] electrolyte abnormalities,[354,374] and lastly, hypotension if administered too rapidly.[72]

An alternative osmotic agent is hypertonic saline (with or without added colloid). Interest in this approach has largely stemmed from the utility of hypertonic saline as a small-volume resuscitant following hemorrhage, and there is little information concerning its use in the operating room. There is no question that it can reduce ICP, sometimes when other measures have failed.[123,453] Whether it is superior to mannitol remains uncertain.

Another alternative (or supplementary) choice is furosemide in doses of 0.3 to 1.0 mg/kg.[365,447] It is not as reliable as mannitol but may be preferable in patients unable to tolerate the transient intravascular volume expansion that

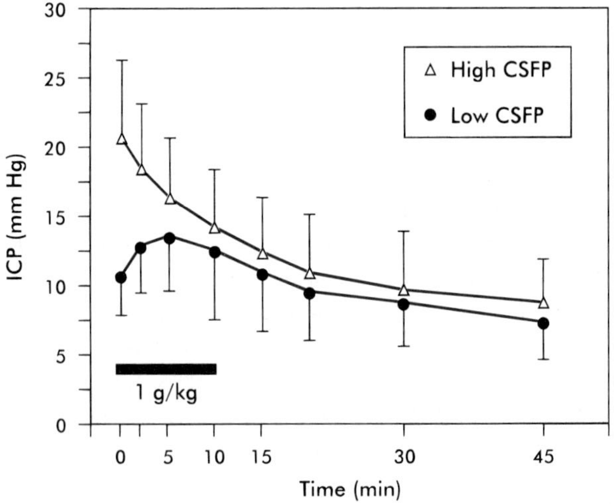

Fig. 67-16. Changes in intracranial pressure (ICP) (actually lumbar cerebrospinal fluid (CSF) pressure) after the administration of 1 g/kg of mannitol. Patients in the "High CSF pressure" group had a mean premannitol ICP of 20.8 mm Hg, while those in the "Low CSF pressure"group had a pressure of 10.5 mm Hg. In the Low CSF pressure group, mannitol resulted in a significant but transient increase in ICP. Nonetheless, no such transient increase was seen in patients with prior intracranial hypertension. All values are mean ± SD. (From recalculated data Ravussin P, Abou-Madi M, Archer D, et al: Changes in CSF pressure after mannitol in patients with and without elevated CSF pressure, *J Neurosurg* 69:869, 1988.)

occurs with mannitol. Its effects are much slower in onset.[447] In situations where brain swelling is severe, a combination of mannitol and furosemide has been used successfully. Under these conditions, the value of furosemide may be related to its unique ability to inhibit the mechanisms that act to maintain normal cell volume in the face of hypertonicity.[256] When normal cells (including neurons and glia) are exposed to a hypertonic environment, they transiently shrink, but rapidly regain their normal volume, largely due to the active importation of chloride. This influx of Cl^- can be blocked by loop diuretics, with the result being a persistant reduction in cell volume. The major problem with a combination of mannitol and furosemide is the often extraordinary diuresis that ensues—a diuresis which can be difficult to distinguish from severe diabetes insipidus.

If this sequence fails to control swelling, the surgeon should be asked to cannulate one of the ventricles to remove CSF, to decompress any cystic lesions or hematomas. At the same time, anesthetic management should be reevaluated. If fluid removal cannot be accomplished, it may be appropriate to discontinue agents with the potential for increasing CBV. We believe that the first drug that should be discontinued is N_2O. It can be replaced with a volatile agent, a narcotic, or a combination of a narcotic and a sedative/hypnotic. If swelling does not resolve, the volatile agent should be discontinued. **Only when these interventions fail should high-dose barbiturates be used *as a therapy of last resort.*** Before starting, every effort should be made to ensure the patient is normovolemic, using whatever isotonic intravenous fluid is desired. Several studies have shown that barbiturates are both venous and arterial vasodilators as well as myocardial depressants,[417,424] and Traeger et al.[424] have shown that hypotension is most commonly related to inadequate cardiac filling pressures. We begin with incremental doses of 150 to 250 mg, repeated as often as hemodynamically tolerated. This is continued until swelling is under control or cardiovascular toxicity becomes a problem. In rare situations, inotropic support may be needed. This use of thiopental should not be confused with "brain protection." We generally have little idea what doses are appropriate. Anecdotal reports of successful control describe the use of huge doses ($<$ 5 g given within a short time).[91,243] This is much more than needed to "suppress the EEG" and is incompatible with rapid postoperative emergence. A postoperative ICP monitor in such cases is advisable because clinical evaluation is impossible.

Anesthesia for Infratentorial Craniectomy: The Sitting Position

Operations in the posterior fossa are unique for several reasons. First, the lesion itself and/or surgical trauma can damage brain areas that control the airway (i.e., pharynx, tongue, larynx), respiration, autonomic function, and consciousness. Second, these operations are performed in unusual positions (i.e., prone, lateral, or sitting, each of which has particular problems). It is the sitting position that has received the bulk of our attention because it poses the greatest management problems. Therefore, we will first discuss the management of the craniectomy performed with the patient in the upright position, and then briefly mention the differences introduced by the alternative positions.

Problems

Despite the concerns about venous air embolization, the sitting position is still in widespread use and offers many advantages over alternative positions. These advantages include excellent surgical exposure, particularly of midline structures and those located in or on the high dorsal brain stem or midbrain (e.g., the pineal). Also there is less pooling of blood and CSF in the surgical field, and blood loss may be less than with nonsitting positions because of lesser venous pressures.[49] This position also is more comfortable for the surgeon. It is often easier to move a large patient into the sitting position than the prone position. Peak airway pressures may be lesser and ventilation/perfusion matching better than those seen in the prone position. The patient's face and airway are accessible, making it easier to monitor facial nerve function. These should be balanced against the disadvantages: (1) venous air embolism; (2) paradoxical air embolism; (3) quadriplegia; (4) hemodynamic deterioration; and (5) pneumocephalus. Other concerns are peripheral nerve injuries and head, neck, or tongue edema. In addition, a serious concern in any posterior fossa procedure is the possibility of injury to the lower cranial nerves and respiratory centers.

Venous air embolization. Venous air embolization (VAE) can occur whenever the pressure within an open blood vessel is subatmospheric. Because normal right atrial pressures range from 2 to 10 mm Hg, this can theoretically occur any time the surgical site is located more than $\approx$ 5 cm above the heart. Experience indicates that clinically significant VAE is rare unless the surgical site is elevated by more than 20 to 40 cm.* The risk of VAE increases dramatically when open veins cannot collapse. This is encountered with injury to the venous sinuses, cerebellar bridging veins, epidural veins, emissary veins, and marrow spaces in the skull or cervical vertebra. This latter possibility explains occasional embolization of air from pin-fixation sites. Another unusual source of air entry is a *ventriculoatrial* (VA) shunt (*not* a ventriculoperitoneal [VP] shunt). If a bubble enters the ventricles, the shunt acts as a direct route to the heart.

It was once believed that VAE was a rare but fatal complication. When more sophisticated monitors were used, a much greater incidence of generally benign events was seen. Standifer et al.[396] evaluated 322 cases (288 with a Doppler)

*VAE can occur in other surgical settings, but many patients undergo procedures where the surgical site is higher than the heart, including supratentorial craniotomies, shoulder repairs, hysterectomies, lumbar laminectomies, and so forth. VAE has been anecdotally described in all of these, as well as during the injection of air during placement of epidural catheters. Clinical experience indicates that the incidence of hemodynamically important emboli in such nonsitting position operations is vanishingly low.

and noted VAE in only 22 patients (7%). Nonetheless, Matjasko et al.[247] reviewed their experience in 554 seated cases and noted air entry in 41% of patients undergoing suboccipital craniectomies and 11.4% of those having cervical laminectomies. Young et al.[456] reported a similar incidence (43%) among 146 patients undergoing suboccipital craniectomies, with an overall incidence of 30% (all procedures combined, 255 patients). Black et al.[46] also noted an incidence of 43%. We conclude that among patients undergoing posterior fossa procedures, the incidence of VAE is ≈ 40%, compared with 10% to 15% for cervical spine surgery.

These four studies include ≈ 1500 reasonably monitored patients, among which VAE was detected in 372. This is probably an underestimate, because some earlier patients were not Doppler monitored, and there are no data regarding Doppler placement in any study. A possible relationship between intraoperative VAE and postoperative morbidity or death could be defined in only six cases (≈ 0.4%). This compares with a "surgical" mortality of ≈ 2%. Although this may be an underestimate, these data still do not support the idea that the sitting position should be abandoned purely because of the risk of VAE. The obvious caveat is that these results were obtained in centers with a great deal of experience and may not be reproducible in hospitals that perform an occasional sitting procedure.

Paradoxic (arterial) air embolization. There is potential for the passage of air from the right to the left atria of the heart, with subsequent entry into the coronary and/or cerebral circulation. This can occur via the pulmonary vascular bed, but more commonly occurs in a patent foramen ovale (PFO). The incidence of clinically significant paradoxic air embolism (PAE) is unknown. A large number of patients are theoretically at risk. Autopsy studies indicate that 25% to 35% of patients have at least a probe-patent foramen ovale. Given a 40% incidence of VAE, one can calculate that ≈ 12% of patients are "at risk" for a PAE (30% of 40%). This value is far greater than the number of patients who suffer a deficit/complication from VAE. Why? First, not everyone with a probe-PFO has a *functional* right-to-left shunt. The number of patients is theoretically reduced even further by the fact that the normal pressure gradient (right atrial pressure less than left atrial pressure) reverses during anesthesia in the sitting position in only ≈ 50% of patients.* Echocardiographic (ECHO) studies demonstrate that right-to-left shunting of contrast material can be produced in up to 18% of normal volunteers[224] but was detected in only 6% to 10% of patients scheduled for surgery.[48] In many cases, shunting was seen only during a Valsalva maneuver performed to increase right atrial pressure. Even in sitting anesthetized patients, ECHO studies revealed right-to-left air passage (either during testing or during a clinical VAE) in 3 of 20 patients (15%). The absence of right-to-left shunting, with or without Valsalva maneuver during preoperative evaluation, does not preclude the occurrence of PAE intraoperatively.

If 15% of patients suffering a VAE also have PAE, why is the incidence of PAE–related complications so low? Most paradoxical emboli should be benign. A review of the anesthetic literature shows a total of seven patients with actual ECHO documented PAE during sitting surgery.[48,80,81,82,136] No sequelae were noted in *any* of these patients. Animal studies in our own laboratory (D. Reasoner and B. Hindman, personal communication) suggest that doses of air on the order of 100 to 150 μl/kg should be directly injected into the rabbit's internal carotid artery to reliably produce a deficit, indicating that tiny bubbles are unlikely to be detrimental (although continuous streams of bubbles, even small ones, may lead to injury).

These arguments are not intended to suggest that PAE is trivial or that the potential for PAE should be ignored. Quite the contrary—it can produce devastating complications. Every bubble entering the arterial circulation does not mean that a stroke will occur, and **the *best* prevention of PAE is still early detection and prevention of VAE.** It has been suggested that all patients considered for a sitting position undergo preoperative echocardiography, an idea unlikely to find wide acceptance in an era of cost consciousness, particularly in view of decades of documented safety of doing the surgery without such studies. A more reasonable approach would be to carry out echocardiographic studies in patients with clinical signs or history suggestive of a functional PFO (e.g., unevaluated murmurs now or in the past). Echocardiographic evaluation should be performed with contrast medium injected before, during, and immediately after a Valsalva maneuver. If shunting is demonstrated, the procedure should probably be carried out in an alternative position, although surgical considerations should be weighed.

Quadriplegia. Episodic cases of unexpected quadriplegia/paresis have been reported over many years after procedures performed in the sitting position.[446] Neither the incidence nor the etiology is known with certainty, but two cases were reported among the ≈ 1500 patients reported in the four studies noted previously. The most likely cause is a combination of cervical cord compression from extreme neck flexion and a reduced arterial perfusion pressure produced by elevating the neck above the heart. In support of this, McPherson et al.[260] have reported major changes in evoked potentials with neck flexion/rotation even in the horizontal position.[260] The risk may be greater in persons with cervical cord compression (i.e., people with similar cervical problems who undergo cervical procedures in the sitting position).[93] Suggested preventive measures included the avoidance of extreme flexion and monitoring of blood pressure at the level of the surgical site, rather than the heart. Somato-

*The importance of this observation has recently been questioned by Black et al.[47] who demonstrated that changes in the gradient may not be as important as believed, largely because transient reversal of the gradient during a single cardiac cycle occurred commonly in pigs with surgically created atrial septial defects (ASD).[47]

sensory-evoked potential (SEP) monitoring is a possible but insufficiently evaluated monitor of such conditions.

Hemodynamic deterioration. Moving an anesthetized patient from the supine to the sitting position results in a number of hemodynamic changes. The most complete study of this is by Marshall et al.,[244] who studied patients receiving one of four anesthetics (enflurane/N_2O, halothane/N_2O, Innovar/N_2O, or morphine/N_2O).[244] Assumption of the sitting position was accompanied by decreased wedge pressure and cardiac output, with increased systemic resistance. The smallest changes were observed in patients receiving a combination of morphine and N_2O, but hemodynamic parameters recorded during surgery were remarkably similar between groups. This study failed to include a "time control" group of patients receiving the same anesthetic but left in the supine position, and some of the changes may simply be related to the duration of anesthesia, not position. Little information is available concerning the hemodynamic consequences of the alternative neurosurgical positions (e.g., prone, lateral). Black et al.[49] found essentially identical 20% incidences of hypotension requiring vasopressors in 330 sitting patients versus 229 horizontal patients.

Pneumocephalus. Pneumocephalus occurs in all craniectomies performed in the sitting position.[423] It is seen in all postoperative craniotomy/craniectomy patients, regardless of position.[340] It is not surprising that tension pneumocephalus is a well-described event after such procedures.[396] CSF drains easily in the sitting position, and air will move upward and collect over the cerebral convexity (the "upside-down bottle" effect). If the wound is then closed and the patient returned to the supine position, CVP and CBV increases and the brain reexpands, potentially compressing the gas. This occurrence alone may be capable of producing a tension pneumocephalus. Artru[13] has argued that the intraoperative use of N_2O may worsen this situation, although experimental studies do not agree.[97,389] A key seems to be whether N_2O administration is delayed until after pathways for air escape has been closed (i.e., whether there is a trapped bubble). Delayed problems can also occur if CSF reaccumulates at a rate faster than the air is absorbed. Tension pneumocephalus may be difficult to diagnose, but should be suspected when a patient fails to awaken after an uneventful procedure, deteriorates after awakening, or suffers some unexplained cardiovascular catastrophe. If clinical changes are mild, simple administration of high concentrations of O_2 will speed resolution.[95] If changes are major, surgical evacuation is indicated.

Other problems. Other complications deserving mention are peripheral nerve injuries[49,255] and severe swelling of the face and tongue.[112,254] Nerve injuries are position-related and probably involve compression and/or stretch of the ulnar nerve at the elbow or peroneal nerve at the knee. Other direct pressure injuries can occur. Sciatic stretch injuries can also occur if excessive flexion at the hip is allowed. Facial or glossal swelling (sometimes so severe as to preclude extubation) is probably related to excessive neck flexion. Similar swelling can also be seen in the prone position.

Preoperative evaluation and premedication

Although intracranial hypertension is a common concern in the patient with a supratentorial tumor, this is less common in those presenting for posterior fossa procedures. The most common cause of elevated ICP in such patients is hydrocephalus, resulting from obstruction of the aqueduct or the fourth ventricle. This is easily recognized on the CT or MRI scan, and in many situations is corrected preoperatively or intraoperatively with a ventricular cannula. Presence of symptomatic hydrocephalus or elevated pressures in the posterior fossa represents contraindication to premedication. Asymptomatic persons with small cerebellopontine angle masses or tumors of the cerebellar hemispheres can usually be premedicated without difficulty.

Monitoring and the physiology of VAE

The principal monitoring challenge of the sitting position is to rapidly detect VAE. Fortunately, extensive clinical and experimental work has removed much of the guesswork from this area.

Slow entrainment of small bubbles is of little significance; either gas dissolves in blood or the bubbles pass into the pulmonary capillaries and are absorbed. If the embolus is larger and/or enters faster than it can be cleared, one sees progressive occlusion of the pulmonary vascular bed. This results in increased pulmonary vascular resistance, increased PA mean pressure, and increased right atrial pressure. If obstruction is severe, cardiac output will decrease, caused by: (1) an "airlock" in the RV; (2) RV failure; or (3) impaired LV filling caused by displacement of the intraventricular septum by a distended RV. In addition, respiratory abnormalities appear. Vascular obstruction results in an increase in the amount of high/lung ("dead space"; see Fig. 67-17). The result is an increased gradient between arterial and end-tidal CO_2 concentrations, manifested by a decreasing $ETCo_2$ and an increasing $Paco_2$.[144] These same V/Q abnormalities will lead to hypoxemia, partially as a result of mechanical occlusion and partially because of the release of vasoactive compounds from either blood or from the vessel walls. In fact, changes in Pao_2 often precede alterations in PA pressure or $ETCo_2$, supporting the idea that vasoactive compounds may be involved. Bubbles of air entering the capillary bed will result in the appearance of N_2O in expired gas, although this is usually detectable only when a patient is breathing 100% O_2.

With sudden massive embolus, these changes occur almost simultaneously. Under such circumstances, "monitoring" is irrelevant; most emboli are not this catastrophic. What typically occurs is a continuous infusion or repeated small boluses of air. In the laboratory, this results in an orderly sequence of hemodynamic/respiratory changes. Several reports have attempted to define this sequence, with

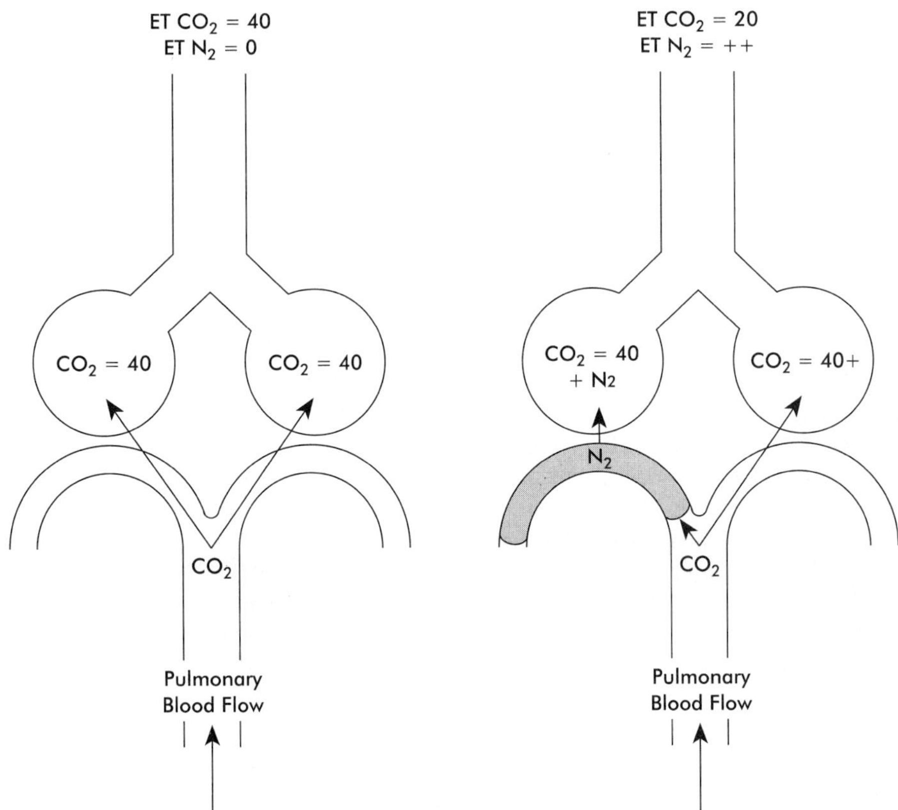

Fig. 67-17. Changes in expired CO_2 and N_2 during VAE. Under normal conditions, alveolar gas is in equilibrium with blood in the pulmonary capillary bed. If the patient has been denitrogenated and is breathing 100% O_2, there should be no N_2 in those alveoli (left diagram). A VAE does two things (right diagram). First, it occludes a portion of the pulmonary circulation, preventing the delivery of CO_2 to the alveoli. As a result, end-tidal CO_2 (which should represent an alveolar gas sample) will decrease (even though $Paco_2$ may rise). In addition, N_2 present in the gas bubble will diffuse into the alveoli and appear in exhaled gas.

the goal of determining which monitoring modality is the most sensitive indicator of air entry. A positive response in the animal laboratory may not accurately reproduce the clinical circumstance. Drummond et al.[102] observed that ≈ 50% of dogs showed an increase in expired N_2O in response to ≈ 0.5 ml/kg of air. A positive response was defined as an increase of 0.04%, and even doses of 1.5 ml/kg resulted in ETN_2 rising from 0 to only 0.25%, a change unlikely to be detected on most clinical gas analyzers, particularly when the anesthetic circuit has any leaks. English et al.[115] noted that 50% of dogs had an increase in PA pressure with 0.25 ml/kg of air, with an increase defined as a change greater than 3 mm Hg. Bedford et al.[39] monitored 100 consecutive patients with a precordial Doppler, capnography, and pulmonary artery catheters. They detected 80 episodes of VAE using Doppler, and in all cases, an effort was made to stop air entrainment at the time a Doppler change was first noted. In ≈ 50% of these episodes, PA pressure increased, with a *mean change* of 11.4 mm Hg. End-tidal CO_2 decreased by 8 to 10 mm Hg (a very large change in hyperventilated patients). Two situations exist. In the first, only Doppler sounds are noted while PA pressure, $PETco_2$, ETn_2, etc. remain unchanged. In the second, everything changes, often to a substantial degree.

Based on the above information, we believe that changes in hemodynamic and respiratory parameters are very *insensitive* monitors of air entrainment. We believe that the only acceptable "early warning" device is the precordial Doppler.[142,267] This device reflects sound waves from moving erythrocytes. Bubbles entering the circulation change the reflectance characteristics of the blood and alter the Doppler frequency. Many studies and clinical experiences have demonstrated the extraordinary sensitivity of this device. Doppler placement should be routinely tested by the injection of 0.25 to 1.0 ml of air (i.e., 0.004 to 0.01 ml/kg) or 3 to 5 ml of agitated saline. Gilgenberg et al.[142] have shown that a Doppler can reliably detect air being infused at a rate of 0.021 ml/kg/min in dogs. This is at least 10 times more sensitive than any hemodynamic/respiratory monitor studied. It also has the advantage of being audible, allowing the anesthesia provider to attend to other duties. The TEE is equally sensitive but requires continuous visual attention (and is far more expensive).[81] There are two difficulties with the Doppler: it should be accurately placed, and it may be *too* sensitive. Doppler placement is not trivial. It is unacceptable to place the transceiver in the fourth intercostal space to the right of the sternum, hear heart sounds, and proceed (this will detect only 90% of air emboli only). One should place the Doppler wherever the right atrium is, and only *after* the patient has been placed in the sitting position, not before, because the heart moves with gravity as the sitting position is assumed. Testing is mandatory and should be repeated at intervals throughout surgery so that operating room personnel become familiar with the sound of air entrainment as well as to confirm that the Doppler is still in the right place. The "gold standard" is air or CO_2 injected through a right atrial catheter. If a catheter cannot be placed, air or agitated saline can be injected through a peripheral IV. If a convincing change in Doppler sounds is not heard, one cannot depend on the instrument as an early warning device. A neurosurgical procedure in the sitting position should not proceed without a properly placed Doppler, despite the presence of respiratory gas monitoring.

The question of excessive sensitivity deserves comment. The Doppler commonly presents its audience with a chorus of chirps and blips, none of which appear to be of consequence. The difficulty lies in deciding which sounds deserve attention. Distinguishing the sounds of air from other sounds is largely a matter of experience, but recognition can be improved by repeated testing of the instrument, by the injection of tiny amounts of air or agitated saline. Determining the amount of air being entrained is a different question, because the Doppler is not quantitative. In some cases, the changed Doppler signal is obvious. In others, one remains uncertain. In the latter, hemodynamic and respiratory monitors become valuable. In our practice, all sitting procedures are monitored with a Doppler, a right atrial catheter, expired CO_2 and expired N_2. If a change in the Doppler signal is noted, attention is shifted to the other monitors. If a change in any of these is noted, the surgeon is notified. A brief Doppler change occurring in isolation rarely indicates action. One should be aware of the possibility that the Doppler may miss an embolus. This should not occur with proper positioning, but this may be more easily said than done. Sudden decreases in $ETco_2$ or the appearance of expired N_2 should quickly prompt one to aspirate from the right atrial catheter. Any sudden decrease in blood pressure should also be considered as a VAE until proven otherwise.

With these comments, what specific monitors are needed for a posterior fossa craniectomy performed in the sitting position? Almost all these patients should have arterial catheterization, for BP control and diagnosis. Blood pressure at the level of the heart is lower than that at the heart. For every 30 of cm of vertical distance between the levels of the heart and that of the brain there are 20 mm Hg difference in mean blood pressure. If the zeroing and calibration of the blood pressure transducer are done at the level of the third or fourth intercoastal space, cerebral perfusion pressure can be estimated by moving the pressure transducer up to the level of the patient's head (the external auditory meatus is a good reference point). Alternatively, one can zero and calibrate the transducer at the level of the head. Probably the most common and serious complications of such operations involve inadvertent injury to cranial nerves or their nuclei, or to other crucial areas on the floor of the fourth ventricle or within the brain stem. Sudden changes in any hemodynamic parameter (BP, heart rate or rhythm) are the most reliable early warning signs of surgical impingement on these crucial structures (although some still believe that respiratory changes in unparalyzed patients are helpful; see following discussion). Beat-to-beat monitoring of arterial pressure provides the necessary early warning. We prefer a right atrial catheter and believe an effort should be made to place one, although failure need not result in cancellation of a case.[263] The greatest value of the right atrial catheter in our opinion is to assist in the accurate placement of the Doppler and to help make the diagnosis of VAE when Doppler changes are unclear. A correctly placed Doppler will readily detect a tiny bubble of air injected into the superior vena cava. If it does not, and the catheter location is known to be correct, then the Doppler position needs to be adjusted. Most centers use multiorifice catheters, which allow more efficient air aspiration.[55,65] The catheter tip should probably be placed just above the right atrium.[55,263] This position can be determined in a number of ways, but the most rapid method is still by ECG. Our practice is to attach the right arm lead of a standard operating room ECG system to the catheter, either via a fluid column (sodium bicarbonate) or via the J-wire used to place the catheter. The catheter is then advanced until a biphasic P-wave is seen, then withdrawn 1 to 3 cm (Fig. 67-18). Some argument exists regarding the site of origin of an ECG signal recorded from a multiorifice catheter.[22] Because no one has ever shown the clinical need for precise catheter positioning, we think this is generally unimportant. Both expired CO_2 and N_2 are monitored.

Some have recommended PA catheterization, because of the diagnostic value of PA pressure monitoring (see previous discussion) and because it allows air to be aspirated from right artery and the PA. PA pressure monitoring offers no advantages over $ETco_2$ monitoring in the average patient.[39] It is difficult to aspirate air from the distal port of the catheter unless a multiorifice pulmonary angiography catheter is used. The middle of the PA may also be the wrong place to find air. PA pressure monitoring does allow one to employ an "N_2O challenge" to determine whether air has been cleared from the pulmonary vasculature after a VAE. If turning on N_2O results in an increase in PA pressure, bubbles still remain. Whether this is sufficient justification for placing this device remains unclear.

Transesophageal echocardiography is a sensitive detector of air and is the only device capable of detecting PAE. It requires constant visual attention. Use of such a device is unlikely cost effective, given the low incidence of PAE–related neurologic injury. Besides, *detection* of PAE is quite different from *prevention.* The latter is best accomplished by the *early detection* of VAE. The early detection via TEE of large

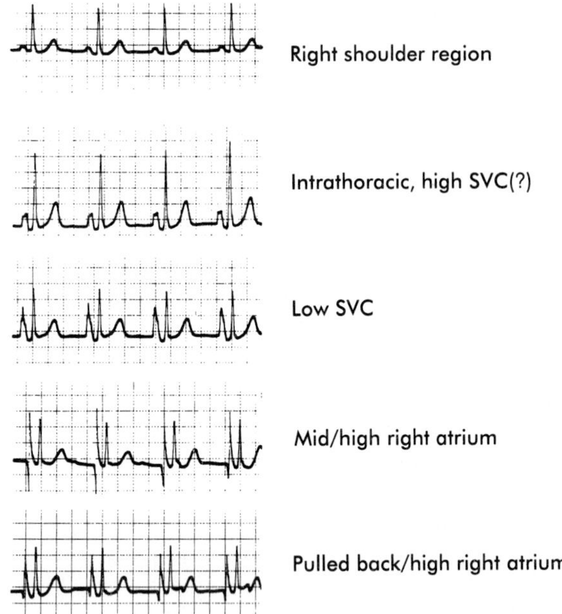

Fig. 67-18. Typical catheter tip ECG signals obtained during placement of a right atrial catheter for a sitting position procedure. The right-arm lead (+) was attached to the catheter, and a lead-2 configuration was used. In the top panel, a typical lead-2 pattern is seen with the catheter tip in an extrathoracic position near the shoulder. As the catheter enters the thorax, the amplitude of all ECG components increases. As the tip nears the right atrium, there is a selective increase in p-wave amplitude, with a relatively sudden change to a biphasic tracing in the high/mid atrium. The bottom tracing was obtained after the catheter was withdrawn 1 to 3 cm from atrial location and was left to reside in the high atrium or low superior vena cava. (From Todd M: Monitoring in neuroanesthesia. In Saidman L, Smith NT, editors: *Monitoring in anesthesia*, ed 3, Boston, 1992, Butterworths.)

or repeated PAE may indicate discontinuation of the sitting position. TEE may also be useful in those few patients in whom Doppler placement is impossible. On balance, we think that it is not justified at present to recommend routine use of TEE, particularly in the absence of any concrete information showing that it can reduce the already low incidence of air-related morbidity.

Anesthesia

As in most neuroanesthetic situations, there are no well-defined indications or contraindications for any particular anesthetic drug combinations. Narcotic/N_2O combinations seem to be associated with fewer hemodynamic changes during assumption of the sitting position, although there are few truly important differences between BP in the anesthetized-supine and anesthetized-sitting groups regardless of anesthetic.[244] Some have argued that N_2O should be avoided in all sitting cases because it will diffuse into and expand the size of any entrained bubble. It has been shown that the use of 50% nitrous oxide did not increase the risk of venous air embolism in patients operated upon in the sitting position.[220] Alternative anesthetic regimens include volatile agent/O_2, high-dose narcotic, or purely intravenous techniques. We feel that nitrous oxide has a major place among the agents used for the anesthetic care of sitting position patients. If air embolization takes place, we feel comfortable (as others did in the past) with discontinuing N_2O when air is detected. In fact, discontinuation of N_2O might even be considered therapeutic. The N_2O-free regimen should be determined before the case starts.

Because some degree of neck flexion is required, we routinely place wire-reinforced ET tubes. An alternative is nasotracheal intubation. Wire reinforced tubes are not risk-free in the postoperative period. These tubes can be indented and obstructed permanently if the patient bites on them. If prolonged postoperative intubation is needed, we recommend changing the wire reinforced tube to a regular ET tube at the conclusion of surgery, but this may not be possible because of airway and tongue swelling. Use of bite blocking devices, good communication with the patient, and vigilance by intensive care personnel is important in preventing this complication.

Some comments on ventilatory management are appropriate. In the early days of posterior fossa surgery, spontaneous ventilation was used as a monitor of brain stem function. This has been supplanted by the use of better hemodynamic monitors combined with controlled ventilation. Most anesthesia providers choose to modestly hyperventilate their patients. Recently Zettner et al.[460] have argued that the risk of VAE may be reduced by modest *hypo*ventilation, and Gelb et al.[253] have reported that respiratory changes can be observed in unparalyzed patients before (or in the absence of) hemodynamic changes. We are still uncomfortable with allowing patients in the sitting position to breathe spontaneously because VAE can trigger a strong inspiratory effort (which can increase the amount of air entrained). A reasonable argument could be made for spontaneous ventilation in horizontal patients, at least after the skull is open and any brain stem compression or hydrocephalus has been relieved.

Positioning and clinical therapy of VAE

We have discussed some of the potential complications of positioning. Another aspect of positioning may be more important. When a major VAE is encountered, initial responses include the surgeon flooding the field or packing it with wet gauze, discontinuing N_2O, and aspirating from the right atrial catheter. Two additional maneuvers can be performed to slow air entry. These are the addition of PEEP and/or bilateral jugular compression.[219,320,321] In both cases, the goal is to increase venous pressure in the head. There are problems with both. Jugular compression is immediately effective and may help identify open veins in the surgical field that might have been the source of air entrainment. This occupies both hands of the anesthesia provider. High levels of PEEP (10 to 15 cm H_2O) are required to elevate venous pressure at the head to values greater than 0,[219] but this may facilitate the right-to-left passage of air through the heart.[320] The latter has

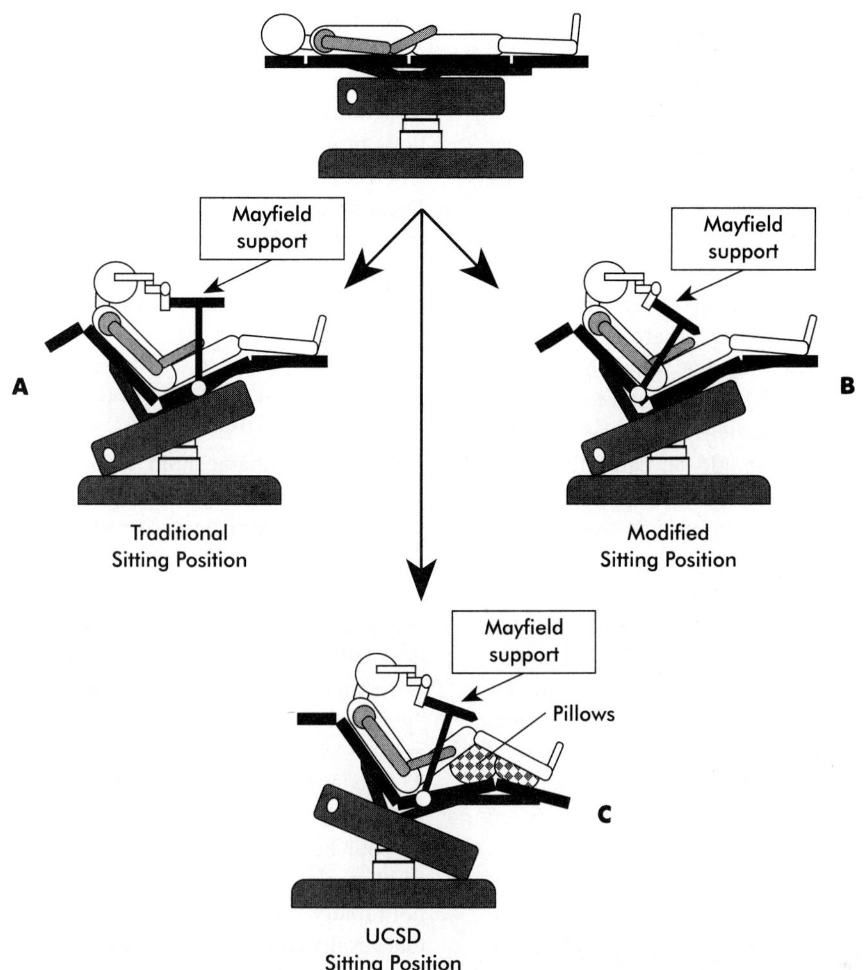

Fig. 67-19. Three variations on the sitting position. **A,** In the "traditional sitting position," the table is placed in steep Trendelenburg, the back elevated, and the Mayfield support attached to the midsection of the table. It is impossible to return the patient to a horizontal position after a severe VAE without removing the head from pin fixation. To facilitate a return to a horizontal position, two alternatives are suggested. **B,** In the first (modified sitting position), the same table position is used, but the Mayfield support is attached to the back section of the table. The horizontal position can now be achieved simply by lowering the back. **C,** In the "UCSD position" the table base is placed in reverse Trendelenburg, the back elevated, and the legs elevated and supported on pillows. In the event of a serious VAE, the horizontal position can be achieved simply by placing the table in the Trendelenburg position.

been disputed.[47,318] Many are uncomfortable with applying PEEP in the face of hemodynamic instability and with the possibility that additional VAE may produce major hemodynamic instability.

If air entrainment continues, or hemodynamic deterioration occurs, the patient should be moved into a horizontal position. With the traditional sitting position (Fig. 67-19, A), this can be accomplished only by removing the patient from pin-fixation. This is time consuming and difficult to perform without contaminating the wound. We believe that the only acceptable sitting position is one that allows the patient to be easily moved. There are two described ways to accomplish this. In one method described by Shapiro at University of California at San Diego, the primary axis of the operating room table is placed in reverse Trendelenburg position, and the legs are supported on pillows (Fig. 67-19, B). A horizontal posture then can be achieved simply by moving the table into a head-down position. An alternative is to place the main axis into steep Trendelenburg position, raise the back, and attach the over-bed support arch and pin-fixation device to the back (cephalad) portion of the table, rather than to the lower (caudad) part (Fig. 67-19, C). A supine position is achieved by lowering the back.

Emergence

In a routine, uncomplicated procedure, the patient can be awakened and extubated at the end of the case. However, two situations alter this.

Air embolism and pulmonary edema. On occasion, a large air embolism will precipitate pulmonary edema. The etiology is unknown, but the condition is usually self-limited. If a patient has suffered a major embolus and has a persistent, large shunt, we prefer to continue mechanical ventilation until a more complete evaluation can be carried out.

Cranial nerve dysfunction. As noted previously, a major complication of posterior fossa surgery (regardless of position) is damage to those cranial nerves that control airway function (i.e., CN IX, X, and XI). There is no reliable intraoperative method for assessing the function of these nerves (although CN VII and VIII can be monitored using facial nerve stimulation and brain stem auditory evoked responses, respectively). Patients should be carefully monitored after emergence to verify that function has been maintained. Patients who have suffered more than two or three transient, sudden hemodynamic or respiratory events during surgical dissection (e.g., hypertension/tachycardia, hypertension/bradycardia, inspiratory effort) are left intubated after awakening. The concern is that these hemodynamic events reflect brain stem injury. These individuals are sedated with fentanyl/droperidol and are generally extubated 24 to 36 hours postoperatively.

There is a small incidence of neurogenic pulmonary edema after posterior fossa surgery, particularly when surgery is performed on the floor of the fourth ventricle. Unlike edema encountered after head trauma, respiratory failure can occur suddenly in fully awake patients. Such an event is most likely to occur in those patients in whom we have seen hemodynamic evidence for brain stem injury, and this provides another reason to be extremely cautious about extubation.

Anesthesia for Infratentorial Craniectomy: the Horizontal Position

Use of horizontal positions (prone or lateral) generally avoids the problems of massive VAE, although Black et al.[49] have shown that Doppler-detected VAE occurs in up to 12% of these cases, reportedly without important consequences. The remaining problems are similar, except for positioning. There is reason to believe that the prone, lateral, and park bench positions are associated with a greater incidence of positioning related injuries.[49,255] These include:

- Brachial plexus injuries: this is a particular problem in the lateral/park bench positions when the "up" arm is pulled caudally to improve access to the retromastoid area, or when the head/neck is excessively rotated; a similar problem can occur in the prone position if the arms are pulled down with excessive force.
- Ulnar nerve injury
- Pressure blisters/skin necrosis of the face caused by inadequate weight distribution on a horseshoe headrest
- Blindness caused by pressure on the eyes in the prone position
- Quadriplegia associated with extreme flexion of the neck (quadriplegia has been described in the prone position as well sitting)

These problems are likely avoidable by careful attention to position, nerve stretch, padding, and so forth. Because these problems are not likely to be fatal, these alternative positions are contended to be "better" than the sitting position. Because VAE/PAE-related fatalities are so rare in the hands of experienced teams, we believe that morbidity may be the more important factor. It is likely that the *overall morbidity* of horizontal approaches is no better than with the sitting position.

Anesthesia for Intracranial Vascular Procedures: Aneurysms

Aneurysmal subarachnoid hemorrhage (SAH) strikes ≈ 30,000 people a year in North America.[44,185] Of this number, 17,000 to 20,000 patients are admitted to hospital, and only 70% of these patients will come to operating room. Of patients entered into the International Cooperative Aneurysm Study, 58% of individuals admitted to the hospital within 3 days after hemorrhage had "good" outcomes; if analysis is restricted to patients who actually undergo surgery, a "good outcome" is seen in ≈ 68%, with death occurring in ≈ 14%.[190,191]

The most common presenting symptom is severe headache, with or without loss of consciousness. The cause of both headache and initial neurologic deterioration is a sudden, severe increase in ICP (Fig. 67-20).[434] If ICP does not rapidly normalize, the patient will die. Severe ischemia that results from shorter or less severe increases in ICP is a major cause of neurologic deficit among survivors. After a patient reaches a medical facility, he/she faces two major problems: (1) "vasospasm" and (2) recurrent hemorrhage. A third problem—hydrocephalus—will not be discussed.

Vasospasm. Strictly speaking, vasospasm is an angiographic diagnosis. Arteries will constrict in response to extravascular blood, but this is transient. By contrast, clinical "vasospasm" typically occurs several days after initial hemorrhage.[98,190,191,444] Acute vasoconstriction is easily reversed by vasodilators (e.g., nitroprusside, nitroglycerin), but delayed vasospasm is not. This led to the hypothesis that vasospasm is actually a form of vessel injury or vasculopathy. Other work indicates that either endothelial relaxing factor (EDRF) or endothelin (a constricting factor) play an important role in this disorder.[68,71,353] In view of uncertainties concerning the etiology of this disorder, many clinicians prefer the term "delayed cerebral ischemia" to define the development or worsening of focal neurologic deficits in patients with subarachnoid hemorrhage (SAH). Such an event occurs in roughly 30% to 40% of patients admitted with SAH.[190,191]

Recurrent hemorrhage. Without therapy, 20% to 30% of patients hospitalized after SAH will rebleed within 2 weeks (and ≈ 7% of patients rebleed within 48 hours).[189,190,191] It can be prevented only by clipping the aneurysm. To reduce presurgical risk, patients are treated with bed rest, sedation, antihypertensives, and antifibri-

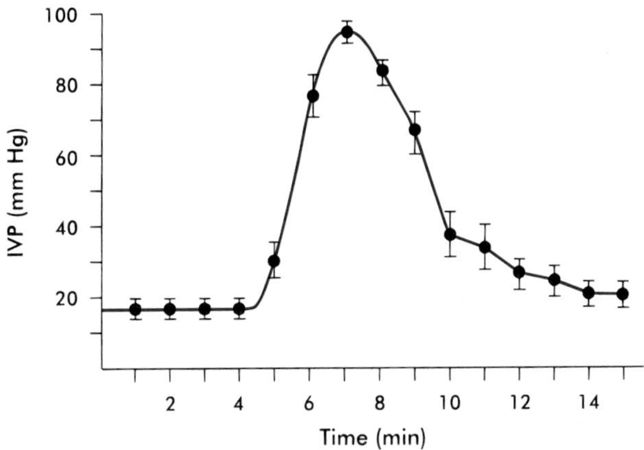

Fig. 67-20. ICPs recorded during and after a recurrent subarachnoid hemorrhage. Data represent the average from seven patients. Note the abrupt increase to near systemic levels (90 to 100 mm Hg) and the rapid decline. (From Voldby B, Enevoldson EM: Intracranial pressure changes follow aneurysm rupture: recurrent hemorrhage, *J Neurosurg* 56:784, 1982.)

nolytic drugs. These therapies are "two-edged swords" that increase risks of respiratory complications and deep vein thrombosis (DVT). Antifibrinolytics can also increase the incidence of vasospasm. Given these problems, surgeons have long advocated early, definitive surgery, despite data obtained in the early 1980s which indicated little difference in morbidity or mortality between patients operated on either early or late,[190,191] with patients undergoing early surgery succumbing to more frequent vasospasm. Sub-sequent introduction of more effective treatments for vasospasm, including nimodipine and hypertensive/hypervolemic therapy has convinced most surgical teams to operate early, at least in good grade patients.

Preoperative evaluation

Special areas of concern in these patients include assessment of: (1) neurologic status; (2) cardiac dysrhythmias and other ECG abnormalities; (3) intravascular volume status; and (4) the use of calcium entry blockers for prevention of vasospasm.

Neurologic status. All patients suffering aneurysmal SAH are assigned a clinical "grade" that provides prognostic information and allows better communication between clinicians. The most widely used system was proposed by Hunt and Hess[176] although the World Federation of Neurologic Surgeons (WFNS) scale may be more objective (Table 67-4).[100] Other grading systems have been proposed, but all follow the same general pattern: The greater the numerical score, the more severely ill the patient.

There are at least three reasons for the anesthesia provider to be aware of the patient's neurologic status. **These patients may deteriorate rapidly, and the anesthesia provider may be the first to identify such a change. Second, the failure of a patient to return to his/her baseline status upon emergence from anesthesia requires distinction between residual anesthetic effects and surgical concerns. Finally, clinical grade correlates well with alterations in intracranial physiology.**[435,436] As grade deteriorates, autoregulation and CO_2 responsiveness become progressively disordered, and the incidence of intracranial hypertension increases. Grade I and II patients typically have near-normal ICP values, and normal vascular responsiveness. Such patients can be approached differently by the anesthesia provider in terms of premedicants, the use of volatile agents and N_2O, the limits of hypotension and so forth, than can grade III through V individuals.

Table 67-4 Neurologic grading system for patients with SAH

Grade	Criteria
Hunt and Hess	
Grade I	Asymptomatic or minimal headache and slight nuchal rigidity
Grade II	Moderate-to-severe headache, nuchal rigidity, no neurologic deficit other than cranial nerve palsy
Grade III	Drowsiness, confusion, or mild focal deficit
Grade IV	Stupor, moderate-to-severe hemiparesis
Grade V	Deep coma, decerebrate rigidity, moribund appearance
World Federation of Neurologic Surgeons	
Grade I	GCS 15, no motor deficit
Grade II	GCS 14–13, no motor deficit
Grade III	GCS 14–13, any motor deficit
Grade IV	GCS 12–7, with or without motor deficit
Grade V	GCS 6–3, with or without motor deficit

Cardiac dysrhythmias and other ECG abnormalities. SAH is associated with an increased incidence of dysrhythmias and ECG morphologic abnormalities.[90,238] Holter monitoring reveals rhythm disturbances in as many as 91% of patients, although retrospective analysis of multiple studies suggest an incidence of ≈ 40% is more accurate.[90,96,212] The most frequent abnormalities are prolongation of the Q-T interval, flattened or inverted T waves, S-T segment depression, and prominent U waves. These may occur in combination or sequentially (Fig. 67-21). The mechanism of these changes remains controversial. Elevated catecholamines, hypercortisolism, and hypokalemia have all been implicated, and evidence also exists that incriminates a hypothalamic neurogenic mechanism. Studies of myocardium-specific enzymes have been inconsistent, but postmortem studies have shown evidence of subendocardial injury. Noninvasive studies of myocardial perfusion (thallium scans) and LV function (echocardiography) show a high incidence of abnormalities, at least in patients with ECG abnormalities.[89,406]

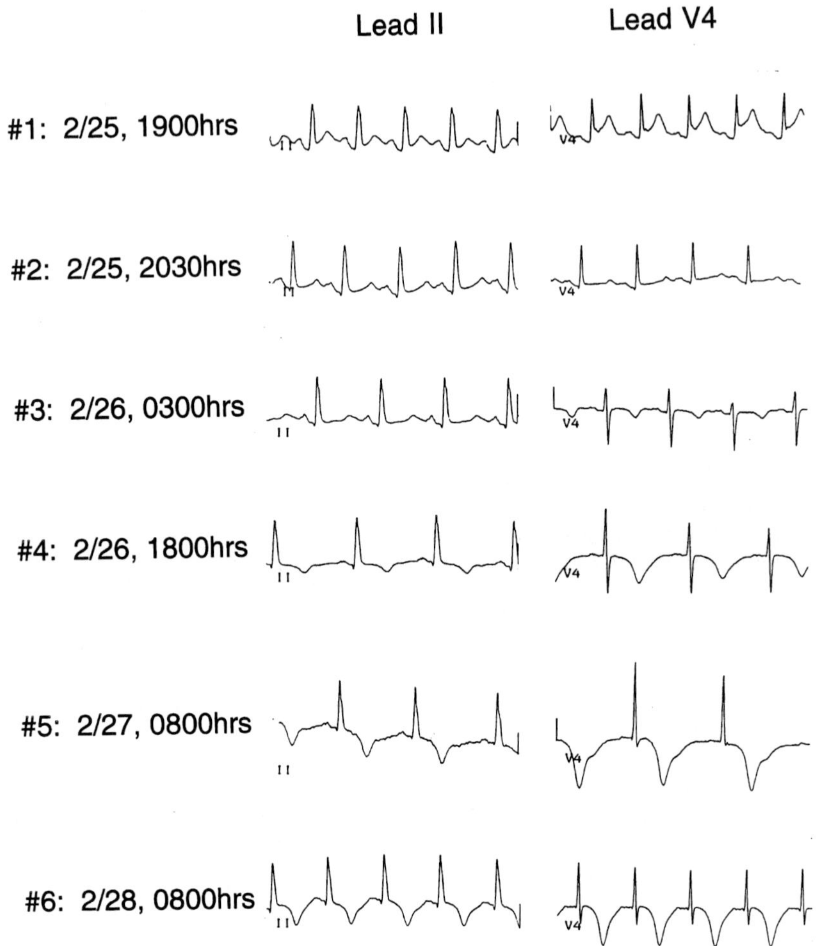

Fig. 67-21. Serial EKG tracings obtained in a young woman with a subarachnoid hemorrhage. The first tracing was obtained ≈ 30 minutes after the onset of headache. Note the sequential appearance of ST-segment elevation, QT prolongation, T-wave inversion and QRS axis changes. There were no changes in serum creatine kinase isoenzymes at any time.

The patient with serious dysrhythmia requires prompt treatment, and patients with SAH should have continuous perioperative ECG monitoring. A difficult dilemma is the patient with ECG changes suggestive of myocardial injury, particularly when the clinical grade is good and early surgery is contemplated. If there is no evidence of congestive heart failure (CHF) or angina and serial enzymes are negative, surgery should proceed. With the patient who has enzymatic evidence of myocardial damage, the dilemma is which represents the greater risk: Anesthesia and surgery in the face of a recent myocardial infarction (MI), or rebleeding because the aneurysm is not clipped? This problem has not been studied systematically. The prognostic implications of a MI precipitated by an SAH is unknown, and cardiovascular diseases are not major causes of death among patients with SAH.[190,191] In the cooperative study, overall hospital mortality from recurrent hemorrhage was 236 of 3521 (6.7%), and the risk of hemorrhage was generally judged to be 1% to 2% per day. In addition, 15% to 20% of patients suffer some degree of serious morbidity caused by vasospasm, which might be alleviated by early surgery combined with aggressive therapy. By contrast, Rao et al.[334] have reported a "best case" risk of reinfarction of ≈ 6% in the first 3 months after MI, with an overall mortality of ≈ 4%,[334] but that low risk has not been confirmed. The Cooperative Aneursym Trial indicated that the actual risk of severe MIs (i.e., severe enough to dictate some change in care) was only ≈ 0.7% overall. This suggests that the risk of postponing surgery long enough to reduce the rate of recurrent MI (e.g., > 3 months) is considerably greater than the risk of death from perioperative reinfarction. We believe that there is little justification for delaying surgery for anything other than in patients undergoing MI with serious LV dysfunction (i.e., cardiogenic shock or nearly that).

Intravascular volume status. The preoperative volume status of untreated patients with SAH is often abnormal. In earlier days, patients were relatively hypovolemic because of bed rest, negative nitrogen balance, decreased erythropoiesis, iatrogenic blood loss, and dysregulation of the autonomic nervous system; this has become less common because of the frequent use of hypervolemia to treat/prevent vasospasm. Hyponatremia is also occasionally observed, caused by either a central salt wasting syndrome or true SIADH.[388]

Calcium antagonists. Although many methods have been used for treatment of vasospasm, most recent work has centered on calcium antagonists, with nimodipine being the first drug released for the specific prophylaxis of vasospasm.[173,349] Like every new drug, nimodipine initially raised concern about whether its preoperative use would make anesthesia more dangerous or difficult. Fortunately, these fears proved unfounded. Patients taking nimodipine do have lesser blood pressures (as well as lower SVRs and greater cardiac outputs), and there are fewer clinical management difficulties as long as anesthetic agents are carefully titrated. An alternative calcium blocker—nicardipine—was initially evaluated as an antivasospastic agent, but trials were halted with the introduction of nimodipine.[153] Nicardipine is now approved only for blood pressure control.

Another drug under evaluation for treatment/prevention of vasospasm (or its ischemic consequences) is the 21-aminosteroid tirilazad.[154,155] This compound is chemically related to methylprednisolone, but has no glucocorticoid activity; primary mode of action appears to be as a free-radical scavenger. Clinical trials in Europe suggest some benefit in men only; U.S. trials are ongoing.[186] The drug appears to pose no anesthetic problems.

Table 67-5 ICP and vascular responsiveness after subarachnoid hemorrhage

Grade	ICP (mm Hg)	CO_2 response: Δ CBF/Δ Pco_2	Autoregulation: Δ CBF/Δ %MABP
II	10 ± 3	1.61 ± 0.67	−0.042 ± 0.194
III	18 ± 6	1.02 ± 0.5	−0.230 ± 0.514
IV–V	29 ± 6	0.61 ± 0.42	−0.344 ± 0.219

*Data are all mean ± SD. Units for CO_2 response are ml/100 g/min change in CBF/mm Hg change in CO_2. Autoregulation is expressed as ml/100 g/min change in CBF/% change in MAP (a value of 0.000 would be perfect autoregulation, and a more negative number indicates progressive autoregulatory impairment). Note that the clinical grading was not consistent between the two reports, and hence the first column was constructed to the best of our ability.

From Voldby B, Enevoldsen EM, and Jensen FT: Cerebrovascular reactivity in patients with ruptured intracranial aneurysm, *J Neurosurg* 62:59, 1985 and Voldby B, Enevoldsen EM: Intracranial pressure changes following aneurysm rupture. Part I: clinical and angiographic correlations, *J Neurosurg* 56:186, 1982.

Premedication

Premedication should balance two factors: (1) risk of anxiety-related hypertension and aneurysmal rerupture; and (2) chance of respiratory depression that may exacerbate intracranial hypertension. Fortunately, it has been possible to generate some guidelines. Voldby et al.[436] have demonstrated a good relationship between clinical grade and ICP, with patients in grades I and II almost uniformly having near-normal ICP values (see Table 67-5). As clinical grade deteriorates, the incidence of intracranial hypertension increases. There is little reason to avoid modest sedation (e.g., with benzodiazepines) in grade I and II individuals, particularly several days after the initial hemorrhage. Patients who are somnolent or who have focal deficits (grades III through V) are transported to the operating room without premedication. Premedication in these cases should be administered intravenously with the anesthesia provider in attendance.

Routine monitoring

Given the potential risks associated with rapid swings in BP (e.g., aneurysmal rupture, profound hypoperfusion) and the need for very accurate beat-to-beat control during profound hypotension, direct arterial cannulation is mandatory (although this can be deferred until after induction if it results in patient agitation). Urinary bladder catheterization yields information on fluid balance, but the near-certain use of mannitol or furosemide will limit the value of urine output as an index of intravascular volume. To improve our assessment of volume status, we favor placement of central venous or PA catheters, at least in older patients and in those with preoperative ECG changes that cannot be readily distinguished from myocardial ischemia, or in patients with a large or relatively inaccessible aneurysm (i.e., where "excess" blood loss is anticipated). Note that this is perhaps the only surgical procedure where pharmacologic hypotension should be maintained in the face of active arterial hemorrhage (from a ruptured aneurysm). Other than central vascular cannulation, there are no reliable methods for rapidly distinguishing normovolemic hypotension from shock in such situations. We recognize that there are risks associated with central catheter placement, and we also realize that many experienced centers do not employ central catheters, particularly those that have abandoned induced hypotension. PA catheterization is reserved for patients with known preexisting cardiac disease, or perhaps for cases where surgery is anticipated to be difficult or prolonged.

Specialized monitoring: EEG and evoked potentials

Because the most feared immediate complication of surgery is a misplaced clip or tissue injury caused by excessive retraction and/or hypotension, many groups have attempted to improve their ability to detect ischemic changes before they become irreversible. Nevertheless, the value of electrophysiologic monitoring remains unclear. EEGs recorded from the perimeter of the craniotomy have yielded contradictory results.[181,413] Because of the uncertainty, most centers probably use EEG monitoring if needed to facilitate drug administration (e.g., barbiturates). Greater attention has been directed at SEPs, because the conduction pathways pass through areas at greatest risk. Symon et al.[130,405] have presented extensive data relating changes in central conduction time with outcome. A correlation with outcome need not necessarily mean that monitoring can prevent a deficit, but several groups have now used SEP monitoring to define the limits of temporary vessel occlusion during surgery.[234,279] Although SEP monitoring has not yet been established as a routine, it may offer some benefits.

Induction and maintenance

We believe that the principal risk is rebleeding. Four reports have shown that the incidence of hemorrhage on induction ranges from 1% to 2%.[140,191,402,426] In one of these studies, hemorrhage was associated with airway difficulties encountered during induction that presumably led to hypertension, coughing, and so forth. Given these considerations, induction is designed to avoid sudden hypertensive events, particularly during laryngoscopy and intubation. We tend to carry patients "deeper" at the time of intubation, using volatile agents, larger doses of narcotics (e.g., fentanyl 12 to 15 μg/kg) or additional thiopental or lidocaine. Arterial pressure is continuously monitored; if BP or heart rate starts to increase with laryngoscopy alone, the laryngoscope is removed and additional anesthetic given. In general, we are far more tolerant of hypotension during induction than we are of hypertension.

Subsequent management is directed at ensuring adequate surgical conditions. Because aneurysms are located around the base of the brain, exposure may be a challenge, particularly with cerebral swelling. This is clearly much worse during "early" surgery (Fig. 67-22).[191] If exposure cannot be facilitated, then the risk of tissue injury from excessive retractor pressures[10,330] or uncontrolled aneurysmal hemorrhage is high. For these reasons, patients may have spinal drains placed, receive mannitol, and be aggressively hyperventilated ($Pa_{CO_2} \approx 25$ mm Hg).

Induced hypotension versus temporary occlusion

To minimize risk of aneurysmal rupture during dissection, one of two interventions is employed: induced hypotension or temporary vessel occlusion (trapping). In both cases, the goal is to reduce intraluminal pressure. With hypotension, a secondary goal is to slow the rate of hemorrhage in the event that rupture occurs.

Hypotension. Induced hypotension has long been a standard component of surgery. Most surgeons believe it to be of value, although this is impossible to "prove," particularly because most surgery performed before the introduction of hypotensive techniques was also done before use of the operating microscope. The argument against hypotension is that SAH and vasospasm may disrupt cerebral autoregulation, particularly in lower-grade patients.[121,435] As a result, the lowest safe MAP that can be employed is unknown, particularly in the face of retraction pressure and other conditions. Hypotension also poses a risk of myocardial ischemia in older patients. Nevertheless, most teams are willing to reduce MAP to values of 70 mm Hg during initial dissection and to pressures as low as 50 mm Hg during direct manipulation of the aneurysm.

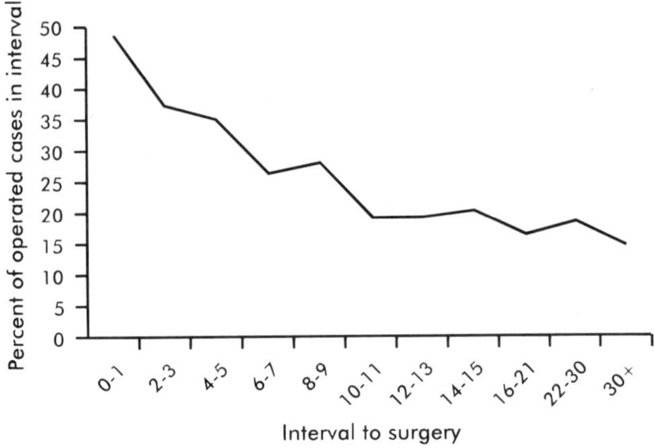

Fig. 67-22. The incidence of a subjectively "tight" brain at craniotomy, relative to the time of surgery after subarachnoid hemorrhage. There is clearly a far greater likelihood of difficult operating conditions with acute aneurysm surgery. (From Kassell NF, Torner JC, Jane JA, et al: The international cooperative study on the timing of aneurysm surgery surgical results, *J Neurosurg* 73:37, 1990.)

Considerable effort has been directed toward determining the ideal agent to produce the hypotension. These efforts have not succeeded. The three agents in most common use are sodium nitroprusside, nitroglycerin, and isoflurane. The first two were discussed above. The use of trimethaphan has been abandoned because of rapid tachyphylaxis. Isoflurane has gained some popularity because it is well tolerated, and some believe it to have some protective effects. Unfortunately, there have been no prospective studies demonstrating an improved (or worsened) neurologic outcome, or altered complication rate, etc. with any agent. The picture is even more complex because polypharmacy is the rule, and these drugs are combined with long-acting nitrates (e.g., hydralazine), beta-blockers, calcium antagonists, preoperative clonidine, etc.

Regardless of the agent used, several points from the earlier discussion of basic physiology/pharmacology should be remembered. Autoregulation is not instantaneous, and abrupt decreases or increases in pressure may lead to transient hypoperfusion during induction of hypotension and hyperperfusion upon discontinuation. Hypotension increases several humoral factors, including norepinephrine, epinephrine, and renin-angiotensin. Recovery from hypotension may then be followed by rebound hypertension that can persist for several hours unless treated. Because hemostasis should be verified before dural closure, blood pressure should be allowed to gradually increase to values on the "high end" of normal (e.g., 140 to 160 mm Hg systolic) during the completion of the intracranial portion of the procedure.

Temporary occlusion. Hypotension has recently become less common, being replaced by the positioning of temporary clips on the parent artery (which effectively produces "regional hypotension"). This avoids many of the systemic problems associated with hypotension and also prevents rupture. If temporary occlusion is prolonged (i.e., >10 to 20 min), it may increase the risk of focal ischemic deficits.[279,364] Despite this risk, the approach is gaining in popularity. In most centers, blood pressure is modestly reduced during initial dissection, and then normalized after temporary clip placement. In some cases, barbiturates are administered to "protect" the brain, although we reserve this for procedures where the duration of occlusion is prolonged.

Emergence and early postoperative care

Rapid return to consciousness permits early clinical assessment and detection of unexpected neurologic deficits (e.g., caused by a clot or misplaced clip). This can lead to either a diagnostic procedure (e.g., angiography and/or reoperation) or the institution of hypertensive-hypervolemic therapy. This emphasis on rapid emergence makes the maintenance of hemodynamic stability more difficult. Kalfas and Little have shown a 2.3% incidence of postoperative intracranial hemorrhage among patients undergoing aneurysm clippings.[183] Their data implicate uncontrolled hypertension as a causative factor. We believe arterial pressure should be monitored without interruption in these patients, including during transportation to the recovery room, and/or to the surgical intensive care unit. Obviously, if such monitoring is to be useful, patients should be accompanied at all times in the early postoperative period by an individual able to administer the pharmacologic agents needed to control hypertensive events.

Treatment of delayed ischemic deficits/symptomatic vasospasm

Despite use of calcium-antagonists, vasospasm remains a major cause of morbidity and death even after otherwise successful clipping. Although there is growing interest in endovascular therapy (e.g., balloon angioplasty) or fibrinolytics (e.g., tPA),[98,300] the only widely accepted acute therapy is hypervolemia or hypertension.[29,98,188,393] The patient with a new focal deficit or decreased level of consciousness is first scanned to rule out infarct, clot, or hydrocephalus. An angiogram may be carried out to verify clip placement. Patients then are moved to an intensive care unit where arterial and central venous/PA pressure monitors are placed, if not already in place. Albumin and/or crystalloids are infused to increase CVP to values of 10 to 12 mm Hg, or pulmonary capillary wedge pressure (PCWP) to 15 to 18 mm Hg. (Initial volume loading can be started before monitoring catheters are in place. Continued therapy is dangerous without such monitors). Hetastarch is avoided because large doses (> 1 to 1.5 l) are associated with coagulation deficits and intracranial hemorrhage.[83,88] If these measures fail to reverse the neurologic deficit, BP is elevated pharmacologically. There are no good guidelines concerning the target BP, but most groups will increase systolic pressure to values as high as 160 to 200 mm Hg if tolerated. The most common drug used is dopamine, but other agents or combinations of agents seem equally efficacious. Many groups think that hematocrit can be modestly decreased (i.e., 33% to 36%), but there is little current enthusiasm for more profound hemodilution.

The major complications are cardiovascular, with a reported incidence of pulmonary edema ranging from 7% to 17%.[29,188,455] Cerebral edema has also been reported.[383] One should beware of the urge to "keep pushing" when initial volume expansion fails to resolve the deficit. Severe pulmonary edema with resultant adult respiratory distress syndrome (ARDS) has been seen. Increasing and maintaining elevated PCWP and BP is strikingly difficult in some patients, particularly the young. They may mount a brisk diuresis in response to volume loading and may be refractory to vasopressors. Vasopressin or DDAVP can be used in such cases, along with more potent alpha- and beta-adrenergic agents, but these in turn further increase the risk of fluid overload, tachyarrhythmias, or myocardial ischemia.

Special problems

Intraoperative hemorrhage. Intraoperative aneurysmal rupture is a potentially catastrophic event reported in 15% to 20% of patients.[33] Hemorrhagic shock and death are not the most likely consequences; instead, one sees cerebral ischemic damage. When brisk bleeding occurs deep within the cranium, the operator is blinded. Ischemia can result from efforts to slow this bleeding, including excessive hypotension (elective or otherwise), more vigorous retraction, or from clips placed on major cerebral vessels.

This is not a rare event, so a plan should exist. The rate of blood loss can usually be handled. Our first response is to increase the rate of IV fluid administration. If bleeding is not stopped within a few minutes, BP is progressively (and smoothly) reduced to mean values as low as 40 to 50 mm Hg (measured at the head). This can be accomplished by any method desired as long as normovolemia is maintained. Manual compression of the carotid arteries in the neck is also effective but it leaves the anesthesia provider unable to perform other tasks. The goal is to slow the rate of hemorrhage so that the source can be found or a feeding vessel identified. If the aneurysm can be directly clipped, there are few problems. More commonly a clip is temporarily applied to a feeding vessel. There is some evidence that prolonged hypotension in the face of ruptures may be more dangerous than temporary clipping.[140] It is probably reasonable to keep duration of hypotension as short as possible.

Intraoperative protection. Barbiturates are the only drugs shown useful in situations of temporary intracranial vessel occlusion (repeated animal studies).[297,395,441] Contrary to popular belief, they need not be given before occlusion but can be administered up to 30 to 60 min after occlusion and still be beneficial. There is no need to subject a hypovolemic patient to the hemodynamic risks of "emergency" barbiturate loading. We ensure adequate vascular volume with hypotension and then begin barbiturate administration with small (100 to 200 mg) boluses of thiopental.

Other anesthetics are progressively reduced as the dose increases. Our goal is to administer a dose of ≈ 15 to 30 mg/kg of drug over a 30-minute period. If vessel occlusion persists, a dose of ≈ g/hr of thiopental will maintain a reasonable degree of EEG and metabolic suppression. Note that although the traditional goal is EEG burst-suppression or isoelectricity, there is data suggesting that lesser doses are equally effective.[37,440]

Recently, etomidate has been advocated as a protective agent, based on its ability to reduce CMR,[34] but two animal studies failed to demonstrate protective efficacy.[101,366] Hence, we do not believe this is reasonable, other than perhaps in the context of a clinical trial.

Renewed interest in use of hypothermia has been generated by recent demonstration of protective value of relatively mild hypothermia 32° to 34° C. Some have argued that patients should simply be allowed to spontaneously cool (as they almost always do) without active warming in the operating room. This may prove reasonable, but in view of the problems associated with awakening a hypothermic patient, as well as the risk of myocardial ischemia,[129] we believe that some concrete demonstration of efficacy is needed before this is done routinely.

Anesthesia for Intracranial Vascular Procedures: Arteriovenous Malformations

Although the care of these patients has many things in common with the care of those undergoing aneurysm clippings, differences do exist. Risk of recurrent hemorrhage is much lower than with an aneurysm; surgery for definitive excision is rarely emergent. Hypertension-induced hemorrhage is almost nonexistent;[407] blood pressure control during induction is probably not as crucial. Vasospasm is rare, so there is little need for calcium antagonists or hypervolemic/hypertensive therapy. The major risks are intraoperative hemorrhage—which can be torrential—and a disorder called *reperfusion breakthrough.*[5,30,284] Hemorrhage is handled by transfusion and induced hypotension. However, reperfusion breakthrough is a much more difficult problem.

An AVM represents a low resistance pathway shunting blood directly from arteries to veins. The result is that perfusion pressure to adjacent normal tissues may be very low, and these tissues may therefore be maximally dilated. If the AVM is suddenly obliterated, perfusion pressure to these tissues may increase dramatically. AVM flow rates in excess of a liter/minute have been estimated; with 50 to 75 mm Hg increases in collateral perfusion pressures after AVM occlusion.[302] This can lead to either rapid formation of cerebral edema or actual physical disruption of vessels with intraparenchymal hemorrhage. The result is a phenomenon often called malignant brain swelling or "reperfusion breakthrough," where the brain begins to rapidly herniate out of the craniotomy site.

To date, the only possibly successful therapy for this is a combination of induced hypotension (to reduce perfusion pressure) and very high doses of barbiturates.[91,243] The doses used are governed by the patient's response, not by some theoretical "EEG suppressant" dose of barbiturate. Thiopental (or pentobarbital) loading is continued until the swelling is controlled or until cardiovascular toxicity occurs. Barbiturate-induced hypotension may actually be beneficial. Of equal importance is the realization that this therapy, particularly the control of blood pressure, may need to be continued for several days postoperatively. This necessitates PA catheterization, mechanical ventilation, heavy sedation, ICP monitoring, and a very skilled intensive care unit team.

There is a theoretical risk that hyperventilation will increase flow throughout the AVM because only normal vessels are responsive. Although there is some experimental support for this idea,[283,459] there is little clinical reason for concern.

Anesthesia for Cervical Spine Disease

Cervical spine disease care does not involve much "neuroanesthetic" physiology or pharmacology and has been well reviewed elsewhere.[77,162] A few comments are in order.

Our greatest fear in patients with cervical spine disease is that of permanent injury to the spinal cord during induction, intubation, and positioning. This is not a trivial concern. Neck extension can compress the cervical cord, at least in patients with cervical stenosis.[231] Quadriplegia/paresis following anesthetic induction has been reported in at least three patients. These patients can be managed safely[77] if we understand the diseases involved and the consequences of various interventions.

Some experts have concluded that all patients with any form of cervical spine disease require awake fiber optic intubation and awake positioning. This is excessively dogmatic. It is preferable to assess spinal column stability and/or spinal cord compression. Usually this determination will have already been made during diagnostic workup. The information may not be present in the chart, and/or there may be no obvious clues, such as Gardner-Wells tongs or halo-fixation devices. In these cases the anesthesia provider should make an evaluation. History and examination of the patient's active range of motion make sense (the patient is asked to do the moving, do not move the neck for him/her). With a full range of motion, an otherwise normal airway, and no displacement on flexion/extension films, general anesthesia can probably be induced in a routine manner, followed by direct laryngoscopy. Axial traction (perhaps applied manually) is probably reasonable in the patient with a normal airway and a stable cervical spine whose only complaint is mild pain on rotation or extension, particularly if the disorder is some form of spondylolisthesis or spinal stenosis. The role of traction in decompressing the cervical cord in such situations has been demonstrated by Magnaes (Fig. 67-23).[231] If a difficult intubation is anticipated; if there is radiologic evidence of instability (even if the patient can move); if there is a serious preexisting neurologic deficit (even if partially resolved); or if neck movement is accompanied by severe pain, we believe

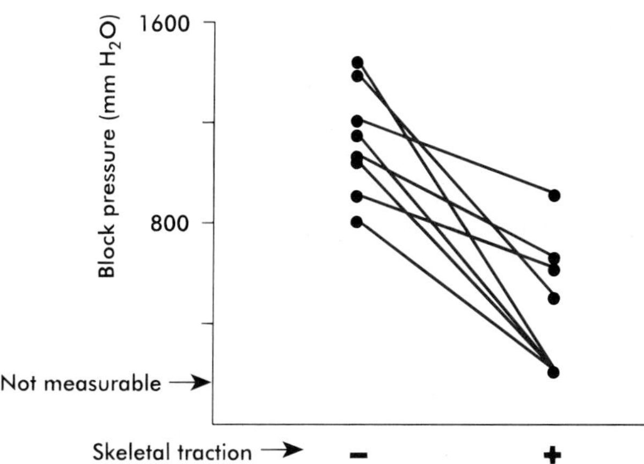

Fig. 67-23. Changes in cervical "block pressure" (y axis) during laryngoscopy before and after the application of neck traction. Data was obtained from eight patients with cervical stenosis. Note that "block pressure" is measured by placing a catheter in the lumbar subarachnoid space and then measuring CSF pressure during a controlled infusion of fluid. With cervical cord compression, lumbar CSF pressure rises rapidly until it exceeds that needed to force fluid around the area of compression, at which point a plateau appears in the pressure trace. Less compression results in lower block pressures. (From Magnaes B: Clinical recording of pressure on the spinal cord and cauda equina. Part 3. Pressure on the cervical spinal cord during endotracheal intubation in patients with cervical spondylosis, *J Neurosurg* 57:64, 1982.)

that some alternative approach is indicated. Our preference remains awake fiber optic intubation, followed by awake positioning. Alternatively, one may employ one of the newer airway management devices (e.g., Bullard laryngoscope, light wand, Augustine intubating airway). In some cases, it may be reasonable to perform the intubation after induction of general anesthesia, at least if the patient can be easily ventilated by mask. Any of the above noted devices can then be used to facilitate intubation. A recently suggested compromise is use of the laryngeal mask airway, which can then serve as both a means of ventilation and a guide for the fiber optic scope. The exact method chosen is often a matter of personal choice; regardless of technique, the obvious goal is to avoid marked extension (or flexion) of the cervical spine.

What is the approach for the patient with a truly unstable neck who will not cooperate with an awake intubation? Some experts might insist on an awake approach, but we disagree, because the cervical cord can be injured either by intubation or by a thrashing patient. Another factor that plays a role in decision-making is the location of the injury. Most cervical spine movement during direct laryngoscopy occurs between the occiput and C2.[163,368] If the airway is determined to be normal, it may be more acceptable to perform direct laryngoscopy with manual stabilization (perhaps after placement of Gardner-Wells tongs) in a patient with a subaxial injury than someone with a C1/C2 fracture/instability. Note that the goal is not to apply traction (which, if applied with excessive vigor, may produce vertebral separation[45]) but to simply prevent neck extension. To further avoid extension, we rarely attempt to obtain full exposure of the glottis, perferring instead to carry out a "directed but semi-blind" intubation. On the other hand, if the airway is judged to be "difficult" (where more movement may occur at lower segments), this may be dangerous, although there may be little choice. Alternatives may include fiber optic intubation after induction of anesthesia, "blind" nasal intubation, or use of newer intubating devices mentioned above.[163] If awake intubation is deemed impossible, if the airway is truly difficult (e.g., massive facial trauma) and if general anesthesia before intubation is felt to be dangerous (e.g., a truly full stomach), there may be little choice but to proceed with tracheostomy (although doing this in an awake, combative patient may produce just as much additional injury. If neurologic assessment after intubation is critical, it is possible to induce anesthesia using thiopental or propofol and a short-acting relaxant, maintain anesthesia with N_2O or propofol, and then reawaken the patient to assess motor function.

One issue we have not discussed concerns the quadriplegic patient with spinal shock. The physiology of this disorder has been well described and is very similar to the hypotension seen during high spinal anesthesia. Usually, such patients are already intubated and should have arterial and central venous/PA catheters in place. Keys to successful care are maintenance of normal intravascular volume without overload and judicious use of vasopressors (e.g., ephedrine, dopamine, phenylephrine).

Transsphenoidal Hypophysectomy

This operation revolutionized the surgical approach to the sella turcica and to the immediate suprasellar region, turning a difficult subfrontal craniotomy into a near-routine operation. Nevertheless, there are a few major problems.

First, the airway is shared with the surgeon. The endotracheal tube should be very well secured to the lower jaw. There is also danger that blood, tissue, and bone fragments can fall into the posterior pharynx. A throat pack minimizes the chance of these items being swallowed, but we believe that laryngoscopy should be performed before extubation, to ensure that the pharynx is clear.

Second, typical neuroanesthetic maneuvers designed to reduce ICP can be counterproductive in these cases because they make the pituitary retreat upward out of the sella. In contrast, many surgeons request that the patient be hypercapnic or that a valsalva maneuver be performed to "deliver" the gland down into the surgical field.

Third, the carotid arteries lie just lateral to the surgical site, particularly in the suprasellar area. If they are damaged, blood loss can be torrential (and, because the bleeding site is often partly intracranial, fatal).

These patients are at risk for developing diabetes insipidus (DI), particularly when the resection involves the suprasellar regions. The diagnosis is usually straightforward; sudden onset of diuresis. The best course is to initially decrease the IV rate to a minimum and wait. If diuresis persists in the face of such restriction, the diagnosis becomes likely; it becomes certain if hypovolemia develops in the face of continuing urine output. If in doubt, paired urine and serum osmolalities will help, although again these may be coincidently "normal" if the patient has received a large volume of IV fluids. In the event that DI does develop, the temptation to reach for an ADH replacement should probably be resisted, at least initially. Most cases are transient and require no therapy other than fluid replacement. We treat only when the volume of urine output begins to exceed 1 l/hr or if it persists for more than a few hours. Drug choice is largely personal, although pitressin in oil is probably obsolete. Intravenous DDAVP is available and is both safer than aqueous pitressin (which can produce intense coronary vasoconstriction) and longer acting.

KEY POINTS

- Most of the physiologic parameters neuroanesthesia providers want to measure are not easy to record in the clinical setting, such as the effect of drugs on CBF, CMR, or ICP.
- Although measurement of CBF and $CMRO_2$ or CMRGlu are not yet within the clinical realm, the anesthesia provider should be familiar with the various methods of measuring CBF and CMR to understand published studies on drug effects.
- To understand ICP, remember the analogy of the brain as a "closed box," out of which something should leave if something else enters.
- Although blood is the smallest of the four kinds of tissues located in the brain, its importance lies in the fact that the CBV—and hence ICP—can be changed very rapidly.
- The five factors that control cerebral flow, CBV, and ICP are $PaCO_2$, PaO_2 plus arterial content, autoregulation, cerebral flow-metabolism coupling, and autonomic nervous system control.
- Although the mechanism(s) controlling flow-metabolism coupling are unknown, it is important to recognize that anesthetics do not actually "uncouple" flow and metabolism.
- Different anesthetics (e.g., barbiturates, propofol, etomidate, the volatile agents, and narcotics) all have somewhat different effects on cerebral flow and CMR. In general, IV drugs reduce CBF, whereas volatile agents are vasodilators. Essentially all agents, except perhaps ketamine, reduce CMR.
- All volatile anesthetics can increase CBF and ICP, in some cases dramatically. These drug-induced ICP increases have never been demonstrated to be detrimental (at least during elective surgery) and are relatively easily counteracted by other ICP control measures, including hyperventilation.
- Nitrous oxide is not benign in its effects on the brain. It can considerably increase CBF.
- In a patient who is severely hypertensive because of intracranial hypertension, it is probably unwise to aggressively lower blood pressure.
- The sitting position, although accompanied by hazards of air embolism and other problems, is still in wide use in neurosurgery. Despite problems with the sitting position, it is not clear that alternative positions are better.
- Cerebrovasospasm, its diagnosis, and its treatment should occupy the attention of the neuroanesthesia provider. The most recent work in the field has centered on the calcium antagonists, specifically nimodipine.
- Reduction of brain swelling, even though the cranium is open, is key to successful neuroanesthesia. "Relaxation" of the brain during the neurosurgical procedure itself not only may require hyperventilation but also osmotic diuretics, such as mannitol, assuming the patient is well anesthetized and the skeletal musculature is paralyzed.
- During cerebral aneurysm surgery, there should be a plan for dealing with a sudden rupture and the blood loss that can occur from such a tiny operative site.

REFERENCES

1. Aaslid R, Newell DW, Stooss R, et al: Assessment of cerebral autoregulation dynamics from simultaneous arterial and venous transcranial doppler recordings in humans, *Stroke* 22:1148–1154, 1991.
2. Adams RW, Cucchiara RF, Gronert GA, et al: Isoflurane and cerebrospinal fluid pressure in neurosurgical patients, *Anesthesiology* 54:97–99, 1981.
3. Adams RW, Gronert GA, Sundt TM, et al: Halothane, hypocapnia, and cerebrospinal fluid pressure in neurosurgery, *Anesthesiology* 37:510–517, 1972.
4. Adler L, Firestone L, Mintun M, et al: Central mechanisms of pain and opioid analgesia elucidated by positron emission tomography, *Anesthesiology* 81:A917, 1994.
5. Al-Rodhan NRF, Sundt TM, Piepgras DG, et al: Occlusive hyperemia—a theory for the hemodynamic complications following resection of intracerebral arteriovenous

malformations, *J Neursurg* 78:167–175, 1993.

6. Albanese J, Durbec O, Viviand X, et al: Sufentanil increases intracranial pressure in patients with head trauma, *Anesthesiology* 79:493–497, 1993.
7. Algotsson L, Messeter K, Rosen I, et al: Effects of nitrous oxide on cerebral haemodynamics and metabolism during isoflurane anaesthesia in man, *Acta Anaesthesiol Scand* 36:46–52, 1992.
8. Alkire MT, Haier RJ, Barker SJ, et al: Cerebral metabolism during propofol anesthesia in humans studied with positron emission tomography, *Anesthesiology* 82: 393–403, 1995.
9. Andersen AR: 99mTc-D,L-hexamethylene-propyleneamine oxime (99mTc-HMPAO): basic kinetic studies of a tracer of cerebral blood flow, *Cerebrovasc Brain Metab Rev* 1:288–318, 1989.
10. Andrews RJ, Bringas JR: A review of brain retraction and recommendations for minimizing intraoperative brain injury, *Neurosurgery* 33:1052–1064, 1993.
11. Archer DP, Labrecque P, Tyler JL, et al: Measurement of cerebral blood flow and volume with positron emission tomography during isoflurane administration in the hypocapnic baboon, *Anesthesiology* 72: 1031–1037, 1990.
12. Archer DP, Labrecque P, Tyler JL, et al: Cerebral blood volume is increased in dogs during administration of nitrous oxide or isoflurane, *Anesthesiology* 67:642–648, 1987.
13. Artru AA: Nitrous oxide plays a direct role in the development of tension pneumocephalus intraoperatively, *Anesthesiology* 57:59–61, 1982.
14. Artru AA: Effects of halothane and fentanyl on the rate of CSF production in dogs, *Anesth Analg* 62:581–585, 1983.
15. Artru AA: Relationship between cerebral blood volume and CSF pressure during anesthesia with halothane or enflurane in dogs, *Anesthesiology* 58:533–539, 1983.
16. Artru AA: Isoflurane does not increase the rate of CSF production in the dog, *Anesthesiology* 60:193–197, 1984.
17. Artru AA: Relationship between cerebral blood volume and CSF pressure during anesthesia with isoflurane or fentanyl in dogs, *Anesthesiology* 60:575–579, 1984.
18. Artru AA: Cerebral metabolism and the electroencephalogram during hypocapnia plus hypotension induced by sodium nitroprusside or trimethaphan in dogs, *Neurosurgery* 18:36–44, 1986.
19. Artru AA: Cerebrospinal fluid dynamics. In Cucchiara RM, Michenfelder JD, editors: *Clinical Neuroanesthesia,* New York 1990, Churchill-Livingstone, pp 41–76.
20. Artru AA: Cerebrospinal fluid. In Cottrell JE, Smith DS, editors: *Anesthesia and neurosurgery,* St. Louis, 1994, Mosby–Year Book, pp 93–116.
21. Artru AA: Intracranial volume/pressure relationship during desflurane anesthesia in dogs: Comparison with isoflurane and thiopental/halothane, *Anesth Analg* 79: 751–760, 1994.
22. Artru AA, Colley PS: The site of origin of the intravascular electrocardiogram recorded from multiorificed intravascular catheters, *Anesthesiology* 69:44–48, 1988.
23. Artru AA, Katz RA: Cerebral blood volume and CSF pressure following administration of ketamine in dogs; modification by pre- or posttreatment with hypocapnia or diazepam, *J Neurosurg Anesthesiol* 1:8–15, 1989.
24. Artru AA, Katz RA, Colley PS: Autoregulation of cerebral blood flow during normocapnia and hypocapnia in dogs, *Anesthesiology* 70:288–292, 1989.
25. Artru AA, Nugent M, Michenfelder JD: Enflurane causes a prolonged and reversible increase in the rate of CSF production in the dog, *Anesthesiology* 57: 255–260, 1982.
26. Artru AA, Shapira Y, Bowdle TA: Electroencephalogram, cerebral metabolic, and vascular responses to propofol anesthesia in dogs, *J Neurosurg Anesthesiol* 4:99–109, 1992.
27. Artru AA, Steen PA, Michenfelder JD: Cerebral metabolic effects of naloxone administered with anesthetic and subanesthetic concentrations of halothane with the dog, *Anesthesiology* 52:217–220, 1980.
28. Artru AA, Wright K, Colley PS: Cerebral effects of hypocapnia plus nitroglycerin-induced hypotension in dogs, *J Neurosurg* 64:924–931, 1986.
29. Awad IA, Carter LP, Spetzler RF, et al: Clinical vasospasm after subarachnoid hemorrhage: response to hypervolemic hemodilution and arterial hypertension, *Stroke* 18:365–372, 1987.
30. Awad IA, Magdinec M, Schubert A: Intracranial hypertension after resection of cerebral arteriovenous malformations—predisposing factors and management strategy, *Stroke* 25:611–620, 1994.
31. Babikian VL, Wechsler LR: *Transcranial doppler ultrasonography,* St. Louis, 1993, Mosby–Year Book.
32. Baron JC, Frackowiak RSJ, Herholz K, et al: Use of PET methods for measurement of cerebral energy metabolism and hemodynamics in cerebrovascular disease, *J Cereb Blood Flow Metab* 9:723–742, 1989.
33. Batjer H, Samson D: Intraoperative aneurysm rupture: incidence, outcome and suggestions for surgical management, *Neurosurgery* 18:701–707, 1986.
34. Batjer HH: Cerebral protective effects of etomidate—experimental and clinical aspects, *Cerebrovasc Brain Metab Rev* 5: 17–32, 1993.
35. Bauer JH, Reams GP: The role of calcium entry blockers in hypertensive emergencies, *Circulation* 75:V174–180, 1987.
36. Baughman VL, Hoffman WE, Miletich DJ, et al: Cerebrovascular and cerebral metabolic effects of N20 in unrestrained rats, *Anesthesiology* 73:269–272, 1990.
37. Baughman VL, Hoffman WE, Thomas C, et al: Comparison of methohexital and isoflurane on neurologic outcome and histopathology following incomplete ischemia in rats, *Anesthesiology* 72:85–94, 1990.
38. Bedford RF, Dacey R, Winn HR, et al: Adverse impact of a calcium entry-blocker (verapamil) on intracranial pressure in patients with brain tumors, *J Neurosurg* 59:800–802, 1983.
39. Bedford RF, Marshall WK, Butler A, et al: Cardiac catheters for diagnosis and treatment of venous air embolism, *J Neurosurg* 55:610–614, 1981.
40. Bedford RF, Morris L, Jane JA: Intracranial hypertension during surgery for supratentorial tumor: correlation with preoperative computed tomography scans, *Anesth Analg* 61:430–433, 1982.
41. Belopavlovic M, Buchthal A: Modification of ketamine-induced intracranial hypertension in neurosurgical patients by pretreatment with midazolam, *Acta Anaesthesiol Scand* 26:458–462, 1982.
42. Berntman L, Dahlgren N, Siesjo BK: Cerebral blood flow and oxygen consumption in the rat brain during extreme hypercarbia, *Anesthesiology* 50:299–305, 1979.
43. Bevan JA: The human adrenergic neurovascular mechanism, *Fed Proc* 44: 317–320, 1985.
44. Biller J, Godersky JC, Adams HP: Management of aneurysmal subarachnoid hemorrhage, *Stroke* 19:1301–1318, 1988.
45. Bivins HG, Ford S, Bezmalinovic Z, et al: The effect of axial traction during orotracheal intubation of the trauma victim with an unstable cervical spine, *Ann Emerg Med* 17:25–29, 1988.
46. Black PM, Tzouras A, Foley L: Cerebrospinal fluid dynamics and hydrocephalus after experimental subarachnoid hemorrhage, *Neurosurgery* 17:57–62, 1985.
47. Black S, Cucchiarra RF, Nishimura RA, et al: Parameters affecting the occurrence of paradoxical air embolism, *Anesthesiology* 71:235–241, 1989.
48. Black S, Muzzi DA, Nishimura RA, et al: Preoperative and intraoperative echocardiography to detect right-to-left shunt in patients undergoing neurosurgical procedures in the sitting position, *Anesthesiology* 72:436–438, 1990.
49. Black S, Ockert DB, Oliver WC, et al: Outcome following posterior fossa craniectomy in patients in the sitting or horizontal positions, *Anesthesiology* 69:49–56, 1988.
50. Bloor BC: General pharmacology of a_2-adrenoceptors, *Anaesth Pharmacol Rev* 1:221–232, 1993.
51. Boarini DJ, Kassell NF, Coester HC, et al: Comparison of systemic and cerebrovascular effects of isoflurane and halothane, *Neurosurgery* 15:400–409, 1984.
52. Bolognese P, Miller JI, Heger IM, et al: Laser-Doppler flowmetry in neurosurgery, *J Neurosurg Anesthesiol* 5:151–158, 1993.
53. Brazy JE: Effects of crying on cerebral blood volume and cytochrome aa3, *J Pediatr* 112:457–461, 1988.
54. Bryson HM, Fulton BR, Faulds D: Propofol, *Drugs* 50:513–559, 1995.
55. Bunegin L, Albin MS, Helsel PE, et al: Positioning the right atrial catheter, *Anesthesiology* 55:343–348, 1981.
56. Burrows FA, Bissonnette B: Cerebral blood flow velocity patterns during cardiac surgery utilizing profound hypothermia with low-flow cardiopulmonary bypass or

circulatory arrest in neonates and infants [see comments], *Can J Anaesth* 40: 298–307, 1993.
57. Busija DW: Sympathetic nerves reduce cerebral blood flow during hypoxia in awake rabbits, *Am J Physiol* 247:H446–H451, 1984.
58. Camm AJ, Garratt CJ: Adenosine and supraventricular tachycardia, *New Engl J Med* 325:1621, 1991.
59. Carl P, Hogskilde S, Lang-Jensen T, et al: Pharmacokinetics and pharmacodynamics of eltanolone (pregnanolone), a new steroid intravenous anesthetic, in humans, *Acta Anaesthesiol Scand* 38:734–741, 1994.
60. Carlsson C, Smith DS, Keykhah MM, et al: The effects of high dose fentanyl on cerebral circulation and metabolism in rats, *Anesthesiology* 57:375–380, 1982.
61. Chan R, Leniger-Follert E: Effect of isovolemic hemodilution on oxygen supply and electrocorticogram in cat brain during focal ischemia and in normal tissue, *Int J Microcirc* 2:297–313, 1983.
62. Chiolero RL, Ravussin P, Anderes JP, et al: The effects of midazolam reversal by RO 15-1788 on cerebral perfusion pressure in patients with severe head injury, *Inten Care Med* 14:196–200, 1988.
63. Cloyd JC, Snyder BD, Cleeremans B, et al: Mannitol pharmacokinetics and serum osmolality in dogs and humans, *J Pharmacol Exp Ther* 236:301–306, 1986.
64. Cold GE, Christensen KJ, Norddentoft J, et al: Cerebral blood flow, cerebral metabolic rate of oxygen and relative CO_2 reactivity during neurolept anaesthesia in patients subjected to craniotomy for supratentorial cerebral tumors, *Acta Anaesthesiol Scand* 32:310–315, 1988.
65. Colley PS, Artru AA: Bunegin-Albin catheter improves air retrieval and resuscitation from lethal venous air embolism in dogs, *Anesth Analg* 66:991–994, 1987.
66. Colley PS, Sivarajan M: Regional blood flow in dogs during halothane anesthesia and controlled hypotension produced by nitroprusside or nitroglycerin, *Anesth Analg* 63:503–510, 1984.
67. Conzen PF, Vollmar B, Kabazettl H, et al: Systemic and regional hemodynamics of isoflurane and sevoflurane in rats, *Anesth Analg* 74:79–88, 1992.
68. Cook DA: Mechanisms of cerebral vasospasm in subarachnoid haemorrhage, *Pharmacol Ther* 66:259–284, 1995.
69. Cook DJ, Anderson RE, Michenfelder JD, et al: Cerebral blood flow during cardiac operations: comparison of Kety-Schmidt and xenon-133 clearance methods [see comments]. *Ann Thorac Surg* 59:614–620, 1995.
70. Cooper KR, Boswell PA, Choi SC: Safe use of PEEP in patients with severe head injury, *J Neurosurg* 63:552–555, 1985.
71. Cosentino F, Katusic ZS: Does endothelin-1 play a role in the pathogenesis of cerebral vasospasm? *Stroke* 25:904–908, 1994.
72. Cote CJ, Greenhow DE, Marshall BE: The hypotensive response to rapid intravenous administration of hypertonic solutions in man and in the rabbit, *Anesthesiology* 50:30–35, 1979.
73. Cottrell JE, Gupta B, Rappoport H, et al: Intracranial pressure during nitroglycerin-induced hypotension, *J Neurosurg* 53: 309–311, 1980.
74. Cottrell JE, Patel K, Turndorf H, et al: Intracranial pressure changes induced by sodium nitroprusside in patients with intracranial mass lesions, *J Neurosurg* 48: 329–331, 1978.
75. Cottrell JE, Robustelli A, Post K, et al: Furosemide- and mannitol-induced changes in intracranial pressure and serum osmolality and electrolytes, *Anesthesiology* 47:28–30, 1977.
76. Cottrell JE, Smith DS: *Anesthesia and neurosurgery,* ed 3, St. Louis, 1994, Mosby–Year Book.
77. Crosby ET, Lui A: The adult cervical spine: implications for airway management, *Can J Anaesth* 37:77–93, 1990.
78. Crumrine RS, Nulsen FE, Weiss MH: Alterations in ventricular fluid pressure during ketamine anesthesia in hydrocephalic children, *Anesthesiology* 42:758–761, 1975.
79. Cucchiara RF, Michenfelder JD: *Clinical neuroanesthesia,* New York, 1990, Churchill-Livingstone.
80. Cucchiara RF, Nishimura RA, Black S: Failure of preoperative echo testing to prevent paradoxical air embolism: Report of two cases, *Anesthesiology* 71:604–607, 1989.
81. Cucchiara RF, Nugent M, Seward JB, et al: Air embolism in upright neurosurgical patients: detection and localization by two-dimensional transesophageal echocardiography, *Anesthesiology* 60:353–355, 1984.
82. Cucchiara RF, Seward JB, Nishimura RA, et al: Identification of patient foramen ovale during sitting position craniotomy by transesophageal echocardiography with positive airway pressure, *Anesthesiology* 63:107–109, 1985.
83. Cully MD, Larson CP, Silverberg GD: Hetastarch coagulopathy in a neurosurgical patient, *Anesthesiology* 66:706–707, 1987.
84. Cunitz G, Danhauser I, Wickbold J: Comparative investigations on the influence of etomidate, thiopentone and methohexitone on the intracranial pressure of the patient, *Anaesthesia* 27:64–70, 1978.
85. D'Alecy LG, Rose CJ, Sellers SA: Sympathetic modulation of hypercapnic cerebral vasodilation in dogs, *Circ Res* 45:771–785, 1979.
86. Dahl A, Russell D, Nyberg-Hansen R, et al: Effect of nitroglycerin on cerebral circulation measured by transcranial doppler and SPECT, *Stroke* 20:1733–1736, 1989.
87. Dam M, Ori C, Pizzolato G, et al: The effects of propofol anesthesia on local cerebral glucose utilization in the rat, *Anesthesiology* 73:499–505, 1990.
88. Damon L, Adams M, Stricker RB, et al: Intracranial bleeding during treatment with hydroxyethyl starch (letter), *New Engl J Med* 317:964–965, 1987.
89. Davies KR, Gelb A, Manninen PH, et al: A comparison of electrocardiographic and echocardiographic abnormalities in subarachnoid hemorrhage, *Can J Anaesth* 37:S25, 1990.
90. Davis TP, Alexander J, Lesch M: Electrocardiographic changes associated with acute cerebrovascular disease: a clinical review, *Prog Cardiovasc Dis* 36:245–260, 1993.
91. Day AL, Friedman WA, Sypert GW, et al: Successful treatment of the normal perfusion pressure breakthrough syndrome, *Neurosurgery* 11:625–630, 1982.
92. Dearden NM, McDowall DG: Comparison of etomidate and althesin in the reduction of increased intracranial pressure after head injury, *Br J Anaesth* 57:361–368, 1985.
93. Deem S, Shapiro HM, Marshall LF: Quadraplegia in a patient with cervical spondylosis after thoracolumbar surgery in the prone position, *Anesthesiology* 75: 527–528, 1991.
94. Deutsch G, Samra SK: Effects of nitrous oxide on global and regional cortical blood flow, *Stroke* 21:1293–1298, 1990.
95. Dexter F, Hindman BJ: Theoretical analysis of cerebral venous blood hemoglobin oxygen saturation as an index of cerebral oxygenation during hypothermic cardiopulmonary bypass. A counterproposal to the "luxury perfusion" hypothesis, *Anesthesiology* 83:406–412, 1995.
96. DiPasquale G, Pinelli G, Andreoli A, et al: Holter detection of cardiac arrhythmias in intracranial subarachnoid hemorrhage, *Am J Cardiol* 59:596–600, 1987.
97. Domino KB, Hemstad JR, Lam AM, et al: Effect of nitrous oxide in intracranial pressure after cranial-dural closure in patients undergoing craniotomy, *Anesthesiology* 77:421–425, 1992.
98. Dorsch NW: Cerebral arterial spasm—a clinical review, *Br J Neurosurgery* 9: 403–412, 1995.
99. Doze VA, Chen BX, Maze M: Dexmedetomidine produces a hypnotic-anesthetic action in rats via activation of central alpha-2 adrenoceptors, *Anesthesiology* 71: 75–79, 1989.
100. Drake CG: Report of World Federation of Neurological Surgeons Committee on a universal subarachnoid hemorrhage grading scale, *J Neurosurg* 68:985–986, 1988.
101. Drummond JC, Cole DJ, Patel PM, et al: Focal cerebral ischemia during anesthesia with etomidate, isoflurane, or thiopental: a comparison of the extent of cerebral injury, *Neurosurgery* 37:742–748, 1995.
102. Drummond JC, Prutow RJ, Scheller MS: A comparison of the sensitivity of pulmonary artery pressure, end-tidal carbon dioxide, and end-tidal nitrogen in the detection of venous air embolism in the dog, *Anesth Analg* 64:688–692, 1985.
103. Drummond JC, Scheller MS, Todd MM: The effect of nitrous oxide on cortical CBF during anesthesia with halothane and isoflurane, with and without morphine, in the New Zealand White rabbit, *Anesth Analg* 66:1083–1089, 1987.
104. Drummond JC, Todd MM: The response of the feline cerebral circulation to Pa_{CO_2} during anesthesia with isoflurane and halothane and during sedation with nitrous oxide, *Anesthesiology* 62:268–273, 1985.
105. Drummond JC, Todd MM, Scheller MS, et al: A comparison of the direct cerebral vasodilating potencies of halothane and

isoflurane in the New Zealand White rabbit, *Anesthesiology* 65:462–467, 1986.

106. Duncan R: Epilepsy, cerebral blood flow, and cerebral metabolic rate, *Cerebrovasc Brain Metab Rev* 4:105–121, 1992.
107. Durward QJ, Amacher L, Maestro RF, et al: Cerebral and cardiovascular responses to changes in head elevation in patients with intracranial hypertension, *J Neurosurg* 59:938–944, 1983.
108. Ebrahim ZY, DeBoer GE, Luders H, et al: Effect of etomidate on the electroencephalogram of patients with epilepsy, *Anesth Analg* 65:1004–1006, 1986.
109. Ebrahim ZY, Schubert A, Vanness P, et al: The effect of propofol on the electroencephalogram of patients with epilepsy, *Anesth Analg* 78:275–279, 1994.
110. Edvinsson L: Sympathetic control of cerebral circulation, *TINS* 0:425–429, 1982.
111. Eintrei C, Leszniewski W, Carlsson C: Local application of (133)Xenon for measurement of regional cerebral blood flow (rCBF) during halothane, enflurane and isoflurane anesthesia in humans, *Anesthesiology* 63:391–394, 1985.
112. Ellis SC, Bryan-Brown CW, Hyderally H: Massive swelling of the head and neck, *Anesthesiology* 42:102–103, 1975.
113. Elwell CE, Cope M, Edwards AD, et al: Quantification of adult cerebral hemodynamics by near-infrared spectroscopy, *J Appl Physiol* 77:2753–2760, 1994.
114. Eng C, Lam AM, Mayberg TS, et al: The influence of propofol with and without nitrous oxide on cerebral blood flow velocity and CO2 reactivity in humans, *Anesthesiology* 77:872–879, 1992.
115. English JB, Westenskow D, Hodges MR, et al: Comparison of venous air embolism monitoring methods in supine dogs, *Anesthesiology* 48:425–429, 1978.
116. Eriksson S, Hagenfeldt L, Law D, et al: Effect of prostaglandin synthesis inhibitors on basal and carbon dioxide stimulated cerebral blood flow in man, *Acta Physiol Scand* 117:203–211, 1983.
117. Estilo AE, Cottrell JE: Naloxone, hypertension, and ruptured cerebral aneurysm, *Anesthesiology* 54:352, 1981.
118. Fanconi S, Duc G: Intratracheal suctioning in sick preterm infants: prevention of intracranial hypertension and cerebral hypoperfusion by muscle paralysis, *Pediatrics* 79:538–543, 1987.
119. Faraci FM, Brian JE: Nitric oxide and the cerebral circulation, *Stroke* 25:692–703, 1994.
120. Faraci FM, Heistad DD: Regulation of cerebral blood vessels by humoral and endothelium-dependent mechanisms. Update on humoral regulation of vascular tone, *Hypertension* 17:917–922, 1991.
121. Farrar JK, Gamache FW, Ferguson G, et al: Effects of profound hypotension on cerebral blood flow during surgery for intracranial aneurysms, *J Neurosurg* 55:857–864, 1981.
122. Fenstermacher JD: Volume regulation of the central nervous system. In Staub NC, Taylor AE, editors: *Edema,* New York, 1984, Raven Press, pp 383–404.
123. Fisher B, Thomas D, Peterson B: Hypertonic saline lowers raised intracranial pressure in children after head trauma, *J Neurosurg Anesth* 4:4–10, 1992.
124. Fleischer JE, Milde JH, Moyer TP, et al: Cerebral effects of high-dose midazolam and subsequent reversal with Ro 15-1788 in dogs, *Anesthesiology* 68:234–242, 1988.
125. Forster A, Juge O, Louis M, et al: Effects of a specific benzodiazepine antagonist (RO 15-1788) on cerebral blood flow, *Anesth Analg* 66:309–313, 1987.
126. Forster A, Juge O, Morel DK: Effects of midazolam on cerebral blood flow in human volunteers, *Anesthesiology* 56: 453–455, 1982.
127. Fortune JB, Feurstel PJ, Weigle CGM, et al: Continuous measurement of jugular venous oxygen saturation in response to transient elevations of blood pressure in head-injured patients, *J Neurosurg* 80:461–468, 1994.
128. Fox PT, Raichle ME, Mintun MA, et al: Nonoxidative glucose consumption during focal physiologic neural activity, *Science* 241:462–464, 1988.
129. Frank SM, Beattie C, Christopherson R, et al: Unintentional hypothermia is associated with postoperative myocardial ischemia, *Anesthesiology* 78:468–476, 1993.
130. Friedman WA, Chadwick GM, Verhoeven FJS, et al: Monitoring of somatosensory evoked potentials during surgery of middle cerebral artery aneurysms, *Neurosurgery* 29:83–88, 1991.
131. Friesen RH, Honda AT, Thieme RE: Changes in anterior fontanel pressure in preterm neonates during tracheal intubation, *Anesth Analg* 66:874–878, 1987.
132. Friesen RH, Thieme RE, Honda AT, et al: Changes in anterior fontanel pressure in preterm neonates receiving isoflurane, halothane, fentanyl, or ketamine, *Anesth Analg* 66:431–434, 1987.
133. From RP, Warner DS, Todd MM, et al: Anesthesia for craniotomy: a double-blind comparison of alfentanil, fentanyl, and sufentanil, *Anesthesiology* 73:896–904, 1990.
134. Frost JJ: Receptor imaging by positron emission tomography and single-photon emission computed tomography, *Invest Radiol* 27:S54–S58, 1992.
135. Fukuda O, Endo S, Kuwayama N, et al: The characteristics of Laser-Doppler flowmetry for the measurement of regional cerebral blood flow, *Neurosurgery* 36: 358–364, 1995.
136. Furuya H, Suzuki T, Okumura F, et al: Detection of air embolism by transesophageal echocardiography, *Anesthesiology* 58:124–129, 1983.
137. Gaab MR, Czech T, Korn A: Intracranial effects of nicardipine, *Br J Clin Pharmacol* (suppl 1)20:67S–74S, 1985.
138. Gaab MR, Haubitz I, Brawanski A, et al: Acute effects of nimodipine on the cerebral blood flow and intracranial pressure, *Neurochirurgia* (*Stuttg*) 281:93–99, 1985.
139. Ghani GA, Sung YF, Winstein MS, et al: Effects of intravenous nitroglycerin on the intracranial pressure and volume pressure response, *J Neurosurg* 58:562–565, 1983.
140. Giannotta SL, Oppenheimer JH, Levy ML, et al: Management of intraoperative rupture of aneurysm without hypotension, *Neurosurgery* 28:531–536, 1991.
141. Giffin JP, Cottrell JE, Shwiry B, et al: Intracranial pressure, mean arterial pressure, and heart rate following midazolam or thiopental in humans with brain tumors, *Anesthesiology* 60:491–494, 1984.
142. Gildenberg PL, O'Brien RP, Britt WJ, et al: The efficacy of precordial doppler monitoring for the detection of venous air embolism, *J Neurosurg* 54:75–78, 1981.
143. Glass PSA, Hardman D, Kamiyama Y, et al: Preliminary pharmacokinetics and pharmacodynamics of an ultra-short-acting opioid—remifentanil (GI87084B), *Anesth Analg* 77:1031–1040, 1993.
144. Glenski JA, Cucchiara RF, Michenfelder JD: Transesophageal echocardiography and trancustaneous O_2 and CO_2 monitoring of neurosurgical patients: detection of air embolism, *Anesthesiology* 64:546–550, 1986.
145. Greenberg JH, Alavi A, Reivich M, et al: Local cerebral blood volume response to carbon dioxide in man, *Circ Res* 43: 324–331, 1978.
146. Grosslight K, Foster R, Colohan AR, et al: Isoflurane for neuroanesthesia: risk factors for increases in intracranial pressure, *Anesthesiology* 63:533–536, 1985.
147. Grubb RL, Raichle ME, Eichling JO, et al: The effects of change in $Paco_2$ on cerebral blood volume, blood flow, and vascular mean transit time, *Stroke* 5:630–639, 1974.
148. Gur D, Yonas H, Good WF: Local cerebral blood flow by xenon-enhanced CT: current status, potential improvements, and future directions, *Cerebrovasc Brain Metab Rev* 1:68–86, 1989.
149. Gyulai F, Firestone L, Mintun M, et al: Loci of N2O analgesia in the human brain. A PET study, *Anesthesiology* 83:A163, 1995.
150. Haberl RL, Heizer ML, Marmarou A, et al: Laser-Doppler assessment of brain microcirculation: effect of systemic alterations, *Am J Physiol* 256:H1247–H1254, 1989.
151. Haberl RL, Villringer A, Dirnagl U: Applicability of laser-Doppler flowmetry for cerebral blood flow monitoring in neurological intensive care, *Acta Neurochirurgica* (Suppl)59:64–68, 1993.
152. Haigh JD, Nemoto EM, DeWolf AM, et al: Comparison of the effects of succinylcholine and atracurium on intracranial pressure in monkeys with intracranial hypertension, *Can Anaesth Soc J* 33:421–426, 1986.
153. Haley EC, Kassell NF, Torner JC, et al: A randomized trial of two doses of nicardipine in aneurysmal subarachnoid hemorrhage—a report of the Cooperative Aneurysm Study, *J Neurosurg* 80:788–796, 1994.
154. Hall ED: Neuroprotective actions of glucocorticoid and nonglucocorticoid steroids in acute neuronal injury, *Cell Molec Neurobiol* 13:415–432, 1993.
155. Hall ED, Yonkers PA, Andrus PK, et al: Biochemistry and pharmacology of lipid antioxidants in acute brain and spinal cord injury, *J Neurotrauma* 9:S425–S442, 1992.
156. Hamar J, Arisztid GB, Kovach AGB, et al: Effect of phenoxybenzamine on cerebral

blood flow and metabolism in the baboon during hemorrhagic shock, *Stroke* 10: 401–407, 1979.
157. Hamill JF, Bedford RF, Weaver DC, et al: Lidocaine before endotracheal intubation: intravenous or laryngotracheal? *Anesthesiology* 55:578–581, 1981.
158. Hansen TD, Warner DS, Todd MM, et al: Distribution of cerebral blood flow during halothane versus isoflurane anesthesia in rats, *Anesthesiology* 69:332–337, 1988.
159. Hansen TD, Warner DS, Todd MM, et al: The role of cerebral metabolism in determining the local cerebral blood flow effects of volatile anesthetics: evidence for persistent flow-metabolism coupling, *J Cereb Blood Flow Metab* 9:323–328, 1989.
160. Hansen TD, Warner DS, Todd MM, et al: Relative cerebral blood flow effects of nitrous oxide and volatile anesthetics, *Br J Anaesth* 63:290–295, 1989.
161. Hartman GS, Fiamengo SA, Riker WF: Succinylcholine: mechanism of fasciculations and their prevention by d-turbocurarine or diphenylhydantoin, *Anesthesiology* 65:405–413, 1986.
162. Hastings RH, Marks JD: Airway management for trauma patients with potential cervical spine injuries, *Anesth Analg* 73: 471–482, 1991.
163. Hastings RH, Vigil AC, Hanna R, et al: Cervical spine movement during laryngoscopy with the Bullard, Macintosh, and Miller laryngoscopes, *Anesthesiology* 82:859–869, 1995.
164. Hatano Y, Nakamura K, Moriyama S, et al: The contractile responses of isolated dog cerebral and extracerebral arteries to oxybarbiturates and thiobarbiturates, *Anesthesiology* 71:80–86, 1989.
165. Heinemeyer G: Clinical pharmacokinetic considerations in the treatment of increased intracranial pressure, *Clin Pharmacokinet* 13:1–25, 1987.
166. Henriksen HT, Jorgensen PB: The effect of nitrous oxide on intracranial pressure in patients with intracranial disorders, *Br J Anaesth* 45:486–492, 1973.
167. Henriksen L, Paulson OB, Lauritzen M: The effects of sodium nitroprusside on cerebral blood flow and cerebral venous blood gases. I. Observations in awake man during and following moderate blood pressure reduction, *Eur J Clin Invest* 12: 383–387, 1982.
168. Herregods L, Mergaert C, Rolly G, et al: Comparison of the effects of the 24-hour propofol or fentanyl infusions on intracranial pressure, *J Drug Dev* 2:99–100, 1989.
169. Heymann MA, Payne BD, Hoffman JIE, et al: Blood flow measurements with radionuclide-labeled particles, *Prog Cardiovasc Dis* 20:55–79, 1977.
170. Hoffman J, Konopka K, Buckhorn C, et al: Ethanol-inducible cytochrome P450 in rabbits metabolizes enflurane, *Br J Anaesth* 63:103–108, 1989.
171. Hoffman JM, Hanson MW, Coleman RE: Clinical positron emission tomography imaging, *Radiol Clin North Am* 31: 935–959, 1993.
172. Hoffman WE, Cunningham F, James MK, et al: Effects of remifentanil, a new short-acting opioid, on cerebral blood flow, brain electrical activity, and intracranial pressure in dogs anesthetized with isoflurane and nitrous oxide, *Anesthesiology* 79:107–113, 1993.
173. Hongo K, Kobayashi S: Calcium antagonists for the treatment of vasospasm following subarachnoid haemorrhage, *Neurological Research* 15:218–224, 1993.
174. Hormann C, Mohsenipour I, Gottardis M, et al: Response of cerebrospinal fluid pressure to continuous positive airway pressure in volunteers, *Anesth Analg* 78:54–57, 1994.
175. Hougarrd K, Hansen A, Brodersen P: The effect of ketamine on regional cerebral blood flow in man, *Anesthesiology* 41: 562–567, 1974.
176. Hunt WE, Hess RM: Surgical risk as related to time of intervention in the repair of intracranial aneurysms, *J Neurosurg* 28: 14–20, 1968.
177. Iadecola C, Pelligrino DA, Moskowitz MA, et al: Nitric oxide synthase inhibition and cerebrovascular regulation, *J Cereb Blood Flow Metab* 14:175–192, 1994.
178. Jennett B, Teasdale G: *Management of head injuries,* Philadelphia, 1981, FA Davis.
179. Jennett WB, Barker J, Fitch W, et al: Effect of anesthesia on intracranial pressure in patients with space-occupying lesions, *Lancet* 1:61–64, 1969.
180. Jobes DR, Kennell EM, Bush GL, et al: Cerebral blood flow and metabolism during morphine-nitrous oxide anesthesia in man, *Anesthesiology* 47:16–18, 1977.
181. Jones TH, Chiappa KH, Young RR, et al: EEG monitoring for induced hypotension for surgery of intracranial aneurysms, *Stroke* 10:292–294, 1979.
182. Kaieda R, Todd MM, Warner DS: The effects of anesthetics and PaCO2 on the cerebrovascular metabolic, and electroencephalographic responses to nitrous oxide in the rabbit, *Anesth Analg* 68:135–143, 1989.
183. Kalfas IH, Little JR: Postoperative hemorrhage: a survey of 4992 intracranial procedures, *Neurosurgery* 23:343–347, 1988.
184. Karlsson BR, Forsman M, Roald OK, et al: Effect of dexmedetomidine, a selective and potent a2-agonist, on cerebral blood flow and oxygen consumption during halothane anesthesia in dogs, *Anesth Analg* 71: 125–129, 1990.
185. Kassell NF, Drake CG: Timing of aneurysm surgery, *Neurosurgery* 10:514–519, 1982.
186. Kassell NF, Haley EC, Apperson-Hansen C, et al: Randomized, double-blind, vehicle controlled trial of tirilazad mesylate in patients with aneurysmal subarachnoid hemorrhage: a cooperative study in Europe, Australia, and New Zealand, *J Neurosurg* 84:221–228, 1996.
187. Kassell NF, Hitchon PW, Gerk MK, et al: Alterations in cerebral blood flow, oxygen metabolism, and electrical activity produced by high dose sodium thiopental, *Neurosurgery* 7:598–603, 1979.
188. Kassell NF, Peerless SJ, Durward QJ, et al: Treatment of ischemic deficits from vasospasm with intravascular volume expansion and induced arterial hypertension, *Neurosurgery* 11:337–343, 1982.
189. Kassell NF, Torner JC: Aneurysmal rebleeding: a preliminary report from the Cooperative Aneurysm Study, *Neurosurgery* 13:479–481, 1983.
190. Kassell NF, Torner JC, Haley EC, et al: The International Cooperative Study on the timing of aneurysm surgery. Part 1: Overall management results, *J Neurosurg* 73: 18–36, 1990.
191. Kassell NF, Torner JC, Jane JA, et al: The International Cooperative Study on the timing of aneurysm surgery, Part 2: Surgical results, *J Neurosurg* 73:37–47, 1990.
192. Kawamura Y, Meyer JS, Hiromoto H, et al: Neurogenic control of cerebral blood flow in the baboon. Effects of alpha adrenergic blockade with phenoxybenzamine on cerebral autoregulation and vasomotor reactivity to changes in $PaCO_2$, *Stroke* 5:747–758, 1974.
193. Kearse LA, Koski G, Husain MV, et al: Epileptiform activity during opioid anesthesia. *Electroencephalogr Clin Neuro* 87:374–379, 1993.
194. Kety S, Schmidt CF: The determination of cerebral blood flow in man by the use of nitrous oxide in low concentrations, *Am J Physiol* 143:53–65, 1945.
195. Keykhah MM, Smith DS, Carlsson C, et al: Influence of sufentanil on cerebral metabolism and circulation in the rat, *Anesthesiology* 63:274–277, 1985.
196. Kim CS, Arnold FJ, Itani MS, et al: Decreased sensitivity to metocurine during long-term phenytoin therapy may be attributable to protein binding and acetylcholine receptor changes, *Anesthesiology* 77:500–506, 1992.
197. Kitaguchi K, Ohsumi H, Kuro M, et al: Effects of sevoflurane on cerebral circulation and metabolism in patients with ischemic cerebrovascular disease, *Anesthesiology* 79:704–709, 1993.
198. Knot HJ, Nelson MT: Regulation of membrane potential and diameter by voltage dependent K^+ channels in rabbit myogenic cerebral arteries, *Am J Physiol* 269: H348–H355, 1995.
199. Knudsen L, Cold GE, Holdgard HO, et al: Effects of flumazenil on cerebral blood flow and oxygen consumption after midazolam anaesthesia for craniotomy, *Br J Anaesth* 67:277–280, 1991.
200. Kobayashi Y, Ochiai R, Takeda J, et al: Serum and urinary inorganic fluoride concentrations after prolonged inhalation of sevoflurane in humans, *Anesth Analg* 74:753–757, 1992.
201. Koenig HM, Pelligrino DA, Albrecht RF: Halothane vasodilation and nitric oxide in rat pial vessels, *J Neurosurg Anesthesiol* 5:264–271, 1993.
202. Koenig HM, Pelligrino DA, Wang Q, et al: Role of nitric oxide and endothelium in rat pial vessel dilation response to isoflurane, *Anesth Analg* 79:886–891, 1994.
203. Kofke WA, Garman RH, Tom WC, et al: Alfentanil-induced hypermetabolism, seizure, and histopathology in rat brain, *Anesth Analg* 75:953–964, 1992.
204. Kosteljanetz M: Acute head injury: pressure-volume relations and cerebrospinal fluid dynamics, *Neurosurgery* 18:17–24, 1986.

205. Kovarik WD, Mayberg TS, Lam AM, et al: Succinylcholine does not change intracranial pressure, cerebral blood flow velocity, or the electroencephalogram in patients with neurologic injury, *Anesth Analg* 78:469–473, 1994.
206. Kuramoto T, Oshita S, Takeshita H, et al: Modification of the relationship between cerebral metabolism, blood flow and the EEG by stimulation during anesthesia in the dog, *Anesthesiology* 51:211–217, 1979.
207. Kurth CD, Steven JM, Nicolson SC: Cerebral oxygenation during pediatric cardiac surgery using deep hypothermic circulatory arrest, *Anesthesiology* 82:74–82, 1995.
208. Kuschinsky W: Coupling between functional activity, metabolism and blood flow in the brain: State of the art, *Microcirc* 2:357–378, 1982.
209. Lam AM, Mayberg TS, Eng CC, et al: Nitrous oxide-isoflurane anesthesia causes more cerebral vasodilation than an equipotent dose of isoflurane in humans, *Anesth Analg* 78:462–468, 1994.
210. Lanier W, Iaizzo P, Milde J: Cerebral function and muscle afferent activity following intravenous succinylcholine in dogs anesthetized with halothane: the effects of pretreatment with a defasciculating dose of pancuronium, *Anesthesiology* 71:87–95, 1989.
211. Lanier WL, Milde JH, Michenfelder JD: Cerebral stimulation following succinylcholine in dogs, *Anesthesiology* 64: 551–559, 1986.
212. Lanzino G, Kongable GL, Kassell NF: Electrocardiographic abnormalities after nontraumatic subarachnoid hemorrhage, *J Neurosurg Anesthesiol* 6:156–162, 1994.
213. Larsen R, Teichmann J, Hilfiker O, et al: Nitroprusside-hypotension: cerebral blood flow and cerebral oxygen consumption in neurosurgical patients, *Acta Anaesthesiol Scand* 26:327–330, 1982.
214. Lauritzen M: Long-lasting reduction of cortical blood flow of the rat brain after spreading depression with preserved autoregulation and impaired CO_2 response, *J Cereb Blood Flow Metab* 4:546–554, 1984.
215. Lebrun-Gandie P, Baron J, Soussaline F, et al: Coupling between regional blood flow and oxygen utilization in the normal human brain, *Arch Neurol* 40:230–236, 1983.
216. Levy ML, Aranda M, Zelman V, et al: Propylene glycol toxicity following continuous etomidate infusion for the control of refractory cerebral edema, *Neurosurgery* 37:363–371, 1995.
217. Lewelt W, Jenkins LW, Miller JD: Effects of experimental fluid-percussion injury of the brain on cerebrovascular reactivity to hypoxia and to hypercapnia, *J Neurosurg* 56:332–338, 1982.
218. Lischke V, Busse R, Hecker M: Selective inhibition by barbiturates of the synthesis of endothelium-derived hyperpolarizing factor in the rabbit carotid artery, *Brit J Pharmacol* 115:969–974, 1995.
219. Lodrini S, Montolivo M, Pluchino F, et al: Positive end-expiratory pressure in supine and sitting positions: Its effects on intrathoracic and intracranial pressure, *Neurosurgery* 24:873–877, 1989.
220. Losasso TJ, Muzzi DA, Dietz NM, et al: Fifty percent nitrous oxide does not increase the risk of venous air embolism in neurosurgical patients operated upon in the sitting position, *Anesthesiology* 77:21–30, 1992.
221. Lou HC, Edvinsson L, MacKenzie ET: The concept of coupling blood flow to brain function: revision required? *Ann Neurol* 22:289–297, 1987.
222. Luce JM, Huseby JS, Kirk W, et al: Mechanism by which positive end-expiratory pressure increases cerebrospinal fluid pressure in dogs, *J Appl Physiol* 52: 231–235, 1982.
223. Lutz LJ, Milde JH, Milde LN: The cerebrospinal functional, metabolic, and hemodynamic effects of desflurane in dogs, *Anesthesiology* 73:125–131, 1990.
224. Lynch JJ, Schuhard GH, Gross CM, et al: Prevalence of right-to-left atrial shunting in a healthy population: detection by valsalva maneuver contrast echocardiography, *Am J Cardiol* 53:1478–1480, 1984.
225. Madden JA: The effect of carbon dioxide on cerebral arteries, *Pharmac Ther* 59: 229–250, 1993.
226. Madsen JB, Cold GE, Eriksen HO, et al: CBF and $CMRo_2$ during craniotomy for small supratentorial cerebral tumours in enflurane anaesthesia: A dose response study, *Acta Anaesthesiol Scand* 30: 633–636, 1986.
227. Madsen JB, Cold GE, Hansen ES, et al: The effect of isoflurane on cerebral blood flow and metabolism in humans during craniotomy for small supratentorial cerebral tumors, *Anesthesiology* 66:323–336, 1987.
228. Madsen JB, Cold GE, Hansen ES, et al: Cerebral blood flow and metabolism during isoflurane induced hypotension in patients subjected to surgery for cerebral aneurysms, *Br J Anaesth* 59:1204–1207, 1987.
229. Madsen PL, Vorstrup S: Cerebral blood flow and metabolism during sleep, *Cerebrovasc Brain Metab Rev* 3:281–296, 1991.
230. Maekawa T, Tommasino C, Shapiro HM, et al: Local cerebral blood flow and glucose utilization during isoflurane anesthesia in the rat, *Anesthesiology* 65:144–151, 1986.
231. Magnaes B: Clinical recording of pressure on the spinal cord and cauda equina. Part 3: Pressure on the cervical spinal cord during endotracheal intubation in patients with cervical spondylosis, *J Neurosurg* 57: 64–66, 1982.
232. Maktabi MA, Elbokl FF, Faraci FM, et al: Halothane decreases the rate of production of cerebrospinal fluid—possible role of vasopressin v1 receptors, *Anesthesiology* 78: 72–82, 1993.
233. Manninen PH, Cuillerier DJ, Nantau WE, et al: Monitoring of brainstem function during vertebral basilar aneurysm surgery—the use of spontaneous ventilation, *Anesthesiology* 77:681–685, 1992.
234. Manninen PH, Lam AM, Nantau WE: Monitoring of somatosensory evoked potentials during temporary arterial occlusion in cerebral aneurysm surgery, *J Neurosurg Anesth* 2:97–104, 1990.
235. Manohar M: Regional brain blood flow and cerebral cortical O_2 consumption during sevoflurane anesthesia in healthy isocapnic swine, *J Cardiovasc Pharmacol* 8:1268–1275, 1986.
236. Marcus ML, Busija DW, Bischof CJ, et al: Methods for measurement of cerebral blood flow, *Fed Proc* 40:2306–2310, 1981.
237. Marin J, Lobato RD, Rico ML, et al: Effect of pentobarbital on the reactivity of isolated human cerebral arteries, *J Neurosurg* 54:521–524, 1981.
238. Marion DW, Segal R, Thompson ME: Subarachnoid hemorrhage and the heart, *Neurosurgery* 18:101–106, 1986.
239. Markus H: Transcranial doppler detection of circulating cerebral emboli—a review, *Stroke* 24:1246–1250, 1993.
240. Marsh ML, Aidinis SJ, Naughton KVH, et al: The technique of nitroprusside administration modifies the intracranial pressure response, *Anesthesiology* 51:538–541, 1979.
241. Marsh ML, Dunlop BJ, Shapiro HM, et al: Succinylcholine-intracranial pressure effects in neurosurgical patients, *Anesth Analg* 59:550–551, 1980.
242. Marsh ML, Shapiro HM, Smith RW, et al: Changes in neurologic status and intracranial pressure associated with sodium nitroprusside administration, *Anesthesiology* 51:336–338, 1979.
243. Marshall LF, U HS: Treatment of massive intraoperative brain swelling, *Neurosurgery* 13:412–414, 1983.
244. Marshall WK, Bedford RF, Miller ED: Cardiovascular responses in the seated position—impact of four anesthetic techniques, *Anesth Analg* 62:648–653, 1983.
245. Martyn JA, White DA, Gronert GA, et al: Up-and-down regulation of skeletal muscle acetylcholine receptors. Effects on neuromuscular blockers, *Anesthesiology* 76: 822–843, 1992.
246. Marx W, Shah N, Long C, et al: Sufentanil, alfentanil and fentanyl: impact on cerebrospinal fluid pressure in patients with brain tumors, *J Neurosurg Anesthesiol* 1:3–7, 1989.
247. Matjasko J, Petrozza P, Cohen M, et al: Anesthesia and surgery in the seated position: analysis of 554 cases, *Neurosurgery* 17:695–702, 1985.
248. Matsumiya N, Dohi S: Effects of intravenous or subarachnoid morphine on cerebral and spinal cord hemodynamics and antagonism with naloxone in dogs, *Anesthesiology* 59:175–181, 1983.
249. Matta BF, Lam AM, Mayberg TS, et al: A critique of the intraoperative use of jugular venous bulb catheters during neurosurgical procedures, *Anesth Analg* 79:745–750, 1994.
250. Matta BF, Mayberg TS, Lam AM: Direct cerebrovasodilatory effects of halothane, isoflurane, and desflurane during propofol-induced isoelectric electroencephalogram in humans, *Anesthesiology* 83:980–985, 1995.
251. Mayberg TS, Lam AM, Matta BF, et al: Ketamine does not increase cerebral blood flow velocity or intracranial pressure during isoflurane/nitrous oxide anesthesia in

patients undergoing craniotomy, *Anesth Analg* 81:84–89, 1995.

252. Maze M, Scheinin M: Molecular pharmacology of a2-adrenergic receptors, *Anaesth Pharm Rev* 1:233–237, 1993.
253. Maze M, Tranquilli W: Alpha-2 adrenoceptor agonists: defining the role in clinical anesthesia, *Anesthesiology* 74:581–605, 1991.
254. McAllister RG: Macroglossia—a positional complication, *Anesthesiology* 40: 199–200, 1974.
255. McAlpine FS, Seckel BR: Complications of positioning. The peripheral nervous system. In Martin JT, editor: *Positioning in anesthesia and surgery,* Philadelphia, 1987, WB Saunders.
256. McManus ML, Churchwell KB, Strange K: Regulation of cell volume in health and disease, *New Engl J Med* 333:1260–1266, 1995.
257. McPherson RW, Kirsch JR, Ghaly RF, et al: Effect of nitric oxide synthase inhibition on the cerebral vascular response to hypercapnia in primates, *Stroke* 26:682–687, 1995.
258. McPherson RW, Kirsch JR, Moore LE, et al: Nw-nitro-L-arginine methyl ester prevents cerebral hyperemia by inhaled anesthetics in dogs, *Anesth Analg* 77:891–897, 1993.
259. McPherson RW, Koehler RC, Traystman RJ: Effect of jugular venous pressure on cerebral autoregulation in dogs, *Am J Physiol* 255:H1516–H1524, 1988.
260. McPherson RW, Szymanski J, Rogers MC: Somatosensory evoked potential changes in positioning-related brain stem ischemia, *Anesthesiology* 61:88–90, 1984.
261. Messeter K, Nordstrom CH, Sundbarg G, et al: Cerebral hemodynamics in patients with acute severe head trauma, *J Neurosurg* 64:231–237, 1986.
262. Michenfelder JD: The interdependency of cerebral functional and metabolic effects following massive doses of thiopental in the dog, *Anesthesiology* 41:231–236, 1974.
263. Michenfelder JD: Central venous catheters in the management of air embolism: whether as well as where, *Anesthesiology* 55:339–341, 1981.
264. Michenfelder JD: *Anesthesia and the brain: Clinical, functional, metabolic, and vascular correlates,* New York, 1988, Churchill Livingstone.
265. Michenfelder JD, Milde JH: Failure of prolonged hypocapnia, hypothermia, or hypertension to favorably alter acute stroke in primates, *Stroke* 8:87–91, 1977.
266. Michenfelder JD, Milde JH: The interaction of sodium nitroprusside, hypotension and isoflurane in determining cerebral vascular effects, *Anesthesiology* 69:870–875, 1988.
267. Michenfelder JD, Miller RH, Gronert GA: Evaluation of an ultrasonic device (precordial Doppler) for the diagnosis of venous air embolism, *Anesthesiology* 36:164–167, 1972.
268. Michenfelder JD, Sundt TM, Fode N, et al: Isoflurane when compared with enflurane and halothane decreases the frequency of cerebral ischemia during carotid end-arterectomy, *Anesthesiology* 67:336–340, 1987.
269. Michenfelder JD, Theye RA: Effects of fentanyl, droperidol, and Innovar on canine cerebral metabolism and blood flow, *Br J Anaesth* 43:630–635, 1971.
270. Michenfelder JD, Theye RA: Canine systemic and cerebral effects of hypotension induced by hemorrhage, trimethaphan, halothane, or nitroprusside, *Anesthesiology* 46:188–195, 1977.
271. Milde LN, Milde JH: The cerebral and systemic hemodynamic and metabolic effects of desflurane-induced hypotension in dogs, *Anesthesiology* 74:513–518, 1991.
272. Milde LN, Milde JH, Gallagher WJ: Effects of sufentanil on cerebral circulation and metabolism in dogs, *Anesth Analg* 70:138–146, 1990.
273. Milde LN, Milde JH, Michenfelder JD: Cerebral functional, metabolic, and hemodynamic effects of etomidate in dogs, *Anesthesiology* 63:371–377, 1985.
274. Miller JD, Smith RR: Transcranial Doppler sonography in aneurysmal subarachnoid hemorrhage, *Cerebrovasc Brain Metab Rev* 6:31–46, 1994.
275. Miller R, Tausk HC, Stark DC: Effect of Innovar, fentanyl and droperidol on the cerebrospinal fluid pressure in neurosurgical patients, *Can Anaesth Soc J* 22: 502–508, 1975.
276. Minton MD, Grosslight K, Stirt JA, et al: Increases in intracranial pressure from succinylcholine: prevention by prior nondepolarizing blockade, *Anesthesiology* 65: 165–169, 1986.
277. Mirski MAZ, Rossell LA, McPherson RW, et al: Dexmedetomidine decreases seizure threshold in a rat model of experimental generalized epilepsy, *Anesthesiology* 81: 1422–1428, 1994.
278. Misfeldt BB, Jorgensen PB, Spotoft H, et al: The effects of droperidol and fentanyl on intracranial pressure and cerebral perfusion pressure in neurosurgical patients, *Br J Anaesth* 48:963–968, 1976.
279. Mizoi K, Yoshimoto T: Permissible temporary occlusion time in aneurysm surgery as evaluated by evoked potential monitoring, *Neurosurgery* 33:434–440, 1993.
280. Monitto CL, Kurth CD: The effect of fentanyl, sufentanil, and alfentanil on cerebral arterioles in piglets, *Anesth Analg* 76:985–989, 1993.
281. Moore L, Kirsch J, Helfaer M, et al: Isoflurane induced cerebral hyperemia: role of prostanoids and nitric oxide in pigs, *J Neurosurg Anesthesiol* 4:304(abstract), 1992.
282. Moorthy SS, Hilgenberg JC: Resistance to non-depolarizing muscle relaxants in paretic upper extremities of patients with residual hemiplegia, *Anesth Analg* 59:624, 1980.
283. Morgan MK, Anderson RE, Sundt TM: The effects of hyperventilation on cerebral blood flow in the rat with an open and closed carotid-jugular fistula, *Neurosurgery* 25:606–612, 1989.
284. Morgan MK, Johnston IH, Hallinan JM, et al: Complications of surgery for arteriovenous malformations of the brain, *J Neurosurg* 78:176–182, 1993.
285. Morris PJ, Heuser D, McDowall DG, et al: Cerebral cortical extracellular fluid H^+ and K^+ activities during hypotension in cats, *Anesthesiology* 59:10–18, 1983.
286. Morris PJ, Todd MM, Philbin D: Changes in canine intracranial pressure in response to infusion of sodium nitroprusside and nitroglycerin, *Br J Anaesth* 54:991–996, 1982.
287. Moss E, Dearden NM, McDowall DG: Effects of 2% enflurane on intracranial pressure and cerebral perfusion pressure, *Br J Anaesth* 55:1083–1087, 1983.
288. Moss E, McDowall DG: ICP increases with 50% nitrous oxide in oxygen in severe head injuries during controlled ventilation, *Br J Anaesth* 51:757–760, 1979.
289. Moszynski K: Dynamic changes in cerebrospinal fluid pressure during neurosurgical operations, *Acta Neurochir* 34: 285–286, 1976.
290. Muizelaar JP, Marmarou A, Ward JD, et al: Adverse effects of prolonged hyperventilation in patients with severe head injury: a randomized clinical trial, *J Neurosurg* 75:731–739, 1991.
291. Murkin JM, Farrar JK, Tweed WA: Sufentanil anaesthesia reduces cerebral blood flow and cerebral oxygen consumption, *Can J Anaesth* 35:S131, 1988.
292. Murkin JM, Farrar JK, Tweed WA, et al: Cerebral autoregulation and flow/metabolism coupling during cardiopulmonary bypass: the influence of $Paco_2$, *Anesth Analg* 66:825–832, 1987.
293. Murkin JM, Moldenhauer CC, Hug CC, et al: Absence of seizures during induction of anesthesia with high-dose fentanyl, *Anesth Analg* 63:489–494, 1984.
294. Muzzi DA, Black S, Losasso TJ, et al: Labetalol and esmolol in the control of hypertension after intracranial surgery, *Anesth Analg* 70:68–71, 1990.
295. Muzzi DA, Losasso TJ, Dietz NM, et al: The effect of desflurane and isoflurane on cerebrospinal fluid pressure in humans with supratentorial mass lesions, *Anesthesiology* 76:720–724, 1992.
296. Nakai M, Tamaki K, Maeda M: Sympathetic and metabolic mechanisms of the cerebrovasomotor function of the caudal ventrolateral medulla in rats, *Neuroscience* 50:655–662, 1992.
297. Nehls DG, Todd MM, Spetzler RF, et al: A comparison of the cerebral protective effects of isoflurane and thiopental during temporary focal ischemia in primates, *Anesthesiology* 66:453–464, 1987.
298. Newell DW, Aaslid R: Transcranial Doppler: clinical and experimental uses, *Cerebrovasc Brain Metab Rev* 4:122–143, 1992.
299. Ngai AC, Winn HR: Modulation of cerebral arteriolar diameter by intraluminal flow and pressure, *Circ Research* 77: 823–840, 1995.
300. Nichols DA, Meyer FB, Piepgras DG, et al: Endovascular treatment of intracranial aneurysms, *Mayo Clin Proc* 69:272–285, 1994.
301. Nishikawa T, Omote K, Namiki A, et al: The effects of nicardipine on cerebrospinal fluid pressure in humans, *Anesth Analg* 65:507–510, 1986.
302. Nornes H, Grip A: Hemodynamic aspects of cerebral arteriovenous malformations, *J Neurosurg* 53:456–464, 1980.

303. Oberg PA: Laser-Doppler flowmetery, *Crit Rev Biomed Eng* 18:125–163, 1990.
304. Obrist WD, Wilkinson WE: Regional cerebral blood flow measurement in humans by xenon-133 clearance, *Cerebrovasc Brain Metab Rev* 2:283–327, 1990.
305. Ogura K, Takayasu M, Dacey RG: Differential effects of pentobarbital on intracerebral arterioles and venules of rats *in vitro. Neurosurgery* 28:537–541, 1991.
306. Ohsumi H, Kitaguchi K, Nakajima T, et al: Internal jugular bulb blood velocity as a continuous indicator of cerebral blood flow during open heart surgery, *Anesthesiology* 81:325–332, 1994.
307. Orlowski JP, Shiesley D, Vidt DG, et al: Labetalol to control blood pressure after cerebrovascular surgery, *Crit Care Med* 16:765–768, 1988.
308. Ornstein E, Matteo RS, Schwartz AE, et al: The effect of phenytoin on the magnitude and duration of neuromuscular block following atracurium or vecuronium, *Anesthesiology* 67:191–196, 1987.
309. Ornstein E, Matteo RS, Young WL, et al: Resistance to metocurine-induced neuromuscular blockade in patients receiving phenytoin, *Anesthesiology* 63:294–298, 1985.
310. Ornstein E, Young WL, Fleischer LH, et al: Desflurane and isoflurane have similar effects on cerebral blood flow in patients with intracranial mass lesions, *Anesthesiology* 79:498–502, 1993.
311. Pandit UA, Mudge BJ, Keller TS, et al: Pneumocephalus after posterior fossa exploration in the sitting position, *Anaesthesia* 37:996–1001, 1982.
312. Pappada G, Formaggio G, Regalia F, et al: Course of intracranial pressure after extirpation of posterior fossa tumours, *Acta Neurochir* (*Wien*) 70:11–19, 1984.
313. Patel PM, Mutch WAC: The cerebral pressure-flow relationship during 1.0 MAC isoflurane anesthesia in the rabbit: the effect of different vasopressors, *Anesthesiology* 72:118–124, 1990.
314. Paulson OB, Strandgaard S, Edvinsson L: Cerebral autoregulation, *Cerebrovasc Brain Metab Rev* 2:161–192, 1990.
315. Paulson OB, Waldemar G: Role of the local renin-angiotensin system in the autoregulation of the cerebral circulation, *Blood Ves* 28:231–235, 1991.
316. Pearce, WJ: Mechanisms of hypoxic cerebral vasodilation, *Pharmacol Ther* 65: 75–91, 1995.
317. Pearce WJ, Dalecy LG: Hemorrhage induced cerebral vasoconstriction in dogs, *Stroke* 11:190–197, 1980.
318. Pearl RG, Larson CP: Hemodynamic effects of positive end-expiratory pressure during continuous venous air embolism in the dog, *Anesthesiology* 64:724–729, 1986.
319. Pelligrino DA, Miletich DJ, Hoffman WE, et al: Nitrous oxide markedly increases cerebral cortical metabolic rate and blood flow in the goat, *Anesthesiology* 60: 405–412, 1984.
320. Perkins-Pearson NAK, Bedford RF: Hemodynamic consequences of PEEP in seated neurological patients-Implications for paradoxical air embolism, *Anesth Analg* 63:429–432, 1984.
321. Pfitzner J, McLean AG: Controlled neck compression in neurosurgery: studies on venous air embolism in upright sheep, *Anaesthesia* 40:624–629, 1985.
322. Phillis JW: Adenosine in the control of the cerebral circulation, *Cerebrovasc Brain Metab Rev* 1:26–54, 1989.
323. Phirman JR, Shapiro HM: Modification of nitrous oxide induced intracranial hypertension by prior induction of anesthesia, *Anesthesiology* 46:150–152, 1977.
324. Pinaud M, Lelausque JN, Chetanneau A, et al: Effects of propofol on cerebral hemodynamics and metabolism in patients with brain trauma, *Anesthesiology* 73:404–409, 1990.
325. Pinaud M, Souron R, Lelausque JN, et al: Cerebral blood flow and cerebral oxygen consumption during nitroprusside-induced hypotension to less than 50 mm Hg, *Anesthesiology* 70:255–260, 1989.
326. Pohl U: Endothelial cells as part of a vascular oxygen-sensing system: hypoxia-induced release of autacoids, *Experientia* 46:1175–1179, 1990.
327. Powers WJ, Raichle ME: Positron emission tomography and its application to the study of cerebrovascular disease in man, *Stroke* 16:361–376, 1985.
328. Prichard JW, Rosen BR: State-of-the-Art review—functional study of the brain by NMR, *J Cereb Blood Flow Metab* 14: 365–372, 1994.
329. Prough DS, Roy R, Bumgarner J, et al: Acute pulmonary edema in healthy teenagers following conservative doses of intravenous naloxone, *Anesthesiology* 60: 485–486, 1984.
330. Proust F, Hannequin D, Langlois O, et al: Causes of morbidity and mortality after ruptured aneurysm surgery in a series of 230 patients. The importance of control angiography, *Stroke* 26:1553–1557, 1995.
331. Pugsley W, Klinger L, Paschalis C, et al: The impact of microemboli during cardiopulmonary bypass on neuropsychological functioning, *Stroke* 25:1393–1399, 1994.
332. Ramani R, Todd MM, Warner DS: The influence of a cryogenic brain injury on the cerebrovascular response to isoflurane in the rabbit, *J Cereb Blood Flow Metab* 11:388–397, 1991.
333. Ramani R, Todd MM, Warner DS: A dose-response study of the influence of propofol on cerebral blood flow, metabolism and the electroencephalogram in the rabbit, *J Neurosurg Anesthesiol* 4:110–119, 1992.
334. Rao TLK, Jacobs KH, El-Etr AA: Reinfarction following anesthesia in patients with myocardial infarction, *Anesthesiology* 59:499–505, 1983.
335. Rao TLK, Mummaneni N, El Etr AA: Convulsions: an unusual response to intravenous fentanyl administrations, *Anesth Analg* 61:1020–1021, 1982.
336. Ravussin P, Abou-Madi M, Archer D, et al: Changes in CSF pressure after mannitol in patients with and without elevated CSF pressure, *J Neurosurg* 69:869–876, 1988.
337. Ravussin P, Archer DP, Tyler JL, et al: Effects of rapid mannitol infusion on cerebral blood volume. A positron emission tomographic study in dogs and man, *J Neurosurg* 64:104–113, 1986.
338. Reasoner D, Warner DS, Todd MM, et al: Effects of nitrous oxide on cerebral metabolic rate in rats anaesthetized with isoflurane, *Brit J Anesthesiol* 65:210–215, 1990.
339. Reasoner DK, Ryu KH, Hindman BJ, et al: Marked hemodilution increases neurologic injury after focal cerebral ischemia in rabbits, *Anesth Analg* 82:61–67, 1996.
340. Reasoner DK, Todd MM, Scamman FL, et al: The incidence of pneumocephalus after supratentorial craniotomy—observations on the disappearance of intracranial air, *Anesthesiology* 80:1008–1012, 1994.
341. Reddy RV, Moorthy SS, Dierdorf SF, et al: Excitatory effects and electroencephalographic correlation of etomidate, thiopental, methohexital, and propofol, *Anesth Analg* 77:1008–1011, 1993.
342. Reicher D, Bhalla P, Rubinstein EH: Cholinergic cerebral vasodilator effect of ketamine in rabbits, *Stroke* 18:445–449, 1987.
343. Reinstrup P, Ryding E, Algotsson L, et al: Effects of nitrous oxide on human regional cerebral blood flow and isolated pial arteries, *Anesthesiology* 81:396–402, 1994.
344. Reinstrup P, Ryding E, Algotsson L, et al: Distribution of cerebral blood flow during anesthesia with isoflurane or halothane in humans, *Anesthesiology* 82:359–366, 1995.
345. Renou AM, Vernhiet J, Macrez P, et al: Cerebral blood flow and metabolism during etomidate anaesthesia in man, *Br J Anaesth* 50:1047–1051, 1978.
346. Roald OK, Steen PA, Milde JH, et al: Reversal of the cerebral effects of diazepam in the dog by the benzodiazepine antagonist Ro15-1788, *Acta Anesthesiol Scand* 30:341–345, 1986.
347. Roald OK, Steen PA, Stangland K, et al: The effects of triazolam on cerebral blood flow and metabolism in the dog, *Acta Anaesthesiol Scand* 30:223–226, 1986.
348. Robertson CS, Narayan RK, Gokaslan ZL, et al: Cerebral arteriovenous oxygen difference as an estimate of cerebral blood flow in comatose patients, *J Neurosurg* 70: 222–230, 1989.
349. Robinson MJ, Teasdale GM: Calcium antagonists in the management of subarachnoid haemorrhage, *Cerebrovasc Brain Metabol Rev* 2:205–226, 1990.
350. Ropper AH, O'Rourke D, Kennedy SK: Head position, intracranial pressure, and compliance, *Neurology* 32:1288–1291, 1982.
351. Rosenwasser RH, Kleiner LI, Krzeminski JP, et al: Intracranial pressure monitoring in the posterior fossa: a preliminary report, *J Neurosurg* 71:503–505, 1989.
352. Rosner MJ, Coley JB: Cerebral perfusion pressure, intracranial pressure, and head elevation, *J Neurosurg* 65:636–641, 1986.
353. Roux S, Loeffler BM, Gray GA, et al: The role of endothelin in experimental cerebral vasospasm, *Neurosurgery* 37:78–86, 1995.
354. Rudehill A, Lagerkranser M, Lindquist C, et al: Effects of mannitol on blood volume and central hemodynamics in patients un-

dergoing cerebral aneurysm surgery, *Anesth Analg* 62:875–880, 1983.

355. Ruta TS, Drummond JC, Cole DJ: The effect of acute hypocapnia on local cerebral blood flow during middle cerebral artery occlusion in isoflurane anesthetized rats, *Anesthesiology* 78:134–140, 1993.
356. Sabatini U, Celsis P, Viallard G, et al: Quantitative assessment of cerebral blood volume by single-photon emission computed tomography, *Stroke* 22:324–330, 1991.
357. Sadoshima S, Fujii K, Kusuda K, et al: Importance of bilateral sympathetic innervation on cerebral blood flow autoregulation in the thalamus, *Brain Res* 413: 297–301, 1987.
358. Safwat AM, Daniel D: Grand mal seizure after fentanyl administration, *Anesthesiology* 59:78, 1983.
359. Saha GB, MacIntyre WJ, Go RT: Cyclotrons and positron emission tomography radiopharmaceuticals for clinical imaging, *Semin Nucl Med* 22:150–161, 1992.
360. Saidman LJ, Eger EI: Changes in cerebral spinal fluid pressure during pneumoencephalography under nitrous oxide anesthesia, *Anesthesiology* 26:67–72, 1965.
361. Sakabe T, Kuramoto T, Kumagae S, et al: Cerebral responses to the addition of nitrous oxide to halothane in man, *Br J Anaesth* 48:957–961, 1976.
362. Sakurada O, Kennedy C, Jehle J, et al: Measurement of local cerebral blood flow with iodo[14C]antipyrine, *Am J Physiol* 3:H59–H66, 1978.
363. Samra SK, Sneyd JR, Ross DA, et al: Effects of propofol sedation on seizures and intracranially recorded epileptiform activity in patients with partial epilepsy, *Anesthesiology* 82:843–851, 1995.
364. Samson D, Batjer HH, Bowman G, et al: A clinical study of the parameters and effects of temporary arterial occlusion in the management of intracranial aneurysms, *Neurosurgery* 34:22–27, 1994.
365. Samson D, Beyer CW: Furosemide in the intraoperative reduction of intracranial pressure in the patient with subarachnoid hemorrhage, *Neurosurgery* 10:167–169, 1982.
366. Sano T, Patel PM, Drummond JC, et al: A comparison of the cerebral protective effects of etomidate, thiopental, and isoflurane in a model of forebrain ischemia in the rat, *Anesth Analg* 76:990–997, 1993.
367. Sawaya R, Ingvar DH: Cerebral blood flow and metabolism in sleep, *Acta Neurol Scand* 80:481–491, 1989.
368. Sawin P, Todd MM, Traynelis V, et al: Cervical spine motion with direct laryngoscopy and orotracheal intubation: an *in vivo* cineflouroscopic study, *Anesthesiology* 1996.
369. Schell RM, Kern FH, Greeley WJ, et al: Cerebral blood flow and metabolism during cardiopulmonary bypass, *Anesth Analg* 76:849–865, 1993.
370. Scheller MS, Nakakimura K, Fleischer JE, et al: Cerebral effects of sevoflurane in the dog: comparison with isoflurane and enflurane, *Br J Anaesth* 65:388–392, 1990.
371. Scheller MS, Tateishi A, Drummond JC, et al: The effects of sevoflurane on cerebral blood flow, cerebral metabolic rate for oxygen, intracranial pressure and the electroencephalogram are similar to those of isoflurane in the rabbit, *Anesthesiology* 68:548–551, 1988.
372. Scheller MS, Todd MM, Drummond JC: Isoflurane, halothane and regional cerebral blood flow at various levels of $Paco_2$ in rabbits, *Anesthesiology* 64:598–604, 1986.
373. Scheller MS, Todd MM, Drummond JC, et al: The intracranial pressure effects of isoflurane and halothane administered following cryogenic brain injury in rabbits, *Anesthesiology* 67:507–512, 1987.
374. Schettini A, Stahurski B, Young HF, et al: Plasma electrolytes and electrolyte excretion during osmotic and combined osmotic loop diuresis in neurosurgery, *Anesth Analg* 61:213–214, 1982.
375. Schmidek HH, Auer LM, Kapp JP: The cerebral venous system, *Neurosurgery* 17:663–678, 1985.
376. Schwedler M, Miletich DJ, Albrecht RF: Cerebral blood flow and metabolism following ketamine administration, *Can Anaesth Soc J* 29:222–226, 1982.
377. Scott JC, Cooke JE, Stanski DR: Electroencephalographic quantitation of opioid effect: comparative pharmacodynamics of fentanyl and sufentanil, *Anesthesiology* 74:34–42, 1991.
378. Severinghaus JW, Lassen N: Step hypocapnia to separate arterial from tissue Pco_2 in the regulation of cerebral blood flow, *Circ Res* 20:272–278, 1967.
379. Shapiro HM, Wyte SR, Harris AB: Ketamine anaesthesia in patients with intracranial pathology, *Br J Anaesth* 44: 1200–1204, 1972.
380. Shapiro K, Fried A, Takei F, et al: Effect of the skull and dura on neural axis pressure-volume relationships and CSF hydrodynamics, *J Neurosurg* 63:76–81, 1985.
381. Shapiro K, Marmarou A, Shulman K: Characterization of clinical CSF dynamics and neural axis compliance using the pressure-volume index: I. The normal pressure-volume index, *Ann Neurol* 7:508–514, 1980.
382. Sheinberg M, Kanter MJ, Robertson CS, et al: Continuous monitoring of jugular venous oxygen saturation in head-injured patients, *J Neurosurg* 76:212–217, 1992.
383. Shimoda M, Oda S, Tsugane R, et al: Intracranial complications of hypervolemic therapy in patients with a delayed ischemic deficit attributed to vasospasm, *J Neurosurg* 78:423–429, 1993.
384. Shinozuka T, Nemoto EM, Winter PM: Mechanisms of cerebrovascular O_2 sensitivity from hyperoxia to moderate hypoxia in the rat, *J Cereb Blood Flow Metab* 9:187–195, 1989.
385. Shiraishi Y, Ikeda K: Update and biotransformation of sevoflurane in humans: a comparative study of sevoflurane with halothane, enflurane, and isoflurane [see comments], *J Clin Anesth* 2:381–386, 1990.
386. Shockley RP, LaManna JC: Determination of rat cerebral cortical blood volume changes by capillary mean transit time analysis during hypoxia, hypercapnia and hyperventilation, *Brain Res* 454:170–178, 1988.
387. Shulman RG, Blamire AM, Rothman DL, et al: Nuclear magnetic resonance imaging and spectroscopy of human brain function, *Proc Nat Acad Sci USA* 90:3127–3133, 1993.
388. Sivakumar V, Rajshekhar V, Chandy MJ: Management of neurosurgical patients with hyponatremia and natriuresis, *Neurosurgery* 34:269–274, 1994.
389. Skahen S, Shapiro HM, Drummond JC, et al: Nitrous oxide withdrawal reduces intracranial pressure in the presence of pneumocephalus, *Anesthesiology* 65:192–195, 1986.
390. Smith I, White PF, Nathanson M, et al: Propofol. An update on its clinical use, *Anesthesiology* 81:1005–1043, 1994.
391. Sokoloff L: Localization of functional activity in the central nervous system by measurement of glucose utilization with radioactive deoxyglucose, *J Cereb Blood Flow Metab* 1:7–36, 1981.
392. Sollevi A, Lagerkranser M, Irestedt L, et al: Controlled hypotension with adenosine in cerebral aneurysm surgery, *Anesthesiology* 61:400–405, 1984.
393. Solomon RA, Fink ME, Lennihan L: Prophylactic volume expansion therapy for the prevention of delayed cerebral ischemia after early aneurysm surgery: results of preliminary trial, *Arch Neurol* 45: 325–332, 1988.
394. Sperry RJ, Bailey PL, Reichman MV, et al: Fentanyl and sufentanil increase intracranial pressure in head trauma patients, *Anesthesiology* 77:416–420, 1992.
395. Spetzler RF, Hadley MN: Protection against cerebral ischemia: the role of barbiturates, *Cerebrovasc Brain Metab Rev* 1:212–229, 1989.
396. Standifer M, Bay JW, Trusso R: The sitting position in neurosurgery: a retrospective analysis of 488 cases, *Neurosurgery* 14: 649–658, 1984.
397. Star RA: Hyperosmolar states, *Am J Med Sci* 300:402–412, 1990.
398. Stirt JA, Grosslight KR, Bedford RF, et al: "Defasciculation" with metocurine prevents succinylcholine-induced increases in intracranial pressure, *Anesthesiology* 67: 50–53, 1987.
399. Stocchetti N, Paparella A, Bridelli F, et al: Cerebral venous oxygen saturation studied with bilateral samples in the internal jugular veins, *Neurosurgery* 34:38–44, 1994.
400. Strebel S, Lam AM, Matta B, et al: Dynamic and static cerebral autoregulation during isoflurane, desflurane, and propofol anesthesia, *Anesthesiology* 83:66–76, 1995.
401. Sturaitis MK, Moore LE, Kirsch JR, et al: A cholinergic agonist induces cerebral hyperemia in isoflurane- but not pentobarbital-anesthetized dogs, *Anesth Analg* 78:876–883, 1994.
402. Stundt TM, Whisnant JP: Subarachnoid hemorrhage from intracranial aneurysms. Surgical management and natural history of disease, *New Engl J Med* 299:116–122, 1978.
403. Sutton LN, McLaughlin AC, Dante S, et al: Cerebral venous oxygen content as a measure of brain energy metabolism with in-

creased intracranial pressure and hyperventilation, *J Neurosurg* 73:927–932, 1990.
404. Suzuki N, Hardebo JE: The cerebrovascular parasympathetic innervation, *Cerebrovasc Brain Metab Rev* 5:33–46, 1993.
405. Symon L, Wang AD, Costa e Silva IE, et al: Perioperative use of somatosensory evoked responses in aneurysm surgery, *J Neurosurg* 60:269–275, 1984.
406. Szabo MD, Crosby G, Hurford WE, et al: Myocardial perfusion following acute subarachnoid hemorrhage in patients with an abnormal electrocardiogram, *Anesth Analg* 76:253–258, 1993.
407. Szabo MD, Crosby G, Sundaram P, et al: Hypertension does not cause spontaneous hemorrhage of intracranial arteriovenous malformations, *Anesthesiology* 70:761–763, 1989.
408. Takayasu M, Dacey RG: Effects of mannitol on intracerebral arteriolar diameter *in vitro:* extraluminal and intraluminal application, *Neurosurgery* 25:747–752, 1989.
409. Takeshita H, Okuda Y, Sari A: The effects of ketamine on cerebral circulation and metabolism in man, *Anesthesiology* 36: 69–75, 1972.
410. Tarkkanen L, Laitenen L, Johansson G: Effects of D-tubocurarine on intracranial pressure and thalamic electrical impedance, *Anesthesiology* 40:247–251, 1974.
411. Tateishi A, Maekawa T, Takeshita H, et al: Diazepam and intracranial pressure, *Anesthesiology* 54:335–337, 1981.
412. Tempelhoff R, Modica PA, Bernardo KL, et al: Fentanyl-induced electrocorticographic seizures in patients with complex partial epilepsy, *J Neurosurg* 77:201–208, 1992.
413. Tempelhoff R, Modica PA, Rich KM, et al: Use of computerized electroencephalographic monitoring during aneurysm surgery, *J Neurosurg* 71:24–31, 1989.
414. Tiecks FP, Lam AM, Aaslid R, et al: Comparison of static and dynamic cerebral autoregulation measurements, *Stroke* 26: 1014–1019, 1995.
415. Todd MM: The effects of $PaCO_2$ on the cerebrovascular response to nitrous oxide in the halothane anesthetized rabbit, *Anesth Analg* 66:1090–1095, 1987.
416. Todd MM, Drummond JC: A comparison of the cerebrovascular and metabolic effects of halothane and isoflurane in the cat, *Anesthesiology* 60:276–282, 1984.
417. Todd MM, Drummond JC, U HS: The hemodynamic consequences of high dose thiopental anesthesia in humans, *Anesth Analg* 64:681–687, 1985.
418. Todd MM, Warner DS, Sokoll MD, et al: A prospective, comparative trial of three anesthetics for elective supratentorial craniotomy, *Anesthesiology* 78:1005–1020, 1993.
419. Todd MM, Weeks JB: Comparative effects of propofol, pentobarbital and isoflurane on cerebral blood flow and blood volume, *J Neurosurg Anesth* 1996, in press.
420. Todd MM, Weeks JB, Warner DS: Cerebral blood flow, blood volume, and brain tissue hematocrit during isovolemic hemodilution with hetastarch in the rat, *Am J Physiol* 263:H75–H82, 1992.
421. Todd MM, Weeks JB, Warner DS: Microwave fixation for the determination of cerebral blood volume in rats, *J Cereb Blood Flow Metab* 13:328–336, 1993.
422. Todd MM, Wu B, Warner DS, et al: The dose-related effects of nitric oxide synthase inhibition on cerebral blood flow during isoflurane and pentobarbital anesthesia, *Anesthesiology* 80:1128–1136, 1994.
423. Toung TJK, McPherson RW, Ahn H, et al: Pneumocephalus: effects of patient position on the incidence and location of aerocele after posterior fossa and upper cervical cord surgery, *Anesth Analg* 65:65–70, 1985.
424. Traeger SM, Henning RJ, Dobkin W, et al: Hemodynamic effects of pentobarbital therapy for intracranial hypertension, *Crit Care Med* 11:697–701, 1983.
425. Trindle MR, Dodson BA, Rampil IJ: Effects of fentanyl versus sufentanil in equianesthetic doses on middle cerebral artery blood flow velocity, *Anesthesiology* 78:454–460, 1993.
426. Tsementzis SA, Hitchcock ER: Outcome from rescue clipping of ruptured intracranial aneurysm during induction anesthesia and endotracheal intubation, *J Neurol Neurosurg Psych* 48:160–163, 1985.
427. Turner JM, Powell D, Gibson RM, et al: Intracranial pressure changes in neurosurgical patients during hypotension induced with sodium nitropresside or trimethaphan, *Br J Anaesth* 49:419–424, 1977.
428. Van Aken H, Puchstein C, Anger C, et al: Changes in intracranial pressure and compliance during adenosine triphosphate-induced hypotension in dogs, *Anesth Analg* 63:381–385, 1984.
429. van der Linden J, von-Ahn H, Ekroth R, et al: Middle cerebral artery flow velocity during coronary surgery: influence of clinical variables, *J Clin Anesthesiol* 2:7–15, 1990.
430. van der Linden J, Wesslen O, Ekroth R, et al: Transcranial Doppler-estimated versus thermodilution-estimated cerebral blood flow during cardiac operations. Influence of temperature and arterial carbon dioxide tension, *J Thorac Cardiovasc Surg* 102: 95–102, 1991.
431. Van Wylen DGL, Sciotti VM, Winn HR: Adenosine and the regulation of cerebral blood flow. In *Adenosine and Adenine Nucleotides as Regulators of Cellular Function,* Boca Raton, CRC Press, 1991, pp 191–202.
432. Vandesteene A, Trempont V, Engelman E, et al: Effect of propofol on cerebral blood flow and metabolism in man, *Anaesthesia* (Suppl)43:42–43, 1988.
433. Veselis R, Reinsel R, Feshchenko V, et al: Cerebral blood flow (CBF) changes during midazolam sedation using O-15 positron emission tomography, *Anesthesiology* 83:A154, 1995.
434. Voldby B, Enevoldsen EM: Intracranial pressure changes follow aneurysm rupture. Part 3: Recurrent hemorrhage, *J Neurosurg* 56:784–789, 1982.
435. Voldby B, Enevoldsen EM, Jensen FT: Cerebrovascular reactivity in patients with ruptured intracranial aneurysm, *J Neurosurg* 62:59–67, 1985.
436. Voldby B, Enovoldsen EM: Intracranial pressure changes following aneurysm rupture: Part 1: Clinical and angiographic correlations, *J Neurosurg* 56:186–196, 1982.
437. Wahl M, Schilling L: Regulation of cerebral blood flow—a brief review, *Acta Neurochirurgica* (Suppl)59:3–10, 1993.
438. Waldemar G, Paulson OB: Angiotensin converting enzyme inhibition and cerebral circulation—a review, *Br J Clin Pharmacol* 28:177S–182S, 1989.
439. Warner DS, Hansen TD, Vust L, et al: Distribution of cerebral blood flow during deep isoflurane vs pentobarbital anesthesia in rats with middle cerebral artery occlusion, *J Neurosurg Anesth* 1:219–226, 1989.
440. Warner TS, Takaoka S, Ludwig P, et al: Low-dose pentobarbital reduces focal ischemic infarct volume in a magnitude similar to burst suppression, *J Neurosurg Anesthesiol* 7:303, 1995.
441. Warner DS, Zhou J, Ramani R, et al: Reversible focal ischemia in the rat: Effects of halothane, isoflurane, and methohexital anesthesia, *J Cereb Blood Flow Metab* 11:794–802, 1991.
442. Wauquier A, Bovill JG, Sebel PS: Electroencephalographic effects of fentanyl, sufentanil and alfentanil anesthesia in man, *Neuropsychobiology* 11:203–206, 1984.
443. Weeks JB, Todd MM, Warner DS, et al: The influence of halothane, isoflurane, and pentobarbital on cerebral plasma volume in hypocapnic and normocapnic rats, *Anesthesiology* 73:461–466, 1990.
444. Weir B, MacDonald L: Cerebral vasospasm, *Clin Neurosurg* 40:40–55, 1993.
445. Werner C, Kochs E, Rau M, et al: Dose-dependent blood flow velocity changes in the basal cerebral arteries following low-dose ketamine, *J Neurosurg Anesth* 2:86–91, 1990.
446. Wilder BL: Hypothesis: the etiology of midcervical quadriplegia after operation with the patient in the sitting position, *Neurosurgery* 11:530–531, 1982.
447. Wilkinson HA, Rosenfeld S: Furosemide and mannitol in the treatment of acute experimental intracranial hypertension, *Neurosurgery* 12:405–410, 1983.
448. Williams SR, Crockard HA, Gadian DG: Cerebral ischaemia studied by nuclear magnetic resonance spectroscopy, *Cerebrovasc Brain Metab Rev* 1:91–114, 1989.
449. Wolff J, Carl P, Hansen PB, et al: Effects of eltanolone on cerebral blood flow and metabolism in healthy volunteers, *Anesthesiology* 81:623–627, 1994.
450. Wollman H, Alexander SC, Cohen PJ, et al: Cerebral circulation of man during halothane anesthesia. Effects of hypocarbia and of d-turbocurarine, *Anesthesiology* 25:180–184, 1964.
451. Wollman H, Smith TC, Stephan GW, et al: Effects of extremes of respiratory and metabolic alkalosis on cerebral blood flow in man, *J Appl Physiol* 24:60–65, 1968.
452. Wood JH, Kee DB: Hemorheology of the cerebral circulation in stroke, *Stroke* 16:765–772, 1985.
453. Worthley LIG, Cooper DJ, Jones N: Treatment of resistant intracranial hypertension with hypertonic saline: Report of two cases, *J Neurosurg* 68:478–481, 1988.
454. Wyper DJL: Functional neuroimaging with single photon emission computed tomogra-

phy (SPECT), *Cerebrovasc Brain Metab Rev* 5:199–217, 1993.
455. Yoshimoto Y, Kwak S: Age-related multifactorial causes of neurological deterioration after early surgery for aneurysmal subarachnoid hemorrhage, *J Neurosurg* 83: 984–988, 1995.
456. Young ML, Smith DS, Murtagh F, et al: Comparison of surgical and anesthetic complications in neurosurgical patients experiencing venous air embolism in the sitting position, *Neurosurgery* 18:157–161, 1986.
457. Young W: H2 clearance measurement of blood flow: a review of technique and polarographic principles, *Stroke* 11:552–564, 1980.
458. Young WL, Prohovnik I, Correll JW, et al: Cerebral blood flow and metabolism in patients undergoing anesthesia for carotid endarterectomy: a comparison of isoflurane, halothane, and fentanyl, *Anesth Analg* 68:712–717, 1989.
459. Young WL, Solomon RA, Prohovnik I, et al: 133Xe blood flow monitoring during arteriovenous malformation resection: a case of intraoperative hyperperfusion with subsequent brain swelling, *Neurosurgery* 22: 765–769, 1988.
460. Zentner J, Albrecht T, Hassler W: Prevention of an air embolism by moderate hypoventilation during surgery in the sitting position, *Neurosurgery* 28:705–708, 1991.
461. Zornow MH, Maze M, Dyck JB, et al: Dexmedetomidine decreases cerebral blood flow velocity in humans, *J Cereb Blood Flow Metab* 13:350–353, 1993.
462. Zornow MH, Scheller MS, Sheehan PB, et al: Intracranial pressure effects of dexmedetomidine in rabbits, *Anesth Analg* 75:232–237, 1992.

CHAPTER 68

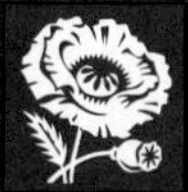

Anesthesia for Adult Cardiac Procedures

ALAN F. ROSS
MARK N. GOMEZ
JOHN H. TINKER

Anesthesia for cardiac surgery involves a breadth of understanding of the circulatory system. Cardiac physiology, invasive cardiovascular monitoring, and vasoactive drugs are standard tools of the trade. Anesthetic agents are selected to optimize cardiac performance for specific cardiac disorders. Working knowledge of cardiopulmonary bypass and its complications are required. New procedures have arisen such as transmyocardial laser revascularization, cardiomyoplasty, and minimally invasive coronary artery revascularization without cardiopulmonary bypass. Focus on cost containment has promoted strategies aimed at early extubation and shortened intensive care unit stays for cardiac surgery. Innovations such as retrograde cardioplegia and modified ultrafiltration have occurred. Transesophageal echocardiography (TEE) has become a standard monitor for procedures as mitral valve reconstruction. New anesthetic and vasoactive drugs continue to be introduced. The student of cardiac anesthesia must be careful not to be too distracted by the above. Instead, the student's focus should be on a core curriculum of circulatory physiology and pharmacology. This dictum holds true for advanced students also. For example, the student who embraces TEE without a solid foundation in hemodynamics will eventually find understanding elusive. Instead, if the core curriculum is understood by the student, the rest will fall into place.

This chapter focuses on cardiac physiology, invasive monitoring, vasoactive drugs, and cardiopulmonary bypass which the authors consider basic to cardiac anesthesia.

These principles must be combined with direct experience in the operating room. Cardiac anesthesia is one specialty of clinical medicine where placement and interpretation of cardiac monitoring modalities and use of vasoactive drugs are routine. This provides a great opportunity for the student to obtain first-hand knowledge and understanding of the principles in this chapter. The real truth is, cardiac anesthesia and surgery provides all of us a unique opportunity to remain students of the circulatory system.

APPROACH TO THE PATIENT WITH CORONARY ARTERY DISEASE

Patient History

Of paramount concern is the degree to which coronary blood flow is restricted and the degree to which previous myocardial infarction (MI) may have impaired ventricular function. In patients with coronary artery disease (CAD), key issues include: (1) history of MI (especially recent); (2) episodes of hospitalization or resuscitation from arrhythmia; (3) history of cardiac medications; and (4) assessment of symptoms indicative of coronary disease severity. Patients may have very different courses after MI which are discernable by history. A patient who required defibrillation and placement of an intra-aortic balloon pump during hospitalization for MI differs greatly from the patient who had a short hospitalization and mild symptoms after MI. A useful means of understanding these differences is a classification scheme for patients with acute MI. Forrester et al.[47] provided a quantitative definition of subsets of MI based on hemodynamics (Table 68-1). Mortality from acute MI was related to the subset.

A related method of characterization of the cardiac patient involves assessment of cardiac medications and other therapies (Table 68-2). The patient whose medication regimen relies on beta-adrenergic blockers is likely to have reasonable myocardial function despite significant CAD. In contrast, a patient who is maintained on digoxin, diuretics, and angiotensin converting enzyme (ACE) inhibitor agents may have marginal myocardial performance. It is likely that prior MI resulted in significant loss of pump function, and resultant congestive heart failure (CHF).

Table 68-1 Hemodynamic subsets of acute myocardial infarction

Class	Clinical definition	Cardiac index	PCWP	Mortality
I	No pulmonary congestion or systemic hypoperfusion	> 2.2	< 18	3%
II	Pulmonary congestion only, good perfusion	> 2.2	> 18	9%
III	Reduced perfusion only, no pulmonary congestion	< 2.2	< 18	23%
IV	Both pulmonary edema and hypoperfusion (shock)	< 2.2	> 18	51%

Cardiac Index number represents cardiac output in l/min/m² body surface and PCWP number represents pulmonary capillary wedge pressure in mm Hg. From Forrester, et al: Medical therapy of acute myocardial infarction by application of hemodynamic subsets, *New Engl J Med* 295:1404, 1976.

A characterization of disease severity can also be made on the basis of symptoms. What is required to provoke typical symptoms of angina? Angina which occurs with significant exertion such as mowing the lawn or shoveling snow is not as ominous as that which occurs with mild activity such as walking or showering, or worse, with no activity at all. How much nitroglycerin is taken? Some patients may take sublingual nitrogclycerin once a month or never. Others with severe disease may take several per day. Does fatigue or dyspnea occur with exertion? These symptoms suggest ventricular failure, either because of a fixed low cardiac output from prior MI or because myocardial ischemia is severe enough to cause acute ventricular dysfunction. Both reasons are indicative of severe disease.

The Cardiac Catheterization

Cardiac catheterization supplies essential information about the patient's cardiac disease. A review should be part of the anesthesia preoperative assessment. Two general kinds of information are included for the patient with CAD. Hemodynamic assessment includes measurement of cardiac pressures, cardiac output, and O_2 saturations; and calculations of systemic (SVR) and pulmonary vascular resistances and in patients with congenital heart disease, the amount of intracardiac shunts. This information can be obtained from the "right heart catheterization." An estimation of left atrial pressure is obtained by the pulmonary capillary wedge pressure (PCWP). Cardiac output is calculated by thermodilution technique or Fick principle. Patient values should be compared with known normal values (Box 68-1).

The second type of information is angiographic data generated by a visually directed "left-heart" catheter which advanced via a major artery to a position directly above the aortic valve. From this position, radiopague contrast dye is injected directly into the right and left coronary arteries, and a cineangiogram created, whereby the location and degree of various coronary stenoses are measured. A different angiogram catheter can be advanced past the aortic valve and into the left ventricle. Here, injection of radiocontrast dye generates the "left ventriculogram" and yields ejection fraction and evidence of myocardial wall motion abnormalities (Table 68-3). Left ventricular end diastolic pressure (LVEDP) can be directly measured when the catheter is in the left ventricle. Often, LVEDP is measured before and after the injection of contrast dye. A significant increase in LVEDP after injection is generally a sign of more severe disease. Radiographic contrast dye may acutely worsen left ventricular function because of decreased O_2 carriage, chelation of calcium, or direct volume effect on the myocardium.[65] To avoid this confounding influence, some re-

Table 68-2 Therapeutic interventions for acute myocardial infarction

Clinical definition	Cardiac index	PCWP	Therapy
Normal or hyperdynamic	> 3	< 12	Beta adrenergic blockers
Reduced perfusion because of hypovolemia	< 2.7	< 9	Volume repletion and reassessment of clinical category
Mild left ventricular failure	< 2.5	18–22	Nitrates, diuretics
Severe left ventricular failure	< 1.8	> 22	(depends on blood pressure)
with satisfactory BP			Nitrates, vasodilators
with hypotension			Balloon pump, nitrate, inotropic drugs such as dopamine, dobutamine

Modified from Pasternak, Braunwald, and Sobel: Acute myocardial infarction. In Braunwald, editor: *Heart disease,* ed 4, Philadelphia, WB Saunders, 1992, p, 1250.

BOX 68-1
NORMAL HEMODYNAMIC MEASUREMENTS

Pressures (mm Hg)	
Right atrium (mean)	2–8
Right ventricle (systolic/diastolic)	15/2–30/8
Pulmonary artery (systolic/diastolic)	15/4–30/12
Left atrium or wedge (mean)	2–10
Left ventricle (systolic/diastolic)	100/3–140/12
Systolic arterial (systolic/diastolic)	100/60–140/90

Blood flows	
Cardiac index (liter/min/m^2)	2.6–4.2
Stroke index (ml/beat/m^2)	30–65
Vascular resistance	
Systemic resistance (dynes · sec · CM^{-5})	
Pulmonary resistance (dynes · sec · CM^{-5})	

From Grossman W, editor: *Cardiac catheterization and angiography,* ed 3, Philadelphia, 1986, Lea & Febiger. The authors note: "Normal values should be determined in each individual laboratory."

Table 68-3 Abnormalities of wall motion on the left ventriculogram

Term	Definition
Hypokinesis	Region of the myocardium contracts during systole, but the contraction is less than that of neighboring regions.
Akinesis	Region of myocardium does not contract during systole.
Dyskinesias	Region of myocardium bulges outward during systole, and thus moves in the opposite direction compared to adjacent regions of myocardium.

Note that typically hypokinetic regions are interpreted as indicative of ischemic areas, akinetic regions as indicative of infarcted myocardium, and dyskinetic areas as either very severe ischemia or ventricular aneurysm.

searchers recommend hemodynamic measurements and left ventriculography before performing coronary angiography in stable patients. This sequence may not be possible in unstable patients in whom coronary anatomy is the priority.

Severity of cardiac disease is assessed from both right and left heart catheterizations. Hemodynamic measurements of good ventricular function include low filling pressures (e.g., right atrial pressure, pulmonary artery [PA] pressures, wedge pressure, LVEDP), normal cardiac output, and satisfactory or even high blood pressure. In contrast, poor or severely ischemic ventricular function is indicated by elevated filling pressures, low cardiac output, and low blood pressure. Of note is that "vascular resistance" is of limited use in this assessment. Occasionally, a patient will have a mixture of favorable and unfavorable hemodynamic variables. The best practice in this case is to focus on problem areas. Thus a normal cardiac output but an LVEDP of 20 mm Hg portends possible ventricle dysfunction. A patient with good ventricular function usually has uniformly favorable hemodynamics. The patient with some indications of abnormality will likely manifest exaggerated versions of those same problems either before or after cardiopulmonary bypass.

Indicators of disease severity by left-heart catheterization include ejection fraction, wall motion abnormalities, and severity of CAD. The ejection fraction is considered a good indicator of myocardial function. Recently, Kay et al.[87] reported a retrospective review of 1354 consecutive patients who underwent coronary artery bypass graft (CABG) surgery. Patients with ejection fraction of 0.40 or greater had the best outcomes in terms of lowest mortality, lowest morbidity, and lowest costs. Patients with ejection fraction less than 0.30 had worse outcomes than patients with ejection fraction that was between 0.30 and 0.39.[87]

Ejection fraction and wall motion abnormalities on ventriculogram generally reflect the hemodynamic findings of the right-heart catheterization. A low ejection fraction (< 40%) or regions of dyskinesis suggest significant ventricular dysfunction. Areas of akinesis or diskinesis of the anterior myocardium are regarded as more severe than similar dysfunction of the inferior wall. It is possible to have a low ejection fraction plus regions of dyskinesis and yet a normal cardiac output in some cases of left ventricular aneurysm. Here, systolic enlargement of the anneurysm region causes the measured ejection fraction to be low. However, if enough surrounding myocardium is normal, a sufficient forward cardiac output is possible. The clinical history of fatigue or exercise intolerance is useful to aid assessment.

Clearly the number and degree of coronary stenoses are related to disease severity. The term "triple vessel disease" indicates severe coronary stenoses of the left anterior descending artery, the left circumflex artery, and the right coronary artery. The term "complete occlusion with collateral filling" indicates that the normal blood supply to a region of myocardium has been lost but that some perfusion remains via connections to distal portions of neighboring vessels. **Most ominous is the description of "left main" coronary stenosis.** The left main coronary artery bifurcates into the left anterior descending artery and the left circumflex artery thus supplies a large portion of the left ventricle. Because such a large portion of the heart is at risk, significant ventricular dysfunction will result if ischemia should occur. Another term indicating disease severity is "*left main equivalent*" coronary disease. An example would be complete occlusions of the left anterior descending and the circumflex arteries and an 80% occlusion of the right coronary which provides collateral flow to regions of the anterior descending and circumflex arteries. Here, despite the fact that the anatomic left main coronary artery is normal, the term indicates that any further diminution in coronary blood flow through the stenotic vessel may be accompanied by a severe compromise of myocardial function.[79] **It should be emphasized that a patient may have very severe CAD but still normal indices of ventricular performance.** Such a patient is likely to have significant angina upon exertion, but no history of MI. In contrast, poor ventricular function is indicative of significant prior MI or severe and *ongoing* myocardial infarction.

Another angiographic term is *right-versus-left coronary dominance.* If the right coronary is seen to continue onto the posterior wall of the heart as a posterior descending coronary, dominance is said to be right. This situation occurs in approximately 85% of patients. This posterior descending coronary supplies the posterior and diaphragmatic portion of the interventricular septum. Also in right-dominant circulations, the right coronary artery gives rise to the arteriovenous (AV) nodal artery. If, instead, the circumflex coronary continues inferiorly down the back of the heart as a major posterior descending coronary artery, then coronary dominance is said to be left. This occurs in approximately 8% of patients. In the remainder, dominance by angiography cannot be ascertained and is said to be indeterminate. An example of the clinical relevance is the fact that air bubbles from the aorta most often enter the right coronary artery (the right coronary artery arises from "anterior" (i.e., uppermost in the supine position on the operating room table) in a right-dominant system, air can enter the AV nodal artery and produce heart block.[142] A left-dominant patient who also has left circumflex and/or left main coronary disease may be expected to have poor perfusion of the left ventricular posterior wall, poor protection via cardioplegia, and difficulty with separation from bypass. Hence, coronary dominance is useful to the anesthesiologist if it can be ascertained.

Although coronary angiography is considered the gold standard by which coronary artery stenosis is assessed, there are major limitations to its ability to predict physiologic significance of the lesions. Measurement of the stenosis may be performance with a single radiographic projection, despite the fact that the lesions are often asymmetric. Assuming that the proximal and distal ends of a stenotic segment open into normal vasculature may also be invalid. Also, marked interobserver variability exists.[199]

Coexisting Diseases

Although assessment of cardiac disease is a priority, various coexisting diseases may have an important influence and must be assessed.

Difficult airway or difficult intubation

Occasionally, a patient will have a history of or the appearance of a potentially difficult airway. Examples include patients with obstructive sleep apnea, anklysoing spondylitis, or prior cervical spine fusion. A difficult airway/intubation poses several problems. A typical anesthetic for cardiac surgery uses significant doses of narcotics and long acting, nondepolarizing muscle relaxant drugs. Such an anesthetic would preclude "allowing the patient to wake up" should airway difficulty be encountered. Techniques such as awake intubation may cause undesirable hypertension, tachycardia, and discomfort; circumstances we are trying to avoid in patients with ischemic heart disease.

The approach to this dilemma begins with thorough review of any prior available anesthetic records for description of airway, laryngoscopy, and intubation. This may even require contacting another hospital to obtain the information. Possible modifications of the anesthetic plan may include (1) brief "awake look" with laryngoscope after topical anesthesia to oropharynx; (2) anesthetic induction which avoids long-acting muscle relaxants and narcotics until it is determined that ventilation and intubation are possible; and (3) awake fiberoptic intubation after topical anesthesia to the airway. If awake fiberoptic intubation is performed, after the patient is anesthetized, the view by direct laryngoscopy should be documented so as to provide that information for the next time general anesthesia is required. The patient who has been a difficult airway/intubation requires that this be clearly communicated to the physicians involved in postoperative care.

Full stomach or gastroesohageal reflux

Although it is unusual for an elective cardiac patient to be considered a "full stomach," there are situations when this must be considered. The patient arriving for cardiac transplantation may not have been "NPO" at all. The patient arriving emergently from the catheter lab may also be at such risk. Other circumstances of risk are patients with delayed gastric emptying such as may occur with diabetes, preoperative anxiety and stress, or medications such as narcotics. The patient with hiatal hernia or symptoms of active gastroesophageal reflux can also present problems. Approaches to these problems may include: preoperative medication with metoclopramide and H_2 antagonists, sodium citrate, cricoid pressure, rapid sequence induction and intubation, and even awake fiberoptic intubation. Incidentally, patients with hiatal hernia are considered relative contraindications for TEE.

Other vascular disease

It is not uncommon for patients to have evidence of other peripheral vascular disease.[150] Of foremost concern is the presence of cerebrovascular disease, because stroke is a persistent cause of morbidity after cardiopulmonary bypass. Finding of a carotid bruit or symptoms of transient ischemic attack (TIA) are important and should be addressed preoperatively. Another issue is whether blood pressure is the same in each arm. This is important for deciding site for arterial line placement. Presence of femoral or aortic vascular disease may preclude placement of intra-aortic balloon pump.

Of note is the recent report by Daily et al.[38] that the combined procedure of carotid endarterectomy (CEA) plus CABG is associated with a significant reduction in medical costs. The authors retrospectively analyzed cases of first-time isolated CEA, isolated CABG, and combined procedures. Although the incidence of mortality or stroke was not different, hospital costs were CEA $4896, CABG $10,959, and combined CEA plus CABG $11,089. When Medicare hospital reimbursement was considered, a potential savings of $10,077 was estimated by combining the procedures.

Renal disease

Cardiac surgery presents several potential stresses to the patient with renal insufficiency. Angiographic dye used for cardiac catheterization may exacerbate renal insufficiency. Various vasopressor drugs and the abnormal circulation of cardiopulmonary bypass may adversely affect renal perfusion. Excessive use of suction in the surgical field contributes to hemolysis and serum free hemoglobin which may adversely affect the kidney.

The patient with renal failure presents a number of challenges. Preoperatively, patients may be anemic despite the use of erythropoietin. Preoperative hemodialysis may render the patient relatively hypovolemic. Platelet dysfunction may contribute to coagulopathy. Care of a dialysis site includes avoiding intravenous (IV) or arterial catheters or blood pressure cuff at the site; positioning and protecting the site during surgery; and verifying the patency (presence of a thrill) in the pre- and postbypass period. The patient with an arteriovenous fistula will predictably have a lower diastolic pressure and higher cardiac output (includes output shunted through the fistula). Mixed venous O_2 saturation is also affected because it contains arterial blood which has been shunted through the fistula.

Without strict attention to fluid and hematocrit balance, major problems with fluid overload plus anemia and coagulopathy may occur by the end of the case. Extra crystalloid fluids should be avoided by both anesthesiologist and perfusionist, and hemoconcentration should occur during cardiopulmonary bypass. Potassium balance is another critical issue. Cardioplegia and each unit of blood transfusion represents a potassium load. Although insulin and dextrose or epinephrine will reduce serum potassium level, this is only temporary and does not remove potassium from the body. Definitive removal of potassium requires exchange-resin enema, or hemodialysis in the postoperative period. When potassium levels are expected to be changing, serial measurements of potassium (e.g., every hour) are necessary. The electrocardiogram (ECG) may not provide adequate warning of hyperkalemia with tall, peaked T waves. Instead, the first sign of dangerous hyperkalemia may be heart block.

Hypertension

The patient with significant hypertension may have altered states of autoregulation in both the cerebral and coronary circulations. Presumably, this means that a higher than normal blood pressure may be required for adequate organ perfusion. Left ventricular hypertrophy may also accompany significant hypertension, resulting in a less compliant ventricle which relies on atrial contraction for optimum filling. This means that rhythms other than sinus are likely to be accompanied by abrupt decreases in blood pressure. A normal blood pressure during a junctional rhythm may abruptly jump to hypertensive levels if sinus rhythm is resumed. Such swings in pressure are particularly disconcerting during cannulation of the aorta. Anecdotal reports indicate that small doses of beta-blocker drugs are useful to restore a junctional rhythm to sinus. Patients who are hypertensive preoperatively are likely to be hypertensive in the postoperative period. This will likely necessitate the availability of a potent vasodilator agent such as nitroprusside for blood pressure control.

Physiologic Principles of Coronary Artery Disease Pertinent to Anesthetic Management

Restriction of coronary blood flow is the physiologic hallmark of CAD.[58] Autoregulation is the normal means by which the coronary arteries match the supply of blood to the metabolic needs of the heart over a wide range of circumstances.[72] Substantial increases in cardiac work are possible because coronary flow increases with metabolic demand.[31] Atherosclerosis of a coronary artery both physically obstructs coronary blood flow and impairs autoregulation. In such circumstances, either an increase in myocardial O_2 demand or a decrease in O_2 supply may cause ischemia. Although postoperative MI may be related to a complex interaction among a number of variables,[93,113,168,171] the anesthesiologist generally assumes that prevention and treatment of intraoperative myocardial ischemia is an important goal.[7,55,108] Goals to this end are efforts to minimize myocardial O_2 demand and efforts to maximize myocardial O_2 supply.

Factors that influence myocardial oxygen demand

Major determinants of myocardial O_2 consumption include myocardial wall tension and the contractile state of the heart.[21,30,160,173] During awake exercise, the combination of a blood pressure rise and increase in heart rate (the "rate-pressure product") has been a clinically useful measure of myocardial O_2 consumption.[153] Because it is well known that the "stress response" of surgery causes hypertension and tachycardia, a major goal is to prevent such increases in myocardial O_2 demand by use of appropriate anesthetic agents.[109] Some have attempted to literally extrapolate the "rate-pressure product" to circumstances of anesthesia and surgery. This strategy has been less useful[8,90] than in the awake, exercising patient likely because of the unusual factors which affect intraoperative heart rate and blood pressure (Table 68-4).

The basic goal of preventing excessive myocardial O_2 demand is valid. The inotropic state of the heart is an important factor in myocardial O_2 demand. Positive inotropic agents will increase myocardial contractility and thus increase O_2 demand. For this reason, inotropic agents are generally avoided *before* coronary revascularization. Unnecessarily high contractility can be reduced by anesthetics, which limit the degree of sympathetic stimulation.[109] In fact, if cardiac function is satisfactory, beta-adrenergic blocking drugs may be administered to reduce contractility.

Table 68-4 Problems with intraoperative rate pressure product

Example	Systolic blood pressure	Heart rate	Rate pressure product
Patient A mild hypertension	150 mm Hg	60	9000
Patient B moderately large blood loss	100 mm Hg	90	9000

The rate pressure product was originally proposed for awake, exercising patients in whom both the heart rate and blood pressure increased with exertion. This association is not necessarily true during operation, and in fact circumstances may be such that the heart rate and blood pressure vary in different directions. Thus although both hypothetical patients have a rate pressure product of 9000, patient B would be considered at much higher risk for myocardial ischemia than patient A.

It is worth noting that anemia can stimulate compensatory responses which increase myocardial O_2 demand when at the same time reducing myocardial O_2 supply. In the anemic patient, it makes little sense to avoid blood transfusion in the prebypass period, knowing that transfusion will be necessary during the bypass or postbypass period.

The net balance of any particular therapy must consider the effects of both demand and supply.[75] Beta-adrenergic blockade limits myocardial O_2 *demand* by reducing increases in contractility that would otherwise occur because of catecholamines and the sympathetic nervous system. Additionally, by maintaining a slow heart rate, beta blockers maximize the period of diastole and thereby act to maintain *supply*. Thus this therapy is favorable for both demand and supply concerns. In contrast, reduction of blood pressure might appear favorable because of the reduced myocardial O_2 consumption. Reduced blood pressure may cause a reduction of coronary blood flow through stenotic lesions. Thus, the balance of such therapy may be unfavorable. In practice, the anesthesiologist seeks both to limit myocardial O_2 demand and maximize supply.[191] Yet, rather than wait for ischemia to occur, the anesthetic is designed to optimize this balance.[82]

Factors that influence myocardial oxygen supply

Normal autoregulation provides relatively constant coronary blood flow despite significant variations in blood pressure.[73] With anemia, autoregulation increases blood flow to maintain necessary O_2 delivery.[73] The maximum ability of the coronary vessel to autoregulate can be experimentally determined by administration of vasodilators. In circumstances of pharmacologic maximal coronary vasodilation, coronary blood flow is thereafter linearly related to the blood pressure. Blood flow in excess of that which would normally occur with intact autoregulation is termed **coronary vascular reserve** (Fig. 68-1).

If a coronary stenosis is present, flow through the artery is restricted. In an effort to maintain normal flow, a portion of the coronary vascular reserve may be expended to counter the effects of the stenosis. As the stenosis increases in severity, more of the vasodilator reserve is used. Finally, all of coronary autoregulation is used simply to maintain resting blood flow to the myocardium. When coronary autoregulation has been maximally used, the coronary blood flow varies directly with the driving blood pressure. In this circumstance, decreased blood pressure may cause decreased coronary blood flow and resultant myocardial ischemia. **Thus a major goal of anesthesia for patients with coronary atherosclerosis is maintenance of arterial pressure.**[55] For similar reasons, the patient with severe coronary stenosis will be unable to compensate for anemia because autoregulation is already maximized.

A second principle for cardiac anesthesia concerns the importance of diastole. A major share of epicardial and virtually all middle cardial and endocardial coronary blood flow occurs during this period. This applies primarily to the left ventricle because significant coronary blood flow also occurs during systole in the right ventricle. The period of diastole establishes the time available for coronary blood flow. Therefore, tachycardia is detrimental because of the shortening of the diastolic interval.[106] Substantial improvement in coronary flow time can be obtained simply by avoiding faster heart rates. Can this be extrapolated to very slow heart rates? Experimentally, there is a limit to the benefits of slow heart rates. Bellamy[13] noted experimentally that epicardial coronary flow ceased during long periods of diastole despite apparently appropriate coronary driving pressure. Explanations of this "zero-flow" phenomenon are controversial.[92]

A third principle is the role of the diastolic ventricular filling pressure.[103] This pressure is considered to be in opposition to coronary blood flow. Typically, blood is considered to move through the myocardium on the basis of a pressure gradient: a proximal coronary driving pressure minus the distal opposing pressure. The proximal driving pressure is often considered to be the aortic pressure throughout diastole. A specific number is not accurate because the pressure decreases throughout diastole. The nature of the distal opposing pressure is a subject of controversy.[14] Coronary sinus pressure, LVEDP, or the pressure within the wall of the ventricular myocardium have all been suggested.[117] Clinically, the LVEDP is used because it can be estimated reasonably and is related physically to the region at greatest risk for ischemia, namely the subendocardium.[74]

The above scheme fails to consider the critical effect of the coronary stenosis. Thus a substantial drop in pressure occurs when blood is forced across a coronary stenosis. **Thus the driving pressure that moves blood across the myocardium is not the aortic diastolic pressure, but rather whatever pressure remains, distal to the critical coronary stenosis.** The significance is that the pressure gradient that exists to provide coronary blood flow may be rather modest, and will be influenced substantially by changes in LVEDP, that is, wedge pressure. For this reason, cardiac anesthesiologists are particularly interested in monitoring ventricular filling pressures via the pulmonary artery (PA) catheter. Nitroglycerin is frequently used to maintain lower filling pressures. In practice, attempts to optimize coronary perfusion pressure gradients involve both raising the diastolic arterial blood pressure and decreasing the LVEDP.

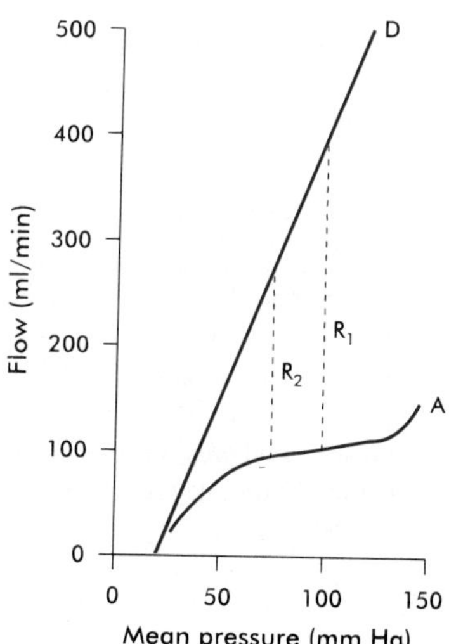

Fig. 68-1. Coronary pressure flow diagram. Diagram of pressure-flow relationships in normal left ventricle during autoregulation (*A*) and maximal vasodilation (*D*). R_1 and R_2 are the coronary flow reserves at mean coronary perfusing pressures of 75 and 100 mm Hg when aortic pressure and heart rate are constant. (From Hoffman JIE: Maximal coronary flow and the concept of coronary vascular reserve, *Circulation* 70:153, 1984.)

A question is often raised regarding the patient who demonstrates both elevated filling pressures with simultaneous hypotension. Can nitroglycerin be safely administered? The answer is yes, but provision must first be made to protect the arterial pressure. Here, judgment is required regarding myocardial contractility. If left ventricular dysfunction is severe, inotropic support with epinephrine or norepinephrine should be initiated prior to nitroglycerin. If left ventricular function is deemed satisfactory, arterial pressure can be augmented with a pure vasoconstricter agent and nitroglycerin added subsequently. A therapy to avoid is to administer fluids in the misguided hope that blood pressure will increase. The likelihood is that blood pressure will remain unchanged but that filling pressures will be further increased (worsened) resulting in even less favorable conditions for coronary blood flow, especially to the subendocardial left ventricular regions.

Another concern is whether therapy with nitroglycerin will reduce preload and cause cardiac output to decrease. The goal of therapy for the coronary patient is to promote conditions which maximize coronary blood flow, not cardiac output. It is not infrequent that therapy which decreases filling pressures (nitroglycerin) plus therapy which increases blood pressure (alpha-adrenergic agonist) will also result in increased cardiac output. A possible explanation is that some level of myocardial ischemia was relieved by the therapy (Box 68-2 and Fig. 68-2).

BOX 68-2
PROBLEMS IN ESTIMATING CORONARY PERFUSION PRESSURE (CPP)

Not valid	Valid
CPP = ADP − LVEDP	CPP = PDS − LVEDP
45 mm Hg = 60 mm Hg − 15 mm Hg	5 mm Hg = 20 mm Hg − 15 mm Hg

*Although aortic diastolic pressure (ADP) is often considered to be the driving pressure for coronary blood flow, the coronary pressure distal to stenosis (PDS) is considerably less. The perfusion pressure gradient across the myocardium is better estimated by using this distal coronary pressure. This method illustrates that elevations of left ventricular end-diastolic pressure (LVEDP) may markedly oppose coronary blood flow. Unfortunately, the coronary pressure distal to any given coronary stenosis is not measurable.

Other variables can also be optimized to improve myocardial O_2 delivery. High concentrations of inspired O_2 and correction of anemia can provide significant increases in O_2 delivery even if no increase in coronary blood flow is possible.

By combining the previous principles, the anesthetic is planned to facilitate O_2 delivery to the myocardium when blocking stressful sympathetic responses that drive the myocardium to overuse limited O_2 supplies. The major goal is to provide O_2 to the heart. Therapy is not directed at increasing cardiac output. Administration of fluids to increase cardiac output makes little sense if existing cardiac output is sufficiently perfusing the body, as evidenced by lack of metabolic acidosis. Increased filling pressure may easily worsen the coronary perfusion pressure gradient. Administration of positive inotropic agents may waste delivered myocardial O_2 if augmented contractility is unnecessary.[75] Table 68-5 summarizes the management goals for CAD.

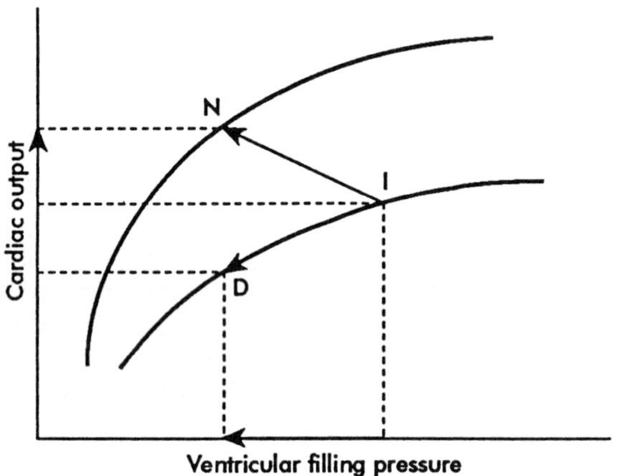

Fig. 68-2. Therapy of myocardial ischemia with nitroglycerin. This figure illustrates two ventricular function curves. A hypothetic patient is placed at point *I* and nitroglycerin is administered. If nitroglycerin acts purely as a venodilator, reduction in filling pressure (wedge pressure) would be accompanied by a reduction in cardiac output, shown as point *D*. If, however, nitroglycerin acts to relieve some degree of myocardial ischemia, an increased cardiac output would occur despite the reduction in filling pressure. This point *N* must lie on a different, more favorable ventricular function curve.

APPROACH TO THE PATIENT WITH VALVULAR HEART DISEASE

The patient with valvular heart disease likely has had a known heart murmur for a number of years. Various abnormalities of cardiac valve function place different demands on the heart. Long-standing abnormalities are likely to have resulted in compensatory myocardial and possibly lung changes. These differences will have implications for anesthetic management.

A basic division can be made between aortic valve versus the mitral valve disease. Pulmonic and tricuspid valvular heart lesions are encountered less frequently. Anticipated responses to tachycardia, bradycardia, hypertension, vasodilation, and the ability of the heart to increase its cardiac output will differ according to which valve is abnormal. Goals of management for any valvular heart lesion may be complicated by the presence of coexisting CAD.

Aortic Stenosis

Despite obstruction to left ventricular outflow because of aortic valve stenosis, cardiac output is maintained for many years by compensatory left ventricular hypertrophy. Symp-

Table 68-5 Summary of management goals for coronary artery disease

Variable	Effect	Goal
Myocardial contractility	Sympathetic stimulation from surgical stress increases myocardial oxygen demand	Appropriate anesthetic agents to block stress response, beta-blocker drugs, avoid inotropic stimulation
	In congestive heart failure, a dilated ventricle increases wall stress and LVEDP	With left ventricular failure, inotropic support may have a favorable net effect on oxygen supply and demand
Blood pressure	Increased blood pressure increases oxygen demand, but also coronary flow, decreased blood pressure risks decreased coronary flow	Maintain blood pressure at or mildly above normal levels, may require alpha adrenergic agonist
Heart rate	Increased heart rates shorten the time available for diastolic coronary blood flow	Avoid heart rate increase with anesthetic agents first, and beta blocker if necessary
Ventricular filling pressure	Elevated filling pressures oppose coronary blood flow especially to subendocardium	Maintain lower filling pressures with nitroglycerin
Blood oxygen content	Interaction of pulmonary function, inspired oxygen, and blood hematocrit	Adequate tidal volume, positive end expiratory pressure, maintain high inspired oxygen treat anemia with blood transfusion

toms of CHF or syncope occur, usually after middle age. Once these symptoms appear, survival is limited without aortic valve replacement. Both the narrowed aortic valve orifice as well as compensatory left ventricular hypertrophy have implications for anesthetic management. The narrowed aortic valve orifice restricts left-ventricle ejection. The patient may be asymptomatic at rest, but is only able to perform limited exercise. Inability to increase cardiac output means that the heart will be unable to compensate for events like intraoperative hemorrhage or arterial vasodilation. Both tachycardia and bradycardia are poorly tolerated. Tachycardia is problematic because (1) decreased ejection time translates into an increase in the stenotic valve gradient; and (2) perfusion (especially subendocardial) of the hypertrophied ventricle is limited at best. Bradycardia may substantially decrease cardiac output. Marked concentric left ventricular hypertrophy also has important implications. The myocardium is considerably less compliant; a normal amount of left ventricular filling results in filling pressures higher than those seen in a normally compliant heart (Fig. 68-3). The necessity of higher filling pressures renders the patient with aortic stenosis particularly vulnerable to hypovolemia as well as loss of sinus rhythm, which provides atrial augmentation to ventricular filling. A junctional tachycardia can be particularly aggravating for such patients (this can occasionally result after sudden vagolysis; e.g., after pancuronium).

Another problem is that left ventricular hypertrophy is a burden for coronary blood flow. Marcus et al.[118] demonstrated that in left ventricular hypertrophy, coronary autoregulation is used to maintain resting blood flow. Clinically, patients with long-standing aortic stenosis may experience angina even without coronary artery stenosis (Fig. 68-4).

Patients with left ventricular hypertrophy from any cause are at great risk if there should be a trigger of ventricular tachycardia or fibrillation. Resuscitation by closed chest massage and defibrillation may be fruitless because (1) the thickened ventricle can be difficult or impossible to defibrillate; (2) cardiopulmonary resuscitation (CPR) produces even worse subendocardial and midendocardial blood flow than usual; and (3) these patients are often older men who have increased A-P chest diameters. Immediately performing a sternotomy with open-chest massage while cannulating for bypass may be lifesaving.

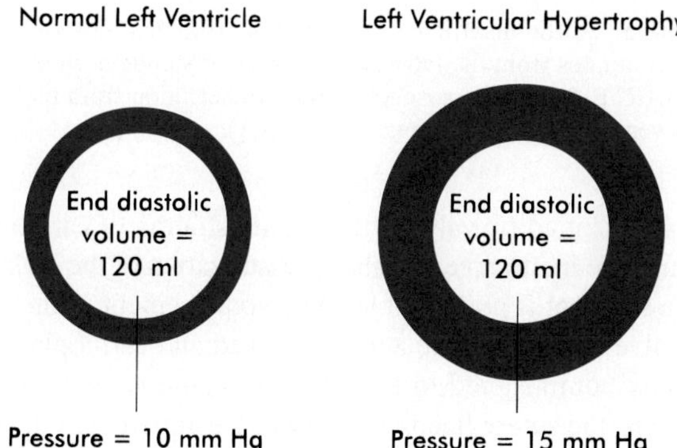

Fig. 68-3. Noncompliance of left ventricular hypertrophy in aortic stenosis. The figure indicates that the end-diastolic volume within each ventricle is similar. Because of the substantial thickening and noncompliance of the left ventricular wall in aortic stenosis, the end-diastolic pressure will be significantly higher than the normal ventricle.

Separation from cardiopulmonary bypass is greatly facilitated by a synchronous atrioventricular cardiac rhythm in such patients. Bleeding and volume replacement are important concerns after bypass in these patients, specifically because of the aortic suture line. Vigilance must also be maintained after bypass because of the potential for intracoronary air embolus, which is always a risk after valve-replacement procedures. The air seems to become trapped in the interstices of the left ventricle and may "break loose" later. Air traveling to the right coronary artery can produce sudden heart block, right ventricular dysfunction, and/or ST segment ischemic changes in the inferior cardiogram leads II, III, and aAF. Such air usually lodges in the right coronary artery because it is uppermost in the supine position, leaving the patient in a head-up tilt position during this critical period risks cerebral air embolus.

Aortic Valvular Insufficiency

Patients with aortic insufficiency present considerations that are distinct from patients with aortic stenosis.[39] Because left ventricular filling occurs forward from the left atrium and backward from the aorta, left ventricular dilatation occurs. The forward stroke volume is larger than normal, which contributes to a higher than normal systolic blood pressure. This is observed on physical examination as a "water-hammer" pulse. The net forward flow from the heart is the difference between the forward stroke volume and the backward regurgitant volume. Measurement of cardiac output by thermodilution technique is as valid as ever because blood flow through the right heart, where the thermodilution measurement is made, must be equal to the net forward flow of the left ventricle.

Regurgitation across the aortic valve during diastole causes diastolic blood pressure to be abnormally low and left ventricular end-diastolic pressure to be abnormally high. The amount of aortic regurgitation depends on the size of the orifice, the length of the diastole, and the diastolic pressure difference between the aorta and left ventricle.[42] Because regurgitation occurs during diastole, slower heart rates provide the opportunity for more backward flow.[64] If the diastolic interval is long enough, an equalization will occur between aortic diastolic blood pressure and left ventricular diastolic blood pressure, a situation known as *diastasis*. As the difference between aortic and left ventricular diastolic pressure decreases, so does the gradient for coronary perfusion. Faster heart rates are preferred to decrease regurgitation. Another factor is diastolic blood pressure. Hypertension can be expected to increase the magnitude of aortic insufficiency and to result in elevation of pulmonary arterial pressures. Systemic arterial vasodilators are advo-

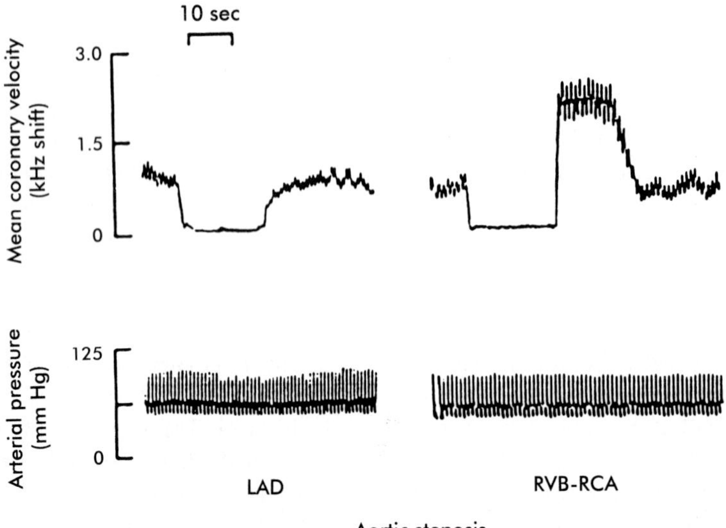

Fig. 68-4. Decreased coronary reserve in left ventricular hypertrophy. Transient occlusion and release of the left anterior descending artery (*LAD*), which supplies hypertrophied left ventricular myocardium in a patient with aortic stenosis, fails to show reactive hyperemia response. In contrast, occlusion and release of a right ventricular branch of the right coronary artery (RVB-BCA), which supplies the normal right ventricle, shows normal reactive hyperemia, indicating the presence of coronary reserve. (From Marcus ML, Doty D, Hiratzka LF, et al: Decreased coronary reserve in a mechanism for angina pectoris in patients with aortic stenosis and normal coronary arteries, *N Engl J Med* 307:1362, 1982.)

cated to increase forward flow in cases of aortic insufficiency, but afterload reduction therapy may be limited if low levels of myocardial perfusion pressure result. Often, vasodilators help the forward flow problem considerably, and do not result in impaired coronary perfusion (i.e., there is no ischemia).

The presence of aortic insufficiency also has implications for cardiopulmonary bypass. During bypass, the left ventricle will continue to fill and to eject blood that regurgitates backward across the incompetent aortic valve (Fig. 68-5). This pumping action of the left ventricle prevents distension. Ventricular fibrillation eliminates the pumping action, and soon the left ventricular pressure will equal the mean aortic pressure. This situation cannot be permitted, and so a left ventricular vent is ideally placed early after institution of cardiopulmonary bypass, usually via the right superior pulmonary vein, through the mitral valve, into the left ventricle. Unfortunately, although the vent may prevent ventricular distension, it provides a short-circuit pathway for blood to return to the bypass pump without perfusion of either the heart or the patient. Net perfusion to the patient is roughly the difference between the forward pump flow and the backward left ventricular vent flow. This situation may also result in low mean arterial pressures. Vasoconstrictors are likely to fail to increase blood pressure because an increase in the amount of aortic regurgitation to the vent may occur instead; that is, even less body perfusion may occur. Application of the aortic cross clamp between the incompetent aortic valve and the aortic inflow cannula from the bypass machine is the remedy. The next problem caused by the incompetent aortic valve is that administration of cardioplegia may be ineffective, because pressurization of the isolated aorta segment is not possible. When replacement of the aortic valve is planned, the aorta is opened and cardioplegia is directly administered to the coronary ostia. As with aortic stenosis, the suture line in the wall of the aorta raises the potential for postoperative bleeding and necessitates vigilant control of blood pressure.

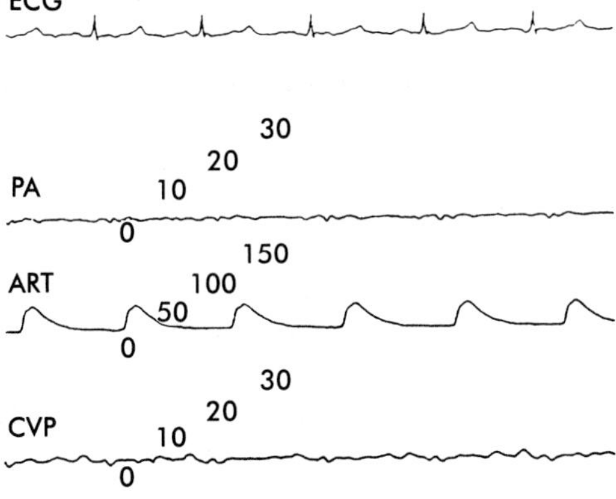

Fig. 68-5. Aortic insufficiency on bypass. Note that pulsatile flow continues from the left ventricle to the systemic aorta pressure (*ART*), despite the absence of pulsatile ejection from the right ventricle to the pulmonary artery (*PA*).

Mitral Stenosis

Narrowing of the mitral orifice (whatever the cause) requires that a significant pressure gradient between the left atrium and the left ventricle be present for blood to flow across the valve. Left ventricular filling is typically inadequate in patients with mitral stenosis, whereas left atrial filling is excessive. The patient thus may suffer from a reduced cardiac output as well as from pulmonary congestion. Dyspnea occurs because increased left atrial and pulmonary venous pressure causes blood to be sequestered in the now-stiffened lung. A key point is that flow across the restrictive mitral orifice occurs during diastole. Tachycardia, which shortens diastole and limits the time available for flow through the mitral valve, can be expected to worsen pulmonary congestion and may cause systemic hypotension (Fig. 68-6).

In early stages of the disease, exercise tolerance is limited by dyspnea of pulmonary congestion. Later, fatigue caused by reduced cardiac output contributes to a severe limitation of activity. Acute onset of atrial fibrillation is particularly problematic because tachycardia and loss of atrial contraction combine to suddenly worsen the ability of the left atrium to empty into the left ventricle. Whether deterioration is primarily caused by loss of atrial contraction or simply by tachycardia has been debated.[138,180] It is clear, however, that sinus tachycardia alone can be detrimental.

Another key point is that a pressure gradient must exist between the left atrium and the left ventricle to drive blood across the stenotic mitral orifice. An elevated pulmonary capillary wedge pressure (PCWP) will be expected. Whereas the PCWP does not accurately measure left ventricular end-diastolic pressure in mitral stenosis, a low PCWP is likely to indicate significantly reduced left ventricular filling. This especially applies to patients who have received preoperative diuretic therapy. Diuretics may have improved dyspnea, but are likely to have reduced the gradient between the left atrium and left ventricle. The induction of anesthesia and positive-pressure ventilation will further reduce venous return and may substantially compromise left ventricle filling. These factors, as well as peripheral vasodilation from anesthesia, may combine to produce a rather spectacular hypotension. The presence of a low PA wedge pressure before the induction of anesthesia may be a warning sign. Although a reduction in PCWP is often considered a goal in cardiac anesthesia, in mitral stenosis this is not necessarily the case. Reduced coronary blood flow is not necessarily related to the PA capillary wedge pressure but more appropriately to left ventricular diastolic pressure, which should be significantly lower. Because patients with mitral stenosis may have pulmonary hypertension and/or right ventricular hypertrophy, the central venous pressure should not be expected to be indicative of the PA wedge pressure.

When left ventricular filling is restricted because of mitral stenosis, it is unlikely that the left ventricle will be able to increase forward cardiac output significantly if peripheral vasodilation occurs. For this reason, "afterload reduction" with nitroprusside is unlikely to improve cardiac output in mitral stenosis; this is in contrast to its demonstrated effectiveness in mitral regurgitation. Although Stone et al.[179] suggested that nitroprusside might be effective for patients with mitral stenosis, this was only true after systemic and pulmonary vasoconstriction had increased as a result of surgical stimulation under "light" anesthesia. Indeed, when hemodynamics under nitroprusside were compared to "preinduction" values, cardiac index actually decreased. A more controlled study by Bolen et al.[19] demonstrated that despite reduction of mean arterial pressure by 10% to 25% with nitroprusside, cardiac output was not augmented in patients with mitral stenosis.

It is always a mistake for the anesthesiologist to think of valvular heart disease in isolated terms; that is, to think only about the valve itself and assume that the ventricle would be normal if only the valve were repaired. This is obvious in aortic stenosis but may not be obvious in mitral stenosis. The latter disease is seldom just mitral disease. Rheumatic disease, for example, is heart disease. The left ventricle is often decidedly abnormal. Using contrast dye ventriculography, Heller and Carleton[70] demonstrated that patients with pure mitral stenosis had significantly lower ejection fractions than normal patients and that contraction was abnormal in the posterobasal region. They hypothesized that a rigid "mitral complex" consisting of the valve leaflets, ring, chordae tendineae, and papillary muscles immobilized this region.[70] This view was previously suggested by autopsy studies.[24,61] To be sure, some or much of the pulmonary con-

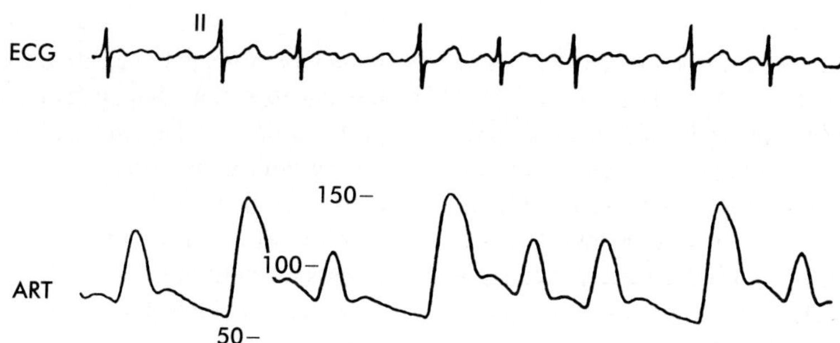

Fig. 68-6. Tachycardia in mitral stenosis. The tracing illustrates that rapid heart rates are poorly tolerated in mitral stenosis. Reduction of diastolic time prevents adequate left ventricular filling and resultant reduction in stroke volume.

gestion is caused by poor valve function, but it is wrong to assume that fixing the valve will solve all problems. In fact, the stenotic valve may have been "protecting" a poorly contractile left ventricle, which, after the valve is repaired or replaced, will fail under the newly increased forward flow/pressure loading.

In longstanding mitral stenosis, chronic left atrial and pulmonary venous pressure elevations seem to produce changes in pulmonary vasculature such that pulmonary resistance is increased. Right ventricular hypertrophy and, later, tricuspid insufficiency occurs. At this point, two sites obstruct left ventricular filling: the stenotic mitral valve and the pulmonary vasculature. The hypertrophied right ventricle may suffer from impaired coronary autoregulation and the warming effects of the operating room lights, which antagonize cardioplegia protection. Severe right ventricular dysfunction may occur at separation from bypass. Whereas younger patients can be managed effectively by anesthetic techniques that avoid tachycardia and excessive myocardial depression, elderly patients with long-standing mitral stenosis and pulmonary hypertension present major challenges. Avoiding the acute onset of atrial fibrillation, yet maintaining relatively high heart rates (because the left ventricle is in failure), and avoiding additional pulmonary vasoconstriction, if possible, are hallmarks. A common error of the postbypass period is to assume that a low PCWP is a sign of hypovolemia. Similarly, evidence of an "empty left ventricle" by TEE is not diagnostic of hypovolemia. Both wedge pressure and left ventricle filling may be decreased because of right ventricular failure or severe pulmonary vasoconstriction. Failure to appreciate these possibilities will prevent appropriate inotrope and/or vasodilator therapy. Worse, presumed hypovolemia may lead to inappropriate fluid infusion, which further aggravates right ventricular dysfunction. Instead, right ventricular function must also be assessed by monitoring the central venous pressure. In patients with pulmonary hypertension and/or right ventricular dysfunction, correction of metabolic acidosis and hypercapnia is important. Consideration should be given to inotropic agents such as isoproterenol whose predominant beta-adrenergic stimulation may aid in dilating the pulmonary vasculature. Intra-aortic balloon counterpulsation may provide support for right ventricular dysfunction by improving coronary perfusion.

Mitral Insufficiency

This valvular heart lesion also presents with a wide spectrum of physiology.[151] Appropriate function requires coordination of six components, including the left atrial wall, annulus, leaflets, chordae tendineae, papillary muscles, and left ventricular wall.[143] The most symptomatic patients are those with acute mitral insufficiency caused by recent disruption of the mitral valve apparatus as a result of endocarditis or worse, MI. In such cases, left ventricular blood regurgitates into a normal, noncompliant left atrium and exposes the lung to high pressures that are capable of causing pulmonary edema. Stress and apprehension from dyspnea is a potent stimulus for sympathetic stimulation, which further aggravates pulmonary congestion by increasing blood pressure. In contrast, patients with long-standing mitral insufficiency have markedly enlarged and compliant left atriums that are capable of accepting the jet of mitral insufficiency without increases in pulmonary venous pressure.[20] Such patients are likely to have atrial fibrillation and reduced cardiac output.[22]

Despite significant mitral regurgitation, these patients may be relatively asymptomatic at rest although limited in their ability to exercise. The degree of mitral insufficiency is often estimated from cardiac catheterization. A qualitative system is based on the degree of opacification of the left atrium when contrast dye is injected into the left ventricle:[65,164]

- Mild (1+): A trace of contrast dye is visible in the atrium but clears during each beat and never opacifies the entire left atrium.
- Moderate (2+): Contrast dye does not clear with each beat and generally opacifies the left atrium after several beats although opacification is not equal to that of the left ventricle.
- Moderately severe (3+): Left atrium is completely opacified and opacification becomes more dense with each cardiac cycle.
- Severe (4+): Contrast agent completely opacifies the atrium during the first cardiac cycle.

In acute mitral insufficiency, giant V waves representing abrupt pressure rises in the left atrium can be demonstrated in the PA wedge tracing. Vasodilator therapy with nitroprusside has been demonstrated to reduce these pressure waves with corresponding improvement in forward cardiac output[31,66,69] (Fig. 68-7). Nitroglycerin therapy for ischemic papillary muscle dysfunction has demonstrated that reduction of these pressure waves accompanied relief of anginal symptoms. Nevertheless, the presence and height of V waves does not necessarily predict the degree of mitral insufficiency for several reasons.[49,63,144]

First, the normal V wave, which represents left atrial filling from the pulmonary veins, may become prominent in circumstances of fluid overload or left ventricular failure (Fig. 68-8). Second, in patients with chronic mitral insufficiency and a large, dilated, and compliant left atrium, a substantial amount of regurgitation can occur without a rise in left atrial pressure.[20] Echocardiography with Doppler techniques is exquisitely sensitive for detecting even trivial mitral regurgitation, but accurate quantification has been a problem.[123,146,174] Biplane TEE can quantify mitral insufficiency with good correlation to that determined at cardiac catheterization.[135,200]

Mortality from valvular heart surgery is typically higher in patients with mitral insufficiency than in those with other valve lesions. Inclusion of patients with acute mitral insufficiency contributes significantly. The state of the myocardium is an important consideration.[36] For example, acute mitral insufficiency presents with abrupt onset of severe pulmonary congestion. If this is caused by a ruptured myxomatous chordae tendineae or endocarditis, and if left ventricu-

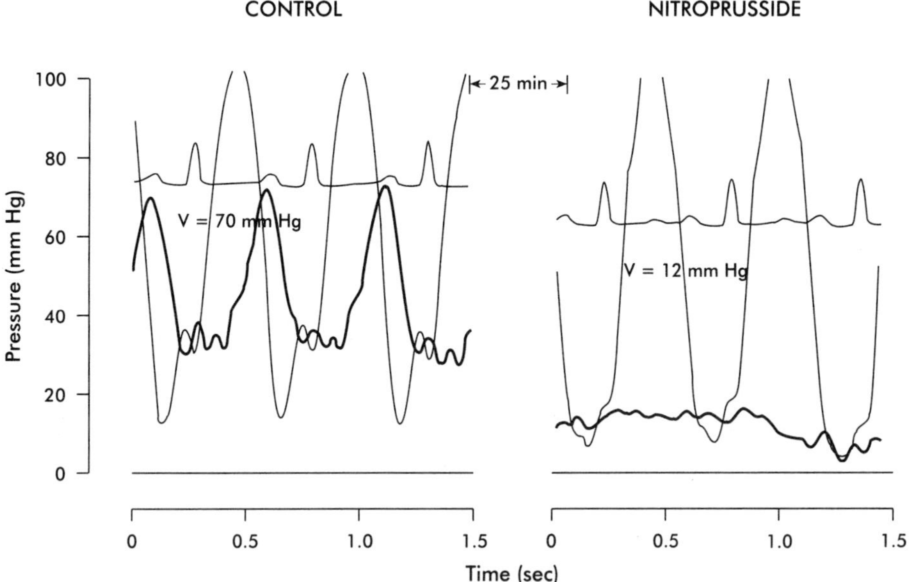

Fig. 68-7. Mitral insufficiency and nitroprusside. Left ventricular (*thin line*) and left atrial (*thick line*) pressures are shown. *Left panel*, a prominent regurgitant wave is present. After vasodilator therapy (*right panel*), the regurgitant wave is gone. (Redrawn from Chatterjeek, Parmley WW, Swan HJC, et al: Beneficial effects of vasodilator agents in severe mitral regurgitation due to dysfunction of subvalvular apparatus, *Circulation* 48:684, 1973.)

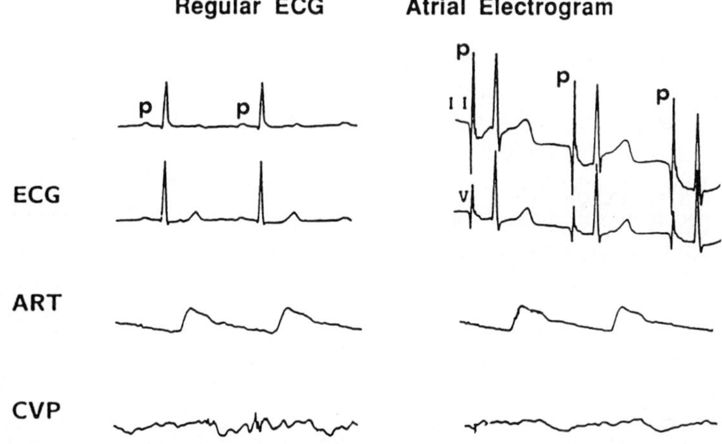

Fig. 68-8. An atrial electrogram. In **A,** the conventional ECG tracing is displayed. The rhythm is sinus but the p waves are difficult to see. In **B,** the same patient is monitored with the atrial electrogram modification of the ECG. Note that the p waves are much more prominent. From Gomez MN, Ross AF, Tinker JH: Special monitoring considerations in cardiac anesthesia. In Blitt CD, Hines RL, editors: *Monitoring in anesthesia and critical care medicine*, ed 3, New York, 1995, Churchill Livingstone.

lar function is otherwise normal, surgery may be well tolerated. In contrast, insufficiency from papillary muscle dysfunction secondary to acute MI represents significant surgical risk because of associated acute injury of the left ventricle. All patients with mitral insufficiency have, in essence, a double outer left ventricle; that is, a low-resistance exit for left ventricular ejection. For this reason, measurement of a "normal" ejection fraction may belie some degree of ventricular dysfunction.[156,192]

An ejection fraction less than 40% in patients with marked mitral regurgitation indicates advanced myocardial dysfunction. Replacement of the mitral valve closes this pathway and forces the left ventricle to eject entirely into the high-pressure aorta.[22,136] Resultant postbypass ventricular failure theoretically should benefit by afterload reduction.[157] Unfortunately, reduction in coronary perfusion may limit the effectiveness of this strategy. The intra-aortic balloon pump simultaneously provides afterload reduction for the left ventricle and augmentation of coronary perfusion pressure; it will often be needed, especially in patients with acute mitral insufficiency.

Another problem with mitral valvular surgery that is relevant to anesthesia involves with the size of the left atrium. Long-standing mitral regurgitation results in a large left atrium, as does mitral stenosis. This large left atrium allows easier mitral replacement or repair because exposure via sternotomy is good. In sharp contrast, the patient with acute mitral regurgitation often does not have an enlarged left atrium. The left atrium lies posterior, and to replace or repair the mitral valve via sternotomy, fairly severe retraction may need to be used. This, in turn, may lead to heart block and relatively inadequate myocardial preservation during cross-clamp. All these factors portend of the difficulty in getting the left ventricle to pump during emergence from bypass.

The presence of coexisting CAD with mitral valve disease significantly affects the prognosis. In the Coronary Artery Surgery Study (CASS), patients undergoing mitral valve replacement and CABG surgery at 15 centers during the years 1975 to 1978 demonstrated an operative mortality of almost 24%.[88] Czer et al.[37] reported on a group of 419 patients who underwent mitral valve replacement. In patients who had no associated coronary disease, the 30-day mortality was 4.2%. In patients who had CAD, the 30-day mortality was 13.9.% if revascularization was performed versus 29.2% when revascularization was not performed. Survival at 8-year follow-up was 68%, 44%, and 15% respectively. Because of the high operative mortality of combined mitral valve replacement and coronary bypass, Arcidi et al.[4] favored coronary bypass surgery alone for a group of 58 patients, the majority of whom had an ischemic basis for mitral insufficiency. A remarkable 3.4% hospital mortality rate and a 5-year survival of 77% were reported. These results were compared with an unmatched group of patients who underwent combined mitral valve replacement and coronary artery bypass surgery at the same institution; these patients had a hospital mortality of 25% and a 5-year survival of 31%.

MONITORING STRATEGIES IN CARDIAC ANESTHESIA

Cardiac anesthesia has pioneered widespread application of several important monitoring techniques for patients with heart disease. The necessity to understand cardiac function during cardiac surgery resulted in the widespread use of PA artery catheters. Popularization of TEE was also due in large part to the efforts of cardiac anesthesiologists. Controversies as to which monitor is better, safer, and/or more cost-effective tend to minimize the progress made in this area. Consider the following 1947 remarks by Hitzig, concerning the value of circulation times:[71]

> In heart failure, the arm-to-lung and the arm-to-tongue times are useful in determining the segment of the circulation in which blood flow is retarded. Thus, in left heart failure . . . the arm-to-lung time was within the normal range whereas the lung-to-tongue time was often enormously increased. Similarly, in right heart failure secondary to left heart failure, both the arm-to-lung and lung-to-tongue times were increased, and the degree of increase paralleled the severity of the heart failure.

The questionable accuracy of these early methods was compounded by questions of safety. Substances used in the past to assess cardiac performance and the anticipated effects of these substances included: (1) histamine causing facial flush, dyspnea, and violent headache; (2) sodium cyanide causing sudden deepening of respiration; (3) radioactive sodium detected by a Geiger counter; (4) saccharine yielding a sweet taste; and (5) IV ether that caused "wavelike" paresthesias if a right-to-left shunt directed the gaseous substance to the brain. Today good outcomes are anticipated and accurate continuous monitoring allows specific therapeutic interventions. Monitoring techniques for cardiac anesthesia include "routine" monitors such as pulse oximetry, capnography, esophageal stethoscope, nerve stimulator, blood pressure cuff, temperature probe, and urinary catheter. More specialized monitoring functions, including multilead computer analyzed ECG, direct arterial pressure, cardiac filling pressures, and ventricular function, will be addressed next.

Electrocardiogram

The electrocardiogram (ECG) is a standard of care for administration of anesthesia. In cardiac anesthesia, the ECG is particularly useful. Abnormalities of ST segment are recognized indicators of ischemia.[194] ST segment and T wave changes frequently occur.[93] Changes in cardiac rhythm and conduction are also noted. The ECG is essential for documenting adequacy of cardioplegia as well as resumption of cardiac rhythm during reperfusion.

Ideally, multiple limb leads as well as precordial leads should be available for analysis. The V_5 electrode has been noted to be most useful in monitoring for ischemia because of its orientation with respect to the anterolateral left ventricular wall. Leads II, III, and aVF are oriented to be better monitors for inferior ischemia. Intraoperative ECG monitoring for cardiac cases should include simultaneous display of V_5 and lead II. Lead II is selected from the inferior leads II, III, and aVF because of its use in assessing cardiac rhythm. Specifically, a sinus node pacemaker mechanism typically produces an upright P wave in limb lead II. This may be helpful to distinguish a sinus node mechanism from a different ectopic atrial focus. Sophisticated computerized ST segment programmed analysis has been advocated to assess ST segment changes. It is not clear whether these sensitive methods are the best monitors for ischemia, because changes in cardiac orientation can occur by sternotomy, internal mammary artery dissection, table rotation, and physical manipulation of the heart. There is no doubt that the ability to make a printed record of the ECG is useful. Comparison of hard copies of various ECG leads clearly facilitates decisions as to whether specific changes in ST segment, T wave, PR interval, or QRS configuration have occurred.

A useful addition to ECG monitoring for cardiac surgical patients is a technique that allows specific monitoring and/or augmentation of atrial electrical activity. Various techniques include use of an esophageal electrode, atrial pacing leads incorporated in some PA catheters, or directly attached atrial pacing wires.[83,193,201] Augmented atrial electrical activity is often useful if the standard ECG fails to clearly demonstrate P waves because it ensures that the patient gets the hemodynamic benefit of atrial contraction if such is possible (Fig. 68-8).

Arterial Pressure Monitoring

Rapid changes in blood pressure and the necessity for arterial blood gas analysis have made monitoring of arterial pressure by an indwelling arterial catheter a standard of practice for cardiac anesthesia. The blood pressure cuff is slow and is useless when cardiopulmonary bypass eliminates pulsatility. The optimal site for arterial cannulation is controversial. Some avoid left-sided radial artery cannulation because internal mammary artery dissection may cause some distortion of the tracing. Our experience suggests that the direction of sternal retraction plays an important role in this problem. Techniques that lift the sternum upward preserve the radial artery tracing, whereas techniques that retract the sternum laterally distort the monitor. Other factors may also influence site of arterial cannulation including presence of previous brachial artery cutdown for cardiac catheterization, known discrepancy in blood pressure between arms, and whether the patient is right- or left-handed. Femoral or dorsalis pedis pedal artery cannulation can be used, as can the brachial or axillary arteries. Because the brachial artery is the only artery supplying the lower arm, this would not be our first choice. The risk of bleeding into the brachial plexus because of systemic heparinization limits enthusiasm for the axillary artery site. Lower-extremity sites are not recommended in circumstances where coarctation of the aorta or aortoiliac vascular disease would render the monitor inaccurate. All direct arterial cannulations should be accompanied by safety considerations, especially the avoidance of cannulation of arteries that supply regions of compromised circulation. The demonstration of a favorable Allen's test before cannulating a radial artery is reassuring although evidence of its importance has been questioned. The catheter diameter, wrist circumference, and duration of use have been related to various risks of radial artery catheterization.[10–12] A radial artery catheter that is "positional" at the beginning of the case *is likely* to be "positional" again, particularly at the time of weaning from bypass or when blood gas analysis is desired. Use of "arm boards" to extend the wrist is avoided because of the likelihood of severely impeding the ulnar circulation to the hand. Instead, our practice is to change "positional" catheters at the beginning of the case. Flushing of arterial catheters must consider that retrograde flow toward the cerebral circulation occurs, so the volumes used must be small and intermittent.

Studies of aortic dynamics have provided information regarding the peripheral pulse.[132] Pressure waves are typically different in a peripheral artery than in the central aorta because of the summation of the forward pressure wave and the backward reflected pressure wave. Specifically, the measured systolic pressure is usually higher and the diastolic pressure is lower in a peripheral arterial site than that measured in the ascending aorta. In contrast, the mean arterial pressure remains relatively constant.[67] Stern et al.[176] have demonstrated that after cardiopulmonary bypass, the relationship between the measured systolic pressure of the radial artery and the ascending aorta is reversed. Specifically, the measured systolic pressure in the ascending aorta may be greater than that of the radial artery. Our experience is that the difference can be substantial and this possibility should be considered when persistent "hypotension" by radial artery pressure monitoring appears inconsistent with other assessments of cardiac performance. The phenomenon resolves over time.

In some circumstances, two separate sites of intra-arterial pressure monitoring are desirable. A specific instance is the repair of a descending thoracic aneurysm. Because of cross-clamping of the descending thoracic aorta, pressure measured in an upper extermity may demonstrate hypertension. However, vasodilator agents such as nitroprusside may not be appropriate because below the cross clamp arterial pressure may be quite low. Because of concern for adequate spinal cord and renal perfusion, placement of an arterial catheter in the dorsal pedal artery or the femoral artery allows monitoring of pressure distal to the cross clamp.[96] When partial, femoral vein to femoral artery cardiopulmonary bypass is used to provide perfusion distal to the thoracic aortic cross clamp, a lower-extremity arterial line in addition to an upper-extremity arterial line is extremely useful to guide the partial bypass flow (Fig. 68-9).

Measures of Cardiac Performance

The pulmonary artery catheter remains a popular method of hemodynamic monitoring.[131] This device makes possible assessment of filling pressures of the right and left ventricles, PA pressures, and cardiac output. The PA catheter allows dependable central venous access for administration of heparin and potent vasoactive drugs. Controversy about the PA catheter has focused on the lack of studies showing statistically significant positive effects on outcomes.[152,185] Many investigations have demonstrated that direct measurements of cardiac filling pressures and cardiac outputs are much more accurate than "clinical judgment." In centers experienced in PA catheter use, the incidence of important complications is remarkably low.[166] Use of the PA catheter has eliminated the complications that formerly occurred as a result of catheters surgically placed in the left and right atria, and the complications associated with the old practice of infusion of potent vasoactive drugs into peripheral veins.

A frequently asked question is whether the monitoring of central venous pressure is as useful as the monitoring of PCWP. Mangano[114] clinically demonstrated that in patients with normal ejection fractions, measurements of central venous pressure (CVP) correlated well with measurements of

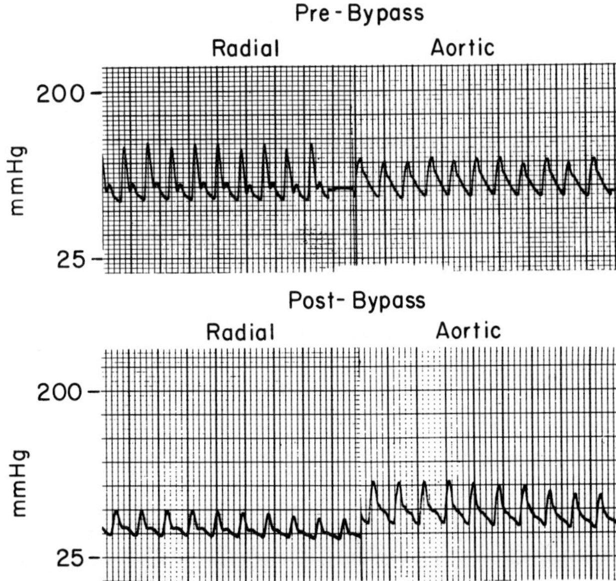

Fig. 68-9. Radial artery versus central aortic blood pressure. Prior to cardiopulmonary bypass (prebypass) the systolic blood pressure is higher when measured in the radial artery than when measured in the central aorta. Immediately after bypass (postbypass), this relationship is reversed and the systolic pressure is higher in the aorta than the radial artery. From Stern DH, Gerson JI, Allen FB, Parker FB: Can we trust the direct radial artery pressure immediately following cardiopulmonary bypass? *Anesthesiology* 62:557, 1985.

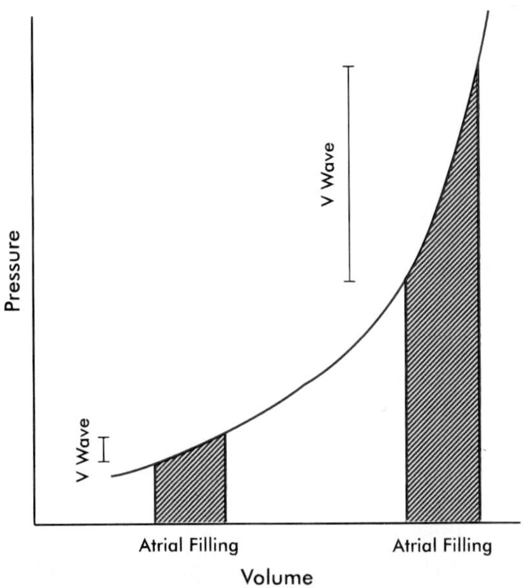

Fig. 68-10. Left atrial pressure-volume relationships. A hypothetic pressure-volume relation of the left atrium is depicted. At the low pressure end of the curve, inflow of blood, represented by the hatched bars, results in a small increase in pressure, i.e., a small V wave; at the high pressure end of the curve, inflow of blood results in a large V wave. (From Grossman W: *Cardiac catheterization and angiography*, ed 3, Philadelphia, 1986, Lea & Febiger.)

PCWP. In patients with poor ejection fractions, measurements of CVP were poorly correlated with measurements of PCWP. These findings have been used to argue that CVP monitoring is as effective as monitoring by the PA catheter, a contention not necessarily intended by the author. Editorial remarks pointed out that unless the exact relationship was known between the CVP and wedge pressure for a particular patient, knowledge of CVP alone would be insufficient to predict the PA wedge pressure.[107] Further, patients may have good ejection fractions preoperatively, whereas after the ischemic cross-clamp required for cardiac surgery, postbypass ventricular function may be severely compromised.

Most cardiac anesthesiologists (not all) strongly believe that monitoring of the PCWP reveals critical information that would not have been available by the measurement of CVP. This is especially true when coronary perfusion pressures are critically important. Another example is the diagnosis of pulmonary vasoconstriction.[100] In this circumstance, PCWP is considerably lower than PA diastolic pressure and may even be lower than the CVP. This will occur in circumstances such as hypercapnia, metabolic acidosis, bronchospasm, blood product administration, and protamine reactions. Systemic hypotension will occur because of inadequate left ventricular filling as indicated by the low wedge pressure. Despite this the CVP is elevated because of the pulmonary vasoconstriction opposing the right ventricular ejection. Monitoring the CVP alone might misleadingly suggest that the systemic hypotension was caused by myocardial failure. Information from the PA catheter would correctly identify the problem as pulmonary vasoconstriction, would dictate an entirely different treatment, and then allow monitoring of the therapy (see Fig. 68-10).

Another such application uses the shape of the PA wedge pressure tracing to provide information. Atrial contraction, mitral valve closure caused by left ventricular contraction, and atrial filling occur in each cardiac cycle and inscribe A, C, and V waves in the wedge pressure tracing.[65] Changes in the appearance of these pressure waves can provide useful information. For example, volume overload or decreased compliance because of left ventricular ischemia[64] typically causes enlargement of these waves (Fig. 68-11). Abnormalities of right ventricular function can similarly alter the appearance of the CVP tracing. A useful fact is that these alterations in the pressure wave tracing exist whether or not the pressure transducer is exactly at the level of the atrium. This facilitates verification that the numeric output from the transducer reflects the condition of the patient. For example, a numeric wedge pressure of 5 mm Hg suggests hypovolemia. However, if the wedge pressure tracing demonstrates large A and V waves, it is likely that the true wedge pressure is considerably higher and that the transducer is incorrectly placed above the level of the right atrium.

Many patients have successfully undergone cardiac surgery with CVP monitoring alone. The CVP monitor also has several specifically useful applications. It can be used as a water manometer to verify and calibrate electronic transducers. Because of the risk of air entrainment, this must be rapid and cannot be used during cardiopulmonary bypass. The CVP is also useful in detection of junctional rhythms and heart block. The onset of junctional rhythm can be heralded by the appearance of distinct "cannon A waves" in the CVP tracing (Fig. 68-12).

The PA catheter allows determinations of cardiac output by thermodilution; these are useful to assess cardiac function and the effects of interventions. Combinations of cardiac output and arterial pressure measurements allow calculations of systemic and pulmonary vascular resistances. Additional functions incorporated into some PA catheters include continuous assessment of mixed venous O_2 saturation or continuous right ventricular stroke volume. Use of these added functions is even more controversial than the use of PA catheters themselves. Mixed venous O_2 saturation changes follow output changes *only* if peripheral (and cardiac) O_2 demand remains constant and blood hemoglobin level is stable. Because this may *not* happen during cardiac surgery or in the immediate recovery period, use of these catheters may be quite misleading. At the least, their considerable extra cost should be taken into account.

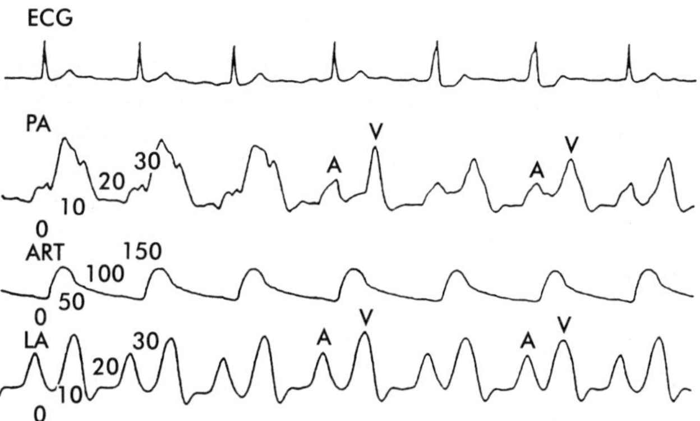

Fig. 68-11. Noncompliant left ventricle. When the pulmonary artery catheter (*PA*) is in wedge position, distinct A and V waves are seen. Simultaneous monitoring of left atrial catheter (*LA*) demonstrates that the wedge tracing is of reasonable fidelity.

The use of the "SVR" calculation also deserves comment. Many physicians insist on this calculation and base therapy on the numerical result. The problem is that considerable variation occurs simply because of the size of the patient. For example, consider two patients both of whom have a blood pressure of 120/60 and CVP of 5. Patient A weighs 100 kg and has a cardiac output of 8 l/min whereas patient B weighs 50 kg and has a cardiac output of 4 l/min. Calculation of the systemic vascular resistance suggests that patient A is vasodilated whereas patient B is vasoconstricted. In fact, neither may be the case! Attempts to standardize the calculation for body size may not improve the situation. Should one calculate an "SVR index" by substituting "cardiac index" for "cardiac output" in the equation? Alternatively, should one calculate an "SVR index" by dividing the "SVR" by the body surface area? Simple arithmetic will demonstrate that very different results are obtained. **Our preference is to use individual trends of blood pressure and cardiac output to assess a particular patient.** Physical examination for warm versus cool extremities is a useful method for determining vasodilation versus constriction and applies to all patients regardless of body size.

A number of researchers have indicated that passage of a PA catheter can be associated with temporary right bundle branch block (RBBB).[42,110] In patients with preexisting left bundle branch block (LBBB), complete heart block has also

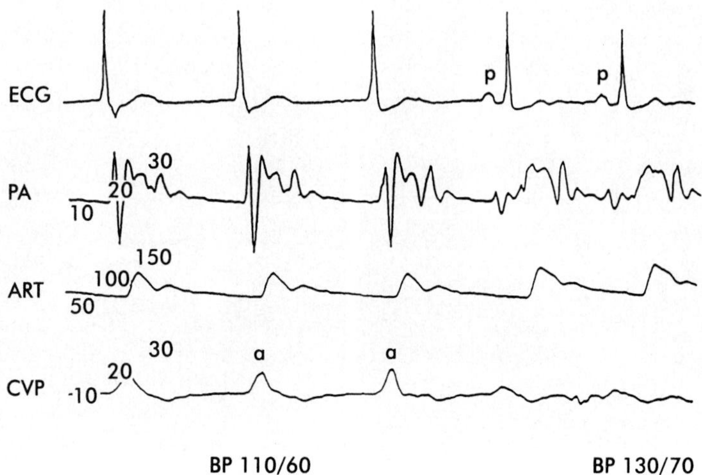

Fig. 68-12. Cannon A waves. A junctional rhythm is accompanied by a low systemic pressure and "cannon A waves" in the central venous pressure tracing. The return to sinus rhythm coincides with disappearance of the cannon waves and a rise in arterial blood pressure. (From Ross A, Roberts SL, Tinker JT: Monitoring in cardiac anesthesia. In Blitt CD, editor: *Monitoring in anesthesia and critical care medecine*, ed 2, New York, 1990, Churchill-Livingstone.)

been reported,[181] leading to the recommendation that temporary prophylactic pacing wires be inserted before introduction of the PA catheter. Recently, Morris et al.[125] reported that PA catheterization in 47 consecutive patients with LBBB resulted in no episode of complete heart block during passage of the catheter, although 5 cases of heart block were noted before or after its removal. The authors concluded that the incidence of complete heart block occurring during introduction of the PA catheter in patients with LBBB is extremely low. However, considering that the incidence of transient RBBB during PA catheterization may be only 6%, the population of Morris et al.[125] may be too small to draw conclusions. Using a PA catheter that includes pacing wires is a sensible option for cardiac patients with preexisting LBBB.[201] Transthoracic Zoll pacing is another alternative.

Transesophageal Echocardiography

This technique uses several exciting developments in assessing cardiac function.[189] The proximity of ultrasonic probe to the left atrium facilitates easy and exquisite monitoring of mitral valve function (Fig. 68-13). Doppler technology with color enhancement of flow velocity patterns has made TEE a sensitive monitor for mitral insufficiency. It is important to remember that *flow velocity* is not the same as *flow.* Indeed, through a large orifice a larger flow can move with a slower velocity. The echocardiogram is also useful for determining regional ventricular wall motion abnormalities. Although it has been contended that this is a more sensitive method for detecting myocardial ischemia than the ECG, unfortunately afterload changes without ischemia also produce wall motion changes. Other applications of TEE include estimates of ventricular volumes, ejection fraction, integrity of the intra-atrial and interventricular septa, and presence of myocardial thrombosis. Major negative aspects of TEE are the enormous cost and complexity of the equipment. It is also problematic to determine the exact cause of the regional wall motion abnormalities detected because these may occur with ischemia, alterations in loading conditions, or circumstances of intraventricular conduction defects and paced rhythms.[170,171] TEE is regarded by some to be a noninvasive monitor, but there have been reports of esophageal injuries in intubated patients.

Applications for TEE include those presented by Katz et al.[84] who reported in 1992 that protruding atheromas of the aortic arch identified by TEE increased the risk of stroke in elderly patients undergoing cardiopulmonary bypass. Atheromas with mobile components were particulary high risk. An exciting potential application of echocardiography is with the use of sonicated albumin as a contrast agent to view tissue perfusion. Kaul et al.[85] compared myocardial contrast echocardiography with radiolabeled microspheres in an animal study. Here blood flow to endocardium versus epicardium as defined by microspheres did not correlate well to myocardial contrast echocardiography.[85] A disadvantage of the TEE has been difficulty in obtaining on line, quantitative information about ventricular function. New technology called automated border detection will allow continuous determination of the left ventricular ejection fraction.[60] This technique has been used in combination with pressure measurements to generate pres-

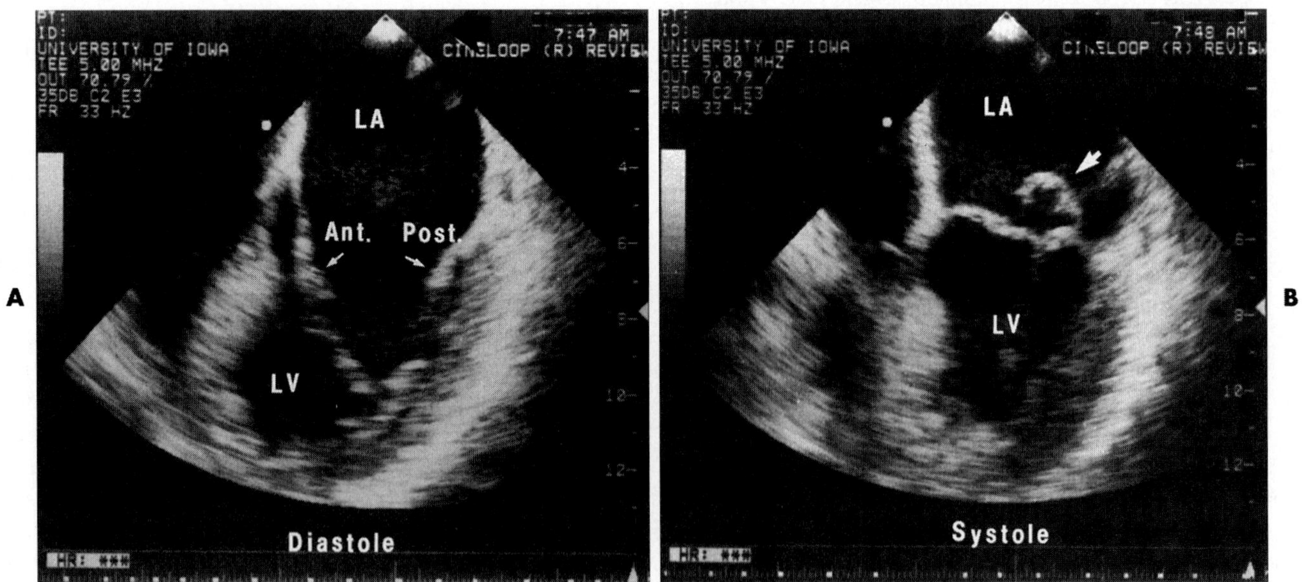

Fig. 68-13. A and B, Transesophageal echocardiography monitoring for surgical repair of the mitral valve. Prior to cardiopulmonary bypass, the posterior leaflet of the mitral valve (post.) prolapses into the left atrium (LA) during systole (arrow). LV = left ventricle. From Gomez MN, Ross AF, Tinker JH: Special monitoring considerations in cardiac anesthesia. In Blitt CD, Hines RL, editors: *Monitoring in anesthesia and critical care medicine*, ed 3, New York, 1995, Churchill-Livingstone.

sure-area relationships as a means to better assess ventricular contractility.[59]

A long-standing debate has been whether the TEE or the PA catheter is a superior monitor. For example, proponents of TEE contend that its ability to provide visual assessment of ventricular volumes results in a better assessment of ventricular filling than do pressure measurements derived from the PA catheter. Specifically, measurement of ventricular filling pressure may be misleading if a change in compliance has occurred. Thus an increase in filling pressure may not be associated with an increase in ventricular volume. TEE that directly visualizes the ventricular chamber would more accurately assess volume status.

Whether or not this translates into better therapy is not clear. Suppose, for example, that myocardial ischemia causes decreased ventricular compliance which results in an increase in wedge pressure. Administration of nitroglycerin would be the likely (and appropriate) response. Would TEE volume measurements, unaffected by pressure and compliance issues, indicate the same need for nitroglycerin? The reason for therapy is precisely because the end-diastolic *pressures* have increased, decreasing subendocardial coronary perfusion.

Rather than establishing the superiority of one method over the other, the TEE and the PA catheter may be seen as having complementary advantages. Comparisons between the two monitoring techniques appear to have been influenced by the biases of the proponents. A recent development in TEE uses a biplane transesophageal imaging transducer, which permits two perpendicular scanning planes that allow perpendicular cross-sections of the heart to be imaged. If two separate views of the heart are possible, in the future computerized assembly of images may provide three dimensional real-time images of cardiac function. Although echo technology is exciting, widespread application may depend on the production of devices that are smaller, less expensive, less complex to operate, and durable enough to withstand the rigors of daily use in the operating room.

Other Monitors

Some aspects of cardiac anesthesia might benefit from additional monitoring techniques. The use of primary narcotic anesthetics has raised the question of the usefulness of an intraoperative awareness monitor. The use of the electroencephalogram (EEG) has been attempted (and disputed) for this purpose as well as to monitor for emboli during cardiopulmonary bypass. Several recent EEG modifications are currently under evaluation. Obviously, therapy for intraoperative awareness is available. Optimal therapy for EEG abnormalities during cardiopulmonary bypass is not understood. Should the full array of EEG electrodes be used or are a few leads sufficient? Can operating room electrical interference be overcome? Transcranial Doppler measurements have been used to facilitate diagnoses of central nervous system (CNS) insults during cardiopulmonary bypass. Like the EEG, the use of transcranial Doppler blood flow would be significantly enhanced if effective therapeutic interventions for the detected abnormalities were understood and proved effective. Stroke following cardiopulmonary bypass is an infrequent but devastating complication.[150]

CARDIOPULMONARY BYPASS

The cardiopulmonary bypass machine supports the respiratory and circulatory functions of the body while surgery is performed upon the heart. The early pioneer of cardiopulmonary bypass, John Gibbon, described that the "ultimate objective" was to be able to operate inside the heart under direct vision. How well this objective was achieved is debatable because his early apparatus maintained a perfused and beating heart. Nonetheless, Gibbon's description indicates that basic cardiorespiratory support goals were essentially the same as in todays practice:

> . . . . support of the cardiorespiratory functions consists in removing venous blood from some peripheral vein continuously, oxygenating the blood and getting rid of the carbon dioxide in it and then injecting the blood continuously in a central direction in a peripheral artery.

The anesthesiologist shares important roles with the perfusionist and surgeon in maintaining safe conduct of this critical life support system. Issues pertinent to the understanding of cardiopulmonary bypass include: knowledge of components and circuitry, anticoagualtion, hemodilution, hypothermia, blood gas management, and what constitutes adequacy of perfusion.

The Bypass Machine Components and Connections

The basic bypass circuit

The basic cardiopulmonary bypass circuit is a group of components connected by tubes for the purpose of converting the patient's low pressure, venous blood (low O_2, high CO_2) into "arterialized" blood (high pressure, high O_2 and lowered CO_2) and returning it to the arterial system of the patient. Typically, large-diameter tubing carries blood from the right atrium or vena cavae to a reservoir from which blood is pressurized by a mechanical pump and passed through an oxygenator that adds O_2 and removes CO_2. Next, a heat exchanger controls perfusate (blood) temperature. The arterialized blood is filtered and returned via plastic tubing and a cannula, which is usually inserted in the proximal aorta. When connected, the patient and the essential components of the bypass machine form a circle (Fig. 68-14). To this basic circuit are added the auxillary functions of the bypass machine which include cardioplegia, suction, and venting functions. These operate intermittently, within the major bypass circuit (Fig. 68-14).

The venous "return"

"Return" here means *to* the bypass machine, *from* the patient (i.e., it is the patient's venous blood returning to the pump-

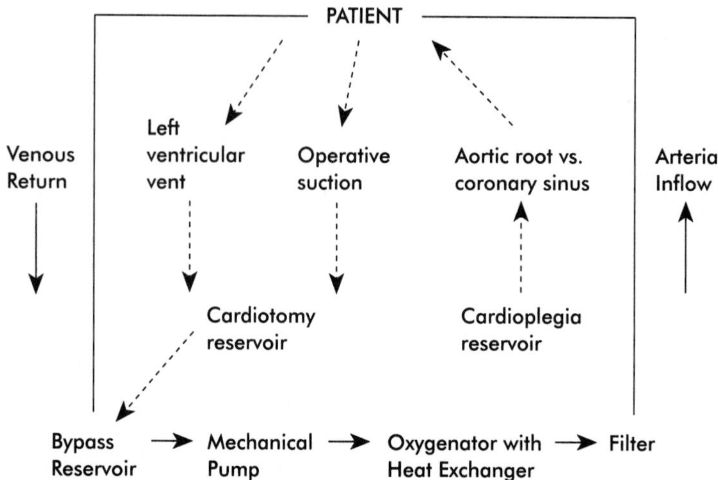

Fig. 68-14. The circuit for full cardiopulmonary bypass. The basic components of venous reservoir, pump, and oxygenator are connected by tubing to the patient so that a circle is formed [solid arrows] through which blood flows continuously. Note that the pump component is illustrated proximal to the membrane oxygenator. If a bubble oxygenator was used, the pump component would be distal to the oxygenator. The lesser, intermittently functioning circuits for suction, left ventricular venting, and cardioplegia are illustrated [dashed arrows] within the basic bypass circle. Note that suction and venting circuits return blood to the bypass machine via the cardiotomy reservoir, while the cardioplegia circuit delivers fluid to the patient. Each auxillary circuit uses a separate pump so as to allow independent flow adjustments.

oxygenator for more O_2). Components which bring the patient's venous blood to the bypass machine include one or more venous cannulae, large-diameter (low-resistance) plastic tubing, and a collection site known as the venous reservoir. The number and sites of venous cannulae are dictated by the planned surgical operation. For coronary artery bypass, a single cannula placed in the right atrium is often sufficient. In contrast, if the surgical procedure requires opening of the right atrium (as in repair of atrial septal defect), air would be entrained, destroying the siphon effect. If the operation requires distortion of the right atrium (such as for mitral valve replacement), a single right atrial cannula would inadequately drain both the superior and inferior vena cava. Thus, in these latter circumstances, two separate venous cannulas are placed, one each in the superior and inferior vena cava. When employing two venous cannulas, several points can be noted. It is worthwhile to initiate cardiopulmonary bypass with only one cannula at a time (other cannula clamped) to demonstrate the adequacy of each. Tourniquets, often of umbilical tape, around each vena cava prevent venous air entrainment if the atrium is opened. One umbilical tape remains loose while the heart is beating, as that coronary sinus blood will not be excluded from the return to the bypass machine.

The venous reservoir is the level of the bypass machine. Due to gravity, venous blood flows passively from the patient to the bypass machine where a reservoir collects the several liters of blood which normally occupy the venous vasculature. This should result in a visibly empty heart, an arterial line tracing without pulsatile ejection, and a CVP that is near or below zero. When adequate venous drainage is achieved, the empty heart will be physically smaller resulting in advancement of the PA catheter. To prevent this, the catheter is withdrawn several centimeters upon initiation of bypass. Without a venous reservoir, flow through the bypass machine would be required to exactly match the amount of venous blood drained from the patient, and reduced venous return would necessitate immediate reductions in pump flow. Without a venous reservoir, venous blood would be incompletely drained from the vena cava causing either the heart to fill, or creating venous congestion of the body's organs.

Poor venous return on bypass will be indicated by a decrease in the volume of blood in the venous reservoir as well as evidence of venous congestion in the patient (i.e., increased) jugular venous pressure and a plethoric appearance of the face. The various causes of reduced venous drainage include: improper positioning of the venous cannula in the patient, a kinked venous return tubing, entrained air in the tubing blocking the siphon, i.e., an "air lock," or an unintended partial clamping of the tubing. Poor venous return has a number of important consequences. The perfusionist is forced to decrease pump flow and thus O_2 delivery to the patient. In an effort to maintain reservoir volume, the perfusionist may add crystalloid fluid which can contribute to an unnecessary decrease in hematocrit. Finally venous congestion of the patient may result in edema creation. Once kinks, clamps, and air locks have been ruled out, minor adjustments of venous cannulae position will markedly improve these problems.

Another situation of failure to adequately empty the heart can occur in patients who have significant CHF, and thus a larger than normal amount of venous blood. Here, the venous reservoir becomes completely filled, but still has not completely emptied the patient's venous system. Blood remaining in the patient continues to enter the heart. It serves no purpose for the perfusionist to increase the pump flow in an effort to "make room" in the reservoir. This action only puts blood back into the patient's venous system. An effective temporary solution is to use the cardiotomy reservoir as an additional venous reservoir chamber. Subsequently, this excess fluid can be removed by ultrafiltration during the course of cardiopulmonary bypass.

The pump and its prime

The next essential component of the bypass machine is the pump which increases the pressure of blood. Historically, a great variety of pumps have been employed for this purpose. Two methods, roller pumps and impeller pumps, constitute the vast majority of pumps used in contemporary cardiopulmonary bypass.

The roller head pump functions by progressively compressing in one direction a plastic tubing which contains blood. The roller head pump is a positive displacement pump (analogous to a piston) which will maintain a constant flow independent of the pressure against which the blood is delivered. This is achieved by a very special (and expensive) electrical motor. This means that arterial vasoconstriction or vasodilation in the patient will result in respectively increased or decreased blood pressure; but pump flow will stay constant unless the perfusionist changes the rheostat on the machine. This is very different from the usual electric motor. Simply pushing harder on an electric drill or sander will greatly decrease the motor speed; this does not occur with these pumps, thus preserving preset pump flow and therefore O_2 delivery.

In contrast, the impeller pump uses a rapidly spinning but nonocclusive turbine-type impeller to create centrifugal force against blood within the pump chamber, which raises the pressure of the blood. The nonocclusive quality of the impeller (analogous to a paddle wheel) means that output flow of the pump will be significantly influenced by the vascular diameter into which the flow is delivered. Thus, vasoconstriction in the patient will be accompanied by a reduction in pump flow. In fact, a clamp can completely occlude the arterial inflow line from an impeller pump, and the impeller will continue to spin. Not so for a roller pump which would burst the arterial tubing if automatic pressure sensors were not present to shut off the pump. Other characteristics differ between these pumps. The impeller pump may be less traumatic to formed elements of the blood, which may be advantageous when prolonged bypass is anticipated. In contrast, the roller pump uses fewer disposable components, giving it an economic advantage. Literally millions of cases have been managed with roller pumps.

Both pumps provide essentially nonpulsatile flow. Originally, the pulsatile nature of blood flow was believed to be an important characteristic. Although contemporary devices are available to provide pulsatile flow during bypass, most efforts to prove superiority over conventional nonpulsatile bypass have not been successful, although in some studies pulsatile flow has been demonstrated as advantageous.[29]

With respect to the pump "prime," as a practical matter, the patient's blood cannot be simply drained into the cardiopulmonary bypass machine and then pumped back into the patient. This would involve an unacceptable period of hypoperfusion while the bypass machine filled, and an unacceptable air-blood interface would exist at the front of the blood returning to the patient. Thus the bypass machine is completely filled or "primed" with fluid prior to connection to the patient. Although early bypass machines were primed with blood, today's prime is largely a crystalloid fluid. In some cases where infants require cardiopulmonary bypass, the "volume" of the bypass machine is large compared with the blood volume of the patient, and a blood prime may be required to maintain a satisfactory hematocrit.

The oxygenator

The oxygenator adds appropriate O_2 and removes excess CO_2 from the venous blood. Early oxygenators simply exposed large surface areas of venous blood to O_2. A more successful approach was to bubble the gaseous O_2 through the venous blood. This type of "bubble oxygenator" required a means to subsequently remove all bubbles remaining to prevent systemic gaseous emboli. The contemporary oxygenator is the membrane oxygenator; a semipermeable membrane that physically separates the blood from gases but allows passage of O_2 and CO_2 according to diffusion gradients. Advantages of the membrane oxygenator include: (1) elimination of bubble creation; (2) lesser trauma to blood elements; and (3) the ability to use N_2O to adjust the percentage of inspired O_2. The cost is higher than the bubble oxygenator but the above advantages are major.

The arterial inflow

After the bypass machine has "arterialized" the blood, it must be returned to the patient's arterial system. Most often the site for arterial cannulation is the ascending aorta. In some circumstances, the femoral artery may be a preferred cannulation site. For example, the ascending aorta may be unsuitable for cannulation in cases of ascending aortic aneurysm, aortic dissection, or severe calcification of the aorta. The femoral arterial site may also be selected in circumstances of second time sternotomy. Here, significant scar tissue is anticipated to increase the risk of bleeding and precludes rapid access to the ascending aorta.

Arterialized blood from the bypass machine should be filtered prior to its return to the patient to prevent systemic emboli to the patient. Measurement of the arterial inflow "line pressure" is performed so as to alert the perfusionist of significantly increased arterial pressure. It is important to ensure that the arterial cannula is positioned correctly in the aorta. Unusually high or low radial arterial pressure may be the result of selective hyperperfusion of one of the head vessels or dissection of the aorta.

Upon initiation of cardiopulmonary bypass, the arterial and venous cannulas are observed for direction of flow and for respective colors of the blood. Although its unlikely that the bypass machine could have been connected backwards or that the perfusionist failed to turn on the O_2, both have occurred. Also upon initiation of bypass, the patient's head is examined for signs of hypoperfusion. Normally, the pink color will transiently disappear because the patient is initially perfused with the crystalloid pume prime. The pink color should rapidly be uniformly restored as the bypass machine pumps oxygenated perfusate to the patient. When it is clear that cardiopulmonary bypass is satisfactory, ventilation of the lungs is discontinued.

Left heart bypass for descending thoracic aneurysm

Left heart bypass is a special arrangement of the bypass machine to provide oxygenated blood to the lower body during repair of a descending thoracic aortic aneurysm. It is instructive to contrast this circumstance to the above description of full cardiopulmonary bypass. As the name implies, only the left heart is "bypassed." Blood comes to the bypass machine from a cannula placed in the left atrium. Because it has already been oxygenated by the patient's lungs, there is no need for an oxygenator in the bypass machine. There also is no need for a venous reservoir because complete drainage of the left atrium is avoided. Instead, the left atrial blood is simply pumped back to the patient usually through a cannula placed in the femoral artery. The minimal components of this bypass machine can be constructed from modern tubing which prevents activation of coagulation, which obviates the need for heparin.

There are several important ways in which management of the patient differs for left heart bypass compared with total cardiopulmonary bypass. The patient's lungs are continually ventilated during bypass. The heart must continue to beat normally throughout the bypass. Thus although a mild decrease in temperature is desirable to reduce O_2 requirements, significant hypothermia and its risk of arrhythmia should be avoided. A means for monitoring the lower-body pressure (femoral artery) as well as the upper-body pressure (right radial artery) should be in place. Also, a measure of left ventricle filling pressure, such as PA diastolic pressure, is useful (Fig. 68-15).

The key to a successful left heart *partial* bypass is to realize that left atrial blood must be distributed both to the lower body by the bypass machine and the upper body by the left ventricle. Vigilant attention to venous return and bypass flow rates is necessary for appropriate balance of the circulations.

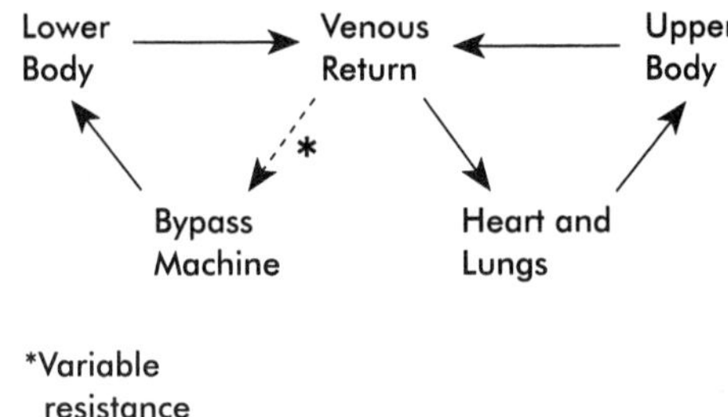

Fig. 68-15. Circuit for "partial" bypass in thoracic aneursym surgery. In this arrangement the venous return must be shared between the bypass pump, which perfuses the body below the aortic cross-clamp, and the heart, which perfuses the body above.

Anticoagulation

Heparin

Systemic anticoagulation by heparin must take place so that the coagulation cascade is not activated when the patient's blood comes into contact with the plastic materials of the heart-lung machine. A typical initial heparin dose is 300 Units/kg. The required dose is significantly higher when aprotinin is used (see below). Because adequate anticoagulation is essential, each step is taken carefully and satisfactory heparin effect is verified. First, heparin is administered via a secure central venous line. Our preference is to use the CVP port of the PA catheter. Blood is withdrawn first to verify patency of the catheter. Several minutes after administration of heparin, verification of its anticoagulation effect is made by measuring the activated clotting time (ACT). Blood for this important test should not be obtained from the same site where the heparin was administered. The best site is a line that is not being flushed with heparin. A commonly accepted ACT value for adequate anticoagulation is more than 400 seconds. When aprotinin is used, the ACT value is recommended to be more than 750 seconds. Cardiopulmonary bypass should not be instituted until this is verified.

Some patients may require additional heparin to attain target ACT. Rarely, a patient with inadequate levels of antithrombin III will be resistant to the anticoagulating effects of heparin and will require administration of fresh frozen plasma (FFP). Heparin levels must be maintained while the patient is on bypass. Systemic cooling will slow the metabolism of heparin. In contrast, periods of normothermia will result in more rapid heparin metabolism. This may become an issue for the patient who requires multiple attempts at separation from bypass. If heparin levels become inadequate, activation of the coagulation system can occur. Although this may not result in macroscopic clotting, microscopic clotting will trigger the fibrinolytic system. This will then interfere with satisfactory coagulation when blood clotting is desirable. Ironically, postbypass bleeding may be blamed on "too much heparin," when in fact the cause of coagulopathy was too little heparin during bypass. In our experience, supplemental doses of heparin do not seem to cause excess bleeding. Instead, the ACT faithfully returns to baseline after protamine.

Protamine

Reversal of the anticogulation effect of heparin is accomplished with protamine. This procedure is performed only after successful separation from cardiopulmonary bypass. If there is a question of hemodynamic stability or further surgery that might require reinstitution of cardiopulmonary bypass, protamine must wait. Protamine is administered slowly and with caution because severe allergic reactions are known to occur. We use a peripheral vein for protamine—the idea is to allow mixing and to further slow delivery. When protamine is administered, suction catheters that return blood to the bypass machine are discontinued. This prevents protamine from entering the bypass machine. After protamine reversal of heparin, activated clotting time should return to normal.

Signs of a protamine reaction are varied. The typical response from too rapid administration is hypotension from vasodilation. This may be countered be temporarily stopping the protamine administration and administering a vasoconstrictor agent. The less typical, more severe protamine reaction is recognized by systemic hypotension accompanied by markedly rising PA pressures. Bronchospasm and O_2 desaturation may also occur. The anesthesiologist must move quickly when such a reaction is identified. The protamine administration is stopped and the surgeon is alerted. The first-line drug is epinephrine infusion to maintain blood pressure, treat bronchospasm, and reduce the allergic response. If blood pressure rises, nitroglycerin is instituted to counter the pulmonary vasoconstriction. If these steps are not rapidly effective, return to cardiopulmonary bypass may be necessary. **A full dose of heparin will again be required.** Of interest are anecdotal reports of resolution of the protamine reaction upon redosing of heparin. If reinstitution of cardiopulmonary bypass was required, the heparin effect will again require reversal. It seems reasonable to attempt to block the allergic response with steroids and diphenhydramine prior to attempting protamine reversal again. Even so, the protamine is administered very slowly.

Other anticoagulation drugs

There are several new drugs whose intent is to reduce bleeding following cardiopulmonary bypass. Of these, aprotinin, a protease inhibitor, has become the most widely used. It is worth recalling that a number of years ago, desmopressin (DDAVP) was hailed as the new agent that significantly reduced bleeding after cardiopulmonary bypass. Rocha et al.[152] compared desmopressin with aprotinin in a randomized study of 109 patients undergoing cardiac surgery with cardiopulmonary bypass. The blood loss was reduced in the aprotinin group but not in the desmopressin group. Aprotinin but not desmopressin was also shown to inhibit fibrinolysis.[155]

Hunt et al.[77] showed in 1992 that aprotinin produces a dose-related prolongation of the ACT and APTT but has no effect on PT. This effect was independent of heparin effect. Because of the prolongation of the ACT, the authors recommended that when aprotinin is used during cardiopulmonary bypass, ACTs should be maintained at times greater than 750 seconds to allow for appropriate levels of heparin.[77] In addition to aprotinin's effect to inhibit fibrinolysis, Mohr et al.[124] determined that aprotinin also contributes to preservation of platelet aggregation function. There continues to be interest in innovative agents to improve the quality of anticoagualtion for cardiopulmonary bypass.[34]

Of interest is also the economic implications of various strategies to improve hemostasis. Harmon et al.[68] reported a cost comparison of desmopressin, tranexamic acid, epsilon-aminocaproic acid (Amicar) and aprotinin. Cost analysis was complex, and included transfusion cost, operating room time, and potential for reoperation. One clear issue was a great difference in the cost of the various drugs. Thus, the drug Amicar costs less than $2 while the cost for aprotinin was $900.

Hemodilution[56,86]

Preparation of the bypass machine necessitates that it be filled, that is, "primed" with fluid. Typically, this is a clear crystalloid solution, although in patients with anemia or in pediatric cases, packed erythrocytes may be added. Several consequences occur from this large volume of clear pump prime including: decreased plasma drug concentrations, and decreased hematocrit blood viscosity and the mean arterial pressure.

As a result of hemodilution, analysis of hematocrit on bypass often reveals values in the low 20s. Such levels of hemodilution anemia can still supply adequate amounts of O_2 delivery because systemic cooling has lowered the metabolic demands of the tissues. The lower blood viscosity which results from hemodilution may actually improve rheologic characteristics of the blood at hypothermic temperatures.

These changes resulting from hemodilution are more pronounced for the pediatric patient, because body size is relatively much smaller compared with the bypass machine, despite efforts to reduce the size and volume of the bypass machine components. A consequence of such hemodilution is that a significant amount of fluid is transferred to the tissues of the patient, and manifest as an increase in total body water (TBW). This excess body water may contribute to tissue edema of the skin, lungs, heart, brain, and bowel, and contribute to organ dysfunction. An effort to counter these problems led to the innovation called "*Modified Ultrafiltration*" (MUF).

Standard ultrafiltration is a filtering process performed during cardiopulmonary bypass which concentrates the blood volume and removes excess water. The limitation to this technique was that total pump volume must remain sufficiently large to completely fill in bypass machine. Recently, a modification of this ultrafiltration process has allowed more complete hemoconcentration. This MUF is used after the patient has been separated from cardiopulmonary bypass so that the volume of the bypass machine is not a limiting factor (see Fig. 68-16).[41,129]

In 1991, an early report by Naik et al.[127] indicated that the modified ultrafiltration technique could reduce the increase in TBW from the 12% rise that occurs with conventional ul-

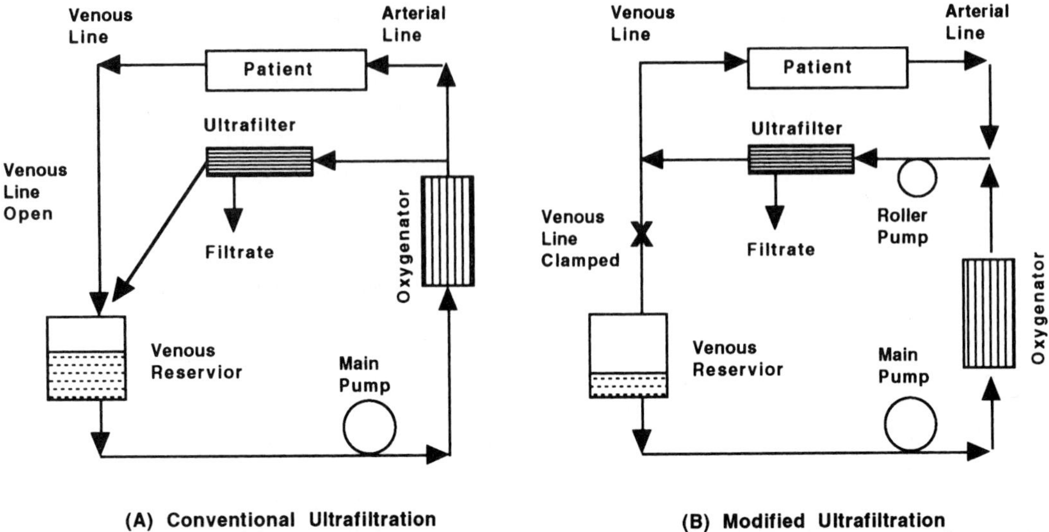

Fig. 68-16. Conventional versus modified ultrafiltration. In **(A)**, conventional placement of the ultrafiltration device is such that the outflow of concentrated blood returns to the venous reservoir. In modified ultrafiltration **(B)**, the ultrafiltration device returns concentrated blood directly to the patient. Note that blood flow is reversed in the aortic and venous cannulas, such that blood is removed from the patient through the aortic cannula and returned to the patient through the venous cannula. Redrawn from Naik SK, Knight A, Elliott MJ: A successful modification of ultrafiltration for cardiopulmonary bypass in children. *Perfusion* 6:41-50, 1991.

trafiltration to 6%. Other findings included higher postoperative hematocrit, less blood loss, and less required blood transfusion in patients treated with MUF. In 1995, Skaryak et al.[167] demonstrated in an animal model of deep hypothermic circulatory arrest that MUF had a benficial effect on the recovery of cerebral O_2 consumption after bypass. Another finding was a significant increase in the systolic and diastolic blood pressures in patients treated with MUF. Possible explanations include greater blood viscosity, removal of myocardial edema, removal of unknown myocardial depressant factors, or conceivably removal of anesthetic agents.[128]

Hypothermia

Early experiments demonstrated that hypothermia without a cardiopulmonary bypass machine could facilitate heart surgery. By lowering the O_2 requirement of the tissues, organs could be excluded from the circulation for prolonged periods of time:

> Such a technic might permit surgeons to operate upon the "bloodless heart" without recourse to extra corporal pumps, and perhaps allow transplantation of organs.[17]

In fact, total body hypothermia was used for human cardiac surgery prior to the advent of the cardiopulmonary bypass machine. Here, an ice bath was used to lower body temperature. This allowed for a limited period of heart surgery, sufficient to repair small abnormalities such as atrial septal defects. Because the heart and lungs were necessary for perfusion and gas exchange, prolonged periods of CPR might be required before normal cardiac activity resumed with norothermia.

The standard practice of current cardiopulmonary bypass is to use a moderate degree of hypothermia to reduce O_2 requirements of the body. The importance of hypothermia has recently again been demonstrated. In 1991, Bellenger et al.[15] reported on the cognitive development of 28 children who had undergone the arterial switch operation for transposition of the great arteries using deep hypothermic circulatory arrest. Although the duration of circulatory arrest was not associated with outcome, the duration of cooling prior to circulatory arrest was. The authors found that shorter periods of cooling were associated with worse developmental scores. The implication was that shorter periods of cooling did not achieve adequate hypothermic protection of the brain.[15]

Another demonstration of the importance of hypothermia arose from the recent interest in continuous, warm blood cardioplegia. In 1991, Lichtenstein et al.[104] reported their experience that continuous 37° blood cardioplegia resulted in superior preservation of cardiac function than did cold cardioplegia. In an effort to test this theory, Martin et al.[119] randomized 1001 elective coronary bypass patients to receive either warm blood cardioplegia or cold crystalloid cardioplegia. The temperature at which cardiopulmonary bypass was conducted also differed. In the warm group, bypass temperature was maintained at greater than 35° and in the cold group, bypass temperature was less than 28°. Overall, the investigators found little difference in indicators of myocardial function. However, the incidence of neurologic events such as stroke and encephalopathy was significantly worse in the warm bypass group.[119] More recently, Singh et al.[165] failed to demonstrate an increased stroke rate for patients undergoing warm cardiopulmonary bypass. Nevertheless, theirs was not a prospective, randomized trial but rather a comparison to a historical control group.[165] Another concern about northermic bypass is that increased temperature may increase neutrophil-endothelium interactions which may increase the risk for postbypass inflammation-mediated organ damage.[121]

Another application of hypothermia is for cerebral protection during operations on the arch of the aorta. In aneurysms of the aortic arch, cardiopulmonary bypass with deep hypothermic circulatory arrest has been the standard method of management. In 1991, Bachet et al.[6] reported their technique of providing cold blood perfusion to the cerebral vessels during the period of circulatory arrest. This technique of "cold cerebroplegia" was used in 54 patients and all patients but one awakened within 8 hours after the operation.[6] Cerebroplegia has also been used in a retrograde fashion by perfusing to the superior vena cava.

Not all hypothermia is necessarily beneficial. Phrenic nerve damage by local hypothermia was reported in 1963.[159] A demyelinating process occurs when temperature is lowered below 4° C, and recovery may take as long as 1 year.[115] In 1992, Allen et al.[2] argued that the application of topical ice to the myocardium is unnecessary and potentially harmful due to phrenic nerve damage. In Allen's retrospective survey, patients who had received topical ice slush had more pleural effusions, atelectasis, and elevated left hemidiaphrams than patients who did not receive topical cooling. There was no apparent difference in myocardial protection for patients who received iced slush.[2]

Blood gas management

Prior to the 1980s, CO_2 was routinely administered via the cardiopulmonary bypass machine during periods of hypothermia. The rationale was that blood should have a pH of 7.4 and PCO_2 of 40 at cold temperatures. Because CO_2 production decreased at hypothermia, it was necessary to add supplemental (about 5%) CO_2 to achieve this goal. This method of management has since been termed the "*pH stat*" method.

During the 1980s, this practice was questioned. It was argued that at cold temperatures, the dissociation of water decreases, so that $[H^+]$ is lower, resulting in a higher pH at electrochemical neutrality. To maintain optimal enzyme function blood pH should also be allowed to rise naturally during hypothermia. To achieve this apparently alkalotic state, CO_2 should not be added during hypothermic cardiopulmonary bypass. This method was called "*alpha stat*" and was rapidly adopted as the accepted means of blood gas management (Table 68-6).[147,149,197,198]

Given the above, it is interesting to review the history of blood gas management. In the early Gibbon cardiopulmonary bypass apparatus, there was no method of determining adequacy of CO_2 removal. Instead, the pH of the blood leaving the oxygenator was measured and CO_2 content inferred. Note, however, that the Gibbon machine operated at

Table 68-6 Carbon dioxide management during cardiopulmonary bypass

Issue	pH-stat	Alpha-stat
Carbon dioxide added during hypothermia	Yes	No
pH/Pco_2 at 37°C	7.28/55	7.4/40*
pH/Pco_2 at 28°C	7.4/40*	7.52/28

*The strategy of alpha-stat is to maintain a pH of 7.4 and Pco_2 at 40 mm Hg at 37°C; the strategy of "pH-stat" adds CO_2 so the pH/Pco_2 is 7.4/40 at hypothermia.

normothermia and assumed that pH changes were "due practically entirely to changes in CO_2 tension."[51] In contrast, Bigelow's early animal experiments used hypothermia but not a bypass machine. His account suggests that a "pH-stat" type management was used during hypothermia:

> When respirations failed at lower temperatures [below 28 degrees C] positive pressure artificial respiration was used. The lungs were inflated with a 5 per cent carbon dioxide in 95 per cent oxygen mixture ten times a minute.[17]

Theoretically, each strategy has advantages and disadvantages. The increased levels of CO_2 occurring with the pH stat strategy may interfere with cerebral autoregulation causing more cerebral blood flow than is necessary.[126] This could potentially result in increased cerebral embolization, brain edema, and intracranial hypertension. In contrast, the alpha stat strategy may cause less cerebral blood flow and shift the oxyhemoglobin dissociation curve to the left preventing the release of O_2 to the tissues. Also controversial was the fact that the alpha stat strategy was related to the physiology of cold blooded vertebrates while the pH stat strategy was more related to physiology of hibernating mammals.[97] During the late 1980s, research for the most part supported the alpha stat strategy. Then in the 1990s, opinion changed again.

In 1993, Jonas et al.[81] reported on the long-term developmental outcome of 16 children who during infancy had undergone a Senning procedure for repair of transposition of the great arteries. All operations were performed under deep hypothermic circulatory arrest after cooling on cardiopulmonary bypass to a tympanic temperature of 16.6°. The strategy for managing pH during the bypass cooling was changed from pH stat to alpha stat in 1985. Developmental testing demonstrated a worse long-term outcome for patients who had received the more alkalotic alpha stat management. The authors concluded that in these circumstances the alpha stat method resulted in less effective cerebral protection.[81] In an animal model of hypothermic circulatory arrest, Aoki et al.[3] demonstrated that the pH stat strategy provided better recovery of brain high-energy phosphates and pH than did the alpha stat strategy.[3]

Although the CO_2 question remains controversial, it is

possible that each strategy has a place. In circumstances where deep hypothermic circulatory arrest is anticipated, the pH stat method may promote more thorough and uniform brain cooling as well as countering the left shift of the oxyhemoglobin curve caused by hypothermia. In circumstances where moderate hypothermia but continuous flow is planned, the alpha stat mechanism may be appropriate. The wide range of local recipes and management strategies can perhaps best be interpreted as a tribute to the remarkable resilience of patients.

Adequacy of Perfusion

Monitoring adequacy of perfusion is a major goal during cardiopulmonary bypass.[148] A pump flow equivilent to a cardiac index of 2.2 l/min m^2 is generally regarded as an adequate pump flow. If however, the patient is markedly anemic or the blood pressure is very low, perfusion may not be adequate. Thus, adequacy of perfusion is assessed by measurement of multiple variables including mean arterial pressure, hematocrit, mixed venous O_2 saturation, blood lactate level, central and peripheral temperatures, urine output, and adequacy of venous drainage.[177,178]

Clowes et al. established an important relationship between bypass machine flow and O_2 uptake by the patient. Basically, as pump flow decreased, O_2 uptake by the patient also decreased. The interpretation was that inadequate O_2 delivery forced some tissues into anerobic metabolism. In contrast, as pump flow was increased, O_2 extraction increased until it leveled off. At this point, further O_2 delivery was not utilized. This work established that adequate pump flow correlates to optimal O_2 extraction. A caveat is that global measures of body perfusion cannot ensure individual organ well-being. For example, a normal O_2 saturation of the venous blood returning to the bypass machine, does not guarantee adequate O_2 delivery to all organs. If anerobic metabolism has occurred, O_2 will not be used but will instead contribute to the venous blood O_2 saturation.

Several reports in the 1990s increased understanding of the adequacy of perfusion. In 1993, Newburger et al.[130] reported on 171 who underwent the arterial switch operation for transposition of the great arteries. In this study, patients were randomized to either deep hypothermic circulatory arrest or low flow bypass for the operation. The authors found that patients treated with circulatory arrest had higher risk of clinical seizures, a longer recovery time until the first reappearance of EEG activity, and a greater release of brain isoenzyme of creatine kinase in the first 6 hours after surgery than did patients treated with low flow bypass.[130] In 1995, Bellinger et al.[16] reported on the developmental outcome of this same group of children at 1 year of age. The authors found that patients treated with circulatory arrest had a higher risk of delayed motor development and neurologic abnormalities than did patients who were treated with low flow bypass.[16]

Together, these reports indicate that higher cardiopulmonary bypass flows are better than lower flows, the extreme being circulatory arrest. Wernovsky et al.[196] reported on the non-neurological aspects of low flow bypass versus circulatory arrest. In 171 patients undergoing the arterial switch procedure, those randomized to low-flow bypass had significantly greater weight gain and positive fluid balance compared with the circulatory arrest patients. Despite this, there was no difference between groups in terms of duration in mechanical ventilation, intensive care unit stay, and hospital stay.[196]

Although hypothermia will reduce O_2 requirements, the limits of what constitutes adequate low flows are not yet described. The practice of monitoring the O_2 saturation of the venous blood returning to the bypass machine as an indicator of adequate perfusion may be questionable.

Cardioplegia

To facilitate surgery, various methods have been employed to render the heart motionless. By reducing O_2 demands of the heart these methods have also reduced ischemic injury to the heart. The standard method of cardiac protection has for many years been a cold, high potassium, crystalloid solution administered to the cross-clamped root of the aorta. More recently, various additives including blood have been used to try to improve effectiveness. This subject was thoroughly reviewed in 1995 by Buckberg.[27]

A major recent change in cardioplegia has been its delivery via a catheter placed in the coronary sinus. The heart is thus perfused in a retrograde fashion. The cardioplegia exits the heart via the coronary ostia and thebesian channels into the right and left ventricles. Proponents of retrograde cardioplegia contend that it provides superior protection to regions of the left ventricle which are supplied by severely stenosed coronary arteries that impede antegrade cardioplegia. The disadvantage of retrograde cardioplegia is that the catheter may not perfuse some branches of the coronary sinus and thus perfusion of the intraventricular septum and right ventricle is less satisfactory. Some experts advocate simultaneous antegrade and retrograde cardioplegia.[80] As a practical matter, the perfusion pressure of the retrograde cardioplegia is monitored. Pressures which are too low may not provide optimum distribution of cardioplegia, and pressures which are too high may be damaging to the coronary sinus.

Another change in cardioplegia techniques involves the temperature at which the solution is administered. A number of proponents suggest that warm, continuously infused cardioplegia provides superior protection. Not all agree. Mehlhorn et al.[120] reported that normothermic blood cardioplegia contributed to myocardial dysfunction by an increased myocardial edema, despite avoidance of ischemia. This occurred because of increased myocardial fluid filtration and decreased lymph flow. Ko et al.[94] reported in an animal model comparing warm versus cold blood cardioplegia that warm cardioplegia did not affect myocardial energetics or performance.[94]

It is of note that cardioplegia is not essential for operation on the heart. Cardiac surgery has many times been performed with cardiopulmonary bypass in which the heart was hypothermic and perfused, but fibrillating. A caveat here is that normal coronary flow occurs during diastole when the myocardium is relaxed. Myocardial wall tension is greater during fibrillation so that driving pressure for coronary perfusion theoretically should also be higher. More recently, interest has focused on the possibility of performing coronary artery bypass grafting on a beating heart. In such circumstances, the heart rate is pharmacologically slowed to facilitate attachment of the distal grafts.

Anesthetic Agents During Bypass

As a consequence of dilution of the patients' blood with the priming volume of the bypass machine, serum levels of drugs must decrease. Thus, supplemental anesthetic agents and muscle-relaxant drugs are administered when cardiopulmonary bypass is instituted. Anesthetic agents may include narcotics, volatile anesthetics administered via the O_2 inflow to the bypass pump, and sedatives such as midazolam. Although the requirement for these drugs is reduced when systemic cooling has lowered brain temperature, they are necessary at the start and conclusion of bypass when the patient is normothermic. The current trend of a lower-dose narcotic anesthetic means more reliance will be placed on sedative agents or volatile anesthetics during cardiopulmonary bypass. Volatile agents, such as isoflurane, are acceptable during cardiopulmonary bypass, provided they are used to induce anesthesia rather than for their side effects, particularly vasodilation. For example, during hypothermia, a steadily increasing blood pressure may require vasodilator therapy. Here, a direct-acting agent, such as nitroprusside, is more appropriate than a high concentration of volatile agent. In contrast, during rewarming, the blood pressure typically decreases. If therapy is required, a direct-acting vasoconstrictor is more appropriate than turning off the inhalation agent. In other words, when volatile inhalation agents are used for their side effects, an overdose of anesthetic may be administered when the patient needs very little (e.g., hypothermia) and an inadequate dose of anesthesia is given when the anesthetic may be "light" (rewarming and normothermia). As a practical point, inhalation agents are often discontinued for a short period prior to the separation from bypass to decrease their depressant effect on the myocardium. During this terminal period of bypass, IV sedative agents are substituted to maintain anesthesia.

The Process of Separation from Cardiopulmonary Bypass

Separation from cardiopulmonary bypass can be divided into three phases: preparation, partial occlusion, and "off bypass." Each phase requires continuous assessment of cardiopulmonary performance.

Preparation

In the preparation phase, certain basic goals are achieved. If cardiac valve replacement has taken place, thorough de-airing of relevant cardiac chambers is essential. Retained intracardiac air is a surprisingly frequent finding and its escape to the systemic circulation can result in cardiac and/or central nervous system (CNS) dysfunction. Using TEE, Oka et al.[134] demonstrated that retained intracardiac air was identified in 79% of patients who had undergone valve replacement despite de-airing maneuvers. These authors recommended that mobilization of intracardiac air be accomplished by filling the heart with blood, stretching the left atrial wall, and ballottement of the cardiac chambers. The mobilized air is removed from the ascending aorta and the left atrium. Others emphasize inflation of the lungs during the de-airing procedure to dislodge bubbles that have become sequestered in the pulmonary veins.[46] Rotation of the table from side to side has also been recommended. Still other experts suggest needle aspiration of various cardiac chambers, including the apex of the left ventricle.[188] Despite these maneuvers, some risk of systemic air release remains. Because of the anterior position of the right coronary artery, air embolism can produce abrupt cardiac dysfunction, which may include ST segment changes, right ventricle dysfunction, and AV block. Occasionally, bubbles can be directly visualized within the right coronary artery. Coronary bypass grafts anastomosed to the anterior ascending aorta also may be a target for retained cardiac air. If cardiac dysfunction occurs secondary to air emboli, the circulation is supported with vasoactive drugs or by the resumption of cardiopulmonary bypass.

Release of the aortic cross-clamp reestablishes myocardial profusion and thus enables a stable cardiac rhythm to become established. Initiation of this often requires electrical defibrillation. Recurrent or resistant ventricular fibrillation may be related to hypothermia, acidosis, myocardial ischemia, or inadequate perfusion pressure.[89] A distended left ventricle will also be resistant to defibrillation. Persistent left ventricular distension following cross-clamp release suggests some degree of aortic insufficiency. In cases of left ventricular hypertrophy, resistant ventricular fibrillation may respond favorably to an increase in the perfusion pressure on bypass. In contrast, persistent asystole is likely to be related to hyperkalemia from cardioplegia and responds to electrical pacing. Therapy for hyperkalemia is usually not indicated unless the patient has renal failure. Potassium levels as high as 6 or 7 mEq/l during bypass will usually drop to prebypass levels without intervention. Treatment of hyperkalemia with insulin often creates worse problems, such as hypokalemia and its associated dysrhythmias and hypoglycemia. Hyperkalemia that interferes with cardiac rhythm generation is best treated by electrical pacing.

In preparation for separation, rhythm should be optimized to include atrial and ventricular synchrony and optimal rate, using electrical pacing if necessary. Adequate rewarming is accomplished with knowledge that warming of the periphery lags well behind nasopharyngeal temperature. Many teams also measure bladder, rectal, or great toe temperatures to verify that peripheral rewarming has occurred.

An important aspect of the preparation phase is a basic assessment of cardiac performance and an anticipation of problems. Factors such as a prolonged ischemic cross-clamp time, difficult CABG because of distal vessel disease, and poor preoperative ventricular function because of recent MI may signal the necessity for inotropic support or other means of mechanical assistance to the circulation. Early estimates can be made by the direct observation of cardiac contractility. Sluggish heart motion often portends the necessity for inotropic support. The right ventricle is most easily observed, but some estimate of left ventricular motion is also possible and should be learned by the student. ST segment elevation may be related to coronary vasoconstriction, air emboli, or myocardial damage, and also suggests that pharmacologic support will soon be needed. Nitroglycerin is begun if ST segment abnormalities are present. Optimization of hematocrit, serum potassium, and acid-base status should also be accomplished in the preparation phase. Considerations of hematocrit level should include the blood present in the bypass circuit. For example, consider a bypass hematocrit of 20. If the bypass reservoir is at low levels during full flow, it is likely that transfusion of packed cells will be necessary. In contrast, if the pump reservoir is full, a hematocrit of 20 probably represents hemodilution rather than lack of erythrocytes. During separation, effort will be required to get these cells into the patient. Leftover perfusate can be hemoconcentrated and transfused before decannulation. Gentle ventilation of the lungs should be tested to detect the infrequent but troublesome occurrence of bronchospasm and to open areas of atelectasis. Early detection of bronchospasm allows therapy to be initiated in the preparation phase.

Partial bypass

To convert full cardiopulmonary bypass to partial bypass, venous return to the bypass pump is partially restricted either by the surgeon or by the perfusionist (Fig. 68-17). Venous blood is, therefore, now directed into the right ventricle. The lungs are inflated and the right ventricle ejects blood into the PA. Oxygenated blood returns to the left atrium and ventricle, and is ejected into the aorta creating a detectable pulse. Continuous assessment of cardiac performance is critical at this time. Modest PA pressures plus good systemic arterial pressures portend successful separation. In contrast, poor systemic pulsatile pressures despite increasing PA pressures indicate that inotropic support will be necessary.

If inotropic and/or vasodilator agents appear necessary, they should be initiated during the partial bypass phase. Administration should be accompanied by discernible improvement in cardiac performance, which is indicated by increased systemic blood pressure with decreased or stable PA pressures. If discernible improvement in performance does not occur immediately, full bypass should be reinstituted and troubleshooting for problems should be begun. An unusually low hematocrit, excessive vasodilation, and/or marked respiratory or metabolic acidosis could be contributing factors. Low radial artery blood pressure compared with central aortic pressure may also be present. Unfortunately, lack of improvement usually means that severe ventricular dysfunction is indeed present. Levels of pharmacologic support should be increased during the partial bypass phase well before attempted separation. A useful monitor is the O_2 saturation sensor on the venous return line of the bypass pump. At a constant partial bypass pump flow, increased mixed venous O_2 saturation suggests improvement in cardiac performance. The drugs used will be discussed later in this chapter.

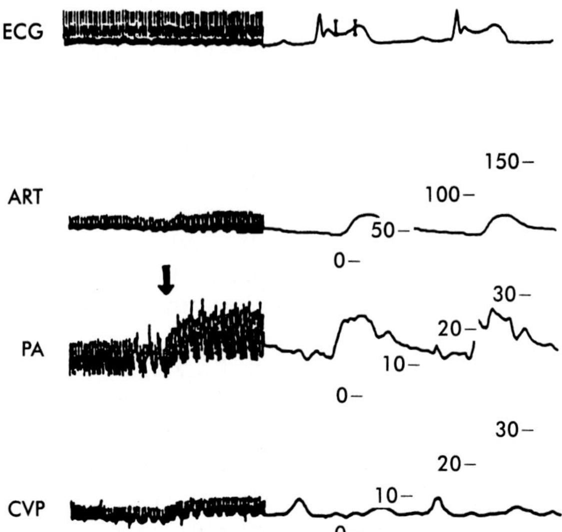

Fig. 68-17. Partial bypass. Partial restriction of venous return to the bypass pump causes blood to fill the heart and by ejected. Note that with moderate pulmonary artery pressure (*PA*), the systemic blood pressure is only modest. This suggests that some myocardial dysfunction may be present.

Off bypass

The final separation from cardiopulmonary bypass is accomplished by progression to complete occlusion of the venous return to the bypass machine. This requires a marked reduction of arterial inflow so as not to empty the reservoir. Balancing decreased venous return with decreased forward pump flow determines the amount of blood volume remaining in the bypass machine reservoir. After venous occlusion, the main pump delivers transfusion.

The perfusionist must carefully balance this critical process to achieve optimal cardiac filling, monitored by PA diastolic or left atrial pressure (if the surgeon has placed a left atrial line). When the patient is "off bypass," continual assessment of cardiopulmonary performance is indicated. This includes consideration of filling pressures, PA and systemic arterial pressures, and cardiac output. The venous blood remaining in the reservoir is transfused in increments such that cardiac filling can be optimized. Overfilling of the heart is deadly at this stage and is counteracted by placing the patient in the reverse Trendelenburg position to aid sequestration of additional blood in lower-body venous capacitance beds. This maneuver may increase the likelihood that air bubbles may enter the cerebral circulation. When separation from bypass appears to have been successful, the venous cannula is removed first. Blood in the venous line is returned to the bypass machine reservoir and transfused as tolerated through the remaining aortic cannula. Blood gas analysis is often useful at this point to assess pulmonary function and acid base balance. The repeated transfusions provide further opportunities to assess cardiac performance. Final steps include protamine reversal of heparin and removal of the aortic cannula. Both these steps can be accompanied by major problems, namely protamine reactions and aortic bleeding.

If complete separation from bypass cannot be accomplished, progressive deterioration in systemic arterial pressure will be accompanied by a progressive increase in filling pressures. This is usually obvious without the need to document a cardiac output. Diagnosis of failure to wean from bypass should be made before the venous cannula is removed. When progressive failure ensues despite pharmacologic support, return to full bypass is indicated. Strategies to facilitate subsequent attempts at separation from bypass include a "rest period" on full bypass and/or institution of mechanical circulatory support such as intra-aortic balloon counter pulsation. If an extended "resting" period is planned, adequate heparinization must be ensured. Consideration should be given to potentially remediable surgical factors such as quality of coronary graft anastomoses. TEE may be useful to identify specific regions of myocardial dysfunction. When additional supportive measures have been instituted, the weaning process begins again.

When separation from bypass produces good systemic arterial pressure, fine tuning of the circulation is relatively easy. More challenging are patients in whom separation from bypass results in systemic hypotension. Table 68-7 illustrates several such patterns. Hypovolemia and/or vasodilation are relatively easy to diagnose and treat. Left ventricular failure is characterized by high wedge pressures and hopefully will respond to inotropic support (Fig. 68-18). More challenging is the occurrence of acute mitral insufficiency. In this case, systemic hypotension is accompanied by very high PA and left atrial pressures. Verification of these pressures can be accomplished by the surgeon's assessment of a tense PA and left arterial appendage. Acute mitral insufficiency may be refractory to inotrope and vasopressor support, and requires reinstitution of cardiopulmonary bypass. If insufficiency is caused by a prolonged period of cross-clamp ischemia, competence may improve with time, and eventually weaning may be accomplished with an intra-aortic balloon pump. Sometimes the mitral valve may need to be repaired or replaced, although a decision to return and perform such a major procedure on such a sick heart is never taken lightly.

Table 68-7 Patterns of hypotension during separation from bypass

Cause of hypotension	ART	LAP	PAP	CVP	Cardiac output*
Hypovolemia	Low	Low	Low	Low	Low
Vasodilation	Low	Normal	Normal	Normal	High
LV failure	Low	High	High	Normal	Low
Pulmonary vasoconstriction	Low	Low	High	High	Low
RV failure	Low	Low	Low	High	Low

*Note that cardiac output is high only in the case of vasodilation. In general, measurement of cardiac output is not the key to diagnosis, but rather a monitor of the effectiveness of therapy.

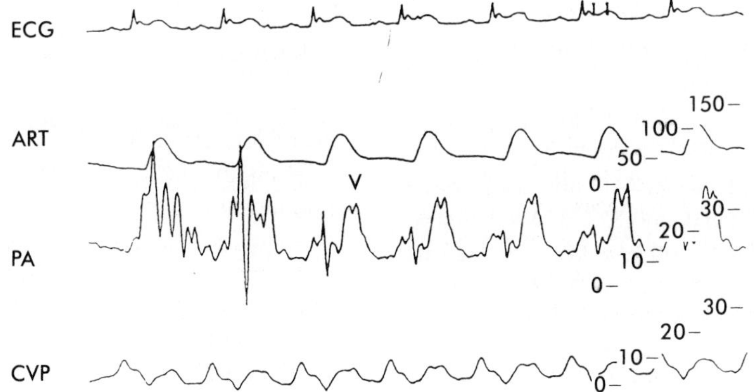

Fig. 68-18. Off bypass, LV dysfunction. The patient from Fig. 68-17 is off bypass. Los systemic pressure (*ART*) and high left ventricular filling pressure (V wave in wedge pressure) indicate left ventricular dysfunction and suggest that more inotropic support is indicated.

An interesting pattern of hypotension during separation from bypass is that which occurs with pulmonary vasoconstriction. In this circumstance, PA pressures are high, but wedge pressure is considerably lower than the PA diastolic pressure.[100] The low wedge pressure suggests that left ventricular failure is not the problem. The high PA pressures indicate adequate right ventricular function. Therapy is directed at the cause of pulmonary vasoconstriction, which may be hypercapnia, metabolic acidosis, or bronchospasm. Vasodilators, especially nitroglycerin, may be useful.

One of the more difficult patterns to diagnose during emergence from bypass is that of right ventricular failure. PA and wedge pressure are low because of poor right ventricular function not hypovolemia. Key to the diagnosis is that the right ventricle is visually contracting poorly and the appearance of the elevated CVP tracing suggests tricuspid insufficiency. The diagnosis is confirmed when attempted transfusion of fluid further raises the CVP, aggravates systemic hypotension, and makes the right ventricle appear grossly distended. Return to cardiopulmonary bypass is then required, and separation is attempted using inotropic support, nitroglycerin, and restriction of transfusion. Improvement of right ventricular function is heralded by increased PA pressures and visible improvement in right ventricular contractility.

PHARMACOLOGIC SUPPORT OF THE CIRCULATION

Anesthetic Agents

The cardiovascular effects of various anesthetic agents have been and continue to be studied by numerous investigators. Despite considerable literature and opinions on the subject, no one anesthetic agent or technique has been conclusively demonstrated to be the best for cardiac surgery. Early admonitions to "avoid hypotension" were replaced by strategies for "afterload reduction." More recently, perfusion pressure has again gained favor.[137,162] A basic dichotomy is between the inhalational anesthetics and IV narcotic agents. Inhalational agents that provide complete general anesthesia usually cause some depression of myocardial contractility.[45] Narcotic agents do not cause myocardial depression, but if used alone may allow some degree of "intraoperative awareness."

The authors use a combination of a narcotic analgetic and a supplemental inhalational agent. The only agent that the authors avoid is N_2O, primarily because it limits the inspired O_2 concentration and may expand any gas bubbles that have gained access to the circulation; others have criticized its circulatory effects.[66] It is worth emphasizing that when choosing an anesthetic, the state of the patient must be considered. For example, the 1969 landmark publication by Lowenstein et al.[109] demonstrated that large-dose IV morphine was a safe anesthetic in patients with minimal circulatory reserve.

Although narcotic agents do not directly cause myocardial depression, it is a mistake to assume that hemodynamics will not be altered. Because of their potent ability to block the sympathetic "stress response," narcotics may well cause hypotension in a hypovolemic, vasoconstricted patient whose level of "sympathetic tone" is increased. Narcotic agents continue to be appropriate for such patients but require careful titration to optimize hemodynamic variables.

Inotropic Agents

Inotropic agents and vasopressors are used frequently in cardiac anesthesia. These agents are some of the most important tools of the cardiac anesthesiologist. Choice of an inotropic agent is influenced by the degree of support needed, the associated effects on blood pressure and heart rate, and the expected incidence of undesirable effects such as arrhythmia or vasoconstriction. Table 68-8 presents the major available inotropic agents according to our impression of their inotropic efficacy.

High-potency inotropic agents include isoproterenol, norepinephrine, and epinephrine. Dopamine, dobutamine, and amrinone are weaker agents.[175,182] The dose ranges listed in Table 68-8 are based on clinical experience and represent doses at which significant inotropic effect can be expected. A number of clinical caveats are important. Although some agents such as norepinephrine or epinephrine can be used at higher doses, agents such as dobutamine or dopamine at higher doses will result in intolerable side effects. For example, this author has seen an advertisement which lists a high dose for dobutamine of 20 μg/kg/min. At this dose marked tachycardia is not just a possibility, it is practically guaranteed! In general when a particular inotrope has failed to achieve the desired hemodynamic effect at the high-dose range, it is reasonable to switch to a different drug. In addition, it is necessary to rule out that some other confounding process may be preventing the expected improvement. Examples of such problems include: metabolic acidosis, hypovolemia, anemia, cardiac tamponade, pneumothorax, and MI. Here, it becomes necessary to balance the various risks. For example, is it reasonable for a patient to receive multiple inotropic drugs and an intra-aortic balloon pump and yet have a hematocrit of 25%?

It may appear paradoxical that efforts during the prebypass period are to avoid elevations in myocardial O_2 con-

Table 68-8 Inotropic agents by relative potency

Agent	Potency	Dose ranges (μg/kg/min)
Isoproterenol	+ + +	.01–.1
Epinephrine	+ + +	.01–.1
Norepinephrine	+ + +	.01–.1
Dobutamine	+ +	1–10
Dopamine	+	1–10
Amrinone*	+	1–10

*A loading dose is recommended for amrinone prior to infusion dose.

sumption, yet in the postbypass period the use of inotropic agents is encouraged. Several considerations may allow these views to be reconciled. In the prebypass period, the coronary blood flow may be limited by atherosclerotic lesions. In the postbypass period, the obstructions to coronary blood flow should have been relieved. Prebypass, a significant period of ischemic cross-clamp time, is anticipated in the near future. Unnecessary prebypass use of limited O_2 supply only adds to the ischemic insult. In the postbypass period, use of O_2 by the myocardium is essential to provide the cardiac function that is necessary to sustain life. Perhaps an ideal circumstance would be to provide intra-aortic balloon pumps for every cardiac patient in the postbypass period. Such devices reduce the requirements for myocardial work while providing augmentation for essential myocardial blood flow. Unfortunately, potential complications of intra-aortic balloon pumping restrict the use of this device to circumstances in which satisfactory hemodynamics cannot be restored by pharmacologic therapy.

Epinephrine

Epinephrine is one of the most valuable and potent inotropes available. Its availability in generic, multidose vials makes it many times less expensive per infusion than some other agents. Benefits of epinephrine include its ability to increase blood pressure as well as cardiac output, without intolerable tachycardia. In addition epinephrine is therapeutic for bronchospasm and is the treatment of choice for allergic reactions. Clinicians should note the tendency of epinephrine to lower serum potassium by stimulation of a $beta_2$-receptor.[26] In cases where some vasoconstriction and powerful inotropy are needed, epinephrine is usually the drug of choice.

Norepinephrine

When persistent vasodilation prevents the restoration of blood pressure to what is perceived as adequate, norepinephrine may be preferable because of its more pronounced vasoconstrictor properties. Unfortunately, the blood pressure desired by the anesthesiologist or surgeon is often quite arbitrary. It should be emphasized that norepinephrine is a potent inotropic agent as well as a vasoconstrictor. As such, it bears no resemblance to phenylephrine, which is devoid of inotropic properties.

Isoproterenol

This inotropic agent is considered a pure beta-adrenergic agent, and the most potent in terms of dP/dt of all inotropic drugs. Its pure beta effects result in markedly increased contractility, increased heart rate and conduction, and vasodilation. Because of its potent inotropic effect, isoproterenol has been used to verify the effectiveness of myomectomy surgery of IHSS. Thus the repair is considered successful if isoproterenol-induced increased contractility does not provoke left ventricular outflow tract obstruction. Although isoproterenol is sometimes valued, sometimes condemned for its ability to stimulate heart rate, it is incorrect to consider its primary effect as a "chronotrope" rather than an inotrope. This misconception seems frequent in circumstances of cardiac transplantation. It is true that the denervated heart benefits from the increased rate stimulation by isoproterenol, but the critical need is for inotropy. If chronotropy was the major primary issue, satisfactory cardiac output could be achieved by electrical pacing. As investigators have demonstrated, pacing alone is ineffective to generate a normal cardiac output in the transplanted heart.

Isoproterenol also has vasodilating activity which can be advantageous in patients with increased pulmonary vascular resistance. One example is longstanding mitral valve disease in which reactive pulmonary vasculature exits. Here, inotropes with significant vasoconstricting properties may cause marked pulmonary vasoconstriction and impair right ventricular function. Drugs such as isoproterenol or dobutamine may be preferable.[52] Another such circumstance is in cardiac transplantation. Here, the recipient of the transplant may have developed increased pulmonary vascular resistance as a consequence of long-standing cardiac disease. In contrast, the donor heart right ventricle is not accustomed to such increased "afterload" and may acutely fail. Here, isoproterenol is ideal as it provides needed inotopy with vasodilation of the pulmonary vasculature.

Clinically, the dose of isoproterenol will require adjustment to optimize the balance between desirable and undesirable effects. Initially when preparing to separate from cardiopulmonary bypass and cardiac contractility is clearly depressed, doses of 0.1 μg/kg/minute are appropriate. However as performance improves, the heart rate will increase and premature atrial contractions will become evident. It will be necessary then to reduce the dose of isoproterenol so as to avoid tachycadia and arrhythmias. Doses of 0.05 μg/kg/minute or less may be satisfactory at this time.

One caveat refers to the use of isoproterenol in circumstance of transient heart block after cardiopulmonary bypass. If the heart block is transient rather than due to structural damage to the conduction system, isoproterenol will work to improve conduction. This may have dramatic consequences. Thus during heart block, ventricular pacing may be necessary to establish a satisfactory ventricular rate, despite atrial rates which may be 120 beats per minute. Restoration of conduction through the AV node will cause an immediate and probably undesirable supraventricular tachycardial because every atrial beat is conducted through to the ventricle. The key to avoiding this situation is to observe carefully for improvement in the AV conduction. This is manifest by the appearance of some early ventricular beats indicating partial recovery of AV node conduction. At this point, it is wise to decrease the dose of isoproterenol so that when full conduction occurs, the heart rate is not intolerably fast.

Dobutamine

Dobutamine is a beta-adrenergic agonist that was designed by alteration of isoproterenol, so as to reduce the chronotropic, arrhythmogenic, and vasodilation effects.[186] In animal experiments, dobutamine was found to have inotropic effects similar to epinephrine because of direct action on beta$_1$-receptors. In contrast to epinephrine, dobutamine's effect of beta$_2$ and alpha receptors was slight. When compared with similar inotropic doses of isoproterenol, dobutamine had less than one fourth the chronotropic effect of isoproterenol.[186]

Clinically, dobutamine is a useful inotropic agent. Applications include circumstances when inotropy is desired but agents such as epinephrine with alpha activity have caused undesireable hypertension. Dobutamine, like isoproterenol, is considered a useful inotrope for right ventricular dysfunction because it provides needed contractility without raising pulmonary vascular resistance. Problems with dobutamine include tachycardia at high doses.[183] Also, although generic dobutamine is available, the cost is still signicantly higher than the standard, multiple-dose bottle of epinephrine.

Dopamine

In cases in which renal or other mesenteric circulation is of concern, low-dose dopamine has an advantage over the other agents.[39,53,141] This is because dopaminergic receptors on the renal and mesenteric vasculature cause vasodilation when stimulated by low-dose ("renal dose") dopamine, 2 to 3 μg/kg/minute. Dopamine has an important role in cardiac anesthesia because of its ability to protect renal perfusion. When a potent vasoconstrictor/inotrope, such as norepinephrine, is used, the addition of low-dose dopamine has been shown to favorably affect renal function.[161]

At higher doses, dopamine is considered to have more beta activity and vasoconstriction occurs at still higher doses. While useful, this concept of multiple receptors for dopamine cannot be taken too literally. At higher doses, dopamine does not "become" a potent beta agent like epinephrine or a vasoconstrictor like norepinephrine. Instead, part of dopamine effects occur because dopamine causes norepinephrine release from nerve terminals.[195] Yet clinically, the most prominent effect from high-dose dopamine in cardiac anesthesia is pronounced and undesirable tachycardia. If beta or alpha effects are desired, better agents are available.

A curious effect of dopamine is its ability to increase cardiac filling pressure. When compared with dobutamine, dopamine increased wedge pressure, whereas dobutamine decreased wedge pressure, although both drugs increased cardiac output. Conceivably, this rise in wedge pressure could adversely affect coronary perfusion, and consideration may be given to the combination of dopamine with nitroglycerin.[105]

Phosphodiesterase inhibitors

Amrinone and milrinone represent newer cardiotonic agents that possess inotropic and vasodilating characteristics.[28,40] Amrinone is listed as a relatively modest inotropic agent. Advertisements for this phosphodiesterase-inhibitor agent suggest that its main advantage is its ability to provide inotropic support without increasing myocardial O_2 consumption. This apparent conflict with principles of thermodynamics may be explained partially by the vasodilating properties at amrinone.[95] The standard vasodilator nitroprusside could also be considered an agent that increases cardic output without increasing O_2 consumption. In fact, nitroprusside can be regarded as an agent that increases cardiac output while *reducing* myocardial O_2 consumption by afterload reduction. Earlier investigations of amrinone had difficulty establishing whether the effects on cardiac performance were the result of inotropic stimulation or simply of vasodilation. In the authors' clinical experience, amrinone is a moderate vasodilator agent, which can be quite useful in improving the peripheral circulation. The vasodilating properties of amrinone have made it a useful agent for patients who have elevated pulmonary vascular resistance and/or right ventricular dysfunction. Such situations may occur in patients undergoing mitral valve replacement or cardiac transplantation.

Milrinone is an analogue of amrinone, reported to be 10 to 30 times more potent. Its action is to inhibit the specific cardiac phosphodiesterase F III, thereby increasing cyclic adenosine monophosphate levels and ultimately increasing the availability of intracellular calcium. Feneck[43] reported the effects of milrinone in 99 adult patients who had a "low cardiac output state" following cardiac surgery. Milrinone was found to produce an increase in cardiac index and heart rate and a fall in PCWP, SVR, and pulmonary vascular resistance. Adverse reactions included some arrhythmia. Although the report concluded that IV milrinone was an effective therapy for low-output states after cardiac surgery, critical examination finds this conclusion overstated. Most remarkable is the definition of low cardiac index given as "less than 2.51 l/min/m^2."[43] Most cardiac anesthesiologists would regard that as normal or moderately high cardiac index following cardiac surgery. Further, no placebo control group was included. This is important because most patients demonstrate continued hemodynamic improvement over time following cardiac surgery. Finally, like amrinone, it is likely that the improvement in cardiac index was caused by systemic vasodilation as well as inotropy.

Royster et al.[158] have studied the combination of the phosphodiesterase inhibitor amrinone plus the conventional catecholamine epinephrine. The finding was that the combination therapy was more effective than either individual agent. Conceivably, this could be attributed to the action of epinephrine to increase levels of cyclic AMP and amrinone's inhibition of cyclic AMP breakdown. Although this synergistic action may be the mechanism, it seems equally plausible that vasodilation by amrinone is the key important contribution. It is well known, for example, that the combination of epinephrine and nitroprusside will result in a greater cardiac output than either drug alone.

Phenylephrine

Phenylephrine (Neosynephrine) and methoxamine (Vasoxyl) are relatively pure vasoconstricting agents; that is, they lack inotropic qualities. Such drugs in modest doses can be useful to adjust systemic blood pressure without increasing cardiac contractility. Use of this drug is helpful in a number of situations. However, in the circumstance of coronary stenosis where capacity for autoregulation is already maximized, blood flow will be dependent on the blood pressure. that is considered optimal by the anesthesiologist. It is true that an increased "afterload" will increase myocardial O_2 consumption. Any pure vasoconstricting agent has the inevitable consequence of reducing peripheral circulation. Use of phenylephrine is restricted to the prebypass and bypass periods. Phenylephrine is not recommended in the postbypass period with the notable exception of IHSS, in which an increase in blood pressure is desirable, but positive inotropic agents may provoke ventricular outflow obstruction.

Thyroid hormone

Recently thyroid hormone has been used to improve ventricular function after cardiopulmonary bypass. This interest was based on the observation that cardiopulmonary bypass results in altered thyroid metabolism.[76,154] Also, hypothyroid patients have reduced cardiac contractility and elevated peripheral vascular resistance.

Klemperer et al.[91] randomized 142 patients undergoing CABG surgery to receive either placebo or IV triiodothyronine after removal of the aortic cross-clamp. Although patients treated with triiodothyronine demonstrated a modestly higher cardiac index (2.97 versus 2.67 l/min/m^2) and lower SVR (1073 versus 1235) in the postoperative period, the amount of necessary cardiovascular support was similar in each group. Thus, epinephrine was required in approximately half the patients in the placebo and thyriod treatment groups. The use of dobutamine, norepinephrine, and nitroprusside was also similar for each group. There was no difference in mortality, postoperative complications, or length of hospital stay between the groups.[91]

A thought-provoking editorial by Utiger[187] acknowledged the finding that serum triiodothyronine levels decreased during coronary bypass surgery. Nonetheless, this decrease also occurs with other illnesses. Perhaps, this decrease is part of the host's defense mechanism and is actually beneficial. Although further study is necessary, it seems that the effects of thyroid hormone are not dramatic for improving cardiac function. In fact, Klemperer et al.[91] were unable to conclude whether the modest thyroid effect on cardiac index was due to inotropic effect or simply vasodilation.

Calcium

Because intracellular calcium is involved in the contractility process, the administration of IV calcium has for a long time been used as a cardiac tonic. However, evidence continues to grow regarding the deleterious effects of calcium administration.[28] These problems include arrthythmia, particularly in patients taking digoxin. One report implicated excess calcium administration in the development of perioperative pancreatic injury following cardiopulmonary bypass.[44]

Vasodilator Agents

Of the vasodilator agents available, nitroglycerin and nitroprusside are currently (still) the most useful. Because of differences in their sites of vasodilation, nitroglycerin and nitroprusside have quite different properties (Table 68-9).[33,122] Nitroprusside is best characterized as a dilator of the entire circulation—arterial and venous—and is particularly useful in promoting peripheral circulation. Conceptually it is useful to view nitroprusside as an agent that tends to convert myocardial pressure work (expensive) into flow work (cheap—in terms of O_2 use). This may or may not be an appropriate goal depending on the individual patient. For example, in the postbypass period, a patient who has undergone CABG surgery and who has a blood pressure of 90/60 may benefit from improved peripheral circulation, but a greater concern is to provide better perfusion pressure to the myocardium. Nitroprusside would improve peripheral circulation at the expense of myocardial perfusion. The theory that afterload reduction in the postbypass period is beneficial to all patients is questionable. Benefits of reduced myocardial work must be balanced against potential consequences of decreased coronary perfusion pressure.

The ability of nitroprusside to dilate small arterial vessels gives it the potential to create the adverse circumstance known as *coronary steal.*[111] By providing a low-resistance pathway within the myocardium—that is, dilating vessels to nonischemic areas while lowering perfusion pressure—perfusion of ischemic areas may actually decrease. For this reason, nitroprusside is generally avoided in the prebypass period in patients with CAD. Hypotension from any cause is undesirable in patients with CAD, especially during the prebypass period before coronary grafting has bypassed the worst stenoses.

Nitroprusside may be useful for the patient with valvular heart disease such as aortic and/or mitral insufficiency. In these cases, systemic arterial dilation may facilitate forward blood flow, thus reducing the regurgitant flow fraction.[31,69]

Table 68-9 Vasodilator agents

Agent	Site of action	Dose ranges (μg/kg/min)
Nitroglycerin	Venous and epicardial coronary artery	1–10
Nitroprusside	Arterial	1–10

In contrast, nitroprusside is useful in circumstances such as aortic stenosis or mitral stenosis, in which the heart is unable to increase forward cardiac output significantly in response to vasodilation. Nitroprusside is most useful during or after bypass when increased systemic blood pressure occurs with evidence of decreased cardiac output or decreased peripheral circulation.[35] Hypertension after bypass, which is commonly seen, not only increases myocardial afterload and O_2 consumption unnecessarily, it also worsens bleeding.

Nitroglycerin is primarily a venodilating agent. Its ability to increase venous capacitance makes it useful for lowering cardiac filling pressures. Increases in venous capacitance can be produced without much decrease in systemic pressure. If this results in lower ventricular filling pressure, then coronary perfusion pressures are improved. Thus, nitroglycerin is an ideal agent for optimizing the coronary perfusion pressure gradient. Nitroglycerin also has the unusual property of dilating epicardial coronary arteries rather than smaller myocardial arteriolar vessels.[25,54,111] This allows nitroglycerin the unique ability to improve perfusion to ischemic areas of the myocardium. Still, reduction of filling pressures to the left ventricle, with consequent improvement in coronary perfusion pressure, may be nitroglycerin's most important effect.[7] If myocardial ischemia is present, administration of nitroglycerin may increase cardiac output if ischemia is relieved (Fig. 68-19).[82]

When ischemia is absent, nitroglycerin may decrease cardiac output because of decreased preload. The usefulness of nitroglycerin is best appreciated when optimization of myocardial perfusion is a goal. One circumstance in which nitroglycerin is undesirable is for treatment of hypertension

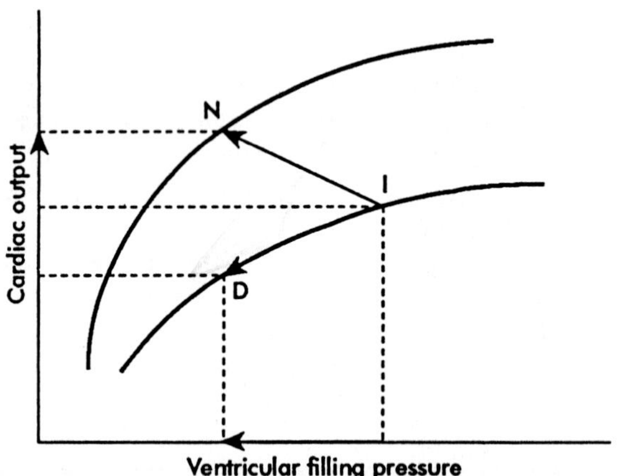

Fig. 68-19. Therapy of myocardial ischemia with nitroglycerin. This figure illustrates two ventricular function curves. A hypothetic patient is placed at point *I* and nitroglycerin is administered. If nitroglycerin acts purely as a venodilator, reduction in filling pressure (wedge pressure) would be accompanied by a reduction in cardiac output, shown as point *D*. If, however, nitroglycerin acts to relieve some degree of myocardial ischemia, an increased cardiac output would occur despite the reduction in filling pressure. This point *N* must lie on a different, more favorable ventricular function curve.

during cardiopulmonary bypass. Although it is true that administration of sufficient quantities of nitroglycerin will cause arterial vasodilation, the marked increase in venous capacitance actually decreases the gradient for venous return to the atrial cannula of the bypass pump; that is, the level of the venous reservoir monitored by the perfusionist drops precipitously. The volume of the bypass machine reservoir has been shifted to the patient. The resulting low level in the bypass pump reservoir may require the perfusionist to reduce systemic perfusion flow and/or add additional fluid to the reservoir.

Other vasodilators may be useful in specific circumstances. Prostaglandin infusions are useful for maintaining a patent ductus arteriosus in a newborn with congenital heart disease and for providing PA vasodilation in adults with right ventricular dysfunction. Anecdotal reports suggest that prostaglandin may be effective in relieving coincidental bronchospasm. Despite metabolism by lung, prostaglandin infusions unfortunately contribute to systemic hypotension, so they should be administered cautiously.

Other Drugs

Antiarrhythmic agents are occasionally needed during the course of some cardiac anesthetics. For ventricular arrhythmias, lidocaine is the usual drug of choice because of its efficacy and lack of adverse effects. Its effectiveness in suppressing ventricular arrhythmia is enhanced by normal potassium levels. More than 1 bolus dose (50 to 75 mg) of lidocaine is often necessary to establish adequate serum level.

When lidocaine is ineffective in suppressing ventricular arrhythmias, hypokalemia, an ischemic dysrhythmogenic focus, or excessive use of arrhythmogenic inotropic agents should be suspected. Electrical defibrillation following release of the aortic cross-clamp may be facilitated by administration of lidocaine. In circumstances in which left ventricular hypertrophy is present, such as aortic stenosis, electrical defibrillation is more likely to succeed after the coronary perfusion pressure has been increased. This may require a vasoconstrictor—for example, phenylephrine—if sufficient bypass pump flow is already present. Alternative antiarrhythmic agents—for example, procainamide or bretylium—may be used when lidocaine is ineffective in controlling ventricular arrhythmias. Both procainamide and bretylium often result in problematic adverse side effects. Overly rapid administration of procainamide can cause persistent hypotension as well as interventricular conduction problems manifested as QRS widening. Bretylium may temporarily provide improvement in myocardial performance because of the release of norepinephrine from nerve endings. Unfortunately this transient effect is followed by decreased cardiac performance because of the now-depleted norepinephrine stores. Bretylium was originally developed as an antihypertensive agent. When confronted with ventricular arrhythmias in a patient who has been receiving digoxin, even greater consideration should be given to raising the serum potassium even if the latest laboratory results show electrolytes to be within limits.

Beta-adrenergic–blocking drugs are often administered during cardiac anesthesia to control excessive heart rates and decrease cardiac contractility. Potential adverse consequences of beta-adrenergic blockade must always be considered. Patients with histories of asthma may exhibit serious bronchospasm when given nonselective beta-adrenergic blockers. Another example of adverse consequence concerns the recommendation that beta-adrenergic blockers be given for dissecting aortic aneurysm to decrease shear forces. If the dissection has caused aortic insufficiency, beta-adrenergic blockade may exacerbate regurgitation by prolonging the diastolic interval. Recently, the short-acting beta-blocker esmolol has received considerable publicity. Its short half-life may necessitate multiple doses or an infusion for sustained effect. Whether esmolol is more or less desirable than propranolol or metoprolol is open to debate; its use is clearly more expensive.

Recent Developments: The Economics of Cardiac Anesthesia

The important consideration of cost containment is rapidly becoming priority in cardiac anesthesia. A particular issue is the trend toward early extubation and shorter intensive care unit stays. Arom et al.[5] reported in 1995 on the cost effectiveness and predictors of early extubation in 645 patients who were admitted to their intensive care unit following CABG surgery. Early extubation was defined as extubation in less than 12 hours and was accomplished in 42% of patients. Factors associated with late extubation (> 12 hours) included older age, preoperative diuretics, female gender, and unstable angina. Of note was the conclusion that the hospital charge per patient was approximately $6000 less in the early extubation group.

At first, the previous economics seem to strongly support early extubation. Nonetheless, it is unlikely that the endotracheal tube alone was responsible for findings. Thus, it seems likely that healthier patients would be extubated early and the sicker ones later. Perhaps it is not so surprising that hospitals costs are less for healthier patients.

Having said this, it is probable that early extubation does contribute to some savings. In fact, some centers would regard 12 hours as a *long* time until patient extubation. The larger question is whether early extubation is physiologically a sound practice. Thus for years, high-dose narcotic anesthesia has been used to try to block the "stress response" of surgery. Suddenly, such doses are no longer considered essential. One must question whether physiology or economics is driving these current trends.

These economic issues are likely to continue to be major concerns. Smith et al.[172] reported in 1994 that postoperative costs associated with CABG surgery could be predicted from preoperative risk factors. Risk factors for increased costs included: older age, lower left ventricular ejection fraction, prior CABG, female gender, no prior percutaneous transluminal coronary angioplasty, increased severity of coronary disease, black race, and diabetes. A similar assessment in 1994 by Mauldin et al.[116] identified higher angina grade, previous MI, older age, CHF, and greater number of diseased vessels as important determinants of costs.

Anesthesiologists (and other physicians) may object to the proliferation of price tags on their practices. However, the era of scarce resources is upon us. The best approach is to use this information to direct our resources to improve patient care.

KEY POINTS

- This chapter includes several clinical case presentations. The beginning anesthesiologist, after gaining experience from a few cardiac cases, will want to return to these case histories for further review.
- Coronary artery regulation is a formidable physiologic factor that is markedly affected by coronary artery stenosis.
- The major determinants of coronary blood flow are myocardial metabolic requirements, diastolic interval, left ventricular end-diastolic pressure, and arterial mean pressure.
- Different kinds of valvular heart disease and their effects on myocardial and coronary physiology require different intraoperative managements.
- Mitral stenosis, especially that caused by rheumatic heart disease, is not just valvular disease; it is also heart disease.
- The ventricular ejection fraction is a useful indicator of ventricular function. It must be recognized that some pitfalls exist for interpretation of the ejection fraction data. Importantly, ejection fraction data should be compatable with other information from the cardiac catheterization and the patient's history and physical findings.
- The value of the ECG should not be underestimated. Beginning cardiac anesthesiologists see all the other numbers being displayed, often in multiple colors, and they forget the usefulness of the ECG, especially with respect to the ST segments in the V5 leads.
- Often, during emergence from bypass, there are dramatic differences between the radial-indicated arterial pressure and that recorded from the base of the aorta. The anesthesiologist should know this and understand why it occurs.
- Monitoring of the PCWP gives the anesthesiologist a chance to monitor coronary perfusion pressure.
- It is wrong to assume that all you need to know to use the PA catheter is how to place it. Students of cardiac anes-

thesia spend years learning the nuances of how to use this important device.

- TEE can supply important and unique information for a variety of cases. The trend appears that its usefulness and indications are increasing.
- Cardiac anesthesia presents the opportunity to study the unique physiology that occurs during cardiopulmonary bypass. This includes hypothermia, hemodilution, viscosity, O_2 transfer, relationship of hypothermia to O_2 requirements, and various sophisticated alarm and measuring systems.
- The separation from cardiopulmonary bypass should be based upon the requirements of the patient rather than the physician's ego. The use of inotropic agents is not a sign of poor surgery or anesthesia. Efforts to avoid appropriate inotropic drugs often result in overtransfusion of the patient, which likely worsens circumstances for a struggling heart.
- The anesthesiologist must remember that phenylephrine is not a positive inotrope and will cause peripheral vasoconstriction. Its use should be temporary and in restricted dosage. Phenylephrine will cause a failing heart to worsen.
- Despite the fact that inotropes should be avoided prebypass, their use is encouraged postbypass. The agent of first choice, almost without exception, is epinephrine.
- The anesthesiologist must understand the differences between nitroprusside and nitroglycerin. Although both are vasodilators, the effects on blood pressure, myocardial perfusion, and cardiac output are quite different.

KEY REFERENCES

Braunwald E: Control of myocardial oxygen consumption, *Am J Cardiol* 7:416, 1971.

Grossman W: Why is left ventricular diastolic pressure increased during angina pectoris? *J Am Coll Cardiol* 5:607, 1985.

Harshaw CW, Grossman W, Munro AB, et al: Reduced systematic vascular resistance as therapy for severe mitral regurgitation of valvular origin, *Ann Intern Med* 83:312, 1975.

Hoffman JIE: Determinants and prediction of transmural myocardial perfusion, *Circulation* 58:381-1978.

Hoffman JIE, Buckberg GD: The myocardial supply: demand ratio—a critical review, *Am J Cardiol* 41:327, 1978.

O'Rourke MF, Yaginuma T: Wave reflections and the arterial pulse, *Arch Intern Med* 144:366, 1984.

Sonnenblick EH, Roos J, Braunwald E: Oxygen consumption of the heart, *Am J Cardiol* 22:328, 1968.

Vandenberg BF, Kerber RE: Transesophageal echocardiography and intraoperative monitoring of left ventricular function, *Anesthesiology* 73:799, 1990.

REFERENCES

1. Atkins CV, Buckley MJ, Daggett WM, et al: Preoperative coronary grafting: changing patient profiles, operative indications, techniques, and results, *Ann Thorac Surg* 58(2):356–364 1994.
2. Allen BS, Buckberg GD, Rosenkrantz ER, et al: Topical cardiac hypothermia in patients with coronary disease, *J Thorac Cardiovasc Surg* 104:626, 1992.
3. Aoki M, Nomura F, Stromski ME, et al: Effect of pH on brain energetics after hypothermic circulatory arrest, *Ann Thorac Surg* 55:1093, 1993.
4. Arcidi JM, Hebeler RF, Craver JM, et al: Treatment of moderate mitral regurgitation and coronary disease by coronary bypass alone, *J Thorac Cardiovasc Surg* 95:951, 1988.
5. Arom KV, Emergy RW, Peterson RJ, Schwartz M: Cost effectiveness and predictors of early extubation, *Ann Thorac Surg* 60(1):127–132, 1995.
6. Bachet J, Goudot B, Teodori G, et al: Cold cerebroplegia, *J Thorac Cardiovasc Surg* 102:85, 1991.
7. Bache RJ: Effect of nitroglycerin and arterial hypertension on myocardial blood flow following acute coronary artery occlusion in the dog, *Circulation* 57(3):557, 1978.
8. Barash PG, Kopriva CJ: The rate-pressure product in clinical anesthesia: boon or bane? *Anesth Analg* 59(4):229, 1980.
9. Becker LC: Conditions for vasodilator-induced coronary steal in experimental myocardial ischemia, *Circulation* 57(6): 1103, 1978.
10. Bedford RF, Wollman H: Complications of percutaneous radial artery cannulation, *Anesthesiology* 38:228, 1973.
11. Bedford RF: Radial arterial function following percutaneous cannulation with 18- and 20-gauge catheters, *Anesthesiology* 47:37, 1977.
12. Bedford RF: Wrist circumference predicts the risk of radial artery occlusion after cannulation, *Anesthesiology* 48:377, 1978.
13. Bellamy RF: Diastolic coronary artery pressure-flow relations in the dog, *Circ Res* 43:92, 1978.
14. Bellamy RJ: Calculation of coronary vascular resistance, *Cardiovasc Res* 14:261, 1980.
15. Bellinger DC, Wernovsky G, Rappaport LA, et al: Cognitive development of children following early repair of transposition of the great arteries using deep hypothermic circulatory arrest, *Pediatrics* 87:701, 1991.
16. Bellinger DC, Jonas RA, Rappaport LA: Developmental and neurologic status of children after heart surgery with hypothermic circulatory arrest or low-flow cardiopulmonary bypass, *N Engl J Med* 332:549, 1995.
17. Bigelow WG, Lindsay WK, Greenwood WF: Hypothermia. Its possible role in cardiac surgery: An investigation of factors governing survival in dogs at low body temperatures, *Ann Surg* 132:849, 1950.
18. Bjork VO, Hultquist G: Brain damage in children after deep hypothermia for open-heart surgery, *Thorax* 15:284, 1960.
19. Bolen JL, Lopes MG, Harrison DC, et al: Analysis of left ventricular function in response to afterload changes in patients

with mitral stenosis, *Circulation* 52:894, 1975.

20. Braunwald E: The syndrome of severe mitral regurgitation with normal left atrial pressure, *Circulation* 27:29, 1963.
21. Braunwald E: Control of myocardial oxygen consumption, *Am J Cardiol* 7:416, 1971.
22. Braunwald E: *Heart disease: a textbook of cardiovascular medicine,* Philadelphia, 1984, WB Saunders.
23. Braunwald E, Kloner RA: The stunned myocardium: prolonged, postischemic ventricular dysfunction, *Circulation* 66: 1146, 1982.
24. Brock RC: The surgical and pathological anatomy of the mitral valve, *Br Heart J* 14(4):89, 1952.
25. Brown BG, Bolson E, Peterson RB, et al: The mechanisms of nitroglycerin action: stenosis vasodilatation as a major component of the drug response, *Circulation* 64(6):1089, 1981.
26. Brown MJ, Brown DC, Murphy MB: Hypokalemia from beta2-receptor stimulation by circulating epinephrine, *N Engl J Med* 209(23):1414, 1983.
27. Buckgerg GD: Update on current techniques of myocardial protection, *Ann Thorac Surg* 60:805, 1995.
28. Butterworth J: Selecting an inotrope for the cardiac surgery patient, *J Cardiothoracic Vasc Anesth* 7:26, 1993.
29. Champsaur G, Parisot P, Martinot S, et al: Pulsatility improves hemodynamics during fetal bypass. Experimental comparative study of pulsatile versus steady flow, *Circulation* 90(5 Pt 2):II47–II50, 1994.
30. Chatterjee K, Parmley WW, Ganz W, et al: Hemodynamic and metabolic responses to vasodilator therapy in acute myocardial infarction, *Circulation* 48:1183, 1973.
31. Chatterjee K, Parmley WW, Swan HJC, et al: Beneficial effects of vasodilator agents in severe mitral regurgitation due to dysfunction of subvalvular apparatus, *Circulation* 48:684, 1973.
32. Cheng DC, Moyers JR, Knutson RM, et al: Dose-response relationship of isoflurane and halothane versus coronary perfusion pressures, *Anesthesiology* 76:113, 1992.
33. Chiariello M, Gold HK, Leinbach RC, et al: Comparison between the effects of nitroprusside and nitroglycerin on ischemic injury during acute myocardial infarction, *Circulation* 54(5):766, 1976.
34. Chomiak PN, Walenga JM, Koza MJ, et al: Investigation of a thrombin inhibitor peptide as an alternative to heparin in cardiopulmonary bypass surgery, *Circulation* 88(5 Pt 2):II407-II412, 1993.
35. Cohn JN, Franciosa JA: Vasodilator therapy of cardiac failure, *N Engl J Med* 297(1):27, 1977.
36. Cohn LH: Surgery for mitral regurgitation, *JAMA* 260:2883, 1988.
37. Czer LSC, Gray RJ, DeRobertis MA, et al: Mitral valve replacement: impact of coronary artery disease and determinants of prognosis after revascularization, *Circulation* 70(suppl I):198, 1984.
38. Daily PO, Freeman RK, Dembitsky WP, et al: Cost reduction by combined carotid endarterectomy and coronary artery bypass grafting, *J Thorac Cardiovasc Surg* 111(6): 1185-1192, 1996.
39. Davis RF, Lappas DG, Kirklin JK, et al: Acute oliguria after cardiopulmonary bypass: renal functional improvement with low-dose dopamine infusion, *Crit Care Med* 10(12):852, 1982.
40. Doyle AR, Dhir AK, Moors AH, Latimer RD: Treatment of perioperative low cardiac output syndrome, *Ann Thorac Surg* 59:S3-11, 1995.
41. Elliott MJ: Ultrafiltration and modified ultrafiltration in pediatric open heart operations, *Ann Thorac Surg* 56:1518, 1993.
42. Elliott CG, Zimmerman GA, Clemmer TP: Complications of pulmonary artery catheterization in the care of critically ill patients: a prospective study, *Chest* 76:647, 1979.
43. Feneck RO, for the European Multicenter Trial Group: effects of variable dose milrinoe in patients with low cardiac output after cardiac surgery, *Am Heart J* 121: 1995–1999, 1991.
44. Fernandez-del Castillo C, Harringer W, Warshaw AL, et al: Risk factors for pancreatic cellular injury after cardiopulmonary bypass, *New Engl J Med* 325:382, 1991.
45. Filner BE, Karliner JS: Alterations of normal left ventricular performance by general anesthesia, *Anesthesiology* 45(6):610, 1976.
46. Fishman NH, Carlsson E, Roe BB: The importance of the pulmonary veins in systemic air embolism following open-heart surgery, *Surgery* 66:655, 1969.
47. Forrester, et al: Medical therapy of acute myocardial infarction by application of hemodynamic subsets, *New Engl J Med* 295:1404, 1976.
48. Frazier OH, Cooley DA, Kadipasaglu KA, et al: Myocardial revascularization with laser. Preliminary findings, *Circulation* 92(9 Suppl):I158-1165, 1995.
49. Fuchs RM, Heuser RR, Yin FCP, et al: Limitations of pulmonary wedge v waves in diagnosing mitral regurgitation, *Am J Cardiol* 49:849, 1982.
50. Gallagher KP, Osakada G, Matsuzaki M, et al: Myocardial blood flow and function with critical coronary stenosis in exercising dogs, *Am J Physiol* 243:H698, 1982.
51. Gibbon JH: Application of a mechanical heart and lung apparatus to cardiac surgery, *Minn Med* 171, 1954.
52. Gillespie TA, Ambos HD, Sobel BE, et al: Effects of dobutamine in patients with acute myocardial infarction, *Am J Cardiol* 39:588, 1977.
53. Goldberg LI: Drug therapy: dopamine—clinical uses of an endogenous catecholamine, *N Engl J Med* 291:707, 1974.
54. Goldstein RE: Coronary vascular responses to vasodilator drugs, *Prog Cardiovasc Dis* 24(6):419, 1982.
55. Gomez MN, Duke PC: Prevention and treatment of intraoperative myocardial ischemia, *Anesthesiol Clin North Am* 9(3):591, 1991.
56. Gordon RJ, Ravin M, Daicoff GR, et al: Effects of hemodilution on hypotension during cardiopulmonary bypass: anesthesia and analgesia, *Curr Res* 54(4):482, 1975.
57. Gotzsche LB, Pedersen EM, Keld D, Paulsen PK: Reduced cardiac reserve in amiodarone-treated pigs after cardiopulmonary bypass and cardioplegic arrest, *JACC* 20(1):236–241, 1992.
58. Gould KL, Lipscomb K: Effects of coronary stenoses on coronary flow reserve and resistance, *Am J Cardiol* 34:48, 1974.
59. Gorcsan J, Gasior TA, Mandarino WA, et al: Assessment of the immediate effects of cardiopulmonary bypass on left ventricular performance by on-line pressure-area relations, *Circulation* 89(1):180–190, 1994.
60. Gorcsan J III, Gasior TA, Mandarino WA , et al: On-line estimation of changes in left ventricular stroke volume by transesophageal echocardiographic automated border detection in patients undergoing coronary artery bypass grafting, *Am J Cardiol* 72(9):721–727, 1993.
61. Grant RP: Architectonics of the heart, *Am Heart J* 46:405, 1953.
62. Greves J, Rahimtoola SH, McAnulty JH, et al: Preoperative criteria predictive of late survival following valve replacement for severe aortic regurgitation, *Am Heart J* 101:300, 1981.
63. Grose R, Strain J, Cohen MV: Pulmonary arterial V waves in mitral regurgitation: clinical and experimental observations, *Circulation* 69:214, 1984.
64. Grossman W: Why is left ventricular diastolic pressure increased during angina pectoris? *J Am Coll Cardiol* 5:607, 1985.
65. Grossman W, editor: *Cardiac catheterization and angiography,* ed 3, Philadelphia, 1986, Lea & Febiger.
66. Grossman W, Harshaw CW, Munro AB, et al: Lowered aortic impedance as therapy for severe mitral regurgitation, *JAMA* 230:1011, 1974.
67. Hamilton WF, Dow P: An experimental study of the standing waves in the pulse propagated through the aorta, *Am J Physiol* 125:48, 1939.
68. Harmon DE: Cost/benefit analysis of pharmacologic hemostasis, *Ann Thorac Surg* 61(2 Suppl):S21-S25, 1996.
69. Harshaw CW, Grossman W, Munro AB, et al: Reduced systematic vascular resistance as therapy for severe mitral regurgitation of valvular origin, *Ann Intern Med* 83:312, 1975.
70. Heller SJ, Carleton RA: Abnormal left ventricular contraction in patients with mitral stenosis, *Circulation* 42:1099, 1970.
71. Hitzig WM: The value of circulation times, *Mod Concepts Cardiovasc Dis* 16(8), 1947.
72. Hoffman JIE: Determinants and prediction of transmural myocardial perfusion, *Circulation* 58:381, 1978.
73. Hoffman JIE: Maximal coronary flow and the concept of coronary vascular reserve, *Circulation* 70(2):153, 1984.
74. Hoffman JIE, Buckberg GD: Pathophysiology of subendocardial ischaemia, *Br Med J* 1:76, 1975.
75. Hoffman JIE, Buckberg GD: The myocardial supply: demand ratio—a critical review, *Am J Cardiol* 41:327, 1978.
76. Holland FW, Brown PS Jr, Weintraub BD, Clark RE: Cardiopulmonary bypass and thyroid function: A "euthyroid sick syndrome," *Ann Thorac Surg* 52:46, 1991.
77. Hunt BJ, Segal H, Yacoub M: Aprotinin and heparin monitoring during cardiopulmonary bypass, *Circulation* 86(5 Suppl): II410-II412, 1992.
78. Horvath KA, Smith WJ, Laurence RG, et al: Recovery and viability of an acute myo-

cardial infarct after transmyocardial laser revascularization, *J Am Coll Cardiol* 25(1):258–263, 1995.

79. Hutter AM Jr: Is there a left main equivalent? *Circulation* 62:207, 1980.
80. Ihnken K, Morita K, Buckberg GD: The safety of simultaneous arterial and coronary sinus perfusion: experimental background and initial clinical results, *J Caardia Surg* 9:15, 1994.
81. Jonas RA, Bellinger DC, Rappaport LA, et al: Relation of pH strategy and developmental outcome after hypothermic circulatory arrest, *J Thorac Cardiovasc Surg* 106: 362, 1993.
82. Kaplan JA, Dunbar RW, Jones EL: Nitroglycerin infusion during coronary artery surgery, *Anesthesiology* 45(1):14, 1976.
83. Kates RA, Zaidan JR, Kaplan JA: Esophageal lead for intraoperative electrocardiographic monitoring, *Anesth Analg* 61:781, 1982.
84. Katz ES, Tunick PA, Rusinek H, et al: Protruding aortic atheromas predict stroke in elderly patients undergoing cardio-pulmonary bypass: experience with intraoperative transesophageal echocardiography, *JACC* 20(1):70–77, 1992.
85. Kaul S, Jayaweera AR, Glasheen WP, et al: Myocardial contrast echocardiography and the transmural distribution of flow: a critical appraisal during myocardial ischemia not associated with infarction, *JACC* 20(4):1005–1016, 1992.
86. Kawashima Y, Yamamoto Z, Manabe H: Safe limits of hemodilution in cardiopulmonary bypass, *Surgery* 76(3):391, 1974.
87. Kay GL, Sun GW, Aoki A, et al: Influence of ejection fraction on hospital mortality, morbidity, and costs for CABG patients, *Ann Thorac Surg* 60(6):1640-1650, 1995.
88. Kennedy JW, Kaiser GC, Fisher LD, et al: Clinical and angiographic predictors operative mortality from the Collaborative Study in Coronary Artery Surgery (CASS), *Circulation* 63:793, 1981.
89. Kerber RE, Sarnat W: Factors influencing the success of ventricular defibrillation in man, *Circulation* 60:226, 1979.
90. Kissin I, Reves JG, Mardis M: Is the rate-pressure product a misleading guide? *Anesthesiology* 52:373, 1980.
91. Klemperer JD, Klein K, Gomez M, et al: Thyroid hormone treatment after coronary-artery bypass surgery, *New Engl J Med* 333:1522, 1995.
92. Klocke FJ, Weinstein IR, Klocke JF, et al: Zero-flow pressures and pressure-flow relationships during single long diastoles in the canine coronary bed before and during maximum vasodilation, *J Clin Invest* 68:970, 1981.
93. Knight AA, Hollenberg M, London MJ, et al: Perioperative myocardial ischemia: importance of the preoperative ischemic pattern, *Anesthesiology* 68:681, 1988.
94. Ko W, Zelano J, Isom OW, Krieger KH: The effects of warm versus cold blood cardioplegia on endothelial function, myocardial function, and energetics, *Circulation* 88(5 Pt 2):II359-II365, 1993.
95. Konstam MA, Cohen SR, Weiland DS, et al: Relative contribution of inotropic and vasodilator effects to amrinone-induced hemodynamic improvement in congestive heart failure, *Am J Cardiol* 57:242, 1986.
96. Kopman EA, Ferguson TB: Intraoperative monitoring of femoral artery pressure during replacement of aneurysm of descending thoracic aorta, *Anesth Analg* 56:603, 1977.
97. Kreienbulh G, Strittmatter J, Ayim E: Blood gas analyses of hibernating hamsters and dormice, *Pflugers Arch* 366:167, 1976.
98. Lange R, Sack FU, Voss B, et al: Treatment of dilated cardiomyopathy with dynamic cardiomyoplasty: the Heidelberg experience, *Ann Thorac Surg* 60(5):1219–1225, 1995.
99. Laniado S, Yellin EL, Yoran C, et al: Physiologic mechanism in aortic insufficiency, *Circulation* 66:226, 1982.
100. Lappas D, Lell WA, Gabel JC, et al: Indirect measurement of left-atrial pressure in surgical patients—pulmonary capillary wedge and pulmonary artery diastolic pressures compared with left atrial pressure, *Anesthesiology* 38:394, 1973.
101. Lappas DG, Buckley MJ, Laver MB, et al: Left ventricular performance and pulmonary circulation following addition of nitrous oxide to morphine during coronary artery surgery, *Anesthesiology* 43(1):61, 1975.
102. LeBoutillier M III, Grossi EA. Steinberg BM, et al: Effect of retrograde warm continuous cardioplegia on right ventricular function, *Circulation* 90(5 Pt 2):II306-II309, 1994.
103. Levine HJ, Gaasch WH: Diastolic compliance of the left ventricle, *Mod Concepts Cardiovasc Dis* 47(8):95, 1978.
104. Lichtenstein SV, Kassam AA, Dalati HE: Warm heart surgery, *J Thorac Cardiovasc Surg* 101:269, 1991.
105. Loeb HS, Ostrenga JP, Gaul W, et al: Beneficial effects of dopamine combined with intravenous nitroglycerin on hemodynamics in patients with severe left ventricular failure, *Circulation* 68(4):813, 1983.
106. Loeb HS, Saudye A, Croke RP, et al: Effects of pharmacologically induced hypertension on myocardial ischemia and coronary hemodynamics in patients with fixed coronary obstruction, *Circulation* 57:41, 1978.
107. Lowenstein E: To (PA) catheterize or not to (PA) catheterize—that is the question, *Anesthesiology* 53:361, 1980.
108. Lowenstein E: Perianesthetic ischemia episodes cause myocardial infarction in humans—a hypothesis confirmed, *Anesthesiology* 62:103, 1985.
109. Lowenstein E, Hallowell P, Frederick HL, et al: Cardiovascular response to large doses of intravenous morphine in man, *N Engl J Med* 281(25):1389, 1969.
110. Luck JC, Engel TR: Transient right bundle-branch block with "Swan-Ganz" catheterization, *Am Heart J* 92:263, 1976.
111. Macho P, Vatner SF: Effects of nitroglycerin and nitroprusside on large and small coronary vessels in conscious dogs, *Circulation* 64(6):1101, 1981.
112. Magilligan DJ: Indications of ultrafiltration in the cardiac surgical patient, *J Thorac Cardiovasc Surg* 89:183, 1985.
113. Mangano DT: Anesthetics, coronary artery disease, and outcome: unresolved controversies, *Anesthesiology* 70:175, 1989.
114. Mangano DT: Monitoring pulmonary arterial pressure in coronary artery disease, *Anesthesiology* 53:364, 1980.
115. Marco JD, Hahn JW, Barner HB: Topical cardiac hypothermia and phrenic nerve injury, *Ann Thorac Surg* 23:235, 1987.
116. Mauldin PD, Weintraub WS, Becker ER: Predicting hospital costs for first-time coronary artery bypass grafting from preoperative and postoperative variables, *Am J Cardiology* 74(8):772–775, 1994.
117. Marcus ML: *The coronary circulation in health and disease,* New York, 1983, McGraw-Hill.
118. Marcus ML, Doty D, Hiratzka LF, et al: Decreased coronary reserve—a mechanism for angina pectoris in patients with aortic stenosis and normal coronary arteries, *N Engl J Med* 307:1362, 1982.
119. Martin TD, Craver JM, Gott JP: Prospective, randomized trial of retrograde warm blood cardioplegia: myocardial benefit and neurologic threat, *Ann Thorac Surg* 57:298, 1994.
120. Mehlhorn U, Allen SJ, Adams DL, et al: Normothermic continuous antegrade blood cardioplegia does not prevent myocardial edema and cardiac dysfunction, *Circulation* 92(7):1940–1946, 1995.
121. Menasche P, Peynet J, Lariviere J, et al: Does normothermia during cardiopulmonary bypass increase neutrophilendothelium interactions? *Circulation* 90(5 Pt 2):II275-II279, 1994.
122. Miller RR, Fennell JB, Young AR, et al: Differential systemic arterial and venous actions and consequent cardiac effects of vasodilator drugs, *Prog Cardiovasc Dis* 24(5):353, 1982.
123. Miyatake K, Izumi K, Okamoto M, et al: Semiquantitative grading of severity of mitral regurgitation by real-time two-dimensional Doppler flow imaging technique, *J Am Coll Cardiol* 7:82, 1986.
124. Mohr R, Goor DA, Lusky A, Lavee J: Aprotinin prevents cardiopulmonary bypass-induced platelet dysfunction. A scanning electron microscope study, *Circulation* 86(5 Suppl):II405-II409, 1992.
125. Morris D, Mulvihill D, Wilbur YWL: Risk of developing complete heart block during bedside pulmonary artery catheterization in patients with left bundle-branch block, *Arch Intern Med* 147:2005, 1987.
126. Murkin JM, Farrar JK, Tweed WA, et al: Cerebral autoregulation and flow/metabolism coupling during cardiopulmonary bypass: the influence of PaCO2, *Anesth Analg* 66:825, 1987.
127. Naik SK, Knight A, Elliot MJ: A successful modification of ultrafiltration for cardiopulmonary bypass in children, *Perfusion* 6:41, 1991.
128. Naik SK, Knight A, Elliot MJ: A prospective randomized study of a modified technique of ultrafiltration during pediatric open-heart surgery, *Circulation* 84 [suppl III]: III-422, 1991.
129. Naik SK, Elliot MJ: Ultrafiltration and paediatric cardiopulmonary bypass, *Perfusion* 8:101, 1993.
130. Newburger JW, Jonas RA, Wernovsky G, et al: A comparison of the perioperative neurologic effects of hypothermic circulatory arrest versus low-flow cardiopulmonary

bypass in infant heart surgery, *N Engl J Med* 329:1057, 1993.
131. Nuchbinder N, Ganz W: Hemodynamic monitoring: invasive techniques, *Anesthesiology* 45(2):146, 1976.
132. O'Rourke MF, Yaginuma T: Wave reflections and the arterial pulse, *Arch Intern Med* 144:366, 1984.
133. Oakley RM, Jarvis JC: Cardiomyoplasty. A critical review of experimental and clinical results [review], *Circulation* 90(4):2085–2090, 1994.
134. Oka Y, Inoue T, Hong Y, et al: Retained intracardiac air–transesophageal echocardiography for definition of incidence and monitoring removal by improved techniques, *J Thorac Cardiovasc Surg* 91:329, 1986.
135. Omoto R: New trend in transesophageal echocardiographic technology: use of biplane transesophageal probe, *Circulation* 82:1507, 1990.
136. Osbakken MD, Bove AA, Spann JF: Left ventricular regional wall motion and velocity of shortening in chronic mitral and aortic regurgitation, *Am J Cardiol* 47:1055, 1981.
137. Paradis NA, Martin GB, Rivers EP, et al: Coronary perfusion pressure and the return of spontaneous circulation in human cardiopulmonary resuscitation, *JAMA* 263: 1106, 1990.
138. Paris TM, McAllister M, Ross JJ, et al: Doppler-echocardiographic evaluation of left atrial contribution to left ventricular filling in mitral stenosis at rest and during exercise, *Am J Cardiol* 64:1058, 1989.
139. Partigton MT, Acar C, Buckberg GD, et al: Studies of retrograde cardioplegia I. Capillary blood flow distribution to myocardium supplied by open and occluded arteries, *J Thorac Cardiovasc Surg* 97:605, 1989.
140. Partigton MT, Acar C, Buckberg GD, Pierre JL: Studies of retrograde cardioplegia II. Advantages of antegrade/retrograde cardioplegia to optimize distribution in jeopardized myocardium, *J Thorac Cardiovasc Surg* 97:613, 1989.
141. Pawlik W, Mailman D, Shanbour LL, et al: Dopamine effects on the intestinal circulation, *Am Heart J* 91(3):325, 1976.
142. Pepine CJ, Hill JA, Lambert CR: *Diagnostic and therapeutic cardiac catheterization,* Baltimore, 1989, Williams & Wilkins.
143. Perloff JK, Roberts WC: The mitral apparatus: functional anatomy of mitral regurgitation, *Circulation* 46:227, 1972.
144. Pichard AD, et al: Large V waves in the pulmonary wedge pressure tracing in the absence of mitral regurgitation, *Am J Cardiol* 50:1044, 1982.
145. Pierce EC: The membrane versus bubble oxygenator controversy, *Ann Thorac Surg* 29(6):497, 1980.
146. Popp RL: Echocardiography, *N Engl J Med* 323:101; 165, 1990.
147. Prough DS, Stump DA, Troost BT: Paco2 management during cardiopulmonary bypass: intriguing physiologic rationale, convincing clinical data, evolving hypothesis, *Anesthesiology* 72:3, 1990.
148. Putnam EA, Manners JM: Vascular resistance during cardiopulmonary bypass, *Anaesthesia* 38:635, 1983.
149. Ream AK, Reitz BA: Temperature correction of P-co2 and pH in estimating acid-base status, *Anesthesiology* 56:41, 1982.
150. Reed GL, Singer DE, Picard EH, et al: Stroke following coronary artery bypass surgery, *N Engl J Med* 319(19):1246, 1988.
151. Roberts WC, Perloff JK: Mitral valvular disease, *Ann Intern Med* 77:939, 1972.
152. Robin ED: The cult of the Swan-Ganz catheter, *Ann Intern Med* 103:445, 1985.
153. Robinson BF: Relation of heart rate and systolic blood pressure to the onset of pain in angina pectoris, *Circulation* 35:1073, 1967.
154. Robuschi G, Medici D, Fesani F, et al: Cardiopulmonary bypass: a low T4 and T3 syndrome with blunted thyrotropin (TSH) response to thyrotropin-releasing hormone (TRH), *Horm Res* 23:151–158, 1986.
155. Rocha E, Hidalgo F, Llorens R, et al: Randomized study of aprotinin and DDAVP to reduce postoperative bleeding after cardiopulmonary bypass surgery, *Circulation* 90(2):921–927, 1994.
156. Ross J Jr: Left ventricular function and the timing of surgical treatment in valvular heart disease, *Ann Intern Med* 94:498, 1981.
157. Ross J, Braunwald E: The study of left ventricular function in man by increasing resistance to ventricular ejection with angiotensin, *Circulation* 29:739, 1964.
158. Royster RL, Butterworth JF IV, Prielipp RC, et al: Combined inotropic efects of amrinone and epinephrin following cardiopulmonary bypass in man, *Anesth Analg* 64:1214, 1985.
159. Scannell JG, Shaw RS, Burke JF, et al: Operative treatment of aortic stenosis in the adult, *Circulation* 27:772, 1963.
160. Sarnoff SJ, Braunwald E, Welch GH, et al: Hemodynamic determinants of oxygen consumption of the heart with special reference to the tension-time index, *Am J Physiol* 192(1):148, 1958.
161. Schaer GL, Fink MP, Parrillo JE: Norepinephrine alone versus norepinephrine plus low-dose dopamine: enhanced renal blood flow with combination pressor therapy, *Crit Care Med* 13(6):492, 1985.
162. Schleien CL, Berkowitz ID, Traystman R, et al: Controversial issues in cardiopulmonary resuscitation, *Anesthesiology* 71:133, 1989.
163. Schranz D, Droege A, Broede A, et al: Uncoupling of human cardiac beta-adrenoceptors during cardiopulmonary bypass with cardioplegic cardiac arrest, *Circulation* 87(2):422–426, 1993.
164. Sellars RD, Levy MJ, Amplatz KW, et al: Left retrograde cardioangiography in acquired cardiac disease, *Am J Cardiol* 14:437, 1964.
165. Singh AK, Bert AA, Feng WC, Rotenberg FA: Stroke during coronary artery bypass grafting using hypothermic versus northermic perfusion, *Ann Thorac Surg* 59:84, 1995.
166. Shah KB, Rao TLK, Laughlin S, et al: A review of pulmonary artery catheterization in 6245 patients, *Anesthesiology* 61:271, 1984.
167. Skaryak LA, Kirshbom PM, DiBernardo LR, et al: Modified ultrafiltration improves cerebral metabolic recovery after circulatory arrest, *J Thorac Cardiovasc Surg* 109: 744, 1995.
168. Slogoff S, Keats AS: Does perioperative myocardial ischemia lead to postoperative myocardial infarction? *Anesthesiology* 62:107, 1985.
169. Slogoff S, Keats AS: Randomized trial of primary anesthetic agents on outcome of coronary artery bypass operations, *Anesthesiology* 70:179, 1989.
170. Smith JS, Cahalan MK, Benefiel DJ, et al: Intraoperative detection of myocardial ischemia in high-risk patients: electrocardiography versus two-dimensional transesophageal echocardiography, *Circulation* 72:1015, 1985.
171. Smith JS, Roizen MF, Cahalan MK, et al: Does anesthetic technique make a difference? Augmentation of systolic blood pressure during carotid endaerectomy: effects of phenylephrine versus right anesthesia and of isoflurane versus halothane on the incidence of myocardial ischemia, *Anesthesiology* 69:846, 1988.
172. Smith LR, Milano CA, Molter BS, et al: Preoperative determinants of postoperative costs associated with coronary artery bypass graft surgery, *Circulation* 90(5 Pt. 2):II24-II28, 1994.
173. Sonnenblick EH, Ross J, Braunwald E: Oxygen consumption of the heart, *Am J Cardiol* 22:328, 1968.
174. Spain MG, Smith MD, Grayburn PA, et al: Quantitative assessment of mitral regurgitation by Doppler color flow imaging: angiographic and hemodynamic correlations, *J Am Coll Cardiol* 13:585, 1989.
175. Steen PA, Tinker JH, Pluth JR, et al: Efficacy of dopamine dobutamine, and epinephrine during emergence from cardiopulmonary bypass in man, *Circulation* 57(2):378, 1978.
176. Stern DH, Gerson JI, Allen FB, et al: Can we trust the direct radial artery pressure immediately following cardiopulmonary bypass? *Anesthesiology* 62:557, 1985.
177. Stockard JJ, Bickford RG, Myers RR, et al: Hypotension-induced changes in cerebral function during cardiac surgery, *Stroke* 5:730, 1974.
178. Stockard JJ, Bickford RG, Schauble JF: Pressure-dependent cerebral ischemia during cardiopulmonary bypass, *Neurology* 23:521, 1973.
179. Stone GJ, Hoar PF, Faltas AN, et al: Nitroprusside and mitral stenosis, *Anesth Analg* 59:662, 1980.
180. Stott DK, Marpole DGF, Bristow JD, et al: The roles of left atrial transport in aortic and mitral stenosis, *Circulation* 61:1031, 1970.
181. Thomson IR, Dalton BC, Lappas DG: Right bundle-branch block and complete heart block caused by the Swan-Ganz catheter, *Anesthesiology* 51(35):9, 1979.
182. Tinker JH, Tarhan S, White RD, et al: Dobutamine for inotropic support during emergence from cardiopulmonary bypass, *Anesthesiology* 44(4):281, 1976.
183. Tinker JH: unpublished observations. (Remarks regarding dobutamine and flat dose response curve.)
184. Tuman KJ, McCarthy RJ, Spiess BD, et al: Does choice of anesthetic agent signifi-

cantly affect outcome after coronary artery surgery? *Anesthesiology* 70:189, 1989.
185. Tuman KJ, McCarthy RJ, Spiess BD, et al: Effect of pulmonary artery catheterization on outcome in patients undergoing coronary artery surgery, *Anesthesiology* 70:199, 1989.
186. Tuttle RR, Mills J: Development of a new catecholamine to selectively increase cardiac contractility, *Circ Res* 36:185, 1975.
187. Utiger RD: Altered thyriod function in nonthyroidal illness and surgery [editorial], *New Engl J Med* 333:1562, 1995.
188. Utley JR, Stephens DB: Air embolus during cardiopulmonary bypass. In *Pathophysiology and techniques of cardiopulmonary bypass,* vol 2, Baltimore, 1983, Williams & Wilkins.
189. Vandenberg BF, Kerber RE: Transesophageal echocardiography and intraoperative monitoring of left ventricular function, *Anesthesiology* 73:799, 1990.
190. van Oeveren W, Kazatchkine MD, Descamps-Latscha B, et al: Deleterious effects of cardiopulmonary bypass, *J Thorac Cardiovasc Surg* 89:888, 1985.
191. Vatner SF, McRitchie RJ, Maroko PR, et al: Effects of catecholamines, exercise and nitroglycerin on the normal and ischemic myocardium in conscious dogs, *J Clin Invest* 54:563, 1974.
192. Vokonas PS, Gorlin R, Cohn PF, et al: Dynamic geometry of the left ventricle in mitral regurgitation, *Circulation* 48:786, 1973.
193. Waldo AL, Machean WAH: *Diagnosis and treatment of cardiac arrhythmias following open heart surgery,* New York, 1980, Futura Publishing.
194. Weiner DA, Ryan TJ, McCabe CH, et al: Correlations among history of angina, ST-segment response and prevalence of coronary artery disease in the coronary artery surgery study (CASS), *N Engl J Med* 301:230, 1979.
195. Weiner N: Norepinephrine, epinephrine, and the sympathomimetic amines. In Gilman AG, Goodman LS, et al, editors: *The Pharmacological Basis of Therapeutics,* ed 7, New York, 1985, MacMillan.
196. Wernovsky G, Wypij D, Jonas RA, et al: Postoperative course and hemodynamic profile after the arterial switch operation in neonates and infants. A comparison of low-flow cardiopulmonary bypass and circulatory arrest, *Circulation* 92(8):2226–2235, 1995.
197. White FN: A comparative physiological approach to hypothermia, *J Thorac Cardiovasc Surg* 82:821, 1981.
198. Williams JJ: A fresh look at an old question, *Anesthesiology* 56(1):1, 1982.
199. Wright C, White C, Furda J, et al: Can the coronary angiogram predict the functional significance of a coronary stenosis? *Circulation* 62:214, 1980.
200. Yoshida K, Yoshikawa J, Yamaura Y, et al: Assessment of mitral regurgitation by biplane transesophageal color Doppler flow mapping, *Circulation* 82:1121, 1990.
201. Zaidan JR, Freniere S: Use of pacing pulmonary artery catheter during cardiac surgery, *Ann Thorac Surg* 35:633, 1983.

CHAPTER 69

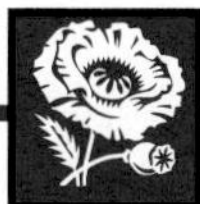

Anesthesia for Treatment of Congenital Heart Disease: A Problem Oriented Approach

PAUL R. HICKEY

The goal of anesthetic management in treatment of patients with congenital heart disease (CHD) is to maintain circulatory homeostasis despite the destabilizing events accompanying therapeutic procedures. Anesthesia for management of congenital heart disease is complicated by the diversity of lesions and the variety of therapeutic approaches. Congenital cardiac defects vary widely in severity, anatomic combinations, and pathophysiologic conditions. Complex cardiovascular pathophysiologic conditions change dynamically with time and also with organ development and therapeutic interventions. In these circumstances, simple formulas for anesthetic management are not valid. The pathophysiology of each lesion and its alteration by previous medical and surgical treatment and by the proposed procedure should be individually considered in planning anesthetic management. Major interventional procedures in the catheterization laboratory are increasingly replacing or supplementing surgical procedures. Their anesthetic management also should be considered. Such transcatheter procedures can cause profound changes in homeostasis and often require anesthesia, particularly in children. Thus, anesthetic considerations for these transcatheter interventional procedures have been included.

Anesthetic management of CHD is first approached by focusing on common pathophysiologic problems related to specific cardiac defects and previous therapeutic interventions. Understanding of these problems is critical for deciding anesthetic management priorities. Knowledge of the effects of anesthetic drugs, manipulations, and adjunctive agents on the pathophysiologic and the therapeutic procedure is essential for anticipating the responses of any patient.

SPECIFIC PROBLEMS RESULTING FROM CONGENITAL HEART DISEASE

Although many different lesions in varying combinations occur in patients with CHD, problems that decrease cardiopulmonary reserve include (1) intracardiac shunting

with increases and decreases in pulmonary blood flow, (2) hypoxemia from inadequate pulmonary blood flow or intracardiac shunting, (3) congestive heart failure from volume or cardiac pressure overload, (4) pulmonary vascular obstructive disease (PVOD) from excessive pulmonary blood flow and pressure, (5) obstruction to left or right heart outflow from stenosis at various sites, and (6) coronary ischemia from congenital defects and iatrogenic intrusions. Of the 8 of 1000 live births with CHD, one third have critical diseases requiring catheterization or surgery in the first year, so anesthetic management for CHD frequently involves immature neonatal circulatory and pulmonary physiology.[67,94] Physiologic limitations of the immature heart, circulation, and lungs are superimposed on CHD problems. Table 69-1 shows problems encountered with CHD patients usually seen in the operating room or catheterization laboratory and frequencies of occurrence. In longstanding or particularly severe lesions, problems may occur more frequently than indicated in this table.

Intracardiac Shunting

Shunting within the heart and between the great vessels gives rise to many of the problems seen in patients with CHD. These include hypoxemia, excessive pulmonary blood flow, high volume loads, and CHD. Control of intracardiac shunting thus is a central issue in CHD and its anesthetic management. The hemodynamics of intracardiac shunts are complex and depend on numerous factors determining shunt magnitude and direction (Fig. 69-1). Complete description of the dynamics of a particular shunt requires more data than are ordinarily clinically available.[19] The determinants of shunting, such as ventricular compliance, may change considerably during anesthesia and operative manipulations without the changes being readily measurable. A simplified view of shunt hemodynamics is useful in clinically assessing the hemodynamic importance of shunts and their probable alterations during therapeutic procedures.

Shunt orifice and outflow resistance are important determinants of shunting. By considering outflow resistance and the size of the shunt orifice, intraoperative changes in shunt magnitude and direction can be predicted in simple and complex shunts. Manipulation of pulmonary or systemic outflow resistances can alter shunt directions and magnitudes, depending on type of shunt. Also important in determining pulmonary and systemic vascular resistances are influences of cytokines, activated complement, and other endogenously released humoral agents such as nitric oxide. Local and circulating levels of such agents can be profoundly altered by surgical procedures and cardiopulmonary bypass.[102] Effects of such agents on vascular resistances may overwhelm clinical efforts to manipulate vascular resistances.

Simple shunts

In simple shunts (without associated obstructive lesions), outflow resistance is equivalent to pulmonary vascular resistance (PVR) on the right and systemic vascular resistance (SVR) on the left. The effects of shunt orifice and vascular resistances on simple shunts are schematically shown in Fig. 69-2. Shunts with small orifices are relatively fixed in magnitude and are restrictive by definition. As the communication becomes larger and nonrestrictive (equal to or exceeding the aortic valve area), shunt direction and magnitude depend more on the ratio of outflow resistances, i.e., the relative resistances of the pulmonary versus systemic vascular beds (PVR/SVR).[177]

In many forms of CHD, hypoxemia requires additional pulmonary blood flow from surgically constructed aortopulmonary anastomoses. Aorta-to-pulmonary artery flow through a small diameter (restrictive) Blalock-Taussig shunt will increase moderately with elevations in systemic arterial pressure when PVR remains constant or alternatively by decreasing PVR with a constant systemic arterial pressure. These changes increase pulmonary blood flow and arterial oxygen saturation and probably will be beneficial in increasing tissue oxygen delivery when oxygen saturations are very low (> 70%). In contrast, when arterial oxygen saturations are greater (e.g., 85% to 90%, approaching the plateau of the oxyhemoglobin dissociation curve), further increases in arterial oxygen saturation require high levels of pulmonary blood flow and may not improve tissue oxygen delivery because of concomitant decreases in systemic flow (Fig. 69-3). High pulmonary flow through large, unrestrictive shunts are required for greater levels of arterial oxygen saturation, and they increase cardiac volume loading. This volume loading often may exacerbate congestive heart failure, producing a net decrease in systemic cardiac output and net oxygen delivery despite the small increases in arterial oxygen saturation produced by increased pulmonary flow. Thus the same relative changes in SVR and PVR could be detrimental with a large, nonrestrictive aortopulmonary shunt. Also, with large, nonrestrictive ventricular septal defects, the same relative changes in PVR/SVR can increase left-to-right shunting, subjecting the heart to further increased volume loads, worsening congestive heart failure.

In contrast, with tetralogy of Fallot, because pathophysiology consists of right-to-left complex shunt flow through a ventricular septal defect, the same changes, namely increasing SVR and decreasing or holding PVR constant, will decrease right-to-left shunting and improve the clinical picture. Arterial oxygen saturation will increase by decreasing systemic venous blood shunted into the left atrium and mixing with pulmonary venous blood, improving the patient's clinical condition. Relative levels of PVR and SVR needed to optimize the patient's clinical status with an intracardiac shunt become clearer when the pathophysiologic condition of the defect is detailed. Characteristics and examples of simple shunts of various sizes are listed in Table 69-2 on page 1704.

Mixing

If the intracardiac communication is sufficiently large, the two cardiac chambers or great vessels effectively become a

Table 69-1 Frequency of hemodynamic problems in various forms of congenital heart disease

Lesion	Hypoxemia	Intracardiac shunting	Excessive pulmonary blood flow	Congestive heart failure	Left-sided obstruction	Coronary ischemia	Immature circulation	Obstruction to pulmonary flow
Atrial septal defect	Rarely	Always (L → R)	Usually	Rarely	Not seen	Not seen	Not seen	Rarely
Patent ductus arteriosus	Rarely	Always (L → R)	Usually	Sometimes	Not seen	Not seen	Sometimes	Rarely
Ventricular septal defect	Rarely	Always (L → R)	Usually	Often	Not seen	Not seen	Often	Late (PVOD)
Tetralogy of Fallot	Often	Always (L ↔ R)	Rarely	Sometimes	Not seen	Rare	Occasionally	Usually
Atrioventricular canal (partial or complete)	Rarely	Always (L → R)	Usually	Often	Not seen	Rare	Often	Late (PVOD)
Transposition of great arteries	Always	Always (mixing)	Sometimes	Sometimes	Rare	Sometimes	Often	Rarely
Coarctation of aorta	Not seen	Occasionally (through PDA)	Not seen	Rarely	Always	Occasionally	Sometimes	Not seen
Interrupted aortic arch	Always (in lower half of body)	Always (through PDA)	Not seen	Rarely	Always	Rarely	Usually	Not seen
Pulmonary atresia	Always	Always (R → L)	Sometimes	Sometimes	Rare	Occasionally	Usually	Always
Truncus arteriosus	Usually	Always (mixing)	Usually	Often	Rare	Sometimes	Usually	Late (PVOD)
Anomalous origin of coronary artery	Not seen	Not seen	Not seen	Often	Not seen	Always	Occasionally	Not seen
Single ventricle	Usually	Always (mixing)	Often	Often	Occasionally	Sometimes	Usually	Occasionally
Aortic stenosis	Not seen	Not seen	Not seen	Occasionally	Always	Not seen	Occasionally	Sometimes
Critical AS		Usually (PDA)	Not seen	Usually	Always	Not seen	Frequently	Always
Pulmonic stenosis	Occasionally	Not seen	Not seen	Occasionally	Not seen	Always	Not seen	Sometimes
Critical PS	Always	Usually (PDA)	Not seen	Usually	Not seen	Always	Not seen	Always
Tricuspid atresia	Always	Always	Frequently	Occasionally	Not seen	Always	Rarely	Frequently
Total anomalous pulmonary venous return	Occasionally	Always	Sometimes	Frequently	Not seen	Frequently	Rarely	Always

PVOD — pulmonary vascular obstructive disease; PDA — patent ductus arteriosus; AS — aortic stenosis; PS — pulmonic stenosis.

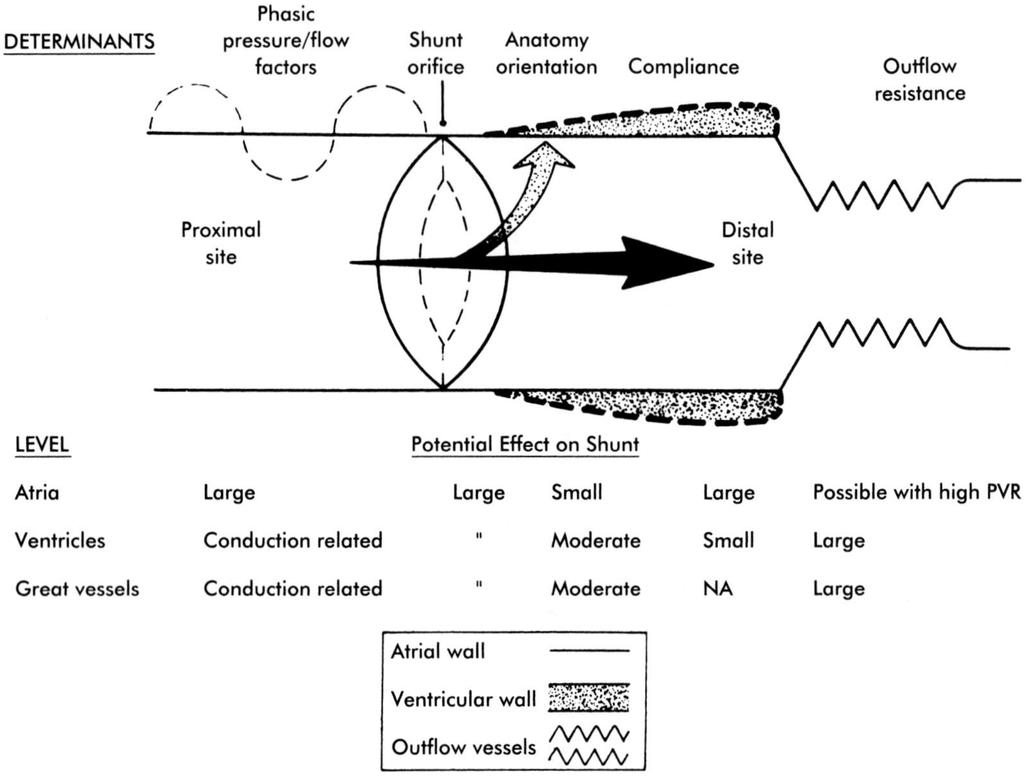

Fig. 69-1. Effects of the many determinants on central cardiac shunting at various levels. PVR, pulmonary vascular resistance. (From Berman W Jr: The hemodynamics of shunts in congenital heart disease. In Johansen K, Burggren WW: *Cardiovascular shunts: phylogenetic, ontogenetic, and clinical aspects*, New York, 1985, Raven Press.)

common chamber. More or less complete mixing (bidirectional shunting) occurs. This usually causes some degree of hypoxemia, despite normal or increased pulmonary blood flow. Mixing implies equal shunting in both directions for any period greater than a few cardiac cycles. If shunting is bidirectional but quantitatively unequal for any long period, there will be a net transfer of blood into the pulmonary or systemic circulation. Continued for more than a few minutes (several hundred cardiac cycles in the infant), this would theoretically put the patient's entire blood volume on one side of the circulation. Actually, this does not occur because changes in compliance resulting from large shifts of blood tend to counteract shunt inequality. Thus, for periods longer than a few cardiac cycles, shunting will be equal in both directions.

With complete mixing in a common chamber and with no outflow obstruction, the amount of pulmonary and systemic blood flow depends on PVR/SVR. Because normal PVR often is much less than SVR (as little as one twentieth of SVR in older children and adults), pulmonary blood flow can become large with a nonrestrictive simple shunt, even in neonates. In these situations, it can become important to limit pulmonary blood flow because pulmonary volume overload can lead to congestive heart failure, inadequate systemic flow, and progressive acidosis. With mixing, arterial oxygen saturation is determined by the relative amount of pulmonary and systemic blood flow (Q_p/Q_s). Because of the shape of the oxyhemoglobin dissociation curve, increasingly large amounts of pulmonary blood flow are required to further increase arterial oxygen saturation as it increases. This is shown in Fig. 69-3 and explains why high arterial oxygen saturations of 90% or greater when CHD is present with mixing physiology can only occur with very high pulmonary blood flows. This high flow frequently leads to congestive heart failure from volume overload, which in turn results in net decreased systemic cardiac output.

Complex shunt lesions

In complex shunts (Fig. 69-4), fixed central outflow obstruction is present at some level on one or the other side of the circulation. Fixed resistance additively increases downstream vascular outflow resistance, which increases shunting to the opposite side. When the fixed resistance is high, it largely dictates total shunting; only part of shunt flow in complex shunts is related to relative resistances in the distal pulmonary and systemic beds. As outflow obstruction in-

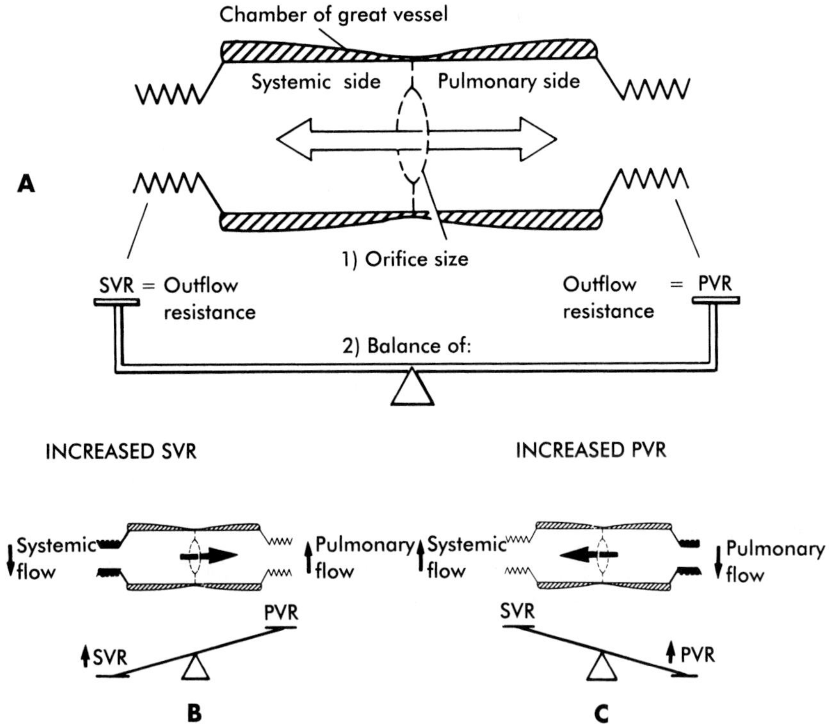

Fig. 69-2. Determinants of magnitude and direction of simple central shunts. *1*, Orifice size is important in determining magnitude of shunting and pressure gradient across shunt and is generally fixed. *2*, Balance of PVR (pulmonary vascular resistance) and SVR (systemic vascular resistance) is dynamic and determines direction of shunt and variations in magnitude around limits fixed by orifice size. **A,** Balanced PVR/SVR. **B,** Increased pulmonary flow with increased SVR. **C,** Increased systemic flow with increased PVR. (From Hickey PR, Wessel DL: Anesthesia for treatment of congenital heart disease. In Kaplan JA, ed: *Cardiac anesthesia*, ed 2, New York, 1987, Grune & Stratton.)

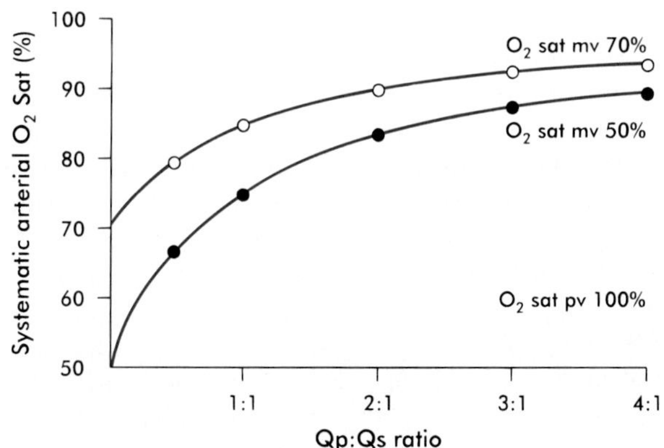

Fig. 69-3. Changes in systemic arterial O_2 saturation with mixing lesions as Qp:Qs (pulmonary-to-systemic flow) ratio changes assuming different levels of mixed venous (*mv*) O_2 saturation. This assumes a pulmonary venous (pv) O_2 saturation of 100%. (From Rudolph AM: *Congenital diseases of the heart*, Chicago, 1974, Year Book Medical Publishers.)

creases and becomes a greater component of total resistance to flow, changes in ipsilateral vascular resistance (PVR or SVR) become progressively less important in determining flow because they become smaller components of total resistance. This is particularly true on the right side, where normal PVR is only a fraction of the resistance offered by most right-sided obstructive lesions seen in CHD. In contrast, changes in vascular resistance (PVR or SVR) contralateral to the fixed obstruction will become relatively more important in determining shunting in complex shunts.

For example, in tetralogy of Fallot with severe pulmonic stenosis, a large component of the right-to-left ventricular septal defect shunting is caused by fixed pulmonary valve stenosis. An additional, variable aspect of shunting may be caused by variations in PVR or dynamic right outflow infundibular obstruction. Dynamic changes in variable portions of the total right ventricular outflow obstruction may increase or decrease total right-to-left shunting, thereby increasing or decreasing

Table 69-2 Simple shunts (no obstructive lesions)

Restrictive shunts (small communications)	Nonrestrictive shunts (large communications)	Common chambers (complete mixing)
Characteristics		
Large Pressure Gradient	Small Pressure Gradient	No pressure gradient
Direction and magnitude more *independent* of PVR/SVR	Direction and magnitude more dependent on PVR/SVR	Bidirectional shunting
Less subject to control	More subject to control	Net Q_p/Q_s totally depends on PVR/SVR
Examples		
Small VSD, small PDA, Blalock shunts, small ASD	Large VSD, large PDA, large Waterson shunts	Single ventricle, truncus arteriosus, single atrium

PVR — pulmonary vascular resistance; SVR — systemic vascular resistance; PDA — patent ductus arteriosus; VSD — ventricular septal defect; Q_p — pulmonary blood flow; Q_s — systemic blood flow.

hypoxemia. At baseline, when dynamic obstructive components are minimal, right-to-left shunting is determined largely by this large, fixed pulmonic obstruction. This presumes constant SVR and cardiac output; large changes in SVR will markedly change shunting by altering the balance contralateral to the final obstruction (Fig. 69-4). Characteristics and examples of complex shunts are listed in Table 69-3.

Complete obstruction

When obstruction to central outflow becomes complete, as in patients with tricuspid atresia, pulmonary atresia, or aortic atresia, shunting across communications proximal to the obstruction becomes total and obligatory and can be considered an extreme type of simple shunt as listed in Table 69-3. This should be associated with another downstream shunt that provides flow to the obstructed side of the circulation. The associated shunt can be a patent ductus arteriosus, which provides pulmonary blood flow in pulmonary valvular atresia or provides systemic blood flow in aortic valvular atresia. Downstream shunting variably depends on PVR/SVR, depending on the restrictive nature of the "compensatory" shunt, i.e., a small patent ductus will constitute most of the resistance when the ductus is the site of the compensatory shunt in pulmonic atresia. In this situation, the small ductus will limit pulmonary blood flow.

Intracardiac shunting and air emboli

Systemic air embolus is a constant danger in patients with CHD, regardless of nominal left-to-right shunting patterns because anesthetic and surgical manipulations can dynamically alter shunts. Air traps are advisable for all intravenous (IV) lines, but these do not substitute for meticulous attention and constant vigilance in the purging of air bubbles. Systemic air emboli are a relative contraindication to use of nitrous oxide in patients with CHD (to be discussed). Right-to-left shunts may occur during some portions of the cardiac cycle or during straining or coughing in patients with open communications and nominal left-to-right shunts because normal transatrial pressure gradients are transiently reversed.[12,79,114] Right-to-left shunting may occur even across functionally "closed" communications. A "probe patent" foramen ovale is common in children (and adults) with and without CHD. Transient right-to-left shunting across such a foramen ovale has even been documented in a healthy child during emergence from anesthesia.[143] In many patients with CHD, direct shunting of microbubbles and macrobubbles of air into the systemic intracerebral arterial circulation from multiple IV lines and injections can be readily documented with transcranial Doppler. "Bubble-free" room temperature solutions may "rain out" bubbles at 37° C. The cerebral effects of such arterial air emboli have not been ascertained except in patients with massive cerebral arterial air emboli.

Severe Hypoxemia

Severe hypoxemia in patients with CHD results from inadequate pulmonary blood flow or defects that allow mixing as defined previously. Chronic hypoxemia requires adaptations to provide adequate tissue oxygen transport. Although moderate hypoxemia is well tolerated in neonates, hypoxemia after infancy produces special problems including polycythemia, increased blood volume, and vasodilation, neovascularization, and alveolar hyperventilation with chronic respiratory alkalosis. Chronic hypoxemia and its accompanying adaptive mechanisms may limit cardiac reserve and oxygen delivery during the stress of anesthetic induction and surgery. Additionally, in such patients, the margin for error and tolerance for loss of airway will be decreased.[193]

Polycythemia increases blood hematocrit and blood viscosity to dangerously high levels that cause vascular stasis and worsen tissue hypoxia.[151] Although an increased hematocrit improves blood oxygen carrying capacity, resultant increased blood viscosity will decrease cardiac output when the hematocrit is greater than 60%. Patients with polycythemia and cyanosis have increased risk for renal or cerebral thrombosis because of increased viscosity, particularly if they become dehydrated.[163] Hematocrits greater than 70% generally are associated with increased risk of cerebrovascular accidents and coagulopathies. These patients may have histories of cerebrovascular accidents and sometimes already have residual neurologic deficits. They require IV hydration starting on the evening before anesthesia and also postoperatively until oral intake is adequate. Some patients may benefit from erythrophoresis before surgery if hematocrits exceed 60% to 70%.

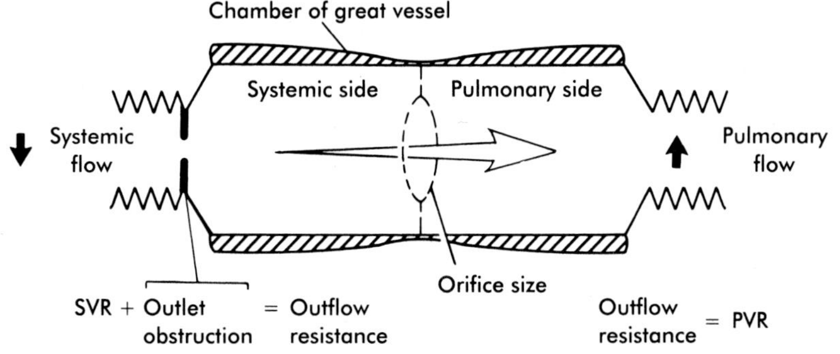

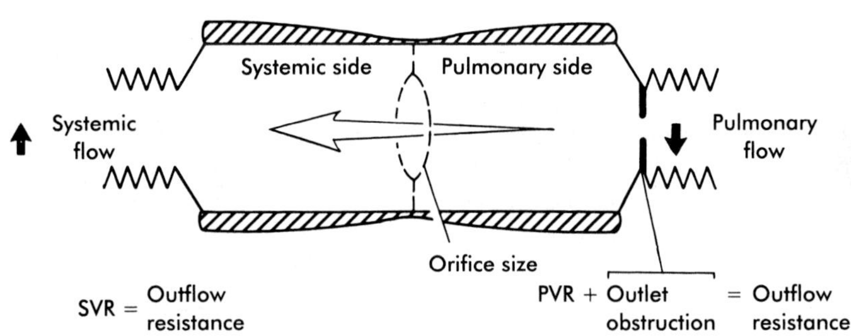

Fig. 69-4. Determinants of complex shunting with systemic or pulmonary outflow obstruction. Orifice size again limits magnitude, but balance of outflow resistances includes outlet obstruction on either side of the circulation in addition to SVR (systemic vascular resistance) or PVR (pulmonary vascular resistance). Addition of outlet obstruction increases flow on the opposite side and decreases flow on the same side. (From Hickey PR, Wessel DL: Anesthesia for treatment of congenital heart disease. In Kaplan JA, ed: *Cardiac anesthesia*, ed 2, New York, 1987, Grune & Stratton.)

Table 69-3 Complex shunts (shunt and obstructive lesions)

Partial outflow obstruction	Total outflow obstruction
Characteristics	
Shunt magnitude and direction largely fixed by obstruction	Shunt magnitude and direction totally fixed
Shunt depends less on PVR/SVR	All flow goes through shunt
Oridice and obstruction determine pressure gradient	Pressure gradient depends on orifice
Examples	
Tetralogy of Fallot, VSD and pulmonic stenosis, VSD with coarctation	Tricuspid atresia, mitral atresia, pulmonary atresia, aortic atresia

Polycythemic CHD patients also have coagulopathies in part because of decreased levels of platelets and fibrinogen.[110] These coagulopathies increase risk of excess intraoperative bleeding, and appropriate arrangements should be made for intraoperative transfusion of clotting factors when necessary.

Patients with severe hypoxemia caused by intracardiac shunting generally undergo anesthesia for procedures designed to improve their pulmonary blood flow and arterial oxygen saturation. Induction of anesthesia itself using a variety of techniques markedly increases arterial saturation.[74,115] This induction-related increase in arterial saturation probably results from greater systemic venous oxygen saturation caused by greater inspired oxygen concentrations plus decreased oxygen consumption with induction of anesthesia and muscle paralysis.[97,130] Systemic venous blood with a greater oxygen saturation is shunted into the systemic circulation, decreasing the degree of hypoxemia seen. Thus, induction of anesthesia itself may be therapeutic for patients with CHD with severe hypoxemia and can sometimes be used to temporize until correction or palliation can be accomplished surgically.

Excessive Pulmonary Blood Flow

Excessive pulmonary blood flow is common in patients with CHD and produces cardiac and pulmonary complications. Volume overload always compromises cardiac reserve, regardless of the presence of frank congestive heart failure. Increased pulmonary artery (PA) pressure and blood flow can limit gas exchange by several mechanisms. Compression of large bronchi by distended pulmonary vessels may obstruct large and small airways and increase the work of breathing. The increased pulmonary venous return distends the left atrium and may obstruct the left main stem bronchus. Most importantly, increased pulmonary blood flow and pressure combine with elevated left atrial pressure to produce pulmonary venous congestion and increased interstitial and alveolar lung water. Resultant lung compliance deterioration and increased airway resistance can produce tachypnea and sometimes wheezing. Regions of the lung with atelectasis and intrapulmonary shunt then will contribute to systemic arterial desaturation, even in a child with "acyanotic" heart disease and left-to-right shunting.

Pulmonary vascular obstructive disease is produced by prolonged high pulmonary flows and pressures. The anatomic lesion is hypertrophy of the medial layer of pulmonary arteries, intimal thickening, with resultant increased pulmonary vascular resistance and reactivity.[82,165] Fig. 69-5 shows normal progression of pulmonary flows, pressures, and vascular resistance during early childhood and alterations in the normal progression with a large VSD. Fig. 69-6 indicates normal evolution of pulmonary arteries during infancy and alteration caused by high pulmonary flows and pressures resulting from left-to-right shunting through a VSD. Smaller pulmonary arteries are anatomic substrates of increased pulmonary vascular reactivity and high PVR seen in patients with pulmonary vascular obstructive disease. When PVR eventually equals or exceeds SVR, a left-to-right shunt then will become a right-to-left shunt (Eisenmenger syndrome). PVOD can occur during the first year of life in patients with some lesions such as an atrioventricular canal but may require decades to develop in patients with atrial septal defects.[83,194] Depending on severity and duration of these changes, correction of the underlying lesion may result in varying degrees of reversal of the pulmonary vascular changes and decreases in pulmonary hypertension.

In neonates with a widely patent ductus arteriosus and a single source of blood supply to the systemic and pulmonary circulations, pulmonary blood flow may become particularly excessive intraoperatively. This is signaled by high systemic arterial saturations (> 90%) in these mixing types of pathophysiologic conditions. It occurs in patients with lesions such as truncus arteriosus or hypoplastic left heart syndrome and results in acute congestive heart failure with ventricular enlargement, low systemic output, high arterial oxygen saturation, and hypotension. This can produce myocardial ischemia in neonates.[216] The myocardial ischemia seen in this situation can be remedied only by acutely increasing PVR by placing a tourniquet on one of the branch pulmonary arteries or by applying a partially occluding PA clamp. These maneuvers mechanically increase PVR, decrease the excessive pulmonary blood flow and arterial saturation, and increase systemic (coronary) perfusion pressure, and at the same time decrease cardiac volume load and reduce ventricular diameter. In patients with CHD with tendencies toward excessive pulmonary blood flow and only mild hypoxemia, anesthetic management is planned to avoid major decreases in PVR because such decreases will exacerbate the increased pulmonary flow and lead to cardiovascular decompensation.

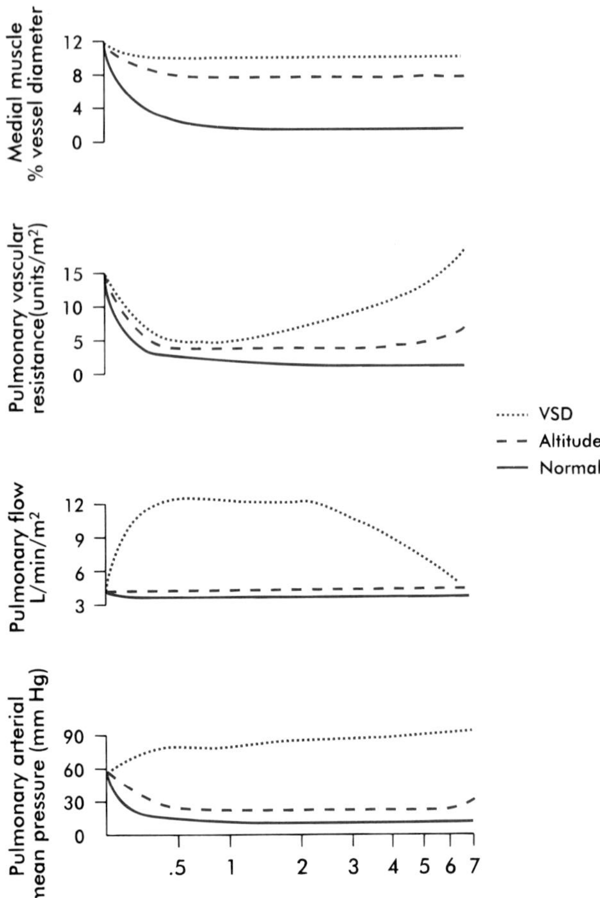

Fig. 69-5. Normal and abnormal developmental changes in pulmonary arterial tree during the first years of life. Pulmonary vascular resistance, percent of arterial smooth muscle, and pressure normally fall in first year of life. A large, nonrestrictive VSD with a large L-R shunt results in an immediate increase in flow and a later increase in vascular resistance. (From Rudolph AM: *Congenital diseases of the heart*, Chicago, 1974, Year Book Medical Publishers.)

Congestive Heart Failure

The child with CHD will develop congestive heart failure because of increased pressure, volume, or combined pres-

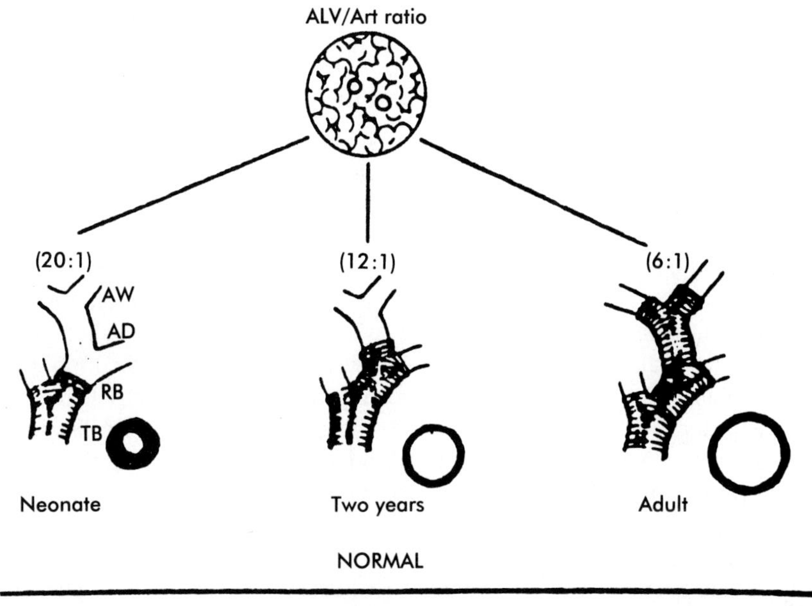

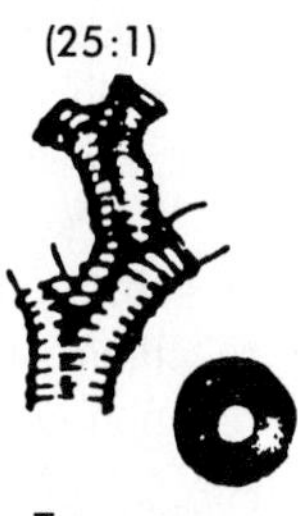

Fig. 69-6. Developmental changes in peripheral pulmonary arterial tree in normal patients and in the presence of VSD with large L-R shunt. Alveolar-to-arteriolar (*ALV/Art*) ratio decreases with age because of extensive arborization of arterial tree as arteriolar lumen increases and muscle layer thins and spreads distally. Pulmonary hypertension with high flow from L-R shunt in a VSD cause pulmonary vascular obstructive disease marked by decreased numbers of pulmonary arterioles (*ALV/Art of 25:1*), decrease in vessel lumen, increase in muscle thickness, and more distal spread of muscle. Letters indicate arterioles from level of the terminal bronchiolus (*TB*) to the alveolar wall (*AW*). (From Rabinovitch MB, Haworth SG, Castaneda AR et al: Lung biopsy in congenital heart disease: a morphometric approach to pulmonary vascular disease, *Circulation* 58:1107,

sure and volume loads. Increased volume loads can result from intracardiac shunting or valvular insufficiency. Increased pressure loads can result from valvular obstruction, stenosis of major systemic or pulmonary arteries, or from diffuse PVOD. Patients compensate by well-known mechanisms. Increased catecholamine production redistributes cardiac output to favored organs, increases heart rate, decreases skin temperature, and frequently induces a catabolic nutritional state.[190] Pulmonary congestion increases the work of breathing and caloric demand, whereas tachypnea limits intake of calories. Derangements vary with severity of congestive heart failure. In the severe cases, growth is retarded, and body weight is well below the third percentile for age. These patients often are tachypneic, tachycardic, and dusky in room air and may have chest wall retractions, expiratory wheezes, and diffuse rhonchi. Capillary refill may be prolonged and extremities cool to the touch, with palpable hepatomegaly. Preoperative chest radiographs demonstrate cardiac enlargement and increased pulmonary vascular markings with areas of atelectasis despite hyperexpansion of the lungs. In severe cases, medical management consisting of administration of digoxin and diuretics is indicated before surgery, which may induce a profound metabolic hypochloremic alkalosis with potassium depletion.

Other children with lesser degrees of congestive heart failure caused by CHD may be only mildly symptomatic but still have substantially decreased cardiovascular reserves.

The additional stress of anesthesia and surgery may result in cardiac decompensation, particularly when compensation depends on maximal sympathetic tone. Reversibility of ventricular dysfunction accompanying congestive heart failure in those with CHD varies depending on severity of the defect, degree of correction, and duration of ventricular dysfunction.

Prolonged congestive heart failure and attendant ventricular dysfunction result in cardiomegaly and ventricular hypertrophy. The amount and location of cardiomegaly or hypertrophy occurring depends on the combination of cardiac pressure and volume loads and intracardiac anatomy. Long-standing cardiomegaly and hypertrophy jeopardize the myocardium in children, particularly in those with chronic hypoxemia. In the young, growing heart, pressure-overload hypertrophy appears to occur in association with myocardial angiogenesis rather than with diminished myocardial capillary density as occurs in adults.[60] Despite the former compensatory mechanism, microscopic areas of myocardial infarction eventually appear over time in young hearts subjected to chronic overload, particularly in those with chronic hypoxemia.[63] This results in progressive ventricular dysfunction in the affected ventricle as working muscle mass is depleted and is replaced by fibrous tissue. Some ventricular dysfunction may be reversible, depending on timing of correction of the underlying defect. For example, ventricular septal defects and tetralogy of Fallot defects repaired during early infancy before myocardial damage occurs subsequently have better ventricular function than those repaired later in childhood.[24,43,98,104,123]

In patients with any degree of congestive heart failure, anesthetic treatment is planned to avoid large doses of myocardial depressants and alterations of PVR or SVR that will exacerbate cardiac failure. Which alterations will be detrimental depend on individual pathophysiology findings. In patients with severe congestive heart failure or in those with detrimental alterations in pathophysiologic conditions that cannot be avoided, appropriate pressor and inotropic support are included in the anesthetic plan.

Obstructions to Systemic Blood Flow

Congenital lesions producing obstruction to left heart outflow include interruption of the aortic arch, coarctation of the aorta, aortic stenosis (subvalvar, valvar, or supravalvar), mitral stenosis and atresia, and hypoplastic left heart syndrome (HLHS). These patients may have left ventricular hypertrophy, coronary ischemia, and limited systemic ventricular reserve. Systemic perfusion in neonates with these problems often depends on a patent ductus arteriosus that may be rapidly narrowing. Such infants usually present with shock and metabolic acidosis, requiring resuscitation with prostaglandin E_1 (PGE_1) preoperatively. Ventricular fibrillation is a distinct risk. Older children with less severe forms of stenosis often are asymptomatic with only mild hypertension in coarctation of the aorta or mild aortic stenosis. They may have dysrhythmias, syncope, fatigue, or chest pain in various forms of aortic stenosis.

Obstructions to Pulmonary Blood Flow

Pulmonary flow obstructions occur at many levels in the right side of the circulation. Right ventricular hypertension, pulmonary hypertension, and hypoxemia may result, depending on where the obstructions occur and the presence of intracardiac shunting. Combinations of these problems are seen in pulmonary valve and subvalvular stenosis, PA stenosis, PVOD, tetralogy of Fallot, and pulmonary atresia. High levels of right ventricular afterload result in a hypertensive, hypertrophied right ventricle that is prone to myocardial ischemia. As right ventricular intracavitary pressures approach and then exceed systemic arterial pressures, coronary perfusion pressures become inadequate, and right ventricular failure results from myocardial ischemia. Acute therapy is aimed at increasing systemic arterial pressure with alpha-adrenergic agents, such as phenylepinephrine, to improve coronary perfusion of the right ventricle.[206] Lowering of pulmonary vascular resistance also is beneficial if it can be accomplished without decreasing systemic (coronary) perfusion pressure.

Patients with right ventricular hypertension resulting from outflow obstruction or obstruction of the larger pulmonary vessels can be effectively treated with balloon dilation in the cardiac catheterization laboratory or with a surgical procedure. Unilateral or segmental pulmonary edema requiring management may be seen after such procedures. When pulmonary vascular resistance at the small vessel level is markedly elevated and irreversible, as in those with end-stage PVOD, therapy is frequently ineffective. Patients with a markedly hypertensive pulmonary circulation of any duration suffer from cor pulmonale or dysrhythmias and are prone to sudden, poorly understood increases in pulmonary vascular resistance. Such pulmonary hypertensive crises may occur without warning, resulting in refractory acute right ventricular failure and sometimes in death. When systemic levels of pulmonary arterial pressure are encountered in the operating room, despite corrective procedures, every effort should be made to find a way to correct this problem because of the associated high risks of sudden decompensation and death.

Coronary Ischemia

Although acquired coronary artery disease is rare in children with CHD, except in those with transplanted hearts, coronary ischemia may occur with left heart outflow obstruction, surgical retraction, "pulmonary steal" in neonates with a single source of pulmonary and systemic flows, or anomalous coronary arteries arising from the PA. In neonates with truncus arteriosus, intraoperative decreases in pulmonary vascular resistance can lead to decreased systemic flow and diastolic pressure, which produces ST segment changes indicative of acute myocardial ischemia. Maneuvers to decrease pulmonary flow, such as temporarily ligating the left or right PA, can increase diastolic pressure and reverse the ischemia and ST segment changes seen on electrocardiography (ECG).[216] In anomalous coronary arteries, retrograde flow into the PA occurs via anastomotic connection with normal coronary arteries when flow is stolen from the greater pressure, normal coronaries originating from the aortic root. Myocardial infarcts and ventricular dysfunction can result; these problems may be preventable or reversible if the anomalous coronary arteries are detected and corrected early in life.

Rarely, patients may have aberrant sinusoidal coronary arteries originating directly from the right ventricular cavity. These arteries provide nutrient, antegrade (albeit hypoxemic) flow into the coronary bed as long as high (systemic) pressures are maintained in the right ventricle. Any intervention that substantially decreases right ventricular intracavitary pressure results in intractable and even fatal coronary ischemia. When perfusion pressure decreases, flow from these vessels becomes retrograde into the right ventricular cavity as flow is "stolen" from adjacent, communicating systemic coronary arterial beds.

Immaturity of the Circulation

Transitional circulation

Transitional circulation consists of a patent ductus arteriosus (PDA), patent foramen ovale, and high pulmonary vascular resistance, as is shown schematically in Fig. 69-7. In neonates with severe, life-threatening CHD, the transitional circulation plays a major role in maintaining viability because its persistence is required to sustain functional circulation until therapeutic interventions can be undertaken. Particularly important in maintaining an intact circulation is patency of the ductus arteriosus. Before anatomic (as opposed to physiologic) closure occurs at several weeks of age in the normal sequence, the ductus may remain open in response to hypoxemia or PGE_1 infusion.[66,146] Reopening of the ductus has been documented in infants aged more than 7 days and in whom the ductus has been kept open with PGE_1 infusions for many weeks when necessary.[37,220]

The patent ductus arteriosus plays a critical role in maintaining life by providing either systemic or pul-

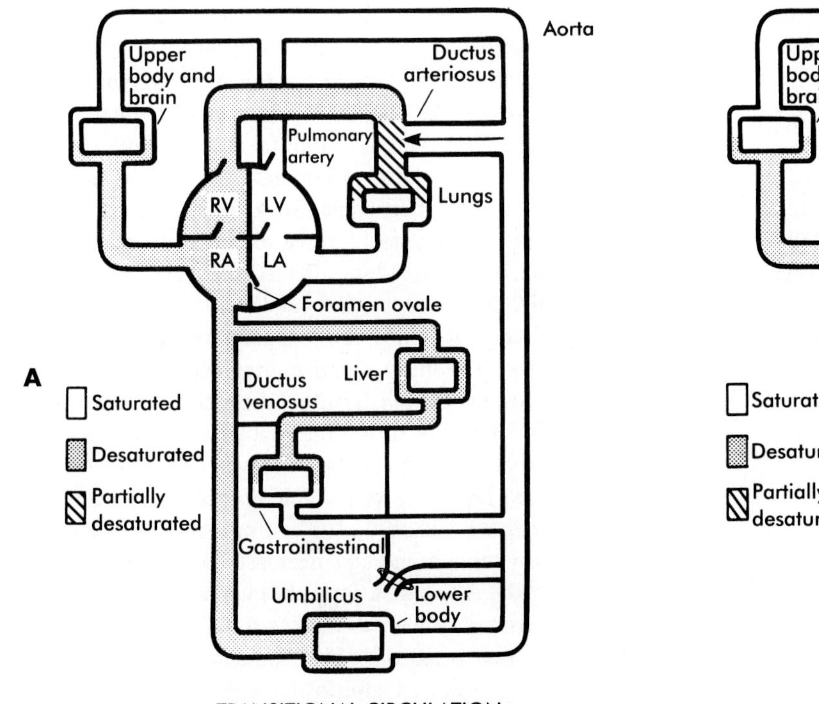

Fig. 69-7. Schematic diagram of central shunting and blood saturations that occur normally in the transitional circulation in the first few hours and days after birth. **A,** In the first few hours, foramen ovale is widely patent and pulmonary vascular resistance is high, leading to right-to-left shunting. **B,** Depiction of a later stage of transitional circulation when pulmonary vascular resistance falls and the ductus remains patent, resulting in left-to-right shunting. Foramen ovale is functionally closed. (From Hickey PR, Crone RK: Cardiovascular physiology and pharmacology in children. In Ryan JR, Todres PS, Coté C et al, eds: *A practice of anesthesia for infants and children*, New York, 1986, Grune & Stratton.

monary blood flow in neonates with severe congenital heart lesions (Box 69-1). Acute decompensation occurs in these infants when the ductus closes. When systemic and coronary perfusion depend on a PDA, closure results in reduction of systemic flow, coronary insufficiency, rapidly progressive metabolic acidosis, and death.[81,100] When pulmonary flow depends on a patent ductus, closure results in acute reduction of pulmonary flow, progressive hypoxemia, and death.[29] In neonates with ductus-dependent lesions who decompensate after closure, therapy with PGE_1 infusion for 24 to 48 hours provides effective resuscitation and correction of metabolic deficits.[218] Side effects of PGE_1 infusion include apnea and vasodilation; many neonates receiving PGE_1 infusions will need intubation and ventilatory support and supplementation of intravascular volume.[128]

High pulmonary vascular resistance in the transitional circulation is particularly important when the congenital defect is one with only a single, nonrestrictive source of pulmonary and systemic blood flow as in truncus arteriosus, HLHS, or pulmonary atresia. When the ductus arteriosus is kept widely patent with PGE_1 or when there is no ductus involved (truncus arteriosus), decreases in high pulmonary vascular resistance from the immediate postnatal levels produce "pulmonary steal" of systemic blood flow and low diastolic blood pressure. This leads to systemic hypoperfusion, coronary ischemia, and progressive metabolic acidosis, despite good arterial oxygen saturations.[81,99]

The immature heart

At birth, the immature heart is markedly different from the mature heart. Right and left ventricles have roughly equal size and wall thickness; the right ventricle is slightly heavier.[174] The increased afterload on the left and decreased afterload on the right, occurring with birth, leads to progressive thickening of the left ventricular wall. By age 4 weeks, the left ventricle weighs more than the right.[57] By age 3 or 4 years, the left ventricle is approximately twice as heavy as the right, the normal adult relationship.

These changes are accompanied by myocyte ultrastructural development. Small immature myocytes with chaotically arranged myofibrils accounting for 30% of gross muscle mass evolve into larger mature myocytes with organized, longitudinally oriented myofibrils that make up 60% of muscle mass.[9,155] The larger mass of noncontractile elements in immature myocytes results in noncompliant cells with lesser contractile capacities. Myocardial contractility and compliance increase with development; immature myocardium develops less force during contraction than does adult myocardium, and velocity and magnitude of shortening also are less in immature myocytes.[154,155]

Other changes include development of the transverse tubular system, essentially absent in the neonatal heart, and development of sarcoplasmic reticulum, increasing its capacity to store and release calcium.[156,203] Contractile proteins, namely myosin, tropomyosin, and troponin T, required for myocardial contraction also change their isoforms during this period.[96]

These changes, taken together, may explain increased sensitivity to inhalation anesthetic agents seen in the immature heart.[64,112,113,166] Ultrastructural changes occurring in maturing myocytes result in improved myocardial function, but until myocytes fully mature, cardiac reserve will be limited. This should be appreciated in anesthetic treatment of infants with CHD, who have additional sources of decreased cardiac reserve in addition to immaturity. Despite these factors, immaturity confers some "advantage" for cardiac function during hemodynamic stress because during acidosis contractile function is less affected,[152,153] and intracellular myocardial pH is better maintained.[154]

Functional capacities of the immature heart have been well defined. The immature, noncompliant ventricle is very sensitive to increases in filling volume and is relatively restricted in its ability to respond with increased stroke volume. Although stroke volume improves with increased filling pressure, the range over which this occurs is narrow. The Starling curve is reached at filling pressures of 4 mm Hg, and stroke volume actually decreases at filling pressures near 7 mm Hg.[195] This Starling plateau may be a result of increased afterload effects as mean arterial pressure increases with increased preload.[200] The immature ventricle is very sensitive to increased afterload. With constant afterload, stroke volume improves with progressive increases in left atrial pressure from 5 to 10 mm Hg. Because the immature heart is noncompliant, small increases in intravascular volume will rapidly increase filling pressures to the plateau of the Starling curve where stroke volume is fixed. At the level of filling pressure where stroke volume is fixed, cardiac output becomes rate-dependent. Additional increases in volume will push filling pressures to the descending portion of the curve, and the ventricle begins to fail. Although the Starling curve of the neonate is clearly shifted to the left compared

BOX 69-1
DUCTUS-DEPENDENT NEONATAL CONGENITAL HEART DEFECTS

PDA provides systemic flow

Critical coarctation of the aorta
Interrupted aortic arch
Hypoplastic left heart syndrome
Critical aortic stenosis

PDA provides pulmonary flow

Pulmonary atresia
Critical pulmonic stenosis
Severe subpulmonic stenosis with VSD
Tricuspid atresia with pulmonic stenosis

PDA — patent ductus arteriosus; VSD — ventricular septal defect.

with older children and adults, it still does apply.[52,109] Because of this, cardiac output is not entirely rate-dependent at lesser filling pressures and rates within neonatal physiologic range. Increases or decreases in heart rate within physiologic ranges result in changes in stroke volume without major changes in cardiac output in the term human fetus and in the lamb.[27,105] It is only when the plateau of the Starling curve is reached that the immature heart becomes truly rate-dependent.

Reduced compliance and similarity in size and wall thickness of the ventricles during the first month leads to an intimate interrelationship between right and left ventricular function.[52] Failure of one immature ventricle quickly causes septal shift, and in contrast to adults, congestive heart failure quickly becomes biventricular. This has important implications for ventilatory management, namely the fact that inadequate ventilation in infants rapidly leads to increased right ventricular afterload and biventricular failure because of the muscular, hyperreactive pulmonary circulation. This also applies to small infants with CHD. As a result of the poor tolerance of the immature heart for increased afterload, right ventricular failure of some degree may result, which, in turn, rapidly compromises function of the left ventricle. Thus, adequacy of ventilation in the infant frequently determines cardiac function even if severe hypoxemia has not yet occurred.

In summary, functional capacity of the immature infant heart and cardiac reserve improve with age. Increasing preload or afterload will result in ventricular failure sooner in neonates and infants than in adults, and failure quickly becomes biventricular. By age 3 or 4, adult levels of systemic arterial pressure and pulmonary vascular resistance are achieved, and the previously mentioned functional limitations probably no longer apply. Additional stresses and loads placed on the immature heart by various forms of CHD will further reduce cardiac reserves in infants, thus reducing their already compromised ability to deal with stresses of anesthesia and surgery.

Combined problems

Combinations of the previously mentioned problems will be found in many patients with CHD. Excessive flows caused by intracardiac shunting and flow obstruction often will lead to congestive heart failure. In older children with long-standing complex lesions that cannot be readily corrected, ventricular function may gradually deteriorate because of long-standing ventricular pressure or volume overload. Chronic volume loading is seen in those with aortic or mitral valve regurgitation or in patients with long-standing pulmonary-to-systemic arterial shunts. The latter patients may have only mild-to-moderate hypoxemia despite complete mixing when there is a large shunt and excessive pulmonary blood flow. The price paid for near-normal levels of arterial oxygen saturation is chronic ventricular dilation and potential development of PVOD. These patients may have combined problems of hypoxemia and mild cyanosis, some degree of PVOD, and left ventricular dilation with progressively decreasing ejection fractions.

In infants and especially neonates, problems of transitional circulation and limited functional capacity of the immature heart are invariably added to physiologic problems created by the CHD itself. Because the most severe forms of CHD generally are present in neonates, such congenital heart problems are complicated by physiologic limitations of the immature heart and lungs.

In patients with complex congenital disease in whom a number of previously discussed problems are present, assessment should be directed at myocardial performance and reserve, quantification of pulmonary blood flow, degree of cyanosis, and evaluation of PVR. For example, a patient with a long-standing Waterston shunt who is only mildly cyanotic but easily fatigued and who has a heaving precordium with bounding pulses may be expected to have a high normal hematocrit with oxygen saturation in the upper 80s. Pulmonary blood flow will be torrential, and PVR is elevated. This patient may not be a candidate for reparative cardiac procedures because of high (and irreversible) PVR resulting from progressive PVOD.

INTRAOPERATIVE PROBLEMS OCCURRING WITH SPECIFIC PROCEDURES OR TECHNIQUES USED IN TREATMENT OF CONGENITAL HEART DISEASE

Complex intracardiac anatomy, incomplete or misdiagnosis of specific lesions, limitations of currently available procedures, and technical errors combine to result in hemodynamic problems in an appreciable fraction of patients who require surgical or transcatheter treatment of CHD. **These problems often present as hemodynamic instability, low cardiac output, or hypoxemia in the operating room or in the catheterization laboratory immediately after the cardiac repair or later in the intensive care unit. Causes may not be readily apparent and may require intraoperative pressure measurements, intraoperative or postoperative echocardiography, and sometimes early postoperative cardiac catheterization before the cause is clearly established and before therapy can be properly directed.**

Problems Associated with Specific Surgical Procedures

The anesthesia care team should deal with such problems until their causes are discovered and corrected. Primary pump failure is only infrequently the cause of difficulties seen in this setting. In the majority of patients, a specific mechanical problem in the circulation system is responsible. Table 69-4 lists the incidence of different problems commonly seen with specific surgical procedures.

Excessive pulmonary flow

In addition to its occurrence in lesions described previously, excessive pulmonary flow may be a result of operative procedures. A surgically created aortopulmonary shunt such as a Blalock-Taussig shunt can be too large, with excessive

Table 69-4 Hemodynamic problems resulting from various cardiac surgical procedures

Procedure	Excessive pulmonary flow	Inadequate pulmonary flow	Intracardial shunting	Obstruction to left heart inflow/outflow
PDA ligation	Rarely (partial ligation)	Rarely (mistaken PA ligation)	Not seen	Rarely (mistaken aortic ligation)
ASD closure	Rarely (residual ASD)	Not seen	Rarely (residual ASD)	Not seen
VSD closure	Occasionally (residual VSD)	Not seen	Occasionally (residual VSD)	Occasionally
Tetralogy of Fallot repair	Occasionally	Rarely	Occasionally (residual VSD)	Not seen
Complete atrioventricular canal repair	Occasionally (residual VSD)	Not seen	Occasionally (residual VSD)	Not seen
Transposition: Mustard or Senning repair	Not seen	Not seen	Rarely	Occasionally (obstruction of pulmonary veins—inflow)
Transposition: Arterial switch repair	Not seen	Not seen	Rarely	Rarely (supraaortic stenosis)
Coarctation repair	Not seen	Not seen	Not seen	Occasionally (residual aortic gradient)
Fontan repair	Not seen	Occasionally	Occasionally (baffle leak)	Not seen
PA banding	Occasionally	Often	Always	Not seen
Blalock-Taussig shunt (classic or modified)	Occasionally	Occasionally	Always	Not seen
Glenn shunt	Not seen	Occasionally	Always	Not seen
Total anomalous pulmonary venous return	Not seen	Occasionally	Rarely	Occasionally (PV obstruction)

PDA—patent ductus arteriosus; ASD—atrial septal defect; VSD—ventricular septal defect; PS—pulmonic stenosis; RV—right ventricle; Des Ao—descending aorta.

pulmonary blood flow and low systemic cardiac output. Residual intracardiac left-to-right shunt can produce excessive pulmonary blood flow as a result of incomplete repair or undiagnosed and unsuspected defect. Increased volume load may result in low cardiac output in a heart that has been injured by a period of hypothermic ischemia with cross-clamping during cardiopulmonary bypass. Measures designed to increase PVR and to provide inotropic support will improve the hemodynamic condition temporarily until a specific diagnosis can be made and until residual problems are corrected (Box 69-2).

Excessive pulmonary flow also can result from failure to ligate an aortopulmonary shunt (e.g., a patent ductus arteriosus or a Blalock-Taussig shunt). In some patients, an extensive series of large and small native aortopulmonary collateral vessels from the descending aorta, bronchial arteries, and the vertebral arterial system can produce excessive pulmonary flow postoperatively. In the absence of a few large collaterals that can be easily approached and ligated surgically, this problem is best approached pre- or postoperatively in the catheterization laboratory where multiple small vessels can be embolized. Until interruption of collateral supply is accomplished, inotropic support often is needed. Presence of such collaterals can jeopardize cerebral blood flow during cardiopulmonary bypass, particularly when the pulmonary collaterals originate from vessels also supplying the head. This problem is more likely when alpha-stat acid–base management is used for hypothermic bypass, and low Pa_{CO_2} levels dilate the pulmonary circulation while constricting the cerebral circulation.

Inadequate pulmonary flow

This occurs also in association with surgically created aortopulmonary shunts, such as the Blalock shunt, that are too small, have clotted, or have partially obstructed anastomoses. These patients may become hypoxemic (SaO_2 <

Obstruction to right heart inflow/outflow	Conronary ischemia	Dysrhythmias	Low cardiac output
Rarely (ligation of PA)	Not seen	Not seen	Rarely
Not seen	Not seen	Rarely	Rarely
Rarely	Not seen	Rarely	Occasionally (residual VSD)
Occasionally (residual PS)	Not seen	Rarely	Occasionally (RV dysfunction and PI)
Not seen	Not seen	Rarely	Occasionally (mitral insufficiency)
Occasionally (SVC or IVC inflow obstruction)	Rarely	Frequently (atrial)	Occasionally
Rarely (suprapulmonary stenosis)	Occasionally (iatrogenic coronary obstruction)	Rarely	Occasionally (2° to coronary ischemia)
Not seen	Not seen	Not seen	Not seen
Occasionally	Not seen	Occasionally (often 2° to high PVR)	Often (2° to high PVR)
Always	Not seen	Rarely	Occasionally (loose PA band)
Not seen	Not seen	Rarely	Occasionally
Often (transient SVC obstruction)	Not seen	Rarely	Occasionally
Often (transient increased PVR)	Not seen	Rarely	Often

70%) immediately after opening the newly constructed shunt after an existing source of pulmonary blood, e.g., patent ductus arteriosis, is ligated. Degree of hypoxemia may not be appreciated until reversal of muscle paralysis and emergence from anesthesia. Increases in oxygen consumption and resultant decreases in mixed venous oxygen saturation accompanying these events can result in substantial decreases in arterial oxygen saturation when pulmonary flow through the shunt is marginal. Anesthesia, hypothermia, and paralysis using muscle relaxants will improve the situation temporarily until increased shunt flow can be established. PA banding procedures also can produce the picture described previously. Inadequate flow and increased right ventricular afterload resulting from excessive tightening usually is immediately apparent as progressive hypoxemia, right ventricular dilation, hypotension, and bradycardia. This is acute right ventricular failure and is managed by immediate loosening of the band.

BOX 69-2
ANESTHETIC MANAGEMENT OF EXCESSIVE PULMONARY BLOOD FLOW

Signs

High arterial saturations in mixing physiology
Oxygen saturation step-up from RA to PA
Elevated pulmonary artery pressures

Therapeutic maneuvers

Low FIO_2
Normocapnia or mild hypercapnia
Positive end-expiratory pressure
Mechanical restriction of pulmonary flow (clamp or band)
Inotropic and pressor support
Ligation or coil embolization of aortopulmonary shunts and collaterals

Inadequate pulmonary flow also may occur after a Fontan procedure. This procedure is used when there is no pulmonary ventricle to pump blood through the lungs; pulmonary blood flow depends on a gradient between central venous pressure and left atrial pressure. Moderate elevations in PVR resulting from cardiopulmonary bypass and associated events or mechanical obstruction to blood flow in the Fontan pathway can severely restrict pulmonary flow, resulting in inadequate left heart filling. Low cardiac output is seen with high central venous pressure (CVP > 17 to 20 mm Hg). These patients generally are not hypoxemic. Inotropic support, "pulmonary" vasodilators, and other manipulations to decrease PVR shown in Box 69-3 are only temporizing measures. Urgent reoperations are needed to avoid progressive low cardiac output, multiorgan dysfunction, and death. When fenestrated Fontan procedures are done, shunting through the fenestration will maintain cardic output even when PVR is high; cardiac output will be maintained, but hypoxemia will result from low pulmonary blood flow. With the fenestrated Fontan, the cardiac output is better maintained, and tolerance for transient increases as PVR improves.

Intracardiac shunting

Intracardiac shunting occurs intentionally in surgical procedures such as creation of aortopulmonary shunts and PA bands because these are palliative procedures wherein no attempt is made to completely correct the anatomy. Residual intracardiac shunting also occurs unintentionally. Residual defects may remain because of inadequacies in the surgical repair or because of undiagnosed additional defects. Any time an intracardiac patch or baffle is placed, there is potential for residual intracardiac shunting. Such residual shunting usually produces either excessive or insufficient pulmonary blood flow, depending on individual pathophysiology. It is handled by manipulating SVR/PVR to minimize detrimental effects.

BOX 69-3
ANESTHETIC MANAGEMENT OF INADEQUATE PULMONARY BLOOD FLOW

Signs

$SaO_2 < 75\%$
Right atrial pressure > 15–17 mm Hg (Fontan)

Therapeutic maneuvers

100% O_2
Increased systemic perfusion pressure with pressors
Hypocapnia to $Paco_2 < 25$ mm Hg with hyperventilation and alkalinization
Maintainance of normal FRC (avoiding hyperexpansion or atelectasis of lungs)
Trial of PEEP (low levels 3–7 cm H_2O)
Reduce oxygen consumption (anesthesia, paralysis, hypothermia)
Drainage of pleural and peritoneal cavities
Trial of pulmonary vasodilators, including nitric oxide

FRC — functional residual capacity; PEEP — positive end-expiratory pressure.

Obstruction to left heart outflow or inflow

When complex reconstructions of the ventricular septum are done inside the heart near the left ventricular outflow tract, subaortic obstructions to flow may be created, which result in low cardiac output and persistent, large inotropic requirement. This problem should be suspected because of the combination of hemodynamic instability and a complex ventricular septal defect repair in the subaortic region. Diagnosis can be made using pullback pressure measurements from the left ventricle to the aortic root and by intraoperative echocardiography. Supportive measures, including inotropic support (Box 69-4), in these patients are no substitute for correction of outflow obstruction.

In other ventricular septal repairs, large degrees of obstruction to right heart outflow producing suprasystemic right ventricular pressures may cause bowing and shift of the intraventricular septum into the left ventricular outflow tract and even obstruction. The obstruction to right ventricular outflow should be corrected and usually will greatly improve left heart function. Again, inotropic support is only a temporizing measure.

Obstruction to left heart inflow (i.e., pulmonary venous return) may occur with atrial baffle repairs of transposition of the great arteries (Mustard or Senning repairs) or occasionally with repair of total anomalous pulmonary venous return. This presents as low cardiac output; pulmonary hypertension; and severe, poorly tolerated pulmonary edema. Immediate relief of the pulmonary venous obstruction is indicated.

Obstruction to right heart outflow or inflow

This occurs most frequently in tetralogy of Fallot repair or other repairs of pulmonic stenosis and PA hypoplasia. Inad-

BOX 69-4
ANESTHETIC MANAGEMENT OF LEFT HEART OUTFLOW OBSTRUCTION

Signs

Large inotropic requirement
Low cardiac output
High LA pressure

Therapeutic maneuvers

High left atrial filling pressures
Maintenance of high coronary perfusion pressures
Minimization of RV afterload
Inotropic and pressor support

equate relief of the pulmonary stenosis leads to right ventricular hypertension and often some degree of right heart failure, which may not be tolerated. In the immature heart, right ventricular failure is always accompanied by some degree of left ventricular dysfunction. Moderate outflow obstruction does not usually cause severe problems but often requires inotropic support intraoperatively and postoperatively. Measures used in these situations are outlined in Box 69-5.

Obstruction to right heart inflow occasionally occurred with complex intraatrial baffle repairs of transposition of the great arteries (Mustard or Senning repairs). Most common is superior vena cava obstruction, intraoperatively seen as low cardiac output and immediately apparent when surgical drapes are removed and severe head and upper body edema and venous stasis are apparent. Similar problems with inferior vena cava obstruction occur less frequently during Mustard and Senning repairs. These repairs are now infrequently done because of the superiority of great vessel switch procedures for transposition repairs.

Coronary ischemia

Coronary ischemia associated with congenital heart procedures usually has iatrogenic origins. The "switch" operation for transposition of the great arteries entails relocation of the coronary arteries in small infants from the right ventricular outflow tract to the left ventricular outflow tract. Technical errors in transplantation of these small cornary arteries may result in stenosis from excessive tension, anastomotic obstruction, or tortion of transplanted coronary arteries. Coronary ischemia may then develop intraoperatively or later. It most often is apparent as ventricular failure and low cardiac output.

In other types of repairs in which dissection and retraction around the aortic root is done, compression, inadvertent suture ligation, and inadvertent transection of coronary arteries can occur. These events may be first signaled by ST-T wave ECG changes. It is important to continuously monitor two ECG leads in congenital heart surgery, preferably leads II and V_5 or V_6. When ischemia is seen, the measures outlined in Box 69-6 are useful until the cause is found and corrected.

The most frequent type of coronary ischemia seen is simply that associated with inadequate coronary perfusion pressures when weaning from bypass. Even in children with normal coronary arteries, stress of high afterload, dilated ventricles, and tachycardia can result in coronary ischemia, particularly during hypotension. Such ischemia usually is easily managed by increasing systemic arterial pressure using a vasopressor or by increasing cardiopulmonary bypass (CPB) flow pump output, slowing heart rate, and correcting overdistension of the ventricle. Nitroglycerine is rarely useful because of the etiology of most coronary ischemia in patients with CHD.

Dysrhythmias

Most dysrhythmias seen in patients with CHD are iatrogenic and are related to mechanical or ischemic injury to conduction pathways. Anesthetic agents can alter or exacerbate existing dysrhythmias but are rarely solely responsible for dysrhythmias seen during cardiac procedures.[121] These dysrhythmias limit cardiovascular reserve and increase operative risk. Some patients with CHD may be receiving antiarrhythmic drugs or have implanted pacemakers. Particular attention should be paid to the patient's intrinsic rate and rhythm plus characteristics of pacemaker function. In patients with surgically induced complete heart block, immediate temporary pacing generally is required. If arteriovenous conduction has not returned in 10 days, permanent pacing is needed because arteriovenous conduction rarely returns after this time.[53]

In patients with CHD with permanent pacemakers undergoing cardiac surgical procedures, asystole will often result if pacemaker failure occurs. Although setting the pacemaker to asynchronous mode will protect against interference from inappropriate sensing caused by electrocautery, cautery use

BOX 69-5
ANESTHETIC MANAGEMENT OF RIGHT HEART OUTFLOW OBSTRUCTION

Signs

Inotropic requirement
Low cardiac output
High RA pressure and RV pressures

Therapeutic maneuvers

Maintenance of high RA filling pressures
Maintenance of high coronary perfusion pressures
Minimization of PVR
Inotropic support

BOX 69-6
ANESTHETIC MANAGEMENT OF CORONARY ISCHEMIA IN CONGESTIVE HEART DISEASE

Signs

ST-T segment changes in ECG levels II or $V_{5\text{-}6}$
Cyanotic demarcation of epicardial coronary distribution
Dyskinetic regional myocardial wall motion
Low cardiac output

Therapeutic maneuvers

Checking of surgical retraction
High coronary perfusion pressures
Minimization of ventricular distension and heart rate
Nitroglycerine rarely useful
Inotropic and pressure support

occasionally has caused complete pacemaker failure in patients with CHD through actual "burnout" of the pacemaker generator from current induced in the pacer lead by high-frequency electrocautery currents. External pacing capabilities or pacing via a temporary wire may be needed. Alternatively, a bipolar cautery may be used until the pacemaker generator is removed. Bipolar pacemakers do not interfere with normal pacemaker function or damage pacemaker generator circuits unlike the radiofrequency currents used by electrocautery.

In patients whose conduction systems have been injured intraoperatively and whose cardiac output is marginal after surgery, synchronous atrioventricular pacing may be useful to increase cardiac output. Ventricular extrasystoles are unusual in children with CHD and usually indicate myocardial damage. They are managed conventionally with normalization of electrolytes and acid–base balance, overdrive pacing, and antidysrhythmic agents.

Low cardiac output

Low cardiac output is the final common pathway and expression of multiple problems associated with surgical treatment of patients with CHD. Supportive management with inotropic and pressor agents, replacement of intravascular volume, pacing, and other measures should be considered only temporary therapy for support until the cause can be accurately diagnosed and corrected (Box 69-7). Primary myocardial injury and pump failure should be a diagnosis of last resort. All other possible residual or undiagnosed and correctable lesions should be sought before this diagnosis is accepted. When all other possibilities have been excluded and when a reversible lesion such as myocardial "stunning" or reversible pulmonary hypertension is diagnosed, maximal medical and ventilatory support is instituted. In extreme cases, extracorporeal membrane oxygenation (ECMO) and ventricular assist devices (VADs) have been successfully used for temporary circulatory and ventilatory support.[8]

BOX 69-7
ANESTHETIC MANAGEMENT OF LOW CARDIAC OUTPUT

Signs

High filling pressures
Poor ventricular function
Progressive metabolic acidosis
Low urine output

Therapeutic maneuvers

Cause should be determined
Discontinuation of inhalation anesthetic agents
Optimizing of ventilatory pattern
Synchronous arteriovenous pacing
Elevation of filling pressures
Period of partial circulatory support on bypass
Maximization of pressor and inotropic support
Ventricular assist devices if indicated
Extracorporeal membrane oxygenation support if indicated

Problems Associated with Cardiopulmonary Bypass for Congenital Heart Disease and Their Management

Management of CPB in children with CHD differs considerably from adults with acquired heart disease. Aortopulmonary communications, abnormal intracardiac anatomy, small body size, and immature cardiovascular systems alter CPB management. Historically, the morbidity of CPB in neonates and small infants has been a major limiting factor in surgical treatment.[107] There is substantial evidence that nonepithelial surface-induced damage to formed blood elements and blood proteins is proportionally greater in small children and infants, who leave large surface area-to-body mass ratios. In recent years, technologic refinements have lowered the contribution of CPB-related problems to pediatric mortality, but CPB remains a substantial issue, particularly in small infants. Growing knowledge about the roles of cytokines, activated leukocytes, platelets, and endothelial cells in the inflammatory response to CPB holds promise for reducing this morbidity rate.[91]

Potential perfusion problems associated with cardiopulmonary bypass in patients with congenital heart disease

Because of the factors of scale related to surface area and blood volume, substantial hemodilution and multiple exchanges of the entire circulating blood volume are required when conventional pediatric CPB circuits are used in small infants. The minimum pump prime required even by current infant-sized pump oxygenator circuits (250 to 500 ml) is very large compared with the neonate native circulating blood volume (approximately 300 ml). CPB results in an exchange of one or more blood volumes in neonates and small infants, plus hemodilution to hematocrits of 20%. This extensive dilutional exchange may make postbypass hemostasis difficult without fresh blood products and also imposes large crystalloid and metabolic loads. CPB priming solution has substantial metabolic consequences because of its large volume. Depending on the constituents of the pump prime solution, large glucose, lactate, and osmotic loads are imposed.[136] These loads can be substantially reduced with modern washing and ultrafiltration techniques.[168] Ultrafiltration techniques likely reduce bypass morbidity in infants by decreasing levels of cytokines and other inflammatory mediators.[102,103]

Pump perfusion in children is regulated primarily by flow rate in most institutions. **Because of the greater relative cardiac output of infants and their greater surface area-to-body mass ratio, pump flow rates as high as 150 to 200 ml/kg/min are used in neonates weighing 2 or 3 kg to provide normal cardiac output. Despite these high flows, mean arterial pressures during bypass often are about**

30 mm Hg in infants, particularly during deep hypothermia when hemodilution markedly decreases blood viscosity. In older children, lesser flows are used, and perfusion pressures increase until the standard adult flows (50 to 70 ml/kg/min) and pressures are achieved in patients weighing more than 50 kg. Because of the low mean arterial pressures frequently used during bypass surgery in infants, unobstructed venous return to the pump–oxygenator reservoir is critically important during bypass surgery, particularly in the superior vena cava. Presence of high venous pressures in the cerebral circulation can markedly hamper cerebral perfusion in children when mean arterial pressures are low during bypass surgery. This is particularly true during deep hypothermia in children when pressure–flow autoregulation of cerebral perfusion may not be present.[77,78] When caval occlusion tapes are tightened around venous cannulae, it is especially important to check for signs of superior or inferior vena caval obstruction or alternatively to monitor pressures in central venous lines positioned superior to the caval tape.

In the absence of inferior or superior vena caval obstructions, with normal venous pressures, low arterial perfusion pressures cause no problem in hemodiluted children receiving adequate flow. Unfortunately, the margin of error is small for proper positioning of inferior and superior vena cava cannulae in the small infant heart. Obstruction of hepatic or jugular veins can easily occur, so signs of caval obstruction should not be ignored, particularly when venous pump return is inadequate.

The frequent presence of aortopulmonary collaterals in patients with CHD makes the definition of adequate bypass flow rates uncertain. In assessing perfusion during CPB in patients with CHD, the potential effect of aortopulmonary shunts or collaterals on systemic perfusion should be considered. A high perfusion rate may be indicated by pump head revolutions, but unless all sources of aortopulmonary shunting are controlled, much of the aortic perfusion from the pump will pass into the lungs through shunts and collaterals and return to the pump from the pulmonary veins through intracardiac defect to the right atrial venous cannula. Blood taking this route does not perfuse the systemic circulation and especially does not perfuse brain. This may constitute a large proportion of apparent pump flow. Although well-defined shunts, such as patent ductus arteriosus, Blalock-Taussig shunts, or Waterston shunts, may be ligated before bypass, many children with cyanotic disease will have extensive aortopulmonary collaterals that are not easily controlled. During these conditions, pump flow rates may bear little relation to actual systemic perfusion.

Abnormally low perfusion pressure during bypass surgery despite high pump flows should suggest open systemic-to-pulmonary shunts. Sources of such shunts should be sought and controlled. Other indices of flow adequacy should be followed to ensure adequate perfusion of vital organs. There is evidence, for example, that systemic arterial collaterals to the lungs originating from the vertebral arteries may "steal" flow from the basilar artery and the brain during CPB, causing cerebral ischemia and choreoathetosis.[215]

During bypass cooling and warming, the rate of change recorded from temperature probes placed in various parts of the body provides an index of regional perfusion. Core temperature, measured by distal esophageal temperature, generally changes most quickly, followed by a lag of several degrees for nasopharyngeal or tympanic temperatures, the latter two better indicating brain perfusion. Rectal or extremity skin temperatures lag farther because these areas reflect more peripheral perfusion. Temperature gradients between these regional beds will decrease as steady state is approached, and generally will be seen in reverse order during warming. Deviations from normal temperature gradients seen on cooling and warming may indicate perfusion problems. Unfortunately, such variations from normal temperature gradients do not predict adequacy of cooling when jugular venous bulb oxygen saturations are measured during bypass cooling in small children.[106] In the absence of bypass warming or cooling, urine output and systemic acid–base balance are reasonable indicators of perfusion. Oxygen saturation of the venous outflow to the pump also is an important indicator of tissue perfusion. This value should be approximately 70% or greater, particularly during hypothermic bypass surgery.

Management of ventilation of the lungs during bypass surgery has been controversial. During partial bypass surgery, some ventilation is probably indicated if the pulmonic ventricle is demonstrably ejecting blood. This serves to oxygenate the small amount of blood being ejected so that the coronary arteries, which will receive the bulk of this blood, will be perfused with saturated blood. Low flow of 100% oxygen into the lungs should continue, even if no mechanical ventilation takes place, so that apneic oxygenation will occur as long as pulmonary blood flow continues. Frequent visual checks of arterial and venous lines at the pump provide estimates of the arteriovenous oxygen saturation difference and oxygen consumption. These estimates are periodically confirmed by measurement of venous and arterial blood gases, along with electrolytes, glucose, hematocrit, ionized calcium, and activated thromboplastin time (ACT) during bypass surgery. Addition of blood, sodium bicarbonate, calcium, heparin, potassium, and crystalloid solutions to the pump reservoir, along with gas flow through the oxygenator, will be guided by these measurements. Instruments that provide continuous Pa_{O_2}, $P\bar{v}_{O_2}$, pH, and P_{CO_2} are available to be used during bypass, but they may not be as accurate as *in vitro* blood gas analysis.

Brain damage from bypass in patients with congenital heart disease

Brain damage associated with repair of CHD in children has been even less well defined and studied than brain damage associated with adult cardiac surgery. Brain cooling and protection are important issues because major incidence of brain injury is associated with deep hypothermia, CPB, and circulatory arrest in children undergoing repair of CHD.[59] The most common problem seen is choreoathetosis,[14,48] which has been reported with deep and moderate hypothermia, with long and short circulatory arrest, and with low and normal bypass flows. Thus, the exact cause of this problem is unclear, but it is almost certainly the result of disturbances of brain perfusion in the basal ganglia. Although it is known that brain blood flow is altered by temperature,[76] $Pa{CO_2}$ levels,[149] and use of prolonged circulatory arrest periods[76] among other factors, it is not known how these factors may interact to produce brain damage, such as choreoathetosis, in the isolated cases in which it occurs. Recent work has identified cerebral steal from systemic arterial collaterals to the pulmonary arteries originating from the vertebral–basilar artery system and short cooling times as possible causes, but this remains to be confirmed.[216] In brain damage other than choreoathetosis, a relationship between high cooling rates and short cooling times before circulatory arrest and subsequent decreases in neurodevelopmental test scores in infants also has been shown.[17] **Even in the absence of overt neurologic injury, studies have shown that periods of hypothermic circulatory arrest greater than 30 minutes during bypass repairs of CHD in infants are associated with a greater incidence of postoperative seizures and lesser neurodevelopmental scores at 1 year age.**[17,157]

Weaning from bypass

During rewarming, air is vented from the heart before ejection of blood into the systemic circulation is allowed. Arterial blood gases, electrolytes, glucose, and coagulation parameters are checked periodically during bypass surgery, but especially during rewarming. Electrolytes, especially ionized calcium, are adjusted to normal ranges before separation from bypass. Adequacy of rewarming is judged by temperature recording from multiple sites, and is particularly important when deep hypothermia has been used.

The need for vasopressor and inotropic support to accomplish weaning from bypass is first estimated by close observation of the heart's behavior during rewarming. Dysrhythmias, coronary perfusion problems, and state of myocardial contractility can be estimated from the appearance of the heart. Separation from bypass should be accomplished in close concert with the surgical team using all available sources of information about hemodynamic status. Monitoring appropriate intracardiac and intraarterial pressures and waveforms and transesophageal echocardiogram may provide good information about the adequacy of the operative repair, myocardial preservation, ventricular function, and the state of the pulmonary circulation.[70] Slavish adherence to numbers produced by intracardiac catheters and pressure monitoring systems without visual confirmation of cardiac performance can lead to numerous errors. Small size and presence of unsuspected congenital defects make interpretation of pressures from monitors difficult.[38,141,185] When rewarming is complete and when cardiac function is judged adequate, weaning from extracorporeal circulation is accomplished by slowly allowing the heart to fill and eject while reestablishing ventilation. Optimal ventricular filling pressures are estimated using filling pressures from preoperative catheterization data, appearance of the heart, and by infusing small volume increments while watching filling and systemic arterial pressures. Using this latter technique, a mental Frank-Starling" curve can be constructed.

If systemic arterial pressure or gas exchange is inadequate, CPB is reinstituted while problems are analyzed. Problems with oxygenation after bypass surgery are as frequently caused by deficiencies in pulmonary blood flow as by deficiencies in ventilation. With low $Pa{O_2}$, adequacy of pulmonary blood flow and ventilation should be critically assessed. Analysis of problems with weaning should start with reassessment of surgical repair, adequacy of ventilation, and verification that inotropic support is reaching the heart. Measurement of PA and atrial and intraventricular pressures often will be helpful, along with pullback pressure gradient measurement across aortic and pulmonic valves if indicated.

In patients who are doing poorly after the bypass period, missed or residual lesions are likely. This should be carefully considered before commiting the child to prolonged inotropic support postoperatively. **Residual defects are by far the most frequent cause of immediate hemodynamic problems and instability after repair, even in institutions with superb diagnostic and surgical expertise in CHD.** Questions of inadequate repair should be resolved using intraoperative echocardiography, including Doppler assessment of intracardiac shunts, with either epicardial or transesophageal approaches.[46,75,198] In complex CHD, a physician specially trained and expert in the echocardiographic assessment of CHD should interpret such studies. When the problem is identified, appropriate corrective measures are taken, and weaning is again attempted. If there are no readily apparent anatomic problems and if the difficultly with weaning appears to be a result of reversible myocardial dysfunction or reversible pulmonary hypertension that cannot be adequately managed, use of a left or right VAD or ECMO should be considered.

Deep hypothermic circulatory arrest and low-flow bypass

In an effort to avoid the high morbidity rate historically associated with CPB in young children undergoing intracardiac repairs for CHD, deep hypothermia with circulatory arrest or with low-flow continuous bypass has been used. Deep hypothermic circulatory arrest (DHCA) with core and cerebral temperatures of less than 20°C in children weighing less than 10 kg and in selected older patients provides ideal operating conditions for the surgeon, reduces bypass time and blood trauma, and maximizes myocardial protection.[85] These advantages are offset by risk of CNS damage from prolonged ischemic times, especially if they are 30 minutes or more. Some centers have abandoned DHCA in favor of hypothermic low-flow CPB techniques because of concerns about subclinical neurologic damage and impairment of intellectual development.

The potential disadvantages of DHCA are prolonged periods of ischemia to vital organs. As a practical matter in the large clinical experience with DHCA during the past 20 years, the only organ at appreciable risk is the brain. Numerous studies of neurologic outcome with DHCA in children and adults have been done; the majority show no overt cerebral damage resulting from DHCA.[22,36,44,51,184,209,217] A minority of these studies have shown some evidence of effects on subsequent intellectual development, but usually only at circulatory arrest periods of more than 45 minutes. Neurologic outcome studies done in DHCA patients have been criticized as being rather poorly controlled, nonrigorous in their assessment of neurologic injuries, and lumping together heterogeneous groups of patients. The most recent study that avoids these problems shows evidence of intellectual impairment at 1-year follow-up evaluations in infants subjected to DHCA periods of 30 minutes or more.[17,157] Other experimental and clinical studies have also found subtle signs of cerebral insult after DHCA, such as occasional transient seizures and minor neurologic deficits.[28,55,140,148,196]

Because mechanisms of ischemic protection of the hypothermic brain are incompletely understood, there are no accepted optimal techniques for cerebral protection and no well-defined "safe" period of circulatory arrest, but circulatory arrest is being less frequently used in favor of low flow bypass techniques. DHCA periods of more than 30 minutes are avoided whenever possible. **Evidence suggests that anesthetic management may be important in cerebral protection. Recovery from cerebral ischemia occurring during hyperglycemia is impaired, suggesting that hyperglycemia in the mature brain should be avoided in DHCA.[116] Children often have hyperglycemic responses to the stress of hypothermic cardiopulmonary bypass surgery,[18,183] and deep levels of anesthesia can markedly attenuate the hyperglycemic stress responses and other hormonal and metabolic stress responses seen with CPB in children.** Experimental evidence and preliminary clinical evidence suggest that hyperglycemia is not harmful in the immature infant brain and that hypoglycemia is a greater risk in this age group.[201]

Anesthetic management should emphasize use of muscle relaxants, barbiturates, and reduction of stress responses to minimize oxygen consumption and hyperglycemia during the ischemic period, but clinical studies of optimal anesthetic management for DHCA have not been done to confirm or refute these suggestions. **Certainly, hypoglycemia should be avoided before, during, and after DHCA, and glucose should be periodically monitored.** Pharmacologic protective agents such as high-dose steroids and barbiturates have not been shown to be protective against DHCA-related brain damage despite theoretical support for their use. Although there are cogent theoretic reasons why acid–base management, through its influences on cerebral blood flow and cerebral intracellular pH in the brain,[207] may affect such damage, clinical studies of its effects during DHCA have not yet been done. Acid–base management has thus far not been shown to have an important effect on the incidence of cerebral complications in hypothermic open heart surgery, at least in adults in whom circulatory arrest has not been used.[15]

The alternative to DHCA, low flow hypothermic CPB, has been shown to be superior to DHCA in terms of neurologic outcome.[17,157] There is no "standard" for "low-flow" bypass. Experimental studies have established that with decreasing total bypass flow during moderately hypothermic CPB surgery, the brain takes an increasingly larger fraction for itself to preserve normal cerebral oxygen consumption levels. When flow becomes sufficiently low, oxygen consumption decreases because of ischemia.[62,139] Low-flow bypass has been demonstrated in several studies to result in loss of somatosensory evoked-potentials and intracellular ATP and to be associated with decreased intracellular pH when flow levels are sufficiently lessened.[167,207,214] In experimental studies measuring brain levels of high energy phosphates *in vivo,* very low flows (down to 10 ml/kg/hr) maintained normal brain creatinine phosphate (CP) and adenosine triphophate levels in sheep during hypothermic low-flow bypass surgery.[189] In contrast, no middle cerebral artery flow has been detected using transcranial Doppler in clinical studies of infants and using greater levels of flow during hypothermic low-flow bypass surgery in one institution. A recent clinical study showed inconsistent perfusion of the middle cerebral artery during hypothermic low-flow bypass surgery in infants in whom flows of less than 30 ml/kg/min were used.[221]

Rossi et al.[175] showed that creatine kinase levels were equally elevated after DHCA and after low-flow hypothermic bypass in infants, suggesting that, by this measure of brain injury, there was no difference between the two techniques. **Thus, without any established "safe" level of low-flow bypass surgery, some degree of cerebral ischemia and damage may occur even when low-flow bypass surgery is used in preference to DHCA.** Continuous low-flow bypass surgery thus may well provide a false sense of security about brain protection. Together with less favorable operating conditions obtained with low-flow bypass surgery, this false security can markedly prolong low-flow bypass time, bypass damage, and potentially cerebral ischemic time that may occur during low-flow bypass surgery. Because the mechanisms of cerebral injury and the physiology of low-flow bypass surgery during hypothermia in infants and children are not well understood, the cerebral protective effects of low-flow bypass surgery may not always be better than DHCA.

Recent cerebral blood flow studies in children undergoing DHCA and low-flow bypass surgery by Greeley et al.[48] have shown that cerebral pressure-flow autoregulation is lost in children during deep hypothermia but that metabolism-flow regulation is retained. After prolonged circulatory arrest, cerebral blood flow and metabolism subsequently remain depressed during and after bypass compared with more normal recovery of metabolic rate and cerebral blood flow with continuous low-flow bypass.[48,77,78] These findings are consistent with delayed recovery of electroencephalograph (EEG) and somatosensory-evoked potentials after prolonged DHCA.[39,208] Despite delayed recovery of these functional measures and low cerebral blood flow and metabolism immediately after DHCA, gross neurologic deficits are seen infrequently.

Deep hypothermic circulatory arrest provides optimal conditions on precise surgical repairs of complex intracardiac problems in tiny hearts, minimizes the formidable morbidity of CPB in small infants, improves myocardial protection, and lessens the incidence of cannulation-related problems and obstruction in the inferior and superior vena cavae. Recent outcome studies have provided support for the concept that DHCA has some detrimental effect on neurologic outcome, at least for circulatory arrest periods of more than 30 minutes. Low-flow CPB, particularly without use of comparable deep hypothermic levels, does not necessarily prevent cerebral ischemia. Its use may prolong total bypass time and related morbidity. At present, evidence suggests low-flow CPB provides better cerebral protection, but knowledge of the optimal levels and conditions for low-flow CPB remains scant.

Anesthetic Problems During Closed Cardiac Procedures

Anesthesia for closed cardiac procedures may be more demanding than those involving CPB because bypass support can temporarily solve many hemodynamic problems that otherwise cause intraoperative deterioration. Monitoring requirements are just as stringent, and venous and arterial access are even more important. Pulse oximetry is invaluable to help evaluate the infant's condition. **Patent ductus arteriosus and coarctation of the aorta are the only lesions corrected with closed surgical procedures;** ductus ligation and other closed procedures can now be done using video-assisted thoracoscopic surgery. Closed palliative procedures are used in patients with hypoxemia to increase pulmonary blood flow by constructing surgical shunts, to decrease excessive pulmonary blood flow using a PA band, and to improve atrial mixing of pulmonary and systemic venous return (Blalock-Hanlon atrial septectomy) in transposition of the great arteries. Palliative surgical procedures now are performed less frequently because early correction of many severe CHDs has become possible with low mortality rate and because of the efficacy and safety of interventional cardiac catheterization. Such palliative procedures, when used in preference to reparative procedures, have appreciable mortality and morbidity rates of their own.[132] Reparative operations that correct the intracardiac pathophysiologic conditions are increasingly feasible and preferable even in newborns.[33,34,108,158]

Acid–base and electrolyte balance are meticulously maintained throughout closed procedures. When these procedures are done via thoracotomy, the operative field is rarely visible to the anesthesia care team. Marked deterioration in cardiopulmonary status may result from surgical manipulation and retraction. Any deterioration of the infant's condition should be immediately communicated to the surgical team, who have a better view of the surgical field. Serious deterioration should prompt solicitation of surgical help. Release of retraction usually results in return to hemodynamic stability. Some compromise of ventilation and pulmonary blood flow inevitably occurs in these procedures, sometimes with severe decreases in arterial oxygen saturations. Inadvertent compression of coronary arteries during these procedures may cause severe cardiac ischemia and dysfunction; that is readily correctable by adjustment of retraction. Anesthetic management using deep levels of anesthesia that minimizes oxygen consumption and supports cardiovascular stability usually minimizes intraoperative problems but may prolong postoperative ventilation. In extreme cases, periods of inotropic and pressor support may be required intraoperatively.

Patent ductus arteriosus and vascular ring interruption using thoracoscopic procedures

Ligation of a patent ductus arteriosus and other procedures such as interruption of vascular rings can now be done thoracoscopically. Such procedures can be done with either one-lung anesthesia or two-lung anesthesia with lung retraction.[119] In either case, transient decreases in arterial oxygen saturation may occur that can be managed with brief reexpansion of the collapsed lung. Visualization of the operative field is superior when thoracoscopy is used. Conversion to open thoractomy may occasionally be required if exposure is not adequate or if bleeding occurs. Transesophageal echocardiographic confirmation of interruption of flow is useful to ensure complete closure of the vessel.[120]

Surgical shunts

Severe hypoxemia occurring in the operating room during or after creation of the shunt implies inadequate pulmonary blood flow. Intrapulmonary shunting should be considered in lungs that are retracted, but mechanical obstruction of flow into the PA because of retraction or actual shunt obstruction (kinking or thrombosis) is the usual cause. Reinflation of the retracted lung segment will eliminate intrapulmonary shunting. If hypoxemia persists, hyperventilation can minimize PVR and optimize gas exchange until pulmonary blood flow can be improved.

Systemic-to-PA shunts are inherently inefficient, recirculating oxygenated blood into the lungs and placing a volume load on the heart. **Pulmonary blood flow should be several times greater than the systemic flow to substantially reduce hypoxemia** (Fig. 69-3). When the surgically created shunt is too large, pulmonary flows are excessive. This is manifested by pulmonary edema (sometimes unilateral) on chest radiography postoperatively. Intraoperatively, large pulse pressures, excessively low diastolic arterial pressures, and sometimes inadequate systemic output result in children whose arterial oxygen saturation is relatively high despite complete mixing of systemic and pulmonary venous return. Maneuvers to increase PVR can compensate to a limited degree for excessive pulmonary flow, but early or late shunt revision often is necessary. Other reported acute complications of systemic-to-PA shunts include Horner's syndrome, chylothorax, and acute ischemia of the ipsilateral arm when the subclavian artery is sacrificed.

The Glenn shunt (superior vena cava to right PA with no pump in between) is limited to patients with low PVR because venous pressure is used to provide pulmonary blood flow. Consequently, use in newborns and infants is excluded. Other problems with Glenn shunts include thrombosis, occlusion, or elevation of PVR leading to SVC syndrome. The Glenn shunt is more efficient than an arterial shunt and is useful in patients who have congestive heart failure stemming from volume overload. In general, for other patients, the Blalock-Taussig shunt has proven the most reliable of the surgical shunts, with good long-term patency rates regardless of age. Early mortality is less than and incidence of late postoperative complications is lesser than for alternative shunt procedures.[10]

PA banding

When pulmonary blood flow is excessive and when high pressure is communicated to the pulmonary vasculature, surgical intervention may be necessary to prevent progressive PVOD or to lessen symptoms of high output congestive heart failure and inadequate systemic output. **When early complete repair is not possible, pulmonary blood flow is restricted by banding the PA. This adds pulmonary outflow resistance, which converts simple, nonrestrictive shunting situations into complex shunts with limited pulmonary flow.** During induction of anesthesia before the band is applied, PVR may occasionally decrease enough to result in massive pulmonary flow and systemic hypotension ("pulmonary steal"). In this case, a partial occlusion of the PA with a clamp will aid in maintaining hemodynamic stability until the band can be applied.

Unfortunately, the banding procedure is unsatisfyingly crude and results are hemodynamically unpredictable.[132] Adequacy of the band in the operating room is assessed by observing an increased systemic blood pressure and an acceptable decrease in systemic oxygen saturation. Direct measurement of PA pressure beyond the band is done, adjusting this pressure to approximately one-half the systemic arterial pressure. Continuous monitoring of arterial oxygen saturation is helpful in rapidly assessing critically low levels of pulmonary blood flow that may occur during band tightening.

Transcatheter Management of Congenital Heart Disease in the Cardiac Catheterization Laboratory and Associated Problems

Congenital heart problems are frequently managed today by transcatheter interventions in the catheterization laboratory.[16,162] Physiologic derangement and complications during such interventions may approach that seen in the cardiac operating room.[92] Anesthesia is often advisable for patient comfort and safety and for monitoring and management of complications.[118] Table 69-5 lists the lesions currently managed using interventional cardiac catheterization, the procedures used, and their effects and complications.

Evolving techniques of nonsurgical management of CHDs have markedly altered pediatric cardiac anesthesia. Atrial septal defects, ventricular septal defects, patent ductus arteriosus, and coarctation of the aorta commonly form the bulk of pediatric cardiac surgery done in many programs. These lesions now can be managed in the interventional catheterization laboratory using nonsurgical transcatheter techniques.[26,131,173,212] A number of these procedures, including closure of atrial septal and patent ductus arteriosus defects, can even be done on an outpatient basis.[92,212] In centers doing large numbers of interventional catheterization procedures, these common congenital heart lesions are seen less frequently in the operating room. Transcatheter closures of ASDs have been successfully done in hundreds of patients. Smaller number of VSDs, including multiple VSDs, have also been closed with these techniques.[118] These and other new interventional techniques are becoming common.[23,172] Interventional catheterization techniques listed in Table 69-5 also are used increasingly in conjunction with surgical procedures to improve the results of surgical management of CHD and to extend therapy to previously unmanageable lesions.

Anesthetic care in the interventional cardiac catheterization laboratory

Catheterization procedures have become more invasive, use larger and multiple catheters, involve more blood loss, and produce more pain in smaller and sicker patients. The cardiac catheterization laboratory has effectively turned into an operating room where major problems and complications can result from increasingly invasive procedures.[92] Although many patients seen in the pediatric catheterization laboratory can be adequately sedated by cardiologists,[92] complex procedures in sick children require anesthetic care. Anesthesia, monitoring, and hemodynamic management are needed for many of these invasive procedures in children and contribute substantially to a successful procedure.[16,133] Many patients can be treated with monitored IV sedation techniques, but others require general endotracheal anesthesia. Indications for using either technique are not yet well defined but depend on patient condition, procedure, and anticipated complications.

Anesthetic management is handicapped by the catheterization laboratory environment. Problems include poor patient access, poor lighting, radiation hazards, and lack of communication with cardiologists. Independent monitoring, independent intravenous and sometimes intraarterial access, independent light sources, and adequate access to the patient's airway should be sought. Prevention or prompt management of complications is a major anesthetic task in this

Table 69-5 Interventional procedures in the cardiac catheterization laboratory affecting pathophysiology of congenital heart disease

Procedure	Structure/lesion	Effects	Complications
Coil embolizations	Aortopulmonary collaterals	Reduce pulmonary flow	Hypoxemia, systemic embolization
	Blalock-Taussig shunts	" " "	
	Anomalous coronary arteries	Increase conronary flow and reduce pulmonary flow	
Transcatheter device closures	Patent ductus arteriosus	Eliminate shunt, reduce pulmonary flow	Air embolization, device embolization, interference with mitral and tricuspid valve function
	Atrial septal defect	Eliminate shunt, reduce pulmonary flow, and prevent paradoxic embolization	
	Ventricular septal defect	Eliminate shunt, reduce pulmonary flow	
Balloon and stent dilations	Pulmonary stenosis	Increase pulmonary flow	Embolization of stent, pulmonary artery disruption, unilateral pulmonary edema, pulmonary insufficiency, aortic insufficiency, mitral insufficiency, tricuspid insufficiency, aortic dissection
	Blalock-Taussig shunts	" " "	
	Pulmonary valve stenosis	" " "	
	Tricuspid valve stenosis	" " "	
	Aortic valve stenosis	Increase systemic flow	
	Mitral valve stenosis	" " "	
	Aorta (coarctations and others)	" " "	
Atrial septostomies (balloon and blade)	Interatrial septum	Increase pulmonary blood flow	Perforation of heart, tamponade
Radiofrequency transcatheter mapping and ablation	Anomalous conduction pathways	Eliminate dysrhythmias, especially supraventricular tachycardia	Complete heart block, supraventricular tachycardia

setting. Without a thorough understanding of transcatheter procedures, their complications, and their management, the anesthesia provider is handicapped in coping with accelerating development of these new techniques.

Problems and hemodynamic complications

Complications of various interventional procedures are related partly to the type of interventional procedure, but all share risks associated with percutaneous access to major veins and arteries. Specific problems that may occur during various interventional transcatheter procedures are listed in Table 69-5. Many problems are sudden, occur without warning, and are potentially life threatening. As in the operating room, successful management of complications depends heavily on prompt action by anesthesia providers cooperating closely with the interventional cardiologists and radiologists.

Loss of control of embolic and closure devices results in systemic and pulmonary arterial embolization. Embolized devices can usually be retrieved using a variety of retrieval catheters, but in a minority of patients, surgical removal is required. If the device is lodged in the heart or a great vessel, CPB may be required for removal. Such device embolizations usually do not cause extreme hemodynamic instability or cardiovascular decompensation requiring emergency surgical removal, but urgent surgical procedures may be necessary. Even after successful transcatheter retrieval, femoral artery and vein reconstructions are occasionally necessary when embolized devices or large dilation balloons are removed through these vessels.[30] When deliberate embolization of aortopulmonary collaterals excessively decreases pulmonary flow and produces severe hypoxemia, general anesthesia and muscle paralysis can increase arterial oxygen saturation to acceptable levels by decreasing oxygen consumption, at least until surgical intervention.

Disruption and avulsion of major blood vessels also occur, particularly PA disruption during balloon dilation procedures.[176] PA disruption is signaled by hemoptysis or appearance of contrast media in the pleural space or major lung fissures. Substantial hemoptysis calls for immediate endotracheal intubation for airway control and ventilation. Positive end-expiratory pressure (PEEP) may be useful. Intrapulmonary hemorrhage often is self-limited, but hemothorax can be severe and can result in death.[176] Transient unilateral pulmonary edema can occur during PA dilation, because of sudden increases in flow after dilation to a previously underperfused lung.[11,176] Unilateral pulmonary edema and disruption of PA integrity can occur abruptly. Both can cause the appearance of frank blood or blood-tinged edema or fluid in substantial quantities in the airway. Management starts with endotracheal intubation and positive pressure ventilation unless symptoms are only minimal.

Intracardiac air embolization may be a particular problem when clamshell devices are used for PDA, ASD, and VSD closures because the large delivery sheath in the heart is transiently open to atmosphere. Transcatheter closure of an ASD using a clamshell device in shown schematically in Fig. 69-8. In patients with intracardiac shunts, air embolization may be life threatening. The large delivery sheath represents a potential space for air accumulation and subsequent delivery into the heart. In addition, when the entry port of the large delivery sheath is open during removal and reinsertion of various catheters and devices, extreme inspiratory efforts may entrain intracardiac air. Air delivered into the right atrium may be shunted across the ASD even in the presence of nominal left-to-right shunting. Left atrial air embolization during these procedures can be seen with fluoroscopy. Resultant ST segment changes, hypotension, arterial desaturation, and bradycardia generally respond to air

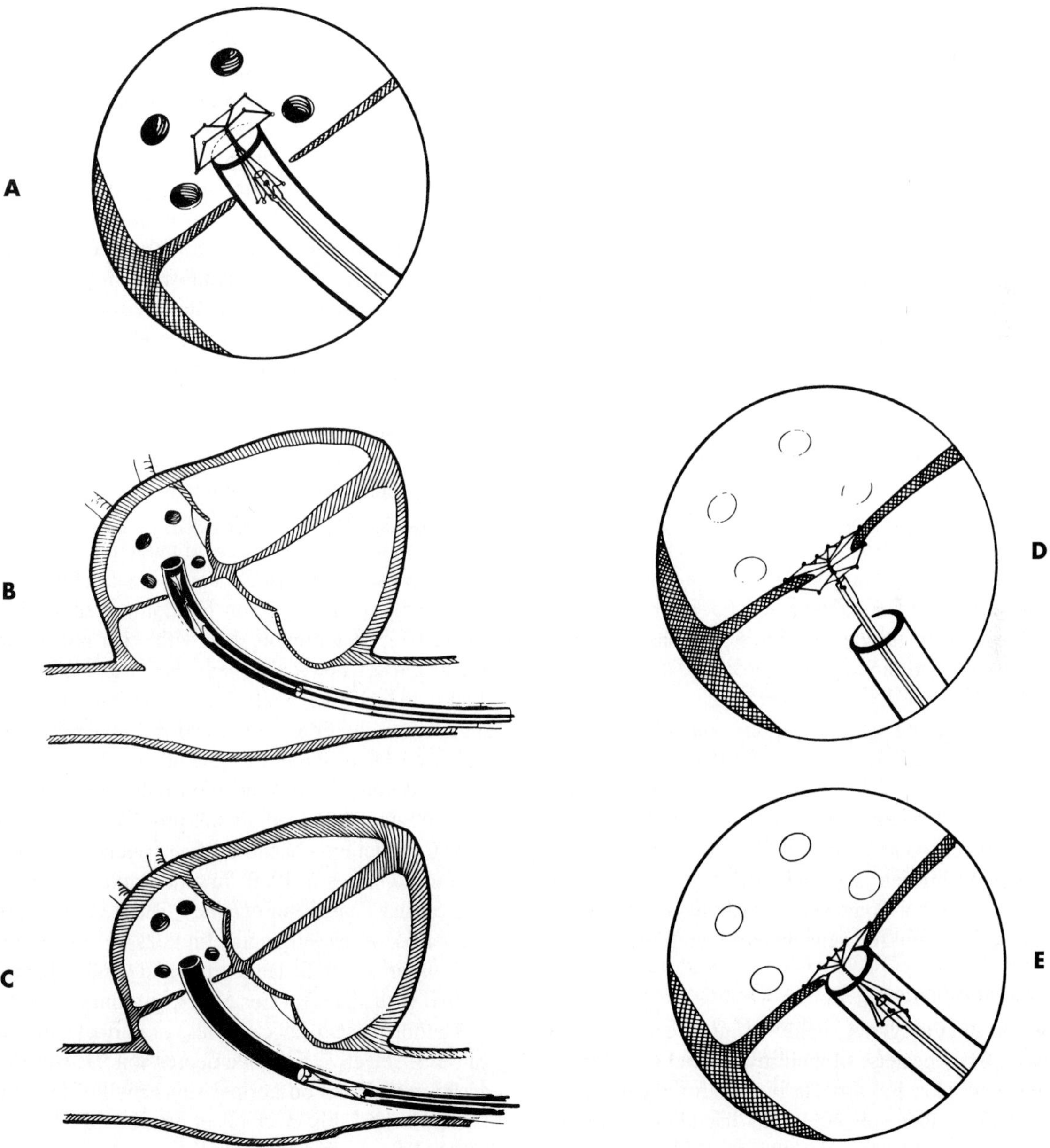

Fig. 69-8. Technique of transcatheter ASD closure. **A,** Collapsed clamshell device is through the sheath. **B,** Device and sheath as a unit are positioned on the left atrial side of the defect using previously determined fluoroscopic landmarks. **C,** Sheath is then pulled partially back, allowing one set of flexible, spring-loaded arms (covered with Dacron mesh) to spring open in the left atrium. **D,** Sheath, delivery system, and the half-opened clamshell device are then pulled back as a unit until the open arms engage the left atrial septal surface. **E,** Sheath is pulled farther back to expose the proximal half of the device, allowing it to spring open and engage the right atrial septal surface. Subsequently the clamshell device is released and the delivery system withdrawn.

aspiration followed by sealing the entry port, along with administration of atropine and inotropic support to maintain coronary perfusion. Meticulous purging of air from the catheter system, sealing open ports, should minimize air embolism. Controlled positive pressure endotracheal ventilation in anesthetized, paralyzed patients may decrease potential for air entrainment.

Tricuspid or mitral regurgitation with hemodynamic compromise also may occur acutely when large catheters impinge on atrioventricular valves. These large catheters can cause dynamic stenosis as they pass across small valves. These problems usually respond to inotropic support and repositioning of the delivery catheter and device. Acute myocardial perforation with tamponade also occurs occasionally during the course of interventional cardiac catheterization procedures. Prompt support of the circulation with volume infusions and pressor support, along with immediate catheter drainage of the pericardial space, are essential.

EFFECTS OF ANESTHESIA AND RELATED MANIPULATIONS ON PATHOPHYSIOLOGY OF CONGENITAL HEART DISEASE

Anesthetic Agents in Congenital Heart Disease

Individual pathophysiology and the proposed therapeutic procedure largely dictate anesthetic management. It is often the skill with which the technique is used that determines how successful the anesthesia team will be in maintaining cardiovascular stability. Several anesthetic techniques provide good cardiovascular stability in children with severe CHD,[69] but cardiovascular stability may not be the only criterion for a successful anesthetic. Stress responses to pain and other noxious stimulation are profound even in the youngest neonates.[3,4,7] Extreme hormonal and metabolic stress responses during cardiac surgery and CPB can be pathologic in magnitude and are associated with poorer outcome in neonates undergoing cardiac surgery, despite hemodynamic stability.[5,6] Anesthetic techniques clearly have an impact on stress responses—metabolic and hormonal. It is important to give children of all ages adequate anesthesia for suppression of the hormonal and metabolic responses to noxious stimulation and for humane considerations.

Inhalational anesthetics

Inhalation anesthetic agents should be used cautiously in children with CHD because of their myocardial and circulatory depression. This is particularly true for induction of anesthesia before adequate access to the circulation and complete hemodynamic monitoring are established. Safe use of conventional inhalation induction with potent anesthetics depends on evaluation of the child's cardiac lesion and understanding the effects in young children with CHD. In children of any age with marginal cardiovascular reserve, myocardial depression caused by potent inhalational agents may produce systemic hypotension, but these agents are still unquestionably useful in small, titrated concentrations to control hypertensive responses after induction when the airway is secure after monitoring and hemodynamic stability are established.

Even in cyanotic children, if there is reasonable functional cardiac reserve, anesthesia can be induced with halothane and oxygen, even with 70% nitrous oxide (the latter relatively contraindicated because of air bubble expansion), without clinically significant decreases in arterial oxygen saturation.[84,145] **Dramatic decreases in arterial pressures occur with these techniques, sometimes to severe degrees. In infants, such induction techniques are of special concern because of the immature circulatory system. Use of these agents may considerably narrow the margin of safety in infants and younger children with severe CHD. At least in those given halothane, the levels tolerated by sick infants provide little suppression of the stress responses to cardiac surgery and CPB.**[5] **Numerous studies have shown that even the normal immature cardiovascular system of infants without CHD does not tolerate halothane or isoflurane well; approximately 50% of infants with normal cardiovascular systems will develop substantial hypotension and bradycardia during induction with these agents unless cardiovascular function is supported.**[50,64–66] Ventricular function declines during halothane and isoflurane induction in normal infants; stroke volume and ejection fraction decrease by as much as 38%, although the depression with isoflurane may be somewhat less than with halothane.[129,137,150] Sevoflurane is becoming popular as a more rapid induction agent in children. It also causes myocardial depression in children, although stroke volume and ejection fraction are somewhat less depressed with sevoflurane than with other potent inhalational agents.[95,126,164] Few published studies of desflurane in children with CHD are available, but studies in healthy children suggest that its effects on ejection fraction and stroke volume are little different from halothane.[222] Isoflurane may be an unwise choice for inhalation induction in cyanotic children because increased airway problems and laryngospasm during induction—because of the agent's pungency—may lead to increases in PVR. In older children, somewhat less myocardial depression occurs.[13] These clinical findings are supported by experimental findings in immature animals, both *in vitro* with isolated atrial and ventricular muscle and *in vivo* with some species of young animals.[25,41,112,113,166]

Halothane also can cause loss of normal sinus rhythm because of selective SA node depression. Because ventricular function depends on normal sinus rhythm in compromised hearts, loss of this mechanism may be especially critical in CHD. This applies to right and left ventricular function in patients in whom right ventricular dysfunction may be expected to be a problem, such as tetralogy of Fallot.[80] Although greater reductive metabolism of halothane has been demonstrated in cyanotic cardiac patients, no increase in postoperative hepatic and renal derangements has been documented, and historically "halothane hepatitis" has not been a problem in cyanotic (or other) children.[166]

Use of nitrous oxide in children with CHD and shunts is controversial because of its potential for enlarging systemic air emboli. Use of nitrous oxide may cause expansion of intravascular air emboli, exaggerating their circulatory effects, even without additional systemic embolization.[138] In patients with systemic embolization of air to the coronary circulation, nitrous oxide has been shown experimentally to be deleterious.[197] In children with intracardiac shunts, the potential exists for systemic shunting of microbubbles and macrobubbles of air from IV lines and from exposure of the left heart to the atmosphere during open cardiac surgical procedures. Although clinical problems have not been reported from enlargement of air emboli by nitrous oxide in this setting, avoidance of its use is prudent in patients in whom systemic air embolization is a strong possibility.

Nitrous oxide in adults decreases cardiac output, systemic arterial pressure, and heart rate and increases PVR, especially in patients with elevated PVR.[93,117,182] In children with right-to-left shunts who have decreased pulmonary flow or pulmonary hypertension, increases in PVR with nitrous oxide would be detrimental, but, at least in one study, no increase in PA pressure or PVR was observed in infants given 50% nitrous oxide, regardless of preexisting PVR.[88] Mild but notable decreases in cardiac output, systemic arterial pressure, and heart rate were seen in these infants. Inhalation induction with 70% nitrous oxide and halothane in cyanotic children does not decrease arterial oxygen saturation, suggesting that pulmonary blood flow is not decreased and that PVR is not substantially increased by nitrous oxide.[74,115] Although use of nitrous oxide prevents use of 100% O_2, this may not actually decrease arterial saturation in cyanotic children without lung disease because increases in FIO_2 have little effect on arterial desaturation caused by large central intracardiac cardiac shunts.[122] The effects of FIO_2 on arterial saturation for different levels of right-to-left shunting are shown in Fig. 69-9.

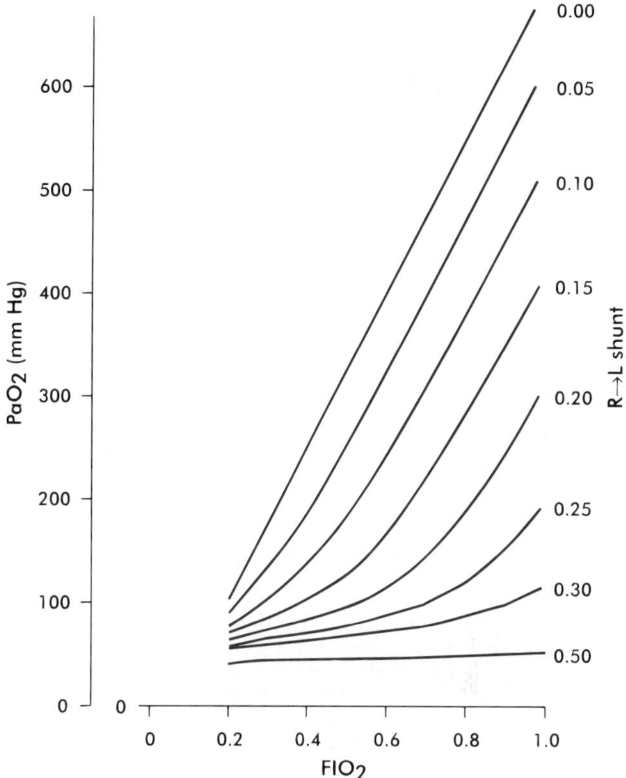

Fig. 69-9. Iso-shunt graph depicting relationship between inspired FIO_2 and arterial Pao_2 with different amounts of R-L shunting. Assumes normal values of pH, $Paco_2$, pulmonary venous saturation, and mixed venous saturation. (Modified from Lawler PGP, Nunn JF: A reassessment of the validity of the iso-shunt graph, *Br J Anaesth* 56:1325, 1984.)

Use of inhalational agents in children with intracardiac shunting is theoretically complicated by differences in uptake and distribution. A complex computer model suggests inhalation induction will be slowed in the presence of central right-to-left shunts, slowed less in mixed shunts, and little changed in pure left-to-right shunts, all in proportion to the size of the shunt.[192] These models assume constant cardiac output and are most marked for insoluble gases such as nitrous oxide. In children with left-to-right shunts, speed of inhalation induction actually is altered little clinically.[191] Experimental data in animals with right-to-left shunts confirm slowing of induction, but data in children with right-to-left shunts are not available.[187] Inhalation induction often seems somewhat slow in children with pure right-to-left shunts, but this effect is not marked, probably because of the effects of multiple other variables affecting uptake. Relatively slow induction of anesthesia in children with pure right-to-left shunts is a consideration in deciding how rapidly to increase the inhaled concentrations of potent anesthetics during induction, without producing severe myocardial depression.

Intramuscular and intravenous anesthetics

Some IV anesthetics, such as ketamine and high-dose opiates, can provide improved safety margins for induction of anesthesia in the immature and compromised cardiovascular system of neonates and infants with severe cardiac disease and in older children with minimal cardiovascular reserve. Very high transient arterial, cardiac, and brain concentrations of IV agents can result from normal IV doses given as a bolus in children with known right-to-left shunts because mixing, uptake, and pulmonary metabolism are bypassed. For example, IV lidocaine in a 1-mg/kg antiarrhythmic bolus dose administered in dogs with right-to-left shunts resulted in arterial concentrations higher than those reported to cause irreversible myocardial toxicity.[40] The potential for transiently high arterial levels of IV anesthetic agents in patients with intracardiac mixing and right-to-left shunts should be considered in planning.

Ketamine. When IV access is a problem, intramuscular ketamine (3 to 5 mg/kg) is well tolerated in sick children with cyanosis or congestive heart failure.[127,202] In contrast to older literature, ketamine has been shown to have a positive inotropic effect in experimental studies of isolated ventricular muscle.[40,169,170] Concomitant intramuscular succinylcholine can be used to facilitate airway control. Atropine or glycopyruvate given with ketamine may be helpful to offset secretions produced by ketamine. A small dose of midazolam (0.1 mg/kg) can be used to attenuate ketamine's dysphoric effects. Although increases in PVR have been reported in adults after ketamine administration, in well-premedicated children, ketamine causes no change in PVR when the airway is maintained and ventilation is supported.[68,87,145] In children with CHD, the ejection fraction has been shown to be well preserved during ketamine anesthesia.[21] Our clinical experience with intramuscular ketamine has been excellent with most forms of heart disease, including those with limited pulmonary blood flow and cyanosis in whom arterial saturation usually improves with ketamine.[74,115] Ketamine has long been used for cardiac catheterization procedures. Ketamine combined with midazolam has been used for interventional cardiac catheterization procedures such as PDA and ASD closures.[16,42]

When IV access is available in patients with marginal cardiac reserve, ketamine (1 or 2 mg/kg, IV), is an excellent induction agent in patients with most forms of CHD. Relative contraindications are coronary insufficiency caused by an anomalous coronary artery, severe critical aortic stenosis, or hypoplastic left heart syndrome with aortic atresia and hypoplasia of the ascending aorta. These patients are at risk for ventricular fibrillation because of relative coronary insufficiency; tachycardia and catecholamine release with ketamine may predispose these patients to ventricular fibrillation.

Opiates. As in adults with severe cardiac disease, high-dose IV opiates, given together with pancuronium and with 100% oxygen, or air and oxygen, are excellent as induction agents in very sick children with all forms of CHD. High-dose opiates in infants and neonates provide excellent hemodynamic stability with suppression of hormonal and metabolic stress responses.[5,7] **Anesthetic techniques based primarily on high doses of opiates have become standard care for infants and small children with severe forms of CHD, especially if they are critically ill.** Hyperglycemic responses to cardiac surgery in children are suppressed by greater doses of fentanyl, so blood glucose measurements are necessary.[56] High-dose fentanyl technique has been reported to be effective in premature neonates undergoing patent ductus ligation and has been shown to effectively attenuate stress responses for this procedure.[7,171] Fentanyl dosages as low as 10 ug/kg may be sufficient for effective baseline anesthesia in neonates, but larger dosages are necessary for prolonged anesthesia.[219] In high-risk, full-term neonates and older infants with severe CHD, use of the high-dose fentanyl in doses up to 75 μg/kg, given with pancuronium, results in minimal hemodynamic changes on induction and intubation; only mild hemodynamic responses to surgical incision generally occur.[86] Additional doses or infusions of potent opiates may be necessary for procedures involving CPB because narcotic levels decrease markedly in children on CPB.[111] **There is evidence that suppression of stress responses and amnesia is better if another anesthetic agent, such as a benzodiazepine (midazolam), is used during high-dose opiate anesthesia.**

With the use of high-dose opiate anesthetic techniques, oxygen saturation levels are well maintained and may actually improve during induction, intubation, and surgical stimulation even in cyanotic children.[115] Changes in cardiac index, SVR, and PVR in infants given 25 μg/kg of fentanyl have been shown to be minimal.[89]

Use of pancuronium with the high-dose fentanyl technique is recommended; the vagolytic effects of pancuronium offset the vagotonic effects of fentanyl. When other muscle relaxants are used with high-dose opiates, hemodynamic stability may not be obtained.[181] When fentanyl or other opiates are used with nitrous oxide, the negative inotropic effects of nitrous oxide may appear, especially in sicker patients.[147] Sufentanil (5 to 20 μg/kg) is an alternative to fentanyl and provides roughly equivalent hemodynamic stability, suppression of stress responses, and postoperative analgesia.[47,142] The use of a high-dose fentanyl or sufentanil technique usually necessitates continuous postoperative ventilatory support. Alfentanil, a shorter-acting potent opiate used as a continuous infusion, can be of use for providing hemodynamic stability and stress suppression in children in whom postoperative ventilatory support is not needed. A loading dosage of 20 μg/kg and an infusion of 1 μg/kg/min as a supplement to nitrous oxide–halothane has been reported in children undergoing surgery for CHD.[49] Renifentanil, an ultrashort-acting opiate, has promise as an anesthetic agent for those with CHD, but no studies of its effects in children with CHD are yet available.

Propofol. Its short duration of action makes propofol attractive for brief procedures in patients with CHD. In the isolated heart, propofol has myocardial depressant properties somewhat greater than thiopental and substantially more than ketamine.[188] Its use in patients with CHD should be restricted to patients with adequate cardiovascular reserve; for those patients with marginal cardiovascular reserve, use of propofol can precipitate cardiovascular decompensation and even collapse.

Successful use of propofol for pediatric patients with CHD undergoing cardiac catheterization and transesophageal echocardiography has been reported,[134] but in one study, a substantial percentage of patients given propofol had decreases in blood pressure of greater than 20% from baseline.[124] These mild deleterious effects on blood pressure are confirmed in other studies.[101] Increased incidences of bradycardia and junctional rhythm have also been reported in children receiving propofol compared with those receiving barbiturates.[179] In one specific study of propofol's effects on cardiac conduction in pediatric patients, no substantial effects were seen.[52] **These data, taken together with clinical experience, suggest that propofol's use in**

patients with CHD should be restricted to those with good levels of cardiovascular reserve because of its cardiac depressant properties.

Thiopental and other intravenous agents. Intravenous induction with thiopental generally is not used in patients with severe cardiac defects, although in a reduced dosage of 1 or 2 mg/kg, it may be safe for induction in patients with moderate defects and may actually result in improved arterial oxygen saturation in cyanosis. In pediatric patients with minimal or mild cardiac defects, IV induction with larger dosages of thiopental (3 to 5 mg/kg) are usually well tolerated, provided the patient is not hypovolemic. Rectally administered barbiturates, notably methohexital, may be an acceptable induction technique in an otherwise uncooperative child with less severe CHD and good cardiac reserve, but absorption is variable, and myocardial depression is possible.[61] Etomidate has not been used extensively enough in children with CHD to be sure of its effects, and no studies of the hemodynamic effects in small children are available.

Muscle relaxants

Pancuronium dosage requirements are unchanged in children with CHD and intracardiac shunts; it produces no heart rate or blood pressure changes when given slowly in these patients.[135] Through its vagolytic effect, a bolus dose of pancuronium can produce tachycardia and hypertension in children, which may sometimes be desirable to support cardiac output in infants with relatively fixed stroke volumes.[32] If tachycardia is undesirable, metubine causes no increase in heart rate, blood pressure, or cardiac rythym changes in small children, even at dosages of 0.5 mg/kg.[72] For those patients in whom a short-acting nondepolarizing muscle relaxant is desirable, atracurium or vecuronium at the lower end of their dose ranges have few cardiovascular side effects in children as does cisatracurium.[71,73] Use of the latter two muscle relaxants rather than pancuronium during induction combined with a high-dose opiate anesthetic may produce clinically significant bradycardia as has been reported in adults.[186] Bradycardia or even sinus arrest can also be a problem with use of succinylcholine in children with CHD, particularly those given large doses of opiates. To avoid these problems in vagotonic young children, atropine should be used with succinylcholine. If potent opiates are used at the same time as succinylcholine, severe bradycardia may be avoided by concomitant use of atropine.

Conduct of the Anesthetic

Anesthetic plan and goals

Virtually all children with CHD will tolerate well-managed anesthetics, but tolerance for events such as loss of airway patency, hypoventilation, inappropriate amounts and choices of anesthetics, and major intraoperative surgical insults is often very limited. The anesthetic plan should be aimed at maintaining or improving existing circulatory homeostasis throughout the procedure, but particularly during induction of anesthesia. **Because resuscitation may be very difficult in patients with CHD once cardiovascular collapse occurs, prevention of circulatory decompensation is the priority.** This makes anticipation of potential problems a particularly important part of the anesthetic plan.

Preoperative assessment

An important aim of preoperative assessment is to identify those patients with CHD who are likely to develop problems. Cardiac catheterization and echocardiogram data are most useful. Box 69-8 lists the critical indices of severe circulatory impairment in CHD. Patients who have any one of these indices are at risk for perioperative hemodynamic problems. If a patient has two or more of the listed criteria of critical impairment, particular care should be taken with planning the anesthetic. In such patients, depending on the experience of the anesthesia team, consultation with the patient's cardiologist to clarify critical aspects of the patient's pathophysiology may be advisable. In patients who have CHD that does not include any of the listed criteria in Box 69-8, the chances of hemodynamic problems with anesthesia are relatively low. Additional risk factors for patients with CHD undergoing anesthesia are listed in Box 69-9.

Preoperative preparation and medication

Before surgery, patients should be in the optimum condition allowed by their underlying disease. Emergency operations

BOX 69-8
INDICES OF CRITICAL IMPAIRMENT IN CONGENITAL HEART DISEASE

Arterial saturation $< 75\%$
$Q_p/Q_s > 2:1$
LV outflow tract gradient > 50 mm Hg
RV outflow tract gradient > 50 mm Hg
PVR > 6 Wood units
Polycythemia with Hct $> 60\%$

Q_p—pulmonary flow; LV—left ventricle; PVR—pulmonary vascular resistance; Q_s—systemic flow; RV—right ventricle; Hct—hematocrit.

BOX 69-9
GENERAL ASSOCIATED RISK FACTORS IN CONGENITAL HEART DISEASE

Severe form of isolated lesion
Complex lesions
Concurrent infectious disease
Metabolic derangements
Congestive heart failure
Previous palliative or corrective procedures
Acute hemodynamic deterioration

in critically ill, severely hypoxemic, and acidotic neonates are rarely necessary because the advent of PGE_1 treatment of ductus-dependent circulation in those with CHD. In most patients, a period of 24 to 48 hours of medical therapy will markedly improve the condition of most critically ill children with CHD and will lessen perioperative morbidity. Such therapy should be considered part of the preoperative preparation of sick children with CHD. Patients with more chronic problems, such as congestive heart failure and chronic pulmonary infections resulting from excessive pulmonary blood flow and congestion, should be at their pulmonary baselines if possible. Children taking cardiac medications should have their medications continued up to and including the morning of surgery, except for diuretics.

Preoperative medication can take many forms. A good preoperative visit may establish sufficient rapport with parents and child to eliminate need for preoperative medication, whereas relatively large doses of IV sedation may be needed for the extremely anxious child. The goal should be a lightly sedated patient without respiratory depression. In patients with severe hypoxemia and cyanosis or with pulmonary hypertension, premedication should be relatively light to avoid depression of ventilation that may exacerbate their decreased hypoxic ventilatory drive or further increase their PVR. When anxiety levels are high and severe hypoxemia, severe congestive heart failure, or pulmonary hypertension preclude heavy premedication before arriving in the preoperative holding area, intramuscular ketamine and midazolam are given just before the child is taken to the operating room. Such premedication is well tolerated by all but critically ill children and can ease the difficulties experienced by children and parents. Properly monitored transport should be available, with an anesthesia caregiver in constant attendance. This combination of drugs is quickly effective so that a deeply sedated child can be separated from anxious parents. Use of portable pulse oximetry and a precordial stethoscope are often advisable for the trip to the operating room. If there is any question of cardiac stability during this period, an IV line is started immediately after sedation is given or in extreme cases even before sedation. With the availability of EMLA cream, preoperative IV insertion for premedication has become much easier.

Alternatively, oral midazolam in a dosage of 0.75 to 1.0 mg/kg can be given to small children in the presence of the anesthesia provider. This will often result in excellent premedication and may be supplemented by intramuscular ketamine, if needed, mixed with atropine or glycopyrolate.

Induction of anesthesia

Because of the potential for rapid and dramatic hemodynamic changes in young patients with CHD, especially infants, complete preparation of anesthetic and monitoring equipment and required drugs is essential. Adequate assistance should be immediately available during induction, particularly if the patient meets a number of the criteria of severe disease listed in Table 69-1. Flexibility is needed in choice of induction techniques because response to premedication and emotional needs of parents and children facing a cardiac procedure can place constraints on choices.

Choice of induction technique will be influenced by response to premedication and the parent–child–anesthesia provider relationship and to the anesthetic management plan. In older patients who are not hypoxemic and who have minimal compromise of their cardiac reserve, choice of induction techniques is large. Rectal, intramuscular, IV, or inhalation induction techniques using various agents can be used with reasonable safety if individual pathophysiologic limitations are respected. With younger, sicker, and less cooperative patients, choices decrease. In older children with only mildly compromised cardiac function, rectal administration of anesthetic agents such as barbiturates can be a useful technique, but lack of control and potential for circulatory depression make this technique unacceptable for sick infants.

In children with good IV access, quick insertion of a small-bore IV needle for induction can be virtually painless, if sufficiently long applications of EMLA cream are used. Cooperative small children who have adequate cardiac reserve but difficult IV access or a morbid fear of needles can be induced cautiously with inhalation anesthetics, even if cyanotic. An IV catheter is then inserted expeditiously to facilitate intubation with adjunctive IV agents, avoiding the risk of deep levels of inhalational anesthesia in circulatory systems with little reserve, particularly in the immature circulation of the infant. Such use of an inhalational anesthesic for induction of patients with severe CHD without presence of a working IV heavily depends on the judgment of the anesthesia provider for safety.

Maintenance of anesthesia

Maintenance of anesthesia in the pediatric heart patient depends on preoperative status and response to induction and on the surgical procedure and intraoperative events. Whether inhalational agents, additional narcotics, or other IV agents are used for maintenance depends on patient tolerance and postoperative plans for ventilatory management.

In children with CHDs, intraoperative changes in cardiac shunting are unique problems during maintenance of anesthesia. Although it is not always clear whether clinical deterioration is caused by changes in shunting or by primary myocardial depression or dysfunction, the intraoperative events and progress of the anesthetic will usually suggest a cause. Hypotension and hypoxemia, particularly during induction of anesthesia, should be aggressively and immediately managed. Decreases in arterial oxygenation or in systemic blood flow may be caused by alterations in intracardiac shunting in these children and can usually be managed by manipulations of PVR/SVR (to be discussed), but in some patients, inotropes will be needed, assuming that circulating blood volume is adequate.

Manipulation of pulmonary and systemic vascular resistance

Manipulation of PVR/SVR allows some control over shunting, depending on specific pathophysiology. PVR is particularly important because of the frequency of disturbances of pulmonary blood flow and right-sided defects in patients with CHD. Usually the goal is to decrease PVR to improve pulmonary flow, right heart function, and oxygenation, but in some lesions, pulmonary flow may be excessively high at the expense of systemic output, requiring increases in PVR.[81] Many intraoperative manipulations tend to alter PVR. Manipulations that increase PVR are frequent problems because of increased reactivity of the abnormal pulmonary vasculature often found in patients with CHD. These manipulations include sympathetic stimulation, encroachments on lung volumes that produce atelectasis (surgical retraction, pleural and peritoneal collections, and abdominal packing), CPB, alveolar hypoxia, and hypoventilation. Manipulations that increase and decrease PVR are shown in Box 69-10. Ventilation is important because it is subject to control by the anesthesia provider and is crucial in attempts to control PVR via airway pressure, lung volumes, alveolar $Paco_2$ and Pao_2, and other, less well-understood variables.

The effects of various anesthetic agents on PVR are poorly understood. Ketamine and nitrous oxide increase PVR in adults, but studies of ketamine and nitrous oxide in infants with normal or elevated PVR have shown no increase in PVR when ventilation and FIO_2 are constant.[88,122,145] Stress responses in the pulmonary circulation of patients with CHD are a primary concern in some patients. Large doses of potent narcotics, such as fentanyl, attenuate pulmonary vascular responses to noxious stimuli, such as endotracheal suctioning in infants, but do not change baseline PVR.[90,199] Reactive pulmonary hypertensive responses are partially mediated by the sympathoadrenal axis and are thus attenuated by an adequate depth of anesthesia. CPB increases PVR through activation of the inflammatory response, cytokine release, and ischemia of the endothelium in the pulmonary circulation. After bypass surgery, elevated PVR can be a substantial problem.

PVR can be controlled independently of SVR by manipulating various aspects of ventilation (Box 69-10). Nitric oxide delivered through to alveoli has been shown to be a pulmonary vasodilator and to be effective in patients with CHD.[45] In contrast to inhaled nitric oxide, even selective infusions of rapidly metabolized vasodilators (e.g., nitroprusside) into the pulmonary circulation can result in systemic drug concentrations and systemic hemodynamic effects without desired effects on PVR.[160] Nitric oxide has been shown effective in selectively reducing PVR in a variety of different CHD lesions accompanied by high PVR; this can be accomplished without altering SVR.[210] Not all patients with CHD with high PVR respond to inhaled nitric oxide, particularly after the neonatal period, but nitric oxide therapy should be tried whenever high PVR is a substantial problem in patients with CHD of any age.[211] High levels of inspired oxygen, especially 100% O_2, also decrease elevated PVR in infants without changing SVR, whereas inspired oxygen levels of 21% or less increase PVR.[1,31,78] Hypoventilation, with associated acidosis and hypercapnia, also increases PVR. Hyperventilation to alkalotic pHs (> 7.50) and low $Paco_2$ reliably decreases PVR in infants and improves right ventricular function.[35,144,204,205] This maneuver increases pulmonary blood flow and decreases right-to-left shunting in neonates, increasing Pao_2.[54,161] Although prolonged hyperventilation to decrease PVR may theoretically cause problems from decreased cerebral blood flow, clinical and experimental studies in hyperventilated infants show no evidence of cerebral damage.[20,20,58,205] The pattern of ventilation and PEEP also can alter PVR. PVR is lowest at normal FRC. At low lung volumes with atelectasis and at high lung volumes with hyperinflation of alveoli, PVR increases.[213] High levels of PEEP increase PVR primarily by hyperinflation of alveoli, but if atelectasis and pulmonary edema are corrected by PEEP, PVR may decrease. Different patterns of ventilation may further reduce PVR by releasing prostacyclin in the pulmonary vasculature.[125,180]

Manipulation of SVR by use of vasopressors is useful when there is a need for increased coronary perfusion pressure or a need to decrease right-to-left shunting that causes severe systemic hypoxemia. Phenylephrine has been shown effective in reducing right-to-left shunting in tetralogy of Fallot and increasing arterial oxygen saturation.[159] A mechanical method for increasing SVR to decrease right-to-left shunting in tetralogy of Fallot is compression of the abdominal aorta. This can be done immediately and can be used to gain time while other pharmacologic therapy is started or while the child is prepared for CPB.

BOX 69-10
MANIPULATION ALTERING PULMONARY VASCULAR RESISTANCE

Increased PVR

Hypoxia
Hypercapnia
Acidosis
Hyperinflation
Atelectasis
Sympathetic stimulation
High hematocrit
Mechanical pulmonary artery constriction

Decreased PVR

Oxygen
Hypocapnia
Alkalosis
Normal FRC
Blockage of sympathetic stimulation
Low hematocrit
Inhaled nitric oxide

PVR—pulmonary vascular resistance; FRC—functional residual capacity.

KEY POINTS

- Congenital heart diseases that decrease cardiopulmonary reserve include intracardiac shunting, hypoxemia from inadequate pulmonary blood flow or intracardiac shunting, congestive failure from volume or pressure overload, vascular obstructive disease from excessive pulmonary blood flow, various kinds of stenoses, and occasional coronary ischemia.
- Many of the determinants of shunting (its magnitude and direction) may change considerably during anesthesia and operative manipulations.
- There are simple shunts, bidirectional shunts, and occasionally complex shunts. The key for the anesthesia providers is to understand the effects of vasodilators, cardiac depressants, and surgical manipulation on these various shunts.
- "Bubble discipline" is an important concept in dealing with anesthesia administration for patients with congenital heart disease.
- Chronic hypoxia leads to polycythemia, which, in turn, leads to dramatic increases in blood viscocity.
- The anesthesia provider should understand the hemodynamic consequences of pulmonary vascular hypertrophy, the end stage of which is the Eisenmenger syndrome.
- Even though a child with congenital heart disease may not have frank failure, cardiac reserves may be dramatically decreased, especially if episodes of prolonged congestive failure have been a part of the history of the patient and have resulted in cardiomegaly or ventricular hypertrophy.
- "Transitional circulation" keeps neonates alive with severe life-threatening congenital heart disease. In this context, therapy with PGE_1 infusion should be understood, especially the possibility of side effects, such as apnea and major vasodilation.
- The functional capacities of the immature heart should be of particular interest to anesthesia providers. The immature noncompliant ventricle is extraordinarily sensitive to increases in volume and is considerably restricted in its ability to respond to same by increasing stroke volume. The Starling curve plateau in neonates is reached at left venticular end-diastolic pressures of 4 mm Hg. Therefore, cardiac compliance values in neonates do not correspond to values for adult patients.
- Adult arterial pressures, especially during bypass, also do not apply to neonates and infants.
- The procedures for weaning from bypass and using deep hypothermic circulatory arrest or low-flow hypothermic bypass are very important. They should be reviewed in detail.
- The anesthesia provider should fully understand the hemodynamic consequences and purpose of various PA banding procedures and various kinds of transcatheter management of congenital lesions. Transcatheter procedures require anesthetic care in the interventional cardiac catheterization laboratory.
- Halothane has been a successful induction anesthetic in children with various kinds of transcatheter treatment of congenital lesions. Transcatheter procedures require anesthetic care in the interventional cardiac catheterization laboratory.
- Intravenous anesthetics, including high-dose opioids or ketamine, may provide increased margins of safety in some infants with congenital heart disease. Intravenous agents, however, have the possibility of very high transients after intravenous bolus doses because of inadequate mixing or shunting.
- Intramuscular ketamine, 3 to 5 mg/kg, is reasonably well tolerated, even in sick children with cyanotic congenital heart disease.
- The manipulation of pulmonary and systemic vascular resistance described in this chapter are worth reviewing for anesthesia providers engaged in the practice of anesthesia for congenital heart disease.
- Inhaled nitric oxide is now a clinically useful and efficacious selective pulmonary vasodilator for many, but not all, patients with CHD.

REFERENCES

1. Abman SH, Wolfe RR, Accurso FJ, et al: Pulmonary vascular response to oxygen in infants with severe bronchopulmonary dysplasia, *Pediatrics* 75:80–84, 1985.
2. Albrecht RF, Miletich DJ, Ruttle M: The effects of prolonged hyperventilation on cerebral metabolism, *Anesthesiology* 61: A247, 1984(abstract).
3. Anand KJS, Aynsley-Green A: Metabolic and endocrine effects of surgical ligation of patent ductus arteriosus in the human preterm neonate: are there implications for further improvement of postoperative outcome? *Mod Probl Paediatr* 23:143–157, 1985.
4. Anand KJS, Brown MJ, Bloom SR, et al: Studies on the hormonal regulation of fuel metabolism in the human newborn infant undergoing anaesthesia and surgery, *Hormone Res* 22:115–128, 1985.
5. Anand KJ, Hansen DD, Hickey PR: Hormonal-metabolic stress responses in neonates undergoing cardiac surgery, *Anesthesiology* 73:661–670, 1990.
6. Anand KJS, Hickey PR: Halothane-morphine compared to high-dose sufentanil anesthesia and postoperative analgesia in neonatal cardiac surgery, *N Engl J Med* 326:1–9, 1992.
7. Anand KJS, Sippell WG, Aynsley-Green A: Randomised trial of fentanyl anaesthesia in preterm babies undergoing surgery: effects on the stress response, *Lancet* 1987:243–248, 1987.
8. Anderson HL, Attorri RJ, Custer JR, et al: Extracorporeal membrane oxygenation for

pediatric cardiopulmonary failure, *J Thorac Cardiovasc Surg* 99:1011–1021, 1990.

9. Anversa P, Olivetti G, Loud AV: Morphometric study of early postnatal development in the left and right ventricular myocardium of the rat. I. Hypertrophy, hyperplasia, and nucleation of myocytes, *Circ Res* 46:495, 1980.
10. Arciniegas E, Farooki ZQ, Hakimi M, et al: Classic shunting operations for cyanotic congenital heart defects, *J Thorac Cardiovasc Surg* 84:88–96, 1982.
11. Arnold LW, Keane JF, Keane JF, et al: Transient unilateral pulmonary edema after successful dilation of peripheral pulmonary stenosis, *Am J Cardiol* 62:327–330, 1988.
12. Banas JS, Meister SG, Gazzaniga AB, et al: A simple technique for detecting small defects of the atrial septum, *Am J Cardiol* 28:467–471, 1971.
13. Barash PG, Glanz S, Katz JD, et al: Ventricular function in children during halothane anesthesia: an echocardiographic evaluation, *Anesthesiology* 49:79–85, 1978.
14. Barratt-Boyes BG. Choreoathetosis as a complication of cardiopulmonary bypass, *Ann Thorac Surg* 50:693–694, 1990.
15. Bashein G, Townes BD, Nessly ML, et al: A randomized study of carbon dioxide management during hypothermic cardiopulmonary bypass, *Anesthesiology* 72:7–15, 1990.
16. Beekman RH, Rocchini AP. Transcatheter treatment of congenital heart disease. Progress in cardiovascular diseases, *Prog Cardiovasc Dis* 32:1–30, 1989.
17. Bellinger DC, Jonas RA, Rappaport LA, et al: A comparison of the developmental and neurological status at one year of children who underwent heart surgery using hypothermic circulatory arrest of low-flow cardiopulmonary bypass, *N Engl J Med* 332:549–555, 1995.
18. Benzing G III, Francis PD, Kaplan S, et al: Glucose and insulin changes in infants and children undergoing hypothermic open heart surgery, *Am J Cardiol* 52:133–136, 1983.
19. Berman W Jr: The hemodynamics of shunts in congenital heart disease. In Johansen K, Burggren WW, editors: *Cardiovascular shunts: phylogenetic, ontogenetic, and clinical aspects.* New York, 1985, pp 399-410, Raven Press.
20. Bernbaum JC, Russell P, Sheridan PH, et al: Long-term follow-up of newborns with persistent pulmonary hypertension, *Crit Care Med* 12:579–583, 1984.
21. Bini M, Reves JG, Berry D, et al: Ejection fraction during ketamine anesthesia in congenital heart diseased patients, *Anesth Analg* 60:186, 1984 (abstract).
22. Blackwood MJA, Haka-Ilse K, Steward DJ. Developmental outcome in children undergoing surgery with profound hypothermia, *Anesthesiology* 65:437–440, 1986.
23. Borow KM, Karp R: Atrial septal defect: lessons from the past, directions for the future, *N Eng J Med* 323:1698–1700, 1990.
24. Borrow KM, Keane JF, Castenada AR, et al: Systemic ventricular function in patients with tetralogy of Fallot, ventricular septal defect and transposition of the great arteries repaired during infancy, *Circulation* 64:878–885, 1981.
25. Boudreaux JP, Schieber RA, Cook DR: Hemodynamic effects of halothane in the newborn piglet, *Anesth Analg* 63:731–737, 1984.
26. Bridges ND, Perry SB, Keane JF, et al: Preoperative transcatheter closure of congenital muscular ventricular septal defects, *N Engl J Med* 324:1312-1317, 1991.
27. Brinkman CR, Johnson GH, Assali NS: Hemodynamic effects of bradycardia in the fetal lamb, *Am J Physiol* 223:1465–1469, 1972.
28. Brunberg JA, Doty DB, Reilly EL: Choreoathetosis in infants following cardiac surgery with deep hypothermia and circulatory arrest, *J Paediatr* 84:232, 1974.
29. Buckley LP, Dooley KJ, Fyler DC: Pulmonary atresia and intact ventricular septum in New England, *Am J Cardiol* 37:124–129, 1976.
30. Burrows PE, Benson LE, Williams WG, et al. Iliofemoral arterial complications of balloon angioplasty for systemic obstructions in infants and children, *Circulation* 82:1697–1704, 1990.
31. Bush A, Busst C, Booth K, et al: Does prostacyclin enhance the selective pulmonary vasodilator effect of oxygen in children with congenital heart disease, *Circulation* 74:135–144, 1986.
32. Cabal LA, Siassi B, Artal R, et al: Cardiovascular and catecholamine changes after administration of pancuronium in distressed neonates, *Pediatrics* 75:284–287, 1985.
33. Castaneda AR, Freed MD, Williams RG, et al: Repair of tetralogy of Fallot in infancy, *J Thorac Cardiovasc Surg* 74:372–381, 1977.
34. Castaneda AR, Mayer JE, Jonas RA, et al: The neonate with critical congenital heart disease: repair—a surgical challenge, *J Thorac Cardiovasc Surg* 98:869–875, 1989.
35. Chang AL, Zucker HA, Hickey PR, et al: Pulmonary vascular resistance after cardiac surgery: the role of carbon dioxide and hydrogen ion, *Crit Care Med* 23:568–579, 1995.
36. Clarkson PM, MacArthur BA, Barratt-Boyes BG, et al: Developmental progress after cardiac surgery in infancy using hypothermia and circulatory arrest, *Circulation* 62:855–861, 1980.
37. Clyman RI, Mauray F, Roman C, et al: Factors determining the loss of ductus arteriosus responsiveness to prostaglandin E, *Circulation* 68:433–436, 1983.
38. Coblentz MG, Criscito MA, Cohn JD: Persistent left superior vena cava complicating hemodynamic monitoring catheterization, *Crit Care Med* 6:32–35, 1978.
39. Coles JG, Taylor MJ, Pearce JM, et al: Cerebral monitoring of somatosensory evoked potentials during profoundly hypothermic circulatory arrest, *Circulation* 70:(I)96–102, 1984.
40. Cook DJ, Carton EG, Housmans PR: Mechanism of the positive inotropic effect of ketamine in isolated ferret ventricular papillary muscle, *Anesthesiology* 74: 880–888, 1991.
41. Cook DR, Brandom BW, Shiu G, et al: The inspired median effective dose, brain concentration at anesthesia, and cardiovascular index for halothane in young rats, *Anesth Analg* 60:182–185, 1981.
42. Coppel DL, Dundee JW: Ketamine anesthesia for cardiac catheterization, *Anaesthesia* 27:25–31, 1972.
43. Cordell D, Graham T Jr, Atwood G, et al: Left heart volume characteristics following ventricular septal closure defects in infancy, *Circulation* 54:417–422, 1976.
44. Coselli JS, Crawford ES, Beall AC, Jr, et al: Determination of brain temperatures for safe circulatory arrest during cardiovascular operation, *Ann Thorac Surg* 45: 638–642, 1988.
45. Curran RD, Mavroudis D, Backer CL, et al: Inhaled nitric oxide for children with congenital heart disease and pulmonary hypertension, *Ann Thorac Surg* 60: 1765–1771, 1995.
46. Cyran SE, Kimball TR, Meyer RA, et al: Efficacy of intraoperative transesophageal echocardiography in children with congenital heart disease, *Am J Cardiol* 63: 594–598, 1989.
47. Davis PJ, Cook DR, Stiller RL, et al: Pharmacodynamics and pharmacokinetics of high-dose sufentanil in infants and children undergoing cardiac surgery, *Anesth Analg* 66:203–208, 1987.
48. DeLeon S, Ilbawi M, Arcill R, et al. Choreoathetosis after deep hypothermia without circulatory arrest, *Ann Thorac Surg* 50:714–719, 1990.
49. den Hollander JM, Hennis PJ, Burm AGL, et al: Alfentanil in infants and children with congenital heart defects, *J Cardiothorac Anes* 2:12–17, 1988.
50. Diaz JH, Lockhart CH: Is halothane really safe in infancy? *Anesthesiology* 51:S313, 1979(abstract).
51. Dickinson DF, Sambrooks JE: Intellectual performance in children after circulatory arrest with profound hypothermia in infancy, *Arch Dis Child* 54:1–6, 1979.
52. Downing SE, Talner NS, Gardner TH: Ventricular function in the newborn lamb, *Am J Physiol* 208:931–937, 1965.
53. Driscoll DJ, Gillette PC, Hallman GL, et al: Management of surgical complete A-V block in children, *Am J Cardiol* 43: 1175–1180, 1979.
54. Drummond WH, Gregory GA, Heymann MA, et al: The independent effects of hyperventilation, tolazine and dopamine on infants with persistent pulmonary hypertension, *J Pediatr* 98:603–611, 1981.
55. Ehyai A, Fenichel GM, Bender HW. Incidence and prognosis of seizures in infants after cardiac surgery with profound hypothermia and circulatory arrest, *JAMA* 252:3165–3167, 1984.
56. Ellis DJ, Steward DJ: Fentanyl dosage is associated with reduced blood glucose in pediatric patients after hypothermic cardiopulmonary bypass, *Anesthesiology* 72: 812–815, 1990.
57. Emery JL, Mithal A: Weights of cardiac ventricles at and after birth, *Br Heart J* 23:313–316, 1961.
58. Ferrara B, Johnson DE, Chang P, et al: Efficacy and neurologic outcome of profound hypocapnia alkalosis for the treatment of persistent pulmonary hypertension in infancy, *J Pediatr* 105:457–461, 1984.

59. Ferry PC: Neurologic sequelae of open-heart surgery in children: an "irritating question," *AJDC* 144:369–373, 1990.
60. Flanagan MF, Fujii AM, Colan SM, et al: Myocardial angiogenesis and coronary perfusion in left ventricular pressure-overload hypertrophy in the young lamb, *Circ Res* 68:1458–1470, 1991.
61. Forbes RB, Murray DJ, Dull DJ, et al: Hemodynamic effects of methohexitone for induction of anesthesia in children, *Can J Anaesth* 36:526–529, 1989.
62. Fox LS, Blackstone EH, Kirklin JW, et al: Relationship of brain blood flow and oxygen consumption to perfusion flow rate during profoundly hypothermic cardiopulmonary bypass, *J Thorac Cardiovasc Surg* 87:658–664, 1984.
63. Franciosi RA, Blanc WA: Myocardial infarction in infants and children. I. A necropsy study in congenital heart disease, *J Pediatr* 73:309, 1968.
64. Friesen RH, Henry DB: Cardiovascular changes in preterm neonates receiving isoflurane, halothane, fentanyl and ketamine, *Anesthesiology* 64:238–242, 1986.
65. Friesen RH, Lichtor JL: Cardiovascular depression during halothane induction in infants: a study of three induction techniques, *Anesth Analg* 61:42–45, 1982.
66. Friesen RH, Lichtor JL: Cardiovascular effects of inhalation induction with isoflurane in infants, *Anesth Analg* 62:411–414, 1983.
67. Fyler DC: Report of the New England Regional Infant Cardiac Program, *Pediatrics* 65(Suppl 2):375, 1980.
68. Gassner S, Cohen M, Aygen M, et al: The effect of ketamine on pulmonary artery pressure: An experimental and clinical study, *Anaesthesia* 29:141–146, 1974.
69. Glenski JA, Friesen RH, Berglund NL, et al: Comparison of the hemodynamic and echocardiographic effects of sufentanil, fentanyl, isoflurane, and halothane for pediatric cardiac surgery, *J Cardiovasc Anesth* 2:147–155, 1988.
70. Gold JP, Jonas RA, Lang P, et al: Transcutaneous intracardiac monitoring lines in pediatric surgical patients: a 10-year-experience, *Ann Thorac Surg* 42: 185–191, 1986.
71. Goudsouzian NG, Liu LMP, Cote CJ, et al: Safety and efficacy of atracurium in adolescents and children anesthetized with halothane. *Anesthesiology* 59:459–462, 1983.
72. Goudsouzian NG, Liu LMP, Savarese JJ: Metocurine in infants and children, *Anesthesiology* 49:266–269, 1978.
73. Goudsouzian NG, Martyn JJA, Liu LMP, et al: Safety and efficacy of vecuronium in adolescents and children, *Anesth Analg* 62:1083–1088, 1983.
74. Greeley WJ, Bushman GA, Davis DP, et al: Comparative effects of halothane and ketamine on systemic arterial oxygen saturation in children with cyanotic congenital heart disease, *Anesthesiology* 65:666–668, 1986.
75. Greeley WJ, Kern FH, Kisslo JA, et al: Intramyocardial air causing right ventricular dysfunction after repair of congenital heart defects, *Anesthesiology* 73:1042–1046, 1990.
76. Greeley WJ, Kern FH, Reves JG, et al: Effect of cardiopulmonary bypass and total circulatory arrest on cerebral metabolism and flow/metabolism coupling in children, *J Thorac Cardiovasc Surg* 101:783–794, 1991.
77. Greeley WJ, Ungerleider RM, Kern FH, et al: Effects of cardiopulmonary bypass on cerebral blood flow in neonates, infants and children, *Circulation* 80:1209–1215, 1989.
78. Greeley WJ, Ungerleider RM, Smith LR, et al: The effects of deep hypothermic cardiopulmonary bypass and total circulatory arrest on cerebral blood flow in infants and children, *J Thorac Cardiovasc Surg* 97: 737–745, 1989.
79. Gross CM, Wann S, Johnson GL: Valsalva maneuver echocardiography: a new technique for improved detection of right-to-left shunting in patients with systemic embolism, *Am J Cardiol* 49:955, 1982 (abstract).
80. Guyton RA, Andrews MJ, Hickey PR, et al: The contribution of atrial contraction to right heart function before and after right heart ventriculotomy, *J Thorac Cardiovasc Surg* 71:1–10, 1976.
81. Hansen DD, Hickey PR: Anesthesia for hypoplastic left heart syndrome: use of high dose fentanyl in 30 neonates, *Anesth Analg* 65:127–132, 1986.
82. Haworth SG: Normal pulmonary vascular development and its disturbance in congenital heart disease. In Godman MJ, editor: *Paediatric cardiology,* vol 4, New York, 1981, pp 46-55, Churchill-Livingstone.
83. Haworth SG: Pulmonary vascular disease in secundum atrial septal defect in childhood, *Am J Cardiol* 51:265–272, 1983.
84. Hensley FA, Larach DR, Stauffer RA, et al: The effect of halothane/nitrous oxide/oxygen mask induction on arterial hemoglobin saturation in cyanotic congenital heart disease, *Anesthesiology* 63:A3, 1985(abstract).
85. Hickey PR, Andersen NP: Deep hypothermic circulatory arrest: a review of pathophysiology and clinical experience as a basis for anesthetic management, *J Cardiothorac Anesth* 1:137–155, 1987.
86. Hickey PR, Hansen DD: Fentanyl and sufentanyl-oxygen-pancuronium anesthesia for cardiac surgery in infants, *Anesth Analg* 63:117–124, 1984.
87. Hickey PR, Hansen DD, Cramolini MD: Pulmonary and systemic responses to ketamine in infants with normal and elevated pulmonary vascular resistance, *Anesthesiology* 62:287–293, 1985.
88. Hickey PR, Hansen DD, Strafford M, et al: Pulmonary and systemic hemodynamic effects of nitrous oxide in infants with normal and elevated pulmonary vascular resistance, *Anesthesiology* 65:374–378, 1986.
89. Hickey PR, Hansen DD, Wessel D, et al: Pulmonary and systemic hemodynamic responses to fentanyl in infants, *Anesth Analg* 64:483–486, 1985.
90. Hickey PR, Hansen DD, Wessel DL, et al: Blunting of stress responses in the pulmonary circulation of infants by fentanyl, *Anesth Analg* 64:1137–1142, 1985.
91. Hickey PR, McGowan FX: Adhesion molecules and inflammation: the next targets for perioperative organ protection? *Anesth Analg* 81:1123–1124, 1995.
92. Hickey PR, Wessel DL, Streitz SL, et al: Transcatheter closure of atrial septal defects: hemodynamic complications and anesthetic management, *Anesth Analg* 74:44–50, 1992.
93. Hilgenberg JC, McCammon RL, Stoelting RK: Pulmonary and systemic vascular responses to nitrous oxide in patients with nitrous oxide and pulmonary hypertension, *Anesth Analg* 59:323–326, 1980.
94. Hoffman JI, Christianson R: Congenital heart disease in a cohort of 19,502 births with long term followup, *Am J Cardiol* 42:641, 1978.
95. Holzman RS, van der Velde ME, Kaus SJ, et al: Sevoflurane depresses myocardial contractility less than halothane during induction of anesthesia in children, *Anesthesiology* 85:1260–1267, 1996.
96. Humphreys JE, Cummins P: Regulatory proteins of the myocardium. Atrial and ventricular tropomyosin and troponin-I in the developing and adult bovine and human heart, *J Mol Cell Cardiol* 16:643, 1984.
97. Irish CL, Murkin JM, Cleland A, et al: Neuromuscular blockade significantly decreases systemic oxygen consumption during hypothermic cardiopulmonary bypass, *J Cardiothorac Vasc Anesth* 5:132–134, 1991.
98. Jamakani J, Graham T Jr, Canent R Jr, et al: The effect of corrective surgery on heart volume and mass in children with ventricular septal defect, *Am J Cardiol* 27:254–258, 1971.
99. Jonas RA, Lang P, Hansen DD, et al: First-stage palliation of hypoplastic left heart syndrome: the importance of coarctation and shunt size, *J Thorac Cardiovasc Surg* 92:6–13, 1986.
100. Jonas RA, Lang P, Mayer JE, et al: The importance of prostaglandin E in resuscitation of the neonate with critical aortic stenosis, *J Thorac Cardiovasc Surg* 89:314–315, 1985.
101. Jones RD, Visram AR, Chan MM, et al: A comparison of three induction agents in paediatric anaesthesia—cardiovascular effects and recovery, *Anesth Int Care* 22(5): 545–555, 1994.
102. Journois D, Israel-biet D, Pouard P, et al: High-volume, zero-balanced hemofiltration to reduce delayed inflammatory response to cardiopulmonary bypass in children, *Anesthesiology* 85:965–976, 1996.
103. Journis D, Pouard P, Greeley WJ, et al: Hemofiltration during cardiopulmonary bypass in pediatric cardiac surgery, *Anesthesiology* 81:1181–1189, 1994.
104. Katz NM, Blackstone EH, Kirklin JW, et al: Late survival and symptoms after repair of tetralogy of Fallot, *Circulation* 65:403–410, 1982.
105. Kenny J, Plappert T, Doubilet P, et al: Effects of heart rate on ventricular size, stroke volume, and output in the normal human fetus: a prospective Doppler echocardiographic study, *Circulation* 76: 52, 1987.
106. Kern FH, Jonas RA, Mayer JE, et al: Temperature monitoring during infant CPB: does it predict efficient brain cooling? *Ann Thorac Surg* 54:749–754, 1992.

107. Kirklin JK, Westaby S, Blackstone EH, et al: Complement and the damaging effects of cardiopulmonary bypass, *J Thorac Cardiovasc Surg* 86:845–857, 1983.
108. Kirklin JK, Blackstone EH, Kirklin JW, et al: Intracardiac surgery in infants under age 3 months: incremental risk factors for hospital mortality, *Am J Cardiol* 48:500–506, 1981.
109. Kirkpatrick SE, Pitlick PT, Naliboff J, et al: Frank-Starling as an important determinant of fetal cardiac output, *Am J Physiol* 231:495-500, 1976.
110. Kontras S, Sirak H, Newton W: Hematologic abnormalities in children with congenital heart disease, *JAMA* 195:611–615, 1976.
111. Koren G, Goresky G, Crean P, et al: Pediatric fentanyl dosing based on pharmacokinetics during cardiac surgery, *Anesth Analg* 63:577–582, 1984.
112. Krane EJ, Su JY: Comparison of the effects of halothane on skinned myocardial fibers from newborn and adult rabbit. I. Effects on contractile proteins, *Anesthesiology* 70:76–81, 1989.
113. Krane EJ, Su JY: Comparison of the effects of halothane on skinned myocardial fibers from newborn and adult rabbit: II. Effects on sarcoplasmic reticulum, *Anesthesiology* 71:103–109, 1991.
114. Kronik G, Mosslacher H: Positive contrast echocardiography in patients with patent foramen ovale and normal right heart hemodynamics, *Am J Cardiol* 49: 1806–1809, 1984.
115. Laishley RS, Burrows FA, Lerman J, et al: Effect of anesthetic induction regimens on oxygen saturation in cyanotic congenital heart disease, *Anesthesiology* 65:673–677, 1986.
116. Lanier WL, Stangland KJ, Scheithauer BW, et al: The effects of dextrose infusion and head position on neurologic outcome after complete cerebral ischemia in primates: examination of a model, *Anesthesiology* 66:39–48, 1987.
117. Lappas DG, Buckley MJ, Laver MB, et al: Left ventricular performance and pulmonary circulation following addition of nitrous oxide to morphine during coronary-artery surgery, *Anesthesiology* 43:61, 1975.
118. Laussen PC, Hansen DD, Perry SB, et al: Transcatheter closure of ventricular septal defects: hemodynamic instability and anesthetic management, *Anesth Analg* 80: 1076–1082, 1995.
119. Lavoie J, Burrows FA, Hansen D: Video-assisted thoracoscopic surgery for the treatment of congenital cardiac defects in the pediatric population: anesthetic considerations, *Anesth Analg* 82:563–567, 1996.
120. Lavoie J, Javorski JJ, Donahue K, et al: Detection of residual flow by transesophageal echocaradiography during video-assisted thoracoscopic patent ductus arteriosus interruption, *Anesth Analg* 80:1071–1075, 1995.
121. Lavoie J, Walsh EP, Burrows FA, et al: Effects of propofol or isoflurane anesthesia on cardiac conduction in children undergoing radiofrequency catheter ablation for tachydysrhythmias, *Anesthesiology* 82(4): 884–887, 1995.
122. Lawler PGP, Nunn JF: A reassessment of the valaidity of the iso-shunt graph, *Br J Anaesth* 56:1325–1335, 1984.
123. Lawrence A, Berger HJ, Johnston DE, et al: Radionuclide assessment of right and left exercise reserve after total correction of Tetralogy of fallot, *Am J Cardiol* 45:1013, 1980.
124. Lebovic S, Reich DL, Steinberg LG, et al: Comparison of propofol versus ketamine for anesthesia in pediatric patients undergoing cardiac catheterization, *Anesth Analg* 74:490–494, 1992.
125. Leffler CW, Hessler JR, Green RS: The onset of breathing at birth stimulates pulmonary vascular prostacyclin synthesis, *Ped Res* 18:938–942, 1984.
126. Lerman J, Oyston JP, Gallagher TM, et al: The minimum alveolar concentration (MAC) and hemodynamic effects of halothane, isoflurane, and sevoflurane in newborn swine, *Anesthesiology* 73: 717–721, 1990.
127. Levin RM, Seleny FL, Streczyn MV: Ketamine-pancuronium-narcotic technique for cardiovascular surgery in infants—a comparative study, *Anesth Analg* 54: 800–805, 1975.
128. Lewis AB, Freed MA, Heyman MA, et al: Side effects of therapy with prostaglandin E1 in infants with critical congenital heart disease, *Circulation* 64:893–899, 1981.
129. Lichtor JL, Beker BE, Ruschhaupt DG: Myocardial depression during induction in infants, *Anesthesiology* 59:A452, 1983 (abstract).
130. Lindahl SGE: Oxygen consumption and carbon dioxide elimination in infants and children during anaesthesia and surgery, *Br J Anaesth* 62:70, 1989.
131. Lock JE, Rome JJ, Davis R, et al: Transcatheter closure of atrial septal defects: experimental studies, *Circulation* 79:1091–1099, 1989.
132. Macartney FJ, Taylor JFN, Graham GR, et al. The fate of survivors of cardiac surgery in infancy, *Circulation* 62:80, 1980.
133. Malviya S, Burrows FA, Johnston AE, et al: Anaesthetic experience with paediatric interventional cardiology, *Can J Anaesth* 36:320-324, 1989.
134. Marcus B, Steward DJ, Khan NR, et al: Outpatient transesophageal echocardiography with intravenous propofol anesthesia in children and adolescents, *J Am Soc Echocardiogr* 6:205–209, 1993.
135. Maunuksela EL, Gattiker RI: Use of pancuronium in children with congenital heart disease, *Anesth Analg* 60:798–801, 1981.
136. McKnight CK, Elliott MJ, Pearson DT, et al:. The effects of four different crystalloid bypass pump-priming fluids upon the metabolic response to cardiac operation, *J Thorac Cardiovasc Surg* 90:97–111, 1985.
137. McNeill AM, Lerman J, Gregory GA: Echocardiographic assessment of ventricular function in children during isoflurane anesthesia, *Anesthesiology* 61:A426, 1984(abstract).
138. Mehta M, Sokoll MD, Gergis SD: Effects of venous air embolism on the cardiovascular system and acid base balance in the presence and absence of nitrous oxide, *Acta Anaesthesiol Scand* 28:266–274, 1984.
139. Miyamoto Y, Kawashima Y, Matusuda H, et al: Optimal perfusion flow rate for the brain during deep hypothermic cardiopulmonary bypass at 20°C: an experimental study, *J Thorac Cardiovasc Surg* 92: 1065–1070, 1986.
140. Molina JE, Einzig S, Mastri AR, et al: Brain damage in profound hypothermia: perfusion versus circulatory arrest, *J Thorac Cardiovasc Surg* 87:596–604, 1984.
141. Moore RA, McNicholas K, Gallagher JD, et al: Migration of pediatric pulmonary artery catheters, *Anesthesiology* 58: 102–104, 1983.
142. Moore RA, Yang SS, McNicholas KW, et al: Hemodynamic and anesthetic effects of sufentanil as the sole anesthetic for pediatric cardiovascular surgery, *Anesthesiology* 62:725–731, 1985.
143. Moorthy SS, Dierdorf SF, Krishna G, et al: Transient hypoxemia from a transient right-to-left shunt in a child during emergence from anesthesia, *Anesthesiology* 66:234–235, 1987.
144. Morray JP, Lynn AM, Mansfield PB: Effect of pH and PCO2 on pulmonary and systemic hemodynamics after surgery in children with congenital heart disease and pulmonary hypertension, *J Pediatr* 113: 474–479, 1988.
145. Morray JP, Lynn AM, Stamm SJ, et al: Hemodynamic effects of ketamine in children with congenital heart disease, *Anesth Analg* 63:895–899, 1984.
146. Moss AJ, Emmanouilides GC, Adams FH, et al: Response of the ductus arteriosus and pulmonary and systemic arterial pressure to changes in oxygen environment in newborn infants, *Pediatrics* 33:937, 1964.
147. Motomura S, Kissin I, Aultman DF, et al: Effects of fentanyl and nitrous oxide on contractility of blood-perfused papillary muscle of the dog, *Anesth Analg* 63:47–50, 1984.
148. Muraoka R, Yokota M, Aoshima M, et al: Subclinical changes in brain morphology following cardiac operations as reflected by computed tomographic scans of the brain, *J Thorac Cardiovasc Surg* 81: 364–369, 1981.
149. Murkin JM, Farrar JK, Tweed WA, et al: Cerebral autoregulation and flow/metabolism coupling during cardiopulmonary bypass. The influence of Paco2, *Anesth Analg* 66:825–832, 1987.
150. Murray D, Forbes R, Murphy K, et al: Nitrous oxide: cardiovascular effects in infants and small children during halothane and isoflurane anesthesia, *Anesth Analg* 67:1059–1064, 1988.
151. Nadas AS, Fyler DC: *Pediatric cardiology.* Philadelphia, 1972, WB Saunders.
152. Nakanishi T, Okuda H, Kamata K, et al: Influence of acidosis on inotropic effect of catecholamines in newborn rabbit hearts, *Am J Physiol* 253:H1441–H1448, 1987.
153. Nakanishi T, Okuda H, Nakazawa M, et al: Effect of acidosis on contractile function in the newborn rabbit heart, *Pediatr Res* 19:482–488, 1985.
154. Nakanishi T, Seguchi M, Tsuchiya T, et al: Effect of acidosis on intracellular pH and calcium concentration in the newborn and adult rabbit myocardium, *Circulation* 67:111, 1990.

155. Nassar R, Reedy MC, Anderson PAW: Developmental changes in the ultrastructure and sarcomere shortening of the isolated rabbit ventricular myocyte, *Circ Res* 61:465, 1987.
156. Naylor WG, Fassold E: Calcium accumulating and ATPase activity of cardiac sarcoplasmic reticulum before and after birth, *Cardiovasc Res* 11:231, 1977.
157. Newburger JW, Jonas RA, Wernovsky G, et al: Comparison of the perioperative neurologic complications of hypothermic arrest versus low flow cardiopulmonary bypass in infant heart surgery, *N Engl J Med* 329: 1057–1064, 1993.
158. Norwood WI, Dobell AR, Freed MD, et al: Intermediate results of the arterial switch repair: a 20-institution study, *J Thorac Cardiovasc Surg* 96:854–863, 1988.
159. Nudel D, Berman N, Talner N: Effects of acutely increasing systemic vascular resistance on arterial oxygen tension in tetralogy of Fallot, *Pediatrics* 58:248, 1976.
160. Pearl RG, Maze M, Rosenthal MH: Pulmonary and systemic hemodynamic effects of central venous and left atrial sympathomimetic drug administration in the dog, *J Cardiothorac Anesth* 1:29–35, 1987.
161. Peckham GJ, Fox WW: Physiologic factors affecting pulmonary artery pressure in infants with persistent pulmonary artery hypertension, *J Pediatr* 93:1005–1010, 1981.
162. Perry SB, Keane JF, Lock JE: Interventional catheterization in pediatric congenital and acquired heart disease, *Am J Cardiol* 61:109G–117G, 1988.
163. Phornphutkul C, Rosenthal A, Nadas A: Cerebrovascular accidents in infants and children with cyanotic congenital heart disease, *Am J Cardiol* 32:329–334, 1973.
164. Piat V, Dubois MC, Johanet S, et al: Induction and recovery characteristics and hemodynamic responses to sevoflurane and halothane in children, *Anesth Analg* 79(5): 840–844, 1994.
165. Rabinovitch M, Haworth SG, Castaneda AR, et al: Lung biopsy in congenital heart disease; a morphometric approach to pulmonary vascular disease, *Circulation* 58:1107–1122, 1978.
166. Rao CC, Boyer MS, Krishna G, et al: Increased sensitivity of the isometric contraction of the neonatal isolated rat atria to halothane, isoflurane and enflurane, *Anesthesiology* 64:13–18, 1986.
167. Rebeyka IM, Coles JG, Wilson GJ, et al: The effect of low-flow cardiopulmonary bypass on cerebral function: an experimental and clinical study, *Ann Thorac Surg* 43:391–396, 1987.
168. Ridley PD, Ratcliffe JM, Alberti KGMM, et al: The metabolic consequences of a "washed" cardiopulmonary bypass pump-priming fluid in children undergoing cardiac operations, *J Thorac Cardiovasc Surg* 100:528–537, 1990.
169. Riou B, Lecarpentier Y, Viars P: Inotropic effect of ketamine on rat cardiac papillary muscle, *Anesthesiology* 71:116–125, 1989.
170. Riou B, Viars P, Lecarpentier Y: Effects of ketamine on the cardiac papillary muscle of normal hamsters and those with cardiomyopathy, *Anesthesiology* 73:910, 1990.
171. Robinson S, Gregory GA: Fentanyl-air-oxygen anesthesia for ligation of patent ductus arteriosus in preterm infants, *Anesth Analg* 60:331–334, 1981.
172. Rocchini AP: Transcatheter closure of atrial septal defects: past, present, and future, *Circulation* 82:1044–1045, 1990.
173. Rome JJ, Keane JF, Perry SB, et al: Double-umbrella closure of atrial septal defects: initial clinical applications, *Circulation* 82:751–758, 1990.
174. Romero T, Covell J, Friedman WF: A comparison of pressure volume relations of the fetal, newborn, and adult heart, *Am J Physiol* 222:1285–1290, 1972.
175. Rossi R, van der Linden J, Ekroth R, et al: No flow or low flow: a study of the ischemic marker creatine kinase BB after deep hypothermic procedures, *J Thorac Cardiovasc Surg* 98:193–199, 1989.
176. Rothman A, Perry SB, Keane JF, et al: Early results and follow-up of balloon angioplasty for branch pulmonary artery stenoses, *J Am Coll Cardiol* 15:1109–1117, 1990.
177. Rudolph AM: *Congenital diseases of the heart.* Chicago, 1974, pp 79-87, Year Book Medical Publishing.
178. Rudolph AM, Yuan S: Response of the pulmonary circulation to hypoxia and H^+ ion changes, *J Clin Invest* 45:399–405, 1966.
179. Saarnivaara L, Hiller A, Oikkonen M: QT interval, heart rate and arterial pressures using propofol, thiopentone or methohexitone for induction of anaesthesia in children, *Acta Anaesth Scand* 37(4):419–23, 1993.
180. Said SI: Pulmonary metabolism of prostaglandins and vasoactive peptides, *Annu Rev Physiol* 44:257–268, 1982.
181. Salmenpera M, Peltola K, Takkunen O, et al: Cardiovascular effects of pancuronium and vecuronium during high-dose fentanyl anesthesia, *Anesth Analg* 62:1059–1064, 1983.
182. Schulte-Sasse U, Hess W, Tarnow J: Pulmonary vascular responses to nitrous oxide in patients with normal and high pulmonary vascular resistance, *Anesthesiology* 57:9–13, 1982.
183. Seifen AB, Schedewie HK, Williams DG: Endocrine functions during deep hypothermia in pediatric cardiac surgery, *Anesthesiology* 57:A419, 1982 (abstract).
184. Settergren G, Ohqvist G, Lundberg S, et al: Cerebral blood flow and cerebral metabolism in children following cardiac surgery with deep hypothermia and circulatory arrest. Clinical course and follow-up of psychomotor development, *Scand J Thorac Cardiovasc Surg* 16:209–215, 1982.
185. Sprague DH, Sherwood HL: Inadvertent retrograde catheterization of persistent left superior vena cava with pulmonary artery catheter, *Anesthesiology* 53:268, 1980 (letter).
186. Starr NJ, Sethna DH, Estefanous FG: Bradycardia and asystole following rapid administration of sufentanil with vecuronium, *Anesthesiology* 64:521–523, 1986.
187. Stoelting RK, Longnecker DE: The effect of right-to-left shunt on the rate of increase of arterial anesthetic concentration, *Anesthesiology* 36:352–356, 1972.
188. Stowe DF, Bosnjak ZJ, Kampine JP: Comparison of etomidate, ketamine, midazolam, propofol, and thiopental on function and metabolism of isolated hearts, *Anesth Analg* 74:547–558, 1992.
189. Swain JA, McDonald TJ, Griffith PK, et al: Low flow hypothermic cardiopulmonary bypass protects the brain, *J Thorac Cardiovasc Surg* 70:(1)96–102, 1984.
190. Talner NS: Heart failure. In Adams FH, Emmanouilides GC, editors: *Moss' heart diseases in infants, children and adolescents*, ed 3, Baltimore, 1983, pp 708-725, Williams and Wilkins.
191. Tanner G, Angers D, Barash PG, et al: Does a left to right shunt speed the induction of inhalational anesthesia in congenital heart disease? *Anesthesiology* 57:A427, 1982(abstract).
192. Tanner GE, Angers DG, Barash PG, et al: Effect of left-to-right, mixed left-to-right, and right-to-left shunts on inhalational anesthetic induction in children, *Anesth Analg* 64:101–107, 1985.
193. Theodore J, Robin ED, Burke CM, et al: Impact of profound reductions of PaO_2 on O_2 transport and utilization in congenital heart disease, *Chest* 293–302, 1985.
194. Thgien G, Maxxucco A, Grisolia EF, et al: Postoperative pathology of complete atrioventricular defects, *J Thorac Cardiovasc Surg* 83:891–900, 1982.
195. Thornburg KL, Morton MJ: Filling and arterial pressure as determinants of RV stroke volume in the sheep fetus, *Am J Physiol* 244:H656–663, 1983.
196. Treasure T, Naftel DC, Conger KA, et al: The effect of hypothermic circulatory arrest time on cerebral function, morphology, and biochemistry, *J Thorac Cardiovasc Surg* 86:761–770, 1983.
197. Tuman KJ, McCarthy RJ, Spiess BD, et al. Effects of nitrous oxide on coronary perfusion after coronary air embolism, *Anesthesiology* 67:952–959, 1987.
198. Ungerleider RM, Greeley WJ, Sheikh KH, et al: Routine use of intraoperative epicardial echocardiography and Doppler color flow imagining to guide and evaluate repair of congenital heart lesions, *J Thorac Cardiovasc Surg* 100:297–309, 1990.
199. Vacanti JP, Crone RK, Murphy JD, et al: The pulmonary hemodynamic response to perioperative anesthesia in the treatment of high-risk infants with congenital diaphragmatic hernia, *J Pediatr Surg* 19:672–679, 1984.
200. VanHare GF, Hawkins JA, Schmidt KG, et al: The effects of increasing mean arterial pressure on left ventricular output in newborn lambs, *Circ Res* 67:78, 1990.
201. Vannucci RC, Mujsce DJ. Effect of glucose on perinatal hypoxic-ischemic brain damage, *Biol Neonate* 62:215–224, 1992.
202. Vaughan RW, Stephen MD: Ketamine for corrective cardiac surgery in children, *South Med J* 66:1226–1230, 1973.
203. Vetter R, Will H, Kuttner I, et al: Developmental changes of Ca^{++} transport systems in chick heart, *Biomed Biochem Acta* 45:S219, 1986.
204. Vitanen A, Salmenpera M, Heinonen J, et al: Pulmonary vascular resistance before and after cardiopulmonary bypass; the effects of $Paco_2$, *Chest* 95:773, 1989.
205. Vitanen A, Salmenpera M, Heinonen J:

Right ventricular response to hypercarbia after cardiac surgery, *Anesthesiology* 73: 393–400, 1990.

206. Vlahakes GJ, Turley K, Hoffman JI: The pathophysiology of failures in acute right ventricular hypertension: hemodynamic and biochemical correlations, *Circulation* 63:87–95, 1981.
207. Watanabe T, Orita H, Kobayashi M, et al: Brain tissue pH, oxygen tension, and carbon dioxide tension in profoundly hypothermic cardiopulmonary bypass: comparative study of circulatory arrest, nonpulsatile low-flow perfusion, and pulsatile low-flow perfusion, *J Thorac Cardiovasc Surg* 97:396–401, 1989.
208. Weiss M, Weiss J, Cotton J, et al: A study of the electroencephalogram during surgery with deep hypothermia and circulatory arrest in infants, *J Thorac Cardiovasc Surg* 70:316–329, 1975.
209. Wells FC, Coghill S, Caplan HL, et al: Duration of circulatory arrest does influence the psychological development of children after cardiac operation in early life, *J Thorac Cardiovasc Surg* 86:823–831, 1983.
210. Wessel DL, Adatia I: Clinical applications of inhaled nitric oxide in children with pulmonary hypertension, *Adv Pharmacol* 34:475-504, 1995.
211. Wessel DL, Adatia I, Thompson JE, et al: Delivery and monitoring of inhaled nitric oxide in patients with pulmonary hypertension, *Crit Care Med* 22:930–938, 1994.
212. Wessel DL, Keane JF, Parness I, Lock JE. Outpatient closure of the patent ductus arteriosus, *Circulation* 77:1068–1071, 1988.
213. West JB, Dollery R, Naimark A: Distribution of blood flow in isolated lung: relation to vascular and alveolar pressures, *J Appl Physiol* 19:713–724, 1964.
214. Wilson GJ, Rebeyka IM, Coles JG, et al: Loss of the somatosensory evoked response as an indicator of reversible cerebral ischemia during hypothermic, low-flow cardiopulmonary bypass, *Ann Thorac Surg* 45:206–209, 1988.
215. Wong PC, Balon CF, Hickey PR, et al: Factors assoicated with choreoathetosis following cardiopulmonary bypass in children with congenital heart disorders, *Circulation* 86:II-118–126, 1992.
216. Wong RS, Baum VC, Sangwan S. Truncus arteriosus: Recognition and therapy of intraoperative cardiac ischemia, *Anesthesiology* 74:378–380, 1991.
217. Wright JS, Hicks RG, Newman DC, et al: Deep hypothermic arrest: observation on later development in children, *J Thorac Cardiovasc Surg* 77:466–468, 1979.
218. Yamaguchi M: Congenital heart disease: diagnostic approaches, surgical indications and operative results, *Prog Cardiovasc Dis* 32:48, 1989.
219. Yaster M: The dose response to fentanyl in neonatal surgery, *Anesthesiology* 63:A471, 1985(abstract).
220. Yokota M, Muraoka R, Aoshima M, et al: Modified Blalock-Taussig shunt following long-term administration of prostaglandin E for ductus-dependent neonates with cyanotic congenital heart disease, *J Thorac Cardiovasc Surg* 90:399, 1985.
221. Zimmerman AA, Burrows FA, Jonas RA, et al: The limits of detectable cerebral perfusion in neonates undergoing deep hypothermic low-flow cardiopulmonary bypass, *J Thorac Cardiovasc Surg* Submitted.
222. Zwass MS, Fisher DM, Welborn LG, et al: Induction and maintenance characteristics of anesthesia with desflurane and nitrous oxide in infants and children, *Anesthesiology* 76:373–378, 1992.

CHAPTER 70

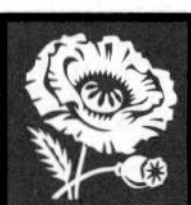

Thoracic Anesthesia

STUART J. WEISS
STANLEY J. AUKBURG

Advances in management of thoracic disease parallel the advances in thoracic anesthesia and surgery. In the early twentieth century, thoracic surgery was limited to rib resection, decortication, and drainage of empyema as management for tuberculosis. During the first part of this century, pulmonary resections were accomplished by tightening a snare or tourniquet around the lesion and subsequently removing the necrotic tissue several days later. These procedures depended on the iatrogenic development of a passive pneumothorax in spontaneously ventilating patients. As expected, the unilateral pneumothorax was poorly tolerated and associated with mediastinal shift, dyspnea, and rapid ineffective spontaneous respiratory movements. A high incidence of perioperative morbidity resulted from infection, hemorrhage, and air leak.

The period of 1930 to 1950 saw major advancements in surgery and anesthesia. In the 1930s, Drs. Gale and Waters in the United States and Magill in the United Kingdom developed the techniques of endobronchial intubation and placement of bronchial blockers, respectively, to selectively ventilate one lung. In addition, the introduction of muscle relaxants and controlled ventilation improved patient safety and surgical operating conditions. The development of single lung isolation techniques accelerated from 1950 to 1960 with the development of double-lumen endotracheal tubes. In addition, patient safety and anesthetic management were markedly improved by the introduction of halogenated inhalational anesthetics and the dramatically increased use of perioperative physiologic monitoring. More recently, use of the fiberoptic bronchoscope greatly increased the success of single lung ventilation by facilitating the placement and confirmation of position of double-lumen endotracheal tubes.

Thoracic surgery and anesthesia continue to evolve. The development of endoscopic surgery has revolutionized thoracic surgery by providing for the relatively noninvasive access to the contents of the thoracic cavity. Although endoscopic surgery has not replaced open thoracotomy for major pulmonary surgical resections, its use has further expanded to nonpulmonary surgery, such as thymectomy, pericardectomy, and sympathectomy. Surgical management of end stage disease by lung reduction and transplantation are additional current challenges for thoracic anesthesiologists.

The following chapter focuses on important perioperative considerations for the patient undergoing thoracic surgery. The initial portion of the chapter presents the relevant anatomy and pathophysiology. The next sections focus on specific anesthetic concerns and perioperative management issues of operative procedures. Our approach to the anesthetic management of these patients should be flexible to allow for either the short diagnostic procedure or the prolonged anatomic tumor resection. Current strategies for staging and management of lung tumors call for sequential bronchoscopy, mediastinoscopy, and pulmonary resection. In addition, nonpulmonary thoracic operations, such as thymectomy, pericardectomy and sympathectomy, use many of the same techniques and management strategies.

ANATOMY/PHYSIOLOGY

Thoracic Cavity

The thoracic cavity is formed by the ribs laterally, sternum anteriorly, vertebral column posteriorly, and by the diaphragm and thoracic inlet inferiorly and superiorly. The thoracic cavity encompasses the lungs, which provide oxygenation of venous blood, excretion of carbon dioxide, and metabolism of endogenous compounds.

Airway

The trachea is the initial conduit for air flow. Its cross-section is outlined by the horseshoe shape of the cartilage anteriorly and the membranous portion posteriorly. The membranous portion consists of a fibrous envelope containing smooth muscle and epithelium. The location of the membranous trachea and the vertical orientation of the exposed muscle fibers guide fiberoptic-assisted placement of double-lumen endotracheal tubes into the appropriate side. The innominate artery lies just anterior to the trachea. Tracheal-innominate fistulae are rare but lethal complications of tracheal resection, tracheostomy, or prolonged intubation.

The trachea initially bifurcates into the right and left mainstem bronchi and then into the lobar and segmental bronchi. The right bronchus is shorter, wider and more in line with the trachea as compared with the left bronchus. Because of the more oblique orientation of the left bronchus, inhaled foreign bodies and aspirated fluid are more likely to go into the right bronchus. The right bronchus provides access to three lobes (the upper, middle, and lower lobes) that are separated by major fissures. On the left, a major fissure separates the lower and upper lobes. The lobes of the lung are subdivided into bronchial pulmonary segments, each of which has its own bronchus, artery, and vein. The movement of air progresses through a series of branching tubes, which become narrower and more numerous as they penetrate deeper into the lung. The conducting airways contain no alveoli and therefore contribute a portion, about 50 ml, of the anatomic dead space.

Mediastinum

The mediastinum is the region between the two pleural sacs extending from the superior aperture of the thorax to the diaphragm inferiorly and from the sternum and costocartilages anteriorly to the thoracic vertebrae posteriorly. The mediastinum contains the heart, the great vessels, and the thymus gland. For purposes of description, the mediastinum is divided into four subdivisions. The middle mediastinum contains the pericardium with the adjacent phrenic nerves, the heart, and the great vessels emanating to and from it. The superior mediastinum lies between the thoracic inlet and the horizontal plane connecting the sternal angle with the lower border of the fourth thoracic vertebrae. The main contents of the superior mediastinum are the thymus; great vessels draining blood from the upper body, head and neck; aortic arch, and several nerves, of which the phrenic and vagal are most prominent. The posterior mediastinum is bounded anteriorly by the pericardium, posteriorly by the vertebral column, and inferiorly by the diaphragm. The posterior mediastinum contains the thoracic aorta, thoracic duct, azygos and hemiazygos veins, esophagus, and bifurcation of the trachea with the two bronchi. The anterior mediastinum lies between the body of the sternum inferiorly and the pericardium posteriorly. It contains lymphatic vessels, lymph nodes, and branches of the internal thoracic artery.

Pulmonary Vasculature

The lungs are blood vessel-rich structures with extensive capillary networks that allow gas exchange. The main pulmonary artery branches and follows the bronchial tree, decreasing in size with each bronchial generation. The arteries branch to supply the respiratory bronchioles and alveolar sacks, which provide for gas exchange. The vascular endothelial surfaces form boundaries of the capillaries and occupy about 50% of the surface of the alveolar wall.

The pulmonary capillary network not only provides an enormous surface area for gas exchange but also for active metabolism, synthesis, and release of stored vasoactive substances. One of the most important synthetic products is pulmonary surfactant. In addition, the pulmonary circulation is responsible for the conversion of the relatively inactive polypeptide, angiotension I, into the potent vasoconstrictor, angiotension II, by angiotension-converting enzyme (ACE). The lung also maintains an active role as a biochemical filter, inactivating exogenous and endogenous substances by metabolic elimination or cellular uptake. The release of vasoactive substances can be stimulated either by manipulation during surgery or by hypo- or hyperinflation. One such example is that of hypoxic pulmonary vasoconstriction, which functions in a homeostatic capacity to normalize the perfusion to ventilation inhomogeneity caused by alveolar hypoxia.

The metabolic functions of the pulmonary circulation also can trigger pathologic consequences. Anaphylactoid response to protamine is of particular importance to the cardiac anesthesiologist. The biologically active substances (histamine, slow-reacting substance of anaphylaxis, prostaglandin E $[PGE]_1$, PGE_2, prostaglandin F $[PGF]_2$, and bradykinin) are released in response to specific biochemical and mechanical triggers.

Bronchial Vessels

The bronchial vasculature normally accounts for about 1% of the cardiac output, but it may increase its flow in response to acute lung disease or injury. The origin of the bronchial arteries is variable, coming from the aorta or intercostal, subclavian, or innominate arteries. The bronchial arteries enter the hilus of the lung and form a communicating arc around the main bronchus. The vessels follow the bronchi distally, supplying the vasovasorum of the pulmonary arteries and bronchi. The dominant deep bronchial venous system drains into the pulmonary veins, and the lesser superficial system of bronchial veins drains into the azygos, hemiazygos, and mediastinal veins.

The clinical importance of the bronchial vasculature system is appreciated under conditions of acute lung stress or injury. Neovascularization and increased blood flow occurs in response to acute and chronic lung disease. This response may help to preserve a normal pulmonary ventilation to perfusion ratio and protect the lung from ischemia. Patients receiving a lung transplant do not have reanastomosis of the bronchial arterial circulation and are believed to be at increased risk of ischemic injury immediately after surgery.

Lymphatic System

The lymphatic circulation has a major role in maintaining the balance of fluids across the endothelial membrane. Transcapillary flow (F) is proportional to the difference between pulmonary capillary hydrostatic pressure (inside pressure − outside pressure) and the difference between the capillary oncotic pressure and the interstitial oncotic pressure ($F\alpha$ [P (inside − outside) − Π (capillary − interstitial)]. Transcapillary flow also depends on the capillary filtration coefficient (K), which is a function of the effective capillary surface area and membrane permeability. Any clinical situation that impedes lymphatic flow increases the risk of pulmonary edema and pleural effusion. Abnormal clinical states that increase capillary permeability increase the flow of fluid into the interstitial space and increase the chance of developing pulmonary edema. In addition, pulmonary interstitial edema also may result from marked increases in negative pleural pressure. Markedly increased negative pressures can result from upper airway obstruction (tumors, laryngospasm, epiglottis), rapid reexpansion of the lung, or aggressive suctioning.

There are two major pulmonary lymphatic plexuses: the superficial and deep plexuses. The lymphatic drainage pattern of these plexuses is from the periphery toward more proximal lymph nodes. Lymph nodes are located at the carina and points of bifurcation of the bronchi and alongside the trachea and great cardiac vessels. The location of the lymph nodes is classified for prognostic assessment of primary pulmonary cancers. The lowest number is assigned to the most central nodes and progresses to greater numbers at the periphery. The pattern of lymphatic drainage impacts on the sensitivity and specificity of mediastinoscopy to diagnose and detect the spread of disease.

Malignant disease of the right lung spreads ipsilaterally up the chain from the pulmonary nodes in the periphery to the paratracheal, scalene, or tracheal nodes more proximally. In contrast, disease from the left lung can either spread ipsilaterally or contralaterally up the chain or proceed subdiaphragmatically to the paraaortic lymph nodes. Biopsying of a lymph node unilateral to the lesion may provide false-negative results if spread occurs contralaterally or subdiaphragmatically.

Work of Breathing

During inspiration, the thorax increases its vertical, transverse, and anterior–posterior diameters. During normal spontaneous inspiration, the major contribution to respiratory mechanics is by the contraction and downward excursion of the diaphragm, which increases the vertical dimension of the thorax. The dimensions of the thorax also are increased by the outward and upward swinging movement of the ribs during inspiration. The importance of diaphragmatic excursion and chest wall movement is most easily appreciated in patients with compromised respiratory function related to positioning. The patient in a flexed lateral decubitus or Trendelenburg position experiences increased abdominal pressure, which limits diaphragmatic excursion and chest wall movement. In addition, patients undergoing thoracic operations are at increased risk of phrenic nerve injury or diaphragmatic dysfunction, which may result in clinically significant postoperative ventilatory compromise.

The mechanics of respiration are divided into the inspiratory and expiratory phases. The work of normal breathing is associated with the inspiratory phase, whereas expiration normally is a passive process related to elastic recoil of the lung and chest cage structures. The work of inspiration depends on overcoming airway resistance and the elastic forces created by the lung and chest wall mechanics. During normal quiet breathing, the work of respiration constitutes only 2% to 3% of total energy expenditure. During heavy exercise, pulmonary ventilation and total body energy expenditure increases some fifteen- to twentyfold, whereas the proportion of energy expended for ventilation increases only slightly to 3% to 4%. Pulmonary disease or dysfunction that alters compliance, airway resistance, lung or chest wall mechanics can dramatically increase the work of breathing to one-third or more of the total body energy expenditure. The excess work associated with respiratory disease can progress to the point where it compromises pulmonary function. For example, the patient with preexisting respiratory disease may exhibit dramatic clinical decompensation postoperatively. Hypoventilation related to diaphragmatic dysfunction and atelectasis can result in respiratory failure in patients with minimal reserve.

Physiology of Lung Collapse

Elastic properties of the lung provide a continual force to collapse the lung away from the chest wall. This elastic tendency is caused by elastic fibers and surface tension. The elastic fibers account for about one third of the elastic recoil, and the phenomenon of surface tension accounts for the remaining two thirds. The elastic recoil of the lungs can be quantitated by measuring the amount of negative pressure in the intrapleural space required to prevent collapse of the lungs. At end expiration, the intrapleural pressure measures about −4 mm Hg, which is sufficient to keep the lungs expanded. With deep respiration, the lungs are stretched, and the intrapleural pressure required to expand the lungs may be as great as −18 mm Hg. During normal respiration, prevention of atelectasis depends on the reduction of alveolar surface tension surfactant. The clinical importance is most easily appreciated by considering newborn babies. Premature infants who have not secreted adequate amounts of surfactant develop respiratory failure based on the inability to open and maintain adequate alveolar expansion.

Cough Reflex

A normal cough reflex is critical for maintenance of pulmonary toilet. Afferent impulses from the respiratory passages are conducted centrally by the vagus nerve. Efferent impulses trigger closure of the epiglottis, apposition of the vocal cords, and contraction of abdominal, chest, and diaphragmatic muscles. Consequently, the pressure within the lungs increases to 100 mm Hg. Opening of the vocal cords and the epiglottis results in explosive exhalation, in which gas velocity in the airway increases to 75 to 100 miles/hour. This high velocity air usually carries with it any foreign material and secretions that may be present in the bronchi and trachea. Patients having postoperative dysfunction related to recurrent laryngeal or phrenic nerve injury, trauma to the diaphragm, or pain and who cannot cough effectively are at risk for serious morbidity. Such patients may benefit from conservative measures to improve pulmonary toilet, such as breathing humidified gases to prevent inspissated secretions, chest physiotherapy, and nasal tracheal suctioning to clear secretions.

PREOPERATIVE EVALUATION OF THE PATIENT UNDERGOING THORACIC SURGERY

The preoperative evaluation of patients undergoing noncardiac thoracic surgery is similar to any patient undergoing general anesthesia. The anesthesiologist should perform a history and physical examination and be familiar with current laboratory studies, electrocardiogram (ECG), and radiologic studies of the chest. The anesthesiologist also should understand the evaluation of pulmonary function and the prediction of postoperative pulmonary function. This knowledge will help formulate a rational anesthetic and perioperative plan.

History

Most patients with lung cancer have a smoking history and therefore have some degree of chronic bronchitis and emphysema. **This history is important because the management of infections and reactive airway disease preoperatively will have a positive impact by decreasing the incidence of postoperative complications.** Exercise tolerance also should be assessed because this will estimate a patient's cardiovascular and pulmonary reserve.[18,38,39,133,142,279,337]

Physical Examination

Along with a routine assessment of the airway and cardiovascular systems, the anesthesiologist should pay particular attention to the respiratory system during the physical examination. Observation of the respiratory rate and pattern may give insight into the pulmonary reserve of the patient. The auscultation of wheezes, rales, or rhonchi indicates abnormalities that can be managed preoperatively. Clubbing of the fingernails may indicate chronic hypoxia or lung cancer. Deviation of the trachea may indicate a mediastinal mass, hemothorax, pneumothorax, or fibrothorax. The anesthesiologist also should assess the patient's ability to tolerate the supine position, because an intolerance to this position may indicate major airway obstruction from a mediastinal mass.

Diagnostic Studies

Laboratory tests should be ordered based on positive findings elicited from history and physical examination. The complete blood count may reveal polycythemia, reflecting prolonged smoking and hypoxia, or leukocytosis, indicating an active infection. Liver function studies may be altered, indicating hepatic metastases or drug or alcohol effects. Renal function can be assessed by measuring blood urea nitrogen (BUN) and creatinine levels.

The ECG should be assessed for the presence of cardiac or pulmonary disease. Signs and symptoms of ischemia indicate the need for further cardiac workup. Additionally, manifestations of cor pulmonale (Box 70-1) may indicate the presence of pulmonary hypertension, which may portend an intolerance to major pulmonary resection.[162]

Abnormal chest radiographs frequently antedate the first sign or symptom of lung cancer by seven or more months. The radiograph may reveal tumor, secondary changes in lung parenchyma distal to an obstructed airway, or other abnormalities caused by intrathoracic and extrapulmonary tumor spread. Radiographic findings that may have implications to perioperative anesthetic management are listed in Table 70-1. The tumor may impinge on the trachea or the mainstem bronchi and thus influence the induction of anesthesia or choice and placement of an endotracheal tube (Fig. 70-1). For example, tumor involvement of the trachea would suggest use of awake sedated fiberoptic intubation, whereas isolated impingement of the left bronchus would suggest the use of a right-sided double-lumen endotracheal tube.

In addition, patients usually have a computer tomographic (CT) scan of the chest, which is helpful in delineating the presence or absence of high level node and extrapulmonary spread of the disease. Further diagnostic workup is guided by these studies. If mediastinal nodes are suspected, mediastinoscopy or parasternal mediastinotomy may be performed to confirm the diagnosis and to determine the extent of tumor spread. If clinical manifestations of distant organ involvement are present, appropriate investigations, such as bone scan and scan of the brain, liver, and upper abdomen, also should be performed.

Assessment of Respiratory Function

Preoperative evaluation of pulmonary functional reserve is used to estimate the patient's ability to tolerate thoracotomy and lung resection.* Patients undergoing thoracotomy for lung resection usually have a long-standing history of smoking and varying degrees of underlying lung disease. Therefore, they have decreased pulmonary reserve and are at increased risk for operative and postoperative morbidity and mortality. **Carcinoma of the lung is associated with an average survival period of 18 months and a mortality rate of 100% after 5 years if not surgically treated. Therefore, every effort should be made to give the patient the benefit of surgical resection.** It is difficult to answer the question, "What is an appropriate risk for rendering the patient a respiratory cripple postoperatively when managing a disease with a mortality rate of almost 100%?" Although most patients do not undergo a complete pneumonectomy, they should be evaluated as potential candidates. It is not uncommon that a more extensive resection is needed than initially anticipated. The next section discusses the tests available to assess respiratory function and the criteria for eligibility to undergo thoracotomy and pulmonary resection (Fig. 70-2).

Arterial blood gas analysis

Arterial carbon dioxide tension of more than 40 mm Hg suggests increased risk for postoperative complications. Because hypercapnia may be reversible, attempts should be made to correct all potential reversible conditions, such as bronchospasm or infection. In contrast, hypoxemia is not a consistent criterion for increased risk. The change in Pao_2 after thoracotomy and lung resection varies. Lung resection beyond the tumor may not be associated with any further decrement in oxygenation, but it may increase oxygenation by improving ventilation perfusion matching. Tumors that

* References 13, 17, 28, 30, 40, 71–74, 127, 162, 164, 184, 234, 287, 288, 298, 321, 328–331

BOX 70-1
CHARACTERISTIC ELECTROCARDIOGRAPHIC CHANGES OF COR PULMONALE

Peaked P waves in leads II, III, and aV_F
Deep s waves in leads V_5 and V_6
Prominent R waves in leads V_1 and V_2
Right bundle branch block (complete or incomplete)
Right axis deviation
ST segment depression in leads II, III, and a V_F ("strain")
T-wave depression in anterior precordial leads

Table 70-1 Radiographic findings with important anesthetic complications

Abnormality	Anesthetic implication
Tracheal deviation	Difficulty with intubation Identify cause: mediastinal mass, nodal metastasis, thyroid gland, aortic aneurysm, or other
Mediastinal mass	Difficulty with intubation Difficulty with ventilation even after successful intubation (see later discussion in chapter) Possibility of superior vena caval syndrome and obstruction Cardiac and vascular compressions
Pleural effusion	Cor pulmonale congestive heart failure Need for additional monitoring Careful assessment of response to myocardial depression from anesthetic drugs
Bullae	Risk of rupture with positive pressure and creation of pneumothorax Wasted ventilation, increased dead space Compression of healthy adjacent lung
Abscess	Need for separation of two lungs to prevent spillage and contamination of healthy lung
Consolidation and atelectasis	Need to manage infections aggressively with antibiotics Ventilation/perfusion mismatch and venous admixture and hypoxemia
Normal chest radiograph	Patient still may have chronic, diffuse infiltrative lung disease with normal chest radiograph Computed tomography is superior to chest radiograph in diagnosing diffuse infiltrative lung disease and should be done before lung biopsy

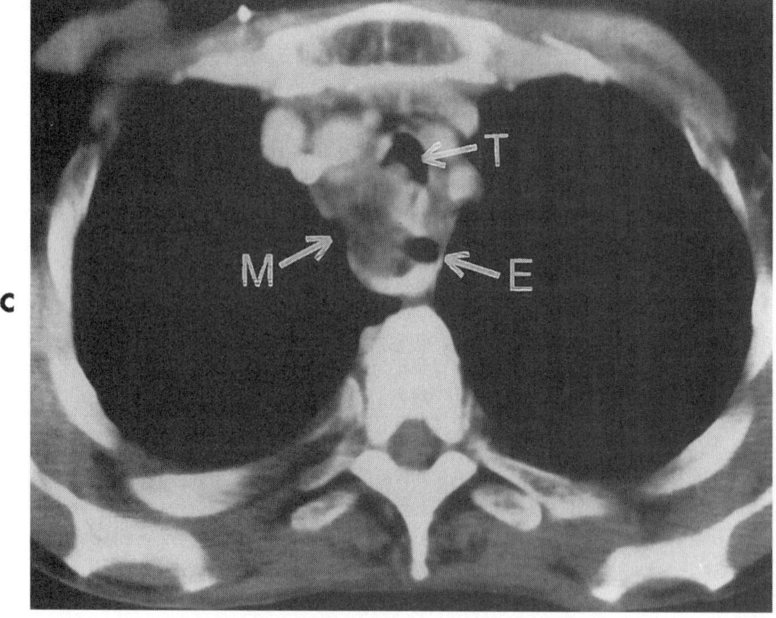

Fig. 70-1. Patient is 62-year-old man with esophageal cancer presented with dysphagia and progressive shortness of breath. Panels **A** and **B** show enlarged lung fields with flattened hemidiaphragms consistent with COPD. A mass, designated by an arrow, arises from a structure posterior to the trachea at the level of the manubrium, causing partial opacification and deviation of the trachea which is better visualized with the lateral chest radiography, panel **B.** The CT scan of the chest, panel **C,** shows a large tumor mass (M) in the mediastinum arising from the esophagus (E) and invading the right side and membranous portion of the trachea (T).

have already occluded the bronchus and the blood supply have already caused a functional resection.

Spirometry

Spirometry has proved to be an effective, inexpensive, and noninvasive way of measuring pulmonary reserve and predicting postoperative pulmonary function. Abnormal spirometry results that suggest an increased risk for postoperative pulmonary complications include forced vital capacity (FVC) less than 50% of predicted, forced expiratory volume in 1 second (FEV_1) less than 2 l, and FEV_1/FVC ratio less than 50%. Other tests having predictive value are the maximum voluntary ventilation (MVV) and diffusing capacity (DLCO). The MVV is effort dependent requiring the patient to breath as fast and as deeply as possible for 6 to 12 seconds. This test is similar to an exercise test because it reflects the entire cardiorespiratory system and the patient's cooperation and motivation. The DLCO is reemerging as an

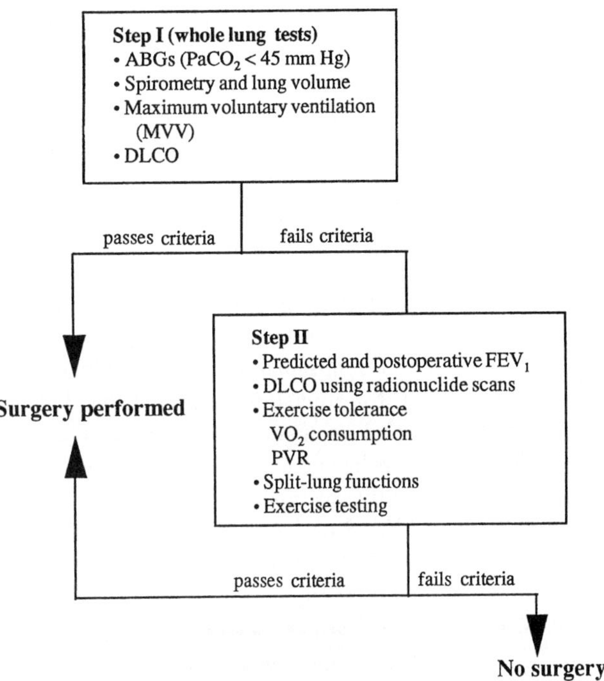

Fig. 70-2. Sequence of tests for lung resection.

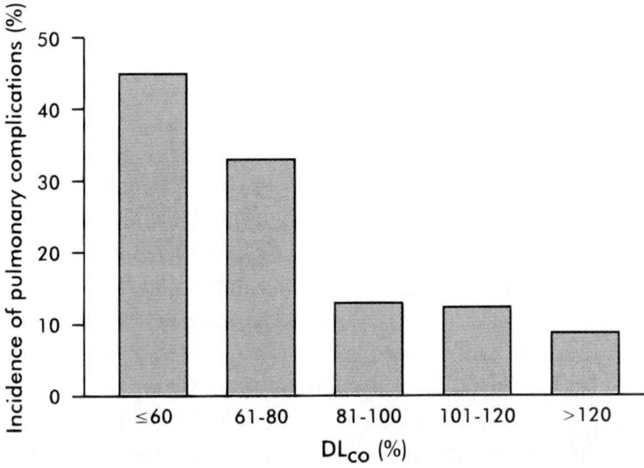

Fig. 70-3. Prevalence of pulmonary complications after major pulmonary resection versus DL_{co}% for 165 patients. (From Ferguson MK, Little L, Rizzo L, et al: Diffusing capacity predicts morbidity and mortality after pulmonary resection, *J Thorac Cardiovasc Surg* 96:894, 1988.)

important predictor of risk in patients undergoing pulmonary resection. Several studies have shown that the DLCO for carbon monoxide is a good predictor of postoperative complications, including death and respiratory failure (Fig. 70-3). DLCO less than 50% to 60% of the predicted value is an indication for further testing with split lung function studies before undertaking major pulmonary resection.

Split lung function and ventilation: perfusion studies

Patients who are deemed to be at increased risk after the initial phase of the pulmonary function evaluation should receive additional testing to assess the effect of lung resection. The goal is to predict the impact of resection on postoperative lung function. The involved lung tissue may contribute little to existing lung function, and therefore its removal may not cause further deterioration of pulmonary function. Thus, some patients who would be denied operations based on the initial results may be considered surgical candidates after more specific evaluation.

The effect of anticipated lung resection can be predicted using radioisotope ventilation scans, perfusion scans, or a combination of both. The radioactive technetium-99 scan yields data about regional perfusion, and the xenon-133 ventilation scan provides data about regional ventilation and lung volumes. The results allow estimation of the fraction of lung function that is contributed by the lung segments to be removed. The equation for calculating the predicted postpneumonectomy lung function is postoperative FEV_1 = preoperative FEV_1 × perfusion (%) to the remaining lung. A modification of this equation has been proposed to predict the decrement in lung function after lobectomy: loss of function = preoperative FEV_1 × functional segments in the lobe to be resected/total number of segments in both lungs.

BOX 70-2
CRITERIA FOR INOPERABILITY USING SPLIT-LUNG FUNCTION STUDIES

Mean pulmonary arterial pressure after balloon occlusion > 35 mm Hg
Pa_{O_2} with temporary unilateral pulmonary artery balloon occlusion < 45 mm Hg
Pa_{CO_2} with balloon occlusion > 60 mm Hg
Predicted postoperative FEV_1 < 800 ml
Predicted postoperative FEV_1 < 30% of expected normal value for patient
Combined predicted postoperative FEV_1 < 35% and predicted postoperative DLCO < 35% of expected normal value for patient

Pa_{O_2}/Pa_{CO_2}—arterial oxygen/carbon dioxide tension; FEV_1—forced expiratory volume in 1 second; DLCO—diffusing lung capacity for carbon monoxide.

Most authorities consider that the minimal predicted postoperative FEV_1 that will be tolerated by a patient is 800 ml (Box 70-2). This is based on the observation that patients with chronic obstructive pulmonary (COPD) disease having an FEV_1 value less than 800 ml had dramatic reduction in their level of daily function.[328] Additionally, patients with COPD start retaining CO_2 and developing hypercapnia when their FEV_1 value is less than 800 ml.[393] These previous studies may have been overly conservative.[70,350] Because an absolute value for FEV_1 does not account for persons of different gender, height, and age, some physicians base their decision on a FEV_1 greater than 30% to 40% of the predicted value.[288]

Exercise studies

In contrast with some previous studies, several recent studies support the use of preoperative maximal and submaximal exercise testing as a good predictor of postoperative pulmonary complications in patients undergoing pulmonary resection.[40,184,324,331] In one study, the patients who either died within 60 days of lung resection or remained ventilator-dependent had a better correlation with the exercise indices of O_2 delivery and maximal O_2 consumption as compared with quantitative lung scans.[329] Exercise testing may better predict adverse outcomes by uncovering deficits in O_2 transport or cardiac function. A maximal oxygen consumption of less than 1 l/min is associated with a 75% mortality rate, whereas death is rare if oxygen consumption is more than 1 l/min. Additional exercise-related criteria indicating increased risk for pulmonary resection include (1) pulmonary vascular resistance more than 190 dynes/ sec/cm^5 (with exercise), (2) arterial oxygen desaturation more than 2% with exercise, and (3) maximal oxygen consumption less than 15 ml/kg/min. Disadvantages of exercise testing are that it depends on patient effort and cooperation, and it requires special equipment and trained personnel to administer the tests.

Pulmonary vascular studies

Preexisting impairment of pulmonary vascular compliance associated with congestive heart failure and cor pulmonale may be exacerbated after extensive lung resection, leading to serious pulmonary hypertension and right-sided heart failure. A recent study examined the predictive value of measured pulmonary vascular resistance (PVR) in patients undergoing pulmonary resection.[162] These authors found that PVR more than 190 dynes/sec/cm^5 was associated with increased risk of complications unless PVR decreased to less than 190 dynes/sec/cm^5 during exercise. In an attempt to simulate the cardiovascular effects of pneumonectomy, patients can undergo a right heart catheterization with occlusion of the affected pulmonary artery. The criteria for inoperability include (1) an increase in mean pulmonary artery pressure to above 35 to 40 mm Hg, (2) an increase in Pa_{CO_2} to greater than 60 mm Hg, and (3) a decrease in Pa_{O_2} to less than 45 mm Hg (Box 70-2).[265]

Right Heart Function

Patients who are to undergo thoracotomy and lung resection frequently have a long-standing history of smoking and underlying COPD, which can lead to pulmonary arterial hypertension and its sequelae. Pulmonary arterial hypertension results from an increase in PVR caused by a reduction of cross-sectional area of the pulmonary vascular bed. This reduction results from the destruction of the alveolar septa and from hypoxemia-induced pulmonary vasoconstriction. Over time, pulmonary hypertension can lead to right ventricular hypertrophy, cor pulmonale, and eventually right ventricular failure. The normal pulmonary vascular bed can tolerate an increase in cardiac output of 250% without an increase in pulmonary artery pressure. In contrast, even a small increase of cardiac output causes a large increase in pulmonary artery pressure in patients with a restricted pulmonary vascular bed. The preoperative evaluation of these patients should assess for signs and symptoms of pulmonary hypertension, right ventricular and right atrial hypertrophy, cor pulmonale, and congestive heart failure (Boxes 70-3 and 70-4 and Fig. 70-4).

One study of left ventricular function in patients with chronic pulmonary hypertension concluded that left ventricular function was normal at rest but impaired during exercise. These patients had an abnormal left ventricular end-diastolic pressure–volume relationship because of septal bulging and septal hypertrophy.[259] Another study confirmed the interrelationship between the two ventricles and

BOX 70-3
CLINICAL SIGNS AND SYMPTOMS OF PULMONARY HYPERTENSION, RIGHT VENTRICULAR HYPERTROPHY, AND COR PULMONALE

Patient has prominent neck veins and prominent A waves, and perhaps prominent V waves are seen on electrocardiogram
Prominent left parasternal heave and rocking motion synchronous with heartbeat may be present
Dullness to percussion over left second intercostal space near sternum may be present, indicating dilatation of main pulmonary artery. However, if too much emphysema is present, entire precordium may be resonant because of hyperinflation of lungs
On auscultation, pulmonary component of second heart sound increases, with narrowing or loss of normal splitting in second heart sound
High-pitched, early systolic ejection click is heard
Systolic ejection murmur is present
Right-sided atrial S_4 gallop usually indicates increased right ventricular end-diastolic pressure and may coincide with prominent A waves in jugular venous pulse. S_4 gallop usually is not ominous
Middiastolic right-sided S_3 gallop usually is evidence of impaired right ventricular function and is usually ominous. Right-sided gallops can be differentiated from left-sided gallops because they increase in intensity with inspiration
Early-diastolic, pulmonary regurgitant murmur may indicate functional pulmonary insufficiency caused by dilation of root of pulmonary artery and pulmonic valve
Right-sided heart failure with chronic, dependent edema; large, tender liver; ascites; positive, hepatojugular reflex; and dilated, distended, pulsating neck veins are signs

BOX 70-4
RADIOGRAPHIC SIGNS OF PULMONARY HYPERTENSION

Dilation of main pulmonary vessels
Attenuation of peripheral pulmonary vasculature, leading to oligemic peripheral lung zones
Radiographic findings characteristic of chronic obstructive pulmonary disease, such as hyperinflated lungs and low, flat diaphragms
Manifestations of right ventricular hypertrophy, clockwise cardiac rotation, and loss of air space behind sternum on lateral chest radiograph
Temporary unilateral pulmonary artery occlusion and measurement of pulmonary vascular resistance (see previous sections)

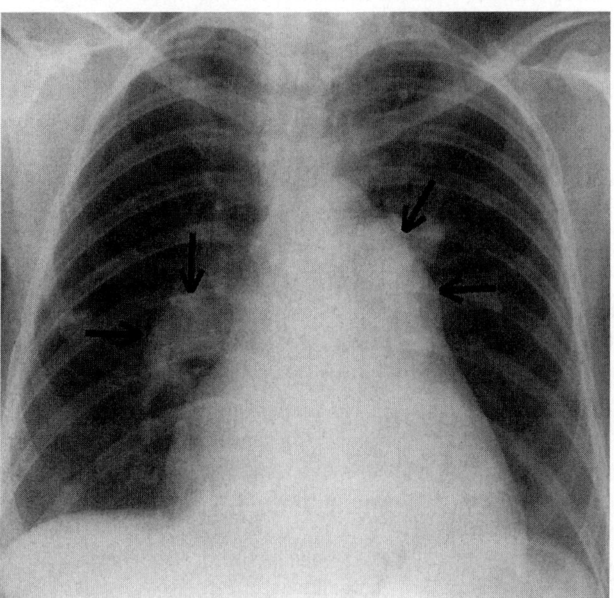

Fig. 70-4. The chest radiograph shows evidence of pulmonary hypertension. The prominent central pulmonary arteries (PA) are markedly enlarged bilaterally. In addition, the radiographic findings of right atrial enlargement and diminished peripheral vascularity are consistent with the diagnosis of cor pulmonale.

demonstrated alterations in left ventricular geometry as a result of right ventricular hypertrophy and septal bulging. The authors suggested that distortion of the interventricular septal curvature results in impingement and narrowing of the left ventricular outflow tract, possibly accounting for concomitant left ventricular hypertrophy. Right heart dysfunction usually is the result of pulmonary hypertension or left ventricular dysfunction. Increased left atrial pressure may result in pulmonary congestion, pulmonary edema, respiratory failure, acidosis and hypoxia, and further increases in pulmonary artery pressure and right ventricular afterload.

PREOPERATIVE PREPARATION OF THE PATIENT UNDERGOING THORACIC SURGERY

The preoperative preparation of the patient for thoracic surgery should focus on treatable conditions.[18,38,39,133,142,279,337]

Available data substantiate that prophylactic measures decrease postoperative complications. Stein et al.[413] found that postoperative complications developed in 4 of 17 well-prepared patients compared with 13 of 17 unprepared patients. Patients undergoing thoracic surgery and lung resection are at increased risk for pulmonary complications because they often have preexisting lung disease, incur injury to the dependent lung because of compression and edema, and suffer surgical trauma to the nondependent lung. Postoperatively, patients fail to breath deeply or generate an adequate cough because of incisional pain. Prophylactic measures, such as bronchodilator therapy, hydration, and chest physical therapy, decrease the incidence of postoperative complications and should be started preoperatively and continued postoperatively. In addition, preoperative patient education about the importance of cessation of smoking, incentive spirometry, and bronchodilator therapy also are beneficial.

Cessation of smoking for at least 4 to 8 weeks before surgery is associated with decreased incidence of postoperative respiratory complications.[356] Although cessation of smoking for 12 to 24 hours preoperatively does not decrease the incidence of postoperative respiratory complications, it still may have a salutary effect by decreasing the concentration of carboxyhemoglobin. A decrease in carboxyhemoglobin would increase the oxygen-carrying capacity of blood and would shift the oxyhemoglobin curve to the right.[123] Other beneficial effects of stopping smoking several weeks before surgery include decreasing sputum production and improving ciliary activity.[238,356]

The chronic wheezing that often is present in patients with COPD results from air flow obstruction caused by bronchial smooth muscle contraction, accumulation of secretions, and mucosal edema. In patients with acute exacerbation, elective operation should be postponed until proper management has been instituted. Sympathomimetic drugs activate beta-2 adrenergic receptors, increasing intracellular cyclic AMP to cause bronchodilation. The preferred route of administration in the management of bronchospasm is via inhaled aerosol because there is less systemic absorption and fewer cardiovascular side effects. Other bronchodilators, such as aminophylline or theophylline, increase intracellular cyclic AMP by inhibition of its breakdown by phosphodiesterase. These drugs have a greater incidence of systemic side effects, in part because of their relatively low toxic-to-therapeutic ratio. In addition to bronchodilation, aminophylline may improve diaphragmatic contractility and resistance to respiratory fatigue.[21] Bronchodilation also can be produced by parasympatholytics, like ipratropium bromide, which inhibit parasympathetic vagal tone of the tracheobronchial tree. When given by inhalation, the therapeutic margin of aerosolized ipratropium is greater than atropine, and severe side effects have not been reported. In patients with chronic bronchitis and emphysema, ipratropium usually is as potent a bronchodilator as the adrenergic agents.[200] Other management for wheezing includes the administration of steroids. Although steroids are not bronchodilators, they suppress inflammation in the tracheobronchial tree and decrease mucosal edema. Because they are slow to act, their benefit in a patient with acute bronchospasm is debatable.

Mobilization of secretions and improved pulmonary toilet improve perioperative pulmonary function. Mobilization of secretions is achieved by a combination of deep breathing, vigorous coughing, postural drainage, hydration, and chest percussion.[204,292,326] Chest physical therapy is relatively contraindicated in patients with lung abscesses, pulmonary metastases, or a history of hemoptysis.

Acute and chronic infection should be managed vigorously before operation. A change in the color and quantity of sputum produced by a patient with COPD may indicate infection. Antibiotics against the usual pathogens found in these patients' respiratory tracts may be used until the results of Gram stain, culture, and sensitivity tests are available. One prospective study reported decreased incidence of postoperative pulmonary complications and mortality rate in patients treated with prophylactic antibiotics before pulmonary operations.[104]

LUNG CANCER

Classification

Most anatomic pulmonary resections are performed in an attempt to cure lung cancer. Lung cancer is divided into three broad categories based on histology: small cell lung cancer (SCLC), nonsmall cell lung cancer (NSCLC), and miscellaneous. Lung cancer is further staged by the TNM system, which is based on cell type (T), the extent of lymph node involvement (N), and metastatic spread (M; Box 70-5). The TNM system is used to group patients into subsets. The TNM subsets are combined in six stages that have implications about treatment options, surgical resectability, and prognosis. The pathologic diagnosis and staging of lung cancer can be determined by bronchoscopy and mediastinoscopy. The biopsy samples usually are analyzed while the patient is still anesthetized, and the results are used to determine utility of further surgical resection.

The approaches to therapy for NSCLS and for SCLC differ. In general, small cell carcinomas have metastized by the time of diagnosis and are managed primarily by chemotherapy without radiotherapy. Nonsmall cell carcinomas often are more localized and thus better candidates for curative re-

BOX 70-5
DEFINITIONS FOR STAGING BRONCHOGENIC CARCINOMA

TO: No evidece of primary tumor
TX: Tumor proved by presence of malignant cells in bronchopulmonary secretions but not visualized radiographically or bronchoscopically, or any tumor that cannot be assessed
TIS: Carcinoma in situ
T1: Tumor 3.0 cm or less in greatest diameter, surrounded by lung or visceral pleura, and without evidence of invasion proximal to lobar bronchus at bronchoscopy
T2: Tumor more than 3.0 cm in greatest diameter or tumor of any size that either invades visceral pleura or has associated atelectasis or obstructive pneumonitis extending to hilar region; at bronchoscopy proximal extent of demonstrable tumor should be within lobar bronchus at least 2.0 cm distal to carina; any associated atelectasis or obstructive pneumonitis should involve less than an entire lung, and no pleural effusion should be present
T3: Tumor of any size with direct extension into an adjacent structure, such as parietal pleura, chest wall, diaphragm, or mediastinum and its contents; or tumor shown bronchoscopically to involve a main bronchus less than 2.0 cm distal to carina; or any tumor associated with atelectasis or obstructive pneumonitis of an entire lung or pleural effusion
N0: No demonstrable metastasis to regional lymph nodes
N1: Metastasis to lymph nodes in peribronchial or ipsilateral hilar region, or both, including direct extension
N2: Metastasis to lymph nodes in mediastinum
M0: No distant metastasis
M1: Distant metastasis, such as in scalene, cervical, or contralateral hilar lymph nodes; brain; bones, liver; or contralateral lung

Occult carcinoma	Stage 1	Stage 2	Stage 3
TX N0 M0	TIS N0 M0	T2 N1 M0	T3 any N or M
	T1 N0 M0		N2 any T or M
	T1 N1 M0		M1 any T or N
	T2 N0 M0		

From Spiro SG: The diagnosis and staging of lung cancer. In Smyth JR, editor: *The management of lung cancer,* London, 1984, Edward Arnold.

section. Patients with early disease may benefit from resection followed by postoperative chemotherapy.

Intrathoracic Metastatic Manifestations

Clinical manifestations of lung cancer are varied. Common symptoms include shortness of breath, chest pain, and increasing dyspnea (Table 70-2). Pleural effusions are a common but nonspecific finding observed on chest radiographs. The effusions result from obstruction of lymphatic drainage or malignant extension of the tumor to the lung surface. Chest pain associated with lung cancer usually is a dull or mild nonspecific pain occurring ipsilateral to the tumor. Metastasis to the chest wall and ribs can result in local tenderness and pleuritic chest pain. Shoulder pain may result from tumor growth at the lung apex and invasion or encroachment of the brachial plexus (such as in Pancoast's tumor). Tumor extension into the pericardium can result in pericarditis, cardiac dysrhythmias, and pericardial effusions that cause tamponade. In addition, superior vena cava obstruction by local growth or lymphatic metastases will impede venous return from the head and upper extremities. Its implications to clinical management will be discussed later in this chapter.

Other manifestations of lung cancer include neurologic symptoms caused by mechanical encroachment or invasion of the nerve plexus. Involvement of the brachial plexus may not only result in shoulder pain but also in upper arm weakness. Involvement of the phrenic nerve can lead to unilateral diaphragmatic dysfunction, and involvement of the recurrent laryngeal nerve can result in hoarseness of voice.

Table 70-2 Incidence of various clinical manifestations on initial examination of patients with bronchogenic carcinoma

Clinical manifestation	Incidence (%)
Asymptomatic	5
Bronchopulmonary	75
Cough	
Hemoptysis	57
Chest pain	40
Dyspnea	30
Wheezing	10
Extrapulmonary intrathoracic	
Hoarseness	5
Superior vena caval syndrome	4
Chest wall pain	5
Pain radiating into upper extremity	< 5
Horner's syndrome	< 5
Dysphagia	1
Pleural effusion	10
Extrathoracic metastatic	3–6
Liver skeleton	
Adrenals	
Gastrointestinal tract	
Kidneys	
Pancreas	
Extrathoracic nonmetastatic (paraneoplastic)	2
Endocrine/metabolic	
Neuromuscular	
Skeletal	
Dermatologic	
Hematologic	
Nonspecific	10–22
Weight loss	
Weakness	
Anorexia	
Lethargy	
Malaise	
Fever	

Based on data from references 237, 398, 408.

Extrathoracic Metastatic Manifestations

Common extrathoracic sites of metastases include lymph nodes, brain, bone, liver, skin, and suprarenal glands (Table 70-3). The neurologic manifestations of metastatic brain tumors include hemiplegia, personality changes, cerebellar disturbances, seizures, headache, and confusion. Metastases to bone occur primarily in ribs, vertebra, humerus, and femur. Although metastases to the spinal cord and vertebral column are less common, they have implications for positioning and postoperative management of pain.

Extrathoracic Nonmetastatic Manifestations

Less than 10% of patients with lung cancer develop a paraneoplastic syndrome. The systemic manifestations of such syndromes impact on the perioperative treatment of these patients. The extrapulmonary manifestations of lung cancer affect the metabolic, neuromuscular, skeletal, dermatologic, vascular, and hematologic systems. The metabolic and neuromuscular manifestations are more likely to affect perioperative management (Box 70-6). In general, the symptoms resolve, and laboratory studies return to normal after a successful tumor resection.

Metabolic manifestations usually result from endocrine secretions by the tumor.

- Cushing's syndrome most often is associated with small cell carcinoma of the lungs; it is characterized by increased elevations in adrenal corticotrophic hormone (ACTH).
- Excessive antidiuretic hormone (ADH) may manifest as nausea, vomiting, anorexia, hyponatremia, seizures, or other neurologic disturbances. This is most commonly found in patients with small cell carcinoma of the lung.
- Carcinoid syndrome is associated with production of serotonin; it is diagnosed by elevated 5-hydroxyindoleacetic acid (5-HIAA).
- Hypercalcemia, which is associated with hypophosphatemia, results from a parathyroid hormone-like polypeptide secreted most often by bronchogenic carcinoma.
- Hypoglycemia and ectopic gonadotropin production are rare manifestations.

Table 70-3 Incidence of organ involvement by metastatic disease from lung carcinoma

Study	Liver (%)	Lung (%)	Skeleton (%)	Adrenals (%)	Kidneys (%)	Brain (%)	Pancreas (%)
Ochsner and De Bakey (1941–1942), 3047 autopsies	33.3	23.3	21.3	20.3	17.5	16.5	7.3
Galluzzi and Payne (1955), 741 autopsies	39.0	—	15.0	33.0	15.0	—	—
Spencer (1968), 1000 autopsies	38.5	—	15.5	26.4	14.3	18.4	—

BOX 70-6
CLASSIFICATION OF EXTRAPULMONARY MANIFESTATIONS OF LUNG CARCINOMA

Metabolic

- Cushing's syndrome
- Excessive antidiuretic hormone
- Carcinoid syndrome
- Hypercalcemia
- Ectopic gonadotropin
- Insulin-like activity

Neuromuscular

- Carcinomatous myopathy
- Peripheral neuropathies
- Subacute cerebellar degeneration
- Encephalomyelopathy

Skeletal

- Clubbing
- Pulmonary hypertrophic osteoarthropathy

Dermatologic

- Acanthosis nigricans
- Scleroderma
- Other dermatoses

Vascular

- Migratory thrombophlebitis
- Nonbacterial verrucal endocarditis
- Arterial thrombosis

Hematologic

- Anemia
- Fibrinolytic purpura
- Nonspecific leukocytosis
- Polycythemia

From Shields TW: Carcinoma of the lung. In *General thoracic surgery,* ed 2, Philadelphia, 1983, Lea & Febiger.

- The neuromuscular manifestations are the most frequent extrathoracic non-metastatic effects of lung cancer, most often small cell carcinoma of the lung.[195] The paraneoplastic myopathy, Eaton-Lambert syndrome, may appear as a myasthenic-like syndrome characterized by proximal muscle weakness, particularly of the pelvic and thigh muscles. The defect in neuromuscular transmission is a result of an antibody-mediated impairment of presynaptic neurocalcium channel activity, which reduces the nerve stimulus-induced release of acetylcholine.[230,338] Patients with this syndrome do not respond as well to anticholinesterase drugs as do patients with myasthenia gravis. These patients exhibit an increased sensitivity to succinylcholine and nondepolarizing muscle relaxants.
- Other neuromuscular manifestations include subacute cerebral degeneration, encephalomyelopathy, and polymyositis. The cause and the pathogenesis of these neuropathies is unclear. The current hypothesis is that they are caused by an autoimmune response to substances produced by tumor cells.[230,320]

MONITORING DURING THORACIC ANESTHESIA

The treatment of patients undergoing thoracic surgery is one of the most challenging aspects of anesthesiology. The patients usually have major underlying respiratory and cardiac disease. Respiratory and cardiovascular function is altered further by surgical manipulations, operative position, and periods of lung collapse and one-lung ventilation, which worsen V/Q mismatches. Thus, it is extremely important to constantly monitor oxygenation and ventilation. There is disagreement about the need for invasive monitoring for patients undergoing thoracotomy.[52,144] Monitoring should be individualized, depending on the extent of operation and the patient's underlying cardiovascular and respiratory condition (Table 70-4).

Anesthetic mishaps related to failure to check equipment are responsible for 22% of critical incidents that occur dur-

Table 70-4 Use of monitoring to detect and diagnose intraoperative events

Respiration	
Pattern, respiratory rate	Apnea, respiratory difficulty, rales
Auscultation	Wheezing, rhonchi, apnea, compliance
Airway pressure	Obstruction, pneumothorax, bronchospasm, secretions
Oxygenation	
FIO_2 analyzer	Inadvertent hypoxia
Pulse oximetry	Hypoxia, integrity of pulse
Arterial blood gas	Acidosis (metabolic, respiratory)
Ventilation	
Capnography	Bronchospasm Hypoventilation and apnea Confirm endotracheal intubation Return of spontaneous ventilation during controlled ventilation
Cardiovascular function	
ECG	Arrhythmia, ischemia
Intraarterial catheter	Hypo- or hypertension Arterial compression
PA catheter	Pulmonary hypertension, filling pressures, assess cardiac performance
SvO_2	Adequacy of cardiac output
TEE	Ischemia, volume status, RV dysfunction

ing anesthesia.[105] Thoracic surgical patients are at increased risk for equipment failure resulting from repositioning and from alterations in ventilatory techniques. Therefore, the function of the anesthesia machine, ventilator, and the anesthesia circuit should be carefully assessed preoperatively in an orderly and systematic manner.[353]

Monitoring for patients undergoing thoracic surgery includes ECG, pulse oximetry, blood pressure, and capnography. Other noninvasive monitors provide crucial information. Auscultation for wheezing, rales, or rhonchi assist in the diagnosis of endotracheal tube malposition, congestive heart failure, airway disconnect, or bronchospasm. Airway pressures give valuable information about changes in lung compliance, the occurrence of bronchospasm, or malposition of the double-lumen endotracheal tube. Perioperatively, pulse oximetry is the most valuable monitor for early diagnosis of problems with oxygenation. Capnography gives a continuous display of the CO_2 waveform and alerts the anesthesiologist to apnea, airway disconnects, and hypoventilation. The end-tidal CO_2 usually correlates well with $Paco_2$, with end-tidal CO_2 about 4 to 6 mm Hg less than the $Paco_2$. Both usually follow the same trend, but the difference between them may increase if ventilation perfusion matching worsens as in the case of one lung ventilation.

The anesthesiologist may require additional monitoring, such as systemic arterial or pulmonary arterial catheters, when caring for patients with a history of pneumonia, cardiac disease, or major anatomic pulmonary resection. Intraarterial catheters are routinely used to monitor arterial blood gases and hemodynamics during major anatomic resections.

The pulmonary artery (PA) catheter is used to monitor cardiac output, left ventricular function, pulmonary artery pressures, and mixed venous oxygenation. It can be used to estimate the effect of pulmonary resection on right ventricular function because patients with preoperative cardiac dysfunction are at risk of acute right ventricular failure after a pulmonary resection. A dramatic increase in pulmonary artery pressures during temporary clamping of vessels would contraindicate such resection. More than 90% of PA catheters float into the right lung.[45] During a right thoracotomy with the patient in the left lateral decubitus position, the PA catheter is in the nondependent lung. This lung is either collapsed if one-lung ventilation is used or is in zone 1 or 2 if the lung is ventilated. When the PA catheter is in zone 1 or 2 of the lung, the pressure recorded during balloon occlusion of the catheter is more indicative of airway pressure than of left atrial pressure, especially if a large tidal volume, positive end-expiratory pressure (PEEP), or constant positive airway pressure (CPAP) is applied to the lung. Also, if hypotension and decreased cardiac output occur, perfusion of the nondependent lung will decrease and may lead to total or near-total collapse of the pulmonary veins. In these patients, airway pressure will be greater than pulmonary venous pressure, and the pressure recorded by the PA catheter will reflect airway pressure and not left atrial pressure. Conversely, when left thoracotomy is performed and when the PA catheter is in the dependent right lung, which is well perfused and functioning in zone 3, the pressures obtained when the PA catheter is occlusive will reflect left atrial pressure.

The mode of ventilation (controlled or spontaneous) and lung compliance have important influences on PEEP/CPAP-induced discrepancies between pulmonary artery occlusion pressure (PAOP) and left atrial pressure.[59] During spontaneous ventilation in compliant lungs with the patient in the lateral decubitus position and the PA catheter in zone 1 or 2 (i.e., in the nondependent lung above the level of the left atrium), the PAOP remains an accurate reflection of left atrial pressure, even with a CPAP as great as 20 mm Hg. During controlled ventilation (as is the usual case during thoracotomy), large PEEP-induced discrepancies occur between PAOP and left atrial pressure.[59] In the noncompliant lung (e.g., pulmonary edema or respiratory distress syndrome), the transmission of PEEP to the pulmonary microvasculature is decreased, and therefore the noncompliant lung moderately protects the accuracy of PAOP measurement as a reflection of left atrial pressure.

The influences of catheter position, surgical manipulation, hypoxic pulmonary vasoconstriction (HPV), and one-lung ventilation on the accuracy of measured cardiac output are debatable. Although one study found that the pulmonary artery catheter in the nondependent lung underestimated measured cardiac output values, other clinical and animal studies found no difference whether the thermistor was located in the main trunk or branches of the pulmonary artery or in the dependent or nondependent lung.[178,209,263]

LATERAL DECUBITUS POSITION

The lateral decubitus position (or some variation of it) is common during thoracic surgery (Table 70-5). It allows for complete access to the hemithorax and permits extending the incision anteriorly and posteriorly. It offers access to the pleural cavity, the hilar vessels, the lateral pericardium, and the descending thoracic aorta. The lateral decubitus position is used for patients undergoing pulmonary surgery and operations on the esophagus, thoracic aorta, thoracic spine, and certain cardiac procedures. This position may affect pulmonary, cardiovascular, and neurologic physiology. Orientation of one lung in a more dependent position alters pulmonary mechanics and increases the risk of contaminating the dependent lung with blood and purulent materials. The dependent lung has decreased functional residual capacity (FRC) and increased airway closure and atelectasis, which may continue postoperatively. Increased pulmonary blood flow and reduced ventilation to the dependent lung results in ventilation and perfusion abnormalities when both lungs are ventilated, although the increased blood flow to the dependent lung is advantageous during single-lung ventilation.

The lateral decubitus position is associated with serious hazards (see Chapter 35). To avoid complications, special attention should be given to the orientation of the cervical spine, positioning of the extremities, and placement of straps to anchor the body. A roll should be placed under the axilla to prevent compression of neurovascular structures by the head of the humerus. The use of a soft contour bag ("bean bag") is advocated because it not only functions as a chest roll but also supports the patient and decreases the risk of pressure necrosis by molding to the patient's body. Slight flexion of the dependent hip and knee help stabilize the patient and decrease stretch of the sciatic nerve. The nondependent leg is positioned on a pillow to avoid pressure on the dependent leg. Positioning of the upper extremities and the head require special attention to avoid compression or stretch injury to the brachial plexus and peripheral nerves. The cervical spine is placed in a neutral position, and the dependent arm is outstretched (Fig. 70-5). The nondependent arm is elevated superiorly on an arm board to bring the vertebral border of the scapula forward. The decubitus position is further stabilized by placing straps or tape across the table at the level of the hip and across the leg, paying attention to avoid compression of tissue (Fig. 70-6).

The standard lateral decubitus position may be modified to facilitate surgical exposure. Patients often are flexed during open thoracotomies and video thoracoscopies to open the intercostal spaces and to facilitate the introduction of cameras or surgical instruments. Slight rotation of the upper chest from 90° permits better access for more anterior or posterior incisions. Positioning of the nondependent arm in a more cephalad and abducted orientation permits surgical

Table 70-5 Various patient positions used during thoracic surgery

Position	Possible surgical incisions	Clinical application
Supine	Median sternotomy	Cardiac surgery, mediastinal, major liver, or vascular trauma
	Bilateral intercostal transverse sternotomy	Repair pectus excavatum, bilateral lung transplant
	Anterior or anterolateral incisions: side to be incised may be slightly elevated	Pericardial tamponade, lung biopsy
Upright	For minor thoracic procedures during local anesthesia	Used in high-risk patients (e.g., open drainage of empyema) and for biopsy of lung or pleura
Lateral decubitus (90° angle to table)	Anterolateral and posterolateral thoracotomy incisions	Standard thoracotomy position
To provide optimal access for cardiac, thoracic, vascular, or gastrointestinal pathology, the obliqueness of the patient's back to the table can vary between 45° to 135°	Anterolateral and posterolateral thoracotomy incisions	To improve exposure in certain cardiothoracic, vascular, or gastroesophageal procedures
	Anterior thoracotomy	
	Posterior thoracotomy	Tracheal or esophageal surgery, thyroid or vascular trauma, penetrating neck injuries
	Cervicothoracic incision	
	Thoracoabdominal incisions	Thoracoabdominal aortic surgery

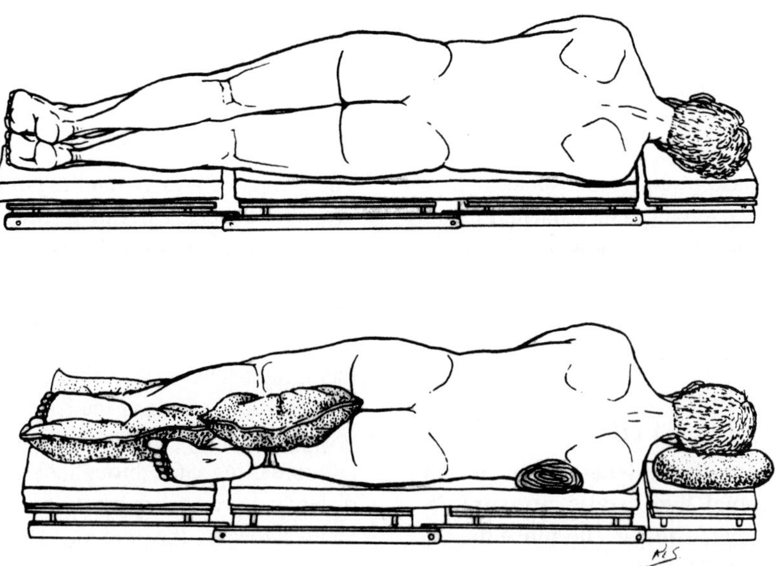

Fig. 70-5. Standard right lateral decubitus position. *Upper figure*, improper head position and inadequate padding. *Lower figure*, proper padding over bony prominences, chest roll to protect axilla, proper alignment of cervical spine. Flexed lower leg stabilizes torso. (From Lawson NW: The lateral decubitus position. In Martin JT, editor: *Positioning in anesthesia and surgery*, Philadelphia, 1987, WB Saunders.)

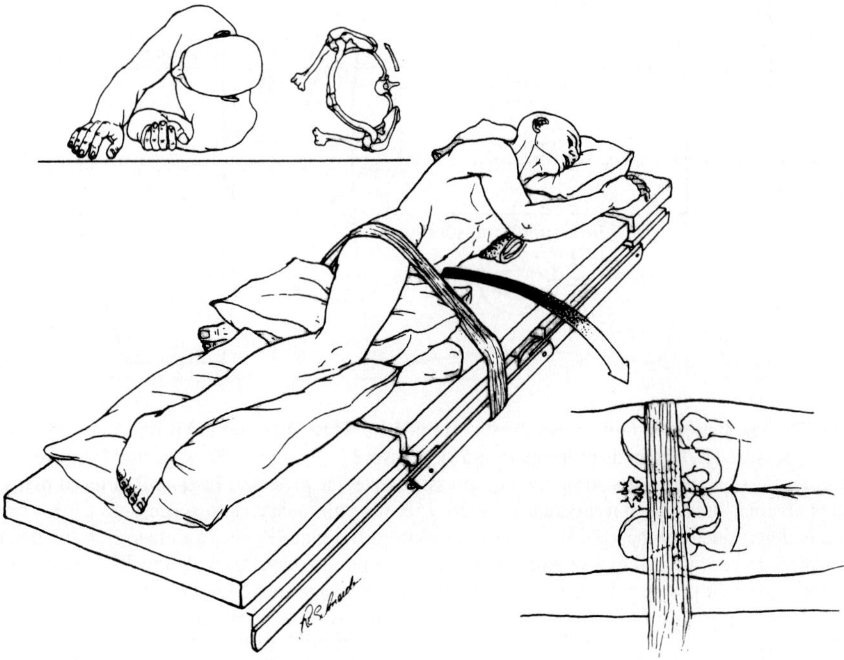

Fig. 70-6. Proper placement of padding restraints and chest roll. *Upper inset*, flexion and extension of the up-side arm will rotate the scapula (*arrow*) out of the thoracotomy field in a manner similar to that achieved by suspension of the arm. *Lower inset*, stabilizing hip straps placed to avoid compression of the up-side femoral head and potential avascular necrosis. (From Lawson NW: The lateral decubitus position. In Martin JT, editor: *Positioning in anesthesia and surgery*, Philadelphia, 1987, WB Saunders.)

approach that preserves the integrity of the latissimus and pectoralis muscles.

Proper positioning of the endobronchial tube should be reconfirmed after the patient is placed in the lateral decubitus position. Repositioning often is associated with slight flexion or extension of the neck, resulting in displacement of the endotracheal tube within the trachea or bronchi. Flexion of the neck moves the endotracheal tube distally, whereas extension of the neck moves the tube proximally. Confirmation of tube position with fiberoptic endoscopy decreases the incidence of inadequate lung isolation.

Physiology: Upright Position

Distribution of perfusion

Distention of vessels in the dependent portion of the lung caused by gravitational hydrostatic pressure results in relatively greater perfusion in the more dependent portion of the lung (Fig. 70-7). The apices of the lung may have little or no perfusion. A decrease in the cardiac output and pulmonary arterial pressure results in an increase in the extent of zone 1, whereas an increase in cardiac output and pulmonary arterial pressure decreases the extent of zone 1.

Distribution of ventilation

The effects of gravity tend to collapse the apex of the lung inward and create a negative intrapleural pressure as the lung tries to pull away from the chest wall, whereas the lower dependent regions tend to push outward toward the chest wall and create a relatively positive pressure. Because the density of the lungs is 25% that of water and because the height of the upright lung is about 30 cm, the difference between the intrapleural pressure at the base of the lung versus the apex is approximately 7.5 cm water.[225] Because the intraalveolar pressure is the same throughout the lung, the transpulmonary distending pressure is greatest at the top of the lung and decreases toward the bottom. Therefore, the alveoli in the apices are largest, and those in the base are the smallest. Approximately a fourfold alveolar volume difference exists between the base and the apex of the lung (Fig. 70-8). The

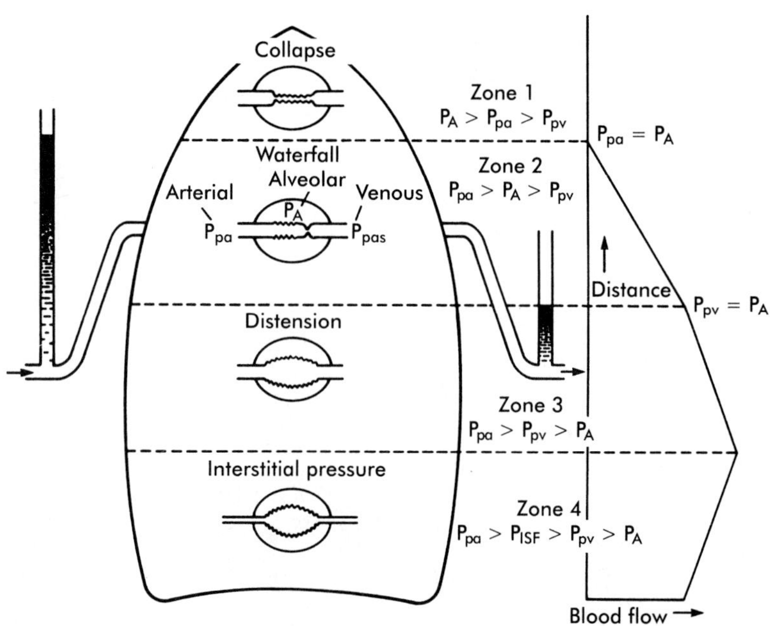

Fig. 70-7. Schematic diagram shows the distribution of blood flow in the upright lung. In *zone 1,* alveolar pressure (P_A) exceeds pulmonary artery pressure (P_{pa}), and no flow occurs because the intraalveolar vessels are collapsed by the compressing alveolar pressure. In *zone 2,* arterial pressure exceeds alveolar pressure, but alveolar pressure exceeds pulmonary venous pressure (P_{pv}). Flow in zone 2 is determined by the arterial-alveolar pressure difference (P_{pa}-P_A) and has been likened to an upstream river waterfall over a dam. Because P_{pa} increases down zone 2, and P_A remains constant, the perfusion pressure increases, and flow steadily increases down the zone. In *zone 3,* pulmonary venous pressure exceeds alveolar pressure, and flow is determined by the arterial-venous pressure difference (P_{pa}-P_{pv}), which is constant down this portion of the lung. The transmural pressure across the wall of the vessel increases down this zone so that the caliber of the vessels increases (resistance decreases), and therefore flow increases. Finally, in *zone 4,* pulmonary interstitial pressure becomes positive and exceeds pulmonary venous pressure and alveolar pressure. Consequently, flow in zone 4 is determined by the arterial-interstitial pressure difference (P_{pa}-P_{ISP}). (Redrawn from West JB: *Ventilation blood flow and gas exchange*, ed 4, Oxford, 1985, Blackwell Scientific and *Journal of Applied Physiology.*)

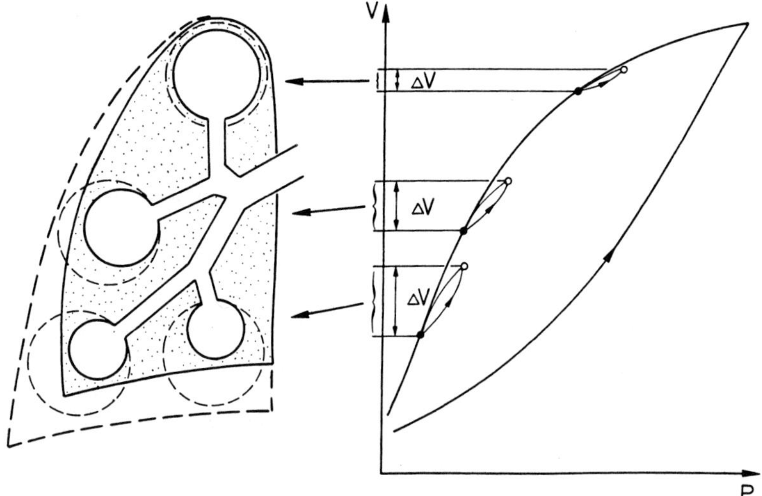

Fig. 70-8. During quiet breathing the lower parts of the lung show greater volume changes (ventilation) than the upper parts. (From Weibel ER, editor: *The pathway for oxygen: structure and function in the mammalian respiratory system*, Cambridge, MA, 1984, Harvard University Press.)

small alveoli in the base of the lung are on the steep portion of their compliance curve, whereas the nondependent alveoli are on the relatively flat, noncompliant portion of the curve. **Therefore, in the upright position, the tidal volume is preferentially distributed to the basilar alveoli, because they expand more per unit pressure change than the apical alveoli.**

Relationship between ventilation and perfusion

Blood flow and ventilation increase linearly moving down the normal upright lung.[225] Because the increase in blood flow (Q) is greater than the increase in ventilation (V), the ventilation-to-perfusion ratio decreases from the lung apex to the base (Figs. 70-9 and 70-10). Other nongravitational determinants of pulmonary vascular resistance and blood flow distribution include cardiac output, alveolar hypoxia, lung volume, and alternate nonalveolar pathways of blood flow through the lung.

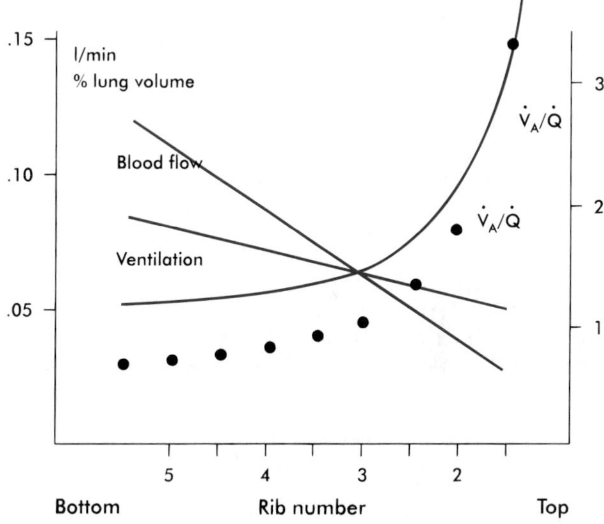

Fig. 70-9. Distribution of ventilation and blood flow (*left-hand vertical axis*) and the ventilation/perfusion ratio (*right-hand vertical axis*) in normal upright lung. Blood flow and ventilation are expressed in l/min percent alveolar volume and have been drawn as smoothed out linear functions of vertical height. The closed circles mark the ventilation-to-perfusion ratios of horizontal lung slices (three of which are shown in Fig. 70-10). A cardiac output of 6 l/min and a total minute ventilation of 5.1 l/min were assumed. (From West JB: *Ventilation/blood flow and gas exchange*, ed 4, Oxford, 1985, Blackwell Scientific.)

Physiology: Lateral Decubitus Position

Patient awake, spontaneously breathing

Gravity causes a vertical gradient in the distribution of pulmonary blood flow in the lateral decubitus position for the same reason it does in the upright position (Fig. 70-11). The vertical hydrostatic gradient is less than it is in the upright position because the distance from the most dependent to the most nondependent part of the lung is less. Consequently, there is less zone 1 and more zone 2 and 3 blood flow in the lateral decubitus position compared with the upright position. Nevertheless, blood flow to the dependent lung still is much greater than blood flow to the nondependent lung. Normally, in the upright position, the right lung because of its larger size receives 55% of the total blood flow, whereas the left lung receives 45% of total blood flow.[373,468] When the right lung is nondependent, it receives approximately 45% of total blood flow, whereas the dependent left lung receives 55% of the total blood flow. When the left lung is nondependent, it receives approximately 35% of the total blood flow, whereas 65% goes to the dependent right lung. As in the upright position, ventilation also is relatively increased in the dependent lung zones (Fig. 70-12).

In addition, in the lateral decubitus position, the dome of the lower diaphragm is pushed higher into the chest than the

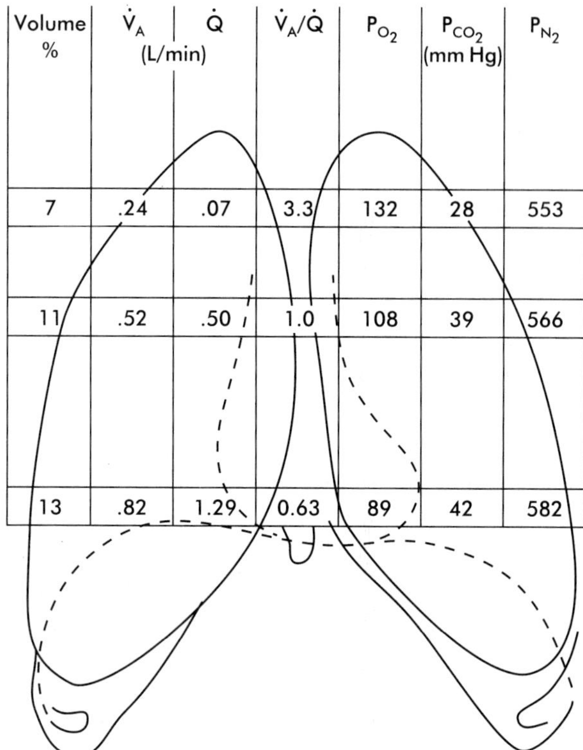

Fig. 70-10. Ventilation-to-perfusion ratio ($\dot{V}/\dot{Q}$) and the regional composition of alveolar gas. Values for the regional flow ($\dot{Q}$), ventilation (V_A), Po_2, and Pco_2 are derived from Fig. 70-9. PN_2 has been obtained by what remains from the total gas pressure (which, including water vapor, equals 760 mm Hg). The volumes (vol [%]) of the three lung slices also are shown. Compared with the top of the lung, the bottom of the lung has a low ventilation-to-perfusion ratio and is relatively hypoxic and hypercapnic. (From West JB: Regional differences in gas exchange in the lung of erect man, *J Appl Physiol* 17:893, 1962.)

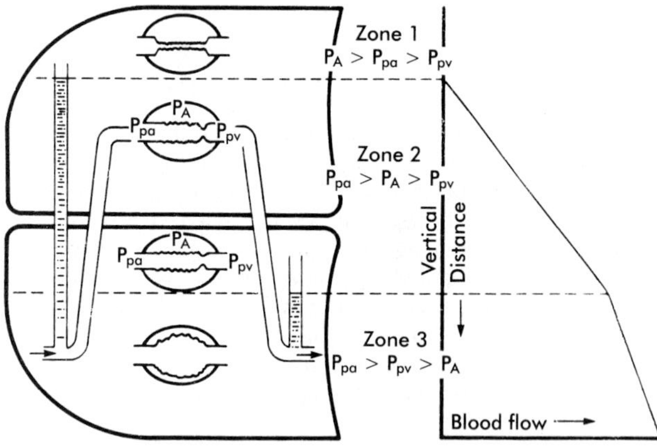

Fig. 70-11. Schematic representation of the effects of gravity on the distribution of pulmonary blood flow in the lateral decubitus position. Vertical gradients in the lateral decubitus position are similar to those in the upright position and cause the creation of zones 1, 2, and 3. Consequently, pulmonary blood flow increases with lung dependency and is largest in the dependent lung and least in the nondependent lung. (Modified from Kaplan JA: Hemodynamic monitoring. In Kaplan JA, editor: *Thoracic anesthesia*, New York, 1983, Churchill-Livingstone.)

dome of the upper diaphragm and is therefore more stretched and sharply curved than the upper diaphragm. This gives the dependent diaphragm more efficiency during spontaneous ventilation. Thus, in the lateral decubitus position with an awake, spontaneously breathing patient, the dependent lung is better ventilated than the nondependent lung, and V/Q still is well matched.[417]

Patient anesthetized, chest closed

In the anesthetized, spontaneously breathing patient in the lateral decubitus position, the dependent lung continues to receive relatively more perfusion than the nondependent lung.

The distribution of ventilation changes after the induction of anesthesia (Fig. 70-13).[362,372] With the induction of general anesthesia, FRC decreases. Both lungs share in the loss of lung volume and move to a lower location on the pressure–volume curve. The dependent lung now occupies the low flat portion of the curve (i.e., is less compliant). The nondependent lung, initially in the noncompliant part, now moves to the steep compliant part of the curve. Compression by the weight of the mediastinum and the abdominal contents contribute to the decrease in FRC of the dependent lung. Therefore, with the induction of anesthesia, little change occurs in perfusion distribution, whereas dramatic change occurs in ventilation distribution. Now the nondependent lung receives most of the ventilation but still is less perfused, whereas the dependent lung receives less ventilation but continues to be more perfused, which leads to an increase in shunt (dependent lung has a low V/Q ratio) and dead space ventilation (nondependent lung has a V/Q ratio greater than 1).

Patient anesthetized, paralyzed, mechanically ventilated

Mechanical ventilation causes further deterioration in the V/Q relationship. Perfusion continues to be more to the dependent lung because of gravitational effects, but now there is even more distribution of ventilation to the nondependent lung. With the institution of mechanical ventilation, the highly curved diaphragm in the dependent hemithorax no longer confers any advantage in ventilation because it is no longer actively contracting.[371] In addition, the weight of the abdominal viscera physically restricts expansion of the dependent lung, leading to further preferential distribution of ventilation to the nondependent, less-perfused lung.

The anesthetized patient in the lateral decubitus position has an unfavorable V/Q ratio that is made worse by muscle relaxation and controlled ventilation. The application of PEEP to both lungs restores their FRC. The lower lung returns to a steeper, more favorable part on the pressure–volume curve, and the upper lung resumes its original position on the flat, unfavorable portion of the curve. This restores most ventilation to the dependent lung.[373]

Patient anesthetized, chest open

In the spontaneously ventilating patient with an open chest, two phenomena can lead to serious impairment in ventila-

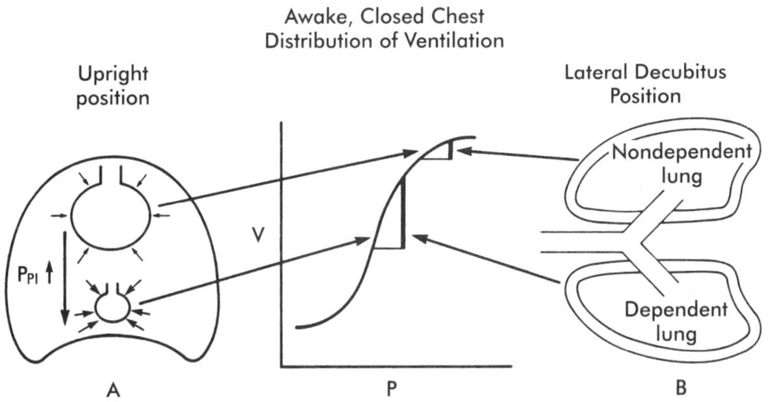

Fig. 70-12. Pleural pressure in the awake patient (closed chest) is most positive in the dependent portion of the lung, and alveoli in this region therefore are most compressed and have the least volume. Pleural pressure is least positive (most negative) at the apex of the lung, and alveoli in this region therefore are least compressed and have the largest volume. When these regional differences in alveolar volume are translated to a regional transpulmonary pressure-alveolar volume curve, the small dependent alveoli are on a steep (*large-slope*) portion of the curve, and the large nondependent alveoli are on a flat (*small-slope*) portion of the curve. In this diagram, regional slope equals regional compliance. Thus, for a given and equal change in transpulmonary pressure, the dependent part of the lung receives a much larger share of the tidal volume than the nondependent part of the lung. In the lateral decubitus position (*right side of diagram*), gravity also causes pleural pressure gradients and therefore similarly affects the distribution of ventilation. The dependent lung lies on a relatively steep portion, and the upper lung lies on a relatively flat portion of the pressure-volume curve. Thus, in the lateral decubitus position, the dependent lung receives the majority of the tidal ventilation. (Modified from Kaplan JA: Hemodynamic monitoring. In Kaplan JA, editor: *Thoracic anesthesia*, New York, 1983, Churchill-Livingstone.)

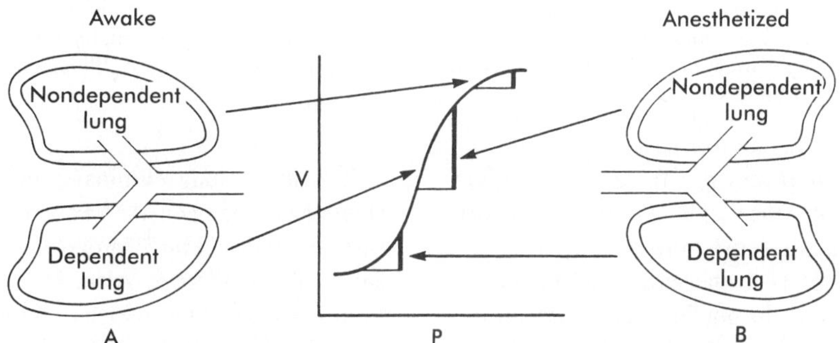

Fig. 70-13. The left side of the schematic shows the distribution of ventilation in the awake patient (closed chest) in the lateral decubitus position, and the right side shows the distribution of ventilation in the anesthetized patient (closed chest) in the lateral decubitus position. The induction of anesthesia has caused a loss in lung volume in both lungs, with the nondependent (up) lung moving from a flat noncompliant portion to a steep compliant portion of the pressure-volume curve and the dependent (down) lung moving from a steep compliant part to a flat, noncompliant part of the pressure-volume curve. Thus, the anesthesized patient in a lateral decubitus position has the majority of the tidal ventilation in the nondependent lung (where there is the least perfusion) and the minority of the tidal ventilation in the dependent lung (where there is the most perfusion). (Modified from Kaplan JA: Hemodynamic monitoring. In Kaplan JA, editor: *Thoracic anesthesia*, New York, 1983, Churchill-Livingstone.)

tion, mediastinal shift, and paradoxical respiration (Fig. 70-14). Mediastinal shift is the up-and-down movement of the mediastinum with respiratory movements caused by changes in the intrapleural pressure in the dependent hemithorax. During inspiration, the tidal volume in the dependent lung is decreased by an amount equal to the downward displacement of the mediastinum, which leads to serious impairment in ventilation to the dependent lung. The mediastinal shift also can cause circulatory changes (decreased venous return) and trigger reflexes associated with sympathetic activation, resulting in a clinical picture similar to shock. The patient is hypotensive, pale, cold, and clammy, with dilated pupils. Local anesthetic infiltration of the pulmonary plexus at the hilum and of the vagus nerve can di-

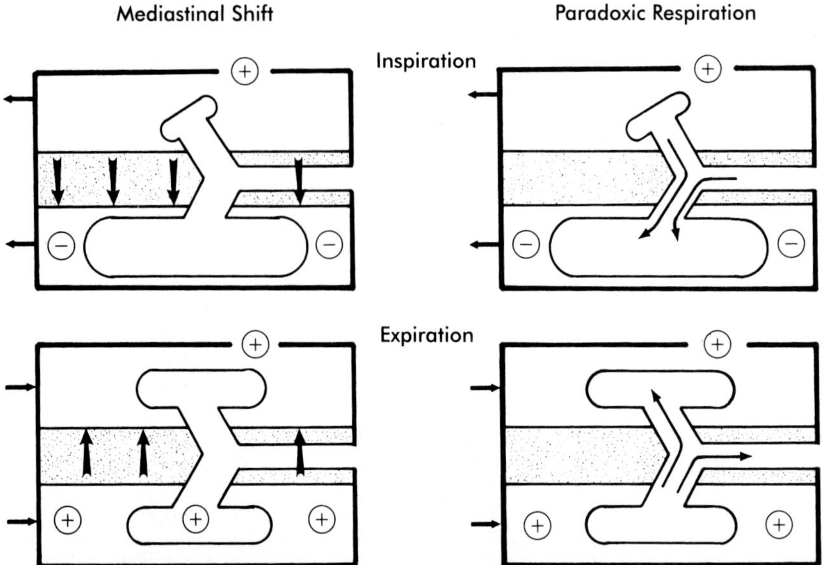

Fig. 70-14. Schematic representation of mediastinal shift and paradoxic respiration in the spontaneously ventilating patient with an open chest and placed in the lateral decubitus position. The open chest is always exposed to atmospheric pressure (+). During inspiration, negative pressure (−) in the intact hemithorax causes the mediastinum to move vertically downward (mediastinal shift). In addition, during inspiration, movement of gas from the nondependent lung in the open hemithorax into the dependent lung in the closed hemithorax and movement of air from the environment into the open hemithorax causes the lung in the open hemithorax to collapse (paradoxic respiration). During expiration, relative positive pressure (+) in the closed hemithorax causes the mediastinum to move vertically upward (mediastinal shift). In addition, during expiration, the gas moves from the dependent lung to the nondependent lung and from the open hemithorax to the environment; consequently, the nondependent lung expands during expiration (paradoxic respiration). (Modified from Benumof JL: Special physiology of the lateral decubitus position, the open chest, and one-lung ventilation. In Benumof JL, editor: *Anesthesia for thoracic surgery*, Philadelphia, 1995, WB Saunders.)

minish these reflexes. More practically, controlled positive-pressure ventilation abolishes the ventilatory and circulatory changes associated with mediastinal shift.

Paradoxic respiration refers to the movement of air between the dependent lung and the nondependent lung during respiration, along with movement of air from the ambient atmosphere in and out of the open chest cavity. Combined with mediastinal shift, it leads to further impairment in ventilation. Paradoxical respiration may be prevented either by manual collapse of the upper lung or more often by controlled positive-pressure ventilation. Because of mediastinal shift and paradoxical respiration, controlled positive-pressure ventilation is the most effective method of providing adequate gas exchange during thoracotomy.

Patient anesthetized, mechanically ventilated, chest open

Opening the chest results in a marked increase in the compliance of the upper lung, with a slight but still important increase in the compliance of the dependent lung. Airway pressure decreases in the dependent and the nondependent lungs. As a result, ventilation of the nondependent lung increases further compared with the closed-chest state.[322] The cardiac index increases dramatically with opening of the chest and pleura, but mean arterial pressure does not change drastically.[458]

The upper lung eliminates more CO_2 shortly after the pleura has been opened.[458] The increased elimination of CO_2 from the upper lung is proportionately greater than the increase in ventilation. Also, the end-tidal P_{CO_2} measured from the upper lung increases more than that of the lower lung, which reflects a marked increase in the blood flow to the upper lung. The decrease in airway pressure on opening the pleura, along with the increase in cardiac index, results in increased blood flow to the nondependent lung.

An exposed lung with normal elasticity does not fill the pleural cavity during most of the respiratory cycle. Thus, the vertical distance between the heart and the uppermost part of the lung decreases, and the effect of hydrostatic pressure on blood flow through the upper lung may be less important with the pleura open than with it closed, which leads to a decreased amount of zone 1 and a decrease in dead space ventilation in the nondependent lung.

Effect of PEEP

Selective PEEP application to the dependent lung can result in an adequate Pa_{O_2} at a lower inspired O_2 concentration and a smaller shunt fraction than when both lungs were ventilated with zero end-expiratory pressure. The explanation is that PEEP to the dependent lung increases the FRC of that lung, moving it to a steeper, more favorable portion on its pressure–volume curve and leading to improved ventilation of the dependent lung. Even if the increase in pulmonary vascular resistance caused by the application of PEEP shifts blood flow from the dependent to the nondependent lung, that portion of the cardiac output diverted to the nondependent lung still participates in gas exchange as long as it is ventilated or exposed to CPAP.

Effects of Surgical Manipulation

With the onset of surgical manipulations, compliance and distribution of ventilation to the upper lung decrease dramatically. End-tidal P_{CO_2} and CO_2 elimination from the upper lung decrease greatly. Changes in Pa_{CO_2} are minimal.[458] Surgical manipulations mechanically restrict the expansion of the upper lung and counteract its tendency to be overventilated.[468]

Summary

The anesthetized, paralyzed patient in the lateral decubitus position with an open chest may have considerable V/Q mismatch. The nondependent lung receives greater ventilation and less perfusion and has a V/Q ratio of more than 1. The dependent lung has more perfusion and less ventilation (i.e., a low V/Q ratio) and therefore acts as a physiologic shunt. The blood flow distribution is mainly determined by effects of gravity. Causes of poor ventilation of the dependent lung are (1) loss of FRC because of induction of general anesthesia, (2) compression of the dependent lung by the mediastinum, (3) upward shift of the abdominal contents and paralysis of the diaphragm, (4) suboptimal positioning effects, (5) impaired ciliary clearance of mucus, and (6) absorption atelectasis from the use of high FIO_2. Consequently, two-lung ventilation in these patients may result in an increased alveolar-to-arterial PO_2 difference and less than optimal oxygenation.

ONE LUNG ISOLATION

Indications

The usual aim of lung isolation techniques is to provide secure ventilation of the lung within one hemithorax while a nearly motionless lung is operated on in the contralateral hemithorax. **Collapse of the nondependent lung produces less trauma than surgical retraction and offers better exposure of structures within the hemithorax.**[16,73,75] The airways of the operated lung can be incised while positive pressure ventilation continues in the other lung. During thoracoscopic surgery, collapse of the operated lung is essential to provide adequate visualization of structures within the pleural cavity. Although many surgical procedures are greatly facilitated by use of isolation techniques, most procedures are feasible without isolation, although there are some absolute indications for isolation techniques.

When one lung contains either blood or infectious secretions, isolation of the lungs becomes imperative to prevent spillage of contents into the unaffected lung. Isolated lung ventilation is essential when a bronchopleural or bronchocutaneous fistula would render positive pressure ventilation difficult or impossible. Further, directing ventilation toward the healthier lung may result in better oxygenation and ventilation.[193] Some procedures require isolated ventilation, including open procedures on the trachea and mainstem bronchi, such as sleeve and carinal resections, and bronchopulmonary lavage for pulmonary alveolar proteinosis.

Design of Double-Lumen Tubes

Isolated lung ventilation usually is accomplished through a double-lumen endotracheal tube. The central shaft of a double-lumen endotracheal tube is cylindrical and contains a septum that divides it into two symmetric "D"-shaped lumens. At the proximal end of each lumen is a short length of tubing that creates a "Y" shape that permits independent attachment for ventilatory apparatus, clamping, or opening to atmospheric pressure. At the distal end, the shaft is surrounded by an inflatable tracheal cuff. The tracheal lumen terminates just below the tracheal cuff. The other lumen has a cylindrical extension, curved to fit into one of the mainstem bronchi, and carries an inflatable circumferential bronchial cuff. After the double-lumen endotracheal tube has been properly placed within the patient's airway, the bronchial cuff permits the bronchial lumen to be used for positive pressure ventilation of the hemithorax in which it resides. The tracheal cuff provides a seal that directs pressurized gas from the tracheal lumen into the other bronchus. Hence, a properly placed double-lumen endotracheal tube permits selective ventilation or collapse of either lung without regard to which bronchus contains the bronchial extension.

Double-lumen endotracheal tubes are manufactured with bronchial extensions intended for placement into either the left or right mainstem bronchus. The left main stem bronchus arises at a more acute angle with reference to the tracheal axis, but it is adequately long to easily accommodate the endobronchial extension with its inflatable cuff.[88] In contrast, the right mainstem bronchus is nearly a direct extension of the trachea, but it contains a branch to the right upper lobe bronchus that arises very close to the tracheal bifurcation (Figs. 70-15, 70-16). A double-lumen endotracheal tube intended for placement within the right mainstem bronchus therefore requires a fenestration within the bronchial extension and an elaborately shaped cuff to permit a seal without airflow obstruction. Because of these considerations, right-sided tubes are more difficult to manufacture, more difficult to insert, and require more care to ensure continuous ventilation of all lobes of the right lung. **In the absence of a specific indication for a right-sided double-lumen endotracheal tube, a left-sided tube is strongly preferred.**

The earliest double-lumen tubes were red rubber with low-volume, high-pressure cuffs. They often were extruded with cylindrical lumens that reduced the available cross-sectional area and elevated breathing pressure and hence, the

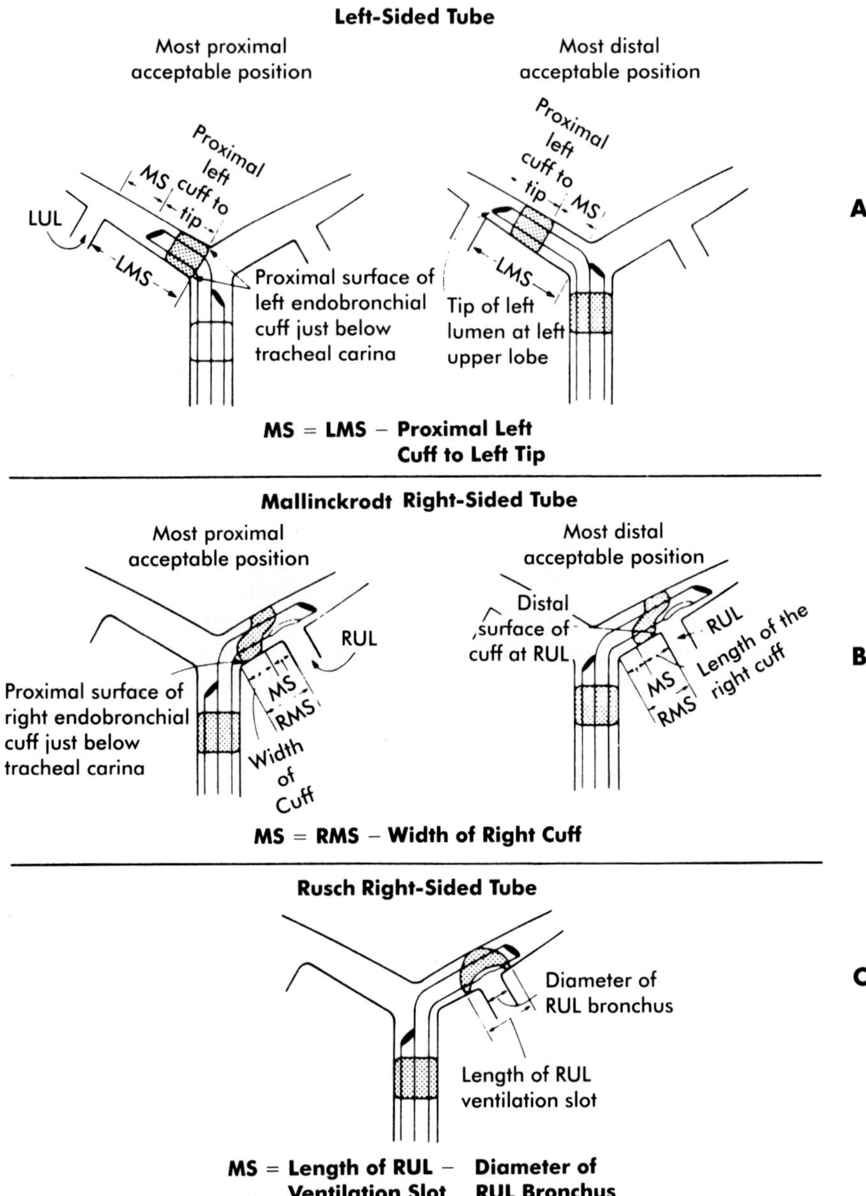

Fig. 70-15. Schematic showing the definitions of the most proximal and most distal acceptable positions of left- and right-sided double-lumen tubes and the margin of safety in positioning double-lumen tubes. **A,** All left-sided double-lumen tubes; **B,** Mallinckrodt right-sided double-lumen tube; **C,** Rusch right-sided double-lumen tube. LMS—length left mainstem bronchus; RMS—length right mainstem bronchus; MS—margin of safety in positioning double-lumen tube; LUL—left upper lobe; RUL—right upper lobe. (From Benumof JL: Separation of the two lungs (double-lumen tube and bronchial blocker intubation). In Benumof JL, editor: *Anesthesia for thoracic surgery*, Philadelphia, 1995, WB Saunders.)

work of breathing. One popular design, the Carlen's tube, had a carinal hook to facilitate the maintenance of correct tube position (Fig. 70-17). This advantage came at the price of increased difficulty of initial tube placement. A tube for right-sided endobronchial placement was introduced by White. Robertshaw improved on the Carlen's tube by replacing the cylindrical lumens with a pair of back-to-back D-shaped lumens and eliminating the carinal hook. Modern double-lumen endotracheal tubes are disposable, made from vinyl chloride, use high-volume flow pressure cuffs, and are similar in design to the Robertshaw tube. Right-sided versions have fenestrated, S-shaped, L-shaped, or dual endobronchial cuffs, depending on the manufacturer (Fig. 70-18).

Placement of Double-Lumen Tubes

Before placement of a double-lumen endotracheal tube, all necessary equipment should be assembled and tested. Direct laryngoscopy with a curved (MacIntosh) laryngoscope

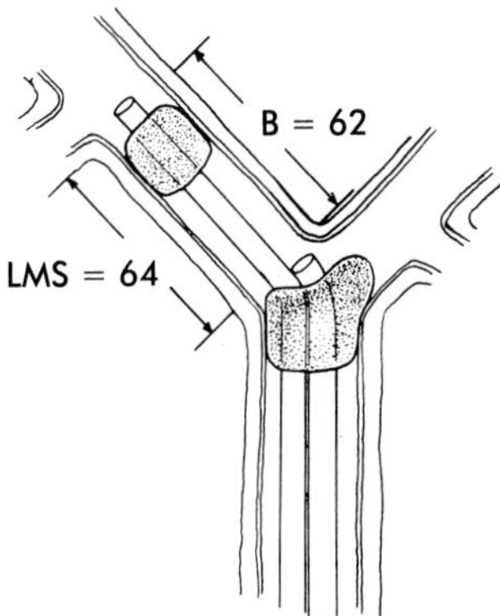

Fig. 70-16. Schematic diagram showing that it is possible for the right lumen to be in the left mainstem bronchus (LMS) when the left lumen is still above the left upper lobe if the LMS is long and length B is short. (From Benumof JL: Separation of the two lungs (double-lumen tube and bronchial blocker intubation). In Benumof JL, editor: *Anesthesia for thoracic surgery*, Philadelphia, 1995, WB Saunders.)

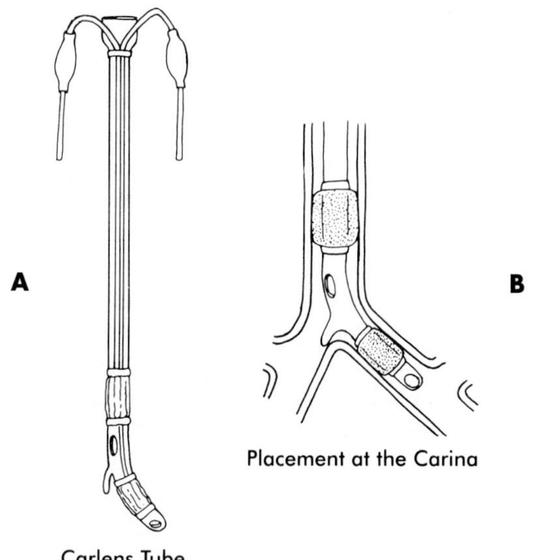

Fig. 70-17. A, Sketch of the red rubber Carlens double-lumen tube. **B,** Close-up of the placement of the red rubber Carlens double-lumen tube at the carina. Note that the left endobronchial lumen and carinal hook straddle the carina. (Modified from Benumof JL: Separation of the two lungs (double-lumen tube and bronchial blocker intubation). In Benumof JL, editor: *Anesthesia for thoracic surgery*, Philadelphia, 1995, WB Saunders.)

blade is preferred because it provides a larger working orifice than a straight blade. The type of tube is chosen based on the surgical procedure, and its size is based on the patient's body habitus (Table 70-6).

After induction of anesthesia and neuromuscular blockade, the glottic opening is exposed. The double-lumen endotracheal tube is held with its bronchial curve oriented anteriorly and its tracheal-pharyngeal curve oriented to the right. The tube is advanced through the glottic opening until the bronchial cuff just passes the vocal cords. If a stylet was used, it is removed with care to neither advance nor withdraw the double-lumen endotracheal tube. The tracheopharyngeal curve is then rotated anteriorly until the proximal end of the double-lumen endotracheal tube just passes the mid-sagittal axis. The bronchial curve should now be oriented to the left and slightly posteriorly. The tube is then advanced until moderate resistance to further insertion is observed. Usually, the appropriate depth is approximately one sixth of the patient's height. A bifurcated connector is attached to the two lumens, and the tracheal cuff is inflated. Intubation of the trachea is then confirmed by capnography, auscultation, and observation. Once it has been determined that both lungs can be adequately ventilated, it is safe to proceed with confirmation that the tube is positioned to allow isolation of the two lungs.

The most efficient method of confirming appropriate anatomic placement of a double-lumen endotracheal tube is direct observation of the endobronchial extension in its intended bronchus via a small diameter fiberoptic bronchoscope. Each lumen of the bifurcated double-lumen endotracheal tube connector is fitted with a fenestrated membrane covered by a removable cap. While the lungs are ventilated with positive pressure, the fenestrated membrane on the tracheal lumen is uncovered, and the bronchoscope is passed through it into the double-lumen endotracheal tube. The bronchoscope is steadily advanced until its tip just exits from the distal opening. If the tube is properly positioned, the carina should be seen just beyond the opening, and the medial wall of the endobronchial extension should be seen entering the contralateral bronchus. The bronchial cuff should be entirely contained within the contralateral bronchus, while an unobstructed view of the opening into the ipsilateral bronchus is enjoyed. Disposable double-lumen tubes usually feature a prominent band around the endobronchial extension several millimeters above the endobronchial cuff to facilitate positioning. When ideally positioned, the band should lie in a plane that contains the edge of the carina. It may be necessary to slightly advance or withdraw the tube to achieve ideal position. Once anatomically correct tube position has been confirmed, it is secured in place using adhesive tape or a specially designed apparatus. Then, the endobronchial cuff is gently inflated under direct bronchoscopic visualization to ensure that the cuff does not herniate into the trachea. Each time the patient is repositioned, it is advisable to verify the position of the double-lumen endotracheal tube.

Although confirmation of position through direct visualization with a fiberoptic bronchoscope usually is rapid and definitive, it is not always feasible. Further, although it assures anatomically correct position, it does not ensure functional isolation of the left and right lungs. Functional isolation is tested by selectively ventilating one lung while the other is vented to the atmosphere, and unilateral ventilation of the intended lung is confirmed by auscultation and visual or tactile observation. The opposite lung then is ventilated, and the test is repeated. A bubble test also may be used

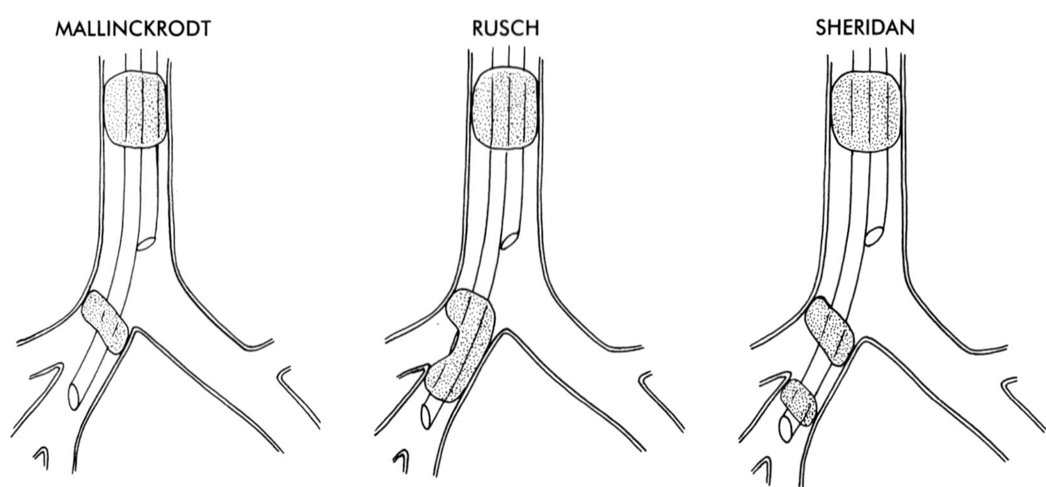

Fig. 70-18. Three designs of a right-sided double-lumen endobronchial tube. (Modified from Slinger P, Triolet W: A clinical comparison of three different designs of right-sided double-lumen endobronchial tubes, *Can J Anaesth* 36:S59, 1989.)

Table 70-6 Choice of double-lumen endotracheal tube

Patient height	Tube size	Depth of insertion
136–164 cm 4′5.5″–5′4.5″	37 Fr	27 cm
165–179 cm 5′5″–5′10.5″	39 Fr	29 cm
180–194 cm 5′11″–6′4.5″	41 Fr	31 cm

Brodsky JB, Benumof JF, Ehenworth J, et al: Depth of placement of left double-lumen endobronchial tubes, *Anesth Analg* 73(5):570–572, 1991.

(Fig. 70-19). A test for functional isolation should always be used when the double-lumen endotracheal tube is placed to prevent spillage of liquid from one lung to the other.

Right-sided tubes demand confirmation of the correct location of the fenestration supplying the right upper lobe bronchus, which is accomplished by passing the bronchoscope into the endobronchial lumen and observing the upper lobe bronchial orifice through the fenestration in the lateral wall of the endobronchial extension (Fig. 70-20).

Occasionally, double-lumen endotracheal tube position may be incorrect. Three possible reasons are (1) the tube is so deeply inserted that the tracheal opening is beyond the carina; (2) the tube is not inserted far enough so that the bronchial cuff is above the carina; or (3) the endobronchial extension has entered the incorrect bronchus so that the tracheal lumen opening is trapped against the lateral wall of the trachea on the ipsilateral side (Fig. 70-21). Gently withdrawing or advancing the tube under direct bronchoscopic visualization should reveal and correct either of the first two causes. If the endobronchial extension is not in the correct bronchus, repositioning of the tube is required.

An alternative method of tube placement eliminates the possibility of placing the endobronchial extension in the wrong bronchus. The tube is passed through the cords and rotated as for the first method. It is advanced only until the tip of the bronchial extension is 20 to 22 cm beyond the central incisors as determined by markings on the shaft. The bronchial cuff is then inflated to seal against the wall of the trachea. An anesthetic circuit is attached to the connector for the bronchial lumen, and intubation of the trachea is confirmed. The bronchoscope is then passed into the bronchial lumen. After the tip of the bronchoscope has entered the trachea, it is advanced under direct visualization past the carina into the desired main stem bronchus (Fig. 70-22). After the bronchoscope is advanced as far as possible, the bronchial cuff is deflated. Using the bronchoscope as a directing stylet, the double-lumen endotracheal tube is advanced until gentle resistance is met. The bronchoscope is withdrawn, the tube is secured, and correct position is ascertained as for the first method.

Complications

Complications associated with double-lumen endotracheal tubes can be divided into two types, those resulting from malposition of the tube and those caused by trauma to the tracheobronchial tree.

Malposition

Malposition may lead to failure to ventilate segments of the dependent lung or failure to collapse the operative lung. A malpositioned double-lumen endotracheal tube may fail to achieve an adequate seal between the two lungs.

Failure to ventilate segments of the ventilated lung can occur if the bronchial lumen obstructs the origin of the upper lobe bronchus, which frequently manifests by hypox-

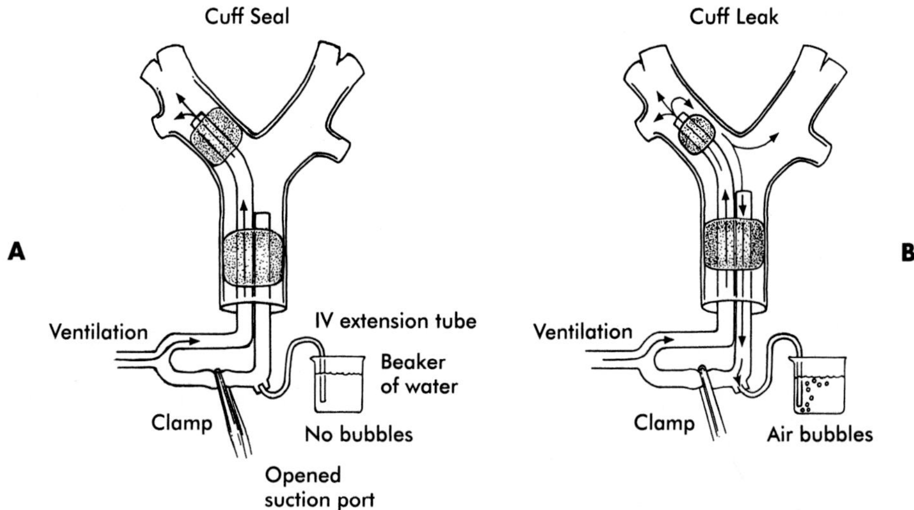

Fig. 70-19. Schematic diagram showing the air bubble detection method for checking adequacy of the seal of the left endobronchial cuff of a left-sided double-lumen tube. **A,** When the left lung is selectively ventilated or exposed to any desired distending pressure and when the left cuff is adequately sealed, no air will escape around the left cuff and out the open right suction port, and thus, no bubbles will be observed passing through the beaker of water. **B,** When the left lung is ventilated or exposed to any desired distending pressure and when the left endobronchial cuff is not adequately sealed, air will escape around the left cuff and out the open right suction port, and thus, air bubbles will be observed passing through the beaker of water. (From Benumof JL: Separation of the two lungs (double-lumen tube and bronchial blocker intubation). In Benumof JL, editor: *Anesthesia for thoracic surgery*, Philadelphia, 1995, WB Saunders.)

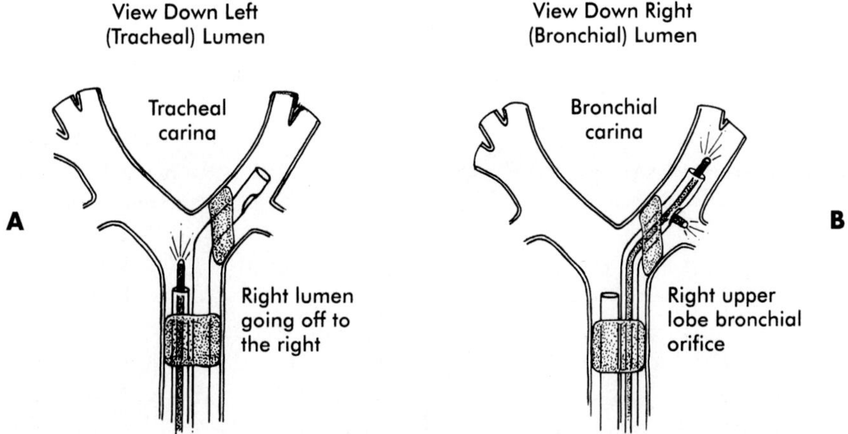

Fig. 70-20. Schematic diagram portraying use of a fiberoptic bronchoscope to determine precise right-sided double-lumen tube position. **A,** When the fiberoptic bronchoscope is passed down the left (tracheal) lumen, the endoscopist should see a clear straight-ahead view of the tracheal carina and the right lumen going off into the right mainstem bronchus. **B,** When the fiberoptic bronchoscope is passed down the right (bronchial) lumen, the endoscopist should see the bronchial carina off in the distance; when the fiberoptic bronchoscope is flexed cephalad and passed through the right upper lobe ventilation slot, the right upper lobe bronchial orifice should be visualized. (From Benumof JL: Separation of the two lungs (double-lumen tube and bronchial blocker intubation). In Benumof JL, editor: *Anesthesia for thoracic surgery*, Philadelphia, 1995, WB Saunders.)

emia and increased peak airway pressures. A common cause of upper lobe obstruction is distal migration of the endobronchial lumen associated with flexion of the neck. Upper lobe obstruction is more common when a right-sided double-lumen endotracheal tube is inserted. Failure to collapse the nonventilated lung may interfere with the operation. Obstruction of the main stem bronchus by either the bronchial cuff or the lateral wall of the tracheal lumen is associated with either too proximal or too distal position of the double-lumen endotracheal tube, respectively.

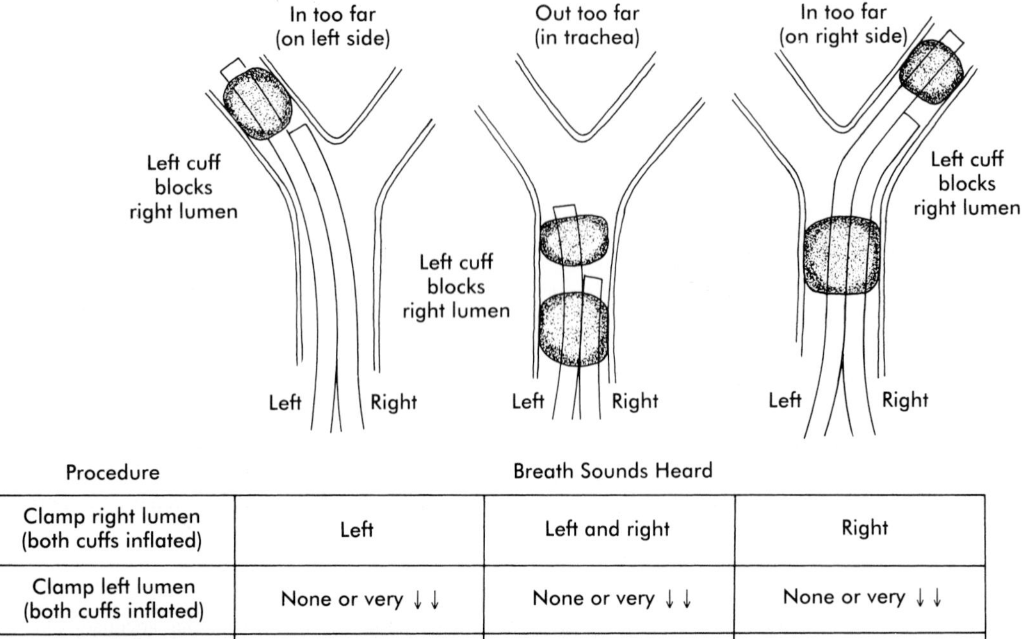

Procedure	Breath Sounds Heard		
Clamp right lumen (both cuffs inflated)	Left	Left and right	Right
Clamp left lumen (both cuffs inflated)	None or very ↓↓	None or very ↓↓	None or very ↓↓
Clamp left lumen (deflate left cuff)	Left	Left and right	Right

Fig. 70-21. There are three major (involving a whole lung) malpositions of a left-sided double-lumen endotracheal tube. The tube can be in too far on the left (both lumens are in the left mainstem bronchus), out too far (both lumens are in the trachea), or down the right mainstem bronchus (at least the left lumen is in the right mainstem bronchus). In each of these three malpositions, the left cuff, when fully inflated, can completely block the right lumen. Inflation and deflation of the left cuff while the left lumen is clamped creates a breath sound—differential diagnosis of tube malposition. (See text for full explanation). L—left; R—right; ↓—decreased. (From Benumof JL: Separation of the two lungs (double-lumen tube and bronchial blocker intubation). In Benumof JL, editor: *Anesthesia for thoracic surgery*, Philadelphia, 1987, WB Saunders.)

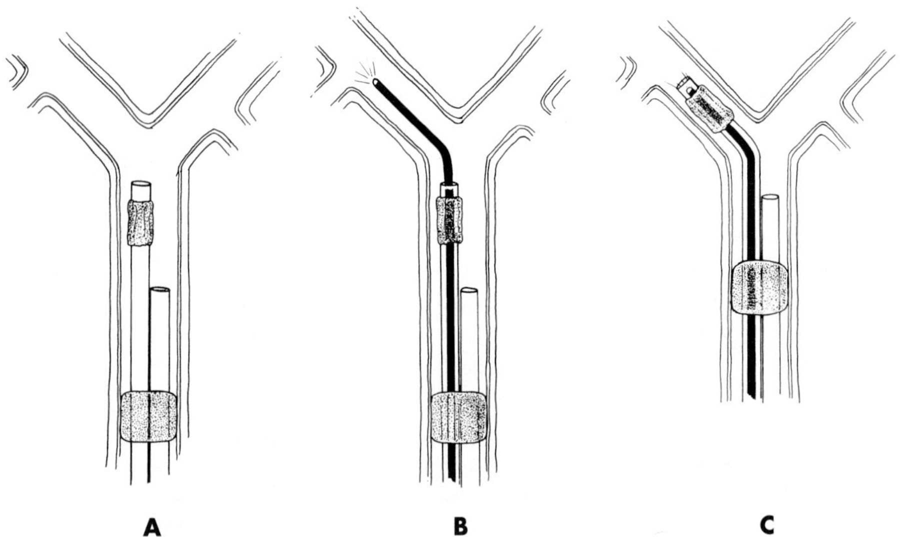

Fig. 70-22. Schematic diagram portraying use of the fiberoptic bronchoscope to insert a left-sided double-lumen tube. **A,** The double-lumen tube can be put into the trachea in a conventional manner, and both lungs can be ventilated by both lumens. The fiberoptic bronchoscope may be inserted into the left lumen of the double-lumen tube through a self-sealing diaphragm in the elbow connector to the left lumen; this allows continued positive pressure ventilation of both lungs through the right lumen without creating a leak. After the fiberoptic bronchoscope has been passed into the left mainstem bronchus **B,** it is used as a stylet for the after-coming left lumen, **C.** The fiberoptic bronchoscope is then withdrawn. Final precise positioning of the double-lumen tube is performed with the fiberoptic bronchoscope in the right lumen. (From Benumof JL: Separation of the two lungs (double-lumen tube and bronchial blocker intubation). In Benumof JL, editor: *Anesthesia for thoracic surgery*, Philadelphia, 1995, WB Saunders.)

Cephalad migration of the double-lumen endotracheal tube can be caused by neck extension or by traction on an inadequately secured tube. As the tube withdraws, the bronchial cuff herniates over the carina into the trachea. When partially herniated, increased cuff pressure may force the cuff further into the trachea. The herniated cuff may partially or fully obstruct the contralateral main stem bronchus, making that lung difficult or impossible to collapse (or ventilate).

Malposition of the tube should be suspected when there is a sudden increase in peak airway pressure, when hypoxemia occurs, or when inflation of the nonventilated lung is detected. Vigilance should be heightened immediately after repositioning the patient and during surgical manipulation near the hilum of the lung. At the first suspicion of a malpositioned double-lumen endotracheal tube, tube position should be confirmed immediately by fiberoptic bronchoscopy. In many patients, the surgeon will be able to manually guide the endobronchial lumen of the double-lumen endotracheal tube into the desired mainstem bronchus.

Traumatic damage

Traumatic damage to the tracheobronchial tree, by double-lumen endotracheal tubes, has been reported.[198] Traumatic injuries include minor insults, such as ecchymosis of the mucous membranes, and more severe ones, like arytenoid dislocation or vocal cord rupture. Catastrophic tracheobronchial rupture has been reported.[77,85,134,170,201,217] The multiple lumen design and relatively large size of double-lumen endotracheal tubes make them stiffer than conventional endotracheal tubes, thus increasing the risk of damage from forceful advancement against resistance. The stiffness is further increased by use of a rigid stylet during tube placement. Therefore, when use of a stylet is required for intubation of the trachea, it should be withdrawn before the bronchial lumen of the double-lumen endotracheal tube is advanced into the mainstem bronchus.

Injuries also may result from excessive pressure in either the tracheal or bronchial cuffs, leading to tissue necrosis or rupture. The small size and high pressure of the bronchial cuff increases the risk of tissue injury from overinflation. Cuff pressure should be regularly monitored by palpation of the pilot balloon or by use of a calibrated device.

Failure to obtain a complete seal is especially hazardous when the double-lumen endotracheal tube is used to protect one lung from liquid contents within the other. The leak may allow spillage of liquid into the unaffected lung. Liquids include saline during bronchopulmonary lavage, pus from unilateral empyema, and blood from airway hemorrhage. In patients in whom a spillage occurs, a failed seal can lead to severe morbidity or death.

Contraindications

The principal contraindication to the use of a double-lumen endotracheal tube is the presence of a luminal airway mass that may be dislodged or may prevent passage of the tube. Relative contraindications include critical dependence on bilateral mechanical ventilation in patients unable to tolerate its interruption, patients requiring rapid placement of an endotracheal tube to avoid aspiration of gastric contents, and patients in whom conventional tracheal intubation is judged to be difficult.

Alternative Methods of Lung Isolation

Endobronchial intubation with a single-lumen tube offers an alternative to the double-lumen endotracheal tube. Disadvantages of using a single-lumen tube include loss of ability to selectively ventilate or suction the contralateral lung and increased difficulty in placing or ascertaining correct placement of the tube. (For pediatric patients, there may be no alternative to an endobronchial intubation using a single-lumen tube.) Endobronchial intubation is especially useful for patients who require emergent tracheal intubation for massive hemoptysis and in whom the only access to the tracheobronchial tree is via a tracheostomy or laryngectomy stoma. For adults, endobronchial intubation requires a tube of adequate length, often more than 31 cm, to ensure that the entire cuff is placed below the carina. Occasionally, it may be necessary to extend the tube using a length of tubing and a connector. Long, low pressure cuffs may offer a disadvantage for endobronchial use.

Although endobronchial intubation of the right side is easier, there is inherent difficulty in preserving ventilation to the right upper lobe. Mainstem intubation is facilitated using a fiberoptic bronchoscope as a directing stylet. Blind left mainstem placement can be achieved with a 92% success rate by turning the head to the right after the tube has passed through the vocal cords and by then rotating the tube 180° so that the convex curve faces posteriorly before advancing it.[359]

When collapse of the left lung and ventilation of the right is required and when use of a double-lumen endotracheal tube is not feasible, a bronchial blocker can be placed in the left main stem bronchus. Use of an appropriately sized Fogarty catheter for endobronchial blockade has been described.[155,327] A styletted and angled Fogarty catheter is placed in the distal trachea under direct vision just before the endotracheal tube is inserted. Then, under radiographic or fiberoptic guidance, the catheter is passed into the desired bronchus, and its balloon is inflated. Absence of a patent lumen extending below the balloon in Fogarty catheters prevents suctioning or oxygen delivery to the occluded lung segment. Also, collapse of the segment depends on uptake of gas from the airways of the occluded segment into its blood supply by "absorption atelectasis," rather than by passive recoil. A pulmonary artery catheter has been used instead of a Fogarty catheter. These catheters contain a transballoon lumen, but the balloon may be too small and high pressure for convenient safe use. The technique offers advantages when the tracheobronchial tree is very small (e.g., in pediatric patients) or when the bronchial lumen is narrowed or distorted by external compression or tumor.

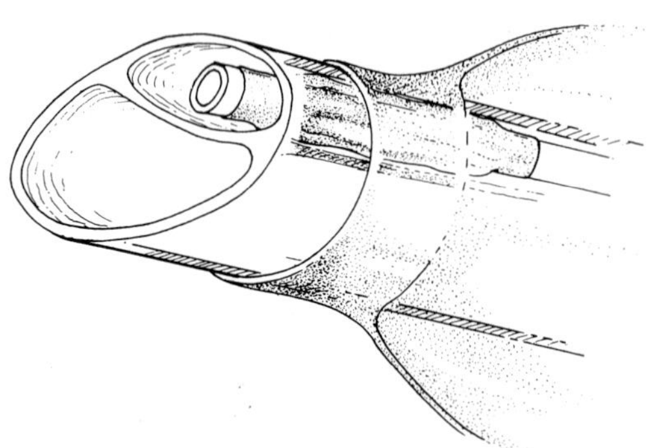

Fig. 70-23. Close-up of the Univent tube shows two lumens. The small tube is retracted into the small lumen before intubation. (Modified from Kamaya H, Krishna PR: New endotracheal tube (Univent tube) for selective blockade of one lung, *Anesthesiology* 63:342, 1985.)

The Univent tube, manufactured in Japan by Fuji Systems, contains a bronchial blocker that passes through a small channel within the anterior wall of an endotracheal tube. The bronchial blocker carries a low-pressure, high-volume cuff and has an internal lumen that can be used for suctioning the collapsed lung or for providing CPAP or high frequency jet ventilation.[460] When the bronchial blocker is fully withdrawn into the wall of the tube, it resembles an ordinary single-lumen endotracheal tube but with a slightly reduced luminal diameter (Fig. 70-23). Initial tube placement in the trachea is accomplished as for any single-lumen tube; then it is rotated 90° toward the lung into which the blocker will be passed and advanced (Fig. 70-24). The blocker then is advanced into the targeted main stem bronchus, after which the tracheal cuff is inflated, and the tube is secured.

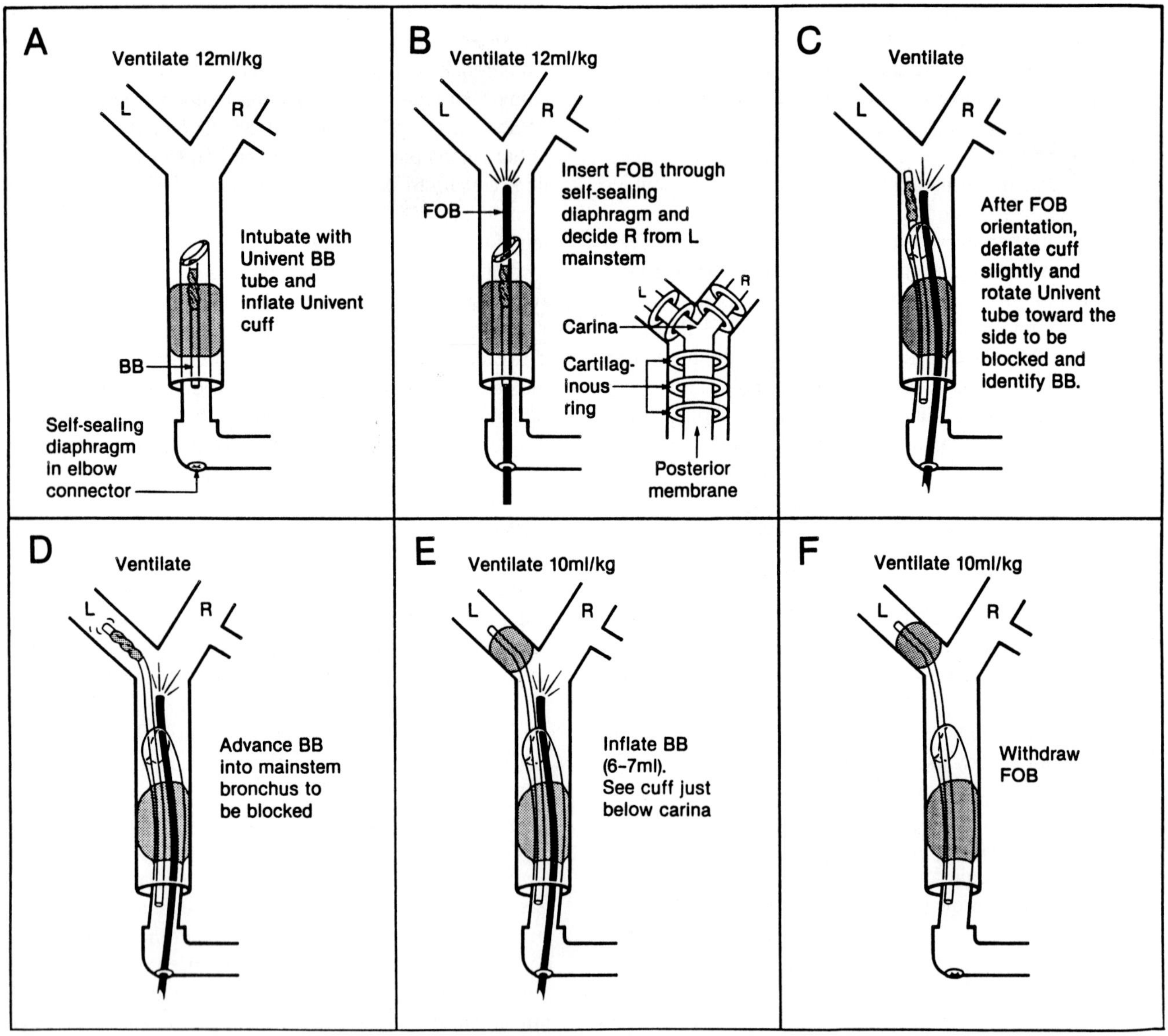

Fig. 70-24. The sequential steps of the fiberoptic-aided method of inserting and positioning the Univent bronchial blocker in the left mainstem bronchus are illustrated. One- and two-lung ventilation is achieved by simply inflating and deflating, respectively, the bronchial blocker balloon. FOB—fiberoptic bronchoscope. (From Benumof JL: Separation of two lungs (double-lumen and bronchial blocker intubation). In Benumof JL, editor: *Anesthesia for thoracic surgery*, Philadelphia, 1995, WB Saunders.)

The depth of the blocker is adjusted and confirmed using a flexible bronchoscope passed through the main lumen of the tube. Additional techniques to assist in placing the blocker include rotation of the head and placing the fiberoptic scope in the opposite lung to divert the blocker into the contralateral side. The tube offers the advantage of allowing easy conversion from single- to two-lung ventilation (and vice versa), and it is suitable for long-term use in an intensive care unit (ICU) setting. The mobility of the blocker and large volume of its cuff increase the likelihood of proximal migration, with herniation of the cuff into the trachea.

HYPOXIC PULMONARY VASOCONSTRICTION

Although total pulmonary blood flow is directly proportional to right ventricular cardiac output, its distribution within the pulmonary vasculature can be altered dynamically. Hypoxia, caused by either atelectasis or ventilation with a hypoxic gas mixture, diverts blood flow to better ventilated, nonhypoxic lung segments. This phenomenon of hypoxic pulmonary vasoconstriction (HPV), first noted by Von Euler and Liljestrand in 1946, is of great importance to the anesthesiologist, particularly during thoracic anesthesia. In the absence of inhibiting factors, HPV can divert blood flow away from nonventilated regions.[290] When a patient is in the lateral decubitus position, the dependent lung receives 60% of the cardiac output, whereas the nondependent lung receives 40%. If the nondependent lung is not ventilated and atelectatic, a maximal HPV response can reduce its blood supply by 50%. As a result, the dependent lung receives 80% of the cardiac output, and the atelectatic nondependent lung receives only 20% of the cardiac output (Fig. 70-25). Therefore, the arterial oxygen tension ($Pa{O_2}$) observed during regional lung hypoxia is much greater than would be expected if the HPV response was not present (Fig. 70-26).

Mechanisms

The precise mechanism for the HPV response is still unclear. Initially, mechanical factors were thought to be important in decreasing blood flow to the atelectatic lung, but several studies found that decreased blood flow to the hypoxic lung was the same whether the lung was atelectatic or ventilated with a hypoxic gas mixture. Therefore, distortion, narrowing, and kinking of the vasculature in an atelectatic lung segment are not the major factors contributing to the diversion of the blood flow to the nonatelectatic lung.[53,297]

The main stimulus for development of HPV is a decrease in alveolar oxygen tension ($P{A}{O_2}$) and, to a lesser extent, a decrease in the mixed venous oxygen tension ($P\bar{v}{O_2}$).[48,357] The postulated site of vasoconstriction is in arterioles that are less than 400 μm in diameter. Mechanisms to explain the HPV response invoke alveolar hypoxia either triggering release of vasoconstrictor substance(s) or altering the cellular metabolic profile of the vascular smooth muscle to favor vasoconstriction (by inhibition of vasodilatation). During the past 15 years, many vasoactive substances have been proposed as mediators of HPV (e.g., leukotriene, prostaglandins, catecholamines, serotonin, angiotension, and bradykinin), but none have proved to be primarily involved in the process. HPV appears to be biphasic. The first phase, initiated within 7 seconds, is localized to vascular smooth muscle and is independent of vascular endothelium.[234] The second phase develops more slowly and depends on the vascular endothelium.[234] Comprehensive discussions of the mechanisms of HPV have recently been published.[258,455]

Hemodynamic variables can influence the magnitude of HPV. **The pulmonary vasoconstrictor response to hypoxia is decreased with increases in PA pressure, cardiac output, left atrial pressure, or central blood volume.**[50] Increases in pulmonary vascular pressures can mechanically open and recruit closed vessels in hypoxic lung regions, overcoming part of the active pulmonary vasoconstriction.[297] An increase in cardiac output can mask the HPV response by recruiting pulmonary vessels or by increasing $P\bar{v}{O_2}$. Alternatively, HPV may increase pulmonary vascular resistance and PA pressures as flow is diverted from a proportionately large section of hypoxic lung to a smaller section of normoxic lung.[297] When flow is diverted from small hy-

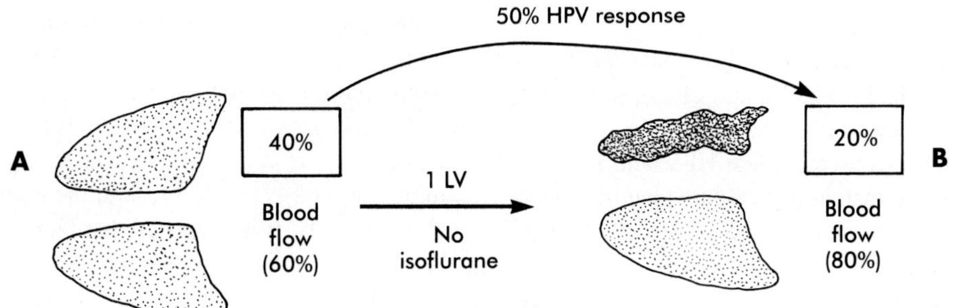

Fig. 70-25. A, Schematic diagram showing that the two-lung ventilation nondependent-to-dependent lung blood flow ratio is 40% to 60%. **B,** When two-lung ventilation is converted to one-lung ventilation (as indicated by atelectasis of the nondependent lung), the HPV response decreases the blood flow to the nondependent lung by 50%, so that the nondependent-to-dependent lung blood flow ratio is now 20% to 80%. (From Wernly JA, et al: Clinical value of quantitative ventilation-perfusion lung scans in the surgical management of bronchogenic carcinoma, *J Thorac Cardiovasc Surg* 80:535, 1980.)

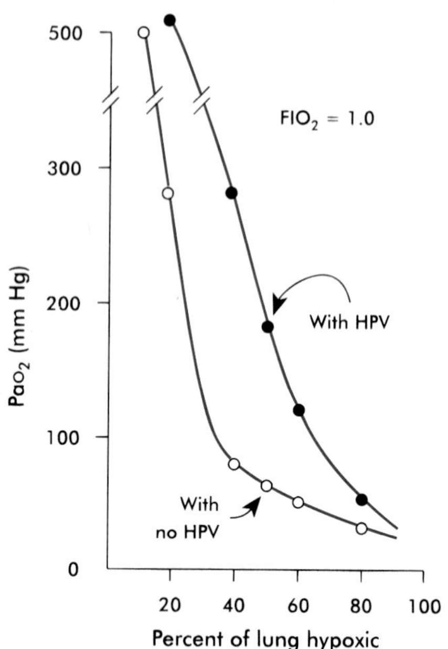

Fig. 70-26. Effect of HPV on Pa_{O_2}. As the percent of lung that is hypoxic increases (*X axis*), the arterial P_{O_2} (Pa_{O_2}) decreases (*y axis*). When the amount of lung that is hypoxic 30% to 70%, which is in the one-lung ventilation/anesthesia range, the decrease in Pa_{O_2} is much greater if there is no HPV compared with the normal expected amount of HPV. HPV—hypoxic pulmonary vasoconstriction. (From Benumof JL: One-lung ventilation and hypoxic pulmonary vasoconstriction: implications for anesthetic management, *Anesth Analg* 64:821, 1985.)

Table 70-7 Effect of vasodilators on hypoxic pulmonary vasoconstriction

Drug	Effect on HPV	References
Hydralazine	No change	63
Nifedipine	Inhibited	62, 368, 400
Verapamil	Inhibited	82, 430
Nitroglycerine	Inhibited	92, 101
Sodium nitroprusside	Inhibited	345, 440

poxic segments, the high compliance of the pulmonary circulation prevents clinically significant changes in pulmonary vascular resistance or PA pressure.

Drugs and anesthetics may modulate HPV and interfere with ventilation perfusion matching. Calcium channel blockers and vasodilators, such as sodium nitroprusside, attenuate the HPV response (Table 70-7). These drugs increase the A-a gradient, often leading to hypoxemia perioperatively. Other perioperative conditions, such as hypocapnia and hypothermia, also decrease the normal HPV response.[50,51]

Effects of Anesthetics

Extensive studies have been performed to examine the effect of inhalation and intravenous anesthetics on HPV. The results and implications of these studies differ according to the type of experimental preparation used. The *in vitro* and *in vivo* isolated preparations (without an intact systemic circulation) demonstrated a dramatic inhibitory effect of inhaled anesthetics on HPV. In human studies and in more physiologic *in vivo* investigations with an intact systemic circulation, inhalation anesthetics produced either no effect or only a mild decrease in HPV.[22,46,370,383] In part, this discrepancy occurs because factors that can modulate the HPV response, such as pulmonary vascular pressure, cardiac output, P_{CO_2}, and temperature are controlled in *in vitro* studies. In the more biologically complex *in vivo* models, these factors seem to greatly decrease the inhibitory effect of inhaled anesthetics on HPV.[44,271]

Intravenous agents such as ketamine and propofol do not dramatically affect HPV.[44,437] Recent studies document that thoracic epidural analgesia does not directly affect HPV. Any changes that were observed during epidural use were attributable to alterations in cardiac function and loading conditions.[232]

Nitric Oxide

Nitric oxide (NO) is a unique endogenous compound that is found in endothelium and smooth muscle cells. NO induces vasodilation by activation of protein kinases and guanylate cyclase and reduction or resequestration of intracellular Ca^+. There is a class of intravenous vasodilators, including nitroglycerine and nitroprusside, that release NO molecules, producing muscle relaxation.

The most common clinical uses of NO are for the management of pulmonary hypertension and ventilation-perfusion mismatching. Intravenous therapy nonselectively produces pulmonary and systemic vasodilation, In contrast, NO administered as an inspired gas is delivered preferentially to well-ventilated areas, selectively dilating the vascular supply to those areas, thereby improving ventilation-to-perfusion matching. In the United States, NO is restricted by the Food and Drug Administration to use as an investigational agent. A number of medical centers are actively investigating the clinical therapeutic potential of NO in various disease states, such as primary pulmonary hypertension, lung transplantation, cardiac transplantation, cardiac disease, adult respiratory distress syndrome (ARDS), acute pulmonary hypertension, congenital heart disease, and idiopathic pulmonary hypertension.

Several groups that use NO in the perioperative and critical care environments have proposed guidelines for its administration.[299,424,473] At present, there are no long-term data about toxicity. It is proposed that NO be administered in the lowest effective dosage for safety and efficiency. Delivery systems require an adequate scavenging system to reduce the risk of occupational exposure and continuous gas concentration monitoring. Concerns about the potential toxicity of NO focus on its conversion from the free radical form to NO_2, which is associated with lung toxicity, and the formation of nitrosylhemoglobin, which is rapidly converted to methemoglobin.[4,190,228,425,462] Clinical reports of NO-associated toxicity include methemoglobin toxicity and paradoxical deterioration in oxygenation related to edema or worsening of right to left shunting.[4,69,325,332,425,460] Discontinuation of NO administration has been associated with rebound pulmonary hypertension.[4,60,189] This effect may be related to development of tolerance or an increase in vascular tone. It is therefore prudent to taper the dose of NO gradually and be vigilant for deterioration in oxygenation or worsening of pulmonary hypertension.

STRATEGIES TO IMPROVE OXYGENATION DURING ONE-LUNG VENTILATION

The occurrence of arterial hypoxemia during one-lung ventilation is unpredictable. There is no correlation between the resting preoperative $Pa{O_2}$ and that measured during one-lung ventilation with the nondependent lung deflated to atmospheric pressure. Neither is there correlation between the extent of intraoperative hypoxemia and the preoperative pulmonary function values or the predicted postoperative FEV_1, although there are strategies to decrease the occurrence of hypoxemia during one-lung ventilation and manage it when present.

The basic principles for management of one-lung ventilation include (1) delay initiation until after turning the patient to the lateral decubitus position, allowing sufficient time for nondependent lung collapse before operation begins, (2) confirm correct positioning of the double-lumen tube by fiberoptic bronchoscopy, (3) use high-inspired O_2 concentrations to decrease the risk of systemic hypoxemia, (4) use a large tidal volume of about 10 ml/kg, and adjust respiratory rate to keep $Pa{CO_2}$ about 40 mm Hg, (5) continuously monitor oxygenation using pulse oximetry, and (6) continuously monitor ventilation by listening to the breath sounds and observing end-tidal CO_2 concentrations.

Measures to improve oxygenation during one-lung ventilation include one or more of the following strategies (1) improve the V/Q distribution in the dependent lung (i.e., PEEP), (2) increase $PA{O_2}$ in the nondependent lung (i.e., CPAP), (3) decrease blood flow to the nondependent lung (i.e., placement of a ligature on the pulmonary artery), and (4) increase blood flow and perfusion to the dependent lung (i.e., nitric oxide).

Prevention of Absorption Atelectasis

Absorption atelectasis, caused by increased FIO_2, can be decreased or prevented by large tidal volumes, PEEP to the dependent lung, and ventilation with an FIO_2 less than 100%.[84] The use of 10% to 20% nitrogen with 80% to 90% O_2 has been suggested to decrease the possibility of absorption atelectasis, because nitrogen splints open the alveoli in areas of low V/Q ratio. The small reduction in the FIO_2 causes only a small decrease in $PA{O_2}$. Nitrogen is more efficacious than N_2O in splinting the alveoli because it is less soluble.

Verification of Tube Position

The most important factor in assuring adequate oxygenation and ventilation is the proper positioning of the double-lumen endotracheal tube. Tube position should be reconfirmed after turning the patient. Secretions that could interfere with ventilation and increase inflation pressure also should be suctioned from the airway.

Employment of Large Tidal Volumes

Small tidal volume ventilation to the dependent lung can decrease FRC and promote airway closure and atelectasis. The development of an hypoxic area in the dependent lung interferes with the overall effectiveness of HPV in the nondependent lung, resulting in decreased arterial oxygenation. The tidal volume at initiation of one-lung ventilation should be about 10 ml/kg, which is relatively large compared with the usual tidal volume during two-lung ventilation of 12 ml/kg. The tidal volume is then adjusted upward or downward according to the airway pressures and arterial blood gas values. Delivering an excessively large tidal volume to the dependent lung can increase airway pressures and the risk of pneumothorax or barotrauma and can increase PVR, thus diverting blood to the nonventilated nondependent lung.[49,165,247,249]

Maintenance of Normocapnia

Respiratory rates should be adjusted to maintain normocapnia. The change from two-lung ventilation to one-lung ventilation usually causes no problem with CO_2 elimination because of the high diffusibility of CO_2 across the alveolar membrane.[26,211,249] Theoretically, hypocapnia should be avoided because it can directly dilate the pulmonary vessels, interfering with HPV in the nondependent lung. Because the tidal volume is decreased with initiation of one-lung ventilation, the respiratory rate should be increased to maintain the same minute ventilation and $Pa{CO_2}$.

Dependent-Lung PEEP

Because the dependent lung often has a decreased volume during one-lung ventilation, several attempts have been made to improve oxygenation by managing the ventilated lung with PEEP. The application of PEEP to the dependent lung results in recruitment of closed alveoli and airways, increased FRC, and increased lung compliance. The disadvantage of applying PEEP to the dependent lung is that the associated increased mean airway pressure and PVR could divert some blood flow to the nondependent, atelectatic, nonventilated lung. Therefore, the effect of using PEEP is a balance between its potential beneficial effects and the possible deleterious effects of decreasing HPV, causing the redistribution of blood flow to the nondependent nonventilated lung. In a patient with a very diseased dependent lung, the positive effect of selective dependent lung PEEP may outweigh its negative effects. In contrast, patients who have a relatively normal dependent lung may have decreased oxygenation if PEEP is selectively applied to that lung (Fig. 70-27).

Selective Nondependent-Lung CPAP

The application of CPAP to the nonventilated nondependent lung improves oxygenation during one-lung ventilation (Fig. 70-28). Even with a maximal HPV response, 20% of

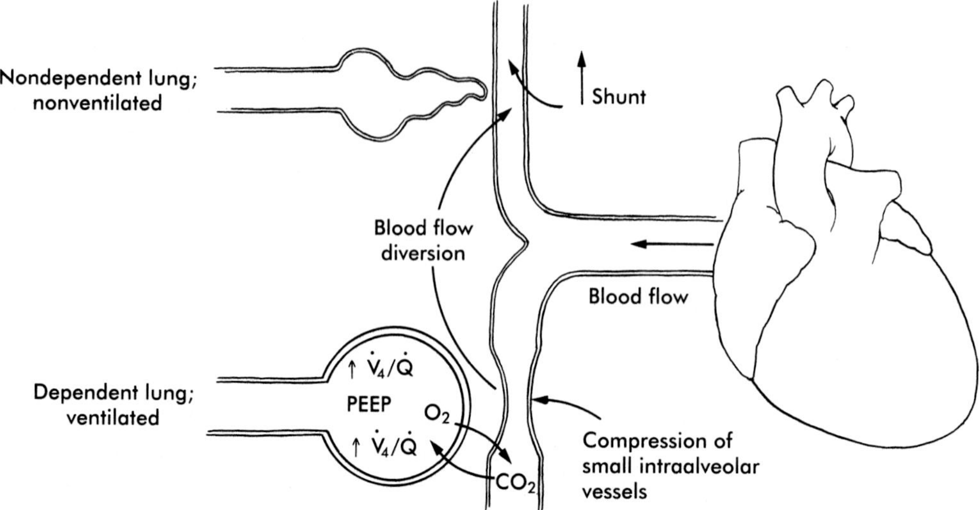

Fig. 70-27. Selective positive end-expiratory pressure (PEEP) to the ventilated-dependent lung can increase dependent lung ventilation-to-perfusion ratios ($\uparrow \dot{V}_A/\dot{Q}$). Dependent lung PEEP also can cause compression of the small intraalveolar vessels in the dependent lung, causing blood flow diversion to the nonventilated nondependent lung, thereby increasing the shunt through the nonventilated nondependent lung. Therefore, the overall arterial oxygenation effect of dependent lung PEEP will be a trade-off between the good effect of an increase in dependent lung $\dot{V}_A/\dot{Q}$ and the bad effect of increased nonventilated lung blood flow. (From Benumof JL, editor: *Anesthesia for thoracic surgery*, Philadelphia, 1987, WB Saunders.)

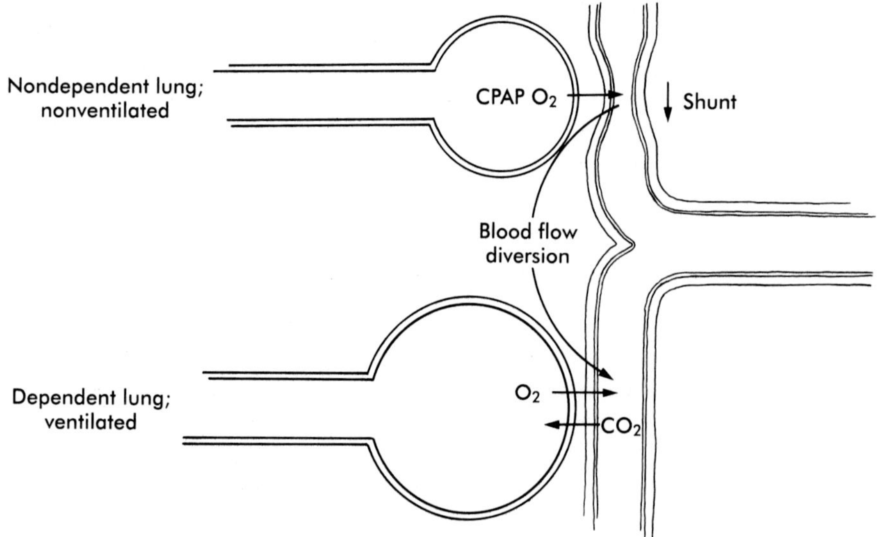

Fig. 70-28. Selective continuous positive airway pressure (CPAP) to the nonventilated nondependent lung (static distension without tidal movement) allows this lung to participate in oxygen uptake and markedly decreases the shunt through the nonventilated nondependent lung. Even if the nonventilated nondependent lung CPAP causes blood flow diversion to the ventilated dependent lung, the diverted flow can still participate in oxygen uptake and CO_2 elimination in the ventilated dependent lung. Usually 5 to 10 cm H_2O of nondependent lung CPAP is all that is clinically needed, and this amount of CPAP does not cause any serious surgical interference. (From Benumof JL, editor: *Anesthesia for thoracic surgery*, Philadelphia, 1995, WB Saunders.)

the cardiac output still flows through the nondependent lung. The use of an inhalation agent, such as isoflurane, may increase the nondependent lung blood flow to 24% of the cardiac output. Application of CPAP during one-lung ventilation leads to the oxygenation of blood that perfuses the nondependent lung and thereby dramatically increases Pa_{O_2}. CPAP is initiated during the deflation phase of a large tidal volume breath to maintain uniform expansion and avoid the need to overcome critical opening pressures of collapsed alveoli. The application of 5 to 10 cm H_2O CPAP usually does not interfere with surgical exposure during open thoracotomies, but it may impede visualization during thoracoscopy. No major hemodynamic effects are observed with CPAP of 5 to 10 cm H_2O applied to the nondependent lung in humans.[99,149] Although CPAP at less than 10 cm H_2O does not compress small intraalveolar vessels, 15 cm H_2O of CPAP causes a decrease in blood flow through the nondependent lung, diverting flow to the dependent lung.[11]

During one-lung ventilation, the nondependent lung does not remain totally unventilated, even with a perfectly positioned double-lumen endotracheal tube. Each time the dependent lung is inflated, the mediastinum is displaced upward into the nondependent thorax. During the exhalation phase, the mediastinum falls away from the nondependent side. The effect of the mediastinal movement created by ventilation produces asynchronous, "pendelluft" ventilation of the nondependent lung. This phenomenon may be observed as a small puff of air emanating from the lumen of nondependent endotracheal tube, which may be misinterpreted as a failed seal of the bronchial cuff. Because the nondependent lung is ordinarily open to the atmosphere, the pendelluft ventilation introduces room air into the tracheobronchial tree. Thus, even in the absence of CPAP, delivering 100% oxygen via T-piece may improve oxygenation of blood flowing through the nondependent lung.

Several selective CPAP systems for the nondependent lung have been described (Figs. 70-29 and 70-30).[1,81,207,423] The conventional method for instituting CPAP during one- lung ventilation uses an O_2 source and a manometer or PEEP valve.[33] Several designs of CPAP systems contain reservoir bags (i.e., Mapelson D circuit) which allow delivery of independent tidal breaths or sighs to the nondependent lung. Delivery of oxygen at high flows via a catheter placed in the main stem bronchus of the nondependent lung produces CPAP without need for a PEEP valve. In most situations, an O_2 flow rate of 5 to 10 l/minute creates CPAP of 5 to 10 cm H_2O, which is sufficient for improving oxygenation. One advantage of this system is that the elimination of CO_2 is proportional to the flow rate of the gas in the CPAP system. A very high O_2 flow rate delivered at or below the carina may even provide adequate gas exchange without any tidal exchange, which is known as "continuous high-flow apneic ventilation."

Differential PEEP/CPAP

The first step to improve arterial oxygenation after confirming proper tube placement involves application of 5 to 10 cm H_2O of CPAP to the nondependent lung. If oxygenation is still inadequate, 5 cm H_2O of PEEP is applied to the dependent lung. If arterial oxygenation remains poor, tube position should be confirmed, and the patient's hemodynamic status should be assessed. A decrease in cardiac output, leading to a decrease in mixed venous oxygen saturation (SvO_2), can magnify the effect of shunt on arterial oxygenation. If hypoxemia is persistent, nondependent lung CPAP should then be increased to 10 cm H_2O. In patients undergoing thoracotomy with one-lung ventilation, sufficient increase in arterial oxygenation can be achieved by combining 10 cm H_2O of CPAP to the nondependent lung and 10 cm H_2O of PEEP to the dependent lung. Serious hemodynamic effects have not been observed from these magnitudes of PEEP and CPAP (Fig. 70-31).[99,149]

Asynchronous Ventilation of the Nondependent Lung

If hypoxemia still persists after differential CPAP/PEEP, the nondependent lung may be intermittently ventilated with

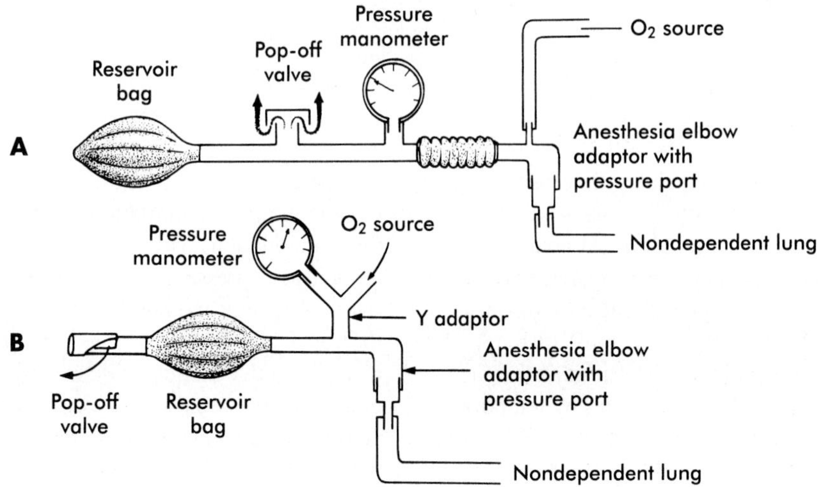

Fig. 70-29. A and **B,** Schematic diagram showing two nondependent lung continuous positive airway pressure (CPAP) systems with reservoir bags. Both of these systems contain an oxygen source, some type of pressure relief valve, and a pressure manometer to measure the CPAP. The presence of a reservoir bag allows for intermittent positive-pressure breathing and sighing, if desired. (From Benumof JL: Conventional and differential lung management of one-lung ventilation. In Benumof JL, editor: *Anesthesia for thoracic surgery*, Philadelphia, 1995, WB Saunders.)

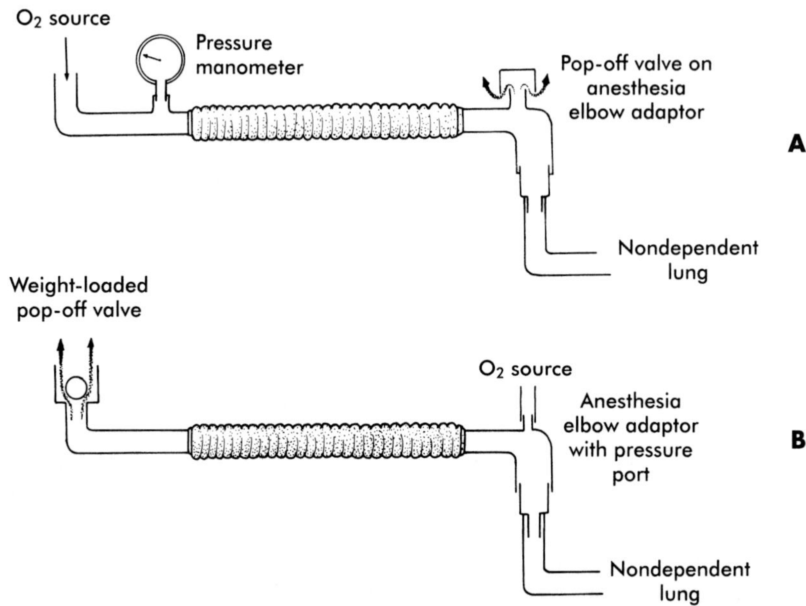

Fig. 70-30. **A** and **B,** Schematic diagram showing two nondependent lung continuous positive airway pressure (CPAP) systems without reservoir bags. Both contain an oxygen source and a pressure relief valve, but **A** has a pressure manometer to measure the CPAP, whereas **B** does not. (From Benumof JL: Conventional and differential lung management of one-lung ventilation. In Benumof JL, editor: *Anesthesia for thoracic surgery*, Philadelphia, 1995, WB Saunders.)

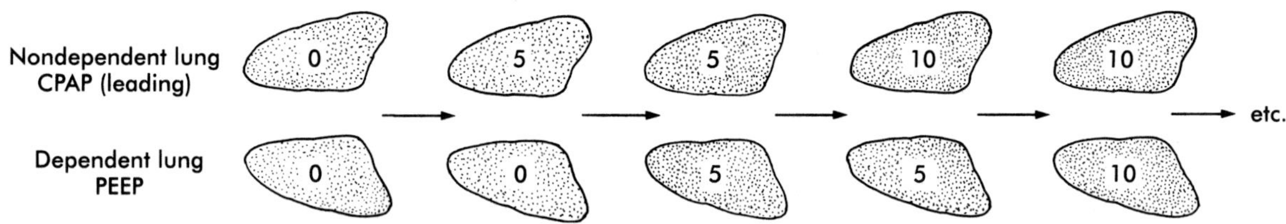

Fig. 70-31. A search for optimal nondependent lung continuous positive airway pressure (CPAP) and dependent lung positive end-expiratory pressure (PEEP) is performed by leading with nondependent lung CPAP and following with dependent lung PEEP. Leading with nondependent lung CPAP removes the deleterious arterial oxygenation blood flow diversion effects of dependent lung PEEP. (Modified from Benumof JL, editor: *Anesthesia for thoracic surgery*, Philadelphia, 1995, WB Saunders.)

positive pressure and 100% O_2. The value of intermittent reinflation of the collapsed lung with O_2 was studied in a group of patients undergoing thoracotomy. Although intermittent reinflation of the nondependent lung resulted in a major improvement in arterial oxygenation, the effects declined with repeated inflations.[285] Finally, most of the V/Q mismatch and arterial hypoxemia can be eliminated by decreasing blood flow to the nondependent lung by temporarily ligating its pulmonary artery (Fig. 70-32).

Selective Nondependent-Lung High-Frequency Ventilation

Any method that results in splinting the alveoli and air spaces of the nondependent lung will lead to an improvement in arterial oxygenation and a decrease in the transpulmonary shunt. High-frequency ventilation of the nondependent lung has been studied in combination with conventional positive-pressure ventilation of the dependent lung. Using this combination, $Pa{O_2}$ was much better than with intermittent positive-pressure ventilation of the dependent lung with total collapse of the nondependent lung.[464] In most patients, the same increase in arterial oxygenation can be achieved using selective nondependent lung CPAP, which requires much simpler equipment compared with high-frequency ventilation apparatus. In some situations, high-frequency ventilation may be more advantageous:

- If the nondependent lung has a major bronchopleural fistula, high-frequency ventilation to the nondependent lung using low airway pressures helps to decrease the air leak and improve oxygenation and ventilation.[31]
- During operation on the major conducting airways, high-frequency ventilation permits the use of small venti-

Reconfirm proper tube placement after turning to the lateral decubitus position.

↓

Initial one-lung ventilation setting
- TV 10 ml/kg
- FIO_2 80% -100% ± nitrogen 0%-20%
- adjust respiratory rate to maintain $PaCO_2 \approx 40$ mm Hg
- PEEP 0-5 mm Hg

↓

↑ FIO_2
↑ TV if too small or ↓ TV if too large
consider malposition of double-lumen tube or balloon
reconfirm position of ETT with bronchoscope

↓

Optimize volume status, cardiac output, and hemoglobin content to improve O_2 delivery and prevent mixed venous O_2 desaturation; the latter will magnify the effect of any given degree of shunt on PaO_2

↓

Start nondependent lung CPAP with 5 cm H_2O; increase as needed

↓

Start dependent lung PEEP to follow, then match CPAP of nondependent lung

↓

Intermittent reinflation of the nondependent lung with positive pressure breaths with 100% FIO_2 every 5 minutes, as needed

↓

Reinstitute two-lung ventilation

↓

Clamping/ligation of the pulmonary artery of the nondependent lung

Fig. 70-32. Algorithm for managing one-lung ventilation and improving oxygenation.

lation catheters that pass through the operating field.[31,340,364,378,415]

- Unilateral high-frequency jet ventilation with contralateral intermittent positive-pressure ventilation has been used in the anesthetic treatment of patients with severely compromised respiratory reserve. The technique provided satisfactory anesthesia, good operating conditions, and adequate gas exchange.[311]

A recent study of eight patients undergoing posterolateral thoracotomy using double-lumen endobronchial tubes compared the effect of high-frequency jet ventilation to the nondependent lung with the application of CPAP. Jet ventilation and CPAP to the nondependent lung were equally effective in improving arterial oxygenation, but the cardiac output was better maintained with jet ventilation. Therefore, O_2 delivery (cardiac output × arterial O_2 content) was greater with jet ventilation than with CPAP. High-frequency jet ventilation provided a quiet surgical field and satisfactory surgical exposure.[315]

ANESTHETIC TECHNIQUES

Although thoracic surgery can be performed during regional block, most thoracotomies are performed during general anesthesia with controlled ventilation. Epidural or other regional anesthetic techniques often are used for postoperative pain control. Recent evidence suggests that use of conduction anesthesia for preemptive analgesia may improve long-term outcomes, and short-term comfort.

General Anesthesia

The choice of induction agent and dosage is influenced by the patient's medical condition. In patients in whom extensive airway instrumentation or manipulation proceed thoracotomy, an antisialogogue, glycopyrrolate, can reduce secretions. Narcotics supplement the inhalational anesthetic, although the dosage of systemic narcotic should be reduced in patients who will receive epidural narcotics. The incidence of postoperative respiratory depression is related to the total dosage of narcotics administered systematically and epidurally. After the induction of general anesthesia, controlled manual ventilation with mask is started using an inhalation anesthetic. N_2O can also be used during the induction phase and during prepping, draping, and positioning of the patient. Because large intrapulmonary shunts are anticipated with initiation of one-lung ventilation, it is prudent to increase the inspired concentration of oxygen. N_2O should be avoided in patients who have marginal preoperative oxygenation or in those with large bullae and emphysematous lungs to avoid expansion of bullae by N_2O.

After the induction of anesthesia, the trachea is intubated

with a single-lumen or double-lumen tube as indicated by the surgical procedure. Position of the endotracheal tube is confirmed by careful auscultation, capnography, and, if indicated, by fiberoptic bronchoscopy.

Volatile, halogenated anesthetic drugs have several desirable properties for use during thoracic procedures. They decrease airway irritability and obtund airway reflexes in patients who usually have reactive airways, and they maintain adequate anesthesia while allowing increased inspired oxygen concentrations. They can be eliminated rapidly, allowing tracheal extubation in the operating room with less concern for postoperative respiratory depression. Although volatile anesthetics allow high inspired O_2 concentrations, they may reduce PaO_2 by increasing the shunt related to partial inhibition of HPV.[46,64,370] The inhibition of HPV by inhaled anesthetics may be of more clinical importance in some patients than in others because substantial variability occurs.

Patients with mediastinal and airway tumors may be at risk for airway obstruction during induction of anesthesia. In such patients, the anesthetic plan and emergency treatment strategies should be discussed with the surgeon preoperatively. If emergent need of tracheostomy, rigid bronchoscopy, or extracorpeal oxygenation are anticipated, the entire operating team should be prepared to act smoothly and efficiently. Patients at increased risk of airway obstruction may require awake fiberoptic intubation or spontaneous ventilation to avoid airway obstruction. Special management concerns for mediastinal tumors are discussed later.

Regional Anesthesia

Epidural anesthesia, paravertebral block, intercostal nerve blocks, or field blocks have been occasionally used as the sole anesthetic for various thoracic procedures, including thoracotomy.

Field block consists of local infiltration of the skin and muscles surrounding the operative site. Intercostal nerve blocks anesthetize the nerves in the intercostal groove along the lower margin of each rib. Paravertebral blocks anesthetize the intercostal nerves as they emerge from the intervertebral foramen; a separate injection is made for each spinal nerve. Epidural block is performed by placing a catheter in the epidural space and local anesthetic is administered to anesthetize the spinal nerves and cord. The spread and intensity of the block are determined by the volume and concentration of drug injected.

Crawford et al.[115] described 677 patients with tuberculosis in whom epidural anesthesia was used for thoracotomy. Epidural anesthesia alone was successful in 95% of the patients, but supplemental anesthesia was required in the other 5% of patients. The most striking finding of this study was the low incidence of postoperative respiratory infections and spread of tuberculosis with this technique when compared with patients who had similar operations during general anesthesia. This was attributed to the ability of patients to expectorate secretions throughout the procedure. Additional advantages of epidural anesthesia were the lower incidence of nausea, rapid resumption of oral intake, and decreased blood loss. A disadvantage involved coughing paroxysms that occurred occasionally with ligation of the bronchus.

Others have described the use of thoracic epidural blockade for open thoracotomies or thoracoscopies in awake sedated patients.[80,210] The most surprising results were the absence of paradoxical respiration and dyspnea. The breathing pattern and speech appeared normal even when an upper lobe bronchus was transsected and held open. Several factors may have contributed to the success of this unorthodox technique: (1) analgesia was complete, and patients were comfortable; (2) the patients were extremely cooperative and had a good rapport with the anesthesiologist; (3) the use of premedication and sedation was minimal; (4) supplemental O_2 was administered by positive pressure mask if the patient reported any shortness of breath; and (5) operation was remarkably gentle and swift.

Combined Epidural Blockade and General Anesthesia

It is unlikely that the routine patient would tolerate the sole use of regional anesthesia. The techniques of general and epidural anesthesia often are combined to achieve the benefits of each. General anesthesia provides amnesia, analgesia muscle, relaxation, and somnolence. During the early recovery from general anesthesia, patients may experience residual sedation, respiratory depression, and inadequate postoperative analgesia. Epidural anesthesia has the advantages of reduction in afterload,[441] improved pulmonary function, decreased incidence of venous thromboembolism,[305,307,342] and suppression of the stress response.[156] Potential disadvantages include the time required to establish the block, increased fluid requirements associated with sympathectomy, and the potential for technical complications such as epidural hematoma.

The relative contribution of each technique to a combined anesthetic can vary. The epidural blockade may either be used for postoperative analgesia or as the major anesthetic, with light general anesthesia used for amnesia and sedation. A prospective, randomized, controlled clinical study examined the effect of epidural anesthesia and postoperative analgesia on postoperative morbidity rate in high-risk surgical patients.[470] When compared with control patients, those who received epidural anesthesia and analgesia had fewer overall complications and fewer cardiovascular or major infectious complications. Urinary cortisol secretion, a marker of the stress response to surgery, was dramatically decreased during the first 24 postoperative hours in those receiving epidural anesthesia. Finally, hospital costs were less for patients who received epidural anesthesia.[470]

Vital capacity and lung compliance decrease after general anesthesia and neuromuscular blockade in patients undergoing thoracotomy.[79] Epidural analgesia with light general anesthesia results in less decrease in static compliance and fewer alterations in postoperative pulmonary function.[78] A comparison of epidural analgesia with general anesthesia noted a decrease in the size of myocardial infarctions, probably related to improved regional subendocardial perfusion.[441] Possible mechanisms include afferent sensory blockade, decreased adrenergic tone, and coronary and systemic vasodilation with a reduction in cardiac preload and afterload.[79,254,360] Patients who received epidural anesthesia had fewer cardiovascular complications, including congestive heart failure.[470]

The use of epidural anesthesia and analgesia is associated with fewer major postoperative infections. This may result from (1) decreased duration of endotracheal intubation and mechanical ventilation, which diminishes many of the defense mechanisms against infection;[388,409] (2) decreased duration of ICU stay postoperatively and reduced risks of nosocomial infection;[19,319] and (3) suppression of the endocrine stress response to operation, which has an inhibitory effect on the immune system.[227] Immune competence is less disturbed postoperatively when epidural anesthesia is used compared with other anesthetic and analgesic techniques.[223,375]

An epidural catheter can be inserted in the high thoracic (C7–T4), mid-thoracic (T4–T9), or low thoracic-lumbar (T9–L2) regions. To date, no studies have demonstrated overwhelming superiority of one approach. In the experience of the authors, the mid-thoracic level, about T7, provides excellent conditions for thoracic and thoracoabdominal procedures. The higher thoracic approach generally is avoided because of the risk of blocking the phrenic nerve (C3, C4, C5) through cephalad extension of epidural local anesthetics. The low thoracic region is suitable for thoracoabdominal procedures, such as gastrectomy or a low thoracoabdominal aneurysm. Use of a lumbar epidural blockade in patients undergoing thoracic surgery requires a greater dosage of local anesthetics or narcotics to provide analgesia in the thoracic regions and is not routinely recommended. A recent study indicates that low thoracic epidural catheter placement is associated with a higher incidence of neurologic complication than either high or mid-thoracic placement. **Because of the multiple advantages conferred by thoracic epidural analgesia, the anesthetic plan for open thoracotomy should always include placement of thoracic epidural catheter unless an absolute contraindication is present.**

THORACOSCOPY VERSUS THORACOTOMY

Evolution of surgical technique and technical advances in electronics and instrumentation have lead to renewed interest in thoracoscopy. In a health care environment that values cost and patient outcome, video-assisted thoracoscopy (VAT) may have advantages beyond open thoracotomy, including decreased postoperative pain, pulmonary impairment, and hospital stay. Thoracoscopy permits the visualization of the pulmonary cavity through several small portals. These portals provide access for the video camera and allow manipulation of thoracic structures and use of surgical instruments such as staplers, dissectors, coagulators, and lasers. Although initially used for only minor surgical procedures, the application of VAT has expanded considerably (Box 70-7). VAT is used for diagnostic and therapeutic procedures. If access is inadequate or if bleeding complications occur, VAT is easily converted to a limited open thoracotomy.

Anesthetic treatment for patients undergoing thoracoscopy is similar to that for open thoracotomy (Table 70-8). Although limited thoracoscopy has been performed in spontaneously breathing, sedated patients, this procedure usually is performed during general anesthesia with placement of a double-lumen endotracheal tube for lung separation. The ability to visualize the contents of the thoracic cavity depends on adequate lung isolation and deflation of the operative lung. Many patients have obstructive lung disease that impedes passive deflation of the nonventilated lung. To foster deflation, the nondependent lung should be carefully suctioned of secretions that may cause air trapping, then denitrogenated by ventilating with 100% oxygen, with single-lung ventilation initiated before skin incision. The tidal volume delivered to the ventilated dependent lung should be decreased to prevent upward shift of the mediastinum during single-lung ventilation. If deflation is inadequate, CO_2 can be insufflated into the nondependent thoracic cavity. Intraoperative hypotension may develop if excessive gas inflation causes mediastinal shift and reduction in venous return to the heart. Advantages of VAT over open thoracotomy are controversial.[100,241,264,280,308,386,447] Analgesic requirements and length of hospital stay are less than those for open thoracotomy.[264,280,308,386,447] Adequate

BOX 70-7
APPLICATIONS OF VIDEO-ASSISTED THORACOSCOPY

- Pulmonary
  - Lung biopsy
  - Resection mass
  - Bleb resection
  - Volume reduction pneumoplasty
- Pleura
  - Diagnostic evaluation
  - Pleurodesis
  - Decortication
- Pericardium
  - Pericardial drainage
  - Pericardectomy
  - Automatic implantable cardiovertor/defibrillator placement
- Mediastinum
  - Lymph node biopsy
  - Biopsy and resection of mediastinal mass
  - Vagotomy
- Esophageal surgery
  - Thoracic duct ligation
- Sympathectomy
  - Microdiscectomy

Table 70-8 Anesthetic guidelines for video-assisted thoracoscopy and thoracotomy

	Video-assisted thoracoscopy	Thoracotomy
Indication	Diagnostic, therapeutic (see Box 70-7)	Same*
Monitors	Standard monitors Optional (arterial, pulmonary artery catheter, Foley catheter)	Same*
Anesthesia	General anesthesia Optional (combined regional/general anesthesia)	Same*
Additional equipment	Fiberoptic bronchoscope Arm board Pillows Bean bag or chest roll	Same*
Ventilation	Double-lumen endotracheal tube Bronchial blockers	
Position	Lateral decubitus position (check and pad pressure points)	Same*
Incision	Several portals for the introduction of equipment	Lateral thoracotomy Anterior thoracotomy Posterior thoracotomy Muscle-sparing incision
Unique considerations	Single-lung ventilation	Same*
Intraoperative complications	Hypoxia Hypercapnia Bleeding	Same*
Estimated blood loss	< 300 ml	Variable
Postoperative analgesia	Parenteral opiates NSAIDs Intrapleural catheter, intercostal nerve block	Epidural $>$ parenteral opiates NSAIDs
Postoperative morbidity	Hypoxia (atelectasis, pneumothorax, PE) Bleeding	Same*
Postoperative care	Adequate analgesia Supplemental O_2 Chest radiograph May require close follow-up evaluation overnight	Same*

*Same as *Video-assisted thoracoscopy.*

postoperative analgesia can be obtained with a combination of parenteral opiates, nonsteroidal antiinflammatories (NSAIDs), intercostal nerve blocks, or an intrapleural catheter. It is not this author's practice to place an epidural catheter for VAT except in patients with severe pulmonary or cardiac disease.

ANESTHESIA FOR PATIENTS UNDERGOING BRONCHOSCOPY

Background

Although introduced in the 1890s, it remained for Chevalier Jackson to perfect the therapeutic application of bronchoscopy for retrieval of foreign bodies and diagnostic use in patients with neoplastic and inflammatory disease. The introduction of the fiberoptic bronchoscope has had a dramatic impact on the use of the technique.

The rigid bronchoscope is a hollow, metal tube with a blunted and beveled distal tip that allows insertion into the airway with minimal trauma. The proximal end is adapted for observation of the airway, maintenance of gas exchange, and introduction of surgical instruments. The proximal side arm is adapted for administration of oxygen or other gases and also enables mechanical ventilation during bronchoscopy. Within the wall of the bronchoscope, there are a series of channels for the illumination of the distal field and for suctioning secretions and blood. The large size of the rigid bronchoscope permits insertion of sponges, snares, knives, scissors, electrodes, and other special devices. The most common uses of a rigid bronchoscope are for retrieval of large foreign bodies, evaluation and debulking of bronchial tumors, access to bleeding sites, and overall evaluation of the airways.

Use of the flexible bronchoscope has supplanted that of the rigid instrument in many patients. The flexible fiberoptic bronchoscope contains clusters of glass fibers that illuminate the airway and transmit the visual image. Several hollow ports or channels are incorporated for suctioning, instillation of medications or lavage fluid, and for the introduction of accessory instruments. Flexion of the distal tip by cables allows the instrument to be directed to all segments of the tracheobronchial tree. Indications for fiberoptic bronchoscopy are listed in Box 70-8. Bronchoscopy often is only the first of several diagnostic or therapeutic procedures. After bronchoscopy, mediastinoscopy or thoracoscopy may be performed to further evaluate the presence of disease or for its management.

BOX 70-8
INDICATIONS FOR FIBEROPTIC BRONCHOSCOPY

Diagnostic indications

Staging and characterization of pulmonary disease
Evaluation of the site and etiology of pulmonary symptoms

Therapeutic indications

Tracheal intubation
Positioning of the double-lumen endotracheal tube
Removal of secrections and bronchial toilet
Laser of tumors

Flexible Fiberoptic Bronchoscopy

Anesthetic management

Flexible fiberoptic bronchoscopy is performed during local anesthesia in sedated spontaneously breathing patients or during general anesthesia with or without placement of an endotracheal tube (Table 70-9).

Awake fiberoptic bronchoscopy is performed after administration of sedation, an antisialagogue, and adequate local anesthesia. If the correct balance of these components is not achieved, serious trauma can result from coughing and movement of the uncomfortable patient. Techniques of anesthetizing the airway, which can be used alone or in combination,[108,213,231,252,454] include

- Topical application of local anesthetic to the nose, mouth, or oral pharynx
- Internal or percutaneous block of the superior laryngeal nerve
- Glossopharyngeal nerve block
- Recurrent laryngeal nerve block either by spraying of the tracheal bronchial mucosa from inside with local anesthetic or percutaneous transcricothyroid membrane injection

Table 70-9 Anesthetic guidelines for fiberoptic bronchoscopy and rigid bronchoscopy

	Fiberoptic bronchoscopy		Rigid bronchoscopy
Indication	Diagnostic, biopsy, lavage, confirm placement ETT		Therapeutic, laser, retrieval foreign body, pulmonary toilet
Monitors	Standard monitors		Same*
Anesthesia	General anesthesia, sedation with block		General anesthesia
Additional equipment			Shoulder roll
Airway	Awake spontaneous ventilation, single-lumen ETT (≥ 8 mm)		Apneic ventilation IPPB Jet ventilation
Position	Semirecumbent (awake patients)		Cervical extension
Unique considerations	Local and nerve blocks, antisialagogue		Lidocaine intravenously or intratracheal, muscle relaxation, antisialagogue
Intraoperative complications	Bronchospasm Bleeding Pneumomediastinum Pneumothorax Subcutaneous emphysema Barotrauma Hypoxia Hypercapnia	Vasovagal (bradycardia) Arrhythmias Fever (bacteremia)	Same* Dental trauma
Analgesia	Minimal pain (parental opiates)		
Postoperative morbidity	Atelectasis Bleeding and hemoptysis Bronchospasm Fever		Same*
Postoperative care	Chest radiography Humidified O_2 No eating or drinking until protective airway reflexes have returned		Same*

*Same as *Fiberoptic bronchoscopy.*

- Instillation of nebulized local anesthetic to the mucous membrane of the mouth, pharynx, larynx, trachea, and bronchi

The use of sedation and an antisialagogue improves bronchoscopic conditions. An anticholinergic, such as glycopyrrolate, is preferred because of the lack of central nervous system (CNS) side effects. A benzodiazepine is useful for anxiolysis and increasing the threshold for CNS toxicity to local anesthetics. Sedation should be used with caution, especially in elderly debilitated patients or in those with serious underlying respiratory compromise. Cardiac and respiratory function should be monitored during the procedure by a person who is not responsible for the endoscopy. After the procedure, the patient should be placed in a monitored environment initially to evaluate for complications from the procedure or the sedation.

Monitoring should follow the principles outlined in the section, "Monitoring During Thoracic Anesthesia." Because capnography often is unreliable during bronchoscopy, pulse oximetry is the most important monitor to assess the adequacy of oxygenation. Anesthetic treatment of patients undergoing bronchoscopy is similar to that for those undergoing lung resection. High fresh gas flow rates are indicated when suction is applied via the bronchoscope.

Ventilation management

In patients during general anesthesia, fiberoptic bronchoscopy usually is performed through an endotracheal tube. The resulting marked reduction in the effective functional internal diameter of the endotracheal tube available for ventilation is associated with increased airway resistance and can result in distal air trapping. To reduce complications, the anesthesiologist should avoid spontaneous ventilation, eliminate PEEP from the circuit, ventilate with a prolonged expiratory phase (inspiratory/expiratory [I/E] ratio of 1:3), and use the largest endotracheal tube possible. Suppression of airway reflexes to prevent laryngospasm and bronchospasm can be accomplished by the use of inhaled anesthetic agents and by the administration of lidocaine. A helium-O_2 mixture will decrease airway resistance.

Rigid Bronchoscopy

Anesthetic management

Maintenance of anesthesia can be achieved with mixtures of oxygen and potent inhalational anesthetics. Intravenous anesthetics and narcotics can either supplement or substitute for inhaled anesthetics. Topical anesthesia with lidocaine suppresses cough reflexes and prevents bronchospasm. Patients undergoing rigid bronchoscopy should be paralyzed to prevent sudden movement or cough, which can result in major morbidity.

Ventilation management

Intermittent positive pressure ventilation can be delivered during rigid bronchoscopy by connecting the standard anesthesia circuit to the ventilating side-port of the rigid bronchoscope (Fig. 70-33). This ventilating technique requires no special equipment, allows for accurate measurement of the FIO_2 and inhaled anesthetic concentration, and provides adequate oxygenation in most patients. The ventilating gases may leak through the space between the bronchoscope and the tracheal wall. To compensate for the leak, gas flows should be increased, and the posterior pharynx and larynx should be packed with gauze. The use of intermittent positive pressure ventilation creates much exposure of personnel to escaped anesthetic gases. Because ventilation is only possible when the eyepiece is in place, the cumulative effect of multiple periods of apnea may result in hypercapnia and cardiac dysrhythmias.

Jet ventilation

The use of Venturi (jet) ventilation has been advocated for prolonged rigid bronchoscopy. The Venturi ventilation technique allows the surgeon an unhurried, undisturbed period of viewing without need for an eyepiece. A potential disadvantage is that jet ventilation can result in spillage of blood and other debris into the tracheobronchial tree.

An intermittent high velocity jet of oxygen entrains air into the bronchoscope, resulting in expansion of the lungs. If the lungs are noncompliant or if the bronchoscope is small in relation to the trachea, large amounts of the tidal volume will escape between the bronchoscope and tracheal wall, resulting in poor alveolar ventilation. Careful observation of the patient's chest movement is necessary to ensure adequate tidal volumes. The adequacy of ventilation, a function of total thoracic compliance, can be monitored by obtaining an arterial blood sample, by transcutaneous CO_2 monitoring, or by intermittent capnography. It is difficult to know the inspired concentration of oxygen because of the variable entrainment of room air, but the adequacy of oxygenation can be monitored by pulse oximetry or arterial blood gas sampling.

The intraluminal pressure is a function of the driving pressure from the in-line reducing valve, size and length of the needle jet, and design of the bronchoscope. In addition, a decrease in the effective intraluminal diameter by the introduction of suction catheters or biopsy forceps can prevent escape of gas introduced by the jet and results in a dramatic increase in intratracheal pressure. If the instruments are tight-fitting, the driving pressure should be decreased to prevent barotrauma.

The apparatus described by Sanders used a high-pressure oxygen source of 50 psi, which was delivered through a 16- or 18-gauge needle located within the rigid bronchoscope (Fig. 70-34). The original jet ventilation system has been improved by connecting the side arm to the anesthesia circuit, thereby entraining an oxygen anesthetic gas mixture. Increasing the size of the jet port (the Carden side arm) results in increased inflation pressure and increased FIO_2 at the distal tip of the bronchoscope.[89] Jet ventilation at low frequencies can provide for adequate oxygenation and ventilation. Commercial high-frequency jet ventilators (HFJV) have been used with the rigid bronchoscope. Rates of 150 to 300 breaths per minute result in ventilation and oxygenation comparable with intermittent low frequency jet ventila-

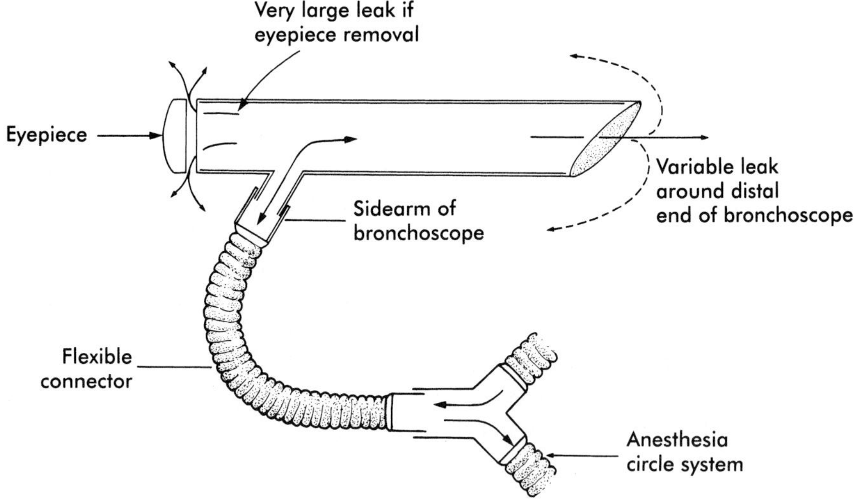

Fig. 70-33. Schematic diagram showing a rigid ventilating bronchoscope system, which consists of the anesthesia circle system attached to a flexible connector that is attached to the sidearm of the bronchoscope. With the proximal eyepiece in place, most of the inspired gas goes into the patient. Because the bronchoscope cannot fully fill the area of the trachea, there is a variable leak around the distal end of the bronchoscope. Exhaled gases are through the anesthesia circle system. When the eyepiece is removed, there is a very large leak out the proximal end of the bronchoscope. (Modified from Benumof JL: Anesthesia for special elective diagnostic procedures. In Benumof JL, editor: *Anesthesia for thoracic surgery*, Philadelphia, 1995, WB Saunders.)

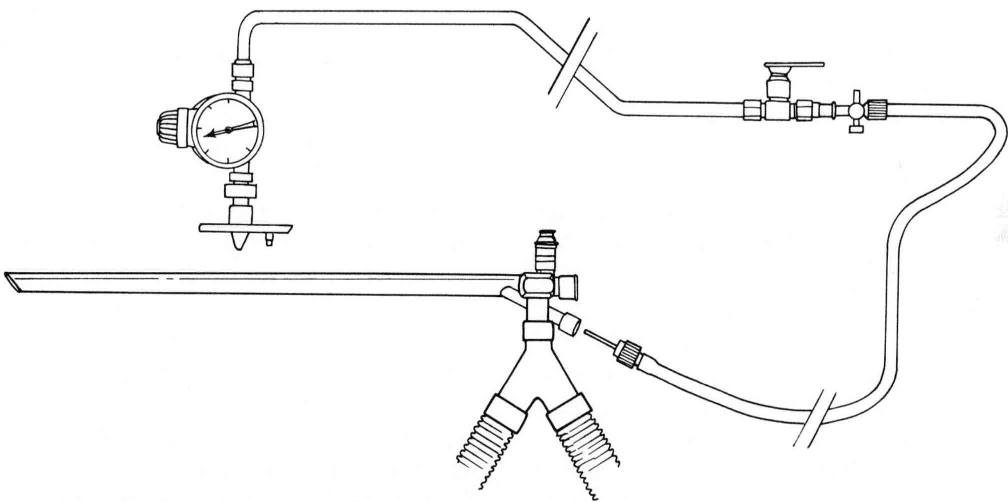

Fig. 70-34. Components needed for jet ventilation through the bronchoscope (Sanders injector). Wall connector for oxygen supply, reducing valve and pressure gauge, high pressure tubing, toggle switch, needle injector jet. (From Eisenkraft JB, Neustein SM: *Problems in anesthesia,* vol 4, Philadelphia, 1990, JB Lippincott.)

tion,[442] but rates greater than 300 breaths per minute result in a decrease in oxygenation and an increase in $Pa{CO_2}$. The major advantage of HFJV over low frequency jet ventilation is that there is less movement of the tracheobronchial tree, providing better surgical conditions for such procedures as laser therapy.

Apneic oxygenation

In the absence of ventilation, adequate oxygenation can be maintained for a prolonged period at the expense of increasing $Pa{CO_2}$. Initially, the patient is ventilated with 100% inspired oxygen until complete denitrogenation is achieved. A small catheter is placed above the carina and insufflated with O_2 at 10 to 15 l/minute. The period of apnea may be associated with a dramatic increase in $Pa{CO_2}$. The arterial concentration of CO_2 increases 6 mm Hg during the first minute followed by a 3 or 4 mm increase for each subsequent minute.[143,365] Therefore, a period of hyperventilation, to a $Pa{CO_2}$ of approximately 30 mm Hg, will increase the period of apnea that can be tolerated before respiratory acidosis ensues. The adequacy of oxygen reserve and generation of CO_2 are functions of pulmonary mechanics and body size.

Only those patients with a predicted FRC-to-body weight ratio of 50 ml/kg or greater should be allowed to remain apneic for more than 5 minutes. Increasing the flow of oxygen from 0.7 l/kg/min to 1.2 l/kg/min decreases the rate of increase of the $Paco_2$ in anesthetized apneic patients.[24,25,404,405]

Complications

Bronchoscopy and local anesthesia of the airway may be associated with perioperative morbidity. Complications of local anesthesia include pulmonary aspiration caused by loss of airway sensation and reflexes and toxic side effects of overdosage. Bronchoscopy alters pulmonary mechanics. Patients may exhibit decreases in FEV_1, FVC, peak expiratory flow rate, and peak inspiratory flow rate. Additional factors that may contribute to decreased lung function or bronchospasm include airway mucosal edema and mechanical activation of irritated airway reflexes.[278] These responses may in part be mediated by the vagus nerve because preoperative administration of an anticholinergic agent, such as glycopyrrolate or atropine, has been shown to prevent or attenuate them.

Rigid bronchoscopy is associated with more trauma than flexible fiberoptic bronchoscopy. Positioning of the patient and placement of the rigid bronchoscope can result in dental trauma or laceration of the mucosa of the larynx, trachea, or bronchi. The trauma has been associated with pneumomediastinum, pneumothorax, and perforation of the esophagus. The cervical hyperextension that is required for placement of the rigid bronchoscope can cause injury to the cervical spine, vasovagal reaction, and cerebral ischemia by occlusion of vertebral arteries.

Hypoxia is a common complication during rigid bronchoscopy.[9,10,135,365] Inadequate ventilation during rigid bronchoscopy can result from large air leaks along the space between the bronchoscope and the tracheal wall or from periods of apnea. There can be a serious loss of lung volume associated with plugging and atelectasis, which may be minimized by pulmonary toilet and ventilation with large tidal volumes. At the end of a procedure during general anesthesia, a single-lumen endotracheal tube should be placed, and the lung should be suctioned and ventilated with large tidal volumes.

Transient cardiac dysrhythmias are common in patients undergoing bronchoscopy.[68,154] Their causes include hypoxia, intense stimulation, hypoventilation with hypercapnia, inadequate depth of anesthesia, vasovagal reaction, and proarrhythmic agents such as halothane, β_2 adrenergic agonists, and bronchodilators.

Postoperative Concerns

Barotrauma with resultant interstitial emphysema, pneumomediastinum, and pneumothorax can occur after fiberoptic and rigid bronchoscopy. To minimize this risk, fiberoptic bronchoscopy should be performed through the largest possible endotracheal tube. Postoperatively, patients may manifest dyspnea or evidence of airway obstruction. Subglottic and mucosal airway edema can result from mechanical irritation.[317,389] In addition, bleeding into the airway can result in reactive bronchospasm. Physical examination should confirm the absence of wheezing or stridor and the presence of bilateral breath sounds. A chest radiograph should be obtained to look for signs of pulmonary emphysema, mediastinal emphysema, or pneumothorax. Initial strategies for management include inhalation of cool moisturized oxygen and use of a bronchodilator. Further specific therapies may entail placement of chest tubes, administration of diuretics, pulmonary toilet, or repeat bronchoscopy.

ANESTHESIA FOR PATIENTS UNDERGOING BRONCHOALVEOLAR LAVAGE

Bronchopulmonary lavage is indicated for management of alveolar proteinosis.[98,124,163,221,274,286,357] The long-term improvements in arterial oxygenation, exercise tolerance, and level of activity vary from patient to patient. Some patients require annual or semiannual lavage, whereas others remain in remission for years.[382] The pathophysiology of the disease is characterized by the abnormal bilateral accumulation of alveolar surfactant.[245,381] Its accumulation is attributed to a failure of clearance mechanisms rather than increased formation. Most patients are diagnosed between the ages of 20 and 50 years and have symptoms of cough, fever, and chest pain. Pulmonary function tests and chest radiographs are abnormal, but definitive diagnosis requires lung biopsy. Indications for lavage include Pao_2 less than 60 mm Hg at rest or hypoxic limitation of normal activity.

Intraoperative Management

Unilateral lung lavage is performed by irrigation of the tracheobronchial tree during general anesthesia (Table 70-10, Fig. 70-35). The preoperative assessment should include ventilation-perfusion scans to characterize the distribution of impairment. Unilateral lung lavage requires placement of a double-lumen endotracheal tube to prevent spillage to the contralateral lung. Monitoring should include placement of an arterial catheter to measure blood gases perioperatively. General anesthesia is induced with intravenous agents and maintained with potent inhaled agents. The trachea then is intubated with the largest left-sided double-lumen endotracheal tube that can be positioned properly.[47] Correct tube position is essential; it should be confirmed with a fiberoptic bronchoscope. Functional isolation should be confirmed using the bubble test previously described (see Fig. 70-19). To prevent leakage of lavage fluid into the contralateral lung, it has been suggested that the bronchial cuff be inflated to functionally separate the lungs at 50 cm/water.[54] The patient should be ventilated with 100% oxygen to minimize the risk of hypoxemia and eliminate nitrogen from the lung. Failure to adequately denitrogenate before lavage may leave peripheral nitrogen bubbles and thus limit effectiveness of the procedure.

The positioning of the patient is somewhat controversial.

Table 70-10 Anesthetic guidelines for bronchial alveolar lavage

Indication	Diagnostic
	Therapeutic (alveolar proteinosis, cystic fibrosis)
Monitors	Standard monitoring, optional (arterial catheter)
Anesthesia	General anesthesia (allows for sequential lavages on both sides)
	Awake, sedated (lavage by bronchoscopy limited to lobe)
Ventilation	Left double-lumen ETT
Position	Lateral decubitus
	Supine
Unique considerations	Single-lung ventilation
	To prevent spillage to the opposite lung, endobronchial balloon should be inflated to functionally separate lungs (about 50 cm water)
	(1) Drain 700–1000 ml warm saline into lung
	(2) Manual chest percussion
	(3) Drainage of fluid in Trendelenburg position
	(4) Repeat until turbidity clears
	(5) Repeat for contralateral lung
	(6) Maintain accurate account of infusion and drainage volumes
	(7) After lavage is completed, suction both lungs thoroughly ventilate with PEEP
Intraoperative complications	Spillage of lavage fluid to contralateral lung
	Hypoxia
	Decrease pulmonary compliance
	Pneumothorax, hydropneumothorax
	Pulmonary edema
Analgesia	None required
Postoperative care	Supplement O_2
	Chest radiography

Lavage of the nondependent lung in the lateral decubitus position has the advantage of improving oxygenation by decreasing blood flow to the nonventilated lung, although this arrangement also increases the risk of spillage from the nondependent to the dependent lung. Lavage of the dependent lung decreases the possibility of spillage, but it may be associated with hypoxia resulting from shunt flow. The supine position balances the risk of aspiration against the risk of hypoxia.

The choice of which lung to lavage first is based on the ventilation and perfusion studies. The lung with the least perfusion is chosen to be lavaged first, to favor gas exchange during single-lung ventilation, and to avoid hypoxia. The procedure is performed by instilling warm, isotonic saline by gravity from a height of 30 cm. The lung will accept 700 to 1000 ml of lavage fluid in the adult.[54] Vigorous manual chest percussion is applied to the hemithorax throughout the lavage.[453] Then, the lavage fluid is drained passively into a collecting system. The lavage procedure is repeated until the drainage decreases in turbidity to near clarity so that it is possible to read fine print through an 0.25-inch diameter column of fluid. Typically, 12 l to 30 l of saline is required. Accurate records of fluid administration and drainage are kept. After the effluent lavage fluid clears, the procedure is terminated, the lavaged lung thoroughly suctioned, and ventilation is reestablished. Because the lavaged lung has decreased compliance, it is ventilated with a large tidal volume (15 to 20 ml/kg) to reexpand the alveoli.[54] To improve compliance during the immediate post-procedure period, the patient should be positioned to enhance drainage, and secretions should be suctioned from the airway. When compliance of the lavaged hemithorax approaches baseline, the neuromuscular blockade is reversed, and the patient is evaluated for extubation.

During the lavage procedure, most patients remain hemodynamically stable, although this procedure may increase right heart strain and decrease left ventricular filling and systemic blood pressure.[418] Arterial oxygen saturation increases during lung filling and decreases with drainage. The increase in intraalveolar pressure, resulting from fluid administration, causes an increase in pulmonary vascular resistance, thereby diverting blood flow to the ventilated side and decreasing the venous admixture. When the lavage fluid is drained, the pulmonary vascular resistance decreases, and the venous admixture increases.

Spillage of lavage fluid into the untreated lung is a serious complication. Leakage is detected by the appearance of bubbles in the lavage fluid, rales or rhonchi in the ventilated lung, discrepancy between the drained lavage fluid volumes, and arterial desaturation. If spillage is suspected, lavage should be stopped, the lung drained, and position of the double-lumen endotracheal tube confirmed. Massive spillage produces acute decreases in lung compliance and severe arterial desaturation (Box 70-9). An unusual but serious com-

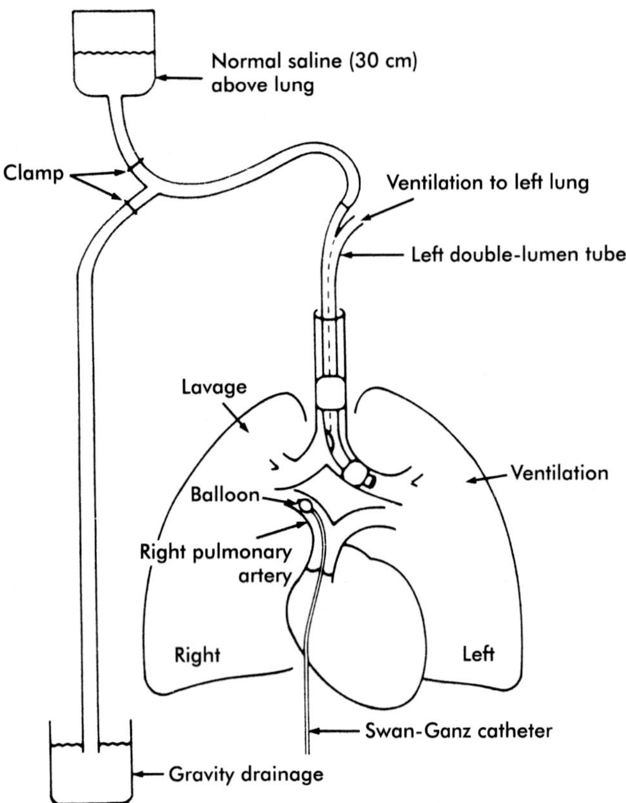

Fig. 70-35. Schematic of the experimental preparation. A canine double-lumen endotracheal tube allows ventilation of the left lung while the right lung is lavaged. Saline is infused at a constant pressure of 23 mm Hg (= 30 cm H_2O) and then drained by gravity pressure. A balloon-tipped catheter is located in the right main pulmonary artery. (From Moazam F, Schmidt JH, Chesrown SE, et al: Total lung lavage for pulmonary alveolar proteinosis in an infant without the use of cardiopulmonary bypass, *J Pediatr Surg* 20:398, 1985.)

BOX 70-9
STEPS TO TAKE AFTER MASSIVE SPILLAGE OF FLUID DURING BRONCHOALVEOLAR LAVAGE

Immediately terminate the lavage procedure
Turn the patient to the lateral decubitus position with the lavaged side dependent
Place the operating table in a head-down position
Perform vigorous suctioning and inflation of both lungs
When arterial oxygenation is improved, replace the double-lumen tube with a single-lumen tube
Do not extubate the patient; provide mechanical ventilation with positive end-expiratory pressure (PEEP) until the functional residual capacity (FRC) and compliance of both lungs are restored

plication of lung lavage is hydropneumothorax. One case report describes increased peak airway pressures and decreased oxygen saturation 20 minutes after an uneventful lung lavage. A chest radiograph revealed mediastinal shift and a left pneumothorax. It was hypothesized that lung lavage decreased lung compliance by washing out surfactants, making it more susceptible to barotrauma. A chest radiograph should be obtained routinely within the first hour after lavage and compared with prelavage examination.[179]

Patients with marginal cardiac or pulmonary reserve or pediatric patients who weigh less than 30 kg who are unable to receive a small double-lumen tube may require an alternate method of bronchial lavage or oxygenation. Alternatives include (1) Extracorporeal membrane oxygenation (ECMO);[14,106,472] (2) Partial venoarterial cardiopulmonary bypass or venovenous bypass;[172,474] (3) Lobar lavage via fiberoptic bronchoscopy (which can be performed in an awake sedated adult during topical anesthesia). This method requires a cuffed bronchoscope inserted into the lobar bronchus through which the lavage is performed.[304] In children too small to place a double-lumen endotracheal tube, lavage may be accomplished either by using a cuffed bronchoscope or a pulmonary artery catheter inserted into the airway via a rigid bronchoscope; and (4) Positioning of a pulmonary artery catheter in the ipsilateral lavaged side.[12] Inflation of the balloon will divert blood toward the ventilated lung, thereby decreasing the venous admixture, although prolonged inflation of a pulmonary artery catheter increases the risk of pulmonary artery rupture.

ANESTHESIA FOR PATIENTS WITH BRONCHOPLEURAL FISTULA

Etiology

The possibility of a bronchopleural fistual should be considered after pneumonectomy, lobectomy, bullectomy, or volume reduction surgery. The symptoms and findings of a clinically significant bronchopleural fistula include dyspnea, subcutaneous emphysema, contralateral deviation of the trachea, expectoration of purulent material, a persistent air leak, and purulent drainage from the chest tube. Diagnosis is confirmed by bronchoscopy and bronchography.

Certain factors predispose patients to develop air leaks after lung resection, including cancer, malnourishment, debilitation, poor general condition, trauma, barotrauma, lung abscesses, immunosuppression, steroid therapy, diabetics, preoperative or postoperative radiation therapy, and pulmonary resection for tuberculosis. Failure of the remaining lung to expand after lung resection to fill the void predisposes to development of bronchopleural fistula. A continued air leak can lead to infection in the pleural space and dehiscence of the bronchial stump.[412]

Surgical Management

When bronchopleural fistula occurs early after resection, prompt resuturing of the bronchial stump may correct it. If the fistula develops later after operation, adequate drainage and reduction of the pleural space constitute initial therapy. Many small fistulas will close spontaneously. If the lung expands to fill the thoracic cavity, the leak usually can be controlled with chest tube drainage. A persistent space indicates a leak from a larger bronchus, usually requiring surgical treatment.[412] Sepsis should be controlled with antibiotics and adequate chest drainage.

Surgical options include (1) decortication if the lung is trapped by a thick purulent layer; (2) shortening of an excessively long bronchial stump, with or without resection of additional lung tissue; (3) closure of the bronchopleural fistula with a pedicled muscle flap, usually in the form of an intercostal flap;[36,128,450] (4) thoracoplasty to obliterate the pleural space, usually combined with a pedicled muscle flap to cover the bronchial stump; and (5) the most recently described method, flexible fiberoptic bronchoscopic application of fibrin glue to seal the communication between the bronchus and the pleural space.

Ventilation

Anesthesiologists care for patients with bronchopleural fistula either in the ICU when respiratory failure and sepsis require ventilator management or in the operating room. Goals include maintenance of adequate ventilation and oxygenation and protection of the contralateral lung from spillage of purulent material. Application of positive pressure by a mask or a mechanical ventilator leads to apparent inadequate ventilation because most of the tidal volume is lost through the fistula. Several methods have been developed to improve the ventilation of patients with bronchopleural fistula and decrease the risk of pneumothorax. Chest tubes with unidirectional valves have been used to prevent air leak during spontaneous inspiration. During positive pressure ventilation, low inflation pressures should be used, and spontaneous ventilation with pressure support should be encouraged to decrease the air leak and to promote closure of the bronchopleural fistula. High-frequency ventilation has been used to manage bronchopleural fistula but with varying results.[8,61,333]

The proposed advantage of high-frequency ventilation is that lower inspiratory pressures and smaller tidal volumes may result in less gas leak through the fistula. Mediastinal or interstitial emphysema may be less with this form of management. To achieve a decrease in air leak through the fistula, the method used for ventilation should provide lower peak and mean airway pressures. Studies performed in animals with healthy lungs show that HFJV was effective in decreasing the air leak through the bronchopleural fistula while maintaining adequate oxygenation and CO_2 elimination. Ultra-HFJV with rates of 450 beats per minute is even more effective than HFJV (120 breaths/minute) in reducing air leaks.[333] Studies in patients who had lung injury, ARDS, and noncompliant lungs produced different results. In these patients, oxygenation and CO_2 elimination were less effective with HFJV than with conventional ventilation. Because the airway pressures were comparable, no difference in air leak across the fistula was found between the two groups. Some patients even had increased air leak with HFJV.[8,12] Adequate oxygenation and CO_2 elimination could have been achieved with HFJV by altering the ventilatory settings, increasing the inspiratory time, and increasing the driving gas pressure, although this would have resulted in greater airway pressures and a further increase in the air leak across the fistula.

Therefore, HFJV may be of benefit only in some patients with bronchopleural fistula. It appears to be less effective when patients have bilaterally diseased, noncompliant lungs. The improvement in the air leak depends on a decrease in peak and mean airway pressures; it is recommended that tracheal pressures and air flow through the leak be measured during HFJV and compared with values obtained during conventional mechanical ventilation. The least airway pressure that allows adequate oxygenation and CO_2 elimination will be most advantageous for these patients.[8] HFJV does not isolate the two lungs, allowing for possible contamination of the contralateral lung by spillage of purulent material from the affected side, especially if an empyema or lung abscess is present.

Anesthetic Management

Intraoperative treatment of patients with bronchopleural fistula presents unique challenges. Management strategies for induction and intubation depend on the severity of the bronchopleural fistula and presence of infection. If a chest tube is not in place or is malfunctioning, a tension pneumothorax may result. Because positive pressure ventilation increases the air leak and risks contaminating the noninfected lung, patients often are induced using rapid sequence induction to minimize the time before tracheal intubation and lung isolation. An alternative approach uses intubation with a double-lumen tube in a spontaneously ventilating patient. Conscious sedation or neuroleptic analgesia has been used to provide a comfortable and cooperative patient.[147] Awake intubation should be considered for patients at increased risk for aspiration of gastric contents caused by full stomach or a bronchopleuroenteric fistula.[96] Once the tube has been positioned, the healthy lung should be isolated immediately, and the head placed slightly raised. The infected lung should be placed in a 30° dependent position to decrease the likelihood of contamination of the healthy lung.

In patients with a small chronic bronchopleural fistula with a minimal air leak and no associated infection or empyema, a standard endotracheal tube can probably be used safely. If intermittent positive pressure ventilation is then found to be inadequate, the tube can be advanced into the bronchus of the healthy side or replaced with a double-lumen tube. If an empyema is present, it should be drained during local anesthesia, and a chest tube should be placed before induction of anesthesia. This decreases the amount of pus in the pleural cavity, decreases the chance of flooding the contralateral lung, and provides a protective measure against the development of a tension pneumothorax. If intermittent positive pressure ventilation using a double-lumen tube provides inadequate oxygenation or ventilation, HFJV to the affected lung through the double-lumen tube is another option.[42] When a double-lumen tube cannot be used, as in pediatric patients or in those with difficult airway anatomy, lung separation can be achieved by endobronchial placement of a single-lumen endotracheal tube or by an endotracheal tube together with a bronchial blocker.

ANESTHETIC IMPLICATIONS OF SPONTANEOUS PNEUMOTHORAX

Patients who develop spontaneous pneumothorax usually are young, healthy, and sometimes athletic, with no preexisting lung disease and no previous lung resections. Surgical treatment for spontaneous pneumothorax includes pleurectomy and chemical pleurodesis.[376]

Surgical treatment is indicated in the following situations: (1) failure of the pneumothorax to resolve with chest tube drainage and suction, which indicates that bronchopleural fistula has formed; (2) if a second ipsilateral or a first contralateral spontaneous pneumothorax occurs; and (3) if the patient's lifestyle is such that a recurrence may be life-threatening or highly inconvenient (recurrence rate for spontaneous pneumothorax is 10% to 25%).

When patients with pneumothorax come to the operating room, they typically have a chest tube in place, and therefore tension pneumothorax usually is not a major concern. Patients usually are treated with a double-lumen endotracheal tube to facilitate surgical exposure for either thoracoscopy or thoracotomy. If a single-lumen tube is placed and if the air leak is too large, a single-lumen tube can be advanced into the bronchus of the unaffected side with the guidance of a fiberoptic bronchoscope or replaced with a double-lumen tube.

ANESTHESIA FOR PATIENTS UNDERGOING BULLECTOMY AND VOLUME REDUCTION PNEUMOPLASTY

There has been a resurgence in the surgical management of bullous disease and emphysema. The rationale for the surgical resection of the diseased lung is to remove areas of nonfunctional lung to permit reexpansion of compressed functional alveoli and to improve diaphragmatic function. Multiple studies have documented the efficacy of this procedure for patents with isolated large bullae, although the benefits of resection of diseased peripheral lung tissue in the presence of bullous emphysema is less certain. Large multicenter trials are under way to assess the efficacy of this therapeutic modality.

Bullae are air-filled spaces within the lung parenchyma. As bullae expand, the volume of the remaining lung is reduced (Fig. 70-36). Plication of large bullae improves lung function by recruiting previously compressed atelectatic lung.[318,324] Preoperative evaluation includes pulmonary function testing, chest radiograph, CT, and ventilation-perfusion scanning to predict which patients will benefit from bullectomy. **Patients most likely to benefit from the plication of large bullae are those in whom the bullae occupies greater than 30% of the hemithorax,[107,275,459] those with progressively enlarging nonfunctional pulmonary units and recurrent pneumothoraces, and those with moderate-to-severe dyspnea that is refractory to conventional medical therapy.[275]** A prospective trial with 20 patients re-

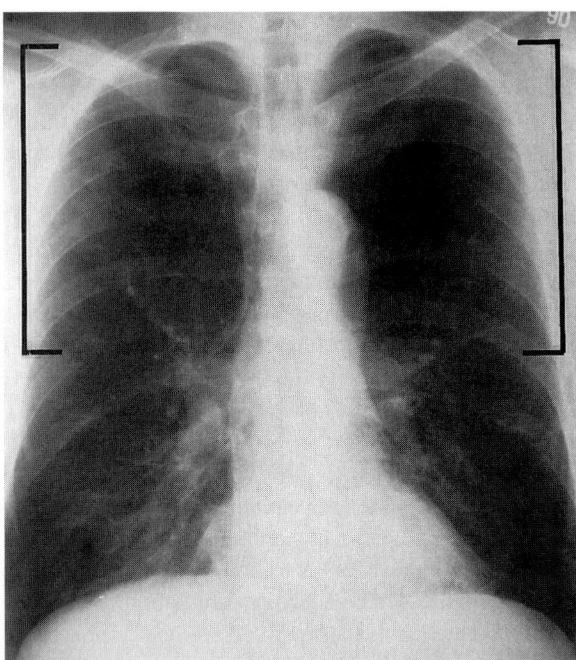

Fig. 70-36. Characteristic radiographic findings of patients with bullous disease. Typical findings in patients with COPD include an increased size of lung fields and flattened hemidiaphragms. The appearance of hyperaeration of both apical lung fields (*bracketed area*), decreased vascular marking in upper lung fields, and compressive atelectasis of the lower lung fields also are consistent with severe bullous lung disease.

ported an increase in FEV_1 (0.77 to 1.4 l), FVC (2.2 to 2.8 l), and arterial oxygenation on inspired room air (64 to 70 mm Hg). The patients experienced less dyspnea and improved quality of life during the next six months. The beneficial effects were attributed to expansion of the remaining lung and improved diaphragmatic function, resulting in improved respiratory mechanics and decreased ventilation to perfusion mismatching. Another study reported more modest improvements in symptoms and pulmonary function analysis (FEV_1, 1.74 to 1.85 l ; FVC, 1.82 to 2.21 l) and was associated with a mortality rate of 5.5%.[448] It is not known whether the difference between these two studies reflected patient selection or a difference in surgical technique. In the first study, resection was performed by open thoracotomy using a stapler, and in the latter study, resection was accomplished by thoracoscopy using laser technology. The goals of future studies will be to improve surgical techniques, ascertain the efficacy of volume reduction surgery, and define the patient population who would benefit most from the procedure.

Surgery

These procedures may be performed as single unilateral, sequential unilateral, or bilateral operations. Single unilateral bullectomy and volume reduction procedures are performed using the lateral decubitus position and video thoracoscopy or open thoracotomy. Sequential unilateral procedures can be performed by repositioning the patient to the contralateral decubitus position after the first side is completed. Bilateral procedures can be performed through a median sternotomy. Median sternotomy does not require repositioning and provides access to the contralateral pleural space in patients with pneumothorax. Plication of bullae and resection of peripheral lung tissue are accomplished with the use of a stapler. A major complicating factor in postoperative recovery is persistent air leaks at the suture line. This problem is decreased by using a stapler with a pericardial buttress.[107]

Anesthetic Considerations

These patients have poor respiratory reserve and challenge the anesthesiologist during induction, single-lung ventilation, and extubation.[266,426] Before operation, the patients often are dyspneic and require supplemental oxygen. Many may have been considered for lung transplantation, but they were excluded because of their age or presence of coexisting diseases. Their tenuous cardiopulmonary status requires judicious use of any benzodiazepines or narcotics. In addition to the standard monitors, an arterial catheter should be placed to assess adequacy of oxygen and ventilation perioperatively.

Either thoracotomy or thoracoscopy require general anesthesia and single-lung ventilation (Table 70-11). The combination of general anesthesia and epidural analgesia decreases the anesthetic requirement intraoperatively, thereby minimizing postoperative residual sedation. Patients with end-stage emphysema tend to have increased endogenous catecholamines caused by hypoxia and hypercapnia, often are hypovolemic, and are at risk for marked hypotension after induction of general anesthesia. General anesthesia can be maintained with either inhalation of intravenous agents or with a combination of techniques. Nitrous oxide should be avoided because of the risk of increasing the size of bullae, further compressing the adjacent lung or causing

Table 70-11 Anesthetic guidelines for bullectomy and volume reduction pneumoplasty

	Bullectomy/volume reduction pneumoplasty	Volume reduction pneumoplasty
Indication	Bullectomy—large bullae > 30% of hemithorax	Severe bullous emphysema
	Volume reduction-severe bullous emphysema	
Preoperative concerns	Review preoperative PFTs and ✔ABG	Same*
	Pulmonary symptoms may mask presence of CAD	
Monitors	Standard monitors and A-line	Same*
Anesthesia	General anesthesia	Same*
	Combined regional/general anesthesia	
Additional equipment	Optional (jet ventilator)	Same*
Ventilation	Double lumen endotracheal tube	Same*
Position	Bullectomy (lateral decubitus)	Lateral decubitus
	Volume reduction pneumoplasty (lateral, supine)	Supine (median sternotomy)
Incision	Bullectomy (thoracotomy, VATS)	Thoracotomy
	Volume reduction pneumoplasty (thoracotomy, VATS, median sternotomy)	VATS
		Median sternotomy
Unique considerations	Single-lung ventilation	Same*
	Avoid PEEP or nitrous oxide	
	Minimize use of long lasting respiratory depressants	
	Restrict administration of intravenous fluids	
Intraoperative complications	Tension pneumothorax	Same*
	Pneumothorax	
	Hypoxia	
	Hypercarbia	
Blood loss	Minimal < 500 ml	Same*
Postoperative analgesia	Epidural	Same*
	Parenteral opiates/NSAIDs	Same*
Postoperative morbidity	Persistent air leak	
	Respiratory dysfunction	Same*
	Hypoxia	
	Hypercarbia	
	Pneumothorax	
	Difficulty weaning from ventilator	
Postoperative care	Monitor respiratory status overnight for signs of decompension	
	O_2 supplement	
	CXR	
	Adequate analgesia	
	Minimize air leak by placing chest tubes to water seal or minimizing suction	

*Same as *Bullectomy/volume reduction pneumoplasty.*

rupture. Communications between bullae and the airway may function as one-way valves, resulting in air trapping with rapid enlargement and compression of the surrounding lung. Initiation of controlled ventilation may be associated with hypoxia and hypercapnia. Acute rupture of bullae with resulting pneumothorax is a constant threat. An acute decrease in blood pressure associated with increased inspiratory pressures and loss of breath sounds should be considered a pneumothorax unless proven otherwise. The prompt placement of a chest tube can avert catastrophe. Low inflation pressures will decrease the risk of pneumothorax.

One-lung ventilation with a double-lumen tube facilitates bilateral volume reduction by providing selective ventilation, yet retaining the capacity for intermittent ventilation of the operative lung to manage hypoxia or hypercapnia or to assist the surgeon in identifying the location of bullae. Initiation of single-lung ventilation is associated with an increase in airway pressure and the concomitant risk of pneumothorax. Jet ventilation has been used to decrease airway pressures. The nonoperated, ventilated lung should be prepped and draped to allow access in case of a pneumothorax. Increased concentrations of halogenated anesthetics may worsen the venous admixture by inhibition of HPV. A continuous infusion of propofol is an excellent adjunct or substitute for inhaled anesthetics.

Postoperative Ventilation

Extubation of the trachea at the end of operation can be accomplished in most patients. The need for continued mechanical ventilation is greater after volume reduction pneumoplasty as compared with plication of bullae. The beneficial effects of operation are not realized immediately after operation. Volume reduction patients may decompensate in response to the usual decrement in postoperative pulmonary function associated with thoracic surgery and pain. They also seem to be more sensitive to residual sedation, respiratory depression from analgesics, residual muscle relaxants, or hypercapnia. The presence of a major air leak can interfere with respiratory function. Criteria for extubation include the presence of a regular respiratory pattern, adequate patient strength, alertness, ability to respond to command, and measurement of an arterial blood gas. If mechanical ventilation is required postoperatively, positive airway pressure should be minimized to decrease the chance of producing pneumothorax from rupture of residual bullae or suture lines. If air leak remains an important factor, airway peak pressure may be minimized by changing the mode of ventilation to pressure control. In addition, the chest tube suction should be put to water seal or at least the suction pressure should be minimal.

ANESTHESIA FOR PATIENTS UNDERGOING DECORTICATION AND PLEURODESIS PROCEDURES

Clinical Features

The pleural space is a virtual cavity between the chest wall and lungs. The visceral and parietal pleura are about two-mm thick and are permeable to fluid and cells. Pleural inflammation, either infectious or noninfectious, increases permeability and results in the collection of high protein pleural fluid. Lymphatic obstruction, altered central venous pressures, and low oncotic pressure contribute to pleural fluid accumulation. Large effusions may dramatically decrease pulmonary function. Additionally, the collection of blood or empyema precipitates deposition of a fibrin layer on the pleura. As the fibrin layer (or peel) matures, the underlying lung is entrapped, and lung expansion is decreased, necessitating surgical intervention to release and expand collapsed lung and to manage infection.

The signs and symptoms of pleural disease include fever, chills, pleuritic chest pain, dyspnea, and hemoptysis. The causative factor for an empyema may be rupture of an abscess into the bronchus and may result in expectoration of foul-smelling purulent sputum or episodes of hemoptysis. Such patients may be cyanotic, hypovolemic, and hypotensive because of bacteremia and release of endotoxins. Preoperative studies include chest radiography and CT scans to locate the site of effusion or empyema.

Patients with a simple nonloculated empyema may be treated conservatively with antibiotic therapy and chest tube drainage. Once the empyema becomes loculated or develops into a fibrous peel, surgical intervention by thoracotomy or thoracoscopy is performed during general anesthesia. The access provided by VAT may be limited, and open thoracotomy is required for more definitive procedure. Perioperative complications include sepsis, wound infection, bronchopleural fistula, and air leaks. Failure to adequately manage a chronic draining empyema may require the placement of an open window thoracostomy for long-term care. This procedure consists of suturing a flap of skin to the pleura, creating an epithelial-lined sinus into the empyema cavity.

Most transudative and noninfected exudative pleural effusions are managed by treatment of the underlying disease. Occasionally, additional intervention is required either because the effusion causes respiratory compromise or is refractory to medical therapy. Management of malignant effusions may require decortication and pleurodesis. A number of agents have been used intrapleurally to produce a chemical pleurodesis that leads to formation of adhesions and obliteration of the pleural space. Common sclerosing agents include tetracycline, talc, and bleomycin. Fever and chest pain are the most common complications of pleurodesis.

Anesthesia Management

Surgical decortication requires the differential ventilation of the healthy and diseased lung to facilitate surgical exposure and to permit complete reexpansion after surgical intervention.[240] After induction and tracheal intubation, patients usually are placed in a lateral decubitus position with the affected lung in the nondependent position. In patients with a lung abscess, placement of an infected lung in the nondependent position increases the risk of contamination to the dependent lung. Most common management issues involve hypovolemia related to bleeding or sepsis and pain associated with decortication and pleurodesis. Inability to remove the fibrous peel may result in failure to reexpand the entrapped lung. After the decortication procedure is completed, positive pressure can be applied to the diseased lung to help break residual fibrous deposition, thus enabling lung reexpansion. Options for postoperative analgesia include patient-controlled analgesia and placement of an epidural catheter.

ANESTHESIA FOR PATIENTS UNDERGOING ESOPHAGEAL SURGERY

Dysphagia is the most common symptom of esophageal disease. **When present for any major length of time, dysphagia can result in dramatic weight loss, dehydration, hypoalbuminemia, anemia, and depressed immune status.** Postprandial heartburn, another common symptom of esophageal disease, is related to reflux of gastric contents into the esophagus. Symptoms may manifest with change in position, exercise, or belching. Patients who experience such symptoms usually are evaluated by barium swallow under fluoroscopy, followed by esophagoscopy and tissue biopsy. Common esophageal lesions are summarized in Box 70-10.

Esophagoscopy

Esophagoscopy is used for tissue biopsy or clarification of esophageal lesions detected after barium contrast studies. In addition, esophagoscopy is used for removal of foreign bodies, dilation of esophageal strictures, sclerotherapy of esophageal varices, diagnosis and management of bleeding lesions, and placement of prosthetic stents across malignant strictures.

Esophagoscopy can be performed using either a rigid or a flexible fiberoptic esophagoscope. Flexible esophagoscopy allows for greater comfort while examining the upper gastrointestinal tract and usually is performed on awake, slightly sedated patients. Although rigid esophagoscopy can be performed on awake, sedated patients, it is more readily accomplished during general endotracheal anesthesia. Rigid esophagoscopy is particularly valuable for removal of foreign bodies and for the examination and management of massive esophageal bleeding.

BOX 70-10
COMMON LESIONS OF THE ESOPHAGUS

- Tumors
  - Squamous cell
  - Adenocarcinoma
- Hiatal hernia
- Benign strictures
  - Reflux esophagitis in the lower one-third of the esophagus
  - Caustic fluid ingestion in the upper one-third of the esophagus
- Motility disorders
  - Achalasia
  - Schatzki's ring
- Collagen diseases (e.g., scleroderma)
- Diverticuli
- Trachea esophageal fistula (congenital or malignant)
- Traumatic perforation or rupture
- Foreign bodies

Anesthetic management

Fiberoptic esophagoscopy can easily be performed during topical anesthesia of the mouth and pharynx combined with mild sedation and an antisialagogue (Table 70-12). Patients should not be allowed to eat or drink until several hours after the procedure when the effect of topical anesthesia has dissipated and when protective airway reflexes have returned.

Rigid esophagoscopy usually is performed on patients during general anesthesia with endotracheal intubation and muscle relaxation. An anticholinergic agent is administered to decrease airway secretions and vagal responses to airway manipulation and gastric distention. Cricoid pressure should be used during induction because many patients are at risk for regurgitation from esophageal diverticuli, stenosis, or obstruction. Awake, sedated endotracheal intubation is an option. To avoid injury to the esophagus during passage of the esophagoscope, a small endotracheal tube is used, and the patient is paralyzed before introduction of the esophagoscope. It also may be necessary to temporarily deflate the endotracheal tube cuff to facilitate passage of the esophagoscope. Complications during esophagoscopy include hemorrhage, cardiac dysrhythmias, aspiration pneumonia, and perforation of the esophagus. Perforation can result in pneumothorax, pneumomediastinum, pneumoperitoneum, or subcutaneous emphysema. At the conclusion of the procedure, the trachea should remain intubated until protective reflexes have returned.

Esophageal Cancer

Patients with esophageal malignancy often are malnourished and have poor nutritional status predictive of poor outcome. Preoperative improvement in nutritional status has been shown to decrease the incidence of wound sepsis and perioperative morbidity and mortality.[306,389] Indications for total parenteral nutrition include inability to swallow food, 10% or greater decrease in body weight, serum albumin less than 3 g, cachexia and anergy, total lymphocyte count less than 1000 cells/mm^3, and transferrin values less than 180 ml.[367]

Patients with esophageal cancer often are treated with chemotherapeutic agents before surgery. The perioperative implications of the previous use of antineoplastic agents for management of esophageal cancer include anemia, leukopenia, and thrombocytopenia. Drugs such as adriamycin, bleomycin, and mitomycin C have additional side effects that are important to the anesthesiologist.

Adriamycin (doxorubicin) can result in acute and chronic toxic cardiac effects. Acute cardiac toxicity from Adriamycin is characterized by supraventricular and ventricular dysrhythmias, abnormal conduction patterns, and ST-T wave changes. These acute changes usually resolve 1 or 2 months after cessation of therapy,[270] although Adriamycin administration also may result in irreversible cardiomyopa-

Table 70-12 Anesthetic guidelines for esophagoscopy

Indication	Diagnostic (biopsy mass, evaluate esophagus) Therapeutic (removal foreign body, arrest bleeding, sclerosis)
Monitors	Standard monitors
Anesthesia	Awake sedated (flexible fiberoptic) General anesthesia (flexible fiberoptic and rigid)
Additional equipment	None
Ventilation	Awake spontaneous respiration Single-lumen ETT (may require small size or deflate cuff to pass scope)
Position	Supine
Incision	None
Unique considerations	Antisialagogue Aspiration precautions
Intraoperative complications	Dysrhythmia Aspiration Hematemesis Pneumomediastinum Pneumoperitoneum Pneumothorax Dental trauma Respiratory compromise Perforation esophagus
Postoperative analgesia	Minimal pain (parenteral opiates, NSAIDs)
Postoperative morbidity	Hematemesis Respiratory distress (vocal cord paralysis)
Postoperative care	Chest radiography No eating or drinking until protective airway reflexes have returned

thy and congestive heart failure. To avoid this complication, the total cumulative dose of Adriamycin usually is limited to a maximum of 300 mg/m^2. Adriamycin-induced cardiomyopathy is diagnosed by obtaining an endomyocardial biopsy and by determining the ejection fraction using a multigated nuclear scan (MUGA scan). If the usual maximal dose is exceeded or if patients demonstrate evidence of cardiomyopathy, then dexazoxane (Zinicard) is given before future Adriamycin therapy.

Bleomycin and mitomycin C[395] can result in pulmonary toxicity. Early symptoms include cough, dyspnea, and rales. The toxic signs may progress to severe hypoxemia at rest and a radiologic picture similar to those with ARDS, followed by pulmonary fibrosis. Predisposing factors include age more than 20 years, dosage greater than 400 U, underlying pulmonary disease, and previous radiation therapy. O_2 in high concentration can predispose the patient to pulmonary toxicity from bleomycin. Because the duration of O_2 sensitivity after the conclusion of bleomycin therapy is unknown, the lowest FIO_2 necessary to maintain adequate arterial saturation should be used perioperatively.

Esophageal Surgery: Esophageal Cancer

Management strategies

Tumors of the lower third of the esophagus are managed by esophagogastrectomy through a left-sided thoracotomy or transhiatal esophagogastrectomy and gastric pull-through technique (Fig. 70-37). Lesions of the middle third of the esophagus are managed by a combined laparotomy and right-sided thoracotomy. Lesions of the upper third of the esophagus may be managed by combined laparotomy and cervical incision (Fig. 70-38). Esophagogastrectomy with colon interposition is a two-stage procedure used for lesions in the upper third of the esophagus when insufficient stomach length or gastric disease prevents performing an esophagogastrostomy. During the first stage, the esophagogastrectomy is performed through a midline laparotomy and right thoracotomy. The patient is then turned supine, and a cervical esophagostomy is performed. During the second stage, an antiperistaltic segment of the colon is passed into the retrosternal space and anastomosed to the cervical esophagus above and to the stomach remnant below (Fig. 70-38).

The approach to surgical management of esophageal cancer is controversial. Major issues involve whether the goal is cure or merely palliation. The transthoracic approach, which involves complete resection of lymph nodes, is potentially curative, whereas the transhiatal approach is considered palliative. Other controversies include whether the patient should undergo immediate reconstruction with colon or stomach to restore continuity or delayed repair. Long-term survival appears to be a function of the stage and aggres-

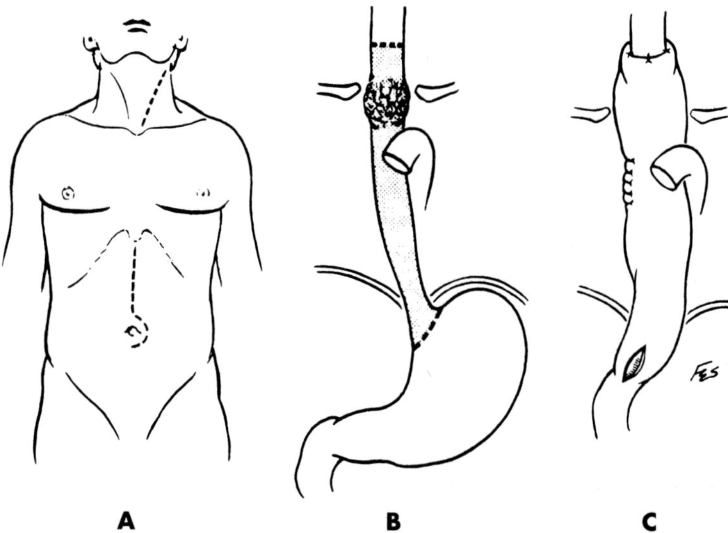

Fig. 70-37. For esophagectomy without thoracotomy, the patient is in the supine position. **A,** Upper midline and left cervical incision (*broken lines*) are made. **B,** The extent of resection (*shaded area*) is shown. **C,** Completed anastomosis. (From Ellis FH Jr: Esophagogastrectomy for carcinoma: technical considerations based on anatomic location of lesion, *Surg Clin North Am* 60:275, 1980.)

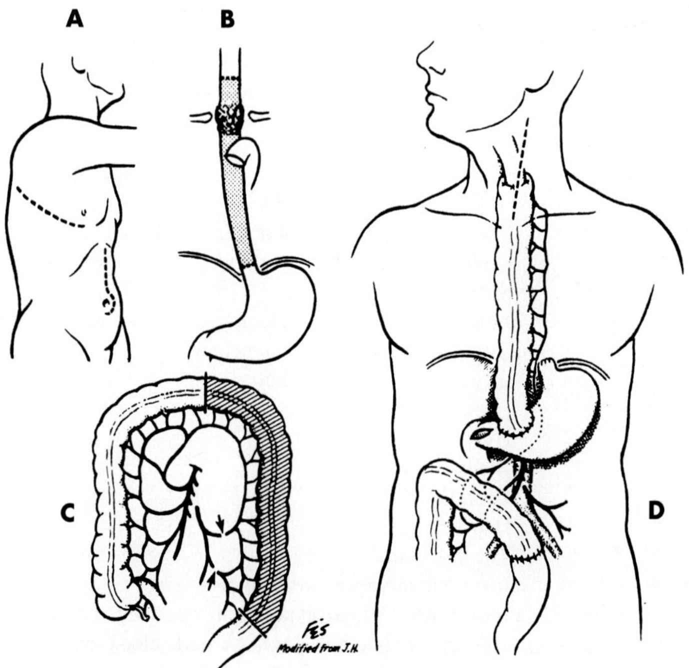

Fig. 70-38. Esophagectomy with interposition of antiperistaltic segment of left colon. **A,** Incisions used in performance of esophagectomy, cervical esophagostomy, pyloromyotomy, and gastrostomy. **B,** Extent of esophageal resection (*shaded area*). **C,** Preparation of segment of left colon (*shaded area*) for interposition based on middle colic artery (note sites of vascular interruption, which maintain the integrity of the vascular arcade). **D,** Completed operation. (From Ellis FH Jr: Esophagogastrectomy for carcinoma: technical considerations based on anatomic location of lesion, *Surg Clin North Am* 60:277, 1980.)

siveness of the tumor at the time of operation rather than the type of operation.

Anesthetic management

Preoperative evaluation should concentrate on the hematologic, nutritional, and cardiopulmonary systems. Preoperative improvement of nutritional status improves outcome dramatically. Hypoalbuminemia, an indicator of poor nutritional status, is associated with increased tissue edema, and anemia may increase the risk of ischemia. Because the operation may be associated with episodes of hemodynamic instability and cardiac arrhythmias, the patient should receive a thorough cardiac evaluation preoperatively. Accompanying respiratory disease should be managed if possible, and strong consideration should be given to placement of an epidural catheter for postoperative analgesia.

Preoperative medication is given according to the patient's general condition to allay anxiety. The use of an anticholinergic drug may be helpful if awake intubation is planned. Guidelines for anesthetic management are presented in Table 70-13. Use of central venous catheterization is encouraged for monitoring of central venous pressure, administration of antiarrhythmics or vasopressors, and fluid

Table 70-13 Anesthetic guidelines for esophagogastrectomy and esophagectomy

Indication	Therapeutic (palliative and curative procedures for esophageal cancer)
Preoperative considerations	Assessment of nutritional status Presence of coexisting cardiopulmonary disease Implications of preoperative chemotherapy
Monitors	Standard monitors, optional (arterial catheter, central venous or pulmonary artery catheters)
Anesthesia	General anesthesia, optional (combined regional and general anesthesia)
Addition equipment	Shoulder roll
Ventilation	Double-lumen ETT or bronchial blocker Single-lumen ETT
Position	Supine Lateral decubitus
Incision	Left thoracotomy—mobilize distal esophagus and stomach without changing positions Right thoracotomy—good exposure of upper and mid-esophagus, easy access to the azygus vein Abdominal transhiatal, abdominal and neck incisions, esophagus mobilized by blunt dissection
Unique considerations	Single-lung ventilation Anticholinergic drug to block carotid sinus reflex (vagal-mediated response) Avoid NO_2 with abdominal surgery Increased risk of aspiration
Intraoperative complications	Aspiration Hypotension Bradycardia Dysrhythmia Hemorrhage Tracheal tears Recurrent laryngeal nerve injury Hypoxia and hypercapnia during one-lung ventilation
Blood loss	1000 cc, but potential for large acute blood loss
Postoperative analgesia	Epidural > parenteral opiates
Postoperative morbidity	Aspiration Pneumothorax Respiratory compromise Hemoptysis Infection Anastomotic leaks
Postoperative care	Chest radiography Elevate head of bed to decrease edema and improve respiratory function Increased fluid requirements during the early postoperative periods

resuscitation. A pulmonary artery catheter should be placed if indicated, based on the patient's cardiopulmonary status; it may prove beneficial postoperatively for optimizing fluid therapy.

Before induction of anesthesia, a large-bore nasogastric tube should be passed, and the proximal esophageal pouch should be emptied. The patient should still be considered to have a full stomach because it is impossible to completely empty the esophagus through an nasogastric tube. Awake intubation during topical anesthesia or induction with cricoid pressure is indicated. If airway compression by large mediastinal lymph nodes is noted, the patient should be treated as described in the section on mediastinal tumors (see Fig. 70-1). Anesthesia is maintained using inhalation anesthetics in O_2, supplemented with intermittent or continuous infusion of narcotics and nondepolarizing muscle relaxants. The combination of epidural and general anesthesia can dramatically decrease inhalation anesthetic and muscle relaxant requirements.

If thoracotomy is planned for esophageal surgery, a double-lumen endobronchial tube and one-lung ventilation to collapse the nondependent lung facilitates surgical exposure. Whether a right-sided or left-sided thoracotomy is performed, a left-sided double-lumen endobronchial tube is recommended because it is easier to position and offers less risk of obstruction of the upper lobe bronchial orifice. **In patients having nonpulmonary surgery, the nondependent lung usually is not severely diseased and thus contributes greatly to normal respiratory function. Paradoxically, this increases the incidence of hypoxemia during single-lung ventilation as compared with that during pulmonary surgery, and the hypoxemia persists as long as the lung is collapsed.**[211]

Marked fluctuating cardiovascular responses are observed frequently during transhiatal esophagectomy. Bradycardia and hypotension may result from stimulation of carotid sinus reflexes during neck dissection and mobilization of the esophagus. They are easily managed with an anticholinergic drug such as atropine. Blunt manual dissection of the esophagus through the diaphragmatic hiatus is associated with hemodynamic lability. Arterial hypertension often occurs during manual dissection of the esophagus and when the stomach is brought up through the posterior mediastinum, whereas hypotension may result from impaired venous return and cardiac function during manual dissection. These relatively long-lasting alterations in hemodynamics could be deleterious to patients with cardiac disease, and they mandate careful intraoperative hemodynamic monitoring. Patients with advanced cardiac dysfunction may not tolerate these manipulations and therefore are not good candidates for a transhiatal esophagectomy. Sudden severe intraoperative hemorrhage also can occur, and therefore large-bore venous access is essential. Other complications include tracheal damage and recurrent laryngeal nerve palsy. Tracheal damage has been reported during transhiatal esophagectomy without thoracotomy and during dissection of the middle third of the esophagus during thoracotomy.

Postoperative concerns

Because esophagogastrectomy is associated with extensive visceral manipulations, difficulty in clearing secretions, advanced patient age with concomitant debilitation, and cardiorespiratory impairment, these patients are commonly left intubated overnight in the ICU. They often have increased fluid requirements during the initial postoperative period, and a pulmonary artery catheter is useful in guiding fluid management. Postoperative complications include pleural effusions, wound infection, pneumonia, and leak from the anastomotic site, resulting in mediastinitis, sepsis, hydrothorax, or pyrothorax.[103] Impaired pulmonary function, airway closure, atelectasis, and hypoxemia typically occur postoperatively because of lung manipulation, residual anesthesia, and postoperative incisional pain. Effective postoperative pain control is essential to facilitate deep breathing, cough, mobilization of secretions, participation in chest physiotherapy, and early ambulation. Postoperative analgesia is most effectively achieved using a thoracic epidural catheter for the infusion of narcotics, with or without local anesthetics.

ANESTHESIA FOR PATIENTS UNDERGOING LASER SURGERY OF THE AIRWAY

Laser technology has been applied extensively for procedures on the upper and lower airways. It has been used successfully in the management of laryngeal tumors, subglottic stenosis, recurrent laryngeal papillomatosis in children, and for the removal and debulking of obstructing airway tumors.[137,177,219,319,346,348,406,407,436,442,443,452,465]

Physics of Lasers

LASER is an acronym for light amplification by stimulated emission of radiation. Laser light is a monochromatic coherent form of electromagnetic radiation that does not occur naturally. To produce a laser beam, atoms are stimulated by electrical, optical, or thermal energy. The stimulated lasing medium radiates energy in the form of light, which is then repeatedly reflected, amplified, and emitted as a laser beam. The lasing medium can be a gas (e.g., helium, argon, CO_2) or a solid medium (e.g., ruby, Nd-YAG). Details of the physics of lasers are beyond the scope of this chapter but can be found in other references.[219,348,407,436]

The effect of the laser beam on tissues depends on its wavelength and its power density. The wavelength depends on the medium from which the laser beam has originated. Laser beams with long wavelengths are strongly absorbed by tissues and therefore are converted into heat energy with a very shallow depth of penetration. Laser light of short wavelength penetrates more deeply into the tissues. Therefore, a CO_2 laser that has a long wavelength (10,600 nm) is absorbed at the very superficial tissue layer, which allows for precise cutting and relatively little edema formation. The neodymium ytrium-aluminum-garnet (Nd-YAG) laser has a short wavelength (1064 nm) and penetrates more deeply into the tissues, allowing use for tumor-debulking procedures.[348] The potassium titanyl-phosphate (KTP) laser emits green light with a wavelength of 552 nm. This lasing medium is produced by adding KTP to Nd-YAG crystals. The KTP laser beam is absorbed by blood and is therefore more effective than an argon laser beam for operation on vascular tumors (e.g., subglottic hemangiomas).

Laser Surgery of the Airway

Malignant tumors of the tracheobronchial tree lead to progressive obstruction of major airways that manifest as progressive stridor. Treatment with external radiation therapy and chemotherapy requires several weeks to produce shrinkage of the tumor and relief of obstructive symptoms. Laser resection has been used in the treatment of partially or totally occluding airway lesions with partial or complete relief of symptoms.[125,187,344] In patients with a totally obstructing airway lesion, lasers can be used to bore through the tumor to reestablish an airway. A serious risk of bronchial perforation and hemorrhage exists. On the other hand, a partially obstructing tumor can be approached tangentially and gradually resected, resulting in widening of the available airway lumen. For partially obstructing lesions, laser resection often provides immediate and dramatic relief of symptoms with a low incidence of bleeding complications. The Nd-YAG laser is the most frequently used laser to resect obstructing tracheobronchial tree tumors.[125,187,343]

The CO_2 laser is used to excise lesions that can be visualized directly in the larynx or that are proximal to the larynx. It is also preferred if minimal penetration and edema formation are desirable, such as in the pediatric airway.[214,446] If a CO_2 laser is to be used for a subglottic lesion, a rigid bronchoscope or laryngoscope is required because the CO_2 laser beam cannot be transmitted along fiberoptic bundles. For supraglottic lesions being managed with a CO_2 laser, a small endotracheal tube can be used for patient ventilation, but the tube should be protected from the laser beam to prevent ignition.

The technique of hematoporphyrin-derivative and laser beam photodynamic therapy has been recently described for the management and possible cure of bronchogenic carcinoma.[112,113,334] Phototherapy in the presence of a sensitizing hematoporphyrin derivative produces light toxicity and destruction of cancer cells. The hematoporphyrin derivative is administered intravenously 3 to 5 days before laser therapy. When tumor cells are sensitized in this manner, a laser beam with a low energy level produces activated O_2 in the tumor cells. The resulting photodynamic chemical reactions impair tumor cell membrane function and cause tumor cell death within 24 to 48 hours. Normal tissue is not harmed by photodynamic therapy. In contrast, a direct thermal laser beam causes coagulation, vaporization, cutting, and excision of tissue. In this case, cellular death is related to the power of the laser beam and is independent of the photochemical reactions mediated by hematoporphyrin derivatives.

Whereas Nd-YAG laser tumor-debulking therapy is palliative, photodynamic therapy can be curative for small lesions. Indications for this technique include patients with small carcinomas *in situ* or early invasive carcinomas, for whom surgery is not feasible technically or physiologically. This modality also can be used after failure of standard therapy and for residual or recurrent local disease. Patients with impaired pulmonary reserve who cannot tolerate extensive pulmonary resection may benefit from photodynamic therapy. Photodynamic therapy can reduce the extent of the surgical resection required, allowing the patient to undergo a less extensive resection. Possible complications include bleeding from the tumor or obstruction of the tracheobronchial tree from sloughing of necrotic tissue.

Intraoperative Considerations

Safety issues

The use of a laser in the operating rooms poses safety hazards for patients and operating room personnel. Warning signs on the operating room door should be clearly visible. Eye injury is a serious hazard of laser surgery. CO_2 laser beams are readily absorbed by the superficial layer of the cornea, leading to corneal opacification. The Nd-YAG laser penetrates the cornea and can result in retinal damage. Protective eye wear with sideguards is therefore required for all operating room personnel. During the use of a CO_2 laser, any pair of eyeglasses, whether plastic or glass and regardless of color, is protective. For use of the Nd-YAG laser, green eyeglasses are needed, whereas for the argon laser, orange eyeglasses should be used. The patient's eyes should be taped closed, covered with moist gauze or towels, and covered with eyeglasses with sideguards. Operating room doors should have opaque coverings, and the windows should be covered with opaque sheets. Because disposable drapes are flammable and difficult to extinguish, patients should be draped with wet towels that are periodically moistened.

Vaporizing tissues with an infrared laser beam (CO_2 and Nd-YAG laser beams are in the infrared spectrum) produces smoke that may be mutagenic, may transmit infectious diseases, and may cause acute bronchial inflammation and impaired pulmonary gas exchange.[173,182] A recent report indicates the presence of papilloma viruses in the vapor of CO_2 laser-treated verrucae,[182] which increases concerns about the vaporization of infected or cancerous tissues during the use of lasers. Noxious fumes should therefore be effectively removed using smoke evacuators. One type of rigid bronchoscope (the Wolfe-Dumon model) especially designed for laser resection has two proximal entrances for the passage of laser fibers and suction catheters. Scavenging the fumes and evacuation of inhalation anesthetics through the suction channel can reduce operating room pollution.

Laser airway surgery may require the use of an endotracheal tube, which increases the risk of explosion or fire, the most common major complication of CO_2 laser surgery.[174,215] The tube should be protected from the laser beam by wrapping it carefully with metallic tape along its entire length down to the proximal end of the cuff. The cuff of a foil-wrapped endotracheal tube remains vulnerable to the laser beam even when the shaft has been protected. The anesthesiologist should therefore limit the O_2 concentration to the minimum needed to maintain adequate oxygenation, even if the endotracheal tube is adequately wrapped and protected. The cuff should be filled with saline solution to act as a heat sink and an automatic sprinkler system if the cuff is perforated. Some clinicians recommend the addition of methylene blue to the saline solution to help detect cuff perforation. A barium stripe in the wall of a PVC tube lowers the ignition threshold, making unmarked tubes preferable. For a more complete discussion the reader is encouraged to review Chapter 84.

Use of helium

The use of helium and O_2 mixtures (60%/40%) during CO_2 laser application has been reported to prevent ignition and fires with unwrapped PVC tubes.[346,347] Helium has greater thermal conductivity, thermal capacity, and thermal diffusivity than nitrogen. These properties of helium inhibit the increase in temperature around the site of laser exposure and thus prevent spontaneous ignition. Besides protecting against airway fire, helium may improve ventilation across an obstructing airway lesion because of its lower density compared with nitrogen, thereby decreasing turbulent gas flow across the stenotic area. O_2-to-N_2O proportioning systems in modern anesthesia machines ensure an O_2 concentration of at least 25% in the fresh gas, although they are not functional for O_2-helium mixtures. Therefore, no protection exists against the delivery of a hypoxic gas mixture when using helium. This can be circumvented by using heliox, a commercially available O_2-helium mixture.

Anesthetic management

Laser surgery often is performed on patients who have underlying respiratory compromise, a long-term history of smoking, and a malignant process encroaching on the airway. Because many of these patients have associated COPD, it is important to evaluate their respiratory function preoperatively and treat with bronchodilators and antibiotics if indicated. Because of the risk of life-threatening airway obstruction during induction of anesthesia or manipulation of the airway, the anesthesiologist should carefully examine the radiologic and other studies (e.g., flow-volume loops) to define precisely the site and extent of airway compromise. Pulmonary function studies and arterial blood gases should be obtained preoperatively. Good communication with the surgeon and other operating room personnel is necessary to plan anesthetic and management strategies in case of emergencies. Choice of endotracheal tube will depend on the size of bronchoscope and type of laser to be used.

Patients at risk of developing airway obstruction or those with severe pulmonary disease should be premedicated with an antisialagogue and minimal sedation only. If the patient is not at risk for airway obstruction, sedative premedications can be administered more liberally. The patient should receive routine monitoring and have large bore venous access for the rapid administration of fluids in case of hemorrhage. Some ventilation techniques described in the next section do not allow the use of capnography. In these patients, monitoring of ventilation is done by careful auscultation of breath sounds, observation of chest movements, or monitoring of arterial blood gases.

The choice of anesthetic induction technique depends on the extent of airway compromise. Patients who have major airway obstruction should maintain spontaneous ventilation during induction. Induction therefore can be achieved by inhalation agents or by administering incremental doses of intravenous hypnotics followed by the gradual introduction of inhalational anesthetics by mask. Alternatively, fiberoptic bronchoscopy can be performed during topical anesthesia to assess the extent and site of airway obstruction (Table 70-14), which may be followed by awake endotracheal intubation with fiberoptic guidance. Patients with minimal or no airway obstruction can receive an ultra–short-acting barbiturate for the induction of anesthesia, followed by muscle relaxation and endotracheal intubation.

Local anesthesia can be used for laser resection of an airway tumor via flexible fiberoptic bronchoscopy. Adequate anesthesia can be achieved by topicalization of the mouth and oropharynx, spraying of the larynx and vocal cords with local anesthetics, superior laryngeal nerve block, or transtracheal injection of a local anesthetic. The hazard of this technique is that unpredictable patient movement can result in disastrous consequences. Therefore, heavy sedation should be maintained when local anesthesia is used. Although local anesthesia can be used for laser airway surgery performed with a rigid bronchoscope, this is not recommended. The degree of discomfort is greater than that with fiberoptic bronchoscopy, and patient movement resulting in trauma and misdirection of the laser beam is more likely to occur.

Use of fiberoptic bronchoscopy during laser therapy

Fiberoptic bronchoscopy for laser resection of airway tumors can be done during local anesthesia and sedation or during general anesthesia with the fiberoptic bronchoscope introduced through the lumen of the endotracheal tube. **The largest endotracheal tube that will pass atraumatically through the glottis should be used to provide a sufficient space for ventilation after the fiberoptic bronchoscope is introduced into the lumen of the tube.** Because resistance to airflow occurs with the introduction of the bronchoscope, patients should not be allowed to breathe spontaneously, but rather ventilation should be controlled. The administration of muscle relaxants may be relatively contraindicated in patients with partial airway obstruction.

Hypercapnia is a common complication of transfiberoptic laser tumor resection, with $Pa{CO_2}$ ranging from 45 to 60

Table 70-14 Anesthetic guidelines for laser ablation

Indication	Therapeutic (palliative of airway obstruction related to tumor)
Monitors	Standard monitors
	Optional (arterial)
Anesthesia	General anesthesia
Additional equipment	Anesthetic ventilator capable of blending an O_2 and air mixture
Ventilation	Rigid bronchoscope
	Single-lumen ETT (special laser tube, but may be less important when using laser way distal to the ETT)
Position	Supine
Unique considerations	Maintain $FIO_2 < 40\%$
	Avoid N_2O (also supports combustion)
Intraoperative complications	Hemoptysis
	Hemorrhage
	Airway fire
	Airway obstruction
	Bronchospasm
	Hypoxia
	Perforation of the tracheobronchial tree
Analgesia	Opiates
Postoperative morbidity	Hemoptysis
	Bronchospasm
	Airway edema
Postoperative care	Humidified O_2

mm Hg.[452] Long-acting narcotics and benzodiazepines should be avoided because of prolonged postoperative somnolence and respiratory depression. Short-action inhalation anesthetics allow for immediate extubation without postoperative respiratory depression or sedation.

Use of rigid bronchoscopy during resection of airway tumors

Many laser resections are performed using a rigid, open-tube bronchoscope.[343,348] There are several advantages to the use of rigid bronchoscopy as opposed to flexible fiberoptic bronchoscopy for Nd-YAG laser resection of airway tumors:

- It allows easy manipulation of the laser beam and provides a greater field of vision, greater access for suction catheters, removal of tumor fragments, or restoration of homeostasis. The rigid bronchoscope can be used to establish an airway. If airway obstruction occurs, the bronchoscope is advanced distally to the site of obstruction, thereby reestablishing airway patency.
- The absence of a combustible endotracheal tube decreases the chance of an airway fire. Although the steel bronchoscope will not burn, carbonized tissue may flare.[336] It is important to use the lowest O_2 concentration needed to maintain adequate arterial saturation.
- The rigid bronchoscope facilitates homeostasis because the bronchoscope can be gradually withdrawn while the endoscopist coagulates bleeding sites as they appear.

Maintenance of ventilation can be achieved using one of several techniques. Conventional intermittent positive pressure ventilation can be maintained by connecting the anesthesia circuit to the ventilating side arm of the rigid bronchoscope, which allows the administration of O_2 and inhalation anesthetics from the anesthesia machine. Anesthesia also can be supplemented with intravneous agents. The patient should be paralyzed to eliminate the risk of sudden unexpected movement. If a major leak occurs around the rigid bronchoscope interfering with the adequacy of ventilation, packing the nose, mouth, and pharynx with gauze is helpful.

The rigid bronchoscope cannot visualize upper lobe lesions. If it is necessary to advance the bronchoscope into the mainstem bronchus, inadequate ventilation to the contralateral lung will result unless the bronchoscope has side holes that allow ventilation of the opposite lung. A method of ventilating the other lung, such as high-frequency ventilation or continuous high-flow apneic ventilation, should be available. In patients with right upper lobe lesions or peripheral lesions that are beyond the range of the rigid bronchoscope, the anesthesiologist should pass a fiberoptic bronchoscope through the lumen of the rigid bronchoscope, with the tip of the rigid bronchoscope kept above the tracheal carina to provide ventilation to both lungs.

Rigid bronchoscopy with low-frequency manual jet ventilation using the Sanders' jet injector at a frequency of 20 breaths per minute has been shown to provide adequate oxygenation and ventilation during bronchoscopy in patients with tracheobronchial stenosis and in those undergoing laser resection of tracheobronchial lesions.[442,443] Total intravenous anesthesia can be achieved with intermittent or continuous infusions of methohexital, etomidate, alfentanil, or sufentanil. Muscle relaxation using short-acting nondepolarizing

BOX 70-11
COMPLICATIONS OF LASER THERAPY

Environmental hazards to patients and operating room personnel
- Eye injuries, skin burns, drape fires, and exposure to noxious fumes

Related to airway maintenance and ventilation techniques
- Obstruction by tumor, edema, blood clots, and tissue debris
- Hypoxemia and hypercapnia

Airway fires

Airway perforation
- Pneumomediastinum, pneumothorax

Hemorrhage and exsanguination

Aspiration of blood, tissue, or infectious debris

agents, such as vecuronium, is recommended. Disadvantages of low-frequency jet ventilation include the lack of precise control of the FIO_2 because of entrainment of ambient air. In addition, Venturi effect can lead to distal migration or aspiration of blood and tissue debris.

Rigid bronchoscopy with HFJV at rates of 150 to 300 breaths per minute can achieve satisfactory surgical conditions and provide adequate gas exchange in patients with tracheobronchial stenosis.[442] At a faster rate, some hypoxemia and hypercapnia are noted. Hypercapnia can occur when the bronchoscope is advanced into a mainstem bronchus from an inadequate ventilation of the contralateral lung. The use of a small tidal volume at a high rate results in an immobile surgical field and decreases the chance of misdirection of the laser beam with trauma to healthy tissues. Additionally, unlike low-frequency ventilation using the Sanders' injector, which creates a Venturi effect, with HFJV, there is continuous egress of gas to the outside, thus decreasing the chance of aspirating blood and tissue debris or forcing it into the distal airway. When arterial desaturation occurs during laser resection, the surgeon should stop the resection and thoroughly suction blood and tissue debris out of the airway, regardless of the ventilation technique being used. The patient should then be hyperventilated with 100% O_2. When adequate arterial oxygenation is reachieved, the O_2 concentration can again be decreased, and the surgeon can resume laser resection.

Complications

Complications of laser surgery are summarized in Box 70-11.

Airway fires are one of the potentially most devastating complications of laser therapy. The sequence of steps necessary for the appropriate management of airway fire is outlined in Table 70-15. Because airway fires can cause severe thermal and chemical injury, the extent of damage should be assessed before the patient is awakened. Bronchoscopic examination reveals the extent of lower airway edema and damage and allows removal of particulate material. Laryngoscopy should be performed to evaluate the proximal extent of injury. If extensive airway damage has resulted from the fire, the trachea should remain intubated, and mechanical ventilation should continue. Severe burns may require a tracheostomy. Chest radiographs should be obtained after surgery, even if the initial postinjury examination showed minimal damage. A 24-hour course of steroids may decrease airway edema. Humidification of inspired gases is recommended to prevent the formation of mucous plugs. The patient should be monitored for at least 24 hours. Severe injury may necessitate a prolonged course of mechanical ventilation and intensive supportive care.

Table 70-15 Management of airway fire

Order of importance	Measure
1	Stop ventilation
2	Disconnect O_2 source; douse with water if needed; remove burned tracheal tube and endoscope
3	Mask ventilate; reintubate
4	Diagnose injury; provide therapy by bronchoscopy and laryngoscopy
5	Monitor patient for at least 24 hours
6	Administer short-term steroids
7	Administer antibiotics and ventilatory support as needed

If surgical drapes catch fire, the anesthesiologist should attempt to remove them from the patient and from the vicinity of any electrical equipment and to extinguish the flames with water or water-based extinguishing agents (class A fire extinguisher). Fires involving electrical equipment should be handled with a class C extinguisher, such as a CO_2 extinguisher.[316]

ANESTHESIA FOR PATIENTS UNDERGOING LUNG TRANSPLANTATION

Lung transplantation is now an established modality for the management of end stage lung and pulmonary vascular disease (Box 70-12). The perioperative treatment of patients undergoing lung transplantation challenges even the most experienced anesthesiologists, surgeons, and intensivists. The following discussion of lung transplantation is an overview; the reader is referred to review articles that address specific management strategies in more detail. There are four types of lung transplantation procedures (single lung, bilateral sequential single lung, double lung, and double lung plus heart transplantation).

Single-lung transplantation provides for efficient organ donor use by increasing the number of recipients from the fixed donor pool. In addition, it is technically easier and requires less ischemic time than two-lung procedures.

BOX 70-12
PATHOLOGIC PROCESSES LEADING TO END-STAGE LUNG DISEASE MANAGED BY LUNG TRANSPLANTATION

Single and double-lung transplantation

- Alpha$_1$-antitrypsin deficiency
- Acquired emphysema
- Primary pulmonary hypertension
- Toxic exposure resulting in acute respiratory failure
- Bilateral septic pulmonary disease
  - Cystic fibrosis
  - Bronchiectasis
- Bronchiolitis obliterans
- Eosinophilic granuloma
- Sarcoidosis

Heart and lung transplantation

- Pulmonary vascular disease associated with right ventricular failure
  - Primary pulmonary hypertension
  - Eisenmenger's syndrome
  - Thromboembolic disease
  - Anatomic developmental anomalies (e.g., complex pulmonary atresia)
  - Venoocclusive disease
- Parenchymal lung disease resulting in chronic respiratory failure associated with cor pulmonale and right ventricular failure
  - Chronic obstructive pulmonary disease
  - Restrictive lung disease (e.g., sarcoidosis, eosinophilic granuloma, cryptogenic fibrosing alveolitis)
  - Septic and destructive lung disease (e.g., cystic fibrosis, bronchiectasis)

Because the site of operation is selected to avoid the difficulties associated with reoperation at a previous surgical site, bleeding is minimized.[284,420,469] Candidates for single-lung transplantation have end stage pulmonary disease resulting from chronic idiopathic pulmonary fibrosis or emphysema. Single-lung transplantation is contraindicated in patients with infected native lungs (cystic fibrosis) or in those with major cardiac dysfunction. Initially, patients with emphysema were not considered suitable recipients. It was believed that hyperventilation of the native lung would compress the transplanted lung,[27,463] although the anticipated imbalance of ventilation to perfusion has not been evident.[284,429,438] The use of single-lung transplantation for patients with pulmonary hypertension and Eisenmenger's syndrome is controversial. The surgical procedure for these patients is complicated by the need to use cardiopulmonary bypass to prevent acute right ventricular failure. Single-lung transplantation in patients with pulmonary hypertension results in a functional pneumonectomy in which both lungs are ventilated, but blood flow is diverted from the native lung, increasing the risk of pulmonary infarction.

Bilateral and bilateral sequential single-lung transplantation are performed in patients with infection in both lungs or with pulmonary hypertension. Bilateral transplantation was performed initially as an *en bloc* procedure with tracheal anastomosis; it required cardiopulmonary bypass. Disadvantages to this approach include the need for anticoagulation, increased use of blood products, use of cardiac arrest, and increased risk of ischemia at the site of tracheal anastomosis. When bilateral transplantation is performed as sequential single-lung transplantation using bronchial anastomoses, the patients do not require cardiopulmonary bypass and are less prone to airway ischemia.[296,352]

Combined transplantation of the heart and both lungs is used for patients with end-stage lung disease combined with severe cardiac dysfunction (Box 70-12). In patients with primary pulmonary hypertension, lung disease may be the primary etiology with cardiac disease resulting from right ventricular failure. Heart–lung transplantation also is applicable for a persistent intracardiac shunt that results in secondary lung disease (Eisenmenger's syndrome). Heart–lung transplantation procedures add the risk of cardiopulmonary bypass.

Pathophysiology of the Transplanted Lung

Lung resection and subsequent allograft implantation results in denervation of the lung and airways, absence of a functional lymphatic system, and loss of the bronchial artery. In the intact lung, afferent information is believed to come from pulmonary stretch receptors and is relayed via the vagus nerve to the medulla,[159] although respiratory timing and tidal volume apparently do not depend on intact vagal innervation of the lungs. Instead, they depend on chest wall afferent signals.[67,428] Denervation of the vagus nerve is associated with loss of cough reflex of the new lung, which results in difficulties with aspiration and maintenance of pulmonary toilet in the early postoperative period. These patients compensate well, and the long-term problems are fewer than expected. Patients undergoing left lung transplantation are at increased risk for surgical damage of the recurrent laryngeal nerve.

Dysruption of lymphatic drainage in the donor lung predisposes to fluid accumulation that manifests as interstitial pulmonary edema. Management includes careful control of fluid administration and judicious use of blood products, combined with diuretics as indicated. Right atrial pressure should be maintained at the least value needed to provide adequate renal perfusion and hemodynamic stability.

Preoperative Assessment and Patient Selection

Selection criteria are continually evolving and are institution-specific. In general, suitable candidates for allograft lung transplantation are those with disabling pulmonary vascular disease or deteriorating chronic respiratory failure. Because of the limited donor population, selection criteria include the potential for full rehabilitation and the absence of serious comorbid disease. Patients with end-stage lung disease resulting from systemic disorders such as systemic lupus have other pathology (e.g., renal dysfunction) that precludes transplantation.

Potential recipients require careful cardiovascular evaluation. Right heart function is assessed to estimate the ability of the recipient's right ventricle to maintain cardiac output during the acute temporary increase in pulmonary vascular resistance associated with the operation. Several groups have used echocardiography and right ventricular ejection fraction obtained from multigated scans and right heart catheterization to assess function. Patients also undergo left heart catheterization and coronary artery angiography to evaluate for the presence of major coronary disease or left ventricular dysfunction. In addition, echocardiography should be used to detect the presence of a patent foramen ovale, which would predispose to paradoxical embolization during increased right heart pressures.

Donor Selection and Procurement

Unfortunately, most potential multiorgan donors are not suitable lung donors because of chest trauma, pulmonary edema, or pulmonary sepsis. Donor criteria are summarized in Box 70-13. Although lungs from nonsmokers are preferred, a smoking history of fewer than 10 pack/years is acceptable. Once a donor has been identified, possible recipients are evaluated for ABO compatibility and size and present pulmonary status. In patients with COPD, a disparity in size between the donor and recipient lungs is less important. Donor lungs increase in size to partially fill an enlarged pleural space, and the recipient's pleural cavity decreases in size. Lungs are excised along with the main bronchus, pulmonary artery, and cuff of the left atrium. The lungs are flushed out *in situ* and subsequently harvested. Total ischemic time should be limited to fewer than six hours.

BOX 70-13
DONOR CRITERIA FOR SINGLE-LUNG AND DOUBLE-LUNG TRANSPLANTATION

Absolute indications

- ABO compatibility
- Radiograph clear
- $Pa_{O_2} > 300$ mm Hg with patient receiving 100% oxygen and positive end-expiratory pressure of 5 cm H_2O
- No evidence of systemic sepsis
- Negative history of pulmonary disease
- Cytomegalovirus serology negative or similar in donor and recipient (indication in case of double-lung transplantation only)

Relative indications

- No lung trauma on side to be transplanted
- Absence of organisms and white cells on Gram stain of bronchial mucus specimen
- Age < or equal of 55 years
- No previous thoracic surgery
- $Pa_{CO_2} < 40$ mm Hg with tidal volume of 15 ml/kg and respiratory rate of 10 – 14/minute
- Peak inspiratory pressure < 20 cm H_2O at tidal volume of 15 ml/kg
- Central venous pressure ≤ 10 mm Hg

$Pa_{O_2}/_{CO_2}$ — arterial oxygen/carbon dioxide tension.
Data from references 67, 76, 439.

Preoperative Preparation

A comprehensive preoperative visit is essential to establish good patient–physician rapport, instill patient confidence, encourage cooperation, and evaluate for associated medical problems. Anesthesia equipment and supplies are similar to those required for thoracic and cardiac surgery. In addition to the usual assortment of airway equipment including PEEP valves, a second ventilator with alternate ventilation modes should be available. Required drugs include heparin, protamine, diuretics, antiarrhythmics (lidocaine, digoxin, procainamide), inotropic, and vasoactive agents (dopamine, dobutamine, epinephrine, nitroglycerin, prostaglandin E1, phenylephrine). Immunosuppressive drugs such as cyclosporin, azothiaprine, or steroids may be indicated on reperfusion of the new lung. Antibiotics and the first dose of immunosuppressive agents frequently are administered immediately before surgery.

Strict technique for protective isolation, including clean scrub suits and shoe covers, should be followed by all personnel. Skin preparation with iodine solution and sterile technique should be used before inserting all intravenous and arterial catheters or before using injection ports. Although the patients often are anxious, preoperative medication should be restricted to an antisialagogue and mild sedation. The patients have tenuous pulmonary and cardiac function, requiring judicious use of benzodiazepines and narcotics. An exception to the use of minimal sedation are patients with primary pulmonary hypertension. These patients tend to have minimal respiratory symptoms, but increased pulmonary vascular resistance caused by anxiety and agitation can increase the load on the right ventricle. Sedated patients should receive limited supplemental oxygen during the preinduction period. In addition to routine standard monitors, an oximetric pulmonary artery catheter is recommended to continuously monitor the adequacy of cardiac function and oxygenation.

Postoperative Analgesia

Postoperative analgesia should be planned before induction. Placement of an epidural catheter for administration of local anesthetic and narcotics provides postoperative analgesia and may be used intraoperatively to decrease the anesthetic requirement. **Thoracic epidural catheters are routinely inserted for single and bilateral sequential single-lung transplantations that do not require cardiopulmonary**

bypass. The benefit of placing an epidural catheter should be balanced against the risk of epidural hematoma related to anticoagulation for cardiopulmonary bypass or antiplatelet therapy. Previous studies of 4483 patients in similar conditions failed to reveal any major neurologic sequelae.[226,323,366] Conversely, there are numerous reports of spontaneous epidural hematomas after anticoagulation in patients without epidural catheters.[208,414]

Operation for Single-Lung Transplantation

Selection of the lung to replace depends on donor and recipient factors. Right pneumonectomy with subsequent reimplantation of the donor lung is easier. Considerations for choice of side depend on the distribution of perfusion between the right and left lung and a history of previous pleurodesis or thoracotomy, which would complicate the operation. If there is marked asymmetry in the arterial perfusion as measured by a radionucleotide lung perfusion scan, transplantation of the lung with the lesser perfusion will allow for additional reserve during the intraoperative and early postoperative periods. Donor considerations influencing the choice include availability and presence of an infiltrate on chest radiograph.

Patients undergoing single-lung transplantation are placed in the anterior lateral decubitus position with the groin exposed for possible cannulation in case cardiopulmonary bypass is required. After entering the chest, the pulmonary artery, vein, and main stem bronchus are isolated and encircled with tapes. Completion of the recipient pneumonectomy is delayed until arrival of a donor lung. The sequence of reanastomoses of the new lung is determined by the surgeon. Revascularization of the lung before the anastomosis of the bronchus results in a major shunt, which may cause marked hypoxia, although this sequence decreases ischemic time and the duration of right ventricular stress. Alternatively, anastomosis of the airway before revascularization avoids the risk of shunt and hypoxia at a time of hemodynamic instability and is the choice of most surgeons. Bronchial anastomosis is facilitated by partial insertion of the smaller bronchus into the larger one.

Anesthesia: induction and maintenance

The induction of general anesthesia can be challenging and dangerous (Table 70-16). To reduce the risk of hypoxia and aspiration, the patient should be preoxygenated and anesthesia induced while cricoid pressure is maintained. Induction of anesthesia can be most easily achieved using a combination of intravenous drugs including fentanyl, sufentanil, midazolam, or etomidate. Narcotics should be administered with caution to avoid truncal rigidity and hypoventilation, which are poorly tolerated. Many of these patients have increased sympathetic tone when awake. Loss of tone on anesthetic induction may cause profound hypotension and hypoxia. A halogenated inhalational agent titrated during anesthetic induction provides some bronchodilation and permits the use of increased inspired oxygen concentrations. The muscle relaxant used to facilitate tracheal intubation should provide hemodynamic stability without histamine release. **Hypercapnia should be avoided to prevent the sudden release of endogenous catecholamines that can increase pulmonary vascular resistance and exacerbate preexisting right ventricular dysfunction. Minimum inflation pressures should be used for controlled ventilation. Many of these patients have pathophysiology that predispose them to having "auto PEEP" or rupture of bullae.**

The use of a balanced anesthetic with a high-dose narcotic supplemented with inhalational agents is common. Isoflurane provides potent analgesia, amnesia, and vasodilation without cardiac depression, although of particular concern during single-lung transplantation, halogenated agents inhibit hypoxic pulmonary vasoconstriction and may impede ventilation-to-perfusion matching. Nitrous oxide should be avoided because it expands air spaces, decreases inspired oxygen concentration, and potentially worsens outcome after embolization of air. Inhalational anesthetics may be contraindicated when using alternate modalities of ventilation, such as jet ventilation. Some people advocate the reduction of inspired concentration of oxygen to lessen the risk of oxygen toxicity and reperfusion injury.[102,185] Presently, there are no data to support this practice, and an increased inspired concentration provides for a greater margin of safety. Epidural analgesia may be used to supplement intraoperative anesthesia. Although the epidural administration of dilute local anesthetics decreases the general anesthetic requirement and smooths the transition to postoperative care, their sympathetic blocking effect may result in hypotension.

Lung separation

Lung transplantation can be performed using either a double-lumen endotracheal tube or bronchial blockers. The type of endotracheal tube chosen is not as important as the anesthesiologist's ability to position it quickly and properly. Left-sided double-lumen endotracheal tubes are most commonly used for left and right lung transplantations. A more comprehensive discussion of double-lumen endotracheal tubes and bronchial blockers has been presented previously.

Intraoperative problems and management strategies

Hemodynamic instability is a frequent problem. The consequences of loss of autonomic tone during induction or with the use of an epidural blockade are accentuated because many lung transplantation recipients are relatively hypovolemic preoperatively. Strategies for managing hypotension include cautious expansion of intravascular volume and administration of alpha adrenergic or mixed adrenergic agonists. Alpha agonists should be used with caution to avoid an increase in pulmonary artery vascular resistance, which tends to worsen right ventricular dysfunction.

Transition from spontaneous ventilation to mechanical ventilation can lead to respiratory and cardiovascular com-

Table 70-16 Anesthetic guidelines for lung transplantation

Monitors	Standard monitors A-line, pulmonary artery catheter with SvO_2 oximetry Foley catheter TEE
Anesthesia	General anesthesia Optional (combined regional and general anesthesia)
Additional equipment	Standard servoventilator (available) Jet ventilator (available) Cardiopulmonary bypass (available)
Ventilation	Double-lumen ETT Bronchial blocker Switch to a single-lumen ETT after surgery
Position	Single-lateral decubitus position and groin accessible for cardiopulmonary bypass Double-supine or sequential lateral decubitus positioning
Incision	Thoracotomy Transverse bilateral thoracotomy
Unique considerations	Single-lung ventilation Clamping PA—improve V/Q mismatching but risk RV failure Increased risk of right-to-left shunt through a patent foramen ovale PA unclamped—release after bronchus is attached to avoid shunt
Intraoperative complications	Bleeding (more common after heparinization) Air embolism Hypoxia Hypercapnia Hypotension Neurologic event Right ventricular failure Cardiac arrhythmias Hyperacute rejection
Blood loss	Variable depending on single versus double transplant and use of anticoagulation for cardiopulmonary bypass
Postoperative analgesia	Epidural, parenteral opiates
Postoperative morbidity	Hypoxia Rejection Infection Bleeding Pulmonary edema Bronchial rupture Pleural effusions Renal insufficiency Diaphragmatic dysfunction
Postoperative care	Monitored in an intensive care unit Immunosuppression Wean FIO_2 Facilitate ventilation and drainage by placing native lung in more dependent position

promise. Positive pressure ventilation transmits pressure to the pleura and pericardium, which may restrict cardiac filling and increase right ventricular afterload. Acute increases in right ventricular afterload and decreases in right ventricular filling can cause displacement of the intraventricular septum and reduce left ventricular compliance. The situation may be further exacerbated in patients with obstructive lung disease. Mechanical ventilation may cause air trapping, leading to "pulmonary tamponade." Administration of intravascular fluids to increase preload and adjustment of the ventilatory parameters by changing the inspiratory-to-expiratory ratio to allow more time for expiration may help lessen the risk of hemodynamic compromise.

Initiation of single-lung ventilation is associated with increased peak airway pressure, which may rupture bullae and cause pneumothorax or air trapping, resulting in pulmonary tamponade. To mitigate against the increase in airway pressure, the set tidal volume is decreased. A compensatory increase in respiratory rate is required to maintain adequate minute ventilation. Pulmonary blood flow through the nonventilated lung contributes to the shunt fraction, resulting in hypercapnia and severe hypoxia. Standard measures to manage hypoxia and hypercapnia, including increasing FIO_2 to 100%, optimizing ventilatory parameters, decreasing inhaled anesthetic concentration to prevent inhibition of hypoxic pulmonary vasoconstriction, and applying PEEP to the dependent lung and CPAP to the nondependent lung, may not result in satisfactory oxygenation and ventilation. In our practice, an alternate mode of ventilation has been effective in managing hypoxia and hypercapnia. Conventional critical care ventilators have markedly improved microprocessor technology, which allows altering ventilator modes (e.g., pressure control), ramp settings, and inspiratory-to-expiratory ratios and permits quantitative adjustment of inspiratory pressures. Circulatory deterioration resulting from ventilatory failure may require partial cardiopulmonary bypass.

Clamping of the pulmonary artery

Completion of the pneumonectomy by clamping the pulmonary artery eliminates the source of venous admixture and improves oxygenation and ventilation, although the right ventricle is sensitive to sudden increases in afterload and does not compensate well. The acute increase in pulmonary artery pressure causes dilation of the right ventricle and concomitant tricuspid regurgitation and right atrial dilation. These alterations in right ventricular geometry affect contractility of the ventricular septum and in turn decrease left-sided function. Inotropic agents, such as dobutamine, amrinone, or milrinone, may improve right ventricular function by pulmonary vasodilation and inotropy. Use of pulmonary arterial vasodilators, such as nitrates or prostaglandin E1, may be helpful. Differential infusion of vasoconstrictive agents into the left side of the heart and vasodilating agents into the right side also have been suggested.[120,222] Inhaled nitric oxide may have a role in decreasing pulmonary artery pressures, but the specific population that would benefit from this therapy has not been identified.[5] TEE provides continuous qualitative assessment of right ventricular function and effectiveness of therapeutic intervention. If these therapeutic interventions fail to alleviate the hemodynamic deterioration, then partial cardiopulmonary bypass should be instituted.

The specific sequence for anastomosis of the pulmonary artery, veins, and bronchus vary according to surgeons preference. Often, the pulmonary veins and artery of the donor lung are anastomosed before the bronchus. As the pulmonary anastomosis is nearing completion, the left atrial clamp is gradually released to produce back bleeding and remove air from the pulmonary vascular bed. Restoring circulation to the transplanted nonventilated lung results in shunting and potentially serious hypoxia. In addition, the acute blood loss associated with back bleeding and the flushing of the preservative solution and metabolites into systemic circulation can lead to acute hypotension. Corrective measures include partial or total reclamping of the pulmonary artery, administration of fluids, jet ventilation, or partial inflation of the transplanted lung. If anastomosis of the bronchus precedes revascularization, the risk of hypoxia related to shunting through nonventilated lung is eliminated.

Bilateral Sequential Single-Lung Versus Double-Lung Transplantation

Bilateral sequential single-lung transplantation has a number of advantages compared with *en bloc* double-lung transplantation. Single-lung transplantation is technically easier; cardiopulmonary bypass is not necessary in most patients, and ischemic arrest of the heart is not required. The *en bloc* transplantation of both lungs is performed through a median sternotomy and requires an abdominal laparotomy for access to the omental flap. In addition, double bronchial anastomosis result in fewer ischemic complications compared with single tracheal anastomosis. The *en bloc* technique through a median sternotomy is used most often for combined heart–lung transplantations.

The surgical approach for sequential bilateral lung transplantation is either through bilateral thoracotomies using the lateral decubitus position or a transverse thoracosternotomy, which extends transversely to both mid-axillary lines. The lung with poorer function, based on ventilation–perfusion scans, is removed first. After the first new lung is implanted, ventilation is switched to the newly transplanted lung, and the second lung is excised. In patients with severe obstructive disease, the contralateral chest cavity is not opened during the first transplantation, because that lung becomes hyperinflated when not confined to the pleural cavity. The resulting air trapping can create serious ventilatory and hemodynamic disturbances.

Postoperative Management

On completion of the procedure the double-lumen tube is replaced with a large single-lumen endotracheal tube. Use of a large diameter tube facilitates endoscopy and pulmonary toilet and minimizes the work of breathing during weaning. During the initial postoperative period, the patient is placed on intermittent mandatory ventilation (IMV). The concentration of oxygen is decreased to avoid oxygen toxicity with the goal of maintaining an arterial oxygen tension of approximately 100 mm Hg.[427] Problems of postoperative ventilation–perfusion mismatch, shunting, and increased dead space are more pronounced in patients undergoing single-lung as compared with bilateral lung transplantation. To improve oxygenation and ventilation, patients receiving a single-lung transplantation are placed in a modified decubitus position with the transplanted side up. When the patients are awake, warm, hemodynamically stable, and without acid–base or electrolyte disturbances, they are slowly weaned from the ventilator.

The newly transplanted lung is susceptible to fluid overload, resulting from disruption of the pulmonary lymphatics. In a recent series of single-lung transplantation recipients, the incidence of early postoperative edema was 60%.[403] In all patients, the pulmonary artery occlusion pressure was normal, suggesting low pressure edema. When the protein concentration of the edema fluid was compared with that of serum, the ratio was greater than 0.5, suggesting increased permeability resulting from endothelial damage. There was an association between the occurrence of pulmonary edema and graft ischemic time.[403] Postoperatively, low-dose vasoconstrictors can be used to support the blood pressure. Judicious use of fluid volume administration, balanced with vasopressor and diuretic therapy, maintains adequate filling pressures and urine output.

Acute pulmonary rejection occurs in 50% to 87% of patients after lung transplantation. Clinical manifestations include cough, breathlessness, low grade fever, and wheezing. There are associated changes in respiratory function (FEV_1 and FVC) and abnormalities on chest radiograph.[218,301] The differential diagnosis of rejection includes postoperative edema, infection, and bronchiolitis obliterans. A bronchial lavage sample should be examined and sent for culture. Administration of steroids can function as a diagnostic test and empirical therapy.

A common first line treatment for transplant rejection is cyclosporin A, a selective reversible inhibitor of immunocompetent T lymphocytes. Its main side effect is nephrotoxicity with acute impairment of renal function that usually recovers with a reduction in dosage. Another side effect is hypertension. Other major forms of immunosuppression therapy include azathioprine, corticosteroids, antitymocyte globulin (ATG), antilymphocyte globulin, and monoclonal antibody to the T3 receptor on lymphocytes (OKT3). Specific immunosuppressive protocols are not detailed here because they vary by institution and are in a continual state of reevaluation and change.

Bronchiolitis obliterans is a devastating complication of lung transplantation. It is characterized by obstruction and destruction of pulmonary airways. Progressive obstruction of airflow leads to arterial hypoxia.[83] Diagnosis can be confirmed by transbronchial biopsy. Therapeutic options are limited because the condition is relatively refractory to increases in immunosuppressant therapy.[83,392] Because of the poor prognosis, retransplantation is frequently the only option.

Infectious complications after a lung transplantation cause morbidity and mortality. Predisposing factors to bacterial infection include use of immunosuppressant therapy, ischemic injury to the lung, presence of pleural effusions, and interruption of lymphatic drainage. Donor-transmitted infections are associated with high mortality rate. Therefore, the airways of the donor lungs are routinely cultured, and the recipient is treated with appropriate antibiotics.

Infections from cytomegalovirus (CMV) have a high mortality rate in lung transplantation recipients. Symptoms of viral pneumonitis are fever and malaise. Laboratory findings include leukopenia, thrombocytopenia, atypical lymphocytosis, and hepatitis.[121,136,401] The recipient may acquire primary infection from a CMV antibody-positive donor or from blood products. Even recipients who are CMV antibody positive before transplantation can experience reactivation of previous infection or be infected with a different strain from the donor.[93,467] Fortunately, most CMV infections and pneumonitis respond to treatment with gancyclovir.[433]

ANESTHESIA FOR PATIENTS UNDERGOING MEDIASTINOSCOPY

Mediastinoscopy and mediastinotomy are performed to diagnose and stage lung cancer to determine resectability.[169,379] These procedures provide access to paratracheal, subaortic, and bronchial lymph nodes to detect metastatic spread of lung carcinomas. Lymphatics of the lung initially drain into the subaortic and paratracheal areas and then to the sides of the trachea, supraclavicular areas, and thoracic ducts. The surgical site is chosen based on likely path for regional spread of metastatic disease. Cervical mediastinal exploration (mediastinoscopy) yields a greater percentage of positive results for tumors affecting the right upper and middle lobes and to a lesser extent left lower lobes. Anterior mediastinotomy is recommended for those patients suspected of tumor in the left upper lobe. Mediastinoscopy is performed in patients in the supine position with the neck extended. Access is gained through an incision in the suprasternal notch, and a tunnel is created by blunt dissection anterior and slightly lateral to the trachea into the mediastinum. The rigid mediastinoscope passes posterior to the inominate and aortic arteries down to the subcarinal area. The mediastinoscope can injure adjacent structures (Fig. 70-39). Increased risk of complications during mediastinoscopy has been noted in patients with major collateral vascular flow and in patients with abnormal or altered anatomy (Table 70-17).[169]

Anesthetic Management

Preoperative assessment should include inspection for the presence of occult airway obstruction or distortion, superior vena cava outlet obstruction, evidence of paraneoplastic syndromes, and cerebral vascular disease. Although mediastinoscopy may be performed during local anesthesia in certain situations (e.g., when a mediastinal mass compromises the airway), most surgeons and anesthesiologists prefer general anesthesia with controlled ventilation (Table 70-18). Muscle relaxants are advantageous for facilitating intubation, controlling ventilation, and preventing sudden movement or coughing that would increase the risk of surgical complications.[444] Intubation and controlled ventilation facilitates dissection, minimizes the potential for air embolism, and assures access to the airway in case of massive hemorrhage. The negative intrathoracic pressure associated with spontaneous ventilation may increase the risk of air

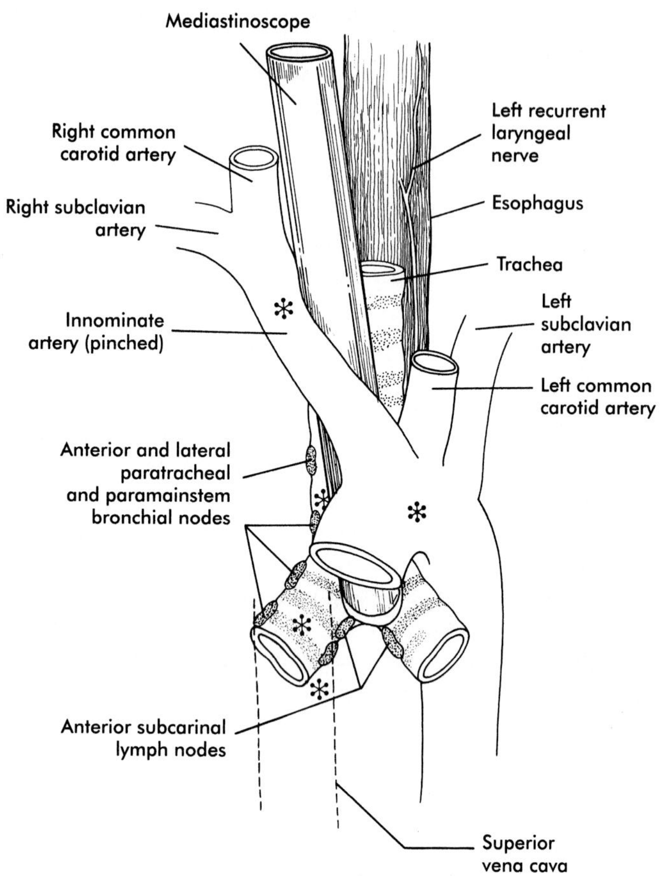

Fig. 70-39. Mediastinoscope within the mediastinum. Note the pinched innominate artery. (Modified from Petty C: Right radial artery pressure during mediastinoscopy, *Anesth Analg* 58:428, 1979.)

Table 70-17 Complications of mediastinoscopy from review of 14 mediastinoscopy series (1968 – 1970)

Complications	Number of patients
Bleeding	
Moderate	15
Necessitating thoracotomy	4
From superior vena cava	1
From brachiocephalic artery	1
Wound hematoma	1
Vocal cord paralysis	
Left vocal cord	7
Side not given	4
Bilateral	4
Hoarseness, possible vocal cord paralysis	1
Pneumothorax	11
Pleural tear	3
Tumor seeding in incision line	1
Perforation of esophagus	1
Myocardial infarction (postoperative)	1
Bradycardia	4
Cardiac arrest (anesthetic error)	1
Wound infection	2
Left hemiparesis (transient)	1
Total	60

From Foster ED, Munro DD, Cobell ARC: Mediastinoscopy: a review of anatomical relationships and complications, *Ann Thorac Surg* 13:273, 1972.

embolism through open venous structures. **Manipulation of the mediastinoscope can compress the innominate artery, thereby decreasing arterial blood flow to the right upper extremity and the right common carotid arteries and obliterating the pulse and pressure in the right arm.**[268] It is recommended that a noninvasive blood pressure cuff be placed on the patient's left arm and either an arterial catheter (if indicated) or pulse oximetry probe be placed in the right upper extremity. Waveform analysis of the arterial pressure or pulse oximeter plethysmograph trace can detect compression.[183]

Complications

The overall complication rate for mediastinoscopies ranges from 1.5% to 3%.[20,35,169,379,457] Appreciation for the surgical risks associated with mediastinoscopy comes from an understanding of the anatomy relevant to the procedure. The most common and potentially serious complications are bleeding, cardiac tamponade, and air embolism. Compromise of other structures such as the trachea, bronchi, esophagus, laryngeal nerve, or innominate artery can lead to temporary or permanent complications. Massive hemorrhage can result from laceration of a pulmonary artery or a thoracic aortic artery.[272,457] Therefore, a large bore IV access catheter should be secured before induction of anesthesia. Clinical situations that increase collateral vascular flow, such as superior vena cava syndrome or aortic coarctation, predispose to bleeding and are relative contraindications to the procedure. Hemorrhage may be temporarily controlled by packing the surgical wound. Immediate thoracotomy may be required to control bleeding. In patients with superior vena cava obstruction, intravenous access should be secured in the lower extremity to avoid distending the thoracic venous vasculature and increasing the risk of bleeding.

Laceration of venous structures in the mediastinum increases the risk of air embolism.[379] Air embolism is associated with a sudden decrease in end tidal CO_2, relative hypotension, tachycardia, and a change in heart sounds heard through an esophageal stethoscope or by precordial Doppler monitor. When air embolism is suspected, nitrous oxide administration should be terminated, the patient placed in the Trendelenburg position, and the concerns communicated to the surgeon. The use of PEEP to increase intrathoracic venous pressure is controversial because of the potential increased risk of paradoxical embolization to the systemic arterial system through a patent foramen ovale.

Table 70-18 Anesthetic guidelines for mediastinoscopy and mediastinotomy

Indication	Diagnostic (biopsy mass, lymph nodes)
Monitors	Standard monitors, optional (arterial catheter)
Anesthesia	General anesthesia
Additional equipment	Shoulder roll
Ventilation	Single-lumen endotracheal tube
Position	Supine with cervical extension
Incision	Mediastinoscopy (suprasternal) Mediastinotomy
Unique considerations	To avoid artifact induced by innominate artery compression, place noninvasive blood pressure cuff on left To detect innominate artery compression, place pulse oximeter on right hand
Intraoperative complications	Dysrhythmia Asthma Hemorrhage Pneumothorax Recurrent laryngeal nerve injury Respiratory compromise Air embolism Perforation esophagus or bronchus Neurologic event (compression innominate artery or hyperextension of the neck)
Blood loss	Usually minimal
Postoperative analgesia	Parenteral opiates
Postoperative morbidity	Pneumothorax Hemoptysis Respiratory distress (vocal cord paralysis)
Postoperative care	Chest radiography Elevate head of bed to decrease edema and improve respiratory function

Compression of the vertebral arteries from hyperextension of the cervical spine or compression of the innominate artery that feeds the right common carotid artery can cause CNS complications.[147,183,358,434] One study documented transient decreases in blood flow for periods ranging from 15 to 35 seconds in 4 of 7 patients.[359] Some authors suggested the use of a Doppler placed over the right carotid artery or a right radial arterial catheter to detect compromise of flow by compression of the innominate artery.

Compression by the mediastinoscope or secondary compression caused by edema or bleeding can compromise the airway.[35] Tracheal laceration can lead to mediastinal emphysema and loss of effective ventilation. If it is suspected, fiberoptic bronchoscopy should be used to define the site and to guide advancement of the endotracheal tube beyond the laceration. Tracheomalacia resulting from long-standing compression of the trachea by mediastinal tumor can predispose to acute tracheal collapse.

Pneumothorax is the second-most common complication of mediastinoscopy. It may be unilateral or bilateral, and use of positive pressure ventilation can rapidly increase its size, causing hemodynamic compromise. It should be suspected if the patient exhibits an increase in peak airway pressures, hypotension, dysrhythmias, deviation of the trachea, or unilateral absence of breath sounds. A chest radiograph can be obtained to confirm the diagnosis if time permits. If the patient exhibits hemodynamic instability, rapid placement of a chest tube is indicated.

Postoperative Concerns

Dyspnea and respiratory difficulty may occur in the initial postoperative period. Intraoperative bleeding or edema can cause compression of the airway, especially in patients with tracheomalacia.[35] Raising the head of the bed improves ventilatory mechanics, facilitates venous return, and decreases edema. Damage to the recurrent laryngeal nerve during mediastinoscopy does not become evident until after extubation. If injury to the recurrent laryngeal is suspected, the vocal cords should be visualized during extubation with the patient breathing spontaneously. Unilateral nerve damage without airway obstruction is managed conservatively.[147,233,363,379] Bilateral nerve injury requires reintubation to prevent airway obstruction. Laryngeal nerve injury during these conditions is permanent in 50% of patients.[203]

ANESTHESIA FOR PATIENTS WITH MEDIASTINAL MASSES

Patients with mediastinal masses may experience catastrophic complications during general anesthesia. Some of the most terrifying moments in the practice of anesthesiology occur while caring for patients who have mediastinal masses and undergo diagnostic procedures, especially those in the pediatric age group.

The mediastinum is divided into the superior, anterior, middle, and posterior mediastina. The most common tumors in the anterior mediastinum are thymomas, mesenchymal tumors, dermoid cysts, thyroid and parathyroid tumors, and lymphomas (Fig. 70-40 and Table 70-19). In the middle and posterior mediastinum, tumor pathologies include pericardial cysts, bronchogenic cysts, lymphomas, neurogenic tumors, and aortic aneurysms.

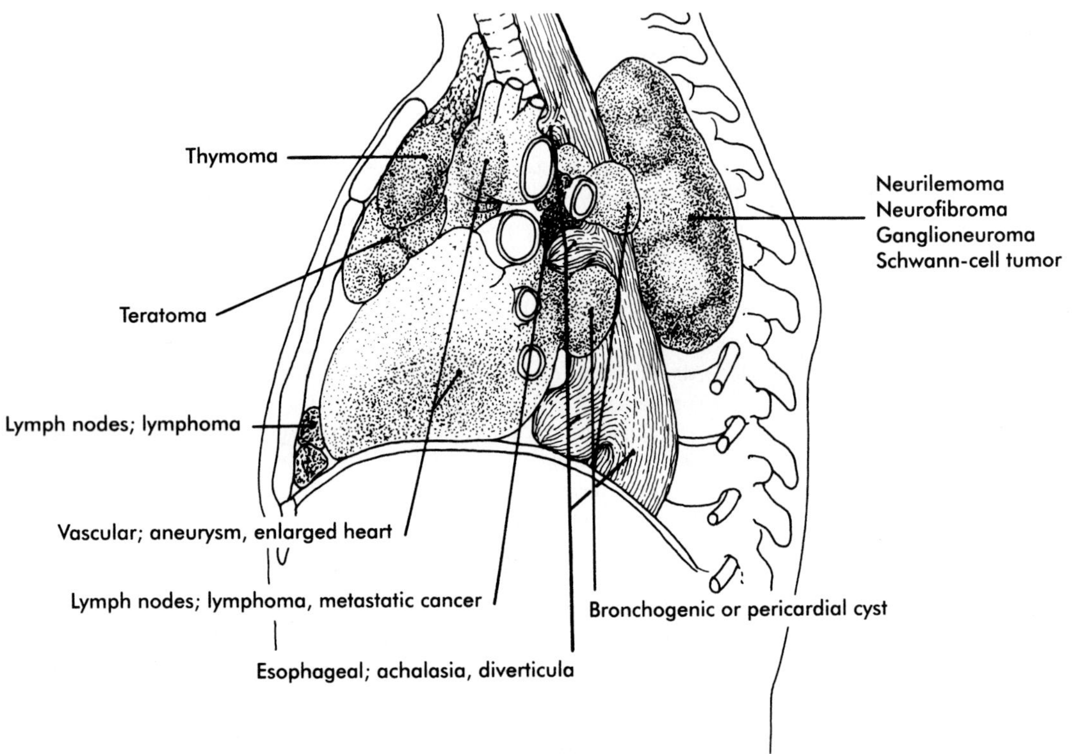

Fig. 70-40. Anatomic location of commonly encountered mediastinal masses. (Modified from Netter FH: *The CIBA collection of medical illustrations*, vol 7, Summit, NJ, 1979, CIBA.)

Table 70-19 Mediastinal mass location

Superior	Anterior	Middle	Posterior
Children			
Lymphoma	Lymphoma	Lymphoma	Neurogenic tumors
Thymoma	Teratoma		Esphageal duplication cysts
Retrosternal thyroid	Cystic hygroma	Tuberculous nodes	Diaphragmatic hernia (Bochdalek)
Parathyroid tumor	Thymoma		
	Pericardial cysts		
	Diaphragmatic hernia (Morgagni)		
Adults			
Lymphoma	Lymphoma	Lymphoma	Neurogenic tumors
Thymoma	Metastatic carcinoma	Metastatic carcinoma	Lymphoma
Restrosternal thyroid	Teratoma	Teratoma	Hernia (Bochdalek)
Metastatic carcinoma	Bronchogenic cyst	Bronchogenic cyst	Aortic aneurysm
Parathyroid tumors	Aortic aneurysm	Aortic aneurysm	
Zenker's diverticulum	Pericardial cyst	Pericardial cyst	
Aortic aneurysm			

Signs and Symptoms

The mechanisms postulated for the clinical symptoms of respiratory and cardiovascular compromise in awake patients include (Table 70-20) (1) progressive airway obstruction caused by compression of the distal trachea or bronchi, (2) loss of lung volume, (3) compression of the pulmonary artery or the heart, (4) superior vena caval obstruction, (5) involvement of the important nervous system elements in the mediastinum (e.g., recurrent laryngeal nerves, sympathetic chain), and (6) spinal cord compression from intraspinal extension of neurogenic tumors of the posterior mediastinum.

The incidence of perioperative complications generally is related to the size of the mediastinal mass and to the extent of disease within the thoracic cavity.[257] In one large series, clinical manifestations included (1) cough and pain, 40% each; (2) weight loss and fever, 24% each; (3) dyspnea and dysphagia, 20% each; (4) superior vena caval obstructions, 16%; (5) tracheal deviation, 12%; (6) Horner's syndrome, 7%; (7) spinal cord compression, 5%; and (8) cyanosis, mediastinal widening, and hoarseness, 3% each. Twenty percent of patients were asymptomatic. Not all patients with mediastinal masses who have acute life threatening airway complications during anesthesia are symptomatic preoperatively. Some are asymptomatic and show no airway compression on chest radiographs. **Therefore, the severity of the patient's preoperative respiratory symptoms may be unrelated to the extent of respiratory or cardiovascular compromise encountered during anesthesia.**[76,130,236]

Diagnostic Evaluation

A careful preoperative diagnostic evaluation should be performed, even in the asymptomatic patient, to determine the extent of mediastinal pathology. A flow chart describing the preoperative evaluation of patients with mediastinal masses is shown in Fig. 70-41. Most patients with mediastinal masses require scans to delineate the tumor size and location (Fig. 70-42). The anesthesiologist should evaluate the extent of compression of the airway, heart, and vascular structures preoperatively.[196,341] The extent of tracheal compression is a reliable predictor of whether difficulty with the airway may be expected. In one series, all of the patients who developed total or near-total airway obstruction during induction or emergence from anesthesia had greater than a 50% decrease in tracheal cross-sectional area as measured by CT scan.[23]

In addition to the chest radiograph and CT scan, a series of noninvasive studies may be performed to evaluate the risk of occult airway or cardiac involvement. Upright and supine flow-volume loops are simple, noninvasive, and sensitive studies for the diagnosis of occult airway obstruction (Fig. 70-43 on page 1806). The dynamic nature of this study makes it an extremely sensitive tool for evaluating obstructive lesions of major airways.[2] The inspiratory limb of the flow-volume loop is useful in diagnosing extrathoracic airway obstruction, whereas the expiratory limb is sensitive to intrathoracic airway obstruction. Maximal inspiratory and expiratory flow-volume loops obtained with the patient in the upright and supine positions enable the extent of functional impairment to be quantitated and help distinguish fixed from variable intrathoracic airway obstruction.[178,300] A disproportionate reduction in maximal expiratory flow should alert the physician to the presence of tracheomalacia and the inherent risk of airway collapse after extubation of the trachea. In addition, echocardiography in the upright and supine positions can reveal encroachment of tumor on the heart and intrathoracic vessels. Flexible fiberoptic bronchoscopy is another method of evaluating dynamic airway obstruction (Fig. 70-44 on page 1806). It allows assessment of the functional anatomy of the entire airway and the response of the airway to variations in intrathoracic pressure and position.

Pretreatment with radiotherapy or chemotherapy to reduce the size of the tumor decreases the risk of perioperative complications. Several investigators have suggested that patients receive empiric treatment of mediastinal pathology for

Table 70-20 Clinical findings in patients with mediastinal masses

History	Physical examination	Laboratory
Airway		
Cough	Decreased breath sounds	Chest radiograph (posteroanterior and lateral to look for tracheal deviation or compression)
Cyanosis	Wheezing	Flow-volume loops, supine and sitting
Dyspnea	Stridor	
Orthopnea	Cyanosis	
Cardiovascular		
Fatigue	Neck or facial edema	Chest radiographic changes in cardiac silhouette
Faintness	Jugular distention	Echocardiogram, supine and sitting
Headache	Papilledema	
Shortness of breath and orthopnea	Blood pressure changes or pallor with postural changes	
Cough	Pulsus paradoxus	

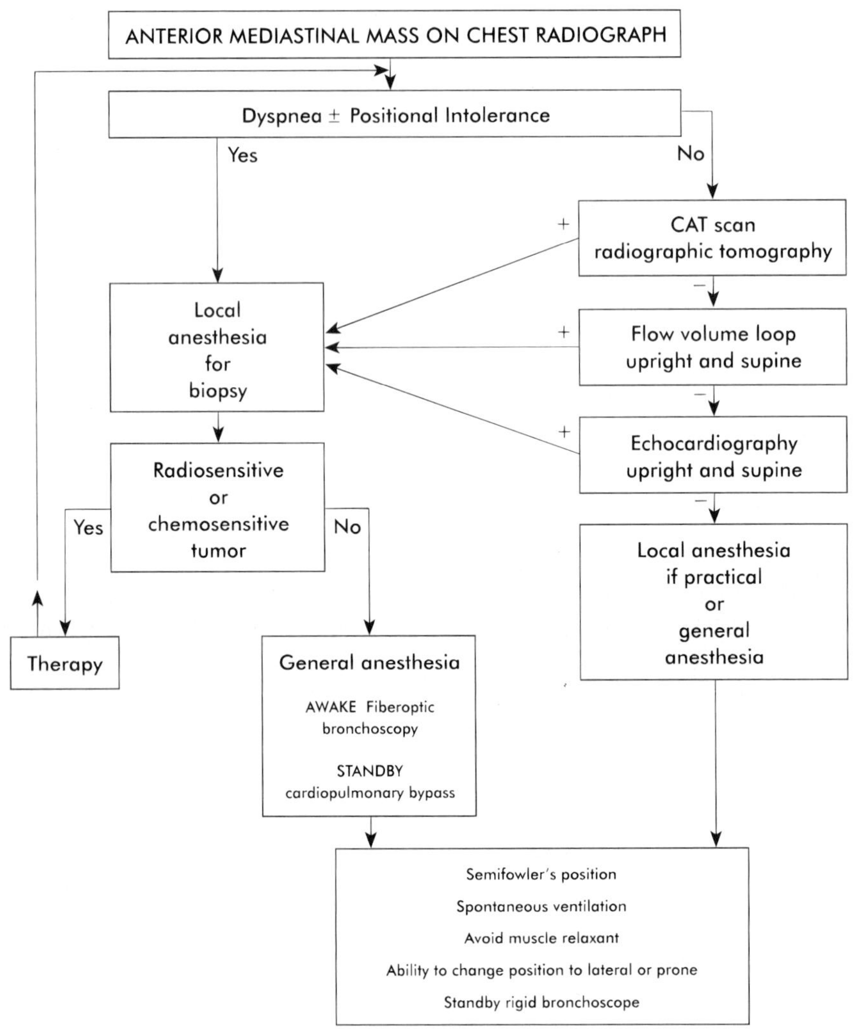

Fig. 70-41. Flow chart describing the preoperative evaluation of the patient with an anterior mediastinal mass. +, positive finding; −, negative work-up. (From Neuman GG, Weingarten AE, Abramowitz RM, et al: The anesthetic management of the patient with an anterior mediastinal mass, *Anesthesiology* 60:144, 1984.)

the presumed diagnosis.[276] Dramatic decrease in postoperative respiratory complications and improvement in risk category were achieved by preoperative radiation therapy for patients with severe clinical or radiologic findings.[432] Such views are controversial, and most clinicians advocate obtaining a biopsy before initiating therapy, even if this requires administration of general anesthesia with its inherent risks. An accurate pathologic diagnosis may be compromised if patients are empirically pretreated. In addition, the option of administering radiotherapy or chemotherapy to reduce the size of the mediastinal mass is not applicable to all patients. Some patients have large, benign mediastinal masses, such as a large dermoid cyst that cannot be managed except by surgical excision. Transcarinal aspiration of a large cystic subcarinal mass can be performed through a fiberoptic bronchoscope. This technique can be used preoperatively in patients who have cystic subcarinal masses to decrease the size of the mass before anesthetic induction. This technique has been reported to facilitate anesthetic management intraoperatively when a patient developed airway obstruction after induction of anesthesia.[293]

Anesthetic Implications and Management

Symptomatic and asymptomatic patients are at risk of developing severe, life-threatening complications after induction of general anesthesia (Table 70-21). Infants and small children may have obstructive symptoms earlier than adults because their small airway size increases the magnitude of airway resistance produced by decreases in airway dimensions. To avoid the risk of complications inherent with general anesthesia, alternate diagnostic techniques can be used. Alternative methods that can be performed in awake, sedated patients include percutaneous needle aspiration of the hilum and mediastinum, mediastinotomy, and thoracoscopy.[7]

When the surgical procedure requires general anesthesia, the anesthesiologist and surgeon should discuss the plan and confirm availability of equipment for emergency airway management (e.g., fiberoptic and

A

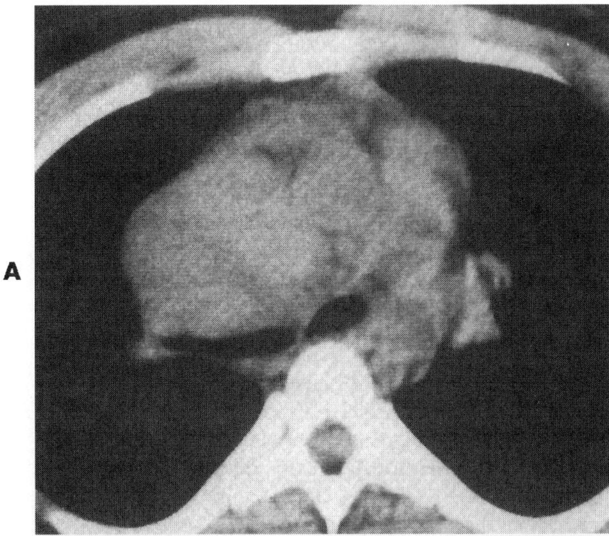

B

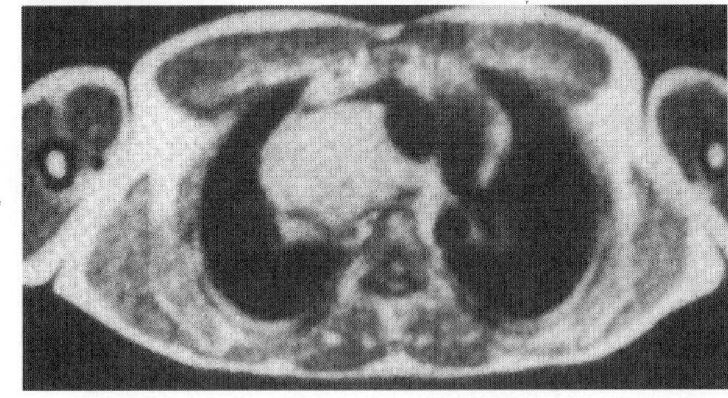

Fig. 70-42. Hodgkin's disease in a 16-year-old boy. **A,** CT scan shows a mediastinal mass anterior to and compressing the right upper lobe bronchus. **B,** T_1-weighted MR image (TR = 500 msec, TE = 30 msec) demonstrates the mediastinal mass and marked narrowing of the mainstem bronchi, especially the right. On MRI, the degree of compression appears much more severe than on CT. The patient was asymptomatic, and the narrowing was thought to be artifactual, caused by respiratory motion volume averaging. (From Siegel MJ, Nadel SN, Glazer HS, et al: Mediastinal lesions in children: comparison of CT and MR, *Radiology* 160:241, 1986.)

rigid bronchoscopes). Difficulties may occur during induction when the patient position is changed, when positive pressure is applied, after the administration of muscle relaxants, after intubation, during emergence, or after extubation.[251] The patient should undergo a slow controlled inhalational induction, with a staged approach that confirms an adequate airway before progressing. Induction may begin in a semirecumbent or seated position and progress to the supine position. After a deep anesthetic plane has been achieved, the anesthesiologist should attempt to gradually control ventilation. If wheezing or stridor ensues, the patient should be returned to spontaneous ventilation. If muscle relaxation is required to facilitate tracheal intubation, an ultrashort-acting relaxant such as succinylcholine should be used. The anesthetic technique should include the use of short-acting agents and avoidance of bolus administration of large doses of drugs. Intubation does not eliminate the risk of complications. Obstruction may even occur distal to a properly placed endotracheal tube that interferes with the normal protective glottic mechanism of physiologic PEEP that increases the tracheal distending pressure and reduces the possibility of dynamic collapse. Dynamic collapse of a tracheal segment also may occur with rapid respirations or cough during awakening from anesthesia.

Compression of the tracheobronchial tree

Neither the presence nor the severity of the patient's preoperative respiratory symptoms reliably predicts the extent of respiratory compromise that could be encountered during anesthesia, although most patients with severe respiratory symptoms have dramatic decreases in tracheal cross-sectional area.[23] The supine position, anesthesia, and muscle paralysis are associated with decreased dimensions of the rib cage, cephalad displacement of the dome of the diaphragm, and a reduction in thoracic volume limiting the space available for the trachea.[56,126,176,260] At low lung volumes, the decreased tracheal distending pressure can lead to tracheal collapse, particularly with tracheomalacia. Spontaneous ventilation is preferred to positive-pressure ventilation because the negative intrapleural pressure of spontaneous ventilation exerts a distending force that opposes bronchial and tracheal collapse. The supine position increases the central blood volume, which can further increase tumor volume and size. Edema, bleeding, and hematoma formation in the tumor as a result of surgical biopsy also can contribute to airway compromise.

Compression of pulmonary artery and heart

Compression of the main pulmonary artery is relatively rare, partly because of the protective effect of the aorta. Compression of the pulmonary trunk or one of the main pulmonary arteries can result in sudden hypoxemia, hypotension, and cardiac arrest. This compression was reported to result in the death of a 6-year-old child undergoing a cervical lymph node biopsy.[272] Another report describes a 14-year-old girl with a large dermoid cyst in the anterior mediastinum who required cardiopulmonary bypass to maintain arterial oxygenation and to counteract severe compression of the pulmonary artery by tumor during anesthesia.[205] Syncope during forced Valsalva maneuvers, such as occurs with a bowel movement, should alert the physician to the possibility of cardiovascular compression. Important factors contributing to a reduction in right ventricular output, hypotension, and severe hypoxemia include patient position, induction of anesthesia, and gravitational effects of the tumor on the heart and pulmonary artery.

Superior Vena Cava Syndrome

Pathophysiology

Superior vena cava syndrome occurs in approximately 6% to 7% of patients with lung carcinoma. Other causes include bronchial carcinoma, malignant lymphoma, and benign conditions that include multinodular goiter, mediastinal granu-

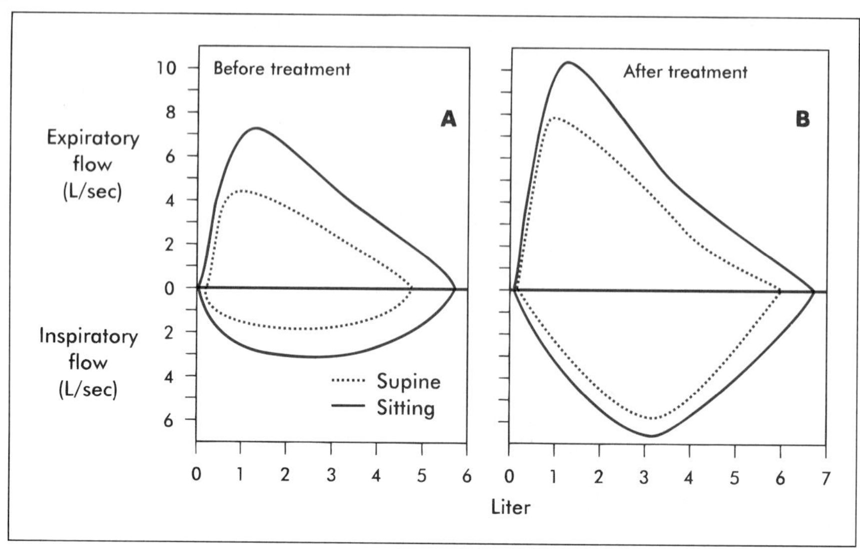

Fig. 70-43. Flow-volume curves obtained in supine and upright (sitting) positions before **(A)** and 4 weeks after **(B)** two courses of chemotherapy in patient with mediastinal Hodgkin's lymphoma. (From Prakash UBS, Abel MD, Hubmayr RD: Mediastinal mass and tracheal obstruction during general anesthesia, *Mayo Clin Proc* 63:1004, 1988.)

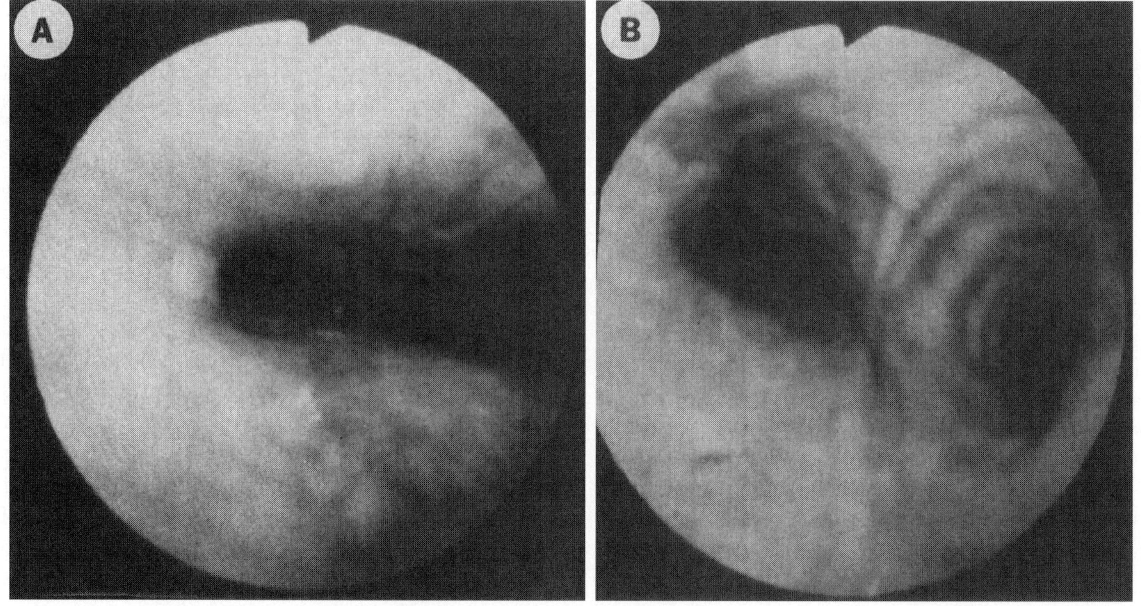

Fig. 70-44. Fiberoptic bronchoscopic appearance of lower trachea with patient in supine position **(A),** exhibiting almost total obstruction of trachea in anteroposterior plane. With patient in sitting position **(B),** lumen appears normal. (From Prakash UBS, Abel MD, Hubmayr RD: Mediastinal mass and tracheal obstruction during general anesthesia, *Mayo Clin Proc* 63:1004, 1988.)

lomas, idiopathic mediastinal fibrosis, and catheter-induced thrombosis of the superior vena cava.[139,321] Obstruction of the superior vena cava impedes venous flow from the head and upper extremities. Clinical features are reviewed in Box 70-14. The symptoms of dyspnea, dysphasia, and stridor may be associated with ruddy complexion and dilated veins across the upper chest and neck (Fig. 70-45). The severity of clinical manifestations depends on the rate at which the SVC is occluded. Slow gradual obstruction is associated with mild signs and symptoms, whereas more severe symptoms occur with rapid onset of obstruction. The severity also depends on the extent of obstruction, site of obstruction (above or below the azygous vein), and integrity of the azygous venous system. Occlusion of the azygous venous system often is symptomatic and may require surgery to bypass the spinal vein and to resect the obstructing lesion.

Choice of therapy depends on etiology. Therapeutic options include radiation, chemotherapy, and thrombectomy.

Table 70-21 Anesthetic guidelines for mediastinal mass

Indication	Biopsy or resection mediastinal mass
Monitors	Standard monitors, arterial catheter
Anesthesia	Preferably awake sedated using local anesthesia
	If general anesthesia is necessary, spontaneous ventilations should be maintained*
Additional equipment	Fiberoptic and rigid bronchoscope
	Multiple-sized ETT
	Standby of cardiopulmonary bypass or ECMO
Ventilation	Spontaneous ventilation preferred
	Intubation does not guarantee a secure patient airway
	Use of flexible bronchoscope to evaluate and intubate airway
Position	As tolerated by patient (sitting, semirecumbent, or supine)
Incision	Depends on location and size of tumor
	Surgical options include biopsy during local anesthesia, mediastinoscopy, mediasternotomy, median sternotomy
Unique considerations	Inability to ventilate
	Risk of cardiovascular collapse
	Superior vera cava syndrome (increased risk of airway edema, bleeding, placement of IV access in lower extremity)
	Avoid use muscle relaxants
	Maintenance of spontaneous ventilation
Intraoperative complication	Hypoxia
	Bleeding
	Hypotension
	Obstruction of airway
Postoperative morbidity	Airway edema, inability to extubate
Postoperative care	Monitored intensive care environment

*Until one can demonstrate that controlled ventilation does not cause airway obstruction or cardiovascular instability.

Once obstruction has produced complete thrombosis, thrombectomy is of little benefit. Patients having total or near total obstruction are at risk for cerebral vascular and airway compromise, both predictors of poor outcome. A tissue diagnosis should be obtained before the institution of therapy if possible. This can be done in most patients, noninvasively by bronchoscopy or lymph node biopsy. Occasionally, an open procedure requiring general anesthesia is necessary. Magnetic resonance imaging (MRI) and contrast venography are used to define the type and location of obstruction. If biopsy of the mediastinal mass is required, an open mediastinotomy should be performed instead of mediastinoscopy because the increased venous pressure increases the risk of bleeding during cervical exploration.

Anesthetic management

Patients with superior vena cava syndrome are at increased risk of airway compromise resulting from acute laryngospasm, bronchospasm, and airway edema caused by tumor edema or surgical manipulation.[117,122] Venous distention and symptoms are exacerbated by changes in positioning (supine or Trendelenburg) and by administration of intravenous fluids, especially through a catheter placed in the upper extremity. All venous access should be placed in the lower extremity, and an arterial catheter should be placed to monitor blood gases and blood pressure. **Venous congestion increases the risk of airway compromise, bleeding, and hypotensive episodes. The preoperative evaluation should include a careful assessment of the airway. Edema of the oral pharynx, larynx, and trachea may be more severe than the external edema and swelling of the face and neck.** Venous engorgement and tumor may involve the recurrent laryngeal nerve and cause external compression of the airway. These patients should be regarded in a manner similar to those with mediastinal masses. Premedication should be limited to the administration of an antisialagogue, and the patients should be transported in a semiseated position to decrease airway edema and facilitate venous drainage. If major airway edema is present, general anesthesia should be induced in a sitting position, and fiberoptic bronchoscopy may be required for airway access. Intraoperative management may be complicated by an abnormal response to the use of muscle relaxants related to a paraneoplastic myasthenic syndrome.[117] Many of these patients remain intubated postoperatively until edema of the airways and laryngeal structures is decreased.

ANESTHESIA FOR PATIENTS WITH THORACIC OUTLET SYNDROME

Thoracic outlet syndrome refers to neurologic and vascular symptoms affecting the upper extremity resulting from com-

BOX 70-14
CLINICAL FEATURES OF SUPERIOR VENA CAVAL SYNDROME

Neurologic

Headache, dizziness, decreased mentation, visual changes, restlessness, agitation, Horner's syndrome, stupor, convulsions

Pathophysiology

Low cardiac output, decreased cerebral perfusion, increased cerebral venous pressure, cerebral edema

Respiratory

Shortness of breath, cough, hoarseness, hypoxemia, tachypnea, stridor

Pathophysiology

Upper airway edema, tracheal obstruction, vocal cord paralysis

Cardiac

Tachycardia; thoracic and cervical venous distention; plethoric face; edema of the face, neck, upper extremities, and trunk; cyanosis; distended veins over chest wall

Pathophysiology

Decreased venous return, development of collateral venous circulation, increased peripheral venous circulation, increased peripheral venous pressure, as high as 40 mm Hg

Gastrointestinal

Nausea, vomiting, dysphagia

Pathophysiology

Fluid imbalance, upper airway edema

Renal

Decreased urine output

Pathophysiology

Low cardiac output

pression of the neurovascular bundle at the thoracic outlet between the first rib and the clavicle or between the anterior scalene muscle and the medial scalene muscle.[118,244,339] The etiology is classified either as noncancerous or cancerous.

The majority of noncancerous causes are related to either trauma or the presence of a cervical rib. A less frequent etiology is hypertrophy of the scalene and subclavian muscles. Clinical manifestations usually are vague and obscure and may be misinterpreted as angina. Pain may be localized to the shoulder or extend along the medial aspect of the arm and forearm, along the proximal shoulder girdle, or to the neck and face. Symptoms may include weakness, numbness, and paresthesias. Conservative management includes rehabilitation exercises, anti-inflammatory drugs, and analgesics. In those with vascular insufficiency or if symptoms are refractory to medical therapy, operation may be indicated. Surgical approaches include resection of the first rib, partial resection of the scalene muscles, or removal of anomalous fibromuscular bands.

General anesthesia is induced with the patient in the supine position. Then, the patient is placed in the lateral decubitus position, and the affected arm is prepped into the surgical field. Noninvasive blood pressure recording and venous access should be placed on the opposite side. The complications of first rib resection include pneumothorax, brachial neuralgia, pleural fusion, temporary phrenic nerve palsy, injury to the subclavian artery, and injury to the long thoracic nerve and T1 roots.

Anesthetic management includes the use of routine monitoring and a double-lumen endotracheal tube to facilitate one-lung isolation (Table 70-22). The patient is placed in the lateral decubitus position, and an incision is made in the lower margin of the anterior axilla. Intraoperative complications include hemorrhage, pneumothorax, brachial nerve injury with resulting nerve dysfunction, and cervical sympathectomy on the ipsilateral side. Because of the position of the nondependent arm and the site of surgery, stretch and surgical trauma to the brachial plexus is a major risk.

The presentation of lung cancer with symptoms of thoracic outlet syndrome is known as Pancoast's syndrome. The most common etiology is a bronchogenic carcinoma originating in or near the superior pulmonary sulcus. These tumors invade the lymphatic system and spread by direct extension to entwine the brachial plexus intercostal arteries, stellate ganglia, and sympathetic chain, thereby producing Horner's syndrome. If the tumor is considered resectable, the pulmonary tumor and extension into the chest wall and brachial plexus should be excised.

ANESTHESIA FOR PATIENTS UNDERGOING THYMECTOMY: MYASTHENIA GRAVIS

Clinical Features

The thymus is a central lymphoid gland that functions in the development and maintenance of immunologic competence. Surgical resection of the thymus most often is performed for myasthenia gravis and less often for primary neoplasm, carcinoid tumor, or multiple endocrine neoplasm syndrome. Seventy-five percent of the patients with myasthenia gravis have associated thymic hyperplasia or thymomas.

Myasthenia gravis is a chronic autoimmune disease involving the neuromuscular junction. The prevalence is 1 per 20,000 to 30,000 population with female patients outnumbering male patients by a ratio of 6:4. The disease is associated with a decrease in the number of acetylcholine receptors and motor endplates, loss of synaptic folds, and widening of the synaptic cleft.[57,119,155,168] The hallmark of this disease is weakness and rapid fatigability of the voluntary muscles with repetitive use. The onset of symptoms usually is slow and insidious and can appear in any group of skeletal muscles, although most patients initially experience the

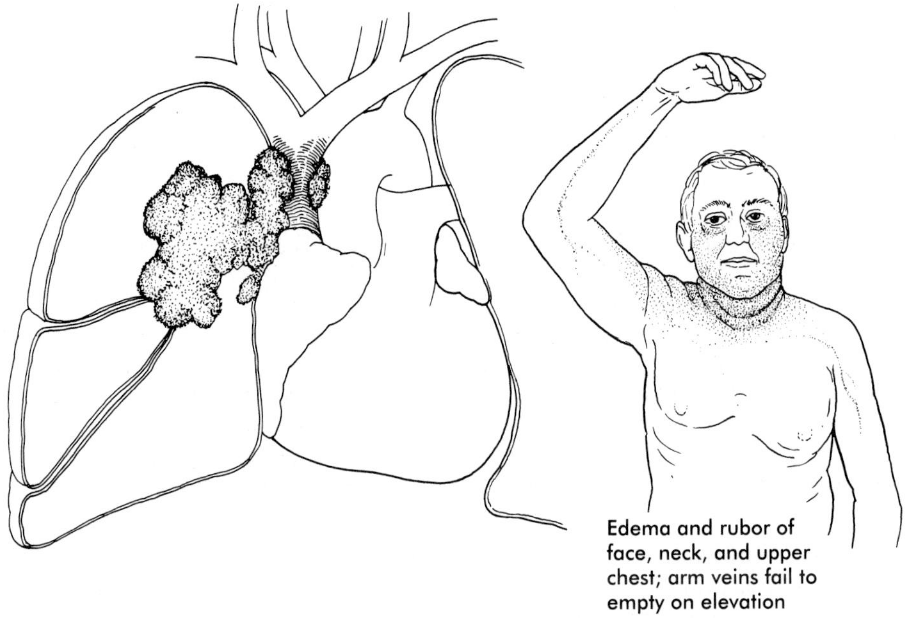

Fig. 70-45. Bronchogenic carcinoma producing superior vena caval obstruction. Superior vena cava syndrome is characterized by edema and rubor of face, neck, and upper chest. Arm veins fail to empty on elevation. (Modified from Netter FH: *The CIBA collection of medical illustrations*, vol 7, Summit, NJ, 1979, CIBA.)

Table 70-22 Anesthetic guidelines for thoracic outlet syndrome

Indication	Therapeutic (syndrome characterized by lateral upper extremity weakness, numbness, paresthesias, pain)
Monitors	Standard monitors
	Noninvasive cuff on opposite side
	Ipsilateral pulse oximetry
Anesthesia	General anesthesia
Ventilation	Single-lumen ETT or double-lumen ETT
Position	Supine or lateral decubitus position, determined by surgical approach
Incision	Cervical region (partial resection of first rib)
	Scalene muscles
Unique considerations	Intravenous access on opposite side
Intraoperative complications	Pneumothorax
	Pleural effusion
	Vascular injury
	Neural injury
	Cervical sympathectomy
Blood loss	Minimal < 500 ml
Postoperative analgesia	Parenteral opiates
Postoperative morbidity	Temporary phrenic nerve palsy
	Pneumothorax
	Brachial plexus neuralgia or palsy
	Injury to long thoracic nerve and T1 roots
Postoperative care	Chest radiography

ocular manifestations, diplopia, and ptosis. One third of myasthenic patients have bulbar symptoms including difficulty swallowing and clearing secretions, which predispose to pulmonary aspiration. The disease has been classified according to severity of debilitation and aggressiveness (Table 70-23). If the symptoms remain limited to ocular manifestations for two years, the likelihood of progression to generalized myasthenia is low, although those patients with rapid onset and generalized symptoms have a poor prognosis and limited response to therapy.

Therapy for myasthenia gravis includes anticholinesterase drugs, corticosteroids, other immunosuppressants such as aza-

Table 70-23 Clinical classification of myasthenia gravis

Stage	Term	Description
I	Ocular myasthenia	Involvement of ocular muscles only; mild symptoms of ptosis and diplopia
II	Mild-to-moderate generalized myasthenia	Slow onset, usually ocular, spreading to skeletal and bulbar muscles; no respiratory involvement; good response to drug
III	Acute fulminating myasthenia	Rapid onset of severe bulbar and skeletal weakness with involvement of muscles of respiration; poor response to therapy
IV	Late severe myasthenia	Severe disease developing 2 years after onset of stage I or II symptoms; poor response to therapy and poor prognosis

thioprine or cyclophosphamide, plasmapheresis, and thymectomy. These therapies may be used individually or in combination. Anticholinesterase drugs, such as neostigmine or pyridostigmine, most often are selected because they provide immediate symptomatic relief. These drugs inhibit the enzyme responsible for hydrolysis of acetylcholine and thereby increase the concentration of neurotransmitter at the neuromuscular junction. The efficacy of corticosteroids in the management of myasthenia is believed to result from interference with the production of antibodies responsible for degradation of the cholinergic receptors. Azathioprine, cyclophosphamide, or plasmapheresis may be effective by virtue of their ability to inhibit production or reduce circulating concentrations of antibodies. Surgical resection of the thymus gland may result in complete remission or dramatic improvement in symptoms.[206]

Anesthetic Considerations

Management of anesthesia for patients with myasthenia gravis should consider the severity of symptoms, presence of other associated disorders (Box 70-15), and preoperative drug therapy. Considerations for the perioperative period are presented in Table 70-24. An assessment of preoperative pulmonary function should be obtained as a baseline for comparison. The patient's preoperative medications should be reviewed for those drugs that could interfere with neuromuscular function (Box 70-16). Drugs that have the potential to exacerbate muscle weakness in these patients include calcium channel blockers, aminoglycosides, and antiarrhythmic agents.[43,132,255,456] Most authors recommend that patients continue their usual dose of anticholinesterase therapy the night before surgery. On the day of operation, patients who are severely symptomatic should receive a full morning dose. Those patients who are only mildly affected should receive half a dose or none at all. The rationale for withholding the morning dose is to prevent antagonism of muscle relaxants that may be used to facilitate tracheal intubation. Patients receiving systemic steroids should continue their steroid supplementation on the day of surgery.

Special attention should be given to the psychological preparation of these patients. They should be told about the increased risk to prolonged muscle weakness and respiratory depression that may require temporary postoperative ventilation. Judicious use of benzodiazepines provides adequate anxiolysis, whereas the use of opiates should be avoided to prevent respiratory depression.

All patients undergoing thymectomy require general anesthesia regardless of the surgical approach. In patients undergoing a transmediastinal approach, the use of an epidural block as an adjunct to general anesthesia has been found to decrease the intraoperative MAC, lessen postoperative analgesic requirements, improve respiratory mechanics, and dramatically decrease the frequency of prolonged intubation.[111,308]

Use of a muscle relaxant is not required but may facilitate tracheal intubation. Anticholinesterase drugs not only inhibit true cholinesterase but also impair activation of

BOX 70-15
DISORDERS ASSOCIATED WITH MYASTHENIA GRAVIS

- Thyroid disease
  - Hyperthyroidism
  - Hypothyroidism
  - Thyroiditis
- Thymoma
- Anemias pernicious
- Multiple sclerosis
- Ulcerative colitis
- Leukemia
- Lymphoma
- Autoimmune disorders
  - Systemic lupus erythematosus
  - Idiopathic thrombocytopenic purpura
  - Rheumatoid arthritis
  - Scleroderma
  - Polymyositis
  - Sjögren's syndrome

Table 70-24 Anesthetic guidelines for thymectomy: myasthenia gravis

Indication	Therapeutic (myasthenia gravis, thymoma, multiple endocrine neoplasm syndrome)
Monitors	Standard monitors
Anesthesia	General anesthesia
Preoperative considerations	Review use of anticholinesterase medications Evaluate strength Assess respiratory function
Ventilation	Usually single-lumen ETT Double-lumen ETT if by video-assisted thoracoscopy
Position	Supine with shoulder roll Occasionally by left lateral decubitus (thoracoscopy)
Incision	Sternotomy, transcervical Portals for video-assisted thoracoscopy
Unique considerations	Myasthenia gravis (increased sensitivity to muscle relaxants, risk of remaining intubated postoperatively, avoid neuromuscular blocking effects of antiarrhythmics, diuretics, and aminoglycosides)
Intraoperative complications	Myasthenia gravis (residual weakness or sedation leading to inability to extubate)
Blood loss	Minimal
Postoperative analgesia	Parenteral opiates, epidural
Postoperative morbidity	Respiratory insufficiency (inadequate reversal of muscle relaxants, excessive sedation, not received daily dose of anticholinesterase)
Postoperative care	Chest radiography Optimize respiratory function (analgesics, raise head of bed) Follow in monitored setting

BOX 70-16
DRUGS THAT CAN EXACERBATE MYASTHENIA GRAVIS

- Acetylcholinesterase in high doses
- Aminoglycosides
- Other antibiotics (e.g., clindamycin, colistin, polymyxin B, tetracycline, trimethaphan)
- Antidysrhythmics (e.g., procainamide, quinidine, propranolol, lidocaine)
- Thyroid hormones
- Quinine (tonic water)
- Lithium
- Phenytoin (Dilantin)
- Oxytocin
- Chlorpromazine
- Chloroquine

plasma cholinesterase. Although patients usually are less sensitive to succinylcholine in the presence of anticholinergic therapy, its duration of action may be extended. Therefore, the dose of succinylcholine should be reduced to avoid prolongation of the response and associated phase two block.[32,95,145,411] Patients with myasthenia gravis have a marked sensitivity to nondepolarizing muscle relaxants, increasing their sensitivity and duration of action.[146,227] If muscle relaxation is required, a small dose of a short-acting nondepolarizing drug, such as atracurium or pipercurium, should be used. Halogenated inhaled anesthetics have muscle relaxing properties. One study found that patients with myasthenia gravis were more sensitive to the neuromuscular depressant effects of isoflurane.[385] Recovery of the electromyographic response was still incomplete 1 hour after terminating isoflurane, despite satisfactory clinical recovery.

The most common surgical approaches are the transcervical and trans-sternal approaches, whereas a minority are performed by thoracotomy or VAT. The transcervical approach has the advantage of avoiding the immediate postoperative alterations in pulmonary mechanics.[148,150,192] Mediastinotomy may be necessary when resecting a hypertrophied thymus that extends substernally. If mediastinotomy or the cervical approach is to be used, a single-lumen tube is appropriate, although if lateral thoracotomy is planned, a double-lumen endotracheal tube is indicated.

Postoperative Concerns

At the end of the operation, neuromuscular transmission is assessed using a nerve stimulator; nondepolarizing muscle relaxants are reversed as necessary, and the patient is allowed to emerge from anesthesia. Residual weakness from isoflurane can cause fade in the response to tetanic stimulation. Suitability for extubation is judged by measuring the patient's pulmonary function and comparing the results with preoperative values. Negative inspiratory force, tidal volume, and vital capacity should be measured immediately before induction and used as the basis for comparison. To improve respiratory mechanics, the patient is placed in a semirecumbent position with the head of the bed raised about 30°, is suctioned for secretions, and receives adequate analgesia without inducing respiratory depression. The patient should be monitored closely for 18 to 24 hours after operation. A chest radiograph is obtained immediately postoperatively to rule out the presence of a pneumothorax. Improvement in myasthenic symptoms after thymectomy may take weeks to months. Therefore, the patient should receive any missed dose of anticholinesterase from the morning of operation.[151]

ANESTHESIA FOR PATIENTS UNDERGOING TRACHEAL RESECTION AND TRACHEOBRONCHIAL RECONSTRUCTION

Indications for tracheal resection include

- Tracheal tumors, most of which are malignant
- Carinal tumors or carinal involvement with a bronchogenic carcinoma
- Tracheal involvement with a thyroid carcinoma
- Traumatic disruption of the trachea and bronchi, which may occur as a result of blunt trauma, penetrating injuries, iatrogenic manipulations, and aspirated sharp foreign bodies
- Tracheal stenosis after prolonged intubation, trauma, etc.

Patients undergoing surgical resection of the trachea, main bronchi, or both impose special anesthetic management problems. The surgical procedure often is prolonged, and episodes of ventilatory insufficiency may be unavoidable. Communication between the anesthesia and surgical teams, with emphasis on the ventilatory treatment of the patient during each phase of the procedure, is imperative. The most challenging aspect of these procedures is to design an effective method of ventilating the lungs during the resection and reconstruction of the airway that does not interfere with surgical exposure and that provides adequate ventilation and oxygenation. Patients with large intratracheal or carinal masses may develop total airway obstruction on the induction of anesthesia. Fortunately, many of these patients undergo laser debulking procedures before undergoing surgical resection. Because an inflated cuff and positive-pressure ventilation adjacent to the suture line may interfere with healing or cause disruption of the anastamosis, after the procedure the patient should breath spontaneously and be extubated in the operating room or shortly thereafter.

Surgical techniques may include resection and primary anastomosis, resection, and reconstruction with prosthetic material or with the insertion of a T-tube stent. Therapeutic adjuncts may include radiotherapy (preoperatively or postoperatively), radioactive seed implantation, and preoperative laser debulking.

Surgical Considerations

Surgery on the trachea and bronchi usually is done through a right thoracotomy to avoid the aortic arch, although if the left bronchus is involved or a left pulmonary resection may be done, a left thoracotomy may be performed. The surgical procedure requires extensive hilar dissection, mobilization of the lungs, and possibly opening of the pericardium. The omentum, serratus muscle, or intercostal muscle may have to be used to wrap the anastomosis or to cover defects in the tracheobronchial tree. Mobilization of the omentum requires an additional abdominal incision. Thoracoabdominal exposure substantially increases fluid requirements. On occasion, pericardium may be used to patch sections of the pulmonary artery involved with tumor. Every effort should be made to maintain normothermia and minimize heat loss. After the procedure, to decrease tension on the anastomosis, it may be necessary to maintain the patient's neck in a flexed position by suturing the skin and soft tissues of the chin to the anterior chest wall. Even in this situation, it is advantageous to extubate the trachea as soon as possible after surgery. Therefore, the anesthetic should be planned with the goal of rapid emergence and recovery from muscle relaxants. Thorough suctioning of the tracheobronchial tree, via a fiberoptic bronchoscope if indicated, should be performed immediately before emergence from anesthesia.

Postoperative complications, particularly pulmonary infections and air leaks through the airway anastomosis, can lead to the development of a bronchopleural fistula and respiratory failure. Factors that predispose to poor healing of the tracheobronchial anastomosis include cancer, previous steroid and antineoplastic chemotherapy, preoperative radiotherapy, extensive dissection and devascularization of the tracheobronchial stump, and poor nutritional status and debilitation. In selecting the technique for airway management, the anesthesiologist should consider the need to provide appropriate surgical conditions. Constant cooperation and communication between the surgical and anesthesia team are extremely important during these procedures.

Perioperative Management Issues

Preoperative assessment and preparation

Patients should be evaluated for airway patency and cardiopulmonary reserve. Unless airway obstruction is imminent, requiring emergency surgery, pulmonary function studies should be obtained (Figs. 70-46 and 70-47). Flow-volume loops are very helpful in detecting fixed or variable intrathoracic or extrathoracic obstructions. Most of these patients have serious underlying pulmonary disease that may further compromise gas exchange intraoperatively and postoperatively. Reversible conditions that alter pulmonary function should be managed with antibiotics and bronchodilators preoperatively. All considerations that apply to patients with airway obstruction resulting from extrinsic compression by mediastinal masses also apply to patients with intrinsic obstruction of the airways. Preoperative ABG values should be obtained. Mucosal edema frequently contributes to airway obstruction in these patients, and preoperative steroids and diuretics may be beneficial.

Monitoring

An intraarterial catheter is indicated for continuous monitoring of blood pressure and for frequent sampling of arterial blood gases. Noninvasive monitoring should include

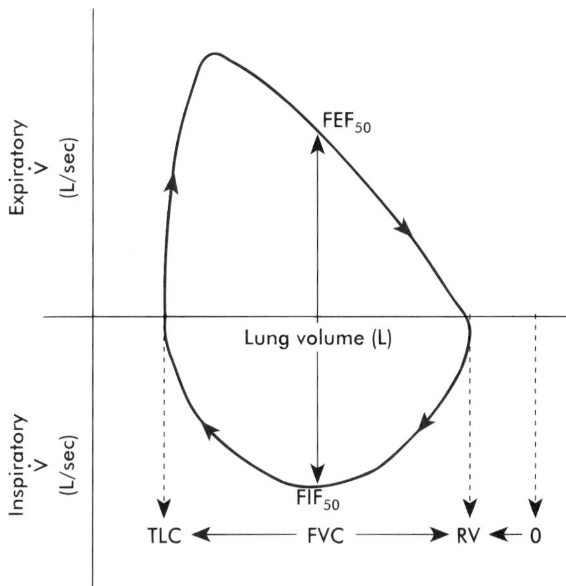

Fig. 70-46. Idealized flow-volume (V̇-V̇) loop. During forced expiration, the rate of airflow increases rapidly at volume close to TLC. As lung volume decreases, flow progressively falls in a near-linear fashion caused by increasing airway resistance. With maximum inspiratory effort, flow normally peaks at a lung volume near the midportion of FVC. At mid-point lung volume, the forced inspiratory flow (FIF_{50}) and forced expiratory flow (FEF_{50}) should normally be equal. When the ratio (FIF_{50}/FEF_{50}) is less than unity, it suggests an extrathoracic obstruction, compromising inspiratory flow. If greater than one, it supports a diagnosis of intrathoracic airway obstruction.

pulse oximetry and capnography. Placement of the pulse oximetry probe on the hand opposite the intraarterial catheter facilitates continuous verification of adequate blood delivery to both upper extremities and can signal the need for adjustment of patient position or surgical retraction.

Induction of anesthesia

Induction of anesthesia follows the same guidelines as discussed in the section on anesthesia for patients with mediastinal masses. The anesthesiologist should know precisely the site and the size of the lesion and the extent of airway lumen compromise before induction of anesthesia. The anesthesiologist should review the chest radiographs, tomograms, CT scans, flow-volume loops, and results of bronchoscopy or bronchography preoperatively. Some patients have such severe airway obstruction that induction of anesthesia would precipitate total airway obstruction. A skilled endoscopist usually can pass a small diameter ventilating bronchoscope past the lesion, allowing ventilation of a least one lung. Once ventilation and oxygenation have been satisfactorily established, intubation of the trachea may be attempted, perhaps over a stylet introduced via the rigid bronchoscope.

Modes of Ventilation

The major challenge during operation for tracheobronchial resection and reconstruction is the maintainance of ventilation. The options include (1) a single-lumen endotracheal tube, (2) a single endobronchial tube or two endobronchial tubes, one into each mainstem bronchus distal to the are of resection, (3) low-frequency jet ventilation, (4) high-frequency ventilation to one or both lungs, above the site of the lesion, or (5) cardiopulmonary bypass through the femoral approach during resection of the carina.[6,235,466] Because of the risk of intrapulmonary hemorrhage with heparinization, cardiopulmonary bypass should be used only in selected patients when absolutely necessary.

Use of conventional ventilation for tracheobronchial reconstruction

When planning to use conventional ventilation during tracheobronchial reconstructive surgery, the anesthesiologist should have several different sizes of armored endotracheal tubes available, some of them still sterile. A long sterile anesthesia circuit is required because it often is necessary for the surgeon to intubate the trachea or bronchus within the sterile field. Airway management depends on the location of the lesion and its distance from the carina.

Resection of a high tracheal lesion

A single-lumen, uncut endotracheal tube is placed above the tracheal lesion after induction of general anesthesia. If the obstruction is mild or if the area of obstruction can be bypassed, mechanical positive-pressure ventilation is safe. The surgeon may help guide the endotracheal tube past the area of stenosis when the trachea is open.[41,243] Alternatively, a sterile tube can be passed through the field into the distal trachea after the trachea has been transsected below the lesion. That tube is then connected, via sterile anesthesia hoses and Y piece, to the anesthesia machine. Armored endotracheal tubes should be used to decrease the possibility of kinking and obstruction. If the distal segment of the trachea is short, the tip of the endotracheal tube can be cut distal to the cuff to allow the tube to remain above the carina (Fig. 70-48).

Repair of a high tracheal lesion usually is done through a cervical incision, possibly combined with a median sternotomy. After excision of the tracheal lesion and placement of the posterior tracheal suture line, the distal endotracheal or endobronchial tube is removed from the trachea. The proximal endotracheal tube then is advanced past the anastomotic lines, reconnected to the anesthesia circuit, and the anastomosis completed.

Resection of a low tracheal lesion

This usually is performed through a right thoracotomy incision. A single-lumen endotracheal tube is placed with its tip above the lesion. If sufficient length of trachea distal to the area of resection is available, a Foley catheter with its tip removed just distal to the balloon may be used as a single-lumen endotracheal tube. It is inserted by the surgeon and maintained in place above the carina, thereby avoiding endobronchial intubation and the need for one-lung ventilation. If the distal tracheal stump is very short, the tube

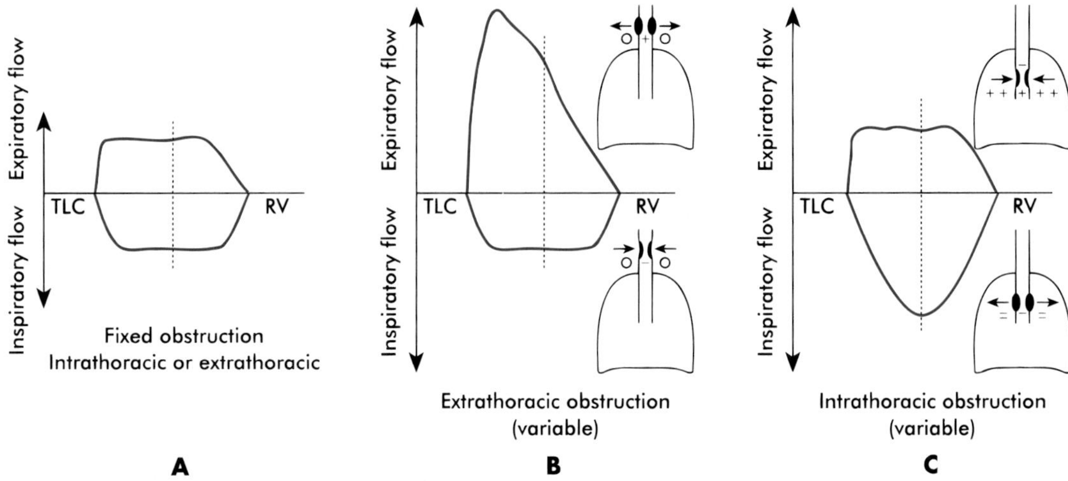

Fig. 70-47. Maximal inspiratory and expiratory flow-volume curves in fixed obstruction (intrathoracic or extrathoracic), in which airway diameter does not change with either inspiration or expiration, extrathoracic variable obstruction, or intrathoracic variable obstruction. The *dotted line* indicates 50% of the vital capacity; the ratio of expired-to-inspired flow at this point is the mid-VC ratio and is normally 0.9 to 1.0. **A,** With a fixed obstruction, expiratory and inspiratory flows are equally altered, and the mid-VC ratio remains normal. **B,** With a variable extrathoracic obstruction, forced expiration results in a slightly positive (+) intratracheal pressure that is greater than the pressure around the airway (atmospheric or 0), resulting in a decrease of the obstruction (airway dilates). During forced inspiration, when pressure around the airway (0) exceeds the intratracheal pressure (−), the obstruction is increased (airway narrows). Because the expiratory curve is normal and the inspiratory curve is altered, the mid-VC ratio is much greater than normal. **C,** With a variable intrathoracic obstruction, forced expiration results in a very positive (++) pleural pressure that is greater than the slightly positive (+) intratracheal pressure, resulting in an increase of the obstruction (airway narrows). During forced inspiration, the intratracheal pressure (−) is greater than the pleural pressure (−−), thus decreasing the obstruction (airway dilates). Because the inspiratory curve is normal and the expiratory curve is attenuated, the mid-VC ratio is much less than normal. A normal flow-volume curve is a composite of the inspiratory curve in **B** and the expiratory curve in **C.** TLC—total lung capacity; RV—residual volume. (Benumof JL: Anesthesia for special elective therapeutic procedures. In Benumof JL, editor: *Anesthesia for thoracic surgery,* Philadelphia, 1995, WB Saunders.)

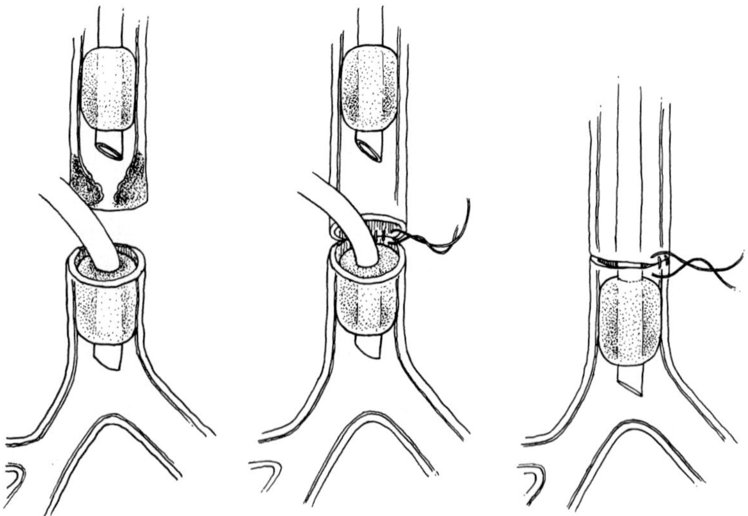

Fig. 70-48. Procedure for resection of high tracheal lesion. (Modified from Geffin B, Bland J, Grillo HC, et al: Anesthetic management of tracheal resection and reconstruction, *Anesth Analg* 48:884, 1969.)

should be advanced into the bronchus of the dependent (usually the left) lung. If oxygenation is inadequate, the shunt can be decreased by temporarily clamping the pulmonary artery of the nondependent side (Fig. 70-49).[186,199,422] When the posterior tracheal suture line has been completed, the distal endobronchial tube or Foley catheter is removed, and the original orotracheal tube is advanced across the suture line into the bronchus of the dependent lung. The anterior suture line then is completed. The endotracheal tube is then pulled proximally so that its tip lies above the suture line.

For carinal resection, a single-lumen endotracheal tube is inserted through the larynx (Fig. 70-50). After the carina is resected, the surgeon places a second endotracheal tube into the bronchus of the dependent lung, usually the left. The tube is connected by a set of sterile anesthesia hoses and Y piece to the anesthesia machine. The left lung is ventilated through the endobronchial tube, whereas the right lung is collapsed as the right bronchus is attached to the trachea. After the right mainstem bronchus has been reattached to the trachea, the original translaryngeal endotracheal tube is

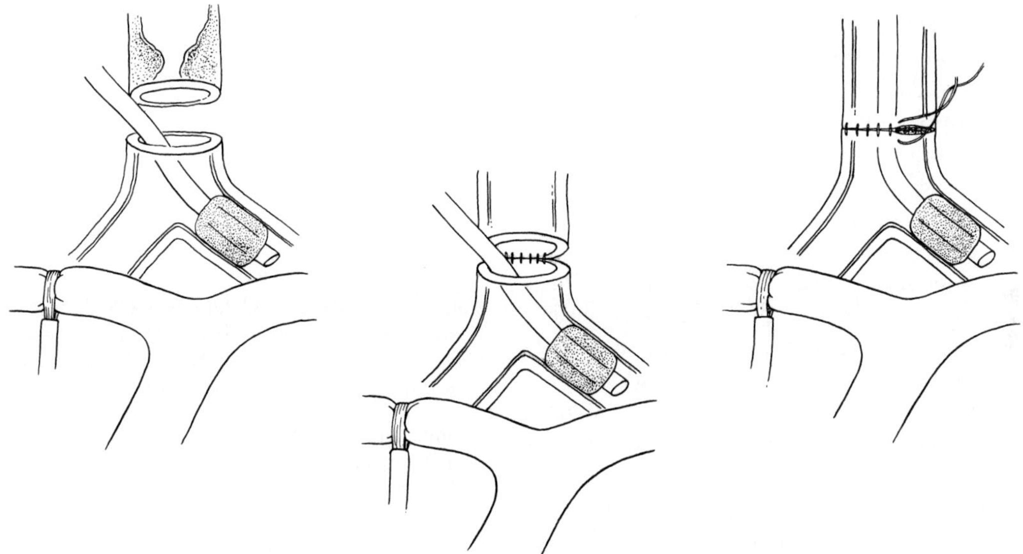

Fig. 70-49. Procedure for resection of lower tracheal lesions. (Modified from Geffin B, Bland J, Grillo HC, et al: Anesthetic management of tracheal resection and reconstruction, *Anesth Analg* 48:884, 1969.)

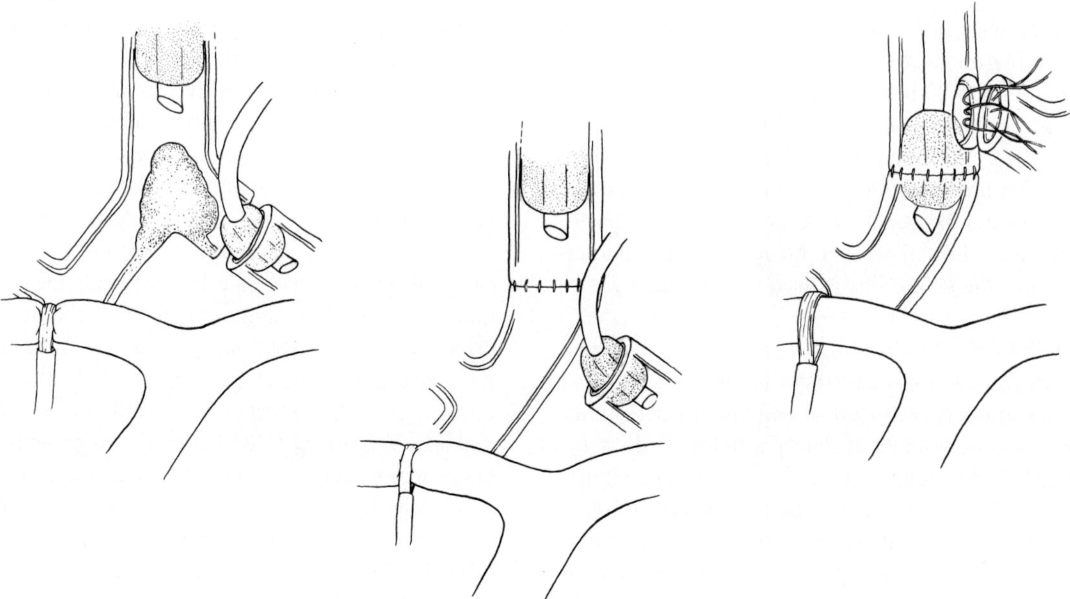

Fig. 70-50. Procedure for resection of carinal lesions. (Modified from Geffin B, Bland J, Grillo HC, et al: Anesthetic management of tracheal resection and reconstruction, *Anesth Analg* 48:884, 1969.)

advanced past the suture line into the right mainstem bronchus. Cutting the tip of this endotracheal tube helps to prevent obstruction of the right upper lobe bronchus. The left endobronchial tube then is removed, and the left mainstem bronchus is attached to the trachea by an end-to-side anastomosis. The endotracheal tube then is pulled proximally so that its tip is above both anastomotic lines.

Alternatively, after the carina is resected, the anesthesiologist can independently ventilate each lung through the distal bronchial stumps. The surgeon places a single-lumen endotracheal tube into each bronchial stump. A plastic Y connector is used to deliver the tidal volume to both endotracheal tubes. A good air seal can be achieved by using stay sutures to pull the bronchial stump against the distal end of the inflated cuff (Fig. 70-51). As the posterior layer of the anastomosis is performed, ventilation is maintained through the accessible distal bronchi. To attach the lateral wall of a bronchus to the trachea, the corresponding endobronchial tube is removed, and one-lung ventilation is used for a limited period. As the anastomosis of the anterior wall nears completion, ventilation from above is restored. The remaining air leak will progressively diminish as the incision is closed. If the air leak is too large, the proximal translaryngeal endotracheal tube may be passed across the anastomotic line into the distal bronchus for short periods. When the anastomosis of one side is complete, that side then is ventilated, and the other endobronchial tube is removed to allow surgical access. Once the second anastomosis is complete, ventilation through the trachea is reestablished.[422] Airway stents may be left in the trachea postoperatively to maintain airway patency.

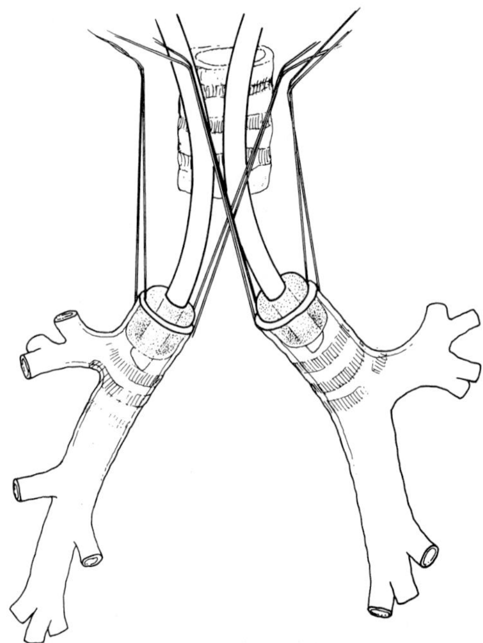

Fig. 70-51. Diagram depicting the method for providing intraoperative endobronchial ventilation. The air seal is achieved by introducing a short length of endobronchial tube into the bronchial stump and by using stay sutures to pull the bronchial stump up against the distal end of the inflated cuff. (Modified from Theman TE, Kerr JH, Nelems JM, et al: Carinal resection. A report of two cases and a description of the anesthetic technique, *J Thorac Cardiovasc Surg* 71:314, 1976.)

Low frequency jet ventilation/low-frequency interrupted high-flow ventilation

Low-frequency jet ventilation has been used to maintain ventilation during tracheal resection.[281,391,396] Intermittent O_2 jets at a rate of 10 to 20 breaths per minute with a pressure of 40 to 60 psi are delivered into the lungs via a small-bore catheter inserted through the endotracheal tube (Fig. 70-52).[281,412] The pressure is regulated to produce adequate chest expansion and oxygenation. After the tracheal anastomosis is complete, the catheter is removed, and the endotracheal tube above the suture line is used conventionally.

High-frequency ventilation

High-frequency positive-pressure ventilation (HFPPV) usually uses a respiratory rate of 60 to 100 breaths per minute administered with a volume-cycled ventilator. It does not depend on gas entrainment. Inspiration is active and expiration is passive. HFJV uses jet pulsations at a rate of 100 to 400 breaths per minute. It depends on gas entrainment. Again, inspiration is active, and expiration is passive. Several reports have described the successful use of HFPPV or HFJV in the treatment of patients having tracheobronchial reconstructions.[116,152,153,194]

HFJV depends on gas entrainment for adequate ventilation and can result in distal aspiration of blood and tumor debris. With HFPPV, a continuous flow of gas occurs to the outside, which protects against distal aspiration of blood and debris. HFPPV provides adequate oxygenation and ventilation by the generation of eddy flows in the airway. It may lead to improved distribution of gas flow compared with conventional mechanical ventilation. Airway pressure during HFPPV is continuously positive. Intrapleural pressure is continuously subatmospheric, with minimal effect on pulmonary and systemic hemodynamics. The principal advantage of HFPPV in tracheobronchial resection is the ability to deliver ventilation through small catheters located either free in the airway or passed through standard endotracheal tubes. These catheters provide less interference with the surgical technique than standard single-lumen or double-lumen endotracheal tubes do. In addition, as soon as the lesion is resected, jet ventilation catheters can be passed into one or both bronchi, providing independent ventilation to both lungs.

HFPPV is likely to be beneficial in patients undergoing (1) carinal resections, (2) sleeve pneumonectomies or sleeve upper lobe resections, (3) tracheal reconstruction supported by Montgomery T tubes, and (4) tracheal resections (Fig. 70-53). For left-sided sleeve pneumonectomy, endobronchial intubation, with a small catheter passed through an endotracheal tube, provides the surgeon with an unobstructed field of vision. The catheter is passed through the operative field and guided by the surgeon into the left mainstem bronchus. The continuous outflow of gas through the

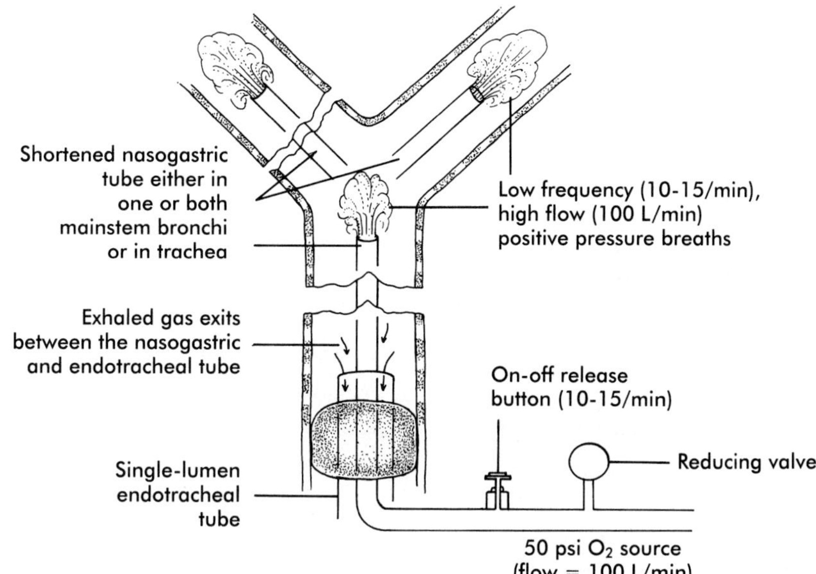

Fig. 70-52. Interruption and release of a very high fresh gas flow (100 l/min) at a low frequency (10 breaths/min) is essentially equivalent to intermittent positive pressure breathing with a very short inspiratory time. A small catheter (nasogastric tube) can be passed through an indwelling single-lumen tube in the trachea and beyond any airway interruption into one or both of the mainstem bronchi and used to ventilate one or both of the lungs. The escape of gas on exhalation is around the small catheter but inside the indwelling single-lumen tube. (Modified from Benumof JL: High-frequency and high-flow apneic ventilation during thoracic surgery. In Benumof JL, editor: *Anesthesia for thoracic surgery*, Philadelphia, 1995, WB Saunders.)

open bronchus during HFPPV minimizes soiling with blood.[129] Ventilation of the right lung with HFPPV via a thin catheter inside the right main bronchus eliminates the problem of right upper lobe collapse associated with the use of right-sided endobronchial tubes.

Carinal resection has been performed using two high-frequency jet ventilators and two catheters, one into each bronchus, to provide independent ventilation to both lungs (Fig. 70-54).[116] This is particularly advantageous when a large carinal tumor dramatically obstructs one or both bronchi, preventing delivery of adequate tidal volume to either lung. In this situation, a catheter is passed into one or both bronchi under fiberoptic bronchoscope guidance. The presence of even two HFJV catheters through the surgical field does not interfere with surgical exposure.

Patients with major tracheal stenosis may not accommodate a large enough endotracheal tube to permit adequate ventilation. Several solutions exist for this problem. First, a special long endotracheal tube that has a small internal diameter can be used; for example, a long 5-mm oral endotracheal tube may pass through the tracheal lesion. Ventilation of an adult through such a small endotracheal tube requires high proximal airway pressures and may not be effective. Second, HFPPV with a small catheter passed through the stenotic area can be used. The anesthesiologist should ensure that enough space exists between the stenotic lesion and the catheter to allow for the adequate outflow of gas; otherwise, barotrauma will occur. Third, the surgeon first can perform laser resection of the stenotic lesion to increase airway diameter.[166]

HFPPV also facilitates tracheal reconstruction supported by a Montgomery tracheal T tube.[243] The Montgomery tracheal T tube is used as a stent to maintain the patency of the upper airway in patients with subglottic and upper tracheal stenosis. The intraluminal limb also maintains the circumference of the airway and supports the tissue graft applied during the reconstruction of the larynx and cervical trachea. Because of the design and shape of the Montgomery endotracheal tube, it is difficult to establish an adequate airway for the administration of conventional mechanical ventilation.[171,309] The use of the extraluminal limb as an airway for delivery of large tidal volumes is associated with a large gas leak through the open, upper intraluminal limb and around the uncuffed tracheal limb. This can be circumvented by two methods. Occlusion of the superior part of the intraluminal limb can decrease the air leak. The occlusion can be accomplished with a Fogarty embolectomy catheter or with a tight pharyngeal pack. Alternatively, the anesthesiologist can perform translaryngeal intubation of the upper intraluminal limb with a small cuffed endotracheal tube. Occlusion of the extraluminal limb then allows the use of positive-pressure ventilation.[269]

HFPPV through a catheter with a 2-mm internal diameter can provide adequate alveolar ventilation and oxygenation during tracheal reconstruction with a tracheal T tube. The T tube and open trachea around it function as expiratory ports for the continuous outflow of gas. If the patient already has a tracheal T tube in place before operation, translaryngeal intubation of the intraluminal limb and trachea can be easily accomplished with the small HFPPV catheter. Alter-

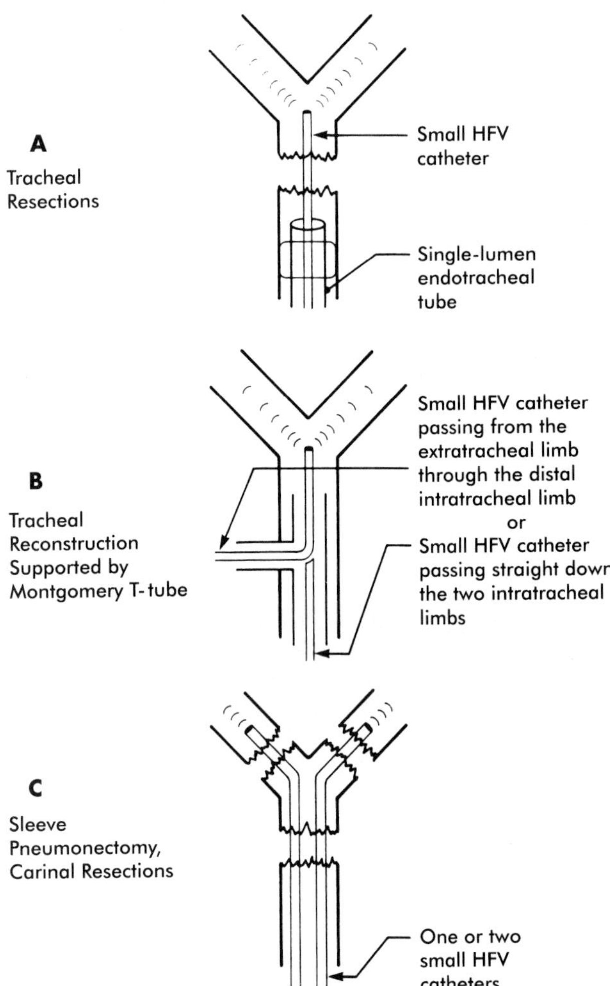

Fig. 70-53. The three types of airway surgery aided by small high-frequency ventilation (HFV) are tracheal resections, tracheal reconstructions that require support by a Montgomery T-tube, and carinal procedures (sleeve pneumonectomy, carinal resections). With tracheal resections **(A),** a simple HFV catheter can be passed beyond the point of airway interruption, but above the tracheal carina, and used to ventilate both lungs with HFV. With tracheal reconstructions supported by a Montgomery T-tube **(B),** the small HFV catheter can be passed from either the extraluminal limb or from the proximal intraluminal trachea limb to the distal intraluminal tracheal limb and can be used to ventilate both lungs with HFV. With carinal procedures **(C),** one or two HFV catheters can be passed into one or both of the mainstem bronchi and can be used to ventilate one or both of the lungs with HFV. (From Benumof JL: High-frequency and high-flow apneic ventilation during thoracic surgery. In Benumof JL, editor: *Anesthesia for thoracic surgery*, Philadelphia, 1995, WB Saunders.)

natively, the catheter can be introduced through the extraluminal limb and gently flexed to direct the catheter to lie above the carina.[152]

Differential lung ventilation with HFJV has been used in patients undergoing tracheobronchial reconstructive surgery, such as pneumonectomy, sleeve lobectomies, and tracheal reconstruction, who have compromised pulmonary reserve. For example, a patient undergoing a right upper sleeve lobectomy is ventilated through an endotracheal tube until resection of the right bronchus and the right upper lobe begins. The endotracheal tube then is advanced into the left mainstem bronchus, and unilateral intermittent positive-pressure ventilation (IPPV) is continued to the left lung. At the same time, HFJV is delivered to the right intermediate bronchus to ventilate the residual right, middle, and lower lobes and thereby maintain better oxygenation.

ANESTHESIA FOR PATIENTS UNDERGOING URGENT SURGERY

Anesthesia for Patients with Massive Hemoptysis

Therapeutic approaches

Massive hemoptysis is an uncommon but life-threatening event that requires rapid management. Massive hemoptysis refers to bleeding that ranges from greater than 200 ml during one episode to 1000 ml within 24 hours.[111,313,471] The most common associated diseases are tuberculosis, bronchiectasis, lung abscesses, and lung cancer (Box 70-17). The cause of hemoptysis is either direct invasion by infection or tumor into blood vessels or trauma (e.g., bleeding after use of a pulmonary artery catheter). Patients at increased risk for perforation of the pulmonary artery by a pulmonary artery catheter include those with pulmonary hypertension, hypothermia, or coagulopathy.[91]

Death from hemoptysis usually results from asphyxia but rarely from exsanguination. The most effective way to stop bleeding from pulmonary sources is definitive pulmonary resection. The site of bleeding can be identified with either a rigid or flexible bronchoscope. Rigid bronchoscopy is preferred because it provides more access for suctioning of blood and removal of clots. The endoscopist may perform therapeutic interventions by the administration of topical saline, vasoconstrictors, laser therapy, or placement of a balloon-tipped Fogarty catheter. Alternative management includes transcatheter embolization of the bronchial and intercostal arteries, but this risks embolization of the spinal cord via collateral circulation. The placement of a pulmonary artery catheter under fluoroscopic guidance may be used in conjunction with other therapies to decrease bleeding by occluding the branch of the pulmonary artery feeding the bleeding site.

Anesthetic management

Management strategies are presented in Table 70-25. Patients with massive hemoptysis often are hemodynamically unstable as a result of hypovolemia and hypoxia. They require resuscitation with fluids, blood products, vasoactive drugs, and correction of any coagulopathies. The major goals of anesthetic management are to prevent contamination of the healthy nonbleeding lung and prevent further hypoxia. A large bore intravenous catheter should be placed for rapid infusion of fluids and blood products. In addition, an arterial catheter should be placed for monitoring of blood pressure and arterial blood gases.

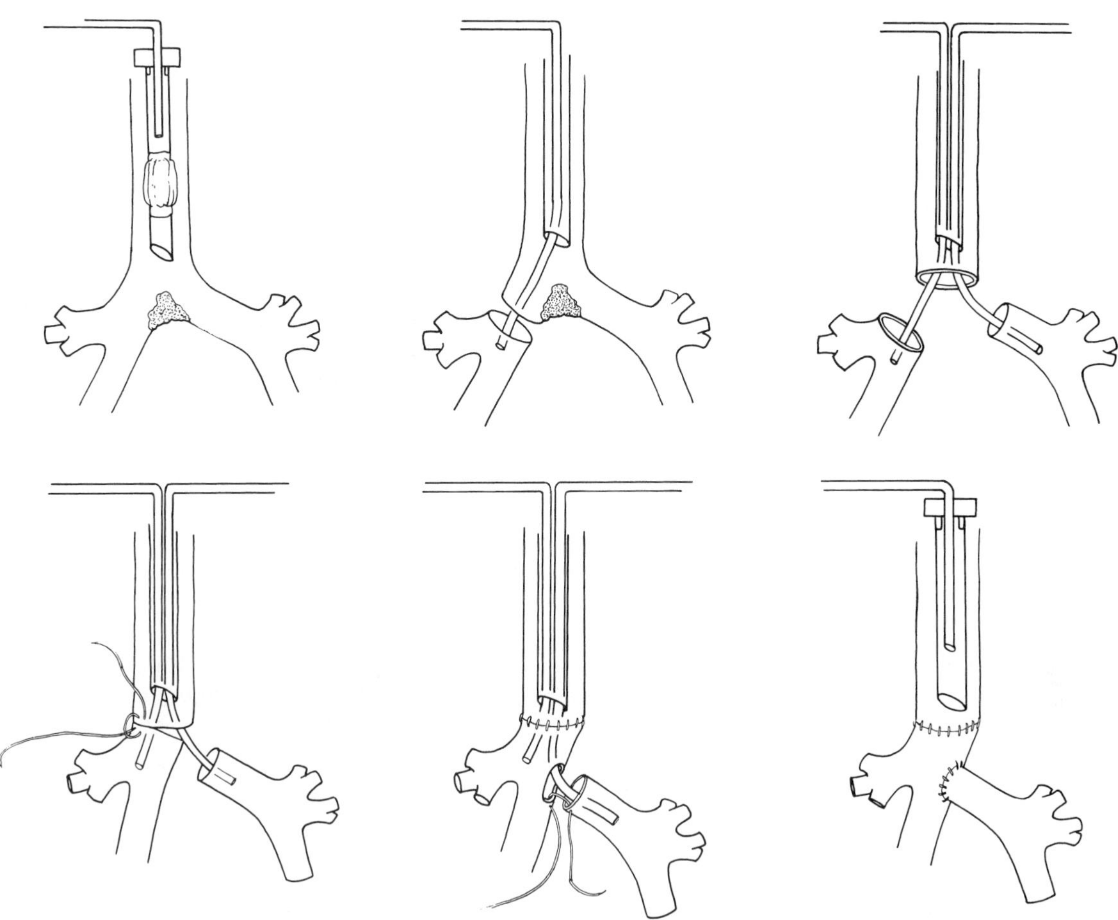

Fig. 70-54. Arrangement of the HFJV catheters during the different phases of the operation. At the end of the right tracheobronchial anastomosis, the left catheter passes between two membranous sutures. It is then withdrawn and introduced into the left main bronchus via the bronchotomy of the right middle bronchus. (Modified from Crinquette V, Wurtz A, Leroy S, et al: Resection et reconstruction de la bifurcation tracheale sous jet ventilation a haute frequence, separee sur les deux poumons, *Ann Chir* 43:673, 1989.)

Patients with massive hemoptysis are at grave risk for aspiration. These patients should undergo either awake intubation or rapid sequence induction followed by tracheal intubation during cricoid pressure. The use of ketamine or etomidate for induction of anesthesia is advocated because the patients are hypovolemic and at risk for cardiovascular collapse. Intubation may be complicated by blood in the airway, obscuring laryngeal structures. Suctioning may be unable to provide adequate visualization. Air bubbles exiting the trachea may serve as the only guide to the site of the glottic orifice. Choice of endotracheal tube depends on the proposed management. Lung separation is best accomplished by placement of a left double-lumen endotracheal tube, but it may be technically difficult in emergency situations. If the bleeding is from the left side, a single-lumen tube can be advanced into the right main stem bronchus. If bleeding originates from the right side, a single-lumen endotracheal tube may be guided into the left mainstem bronchus with the assistance of a fiberoptic bronchoscope.

Once the airway has been secured with a double-lumen tube, the patient is placed in a lateral decubitus position for resection of the bleeding lung segment. Placement of the bleeding lung in a nondependent position mandates complete separation of the lungs to prevent soilage of the dependent nonbleeding lung. Aggressive suctioning of the tracheobronchial tree improves ventilation and oxygenation of the dependent nonbleeding lung. At the end of operation, the endotracheal tube should be left in place, and the patient should be mechanically ventilated. Patients should be observed for recurrent bleeding and impaired oxygen exchange during the early postoperative period.

Anesthesia for Patients Undergoing Removal of Foreign Body from the Airways

Aspiration of foreign bodies is a common problem, particularly in children, and is associated with considerable morbidity and mortality rates.[29] In adults, acute alcoholism, dementia, bulbar muscle dysfunction, and previous history of aspiration are common predisposing factors.[65,68,250] The location of the aspirated object depends on the patient's posture

BOX 70-17
CAUSES OF MASSIVE HEMOPTYSIS

Infection
Tuberculosis
Bronchiectasis
Bronchitis
Lung abscess
Necrotizing pneumonia
Neoplasm
Bronchogenic carcinoma
Metastatic carcinoma
Mediastinal tumor
Endobronchial polyp
Cardiovascular disease
Mitral stenosis
Pulmonary arteriovenous malformation
Pulmonary embolus
Pulmonary vasculitis
Miscellaneous causes
Pulmonary artery catheterization
Exploratory needling
Cystic fibrosis
Pulmonary contusion, laceration
Reperfusion of pulmonary vasculature after pulmonary embolectomy and after cardiopulmonary bypass

From Benumof L: *Anesthesia for thoracic surgery,* Philadelphia, 1987, WB Saunders.

at the time of aspiration. The right lung most often is involved because the axis of the right mainstem bronchus is more in line with the trachea. If the patient is upright at the time of aspiration, the right lower lobe most frequently is affected. The right upper lobe most often is involved in patients in the supine position.

More than 80% of the aspirated foreign bodies are organic material. Organic material, particularly peanuts and other nuts, produce severe mucosal irritation and swelling around the foreign body. The clinical sequelae of foreign body aspiration include acute airway obstruction, atelectasis, inflammation, pneumonia, and abscess formation (Fig. 70-55). The foreign body may act as a one-way valve, resulting in air trapping and regional hyperinflation.

Clinical features and diagnosis

Acute signs and symptoms of aspiration include cough, wheezing, dyspnea, stridor, fever, cyanosis, and hemoptysis. Alternatively, there may be a history of recurrent or intractable pneumonia, unexplained atelectasis, or emphysema.[68,250] Physical examination may reveal unilateral decreased air entry, unilateral localized wheezing, or aphonia.[34,68,157,250] Most foreign bodies are radiolucent but are associated with an abnormal chest radiograph. Findings may include atelectasis, localized hyperinflation, pneumonia, or mediastinal shift.[65] Fluoroscopy may reveal a shift of the mediastinum to the opposite side with exhalation, resulting from air trapping on the affected side.

Therapeutic approach

The urgency of proceeding to bronchoscopy is dictated by the severity of the patient's respiratory distress. If the object is in the larynx or the proximal trachea, it causes considerably more distress and is associated with greater mortality than with objects lodged more peripherally.[157,216] Foreign bodies are removed within the first 24 hours to avoid dislodging them into a more critical position and to decrease the incidence of secondary pneumonia. If possible, removal should be delayed long enough to allow for gastric emptying and patient preparation.[267] An initial trial of bronchodilators, postural drainage, and chest physiotherapy was used formerly in an attempt to dislodge and expel the foreign body. These procedures occasionally resulted in total airway obstruction and cardiac arrest and are no longer recommended.[87,256,267]

Removal of the foreign body with the aid of a bronchoscope is successful about 95% of the time, although bronchoscopy may need to be repeated either because the foreign body was not found initially or because it was incompletely removed.[68,267] Fluoroscopic guidance during bronchoscopy can aid in the removal of small radiopaque objects.[302] Rarely, thoracotomy and bronchotomy are necessary for retrieval of the foreign body.

Anesthetic management

The anesthetic management depends on the patient's age, presence of a full stomach, the severity of respiratory distress, and the location of the foreign body. All patients should be premedicated with an anticholinergic to decrease airway secretions, H2-antagonists to decrease gastric acid secretion, and metoclopramide to promote gastric emptying (Table 70-26). The endoscopist should be prepared for immediate rigid bronchoscopy in case of total airway obstruction.

Adults receive preoxygenation, intravenous induction and direct laryngoscopy. If the foreign body is in the larynx, it often can be removed during direct laryngoscopy, and the patient is allowed to emerge from anesthesia. A foreign body in the trachea or the bronchus requires rigid or fiberoptic bronchoscopy for removal. When a rigid bronchoscope is introduced into the airway, its ventilating side arm is attached to the anesthesia circuit to provide O_2 and inhaled anesthesia. The use of a helium-O_2 mixture can be helpful in patients with partial airway obstruction because the decreased density of the inhaled mixture decreases turbulence and improves flow across the stenotic airway. The maximal effect is obtained with a helium-O_2 mixture of 80% to 20%, but helium also is therapeutic when used in lesser concentrations. After the trachea is intubated, a large-bore nasal or oral gastric tube is inserted into the stomach, and the gastric contents are thoroughly suctioned.

Children are more difficult to manage because of their small airway, which makes them more susceptible

Table 70-25 Anesthetic guidelines for patients with massive hemoptysis

Indication	Hemoptysis
Monitors	Standard monitors, arterial catheter
Anesthesia	General anesthesia
Additonal equipment	Shoulder roll or bean bag
Ventilation	Double-lumen endotracheal tube (if possible)
Position	Lateral decubitus, supine
Incision	Thoracotomy, median sternotomy
Unique considerations	Frequently hypoxic, "full stomach" precautions, hypotensive, tachycardic
	Infectious precautions
	Type and cross for blood products
	Check coagulation status
Intraoperative complications	Hypoxia
	Hypotension
	Hemorrhage
	Dysrhythmia
	Hypotension
	Possibility of extensive lung resection
Blood loss	Variable > 500 ml
Analgesia	Epidural thoracotomy
Postoperative morbidity	Respiratory insufficiency
	Aspiration pneumonia
	Hemoptysis
	ARDS
	Hypoxia
Postoperative care	Chest radiography
	Monitored in intensive care environment

to major airway obstruction. In children with severe respiratory distress, the risks of total airway obstruction that can occur during rapid-sequence induction should be weighed against the risk of aspiration during a slow inhalation induction with spontaneous ventilation. Attempting to place an intravenous catheter before induction can trigger violent struggling, straining, and crying and can precipitate total airway obstruction. A gentle inhalation induction with halothane, using cricoid pressure, can be used even in children with a full stomach.[312] In the absence of intravenous access, intramuscular ketamine may be used for induction. As soon as the child becomes sleepy, cricoid pressure is applied, and inhalation of anesthetic agents is started while continuing spontaneous ventilation.

If the patient is minimally symptomatic with no serious respiratory distress and if the foreign body is thought to be peripherally located, the anesthesiologist can wait 6 to 8 hours before bronchoscopy, although some surgeons or endoscopists do not agree with this approach and prefer to proceed immediately to prevent a local inflammatory reaction to the foreign body. In the absence of a full stomach and if symptoms are minimal, the child may be heavily premedicated to facilitate a smooth inhalation induction. After induction, many anesthesiologists then administer muscle relaxants because spontaneous ventilation is not crucial once deep anesthesia is achieved. When using a rigid bronchoscope, movement can result in major airway trauma or dislodge the entrapped foreign body allowing it to fall farther back into the airway. Spontaneous ventilation can facilitate detection of airway obstruction and prevents distal migration of the foreign body caused by positive-pressure ventilation.

Some objects, such as beads, are hard to grip and may slip during removal, resulting in occlusion more proximally. The object should then be pushed back to its original location to allow adequate ventilation. Multiple instrumentations of the airway may produce mucosal edema and respiratory distress postoperatively. Therapy includes the administration of steroids (dexamethasone, 0.5 to 1.5 mg/kg), humidification of inspired gases, nebulized racemic epinephrine, and initiation of broad-spectrum antibiotic therapy.

Bronchography

After bronchoscopy, diagnostic bronchography may be necessary to define and localize airway lesions. The contrast medium is selectively instilled into the tracheobronchial tree during fluoroscopic guidance. Bronchography is helpful to define congenital anomalies of the airway, cysts communicating with the lower airway, bronchiectasis, and airway compression. Installation of the contrast medium can result in small airway obstruction with diminished pulmonary function in patients with preexisting pulmonary disease.[94] The procedure can be performed during topical anesthesia in awake, sedated adults, but it requires general anesthesia in

A

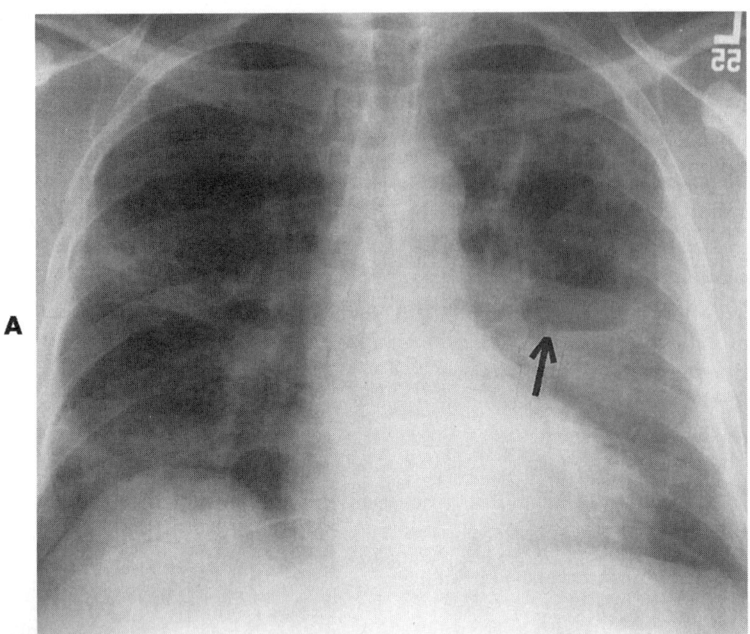

B

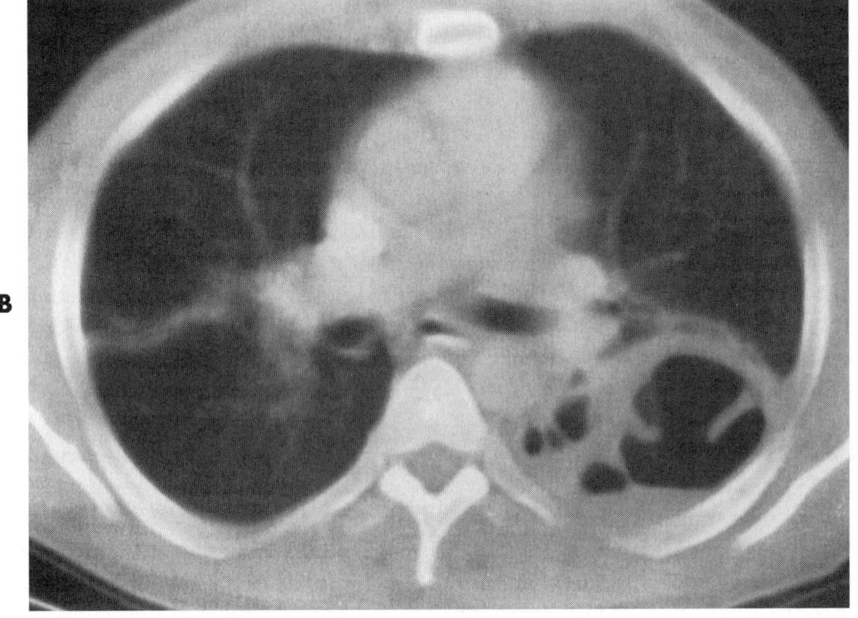

Fig. 70-55. An aspiration pneumonia in 58-year-old man with a history of alcohol abuse progressed to a suppurative cavitary lesion. The patient presented with progressive shortness of breath, fevers, and foul-smelling sputum. The chest radiograph, *panel A,* shows cavitary lesion with an air fluid level in the left lung and several pneumonic infiltrates in the right lung. The chest CT, *panel B*, shows that the large cavitation in the left lower lobe that is consistent with a diagnosis of abscess or tumor. The patient subsequently underwent pulmonary resection that required placement of a double-lumen endotracheal tube to prevent soilage of the contralateral lung.

children. Spontaneous ventilation should be maintained while the contrast medium is slowly injected and deposited on the walls of the bronchi to image bronchial defects. Controlled ventilation or inadvertent coughing results in rapid alveolarization of the dye, complicating the interpretation. At the end of the procedure, as much of the dye as possible should be removed by suctioning and postural drainage, and pulmonary toilet should be encouraged after extubation.

Anesthesia for Patients Undergoing Endoscopy for Ingested Foreign Bodies

The incidence of occurrence of ingested foreign bodies in the hypopharynx or esophagus in young children is as common as aspirations in the airway. Coins and fish bones are the most frequent foreign bodies in the esophagus.[314] Most foreign bodies initially cause laryngeal irritation, coughing, or choking. Subsequent signs and symptoms include refusal to eat, increased salivation, pain or discomfort during swallowing, and vomiting.

The anesthesiologist should determine the nature and the location of the foreign body. Lateral neck radiographs should be obtained to determine the extent of impingement on the airway. In the absence of respiratory distress or airway compression, the anesthesiologist should consider waiting 4 to 8 hours for gastric emptying.[312] The child then is sedated, and anesthesia is induced with either inhalation or intravenous anesthetic agents. Emergency endoscopy should be performed in patients with respiratory distress and airway compression. In spontaneously ventilated patients, preoperative sedation is omitted, and general anesthesia is induced. For patients with foreign bodies located in the hypopharynx or in the upper esophagus, cricoid pressure is contraindi-

Table 70-26 Anesthetic guidelines for retrieval of foreign body

Indication	Aspiration of foreign body
Monitors	Standard monitors
Anesthesia	Pediatric (general anesthesia) Adult (awake sedated, general anesthesia)
Additional equipment	Fiberoptic bronchoscope Rigid bronchoscope
Ventilation	Usually try to maintain spontaneous ventilation Controlled ventilation may be appropriate if mass is distal in tracheobronchial tree
Position	Seated or semirecumbent (Positioned to optimize respiratory status)
Unique considerations	Respiratory status Sedation as tolerated Antisialagogue Precautions for "full stomach" H_2 blocker, metoclopramide, cricoid pressure Anesthetize airway for awake, sedated approach Availability of additional support personnel Place gastric tube to empty stomach after airway is secured
Complications	Loss of airway Hypoxia Cardiac arrest Aspiration Hemoptysis Soilage from contents distal to obstruction
Postoperative morbidity	Hemoptysis Postoperative edema (steroids, raise head of bed) Bronchospasm (racemic epinephrine, bronchodilators) Pneumonia Atelectasis
Postoperative care	Observe in monitored environment Aggressive pulmonary toilet physical therapy Supplemental O_2 Chest radiography

cated. The endotracheal tube size chosen should be slightly smaller than usual to facilitate endoscopy and decrease subsequent subglottic swelling.[312] In addition, a prophylactic dose of dexamethasone (0.5 to 1.0 mg/kg) may be given to decrease laryngeal edema.

A foreign body that is located high in the esophagus may dislodge into the larynx and produce an airway obstruction. Therefore, children with high esophageal foreign bodies should be heavily sedated, intravenous access obtained, and anesthesia induced. In the absence of major airway compression, an intravenous induction with muscle relaxants may be used.

ANESTHESIA FOR PATIENTS WITH ZENKER'S DIVERTICULUM

Clinical Features

Zenker's diverticulum is an outpouching of the pharyngeal mucosa between the inferior constrictor muscles of the pharynx, the thyropharyngeus, and the cricopharyngeus muscles. The etiology is believed to result from dysfunction or spasm of the cricopharyngeus muscle. Patients complain of food sticking in the throat, difficulty swallowing, noisy swallowing, regurgitation of food, and bouts of coughing when lying supine. Neck radiographs may reveal a collection of air anterior to C5 and C6, but diagnosis is confirmed with a barium swallow. Physical examination may reveal a compressible swelling as the sac enlarges. Patients usually are elderly, malnourished,[355] debilitated with coexisting cardiac and respiratory diseases, and susceptible to recurrent pneumonias and lung abscesses from aspiration. Symptomatic lesions are managed by surgical resection.

Intraoperative Management

Oral premedications are not suitable because tablets may lodge in the pouch or be aspirated into the lungs.[37] The risk of regurgitation and aspiration of diverticular contents into the lungs during the immediate preoperative and intraoperative periods is a major concern for the anesthesiologist. The contents of the pouch usually have an alkaline pH and therefore are unlikely to benefit from H_2-receptor antagonists, antacids, or metaclopramide. Regurgitation and aspiration may occur even after successful tracheal intubation because of seepage of fluid around the endotracheal tube cuff during surgical manipulation. Measures to decrease the risk of aspiration during anesthesia include fasting overnight, preoperative emptying of the pouch by manual external pressure, and tilting the head of the bed upward 10° to 30°.

Awake intubation is an option, but coughing and straining may result in regurgitation and aspiration. The risk of aspiration may be increased by topical anesthesia and sedation, which blunt airway reflexes. Therefore, some authors advise against awake intubation.[109] Use of topical anesthesia should be limited to either the supraglottic or infraglottic part of the airway, leaving part of the airway responsive as a protection against aspiration. Transtracheal administration of local anesthetics is relatively contraindicated.

Use of cricoid pressure may precipitate aspiration in some patients. Careful preoperative examination of the barium swallow image may help determine whether cricoid pressure will be beneficial or harmful by defining the size and location of the pouch. If the sac is large, extending down into the mediastinum with its orifice at the level of the cricoid cartilage, cricoid pressure should obliterate the opening and protect against regurgitation. If the sac is small and the opening is cephalad to the cricoid cartilage, the application of cricoid pressure may actually squeeze the sac, resulting in regurgitation of its contents into the hypopharynx (Fig. 70-56).

The preferred approach is a smooth induction with a 30° upward head tilt and avoidance of coughing, bucking, and straining. The combination of intravenous hypnotics (i.e., thiopental or etomidate) supplemented with narcotics and lidocaine and slow, gentle manual mask ventilation should result in a smooth uneventful induction. A nondepolarizing muscle relaxant is administered, and endotracheal intubation is performed after complete relaxation has been achieved. The pharynx around the endotracheal tube can be packed with gauze to prevent seepage of the contents of the diverticulum into the hypopharynx with collection above the endotracheal tube cuff. Surgical access usually is through a cervical incision. A large diverticulum may extend into the mediastinum. Great care and gentleness should be exercised when inserting a nasogastric tube because of the potential for perforation of the diverticulum. Likewise in patients with a difficult airway, blind attempts at intubation of the trachea risk perforating the pouch. Perforation of the diverticulum results in mediastinitis and sepsis. Other complications include air embolism if major vessels are opened during the dissection or bradycardia and hypotension resulting from stimulation of baroreceptors during retraction near the carotid bifurcation.

An alternative is to perform the procedure during regional anesthesia using deep and superficial cervical plexus blocks.[3,114,220] A recent report describes the use of this approach in 58 patients undergoing repair of a Zenker's diverticulum. The risk of aspiration is minimized by preserving protective airway reflexes. Provided the block is limited to one side, the awake, sedated patient is able to cooperate with the surgeon and to swallow on command, allowing the surgeon to view the pathology and assess the adequacy of repair.

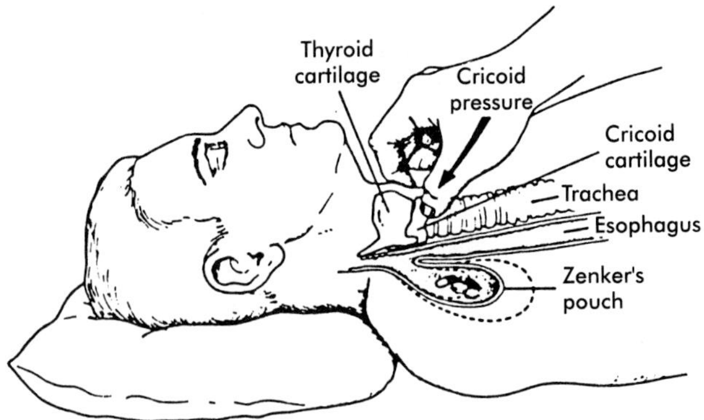

Fig. 70-56. Zenker's pouch in the hypopharynx, with the opening at the level of cricoid cartilage. (From Thiagarajah S, Lear E, Keh M: Anesthetic implications of Zenker's diverticulum, *Anesth Analg* 70:709, 1990.)

COMPLICATIONS OF THORACIC SURGERY AND THEIR MANAGEMENT STRATEGIES

The postoperative complications of thoracic surgery can be characterized as either pulmonary, cardiovascular, neurologic, or miscellaneous (Box 70-18). Some of these are medical and surgical emergencies that require prompt diagnosis and management. Conditions requiring emergent intervention include pneumothorax, pulmonary edema, torsion of a residual lobe, herniation of the heart, malignant arrhythmias, or major hemorrhage. Early diagnosis and efficient management depends on the cooperative efforts of the anesthesia, surgical, and nursing staff. In the following section, the order of presentation is based on the system involved and the severity of symptoms.

Cardiovascular

Herniation of the heart

Cardiac herniation is a rare and rapidly fatal injury if not immediately diagnosed and managed. This complication occurs more often after right pneumonectomy in which the pericardium was opened to gain better access to the pulmonary vessels. It may occur after the creation of a pericardial window for management of a pericardial effusion. This complication has been associated with changing of patient position (lateral decubitus to supine position or placement of the operative lung in the dependent position) or a differential change in intrapleural pressures caused by suctioning of the chest tube after pneumonectomy or vigorous coughing.[180,197,294]

BOX 70-18
COMPLICATIONS OF THORACIC SURGERY

Hemodynamic

- Arrhythmias
- Cardiac herniation
- Right-sided failure
- Tension pneumothorax
- Bleeding

Pulmonary

- Pneumothorax
- Atelectasis
- Shunting
- Pulmonary edema
- Torsion of lobe
- Damage phrenic nerve
- Damage recurrent laryngeal nerve
- Pain

Neurologic

- Positioning injuries
    - Brachial plexus, ulnar nerve, peroneal nerve
- Phrenic nerve
- Recurrent laryngeal nerve
- Paradoxical embolization
- Spinal cord

Miscellaneous

- Alopecia
- Necrosis ear, nose
- Infection

The clinical features of cardiac herniation include acute cardiovascular collapse, evidence of superior vena cava obstruction (distention of neck veins, facial flushing, and edema), altered axis of ECG, bulging of cardiac silhouette, and unusual positioning of pulmonary artery catheter on chest radiograph. A differential diagnosis includes tension pneumothorax, cardiac tamponade, dysrhythmia, pulmonary emboli, and massive hemorrhage. These patients require immediate operation, but they may be stabilized by performing certain therapeutic maneuvers. When the diagnosis is first considered, the patient should be positioned with the operated lung in the nondependent position.[90,273] Even if the heart does not fall back into its normal position, repositioning may relieve aortocaval kinking and increase cardiac output. The tidal volume should be decreased and use of PEEP should be discontinued to decrease any mediastinal shift. Additionally, suctioning of the chest tubes should be discontinued, and injection of air to counter cardiac herniation should be considered.

The patient should be taken to the operating room, and anesthesia should be induced with either ketamine or etomidate and a muscle relaxant. To decrease mediastinal shift, the lungs should be ventilated with small tidal volumes. The surgical procedure consists of reexploring the thorax and repairing the pericardial defect with primary closure, autograft, or prosthetic material.[58]

Cardiac dysrhythmias

Supraventricular dysrhythmias, primarily sinus tachycardia and atrial fibrillation or flutter, occur more often after pneumonectomy then after segmental resections.[261,397] These dysrhythmias are associated with a major increase in morbidity and mortality rates.[253] Dysrhythmias after pneumonectomy are associated with a 25% mortality rates compared with 7% for those patients with normal rhythms.[180] In addition, dysrhythmias prolong the duration of hospitalization in the ICU.[445]

Postoperative cardiac rhythm disturbances do not correlate with preoperative pulmonary function.[259,261] Potential causes include retraction and trauma of the heart (intrapericardial dissection, increase in pulmonary vascular resistance related to reduction of the pulmonary vascular bed), increased sympathetic tone related to inadequate postoperative analgesia, and postoperative respiratory or metabolic imbalance (hypoxia, hypercapnia, respiratory acidosis, and electrolyte imbalances). Some authors have reported decreased postoperative cardiac complications after prophylactic digitalis,[84,234] although the use of preoperative digitalis in patients without cor pulmonale or congestive heart failure remains controversial.[84,239,377,397,461]

The appropriate management strategies for a new dysrhythmia are directed to stabilizing hemodynamics and managing the underlying problem. Hemodynamic instability resulting from new dysrhythmias may require emergent cardioversion, although normotensive patients having either atrial fibrillation or flutter with a rapid ventricular response should be treated with digitalis, calcium channel blocker, or cardioversion. In patients with other supraventricular dysrhythmias, appropriate treatment may include the use of beta blockers (e.g., esmolol), verapamil, phenylephrine, edrophonium, or adenosine. The administration of supplemental oxygen, correction of metabolic and electrolyte abnormalities, and more aggressive management of postoperative analgesia also may be required.

Right ventricular failure

The postoperative course after anatomic pulmonary resection may be complicated by right ventricular failure and acute cor pulmonale. Decreases in the vascular cross-sectional area caused by pulmonary resection increase the pulmonary vascular resistance and right ventricular afterload. Preoperative right heart catheterization or echocardiography may predict patients at risk for this postoperative complication. Operative risk is increased if the pulmonary vascular resistance is greater than 190 dynes/sec/cm^{-5} or if the pulmonary artery pressure increases by more than

40 mm Hg in response to balloon occlusion. In addition, hypercapnia, acidosis, and increases in airway pressure may increase the risk of developing right heart failure. Patients with right heart failure have distended neck veins, peripheral edema, and new onset of atrial dysrhythmias. Echocardiography may be helpful in differentiating right heart failure from cardiac tamponade. Increased right heart volume and ventricular dysfunction can lead to a shift of the intraventricular septum and impede left ventricular filling and function. A decrease in left ventricular preload caused by the increased pulmonary vascular resistance and abnormal septal wall motion will result in a decreased cardiac output and peripheral perfusion pressure. Additionally, the right ventricle may develop ischemia as a result of the increased oxygen demand related to wall stress and the decreased coronary perfusion resulting from decreased cardiac output. Patients who have chronic right-sided heart failure with right ventricular hypertrophy may be at increased risk for developing myocardial ischemia and dysfunction related to decreased coronary perfusion.

The treatment strategies differ for patients having right ventricular failure with either normal or increased pulmonary vascular resistance. Volume expansion in patients with increased pulmonary vascular resistance will further exacerbate right ventricular dysfunction and increase wall stress. The management goals are to improve right ventricular function, decrease pulmonary vascular resistance, and maintain coronary perfusion. Vasodilating agents, such as nitroglycerin, sodium nitroprusside, prostaglandin E1, and nitric oxide, have been used to decrease pulmonary vascular resistance. Often agents such as dobutamine or milronone are chosen for their combined inotropic and vasodilator properties. In patients with decreased systemic blood pressure and inadequate coronary perfusion, vasopressors such as dopamine, phenylephrine, or norepinephrine can be added to enhance coronary perfusion.

Intracardiac shunting

The incidence of a probe-patent foramen ovale is about 25% in adults. During normal conditions, there is negligible right-to-left shunt across the atrial septal defect because the left atrial pressure exceeds that of the right. If the gradient between the right atrium and left atrium is reversed, oxygenated blood can flow from right to left, resulting in paradoxical embolization and hypoxia. The reversal of atrial pressures can occur during conditions of increased peripheral vascular resistance related to the use of PEEP or during the occurrence of pulmonary emboli, pulmonary hypertension, valvular stenosis, ARDS, or even coughing. Reversal of pressures may occur after pneumonectomy or lobectomy.[131,224,410,435] The occurrence of intracardiac shunt should be suspected in those with unexplained postoperative dyspnea and systemic oxygen desaturation. Transesophageal echocardiography can confirm the diagnosis and visualize the atrial septal defect.

Management goals are to decrease shunt flow by decreasing right-sided pressures and pulmonary vascular resistance. Initial management should involve correction of hypoxia, hypercapnia, acidosis, and increased sympathetic tone related to inadequate postoperative analgesia. In addition, the administration of pulmonary vasodilators and preload reduction can be used to decrease right heart pressures. In patients who are mechanically ventilated, the use of PEEP should be avoided if possible. When conservative measures fail, surgical closure of the atrial septal defect may be necessary. Because the presence of an intracardiac shunt predisposes to paradoxical embolization, all intravenous solutions should be rigorously free of air bubbles, and blood products should be administered through micropore filters to exclude particulate matter.

Major hemorrhage

Postoperative bleeding that requires surgical intervention is uncommon. Most major hemorrhage results from slippage of ligatures around major pulmonary vessels. Bleeding from raw pleural surfaces is likely when vascular adhesions between the visceral and parietal pleura have been divided. Other sites of potential bleeding include the bronchial and intercostal arteries. Although chest tube drainage is an indicator of the extent of bleeding, the absence of chest tube drainage does not rule out major hemorrhage. Chest tubes may be malpositioned or occluded by clot, thus hiding the resulting hemothorax. If suspected, repositioning the patient and obtaining a chest radiography will confirm presence of serious pleural effusion with blood.

Pulmonary

Pneumothorax

Pneumothoraces are common complications occurring intraoperatively and postoperatively. The factors that predispose to their development are listed in Box 70-19. The presence of a large pneumothorax is a medical emergency. Clinical signs and symptoms include respiratory distress, decreased breath sounds unilaterally, increased airway pressure with decreased chest compliance, and decreased arterial oxygen saturation. Pneumothorax can expand to the point of tension pneumothorax, which is characterized by hypotension, tracheal shift, and cardiovascular collapse. If sufficient time is available, a chest radiograph is obtained to confirm diagnosis.

Management entails placement of a chest tube for evacuation of intrapleural air. In a spontaneously ventilating patient, the indications for placement of a chest tube are for pneumothorax occupying 15% or more of the hemithorax or for the presence of symptoms. Because mechanically ventilated patients are at risk of increasing size of the pneumothorax, they usually require placement of a chest tube. In emergency situations, decompression of the hemothorax can be accomplished by placement of a 14-gauge intravenous catheter into the intercostal space in the anterior axillary line.

BOX 70-19
FACTORS PREDISPOSING TO DEVELOPMENT OF PNEUMOTHORAX

Preexisting lung disease
Barotrauma
  PEEP, jet ventilation
Procedural complication
  Surgery
    Unintentional violation of pleura space
    Surgical dissection
    Bronchoscopy
    Percutaneous needle biopsy
  Central line placement
  Analgesic technique
    Intrapleural catheter
    Intercostal block
Malfunction of chest tubes
Trauma
Bronchopleural fistula
  Rupture of bronchial stump or anastomosis infection
  Poor wound healing

Torsion of residual lobe

Pulmonary torsion refers to lung rotation on its bronchovascular pedicle. If uncorrected, it will result in pulmonary infarction. Patients undergoing lung resection are at increased risk for torsion of the remaining lobe. The right middle lobe and lingula are at greatest risk for torsion after right upper or left upper lobectomy.[351] Chest radiograph reveals an area of atelectasis or an expanding intrathoracic mass. If suspected, bronchoscopy should be performed followed by immediate surgical reexploration. A double-lumen endotracheal tube should be placed to allow for complete pneumonectomy or untwisting of the rotated bronchial vascular pedicle.

Postoperative respiratory failure

Preexisting lung disease increases the risk for postoperative pulmonary complications. Patients with chronic lung disease have an increased incidence of pulmonary complications. The increase in risk is related to the decrement in preoperative pulmonary function. In addition, smoking increases the risk of postoperative respiratory complications independent of its association with chronic obstructive lung disease.[167,303] Reductions in postoperative complications have been noted with cessation of smoking at least 8 weeks before operation.[451]

The importance of such factors as age, obesity, and malnutrition are less clear. Advanced age alone does not appear to be a risk factor, but it may be a confounding variable. The importance of obesity as a risk factor for postoperative pulmonary complications also is unclear.[462] Respiratory mechanics and pulmonary functions are altered in obese patients.[277,349] The accumulation of fat in respiratory structures reduces compliance and increases the work of breathing. Although obesity may influence the risk of postoperative pulmonary complications, its importance is minor except with morbid obese patients. Malnutrition is not a major risk factor for postoperative pulmonary complications, although it impairs immunity, decreases diaphragmatic muscle function, and diminishes the ventilation response to hypoxia.[361] Even though aggressive nutritional support improves biochemical parameters, it has not been shown to improve pulmonary function.[86,421]

Pulmonary edema

Pulmonary edema occurs because of altered balance of the Starling forces, resulting in a net movement of fluid into the interstitial space. Risk factors for pulmonary edema include cardiac, pulmonary, and anatomic reasons.

Pulmonary edema after lung transplantation may be related to an acute reperfusion injury or graft rejection that alters membrane permeability. These patients are more susceptible because of loss of effective lymphatic drainage of the transplanted lung(s).

Pneumonectomy or reexpansion of atelectatic lung is associated with postoperative pulmonary edema. The etiology of these complications most likely is multifactorial and involves changes in hydrostatic pressure, oncotic pressure, and vascular permeability. Reexpansion pulmonary edema is unilateral and follows the reinflation of atelectatic lungs caused by removal of effusions, evacuation of a pneumothorax, or reinflation after use of a double-lumen endotracheal tube. This type of edema has been related to increased vascular permeability caused by anoxic damage to the endothelium and mechanical changes to the blood vessels.[289,354,462] To avoid mechanical damage caused by excess stretching and increased pressure gradients, the lung should be expanded slowly and gradually.[282,410,449] The factors associated with postoperative pulmonary edema are more complicated. Postpneumonectomy pulmonary edema was initially attributed to fluid overload. Pneumonectomy dramatically decreases the cross-sectional area of the vascular bed, increasing hydrostatic pressure. During normal conditions, the vascular bed can accommodate, although the presence of preexisting cardiac disease combined with aggressive fluid replacement and reduction of lymphatic drainage may predispose to the transudation of edema fluid. Use of a pulmonary artery catheter to evaluate filling pressure may not accurately reflect left ventricular preload. Balloon occlusion of the pulmonary artery may dramatically decrease the remaining cross-sectional area of the pulmonary circulation, rendering a falsely decreased estimation of left atrial pressures. To avoid this, the noninflated catheter can be advanced and wedged briefly in a small peripheral pulmonary vessel. More recently, it has been recognized that a change in permeability is a major contributing factor to edema after pneumonectomy.

Nerve Injuries

Phrenic nerve injury

The phrenic nerve originates from C3, C4, and C5, passing into the chest anterior to the hilum of the lung within the pericardium. It is susceptible to damage during median sternotomy or thoracotomy. Phrenic nerve injury manifests as respiratory failure or failure to wean from mechanical ventilation. Diagnostic tests include chest radiography and fluoroscopic examination of diaphragmatic movement. Chest radiography shows a clear lung with an elevated hemidiaphragm, whereas fluoroscopy documents paradoxical movement of the diaphragm during inspiration. Most patients with normal lung function can tolerate unilateral phrenic nerve injury, although those patients with preexisting lung disease or those who have undergone extensive pulmonary resection may be debilitated. If lung function does not return within 2 to 9 months, alternative therapies, including diaphragmatic pacing and diaphragmatic plication, may be considered.[110,212]

Recurrent laryngeal nerve injury

The left recurrent laryngeal nerve is susceptible to injury during hilar dissection and mediastinoscopy. Unilateral laryngeal nerve injury usually is asymptomatic or manifests by hoarseness of voice, although bilateral nerve injury could result in apposition of the vocal cords and inspiratory obstruction requiring emergent reintubation of the trachea. If vocal cord function does not return after several months, the involved vocal cord may be injected to improve its function.

Spinal cord injury

Spinal cord injury is a rare complication after thoracic surgery.[291] The mechanisms of injury include nerve compression and vascular ischemia. Epidural hematomas and nerve compression can result from placement of epidural catheters or from surgical bleeding into the epidural space. Disruption of the major intercostal artery supplying the anterior spinal artery can result in anterior spinal artery syndrome, leading to paralysis.

Brachial plexus injury

The brachial plexus is susceptible to injury caused by surgical trauma and indirectly caused by positioning.[97,160] Stretch injury of the plexus can occur with extreme abduction, external rotation, and dorsal extension of the arm. For further discussion, the reader is referred to Chapter 35.

POSTOPERATIVE PAIN MANAGEMENT

Postoperative pain control is one of the most important management goals for preventing postoperative respiratory complications. Inadequate pain control leads to shallow respirations, tachypnea, inability to cough effectively, retention of secretions, and atelectasis. These symptoms contribute to postoperative hypoxia, hypercapnia, and respiratory failure in post-thoracotomy patients. Effective postoperative pain management decreases these deleterious effects and abates the increase in norepinephrine levels associated with sympathetic outflow. The associated tachycardia, hypertension, and postoperative hypercoagulability increase the risk for adverse cardiac events in patients with ischemic heart disease. The common approaches use a combination of pharmacologic agents such as NSAIDs, opioids, local anesthetics, and $alpha_2$ adrenergic agonists to manage the dynamic pain associated with pulmonary exercise and ambulation postoperatively. Common routes of administration include intermittent intramuscular or intravenous injections, patient-controlled analgesia (PCA), intercostal nerve blocks, cryoanalgesia, intrapleural catheters, paravertebral block, and epidural or spinal routes.

The mainstay of pharmacologic therapy is the administration of opioids. Many years of clinical use have established the safety and efficacy of these drugs when properly administered. Common side effects include nausea, vomiting, and more importantly, respiratory depression. Opioids are routinely administered intramuscularly, intravenously, or centrally by epidural or intrathecal routes.

Local anesthetics may be administered alone or in combination with opioid agonists. Common routes of administration include epidural, paravertebral, or intrapleural catheters. Side effects of local anesthetics are related to their inhibition of nerve transmission, causing hypotension from sympathetic blockade, numbness, and muscle weakness.

Nonsteroidal antiinflammatory drugs often are used as an adjunct therapy to inhibit peripheral pain and inflammation. They are associated with various side effects, including decreased platelet aggregation, gastrointestinal bleeding, and decreased renal flow in dehydrated patients.

Intercostal Nerve Blocks

Intercostal nerve block is an effective technique to provide postoperative analgesia without central respiratory depression and to attenuate the decrease in pulmonary function after thoracic surgery.[387] Post-thoracotomy pain is not completely managed with intercostal analgesia; it requires supplemental use of parenteral narcotics or NSAIDs. Complications of this technique are few, but they include pneumothorax, local anesthetic toxicity, and neuroaxonal spread of local anesthetics that can result in unintentional hypotension.[310,431]

The intercostal nerve block can be performed intraoperatively by intrathoracic injection or percutaneously by the anesthesiologist after the operation. Nerve blocks are performed at the levels above and below the site of chest tube insertion and incision (Fig. 70-57). Nerve blocks are per-

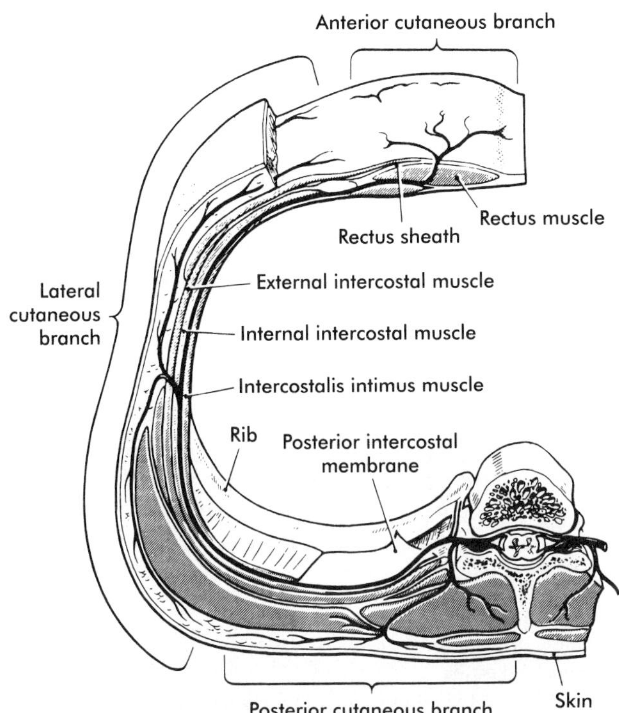

Fig. 70-57. An intercostal nerve and its branches. Approximate area of skin supplied by branches also is shown. There is evidence that local anesthetic injected near the lateral cutaneous branch diffuses posteriorly to reach the posterior cutaneous branch. Note also the spinal nerves and dorsal root ganglia in the region of intervertebral foramen, with risk of perineural spread into spinal fluid after intraneural injection in this region. Direct injection into an intervertebral foramen may reach spinal fluid by means of a dural cuff. Local anesthetic may gain access to epidural space by diffusing into an intervertebral foramen; close to the midline, the intercostal nerve lies directly on the posterior intercostal membrane and pleura. (From Cousins MJ, Bindenbough PO, editors: *Neural blockade*, ed 2, Philadelphia, 1988, JB Lippincott.)

formed at the mid-axillary line by injection of 2 or 3 ml of bupivacaine, 0.5%, with epinephrine (1:200,000 concentration). Because the average duration of these nerve blocks is 4 to 8 hours, placement of indwelling catheters in the intercostal space is used to provide analgesia up to 6 days.[327]

A variation in providing postoperative intercostal analgesia is that of cryogenic analgesia. The efficacy of this technique is debatable compared with epidural or intravenous anesthesia.[246,283,385] Problems associated with cryoanalgesia of the intercostal nerves include long-term neuralgias, prolonged paresthesia, dysesthesias, and loss of intercostal muscle tone. Other possible options are paravertebral and intrapleural analgesia, which are variations of intercostal nerve block.

Intrapleural Analgesia

Intrapleural local anesthetic administration has been used for management of pain after chest and upper abdominal operation, trauma, or pancreatic pain.[66,138,175,262,374,380,394] Intrapleural analgesia is accomplished through placement of a catheter into the space between the parietal and visceral pleura. The catheter may be placed near the posterior medial aspect of the incision by the surgeon at the end of the procedure or by a transcutaneous technique postoperatively. The analgesic effects are produced by the diffusion of local anesthetic through the parietal pleura to produce multiple intercostal nerve blocks. Dosing regimens are either by intermittent bolus injections of 20 to 30 ml of bupivacaine (0.25% to 0.5%) or by continuous infusion.[374] The addition of epinephrine at a concentration of 1:200,000 dramatically decreases blood levels of bupivacaine to nontoxic levels,[242] although the quality of postoperative analgesia appears to be unpredictable.[161,242,369,419] This variability of efficacy depends on correct placement, patient positioning, and prevention of the loss of local anesthetic by chest tube drainage. Except for one study that showed a modest improvement in FVC, intrapleural analgesia has not been shown to have advantages in restoration of pulmonary function, compared with administration of intramuscular or intravenous narcotics.[161,384] Complications with this technique include pneumothorax, infection, and ipsilateral Horner's syndrome from sympathetic blockade.[15,416]

Thoracic Paravertebral Block

An alternate method of achieving multiple intercostal nerve blockade is placement of a thoracic paravertebral block, either by single injection or continuous catheter.[88,141,191] Unilateral analgesia is achieved by depositing local anesthetic in the paravertebral space, which is the locus of the primary ramus of the intercostal nerve. Although this technique avoids some of the disadvantages of intrapleural analgesia, such as loss through chest tube and risk of rapid absorption, it has not gained widespread popularity. No studies to date have documented an improvement in respiratory function equal to or exceeding that reported with use of epidural analgesia.

Epidural Anesthesia

Epidural anesthesia is a commonly used technique for management of post-thoracotomy pain; it has potential benefits for pulmonary and cardiovascular systems. Epidural analgesia has been shown to lessen the postoperative reduction in pulmonary function (FVC, FEV_1, peak exploratory flow rate) and improve arterial oxygenation compared with the use of parenteral narcotics. In addition, administration of epidural narcotics attenuates postoperative sympathetic stimulation and consequent hypertension and tachycardia.[248] The use of local anesthetics also may be cardioprotective by producing sympathetic blockade, resulting in vasodilation of epicardial vessels, improving left ventricular function during ischemia, and decreasing adrenergic outflow.[181,402] Animal studies that evaluated the effects of thoracic epidural have shown a lessening of myocardial ischemia and a reduction in the area of infarction.[335]

Effective postoperative analgesia can be obtained by placing the epidural catheter in either the thoracic or lumbar regions.[140,188,399] The optimal site for placement is controversial.[55,202,229,390] Although technically more difficult, thoracic epidural blockades provide segmental analgesia and theoretically decrease the risk of local anesthetic toxicity and unnecessary block of the lumbar region. The efficacy of the site of epidural narcotic administration may depend in part on the hydrophobicity of the opioid. Some investigators have proposed that epidural administration of lipophilic opioids produces analgesia by systemic absorption predominantly, not at the level of the spinal cord.[390]

It is the clinical practice in many institutions to combine the use of epidural opioids with local anesthetics. Theoretically, the combination of the two agents would act synergistically to provide better analgesia while minimizing the side effects of either agent. The combination of epidural bupivacaine plus morphine or fentanyl provides better analgesia than local anesthetic alone.[27] Addition of bupivacaine to an opioid epidural infusion did not improve post-thoracotomy analgesia when compared with an epidural infusion of narcotic alone. Epidural narcotics appear to provide the predominant analgesic effect.

Side effects associated with neuroaxonal administration of local anesthetics include hypotension and bradycardia, caused by sympathectomy and peripheral vasodilation, and blockade of the cardiac accelerator nerve fibers at T1 to T4. Administration of opioids are associated with the side effects of nausea, vomiting, pruritus, urinary retention, central narcosis, and respiratory depression. The incidence of respiratory depression from neuroaxonal administration of opioids varies from 0.1% to 3%.[295] Depending on the agent used, respiratory depression from opioids may peak from 4 to 10 hours, but may persist up to 24 hours. Patients at increased risk for developing respiratory depression include older, sicker patients having lengthy surgical procedures and those receiving major parenteral narcotics perioperatively or more than 6 mg of epidural morphine or 0.5 mg of intrathecal morphine (Box 70-20).[158] To decrease complications associated with respiratory depression, the patient should be monitored and cared for by knowledgeable staff with clear instructions for management of respiratory depression. Details about appropriate monitoring environment and management strategies for postoperative epidural analgesia are addressed in Chapter 89.

BOX 70-20
FACTORS PREDISPOSING TO DEVELOPMENT OF RESPIRATORY DEPRESSION AFTER EPIDURAL OPIOIDS

Drug factor
Hydrophilic drug (i.e., morphine)
Large doses
Repeated doses
Concomitant administration of parenteral opioids or other CNS depressants
Patient factors
Elderly or debilitated
Coexisting respiratory disease
Thoracic epidural
High sensitivity to opioids (i.e., no previous exposure to opioids)
Intrathecal administration
Increased intrathoracic pressure (e.g., controlled ventilation, coughing, vomiting)

From Etches RC, Sandler AN, Daley MD: Respiratory depression and spinal opioids, *Can J Anaesth* 36:165, 1989.

KEY POINTS

- Patients undergoing thoracic surgical procedures often have preexisting lung disease. One goal of preoperative preparation is to improve pulmonary function by use of bronchodilators for reactive airway disease, antibiotics for infection, and education to promote the cessation of smoking. The heavy smoker should stop smoking 4 to 8 weeks before operation.
- Thoracic surgery is being performed on patients with more severe pulmonary disease than in previous years. Previous exclusion criteria for undergoing general anesthesia now are considered overly conservative.
- Because the mortality rate of untreated lung cancer is great, it is difficult to assign definitive exclusion criteria for lung resection. Parameters used to predict patients at increased risk for postoperative complications include FVC, FEV_1, split lung functions, and exercise tolerance.
- Routine diagnostic procedures that are performed to confirm and evaluate the extent of pulmonary and thoracic disease include bronchoscopy, mediastinoscopy, and VAT. Although often performed during general anesthesia, these procedures may be tolerated in selected awake, sedated patients.

- The preoperative symptoms of dyspnea, shortness of breath, and hoarseness of voice may be related to thoracic tumor pathology. Possible etiologies include superior vena cava obstruction, mediastinal mass, tracheal compression, tracheomalacia, and malignancy. Anesthetic management should include an adequate preoperative evaluation to assess extent of disease, severity of symptoms, and effects of supine positioning on respiratory and cardiac function. The anesthetic plan should be coordinated with the surgeon and support staff to limit perioperative risk. In high-risk patients, anesthesia may proceed with a slow, controlled, and staged induction to cease if respiratory difficulties ensue.
- Topical anesthesia of the upper airway, superior laryngeal nerves, and trachea is required for awake sedated fiberoptic bronchoscopy or endotracheal intubation.
- Lateral decubitus position impacts negatively on the physiology of ventilation and circulation and is associated with position-related injuries.
- Fiberoptic bronchoscopy is the most reliable method for ascertaining correct positioning of the double-lumen endotracheal tube and assuring pulmonary toilet. The anesthesiologist should be facile with its use in the supine and lateral decubitus positions.
- When using single-lung ventilation, the anesthesiologist should be especially alert to problems with ventilation or oxygenation. The majority of problems are related to malposition of the double-lumen tube. Once proper position of the tube is confirmed, management strategies include (1) increased oxygenation to dependent lung (PEEP, increased Vt, increased FIO_2), (2) increased oxygenation of blood flowing to the nondependent lung (CPAP, intermittent ventilation), (3) decreased blood perfusion to nondependent lung (discontinue drugs that inhibit HPV, ligature to PA), increased oxygen content of blood (transfusion, improve SvO_2), and (4) increased perfusion of the dependent lung (increased cardiac output, pulmonary vasodilator, nitric oxide).
- Hypoxic pulmonary vasoconstriction is a homeostatic mechanism that limits perfusion of unventilated nonoxygenated atelectatic alveoli, thereby decreasing the shunt admixture. Hypoxic pulmonary vasoconstriction is activated by decreased alveolar oxygen tension, but is inhibited by certain anesthetic agents and vasodilators.
- Lung transplantation, volume reduction surgery, and other sophisticated intrathoracic operations require extraordinarily careful and complex planning and constant vigilance to maintain adequate ventilation, oxygenation, and hemodynamic stability.
- Video-assisted thoracoscopic procedures are being performed more frequently for diagnostic and therapeutic purposes. These procedures require meticulous single-lung isolation.
- Management after thoracotomy or thoracoscopy is directed to the delicate balance between pain relief and respiratory depression associated with systemic opioids. Epidural analgesia is especially valuable in these patients.

KEY REFERENCES:

Benumof JL, Partridge BL, Salvatierra C, et al: Margin of safety in positioning modern double-lumen endotracheal tubes, *Anesthesiology* 67(5):729, 1987.

Cooper JD, Trulock EP, Triantafillou AN, et al: Bilateral pneumectomy (volume reduction) for chronic obstructive pulmonary disease, *J Thorac Cardiovas Surg* 109(1):106, 1995.

Naunheim KS, Ferguson MK: The current status of lung volume reduction operations for emphysema, *Ann Thorac Surg* 62(2):601, 1996 (review).

O'Connor CJ: Thoracic epidural analgesia: physiologic effects and clinical applications, *J Cardiothorac Vasc Anesth* 7(5):595, 1993 (review).

Pate P, Tenholder MF, Griffin JP, et al: Preoperative assessment of the high-risk patient for lung resection, *Ann Thorac Surg* 61(5):1494, 1996.

Reilly J Jr, Mentzer SJ, Sugarbaker DJ: Preoperative assessment of patients undergoing pulmonary resection, *Chest* 103(4 Suppl):342, 1993 (review).

Triantafillou AN, Heerdt PM: Lung transplantation, *Int Anesth Clin* 29(3):87, 1991 (review).

Weir EK, Archer SL: The mechanism of acute hypoxic pulmonary vasoconstriction: the tale of two channels, *FASEB J* 9(2):183, 1995 (review).

REFERENCES

1. Aalto-Setala M, Heinonen J, Salorinne Y: Cardiorespiratory function during thoracic anesthesia: comparison of two-lung ventilation and one-lung ventilation with and without PEEP, *Acta Anaesthesiol Scand* 19:287, 1975.
2. Abramson AL, Goldstein M, Stenzler A, et al: The use of the tidal breathing flow volume loop in laryngotracheal disease of neonates and infants, *Laryngoscope* 92: 922, 1982.
3. Adams CF: Regional anesthesia for repair of Zenker's diverticulum, *Anesth Analg* 70:676, 1990 (letter).
4. Adatia I, Lillehei C, Arnold JH, et al: Inhaled nitric oxide in the treatment of postoperative graft dysfunction after lung transplantation, *Ann Thorac Surg* 57(5): 1311, 1994.
5. Adatia I, Wessel DL: Therapeutic use of inhaled nitric oxide, *Curr Opin Pediatr* 6(5):583, 1994 (review).
6. Adkins PC, Izawa EM: Resection of tracheal cylindroma using cardiopulmonary bypass, *Arch Surg* 88:405, 1964.
7. Adler OB, Rosenberger A, Peleg H: Fine-needle aspiration biopsy of mediastinal masses: evaluation of 136 experiences, *Am J Radiol* 140:893, 1983.
8. Albelda SM, Hanson-Flaschen JH, Taylor E, et al: Evaluation of high-frequency jet ventilation in patients with bronchopleural fistulas by quantitation of the airleak, *Anesthesiology* 63:551, 1985.
9. Albertini RE, Harrell JH, Moser KM: Management of arterial hypoxemia induced by fiberoptic bronchoscopy, *Chest* 67:134, 1975.
10. Albertini RE, Harrell JH, Kurihar N, et al: Arterial hypoxemia induced by fiberoptic bronchoscopy, *JAMA* 320:1666, 1974.
11. Alfery DD, Benumof JL, Trousdale FR: Improving oxygenation during one-lung ventilation: the effects of PEEP and blood flow restriction to the nonventilated lung, *Anesthesiology* 55:381, 1981.
12. Alfery DD, Zamost BG, Benumof JL: Unilateral lung lavage: blood flow manipulation by ipsilateral pulmonary artery balloon inflation in dogs, *Anesthesiology* 55:376, 1981.
13. Ali MK, Mountain CF, Ewer MS, et al: Predicting loss of pulmonary function after pulmonary resection for bronchogenic carcinoma, *Chest* 77(3):337, 1980.
14. Altose MD, Hicks RE, Edwards MW: Extracorporeal membrane oxygenation during bronchopulmonary lavage, *Arch Surg* 111:1148, 1976.
15. Ananthanarayan C, Kashtan H: Pneumothorax after interpleural block in a spontaneously breathing patient, *Anaesthesia* 45:342, 1990 (letter).
16. Anderson HW, Benumof JL: Intrapulmonary shunting during one-lung ventilation and surgical manipulation, *Anesthesiology* 55:A377, 1981.
17. Anderson WG: Respiratory aspects of the preoperative examination, *Br J Anaesth* 46:549, 1974.
18. Anderson WH, Dossett BE Jr, Hamilton GL: Prevention of postoperative pulmonary complications: use of isoproterenol and intermittent positive pressure breathing on inspiration, *JAMA* 186:763, 1963.
19. Applefeld JJ, Caruthers TE, Reno DJ, et al: Assessment of the sterility of long-term cardiac catheterization using a thermodilution Swan-Ganz catheter, *Chest* 74:337, 1978.
20. Ashbaugh DG: Mediastinoscopy, *Arch Surg* 100:568, 1970.
21. Aubier M, DeTroyer A, Sampson M, et al: Aminophylline improves diaphragmatic contractility, *N Engl J Med* 249:305, 1981.
22. Augustine SD, Benumof JL: Halothane and isoflurane do not impair arterial oxygenation during one-lung ventilation in patients undergoing thoracotomy, *Anesthesiology* 61:A484, 1984 (abstract).
23. Azizkhan RG, Dudgeon DL, Buck JR, et al: Life-threatening airway obstruction as a complication to the management of mediastinal masses in children, *J Pediatr Surg* 20: 816, 1985.
24. Babinski MF, Sierr OG, Smith RB, et al: Clinical application of continuous flow apneic ventilation, *Acta Anaesthesiol Scand* 29:750, 1985.
25. Babinski MF, Smith RB, Bunegin L: Continuous flow apneic ventilation during thoracotomy, *Anesthesiology* 65:399, 1986.
26. Bachand RR, Audet J, Meloche R, et al: Physiological changes associated with unilateral pulmonary ventilation during operations on one lung, *Can Anaesth Soc J* 22: 659, 1975.
27. Badner NH, Komar WE: Bupivacaine 0.1% does not improve post-operative epidural fentanyl analgesia after abdominal or thoracic surgery, *Can J Anaesth* 39:330, 1992.
28. Bagg LR: The 12-min walking distance; its use in the pre-operative assessment of patients with bronchial carcinoma before lung resection, *Respiration* 46:342, 1984.
29. Baker SP, Fisher RS: Childhood asphyxiation: choking or suffocation? *JAMA* 244:1343, 1980.
30. Baldi S, Scappanticci E, Rapellino M, et al: Effect of lung resection on pulmonary function: a comparative study in different surgical procedures, *Panminerva Med* 31(1):19, 1989.
31. Banjaminsson E, Klain N: Intraoperative dual-mode independent lung ventilation of a patient with bronchopleural fistula, *Anesth Analg* 60:118, 1981.
32. Baraka A, Afifi A, Muallem M, et al: Neuromuscular effects of halothane, suxamethonium and tubocurarine in a myasthenic undergoing thymectomy, *Br J Anaesth* 43:91, 1971.
33. Baraka A, Sibai AN, Muallem M, et al: CPAP oxygenation during one-lung ventilation using an underwater seal assembly, *Anesthesiology* 65:102, 1986.
34. Baraka A: Bronchoscopic removal of inhaled foreign bodies in children, *Br J Anaesth* 46:124, 1974.
35. Barash PG, Tsai B, Kitahata IM: Acute tracheal collapse following mediastinoscopy, *Anesthesiology* 44:67, 1976.
36. Barker WL, Faber LP, Ostermiller WE, et al: Management of persistent bronchopleural fistulas, *J Thorac Cardiovasc Surg* 62:393, 1971.
37. Baron SH: Zenker's diverticulum as a cause for loss of drug availability: a new complication, *Am J Gastroenterol* 77:152, 1982.
38. Bartlett RH, Krop P, Hanson EL, et al: Physiology of yawning and its application to postoperative care, *Surg Forum* 21:222, 1970.
39. Bartlett RH, Gazzaniga AB, Geraghty TR: The yawn maneuver: prevention and treatment of postoperative pulmonary complications, *Surg Forum* 22:196, 1971.
40. Bechard D, Wetstein L: Assessment of exercise oxygen consumption as preoperative criterion for lung resection, *Ann Thorac Surg* 44:344, 1987.
41. Belsey R: Resection and reconstruction of the intrathoracic trachea, *Br J Surg* 38:200, 1950.
42. Benjaminsson E, Klain N: Intraoperative dual-mode independent lung ventilation of a patient with bronchopleural fistula, *Anesth Analg* 60:118, 1981.
43. Bennett EJ, Schmidt GB, Patel KP, et al: Muscle relaxants, myasthenia, and mustards? *Anesthesiology* 46: 220, 1977.
44. Benumof JL: One-lung ventilation and hypoxic pulmonary vasoconstriction: implications for anesthetic management, *Anesth Analg* 64:821, 1985.
45. Benumof JL, Saidman LJ, Arkin DB, Diamart M, et al: Where pulmonary arterial catheters go: intrathoracic distribution, *Anesthesiology* 46:336, 1977.
46. Benumof JL, Augustine SD, Gibbons JA: Halothane and isoflurane only slightly impair arterial oxygenation during one-lung ventilation in patients undergoing thoracotomy, *Anesthesiology* 67:910, 1987.
47. Benumof JL, Partridge BL, Salvatierra C, et al: Margin of safety in positioning modern double-lumen endotracheal tubes, *Anesthesiology* 67:729, 1987.
48. Benumof JL, Pirlo AF, Johanson I, et al: Interaction of Pvo^2 with Pao^2 on hypoxic pulmonary vasoconstriction, *J Appl Physiol* 51:871, 1981.
49. Benumof JL, Rogers SN, Moyce PR, et al: Hypoxic pulmonary vasoconstriction and whole-lung PEEP in the dog, *Anesthesiology* 51:503, 1979.
50. Benumof JL, Wahrenbrock EA: Blunted hypoxic pulmonary vasoconstriction by increased lung vascular pressures, *J Appl Physiol* 38:846, 1975.
51. Benumof JL, Wahrenbrock EA: Dependency of hypoxic pulmonary vasoconstriction on temperature, *J Appl Physiol* 72:56, 1977.
52. Benumof JL: Monitoring respiratory function during anesthesia. In Saidman LJ, Smith NT, editors: *Monitoring in anesthesia,* Boston, 1984, Butterworths.
53. Benumof JL: Mechanism of decreased blood flow to atelectatic lung, *J Appl Physiol* 46:1047, 1978.
54. Benumof, JL: Anesthesia for special elec-

tive therapeutic procedures. In Benumof JL, editor: *Anesthesia for thoracic surgery,* Philadelphia, 1995, WB Saunders.

55. Benzon HT: Post-thoracotomy epidural analgesia: lumbar or thoracic placement? *J Cardiothorac Vasc Anesth* 7:515, 1993 (editorial).
56. Bergman NA: Reduction in resting and end-expiratory position of the respiratory system with induction of anesthesia and neuromuscular paralysis, *Anesthesiology* 57:14, 1982.
57. Bergmans J, Fannes-Breselow C, Gribomont B: A reassessment of the neurophysiological evidence for a presynaptic defect in myasthenia gravis, *Electromyogr Clin Neurophysiol* 16:337, 1976.
58. Bergsland J, Battaglia R, Takita H: Modification of the technique of radical intrapericardial pneumonectomy, *Scand J Thorac Cardiovasc Surg* 19:89, 1985.
59. Berryhill RE, Benumof JL: PEEP-induced discrepancy between pulmonary arterial wedge pressure and left atrial pressure: the influence of controlled vs. spontaneous ventilation and compliant vs. noncompliant lungs in the dog, *Anesthesiology* 46:303, 1979.
60. Bigatello LM, Hurford WE, Kacmarek RM, et al: Prolonged inhalation of low concentrations of nitric oxide in patients with severe adult respiratory distress syndrome. Effects on pulmonary hemodynamics and oxygenation, *Anesthesiology* 80:761–770, 1994.
61. Bishop MJ, Benson MS, Sato P, et al: Comparison of high-frequency jet ventilation with conventional mechanical ventilation for bronchopleural fistula, *Anesth Analg* 66:833, 1987.
62. Bishop MJ, Cheney FW: Minoxidil and nifedipine inhibit hypoxic pulmonary vasoconstriction, *J Cardiovasc Pharmacol* 5:184, 1983.
63. Bishop MJ, Kennard S, Artman LD, et al: Hydralazine does not inhibit canine hypoxic pulmonary vasoconstriction, *Am Rev Resp Dis* 128:998, 1983.
64. Bjertnaes LJ: Hypoxia-induced vasoconstriction in isolated perfused lungs exposed to injectable or inhalation anesthetics, *Acta Anaesthesiol Scand* 21:133, 1977.
65. Black RE, Choi KJ, Syme WC, et al: Bronchoscopic removal of aspirated foreign bodies in children, *Am J Surg* 148: 778, 1984.
66. Blake DW, Donnan G, Novella J: Interpleural administration of bupivacaine after cholecystectomy: a comparison with intercostal nerve block, *Anaesth Intensive Care* 17:269, 1989.
67. Bland S, Laserov L, Dyck G, et al: The influence of the chest wall on respiratory rate and depth, *Respir Physiol* 3:47, 1967.
68. Blazer S, Naveh Y, Friedman A: Foreign body in the airway, *Am J Dis Child* 134:68, 1980.
69. Bocchi EA, Bacal F, Auler JOC, et al: Inhaled nitric oxide leading to pulmonary edema in stable heart failure, *Am J Cardiol* 74:70, 1994.
70. Bolliger CT, Soler M, Stulz P, et al: Evaluation of high-risk lung resection candidates: pulmonary haemodynamics versus exercise testing. A series of five patients, *Respiration* 61(4):181, 1994.
71. Boysen PG, Harris JO, Block AJ, et al: Prospective evaluation for pneumonectomy using perfusion scanning, *Chest* 80:163, 1981.
72. Boysen PG, Block AJ, Olsen GN, et el: Prospective evaluation for pneumonectomy using the 99m technetium quantitative perfusion lung scan, *Chest* 72:422, 1977.
73. Boysen PG, Block AJ, Moulder PV: Relationship between preoperative pulmonary function and complications after thoracotomy, *Surg Gynecol Obstet* 152: 813, 1981.
74. Boysen PG: Preoperative assessment of the candidate for thoracotomy and lung resection, *Am Rev Respir Dis* 140:1175, 1989.
75. Boysen PG: Pulmonary resection and postoperative pulmonary function, *Chest* 77:718, 1980.
76. Bray RJ, Fernandes FJ: Mediastinal tumour causing airway obstruction in anaesthetized children, *Anaesthesia* 37:571, 1983.
77. Brodsky JB, Adkins MO, Gaba DM: Bronchial cuff pressures of double-lumen tubes, *Anesth Analg* 69: 608, 1989.
78. Bromage PR: Spirometry in assessment of analgesia after abdominal surgery, *BMJ* 2:589, 1955.
79. Bromage PR: Physiology. In Bromage PR, editor: *Epidural analgesia,* Philadelphia, 1978, WB Saunders.
80. Bromage PR: Surgical applications. In Bromage PR, editor: *Epidural analgesia,* Philadelphia, 1978, WB Saunders.
81. Brown DL, Davis RS: A simple device for oxygen insufflation with continuous positive airway pressure during one-lung ventilation, *Anesthesiology* 61:481, 1984.
82. Brown SE, Linden GS, King RR, et al: Effect of verapamil on pulmonary haemodynamics during hypoxaemia at rest, and during exercise in patients with chronic obstructive pulmonary disease, *Thorax* 38:840, 1983.
83. Burke CM, Theodore J, Dawkins KD, et al: Post-transplant obliterative bronchiolitis and other late lung sequelae in human heart-lung transplantation, *Chest* 86:824, 1984.
84. Burman SO: The prophylactic use of digitalis before thoracotomy, *Ann Thorac Surg* 14:359, 1972.
85. Burton NA, Fall SM, Lyons T, et al: Rupture of the left main-stem bronchus with a polyvinylchloride double-lumen tube, *Chest* 83:928, 1983.
86. Busby BP, Williford WD, Peterson OL, et al: A randomized clinical trial of total parenteral nutrition in malnourished surgical patients: the rationale and impact of previous clinical trials and pilot study on protocol design, *Am J Clin Nutr* 47:357, 1988.
87. Campbell D, Cotton EK, Lilly JR: A dual approach to tracheobronchial foreign bodies in children, *Surgery* 91:178, 1982.
88. Canacher ID, Kokri M: Postoperative paravertebral blocks for thoracic surgery, *Br J Anaesth* 59:155, 1987.
89. Carden E: Recent improvements in anesthetic technique for use during bronchoscopy, *Otol Rhinol Laryngol* 83:777, 1974.
90. Cassorla L, Katz JA: Management of cardiac herniation after intrapericardial pneumonectomy, *Anesthesiology* 60:362, 1984.
91. Cervenko FW, Shelley SE, Spence DG, et al: Massive endobronchial hemorrhage during cardiopulmonary bypass: treatable complication of balloon-tipped catheter damage to the pulmonary artery, *Ann Thorac Surg* 35:326, 1983.
92. Chick TW, Kochukoshy KN, Matsumoto S, et al: The effect of nitroglycerin on gas exchange, hemodynamics and oxygen transport in patients with chronic obstructive pulmonary disease, *Am J Med Sci* 276:105, 1978.
93. Chou S: Acquisition of donor strain of cytomegalovirus by renal- transplant recipients, *N Engl J Med* 314:1418, 1986.
94. Christofordis AJ, Nelson SW, Tomashefski JF: Effects of bronchoscopy on pulmonary function, *Am Rev Respir Dis* 85:127, 1962.
95. Churchill-Davidson HC: Abnormal response to muscle relaxants, *Proc R Soc Med* 48:621, 1955.
96. Clarke HJ, Kwan A, Wright ES, et al: Enterobronchial fistula, *Can J Surg* 27:185, 1984.
97. Clausen EG: Postoperative paralysis of the brachial plexus, *Surgery* 12:933, 1942.
98. Cohen E, Eisenkraft JB: Bronchopulmonary lavage: effects on oxygenation and hemodynamics, *J Cardiothorac Anesth* 4:609, 1990.
99. Cohen E, Thys DM, Eisenkraft JB, et al: Effect of CPAP and PEEP during one lung anesthesia: left versus right thoracotomies, *Anesthesiology* 63:A564, 1985.
100. Cole F Jr, Cole FH, Khandekar A, et al: Video-assisted thoracic surgery: primary therapy for spontaneous pneumothorax? *Ann Thorac Surg* 60(4):931, 1995.
101. Colley PS, Cheney FW, Hlastala MP: Pulmonary gas exchange effects of nitroglycerin in canine edematous lungs, *Anesthesiology* 55:114, 1981.
102. Conacher D, McNally A, Chordhry K, et al: Anaesthesia for isolated lung transplantation, *Br J Anaesth* 60: 588, 1988.
103. Condon HA: Anaesthesia for pharyngolaryngo-esophageactomy with pharyngogastrostomy, *Br J Anaesth* 43:1061, 1971.
104. Cooper DK: The incidence of postoperative infection and the role of antibiotic prophylaxis in pulmonary surgery: a review of 221 consecutive patients undergoing thoracotomy, *Br J Dis Chest* 75:154, 1981.
105. Cooper JB, Newbower RS, Kitz RJ: An analysis of major errors, *Anesthesiology* 60:34, 1984.
106. Cooper JD, Duffin J, Glynn MFX, et al: Combination of membrane oxygenator support and pulmonary lavage for acute respiratory failure, *J Thorac Cardiovasc Surg* 71:304, 1976.
107. Cooper JD, Trulock EP, Triantafillou AN, et al: Bilateral pneumectomy (volume reduction) for chronic obstructive pulmonary disease, *J Thorac Cardiovas Surg* 109(1): 106, 1995.
108. Cooper M, Watson R: An improved regional anaesthetic technique for perioral endoscopy, *Anesthesiology* 43:372, 1975.
109. Cope R, Spargo P: Anesthesia for Zenker's diverticulum, *Anesth Analg* 71:312, 1990 (letter).
110. Cordel AR, Ellison RE: *Complications of intrathoracic surgery,* Boston, 1979, Little Brown.

111. Corey R, Hla MK: Major and massive hemoptysis: Reassessment of conservative management, *Am J Med Sci* 294:301, 1987.
112. Cortese DA, Kinsey JH: Hematoporphyrin derivative phototherapy in the treatment of bronchogenic carcinoma, *Chest* 86:8, 1984.
113. Cortese DA, Kinsey JH: Bronchoscopic phototherapy using hematoporphyrin derivative, *Surg Clin North Am* 64:941, 1984.
114. Cousins MJ, Bridenbaugh PO, editors: *Neural blockade in clinical anesthesia and management of pain,* ed 2, Philadelphia, 1988, JB Lippincott.
115. Crawford OB, Ottosen P, Buckingham WW, et al: Peridural anesthesia in thoracic surgery, a review of 677 cases, *Anesthesiology* 12:73, 1951.
116. Crinquette V, Wurtz A, Leroy S, et al: Resection et reconstruction de la bifurcation tracheale sous jet ventilation a haute frequence, separee sur les deux poumons, *Ann Chir* 43:673, 1989.
117. Croft PB: Abnormal responses to muscle relaxants in carcinomatous neuropathy, *BMJ* 1:181, 1958.
118. Cuetter AC, Bartoszek DM: The thoracic outlet syndrome: controversies, overdiagnosis, overtreatment, and recommendations for management, *Muscle Nerve* 13: 362, 1990.
119. Cull-Candy SG, Miledi R, Trautmann A, et al: On the release of transmitter at normal, myasthenia gravis, and myasthenic syndrome affected human end-plates, *J Physiol (Lond)* 299:621, 1980.
120. Curling PE, Zaidan JR, Murphy DA, et al: Treatment of pulmonary hypertension after human orthoptic heart transplantation, *Anesth Analg* 66:S37, 1987.
121. Dauber JH, Paradis IL, Dummer JS: Infectious complications in pulmonary allograft recipients, *Clin Chest Med* 11:291, 1990.
122. Davenport D, Ferree C, Blake D, et al: Radiation therapy in the treatment of superior vena caval obstruction, *Cancer* 42: 2600, 1978.
123. Davies JM, Latto IP, Jone JG, et al: Effects of stopping smoking for 48 hours on oxygen availability from the blood: a study on pregnant women, *BMJ* 2:355, 1979.
124. deBlic J, Blanche S, Danel C, et al: Bronchoalveolar lavage in HIV infected patients with interstitial pneumonitis, *Arch Dis Child* 64:1246, 1989.
125. Dedhia HV, Leroy L, Jain PR, et al: Endoscopic laser therapy for respiratory distress due to obstructive airway tumors, *Crit Care Med* 12:464, 1985.
126. DeGraff AC, Bouhuys A: Mechanisms of air flow in airway obstruction, *Annu Rev Med* 24:111, 1973.
127. DeMeester TR, Van Heertum RL, Karas JR, et al: Preoperative evaluation with differential pulmonary function, *Ann Thorac Surg* 18:61, 1974.
128. Demos NJ, Timmes JJ: Myoplasty for closure of tracheobronchial fistula, *Ann Thorac Surg* 15:88, 1973.
129. Deslauriers J, Beaulieu M, Benzera A: Sleeve pneumonectomy for bronchogenic carcinoma, *Ann Thorac Surg* 28:465, 1979.
130. DeSoto H: Direct laryngoscopy as an aid to relieve airway obstruction in a patient with a mediastinal mass, *Anesthesiology* 67:116, 1987.
131. Dlabel PW, Stutts BS, Jenkins DW, et al: Cyanosis following right pneumonectomy, *Chest* 81:370, 1982.
132. Drachman DA, Skom JH: Procainamide—a hazard in myasthenia gravis, *Arch Neurol* 13:316, 1965.
133. Dripps RD, Deming MVN: Postoperative atelectasis and pneumonia: diagnosis, etiology and management based upon 1240 cases of upper abdominal surgery, *Ann Surg* 124:94, 1946.
134. Dryden GE: Circulatory collapse after pneumonectomy (an unusual complication from the use of a Carlens catheter): case report, *Anesth Analg* 56:451, 1977.
135. Dubrawsky C, Awe RJ, Jenkins DG: The effect of bronchofibrescopic examination on oxygenation status, *Chest* 67:137, 1975.
136. Dummer JS, White LT, Ho M, et al: Morbidity of cytomegalovirus infection in recipients of heart or heart-lung transplants who received cyclosporine, *J Infect Dis* 152:1182, 1985.
137. Dumon JF, Shapshay S, Bourcereau J, et al: Principles for safety in application of neodymium-YAG laser in bronchoscopy, *Chest* 86:163, 1984.
138. Durrani Z, Winnie AP, Ikuta P: Interpleural catheter analgesia for pancreatic pain, *Anesth Analg* 67:479, 1988.
139. Dyet JF, Naghissi K: Role of venography in assessing patients with superior caval obstruction caused by bronchial carcinoma for bypass operation, *Thorax* 35:628, 1980.
140. E-Baz NM, Faber LP, Jensik RJ: Continuous epidural infusion of morphine for treatment of pain after thoracic surgery: a new technique, *Anesth Analg* 63:757, 1984.
141. Eason MJ, Wyatter R: Paravertebral thoracic block—a reappraisal, *Anesthesia* 34:638, 1979.
142. Egbert LD, Battit GE, Welch CE, et al: Reduction of postoperative pain by encouragement and instruction of patients, *N Engl J Med* 270:825, 1964.
143. Eger EI, Severinghaus JW: The rate of rise of PaCO2 in the apneic anesthetized patient, *Anesthesiology* 22:419, 1961.
144. Ehrenwerth J, Urban MK: Monitoring during thoracic surgery, *Probl Anesth* 4(2):306, 1990.
145. Eisenkraft JB, Book WJ, Mann SM, et al: Resistance to succinylcholine in myasthenia gravis: a dose-response study, *Anesthesiology* 69:760, 1988.
146. Eisenkraft JB, Brooks WJ, Papatestas AE: Sensitivity to vecuronium in myasthenia gravis: a dose-response study, *Can J Anaesth* 37:301, 1990.
147. Eisenkraft JB, Neustein SM: Anesthesia for special problems in thoracic surgery, *Probl Anesth* 4:326, 1990.
148. Eisenkraft JB, Papatestas AE, Kahn CH, et al: Predicting the need for postoperative mechanical ventilation in myasthenia gravis, *Anesthesiology* 65:79, 1986.
149. Eisenkraft JB, Thys DM, Cohen E, et al: Hemodynamic effects of CPAP and PEEP during one-lung anesthesia with isoflurane, *Anesthesiology* 61:A520, 1984.
150. Eisenkraft JB: Anaesthesia for trans-sternal thymectomy in myasthenia gravis, *Ann R Coll Surg Engl* 70:257, 1988 (letter).
151. Eisenkraft JB: Myasthenia gravis and thymic surgery–anaesthetic considerations. In Gothard JWW, editors: *Bailliere's clinical anaesthesiology,* London, 1987, Balliere Tindall.
152. El-Baz N, El-Ganzouri A, Gottschalk W, et al: One-lung high-frequency positive pressure ventilation for sleeve pneumonectomy: an alternative technique, *Anesth Analg* 60:683, 1981.
153. El-Baz N, Holinger L, El-Ganzouri A, et al: High-frequency positive-pressure ventilation for tracheal reconstruction supported by tracheal T-tube, *Anesth Analg* 61:796, 1982.
154. Elguindi AS, Harrison GN, Abdulla AM, et al: Cardiac rhythm disturbances during fiberoptic bronchoscopy: a prospective study, *J Thorac Cardiovas Surg* 77(4):557, 1979.
155. Engel AG: Myasthenia gravis and myasthenic syndromes, *Ann Neurol* 16:516, 1984.
156. Enquist A, Brandt MR, Fernandes A, et al: The blocking effect of epidural analgesia on the adrenocortical and hyperglycaemic response to surgery, *Acta Anaesthesiol Scand* 21:330, 1977.
157. Esclamado RM, Richardson MA: Laryngotracheal foreign bodies in children, *Am J Dis Child* 141:259, 1987.
158. Etches RC, Sandler AN, Daley MD: Respiratory depression and spinal opioids, *Can J Anaesth* 36:165, 1989.
159. Euler C Von: On the central pattern generator for the basic breathing rhythmicity, *J Appl Physiol* 55:167, 1983.
160. Ewing MR: Postoperative paralysis in the upper extremity, *Lancet* 1:99, 1950.
161. Faffin L, Fletcher D, Sperandio M, et al: Interpleural infusion of 2% lidocaine with 1:200,000 epinephrine for post-thoracotomy analgesia, *Anesth Analg* 79:328, 1994.
162. Fee JT, Holmes EC, Gewirtz HS, et al: Role of pulmonary vascular resistance measurements in preoperative evaluation of candidates for pulmonary resection, *J Thorac Cardiovasc Surg* 75(4):519, 1978.
163. Felicetti SA, Silbaugh SA, Muggenburg BA: Effect of flow rate of lavage fluid on the removal of radioactive particles from the lung by bronchopulmonary lavage, *Health Physics* 28(4):399, 1975.
164. Ferguson MK, Little L, Rizzo L, et al: Diffusing capacity predicts morbidity and mortality after pulmonary resection, *J Thorac Cardiovasc Surg* 96:894, 1988.
165. Finley TN, Hill TR, Bonica JJ: Effect of intrapleural pressure on pulmonary shunt to atelectatic dog lung, *Am J Physiol* 205: 1187, 1963.
166. Fischler M, Troche G, Guerin Y, et al: Evolution des techniques d'anesthesie pour resection-anastomose de trachee, *Ann Fr Anesth Reanim* 7:125, 1988.
167. Reference deleted in proofs.
168. Fleetwood-Walker SM, Mitchell R, Hope PJ, et al: An α_2 receptor mediates the selective inhibition by noradrenaline of nociceptive responses of identified dorsal horn neurons, *Brain Res* 334:243, 1985.
169. Foster ED, Munro DD, Dobell ARC:

Mediastinoscopy: a review of anatomical relationships and complications, *Ann Thorac Surg* 13:273, 1972.

170. Foster JMG, Lau OJ, Alimo EB: Ruptured bronchus following endobronchial intubation: a case report, *Br J Anaesth* 55:687, 1983.
171. Fredrickson JM: Reinforced T-tube tracheal stent, *Arch Otolaryngol* 90:120, 1969.
172. Freedman AP, Pelias A, Johnston RF, et al: Alveolar proteinosis lung lavage using partial cardiopulmonary bypass, *Thorax* 36:543, 1981.
173. Freitag L, Chapman GA, Sielcak M, et al: Laser smoke effect on the bronchial system, *Lasers Surg Med* 7:283, 1987.
174. Fried MP: A survey of the complications of laser laryngoscopy, *Arch Otolaryngol* 110:31, 1984.
175. Friedel H: Importance of bronchiological examination in cases of pleural diseases, *Bronches* 20:77, 1970.
176. Froese AB, Bryan AC: Effects of anesthesia and paralysis on diaphragmatic mechanics in man, *Anesthesiology* 41:242, 1974.
177. Froese AB, Bryan AC: High-frequency ventilation: uses and abuses, *Am Rev Respir Dis* 135:1363, 1987.
178. Fry DL, Hyatt RE: Pulmonary mechanics: a unified analysis of the relationship between pressure, volume and gas flow in the lungs of normal and diseased human subjects, *Am J Med* 29:672, 1960.
179. Gale ME, Karlinsky JB, Robins AG: Bronchopulmonary lavage in pulmonary alveolar proteinosis: chest radiograph observations, *AJR Am J Roentgenol* 146(5): 981, 1986.
180. Gallagher C, Sladen RB, Lubarsky D: Thoracotomy: postoperative complications, *Probl Anesth* 4:393, 1990.
181. Gamulin Z, Forster A, Morel D, et al: Effects of infrarenal aortic cross-clamping on renal hemodynamics in humans, *Anesthesiology* 61:394, 1984.
182. Garden JM, O'Banion MK, Shelnitz LS, et al: Papillomavirus in the vapor of carbon dioxide-treated verrucae, *JAMA* 259:1199, 1988.
183. Garry BP, Bivens HE: Blood pressure monitoring during mediastinoscopy, *Can J Anaesth* 36:365, 1989 (letter).
184. Gass GD, Olsen GN: Preoperative pulmonary function testing to predict postoperative morbidity and mortality, *Chest* 89:127, 1986.
185. Gayes JM, Giron L, Nissen MD, et al: Anesthetic considerations for patients undergoing double-lung transplantation, *J Cardiothorac Anesth* 4:486, 1990.
186. Geffin B, Bland J, Grillo HC: Anesthetic management of tracheal resection and reconstruction, *Anesth Analg* 48:884, 1969.
187. Gelb AF, Epstein JD: Laser in treatment of lung cancer, *Chest* 86:662, 1984.
188. George KA, Wright PM, Chisakuta A: Continuous thoracic epidural fentanyl for post-thoracotomy pain relief: with or without bupivacain? *Anaesthesia* 46:732, 1991.
189. Gerlach H, Pappert D, Lewandowski K, et al: Long-term inhalation with evaluated low doses of nitric oxide for selective improvement of oxygenation in patients with adult respiratory distress syndrome, *Intensive Care Med* 19:443–449, 1993.
190. Gibson QH, Roughton FJW: The kinetics of equilibria of the reactions of nitric oxide with sheep haemoglobin, *J Physiol (Lond)* 136:507, 1957.
191. Gilbert J, Hultman J: Thoracic paravertebral block: a method of pain control, *Acta Anaesthesiol Scand* 33:142, 1989.
192. Girnar DS, Weinreich AI: Anesthesia for transcervical thymectomy in myasthenia gravis, *Anesth Analg* 55:13, 1976.
193. Glass DD, Tonnesen AS, Gabel JC, et al: Therapy of unilateral pulmonary insufficiency with a double lumen endotracheal tube, *Crit Care Med* 4:323, 1976.
194. Glenski JA, Crawford M, Rehder K: High-frequency, small-volume ventilation during thoracic surgery, *Anesthesiology* 64:211, 1986.
195. Goodman GE, Livingston RB: Small cell lung cancer, *Curr Probl Cancer* 13(1):1, 1989.
196. Graeber GM, Shriver CD, Albus RA, et al: The use of computed tomography in the evaluation of mediastinal masses, *J Thorac Cardiovasc Surg* 91:662, 1986.
197. Gravel JA: Herniation of the heart—a hazard of thoracic surgery: report of two fatal cases, *Can J Surg* 9:72, 1966.
198. Green ER Jr, Gutierrez FA: Tip of polyvinyl chloride double-lumen endotracheal tube inadvertently wedged in left lower lobe bronchus, *Anesthesiology* 64:406, 1986.
199. Grillo HC, Bendixen HH, Gephart T: Resection of the carina and lower trachea, *Ann Surg* 158:889, 1963.
200. Gross NJ: Ipratropium bromide, *N Engl J Med* 319(8):486, 1988.
201. Guernelli N, Bragaglia BB, Briccoli A, et al: Tracheobronchial ruptures due to cuffed Carlens tubes, *Ann Thorac Surg* 28:66, 1979.
202. Guinard J-P, Mavrocordatos P, Chiolero R, et al: A randomized comparison of intravenous versus lumbar and thoracic epidural fentanyl for analgesia after thoracotomy *Anesthesiology* 77: 1108, 1992.
203. Gunstensen J, Wade JD: Mediastinoscopy: an analysis of 320 consecutive cases, *Br J Surg* 59:209, 1972.
204. Haas A, Pineda H, Haas F, Axen K, et al: Therapeutic modalities. In *Pulmonary therapy and rehabilitation: principles and practice,* Baltimore, 1979, Williams & Wilkins.
205. Hall KD, Friedman M: Extracorporeal oxygenation for induction of anesthesia in a patient with an intrathoracic tumor, *Anesthesiology* 42:493, 1975.
206. Hankins JR, Mayer RF, Satterfield JR, et al: Thymectomy for myasthenia gravis: fourteen-year experience, *Ann Surg* 201: 618, 1985.
207. Hannenberg AA, Satwicz PR, Piens RS Jr, et al: A device for applying CPAP to the nonventilated upper lung during one lung ventilation. II, *Anesthesiology* 60:254, 1984.
208. Harik SI, Raichele ME, Reis DJ: Spontaneous remitting spinal epidural hematoma in a patient on anticoagulants, *N Engl J Med* 284:1355, 1971.
209. Hasan FM, Malanga A, Corrao WM, et al: Effect of catheter position on thermodilution cardiac output during continuous positive-pressure ventilation, *Crit Care Med* 12:387, 1984.
210. Hasenbos MA, Gielen MJ: Anaesthesia for bullectomy. A technique with spontaneous ventilation and extradural blockade, *Anaesthesia* 40(10):977, 1985.
211. Hatch D: Ventilation and arterial oxygenation during thoracic surgery, *Thorax* 21:310, 1966.
212. Hatcher CR, Miller JI: Operative injuries to nerves during intrathoracic procedures. In Cordell RA, Ellison RG, editors: *Complications of intrathoracic surgery,* Boston, 1979, Little Brown.
213. Hay J, Clague J, Nasar M, et al: Local anaesthesia for fibreoptic bronchoscopy, *Thorax* 44:890P, 1989 (abstract).
214. Healy G, McGill T, Strong M: Surgical advances in the treatment of lesions of the pediatric airway: the role of the carbon dioxide laser, *Pediatrics* 61:380, 1978.
215. Healy GB, Strong MS, Shapshay S et al: Complications of CO_2 laser surgery of the aerodigestive tract: experience of 4,416 cases, *Otolaryngol Head Neck Surg* 92:13, 1984.
216. Healy GB: Foreign bodies of the air and food passages in children, *Am J Dis Child* 141:249, 1987.
217. Heiser M, Steinberg JJ, MacVaugh H, et al: Bronchial rupture, a complication of use of the Robertshaw double-lumen tube, *Anesthesiology* 51:88, 1979.
218. Heritier F, Madden B, Hodson ME, et al: Lung allograft transplantation: indications, preoperative assessment and postoperative management, *Eur Respir J* 5(10):1262, 1992 (review).
219. Hermens JM, Bennett MJ, Hirshman CA: Anesthesia for laser surgery, *Anesth Analg* 62:218, 1983.
220. Hiebert CA: Surgery for cricopharyngeal dysfunction under local anesthesia, *Surgery* 131:423, 1976.
221. Hiratzka LF, Swan DM, Rose EF, et al: Bilateral simultaneous lung lavage utilizing membrane oxygenator for pulmonary alveolar proteinosis in an 8-month-old infant, *Ann Thorac Surg* 35:313, 1983.
222. Hochberg MS, Gielchinsky I, Parsonnet V, et al: Pulmonary inactivation of vasopressors following cardiac operations, *Ann Thorac Surg* 41:200, 1986.
223. Hole A, Unsgaard G: The effect of epidural and general anaesthesia on lymphocyte functions during and after major orthopaedic surgery, *Acta Anaesthesiol Scand* 27:135, 1983.
224. Holtzman H, Lippman M, Nakhjaran F, et al: Post-pneumonectomy intraatrial right-to-left shunt, *Thorax* 35:307, 1980.
225. Hoppin FJ Jr, Green ID, Mead J: Distribution of pleural surface pressure, *J Appl Physiol* 27:863, 1969.
226. Horlocker TT, Wedel DJ, Offord KP: Does preoperative antiplatelet therapy increase the risk of hemorrhagic complications associated with regional anesthesia? *Anesth Analg* 70:631, 1990.
227. Howard RJ, Simmons R: Acquired immunologic deficiencies after trauma and surgical procedures, *Surg Gynecol Obstet* 139:771, 1974.

228. Hugod C: Ultrastructural changes of the rabbit lung after a 5 ppm nitric oxide exposure, *Arch Environ Health* 34:12, 1979.
229. Hurford WE, Dutton RP, Alfille PH, et al: Comparison of thoracic and lumbar epidural infusions of bupivacaine and fentanyl for post-thoracotomy analgesia, *J Cardiothorac Vasc Anesth* 7:521, 1993.
230. Irita K, Satoh M, Akata T, et al: Lambert-Eaton myasthenic syndrome, *Can J Anaesth* 37:944, 1990 (letter).
231. Isaac P, Barry JE, Vaughan RS, et al: A jet nebulizer for delivery of topical anaesthesia to the respiratory tract: a comparison with cricothyroid puncture and direct spraying for fiberoptic bronchoscopy, *Anaesthesia* 45:46, 1990.
232. Ishibe Y, Shiokawa Y, Umeda T, et al: The effect of thoracic epidural anesthesia on hypoxic pulmonary vasoconstriction in dogs: an analysis of the pressure-flow curve, *Anesth Analg* 82(5):1049, 1996.
233. Jahangiri M, Taggart DP, Goldstraw P: Role of mediastinoscopy in superior vena cava obstruction, *Cancer* 71(10):3006, 1993.
234. Jarvinen A, Mattila T, Appelqvist P, et al: Cardiac disturbance after pneumonectomy—the value of prophylactic digitalization, *Ann Chir Gynaecol* 67:77, 1978.
235. Jensen V, Milne B, Salerno T: Femoral-femoral cardiopulmonary bypass prior to induction of anaesthesia in the management of upper airway obstruction, *Can Anaesth Soc J* 30:270, 1983.
236. John RE, Narang VPS: A boy with an anterior mediastinal mass, *Anaesthesia* 43:864, 1988.
237. Jones DP: Diagnostic work-up of chest disease, *Surg Clin North Am* 60:743, 1980.
238. Jones RM: Smoking before surgery: the case for stopping smoking, *BMJ* 290:1763, 1985.
239. Juler GL, Stemmer EA, Connolly JE: Complications of prophylactic digitalization in thoracic surgical patients, *J Thorac Cardiovasc Surg* 58:352, 1969.
240. Kaiser D: Indications for thoracoscopy in pleural empyema, *Pneumologie* 43:76, 1989.
241. Kaiser LR, Daniel TM: *Thoracoscopic surgery,* 1993. Little Brown and Co., Boston, 1993.
242. Kambam JR, Hammon J, Parris WC, et al: Intrapleural analgesia for post-thoracotomy pain and blood levels of bupivacaine following intrapleural injection, *Can J Anaesth* 36:106, 1989.
243. Kamvyssi-Dea S, Kritikon P, Exarhos N, et al: Anaesthetic management of reconstruction of the lower part of the trachea, *Br J Anaesth* 47:82, 1975.
244. Karas SE: Thoracic outlet syndrome, *Clin Sports Med* 9:297, 1990.
245. Kariman K, Kylstra JA, Spock A: Pulmonary alveolar proteinosis: prospective clinical experience in 23 patients for 15 years, *Lung* 162:223, 1984.
246. Katz J, Nelson W, Forest R, et al: Cryoanalgesia for post-thoracotomy, *Lancet* 1:512, 1980.
247. Katz JA, Laverne RG, Fairley HB, et al: Pulmonary oxygen exchange during endobronchial anesthesia: effects of tidal volume and PEEP, *Anesthesiology* 56:164, 1982.
248. Kennedy WF Jr, Sawyer TK, Gerbershagen HY, et al: Systemic cardiovascular and renal hemodynamic alterations during peridural anesthesia in normal man, *Anesthesiology* 31:414, 1969.
249. Kerr JH: Physiological aspects of one lung (endobronchial) anesthesia, *Int Anesth Clin* 10:61, 1972.
250. Kim IG, Brummitt WM, Humphry A, et al: Foreign body in the airway: a review of 202 cases, *Laryngoscope* 83:347, 1973.
251. King RM, Telander RL, Smithson WA, et al: Primary mediastinal tumors in children, *J Pediatr Surg* 17:512, 1982.
252. Kinnear WJM, Reynolds L, Gaskin D, et al: Comparison of transcricoid and bronchoscopic routes for administration of local anaesthesia before fiberoptic bronchoscopy, *Thorax* 43:805P, 1988 (abstract).
253. Kirsh MM, Rotman H, Behrendt DM, et al: Complications of pulmonary resection, *Ann Thorac Surg* 20:215, 1975.
254. Klassen GA, Bramwell RS, Bromage PR, et al: Effect of acute sympathectomy by epidural anesthesia on the canine coronary circulation, *Anesthesiology* 52:8, 1980.
255. Kornfeld P, Horowitz SH, Genkins G, et al: Myasthenia gravis unmasked by antiarrhythmic agents, *Mt Sinai J Med* 43:10, 1976.
256. Kosloske A: Tracheobronchial foreign bodies in children: back to the bronchoscope and a balloon, *Pediatrics* 66:321, 1980.
257. Koss MN, Hocholzer L, Nichols PW, et al: Primary non-Hodgkin's lymphoma and pseudolymphoma of lung: a study of 1621 patients, *Hum Pathol* 14:1024, 1983.
258. Kozlowski RZ: Ion channels, oxygen sensation and signal transduction in pulmonary arterial smooth muscle, *Cardiovas Res* 30(3):318, 1995.
259. Krayenbuehl HP, Turina J, Hess O: Left ventricular function in chronic pulmonary hypertension, *Am J Cardiol* 41:1150, 1978.
260. Krayer S, Rehder K, Beck KC, et al: Quantification of thoracic volumes by three-dimensional imaging, *J Appl Physiol* 62:591, 1987.
261. Krowka MJ, Pairolero PC, Trastek VF, et al: Cardiac dysrhythmia following pneumonectomy. Clinical correlates and prognostic significance, *Chest* 91:490, 1987.
262. Kvalheim L, Reiestad F: Intrapleural catheter in the management of postoperative pain, *Anesthesiology* 61:A231, 1984.
263. Landais A, Marin JP, Roche A, et al: Measurement of cardiac output by the thermodilution method during left thoracotomy in the lateral position in the dog, *Acta Anaesthesiol Scand* 34:158, 1990.
264. Landreneau RJ, Hazelrigg SR, Mack MJ, et al: Postoperative pain-related morbidity: video-assisted thoracic surgery versus thoracotomy, *Ann Thorac Surg* 56(6):1285, 1993.
265. Laros CD, Swierenga J: Temporary unilateral pulmonary artery occlusion in the preoperative evaluation of patients with bronchial carcinoma, *Med Thorac* 24(5): 269, 1967.
266. Laurenzi GA, Turino GM, Fishman AP: Bullous disease of the lung, *Am J Med* 32:361, 1962.
267. Law D, Kosloske A: Management of tracheobronchial foreign bodies in children: a reevaluation of postural drainage and bronchoscopy, *Pediatrics* 58:362, 1976.
268. Lee JH, Salvatore A: Innominate artery compression simulating cardiac arrest during mediastinoscopy: a case report, *Anesth Analg* 55:748, 1976.
269. Lee P, English ICW: Management of anaesthesia during tracheal resection, *Anaesthesia* 29:305, 1974.
270. Lefrak EA, Pitha J, Rosenheim S, et al: Adriamycin (NSC-12317) cardiomyopathy, *Cancer Chemother Rep* 6:203, 1975.
271. Lennon PF, Murray PA: Attenuated hypoxic pulmonary vasoconstriction during isoflurane anesthesia is abolished by cyclooxygenase inhibition in chronically instrumented dogs, *Anesthesiology* 84(2): 404, 1996.
272. Levin H, Bursztein S, Heifetz M: Cardiac arrest in a child with an anterior mediastinal mass, *Anesth Analg* 64:1129, 1985.
273. Levin PD, Faber LP, Carleton RA: Cardiac herniation after pneumonectomy, *J Thorac Cardiovasc Surg* 61:104, 1971.
274. Lippmann M, Mok MS, Wasserman K: Anaesthetic management for children with alveolar proteinosis using extracorporeal circulation: report of two cases, *Br J Anaesth* 49:173, 1977.
275. Little AG, Swain JA, Nino JJ, et al: Reduction pneumonoplasty for emphysema. Early results, *Ann Surg* 222(3):365, 1995.
276. Loeffler JS, Leopold KA, Recht A, et al: Emergency prebiopsy radiation for mediastinal masses: impact on subsequent pathologic diagnosis and outcome, *J Clin Oncol* 4:716, 1986.
277. Luce JM: Respiratory complications of obesity, *Chest* 78:626–631, 1980.
278. Lukomsky GI, Ovchinnikov AA, Bilal A: Complications of bronchoscopy: comparison of rigid bronchoscopy under general anesthesia and flexible fiberoptic bronchoscopy under topical anesthesia, *Chest* 79:316, 1981.
279. Lundy JS, Gage RP: P.A.R. spells better care for postanesthesia patients, *Mod Hosp* 63:63, 1944.
280. Mack MJ, Regan JJ, McAfee PC, et al: Video-assisted thoracic surgery for the anterior approach to the thoracic spine, *Ann Thorac Surg* 59(5):1100, 1995.
281. MacNaughton FI: Catheter inflation ventilation in tracheal stenosis, *Br J Anaesth* 47:1225, 1975.
282. Mahfood S, Hix WR, Aaron BL, et al: Reexpansion pulmonary edema, *Ann Thorac Surg* 45:340, 1988.
283. Maiwand O, Makey AR, Rees A: Cryoanalgesia after thoracotomy: improvement of technique and review of 600 cases, *J Thorac Cardiovasc Surg* 92:291, 1986.
284. Mal H, Andreassian B, Pamela F, et al: Unilateral lung transplantation in end-stage pulmonary emphysema, *Am Respir Dis* 140:797, 1989.
285. Malmkvist G: Maintenance of oxygenation during one-lung ventilation effect of intermittent reinflation of the collapsed lung with oxygen, *Anesth Analg* 68:763, 1989.
286. Mann JM, Altus CS, Webber CA, et al: Nonbronchoscopic lung lavage for diagnosis of opportunistic infection in AIDS, *Chest* 91:319, 1987.

287. Marion JM, Alderson PO, Lefrak SS, et al: Unilateral lung function, *Chest* 69:5, 1976.
288. Markos J, Mullan BP, Hillman DR, et al: Preoperative assessment as a predictor of mortality and morbidity after lung resection, *Am Rev Respir Dis* 139(4):902, 1989.
289. Marland AM, Glauser F: Hemodynamic and pulmonary edema protein measurements in a case of reexpansion pulmonary edema, *Chest* 81:250, 1982.
290. Marshall BE, Marshall C: Continuity of response by hypoxic pulmonary vasoconstriction, *J Appl Physiol* 59:189, 1980.
291. Matthew NT, John S: Iatrogeanic ischaemic paraplegia, *Med J Aust* 1:29, 1970.
292. May DB, Munt PW: Physiologic effects of chest percussion and postural drainage in patients with stable chronic bronchitis, *Chest* 75:29, 1979.
293. McDougall JC, Fromme GA: Transcarinal aspiration of a mediastinal cyst to facilitate anesthetic management, *Chest* 97:1490, 1990.
294. McElveen JR, Urgena RB, Rossi NP: Herniation of the heart following radical pneumonectomy: a case report, *Anesth Analg* 51:680, 1972.
295. Mehnert JH, Dupont TJ, Rose DH: Intermittent epidural morphine instillation for control of postoperative pain, *Am J Surg* 146:145, 1983.
296. Metras D, Noirclerc M, Vaillant A, et al: Double-lung transplant: the role of bilateral bronchial suture, *Transplant Proc* 22:1477, 1990.
297. Miller FL, Chen L, Malmkvist G, et al: Mechanical factors do not influence blood flow distribution in atelectasis, *Anesthesiology* 70:481, 1989.
298. Miller JI, Grossman GD, Hatcher CR: Pulmonary function test criteria for operability and pulmonary resection, *Surg Gynecol Obstet* 153:893, 1981.
299. Miller OI, Celermajer DS, Deanfield JE, et al: Guidelines for the safe administration of inhaled nitric oxide, *Arch Dis Child* 70:F47, 1994.
300. Miller RD, Hyatt RE: Obstruction lesions of the larynx and trachea: clinical and physiologic characteristics, *Mayo Clin Proc* 44:145, 1969.
301. Millet B, Higenbottam TW, Flower CDR, et al: The radiographic appearances of infection and acute rejection of the lung after heart-lung transplantation, *Am Rev Respir Dis* 140: 62, 1989.
302. Mills LJ, Lolley DM, Estrera AS, et al: Use of fluoroscopy in the removal of aspirated foreign bodies, *JAMA* 237:1077, 1977 (letter).
303. Mitchell C, Garrahy P, Peake P: Postoperative respiratory morbidity: Identification and risk factors, *Aust NZ J Surg* 52:203, 1982.
304. Moazam F, Schmidt JH, Chesrown SE, et al: Total lung lavage for pulmonary alveolar proteinosis in an infant without the use of cardiopulmonary bypass, *J Pediatr Surg* 20:398, 1985.
305. Modig J, Borg T, Karlstom G, et al: Thromboembolism after total hip replacement: role of epidural and general anesthesia, *Anesth Analg* 62:174, 1983.
306. Moghissi K, Hornshaw J, Teasdale PR, et al: Parenteral nutrition in carcinoma of the esophagus treated by surgery: nitrogen balance and clinical studies, *Br J Surg* 64:125, 1977.
307. Moir DD: Blood loss during major vaginal surgery: a statistical study of the influence of general anaesthesia and epidural analgesia, *Br J Anaesth* 40:233, 1968.
308. Molin LJ, Steinberg JB, Lanza LA: VATS increases costs in patients undergoing lung biopsy for interstitial lung disease, *Ann Thorac Surg* 58(6):1595, 1994.
309. Montgomery WW: Manual of the care of the Montgomery silicone tracheal T-tube, *Ann Otol Rhinol Laryngol* 73:89, 1980.
310. Moore DC: Intercostal nerve block for postoperative somatic pain following surgery of thorax and upper abdomen, *Br J Anaesth* 47(Suppl):284, 1975.
311. Morgan BA, Perks D, Conacher ID, et al: Combined unilateral high frequency jet ventilation and contralateral intermittent positive pressure ventilation, *Anaesthesia* 42:975, 1987.
312. Motoyama EK, Davis PJ: *Anesthesia for infants and children,* ed 5, St. Louis, 1990, Mosby–Year Book.
313. Muthuswamy PP, Akbik F, Franklin C, et al: Management of major or massive hemoptysis in active pulmonary tuberculosis by bronchial arterial embolization, *Chest* 92:77, 1987.
314. Nadi P, Ong GB: Foreign body in the oesophagus: review of 2394 cases, *Br J Surg* 65:5, 1978.
315. Nakatsuka M, Wetstein L, Keenan R: Unilateral high-frequency jet ventilation during one-lung ventilation for thoracotomy, *Ann Thorac Surg* 46:654, 1988.
316. National Fire Protection Association: *NFPA 99: health care facilities,* Quincy, MA, 1984, NFPA.
317. Neuhaus A, Markowitz D, Rotman HH, et al: The effects of fiberoptic bronchoscopy with and without atropine premedication on pulmonary function in humans, *Ann Thorac Surg* 25:393, 1978.
318. Neunheim KS, Ferguson MK: The current status of lung volume reduction operations for emphysema, *Ann Thorac Surg* 62:601, 1996.
319. Neustein SM, Eisenkraft JB: Anesthetic considerations during thoracic procedures using the laser. In *Cardiothoracic and vascular anesthesia update,* vol 1, Philadelphia, 1990, WB Saunders.
320. Newsom-Davis J, Murray NMF: Plasma exchange and immunosuppressive drug treatment in the Lambert-Eaton myasthenic syndrome, *Neurology* 34:480, 1984.
321. Nogeire C, Mincer F, Botstein C: Long-term survival in patients with bronchiogenic carcinoma complicated by superior vena caval obstruction, *Chest* 75:325, 1979.
322. Nunn JF: The distribution of inspired gas during thoracic surgery, *Ann R Coll Surg Engl* 28:223, 1961.
323. Odoom JA, Aih IL: Epidural anaesthesia and anticoagulant therapy: experience with one thousand cases of continuous epidurals, *Anaesthesia* 38:254, 1983.
324. Ohta M, Nakahara K, Yasumitsu T, et al: Prediction of postoperative performance status in patients with giant bulla, *Chest* 101(3):668, 1992.
325. Okamoto K, Sato T, Kurose M, et al: Successful use of inhaled nitric oxide for treatment of severe hypoxemia in an infant with total anomalous pulmonary venous return, *Anesthesiology* 81:256, 1994.
326. Oldenburg FA Jr, Dolovich MB, Montgomery JM, et al: Effects of postural drainage, exercise, and cough on mucus clearance in chronic bronchitis, *Am Rev Respir Dis* 120:739, 1979.
327. Olivet RT, Nauss LA, Payne WS: A technique for continuous intercostal nerve block analgesia following thoracotomy, *J Thorac Surg* 80:308, 1980.
328. Olsen GN, Block AJ, Swenson EW, et al: Pulmonary function evaluation of the lung resection candidate: a prospective study, *Am Rev Respir Dis* 111:379, 1975.
329. Olsen GN, Weiman DS, Bolton JW, et al: Submaximal invasive exercise testing and quantitative lung scanning in the evaluation for tolerance of lung resection, *Chest* 95(2):267, 1989.
330. Olsen GN, Blok AJ, Tobias JA: Prediction of postpneumonectomy pulmonary function using quantitative macroaggregate lung scanning, *Chest* 66:13, 1974.
331. Olsen GN: The evolving role of exercise testing prior to lung resection, *Chest* 95:218, 1989.
332. Oriot D, Boussemart T, Berthier M, et al: Paradoxical effect of inhaled nitric oxide in a newborn with pulmonary hypertension, *Lancet* 342:364, 1993 (letter).
333. Orlando R, Gluck EH, Cohen M, et al: Ultra-high-frequency jet ventilation in a bronchopleural fistula model, *Arch Surg* 123:591, 1988.
334. Ossoff RH, Karlan MS: Instrumentation for CO_2. laser surgery of the larynx and tracheobronchial tree, *Surg Clin North Am* 64:973, 1984.
335. Ottesen S, Renck H, Jynge P: Cardiovascular effects of epidural analgesia. II. Haemodynamic alterations secondary to lumbar epidural analgesia and their modification of plasma expansion and adrenaline administration. An experimental study in the sheep, *Acta Anaesth Scand* 69:17, 1978.
336. Paes M: General anesthesia for carbon dioxide laser surgery within the airway, *Br J Anaesth* 59:1610, 1987.
337. Palmer KNV, Sellick BA: The prevention of postoperative pulmonary atelectasis, *Lancet* 1:164, 1953.
338. Pancrazio JJ, Viglione MP, Tabbara IA, et al: Voltage-dependent ion channels in small cell lung cancer cells, *Cancer Res* 49:5901, 1989.
339. Pang D, Wessel HB: Thoracic outlet syndrome, *Neurosurgery* 22:105, 1988.
340. Parish JM, Gracey DR, Southorn PA, et al: Differential mechanical ventilation in respiratory failure due to severe unilateral lung disease, *Mayo Clin Proc* 59:822, 1974.
341. Parish JM, Rosenow EC, Muhm JR: Mediastinal masses: clues to interpretation of radiologic studies, *Postgrad Med* 76:173, 1984.
342. Parks WY, Poon KC, MacNamara YW: Epidural block for lumbar laminectomy, *Reg Anaesth* 12:48, 1987.
343. Parr GVS, Unger M, Trout RG, et al: One

hundred neodymium-YAG laser ablations of obstructing tracheal neoplasma, *Ann Thorac Surg* 38:374, 1984.
344. Parr GVS, Unger N, Trout RG, et al: One hundred neodymium-YAG (Nd-YAG) laser resections of major airway obstructing tumors, *Anesthesiology* 60:230, 1984.
345. Parsons GH, Leventhal JP, Hansen MM, et al: Effect of sodium nitroprusside on hypoxic pulmonary vasoconstriction in the dog, *J Appl Physiol* 51:288, 1981.
346. Pashayan AG, Gravenstein JS, Cassisi NJ, et al: The helium protocol for laryngotracheal operations with CO_2 laser: a retrospective review of 523 cases, *Anesthesiology* 68:801, 1988.
347. Pashayan AG, Gravenstein JS: Helium retards endotracheal tube fires from carbon dioxide lasers, *Anesthesiology* 62:274, 1985.
348. Pashayan AG: Anesthesia for laser surgery. In Barash PG, Stanley D, Tinker J, editors: *ASA Annual Refresher Course Lectures,* Philadelphia, 1988, JB Lippincott.
349. Pasulka PS, Bistrian BR, Benotti PN, et al: The risk of surgery in obese patients, *Ann Intern Med* 104:540, 1986.
350. Pate P, Tenholder MF, Griffin JP, et al: Preoperative assessment of the high-risk patient for lung resection, *Ann Thorac Surg* 61:1494, 1996.
351. Patterson GA, Cooper JD: Complications of thoracotomy. In Marshall BD, Longnecker DE, Fairley HB, editors: *Anesthesia for thoracic procedures,* Boston, 1988, Blackwell Scientific.
352. Patterson GA, Todd TR, Cooper JD, et al: Airway complications after double lung transplantation, *J Thorac Cardiovasc Surg* 99:14, 1990.
353. Reference deleted in proofs.
354. Pavlin DJ, Nessly ML, Cheney FW: Increased pulmonary vascular permeability as a cause of reexpansion edema in rabbits, *Am Rev Respir Dis* 124:422, 1981.
355. Payne WS, King RM: Pharyngoesophageal (Zenker's) diverticulum, *Surg Clin North Am* 63:815, 1983.
356. Pearce AC, Jones RM: Smoking and anesthesia: preoperative abstinence and perioperative morbidity, *Anesthesiology* 61:576, 1984.
357. Pedersen B, Dahl R: Fiberbronkoskopi og bronkoalveolaer lavage af asthmapatienter, *Ugeskr Laeger* 48:3229, 1989.
358. Petty C: Right radial artery pressure during mediastinoscopy, *Anesth Analg* 58:428, 1979.
359. Petty C: Right radial artery pressure during mediastinoscopy, *Anesth Analg* 58:428–430, 1979.
360. Pflug AE, Halter JB: Effects of spinal anesthesia on adrenergic tone and the neuroendocrine responses to surgical stress in humans, *Anesthesiology* 55:120, 1981.
361. Pingleton SK: Nutritional support in the mechanically ventilated patient, *Clin Chest Med* 9:101, 1988.
362. Potgieter SV: Atelectasis: its evolution during upper urinary tract surgery, *Br J Anaesth* 31:472, 1959.
363. Puhakka HJ: Complications of mediastinoscopy, *J Laryngol Otol* 103:312, 1989.
364. Rafferty TD, Palma J, Motoyama EK, et al: Management of a bronchopleural fistula with differential lung ventilation and positive end-expiratory pressure, *Respir Care* 25:654, 1980.
365. Randazzo GP, Wilson AF: Cardiopulmonary changes during flexible fibreoptic bronchoscopy, *Respiration* 33:143, 1976.
366. Rao TLK, El-Etr AA: Anticoagulation following placement of epidural and subarachnoid catheters: an evaluation of neurologic sequelae, *Anesthesiology* 55:618, 1981.
367. Rao TLK, El-Etr AA: Esophageal and mediastinal surgery. In Kaplan JA, editor: *Thoracic anesthesia,* New York, 1983, Churchill-Livingstone.
368. Redding GJ, Tuck R, Escourrou P: Nifedipine attenuates hypoxic pulmonary vasoconstriction in awake piglets, *Am Rev Respir Dis* 129:785, 1984.
369. Reddy KJ, Hammon J, Parris WCV, et al: Intrapleural analgesia for postthoracotomy pain and blood levels of bupivacaine following intrapleural injection, *Can J Anaesth* 36:106, 1989.
370. Rees DI, Gaines GY: One-lung anesthesia—a comparison of pulmonary gas exchange during anesthesia with ketamine or enflurane, *Anesth Analg* 63:521, 1984.
371. Rehder K, Hatch DJ, Sessler AD, et al: The function of each lung of anesthetized and paralyzed man during mechanical ventilation, *Anesthesiology* 37:16, 1972.
372. Rehder K, Sessler AD: Function of each lung in spontaneously breathing man anesthetized with thiopental-meperidine, *Anesthesiology* 38:320, 1973.
373. Rehder K, Wenthe FM, Sessler AD: Function of each lung during mechanical ventilation with ZEEP and with PEEP in man anesthetized with thiopental-meperidine, *Anesthesiology* 39:597, 1973.
374. Reiestad F, Stromskag KE: Intrapleural catheter in the management of postoperative pain: a preliminary report, *Reg Anesth* 11:89, 1986.
375. Rem J, Brandt MR, Kehlet H: Prevention of postoperative lymphopenia and granulocytosis by epidural analgesia, *Lancet* 1:283, 1980.
376. Riordan JF: Management of spontaneous pneumothorax, *BMJ* 189:71, 1984.
377. Ritchie AJ, Bowe P, Gibbons RP: Prophylactic digitalization for thoracotomy: a reassessment, *Ann Thorac Surg* 50:86, 1996.
378. Rivara D, Bourgaim L, Rieuf P, et al: Differential ventilation in unilateral lung disease: effects of respiratory mechanics and gas exchange, *Intensive Care Med* 5:189, 1979.
379. Roberts JT, Gissen AJ: Management of complications encountered during anesthesia for mediastinoscopy, *Anesth Rev* 6:31, 1979.
380. Rocco A, Reiestad F, Gudman J, et al: Intrapleural administration of local anesthetics for pain relief in patients with multiple rib fractures: a preliminary report, *Reg Anaesth* 12:10, 1986.
381. Rogers RM, Levin DC, Gray BA, et al: Physiological effects of bronchopulmonary lavage in alveolar proteinosis, *Am Rev Respir Dis* 118:255, 1978.
382. Rogers RM, Levin DC, Gray BA, et al: Physiologic effects of bronchopulmonary lavage in alveolar proteinosis, *Am Rev Respir Dis* 118(2):255–264, 1978.
383. Rogers SN, Benumof JL: Halothane and isoflurane do not impair arterial oxygenation during one lung ventilation in patients undergoing thoracotomy, *Anesthesiology* 59:A532, 1983 (abstract).
384. Rose U, Attar Z: Interpleurales Bupivacain und parenterales opioid zur postoperativen analgesie. Eine Vergleichende studie, *Anaesthesist* 41:53, 1992.
385. Rowbottom SJ: Isoflurane for thymectomy in myasthenia gravis, *Anaesth Intensive Care* 17:444, 1989.
386. Rubin JW, Finney NR, Borders BM, et al: Intrathoracic biopsies, pulmonary wedge excision, and management of pleural disease: is video-assisted closed chest surgery the approach of choice? *Am Surg* 60:860, 1994.
387. Sabanathan S, Mearns AJ, Bickford-Smith PJ, et al: Efficacy of continuous extrapleural intercostal nerve block on post-thoracotomy pain and pulmonary mechanics, *Br J Surg* 77: 221, 1990.
388. Sackner MA, Hirsch J, Epstein S: Effect of cuffed endotracheal tubes on tracheal mucous velocity *Chest* 68:774, 1975.
389. Salisbury BG, Metzger CF, Altose MD, et al: Effect of fiberoptic bronchoscopy on respiratory performance in patients with chronic airway obstruction, *Thorax* 30:441, 1975.
390. Sandler AN, Stringer D, Panos L, et al: A randomized, double-blind comparison of lumbar epidural and intravenous fentanyl infusions for post-thoracotomy pain relief. Analgesic, pharmacokinetic, and respiratory effects, *Anesthesiology* 39:330, 1992.
391. Scamman FL, Choi WW: Low frequency jet ventilation for tracheal resection, *Laryngoscope* 96:678, 1986.
392. Scott JP, Higenbottam TW, Clelland C, et al: The natural history of obliterative bronchiolitis and occlusive vascular disease of patients following heart-lung transplantation, *Transplant Proc* 21:2592, 1989.
393. Segall JJ, Butterworth BA: Ventilatory capacity in chronic bronchitis in relation to carbon dioxide reduction, *Scand J Respir Dis* 47:215, 1966.
394. Seltzer JL, Larijani GE, Goldberg ME, et al: A kinetic and dynamic evaluation of intrapleural bupivacaine for subcostal incision pain, *Anesthesiology* 65:A213, 1986.
395. Selvin B: Cancer chemotherapy: implications for the anesthesiologist, *Anesth Analg* 60:425, 1981.
396. Shibata K, Matsuzaki Y, Yoshioka M: Omentum in the management of thoracic surgery, *Jpn J Thorac Surg* 13:1078, 1989.
397. Shields TW, Ujiki GT: Digitalization for prevention of arrhythmias following pulmonary surgery, *Surg Gynecol Obstet* 126:743, 1968.
398. Shields TW: Carcinoma of the lung. In Shields TW, editor: *General thoracic surgery,* ed 2, Philadelphia, 1983, Lea & Febiger.
399. Shulman M, Sanler AN, Bradley JW, et al: Post-thoracotomy pain and pulmonary function following epidural and systemic morphine, *Anesthesiology* 61:569, 1984.
400. Simonneau J, Escourrou P, Duroux P, et al:

Inhibition of hypoxic pulmonary vasoconstriction by nifedipine, *N Engl J Med* 304:1582, 1981.

401. Sissons JGP, Borysiewicz LK: Human cytomegalovirus infection, *Thorax* 44:241, 1989.
402. Sivarajan M, Amory DW, Lindbloom LE, et al: Systemic and regional blood-flow changes during spinal anesthesia in the rhesus monkey, *Anesthesiology* 43:78-88, 1975.
403. Sleiman C, Mal H, Fournier M, et al: Pulmonary reimplantation response in single-lung transplantation, *Eur Respir J* 8:5, 1995.
404. Smith RB, Babinski MF, Angell KE: Apneic diffusion oxygenation with high flows of intratracheal oxygen, *Respir Care* 30:26, 1985.
405. Smith RB, Babinski MF, Bunegin L, et al: Continuous flow apneic ventilation, *Acta Anaesthesiol Scand* 28: 631, 1984.
406. Sosis M, Dillon F: Hazards of a new specially designed plastic endotracheal tube for use with the Nd-YAG laser, *Can J Anaesth* 36:S91, 1989 (abstract).
407. Sosis M: Anesthesia for laser surgery, *Int Anesthesiol Clin* 28:119, 1990.
408. Spiro SG: The diagnosis and staging of lung cancer. In Smyth JF, editor: *The management of lung cancer,* London, 1984, Edward Arnold.
409. Spray SB, Zuidema GD, Cameron JL: Aspiration pneumonia, incidence of aspiration with endotracheal tubes, *Am J Surg* 131:701, 1976.
410. Sprung CL, Loewenherz JW, Baier H, et al: Evidence for increased permeability in reexpansion pulmonary edema, *Am J Med* 71:497, 1981.
411. Stanski DR, Lee RG, MacCannell KL, et al: Atypical cholinesterase in a patient with myasthenia gravis, *Anesthesiology* 46:298, 1977.
412. Steiger Z, Wilson RF: Management of bronchopleural fistulas, *Surg Gynecol Obstet* 158:267, 1984.
413. Stein M, Koota GM, Simon M, et al: Pulmonary evaluation of surgical patients, *JAMA* 181:765, 1962.
414. Stow PJ, Burrows FA: Anticoagulants in anaesthesia, *Can J Anaesth* 34:632, 1987.
415. Stow PJ, Grant I: Asynchronous independent lung ventilation: its use in the treatment of acute unilateral lung disease, *Anaesthesia* 40:163, 1985.
416. Stromskag KE, Hauge O, Steen PA: Distribution of local anesthetics injected into the interpleural space, studied by computerized tomography, *Acta Anaesthesiol Scand* 34:323, 1990.
417. Svanberg L: Influence of posture on lung volumes, ventilation and circulation in normals, *Scand J Clin Lab Invest* 9(suppl 25):1, 1957.
418. Swenson JD, Astle KL, Bailey P: Reduction in left ventricular filling during bronchopulmonary lavage demonstrated by transesophageal echocardiography, *Anesth Analg* 81:634, 1995.
419. Symreng T, Gomez MN, Rossi N: Intrapleural bupivacaine and saline after thoracotomy effects on pain and lung function—a double blind study, *J Cardiothorac Anesth* 3:144, 1989.
420. The Toronto Group Transplant Group: Experience with single-lung transplantation for pulmonary fibrosis, *JAMA* 259: 2258, 1988.
421. The Veterans Affairs Total Parenteral Nutrition Cooperative Study Group: Perioperative total parenteral nutrition in surgical patients, *N Engl J Med* 325:525, 1991.
422. Theman TE, Kerr JH, Nelems JM, et al: Carinal resection: a report of two cases and a description of the anesthetic technique, *J Thorac Cardiovasc Surg* 71:314, 1976.
423. Thiagarajah S, Job C, Rao A: A device for applying CPAP to the nonventilated upper lung during one lung ventilation. I, *Anesthesiology* 60:253, 1984.
424. Tibballs J, Hochmann M, Carter B, et al: An appraisal of techniques for administration of gaseous nitric oxide, *Anaesth Intensive Care* 21:844, 1993.
425. Tibballs J: Clinical applications of gaseous nitric oxide, *Anaesth Intensive Care* 21:866, 1993.
426. Ting EY, Klopstock R, Lyons HA: Mechanical properties of pulmonary cysts and bullae, *Am Rev Respir Dis* 87:538, 1963.
427. Triantafillou AN, Heerdt PM: Lung transplantation, *Int Anesth Clin* 29:87, 1991 (review).
428. Trippenoch T: Chest wall reflexes in the newborn, *Clin Respir Physiol* 21:115, 1987.
429. Trulock EP, Egan TM, Kouchoukos NT, et al: Single lung transplantation for severe chronic obstructive pulmonary disease, *Chest* 96:738, 1989.
430. Tucker A, McMurtry IF, Grover RF, et al: Attenuation of hypoxic pulmonary vasoconstriction by verapamil in intact dogs, *Proc Soc Exp Biol Med* 151:611, 1976.
431. Tucker GT, Moore DC, Bridenbaugh PO, et al: Intraoperative intercostal nerve blocks, *Anesthesiology* 43:124, 1975.
432. Turoff RD, Gomez GA, Berjian E, et al: Postoperative respiratory complications in patients with Hodgkin's disease: relationship to the size of the mediastinal tumor, *Eur J Cancer Clin Oncol* 21:1043, 1985.
433. Tyms AS, Davis JM, Jeffries DJ, et al: BWB759U, an analogue of acyclovir, inhibits human cytomegalovirus in vitro, *Lancet* 2:924, 1984.
434. Urschel JD, Vretenar DF, Dickout WJ, et al: Cerebrovascular accident complicating extended cervical mediastinoscopy, *Ann Thorac Surg* 57:740, 1994.
435. Vacek J, Foster J, Quinton RR, et al: Right-to-left shunting after lobectomy through a patent foramen ovale, *Ann Thorac Surg* 39:576, 1985.
436. Van Der Spek AFL, Spargo PM, Norton M: The physics of lasers and implications for their use during airway surgery, *Br J Anaesth* 60:709, 1988.
437. Van Keer L, Van Aken H, Vandermeersch E, et al: Propofol does not inhibit hypoxic pulmonary vasoconstriction in humans, *J Clin Anesth* 1:284, 1989.
438. Veith FJ, Koerner SK, Siegelman SS, et al: Single lung transplantation in experimental and human emphysema, *Ann Surg* 178:463, 1973.
439. Veith FJ, Montefusco CM: Long-term fate of lung autografts charged with providing total pulmonary function. II. Hemodynamic, functional and angiographic studies, *Ann Surg* 190:654, 1979.
440. Veltzer JL, Doto JO, Jacoby J: Depressed arterial oxygenation during sodium nitroprusside administration for intraoperative hypertension, *Anesth Analg* 55:880, 1976.
441. Vik-Mo H, Ottensen S, Renck H: Cardiac effects of thoracic epidural analgesia before and during acute coronary artery occlusion in open chest dogs, *Scand J Clin Lab Invest* 38:737, 1978.
442. Vourc'h G, Fischler M, Michon F, et al: Manual jet ventilation v. high frequency jet ventilation during laser resection of tracheo-bronchial stenosis, *Br J Anaesth* 55:973, 1983.
443. Vourc'h G, Tannieres ML, Toty L, et al: Anaesthetic management of tracheal surgery using the neodymium-yttrium-aluminum-garnet laser, *Br J Anaesth* 52: 993, 1980.
444. Vueghs PJ, Schurink GA, Vaes L, et al: Anesthesia in repeat mediastinoscopy: a retrospective study of 101 patients, *J Cardiothorac Vasc Anesth* 6:193, 1992.
445. Wahi R, McMurtrey MJ, DeCaro LF, et al: Determinants of perioperative morbidity and mortality after pneumonectomy, *Ann Thorac Surg* 48:33, 1989.
446. Wainwright A, Moody R, Carruth J: Anesthetic safety with the CO2 laser, *Anaesthesia* 36:411, 1981.
447. Waller DA, Forty J, Morritt GN: Video-assisted thoracoscopic surgery versus thoracotomy for spontaneous pneumothorax, *Ann Thorac Surg* 58:372, 1994 (see comments).
448. Waller DA, Forty J, Morritt GN: Video-assisted thoracoscopic surgery versus thoracotomy for spontaneous pneumothorax, *Ann Thorac Surg* 58:372, 1994.
449. Waller DA, Turner N: Re-expansion pulmonary oedema, *Anaesthesia* 44:446, 1989.
450. Wangensteen OH: The pedicled muscle flap in the closure of persistent bronchopleural fistulas, *J Thorac Surg* 5:27, 1935.
451. Warner MA, Divertie MB, Tinker JH: Preoperative cessation of smoking and pulmonary complications in coronary artery bypass patients, *Anesthesiology* 60:380, 1984.
452. Warner ME, Warner MA, Leonard PF: Anesthesia for neodymium-YAG (Nd-YAG) laser resection of major airway obstructing tumors, *Anesthesiology* 60: 230–232, 1984.
453. Wasserman K, Costley B: Advances in the treatment of pulmonary alveolar proteinosis, *Am Rev Respir Dis* 111:361, 1975.
454. Webb AR, Fernando SSD, Dalton HR, et al: Local anesthesia for fibreoptic bronchoscopy: transcricoid injection or the "spray as you go" technique? *Thorax* 45:474, 1990.
455. Weir EK, Archer SL: The mechanism of acute hypoxic pulmonary vasoconstriction: the tale of two channels, *FASEB J* 9:183, 1995.
456. Weisman SJ: Masked myasthenia gravis, *JAMA* 141:917, 1949.
457. Weissberg D, Herczeg E: Perforation of thoracic aortic aneurysm: a complication of mediastinoscopy, *Chest* 78:119, 1980.
458. Werner O, Malmkvist G, Beckman A, et al:

Gas exchange and haemodynamics during thoracotomy, *Br J Anaesth* 56:1343, 1984.

459. Wesley JR, Macleod WM, Mullard KS: Evaluation and surgery of bullous emphysema, *J Thorac Cardiovasc Surg* 63:945, 1972.
460. Wessel DL, Adatia I, Thompson JE, et al: Delivery and monitoring of inhaled nitric oxide in patients with pulmonary hypertension, *Crit Care Med* 22:930, 1994.
461. Wheat MW, Burford TH: Digitalis in surgery: extension of classical indications, *J Thorac Cardiovasc Surg* 41:162, 1961.
462. Wightman JA: A prospective survey of the incidence of postoperative pulmonary complications, *Br J Surg* 55:85, 1968.
463. Wildevuur CRH, Benfield JR: A review of 23 human lung transplantations by 20 surgeons, *Ann Thorac Surg* 9:489, 1970.
464. Wilks D, Schumann T, Riley R, et al: Selective high-frequency jet ventilation of the operative lung improves oxygenation during thoracic surgery, *Anesthesiology* 63:A568, 1985.
465. Wolf GL, Simpson JI: Flammability of endotracheal tubes in oxygen and nitrous oxide enriched atmospheres, *Anesthesiology* 67:236, 1987.
466. Woods F, Neptune W, Palatchi A: Resection of the carina and mainstem bronchi with extracorporeal circulation, *N Engl J Med* 264:492, 1961.
467. Wreghitt T: Cytomegalovirus infections in heart and heart-lung transplant recipients, *J Antimicrob Chemother* 23:49, 1989.
468. Wulff KE, Aulin I: The regional lung function in the lateral decubitus position during anesthesia and operation, *Acta Anesthesiol Scand* 16:195, 1972.
469. Yacoub MH, Banner NR: Recent developments in lung and heart-lung transplantation. In: PJ Morris, NL Tilney editors: *Transplantation reviews,* London, Bailliere Tindall. 3:1, 1989.
470. Yeager MP, Glass DD, Neff RK, et al: Epidural anesthesia and analgesia in high-risk surgical patients, *Anesthesiology* 66:729, 1987.
471. Yeoh CB, Hubaytar RT, Ford JM: Treatment of massive hemorrhage in pulmonary tuberculosis, *J Thorac Cardiovasc Surg* 54:503, 1967.
472. Zapol WM, Snider MT, Schneider RC: Extracorporeal membrane oxygenation for acute respiratory failure, *Anesthesiology* 46:272, 1977.
473. Zapol WM, Rimar S, Gillis N, et al: Nitric oxide and the lung, *Am J Respir Crit Care Med* 149:1375, 1994.
474. Zapol WM, Wilson R, Hales C, et al: Venovenous bypass with a membrane lung to support bilateral lung lavage, *JAMA* 51:3269, 1984.

CHAPTER 71

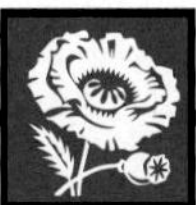

Anesthesia for Major Vascular Surgery

CHARLES BEATTIE
STEVEN M. FRANK
GARRY V. WALKER
NEAL W. SIEX

Surgery of the aorta and its major branches, including carotid endarterectomy, aortic aneurysm and occlusive repair, and lower extremity vascular bypass grafting are considered by many to be the premier anesthetic challenge. Dramatic physiologic changes are superimposed on complex disease states. Vascular surgery necessitates the temporary interruption of arterial blood flow by isolation of the diseased vessel segment with occluding clamps. The resulting tissue ischemia can cause organ damage and production of anaerobic metabolites. Changes in left ventricular afterload, activation of cardiovascular reflexes, and release of vasoactive substances with application and removal of vessel clamps, dispose to cardiac dysfunction and hemodynamic extremes.

The pathologic processes that give rise to aneurysmal and occlusive disease are largely systemic, and thus patients presenting for major vascular surgery usually have either overt or occult involvement of several organ systems. Coexisting coronary artery disease (CAD) is of particular concern because myocardial ischemia, myocardial infarction (MI), and myocardial failure constitute most of the perioperative morbidity. The stress response of surgery must be aggressively controlled in both the intraoperative and the postoperative periods to minimize complications.

This chapter details the fundamental considerations surrounding the perioperative evaluation, preparation, and management for major vascular surgery. As with anesthesia for other specialized procedures, many techniques have been suggested and used to handle the difficulties posed by major vascular surgery. Controversies are common. Alternate viewpoints are presented, especially when their resolution might benefit patient care.

PATHOPHYSIOLOGY OF VASCULAR DISEASE

Theories of Atherogenesis

Although the clinical manifestations of atherosclerosis are obvious, the epidemiology is clearly described, and the light microscopic appearance of the plaque has been known for some time, the pathophysiology of atherosclerosis on the cellular level remains unknown. The arterial wall response to hypertension, diabetes, and the stimuli of elevated blood lipids and cigarette smoke occurs predominantly in men and demonstrates a genetic susceptibility. The cellular response includes macrophage migration from blood to intima, intimal macrophage lipid accumulations, smooth muscle cell migration from media to intima, intimal smooth muscle cell proliferation, lipid-laden macrophage necrosis, and organic calcium precipitation. In addition to these considerations, complexities of the blood-surface arterial interface implicate the factors of velocity, shear stress, pulsatility, elasticity, and microbiochemical environment at the endothelial surface.[370] The "response to injury" hypothesis proposed by Virchow in the nineteenth century has been reviewed in light of modern evidence.[295,296,297] This analysis suggests that atherosclerotic lesions arise through a common pathway of endothelial injury, regardless of the risk factor manifested. Endothelial injury allows blood constituents to contact the ordinarily protected subendothelium. Platelet adherence and degranulation with elaboration of growth factors stimulate arterial smooth muscle cell migration into the intima from the media and promote intimal smooth muscle cell proliferation. Other theories include the monoclonal hypothesis, which proposes that separate atherosclerotic lesions are derived from a single smooth muscle cell at each site acting as a proliferative focus.[26] The clonal senescence hypothesis[238] suggests that smooth muscle cell replication in the arterial wall is maintained by smooth muscle stem cells that are controlled through local feedback by inhibitory hormones. The latter is presumed to emanate from the smooth muscle cells in the arterial media and would decrease with cell senescence, thus causing proliferation of the neighboring intima due to the diminution of feedback inhibition.

Pathophysiology of Atherosclerosis

Atherosclerosis is the primary process leading to MI, stroke, chronic mesenteric ischemia, renovascular hypertension, extremity ischemia, and aneurysmal disease. These pathologic states occur years after the slow onset of plaque formation in the vascular wall. The precise mechanism of final injury is one or more of the following: (1) plaque enlargement reducing blood flow; (2) arterial embolism of plaque-associated platelet thrombi or atheromatous debris; and (3) complete occlusion of arteries at sites of advanced plaques. Currently, accepted risk factors include hyperlipidemia, cigarette smoking, diabetes, hypertension, family history, and the male gender. Correction or modification of some of these may arrest or lessen the progression of disease. The principal risk factor for atherosclerotic brain infarction is hypertension, and there is evidence that improved blood pressure control may be associated with a decreased incidence of stroke.[5] It has also been recognized that lowering serum cholesterol to less than 150 mg/ml may lead to the regression of atherosclerotic plaque.[318]

There are three types of atherosclerotic lesions, which presumably form a progression: (1) the fatty streak; (2) the fibrous plaque; and (3) the complicated lesion (Fig. 71-1). Fatty streaks are elevated intimal lesions that are ubiquitous but minimally impinge on the arterial lumen. They are composed of lipid-laden macrophages, smooth muscle elastic and collagen fibers, and glycosaminoglycan extracellular matrix, all lying beneath an intact and structurally normal endothelium.[370] Fatty streaks are commonly observed in young adults and have been identified in the coronary artery intima of children. Isolated lipid-laden monocytes and macrophages called foam cells have been identified in the intima of infants as young as 1 month of age.[245] Fibrous plaques are accumulations of degenerated foam cells that form a necrotic center and are covered by a thick layer of proliferated smooth muscle cells. Although fatty streaks do not impede flow, enlarging fibrous plaques and complicated lesions may produce flow re-

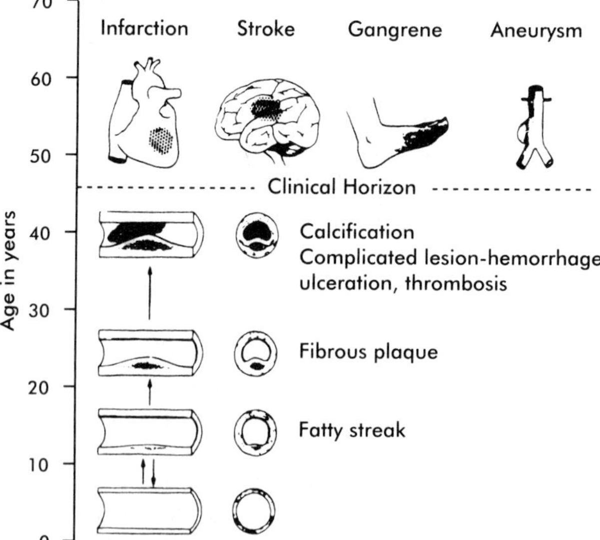

Fig. 71-1. Progression and consequences of atherosclerotic lesions. (From McGill HC Jr: Persistent problems in the pathogenesis of atherosclerosis, *Arteriosclerosis* 4:443, 1984.)

striction, embolization, or thrombosis of extremities or major organs. Complicated lesions of atherosclerosis represent a progression of the fibrous plaque with expansion of the lipid-rich core, precipitation and accumulation of calcium, deterioration of endothelial integrity, platelet aggregation, and hemorrhage into the core.

Atherosclerotic plaques tend to occur in several specific anatomic locations, and plaque development at other sites is uncommon.[143] The coronary arteries, the carotid bifurcation, the infrarenal abdominal aorta, the iliac arteries, and the superficial femoral artery are the most usual sites of development (Fig. 71-2). Patients with diabetes mellitus are often believed to have a unique type of small vessel disease. Although one paper describing a characteristic diabetic atherosclerosis[140] was published, later investigations have not identified a specific diabetic microvascular arterial occlusive disease.[223] The primary cause of amputation in diabetics is conventional large vessel atherosclerosis.[102] However, diabetics who develop atherosclerosis at the femoral-popliteal segment (a common site for nondiabetics) more often have extension into the tibial artery.[370] Peripheral sensory neuropathy in diabetic patients with occlusive disease disposes to an accelerated incidence of limb loss. Arterial emboli vary in significance depending on the size of the embolus, the development of collateral circulation, and the metabolic rate of the ischemic tissue. Common sources of the embolic material are cardiac thrombosis (90%) from the left atrium or ventricle or atherosclerotic debris (10%) from an arterial plaque.[370] Emboli tend to lodge at bifurcations or at sites of vessel narrowing.

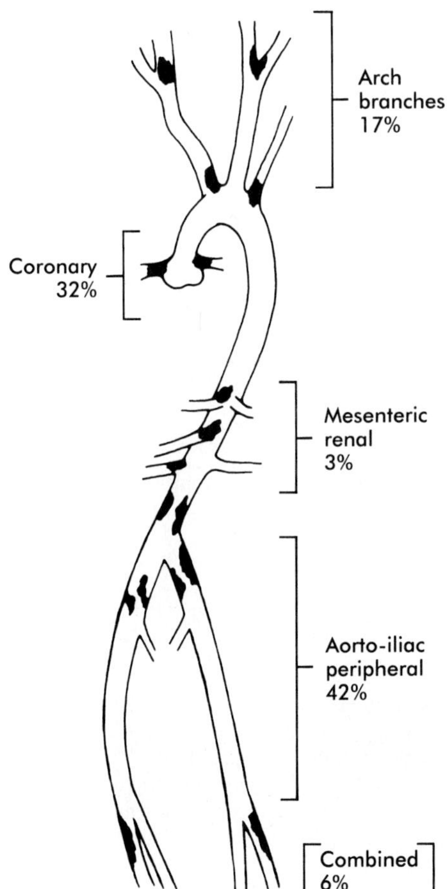

Fig. 71-2. Distribution of atherosclerotic lesions. (From Zwolak RM, Cronenwett JL: Pathophysiology of vascular disease. In Yeager MP, Glass DP, editors: *Anesthesiology and vascular surgery,* Norwalk, 1990, Appleton & Lange.)

Additional comments on pathophysiology are presented at the beginning of the separate sections on carotid, lower extremity, and aortic surgery.

PREOPERATIVE EVALUATION OF THE VASCULAR SURGERY PATIENT

Although occasionally the atherosclerotic process manifests itself in a discrete vascular segment, the more common presentation is diffuse involvement of several organ systems.[231] An appropriate work-up will attend to the possibilities of blood flow limitation to the brain, kidneys, and heart. In addition, vascular patients often report a heavy smoking history, and some degree of pulmonary compromise is expected. Diabetes mellitus is frequently associated with vascular disease, necessitating appropriate evaluation and treatment in the preoperative period. Hypertension is both a predisposing factor for vascular disease and a consequence of its development.

It is well to define the purpose of preoperative evaluation.[184] Risk assessment will have value only if it leads to risk modification or otherwise influences the decisions regarding surgical or anesthetic procedures. A great deal of investigational activity has been conducted to evaluate preoperative testing procedures with the highest degree of sensitivity and specificity that identify patients at risk for perioperative cardiac morbidity and mortality.[21,99,207,237,273,274,282]

These risk-assessment models are based on findings from the history, physical, and electrocardiogram (ECG), and/or additional information from diagnostic studies. The continuing debate concerns the appropriate management sequence to be followed once the risk is predicted. That is, should other tests, such as dipyridamole-thallium imaging (DTI) or dobutamine stress echo cardiography (DSE), be performed toward selection of a subset of patients to be revascularized (percutaneous transluminal angioplasty [PTA] or coronary artery bypass graft [CABG]) prior to vascular surgery, or rather, should the patient proceed directly to vascular surgery with aggressive perioperative medical management in an attempt to reduce risk.[234,235,141] Recent efforts have attempted to put this matter on a rational basis. Two studies[118,241] perform a "decision analysis" wherein each step in the decision process is assigned a probability for one of two potential outcomes. The pathway with the highest probability of a good outcome may be identified, essentially reaching the appropriate decision of whether to conduct a test prior to surgery or proceed directly to surgery. As an example of the application of this methodology, we consider whether to perform DTI on patients requiring abdominal aortic aneurysm (AAA) repair. The decision analysis variables for AAA repair (Fig. 71-3) with their assumed values are shown below:

- BASELINE—Perioperative mortality of AAA in patients *without* CAD (0.5%)
- MSCAD—Mortality of AAA in Patients *with* CAD (9.5%)
- RSM—Mortality of AAA in patient with prior CABG (0.5%)
- MCR—Mortality of patients undergoing coronary revascularization (6.4%)

Also relevant are: prior probability (PP), the probability of CAD in the AAA population (36%); the sensitivity (86%) and specificity (74%) of DTI; and AM, the mortality associated with coronary angiography (0.1%). Fig. 71-4 shows the results of a two-way sensitivity analysis holding all of the above variables constant, except MCR and MSCAD. As an example, for a given MCR of 7.9%, the institution should proceed to AAA repair without further testing if the MSCAD is less than 9.5%. Conversely, the institution should precede AAA repair with testing (leading to angiography, then leading to CABG, as indicated) if the MSCAD is greater than 9.5%. The appeal of this approach is that it emphasizes the local risks at each step which, in turn, are dependent on perioperative management and therefore, presumably modifiable. It is noteworthy that the BASELINE is drawn from reports that included data from only one or two institutions. A review of AAA mortality throughout New York state[157] showed rates of 5.8% to 10.4% depending on the volume of operations performed by the surgeon and the institution. These data blend BASELINE with MSCAD and suggest that BASELINE is probably greater than 0.5%.

The above issues have been extensively reviewed by a task force of the American Heart Association (AHA) and the American College of Cardiology (ACC), culminating in a publication entitled *Guidelines for Perioperative Cardiovascular Evaluation for Non-Cardiac Surgery.*[101] Much of this document directly addresses vascular surgery as the principal class of procedures whose subjects have the highest probability of CAD. Both preoperative findings or "predictors" (Box 71-1) and surgical procedures (Box 71-2) are stratified by levels of severity.

Note that aortic procedures and lower extremity bypass grafting are both in the high-risk procedure list, while carotid endarterectomy (CEA) is considered to be of intermediate risk (Box 71-2). As an example, consider a 65-year-old man presenting for elective infrarenal AAA repair. He has inferior lead Q-waves on his ECG reflecting an old MI, is taking medication for hypertension, and has good exercise tolerance, walking 1 mile each day. This patient has intermediate clinical predictors, good exercise tolerance, and is to undergo a high-risk surgical procedure. Following the algorithm of Fig. 71-5 on page 1848, he would not undergo further noninvasive procedures but would proceed direct to surgery, where, it is assumed, optimum management would

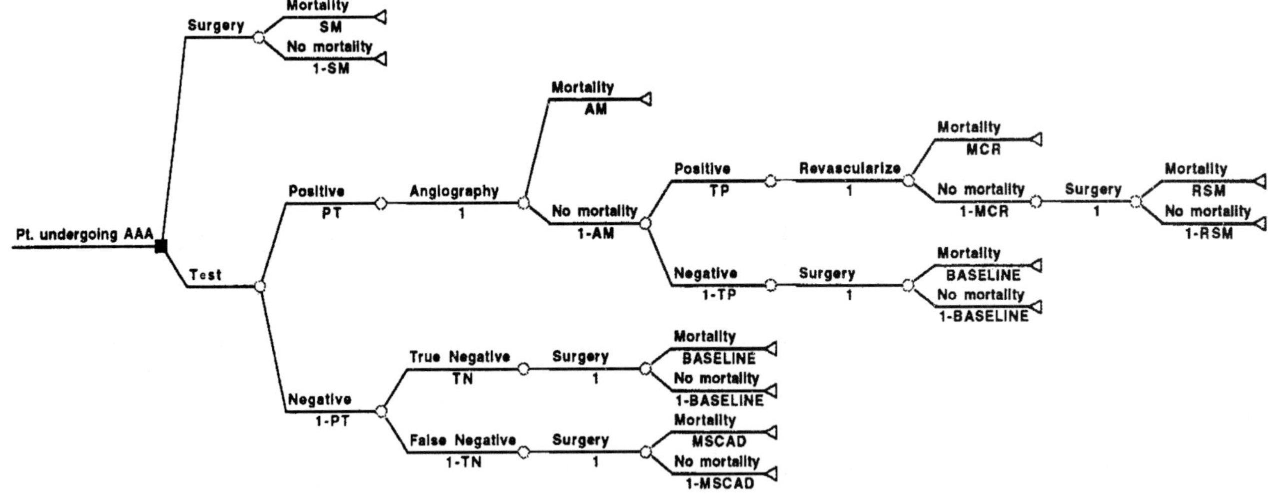

Fig. 71-3. Decision-tree model. The two options are preoperative testing and coronary revascularization versus abdominal aortic aneurysm (AAA) surgery alone. The probability of a possibility for any limb of the model is defined by the variable listed below the line denoting that possibility. The optimal decision is the one with the highest probability of survival. SM—cardiac mortality related to AAA surgery if no testing or revascularization is performed; AM—mortality from coronary angiography; PT—probability of a positive dipyridamole thallium imaging (DTI) test in the study population; TN—probability that a negative DTI test is a true negative; TP—true positive; BASELINE—baseline cardiac mortality of AAA surgery; MSCAD—cardiac mortality related to AAA surgery in patients with significant uncorrected coronary disease; MCR—mortality for coronary revascularization; RSM—cardiac mortality related to AAA surgery in patients who have undergone coronary revascularization. (From Fleisher LA, Skolnick ED, Holroyd KJ, et al: Coronary Artery Revascularization before abdominal aortic aneurysm surgery: A decision analytic approach, *Anesth Analg* 79:663, 1994.)

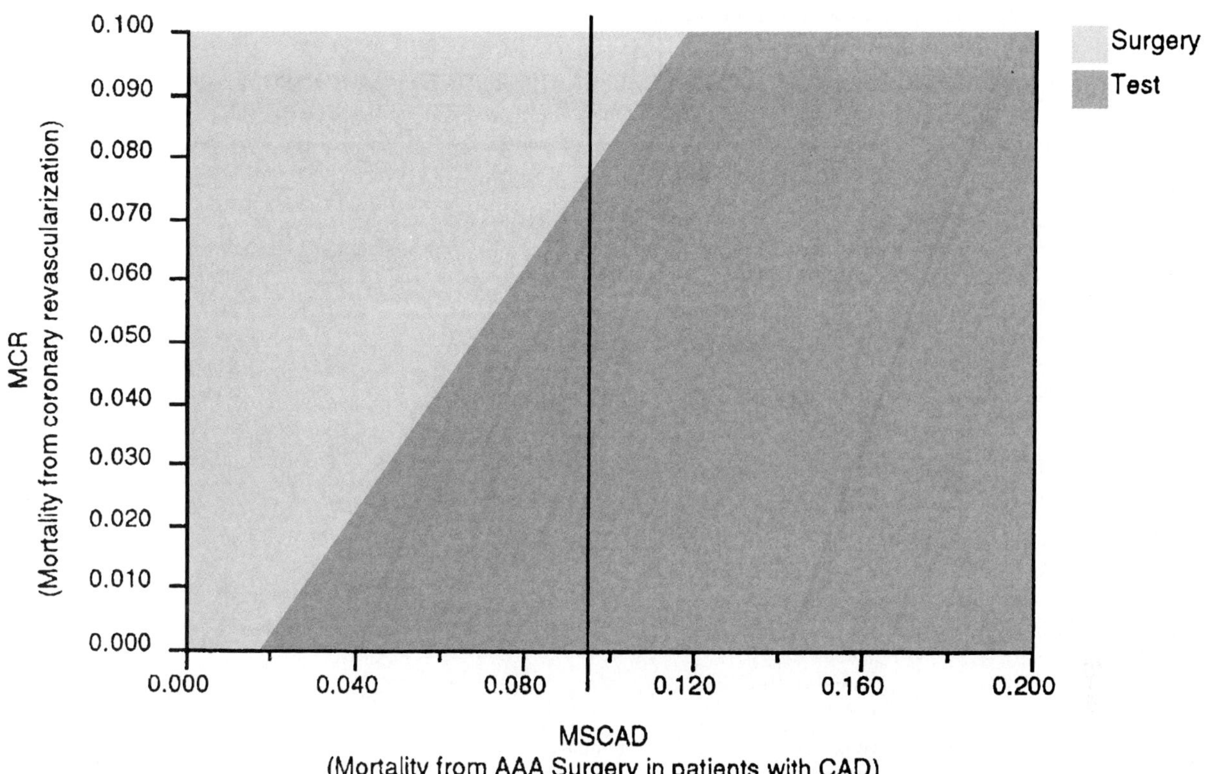

Fig. 71-4. Two-way sensitivity analysis of mortality from abdominal aortic aneurysm (AAA) surgery in patients with coronary artery disease (CAD) versus mortality from coronary revascularization. The vertical line is placed at 9.5% probability of mortality from AAA surgery in patients with CAD. (From Fleisher LA, Skolnick ED, Holroyd KJ, et al: Coronary artery revascularization before abdominal aortic aneurysm surgery: a decision analytic approach, *Anesth Analg* 79:665, 1994.)

occur. Note especially the importance of exercise tolerance in this scheme. This is not based on well-established investigations, but rather derives from the experience of "domain experts" on the task force. Application of these guidelines will result in approximately 50% of all major vascular surgery patients undergoing noninvasive testing.[220] The results of such testing then lead to either the original vascular procedure if the test is negative, or to angiography if the test is positive, with some patients receiving coronary revascularization prior to vascular surgery. As noted in the earlier discussion on decision analysis, the mortality for patients having AAA surgery who have had a prior CABG is very low (0.5%).[105,266]

Many procedures have been both suggested and refuted over time as valuable predictors of perioperative cardiac morbidity. Although recent investigations have enthusiastically promoted DTI[100] and ambulatory ECG monitoring (AECG),[282] cardiologists, surgeons, and anesthesia providers have not reached agreement. Clearly, the cost of these tests is a limiting feature. Mangano[232] estimates that annual medical costs would rise $100 million should DTI be used in only half of vascular surgery patients. Further, appropriate therapeutic decisions based on the results of diagnostic testing have not been evaluated.

If peripheral vascular disease or other physical limitation does not prevent exercise, then an exercise stress test is generally believed to be most appropriate. This is because the procedure not only detects myocardial ischemia, but also establishes functional capacity. The development of dyspnea or syncope during testing suggests the need for coronary angiography and/or extreme caution in perioperative management. A significant number of patients will not be able to undergo an exercise test and these may receive DTI, DSE, radionuclide ventriculography (RNV), or AECG. These are described in some detail later in this section.

A meta-analysis[237] found DSE to be the best predictor (6.2 relative risk), followed by DTI (4.6), RNV (3.7), and AECG (2.7). Conversely, Baron et al.[21] reported on a large number of patients undergoing aortic surgery and found that DTI was not predictive of cardiac mortality, but a clinical history of CAD was predictive. This finding demonstrates the limited value of routine testing and revalidates the proposals[100,101] suggesting testing only by criteria.

Morbidity and Mortality in Vascular Surgery

Overall considerations

Historically, CAD was primarily responsible for 50% of early and late mortality in surgical patients with peripheral

BOX 71-1
CLINICAL PREDICTORS OF INCREASED PERIOPERATIVE CARDIOVASCULAR RISK (MYOCARDIAL INFARCTION, CONGESTIVE HEART FAILURE, DEATH)

Major

- Unstable coronary syndromes
  - Recent myocardial infarction* with evidence of important ischemic risk by clinical symptoms or noninvasive study
  - Unstable or severe† angina (Canadian class III or IV)‡
- Decompensated congestive heart failure
- Significant arrhythmias
  - High-grade atrioventricular block
  - Symptomatic ventricular arrhythmias in the presence of underlying heart disease
  - Supraventricular arrhythmias with uncontrolled ventricular rate
- Severe valvular disease

Intermediate

- Mild angina pectoris (Canadian class I or II)
- Prior myocardial infarction by history or pathological Q waves
- Compensated or prior congestive heart failure
- Diabetes mellitus

Minor

- Advanced age
- Abnormal electrocardiogram (left ventricular hypertrophy, left bundle branch block, ST-T abnormalities)
- Rhythm other than sinus (e.g., atrial fibrillation)
- Low functional capacity (e.g., inability to climb one flight of stairs with a bag of groceries)
- History of stroke
- Uncontrolled systemic hypertension

*The American College of Cardiology National Database Library defines *recent* myocardial infarction as greater than 7 days but less than or equal to 1 month (30 days).
†May include "stable" angina in patients who are unusually sedentary.
‡From Cameau L: Grading of angina pectoris, *Circulation* 54:522–523, 1976.
(From Eagle KA, et al: ACC/AHA Task Force: Guidelines for perioperative cardiovascular evaluation for noncardiac surgery, *JACC* 27(4):918, 1996).

vascular disease.[72,93,108,165,183,343,362] Hertzer[163] showed that only 8% of 1000 vascular surgery patients in whom coronary angiography was performed had normal coronary arteries. Severe and surgically correctable CAD was documented in 14% of patients who had no clinical criteria to suggest this degree of disease. DTI in 100 patients admitted for elective abdominal aortic or lower limb vascular surgery showed that half of the patients had thallium redistribution in at least one segmental defect, suggesting a clinically important coronary stenosis.[214] Depending on the screening test employed, the incidence of significant CAD in patients with abdominal aneurysms, claudication, or carotid artery disease varies from 25% to 90%.[80,163,214,265] Better perioperative care at many institutions has decreased relative mortality due to cardiac complication. Multisystem organ failure has recently been reported as the primary cause of death in elective infrarenal AAA repair.[174]

The mortality rate for elective AAA repair varies from 1.5% to 8%.[17,37,72,83,93,171,276,285] Studies indicate the mortality rate for aortoiliac revascularization to be slightly lower than AAA repair at the same institution.[276] Although many series indicate mortality rates of 25% to 50% for emergency repair of a ruptured AAA, one report indicates that if the aneurysm is contained, the mortality rate is not significantly higher than that of an elective case.[17] Nonlethal MI after abdominal aortic surgery ranges from 4% to 6%.[17,93,183,362] However, a more careful surveillance by prospective evaluation of ECG and CPK MB isoenzymes demonstrates a 17% incidence of MI.[214]

Perioperative risks for patients undergoing lower-extremity vascular bypass grafting may be similar to risks for patients receiving the more invasive surgery required for AAA repair. On the other hand, the 5-year survival rate for patients having isolated aortoiliac disease is approximately 90%, whereas patients with femoral, popliteal, or tibial disease have only a 65% 5-year survival rate.[260] Further, MIs were responsible for 11% of the late mortality in patients with primary aortic disease, compared with 20% in patients with femoral, popliteal, and tibial-peroneal disease.[239]

Previous myocardial infarction

Patients with prior MI are at greater risk for perioperative reinfarction (5% to 8%)[183,323,337] than those without prior MI (0.1% to 0.7%)[277,337] and have a reinfarction mortality rate of

BOX 71-2
CARDIAC RISK* STRATIFICATION FOR NONCARDIAC SURGICAL PROCEDURES

High (report cardiac risk often > 5%)

- Emergent major operations, particularly in the elderly
- Aortic and other major vascular
- Peripheral vascular
- Anticipated prolonged surgical procedures associated with large fluid shifts and/or blood loss

Intermediate (reported cardiac risk generally < 5%)

- Carotoid endarterectomy
- Head and neck
- Intraperitoneal and intrathoracic
- Orthopedic
- Prostate

Low† (reported cardiac risk generally < 1%)

- Endoscopic procedures
- Superficial procedure
- Cataract
- Breast

*Combined incidence of cardiac death and nonfatal myocardial infarction.
†Do not generally require further preoperative cardiac testing.
(From Eagle KA, et al: ACC/AHA Task Force: Guidelines for perioperative cardiovascular evaluation for noncardiac surgery, *JACC* 27(4):919, 1996).

36% to 70%. The more recent the previous MI, the more likely the reinfarction. Substantial literature over the past 30 years has established the risk as follows: within 3 months of prior MI, the reinfarction rate exceeds 30%; at 3 to 6 months the rate is approximately 15%; and after 6 months the rate is approximately 6%.[232,323,337] Rates of 1% to 17% are given[165,183,303,367] for those who experience infarction after vascular surgery without an identified prior MI. Most perioperative MIs seem to occur postoperatively and silently, making them difficult to detect and their precise onset difficult to determine.

The increased perioperative risk in patients with previous MI has been long appreciated. The fact that risk diminishes with time between operation and infarct and stabilizes after 6 months has led most authorities to recommend that surgery be postponed for this interval, if at all possible. Clearly, this practice could conflict with operative indications based on aneurysm size or symptoms of cerebral or peripheral ischemia. Recent studies[283,309,354] suggest that it may be possible to reduce the incidence of reinfarction in patients who have had a preoperative MI. These investigations have employed a special anesthetic protocol with invasive monitoring, aggressive hemodynamic control, and extended intensive care unit management. Results include reinfarction rates of 5.7%, and 4.3% for previous infarctions of 3 to 6 months and less than 3 months before surgery, respectively.[309] These studies establish that careful perioperative management of patients with CAD and preoperative MI may dramatically improve outcome.

Angina and myocardial ischemia

Although preoperative angina should reasonably be expected to correlate with perioperative morbidity, it has proved to be surprisingly difficult to document a relationship.[55,214] Detsky et al. were able to identify a higher incidence of cardiac morbidity in patients with class III or class IV angina in the 2 weeks before surgery or with unstable angina within 3 months of surgery. Silent ischemia, as diagnosed by ambulatory monitoring in the preoperative period, has been suggested to be predictive of postoperative cardiac morbidity and mortality.[272,282]

Myocardial ischemia as diagnosed by ECG, transesophageal echocardiography (TEE), cardiokymography, or lactate changes is noted in 18% to 74% of patients with CAD during noncardiac surgery. ST segment changes most commonly occur in the lateral leads (V_4, V_5). London et al.[224] demonstrated a 90% sensitivity for the simultaneous monitoring of V_4 and V_5 leads with a drop to 80% for V_5 combined with limb lead II.

Intraoperative myocardial ischemia could be caused by increases in myocardial oxygen demand secondary to tachycardia, hypertension, anemia, elevated preload, or increased contractility.[357] However, the majority of the ischemic episodes are probably related to decreased oxygen supply.[217] Factors leading to decreased supply include hypotension, tachycardia, increased filling pressure, anemia, hypoxemia, and obstructed coronary blood flow due to acute thrombosis or spasm.[62,111,144,233]

The postoperative period has not been systematically investigated. There is some indication that the incidence of postoperative myocardial ischemia may be much higher than that of either the intraoperative or preoperative periods.[58,198,272] Postoperative episodes appear to be largely silent and are apt to occur up to several days after surgery.[112,361] A chronically elevated heart rate has been suggested as the primary cause.

Diabetes

Diabetes has been strongly suggested as a predictor for perioperative cardiac morbidity.[100,207] Altered autonomic function in diabetes may predispose to greater intraoperative risk of blood pressure lability.[51] Diabetic autonomic neuropathies can obscure symptoms of myocardial ischemia, thus adding to the already high incidence of "silent" ischemia seen in the perioperative period. The presence of diabetes in vascular surgery patients may identify a population in whom DTI is useful.[100]

Assessment of pulmonary status

Respiratory complications are potentially serious in patients undergoing vascular procedures that involve intra-abdominal and intrathoracic surgery.[129] Cigarette smoking is the etiology for most pulmonary disease.[367] Only when clinical assessment suggests severe compromise of pulmonary function are pulmonary function tests indicated.[129,196,304]

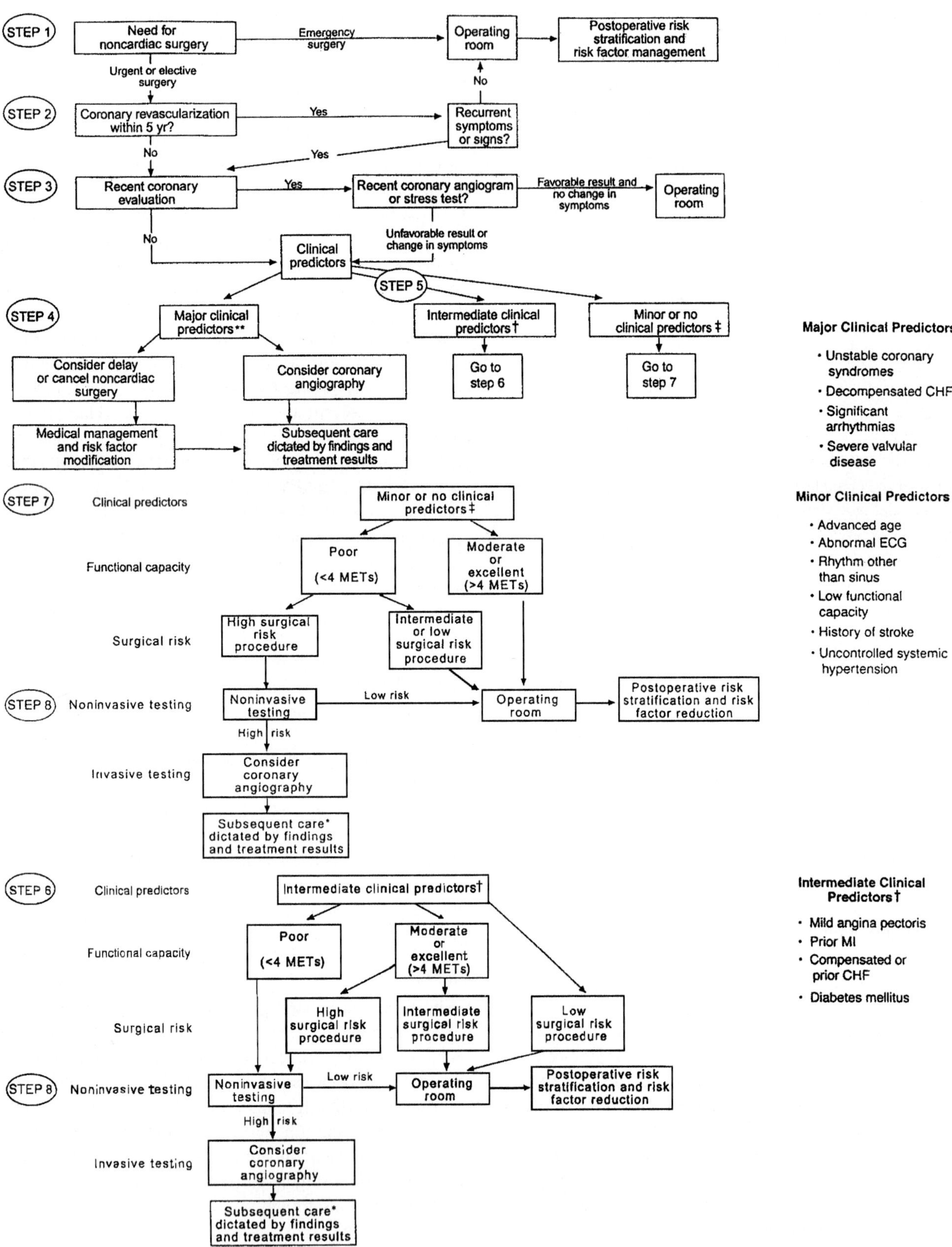

Fig. 71-5. Stepwise approach to preoperative cardiac assessment. Steps are discussed in text. *Subsequent care may include cancellation or delay of surgery, coronary revascularization followed by noncardiac surgery, or intensified care. (From Eagle KA, et al, ACC/AHA Task Force: Guidelines for perioperative cardiovascular evaluation for noncardiac surgery, *JACC* 27(4):921, 1996.)

Pulmonary function tests may be useful for identifying patients who would benefit from perioperative respiratory care and those who are likely to require mechanical ventilation postoperatively. Even patients with severe pulmonary compromise, however, may undergo surgery with an acceptable morbidity and mortality.[363] Arterial blood gases may be used to evaluate the degree of pulmonary insufficiency and provide a baseline for subsequent clinical decisions. Hypercapnia ($Pa{CO_2} > 45$ mm Hg) indicates a higher risk of postoperative morbidity.[342] Lower limits of forced expiratory volume in 1 second (FEV_1) and forced vital capacity (FVC) that would preclude surgery have not been defined.

Assessment of renal function

Patients undergoing aortic surgery are at risk for renal failure. Underlying disease can decrease renal perfusion, and surgical manipulation may exacerbate this condition. Evaluation of the kidney before major vascular surgical procedures involving the aorta is mandatory. Causes of baseline renal insufficiency include atherosclerosis of the renal arteries, hypertension, diabetic nephropathy, and depressed myocardial function. Arterial dye studies performed before the surgery also alter renal function by both a direct toxic effect and by a hyperosmolar-induced diuresis that reduces the intravascular volume.[53] Intravascular volume expansion before, during, and after the angiographic study minimizes renal effects. During abdominal aortic surgery, there are several causes of impaired renal perfusion, which include wide fluctuations in intravascular volume and cardiac output[52] and dysfunctional effects on renal hemodynamics from infrarenal aortic cross-clamping.[128] Also, emboli may shower the kidney when debris is dislodged proximal to an aortic clamp.[252] Suprarenal aortic clamping substantially increases these risks.[48,74] Progress in surgical and anesthetic management (discussed in detail in another section) has decreased the incidence of renal failure. Studies evaluating more than 500 patients have shown that postoperative acute renal failure occurred in less than 6%[17,93] after aortic reconstruction surgery.

Other risk factors

Patients with clinical or radiographic evidence of congestive heart failure (CHF) are more likely to suffer from acute postoperative pulmonary edema, especially those undergoing aortic surgery.[185] Goldman et al. also found a higher incidence of cardiac morbidity in patients with preoperative clinical signs of CHF.[142] Other factors associated with poor outcome in this study were ECG rhythm other than sinus, ventricular ectopic beats, valvular aortic stenosis, recent MI, emergency operation, or poor general medical condition.[142] Detsky et al. extended the Goldman findings to include old MI and severe angina.[92] Adequately controlled hypertension does not apparently increase patient risk.

Patient age is important in major vascular surgery, only because it indicates the possible presence of other risk factors associated with age. That is, age itself is not a contraindication to major vascular surgery,[158,264] although on an overall basis, the risk is higher in older patients.[55,142] The ACC/AHA guidelines[101] list "advanced age" as a minor clinical predictor.

Diagnostic Testing

Diagnostic techniques and vascular surgery

Patients presenting for vascular surgery will have undergone radiographic diagnostic procedures to determine the extent of vascular pathology. This is of concern to the anesthesia provider for three reasons: **(1) lesions of the vasculature identified by these techniques may have bearing on appropriate sites of arterial cannulation for blood pressure monitoring; (2) radiographic contrast media have physiologic effects that may last to the time of operation; and (3) physical trauma at the catheterization site may limit or dictate the sites of cannulation at the time of surgery.**

The complications of the angiographic procedure include hemorrhage, thrombosis or occlusion, pseudoaneurysm formation, and the formation of arterial fistulae, all occurring for a total incidence of about 0.5% for the femoral artery and 1.7% for the axillary artery. Complications related to the contrast media include nonidiosyncratic reactions involving the heart and vascular system and renal failure, for an overall incidence of approximately 3.5%. The total complication rate is approximately 4% for catheterization at the femoral artery and 5.2% at the axillary artery.[168,189,310]

Electrocardiogram

Preoperative ECG abnormalities are observed in 40% to 70% of patients with CAD undergoing noncardiac surgery. ST segment and T-wave abnormalities are noted (65% to 90%) and Q waves in 0.5% to 8%. In a study of 200 patients (age > 40 years) undergoing elective noncardiac surgery, an abnormal preoperative ECG was the only significant independent predictor of cardiac morbidity,[55,56] although both the specificity and sensitivity were low.

Exercise electrocardiography

Stress ECG is a reasonably inexpensive test routinely used to evaluate chest pain and determine prognosis for individuals with known CAD.[82,302,353] Preoperatively, a positive ischemic response and low exercise capacity correlate with cardiac morbidity after noncardiac surgery. Of vascular surgery patients with a positive stress ECG, 37% suffered a perioperative MI versus 1.5% with a negative ECG.[81] In this study, stress testing was a more sensitive indicator than the clinical history or resting ECG. Another investigation[55] failed to establish the stress ECG as an independent predictor of cardiac risk, although it did not study vascular patients alone. The use of stress ECGs in many vascular surgery patients is not feasible due to the limitation in mobility caused by lower extremity ischemia.

Holter monitoring

Holter monitoring is a promising tool for the preoperative assessment of vascular surgery patients. Two studies have correlated the duration and severity of preoperative ST-segment depression as recorded by AECG with perioperative cardiac morbidity in patients undergoing vascular surgery.[272,282] AECG has been previously shown to be a reliable method for detecting myocardial ischemia,[60] and there is evidence to suggest that silent ischemia detected by AECG monitoring is associated with unfavorable outcomes in patients with unstable angina.[40,146] Raby et al.[282] showed that 12 of 32 (37%) patients with preoperative ischemia detected by AECG suffered a MI, unstable angina, or pulmonary edema during or after major vascular surgery. Only one postoperative myocardial event occurred among 144 patients who did not exhibit preoperative ischemia. Pasternak[272] studied 200 major vascular patients and showed that the occurrence of preoperative silent myocardial ischemia and angina were the only significant predictors of perioperative MI. Baseline ECG changes are found in a significant portion of vascular patients and limit the use of this test. Further, the test only provides binary outcome and cannot further stratify high-risk patients to identify a subset who should receive angiography.[117]

Dipyridamole-thallium imaging

Dipyridamole-thallium imaging is noninvasive, fairly sensitive, specific, and can be used to assess risk for cardiac morbidity.[215] It is especially useful in the evaluation of patients who are unable to perform physical activity due to claudication or arthritic conditions. Thallium-201 is taken up by cells similarly to potassium.[352] It is readily assimilated by healthy myocardial cells and thus infarcted, ischemic, or hypoprofused areas appear as defects in the scan.[13]

Preceding the thallium injection with the coronary dilator, dipyridamole produces a coronary-steal phenomenon and creates reversible defects in myocardium supplied by stenosed coronaries. After dissipation of the dilatory effect, defects caused by ischemia will resolve, but those caused by infarcted tissue will persist. DTI locates and quantifies myocardium at risk with appropriate reliability.[147,213] DTI has been proposed for the preoperative work-up of vascular surgery patients.[41,79,99,214] Thallium redistribution was first correlated with postoperative ischemia by Boucher et al.[41] They found that 50% of the patients who had a preoperative redistribution subsequently experienced a postoperative cardiac event. Nonetheless, the incidence of perioperative cardiac morbidity is lower in recently published studies, which showed that 75% of patients with redistribution did not experience any postoperative complications.[79,99,214]

Dipyridamole-thallium imaging may show redistribution with only 40% to 60% narrowing of a vessel.[186] Eagle et al.[100] studied 200 patients undergoing vascular surgery. They found that DTI was most helpful in stratifying patients who had already been identified as high risk by clinical markers alone (e.g., angina, age > 70, ventricular ectopy, diabetes, Q waves on ECG). These experts suggest using DTI to further delineate risk in patients with one or two of these clinical markers. In this subset of patients, a positive DTI was associated with a tenfold higher incidence of cardiac morbidity. Eagle et al.[100] recommend proceeding with coronary angiography in these patients as well as in any patient with three or more markers, in which case the DTI is unnecessary. Conversely, Leppo et al.[214] found that clinical findings correlated with neither redistribution nor postoperative MI. Thus the controversy continues.

Dobutamine stress echocardiography

Incremental infusion of dobutamine during two-dimensional echocardiography has been shown to be a safe and accurate method for detection of CAD in patients who are unable to undergo conventional exercise testing.[301] Clearly, the ability of DTI to identify patients with CAD is limited because its methodology does not create increases in myocardial oxygen consumption, which would unmask significant lesions. The administration of dobutamine causes such an elevation of metabolic demand and any induced ischemia is manifested as segmental wall motion abnormalities, ST-segment depression or angina.[205] Recent reports[237] suggest that DSE is superior in its ability to predict morbidity in vascular surgery but, unfortunately, the test is also the most expensive noninvasive technique.

Angioscintigraphy

Gated blood pool images provide a reproducible and accurate measure of left ventricular function. Patients who have a decreased ejection fraction (EF) as demonstrated by angioscintigraphy also have a high incidence of severe CAD.[3,182] Patients with a decreased calculated EF may benefit from pulmonary artery (PA) pressure monitoring. Pasternak et al.[273,274] found that an EF of less than 0.35 was associated with a much higher incidence of perioperative MI in vascular surgery patients. Subsequent work has shown that depressed function predicts postoperative failure but not infarction.[21]

Coronary angiography

Many authors have recommended coronary angiography for further evaluation of patients with positive findings obtained from less-invasive procedures or as routine work-up for patients having aortic surgery.[33,161,299] The largest series addressing the value of coronary angiography before vascular surgery is that of Hertzer et al.,[167] who studied 1000 patients from 1978 to 1982. They found that of 250 patients with severe correctable CAD, the combined perioperative and 5-year mortality rate was 12% in patients who had CABG before their vascular surgery and 26% in those who did not. Unfortunately, the study was not randomized and the patients not receiving CABG were those who either refused or were not candidates because of other medical considerations. Hertzer et al.[167] recommended routine coronary angiography before major vascular surgery and surgical correction of coronary lesions in selected patients. It is important to reiterate that no large-scale randomized trial has been performed to resolve these issues, which are of the greatest medical and economic importance.

The morbidity and mortality associated with coronary angiography and coronary artery bypass surgery deserve consideration.[116] In one recent investigation, Leppo et al.[214] reviewed 11 of 100 patients scheduled for vascular surgery who underwent coronary angiography on the basis of a strongly positive DTI and exercise test results. Two patients died, one had a cerebrovascular accident, and another had a fatal MI after CABG. Because careful perioperative management may result in a mortality rate below 3%[55,84,341] for AAA repair, it could be argued that angiography and the succeeding CABG surgery actually increased the complication rate.

Chest radiography

In patients with CAD, chest radiographic abnormalities are predictive of ventricular function abnormalities detectable by ventriculography. For example, more than 70% of CAD patients with cardiomegaly on chest radiograph were found to have a low EF (< 40%).[232] Because a low preoperative EF predicts perioperative cardiac morbidity,[207,273,274] preoperative radiographic cardiomegaly may well be similarly associated.

PREOPERATIVE THERAPY

Preoperative CABG

Some patients presenting for major surgery have unstable coronary syndromes that are sufficiently high risk to mandate coronary revascularization. For most patients, the issue is considerably less clear. As previously noted, the local morbidity rates for all aspects of clinical care are critical determinants of the decision process. It is quite clear that those who survive the testing-revascularization (CABG) sequence have much lower risk for the vascular surgery itself. From a broader perspective, the long-term survival of patients with CAD and vascular disease has been studied. It is also clear that patients who have coronary revascularization have much better long-term survival.[266] Thus, it has been suggested that the proposed vascular surgery be viewed as an event which initiates an appropriate process to prepare for the extended lifetime beyond surgery.[101,141]

Preoperative coronary angioplasty

No formal trials evaluating the efficacy of PCTA in reducing perioperative cardiac events in vascular surgery have been reported. Small numbers of patients have been observed retrospectively[8,105,173] and the benefit has been apparently substantial. An unresolved issue is the optimal delay period after PCTA, before vascular surgery. Several days' wait is suggested for coronary plaque and/or for myocardial stabilization.[101]

Medical therapy

Nitrates, beta blockers, and calcium channel blockers are common chronic medications in vascular surgery patients. Perioperative discontinuation of these therapies may lead to perioperative ischemia, dysrhythmias, MI, and cardiac death,[48,106,120,191,249] and therefore it is recommended to continue all significant cardiovascular medications up to and including the morning of surgery. Institution of these medications immediately preoperatively is under consideration in high-risk patients who are otherwise not receiving treatment. Studies suggest that preoperative oral beta-blocker therapy or preinduction IV beta-blocker administration may lessen intraoperative ischemia in both cardiac and noncardiac surgical patients.[76,230,315,328] Also, beta-blocker therapy has been shown to be more effective prophylactically than calcium channel blocker therapy.[59,317] Preoperative clonidine has decreased the anesthetic requirements,[115,136] serum catecholamines,[115] and perioperative blood pressure lability in CABG patients.[115] Clonidine may also reduce the incidence of hypertension in patients undergoing noncardiac surgery.[136] Some complications were observed in these studies, and more work is necessary before identifying a subset of patients in whom prophylactic therapy is appropriate.

Intensive care

Preoperative admission to an intensive care unit with PA catheterization and "optimization" of hemodynamics has been employed and is associated with the lowest morbidity and mortality for the highest-risk patients.[29,139] It is entirely possible, however, that the same results would be obtainable with the initiation of invasive monitoring immediately prior to surgery and aggressive therapy during the case. Obviously, this latter method would be much less expensive and there is no intrinsic physiologic reason why it should not produce equivalent results. Also, intraoperative techniques which ablate the surgical stress response may produce conditions in which the physiologic manipulations can be appropriately carried out without a PA catheter.[58,345]

Overall goals and considerations

Modern developments in risk assessment, surgical risk modification, physiologic monitoring anti-ischemic therapies, stress-ablating techniques of anesthesia and analgesia, and postoperative intensive care and rehabilitation can produce clinical pathways which truly optimize patient care. Full realization of this potential requires collaboration between vascular surgery, cardiac surgery, cardiology, anesthesiology, and critical care medicine to a degree not easily achievable in most institutions. Conceivably, the current pressure to standardize care and control costs by the development of practice guidelines will stimulate an integrated approach.

Vascular surgery patients require intensive perioperative monitoring for two primary reasons: **(1) these patients often have systemic manifestations of atherosclerotic vascular disease and are at risk for cardiac, cerebral, renal, and spinal cord ischemia, all of which can be diagnosed and treated using the appropriate monitors; and (2) vascular procedures involve major physiologic changes, including significant third-space losses, blood loss, and the complications of transfusion (coagulopathies, hypocalcemia, hypothermia, and acidosis).**

Also, there can be significant changes in the hemodynamic profile associated with the application and release of vascular clamps.

The fluid shifts and blood loss may continue into the postoperative period and along with hypertension and tachycardia associated with postoperative pain, can adversely affect the determinates of myocardial oxygen supply and demand. For this reason, one of the primary goals of monitoring in this patient population is to reduce cardiac morbidity. Cerebral ischemia during carotid surgery as well as spinal cord ischemia during thoracic aortic surgery may be diagnosed using appropriate monitors, which can lead to specific therapies. Renal perfusion may also be compromised, especially during aortic reconstruction, thus the importance of monitoring indices of volume status.

Appropriate ECG monitoring during vascular surgery is mandatory. Clinical practice has evolved from single-lead systems to multiple-lead systems capable of sophisticated online computer analysis of the ST segment. The V_5 lead is the single most important lead because of its high sensitivity for detecting ischemic changes.[192,224] An inferior limb lead is commonly displayed as well and increases the detection of ischemia.[125]

The following discussions presume that all standard monitoring devices are employed, including pulse oximetry, capnography, ECG, and body temperature measurement.

CAROTID ENDARTERECTOMY

Pathophysiology of Carotid Disease

Occlusive disease of the carotid system is commonly caused by atherosclerosis and involves the origins of both the internal and external carotid arteries as well as the bifurcation of the common carotid artery.[228] Various theories have been proposed to explain atheromatous plaque formation at the carotid bifurcation. Impedance mismatch, with the associated altered hemodynamic conditions that accompany division of a vessel into conduits of substantially different sizes, may be implicated in the vessel injury.[297] Plaque formation may produce symptoms either by gradually occluding brain blood flow or by exhibiting degenerative changes that lead to atheromatous emboli or thromboemboli. Intraplaque hemorrhage and ulcerative breakdown may result in symptoms of cerebral ischemia.[180,229] The severity of cerebral ischemia is influenced by the degree of blood flow collateralization including the development of the circle of Willis. CEA directly removes the vascular pathology that has produced either occlusion or distal emboli.

Indications

Although successful CEA may reduce the risk of stroke in selected patients, it is always important to balance the risk of operation with the risk of stroke from the unoperated lesion.[340] The issue of which patients are appropriate candidates for CEA continues to be debated in the medical literature.[19,45,54,169,257,340,344] A recent, multicenter randomized trial studying patients with asymptomatic carotid disease (> 60% stenosis) showed a 53% relative risk reduction for stroke or death over a 5-year period if CEA is added to aggressive medical management of modifiable risk factors.[344] Although statistically significant, the *clinical* significance of this result was questioned given the modest 6% absolute risk reduction.[45] In patients with symptomatic carotid stenosis of at least 70%, CEA reduced the absolute risk of stroke by 17% over 2 years compared with medical management alone.[18,257]

Nevertheless, asymptomatic patients are potential candidates for CEA if they have greater than 70% occlusion of the common or internal carotid artery by angiography or duplex imaging or greater than 50% occlusion with positive ocular plethysmography. Studies have shown that asymptomatic carotid bruits in patients with AAA do not indicate an increased risk for postoperative stroke.[185] Therefore, the criteria for CEA should not be altered for patients undergoing peripheral vascular surgery.[360] Other indications for considering operation include a previous atherothrombotic stroke, stroke-in-evolution, crescendo transient ischemic attacks (TIAs), and recurrent global or nonspecific cerebral symptoms despite antiplatelet or anticoagulant therapy.[91] With TIAs or stroke, carotid lesions that are left untreated produce an annual incidence of stroke of approximately 5%, approaching a maximum of 15% the first year.[355] It is generally accepted that the overall rate of surgical morbidity and mortality for a hospital or a surgeon should be less than 5% to justify surgery for symptomatic patients.[228]

Carotid endarterectomy is associated with a relatively low incidence (about 2%) of MI, although cardiac complications are responsible for most early postoperative deaths.[108,164,165,265,360]

Risk

Stroke is the most common and expected major complication during and after CEA. The incidence of stroke varies with the indication for surgery. Combined death and stroke rate in one series ranged from 5.3% when the indication was "asymptomatic bruit" to 9.5% when the indication was "major stroke."[119]

In 295 patients scheduled for CEA undergoing coronary angiography, 27% had advanced CAD, 26% severe correctable coronary stenosis, and 6% severe inoperable CAD.[165] MI is associated with 25% to 50% of all mortality after CEA.[265] The presence of symptoms of CAD increases the proportion of mortality that is cardiac related to 75%.[108] Hypertension occurs in approximately 70% of patients undergoing CEA and is associated with an increase in the risk of stroke, because cerebral blood flow may be reduced and autoregulation impaired.[339]

Monitoring

Monitoring for cerebral ischemia during CEA is controversial. The advent of electroencephalographic (EEG) monitoring and, most recently, compressed spectral array and somatosensory-evoked potentials (SEP) has introduced new possibilities in the detection of cerebral ischemia during surgery. Many centers advocate the routine use of these devices.[288] An older technique uses the measurement of carotid artery stump pressure as an assessment of collateral flow from the circle of Willis.[170] Alternatively, some surgeons choose to bypass the occluded segment with a temporary shunt during the time of occlusion.[162]

Debate continues as to the best method of assessing or preventing cerebral ischemia because none of the aforementioned techniques is without difficulty or complications. Regional anesthesia may not only obviate the need for shunting but carotid clamping for 2 to 3 minutes in the awake patient serves as a useful monitor of neurologic status[96] and may allow for prompt identification of patients who would benefit from shunt placement.[27] Change in contralateral grip strength or consciousness in the setting of adequate mean arterial pressure is an indication for shunt placement. Intraoperative neurologic changes in the awake patient may predict a sixfold increase in the incidence of postoperative stroke (Fig. 71-6).[87]

Shunt insertion may incur an embolism-associated stroke rate of 0.7%.[329] Shunts can also be associated with intimal dissection leading to acute occlusion. By limiting the exposure of the plaque, shunts may affect the adequacy of the endarterectomy.[113] Several authorities argue that any monitoring modality that could reliably indicate inadequate cerebral blood flow would allow a more conservative use of the shunting procedure. However, EEG techniques are associated with both false-positive and false-negative results, and no study to date has demonstrated satisfactorily that the use of these methods improves outcome.[288] Interestingly, patients who have suffered strokes or TIAs are at no greater risk of having EEG evidence of cerebral ischemia during carotid artery cross-clamp than patients without symptoms and with normal baseline EEG.[195] Transcranial Doppler can reliably monitor cerebral blood flow and may benefit patients undergoing CEA.[1,28,269] One series showed that perioperative stroke can be prevented by using transcranial Doppler together with stump pressure monitoring when CEA is performed under general anesthesia.[25]

Caution is especially indicated when monitoring patients who have preexisting neurologic deficits. One study has shown that 4 of 124 patients who had strokes or reversible neurologic deficits before CEA awoke with new deficits despite an unchanged EEG during the procedure.[293]

False-positive results occur and may be secondary to the brain's tolerance for brief periods of ischemia without proceeding to infarction. Additionally, the EEG is affected by anesthetic agents and changes in temperature and blood pressure. One study has shown a sensitivity of 55% and a specificity of 98.5% in 380 patients indicating a high incidence of false-negative results.[244] Finally, the value of EEG monitoring is limited by the fact that the majority of neurologic deficits after CEA are caused by thromboembolism rather than occlusion of blood flow during carotid clamping.[38,251] These objections notwithstanding, if EEG monitoring were limited to patients without preexisting neurologic deficits, thereby eliminating the major cause of false-negative findings, it is quite possible that the use of this monitoring modality would allow for maintenance of lower blood pressure during cross-clamp and more time for surgical repair.[288]

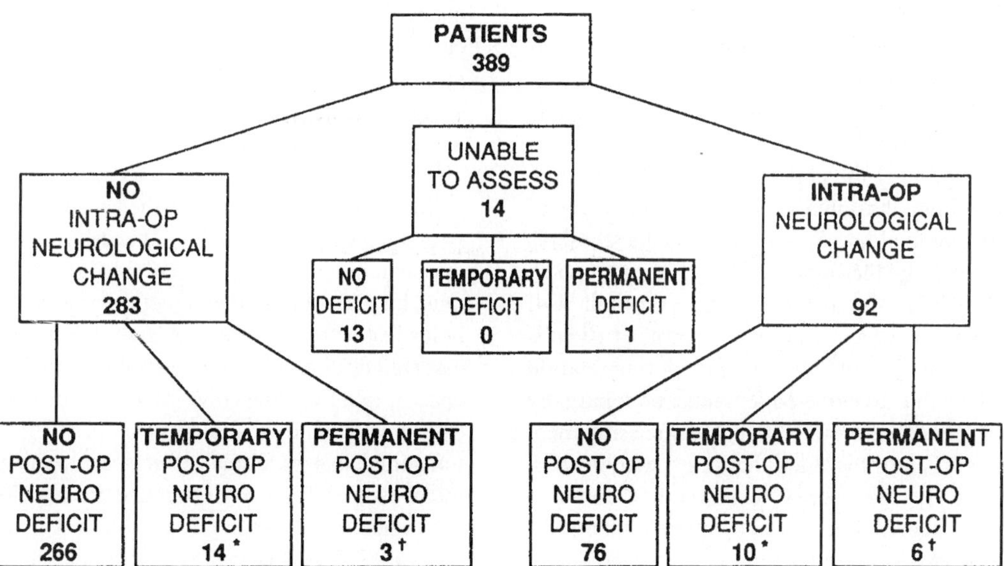

Fig. 71-6. Correlation of intraoperative neurologic change and postoperative neurologic outcome. Number of patients is shown in each box. *$p < 0.05$ for temporary neurologic complication. †$p < 0.01$ for permanent neurologic complication. (From Davies MJ, Mooney PH, Scott DA, et al: Neurologic changes during carotid endarterectomy under cervical block predict a high risk of postoperative stroke, *Anesthesiology* 78(5):832, 1993.)

All patients undergoing CEA should have an arterial catheter for continuous measurement of arterial blood pressure. It is important to carefully measure blood pressure in both arms because differences can be profound,[123] and monitoring in the arm with the lower reading can lead to serious clinical mismanagement. Patients with carotid disease are especially given to this lateral discrepancy.

Intravenous access for volume administration may be limited to one medium-bore (16-gauge) IV line, because significant blood loss is uncommon.

A central venous line is valuable, although not necessary for assuring the expeditious infusion of vasoactive drugs. Its use may be more appropriately reserved for patients with documented or suspected CAD or valvular heart disease. Many clinicians find it desirable to insert a PA catheter in patients with significant cardiac disease. Others point to the relative insensitivity of changes in pulmonary capillary wedge pressure as indication of MI and advocate continuous TEE.[320] Appropriate sites for central access and PA catheters include the antecubital fossa and subclavian or femoral veins. Use of the contralateral side for internal jugular access should proceed with extreme caution to avoid carotid puncture with the possibility of compromised flow and subsequent cancellation of surgery.

Anesthetic Techniques

The goals of anesthesia,[109] which balance concerns for both brain and heart, may be summarized as:

- Hemodynamic extremes should be avoided during induction, incision, surgical manipulation, emergence, and extubation.
- The patient should be sufficiently responsive immediately after surgery to obey commands and thereby facilitate neurologic evaluation.

Clearly, these two objectives narrow the range of acceptable anesthetic options and require clinical expertise. Premedication is used cautiously, if at all, to avoid interference with the second goal.

The question regarding the impact of the anesthetic technique on outcome remains controversial with proponents of both regional and general anesthesia. Regional anesthesia is performed by blocking the superficial and deep cervical plexus formed from spinal nerves C1 through C4. Proponents of this technique believe that an awake patient is the best monitor of neurologic function during carotid surgery. To achieve this goal, the patient must be minimally sedated and the procedure requires a high degree of patient cooperation, a profound blockade, and an expeditious surgeon. Intraoperatively, the internal, external, and common carotid arteries are clamped, followed by neurologic assessment. The clamps are released if a deficit occurs, and one of several options is invoked: (1) case cancellation; (2) elevation of systemic blood pressure and reocclusion; or (3) placement of a shunt that bypasses the operative area.[248] Disadvantages of regional anesthesia include patient discomfort and loss of cooperation, confusion, panic, or seizures. Management of intraoperative problems arising during regional anesthesia may be more difficult and theoretically associated with increased morbidity. Some investigators have found that regional anesthesia by cervical block obviates the use of a shunt in greater than 80% of patients, and facilitates safe, simple, and effective intraoperative cerebral function monitoring.[96,211,308] Regional anesthesia may be associated with shorter hospital stays, decreased intensive care costs, and less cardiovascular morbidity.[7,219,254] Some experts believe it is a safe, effective, and satisfactory technique for elderly and high-risk patients.[68,152] In only one prospective evaluation of CEA conducted under regional anesthesia, the selective use of the intensive care unit and early discharge were concluded to be safe and cost effective.[61] In this study, there was no randomization to any particular anesthetic technique or strict criteria for shunt placement between the groups. One group reported 92% of patients preferred a repeat cervical plexus block for a future CEA.[86] Yet, other studies show similar incidences of neurologic and cardiovascular morbidity regardless of anesthetic technique.[25,271,280] ECG signs of myocardial ischemia in patients undergoing CEA conducted under cervical plexus block were highly predictive of postoperative cardiac events.[204] Thus, in an evolving health care environment, a well-conducted regional anesthetic for CEA may be superior in terms of morbidity, mortality, patient satisfaction, and cost-effectiveness.

Obviously, general anesthesia allows better control of ventilation and thus nearly eliminates the possibility of hypoxemia and dyscapnia—an obvious risk with regional techniques. General anesthesia for CEA may also be associated with reduction in hospital stay and cost.[124] Cardiac morbidity may be independent of anesthetic type. With negligible change in hemodynamics, 25% of patients who have their carotid artery clamped develop immediate myocardial wall motion abnormalities. This effect is reproducible and responds to nitroglycerin. A potential benefit of using general anesthesia is that it allows monitoring with TEE to detect wall motion abnormalities and to guide therapy.

Induction of general anesthesia should proceed slowly with medications titrated to the desired effect. Some use thiopental up to 10 mg/kg in divided doses[206] or as a continuous infusion during the induction process and administer a bolus just before carotid occlusion.[248] This technique may be associated with delayed emergence, especially in the presence of additional sedative-hypnotics or narcotics. In addition to the standard desirable property of rapid hypnosis, thiopental has beneficial effects on brain blood flow and metabolism, which may minimize the severity of brain damage when focal areas of the brain are subjected to ischemia.[247,248,261] However, one study has shown that the protective effects of a 4-mg/kg bolus of thiopental are not comparable in duration to the time of carotid cross-clamping.[250] The role of barbiturates in protection or treatment of cerebral ischemia and their use for that purpose in CEA remains controversial.[197] Addition of a short- or intermediate-acting narcotic, depending on the proposed duration of surgery, is recommended. Moderate doses of narcotic allow for better hemodynamic control during intubation and incision and permit a lower dose of inhalational agent to be used during anesthetic maintenance.[206] Vecuronium seems to be the ideal muscle relaxant for procedures lasting 90 minutes or less. Maintenance of anesthesia may proceed with the addition of nitrous oxide, which promotes hemodynamic stability. Although nitrous oxide has the potential to worsen cerebral ischemia, this has not been proved. Historically, isoflurane emerged as the inhalational agent of choice based on studies that demonstrate a lower critical regional cerebral blood flow when compared with halothane.[246] New agents with low solubility (sevoflurane and desflurane) may facilitate smoother and more rapid emergence. Their use in CEA has not been reported. With nitrous oxide up to 60%, a basal level of analgesia from the narcotic, and hypnosis from the thiopental, it is generally necessary to administer the inhalational agent at a concentration considerably less than 1 minimum alveolar concentration (MAC). The use of a laryngeal mask airway may lessen perioperative hemodynamic responses to airway management, a concept under investigation. Whereas the actual surgical procedure is minimally stimulating, hemodynamic fluctuations can occur secondary to neural reflexes. Blood pressure and heart rate changes during and after carotid surgery are quite variable.[248] Surgical manipulation of the carotid sinus can cause an increase in afferent impulses to the brain stem and trigger an abrupt bradycardia and hypotension. This may be prevented by infiltration of the sinus with local anesthetic by the surgeon. If infiltration has not been performed, then clamp application may cause hypertension and tachycardia because the sinus is now sensing a low pressure. The reverse may or may not be observed with unclamping. The high degree of variability between individuals in this reflex behavior may be due to differing degrees of sinus insensitivity secondary to the atherosclerotic process.

Control of the partial pressure of carbon dioxide in arterial blood ($Pa{CO_2}$) is a matter of some controversy. Hypocapnia produces cerebral vasoconstriction, whereas hypercapnia has been suggested to induce a "steal" phenomenon.[159] Thus most authors recommend the maintenance of normocarbia during CEA. Others continue to recommend maintaining a mild degree of hypocapnia.[206] Given the impact of hypergylcemia on worsening cerebral ischemic injury, the perioperative management of glucose is vital in these patients. Yet, there are no good outcome studies to support the tight control of glucose in diabetic patients undergoing carotid surgery. Glucose should be monitored carefully in the diabetic and maintained in an acceptable range.

It is universally accepted that the blood pressure during carotid occlusion should be maintained at or up to 20% higher than the patient's highest recorded resting blood pressure when awake.[206,248,288] Although many authorities recommend using dilute continuous infusions of an alpha agonist to achieve this goal, a recent investigation has found that the use of phenylephrine in patients receiving "deep" inhalational anesthesia caused a higher incidence of myocardial ischemia than was seen in patients who were allowed to achieve their blood pressure goals by using "light" anesthesia alone, without a vasoconstrictor.[319] Interestingly, despite the high incidence of intraoperative myocardial ischemia, no patient in this study suffered perioperative MI. It is noteworthy that this investigation used an anesthetic procedure that did not employ short-acting narcotics as a supplement to the inhalational agent. Elevation of blood pressure by increasing afterload, superimposed on a myocardium depressed by a potent inhalational agent, should result in deleterious effects. It is doubtful that these findings would apply to a technique in which the concentration of inhalational anesthetic was reduced by supplementation with a narcotic base.

The induction phase of general anesthesia has been extensively studied, and many modalities have been suggested for reducing the stress of intubation and incision.[35,85,336] Nonetheless, considerably less attention has been paid to the equally stressful and complicated process of emergence and extubation.[356] Nowhere are emergence issues more important and complex than in CEA. Although it is desirable to have the patient alert and responsive immediately after the procedure to permit neurologic assessment, hypertension, which can stress and rupture the surgical anastomosis, is an ever-present threat. Patients are frequently smokers with hyperreactive airways and are either treated or untreated hypertensives. Unless thorough precautions are taken, stimulation from the endotracheal (ET) tube at the time of emergence from general anesthesia will cause coughing and straining and can result in severe hypertension.[325] Residual effects from previously administered narcotics are particularly helpful at this time. If recurrent laryngeal nerve injury has been ruled out and the muscle relaxants completely reversed, then early extubation should be considered after careful evacuation of oropharyngeal secretions. Instillation of 60 to 80 mg of 2% lidocaine in the (ET) tube during the surgical closure and careful adjustment to minimal pressure in the (ET) cuff are partially effective techniques to blunt hypertension caused by the presence of the (ET) tube. Aggressive pharmacologic intervention may be necessary. Nitroprusside, nitroglycerine, propranolol, esmolol, and labetalol are potentially useful agents and should be immediately available for administration.[31,127,138,300,326,347]

Postoperative Considerations

There are several potential complications that may occur postoperatively. Intense surveillance is essential, especially given the interest in decreased use of intensive care units.[126,254] Hypertension is common postoperatively and is associated with an increased incidence of cardiac and neurologic complications.[212,314] An avoidable consequence of poorly controlled hypertension is wound hematoma necessitating prompt evaluation and wound exploration. Compared with general anesthesia, regional anesthesia may decrease the need for postoperative IV vasodilators and, therefore, decrease the risk of hypertension-associated complications.[67] Hypotension may occur secondary to carotid hypersensitivity. If not promptly treated, hypotension may result in cerebral or myocardial ischemia or MI.

Bradycardia may occur after carotid sinus plaque removal but is usually mild and self-limited. Thrombosis or emboli are the most common causes of postoperative neurologic deficit. Neurologic complications postoperatively may require reoperation to rule out carotid occlusion. Carotid body injury may persist for up to 10 months postoperatively. Thus, bilateral CEA may require prolonged supplemental oxygen. Recurrent laryngeal, hypoglossal, and marginal mandibular nerve injury may result in hoarseness, tongue deviation on protrusion, and drooping of the corner of the mouth, respectively.[334] Superior laryngeal nerve injury may present as impaired phonation. Spinal accessory nerve injury may result in ipsilateral shoulder weakness.[160,334]

LOWER EXTREMITY VASCULAR SURGERY

Peripheral Vascular Insufficiency

Atherosclerosis affects the lower extremities as aortoiliac, infrainguinal, and a mixed distribution of lesions.[89] Patients are candidates for elective surgery to correct peripheral occlusive disease if they exhibit: (1) intermittent, activity-limiting claudication; (2) ischemic rest pain; (3) ischemic ulceration; or (4) gangrene. Procedures are classified as either inflow or outflow reconstruction. Inflow procedures alleviate obstruction in the aortoiliac segment, and outflow procedures bypass femoral, popliteal, or distal obstruction. The former consists of replacement of the diseased segment by a Y-shaped prosthetic graft, whereas the latter may be performed with reversed saphenous vein, in situ saphenous vein, or a prosthetic graft.[348]

Acute embolic occlusion may necessitate emergency vascular surgery. Such emboli commonly originate in the heart in patients with cardiac dysrhythmias, recent MI, or ventricular aneurysms. These constitute 90% of the cases of embolism to the lower extremities. If ischemia is not reversed within a few hours, limb loss may occur.

Individuals undergoing lower extremity vascular bypass grafting (LEVBG) present the anesthesia provider with a dilemma. The procedure itself is associated with far less (intraoperative and postoperative) nociceptive stimulation than aortic surgery, less hemodynamic fluctuation than carotid or aortic surgery, and can be performed with a pure regional anesthetic. On the other hand, the patients may have severe CAD and other systemic disorders, the former undiscovered because of mobility limitations.[220] Recent data[202,220,226] confirm the remarkable and important fact that cardiac morbidity and mortality for patients undergoing LEVBG is equivalent to, or greater than, patients having AAA repair. Thus, the perioperative management of this group, including the anesthetic technique, must proceed with considerable caution.[320]

Monitoring

It is advisable to assure accurate placement of ECG leads, choice of system (or mode) for monitoring (diagnostic), and the intensity of intra- and postoperative surveillance. Ischemic ECG changes are common and warrant treatment.

Arterial cannulation and continuous pressure monitoring are considered standard. If a radial line is not technically feasible, the axillary approach is recommended. Central venous pressure (CVP) monitoring is frequently helpful. Volume status can be difficult to judge, especially in long, complicated cases which can evolve unexpectedly. Improved response time to the administration of vasoactive agents is often sufficiently important to justify central cannulation.

Pulmonary artery catheterization is not routinely employed by most centers. However, two important investigations of patients undergoing LEVBG used PA catheters before, during, and after surgery and obtained the lowest reported rates of cardiac morbidity (approximately 4%) and reoperation (22%) for vascular occlusion.[29,39] The additional expense of this management scheme will deter its widespread adoption unless the better results fit a favorable cost/benefit analysis.

It is possible that the same results may be achieved less expensively using a treatment plan that features regional anesthesia and analgesia (see following paragraphs). Until resolution of this issue, PA catheters use should be reserved for the 25% of patients with severe left ventricular dysfunction, renal failure, diabetic autonomic neuropathy, or cor pulmonale.[104]

Anesthetic Techniques

Because of their especially high-risk status, and because the nature of the surgery permits a pure regional technique, LEVBG patients have been the subject of several studies comparing regional and general anesthesia.[39,58,345] The results of these clinical trials are worth reviewing, both for guidance in the perioperative management of vascular surgery patients and for insight into the conduct of clinical trials.

Spinal and epidural anesthesia using local anesthetic agents have long been believed to provide overall better operative conditions for a variety of reasons, including avoidance of exposure to airway and pulmonary morbidity, lower blood loss, and most recently, ablation of the surgical stress response. The latter effect presumably produces more stable hemodynamics, reduced hypercoagulability, better wound healing and less immune suppression. Further, vasodilatation, secondary to sympathetic blockade, should be particularly helpful in sustaining graft patency.

Serious difficulties have plagued many published investigations, including both prospective, randomized clinical trials and retrospective studies. The failure to adequately specify a "control" treatment is the most common serious deficiency. An anesthetic technique cannot be characterized by a single label. In addition to the myriad of manipulations and judgments that go into drug choice, dosage, and timing, there are nonuniform assumptions regarding the definition of abnormal or undesirable conditions (hypertension, tachycardia, etc.) and how to treat such conditions if they arise. The term "general anesthesia" conveys no certain information because the mode, means, and mechanisms of the various classes (and entities within each class) of agents permit a virtually infinite combination of possibilities. Further, few studies have taken the trouble or had the necessary cooperation between surgical, anesthesia, and critical care colleagues to design and conduct optimal anesthetic plans that defined and adhered to protocols throughout the perioperative period, including the definition of hemodynamic extremes and their treatment. Moreover, communication of the details of management in published manuscripts are usually inadequate to permit readers to adequately compare study procedures with their own practice.[22,24]

The failure to adequately address these issues has produced findings which vary widely and which must be interpreted carefully. The landmark study by Yeager and colleagues[363] showed much less morbidity and mortality in a group of patients undergoing diverse major surgical procedures who received regional anesthesia (and analgesia) compared with those who received general anesthesia followed by on-demand parenteral narcotics. Only a few vascular surgery subjects were included in this study and the morbidity and mortality in the general anesthesia group was much higher than reported in other studies. No management techniques were specified and the general anesthesia group actually received a wide variety of techniques. Tuman et al.[345] randomized LEVBG and AAA patients to receive epidural supplemented general anesthesia followed by postoperative epidural analgesia or general anesthesia followed by on-demand parenteral narcotics. The anesthetic management in each group was apparently reasonably protocolized, although few management details were given. Tuman et al.[345] found somewhat higher cardiac morbidity in the general group, but the difference was much less dramatic than in Yeager et al.[363] The most remarkable outcome was a larger number of reoperations for inadequate lower extremity flow in the general anesthesia group (20%). Tuman was able to offer a mechanism for this morbidity by observing (using thromboeslatography) a perioperative hypercoagulability in the general anesthesia group not seen in the regional anesthesia group. It has been long believed, with some hard data, that regional blockade with local agents blunts or ablates certain components of the surgical stress response. It is teleologically tenable to view procoagulant activity as an appropriate adaptation to tissue injury (surgery) which, in turn, is potentially detrimental in the setting of vascular stenotic lesions (to heart or legs). Establishing the ability of regional anesthesia to attenuate this phenomenon would be significant.

Caution is warranted in the attribution of prevention of hypercoagulability to the reduced revascularization rates because other possibilities include sympathetic blockade or other aspects of management. Christopherson et al.[58] conducted a randomized trial, called the Perioperative Ischemia Randomized Anesthesia Trial (PIRAT), of 100 patients undergoing LEVBG. Protocols for care in each group were carefully designed to yield optimal outcome. Postoperative analgesia included epidural fentanyl in the regional group and IV patient-controlled analgesia (PCA) in the general group. Cardiac morbidity and mortality in each group was low, and the revascularization rate was high in the general anesthetic group. Rosenfeld et al.[292] using patients from the PIRAT study, reported an increase in plasminogen activator inhibitor (PA I-1) in the general patients but not the regional patients on the morning after surgery (Fig. 71-7). This finding confirms the hypercoagulable state found by Tuman and coworkers postoperatively in the general anesthesia group as well as the ability of regional anesthesia and analgesia to prevent the phenomenon. Also reporting from the PIRAT study, Breslow[43] showed norepinephrine levels to rise at the end of surgery in the general, but not the regional, group and remain elevated through the postoperative period. Clearly, in this study as designed, regional anesthesia/analgesia was effective in blocking the stress response after surgery.

Bode et al.[39] conducted a randomized trial considerably larger than the previous studies. They found low values of cardiac morbidity and mortality and low revascularization rates in both groups. Of note, unlike the previous reports, Bode's methods called for PA catheterization in all patients and prolonged intensive care management. This permitted aggressive optimization of hemodynamic status and probably contributed to the excellent results which were similar in both groups. This methodology would add a very significant cost to LEVBG, if widely adopted.

To summarize the results of published investigations at this time: regional anesthesia may have stress ablation properties which confer the best outcome with the most conservative use of resources. On the other hand, general anesthesia may be quite safely employed with sufficient attention to detail throughout the perioperative period.

ANEURYSMS

Pathophysiology

Aneurysms are arterial expansions that occur as the vascular wall becomes weakened from atherosclerosis or other degenerative processes. The infrarenal abdominal aorta is the most common aneurysmal site, but significant lesions also occur in the iliac, femoral, popliteal, renal, splenic, and carotid arteries. The natural progression of untreated AAAs is expansion and eventual rupture. Laplace's law states that the tension (T) sustained by a vessel wall due to blood pressure (P) is directly proportional to the vessel radius (R) as given by the relationship $T \propto P \times R$.

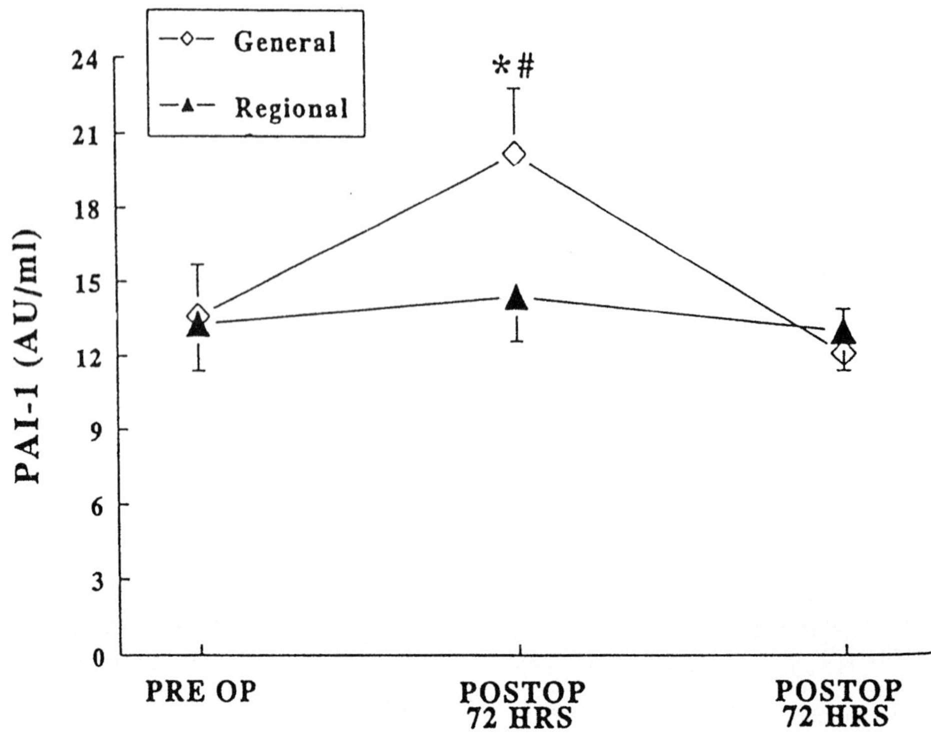

Fig. 71-7. Plasminogen activator inhibitor-1 levels in activity units/milliliter for general and regional anesthesia groups over time. Values are mean ± SEM. #*p*, 0.001 compared to preoperative and 72 h. **p* = 0.05 general anesthesia (GA) compared to regional anesthesia (RA). (From Rosenfeld BA, Beattie C, Christopherson R, et al: The effects of different anesthetic regimens on fibrinolysis and the development of postoperative arterial thrombosis, *Anesthesiology* 79(3):438, 1993.)

Thus the tension is ever increasing (with expansion) as the smooth muscle, collagen, and elastin are ever weakening. The mean radial expansion rate has been estimated at 4 mm/year by sequential ultrasound, although the individual rate varies widely. In general, aneurysm rupture rate corresponds to size. A 5-cm AAA has an annual incidence of rupture of slightly over 4%, whereas the annual risk at 7 cm exceeds 19%, and may exceed 50% at 5 years.[75,130,338]

Because multiple reviews of elective surgical repair for AAA have reported an average operative mortality of about 3.5%,[70,338] the yearly incidence of rupture exceeds the elective surgical mortality when an infrarenal aortic aneurysm approaches 5 cm in diameter. Therefore, the issue of operative timing becomes crucial. The overall mortality of patients with ruptured AAAs is probably 70% to 80%.[338] In patients with increased operative risk due to recent MI, CHF, severe pulmonary insufficiency, renal failure, or age greater than 80 years, Bernstein and Chan[30] suggested individualized management based on AAA size and expansion rates. Their algorithm, which resulted in a combined mortality of only 4% from elective aneurysm surgery and aneurysm rupture, followed patients with ultrasound or computed tomography (CT) scans at 3-month intervals and used a maximum diameter greater than 6 cm, expansion rate greater than 0.4 cm/year, or the development of symptoms as the basis on which to recommend surgical intervention.

Other aneurysms involve the thoracoabdominal aorta, popliteal artery, renal artery, splenic artery, and extracranial carotid artery.[369] Thoracoabdominal aneurysms involve the thoracic and abdominal aorta together. Although the infrarenal portion may exhibit typical atherosclerosis, the suprarenal aorta often shows degenerative changes of the media called mucoid degeneration, myxomatous degeneration, or cystic medial necrosis.[73]

The etiology of the medial degeneration has not been determined. True thoracoabdominal aortic aneurysms have a single-enlarging lumen in contrast to aortic dissection, where the increased aortic diameter is due to a second flow channel.

Monitoring

Aortic aneurysm and aorto-occlusive disease

All patients undergoing aortic surgery should have continuous intravascular monitoring of arterial pressure. As with other types of surgery, the first site considered is the radial artery of the arm with the highest pressure, determined by cuff. Reasons for choosing other sites include inadequate collateral flow to the hand (Allen's test), poor radial pulsations due to previous trauma or proximal vascular disease, and site of cross-clamping above the left subclavian. The axillary artery offers an excellent alternative. Cannulation of the axillary artery is usually performed with the Seldinger technique and an 18- or 20-gauge pediatric CVP catheter. The procedure is quite straightforward and should be performed more commonly.[50] Caution is warranted in flushing an axillary artery catheter because the tip is rather more proximate to the carotid and vertebral system, and air or particulate matter could enter these vessels.

In addition to radial or axillary pressure monitoring, a femoral arterial cannula should be strongly considered in thoracic or thoracoabdominal aneurysm surgery where shunt or bypass procedures are employed. Knowledge of arterial pressure distal to the cross-clamp permits a considerably more rational approach to hemodynamic manipulations during surgery.

Although some clinicians advocate the use of PA catheters in all patients undergoing an aortic cross-clamp procedure,[365] others moderate their use based on the cross-clamp level and extent of ancillary diseases. A rational approach is to use a PA catheter in those cases requiring a suprarenal (or above) cross-clamp and reserve its use in infrarenal aneurysms and occlusive disease to those individuals with significant cardiac, renal, or pulmonary pathology.[88,203] Certainly the rapid, large changes in loading conditions that occur during the procedure and problems of fluid mobilization and renal dysfunction postoperatively combine to make PA catheterization helpful in all but the healthiest patient having a minimal procedure.[52,90,283,313] This endorsement presumes that the venous cannulation and balloon flotation are initiated safely; the pressure transducers are properly leveled, zeroed, and calibrated; thermodilution cardiac outputs are technically sound; calculated and measured parameters are interpreted correctly; and therapeutic interventions reflect appropriate understanding of physiology and pharmacology. If any one of these requisites is missing, PA catheterization is best omitted.[179] Recent modifications of the PA catheter include the ability to continuously measure mixed venous oxygen saturation and, most recently, estimate right ventricular EF and right ventricular end-diastolic volume.[178] These features are potentially valuable in selected cases. Mixed venous saturation is responsive to changes in metabolic rate at constant cardiac output or to changes in cardiac output at constant metabolic rate. Both cardiac output and metabolic rate can fluctuate widely during aneurysm surgery (see section on physiology of aortic cross-clamping). Frequent cardiac output determinations diminish the theoretic value of continuous saturation determination. The right ventricular EF catheter may prove useful in right ventricular failure and/or pulmonary hypertension as a guide to therapy or as a signal of deterioration.[178] This issue remains to be addressed.

Advances in echocardiography, especially the development of two-dimensional probes designed for use in the esophagus, have resulted in progressively increasing the popularity of this monitoring modality during anesthesia and surgery. Left ventricular wall motion abnormalities and abnormal systolic thickening may occur before changes in ST-segment morphology when ischemia is present.[88,320] Smith et al.[320] showed that echocardiography detected myocardial ischemia in 24 of 50 patients requiring cardiovascular surgery, whereas standard ECG monitoring detected only six. Disadvantages of TEE include difficulties in online assessment of subtle changes in the video image. Attention may be diverted away from the patient. The devices are costly, and special technical support and education are necessary.[88,206] Transesophageal echocardiography may prove particularly useful in patients undergoing supraceliac cross-clamping procedures as suggested by Roizen.[290]

Procedures that require aortic cross-clamping above the celiac axis or more cephalad incur a progressively higher risk of major neurologic sequelae.[193,216] The incidence of paraplegia ranges from less than 1% for intrarenal abdominal aneurysms to 40% in thoracic aneurysms.[71,72,335]

Assessment of intraoperative spinal cord ischemia using SEP and motor-evoked potentials (MEP) are promising techniques.[11,77,78,98,208,259,346] Interventions to minimize spinal cord ischemia include the drainage of cerebrospinal fluid (CSF) and continuous measurement of CSF pressure.[172,243] This necessitates placement of a subarachnoid catheter with appropriate measures instituted to ensure sterility and prevention of inadvertent drug injection into the intrathecal space.

Blood loss during aneurysm surgery is highly variable, ranging from less than two units for an uncomplicated infrarenal aneurysm or aortoiliac repair to massive amounts for a difficult thoracoabdominal aneurysm.[262,322] IV access for the rapid administration of large blood volumes is necessary. At least two well-running, large-bore peripheral IV cannulae (16- or 14-gauge) should be placed. For supraceliac cross-clamps or other potentially high blood loss procedures such as reoperation or graft removal, even larger-bore access should be established. Two 8.5-French catheter sheaths placed centrally or at the antecubital fossa are useful when using a rapid transfusion system, which can deliver up to 1500 ml/min of warmed fluids. This device, which was originally manufactured for use in liver transplantation, is well designed and requires minimal training for its use.[300]

Blood-scavenging techniques for autotranfusion have proved useful in AAA repair. The equipment is expensive and requires a certain minimal level of use to be cost effective.[64] Major vascular surgery offers the best opportunity for appropriate employment of blood-scavenging units.[156] Although no randomized, prospective studies of efficacy have been reported, it is obvious that the use of these devices would decrease the exposure to multiple donors. One study[156] showed a 25% to 57% reduction in the number of different donors for patients having vascular procedures.

Some degree of hypothermia is commonly observed in patients undergoing aneurysm surgery.[206] This is caused by the exposure of abdominal contents, the administration of large amounts of fluid, and disturbances in thermoregulatory mechanism caused by anesthesia. All IV fluids, including those given during induction, should be administered through warming devices. Warming blankets are routinely used in some centers.[206] A heated vaporizer should be connected to the breathing circuit, and the room temperature set as high as possible commensurate with reasonable comfort for the surgical personnel. Frank et al.[122] have demonstrated that patients over 65 years of age receiving general anesthetics are more likely to develop inadvertent hypothermia. A warm ambient temperature (24° C), however, was shown to reduce intraoperative heat loss in this study.

PHYSIOLOGY OF AORTIC CROSS-CLAMPING

The extraordinary aspects of anesthetic management in patients having aneurysm and occlusive repair relate to application and release of the aortic clamp.

The hemodynamic and metabolic alterations caused by acute interruption of aortic blood flow have been the subject of both animal and human investigations for many years.[10,49,132,313,327] Features of particular relevance to anesthetic management include changes in arterial blood pressure, cardiac function, myocardial perfusion, and acid-base status, as well as tissue integrity of the kidneys, viscera, and spinal cord. Conflicting findings have been obtained and likely reflect species variation, patient characteristics, degree of collateralization, location of the cross-clamp, baseline cardiac function, type of anesthesia, the use and type of vasodilators, and the presence or absence of CAD. In this section, we review the classic and conflicting findings from the literature and present plausibility arguments for making rational clinical decisions.

Blood Pressure

The degree of hypertension caused by application of an aortic cross-clamp depends on the location of the clamp, the degree of collateralization, and the preocclusion aortic flow. Thus, an infrarenal clamp in a patient with aortic occlusive disease may cause virtually no elevation in the blood pressure because preclamp flow was nil. Also, aortic clamping above a thoracic coarctation may result in no pressure change proximal (or distal) to the clamp because of fully developed collateral flow. In the case of AAA repair, runoff is usually good and collateralization minimal, and therefore, an increase in blood pressure may be expected, the magnitude of which is a direct function of clamp proximity to the heart. Clamping below the renal arteries is the most common clinical circumstance and usually produces only a small increase in blood pressure,[313] but supraceliac occlusion can result in prodigious hypertension.[49] The following discussion analyzes blood pressure changes caused by aortic cross-clamping from a holistic perspective that accounts for changes in venous return and cardiac output.

Venous Return and Cardiac Output

Although it may seem intuitive that cardiac output should decrease with acute occlusion of a major arterial conduit caused by an increase in resistance, there are levels of physiologic complexity involving reflex mechanisms, venous return, and left heart function that modify this expectation.[132] For example, placement of the cross-clamp is important. If the clamp is placed in the supraceliac region, evidence has suggested that venous return and cardiac output actually increase. This result is probably due to blood volume redistribution and splanchnic venous collapse.[324] However, an infrarenal cross-clamp may redistribute blood volume back to the splanchnic bed, decrease preload and cause cardiac output to fall.[130] Because these same issues bear on hemodynamic findings of ventricular preload and pump function, it is well to consider them now. A simple thought experiment will illustrate the basic physical concepts.

Fig. 71-8, condition *A,* shows an idealized schematic of the heart and circulation, the latter split into two parallel vascular beds, each carrying one half of the cardiac output, approximately representing the body above and below the diaphragm. In the normal situation (condition *A*), we assume a total cardiac output of 6 l/min with a filling pressure of 4 mm Hg, a mean arterial pressure of 100 mm Hg, and a calculated systemic vascular resistance (SVR) of 16 peripheral resistance units (PRUs). Now suppose that *both* the arterial outflow and the venous return serving the lower circulation were simultaneously occluded as shown in Figure 71-8, condition *B*. The cardiac output would immediately fall by one half because half of the venous return has been eliminated. Meanwhile, the arterial bed has only half the number of vessels to accept flow, and its resistance to flow will double. The net result of half the cardiac output flowing into twice the resistance is an unchanged blood pressure. Notice, in this scenario, the stroke volume and stroke work are also halved, whereas the effect on filling pressure would be determined by the diastolic and systolic characteristics of the heart. Presumably, the filling pressure would decrease because the ventricle is pumping less blood. This simplified model does not account for the pulmonary circulation or neural reflexes (extrinsic or intrinsic), but it is valuable in illustrating a major point about directional changes in hemodynamic parameters during aortic cross-clamping—by no means do such changes relate solely to the effect of "afterload" on ventricular ejection. In fact, it is probable that "preload" or venous return dominates in many circumstances.[187] In condition *B,* there is no rational concern regarding the decrease in stroke volume and stroke work, because these are clearly appropriate for the remaining tissue (half the original) to be perfused.[132] We shall return to this topic when discussing strategies for hemodynamic control during aortic cross-clamping in the absence of venous occlusion.

The stable hemodynamic situation of condition *B* is not achieved in condition *C* where only venous return is occluded. Clinically, this circumstance arises during orthotopic liver transplantation when performed without venous extracorporeal shunts and during other operations involving the inferior vena cava.[190] In condition *C* in Fig. 71-8, cardiac

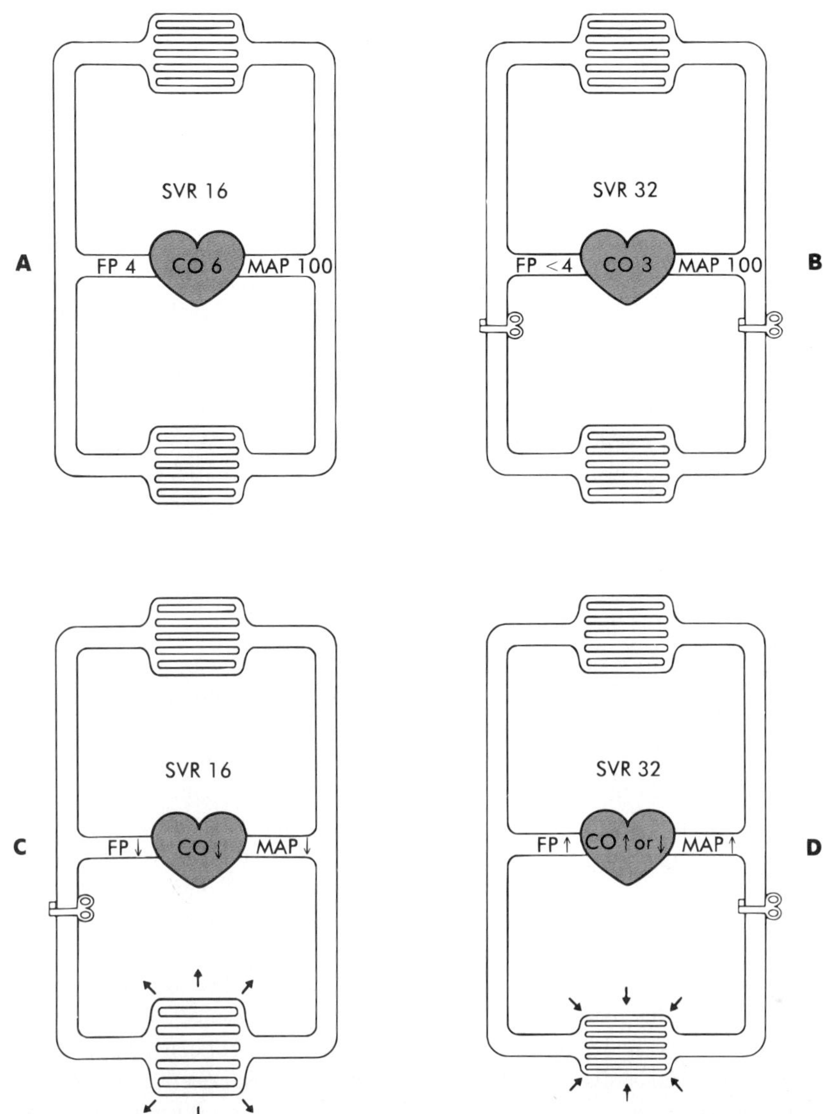

Fig. 71-8. Simplified schematic of the cardiovascular system. Upper and lower vascular beds represent organs and tissues above and below the diaphragm. Neither the pulmonary circulation nor reflex mechanisms are depicted. **A,** In the normal patient, filling pressure (*FP*) is 4 mm Hg, cardiac output (*CO*) is 6 l/min, mean arterial pressure (*MAP*) is 100 mm Hg, and the computed systemic vascular resistance (*SVR*) is 16 peripheral vascular units (PRUs). **B,** Simultaneous clamping of both the aorta and the vena cava (at the diaphragm) causes a 50% reduction in cardiac output because of the drop in venous return. However, SVR exactly doubles (since half the arterial bed is excluded) and the blood pressure remains unchanged. **C,** Vena caval occlusion alone immediately drops venous return by half. Additionally, the capacitive vasculature will continue to sequester blood, further depleting above-clamp circulation. **D,** Aortic occlusion alone may increase or decrease cardiac output although MAP will rise in either case (see text for discussion of alternatives.)

output is decreased by 50% and because SVR is initially unchanged, blood pressure falls. Moreover, blood is sequestered in the capacitance vessels (principally the splanchnic viscera) below the venous clamp, further depleting the circulatory volume above the clamp. In vivo, venous collaterals may exist that partially decompress the below-clamp vasculature, but intravascular volume and/or pressor infusion is usually necessary to sustain an acceptable blood pressure.

Condition *D* in Fig. 71-8 represents a supraceliac aortic cross-clamp. Identical arguments apply to lower cross-clamps, although of course, the magnitude of changes will be different. Clearly, aortic occlusion in condition *D* causes an acute doubling of SVR, and because venous return and cardiac output are not immediately affected, unlike condition *B*, blood pressure must rise substantially. The only physiologic phenomenon preventing blood pressure from doubling would be an inability of the ventricle to eject its former stroke volume against this elevated systemic resistance, or perhaps immediate reflex feedback inhibition. Not only is venous return initially unimpeded, there also is evidence that it may be *increased* with clamp application. Some animal studies[324] and individual patients from clinical reports over the years have shown an increase in cardiac output after clamping the thoracic aorta.[16,49,327]

Several phenomenon may contribute to this observation. An "autotransfusion" of volume from the below-clamp vasculature discharges into the active circulation. Blood in the capacitance vasculature below the clamp may be thought of as having an initial pressure equal to the mean systemic pressure,[107] which is higher than the right atrial pressure and which constitutes the driving force for venous return. If arterial inflow stops at the time of aortic occlusion, the capacitance vessels below the clamp will continue to discharge its contents into the active circulation until its pressure is equal to the right atrial pressure (or intervening vascular waterfall) (Fig. 71-8, D). This constitutes an incremental volume infusion and should serve to temporarily maintain cardiac output if the ventricle was capable of such performance in the face of the elevated afterload. Clearly, the plausibility of this argument depends on maintenance of vascular tone below the clamp. If inhibition of arterial inflow continued, tissue anoxia could supervene, eventually causing relaxation of vascular tone and reuptake of volume.

Other mechanisms[133] have been suggested to explain an increase in cardiac output with thoracic aortic clamping, including an aortic-cardiac reflex,[270] which increases contractility, and elimination of slow time-constant vascular beds (splanchnic) from the circulation.[324,327] Conversely, an increase in aortic pressure should stimulate baroreceptors to depress heart rate, contractility, and vascular tone. Many previous studies have shown a decreased cardiac output with aortic occlusion, and this finding has come to represent the common understanding.[10,278,290,315] How is it possible to obtain such opposing results? Paradoxically, infrarenal and suprarenal cross-clamps eliminate fast time-constant vascular beds (lower extremities, kidneys) and thus could reduce cardiac output while higher thoracic clamps remove the slow time-constant visceral circulation as well, thereby tending to increase cardiac output. Neurohumoral effects also play a role. Gelman et al.[131] have shown increases in blood pressure and computed SVR occurring several minutes following application of a supraceliac aortic cross-clamp in animals. These changes were blunted by various antagonists of adrenoreceptors and angiotensin. Fig. 71-9 summarizes the issues surrounding blood volume distribution during application of supra- and infraceliac cross-clamps.[130]

Myocardial Effects

The effects of aortic cross-clamping on cardiac function and myocardial perfusion have been the subject of several investigations.[10,188,287,290] In the absence of any underlying disorder of contractility or coronary flow, the heart can generate and withstand very high arterial pressures. Although ventricular end-diastolic pressure increases in response to an elevated afterload (the "preload reserve mechanism"),[294] coronary perfusion pressure also increases, and dysfunction of pumping characteristics or myocardial ischemia does not occur in isolated ventricle experiments in healthy hearts (Kiichi Sagawa, personal communication). In practice, ventricular dilatation causing valve incompetence and elevated diastolic pressures promoting pulmonary edema are the natural consequences of extreme left ventricular overload.[177] Obviously, serious deterioration of pump function could be produced if a high afterload is superimposed on a myocardium depressed by cardiomyopathic processes. Moreover, myocardial ischemia itself could be precipitated during clamping, leading to regional wall motion abnormalities or infarction, if afterload elevation occurs in the presence of coronary artery stenosis.[10,47,290] The presumed mechanism for this ischemia is subendocardial hypoperfusion caused by the high intercavitary pressures during diastole and systole, in conjunction with impaired inflow due to stenotic coronary lesions.

One investigation has reported the onset or worsening of regional wall motion abnormalities (by TEE) during aortic occlusion, which did not resolve with moderation of the loading conditions using vasodilators, fluids, and inhalational agents.[290] Unfortunately, the systemic arterial blood pressure and pulmonary capillary wedge pressures in this investigation were only reported as being maintained within a "normal range." Thus, it is unknown whether the apparent ischemic changes would have been alleviated by actually returning loading conditions to their preclamp state. With respect to normalization of loading conditions, it seems reasonable to propose that pharmacologic and mechanical interventions that control hypertension by preload reduction would be most effective in minimizing both dysfunction and ischemia of the left ventricle. End-diastolic volume and thus wall stress are lower in comparison with the afterload-reducing methods, provided the same arterial blood pressure is achieved.

It is quite possible that aortic occlusion could have effects on ventricular function even if mean arterial pressure and computed SVR were normalized to baseline. The blood pressure wave form, as observed in the ascending aorta, is created by characteristics of ventricular ejection and vascular resistance and compliance, as well as by pressure waves returning retrograde from major reflecting sites in the periphery. If sufficiently delayed, reflected waves may appear in diastole, thus augmenting myocardial perfusion. Return during systole, however, would add to wall stress during ejection and increase myocardial oxygen demand.[209] By moving the major reflecting site closer to the heart, aortic cross-clamping could thus cause myocardial dysfunction in the face of a mean aortic pressure normalized by therapy. Roizen et al.[290] found new and worsening wall motion abnormalities more frequently during supraceliac occlusion than with supra- or infrarenal occlusion.

Assessment of myocardial function during the presence of an aortic cross-clamp using the usual measured and de-

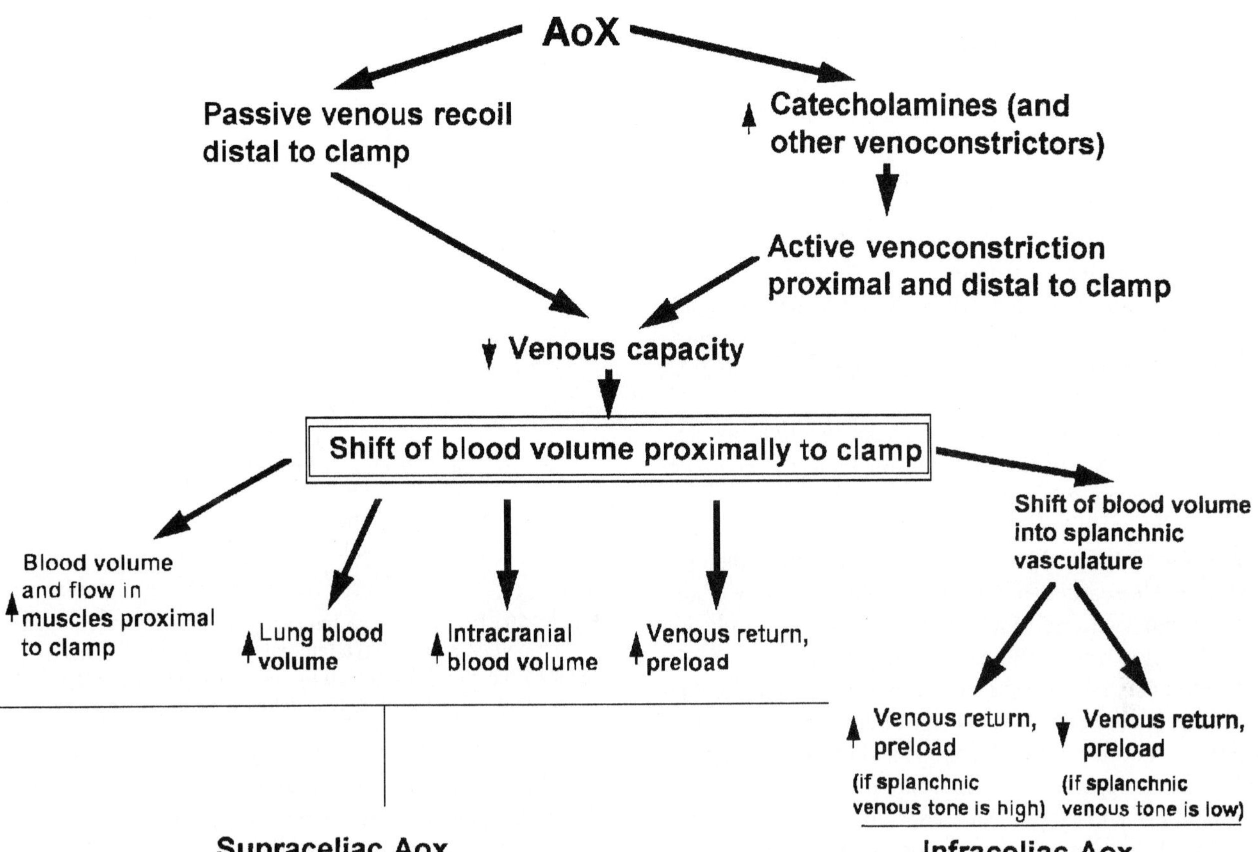

Fig. 71-9. Blood volume redistribution during aortic cross-clamping. This scheme depicts the reason for the decrease in venous capacity, which results in blood volume redistribution from the vasculature distal to aortic occlusion to the vasculature proximal to aortic occlusion. If the aorta is occluded above the splanchnic system, the blood volume travels to the heart, increasing preload and blood volume in all organs and tissues proximal to the clamp. However, if the aorta is occluded below the splanchnic system, blood volume may shift into the splanchnic system or into the vasculature of other tissues proximal to the clamp. The distribution of this blood volume between the splanchnic nonsplanchnic vasculature determines changes in preload. AoX—aortic cross-clamping; ↑ and ↓—increase and decrease, respectively. Reproduced with permission. (From Gelman S: The pathophysiology of aortic cross-clamping and unclamping, *Anesthesiology* 82(4):1029, 1995.)

rived hemodynamic parameters is problematic. If maneuvers are employed that reduce preload, the stroke work and cardiac index are lowered in proportion to the decrease in metabolizing tissue available to the circulation above the cross-clamp.[132] Conversely, afterload-reducing methods may allow an increase in pump function indices—a change that is not necessarily desirable. Knowledge of the expected magnitude of metabolic depression along with insight into the physiologic and pharmacologic mechanisms of the chosen therapy may allow the clinician to differentiate between appropriate and pathologic reductions in pump function. TEE seems most likely to allow accurate evaluation of myocardial function in these potentially confusing circumstances.

Therapeutic Strategies

Most clinicians have viewed the physiologic problem of aortic cross-clamping to be a consequence of increased left ventricular afterload and have proposed interventions that reverse this effect. Vasodilators, notably sodium nitroprusside, are routinely used to control hypertension.[311,312] For thoracic cross-clamps, passive or active shunts (from proximal to distal aorta) have been advocated to reduce afterload.

Arteriolar dilation in vessels supplying organs proximal to the clamp can, in most circumstances, cause them to accommodate a sufficient increase in blood flow to maintain blood pressure within an acceptable range. Obviously, this produces a relative overperfusion of the affected organs. Problems with this method include: (1) partial failure (e.g., inability to adequately control pressure); (2) requirement for high doses of sodium nitroprusside; and (3) exceedingly low pressures in the circulation distal to the lowest clamp. The latter issue is addressed later in this chapter.

Alternate strategies are suggested by the previous discussion on venous return. During the period of cross-clamp, that portion of the body supplied by the occluded arterial flow is unavailable for oxidative metabolism. Thus, the heart does not need to maintain its preclamp output, and interventions that would reduce output seem appropriate.[132] Simultaneous blockage of proportional venous return would solve the problem exactly (condition *B* in Fig. 71-8), and although difficult, the procedure has been attempted.[187] **Venodilation with nitroglycerine, sufficient to lower filling pressure and reduce cardiac output, appears to be the most attractive alternative.** A moderate level of systemic intravascular volume depletion would be synergistic in this regard, but is not recommended, because declamping hypotension must be anticipated and minimized by maintenance of intravascular volume.

Nitroglycerin is already routinely used by clinicians during aortic surgery, but the rationale for its use is generally given as afterload reduction or coronary vasodilation.[176,368]

Although preload reduction with nitroglycerine alone is adequate for infrarenal and suprarenal clamp sites, the drug may not reduce cardiac output sufficiently to achieve a suitable proximal arterial pressure during aortic occlusion above the celiac axis.[203] Note that a full 50% decrease in cardiac output may be necessary. Use of agents that reduce contractility might be effective, but legitimate concerns exist regarding left ventricular decompensation or dysfunction when the inotropic state is reduced in the setting of increased afterload. The logical compromise is to use a combination of low-dose nitroprusside along with nitroglycerine, as a titratable technique to control pressure, acknowledging the dual issues of preload and afterload.[203] Isoflurane, which mildly depresses contractility and causes vasodilatation of both resistance and capacitive vessels, has been safely used for anesthesia and blood pressure control in patients with good myocardial function undergoing thoracic aneurysm repair.[137]

Preload reduction is the underlying principle employed to control cross-clamp hypertension when using partial cardiopulmonary bypass during thoracic aneurysm repair. This method uses femoral venous inflow by gravity to a reservoir/oxygenator, and roller-pump-generated outflow to a femoral artery, thus perfusing retrograde vasculature below the most distal clamp (femoral-femoral bypass, Fig. 71-10). Hypertension caused by clamp application is quickly resolved by taking up volume into the venous reservoir, which reduces venous return to the heart and lowers cardiac output.[194]

Bypass and shunting techniques that divert flow from the left atrium, left ventricle, or proximal aorta to the aorta distal to the lowest clamp have been used to blunt the effects of cross-clamping.[57] Because these methods are not devoid of complications, they are usually reserved for surgery that necessitates thoracic aortic clamping. Femoral-femoral bypass, mentioned previously, suffers from the need for full systemic anticoagulation. The Gott shunt removes the coagulation problem by using a heparin-impregnated, inert, woven graft[145] introduced into either the apex of the left ventricle or the proximal aorta, which passively transfers

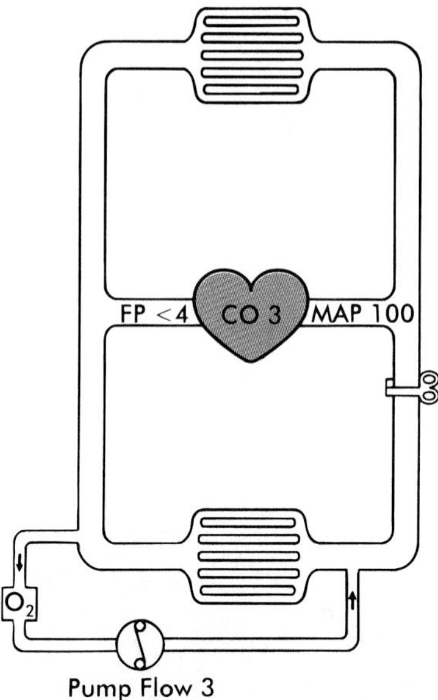

Fig. 71-10. Partial cardiopulmonary bypass using inferior vena caval blood obtained from a femoral venous cannula. After oxygenation the blood is returned by roller pump to the femoral artery, thereby perfusing organs below the aortic clamp.

blood to an insertion site in the lower aorta. Unfortunately, size constraints limit flow and adjustment during surgery is not possible. Recently, interest has been renewed in shunting techniques that use an in-line centrifugal pump (Biomedicus; Medtronic, Eden Prairie, MN) to augment flow[64,175,267] (Fig. 71-11, *A* and *B*). This pump was originally designed as a left ventricular assist device or artificial heart and has the desirable characteristics of atraumatic blood handling, lack of stasis, and low reactivity with elements of the coagulation system. The device allows choice of a low-pressure source for shunt flow, notably the fully oxygenated pulmonary venous or left atrial blood (Fig. 71-11, *B*). Because the pump speed is adjustable, flow may be changed to suit hemodynamic and metabolic needs.

The physiologic principle by which bypass and shunt methods achieve blood pressure control differs according to type. Femoral-femoral bypass and left atrial shunts reduce venous return to the left ventricle and therefore lower its preload, while left ventricular and aortic shunts reduce afterload, in effect presenting a larger cross-sectional area to ventricular ejection.

Metabolic Changes

Two fundamental interconnected metabolic effects characterize aortic cross-clamping: (1) lowered total-body oxidative metabolism (VO_2); and (2) conversion to anaerobic metabolism of the hypoperfused body mass distal to the clamp. Gelman et al.[132] showed that application of an infrarenal cross-clamp caused a 16% decrease in VO_2, whereas other studies have shown that supraceliac cross-clamping causes 55% reduction[305] (Fig. 71-12). Presumably, a suprarenal occlusion would cause a reduction similar to

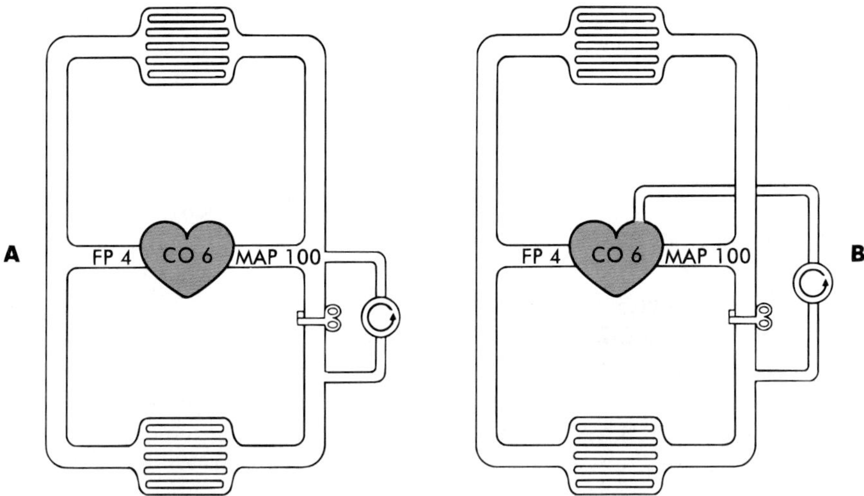

Fig. 71-11. Augmented shunting schemes to "unload" the heart and perfuse below-clamp organs. **A,** Source cannula in the aorta (descending) unloads heart by reducing afterload. **B,** Source cannula in the left atrium unloads heart by reducing left ventricular preload.

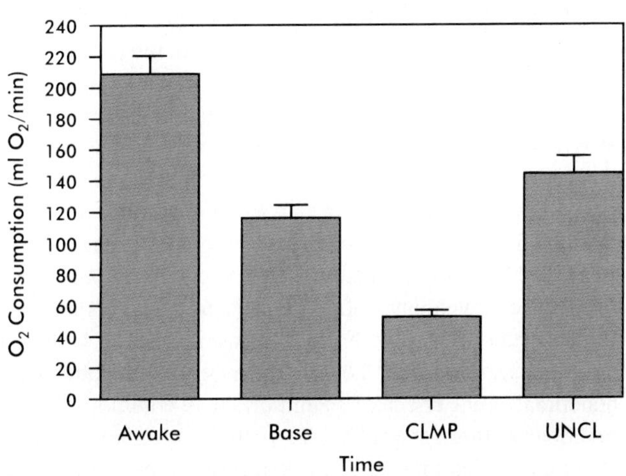

Fig. 71-12. Total-body oxygen consumption (ml O_2/min) in a group of patients undergoing supraceliac aortic cross-clamping. *Awake,* preoperative measurement; base, just before clamping; *CLMP,* during cross-clamping; *UNCL,* within 5 minutes of clamp release. CLMP is only 55% of base value. (From Schurlknight S, Beattie C, O'Rourke K: Metabolic changes during high aortic cross-clamp surgery. Abstracts of the Eighth Annual Meeting of the Society of Cardiovascular Anesthesiologists, p. 72, 1986.)

the infrarenal value because the kidneys do not consume oxygen in proportion to their flow.

The effects of aortic cross-clamping on mixed venous oxygen saturation and partial pressure depend on the therapeutic modalities used to control blood pressure. If arteriolar dilatation is the dominant therapy, then aerobically functioning tissue will be overperfused, its extraction will decrease, and the saturation and partial pressure of oxygen of mixed venous blood will increase substantially. Conversely, preload reduction techniques maintain both oxygen extraction ratio and mixed venous saturation at approximately their preclamp values.

Table 71-1 Single patient data-thoracoabdominal aneurysm repair

	Awake	Post-induction	Aortic cross-clamp	Aortic cross-clamp off
Pao_2 (mm Hg)	61	393	360	168
Pvo_2 (mm Hg)	34	2.6	111	65
A-Vo_2 content (ml O_2/100 ml)	4.8	2.6	0.8	2.1
Vo_2 (ml o_2/min)	216	92	33	71
DIS o_2 (%)	3.8	45	100	24

Table 71-1 shows the partial pressure of oxygen in the arterial (Pao_2) and venous blood (Pvo_2), the cardiac output, arteriovenous oxygen content difference (A-Vo_2), and total body oxygen consumption (Vo_2) for a patient undergoing repair of a thoracic aneurysm. The values are given preoperatively while the patient is breathing room air, after induction of general anesthesia, while the thoracic aorta is cross-clamped, and with unclamping. Note that Vo_2 is much lower after induction, a consistently observed phenomenon caused by both direct metabolic depressant effects of the anesthetic agents and the diminution of central autonomic control. Upon application of the cross-clamp, Vo_2 decreases by 57% compared with preclamp values. Meanwhile, the delivery of 100% O_2 and maintenance (or increase) of cardiac output by nitroprusside combine with the lower Vo_2 to yield a remarkable mixed venous Po_2 of 111 mm Hg—that is, the hemoglobin returning to the heart is fully saturated. This implies that the overall oxygen needs of the aerobically metabolizing tissue (above the clamp) are being met by dissolved oxygen.

Figure 71-13 shows $Paco_2$, lactate, Hco_3^-, and pH at selected times for 13 patients undergoing repair of an AAA which necessitated cross-clamping just above the celiac axis.

Anaerobic metabolism by tissue below the aortic cross-clamp produces lactic acid and a progressive rise in blood lactate (Fig. 71-13) presumably reaching the proximal circulation by collaterals. For infrarenal cross-clamps, the buildup in systemic lactate during occlusion, as well as its release with unclamping, is noticeable but rarely clinically significant.[313] Exceptions to this occur with grossly prolonged ischemic times.

Cross-clamps above the celiac axis not only produce a larger anaerobically functioning tissue mass but also, by excluding the liver and kidneys, greatly attenuate the elimination of lactate. Lactate concentration rises promptly and progressively during high thoracic cross-clamps.[268] The metabolic acidosis thus created may deserve attention, and some authors have recommended a continuous infusion of bicarbonate during the clamping period.[15] Paradoxically, arterial blood samples taken during the cross-clamp period may not show changes in pH. If normocarbia was established before aortic occlusion, then maintenance of the same minute-ventilation after clamping will produce a relative hyperventilation because CO_2 production has substantially diminished. This respiratory alkalosis, which is reflected by hypocarbia (Fig. 71-13) can so closely balance the metabolic acidosis, that pH will be unchanged. Release of the cross-clamp will unmask the base deficit, and a precipitous decrease in pH will be observed.[268]

Ischemic organ damage during the period of aortic occlusion is always of concern, and maintenance of variable degrees of below-clamp flow is addressed in two ways. First, studies have shown that **the distal aorta actually maintains some pressure during cross-clamp because of arterial collaterals.**[137] These investigations conclude that (1) the small flow created by this pressure could contribute to organ protection; (2) the use of nitroprusside lowers the distal aortic pressure considerably, and therefore; (3) therapy other than nitroprusside (e.g., isoflurane) should be used to control blood pressure.[137] Second, the shunting and bypass techniques previously discussed for their control of ventricular loading also maintain below-clamp flow and aerobic metabolism.

This is accomplished by the passive flow through a Gott-type shunt or by flow adjustment when using femoral-femoral bypass or the Biomedicus centrifugal pump to augment shunt flow.[64] Although appropriate flow requirements have not been established, clearly this determination depends on the body mass to be perfused. By far, the most common use of shunting methods is for thoracic aneurysm repair or during the thoracic anastomosis of thoracoabdominal aneurysm repair. Because approximately 50% of total cardiac output goes to organs below the diaphragm,[151] some clinicians routinely set pump flow to 2 to 3 l/min. Some clinicians monitor below-clamp pressure via a femoral arterial cannula and titrate flow to achieve a suitable pressure above and below the clamps. Although either technique will probably suffice for visceral organ protection, maintenance of spinal cord viability is quite another matter and is the subject of a later section. The effectiveness of shunting may be grossly assessed by systemic lactate levels that increase by only half compared with similar operations without shunts (1990, B Drenger, unpublished data). **It is important to note that shunt and bypass procedures are not universally employed.** Most studies have shown no improvement in outcome using these methods compared with "clamp-and-sew" techniques, provided occlusion times are minimized (< 30 min).[69,222]

Renal Protection

Preservation of renal function is a primary concern during aortic aneurysm surgery. Clearly, procedures that require cross-clamping of the aorta above the renal arteries will result in a temporary period of ischemia, with the potential for inducing some degree of renal failure. In animal experiments, preischemia administration of mannitol exerts a protective effect on renal function.[2] Because the mechanisms that produce acute tubular necrosis (ATN) are complex,[255] it is not surprising that controversy exists regarding the exact manner in which mannitol or other agents might prevent ATN.[46,128] It is possible that mannitol exerts its protective effect by the scavenging of free radicals produced upon reperfusion of the kidney with cross-clamp release.[275] Although no human studies have been performed that demonstrate a beneficial renal effect of mannitol,[6] it is common clinical practice to administer 12.5 g/70 kg 10 to 15 minutes before aortic cross-clamping.[288] The use of furosemide is more controversial. Although a protective effect for furosemide has not been established per se, it is generally believed that this agent may result in a conversion of low output–to–high output renal failure, the latter being much easier to manage in the postoperative period. Thus, some clinicians administer the drug routinely for high cross-clamp cases.[15] When diuretics are used, increased fluid requirements and hypokalemia should be anticipated throughout the perioperative period. For the more common infrarenal aneurysms, where cross-clamp application would not seem to impede renal perfusion, renal vascular resistance increases and renal blood flow decreases.[2,128,130] The distribution of renal blood flow is altered during infrarenal aortic cross-clamping, and this phenomenon can result in impairment of function.[128] Renal blood flow is reduced not only during cross-clamp, but post–cross-clamp blood flow does not immediately return to normal.[130] All of these factors combine to increase the risk of postoperative renal dysfunction. Patients with preoperative renal insufficiency, elevated blood urea nitrogen (BUN), and increased creatinine are at increased risk of developing postoperative renal failure.[358]

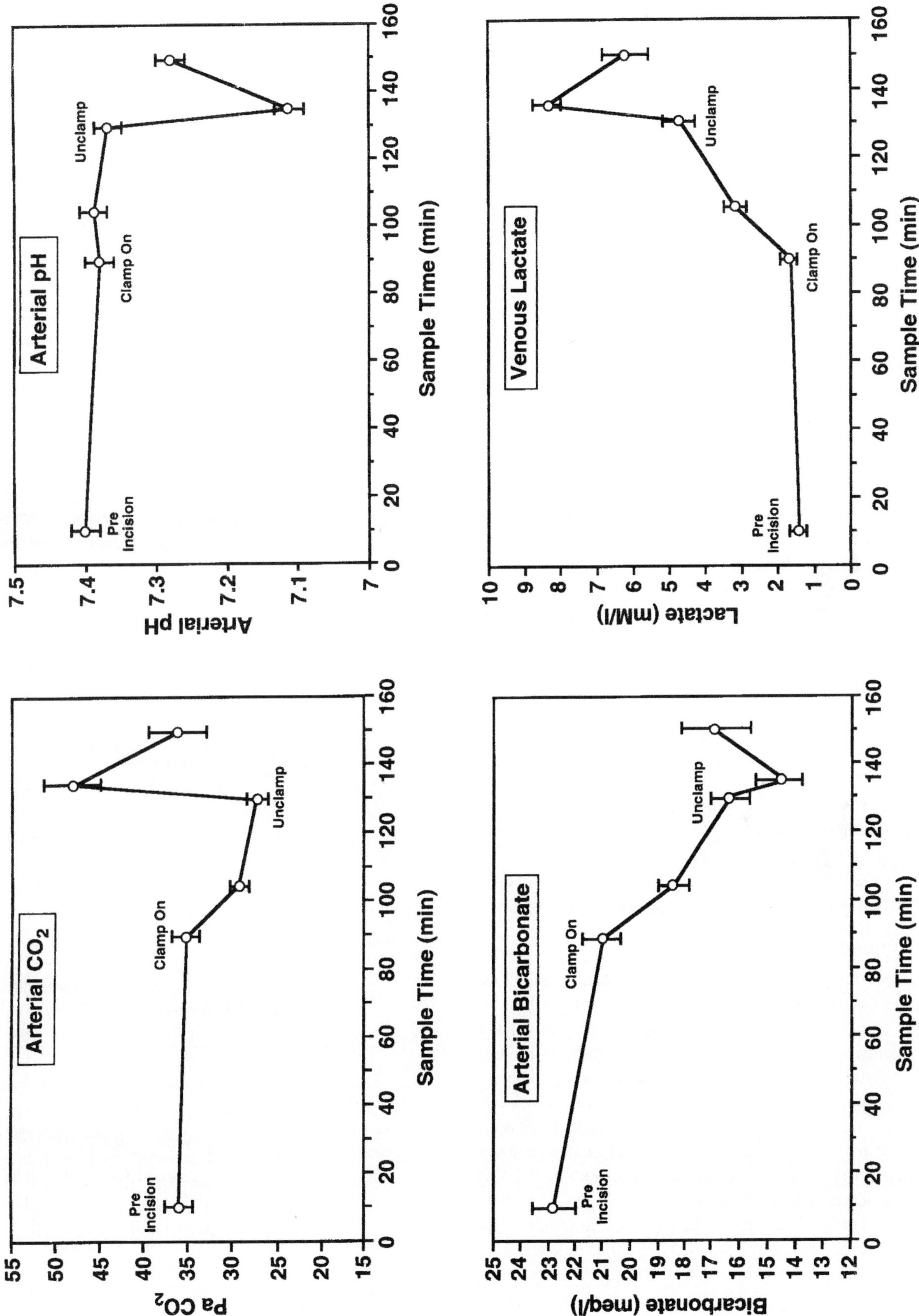

Fig. 71-13. Data from 13 patients undergoing aortic aneurysm repair necessitating supraceliac cross-clamping. *Preincision,* just before surgical incision. *Clamp On,* just prior to cross clamp. *Unclamp,* just before and just after clamp release. Other points are 15 minutes after clamping and 15 minutes after unclamping. Mean ± SEM. (From Beattie C, Unpublished data.)

Maintenance of adequate intravascular volume[358] and a short cross-clamp time, usually less than 30 minutes,[88] has been shown to be the most important factor in avoiding renal dysfunction postoperatively.[52] Many clinicians advocate the use of mannitol,[288] as well as "renal dose" dopamine (3 mcg/kg/min) to increase renal blood flow during aneurysm surgery,[365] especially if some element of renal dysfunction exists preoperatively. Again, clinical practice varies widely.

Spinal Cord Ischemia and Protection

Blood supply to the spinal cord is complex with a large "critical" radicular vessel, the artery radicularis magna (ARM), formed from a segmental intercostal or lumbar artery that supplies blood, from its entry point in the thoracic or lumbar region, to the caudal spinal cord.[10,330] The cord cephalad to the ARM is fed by other segmental vessels[210] but also by longitudinal arteries, notably the anterior spinal artery (ASA), descending from its origin in the brain stem.[331]

Aortic cross-clamping, which either incorporates the ARM between clamps or exposes it to hypoperfusion, may lead to paraplegia or paraparesis.[172] The origin is variable, but it is uncommon for the ARM to be found lower than L2.[95] Low abdominal aortic aneurysm repair is associated with less than a 1% incidence of these dreaded complications. The incidence rises to 7% to 40% for thoracic and thoracoabdominal aneurysm repair,[73,208] stimulating the development of several modalities to provide spinal cord protection.[256] These include identification and reimplantation of segmental vessels,[359] increasing distal aortic perfusion,[149,321] spinal fluid drainage,[243] intrathecal papaverine,[332,333] and hypothermic cardiopulmonary bypass and circulatory arrest.[200] This topic is beyond the scope of this chapter but is covered more extensively in the chapter on thoracic anesthesia.

Unclamping

Release of the aortic cross-clamp results in metabolic and hemodynamic changes that vary in magnitude according to: (1) the extent and nature of the tissue reperfused; (2) the total occlusion time; (3) administration of fluids and therapeutic agents during the cross-clamp period and at the moment of unclamping; and (4) the use of shunts or bypass. The most consistent observation of cardiovascular behavior on clamp release in the absence of shunts or bypass is an acute fall in systemic blood pressure. The dominant influence is a decrease in SVR due to opening of the previously minimally perfused vascular beds. The latter, in turn, may be maximally dilated due to reactive hyperemia. Release of an infrarenal clamp usually causes a small drop in blood pressure that is transient and well tolerated, although treatment with fluid infusion or small increments of a vasopressor occasionally may be necessary. Removal of a supraceliac cross-clamp can result in profound hypotension, which: (1) should be anticipated by vigorous prerelease intravascular volume administration; and (2) frequently requires transient vasopressor support. Fig. 71-14 shows a continuous recording of systemic arterial pressure, PA pressure, right atrial pressure, and end-tidal CO_2 during release of a supraceliac clamp. Note the stability during clamping. Two to three minutes before release, the pressures are observed to rise as vasodilators are discontinued and volume infusion is increased. The decrease in systemic pressure at the moment of release is profound. The subsequent normalization of systemic arterial pressure is due to phenylephrine and volume administration.

Several different mediators have been suggested as being responsible for the hemodynamic effects seen after the release of the aortic cross-clamp including acidosis, lactate

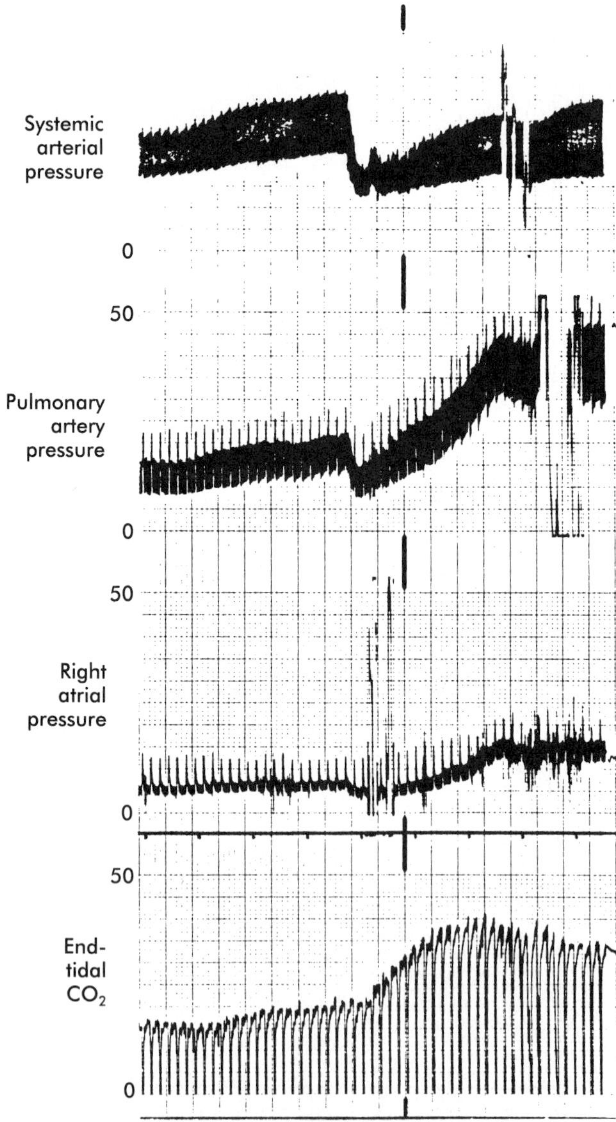

Fig. 71-14. Continuous chart recording of arterial, pulmonary artery (PA), and right arterial pressures and end-tidal CO_2 around the time of release of a supraceliac cross-clamp. NOTE: There is prerelease rise in pressures as vasodilation is reduced. Fall of pressures with releases is followed by rapid return resulting from administration of vasopressors and volume. Elevation of CO_2 (see text) may contribute to rise in PA pressures.

production, renin-angiotensin system, oxygen-free radicals, prostaglandins, compliment activation, and myocardial depressant factors.[130] Myocardial depressant factors have been circumstantially proposed but never specifically identified. Acidosis may be significant as discussed following and could contribute to myocardial depression and systemic vasodilation. Vasoactive intestinal polypeptide (VIP), as measured in mixed venous blood, doubles with reperfusion of the splanchnic organs after supraceliac cross-clamp release (1988, C. Beattie, unpublished data) and could cause vasodilation in vascular beds that were not hyperemic. Unless myocardial ischemia and/or failure appears, stability usually returns within several minutes using conservative therapy. Disseminated intravascular coagulation is an unusual but devastating complication.[174,253] The etiology of the condition is unknown but it is most likely related to cross-clamp duration and intestinal ischemia.

Total-body oxygen consumption increases with unclamping as below-clamp tissues return to aerobic metabolism. Mixed venous blood shows an abrupt desaturation within minutes after release of a supraceliac clamp and rapidly returns to preclamp values (Fig. 71-15). The transient rise in oxygen extraction implied by this finding may only reflect "reloading" of oxygen-depleted hemoglobin, myoglobin, and cytochromes rather than actual energy production. Investigators have addressed the issue of "oxygen debt," wherein reperfusion of a previously ischemic tissue mass may result in an overshoot of oxygen consumption to "repay" a deficit incurred during the anaerobic period.[4] The concept originated in exercise physiology to describe performing muscle that exceeded its aerobic metabolic capacity, and may not apply to tissue made ischemic by obstructed inflow. Some clinical studies have shown a small but significant increase in postclamp V_{O_2} compared with immediate preclamp V_{O_2} (see Fig. 71-11), but the consistency or importance of this finding is unexplored.

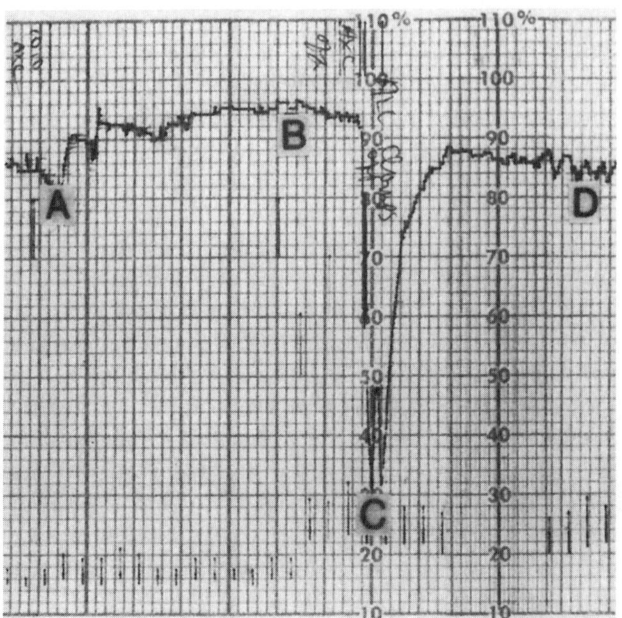

Fig. 71-15. Continuous recording of mixed venous O_2 saturation (from a pulmonary artery catheter, Oximetrix, Inc) during thoracoabdominal aortic aneurysm surgery. **A,** aortic clamp applied. O_2 saturation is 85% before clamping. **B,** O_2 saturation increases to 96% in the patient during cross-clamping. **C,** Saturation falls to 30% transiently during unclamping with return to preclamp values at **D**.

Carbon dioxide is elevated in arterial and venous blood within moments of unclamping, and this is reflected in the end-tidal partial pressure (see Fig. 71-14). Two principal sources contribute to the appearance of CO_2: (1) as the end product of aerobic metabolism; and (2) from the buffering (through carbonic acid) of organic acids that are washed out during reperfusion. The rise in Pa_{CO_2} eliminates the respiratory alkalosis that had stabilized pH during aortic occlusion (see previous section on metabolic changes) and reaches a peak with the bolus of lactic acid (Fig. 71-12) to produce a clinically important rise in hydrogen ion concentration. It was formerly common clinical practice to administer a bolus of sodium bicarbonate just before unclamping in an attempt to buffer the expected fall in pH. Unfortunately, additional CO_2 produced by the exogenous NCO_3 buffering adds to the CO_2 produced by aerobic metabolism dramatically increases Pa_{CO_2}. Carbon dioxide readily diffuses across cell membranes and could worsen intracellular acidosis, resulting in organ dysfunction (e.g., cardiac conduction and contractility disturbances).[34] Bicarbonate should be administered, if desired, during occlusion, well before unclamping.

Lactate increases measurably on release of an infrarenal clamp, but the change is clinically irrelevant. Supraceliac unclamping produces a lactate increase of 3.6 mmol/l for a mean clamp time of 45 minutes[268] (Fig. 71-12). Longer occlusion periods result in higher concentrations. Lactate concentrations rapidly return to normal after complete restoration of hepatic and liver flow and elimination of continued excess production. It is uncommon for significant lactate elevation to persist into the postoperative period.

Partial bypass and shunt techniques maintain near-adequate perfusion of most below-clamp structures, and the lactate bolus with unclamping is diminished when using these methods.

ANESTHETIC TECHNIQUE

For the most part, the premedication, induction, and maintenance of general anesthesia for aortic surgery can be chosen on the same basis as for any major surgery in which patients have known or suspected vascular pathology involving multiple organ systems. Topics of anesthetic relevance, which are discussed in this section, include proposal of a general anesthetic regimen for the critically ill and a critical evaluation of general anesthesia combined with either epidural or subarachnoid local anesthetic, narcotic, or both.

The choice of technique and drug dosages must be governed by specific plans for pulmonary and pain management in the postoperative period as well as by knowledge of intraoperative physiologic changes. Early postoperative extubation is favored by some, but others adopt a more conservative approach and routinely leave patients intubated and mechanically ventilated overnight. If early extubation is planned, then much more clinical finesse is required in the anesthetic management. This issue is repeatedly addressed in the discussion of anesthetic methods and again in the section on postoperative care.

General Anesthesia

After institution of appropriate monitoring and correction of hemodynamic abnormalities with fluids and pharmacologic therapy, induction of general anesthesia should proceed with incremental doses of a sedative hypnotic (e.g., short-acting barbiturate, etomidate, propofol) or a continuous infusion of the chosen agent titrated to effect. A short-acting, potent narcotic, such as fentanyl 5 to 10 μg/kg (or equivalent) in the average adult, should be administered during the induction. Ventilation should be assisted and then controlled as unconsciousness supervenes. Graded stimulation (oral airway, Foley catheter, gentle laryngoscopy with endotracheal lidocaine administration) guides additional narcotic and sedative delivery. Neuromuscular blockade may be introduced at any time during this process after the loss of consciousness. This technique provides for a smooth laryngoscopy and intubation. Residual narcotic effects, with added N_2O or low-dose inhalational agent, covers surgical incision, which may also be preceded by an additional small bolus of narcotic or sedative. Brisk fluid administration (one or more liters of crystalloid) may be necessary during induction to prevent hypotension. Pharmacologic therapy, recent dye studies, and nothing-by-mouth status can produce an intravascular volume depletion upon which is superimposed the generalized withdrawal of sympathetic tone that accompanies anesthetic induction.[307] Anesthetic maintenance may proceed after intubation, with unconsciousness maintained by less than 1 MAC of halogenated agent supplemented by N_2O, additional narcotic, or both. Choice between the halogenated agents may be based on desirable variations in their secondary effects.[32] This technique, which is applicable to any procedure of substantial length, allows the use of minimal doses of inhalational agent, thus ensuring a prompt emergence, yet it establishes a narcotic blood level that affords the basis of postoperative analgesia. The technique permits early extubation, unlike high-dose narcotic or deep inhalational methods, should this option be judged desirable based on the patient's physiologic status at the end of surgery.

Combined Techniques

The introduction of subarachnoid and epidural narcotics for both intraoperative supplementation of general anesthesia and provision of postoperative pain relief has proved to be a major advance in perioperative anesthetic management. Postoperative acute pain management has further refined principles of PCA for both the neuraxial narcotics and IV narcotics. When PCA is combined with classic methods of regional anesthesia, using a variety of local anesthetic agents, a sizeable array of intraoperative and postoperative possibilities emerge. A discussion of the permutations and combinations that may be created is beyond the scope of this chapter, but it is useful to address certain pertinent issues as they relate to major vascular surgery. First, intraoperative and postoperative management issues clearly should be separated. Studies that purport to demonstrate improved clinical outcome for regional or combined regional/general techniques compared with general anesthesia may well have their findings attributed to differences in postoperative pain management rather than intraoperative technique.[24,203] Recent reports[20,345] have reached conflicting conclusions about the influence of anesthetic technique on perioperative morbidity in this patient population. Second, although the value of neuraxial narcotics in moderating postoperative stress is becoming increasingly clear, intraoperative use of this modality dictates important modification of anesthetic management.[150] Any significant dose of parenteral opiates given to blunt the stimuli of intubation and incision may act synergistically with the neuraxial narcotic to produce prolonged or delayed respiratory depression at the end of the procedure. Immediate postsurgery extubation may not be possible without the planned administration of narcotic antagonists. Epidural anesthesia using local anesthetic agents is a theoretically attractive adjunct to general anesthesia and is advocated for vascular surgery by some clinicians.[363] With noxious stimuli blocked at the level of somatic afferents, only those systemic agents necessary to produce unconsciousness, amnesia, and tolerance of an ET tube will be required. Experience has shown, however, that hypotension can be severe when using combined regional and general anesthesia in patients undergoing aortic surgery.[203] The drop in blood pressure that accompanies removal of an aortic cross-clamp is exacerbated by any degree of sympathetic blockade. Excessive fluid administration before cross-clamp[227] or the use of vasopressors[15] with declamping may be required. The former predisposes to hypervolemia in the postoperative period, whereas the latter can be especially awkward if there is any doubt about organ or limb perfusion. Hypotension can be minimized by optimizing intravascular volume and by administering much smaller volumes of local anesthetics in the epidural space than normally required for a "pure" regional anesthetic. Placement of the epidural catheter tip at the appropriate dermatomal level will allow a segmental blockade and maximize the benefit while minimizing the drawbacks of this technique. For low thoracic placement, it may be desirable to inject only 6 to 8 ml of the local anesthetic.

Regardless of the anesthetic method chosen, intraoperative considerations focus on those special issues found only in aortic surgery. The physiology of aortic clamping is discussed at length in a previous section of the chapter.

Emergence

It is becoming increasingly apparent that the postoperative period is associated with the highest incidence of morbidity in patients with cardiac disease undergoing noncardiac surgery.[93,232,233] The appropriate concerns when terminating an aortic procedure are to balance the factors that favor early extubation with those that do not. Ideally, the goal is to produce an extubated, comfortable, well-oxygenated, ventilating patient who is normothermic and normovolemic, has good renal function, and has stable vital signs. For a straightforward infrarenal aneurysm repair in an individual without significant coexisting disease, early extubation should be possible in the majority of cases.[15]

Few investigations have systematically addressed alleviation of the considerable stress that is potentially associated with emergence from general anesthesia.[356] The induction and maintenance regimen previously suggested can be followed by emergence procedures that permit a smooth transition to consciousness and vital reflex function. As surgical closure commences, the inhalational agent is discontinued and N_2O is increased to 60% to 70%. As the end-tidal inhalation agent concentration decreases and the peritoneum is closed, the muscle relaxant is reversed and the patient is allowed to retain CO_2 (up to 55 mm Hg) to stimulate respiratory drive. Increased blood pressure or heart rate may be treated with vasodilators and beta-blocking agents. As respirations return, narcotics are administered in increments (morphine 1 to 2 mg) to keep respiratory rate at 8 to 12 breaths/min. Essentially the goal is to administer as much narcotic as necessary to achieve the given respiratory parameters. As closure is completed, the N_2O is discontinued and the patient is generally extubated within a short time. This technique usually produces a comfortable, spontaneously breathing patient. However, return to an alert state can be delayed and airway adjuncts should be used if required to minimize functional airway obstruction.

Experimental animal work has been reported using perioperative administration of alpha-$_2$ adrenergic agonists to attenuate the hemodynamic response to emergence from anesthesia.[103,279] Confirmation of this salutary effect in humans would be valuable, if it is not accompanied by significant side effects.

Combined regional/general methods may promote early extubation if carefully performed, but studies that seem to demonstrate their superiority in this regard have not used optimal techniques for their comparison general anesthesia group.[22,236,363]

Several possible sequelae of major vascular surgery may render extubation problematic, including fluid "third-spacing," postoperative reduction in pulmonary function, coagulopathies, hypothermia, and renal failure.

POSTOPERATIVE CARE

Decisions regarding the termination of anesthetic care, including emergence methodology, the need for mechanical ventilation and intubation, and techniques for providing postoperative analgesia, are potentially critical determinates of patient morbidity. Clinical practice varies widely. **Relevant factors include the anesthetic technique, extent of aneurysm repair, and patient stability with regard to certain physiologic parameters, including body temperature, pulmonary function, urine output, blood loss, and intravascular volume.**

Many patients will be ready to extubate by all standard criteria at the termination of surgery. However, several factors conspire to complicate what would otherwise appear to be a simple decision. Many of these individuals have a significant smoking history with resulting respiratory compromise. The usual and expected postoperative deterioration of pulmonary function superimposed on a marginal baseline state can result in poor oxygenation developing in the hours immediately after surgery.[97] Further, varying degrees of fluid third-spacing occur commonly during aortic aneurysm repair and continue postoperatively. Even if intravascular volume has been carefully maintained, this fluid must be mobilized and eliminated over time. It is not always possible to monitor and control this process with a sufficient degree of precision. Thus patients who seem to be doing well may develop problems several hours after the procedure and require reintubation.

It is generally conceded that control of the stress response is necessary to reduce the incidence of postoperative cardiac morbidity.[291] Because pain is a major component of stress, its alleviation is an important part of postoperative management considerations. Surgeons and intensivists seem to be gaining an appreciation of this issue. An impressive array of options are available, each of which has its proponents. At one extreme, patients may be given large doses of narcotics with sedative supplementation and planned overnight ventilation, as is commonly done after coronary artery bypass grafting. This approach may be associated with a smoother course for both the intensive care staff and the patient for as long as sedation is maintained. Weaning from mechanical ventilation, or course, must eventually occur, and this begins a period of delicate balance between adequate analgesia for both the surgical incision and presence of the endotracheal tube, and too much sedation, causing respiratory depression. Postoperative mechanical ventilation is associated with bacterial colonization of the respiratory system and could predispose the patient to pneumonia, so extubation is desirable. However, the stress of weaning from ventilatory support may be detrimental to the patient with CAD. The need for continued mechanical ventilation must be considered for each individual case, taking into account the risks and benefits of each alternative.

Several authors have recommended the use of epidural narcotics or local anesthetics as adjunct to postoperative pain relief in aneurysm patients.[23,42,363] One investigation showed that the preoperative administration of morphine (0.1 mg/kg) in the epidural space resulted in significantly lower levels of epinephrine, norepinephrine, and arterial blood pressure in the postoperative period.[42] Some of these patients were extubated and some were not. Another study using a small number of patients has shown that epidural narcotics may also reduce the incidence of postoperative tachycardia, ventricular ectopy, and possibly cardiac ischemia.[23] Conversely, two recent investigations, one using aneurysm surgery[154] and the other using major upper-abdominal surgery (including aneurysm repair)[306] found no difference in morbidity or mortality rates when pure general anesthesia was compared with a combined regional/general technique.

If overnight postoperative intubation is planned, then it is not clear that regional techniques offer any advantage, at least during the time of intubation. If an epidural catheter has been left in place, then it is likely that postextubation analgesia will be superior using neuraxial narcotics. The role of IV PCA versus epidural narcotics in postoperative aneurysm patients has not been investigated in this patient population. A well-conducted study evaluating these two techniques would be helpful. If early extubation is planned, then the use of intraoperative opiates or local anesthetics in the epidural space becomes quite reasonable. Considerably lower doses of inhalational agents may be used during the procedure, and thus the return to mental acuity and reflex-responsiveness is potentially more prompt. As previously noted, supplementation of general anesthesia with epidural local anesthetics can produce serious problems with hypotension that will require administration of excess fluids and/or vasoconstrictors.[227] Provided this effect is either minimized or accounted for, neuraxial techniques may produce the minimal possible stress response.

Myocardial ischemia is common in the postoperative period, although much of it may be "silent" and otherwise require careful surveillance to detect.[101,121,233,272] Although the prognostic significance of preoperative and intraoperative ischemia (to predict major cardiac morbidity) has been proposed,[272,316] significant recent evidence strongly associates the presence of postoperative ischemia with negative outcome.[233] This important finding sets the stage for further interventional studies to define the etiology of this ischemia (tachycardia, vasospasm, platelet thrombi, etc.) and to assess the clinical effect of alternate therapies.

Postoperative care of vascular surgery patients can be complicated. In addition to the issues discussed previously, several other problems may be encountered. Coagulopathies may continue from the operative period or develop anew. Hypothermia may persist and require treatment with heating blankets. Electrolytes and blood gases should be followed closely and complete hemodynamic profiles determined frequently to ensure optimal control. Patients who have experienced a ruptured aneurysm and/or prolonged suprarenal cross-clamping are prime candidates for renal failure. Knowledge of all hemodynamic parameters is necessary to provide adequate therapy and avoid intravascular volume overload.

From preoperative evaluation through intraoperative management and postoperative care, major vascular surgery offers rich and varied opportunities to influence patient morbidity. Laboratory investigations, along with clinical studies and practical experience, continue to change the efficacy of our practice.

KEY POINTS

- Patients presenting for major vascular surgery usually have either overt or occult involvement of several organ systems.
- Atherosclerosis risk factors include hyperlipidemia, tobacco use, diabetes, hypertension, positive family history, and male gender.
- The principal risk factor for brain infarct is hypertension.
- The pathophysiology of atherosclerosis on the cellular level remains unknown.
- Indications for CEA continue to be debated in the literature.
- Laplace's Law is $T \alpha P \times R$. A 5-cm AAA has an annual incidence of rupture of approximately 4%; at 7 cm, the incidence is approximately 19%.
- Preoperative risk assessment will have value only if it leads to risk modification or otherwise influences decisions regarding surgical or anesthetic procedures.
- Coronary artery disease is primarily responsible for approximately 50% of early and late mortality in peripheral vascular surgery patients.
- Most perioperative MI seem to occur postoperatively and silently.
- Current studies seem to indicate that aggressive perioperative management of patients with CAD may make a difference in the overall outcome.
- Patients with diabetes may show changes in autonomic tone predisposing them to greater blood pressure liability and autonomic neuropathies and therefore increased incidence of silent ischemia.
- Many procedures have been suggested and refuted over time as predictors of perioperative cardiac morbidity. Recent studies have promoted: (1) exercise ECG; (2) Holter ambulatory monitoring; (3) DTI; (4) angioscintigraphy; and (5) coronary angiography.
- It is imperative to continue all significant cardiovascular medications perioperatively.
- Invasive monitoring should be chosen and implemented based on patient condition, ancillary diseases, and anticipated hemodynamic changes associated with the surgical procedure.
- For CEA, hemodynamic extremes should be avoided; the goal is to have a responsive patient immediately after surgery to allow assessment of neurologic status. Blood pressure should be maintained at or up to 20% above

baseline at the time of carotid occlusion, the patient should be normocapnic, and there should be a smooth emergence from the anesthesia.

- Induction and maintenance of general anesthesia can be performed quite safely and smoothly in severely ill patients by careful titration of anesthetics combined with aggressive manipulation of hemodynamic parameters.
- The physiology of aortic cross-clamping includes changes in blood pressure, cardiac output, myocardial perfusion, pH, and tissue perfusion of the spinal cord, kidneys, and viscera.
- Hemodynamic changes during aortic cross-clamping relate to the effect of "afterload" on ventricular ejection *but also,* significantly, on venous return.
- Multiple studies of the physiologic effects of aortic cross-clamping have shown opposing results presumably based on interinvestigation differences in: (1) the administration of vasodilators; (2) types of anesthesia used; and (3) intrinsic myocardial function.
- There have been multiple proposed interventions to reverse the effect of increased left ventricular afterload secondary to aortic cross-clamping; these include passive or active shunts, arteriolar dilatation, venodilation, and myocardial depressants.
- Two fundamental metabolic effects of aortic cross-clamping are: (1) decreased total-body oxygen metabolism; and (2) conversion to anaerobic metabolism of the body mass distal to the clamp.
- Renal protection is a primary concern during aortic surgery.
- Several modalities are aimed at spinal cord protection: (1) identification and reimplantation of segmental vessels; (2) increased distal aortic perfusion; (3) CSF drainage; (4) intrathecal papaverine; and (5) circulatory arrest.
- Monitoring for cord ischemia involves stimulation and recording of cortical evoked or MEP, *but* when ischemia is detected, there is no accepted procedure for its alleviation.
- Unclamping leads to an acute fall in blood pressure produced by a decrease in SVR. This can be anticipated by vigorous volume administration before release, discontinuation of vasodilators, "lightened" anesthesia, and use of aggressive fluid resuscitation with or without vasopressors if needed to facilitate release. If blood pressure does not respond within several minutes of conservative therapy, reapplication of the aortic cross-clamp is another option.
- Postoperative care must focus on the same issues as discussed preoperatively and intraoperatively in an attempt to control the stress response.

KEY REFERENCES

Baron J, Bertrand M, Barre E, et al: Combined epidural and general anesthesia versus general anesthesia for abdominal aortic surgery, *Anesthesiology* 75:611, 1991.

Fleisher LA, Barash PG: Preoperative cardiac evaluation for noncardiac surgery: A functional approach, *Anesth Analg* 74:586, 1992.

Tuman K, McCarthy R, March R, et al: Effects of epidural anesthesia and analgesia on coagulation and outcome after major vascular surgery, *Anesth Analg* 73:696, 1991.

Beattie C: Regional versus general anesthesia. In Breslow MJ, Miller CF, Rogers MC, editors: *Perioperative management,* Washington, 1990, Mosby–Year Book.

Gelman S: The pathophysiology of aortic cross-clamping and unclamping, *Anesthesiology* 82(4):1026, 1995.

Gelman S, Rabbani S, Bradley EL: Inferior and superior vena caval blood flows during cross-clamping of the thoracic aorta in pigs, *J Thorac Cardiovasc Surg* 96:387, 1988.

Crawford ES, Stowe CL: True aneurysms of the aorta and iliac arteries. In Moore WS, editor: *Vascular surgery, a comprehensive review,* Orlando, 1986, Grune & Stratton.

Cunningham JN, Laschinger JC, Spencer FC: Monitoring of somatosensory-evoked potentials during surgical procedures on the thoracoabdominal aorta. IV. Clinical observations and results, *J Thorac Cardiovasc Surg* 94:275, 1987.

Hertzer NR, Bevan EG, Young JR, et al: Coronary artery disease in peripheral vascular patients. A classification of 1000 coronary angiograms and results of surgical management, *Ann Surg* 199:223, 1984.

REFERENCES

1. Aaslid R, Markwalder TM, Nornes H: Noninvasive transcranial Doppler ultrasound recording of flow velocity in basal cerebral arteries, *J Neurosurg* 57:769, 1982.
2. Abbott WM, Austen WG: The reversal of renal cortical ischemia during aortic occlusion by mannitol, *J Surg Res* 16:482, 1974.
3. Acinapura AJ, Rose DM, Kramer MD, et al: Role of coronary angiography and coronary artery bypass surgery prior to abdominal aortic aneurysmectomy, *J Cardiovasc Surg* 28:552, 1987.
4. Adams RP, Cain SM: Total and hindlimb oxygen deficit and "repayment" in hypoxic anesthetized dogs, *J Appl Physiol* 55(3): 913, 1983.
5. Ahmed OL, Orchar TJ, Sharma R, et al: Declining mortality from stroke in Allegheny County, Pennsylvania, *Stroke* 19: 181, 1988.
6. Albert RA, Roizen MF, Hamilton WK, et al: Intraoperative urinary output does not predict postoperative renal function in patients undergoing abdominal aortic revascularization, *Surgery* 95:707, 1983.
7. Allen BT, Anderson CB, Rubin BG, et al: The influence of anesthetic technique on perioperative complications after carotid endarterectomy, *J Vasc Surg* 19(5):834, 1994.
8. Allen JR, Helling TS, Hartzler GO: Operative procedures not involving the heart after percutaneous transluminal coronary angioplasty, *Surg Gynecol Obstet* 173:285, 1991.
9. Reference deleted in proofs.
10. Attia RR, Murphy JD, Snider M, et al: Myocardial ischemia due to infrarenal aortic cross-clamping during aortic surgery in patients with severe coronary artery disease, *Circulation* 53:961, 1976.
11. Bachenheimer LC, Kim YD: Anesthetic management of patients undergoing thoracic aortic reconstruction, *Anesthesiol Clin North Am* 13(1):115, 1995.
12. Reference deleted in proofs.
13. Bailey RS, Griffith LSC, Rouleau J, et al: Thallium-201 myocardial perfusion imaging at rest and during exercise: comparative sensitivity to electrocardiography in coronary artery disease, *Circulation* 55:79, 1977.
14. Reference deleted in proofs.
15. Baldwin L, Henderson A, Hickman P: Effect of postoperative low-dose dopamine on renal function after elective major vascular surgery, *Ann Intern Med* 120(9):744, 1994.
16. Barcroft H, Samaan A: The explanation of the increase in systemic flow caused by occluding the descending thoracic aorta, *Am J Physiol* 85:47, 1935.
17. Barnes RW, Lievman PR, Marszlek PB, et al: The natural history of asymptomatic carotid disease in patients undergoing cardiovascular surgery, *Surgery* 12:750, 1981.
18. Barnett HJM, Barnes RW, Robertson JT: The uncertainties surrounding carotid endarterectomy, *JAMA* 268(21):3120, 1992.
19. Barnett HJM, Meldrum HE, Eliasziw M: The dilemma of surgical treatment for patients with asymptomatic carotid disease, *Ann Intern Med* 123(10):723, 1995.
20. Baron J, Bertrand M, Barre E, et al: Combined epidural and general anesthesia versus general anesthesia for abdominal aortic surgery, *Anesthesiology* 75:611, 1991.
21. Baron JF, Mundler O, Bertrand M, et al: Dipyridamole-thallium scintigraphy and gated radio nuclide angiography to assess cardiac risk before abdominal aortic surgery, *N Engl J Med* 330:663, 1994.
22. Beattie C: Con: Regional anesthesia is not preferable to general anesthesia for the patient with heart disease, *J Cardiothorac Anesth* 3(6):797, 1989.
23. Beattie C, Buckley DM, Forrest JB: Reduction of significant cardiac morbidity by epidural morphine in non-cardiac surgery, *Anesthesiology* 73(3A)A71, 1990.
24. Beattie C: Regional versus general anesthesia. In Breslow MJ, Miller CF, Rogers MC, editors: *Perioperative management,* Washington, 1990, Mosby–Year Book.
25. Becquemin JP, Paris E, Valverde A, et al: Carotid surgery - Is regional anesthesia always appropriate? *J Cardiovasc Surg,* 32(5):595, 1991.
26. Benditt EP, Benditt JM: Evidence for a monoclonal origin of human atherosclerotic plaques, *Proc Natl Acad Sci USA* 70:1753, 1973.
27. Benjamin ME, Silva MB Jr, Watt C, et al: Awake patient monitoring to determine the need for shunting during carotid endarterectomy, *Surgery* 114:673, 1993.
28. Bergeron P, Benichou H, Rudondy P, et al: Stroke prevention during carotid surgery in high risk patients [value of transcranial doppler and local anesthesia], *J Cardiovasc Surg* 32(6):713, 1991.
29. Berlauk JF, Abrams JH, Gilmour IJ, et al: Preoperative optimization of cardiovascular hemodynamics improves outcome in peripheral vascular surgery: a prospective, randomized clinical trial, *Ann Surg* 214: 289, 1991.
30. Bernstein EF, Chan EL: Abdominal aortic aneurysm in high-risk patients: outcome of selective management based on size and expansion rate, *Ann Surg* 200:255, 1984.
31. Bernstein JS, Ebert TJ, Stowe DF, et al: Partial attenuation of hemodynamic responses to rapid sequence induction and intubation with labetalol, *J Clin Anesth* 1(6)444, 1989.
32. Bertha BG, Folts JD, Nugent M, et al: Halothane, but not isoflurane or enflurane, protects against spontaneous and epinephrine-exacerbated acute thrombus formation in stenosed dog coronary arteries, *Anesthesiology* 71:96, 1989.
33. Bevan EG: Routine coronary angiography in patients undergoing surgery for abdominal aortic aneurysm and lower extremity occlusive disease, *J Vasc Surg* 3:682, 1986.
34. Bishop RL, Weisfeldt ML: Sodium bicarbonate administration during cardiac arrest, *JAMA* 235:506, 1976.
35. Black TE, Kay B, Healy TEJ: Reducing the haemodynamic responses to laryngoscopy and intubation. A comparison of alfentanil with fentanyl, *Anaesthesia* 39:883, 1984.
36. Blaisdell FW, Cooley DA: The mechanism of paraplegia after temporary thoracic aorta occlusion and its relationship to spinal fluid pressure, *Surgery* 351, 1962.
37. Blombery PA, Ferguson IA, Rosengarten DS, et al: The role of coronary artery disease in complications of abdominal aortic aneurysm surgery, *Surgery* 101:150, 1987.
38. Blume WT, Ferguson GG, McNeil DK: Significance of EEG changes at carotid endarterectomy, *Stroke* 17:891, 1986.
39. Bode RH Jr, Lewis KP, Zarich SW, et al: Cardiac outcome after peripheral vascular surgery: Comparison of general and regional anesthesia, *Anesthesiology* 84:3, 1996.
40. Bonow RO, Bacharach SL, Green MV, et al: Prognostic implications of symptomatic versus asymptomatic (silent) myocardial ischemia induced by exercise in mildly symptomatic and in asymptomatic patients with angiographically documented coronary artery disease, *Am J Cardiol* 60:778, 1987.
41. Boucher CA, Brewster DC, Darling RC, et al: Determination of cardiac risk by dipyridamole-thallium imaging before peripheral vascular surgery, *N Engl J Med* 312:389, 1985.
42. Breslow MJ, Jordan DA, Christopherson R, et al: Epidural morphine decreases postoperative hypertension by attenuating sympathetic nervous system hyperactivity, *JAMA* 261(24):3577, 1989.
43. Breslow MJ, Parker SD, Frank SM, et al: Determinants of catecholamine and cortisol responses to lower extremity revascularization, *Anesthesiology* 79:1202, 1993.
44. Reference deleted in proofs.
45. Brott T, Toole JF: Medical compared with surgical treatment of asymptomatic carotid artery stenosis, *Ann Intern Med* 123(9): 720, 1995.
46. Brown CB, Ogg CS, Camerson JS: High dose furosemide in acute renal failure: A controlled trial, *Clin Nephrol* 15:90, 1981.
47. Brown OW, Hollier LH, Pairolero PC, et al: Abdominal aortic aneurysm and coronary artery disease, *Arch Surg* 116:1484, 1981.
48. Bruce DL, Crowley TF, Lee JS: Preoperative clonidine withdrawal syndrome, *Anesthesiology* 51:90, 1979.
49. Brusoni A, Colombo A, Merlo L, et al: Hemodynamic and metabolic changes induced by temporary clamping of the thoracic aorta, *Eur Surg Res* 10:206, 1978.
50. Bryan-Brown CW, Kwun KB, Lumb PD, et al: The axillary artery catheter, *Heart Lung* 12:492, 1983.
51. Burgos LG, Ebert TJ, Asiddao C, et al: Increased intraoperative cardiovascular morbidity diabetics with autonomic neuropathy, *Anesthesiology* 70:591, 1989.
52. Bush HL, Huse JB, Johnson WL, et al: Prevention of renal insufficiency after abdominal aortic aneurysm resection by optimal volume loading, *Arch Surg* 116:1517, 1981.

53. Byrd L, Sherman RL: Radiocontrast-induced acute renal failure: a clinical and pathophysiologic review, *Medicine* 58:270, 1979.
54. Callow AD, Mackey WC: Long term follow-up of surgically managed carotid bifurcation atherosclerosis—justification for an aggressive approach, *Ann Surg* 210:308, 1989.
55. Carliner NH, Fischer ML, Plotnick GD, et al: Routine preoperative exercise testing in patients undergoing major non-cardiac surgery, *Am J Cardiol* 56:51, 1985.
56. Carliner NH, Fischer ML, Plotnick GD, et al: The preoperative electrocardiogram as an indicator of risk in major non-cardiac surgery, *Can J Cardiol* 2:134, 1986.
57. Cartier R, Orszulak TA, Pairolero PC, et al: Circulatory support during cross-clamping of the descending thoracic aorta, *J Thorac Cardiovasc Surg* 99:1038, 1990.
58. Christopherson R, Beattie C, Frank SM, et al: Perioperative morbidity in patients randomized to epidural or general anesthesia for lower extremity vascular surgery, *Anesthesiology* 79(3):422, 1993.
59. Chung F, Houston PL, Cheng DCH, et al: Calcium channel blockade does not offer adequate protection from perioperative myocardial ischemia, *Anesthesiology* 69:343, 1988.
60. Cohn PF: Silent myocardial ischemia: classification, prevalence, and prognosis, *Am J Med* 79(Suppl 3A):2, 1985.
61. Collier PE: Carotid endarterectomy: a safe cost-efficient approach, *J Vasc Surg* 16(6):926, 1992.
62. Conti CR, Mehta JL: Acute myocardial ischemia: role of atherosclerosis, thrombosis, platelet activation, coronary vasospasm, and altered arachidonic acid metabolism, *Circulation* 75(suppl V):84, 1987.
63. Reference deleted in proofs.
64. Cordell AR, Lavender SW: An appraisal of blood salvage techniques in vascular and cardiac operations, *Ann Thorac Surg* 31: 421, 1981.
65. Reference deleted in proofs.
66. Reference deleted in proofs.
67. Corson JD, Chang BB, Leopold PW, et al: Perioperative hypertension in patients undergoing carotid endarterectomy: shorter duration under regional block anesthesia, *Circulation* 74(S1):I–1, 1986.
68. Corson JD, Chang BB, Shah DM, et al: The influence of anesthetic choice on carotid endarterectomy outcome, *Arch Surgery* 122:807, 1987.
69. Crawford ES, Fenstermacher JM, Richardson W, et al: Reappraisal of adjuncts to avoid ischemia in the treatment of thoracic aortic aneurysms, *Surgery* 67:182, 1970.
70. Crawford ES, Saleh SA, Bobb JW III, et al: Infrarenal abdominal aortic aneurysms: factors influencing survival after operation performed over a 25-year period, *Ann Surg* 193:699, 1981.
71. Crawford ES, Stowe CL: True aneurysms of the aorta and iliac arteries. In Moore WS, editor: *Vascular surgery, a comprehensive review,* Orlando, 1986, Grune & Stratton.
72. Crawford ES, Mizrahi EM, Hess KR, et al: The impact of distal aortic perfusion and somatosensory-evoked potential monitoring on prevention of paraplegia after aortic aneurysm operation, *J Thorac Cardiovasc Surg* 95:357, 1988.
73. Crawford ES, Crawford JL, Safi HJ, et al: Thoracoabdominal aortic aneurysms: perioperative and intraoperative factors determining immediate and long term results of operations in 605 patients, *J Vasc Surg* 3:389, 1986.
74. Cronenwett JL, Lindenauer SM: Distribution of intrarenal blood flow following aortic clamping and declamping, *J Surg Res* 22:469, 1977.
75. Cronenwett JL, Murphy TF, Zelenock GB, et al: Actuarial analysis of variables associated with rupture of small abdominal aortic aneurysms, *Surgery* 98:472, 1985.
76. Cucchiara RF, Benefiel DJ, Matteo RS, et al: Evaluation of esmolol in controlling increases in heart rate and blood pressure during endotracheal intubation in patients undergoing carotid endarterectomy, *Anesthesiology* 65:528, 1986.
77. Cunningham JN, Laschinger JC, Merkin HA, et al: Measurement of spinal cord ischemia during operations upon the thoracic aorta, *Ann Surg* 196:285, 1982.
78. Cunningham JN, Laschinger JC, Spencer FC: Monitoring of somatosensory-evoked potentials during surgical procedures on the thoracoabdominal aorta. IV. Clinical observations and results, *J Thorac Cardiovasc Surg* 94:275, 1987.
79. Cutler BS, Wheeler HB, Paraskos JA, et al: Assessment of operative risk with electrocardiographic exercise testing in patients with peripheral vascular disease, *Am J Surg* 137:484, 1979.
80. Cutler BS, Wheeler HB, Paraskos JA, et al: Applicability and interpretation of electrocardiographic stress testing in patients with peripheral vascular disease, *Am J Surg* 141:501, 1981.
81. Cutler BS, Leppo JA: Dipyridamole thallium-201 scintigraphy to coronary artery disease before abdominal aortic surgery, *J Vasc Surg* 5:91, 1987.
82. Dagenais GR, Rouleau JR, Christen A, et al: Survival of patients with strongly positive exercise electrocardiogram, *Circulation* 65:452, 1982.
83. Damask MC, Weissman C, Todd G: General versus epidural anesthesia for femoral-popliteal bypass surgery, *J Clin Anesth* 2(2):71, 1990.
84. Darling RC, Brewster DC: Elective treatment of abdominal aortic aneurysm, *World J Surg* 4:661, 1981.
85. Davies MJ, Cronin KD, Cowie RW: The prevention of hypertension at intubation: a controlled study of intravenous hydralazine on patients undergoing intracranial surgery, *Anaesthesia* 36:147, 1981.
86. Davies MJ, Murrell GC, Cronin KD, et al: Carotid endarterectomy under cervical plexus block—a prospective clinical audit, *Anaesth Intensive Care* 18(2):219, 1990.
87. Davies MJ, Mooney PH, Scott DA, et al: Neurologic changes during carotid endarterectomy under cervical block predict a high risk of postoperative stroke, *Anesthesiology* 78(5):829, 1993.
88. Davis DW, Isaacson IJ: Anesthetic management of patients undergoing abdominal aortic reconstruction, *Anesth Clin North Am* 13(1):131, 1995.
89. Debakey ME, Lawrie GM, Glaeser DH: Patterns of atherosclerosis and their surgical significance, *Ann Surg* 201:115, 1985.
90. Del Guercio LRM, Cohn JD: Monitoring operative risk in the elderly, *JAMA* 243:1350, 1980.
91. Delmarva Corporation for Medical Care, Inc (peer review organization for Delaware, Maryland and Virginia): Indications for carotid endarectomy 1989, 341B N Aurora St, Easton, MD, 21601.
92. Detsky AS, Abrams HB, McLaughlin JR, et al: Predicting cardiac complications in patients undergoing non-cardiac surgery, *J Gen Intern Med* 1:211, 1986.
93. Diehl JT, Cali RF, Hertzer NR, et al: Complications of abdominal aortic reconstruction. An analysis of perioperative risk factors in 557 patients, *Ann Surg* 197:49, 1983.
94. Reference deleted in proofs.
95. Dommisse GF: The blood supply of the spinal cord: a critical vascular zone in spinal surgery, *J Bone Joint Surg* 56B:225, 1975.
96. Donato AT, Hill SL: Carotid arterial surgery using local anesthesia: a private practice retrospective study, *Am Surg* 58(8):446, 1992.
97. Downs JB: Postoperative respiratory care. In Kaplan JA, editor: *Thoracic anesthesia,* New York, 1983, Churchill-Livingstone.
98. Drenger B, Parker SD, McPherson RW, et al: Spinal cord stimulation evoked potentials during thoracoabdominal aortic aneurysm surgery, *Surgery* 76:689, 1992.
99. Eagle, et al: ACC/AHA Task Force. Guidelines for Perioperative Cardiovascular Evaluation for Noncardiac Surgery. Report of the American College of Cardiology/American Heart Association Task Force on Practice Guidelines (Committee on Perioperative Cardiovascular Evaluation for Noncardiac Surgery). *JACC* 27(4):910, 1996.
100. Eagle KA, Coley CM, Newell JB, et al: Combining clinical and thallium data optimizes preoperative assessment of cardiac risk before major vascular surgery, *Ann Intern Med* 110:859, 1989.
101. Eagle KA, Singer DE, Brewster DC, et al: Dipyridamole-thallium scanning in patients undergoing vascular surgery, *JAMA* 257:2185, 1987.
102. Edmonds ME, Roberts VC, Watkins PJ: Blood flow in the diabetic neuropathic foot, *Diabetologia* 22:9, 1982.
103. Ellis JE, Drijvers G, Pedlow S, et al: Premedication with oral and transdermal clonidine provides safe and efficacious postoperative sympatholysis, *Anesth Analg* 79:1133, 1994.
104. Ellis JE, Klock PA, Klafta JM, et al: Choice of anesthesia and intraoperative monitoring for lower extremity revascularization, *Surg Clin North Am* 75(4):665, 1995.
105. Elmore JR, Hallett J Jr, Gibbons RJ, et al: Myocardial revascularization before abdominal aortic aneurysmorrhaphy: effect of coronary angioplasty, *Mayo Clin Proc* 68:637, 1993.
106. Engelman RM, Hadji-Rousou I, Breyer

RH, et al: Rebound vasospasm after coronary revascularization in association with calcium antagonist withdrawal, *Ann Thorac Surg* 37:469, 1984.

107. Engler RL, Covell JW: Influence of the venous system on ventricular/arterial coupling. In Yin FCP, editor: *Ventricular/vascular coupling,* New York, 1987, Springer-Verlag.
108. Ennix CL, Lawrie GM, Morris GC, et al: Improved results of carotid endarterectomy in patients with symptomatic coronary disease: an analysis of 1546 consecutive carotid operations, *Stroke* 10:122, 1979.
109. Erwin D, Pick MJ, Taylor GW: Anesthesia for carotid surgery, *Anesthesia* 35:246, 1980.
110. Reference deleted in proofs.
111. Falk E: Morphologic features of unstable atherothrombotic plaques underlying acute coronary syndromes, *Am J Cardiol* 63: 114E, 1989.
112. Fegert G, Hollenberg M, Browner W, et al: Perioperative myocardial ischemia in the noncardiac surgical patient (abstract), *Anesthesiology* 69:49, 1988.
113. Ferguson GG: Intra-operative monitoring and internal shunts: are they necessary in CEA? *Stroke* 13(3):287, 1982.
114. Reference deleted in proofs.
115. Flacke JW, Bloor BC, Flacke WE, et al: Reduced narcotic requirement by clonidine with improved hemodynamic and adrenergic stability in patients undergoing coronary bypass surgery, *Anesthesiology* 67:11, 1987.
116. Fleisher LA, Barash PG: Preoperative cardiac evaluation for noncardiac surgery: a functional approach, *Anesth Analg* 74:586, 1992.
117. Fleisher LA, Rosenbaum SH, Nelson, et al: Preoperative dipyridamole thallium imaging and Holter monitoring as a predictor of perioperative cardiac events and long term outcome, *Anesthesiology,* In press.
118. Fleisher LA, Skolnick ED, Holroyd KJ, et al: Coronary artery revascularization before abdominal aortic aneurysm surgery: a decision analytic approach, *Anesth Analg* 79:661, 1994.
119. Fode NC, Sundt TM Jr, Robertson JT, et al: Multicenter retrospective review of results and complications of carotid endarterectomy in 1981, *Stroke* 17:370, 1986.
120. Foex P: Beta-blockade in anesthesia, *J Clin Hosp Pharm* 8:183, 1983.
121. Frank SM, Beattie C, Christopherson R, et al: Perioperative rate-related silent myocardial ischemia and postoperative death, *J Clin Anesth* 2:326, 1990.
122. Frank SM, Norris E, Christopherson R, et al: Right and left arm blood pressure discrepancies in vascular surgery patients, *Anesthesiology* 75:457, 1991.
123. Frank SM, Beattie C, Christopherson R, et al: Epidural vs. general anesthesia, ambient operating room temperature, and patient age as predictors of inadvertent hypothermia, *Anesthesiology* 77:252, 1992.
124. Friedman SG, Tortolani AJ: Reduced length of stay following CEA under general anesthesia, *Am J Surg* 170(8):235, 1995.
125. Fuchs RM, Achuff SC, Grunwald L, et al: Electrocardiographic localization of coronary artery narrowings: studies during myocardial ischemia and infarction in patients with one-vessel disease, *Circulation* 66: 1168, 1982.
126. Gabelman CG, Gann DS, Ashworth CJ, et al: One hundered consecutive carotid reconstructions: local versus general anesthesia, *Amer J Surg* 145:477, 1983.
127. Gallagher JD, Moore RA, Jose AB, et al: Prophylactic nitroglycerin infusions during coronary artery bypass surgery, *Anesthesiology* 64:785, 1986.
128. Gamulin Z, Forster A, Morel D, et al: Effects of infrarenal aortic cross clamping on renal hemodynamics in humans, *Anesthesiology* 61:394, 1984.
129. Gass GD, Olsen GN: Preoperative pulmonary function testing to predict postoperative morbidity and mortality, *Chest* 89:127, 1986.
130. Gelman S: The pathophysiology of aortic cross-clamping and unclamping, *Anesthesiology* 82(4):1026, 1995.
131. Gelman S, Curtis SE, Bradley WE, et al: Angiotensin and adrenoceptors role in hemodynamic response to aortic cross-clamping, *Am J Physiol* 264:H14, 1993.
132. Gelman S, McDowell H, Varner PD, et al: The reason for cardiac output reduction after aortic cross-clamping, *Am J Surg* 155:578, 1988.
133. Gelman S, Rabbani S, Bradley EL: Inferior and superior vena caval blood flows during cross-clamping of the thoracic aorta in pigs, *J Thorac Cardiovasc Surg* 96:387, 1988.
134. Reference deleted in proofs.
135. Reference deleted in proofs.
136. Ghignone M, Calvillo O, Quintin KL: Anesthesia and hypertension: the effect of clonidine on perioperative hemodynamics and isoflurane requirements, *Anesthesiology* 67:3, 1987.
137. Godet G, Bertrand M, Coriat P, et al: Comparison of isoflurane with sodium nitroprusside for controlling hypertension during thoracic aortic cross-clamping, *J Cardiothorac Anesth* 4(2):177, 1990.
138. Gold MI, Brown M, Coverman S, et al: Heart rate and blood pressure effects of esmolol after ketamine induction and intubation, *Anesthesiology* 64:718, 1986.
139. Golden MA, Whittemore AD, Donaldson MC, et al: Selective evaluation and management of coronary artery disease in patients undergoing repair of abdominal aortic aneurysms, *Ann Surg* 212(4):415, 1990.
140. Goldenberg SG, Alex M, Joshi RA, et al: Nonatheromatous peripheral vascular disease of the lower extremity in diabetes mellitus, *Diabetes* 8:261, 1959.
141. Goldman L: Cardiac Risk for vascular surgery, *JACC* 27(4):799, 1996.
142. Goldman L, Caldera D, Nusbaum S, et al: Multifactorial index of cardiac risk in noncardiac surgical procedures, *N Engl J Med* 197:845, 1977.
143. Gordon T, Kannel WB: Predisposition to atherosclerosis in the head, heart, and legs. The Framingham Study, *JAMA* 221:661, 1972.
144. Gorlin R, Fuster V, Ambrose JA: Anatomatic-physiologic links between acute coronary syndromes (editorial), *Circulation* 74:6, 1986.
145. Gott VL: Heparinized shunts for thoracic vascular operations, *Ann Thorac Surg* 14:(2)219, 1972.
146. Gottlieb SO, Weisfeldt ML, Ouyang P: Silent ischemia as a marker for early unfavorable outcomes in patients with unstable angina, *N Engl J Med* 314:1214, 1986.
147. Gould KL: Noninvasive assessment of coronary stenosis by myocardial perfusion imaging during pharmacologic coronary vasodilatation. I. Physiologic basis and experimental validation, *Am J Cardiol* 41:267, 1978.
148. Reference deleted in proofs.
149. Grossi EA, Krieger KH, Cunningham JN, et al: Venoarterial bypass: a technique for spinal cord protection, *J Thorac Cardiovasc Surg* 89:228, 1985.
150. Gustafsson LL, Schildt B, Jacobsen KJ: Adverse effects of extradural and intrathecal opiates: report of a nationwide survey in Sweden, *Br J Anaesth* 54:479, 1982.
151. Guyton AC: *Textbook of medical physiology,* ed 6, Philadelphia, 1981, WB Saunders.
152. Hafner CD, Evans WE: Carotid endarterectomy with local anesthesia: results and advantages, *J Vasc Surg* 7(2):232, 1988.
153. Reference deleted in proofs.
154. Haku E, Hayashi M, Kato H: Anesthetic management of abdominal aortic surgery: a retrospective review of perioperative complications, *J Cardiothoracic Anesth* 3(5): 57, 1989.
155. Reference deleted in proofs.
156. Hallett JW Jr, Popovsky M, Ilstrup D: Minimizing blood transfusions during abdominal aortic surgery: recent advances in rapid autotransfusion, *J Vasc Surg* 5:601, 1987.
157. Hannan EL, Kilburn H Jr, O'Donnell JF, et al: A longitudinal analysis of the relationship between in-hospital mortality in New York State and the volume of abdominal aortic aneurysm surgeries performed, *Health Serv Res* 27:4, 1992.
158. Harris KA, Ameli FM, Lally M, et al: Abdominal aortic aneurysm resection in patients more than 80 years old, *Surg Gynecol Obstet* 162:536, 1986.
159. Heifetz M, Shramek A, Yahel M, et al: Hypercarbic anesthesia in carotid endarterectomy, *Anaesthesia* 28:82, 1973.
160. Hertzer NR, Beven EG: A retrospective comparison of the use of shunts during carotid endarterectomy, *Surg Obstet Gynecol* 151:81, 1980.
161. Hertzer NR, Bevan EG, Young JR, et al: Coronary artery disease in peripheral vascular patients. A classification of 1000 coronary angiograms and results of surgical management, *Ann Surg* 199:223, 1984.
162. Hertzer NR, Bevan EG, Young JR, et al: Incidental asymptomatic carotid bruits in patients scheduled for peripheral vascular reconstruction: results of cerebral and coronary angiography, *Surgery* 96:535, 1984.
163. Hertzer NR, Feldman BJ, Beven EG, et al: A prospective study on the incidence of CN injury during CEA, *Surg Gynecol Obstet* 151:781, 1980.
164. Hertzer HR, Lees CD: Fatal myocardial infarction following carotid endarterectomy. Three hundred thirty-five patients followed

6-11 years after operation, *Ann Surg* 194:212, 1981.
165. Hertzer NR, Young JR, Bevan EG, et al: Late results of coronary bypass in patients with infrarenal aortic aneurysms. The Cleveland Clinic Study, *Ann Surg* 205:360, 1987.
166. Reference deleted in proofs.
167. Hertzer NR, Young JR, Kramer JR, et al: Routine coronary angiography prior to elective aortic reconstruction: results of a selective myocardial revascularization in patients with peripheral vascular disease, *Arch Surg* 114:1336, 1979.
168. Hessel SJ, Adams DF, Abrams HL: Complication of angiography, *Radiology* 138:273, 1981.
169. Hobson RW, Wright CB, Sublett JW, et al: Carotid artery back pressure and endarterectomy under regional anesthesia, *Arch Surg* 109:682, 1974.
170. Hobson RW, Weiss DG, Fields WS, et al: Efficacy of CEA in asymptomatic carotid stenosis, *N Engl J Med* 328:221, 1993.
171. Hollier LH: The case against prophylactic coronary bypass. Mills NL: The case for prophylactic coronary bypass, *Surgery* 96:78, 1984.
172. Hollier LH, Money SR, Naslund TC, et al: Risk of spinal cord dysfunction in patients undergoing thoracoabdominal aortic replacement, *Am J Surg* 164:210, 1992.
173. Huber KC, Evans MA, Bresnahan JF, et al: Outcome of noncardiac operations in patients with severe coronary artery disease successfully treated preoperatively with coronary angioplasty, *Mayo Clin Proc* 67:15, 1992.
174. Huber TS, Harward TRS, Flynn TC, et al: Operative mortality rates after elective infrarenal aortic reconstructions, *J Vasc Surg* 22:287, 1995.
175. Hug HR, Taber RE: Bypass flow requirements during thoracic aneurysmectomy with particular attention to the prevention of left heart failure, *J Thorac Cardiovasc Surg* 57(2)203, 1969.
176. Hummel BW, Raess DH, Gewertz BL, et al: Effect of nitroglycerin and aortic occlusion on myocardial blood flow, *Surgery* 155:159, 1982.
177. Hunter PR, Endrey-Waler P, Bauer GE, et al: Myocardial infarction following surgical operations, *Br Med J* 4:725, 1968.
178. Hurford WE, Zapol WM: The right ventricle and critical illness: a review of anatomy, physiology, and clinical evaluation of its function, *Inten Care Med* 14:448, 1988.
179. Iberti TJ, Fischer EP, Leibowitz AB, et al: Pulmonary artery catheter study group. A multicenter study of physicians' knowledge of the pulmonary artery catheter, *JAMA* 264(22):2928, 1990.
180. Imparato AM, Riles TS, Mintzer R, et al: The importance of hemorrhage in the relationship between gross morphologic characteristics and cerebral symptoms in 376 carotid artery plaques, *Ann Surg* 197:195, 1983.
181. Reference deleted in proofs.
182. Jain KM, Patil KD, Doctor US, et al: Preoperative cardiac screening before peripheral vascular operation, *Ann Surg* 51:77, 1985.
183. Jamieson WRE, Janusz MT, Miyagishima RT, et al: Influence of ischemic heart disease on early and late mortality after surgery for peripheral occlusive vascular disease, *Circulation* 66(suppl I):I92, 1982.
184. Jeffrey CC, Kunsman J, Cullen DJ, et al: A prospective evaluation of cardiac risk index, *Anesthesiology* 58:462, 1983.
185. Johnston KW, Scobie TK: Multicenter prospective study of non-ruptured abdominal aortic aneurysms. I. Population and operative management, *J Vasc Surg* 7:69, 1988.
186. Josephson MA, Brown BG, Hecht HS, et al: Noninvasive detection and localization of coronary stenoses in patients: comparison of resting dipyridamole and exercise thallium-201 myocardial perfusion imaging, *Am Heart J* 103:1008, 1982.
187. Kainuma M, Katsuragawa K: An attempt to avoid changes in blood pressure resulting from aortic clamping or declamping, by the use of a balloon catheter placed in inferior vena cava, *Jap J Anesth* 34:94, 1985.
188. Kalman PG, Wellwood MR, Weisel RD, et al: Cardiac dysfunction during abdominal aortic operation: the limitations of pulmonary wedge pressures, *J Vasc Surg* 3(5):773, 1986.
189. Kandarpa K: *Handbook of cardiovascular and interventional radiologic procedures,* Boston, 1989, Little, Brown and Company.
190. Kang YG, Gelman S: Liver transplantation. In Gelman S, editor: *Anesthesia and organ transplantation,* Philadelphia, 1987, WB Saunders.
191. Kaplan JA, Dunbar RW, Bland JW Jr: A problem for the anesthesiologist, *Anesth Analg* 54:571, 1975.
192. Kaplan JA, King SB III: The precordial electrocardiographic lead (V_5) in patients who have coronary-artery disease, *Anesthesiology* 45:570, 1976.
193. Katz NM, Blackstone EH, Kirklin JW, et al: Incremental risk factors for spinal cord injury following operation for acute traumatic aortic transection, *J Thorac Cardiovasc Surg* 81:669, 1981.
194. Kazui T, Komatsu S, Yokoyama H: Surgical treatment of aneurysms of the thoracic aorta with the aid of partial cardiopulmonary bypass: an analysis of 95 patients, *Ann Thorac Surg* 43:622, 1987.
195. Kearse LA, Lopez-Bresnahan M, McPeck K, Zaslavsky A: Preoperative cerebrovascular symptoms and EEG abnormalities do not predict cerebral ischemia during carotid endarterectomy, *Stroke* 26:1210, 1995.
196. Keith W, Morgan C: Clinical significance of pulmonary function tests, *Chest* 75:712, 1979.
197. Kennedy SK, Wasnick JD: Cerebrovascular surgery. In Yeager MP, Glass DD, editors: *Anesthesiology and vascular surgery,* Norwalk, 1990, Appleton & Lange.
198. Korenaga GM, Kirkpatrick A, Lord JG, et al: Effect of esmolol on tachycardia induced by endotracheal intubation, *Anesth Analg* 64:238, 1985.
199. Reference deleted in proofs.
200. Kouchoukos NT, Wareing TH, Izumoto H, et al: Elective hypothermic cardiopulmonary bypass and circulatory arrest for spinal cord protection during operations on the thoracoabdominal aorta, *J Thorac Cardiovasc Surg* 99:659, 1990.
201. Reference deleted in proofs.
202. Krupski WC, Layug EL, Reilly LM, et al: Comparison of cardiac morbidity rates between aortic and infrainguinal operations: two-year follow-up. Study of Perioperative Ischemia Research Group, *J Vasc Surg* 18:609, 1993.
203. Lampe GH, Mangano DT: Anesthetic management for abdominal aortic reconstruction. In Roizen MF, editor: *Anesthesia for vascular surgery,* New York, 1990, Churchill-Livingstone.
204. Landesberg G, Erel J, Anner H, et al: Perioperative myocardial ischemia in CEA under cervical plexus block and prophylactic nitroglycerin infusion, *J Cardiothorac Vasc Anesth* 7(3):259, 1993.
205. Lane RT, Sawada SG, Segar DS, et al: Dobutamine stress echocardiography for assessment of cardiac risk before noncardiac surgery, *Am J Cardiol* 68:976, 1991.
206. Larsen SF, Olesen KH, Jacobsen E, et al: Prediction of cardiac risk in non-cardiac surgery, *Eur Heart J* 8:179, 1987.
207. Larson CP Jr: Anesthesia and surgery for cerebrovascular insufficiency: one approach at Stanford. In Roizen MF, editor: *Anesthesia for vascular surgery,* New York, 1990, Churchill-Livingstone.
208. Laschinger JC, Owen J, Rosenbloom M, et al: Direct non-invasive monitoring of spinal cord motor function during thoracic aortic occlusion: use of motor-evoked potentials, *J Vasc Surg* 7:161, 1988.
209. Latson TW, Yin FCP, Hunter WC: The effects of finite wave velocity and discrete reflections on ventricular loading. In Yin FCP, editor: *Ventricular/vascular coupling,* New York, 1987, Springer-Verlag.
210. Laxorthes G, Gouaze A, Zadeh Jo, et al: Arterial vascularization of the spinal cord. Recent studies of the anastomotic substitution pathways, *J Neurosurg* 35:253, 1971.
211. Lee KS, Courtland HD, McWhorter JM: Low morbidity and mortality of carotid endarterectomy performed with regional anesthesia, *J Neurosurg* 69:483:1988.
212. Lehv MS, Salzman EW, Silen W: Hypertension complicating CEA, *Stroke* 1(5):307, 1970.
213. Leppo J, Boucher CA, Okada RD, et al: Serial thallium-201 myocardial imaging after dipyridamole infusion: diagnostic utility in detecting coronary stenoses and relationship to regional wall motion, *Circulation* 66:649, 1982.
214. Leppo J, Plaja, J, Gionet M, et al: Noninvasive evaluation of cardiac risk before elective vascular surgery, *J Am Coll Cardiol* 9:269, 1987.
215. Leppo J, Yipintsoi T, Blankstein R, et al: Thallium-201 myocardial scintigraphy in patients with triple-vessel disease and ischemic exercise stress tests, *Circulation* 59:714, 1979.
216. Lesser RP, Raudzens P, Luders H: Postoperative neurological deficits may occur despite unchanged intraoperative somatosensory evoked potentials, *Ann Neurol* 19:22, 1986.
217. Leung JM, O'Kelly BF, Mangano DT, et al: Relationship of regional wall motion ab-

normalities to hemodynamic indices of myocardial oxygen supply and demand in patients undergoing CABG surgery, *Anesthesiology* 73:802, 1990.
218. Reference deleted in proofs.
219. Lipsett PA, Tierney S, Gordon TA, et al: CEA-Is intensive care unit care necessary? *J Vasc Surg* 20:403, 1994.
220. L'Italien GJ, Cambria RP, Cutler BS, et al: Comparative early and late cardiac morbidity among patients requiring different vascular surgery procedures, *J Vasc Surg* 21:935, 1995.
221. Reference deleted in proofs.
222. Livesay JJ, Cooley DA, Ventemiglia RA, et al: Surgical experience in descending thoracic aneurysmectomy with and without adjuncts to avoid ischemia, *Ann Thorac Surg* 39:37, 1985.
223. LoGerfo FW, Coffman JD: Vascular and microvascular disease of the foot in diabetics, *N Engl J Med* 311:1615, 1984.
224. London MJ, Hollenbert M, Wong MG, et al: Intraoperative myocardial ischemia: localization by continuous 12-lead electrocardiography, *Anesthesiology* 69:232, 1988.
225. Reference deleted in proofs.
226. London MJ, Tubau JF, Wong MG, et al: The "natural history" of segmental wall motion abnormalities in patients undergoing noncardiac surgery, *Anesthesiology* 73:644, 1990.
227. Lunn JK, Dannemiller FJ, Stanley TH: Cardiovascular responses to clamping of the aorta during epidural and general anesthesia, *Anesth Analg* 58:372, 1979.
228. Lusby RJ: Surgery for cerebrovascular disease: surgical goals and methods. In Roizen MF, editor: *Anesthesia for vascular surgery*, New York, 1990, Churchill-Livingstone.
229. Lusby RJ, Ferrell LD, Ehrenfeld WK, et al: Carotid plaque hemorrhage. Its role in production of cerebral ischemia, *Arch Surg* 117:1479, 1982.
230. Magnusson J, Thulin T, Werner O, et al: Hemodynamic effects of pretreatment with metoprolol in hypertensive patients undergoing surgery, *Br J Anesth* 58:251, 1986.
231. Mangano DT: Preoperative assessment. In Kaplan JA, editor: *Cardiac anesthesia,* vol 1, ed 2, New York, 1987, Grune & Stratton.
232. Mangano DT: Preoperative risk assessment. Many studies, few solutions: is a Cardiac risk assessment paradigm possible? *Anesthesiology* 83:897, 1995.
233. Mangano DT, Goldman L: Preoperative assessment of patients with known or suspected coronary disease, *N Engl J Med* 333(26):1750, 1995.
234. Mangano DT: Perioperative cardiac morbidity, *Anesthesiology* 72:153, 1990.
235. Mangano DT, Browner WS, Hollenberg M, et al: Association of perioperative myocardial ischemia with cardiac morbidity and mortality in men undergoing non-cardiac surgery, *N Engl J Med* 323(26):1781, 1990.
236. Reference deleted in proofs.
237. Mantha S, Roizen M F, Barnard J, et al: Relative effectiveness of four preoperative tests for predicting adverse cardiac outcomes after vascular surgery: a meta-analysis, *Anesth Analg* 79:22, 1994.
238. Martin GM, Sprague CA: Symposium on *in vitro* studies related to atherogenesis: life histories of hyperplastoid cell lines from aorta and skin, *Exp Mol Pathol* 18:125, 1973.
239. Martinez BD, Hertzer NR, Beven EG: Influence of distal arterial occlusive disease on prognosis following aortobifemoral bypass, *Surgery* 88:795, 1980.
240. Masaryk TJ, Ross JS, Modic MT, et al: Carotid bifurcation: MR imaging, work in progress, *Radiology* 166:461, 1988.
241. Mason JJ, Owens DK, Harris RA, et al: The role of coronary angiography and coronary revascularization before noncardiac vascular surgery, *JAMA* 273:1919, 1995.
242. Reference deleted in proofs.
243. McCullough JL, Hollier CH, Nugent M: Paraplegia after thoracic aortic occlusion: influence of cerebral spinal fluid drainage, *J Vasc Surg* 7:153, 1988.
244. McFarland HR, Pinkerton JA Jr, Frye D: Continuous electroencephalographic monitoring during carotid endarterectomy, *J Cardiovasc Surg* 29:12, 1988.
245. McGill HC Jr: Persistent problems in the pathogenesis of atherosclerosis, *Arteriosclerosis* 4:443, 1984.
246. Messick JM, Casement B, Sharbrough FW, et al: Correlation of regional cerebral blood flow with EEG changes during isoflurane anesthesia for carotid endarterectomy, *Anesthesiology* 66:344, 1987.
247. Michenfelder JD: Anesthesia and surgery for cerebrovascular insufficiency: one approach at the Mayo Clinic. In Roizen MF, editor: *Anesthesia for vascular surgery,* New York, 1990, Churchill-Livingstone.
248. Michenfelder JD, Milde JH, Sundt TM Jr: Cerebral protection by barbiturate anesthesia. Use of middle cerebral artery occlusion in Java monkeys, *Arch Neurol* 33:345, 1976.
249. Miller RR, Olson HG, Amsterdam EA, et al: Propranolol-withdrawal rebound phenomenon. Exacerbation of coronary events after abrupt cessation of anti-anginal therapy, *N Engl J Med* 293:416, 1975.
250. Moffat JA, McDougall MJ, Brunet D, et al: Thiopental bolus during carotid endarterectomy: rational drug therapy? *Can Anaesth Soc J* 30:615, 1983.
251. Morawetz RB, Zeiger HE, McDowell HA Jr, et al: Correlation of cerebral blood flow and EEG during carotid occlusion for endarterectomy (without shunting) and neurologic outcome, *Surgery* 96:184, 1984.
252. Mowlan A, McClintock JT, Campbell GS: Effect on renal function of occlusion of the aorta inferior to the renal vessels, *Surg Gynecol Obstet* 111:423, 1960.
253. Mulcare RJ, Royster TS, Weiss HJ, et al: Disseminated intravascular coagulation as a complication of abdominal aortic aneurysm repair, *Ann Surg* 180:343, 1974.
254. Muskett A, McGreevy J, Miller M: Detailed comparison of regional and general anesthesia for carotid endarterectomy, *Am J of Surgery* 152:691, 1986.
255. Myers BD, Miller DC, Mehigan JT, et al: Nature of the renal injury following total renal ischemia in man, *J Clin Invest* 73:329, 1984.
256. Naslund TC, Hollier LH, Money SR, et al: Protecting the ischemic spinal cord during aortic clamping, *Ann Surg* 215:409, 1992.
257. N Engl J Med, NASCET: Beneficial effect of CEA in symptomatic patients with high grade carotid stenosis, *N Engl J Med* 325(7):445, 1991.
258. Reference deleted in proofs.
259. North RB, Drenger B, Beattie C, et al: Spinal cord stimulation evoked potential monitoring during throacoabdominal aneurysm surgery, *Neurosurgery* 28:325, 1991.
260. Novelsteen A, Suy R, Daenen W, et al: Aortofemoral grafting: factors influencing late results, *Surgery* 88:962, 1980.
261. Nussmeier NA, Arlund C, Slogoff S: Neuropsychiatric complications after cardiopulmonary bypass: cerebral protection by a barbiturate, *Anesthesiology* 64:165, 1986.
262. O'Connor CJ, Rothenberg DM: Anesthetic considerations for descending thoracic aortic surgery: part I, *J CarVasc Anesth* 9(5):581, 1995.
263. O'Connor CJ, Rothenberg DM: Anesthetic considerations for descending thoracic aortic surgery: part II, *J Car Vasc Anesth* 9(6):734, 1995.
264. O'Donnel TF, Darling RC, Linton RR: Is 80 years too old for aneurysmectomy? *Arch Surg* 111:1250, 1976.
265. O'Donnel TF, Callow AD, Willet C, et al: The impact of coronary artery disease on carotid endarterectomy, *Ann Surg* 198:705, 1983.
266. O'Hara PJ, Hertzer NR, Krajewski LP, et al: Ten-year experience with abdominal aortic aneurysm repair in octogenarians: early results and late outcome, *J Vasc Surg* 21:830, 1995.
267. Olivier HF, Maher TD, George AL, et al: Use of the Bio-Medicus centrifugal pump in traumatic tears of the descending aorta, *Ann Thorac Surg* 38:586, 1984.
268. O'Rourke K, Beattie C, Walman AT, et al: Acidosis during high cross-clamp surgery, *Anesthesiology* 63:266, 1985.
269. Padayachee TS, Bishop CCR, Gosling RG, et al: Monitoring cerebral perfusion during carotid endarterectomy, *J Cardiovasc Surg* 31:112, 1990.
270. Pagani M, Pizzinelli P, Bergamaschi M, et al: A positive feedback sympathetic pressor reflex during stretch of the thoracic aorta in conscious dogs, *Circ Res* 50(1):125, 1982.
271. Palmer MA: Comparison of regular and general anesthesia for carotid endarterectomy, *Am J Surg* 157:329, 1989.
272. Pasternak PF, Grossi EA, Baumann FG, et al: The value of silent myocardial ischemia monitoring in the prediction of perioperative myocardial infarction in patients undergoing peripheral vascular surgery, *J Vasc Surg* 10:617, 1989.
273. Pasternak PF, Imparato AM, Bear G, et al: The value of radionuclide angiography as a predictor of perioperative myocardial infarction in patients undergoing abdominal aortic aneurysm resection, *J Vasc Surg* 1:320, 1984.
274. Pasternak PF, Imparato AM, Riles TS, et al: The value of radionuclide angiogram in the prediction of perioperative myocardial infarction in patients undergoing lower extremity revascularization procedures, *Circulation* 72(suppl II):13, 1985.
275. Paterson IS, Klausner JM, Goldman G, et

al: Pulmonary edema after aneurysm surgery is modified by mannitol, *Ann Surg* 210:796, 1989.
276. Plecha FR, Avellone JC, Bevan EG, et al: A computerized vascular registry: Experience of the Cleveland vascular society, *Surgery* 86:826, 1979.
277. Plumlee JE, Boettner RB: Myocardial infarction during and following anesthesia and operation, *South Med J* 65:886, 1972.
278. Priano LL: Infrarenal aortic reconstruction. In Yeager MP, Glass DD editors: *Anesthesiology and vascular surgery,* Norwalk, 1990, Appleton & Lange.
279. Proctor LT, Schmeling WT, Roerig D, et al: Oral dexmedetomidine attenuates hemodynamic responses during emergence from general anesthesia in chronically instrumented dogs, *Anesthesiology* 74:108, 1991.
280. Prough DS, Scuderi PE, Stullken E, et al: Myocardial infarction following regional anaesthesia for carotid endarterectomy, *Can Anesth Soc J* 31(2):192, 1984.
281. Reference deleted in proofs.
282. Raby KE, Goldman L, Creager MA, et al: Correlation between preoperative ischemia and major cardiac events after peripheral vascular surgery, *N Engl J Med* 321(19): 1296, 1989.
283. Rao TK, Jacobs KH, El-Etr AA: Reinfarction following anesthesia in patients with myocardial infarction, *Anesthesiology* 59:499, 1983.
284. Reference deleted in proofs.
285. Reigel MM, Hollier LH, Kazmier FJ, et al: Late survival in abdominal aortic aneurysm patients: the role of selective myocardial re-vascularization on the basis of clinical symptoms, *J Vasc Surg* 2:222, 1987.
286. Reference deleted in proofs.
287. Roberts AJ, Nora JD, Hughes A, et al: Cardiac and renal responses to cross-clamping of the descending thoracic aorta, *J Thorac Cardiovasc Surg* 86:732, 1983.
288. Roizen MF: Anesthetic goals for operations to relieve or prevent cerebrovascular insufficiency. In Roizen MF, editor: *Anesthesia for vascular surgery,* New York, 1990, Churchill-Livingstone.
289. Reference deleted in proofs.
290. Roizen MF, Beaupre PN, Alpert RA, et al: Monitoring with two-dimensional transesophageal echocardiography: comparison of myocardial function in patients undergoing supraceliac, suprarenal-infraceliac, or infrarenal aortic occlusion, *J Vasc Surg* 1:300, 1984.
291. Roizen MF, Lampe GH, Benefiel DJ, et al: Is increased operative stress associated with worse outcome? *Anesthesiology* 67(3A):A1, 1987.
292. Rosenfeld BA, Beattie C, Christopherson R, et al: The effects of different anesthetic regimens on fibrinolysis and the development of postoperative arterial thrombosis, *Anesthesiology* 79(3):435, 1993.
293. Rosenthal D, Stanton PE Jr, Lamis PA: Carotid endarterectomy. The unreliability of intraoperative monitoring in patients having had stroke or reversible ischemic neurological deficit, *Arch Surg* 116:1569, 1981.
294. Ross J Jr: Afterload mismatch and preload reserve: a comceptual framework for the analysis of ventricular function, *Prog Cardiovasc Dis* 18(4):255, 1976.
295. Ross R, Glomset JA: The pathogenesis of atherosclerosis. Part 1. *N Engl J Med* 295:369, 1976.
296. Ross R, Glomset JA: The pathogenesis of atherosclerosis. Part 2. *N Engl J Med* 295:420, 1976.
297. Ross R: The pathogenesis of atherosclerosis—an update, *N Engl J Med* 314:488, 1986.
298. Reference deleted in proofs.
299. Ruby ST, Whittemore AD, Couch NP, et al: Coronary artery disease in patients requiring abdominal aortic aneurysm repair: selective use of a combined operation, *Ann Surg* 201:758, 1985.
300. Sassano JJ: The rapid transfusion system. In Winter P, Kang YG, editors: *Transplantation: anesthetic and perioperative management,* New York, 1986, Praeger.
301. Sawada SG, Segar DS, Ryan T, et al: Echocardiographic detection of coronary artery disease during dobutamine infusion, *Circulation* 83:1605, 1991.
302. Schneider RM, Seaworth JF, Dohrmann ML, et al: Anatomic and prognostic implications of an early positive treadmill exercise test, *Am J Cardiol* 50:682, 1982.
303. Schoeppel LS, Wilkinson C, Waters J, et al: Effects of myocardial infarction on perioperative cardiac complications, *Anesth Analg* 62:493, 1983.
304. Schoonover GA, Olsen GN: Pulmonary function testing in the perioperative period: a review of the literature, *J Clin Surg* 1:125, 1982.
305. Schurlknight S, Beattie C, O'Rourke K, et al: Metabolic changes during high aortic cross-clamp surgery. *Abstracts of the Eighth Annual Meeting of the Society of Cardiovascular Anesthesiologists,* p 72, Richmond, 1986.
306. Seeling W, Bruckmooser K-P, Hufner C: Continuous thoracic epidural analgesia does not diminish postoperative complications after abdominal surgery in patients at risk, *Anaesthesist* 39:33, 1990.
307. Sellgren J, Ponten J, Wallin G: Percutaneous recording of muscle nerve sympathetic activity during propofol, nitrous oxide, and isoflurane anesthesia in humans, *Anesthesiology* 73:20, 1990.
308. Shah DM, Darling RC, Chang BB, et al: Carotid Endarterectomy in awake patients: its safety, acceptability and outcome, *J Vasc Surg* 19:1015, 1994.
309. Shah KB, Kleinman BS, Hafez S: Re-evaluation of perioperative myocardial infarction in patients with poor myocardial infarction undergoing non-cardiac operations, *Anesth Analg* 71:231, 1990.
310. Shehadi WH: Contrast media adverse reactions: occurrence, recurrence and distribution patterns, *Radiology* 143:11, 1982.
311. Shenaq SA: Anesthesia for resection of abdominal aortic aneurysm: one approach at Baylor College of Medicine. In Roizen MF, editor: *Anesthesia for vascular surgery,* New York, 1990, Churchill-Livingstone.
312. Shenaq SA, Chelly JE, Kalberg, et al: Use of nitroprusside during surgery for thoracoabdominal aortic aneurysm, *Circulation* 70(suppl 1):7, 1984.
313. Silverstein PR, Caldera DL, Cullen DJ, et al: Avoiding the hemodynamic consequences of aortic cross-clamping and unclamping, *Anesthesiology* 50:462, 1979.
314. Skydell SL, Machleder HI, Baker JD, et al: Incidence and mechanism of post-carotid endarterectomy hypertension, *Arch Surgery* 122:1153, 1987.
315. Slogoff S, Keats AS, Ott E: Preoperative propranolol therapy and aortocoronary bypass operation, *JAMA* 240:1487, 1978.
316. Slogoff S, Keats AS: Does perioperative myocardial ischemia lead to postoperative myocardial infarction? *Anesthesiology* 62:107, 1985.
317. Slogoff S, Keats AS: Does chronic treatment with calcium entry blocking drugs reduce perioperative myocardial ischemia? *Anesthesiology* 68:676, 1988.
318. Small DM: Progression and regression of atherosclerotic lesions. Insights from lipid physical biochemistry, *Atherosclerosis* 8:103, 1988.
319. Smith JS, Cahalan MK, Benefiel DJ, et al: Intraoperative detection of myocardial ischemia in high-risk patients: electrocardiography versus two-dimensional transesophageal echocardiography, *Circulation* 72:1015, 1985.
320. Smith JS, Roizen MF, Cahalan MK, Benefiel DJ, et al: Does anesthetic technique make a difference? Augmentation of systolic blood pressure during CEA: Effects of phenylephrine versus light anesthesia and isoflurane versushalothane on the incidence of myocardial ischemia, *Anesthesiology* 69:846, 1988.
321. Stallone RJ, Inverson CK, Young JN: Descending thoracic aortic aneurysm, *Am J Surg* 142:106, 1981.
322. Stanton PE Jr, Shannon J, Rosenthal D, et al: Intraoperative autologous transfusion during major aortic reconstructive procedures, *South Med J* 80:315, 1987.
323. Steen PA, Tinker JH, Tarhan S: Myocardial reinfarction after anesthesia and surgery, *JAMA* 239:2566, 1978.
324. Stene JK, Burns B, Permutt S, et al: Increased cardiac output following occlusion of the descending thoracic aorta in dogs, *Am J Physiol* 243:R152, 1982.
325. Stoelting RK: Circulatory changes during direct laryngoscopy and tracheal intubation: influence of duration of laryngoscopy with or without prior lidocaine, *Anesthesiology* 47:381, 1977.
326. Stoelting RK: Attenuation of blood pressure response to laryngoscopy and tracheal intubation with sodium nitroprusside, *Anesth Analg* 58:116, 1979.
327. Stokland O, Miller MM, Ilebekk A: Mechanism of hemodynamic responses to occlusion of the descending thoracic aorta, *Am J Physiol* 238:H423, 1980.
328. Stone JG, Foex P, Sear JW, et al: Myocardial ischemia in untreated hypertensive patients: effect of a single small oral dose of a beta-adrenergic blocking agent, *Anesthesiology* 68:495, 1988.
329. Sundt TM, Houser OW, Sharbrough FW, et al: Carotid endarterectomy: Results, complications and monitoring techniques, *Adv Neurol* 16:97, 1977.
330. Svensson LG, Rickards E, Coull A, et al: Relationship of spinal cord blood flow to

vascular anatomy during thoracic aortic cross-clamping and shunting, *J Thorac Cardiovasc Surg* 91:71, 1986.

331. Svensson LG, Klepp P, Hinder RA, et al: Spinal cord anatomy of the baboon: comparison with man and implications on spinal cord blood flow during thoracic aortic cross-clamping, *S Afr J Surg* 24:32, 1986.
332. Svensson LG, Von Ritter CM, Groeneveld HT, et al: Cross-clamping of the thoracic aorta; influence of aortic shunts, laminectomy, papaverine, calcium channel blocker, allopurinol, and superoxide dismutase on spinal cord blood flow and paraplegia in baboons, *Ann Surg* 204:38, 1986.
333. Svensson LG, Stewart RW, Cosgrove DM, et al: Intrathecal papaverine for the prevention of paraplegia after operation on the thoracic or thoracoabdominal aorta, *J Thorac Cardiovasc Surg* 96:823, 1988.
334. Sweeney PJ, Wilbourn AJ: Spinal accessory (11th) nerve palsy following carotid endarterectomy, *Neurology* 42:674, 1992.
335. Szilagyi DE, Hageman JH, Smith RF, et al: Spinal cord damage in surgery of the abdominal aorta, *Surgery* 83:38, 1978.
336. Tam S, Chung F, Campbell M: Intravenous lidocaine: optimal time of injection before tracheal intubation, *Anesth Analg* 66:1, 1987.
337. Tarhan S, Moffitt E, Taylor WF, et al: Myocardial infarction after general anesthesia, *JAMA* 1451, 1972.
338. Taylor LM, Porte JM: Basic data related to clinical decision-making in abdominal aortic aneurysms, *Surgery* 98:472, 1985.
339. Thompson JE: Complications of carotid endarterectomy and their prevention, *World J Surg* 3:155, 1979.
340. Thompson JE, Hollier LH, Paman RD, et al: Surgical management of abdominal aortic aneurysms: factors influencing mortality and morbidity—a 20-year experience, *Ann Surg* 181:654, 1875.
341. Thompson JE: Don't throw out the baby with the bath water—a perspective on carotid endarectomy (editorial), *J Vasc Surg* 4:543, 1986.
342. Tisi GM: Preoperative evaluation of pulmonary function: validity, indications, and benefits, *Am Rev Respir Dis* 119:293, 1979.
343. Tomatis LA, Fierens EE, Verbrugge GP: Evaluation of surgical risk in peripheral vascular disease by coronary arteriography: a series of 100 cases, *Surgery* 71:429, 1972.
344. Toole JF, Executive Committee for the Asymptomatic Carotid Atherosclerosis Study: Endarterectomy for asymptomatic carotid artery stenosis, *JAMA* 27(18):1421, 1995.
345. Tuman K, McCarthy R, March R, et al: Effects of epidural anesthesia and analgesia on coagulation and outcome after major vascular surgery, *Anesth Analg* 73:696, 1991.
346. Uematsu S, Tolo VT: Recording of the somatosensory evoked potentials during surgery for scoliosis and midline myelotomy to monitor spinal cord function, *Electromyo Clin Neurophysiol* 21:253, 1981.
347. Van Aken H, Puchstein C, Hidding J: The prevention of hypertension at intubation, *Anaesthesia* 37:82, 1982.
348. Veith FJ, Gupta SK, Ascer E: Femoral popliteal and tibial occlusive disease. In Wilson SE, Veith FJ, Hobson RW et al, editors: Vascular principles and practice, New York, 1987, McGraw-Hill.
349. Reference deleted in proofs.
350. Reference deleted in proofs.
351. Reference deleted in proofs.
352. Weich HF, Strauss HW, Pitt W: The extraction of thallium-201 by the myocardium, *Circulation* 56:188, 1977.
353. Weiner DA, McCabe CH, Ryan TJ: Prognostic assessment of patients with coronary artery disease by exercise testing, *Am Heart J* 105:749, 1983.
354. Wells PH, Kaplan JA: Optimal management of patients with ischemic heart disease for non-cardiac surgery by complementary anesthesiologist and cardiologist interaction, *Heart J* 102:1029, 1981.
355. West H, Burton R, Roon AJ, et al: Comparative risk of operation and expectant management of carotid artery disease, *Stroke* 10:117, 1979.
356. Willenkin RL: Management of general anesthesia. In Miller RD, editor: *Anesthesia,* ed 3, New York, 1990, Churchill-Livingstone.
357. Willerson JT, Hillis LD, Winniford M, et al: Speculation regarding mechanisms responsible for acute ischemia heart disease syndromes (editorial), *J Am Coll Cardiol* 8:245, 1986.
358. Williams GM: Complications of vascular surgery, *Surg Clin North Am* 73(2):323, 1993.
359. Williams GM: Thoracoabdominal aneurysm. In Camera JL, editor: *Current surgical therapy-3,* Toronto, 1989, BC Decker.
360. Winslow CM, Solomon DH, Chassin MR, et al: The appropriateness of carotid endarterectomy, *N Engl J Med* 318:721, 1988.
361. Wong MG, Wellington YC, London MJ, et al: Prolonged postoperative myocardial ischemia in high-risk patients undergoing noncardiac surgery (abstract), *Anesthesiology* 69:A56, 1988.
362. Yasher JJ, Indeglia RA, Yasher J: Surgery for abdominal aortic aneurysms—factors affecting survival and long-term results, *Am J Surg* 123:398, 1972.
363. Yeager MP, Glass D, Neff K, et al: Epidural anesthesia and analgesia in high risk surgical patients, *Anesthesiology* 66:729, 1987.
364. Reference deleted in proofs.
365. Yeager MP, Glass DD: Anesthesia for abdominal aortic reconstruction: one approach at Dartmouth Medical School. In Roizen MF, editor: *Anesthesia for vascular surgery,* New York, 1990, Churchill-Livingstone.
366. Reference deleted in proofs.
367. Young AE, Sandberg GW, Couch NP: The reduction of mortality of abdominal aortic aneurysm resection, *Am J Surg* 134:585, 1977.
368. Zaidan JR, Guffin AV, Perdue G, et al: Hemodynamics of intravenous nitroglycerin during aortic clamping, *Arch Surg* 117:1285, 1982.
369. Zarins CK: Peripheral vascular insufficiency: surgical goals and methods. In Roizen MF, editor: *Anesthesia for vascular surgery,* New York, 1990, Churchill-Livingstone.
370. Zwolak RM, Cronenwett JL: Pathophysiology of vascular disease. In Yeager MP, Glass DP, editors: *Anesthiology and vascular surgery,* Norwalk, 1990, Appleton & Lange.

CHAPTER 72

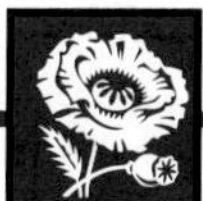

Anesthesia for Gastrointestinal Surgery

WILLIAM T. MERRITT

The gastrointestinal (GI) tract is a fascinating organ system with a complex neurochemical organization.[108] GI surgery occupies a major percentage of the operative time in any general hospital setting. Anesthesia for such procedures likewise represents a major portion of the anesthesiologist's responsibilities. Many of these procedures are done so frequently that they may become routine. Others are sufficiently sophisticated that they are done only in tertiary care and teaching institutions. This chapter includes illustrations of some typical procedures and discusses preoperative, intraoperative, and postoperative considerations. It begins with a discussion of issues pertinent to the effects of anesthesia administration on GI function. Subsequent sections deal with surgical and anesthetic considerations of specific areas regarded as GI in nature.

GASTROINTESTINAL FUNCTION AND THE ADMINISTRATION OF ANESTHESIA

Esophagus and Stomach

Proper function of the esophagus and the lower esophageal sphincter (LES) is a serious concern to the anesthesiologist. If the esophagus is dilated because of obstruction by tumor, destruction of neural mechanisms (e.g., achalasia), or existence of a diverticulum, particulate matter will remain for hours (if not days) after ingestion, and secretions will not pass normally to the stomach. **If the LES is not functioning properly or if a hiatal hernia exists, stomach contents may reflux into the esophagus and pharynx during anesthesia and surgery, increasing the potential for serious aspiration pneumonia.** Placement of a cuffed endotracheal tube during surgical procedures largely protects the airway from such materials. When obstructions are present, endotracheal intubation should occur with the patient awake (e.g., direct oral, blind nasal, or fiberoptic bronchoscopy) or via a rapid-sequence method with the patient anesthetized. With the awake method, sedation should be limited or avoided altogether, especially in patients with a "full" stomach, proximal obstruction, esophageal diverticulum, or altered consciousness. Emptying the gastric or esophageal contents (e.g., nasogastric tube, Sengstaken-Blakemore tube) should decrease the volume and nature of any refluxed material.[41,122] In any patient with known hiatal hernia or LES dysfunction or when the stomach or esophagus is suspected to contain fluid or particulate matter, an attempt should be made to aspirate the material before emergence from anesthesia. In addition, extubation should occur only after swallowing, adequate strength, and the ability to follow commands are apparent.

Many surgical approaches to the esophagus require a thoracotomy and a laparotomy, the lateral position, and a method of collapsing one lung. In addition, an esophageal dilator or a nasogastric or naso-"intestinal" tube often should be positioned at some point during the procedure (the latter should be securely fixed to maintain continuity above and below the anastomosis). Such procedures can be demanding and require considerable preoperative planning.

Management of Acid Reflux

Abdominal surgery has been associated with as much as 75% of the perioperative mortality related to aspiration pneumonitis.[87] In addition, fasting gastric volume can be high in patients with GI disorders, especially duodenal ulcer disease.[40] Many other conditions, some directly related to the GI tract, are associated with some risk of regurgitation of esophageal or stomach contents and ultimate pulmonary aspiration (Box 72-1). In these conditions, an inadequate initial clearance or the return of a substance to the pharynx is followed by ineffective removal with subsequent passage through the glottic opening into the lungs.[43] Mortality associated with aspiration ranges from 3% to 70%,[9,11,47,164] and the true incidence and morbidity are not well quantified. A recent large European study suggests the actual incidence is considerably lower, about 0.05%.[176] Unrecognized or "silent" regurgitation typically occurs, as does subsequent aspiration.[30,34,48,240]

The volume, pH, and presence or absence of particulate matter appear to be the three most important factors determining the severity of the pulmonary insult. Particulate matter obstructs airways and quickly leads to ventilation and perfusion mismatching, hypoxia, hemorrhagic edema, and sometimes acute pulmonary hypertension.[211] Traditionally, gastric volumes greater than 25 ml and pH below 2.5 have been associated with the most severe pneumonitis,[203a,227a] although more recent data suggest that greater volumes of nonparticulate aspirated fluid would be tolerated if the pH were higher than 2.5.[102,132,211]

In addressing the problem of aspiration during the delivery of anesthesia, anesthesiologists have focused on four areas: (1) reduction of the acid content and volume of the stomach contents, (2) improvement of intestinal motility, (3) prevention of reflux into the pharynx, and (4) a better understanding of gastric emptying.

Although antacids increase gastric pH, particulate (i.e., opaque) antacids produce severe aspiration damage similar to that of gastric acid.[102] The use of clear antacids is just as effective in increasing pH but is associated with only mild pulmonary changes if aspirated.[53,90,235]

Histamine-2 (H_2) blocking agents are effective in reducing the acidity and, to a lesser extent, the volume of gastric fluid. Three agents are currently used: cimetidine and ranitidine are backed by extensive clinical experience; famotidine is a more recent introduction.[1,83] None of these agents has much effect on the acidity of material already present in the stomach (e.g., that found in the trauma patient or patients requiring other emergency surgery) but may decrease intraoperative acid production if given before surgery. Oral therapy seems to be as effective (and considerably less expensive) as intravenous (IV) or intramuscular forms when premedication by the oral route is suitable. Administration the night before and the morning of surgery consistently increases gastric pH to above 2.5. Rapid administration of cimetidine has been associated with hypotension,[62,63,95] bradycardia,[200] and cardiac arrest.[216] Ranitidine appears to have a lower incidence of similar side effects.[15,46] Mechanisms may include blockage of the inotropic and chronotropic responses of stimulation of myocardial H_2 receptors.[64,104] These agents alter metabolism or kinetics of various drugs, including the cytochrome P-450 system,[28,166] lidocaine,[21] nifedipine,[222] theophylline,[101,239] warfarin,[219] and phenytoin.[20] Although atropine and glycopyrrolate decrease gastric acid production somewhat, they generally are not used for this specific purpose because they also decrease LES tone.

Gastric and intestinal motility are stimulated by metoclopramide, which acts centrally by inhibiting dopamine and in the gut by releasing acetylcholine. LES tone also increases, but the pylorus and duodenum relax.[39,210] Metoclopramide usually is administered concurrently with an H_2 blocker. For those undergoing emergency surgery and in patients with suspected full stomachs, clear-liquid antacids are given before anesthesia induction in an attempt to bring the pH to above 2.5.

Preventing refluxed material from reaching the pharynx is the goal of cricoid pressure (Sellick's maneuver) and rapid-sequence intubation. When properly performed, cricoid pressure should provide a barrier for at least 100 cm

BOX 72-1
CONDITIONS ASSOCIATED WITH ASPIRATION PNEUMONIA

- Altered state of consciousness
- Inadequate pharyngeal reflexes
- Anesthesia induction, intubation
- "Full" stomach
- Abnormal esophageal function
- Abnormal LES
- Intestinal obstruction
- Abdominal distension
- Pregnancy
- Obesity
- Inadequate muscle relaxant reversal
- Poor cough
- Abdominal infection
- Abdominal trauma
- Pain
- Recent extubation

H_2O of esophageal pressure.[214] Pressure should not be released until the cuff is inflated and until correct placement has been verified by appropriate observations, including auscultation and capnometry.

As more is learned about the physiology of gastric emptying, the tradition of overnight fasting for elective surgery has come into question.[66,127,154,160,227] Residual gastric volumes may be acceptable after 2 to 4 hours of fasting, and the addition of H_2 blockers lowers pH. Such information should not be extrapolated directly to the emergency patient or the patient with a full stomach. **The aspiration of particulate matter produces such a devastating insult in the lung that, except for the most urgent situations, 6 to 8 hours of fasting after solid foods is recommended.** Even after this waiting period, the stomach often still contains food and large amounts of fluid.

Bowel Distension

Nitrous oxide (N_2O) administration is associated with an increase in intraluminal gas volume. Experimentally, in dogs, bowel gas volume increases about 75% to 100% after 2 hours of 70% to 80% N_2O and by 100% to 200% after 4 hours.[88] Normally, luminal contents include approximately 100 ml of gas, mostly swallowed air; aerophagia or bowel obstruction greatly increases this volume. Clinically, N_2O use results in a slow increase in bowel distension and intraluminal pressure. The chief surgical effect is difficulty with abdominal closure at the completion of a procedure. During extreme conditions (e.g., obstruction with distended bowel), increased intraluminal pressure may lead to bowel ischemia. N_2O use during abdominal surgery should probably be limited to the initial 10 to 15 minutes at induction and intubation and to the period of wound closure at the completion of the surgical procedure. (See Endoscopic Procedures section for issues regarding N_2O during laparoscopy.)

Bowel Motility

Neostigmine is representative of anticholinesterase drugs necessary for the reversal of residual nondepolarizing muscular blockade. These drugs have a history of relative safety, although their parasympathetic stimulation leads to undesirable side effects. Bradycardia occurs so often that it is anticipated and managed before its occurrence with the administration of a parasympatholytic drug (e.g., atropine or glycopyrrolate) at reversal of neuromuscular blockade. This parasympathetic stimulation also affects intestinal motility, increasing the frequency and pressure of peristaltic waves, especially in the colon. For unknown reasons, diseased colon (e.g., from ulcerative colitis, diverticulitis[182]) appears to be more susceptible to this effect. This has led to considerable debate over the potential for cholinesterase inhibitors to cause breakdown of colonic anastomoses.[3,27,58,245] Fortunately, residual anesthetic agents and pretreatment with parasympatholytic agents (atropine, glycopyrrolate) attenuate this response. Inadequate perfusion of the anastomotic site, infection, and underlying tissue abnormality are now thought to be more important issues.

Thiopental increases electrical and mechanical activity of the duodenum and jejunum in experimental studies, and atropine premedication decreases the response.[115] Ketamine has little effect on GI motility, and oral diazepam reduces gastric emptying and increases small bowel transit time.[33]

Narcotics have intestinal side effects that are well recognized. LES tone is decreased.[82] Gastric emptying is impaired[149] because of decreased propulsive motility and increased tone in the antrum of the stomach. The duodenum and the small intestine undergo a decrease in propulsive contractions, whereas the amplitude of rhythmic segmental nonpropulsive contractions often is enhanced, which results in an increase in resting tone and can cause peristaltic spasms. The proximal small bowel is more affected than the distal part, and the tone of the ileocecal valve is increased. Parasympatholytic agents can partially abolish these effects. In the large intestine, the effects can be more pronounced; peristaltic waves are decreased or absent. The amplitude of rhythmic nonpropulsive contractions is increased, often to the point of spasm. Anal tone also is increased. Again, diseased bowel appears more susceptible to such effects.[181]

High spinal and epidural anesthesia promote hyperperistaltic activity because of blockade of sympathetic innervation. The unopposed parasympathetic activity may cause nausea and vomiting in about 20% of patients, for whom atropine may be effective.[238] Because of the increased peristaltic activity, controversy has arisen about the effects of spinal or epidural anesthesia on anastomotic breakdown, especially in colon surgery. Some data suggest that this problem is not dramatically increased with regional anesthesia[5] and that colonic blood flow is improved by spinal or epidural anesthesia.[4] Others have disagreed with these findings.[32,230]

Postoperative ileus probably is related to the manual trauma during laparotomy or from increased splanchnic nerve discharge in other procedures. Gastric peristalsis returns within 24 to 48 hours, and colonic activity returns after 48 hours, beginning at the cecum and progressing caudally. Small bowel motility returns more rapidly, and sometimes enteral tube feedings can be initiated within 24 hours. This ileus can lead to mild abdominal distention and absent bowel sounds for as long as 48 to 72 hours. Passage of flatus, cramping, and return of appetite suggest the return of normal peristaltic activity.[169,251]

Although axial narcotics generally are recommended for pain relief in most patients, the side effects of pruritus, urinary retention, and especially respiratory depression are problematic in some. Effects are presumably through local spinal cord receptors and via more central mechanisms after rostral spread in the cerebrospinal fluid or systemic absorption. Although used extensively and successfully in patients undergoing all forms of surgery, including many varieties of abdominal surgery,[64,198] data have shown side effects of axial narcotics on intestinal motility[17] and at least one note of caution.[207]

Biliary Effects

Therapeutic doses of the opioids can cause a marked increase in biliary tract pressure in susceptible patients. For example, 10 mg of subcutaneous morphine can produce a tenfold increase in common bile duct pressure within 15 minutes that can last 2 or more hours.[131] This effect results from opiate receptor-mediated mechanisms that cause spasm of the sphincter of Oddi. Fentanyl and alfentanil also increase common bile duct pressure.[128,194] The general importance of this effect on intraoperative cholangiograms is uncertain, but fentanyl-supplemented anesthesia is associated with a 3% surgical failure rate.[138] Meperidine increases biliary tract pressure via mechanisms that are not receptor-mediated.[107] Opiate antagonists (e.g., naloxone) can reverse this opiate-related increase in biliary tract pressure (except for that caused by meperidine)[158] but also may reverse general analgesic effects. Sublingual nitroglycerin (0.6 mg) decreases the elevated intrabiliary pressure, but atropine only partially attenuates the response. Glucagon (1 to 3 mg), titrated to effect, also reverses opiate-related biliary spasm.[14]

Respiratory Function

Because abdominal surgery is performed with the patient in the supine position, the anesthesiologist should remember several points. Functional residual capacity (FRC) is decreased by 0.5 to 1.0 l in the supine position, and the relationship of FRC to closing volume contributes to the alveolar–arterial oxygen difference and shunt.[65,163,173] This augments the 15% to 20% decrease in FRC associated with general anesthesia,[81] which continues postoperatively.[6] The Trendelenburg position aggravates this problem even further[221] because more of the lung assumes zone III conditions. Patients with elevated pulmonary arterial pressure (e.g., mitral stenosis) generally do not tolerate the Trendelenburg position. Diaphragmatic impairment and abdominal pain contribute to the potential for major respiratory embarrassment after abdominal surgery and, at least initially, are intensified by any negative effects from residual inhalation agents, IV anesthetics, and neuromuscular blockade. After upper abdominal surgery, vital capacity remains abnormal for more than 1 week.[7,94] Experimental data demonstrate that excessive fluid administration contributes to hypoxemia by accumulating in the lungs and increasing arteriovenous shunting.[199]

Endoscopic Procedures

Endoscopic abdominal procedures have gained favor because of inconspicuous scars, less postoperative pain, shorter hospitalizations, and decreased hospital costs.[224] More recently, adrenalectomy has been undertaken through retroperitoneoscopic exposure.[159] As "minimally invasive" surgical techniques, reduced risk is implied, but such endoscopic surgery involves the instillation of gas under pressure into a "closed" cavity, a process that may initiate unique physiologic responses and potential complications.

Diagnostic examination, cholecystectomy, vagotomy, appendectomy, adrenalectomy, colectomy and hiatal, diaphragmatic, and inguinal hernia repair are among the abdominal procedures being performed with laparoscopic equipment. Each procedure has its own indications and conversion rates to an open method (e.g., 1.0% to 6.9% conversion to laparotomy with laparoscopic cholecystectomy).[69]

The physiologic changes associated with laparoscopy include those associated with tilting the patient to facilitate instrumentation and surgery, the pressure effects of instilled gas, and the systemic effects of the gas instilled (and absorbed)—almost universally CO_2.

The head-down position (i.e., Trendelenburg) reduces vital capacity because of the increased weight of the abdominal contents on the diaphragm.[244] This effect is more pronounced in elderly, obese, and debilitated patients. In those undergoing *open* procedures, it is made worse by the placement of retractors and surgical packing under the diaphragm. In addition to this encroachment on lung expansion, right mainstem intubation can occur. Either of these can be associated with hypoxemia.[44] In contrast, the head-up position redistributes central blood volume peripherally and further aggravates any impairment of venous return created by the pneumoperitoneum.

The instillation of CO_2 to create an intentional pneumoperitoneum carries with it a number of physiologic side effects and complications (Box 72-2). Mechanical injury at the time of trocar insertion can lead to bleeding or bowel perforation. Bleeding also can occur from injury to vessels encountered during surgical instrumentation and dissection. With current laparoscopic equipment, intraabdominal pressure is maintained between 12 to 15 mm Hg (17 to 22 cm

BOX 72-2
REPORTED COMPLICATIONS WITH LAPAROSCOPY

Hemorrhage
Hypotension, decreased cardiac output
Acidosis
Pneumothorax
Pneumomediastinum
Mainstem intubation
Subcutaneous emphysema
Airway obstruction
Retroperitoneal CO_2
Venous stasis
Bradycardia, increased vagal tone
Cardiac arrest
Venous CO_2 embolism, fatal
Regurgitation and aspiration

H_2O). Because of leaks around the various cannulae, enormous gas volumes ($\geq$ 50 l)[70] may be required during the course of the procedure to generate this relatively low pressure. Such pressures and the resulting abdominal distention may disturb the protective function of the gastroesophageal junction. The hemodynamic changes associated with this pneumoperitoneum depend on a number of factors, including the pressure of gas obtained, the amount of CO_2 absorbed, the patient's level of hydration, the type of ventilation, and the nature of the surgery. Cardiac function during insufflation of peritoneal CO_2 has been studied primarily in healthy (e.g., no known cardiac disease) patients using a variety of cardiac function measurements (dye dilution, impedance cardiography, transesophageal echocardiography, and pulmonary artery catheters). Unfortunately, none of the studies have controlled well for the level of anesthesia at the various stages of the procedures and have managed hypercapnia differently. Most studies have reported a decrease in left ventricular function and cardiac output (cardiac output decreased 7% to 24%),[67,135,139,162,209] but not all.[89,143a,156,174] Most studies have likewise found an increase in central venous pressure (CVP) (redistribution of abdominal blood volume?), with an increase in systemic vascular resistance and mean arterial pressure. In addition, with assumption of the reverse Trendelenburg position, cardiac index may decrease by 50% of preanesthesia and preinsufflation values.[114,139] Left ventricular end-diastolic, right atrial, and pulmonary capillary wedge pressures dramatically decrease after assumption of reverse Trendelenburg position.[71] Venous stasis of the lower extremities also occurs, with attendant concerns for embolic phenomenon.[52,165] Patients with cardiovascular disease will have responses to laparoscopy that are affected by their degree of cardiac reserve, baseline medications, level of hydration, and their response to the anesthesia used.[114,249] The potential deleterious effects of hypercapnia on cardiac function (e.g., increased sympathetic activity, myocardial depression) may further complicate laparoscopy in those with cardiovascular disease.[197]

During retroperitoneoscopic adrenalectomy (prone–jackknife position or lateral), a small (< 10 cm) cavity in the lumbodorsal fascia is created with a distension balloon trocar. CO_2 is insufflated to a pressure of 15 to 20 mm Hg. A recent report suggests, that unlike laparoscopy, stroke volume and cardiac output appear to increase with insufflation, as do mean arterial pressure, central venous pressure, and pulmonary artery pressure. No change was noted in pulmonary capillary wedge pressure, heart rate and systemic vascular resistance.[103]

Relatively small CO_2 emboli have been detected in 69% of American Society of Anesthesiologists physical status (ASA) I to III patients undergoing laparoscopic cholecystectomy when studied with transesophageal echocardiography.[78] Fatal massive CO_2 embolism has been reported,[152] including a report of death from delayed CO_2 embolism associated with gas trapping in the portal circulation.[204] With time, subcutaneous or mediastinal emphysema and pneumothorax may develop, with associated hypoxemia, hypotension, and cardiovascular collapse. The incidence of extraperitoneal insufflation of CO_2 has been reported to range from as little as 0.4% to 2%[141] to 20% to 64%[236] and is more likely during lengthy procedures, e.g., fundoplication.[57] **The development of pneumothorax and/or pneumomediastinum is a serious and/or potentially life-threatening complication. When either is suspected, from hemodynamic deterioration or from the presence of subcutaneous emphysema, especially of the neck and face, aggressive investigation (auscultation, chest radiograph) and management (e.g., chest tube for tension pneumothorax) should be undertaken. Procedures on the lower esophagus may be more likely to result in these complications.**[236]

Ventilation and pulmonary function are important issues. With conventional open laparotomy, it is well accepted that upper abdominal surgery is associated with postoperative pulmonary dysfunction in approximately 50% of patients.[116] This dysfunction is related to impaired diaphragmatic function, pain, type of incision, and decreased FRC.[24,137,193] **Pulmonary function is also impaired after laparoscopic cholecystectomy, with sustained decreases in forced vital capacity (FVC), peak expiratory flow, and forced expiratory volume in 1 second (FEV1) noted 24 hours after surgery; fortunately, these changes are only about 50% of those seen in conventional open cholecystectomy.**[192]

The exogenous CO_2 insufflated during laparoscopy is soluble in blood and after transperitoneal absorption is presented to the lungs for excretion. End-tidal CO_2 ($ETCO_2$) increases from 0% to 30%[79,124,161] when minute ventilation is held constant. Increasing ventilation by as much as 30% may be necessary to keep the $ETCO_2$ in the mid-30s (mm Hg) range.[121]

The overriding anesthetic concern is the preservation of ventilation, which tends to be impaired by surgical positioning and abdominal distention. This almost always means general anesthesia with intubation.[86,246] Not only does this provide protection for the airway,[92] but it permits adequate measurement of end-tidal CO_2 and manipulation of ventilation as needed. Routine intraoperative monitoring ($ETCO_2$, pulse oximetry, blood pressure, airway pressure) should be adequate for the expected physiologic changes encountered in most patients. The anesthesiologist should be aware of the insufflating pressure being used and should be alerted if an unusual amount of CO_2 is being required.

It is theoretically sound to avoid N_2O for at least two reasons. It diffuses into the abdominal cavity in concentrations sufficient to support combustion of intestinal gas.[80,172] Nitrous oxide also will diffuse into CO_2 bubbles and emboli, increasing their size and potential for obstructive event.

It is important to maintain sufficient muscle relaxation so that spontaneous respiratory effort does not impair the surgical procedure or risk increasing the gradient for embolic gas to enter the central circulation.

Despite the limited surgical scarring, postoperative muscle pain remains a problem, even in children.[153] This has not been eliminated by avoiding succinylcholine or by manipulation of other anesthetic regiments.[221a] Nausea and vomiting is common after laparoscopy, especially in women, and it appears that women are at increased risk for this during their menses.[23] Droperidol, a dopamine receptor antagonist, has been found to decrease nausea and vomiting in nonmenstruating women, but not during menses. Because serotonin has been implicated in several premenstrual syndromes, serotonin antagonist therapy (e.g., ondansetron) may be of benefit.

In the rare event of catastrophic hemodynamic collapse, several conditions should be kept in mind. **Hemorrhage can be obvious or occult (e.g., retroperitoneal). Pneumothorax, massive CO_2 embolus, and pneumomediastinum should be considered. Initial therapy includes releasing the pressurized pneumoperitoneum (i.e., conversion to open procedure). For pneumothorax, a thoracentesis should be performed. If massive embolization is to be managed, any N_2O should be discontinued, and cardiopulmonary resuscitation should be performed.** The patient should be placed in the left lateral position. Attempts at embolus retrieval can be made through a central venous access. If none of this provides sustained benefit, cardiopulmonary bypass may be necessary.

MEDICAL AND SURGICAL CONCERNS IN GI ILLNESS

The Esophagus

The esophagus extends from the pharynx at the level of C6 to the gastroesophageal junction. The hypopharynx courses from the level of the epiglottis to the upper border of the esophagus and funnels food into the esophagus. Swallowing begins as a voluntary process as food and liquid pass through the mouth, which initiates a complex and normally coordinated sequence of involuntary discharges through cranial nerves V, VII, X, and XII to the oropharynx and the esophagus. The upper third of the esophagus contains striated musculature; the lower third has smooth muscle, and the middle third has a mixed muscular supply. Motor innervation is supplied by the vagus nerves. Striated muscle is innervated by preganglionic fibers and smooth muscle by postganglionic fibers from Auerbach's plexus.

In adults, the upper esophageal sphincter (UES) is about 3 cm in length and consists of the cricopharyngeal muscle (striated), a portion of the inferior constrictor muscle superiorly, and circular esophageal muscles inferiorly.[126,183] The primary function of the UES is controlled by the swallowing mechanism in general, but its resting tone is increased in response to esophageal distension or acid from gastroesophageal reflux[248] and decreases during sleep.[140]

The lower end of the esophagus (3 to 5 cm in length) acts as a functional LES. Thickness of the smooth muscle layers increases in this area, and circular fibers develop considerable tension. Control of the LES tone is complex and chiefly results from vagal cholinergic and myogenic mechanisms, although prostaglandins,[26] neuropeptides (e.g., vasoactive intestinal peptide),[31] GI hormones (e.g., gastrin, motilin),[112] the progesterones and estrogens of pregnancy, and thyroid-stimulating hormone[2] are among substances known or suspected of affecting LES tone. Material enters the esophagus after voluntary propulsion by the tongue into the hypopharynx. With relaxation of the UES (resting tone, approximately 20 to 60 mm Hg), food enters the esophagus and is moved along by primary peristaltic waves (25 to 80 mm Hg). LES relaxation (resting tone, 10 to 20 mm Hg) occurs, and the bolus enters the stomach. This whole process takes only 4 to 8 seconds. Secondary peristaltic waves serve to move residual matter through and into the stomach. Normal esophageal motility is depicted in Fig. 72-1.

Acid reflux and hiatal herniation

Reflux of material from the stomach into the esophagus is a complex topic and is covered in depth in other texts.[74] Criteria for diagnosis include those of reflux symptoms (Box 72-3) and the results of various tests, including radiographic studies, endoscopy, biopsy, manometry, and prolonged esophageal pH monitoring. The pH test demonstrates

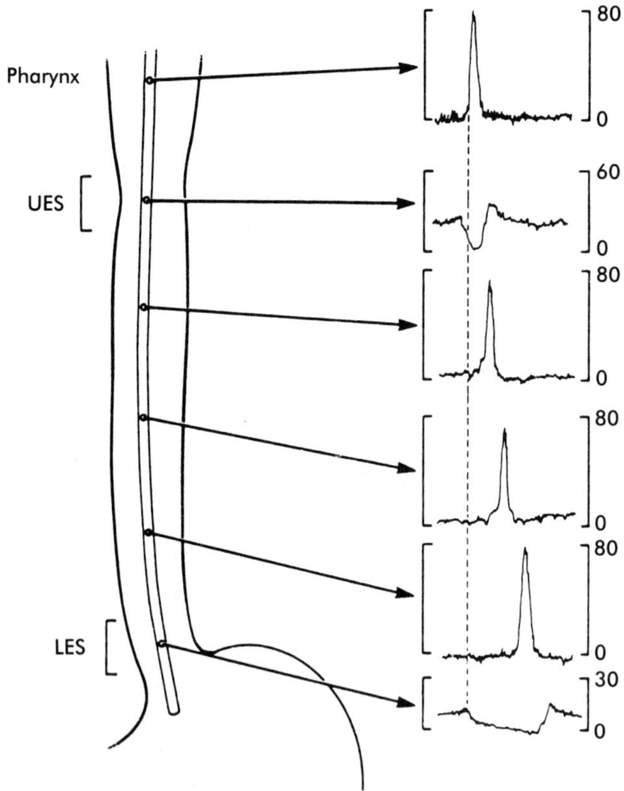

Fig. 72-1. Esophageal manometry. Simplified representation of normal physiologic pressures in pharynx, upper esophageal sphincter (*UES*), esophagus, and lower esophageal sphincter (*LES*). **On right,** high pressure zones are noted as the pressure catheter is withdrawn from stomach. **On left,** normal peristalsis occurs after a swallow, with relaxation followed by contraction and return to resting tone for UES and LES. (Modified from Payne WS, Ellis FH: Esophagus and diaphragmatic hernias. In Schwartz SI, editor: *Principles of surgery,* ed 4, New York, 1984, McGraw-Hill.)

that virtually all healthy subjects have episodes during daily activity when their esophagus is exposed to pH less than 4. This exposure is increased during awake upright activity, especially after eating, and during supine sleep activity,[77] when swallowing is inhibited (Table 72-1). This is largely caused by pressure gradients between the abdomen (+) and the thorax (intermittently −) while the patient is upright and by the normally higher LES tone in those in the supine position.[12,16,136,179,252] pH testing also detects those patients with reflux of alkaline duodenal material into the stomach and esophagus.[98]

The etiology for increased exposure of the esophagus to acid material and ultimately to the risks of acid and particulate matter aspiration can involve one of several mechanisms (Box 72-4). The mechanical competence of the LES depends on intrinsic tone (normally greater than 5 mm Hg[73]), the overall length of the LES muscular segment (normally 3 cm or longer), the portion of that segment that is intraabdominal (at least 1 cm), and interaction with the cardia of the stomach, which should transmit intraabdominal pressure to the distal LES.[36,73,180,185] The most common abnormality is decreased LES tone, but even normal LES tone can be affected by the other mechanisms.

Esophageal clearance of reflux material depends on gravity, intrinsic motor activity, salivation, and whether a hiatal hernia is present. Although the frequency of acid reflux may be greater during the day, the duration of episodes is longer when the patient is in the supine position because of loss of gravitational effects. Additionally, any disease that affects the motor activity of the esophagus may lead to impaired clearance of acid material (Box 72-5) with resultant effects on the esophageal mucosa and potential for aspiration.[123] Saliva is important in neutralizing the small amounts of acid refluxed with peristalsis even in healthy persons, and clearance of this acid is prolonged when saliva is removed by suctioning.[118] The salivation stimulated by heartburn (termed *waterbrash*) can lead to repetitive swallowing, aerophagia, and gastric distension with further reflux.[117]

The presence of a hiatal hernia is associated with additional abnormalities (Fig. 72-2). The hernia produces a defect in esophageal propulsion that results in inadequate acid clearance and longer transit time.[167] The retreat of all or part of the distal LES into the chest impairs the ability of the lower third of the LES, in concert with the cardia of the stomach, to impart extrinsic abdominal pressure and enhance sphincter function. If intrinsic LES tone also is decreased, a setup exists for major reflux of acid material and ultimately for the development of aspiration pneumonia. Despite this, most patients with hiatal hernias are asymptomatic.[68]

Certain abnormalities of gastric function also can result in acid reflux through a normal gastroesophageal junction or exacerbate preexisting LES abnormalities (Box 72-6). Normally, the body and fundus of the stomach are able to adapt to a large volume of material with minimal increases in pressure, although a previous vagotomy interferes with the active relaxation necessary for this to occur, and greater intragastric pressures occur with lesser volumes.[72] Outlet

BOX 72-3
SYMPTOMS OF ACID REFLUX

Heartburn
Anginal type of chest pain
Dysphagia
Regurgitation with bending or in supine position
Cough or wheezing from aspiration
Vagally induced bronchoconstriction

Table 72-1 Times in healthy subjects when esophagus is exposed to pH < 4 (n = 50)

Component	Mean	SD	95%
Upright time	2.34	2.34	8.42
Supine time	0.63	1.0	3.45
Number of episodes	19.00	12.76	46.90
Number > 5 min	0.84	1.18	3.45
Longest episode	6.74	7.85	19.80

Modified from DeMeester TR, Stein HJ: Gastroesophageal reflux disease. In Moody FG, editor: *Surgical treatment of digestive disease,* Chicago, 1990, Year Book Medical Publishers.

BOX 72-4
ETIOLOGY OF ACID REFLUX

Mechanically incompetent lower esophageal sphincter
Ineffective esophageal clearance of refluxed material
Abnormal gastric function

BOX 72-5
DISEASES AFFECTING ESOPHAGEAL MOTILITY

Achalasia
Alcoholic neuropathy
Brainstem lesions
Chagas' disease
Diabetes mellitus
Familial dysautonomia
Myotonia dystrophica
Polymyositis and dermatomyositis
Scleroderma

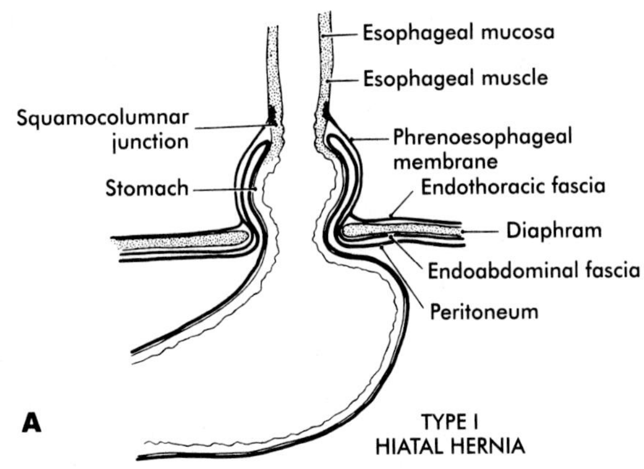

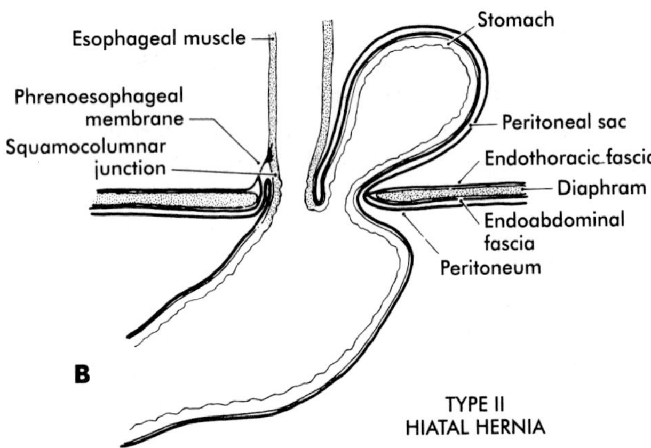

Fig. 72-2. Types of hiatal hernia. **A,** Type I sliding, or axial, hiatal hernia. **B,** Rarer type II rolling, or paraesophageal, hernia. (Modified from Skinner, DB: Hiatal hernia. In Keen G, editor: *Operative surgery and management,* ed 2, New York, 1987, Macmillan.)

BOX 72-6
ABNORMAL GASTRIC FUNCTION AND ACID REFLUX

Increased intragastric pressure
Delayed gastric emptying
Gastric dilation
Increased acid secretion

obstruction of the stomach more obviously leads to increases in pressure, which occurs normally with vomiting, but also with pyloric stenosis in newborns and obstructing ulcers or tumors in patients of any age.

Delayed gastric emptying leads to persistence of gastric acid and foodstuffs. The causes are varied[74] (Box 72-7) but yield a similar effect. As larger volumes accumulate and persist for a longer period, the potential for reflux through either a normal or abnormal LES increases. **Approximately 40% of patients with gastroesophageal reflux have delayed gastric emptying,[157,213] and in approximately one third of these, the delay is clinically significant.** Those rare patients with postviral gastroparesis also may have serious autonomic neuropathy.[175] Patients with various neurologic illnesses may manifest a variety of GI motility abnormalities.[100]

BOX 72-7
DELAYED GASTRIC EMPTYING

Myogenic abnormalities
- Diabetic gastric atony
- Diffuse neuromuscular disorders
- Postviral gastroparesis
- Postvagotomy

Pyloric dysfunction
Altered duodenal motility

As the stomach dilates from any cause, the relationship between the cardia and abdominal portion of the LES changes, which results in decreased maintenance of proper LES tone and increased risk of reflux. In addition to the conditions already mentioned, aerophagia from several causes also may lead to gastric distension. Normally, each pharyngeal swallow results in several cubic centimeters of swallowed air. Patients with reflux may habitually swallow (some even chew gum to stimulate saliva) to clear acid and can develop air-induced gastric distension, which can exacerbate their reflux. Other patients with decreased saliva formation (e.g., with Sjögren's syndrome) or after head and neck irradiation may swallow excessively with resultant aerophagia. Loss of secondary peristalsis, which can occur with diabetes mellitus and collagen vascular diseases, also leads to inordinate swallowing in an effort to propel food along, again with resultant aerophagia.

Gastric acid hypersecretion plays a role in some patients with gastroesophageal reflux who have a mechanically normal LES and is a complicating factor in other patients with abnormal LES function.[18,51,134]

The most serious acute consequence of acid reflux is the risk of aspiration of stomach contents. Chronic complications include esophagitis, stricture formation, and ultimately Barrett's esophagus, and chronic pulmonary disease from repeated episodes of aspiration. Aspects of surgical management are discussed next. Prophylaxis is covered later under anesthesia considerations.

Surgical procedures

Several surgical procedures for patients with esophageal disease are worthy of specific mention, but an extensive discussion is beyond this text.[168,212] Patient positioning, site of incision, and whether the esophagus will be transected are important to the anesthesiologist in all esophageal procedures.

Several approaches exist for the management of reflux disease. The Nissen-type (360° gastric fundoplication) procedure may be approached abdominally or through a left posterolateral thoracotomy. During the abdominal approach, severe liver retraction typically occurs, and the reverse Trendelenburg position is useful to the surgeon. The transthoracic approach may be used for repeat procedures, in obese patients, and when esophageal shortening is suspected. The Belsey-type (240° fundoplication) procedure also is approached from a left lateral chest incision. For any of these procedures, the anesthesiologist may be asked to pass a bougie through the pharynx into the distal esophagus to the area of surgical manipulation so that the repair can be sized. Should the restoration tend to slide back into the chest because the esophagus is too short, a lengthening procedure (e.g., colon interposition) may be required. Except for this latter maneuver, the esophagus is not transected for these procedures.

Several techniques are used for patients with esophageal cancer. For lesions of the distal esophagus, the Ivor-Lewis/McKeown-type repair (Fig. 72-3) includes an anterior abdominal incision followed by a right thoracotomy. The McKeown-type is similar but adds a right neck incision to facilitate the anastomosis of the stomach to the cervical esophageal remnant. Either procedure may include extensive node dissection in the chest, entry into the pericardium or the opposite chest, and thoracic duct ligation. Single-lung ventilation may facilitate operative exposure. Blunt esophagectomy (Fig. 72-4) is used for cervical esophageal disease, for lower-third esophageal carcinoma, and in early noninvasive disease. Abdominal and left cervical incisions are made, and extensive, "blind" bimanual dissection through the chest is performed. Bleeding or tracheal injury may necessitate an emergent thoracotomy. Postoperative recurrent nerve injury is described in 10% of patients.[231]

Peptic Ulcer Disease and Duodenal and Gastric Carcinoma

Millions of Americans have symptoms of acid and peptic ulcer disease.[228] Duodenal ulcer disease (DUD) occurs two to three times more often in men, and mortality rates may be somewhat higher in nonwhites aged to about 65 years. Genetic (e.g., family history, blood group O, HLA types B_5 and B_{12}) and environmental (e.g., smoking, aspirin, nonsteroidal anti-inflammatory drugs [NSAIDs]) factors are involved in DUD. Chronic pulmonary disease, cirrhosis, renal transplantation, and possibly high psychologic stress also may increase the incidence of ulcer disease. Resting and stimulated secretion of acid are increased[19,91] in common DUD, and in patients with gastrinoma (Zollinger-Ellison syndrome). The number of parietal cells secreting acid may be increased. The rapid emptying of stomach contents in some patients with DUD may overwhelm duodenal buffering and clearance mechanisms. Because these patients appear to have reduced duodenal bicarbonate secretion,[130] they are predisposed to ulceration.[147]

Gastric ulcers occur only one third to one fifth as often as duodenal ulcers, and causal factors in gastric ulcer disease (GUD) are largely unrelated to those for DUD. Genetic, psychologic, and hypersecretion of acid are not factors for most patients. The largest group of patients with GUD have normal-to-low secretion of acid and evidence of decreased gas-

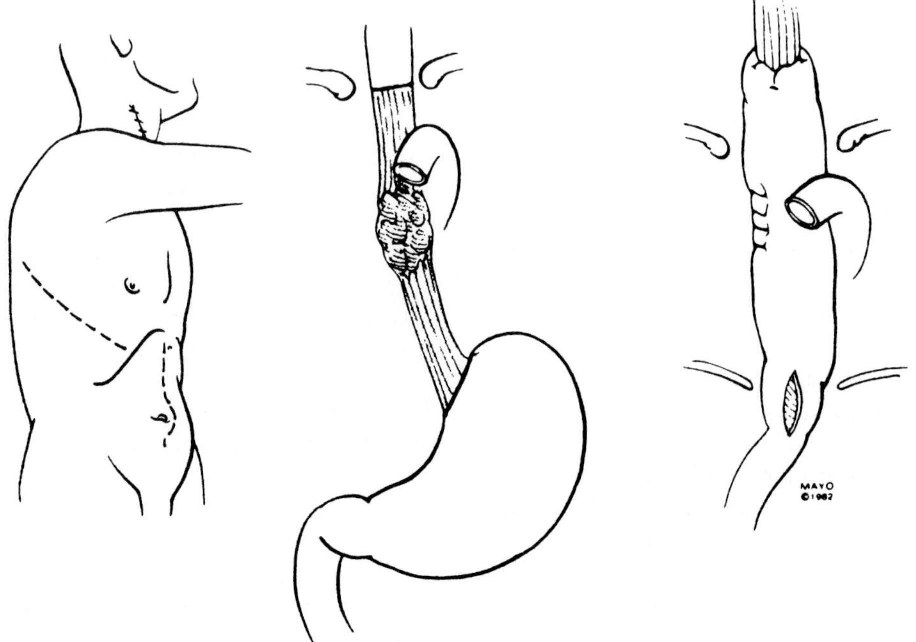

Fig. 72-3. Ivor-Lewis/McKeown-type esophagectomy. After abdominal mobilization of stomach, the chest and neck are explored concurrently to allow total esophagectomy and cervical esophagogastrostomy. (Modified from Payne WE, Ellis FH: Esophagus and diaphragmatic hernias. In Schwartz SI, editor: *Principles of surgery,* ed 4, New York, 1984, McGraw-Hill.)

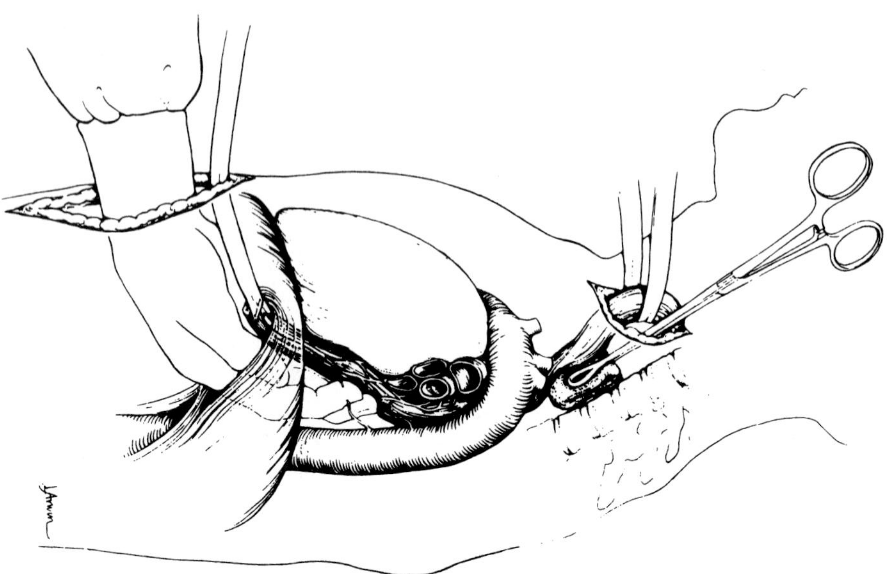

Fig. 72-4. Blunt esophagectomy. Maneuvers necessary for this procedure are capable of causing serious hemodynamic and ventilatory compromise and require appropriate monitoring of blood pressure and respiration. (Modified from Orringer MB, Sloan H: *J Thorac Cardiovasc Surg* 76:643, 1978.)

tric mucosal defenses against acid and pepsin-related endothelial injury. GUD tends to occur in older patients, and possibly as a result, this mortality rate is higher. GUD is associated with gastritis and with gastric carcinoma. Aspirin is clearly a risk factor,[203] as may be NSAIDs; both are thought to work via inhibition of prostaglandin synthesis. Pyloric function may be defective in patients with GUD, permitting reflux of duodenal, biliary, and pancreatic secretions into the stomach, initiating gastritis and ultimately ulcerations.[93] Smoking has been shown to reduce pyloric sphincter tone and increase the risk of bleeding from ulcers.[56] DUD and GUD have been associated with *Helicobacter pylori* infection.[178]

Medical treatment

The medical treatment of patients with ulcer disease involves dietary and environmental restrictions (e.g., avoiding aspirin, NSAIDs, smoking, alcohol; limiting caffeine, anxiety) and medication. Antacids, H_2-receptor antagonists, and coating agents (e.g., sucralfate) are useful in patients with DUD or GUD. Protein pump (H^+, K^+-ATPase) inhibition (e.g., omeprazole) has become important as an extremely potent inhibitor of gastric acid secretion in the patient with DUD. Exogenous prostaglandins ultimately may have a role. Bleeding patients undergo endoscopic procedures with the potential for cauterization. At arteriography, selective administration of vasopressor (e.g., vasopressin into the left gastric artery) or embolization may be warranted.

Surgical treatment

Several procedures and variations are performed for the management of DUD (Box 72-8). Duration of symptoms, gastric outlet obstruction, perforation,[35] and hemorrhage impose specific considerations, as do various known complications of these procedures (Box 72-9). For example, after a truncal or selective vagotomy, about 20% of patients will have clinically impaired gastric emptying if a drainage procedure also is not performed.[96]

BOX 72-8
SURGICAL MANAGEMENT OF DUODENAL ULCER DISEASE

- Vagotomy with drainage via pyloroplasty or gastrojejunostomy
- Vagotomy with antrectomy (hemigastrectomy) and gastroduodenostomy (Billroth I) or gastrojejunostomy (Billroth II)
- Subtotal gastrectomy and Billroth I or II

BOX 72-9
COMPLICATIONS OF PROCEDURES FOR DUODENAL ULCER DISEASE

- Abdominal fullness and pain
- Nausea
- Heartburn
- Reflux and regurgitation
- Bile and food emesis
- Dumping syndrome
- Diarrhea

Erosive gastritis is a common problem. Therapy involves appropriate blood and volume resuscitation, gastric irrigation with saline, and instillation of antacids. When bleeding does not stop or recurs, endoscopic evaluation and cauterization may suffice. If not, angiography may allow visualization of the damaged vessel for embolization or continuous infusion of intraarterial vasopressin.[10] Surgical procedures for hemorrhagic gastritis are required in 10% to 20% of patients. No single technique is considered the procedure of choice, and decisions regarding the nature of the procedure selected may require open visualization of the focal versus diffuse nature of the bleeding. Total gastrectomy, partial gastrectomy with vagotomy, vagotomy and pyloroplasty, devascularization, and simple oversew procedures all have advocates.[61,125,247]

Surgical therapy for patients with gastric ulcer generally involves ulcer removal and antrectomy (i.e., distal gastrectomy) with direct anastomosis to the duodenum (Billroth I procedure). Unless features of hypersection of acid exist, a vagotomy generally is not performed. Perforation can be managed with excision and simple closure in debilitated elderly patients or more definitively in younger stable patients. If malignancy is encountered, an appropriate procedure should be performed.

Gastric carcinoma generally is divided into two broad categories. Early carcinoma is confined to the gastric mucosa or submucosa, regardless of size or of lymph node seeding. Many of these patients are curable surgically. A subtotal gastrectomy is warranted for localized disease, and a total gastrectomy is needed for more extensive involvement. Surgical therapy for advanced gastric carcinoma is generally less successful because less than 10% of patients survive 5 years.[84] Procedures vary as to the extent of gastric resection and to the aggressiveness of lymph node and adjacent organ resection.[76,144,145,218] Some studies have suggested improved survival for patients undergoing palliative resections even when a cure is not possible.

Cholecystitis, Gallstone Disease, Cholecystectomy, and Biliary Disease

Approximately 20 million Americans have cholelithiasis, and another 800,000 are diagnosed each year.[206] Many predisposing factors exist (Box 72-10). The three basic types of gallstones are cholesterol, pigment, and mixed. The last category represents about 75% of all affected patients. Catalysts for stone formation include decreased gallbladder motility with stasis, increased gallblader mucous secretion, altered epithelial ion transport, and possibly increased gallbladder synthesis of prostaglandins,[150] and increased biliary calcium.[25,217]

Diagnosis. Clinical cholecystitis is classically associated with obstruction of the cystic duct (e.g., from stone, edema, sludge, fibrosis) and subsequent epithelial injury, enzyme release, and inflammatory response.[220] In about 75% of patients, cholecystitis is self-limiting and resolves over approximately 1 week, but 5% to 10% of patients develop serious complications, including empyema, cholangitis, gangrene, or perforation. Positive cultures are found in about 20% to 30% of patients aged less than 50 years, in greater than 50% of patients aged more than 70 years,[201] in 20% to 40% of those with chronic disease, and in 60% to 70% of those with acute cholecystitis.[54,99] Gram-negative organisms predominate. An overriding focus in evaluating patients is detecting cystic duct obstruction. Abdominal ultrasonography is extremely useful in detecting cholelithiasis and technetium scans in detecting cystic duct obstruction (even in patients with elevated bilirubin levels). Plain abdominal films, oral cholecystography, and IV cholangiography are more limited as diagnostic tools.

BOX 72-10
FACTORS ASSOCIATED WITH INCREASED INCIDENCE OF GALLBLADDER DISEASE

Increased age
Female sex
Pregnancy
Obesity
Hemolysis
After truncal vagotomy
Long-term parenteral nutrition
Pima Indians

Treatment. Oral therapy using deoxycholic acid analogs results in cholelitholysis because of their ability to decrease the rate-limiting enzyme in cholesterol synthesis coenzyme A reductase.[65] This is effective in some patients. Although it is recognized that asymptomatic gallstones frequently exist, management options are debated. Some studies document that about one third of these patients will develop complications requiring urgent surgery.[60,243] Others note that morbidity and mortality are lower after elective procedures in younger patients,[100,105] although most suggest that routine prophylactic cholecystectomy for asymptomatic disease is not required.[109]

Cholecystectomy generally is performed within several days of onset of symptoms. Approximately 25% of patients develop recurrent cholecystitis if surgery is delayed, and one in eight will require emergency cholecystectomy.[133,146,234] Despite the risks associated with older patients, conservative management (e.g., delayed surgery) in the elderly population may not be advisable; gallbladder empyema, perforation, sepsis, and cardiovascular complications occur more often in this group.[106,170,205]

Recently, several advances have permitted departure from standard laparotomy for uncomplicated gallstone management or gallbladder removal. Lithotripsy with high-frequency shock waves disintegrates some gallstones. General anesthesia usually is not needed, but sedation and analgesia with appropriate monitoring are required.[208] Laparoscopic techniques[83] have become extremely common and are discussed previously (Box 72-11).

BOX 72-11
EFFECTS AND COMPLICATIONS ASSOCIATED WITH LAPAROSCOPY

Altered ventilatory dynamics caused by large volume of intraabdominal carbon dioxide (CO_2)
Hypercapnia from CO_2 absorption
Decreased venous return from increased intraabdominal pressure
Venous CO_2 embolism, intraoperatively and in early postoperative period
Abnormal gastroesophageal junction competence from high intraabdominal pressure

The traditional approach to gallbladder removal (i.e., laparotomy) eventually may be relegated to patients with special considerations (e.g., abscess, perforation, need for intraoperative cholangiogram or bile duct exploration, suspected anatomic abnormalities, obesity). In addition, laparotomy remains the back-up procedure for other procedures that fail or for patients with complications. Surgical manipulation of the abdominal viscera has been associated with various circulatory changes, including bradycardia and hypotension.

Biliary tract cancer

As many as 2000 new cases of gallbladder carcinoma may be seen in the United States annually. Patients are likely to be elderly women who have associated gallstones. Because of early metastasis, most patients are unresectable at presentation, and their 5-year survival rate is extremely low. Patients with microscopic disease have a much better prognosis. Palliative procedures are difficult for those with advanced disease; biliary decompression stents are placed for bile drainage.

Extrahepatic bile duct cancer survival rate depends on the location of the tumor. Survival improves from proximal to distal common duct sites and is best with a papillary morphology. Most patients undergo one or more laparotomies before arrival at a tertiary center. Surgical management generally involves some form of biliary-enteric anastomosis (e.g., Roux-en-Y hepaticojejunostomy, Roux-en-Y choledochojejunostomy, Whipple procedure, palliative Silastic tube drainage) depending on the tumor's location.

Strictures of the biliary tract and sclerosing cholangitis

Benign strictures of the biliary tract result from various causes, including surgical trauma, inflammation from calculi, biliary tract infection (e.g., bacterial cholangitis), blunt or penetrating abdominal trauma, toxic injury during hepatic arterial infusion therapy, and sclerosing cholangitis. Eighty percent of patients have symptoms within 1 year of the associated surgery or trauma.[188] Symptoms and signs include abnormal biliary drainage or bile leakage immediately postoperatively and variable evidence of biliary obstruction and abnormal liver function in all patients. Painless jaundice and cholangitis are seen less often. Cholangiography should define biliary tree anatomy, and the placement of a ring catheter permits drainage and management of infection preoperatively.

When patients have an acute stricture after surgery, operative treatment may consist of the resection of a short segment of bile duct or a segmental duct ligation. More involved injuries usually demand creation of a Roux-en-Y jejunal limb and T-tube of transhepatic drainage catheters. Later in the postinjury period, extensive adhesions often are present, necessitating tedious dissection. Again, surgical management requires creation of a Roux-en-Y loop and decompression via T-tube, ring catheter, or a transhepatic Silastic stent. Sclerosing cholangitis is briefly covered in Chapter 73.

Pancreatic Procedures

Although laparotomy occasionally may be required in the patient with acute pancreatitis (e.g., for draining an abscess), the primary treatment is medical. Patients with pancreatitis are extremely ill with severe abdominal pain and may have fever, nausea and vomiting, jaundice, hypotension, ileus, and external distortion of the stomach on radiographs. Management includes nasogastic suction, maintenance of intravascular volume, anticipation of respiratory insufficiency,[129,151,196] analgesia, and nutritional support.

The patient with chronic pancreatitis may have incapacitating upper abdominal pain radiating to the back, which can be continuous or intermittent, especially after eating. Forty percent of patients have diabetes from loss of pancreatic tissue.[190] Exocrine function may be sufficiently abnormal to require pancreatic enzyme replacement. Obstructions, strictures, and dilations of the pancreatic ductal system are thought to produce the pain through sympathetic pathways. Several surgical procedures have evolved to decompress the ducts and remove damaged pancreas. A caudal pancreatojejunostomy[85] uses a Roux-en-Y loop to decompress the tail of the pancreas. With the Puestow-type[191] procedure (Fig. 72-5), the Roux-en-Y limb envelops the pancreas distally, allowing pancreatic ducts to be opened longitudinally for drainage into the loop. For both of these procedures, a splenectomy and excision of the tail of the pancreas are necessary for technical reasons. A modification of the Puestow procedure[184] (Partington procedure) allows the tail of the pancreas and the spleen to be spared. Postoperatively, some patients require insulin and pancreatic enzyme replacement. Other patients with severe chronic pancreatitis require a near-total pancreatectomy or a pancreatoduodenectomy to remove sufficient tissue to relieve pain. Patients with pseudocyst of the pancreas require drainage of the cyst through a Roux-en-Y loop or directly into the stomach. Alternatively, a distal cyst may be removed by a partial pancreatectomy.

Cancer of the pancreas and periampullary area is a frequently diagnosed problem with, unfortunately, an increasing incidence. Approximately 25,000 patients are diagnosed

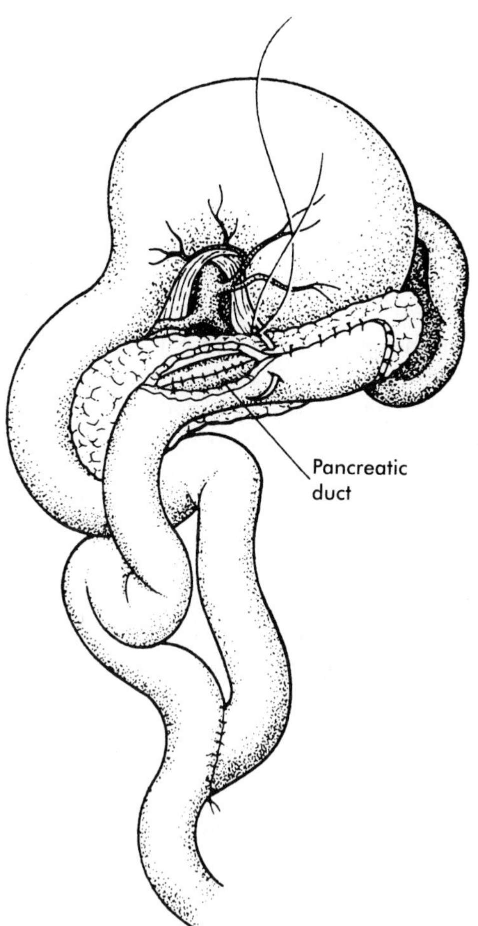

Fig. 72-5. Puestow procedure: lateral or longitudinal pancreatojejunostomy. Roux-en-Y limb of jejunum is sutured to open pancreatic duct along its length. (From Way L: *Current surgical diagnosis and treatment,* Los Altos, CA, 1985, Lange Medical Books.)

each year in the United States. Diagnosis usually is suggested by ultrasonography or computed tomography (CT). Magnetic resonance imaging (MRI), endoscopic retrograde cholangiopancreatography (ERCP), or percutaneous transhepatic cholangiography (PTC) may yield information concerning the site and etiology of bile duct obstruction. Percutaneous fine-needle aspiration biopsy may be performed with the aid of ultrasound examination or CT. Despite this array of tests, determination of the extent of disease and often the tissue diagnosis should await a thorough intraoperative examination. Only then can the necessary procedure be decided. The cure rate is 5% or less, largely because of relatively vague and general symptoms before the onset of jaundice, which greatly narrows the diagnostic possibilities. By the time the diagnosis is suspected, the lesion usually is unresectable. Because only small lesions of the head of the pancreas or ampullary area are resectable and because many of the remaining patients still require a palliative procedure to relieve obstructive jaundice, a considerable number of these patients undergo laparotomy.

Most procedures aimed at a cure are termed a *pancreatoduodenectomy* (Fig. 72-6; i.e., Whipple procedure). Variations include total pancreatectomy, regional pancreatectomy, and similar procedures that preserve the pylorus of the stomach. **These are long, extensive bowel resections that cause considerable morbidity. Serious postoperative complications include hemorrhage, coagulopathy, and hepatic, renal, pulmonary, and cardiovascular failure.**

Endocrine disease of the pancreas also is managed surgically. An insulinoma is the most common of these diseases. Because this tumor secretes insulin autonomously, spontaneous hypoglycemia is seen, with symptoms caused by decreased blood sugar levels and the resultant burst of catecholamine release. The differential diagnosis for hypoglycemia is extensive, but once insulinoma is diagnosed,

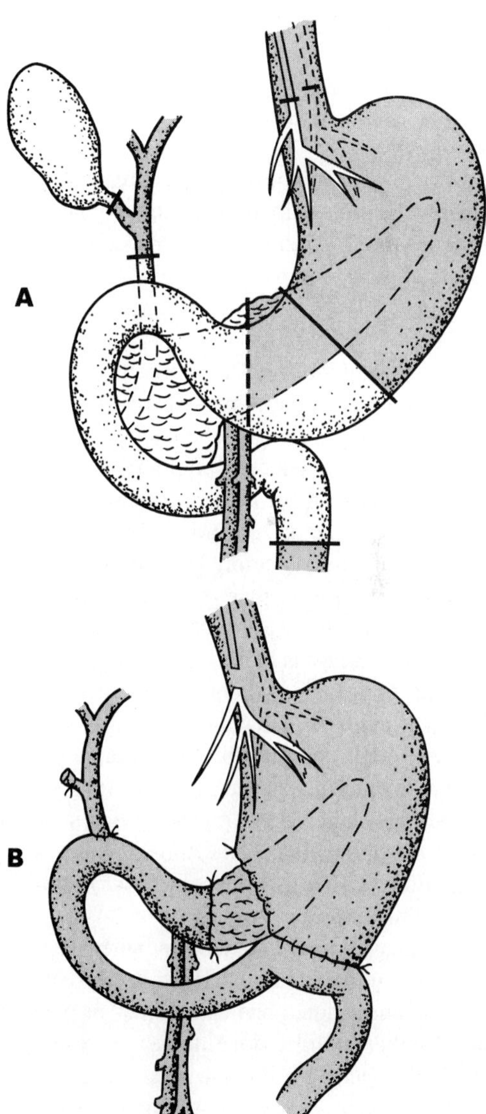

Fig. 72-6. Pancreatoduodenectomy (Whipple procedure). **A,** Presurgical anatomic relationships. **B,** Reconstruction demonstrating biliary, pancreatic, and gastric anastomoses. If distal stomach and pylorus are preserved, truncal vagotomy is unnecessary. Gallbladder is removed if diseased. (Modified from Way L: *Current surgical diagnosis and treatment,* Los Altos, CA, 1985, Lange Medical Books.)

management is surgical. Benign tumors are either enucleated or resected with a margin of pancreas. When no tumor is found at laparotomy, a distal or near-total pancreatectomy is performed, depending on the histology. Malignant disease may be surgically debulked with subsequent chemotherapy.

The Zollinger-Ellison syndrome results from a pancreatic or duodenal tumor (gastrinoma) that secretes excessive gastrin. Symptoms usually are abdominal pain and possibly diarrhea. Associated endocrinopathies include multiple endocrine neoplasia syndrome, type 1 (MEN 1: parathyroid, pituitary, adrenal) and MEN 2 (medullary carcinoma of the thyroid, parathyroid adenoma, pheochromocytoma). Medical management involves H_2-receptor antagonists or omeprazole (parietal cell proton pump blocker) therapy. Surgical management involves vagotomy and pyloroplasty when no tumor is discovered at laparotomy or major resection procedures when a localized tumor is found. The presence of metastatic disease and MEN syndromes dictates medical therapy.

Other endrocrine tumors of the pancreas include vasoactive intestinal peptide (vipoma), glucagonoma, and somatostatinoma. Surgical considerations are similar to those for insulinoma and gastrinoma.

Pancreas transplantation

Pancreas transplantation (PTX) is an emerging therapy for some diabetic patients but remains experimental despite almost 25 years of clinical experience.[143] Most patients receive their PTX with or shortly after a renal transplantation, although some have received a pancreas before becoming uremic (such treatment is controversial).[223]

Evaluation of patients before PTX includes extensive assessment of the cardiovascular system because the incidence of coronary artery disease in young diabetic patients with end-stage renal disease is high.[177] Active infection (e.g., dental abscess, peritonitis, osteomyelitis, decubitus ulcers) should be sought and managed before transplantation. Secondary diabetic complications (e.g., retinopathy) should be documented and quantified in an effort to gauge the effects of the transplant process on their progression. Absolute recipient contraindications include malignancy, active infection (including AIDS), blindness, advanced cardiovascular disease, and major amputation.

Donor organs typically come from patients aged less than 55 years without major atherosclerosis of the celiac axis, abdominal contamination, pancreatic injury or pancreatitis, or diabetes. Neither donor serum glucose nor amylase appear to have predictive value for ultimate function in the recipient.[120] Earlier competition between harvesting teams for the liver or pancreas has been largely resolved by techniques permitting simultaneous retrieval of the liver and the pancreas.[155,229]

The operative technique for PTX is not standardized. One European group with extensive experience drains the implanted pancreas enterically via a Roux-en-Y loop.[113,232] Reexploration is frequent with this procedure because of a high incidence of complications. Assessment of organ function and rejection is difficult.[233] Other centers perform PTX via a bladder drainage procedure (Fig. 72-7). Some have used direct draining of the pancreatic duct into the ureter or bladder, whereas others used a small "button" of duodenum or a closed duodenal segment for union with the bladder. Vascular anastomoses are with the iliac vessels, similar to a renal transplantation. Hypertension, abnormal renal function, and all the sequelae of diabetes mellitus and its management make this a challenging group of patients.

Perioperatively, patients undergoing PTX need to have appropriate cardiovascular monitoring and a regimented approach to managing serum glucose levels. This often entails insulin infusion protocols and frequent (every 30 minutes) intraoperative glucose determinations in an attempt to keep the blood sugar level in the 70 to 100 mg/dl range and to prevent hypoglycemia and hyperglycemia. Glucose-containing solutions are avoided unless the glucose level is lowered to less than 60 mg/dl. With reperfusion of the new pancreas, a dramatic increase occurs in blood sugar levels for reasons not entirely understood. It has been recommended that glucose levels be monitored frequently for the first hour or so after reperfusion. Postoperatively, the patient is treated in an intensive care setting.[97,186,225]

Gastrointestinal Bleeding

GI bleeding often represents a major diagnostic and therapeutic challenge. Initial signs may be hematemesis, melena,

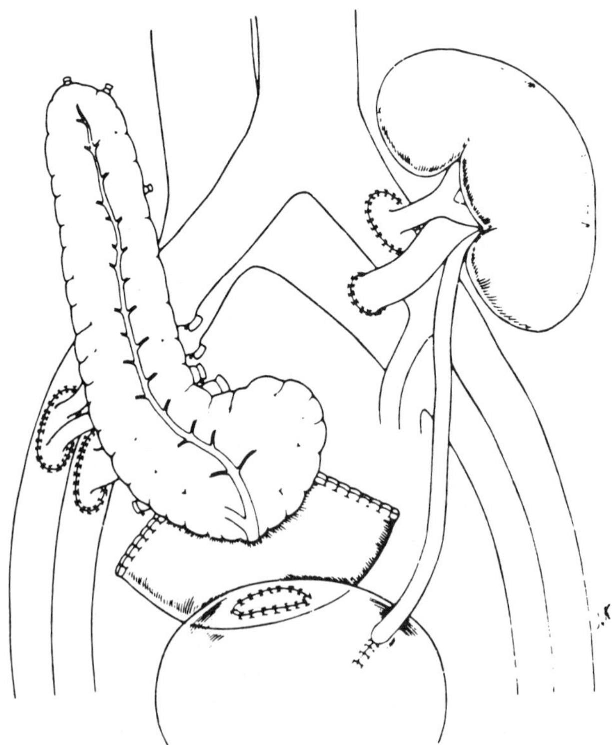

Fig. 72-7. Pancreas transplantation. Pancreas transplanted with bladder drainage via a pancreaticoduodenocystostomy. Concurrent renal transplantation also is depicted. (Modified from Sollinger HW: Pancreas transplantation in humans. In Moody FG, editor: *Surgical treatment of digestive disease,* ed 2, Chicago, 1990, Mosby–Year Book.)

hematochezia, or occult blood in the stool. As little as 60 ml loss per day can result in a black stool, and less than 10 ml can result in a positive Hemoccult test. Many patients with GI bleeding are elderly or debilitated, and symptomatic hemorrhage causes major stress to other organ systems (e.g., cardiac, renal, central nervous).

Upper tract bleeding

The list of potential etiologies for upper GI hemorrhage is lengthy, but the four most common causes appear to be peptic ulcer disease, erosive gastritis, esophageal varices, and Mallory-Weiss tears of the esophagus.[111] Other causes include malignancy, blood dyscrasias, hemostatic disorders, aortoenteric fistulas, Dielafoy's syndrome, and collagen vascular diseases. In one series, 12% of patients with upper GI bleeding had chronic renal failure and bled from angiodysplastic lesions of the stomach and duodenum.[253] **It usually is stated that if the patient's systolic pressure is less than 100 mm Hg, with a pulse greater than 100 (i.e., 2 or 3 units of blood loss or more), and with red or maroon stools, mortality rate is greater than 20%, and surgical intervention is necessary in more than 50% of patients.**[110] Chronic lung, renal, cardiac, and liver disease and age over 60 years add to this burden.

Diagnosis is aided by esophagogastroduodenoscopy in the first 24 hours. Management includes volume replacement and attention to illness in other systems. Some patients may receive parenteral vasopressin, such as an arterial infusion after angiography locates a bleeding ulcer or Mallory-Weiss tear, or an IV infusion for variceal bleeding. Varices often can be controlled with a Sengstaken-Blakemore tube, usually in preparation for more definitive management, such as sclerotherapy. Vasopressin often is still infusing when patients arrive for surgery to control bleeding. Vasopressin has been shown to increase splanchnic and hepatic arteriolar resistance while decreasing portal venous pressure and hepatic blood flow. After a bolus dose, effects may last for approximately 1 hour.[215] Worrisome side effects of vasopressin include coronary artery vasoconstriction with myocardial infarction, a potential complication of its use in patients with myocardial ischemia.[29] Intestinal and extremity ischemia also can occur.[8,148] Sclerotherapy and surgery for esophageal varices is covered in Chapter 73.

Lower tract bleeding

The more frequent causes of lower GI bleeding are anorectal polyps, colonic polyps, colorectal cancer, inflammatory bowel disease, submucosal angiodysplasia, and diverticular disease. In children, juvenile polyps, Meckel's diverticulum, and anteriovenous malformations are additional causes. Because the bleeding often is intermittent, diagnostic evaluation may be frustratingly negative. Endoscopy, radiographic examinations, and selective angiography are among the diagnostic and therapeutic (e.g., electrocoagulation, embolization) modalities. Technetium-99m-labeled erythrocyte scans appear to be useful for slow, recurrent lower GI bleeding.[142] Surgical procedures are directed toward the suspected diagnosis. Infrequently, when troublesome and symptomatic bleeding persists without a diagnosis, laparotomy may be undertaken for intraoperative endoscopy.

Obstructive Disease

Impaired GI transit results from various conditions causing pseudoobstruction (i.e., decreased motility) and paralytic ileus and those producing varying degrees of mechanical obstruction (Box 72-12). Considerable variation exists within each of these broad categories, and associated illness can be extensive.

Pseudoobstruction and paralytic ileus generally represent intestinal motility disorders, and the list of causes is long (Box 72-13).[59] Patients with pseudoobstruction usually have an insidious clinical course that evolves over months and years for the primary disease and for any coexisting GI manifestations. In general, remissions and exacerbations often occur.

Paralytic ileus tends to be acute in onset and to develop in patients with no suspected predisposing disease process. Although probably caused by neurohumoral mechanisms, paralytic ileus is not well understood. **The most common ileus is seen after intraabdominal operations, but this type is apparently not caused by "handling" at surgery.**[3] **The small intestine usually recovers motility within a few hours.**[202] **The stomach resumes its ability to empty after about 24 hours, but the colon may not regain effective motility for 48 hours or longer.** Strangely, it is known that electrical activity and smooth muscle contraction are not impaired postoperatively.[49,171,237] Other abdominal causes include blunt trauma, bowel perforation, bile peritonitis, and intraabdominal sepsis. Nonabdominal causes include lobar pneumonia, myocardial infarction, massive trauma, generalized sepsis, and electrolyte abnormalities such as hypophosphatemia and hypokalemia.

Mechanical obstruction is a vexing diagnostic problem that generally requires surgical intervention. Simple obstruction implies adequate blood flow to the obstructed area, whereas strangulation connotes insufficient circulation to the area. Obturated obstruction is caused by an intraluminal foreign body. Mechanical obstruction tends to be acute, with fairly rapid progression to complete obstruction.

Approximately 60% to 80% of obstruction occurs in the small intestine.[241] Pain, distension, emesis, and obstipation typically are present. Volume loss, tachycardia, and electrolyte disturbances can occur from severe vomiting and the massive volumes that are sequestered in strangulated bowel.

BOX 72-12
CAUSES OF IMPAIRED INTESTINAL TRANSIT

Pseudoobstruction
Paralytic ileus
Mechanical obstruction

BOX 72-13
PSEUDOOBSTRUCTION SYNDROMES

I. Primary idiopathic pseudoobstruction
  A. Familial syndromes
    1. Visceral myopathies
    2. Visceral neuropathies
  B. Sporadic syndromes
    1. Visceral myopathies
    2. Visceral neuropathies
II. Secondary pseudoobstruction
  A. Diseases of GI muscle
    1. Collagen disease
      a. Scleroderma
      b. Dermatomyositis and polymyositis
      c. Systemic lupus erythematosus
    2. Amyloidosis
    3. Generalized muscle disease
      a. Myotonic dystrophy
      b. Progressive muscular dystrophy
  B. Diseases of GI nerves
    1. Parkinson's disease
    2. Hirchsprung's disease
    3. Chagas' disease
    4. Primary autonomic dysfunction
  C. Endocrine diseases involving GI tract
    1. Myxedema ileus
    2. Diabetes mellitus
    3. Hypoparathyroidism
    4. +/− pheochromocytoma
  D. Drug-induced syndromes
    1. Opiates
    2. Psychotropic drugs
    3. Antiparkinsonian drugs
    4. Cathartics
  E. Miscellaneous
    1. Jejunoileal bypass
    2. Jejunal diverticulosis
    3. Inflammatory bowel disease
    4. Paraneoplastic neuropathy
III. Paralytic ileus
  A. Intraabdominal disease
  B. Extraabdominal disease

Modified from Christensen J: Intestinal pseudo-obstruction and paralytic ileus. In Moody FG, editor: *Surgical treatment of digestive disease,* ed 2, Chicago, 1990, Mosby–Year Book.

Approximately 7 to 9 l of fluid are presented to the gut daily[187] from varied sources (Table 72-2). With obstruction, not only is reabsorption hindered, but intestinal fluid secretion may be increased.[119] In addition, rapid infusion of IV fluids, which may be necessary for hemodynamic support, has been reported to increase secretion.[226] Once intraluminal pressure exceeds approximately 20 cm H_2O, reabsorption fails.[250]

Because intestinal fluid has a tonicity and electrolyte composition similar to extracellular fluids, acid–base and electrolyte disturbances generally are not severe. Duodenal obstruction can lead to hypokalemic alkalosis resulting from

Table 72-2 Fluids entering bowel daily

Source	Volume (ml)
Diet	2000
Saliva	1000
Gastric juice	2000
Bile	1000
Pancreatic juice	2000
Succus entericus	1000

BOX 72-14
CONDITIONS MIMICKING SMALL BOWEL OBSTRUCTION

Diabetic ketoacidosis
Sickle crisis
Porphyria
Pancreatitis
Ureteral and biliary colic
Food poisoning
Pseudoobstruction

severe emesis. In addition, once strangulation occurs (and no definitive criteria exist for this diagnosis), necrosis of bowel and bacterial proliferation contribute to rapid sequestration of fluid and colloid in the affected bowel and peritoneal cavity. Together with vomiting, this can produce marked depletion of intravascular volume and the potential for renal and cardiovascular instability.

Other conditions can mimic small bowel obstruction (Box 72-14), making the diagnosis difficult. This especially applies to elderly patients, who often have only minimal evidence of peritoneal irritation.

Acute large bowel obstruction is associated with pain, distension, vomiting, and obstipation, although large bowel obstruction can be more insidious than small bowel obstruction and may present without pain but with "overflow" diarrhea. Fifty percent or more results from colorectal cancer, with much of the rest caused by diverticulitis, volvulus, and fecal impaction.[242] Small bowel obstruction may occur concurrently. An incompetent ileocecal valve may permit the eventual development of feculent vomiting.

Management includes decompression of the stomach, appropriate IV fluids, and attention to conditions in other systems (e.g., infection, renal and cardiovascular problems). Depending on the patient's age and the severity of illness or suspected intervention, invasive hemodynamic monitoring may be warranted.

Patients with GI motility disorders and those with obvious obstruction are at risk for regurgitation and aspiration during the induction and maintenance of anesthesia and postoperatively. The anesthesiologist should be aware of the potential for such difficulty with this group of patients and treat appropriately. At the least, this would include the omission of oral premedication and the use of postoperative (and preoperative when indicated) nasogastric suctioning. Anesthesia should be induced using awake intubation or rapid-sequence or cricoid pressure considerations.

Splanchnic Ischemia and Systemic Inflammatory Response and Multiple Organ Dysfunction

Many severely ill patients require emergency surgical intervention for life-threatening conditions such as abdominal trauma, resection of nonviable bowel, relief of obstruction or strangulation, drainage of an abscess, or removal of a severely inflamed gallbladder. In addition to their abdominal disorder, they may be intubated in an intensive care unit, may have evidence of organ system failure (e.g., pulmonary, renal, central nervous system and major metabolic changes), or may be older with serious cardiac and vascular disease. Many behave as if they have a severe infection whether or not one is eventually discovered. In the past, varying etiologies have been suggested, including gram-negative sepsis, endotoxemia, sepsis syndrome, and multiple system organ failure. Because of the many similarities among such patients, even for those whose clinical course falls outside these diagnoses (e.g., patients with gram-positive sepsis, viral or fungal infection, or no infection at all), other explanations have been sought.

Common to many of these patients is evidence of major inflammatory mediator production and release by macrophages, primarily, but also from platelets, polymorphonuclear leukocytes, and the endothelium. The cyclooxygenase pathway has important effects. More than 30 such mediators have been identified, with cytokines such as tumor necrosis factor (TNF), interleukins 1 and 6, and platelet-activating factor among the most studied.[22]

Such findings have resulted in a new perspective on these conditions, now termed the *systemic inflammatory response syndrome* (SIRS). Currently, the diagnosis of this syndrome requires that two of the findings in Box 72-15 be present.[37] As the process evolves, organ dysfunction may ensue, and if more than one organ system becomes affected, multiple organ dysfunction syndrome (MODS) has developed. **SIRS and MODS appear to be the ends of a hierarchical continuum with an increasing inflammatory response to infectious and noninfectious stimuli;[195] end organ dysfunction and mortality rate increase with increasing inflammatory response.[50]**

Any insult to adequate core tissue perfusion (e.g., cardiac arrest, cardiopulmonary bypass) may result in severe or relative hypotension, with ensuing GI mucosal ischemia. Endogenous vasoconstrictors may be released[189] (Box 72-16), which may affect the splanchnic bed more consistently than others.[13,38,42,45,55] Reperfusion after shock may be associated with oxygen and free radical mucosal damage. In addition, so-called myocardial depressant factors can be released from the pancreas and possibly the small intestine, which further contribute to tissue hypoperfusion and low cardiac output syndrome. As much as 15% to 65% of the circulating volume can redistribute to damaged bowel during this process. Fig. 72-8 illustrates some of the salient features of splanchnic ischemia and the SIRS/MODS complex.

Although the systemic cardiovascular response demanded by these conditions usually is hyperdynamic, it

BOX 72-15
DIAGNOSTIC FINDINGS IN SIRS*

Systemic Inflammatory Response Syndrome

Temperature $> 38°$, $< 36°$
Heart rate > 90
Respiration rate > 20 or $Pa_{CO_2} < 32$ mm Hg
Leukocyte $> 12.0 \times 10^9$/l or $< 4 \times 10^9$/l or > 0.10 immature cells

*Two or more should be present for a diagnosis to be made

BOX 72-16
VASOACTIVE SUBSTANCES AFFECTING SPLANCHNIC BED

Vasoconstrictors

Endogenous

- Angiotensin II
- Vasopressin
- Catecholamines
- Certain prostaglandins
  - $PGF_{2\alpha}$
  - PGB_2
  - PGD_2
- Certain leukotrienes
  - C_4
  - D_4
  - E_4
- Certain thromboxanes
  - TxA_2
- ? Serotonin

Exogenous

- Digoxin
- Atropine
- Physostigmine

Vasodilators

Endogenous

- Vasoactive intestinal peptide
- Histamine
- Glucagon
- Cholecystokinin
- Other eicosanoids
  - PGI_2 (prostacyclin)
  - PGE_2
- Serotonin
- Nitric oxide

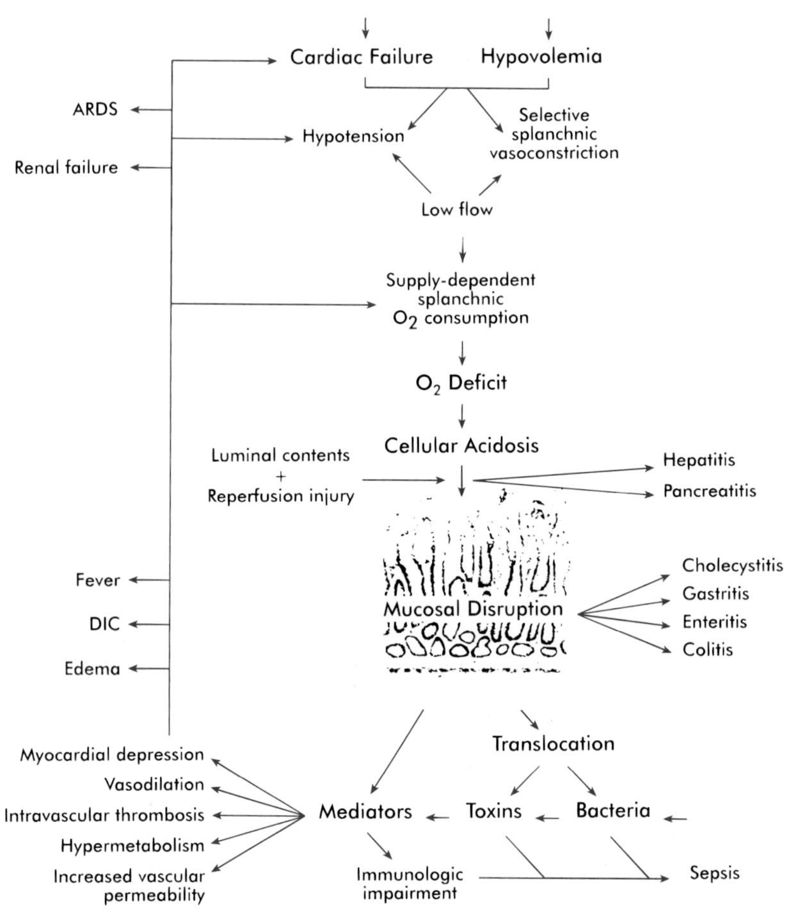

Fig. 72-8. Splanchnic ischemia and multiple organ dysfunction syndrome (MODS). (From Marston A, Bulkley G, Fiddian-Green R, et al, editors: *Splanchnic ischemia and multiple organ failure,* London, 1989, Edward Arnold.)

often is inadequate, either because metabolic requirements are too high (end organ inability to use oxygen) or because of limitations imposed by evolving or underlying myocardial dysfunction. When the anesthesiologist encounters these patients, they frequently are already receiving vasopressor and inotropic support. Management includes intensive evaluation of oxygenation, optimization of volume and cardiovascular function, and avoidance of drugs and agents that will further compromise their already tenuous status.

SUMMARY

The complex physiologic and metabolic interactions of the GI tract and other organ system functions can present fascinating challenges for the anesthesiologist. Because GI surgery often can seem so benign, it is perhaps more difficult to remain "tuned in" to such concerns. The rewards of good patient care should be sufficient incentive to re-examine important issues in GI surgery and anesthesia from time to time.

KEY POINTS

- Diseases of the gastrointestinal system frequently result in abnormal gastric function, with potentially increased anesthetic risk caused by increased intragastric pressure, delayed gastric emptying, gastric dilation, and increased gastric secretion.
- The volume, pH, and presence or absence of particulate matter are the three most important factors determining the severity of the pulmonary insult that occurs with aspiration.
- Extensive bowel, pancreatic, or esophageal resections entail considerable morbidity, with potential serious postoperative complications such as hemorrhage, coagulopathy, and hepatic, renal, pulmonary, or cardiovascular failure.
- Laparoscopy entails the installation of gas into the peri-

toneal cavity with physiologic changes resulting from this gas under pressure and subsequent surgical positioning. Hemodynamic compromise can occur, which, although rare, can be catastrophic.

- Patients with the SIRS/MODS complex usually are ill and will require considerable attention to systemic issues and to their surgical condition.
- If the LES is not functioning properly or if a hiatal hernia exists, stomach contents may reflux into the esophagus and pharynx during anesthesia and surgery, increasing the potential for serious aspiration pneumonia.
- Narcotics have intestinal side effects that are well recognized. LES tone is decreased. Gastric emptying is impaired because of decreased propulsive motility and increased tone in the antrum of the stomach.
- The development of pneumothorax and/or pneumomediastinum is a serious and/or potentially life-threatening complication. When either is suspected, from hemodynamic deterioration or from the presence of subcutaneous emphysema, especially of the neck and face, aggressive investigation (auscultation, chest radiograph) and management (e.g., chest tube for tension pneumothorax) should be undertaken. Procedures on the lower esophagus may be more likely to result in these complications.
- Approximately 40% of patients with gastroesophageal reflux have delayed gastric emptying, and in approximately one third of these, the delay is clinically significant.
- Maneuvers necessary for this blunt esophagectomy are capable of causing serious hemodynamic and ventilatory compromise and require appropriate monitoring of blood pressure and respiration.

KEY REFERENCES

Goyal RK, Hirano I: The enteric nervous system, *N Engl J Med* 334:1106–1115, 1996.

Marston A, Bulkley G, Fiddian-Green R, et al, editors: *Splanchnic ischemia and multiple organ failure,* London, 1989, Edward Arnold.

Rangel-Frausto MS, Pittet D, Costigan M, et al: The natural history of the systemic inflammatory response syndrome (SIRS). A prospective study, *JAMA* 273:117–123, 1995.

Sollinger HW: Pancreas transplantation in humans. In Moody FG, editor: *Surgical treatment of digestive disease,* ed 2, Chicago, 1990, Mosby–Year Book.

REFERENCES

1. Abe K, Shibata M, Demizu A, et al: Effect of oral and intramuscular famotidine on pH and volume of gastric contents, *Anesth Analg* 68:541, 1989.
2. Aggestrup S: Effect of thyrotropin-releasing hormone on the human lower esophageal sphincter pressure, *Scand J Gastroenterol* 19:631, 1984.
3. Aitkenhead AR: Anaesthesia and bowel surgery, *Br J Anaesth* 56:95, 1984.
4. Aitkenhead A, Gilmour D, Hothersall A, et al: Effects of subarachnoid nerve block and arterial Pco_2 on colon blood flow in the dog, *Br J Anaesth* 52:1071, 1980.
5. Aitkenhead AR, Wishart HY, Peebles-Brown DA: High spinal nerve block for large bowel anastomosis, *Br J Anaesth* 50:177, 1978.
6. Alexander J, Spence A, Parikh R, et al: The role of airway closure in postoperative hypoxemia, *Br J Anaesth* 45:34, 1973.
7. Ali J, Weisel R, Layug A, et al: Consequences of postoperative alterations in respiratory mechanics, *Am J Surg* 128:376, 1974.
8. Anderson J, Johnston G: Development of cutaneous gangrene during continuous peripheral infusion of vasopressin, *BMJ* 287:1657, 1983.
9. Arms R, Dines D, Tinstman T: Aspiration pneumonia, *Chest* 65:136, 1974.
10. Athanasoulis C: Medical progress: therapeutic application of angiography, *N Engl J Med* 302:1117, 1980.
11. Awe WC, Fletcher WS, Jacob SW: The pathophysiology of aspiration pneumonitis, *Surgery* 60:232, 1966.
12. Babka J, Hagar G, Castell D: The effect of body position on lower esophageal sphincter pressure, *Am J Dig Dis* 18:441, 1973.
13. Bailey R, Bulkley G, Hamilton S, et al: Pathogenesis of nonocclusive ischemic colitis, *Ann Surg* 203:590, 1986.
14. Bailey PL, Stanley TH: Narcotic intravenous anesthetics. In Miller RD, editor: *Anesthesia,* ed 3, New York, 1990, Churchill-Livingstone.
15. Balestrazzi P, Gregori G, Bernasconi S, et al: Bradycardia and neurologic disorders associated with ranitidine in a child, *Am J Dis Child* 139:442, 1985.
16. Banchero N, Schwartz PE, Wood E: Intraesophageal pressure gradient in man, *J Appl Physiol* 22:1066, 1967.
17. Bardon T, Ruckebusch Y: Comparative effects of opiate agonists on proximal and distal colonic motility in dogs, *Eur J Pharmacol* 110:329, 1985.
18. Barlow AP, DeMeester T, Ball C, et al: The significance of the gastric secretory state in gastroesophageal reflux disease, *Arch Surg* 124(8):937–940, 1989.
19. Baron JH: Current views on pathogenesis of peptic ulcer, *Scand J Gastroenterol* 17(Suppl 80):1, 1982.
20. Bartle W, Walker S, Shapero T: Dose-dependent effect of cimetidine on phenytoin kinetics, *Clin Pharmacol Ther* 33: 649, 1983.
21. Bauer L, Edwards A, Randolph F, et al: Cimetidine-induced decrease in lidocaine metabolism, *Am Heart J* 198:413, 1984.
22. Beal AL, Cerra FB: Multiple organ system failure syndrome in the 1990s. Systemic inflammatory response and organ dysfunction, *JAMA* 271:226, 1994.
23. Beattie WS, Lindblad T, Buckley DN, et al: Menstruation increases the risk of nau-

sea and vomiting after laparoscopy, *Anesthesiology* 78:272, 1993.

24. Becquemin JP, Piquet J, Becquemin MH, et al: Pulmonary function after transverse or midline incision in patients with obstructive pulmonary disease, *Intensive Care Med* 11:247, 1985.
25. Been J, Bills P, Lewis D: Microstructure of gallstones, *Gastroenterology* 76:548, 1979.
26. Behar J: Gastroesophageal reflux disease and its complications with a critical analysis of treatment. In Cohen S, Soloway R, editors: *Diseases of the esophagus,* Edinburgh, 1982, Churchill-Livingstone.
27. Bell CM, Lewis CB: Effect of neostigmine on integrity of ileorectal anastomoses, *BMJ* 3:587, 1968.
28. Bell J, Gower A, Martin L, et al: Interaction of H2-receptor antagonists with drug metabolizing enzymes, *Biochem Soc Trans* 9:113, 1981.
29. Beller B, Trevino A, Urban E: Pitressin induced myocardial injury and depression in a young woman, *Am J Med* 51:675, 1971.
30. Berson W, Adriani J: "Silent" regurgitation and aspiration during anesthesia, *Anesthesiology* 15:644, 1954.
31. Biancani P, Walsh J, Behar J: Vasoactive intestinal peptide: a neurotransmitter for lower esophageal sphincter relaxation, *J Clin Invest* 73:963, 1984.
32. Bigler D, Hjortsø N-C, Kehlet H: Disruption of colonic anastomosis during continuous epidural analgesia: an early postoperative complication, *Anaesthesia* 40:278, 1985.
33. Birnbaum D, Ben-Menachem J, Schwartz A: The influence of oral diazepam on gastrointestinal motility, *Am J Proctol* 21:263, 1970.
34. Blitt CD, Gutman HL, Cohen DD, et al: "Silent" regurgitation and aspiration during general anesthesia, *Anesth Analg* 40:707, 1970.
35. Boey J, Choi S, Alagaratnam T: Risk stratification in perforated duodenal ulcers, *Ann Surg* 205:22, 1987.
36. Bonavina L, Evander A, DeMeester T, et al: Length of the distal esophageal sphincter and competency of the cardia, *Am J Surg* 151:25, 1986.
37. Bone RC: Sepsis, sepsis syndrome, and the systemic inflammatory response syndrome (SIRS). Gulliver in Laputa, *JAMA* 273:155, 1995.
38. Bounous G: Acute necrosis of the intestinal mucosa, *Gastroenterology* 82:1457, 1982.
39. Brock-Utne J, Dow T, Dimopoulos G, et al: The effect of metoclopramide on the lower oesophageal sphincter in late pregnancy, *Anaesth Intensive Care* 6:26, 1978.
40. Brock-Utne J, Moshal M, Downing J, et al: Fasting volume and acidity of stomach contents associated with gastrointestinal symptoms, *Anaesthesia* 32:749, 1977.
41. Brock-Utne J, Rout C, Moodley J, et al: Does pre-operative gastric emptying decrease the risk of acid aspiration in obstetrical anesthesia? A study of gastric acidity and volume at emergency cesarean section, *Anesth Analg* 68:S39, 1989.
42. Bulkley GB: Mediators of splanchnic organ injury: overview and perspective. In Marston A, Bulkley G, Fiddian-Green R, et al, editors: *Splanchnic ischemia and multiple organ failure.* London, 1989, Edward Arnold.
43. Burgess G, Cooper J, Marino R, et al: Laryngeal competence after tracheal extubation, *Anesthesiology* 51:73, 1979.
44. Burton A, Steinbrook RA: Precipitous decrease in oxygen saturation during laparoscopic surgery, *Anesth Analg* 76:1177, 1993.
45. Bynum T, Gallavan R, Jacobson E: The pathophysiology of nonocclusive ischemia. In Shepherd A, Granger D, editors: *Physiology of the intestinal circulation,* New York, 1984, Raven Press.
46. Camarri E, Chirone E, Fanteria G, et al: Ranitidine induced bradycardia, *Lancet* 2:160, 1982.
47. Cameron J, Mitchell W, Zuidema G: Aspiration pneumonia: clinical outcome following documented aspiration, *Arch Surg* 106:49, 1973.
48. Carlsson C, Islander G: Silent gastropharyngeal regurgitation during anesthesia, *Anesth Analg* 60:655, 1981.
49. Carmichael MJ, Weisbrodt NW, Copeland EM: Effect of abdominal surgery on intestinal myoelectrical activity in the dog, *Am J Surg* 133:34, 1977.
50. Casey LC, Balk RA, Bone RC: Plasma cytokine and endotoxin levels correlate with survival in patients with the sepsis syndrome, *AIM* 119:771, 1993.
51. Casten DF: Esophageal hiatal hernia and gastric acid secretion, *Arch Surg* 88:255, 1964.
52. Celli BR, Rodriques KS, Snider GL: A controlled trial of intermittent positive pressure breathing, incentive spirometry, and deep breathing exercises in preventing pulmonary complications after abdominal surgery, *Am Rev Respir Dis* 130:12, 1984.
53. Chen C, Toung T, Haupt H, et al: Evaluation of the efficacy of Alka-Seltzer effervescent in gastric acid neutralization, *Anesth Analg* 63:325, 1984.
54. Chetlin S, Elliott D: Biliary bacteremia, *Arch Surg* 102:303, 1971.
55. Cheung L: Gastric mucosal blood flow: its measurement and importance in mucosal defense mechanisms, *J Surg Res* 36:282, 1984.
56. Cheung LY, Ashley SW: The pathogenesis of acid-peptic disease. In Moody FG, editor: *Surgical treatment of digestive disease,* ed 2, Chicago, 1990, Mosby–Year Book.
57. Chice JD, Joris J, Lamy M: Respiratory changes induced by subcutaneous emphysema during laparoscopic fundoplication. *Br J Anaesth* 72:A37, 1994.
58. Child CS: Prevention of neostigmine-induced colonic activity: a comparison of atropine and glycopyrronium, *Anaesthesia* 39:1083, 1984.
59. Christensen J: Intestinal pseudo-obstruction and paralytic ileus. In Moody FG, editor: *Surgical treatment of digestive disease,* ed 2, Chicago, 1990, Mosby–Year Book.
60. Clagett OT: Diseases of the gallbladder: diagnosis and management, *Surg Clin North Am* 25:929, 1945.
61. Cody H, Wichern W: Choice of operation for acute gastric mucosal hemorrhage: report of 36 cases and review of the literature, *Am J Surg* 134:322, 1977.
62. Cohen J, Weetman A, Dargie J, et al: Life-threatening arrhythmias and intravenous cimetidine, *BMJ* 2:768, 1979.
63. Coursin D, Farin-Rusk C, Springman S, et al: The hemodynamic effects of intravenous cimetidine versus ranitidine in intensive care unit patients: a double-blind, prospective, cross-over study, *Anesthesiology* 69:975, 1988.
64. Cousins M, Mather L: Intrathecal and epidural administration of opioids, *Anesthesiology* 61:276, 1984.
65. Coyne M, Bonorris G, Goldstein L, et al: Effect of chenodeoxycholic acid and phenobarbital on the rate-limiting enzymes of hepatic cholesterol and bile acid sythesis in patients with gallstones, *J Lab Clin Med* 87:281, 1976.
66. Crawford M, Lerman J, Christensen S, et al: Effects of duration of fasting on gastric fluid pH and volume in healthy children, *Anesth Analg* 71:400, 1990.
67. Critchley LAH, Critchley AJH, Gin T: Haemodynamic changes in patients undergoing laparoscopic cholecystectomy: measurement by transthoracic electrical bioimpedance, *Br J Anaesth* 70:681, 1993.
68. Crozier R, Jonasson H: Symptomatic esophageal hiatus hernias: study of 105 patients, *Arch Intern Med* 113:737, 1964.
69. Cunningham AJ: Laparoscopic surgery—anesthetic implications, *Surg Endosc* 8:1271, 1994.
70. Cunningham AJ: Laparoscopic surgery—anesthetic implications, *Surg Endosc* 8:1272, 1994.
71. Cunningham AJ, Turner J, Rosenbaum S, et al: Transesophageal echocardiographic assessment of haemodynamic function during laparoscopic cholecystectomy, *Br J Anaesth* 70:621, 1993.
72. Davenport HW: *Physiology of the digestive tract,* ed 5, Chicago, 1982, Mosby–Year Book.
73. DeMesster T, Lafontaine E, Joelsson B, et al: The relationship of a hiatal hernia to the function of the body of the esophagus and the gastroesophageal junction, *J Thorac Cardiovasc Surg* 82:547, 1981.
74. DeMeester TR, Stein HJ: Gastroesophageal reflux disease. In Moody FG, editor: *Surgical treatment of digestive disease,* ed 2, Chicago, 1990, Mosby–Year Book.
75. DeMeester TR, Wernly J, Bryant G, et al: Clinical and in vitro analysis of determinants of gastroesophageal competence: a study of the principles of antireflux surgery, *Am J Surg* 137:39, 1979.
76. Dent D, Madden M, Price S: Randomized comparison of R1 and R2 gastrectomy for gastric cancer, *Br J Surg* 75:110, 1988.
77. Dent J, Dodds W, Friedman R, et al: Mechanism of gastroesophageal reflux in recumbent asymptomatic human subjects, *J Clin Invest* 65:256, 1980.
78. Derouin M, Couture P, Boudreault D, et al: Detection of gas embolism by transesophageal echocardiography during laparoscopic cholecystectomy, *Anesth Analg* 82:119, 1996.
79. Desmond J, Gordon RA: Ventilation in patients anaesthetized for laparoscopy, *Can Anaesth Soc J* 17:378, 1970.

80. Diemunsch P, Van Dorsselaer T, Mutter D, et al: Evolution of the nitrous oxide fraction in the carbon dioxide pneumoperitoneum during laparoscopy under general anesthesia. *Anesthesiology* A1085, 1995.
81. Don H: The mechanical properties of the respiratory system during anesthesia, In Kafer E, editor: *Anesthesia and respiratory function,* Boston, 1977, Little Brown.
82. Dowlatshahi K, Evander A, Walther B, et al: Influence of morphine on the distal oesophagus and the lower oesophageal sphincter—a manometric study, *Gut* 26:802, 1985.
83. Dubois F, Icard P, Berthelot G, et al: Coelioscopic cholecystectomy: preliminary report of 36 cases, *Ann Surg* 211:60, 1990.
84. Dupont J, Cohn I: Gastric carcinoma, *Curr Probl Cancer* 4:1, 1980.
85. DuVal MK: Caudal pancreatico-jejunostomy for chronic relapsing pancreatitis, *Ann Surg* 140:775, 1954.
86. Edelman DS: Laparoscopic cholecystectomy under continuous epidural anesthesia in patients with cystic fibrosis, *Am J Dis Children* 145:723, 1991.
87. Edwards G, Morton H, Pask E, et al: Deaths resulting from anaesthesia: a report on 1,000 cases, *Anaesthesia* 50(5): 440–453, 1995.
88. Eger EI, Saidman LJ: Hazards of nitrous oxide anesthesia in bowel obstruction and pneumothorax, *Anesthesiology* 26:61, 1965.
89. Ekman LG, Abrahamsson J, Biber B, et al: Hemodynamic changes during laparoscopy with positive end-expiratory pressure ventilation, *Acta Anaesthesiol Scand* 32:447, 1988.
90. Eyler S, Cullen B, Murphy M, et al: Antacid aspiration in rabbits: a comparison of Mylanta and Bicitra, *Anesth Analg* 61:288, 1982.
91. Feldman M, Richardson CT: Total 24-hour gastric acid secretion in patients with duodenal ulcer: comparison with normal subjects and effects of cimetidine and parietal vagotomy, *Gastroenterology* 90:540, 1986.
92. Filipi CJ, Fitzgibbons RJ, Salerno GM, et al: Laparoscopic herniorrhaphy, *Surg Clin N Am* 75:1109, 1992.
93. Fisher R, Cohen S: Pyloric sphincter dysfunction in patients with gastric ulcer, *N Engl J Med* 288:273, 1976.
94. Ford G, Whitelaw W, Rosenal T, et al: Diaphragm function after upper abdominal surgery in humans, *Am Rev Respir Dis* 127:431, 1983.
95. Freston J: Cimetidine II: adverse reactions and patterns of use. *Ann Intern Med* 97:728, 1982.
96. Fromm D: Duodenal ulcer. In Moody FG, editor: *Surgical treatment of digestive disease,* ed 2, Chicago, 1990, Mosby–Year Book.
97. Fromme G, Janossy T: Glucose changes during pancreas transplantation, *Anesth Analg* 68:S92, 1989.
98. Fuchs KH, DeMeester TR, Schwizer W, et al: Concomitant duodenogastric and gastroesophageal reflux: the role of twenty-four hour gastric pH monitoring. In Siewert JR, Hölscher AH, editors: *Diseases of the esophagus,* New York, 1988, Springer-Verlag.
99. Fukunaga F: Gallbladder bacteriology, histology and gallstones: study of unselected cholecystectomy specimens in Honolulu, *Arch Surg* 106:169, 1973.
100. Ganey J, Johnson P, Prillaman P, et al: Cholecystectomy: clinical experience with a large series, *Am J Surg* 151:352, 1986.
101. Gardner M, Sikorski G: Ranitidine and theophylline, *Ann Intern Med* 102:559, 1985.
102. Gibbs C, Schwartz D, Wynne J, et al: Antacid pulmonary aspiration in the dog, *Anesthesiology* 51:380, 1979.
103. Giebler RM, Walz MK, Peitgen K, et al: Hemodynamic changes after retroperitoneal CO_2 insufflation for posterior retroperitoneoscopic adrenalectomy, *Anesth Analg* 82:827, 1996.
104. Ginsburg R, Bristow M, Stinson E, et al: Histamine receptors in the human heart, *Life Sci* 26:2245, 1980.
105. Glenn F: Silent gallstones, *Ann Surg* 193:251, 1981.
106. Glenn F: Surgical management of acute cholecystitis in patients 65 years of age and older, *Ann Surg* 193:56, 1981.
107. Goldberg M, Vatashsky E, Haskel Y, et al: The effect of meperidine on the guinea pig extrahepatic biliary tract, *Anesth Analg* 66:1282, 1987.
108. Goyal RK, Hirano I: The enteric nervous system, *N Engl J Med* 334:1106, 1996.
109. Gracie W, Ransohoff D: The natural history of silent gallstones: the innocent gallstone is not a myth, *N Engl J Med* 307:798, 1982.
110. Greenberger NJ: Gastrointestinal bleeding. In Moody FG, editor: *Surgical treatment of digestive disease,* ed 2, Chicago, 1990, Mosby–Year Book.
111. Greenberger NJ: *Gastrointestinal disorders: a pathophysiologic approach,* ed 4, Chicago, 1990, Mosby–Year Book.
112. Grossman M: Chemical messengers: a view from the gut, *Fed Proc* 38:2341, 1979.
113. Groth C, Lundgren G, Ostman J, et al: Experience with nine segmental pancreatic transplantations in pre-uremic diabetic patients in Stockholm, *Transplant Proc* 12:68, 1980.
114. Harris SN, Luther MA, Ballantyne GH, et al: Alterations of cardiovascular performance during laparoscopic colectomy, *Anesthesiology* 83:A75, 1995.
115. Healy T, Foster GE, Evans DF, et al: Effect of some IV anaesthetic agents on canine gastrointestinal motility, *Br J Anaesth* 52:229, 1981.
116. Hedenstierna G: Mechanisms of postoperative pulmonary dysfunction, *Acta Chir Scand* (Suppl) 550:152, 1989.
117. Helm J, Dodds W, Hogan W: Salivary reponses to esophageal acid in normal subjects and patients with reflux esophagitis, *Gastroenterology* 93:1393, 1982.
118. Helm J, Dodds W, Pelc L, et al: Effect of esophageal emptying and saliva on clearance of acid from the esophagus, *N Engl J Med* 310:284, 1984.
119. Herrin R, Meek W: Distention as a factor in intestinal obstruction, *Arch Intern Med* 51:152, 1933.
120. Hesse U, Sutherland D: Influence of serum amylase and plasma glucose levels in pancreas cadaver donors on graft function in recipients, *Diabetes* 38(Suppl 1):1, 1989.
121. Hirvonen EA, Nuutinen LS, Kauko M: Ventilatory effects, blood gas changes, and oxygen consumption during laparoscopic hysterectomy, *Anesth Analg* 80: 961, 1995.
122. Holdsworth J, Furness R, Roulston G: A comparison of apomorphine and stomach tubes for emptying the stomach before general anaesthesia in obstetrics, *Br J Anaesth* 46:526, 1974.
123. Holloway R: The oesophagus. In Shearman D, Finlayson N, editors: *Diseases of the gastrointestinal tract and liver,* ed 2, Edinburgh, 1989, Churchill-Livingstone.
124. Hsing CH, Hseu SS, Tsai SK, et al: The physiologic effect of CO_2 pneumoperitoneum in pediatric laparoscopy, *Acta Anaesthesiol Sin* 33:1, 1995.
125. Hubert J, Kiernan P, Welch J, et al: The surgical management of bleeding stress ulcers, *Ann Surg* 191:672, 1980.
126. Hurwitz A, Duranceau A: Upper-esophageal sphincter dysfunction: pathogenesis and treatment, *Am J Dig Dis* 23:275, 1978.
127. Hutchinson A, Maltby J, Reid C: Gastric fluid volume pH in elective inpatients. I. Coffee or orange juice versus overnight fast, *Can J Anaesth* 35:12, 1988.
128. Hynynen MJ, Turanen M, Kortilla KT: Effects of alfentanil and fentanyl on common bile duct pressure, *Anesth Analg* 65:370, 1986.
129. Imrie CW, Ferguson JC, Murphy D, et al: Arterial hypoxia in acute pancreatitis, *Br J Surg* 64:185, 1977.
130. Isenberg JI, Selling JA, Hogan D, et al: Impaired proximal duodenal mucosal bicarbonate secretion in patients with duodenal ulcer, *N Engl J Med* 316:374, 1987.
131. Jaffe JH, Martin WR: Opioid analgesics and antagonists. In Gilman AG, Goodman LS, Rall TW, et al, editors: *The pharmacological basis of therapeutics,* ed 7, New York, 1985, Macmillan.
132. James C, Modell J, Gibbs C, et al: Pulmonary aspiration: effects of volume and pH in the rat, *Anesth Analg* 63:665, 1984.
133. Jarvinen H, Hastabacka J: Early cholecystectomy for acute cholecystitis, a prospective randomized study, *Ann Surg* 191:501, 1980.
134. Johansson K, Ask P, Boeryd B, et al: Oesophagitis, signs of reflux and gastric acid secretion in patients with gastro-oesophageal reflux disease, *Scand J Gastroenterol* 21:837, 1986.
135. Johannsen G, Anderson M, Juhl B: The effect of general anesthesia on the haemodynamic events during laparoscopy with CO_2-insufflation, *Acta Anaesthesiol Scand* 33:132, 1989.
136. Johnson L, Lin T, Hong S: Gastroesophageal dynamics during immersion in water to the neck, *J Appl Physiol* 38:449, 1975.
137. Johnson WC: Postoperative ventilatory performance: dependence upon surgical incision, *Am Surg* 41:15, 1975.

138. Jones R, Detmer M, Hill A, et al: Incidence of choledocho-duodenal sphincter spasm during fentanyl-supplemented anesthesia, *Anesth Analg* 60:638, 1981.
139. Joris JL, Noirot DP, Legrand MJ, et al: Hemodynamic changes during laparoscopic cholecystectomy, *Anesth Analg* 76:1067, 1993.
140. Kahrilas P, Dodds W, Dent J, et al: Effect of sleep, spontaneous gastroesophageal reflux, and a meal on upper esophageal sphincter pressure in normal human volunteers, *Gastroenterology* 92:466, 1987.
141. Kalhan SB, Reaney JA, Collins RL: Pneumomediastinum and subcutaneous emphysema during laparoscopy, *Cleve Clin J Med* 57:639, 1990.
142. Kalloo A, Ciarleglio C, Stanczak V, et al: Technetium-99m labeled red blood cell scans: are they really useful in the diagnosis of lower gastrointestinal bleeding? *Gastroenterology* 95:A213, 1988.
143. Kelly W, Lillehei R, Merkel F, et al: Allotransplantation of the pancreas and duodenum along with the kidney in diabetic nephropathy, *Surgery* 61:827, 1967.
143a. Kelman G, Swapp G, Smith I, et al: Cardiac output and arterial blood-gas tension during laparoscopy, *Br J Anaesth* 44:1155–1162, 1972.
144. Kodama Y, Sugimachi K, Soejia K, et al: Evaluation of extensive lymph node dissection for carcinoma of the stomach, *World J Surg* 5:241, 1981.
145. Korenaga D, Okamura T, Baba H, et al: Results of resection of gastric cancer extending to adjacent organs, *Br J Surg* 75:12, 1988.
146. Lahtinen, Alhava E, Aukee S: Acute cholecystitis treated by early and delayed surgery: a controlled clinical trial, *Scand J Gastroenterol* 13:673, 1978.
147. Lam SK, Isenberg JI, Grossman MI, et al: Rapid gastric emptying in duodenal ulcer patients, *Dig Dis Sci* 27:598, 1982.
148. Lambert M, de Peyer R, Muller A: Reversible ischemic colitis after intravenous vasopressin therapy, *JAMA* 247: 666, 1982.
149. Lamki L, Sullivan S: A study of gastrointestinal opiate receptors: the role of the mu receptor on gastric emptying: concise communication, *J Nucl Med* 24:689, 1983.
150. LaMorte W, Booker M, Scott T, et al: Increases in gallbladder prostaglandin synthesis before the formation of cholesterol gallstones, *Surgery* 98:445, 1985.
151. Lankisch P, Rahlf G, Koop H: Pulmonary complications in fatal acute hemorrhagic pancreatitis, *Dig Dis Sci* 28:111, 1983.
152. Lantz PE, Smith JD: Fatal carbon dioxide embolism complicating attempted laparoscopic cholecystectomy: case report and literature review, *J Forensic Sci* 39:1468, 1994.
153. Lejus C, Delile L, Plattner V, et al: Randomized, single-blinded trial of laparoscopic versus open appendectomy in children: effects on postoperative analgesia, *Anesthesiology* 84:801, 1996.
154. Maltby J, Reid C, Hutchinson A: Gastric fluid volume and pH in elective inpatients. II. Coffee or orange juice with ranitidine, *Can J Anaesth* 35:16, 1988.
155. Marsh C, Perkins J, Sutherland D, et al: Combined hepatic and pancreatico-duodenal procurement for transplantation, *Surg Gynecol Obstet* 168:254, 1989.
156. Marshall RL, Jebson PJR, Davie IT, et al: Circulatory effects of carbon dioxide insufflation of the peritoneal cavity for laparoscopy, *Br J Anaesth* 44:680, 1972.
157. McCallum R, Berkowitz D, Lerner E: Gastric emptying in patients with gastroesophageal reflux, *Gastroenterology* 80:285, 1981.
158. McCammon R, Stoelting R, Madura J: Effects of butorphanol, nalbuphine and fentanyl on intrabiliary tract dynamics, *Anesth Analg* 63:139, 1984.
159. McDougall EM, Clayman RV, Fadden PT: Retroperitoneoscopy: the Washington University Medical School experience, *Urology* 43:446, 1994.
160. McGrady E, MacDonald A: Effect of the preoperative administration of water on gastric volume and pH, *Br J Anaesth* 60:803, 1988.
161. McKinstry LJ, Perverseff RA, Yip RW: Arterial and end-tidal carbon dioxide in patients undergoing laparoscopic cholecystectomy, *Anesthesiology* A108, 1992.
162. McLaughlin JG, Bonnell BW, Scheeres DE, et al: The adverse hemodynamic effects related to laparoscopic cholecystectomy, *Anesthesiology* 77:A70, 1992.
163. Mead J, Agostoni E: Dynamics of breathing. In Fenn W, Rahn H, editors: *Handbook of physiology,* vol 1, Baltimore, 1964, Williams & Wilkins.
164. Mendelson C: The aspiration of stomach contents into the lungs during obstetric anesthesia, *Am J Obstet Gynecol* 52:191, 1946.
165. Millard JA, Hill BB, Cook PS, et al: Intermittent sequential pneumatic compression in prevention of venous stasis associated with pneumoperitoneum during laparoscopic cholecystectomy, *Arch Surg* 128:914, 1993.
166. Mitchard M, Harris A, Mullinger B: Ranitidine drug interations—a literature review, *Pharmacol Ther* 32:293, 1987.
167. Mittal R, Lange R, McCallum R: Identification and mechanism of delayed esophageal acid clearance in subjects with hiatus hernia, *Gastroenterology* 92:130, 1987.
168. Moody FG, editor: *Surgical treatment of digestive disease,* ed 2, Chicago, 1990, Mosby–Year Book.
169. Moossa AR, Mayer AD, Lavelle-Jones M: Surgical complications. In Sabiston DC, editor: *Textbook of surgery: the biological basis of modern surgical practice,* ed 14, Philadelphia, 1991, WB Saunders.
170. Morrow D, Thompson J, Wilson S: Acute cholecystitis in the elderly: a surgical emergency, *Arch Surg* 113:1149, 1978.
171. Neely J, Catchpole B: Ileus: the restoration of alimentary-tract motility by pharmacological means, *Br J Surg* 58:21, 1971.
172. Neukman GG: Laparoscopy explosion hazards with nitrous oxide, *Anesthesiology* 78:875, 1993.
173. Nunn J: Mechanisms of pulmonary ventilation. In *Applied respiratory physiology,* ed 2, London, 1977, Butterworth.
174. Odeberg S, Ljungqvist O, Svenberg T, et al: Haemodynamic effects of pneumoperitoneum and the influence of posture during anaesthesia for laparoscopic surgery, *Acta Anaesthesiol Scand* 38:276, 1994.
175. Oh JJ, Kim CH: Gastroparesis after a presumed viral illness: clinical and laboratory features and natural history, *Mayo Clin Proc* 65:636, 1990.
176. Olsson GL, Hallen B, Hambraeus-Jonzon K: Aspiration during anaesthesia: a computer-aided study of 185,358 anaesthetics, *Acta Anaesthesiol Scand* 30:84, 1986.
177. Orie J, Jabi H, Besozzi M, et al: Thallium-201 myocardial perfusion imaging and coronary arteriography in asymptomatic patients with end stage renal disease secondary to juvenile onset diabetes mellitus, *Transplant Proc* 18:1709, 1986.
178. Ormand J, Talley N: Helicobacter pylori: controversies and an approach to management, *Mayo Clin Proc* 65:414, 1990.
179. Orr W, Robinson M, Johnson L: Acid clearing during sleep in patients with esophagitis and controls, *Dig Dis Sci* 26:423, 1981.
180. O'Sullivan G, DeMeester T, Joelsson B, et al: The interaction of the lower esophageal sphincter pressure and length of sphincter in the abdomen as determinants of gastroesophageal competence, *Am J Surg* 143:40, 1982.
181. Painter NS, Truelove SC: The intraluminal pressure patterns in diverticulosis of the colon. Part II. The effect of morphine, *Gut* 5:201, 1964.
182. Painter NS, Truelove SC: The intraluminal pressure patterns in diveritculosis of the colon. Part III. The effect of prostigmine, *Gut* 5:365, 1964.
183. Palmer E: Disorders of the cricopharyngeus muscle: a review, *Gastroenterology* 71:510, 1976.
184. Partington P, Rochelle R: Modified Puestow procedure for retrograde drainage of the pancreatic duct, *Ann Surg* 152: 1037, 1960.
185. Pellegrini C, DeMeester T, Skinner D: Response of the distal esophageal sphincter to respiratory and positional maneuvers in humans, *Surg Forum* 27:380, 1976.
186. Perkins J, Fromme G, Narr B, et al: Pancreas transplantation at Mayo. II. Operative and perioperative management, *Mayo Clin Proc* 65:483, 1990.
187. Phillips SF: Diarrhea: a current view of the pathophysiology, *Gastroenterology* 63:495, 1972.
188. Pitt HA, Miyamoto T, Parapatis SK, et al: Factors influencing outcome in patients with postoperative biliary strictures, *Am J Surg* 144:14, 1982.
189. Porter J, Sussman M, Bulkley G: Splanchnic vasospasm in circulatory shock. In Marston A, Bulkley G, Fiddian-Green RG, et al, editors: *Splanchnic ischemia and multiple organ failure,* London, 1989, Edward Arnold.
190. Prinz RA, Greenlee HB: Pancreatic duct drainage in 100 patients with chronic pancreatitis, *Ann Surg* 194:313, 1981.
191. Puestow CB, Gillesby WJ: Retrograde surgical drainage of the pancreas for chronic relapsing pancreatitis, *Arch Surg* 76:898, 1958.
192. Putensen-Himmer G, Putensen C, Lammer H, et al: Functional residual capacity, post-operative lung function, and gas exchange following open laparotomy or laparoscopy for cholecystectomy, *Anesthesiology* 77:A1253, 1992.
193. Rademaker BM, Ringers J, Odoom JA, et al: Pulmonary function and stress response after laparoscopic cholecystectomy: comparison with subcostal incision and influence of thoracic epidural analgesia, *Anesth Analg* 75:381, 1992.
194. Radnay PA, Duncalf D, Novakoric M, et

al: Common bile duct pressure changes after fentanyl, morphine, meperidine, butorphanol and naloxone, *Anesth Analg* 63:441, 1984.

195. Rangel-Frausto MS, Pittet D, Costigan M, et al: The natural history of the systemic inflammatory response syndrome (SIRS): a prospective study, *JAMA* 273:117, 1995.
196. Ranson JH, Turner J, Roses D, et al: Respiratory complications in acute pancreatitis, *Ann Surg* 179:557, 1974.
197. Rasmussen JP, Dauchot PJ, DePalma RG, et al: Cardiac function and hypercarbia, *Arch Surg* 113:1196, 1978.
198. Rawal N, Coombs DW, editors: *Spinal narcotics,* Boston, 1990, Kluwer Ascademic.
199. Ray J, Yost L, Moallem S, et al: Immobility, hypoxemia, and pulmonary arteriovenous shunting, *Arch Surg* 109: 537, 1974.
200. Reding P, Devroede C, Barbier P: Bradycardia after cimetidine, *Lancet* 2:1227–1228, 1977.
201. Reiss R, Eliashiv A, Deutsch A: Septic complications and bile cultures in 800 consecutive cholecystectomies, *World J Surg* 6:192, 1982.
202. Rennie JA, Christofides ND, Mitchenere P, et al: Neural and humoral factors in postoperative ileus, *Br J Surg* 67:694, 1980.
203. Richardson C: Gastric ulcer. In Sleisenger MH, Fordtran J, editors: *Gastrointestinal disease: pathophysiology, diagnosis, management,* Philadelphia, 1983, WB Saunders.

203a. Roberts R, Shirley M: Reducing the risk of acid aspiration during cesarean section, *Anesth Analg* 53:859, 1974.

204. Root B, Levy M, Pollack S, et al: Gas embolism death after laparoscopy delayed by "trapping" in portal circulation, *Anesth Analg* 57:232, 1978.
205. Roslyn J, Busuttil R: Perforation of the gallbladder: a frequently mismanaged condition, *Am J Surg* 137:307, 1979.
206. Roslyn J, DenBesten L: Gallstones and cholecystitis. In Moody F, editor: *Surgical treatment of digestive disease,* ed 2, Chicago, 1990, Mosby–Year Book.
207. Ryan P, Schweitzer S, Collopy B, et al: Combined epidural and general anesthesia versus general anesthesia in patients having colon and rectal anastomoses, *Acta Chir Scand Suppl* 550:146, 1988.
208. Sackmann M, Delius M, Sauerbruch T, et al: Shockwave lithotripsy of gallbladder stones: the first 175 patients, *N Engl J Med* 318:393, 1988.
209. Safran D, Sgambati S, Orlando R: Laparoscopy in high-risk cardiac patients, *Surg Gynecol Obstet* 176:548, 1993.
210. Schulze-Delrieu K: Metoclopramide, *Gastroenterology* 77:768, 1979.
211. Schwartz D, Wynne J, Gibbs C, et al: The pulmonary consequences of aspiration of gastric contents at pH values greater than 2.5, *Am Rev Respir Dis* 121:119, 1980.
212. Schwartz SI, Ellis H, editors: *Maingot's abdominal operations,* ed 9, Norwalk, CT, 1989, Appleton & Lange.
213. Schwizer W, Hinder R, DeMeester T: Does delayed gastric emptying contribute to gastroesophageal reflux disease? *Am J Surg* 157(1):74–81, 1989.
214. Sellick BA: Cricoid pressure to control regurgitation of stomach contents during induction of anesthesia, *Lancet* 2:404, 1961.
215. Shaldon S, Dolle W, Guevara L, et al: Effect of pitressin on the splanchnic circulation in man, *Circulation* 24:797, 1961.
216. Shaw R, Mashford M, Desmond P: Cardiac arrest after intravenous injection of cimetidine, *Med J Aust* 2:629, 1980.
217. Shiffman J, Moore E: Acidification of gallbladder bile is defective in patients with all types of gallstones: a selective defect, *Gastroenterology* 94:591, 1988.
218. Shiu M, Moore E, Sanders M, et al: Influence of the extent of resection on survival after curative treatment of gastric carcinoma, *Arch Surg* 122:1347–1351, 1987.
219. Silver B, Bell W: Cimetidine potentiation of the hypoprothrombinemic effects of warfarin, *Ann Intern Med* 90:348, 1979.
220. Sjodahl R, Tagesson C, Wetterfors J: Lysolecithin-mediated inflammatory reaction in rabbit gallbladder, *Acta Chir Scand* 141:403, 1975.
221. Slocum H, Hoeflich E, Allen CR: Circulatory and respiratory distress from extreme positions on the operating table, *Surg Gynecol Obstet* 84:1065, 1947.

221a. Smith I, Ding Y, White PF: Muscle pain after outpatient laparoscopy: influence of propofol versus thiopental and enflurane, *Anesth Analg* 76:1181, 1993.

222. Smith S, Kendall M, Lobo J, et al: Ranitidine and cimetidine: drug interactions with single dose and steady-state nifedipine administration, *Br J Clin Pharmacol* 23:311, 1987.
223. Sollinger HW: Pancreas transplantation in humans. In Moody FG, editor: *Surgical treatment of digestive disease,* ed 2, Chicago, 1990, Mosby–Year Book.
224. Southern Surgeons Club: A prospective analysis of 1518 laparoscopic cholecystectomies, *N Engl J Med* 324:1073, 1991.
225. Squifflet J, Carlier M, Pirson Y, et al: Six human pancreas transplants: results and perioperative management, *Acta Anaesthesiol Belg* 37:107, 1986.
226. Sung D, Williams L: Intestinal secretion after intravenous infusion in small bowel obstruction, *Am J Surg* 121:91, 1971.
227. Sutherland A, Maltby J, Sale JP, et al: The effect of preoperative oral fluid and ranitidine on gastric fluid volume and pH, *Can J Anaesth* 34:117, 1987.

227a. Teabeaut JR: Aspiration of gastric contents: an experimental study, *Am J Pathol* 28:51, 1952.

228. Third International Symposium on Gastroenterology. In *Peptic ulcer disease: an update,* New York, 1979, Biomedical Information.
229. Thistlethwaite J, Lloyd D, Broelsch C, et al: Whole-pancreas and liver procurement from single-cadaver organ donors: where should vascular structures be divided? *Diabetes* 38(Suppl 1):232, 1989.
230. Threissman DA: Disruption of colonic anastomosis associated with epidural anesthesia, *Reg Anaesth* 5:22, 1980.
231. Tryzelaar JF, Neptune WB, Ellis FA, et al: Esophagectomy without thoracotomy for carcinoma of the esophagus, *Am J Surg* 143:486, 1982.
232. Tyden G, Groth CG: Vascularized pancreatic transplantation. In Morris PT, Tilney N, editors: *Progress in transplantation,* London, 1986, Churchill-Livingstone.
233. Tyden G, Reinholt F, Brattstrom C, et al: Diagnosis of rejection in recipients of pancreatic grafts with enteric exocrine diversion by monitoring pancreatic juice cytology and amylase secretion, *Transplant Proc* 19:3892, 1987.
234. van der Lindenden W, Sunzel H: Early versus delayed operation for acute cholecystitis: a controlled clinical trial, *Am J Surg* 120:7, 1970.
235. Viegas O, Ravindran R, Stoops C: Duration of efficacy of sodium citrate as an antacid, *Anesth Analg* 61:220, 1982 (abstract).
236. Wahba RWM, Tessler MJ, Kleiman SJ: Acute ventilatory complications during laparoscopic upper abdominal surgery, *Can J Anaesth* 43:77, 1996.
237. Wangensteen OH: In *Intestinal obstruction,* ed 3, Springfield, IL, 1955, Charles C Thomas.
238. Ward R, Kennedy W, Bonica J, et al: Experimental evaluation of atropine and vasopressors for the treatment of hypotension of high subarachnoid anesthesia, *Anesth Analg* 45:621, 1966.
239. Weinberger M, Smith G, Milavetz G, et al: Decreased theophylline clearance due to cimetidine, *N Engl J Med* 304:72, 1981.
240. Weiss WA: Regurgitation and aspiration of gastric contents during inhalation anesthesia, *Anesthesiology* 11:102, 1950.
241. Welch J: *Bowel obstruction: differential diagnosis and clinical management,* Philadelphia, 1989, WB Saunders.
242. Welch J: Mechanical obstruction of the small and large intestines. In Moody FG, editor: *Surgical treatment of digestive disease,* ed 2, Chicago, 1990, Mosby–Year Book.
243. Wenckert A, Robertson B: The natural course of gallstone disease: eleven-year review of 781 nonoperated cases, *Gastroenterology* 50:376, 1966.
244. Wilcox S, Vandam LD: Alas, poor Trendelenburg and his position! A critique of its uses and effectiveness, *Anesth Analg* 67:574, 1988.
245. Wilkins JL, Hardcastle JD, Mann CV, et al: Effects of neostigmine and atropine on motor activity of ileum, colon, and rectum of anaesthetized subjects, *BMJ* 1:793, 1970.
246. Williamson R: Clinical freedom, clinical behaviour, and anesthesia for laparoscopy, *Anesthesia* 44:999, 1988.
247. Wilson W, Gadacz T, Olcott C, et al: Superficial gastric erosions: response to surgical treatment, *Am J Surg* 126:133, 1973.
248. Winship D: Upper esophageal sphincter: does it care about reflux? *Gastroenterology* 85:470, 1983.
249. Wittgen CM, Andrus CH, Fitzgerald SD, et al: Analysis of the hemodynamic and ventilatory effects of laparoscopic cholecystectomy, *Arch Surg* 12:997, 1991.
250. Wright H, O'Brien J, Tilson M: Water absorption in experimental closed segment obstruction of the ileum in man, *Am J Surg* 121:96, 1971.
251. Yamada T, Alpers DH, Owyang C, et al, editors: *Textbook of gastroenterology,* Philadelphia, 1991, JB Lippincott.
252. Zaninotto G, DeMeester T, Schwizer W, et al: The lower esophageal sphincter in health and disease, *Am J Surg* 155:104, 1988.
253. Zuckerman GR, Cornette GL, Clouse RE, et al: Upper gastrointestinal bleeding in patients with chronic renal failure, *Ann Intern Med* 102:588, 1985.

CHAPTER 73

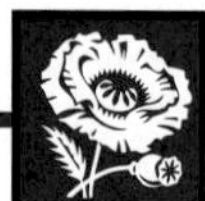

Anesthesia for Liver Surgery

WILLIAM T. MERRITT
SIMON GELMAN

Because the liver has such an important role in metabolism and distribution of most medications and toxins, the adequacy of liver function is extremely important to anesthesiologists. It is often difficult, however, to know which patients have liver disease or the severity of any derangements. As an indication of the importance of liver disease in U.S. society, the Centers for Disease Control (CDC) consistently reports that the age-adjusted death rates for chronic liver disease and cirrhosis are approximately 9 deaths per 100,000 population, enough to rank as the ninth leading cause of death in the United States. Also, the male/female and black/white ratios for liver disease are both 2:1.[185]

As newer medications and treatments prolong the lives of those with the most severe liver disease, and as liver transplantation becomes more prevalent, many more patients arrive in our operating rooms and intensive care units for definitive and palliative care. Therefore, anesthesiologists must have a reasonable understanding of the anatomy, biochemistry, physiology, and pharmacology of normal liver function; the common liver diseases; and the effects of liver disease on general homeostasis. Within the context of these topics, this chapter discusses specific anesthetic considerations. In addition, certain surgical procedures (performed only on patients with liver disease) and their anesthetic implications are covered as well. Such a background provides the basis for the prudent delivery of anesthesia and appropriate adjunctive therapy to those who have, or are suspected of having, liver disease.

ANATOMY AND PHYSIOLOGY

The liver is the largest organ of the body. In the adult it weighs approximately 1500 g and represents 2% of body weight; in the newborn, however, it is 5% of total body weight. The liver is traditionally divided into two major lobes, which are supplied by right and left branches of the hepatic artery and portal vein. Based on the location of the portal triad vessels and the hepatic veins, the liver can be further subdivided into eight segments (Fig. 73-1), which facilitates surgical resection procedures.[27] Bile drains into right and left hepatic ducts. A thin covering of connective tissue, Glisson's capsule, encloses the liver. The small amount of connective tissue within the normal liver provides a supporting framework for the hepatic parenchyma and the vessels and nerves within the liver.

Blood supply to the liver is via the hepatic artery and the portal vein. Both enter the liver substance through the porta hepatis, a fissure on the undersurface of the right lobe. **The hepatic artery is richly invested with smooth muscle capable of altering arterial flow. The portal vessels have less myogenic control, which results in more passive changes in portal blood flow.** Sympathetic nerve fibers from the seventh to tenth thoracic vertebrae (T7 to T10) synapse within the celiac plexus along with both the right and the left vagus nerves and the phrenic nerve. Neural fibers then travel by way of the arteries and bile ducts into the liver parenchyma and capsule.[26] Venous drainage from the liver is via short hepatic veins that enter the suprahepatic inferior vena cava (IVC). These veins maintain high flows and are quite difficult to expose surgically, especially in the patient with traumatic bleeding.

Approximately 25% of the cardiac output courses through the liver, which represents a blood flow of about 100 ml/100 g of tissue. The hepatic artery distributes approximately 25% of total liver blood flow and supplies approximately 45% to 50% of hepatic oxygen (O_2). The portal vein delivers approximately 75% of hepatic blood flow, and although partially deoxygenated from transit through the stomach, pancreas, spleen, and intestines, provides the remaining 50% to 55% of hepatic O_2 requirements. The portal blood, however, is rich in nutrients absorbed within the gastrointestinal (GI) tract.

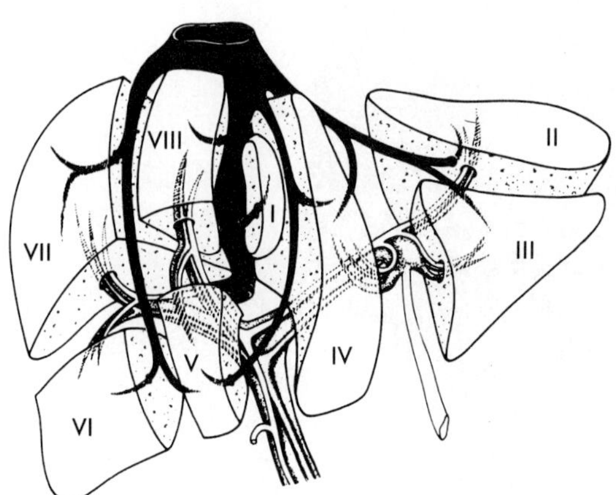

Fig. 73-1. Stylized depiction of hepatic segments I to VIII with their respective blood supplies. (From Bismuth H: Surgical anatomy and anatomical surgery of the liver, *World J Surg* 6:3, 1982.)

Portal flow is regulated primarily by arterioles in the preportal splanchnic organs and to a limited extent by resistance within the liver, resulting in normal portal pressures of 7 to 10 mm Hg. Presinusoidal sphincters determine the relatively uniform distribution of flow through the liver and play a limited role in the regulation of portal flow. Some data strongly suggest that the major site of venous resistance within the liver is postsinusoidal. The sinusoidal pressure is determined by the tone of presinusoidal and postsinusoidal sphincters and blood flow. Smooth muscles in the wall of the venules regulate venous compliance and blood volume. Both resistance and compliance are predominantly controlled by the sympathetic innervation mediated through alpha-adrenergic receptors. Changes in hepatic venous compliance play an essential part in the overall regulation of cardiac output. However, metabolic and vascular smooth muscle regulation of hepatic venous compliance plays a very small role, if any, in controlling hepatic venous resistance. The primary regulating mechanism seems to be mediated via sympathetic alpha-adrenergic receptors. This results in the liver serving as a substantial reservoir of blood volume. For example, during hemorrhage, the liver may be capable of "discharging" about 500 ml of blood into the adult systemic circulation. Unfortunately, disease and various drugs can modify this protective response. Patients with liver disease have a decreased sensitivity to catecholamines, probably because of an increase in the concentration of glucagon (and other vasodilating compounds). This results in a decreased ability to elicit such sympathetic nervous system defenses as constriction of resistive vessels in the musculature and splanchnic areas and constriction of capacitance vessels to divert blood volume to the systemic circulation in patients with hypovolemia or hemorrhage.

The major site of resistance in the hepatic arterial vasculature is the arterioles. **Regulation of the hepatic arteriolar tone is mainly achieved by local and intrinsic mechanisms that adjust hepatic arterial flow to compensate for changes in portal blood flow. This buffer response results in an increase in hepatic arterial flow when portal flow decreases.**[96,152] This increase in arterial flow is an attempt to maintain hepatic O_2 supply and probably total blood flow. This is important for the clearance of both endogenous and exogenous compounds, depending on enhanced, or at least normal, liver blood flow for high extraction rates. Hepatic arterial autoregulation is complex. Neural, metabolic, and myogenic factors are important, as are the effects of substances within portal blood.[96,152] For example, a decrease in portal O_2 content or pH is associated with an increase in hepatic arterial blood flow, even if portal flow is experimentally maintained.[96] The "washout theory" implies that a vasodilating chemical, probably adenosine, is formed within liver cells. When portal flow decreases, this substance is not removed and therefore accumulates, leading to hepatic arterial vasodilatation. On the other hand, an increase in portal flow permits more effective washout of this compound and results in decreased vasodilatation in the hepatic arterial system.

Lymphatic drainage of the liver is accomplished through vessels exiting at the porta hepatis and accompanying the IVC into the thorax. Lymph outflow from the liver is directly related to pressures within the hepatic sinusoids. The sinusoids are lined by a discontinuous layer of endothelium, and the pore structure is not covered by a basement membrane. This results in an inefficient physical barrier to loss of sinusoidal fluid. Normally, fluid is retained within the sinusoid by a favorable protein-oncotic gradient and a low sinusoidal outflow resistance. With the development of higher outflow resistance (e.g., cirrhosis), large amounts of fluid transude into the hepatic lymph system. With sufficiently high pressures, fluid leaks through the liver capsule into the peritoneal cavity as ascites. Normally, hepatic lymph has approximately 90% of the protein content of plasma. In cirrhotic patients, the hepatic lymph concentration falls to approximately 60% of plasma.[286]

Bile ducts accompany the hepatic arteries and the portal veins, forming the portal triad. Bile flows from the bile canaliculi of the liver to enter terminal bile ductules, larger interlobular bile ducts, and finally the right and left hepatic bile ducts, which ultimately form the common hepatic duct (Figs. 73-2 to 73-4). This duct is approximately 3 cm in length and is joined by the cystic duct from the gallbladder to form the common bile duct, which empties into the duodenum. The gallbladder is tucked under the edge of the right lobe of the liver. It is distensible and can hold 30 to 50 ml of bile. Arterial supply to the gallbladder is through the cystic artery, which typically arises from the right hepatic artery. The venous drainage of the gallbladder is through the cystic vein, which empties into the right portal vein.

HISTOLOGIC ORGANIZATION OF LIVER LOBULE

As early as the 1600s, the basic histologic pattern or lobule was recognized. The unit can be viewed from two moderately different structural and functional perspectives.

Classically, the lobule is pictured as a roughly hexagonal prism of tissue approximately 1 × 2 mm in size. At the angles of the hexagon are the portal canals containing connective tissue and the portal triad vessels (i.e., hepatic artery, portal vein, bile ducts). At the center of this lobule lies the central vein, which is actually a terminal venule. The liver parenchyma is arranged in single cell plates between the blood-carrying channels termed *sinusoids* (Figs. 73-2 and 73-3). These platelike, glandular, epithelial cells radiate from the central vein to the portal canals at the periphery of

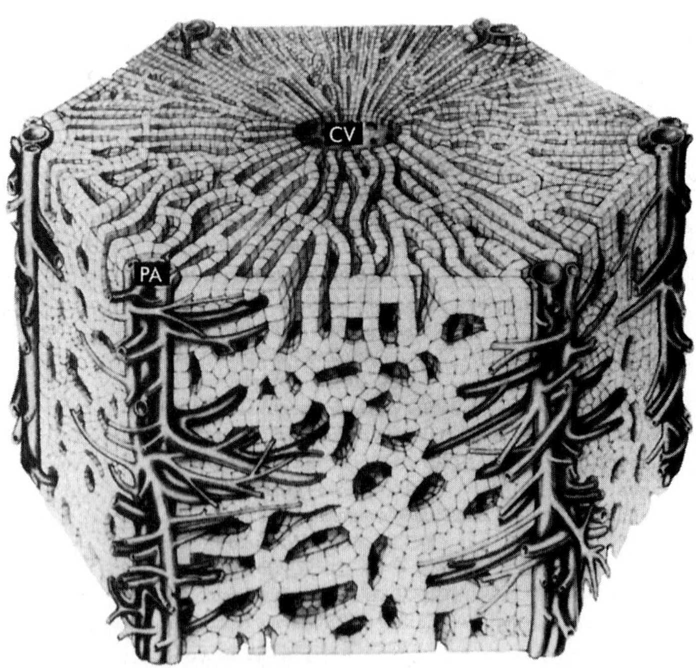

Fig. 73-2. Liver lobule, schematic view. Central vein (*CV*) lies in center of lobule, surrounded by anastomosing cords of blocklike hepatocytes. Around periphery of this schema are six portal areas (*PA*), consisting of branches of portal vein, hepatic artery, and bile duct. (From Zakim D, Boyer TD, editors: *Hepatology: A textbook of liver disease,* ed 2, Philadelphia, 1990, WB Saunders.)

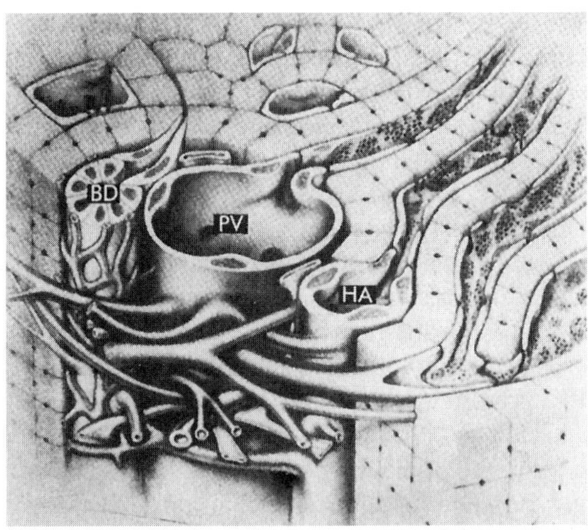

Fig. 73-3. Relationships of branches of portal vein (*PV*), hepatic artery (*HA*), and bile duct (*BD*). (Modified from Jones A, Spring-Mills E: In Weiss L, Greep R, editors: *Histology,* ed 4, New York, 1977, McGraw-Hill.)

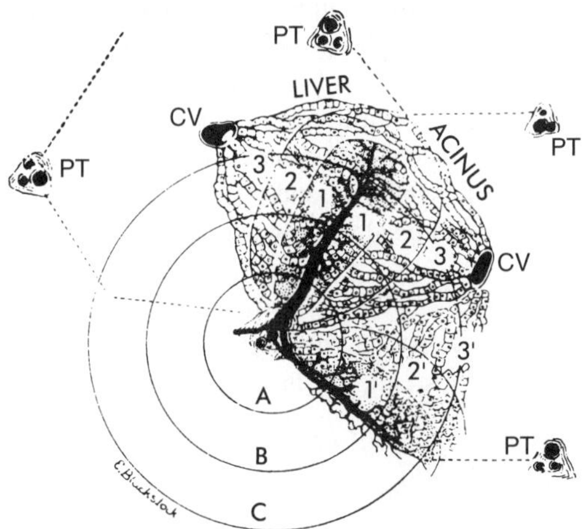

Fig. 73-4. Blood supply of hepatic structural unit, or acinus. Supply of O_2 and nutrients decreases from zone 1 to zone 3. Zones 1′, 2′, and 3′ represent areas of an adjacent acinus. Circle A is periportal, whereas B and C are more peripheral. PT—Portal triad; CV—central vein. (Modified from Rappaport AM, Borowy ZJ, Lougheed WM, et al: Subdivision of hexagonal liver lobules into a structural and functional unit: role in hepatic physiology and pathology, *Anat Rec* 119:11, 1954.)

the lobule. Each lobule represents a three-dimensional labyrinth of cell plates, with interconnected and subdivided spaces, or lacunae.

Another perspective of liver organization[211] (Fig. 73-4) views the liver lobule as an acinus. According to this model, liver cells are grouped into concentric zones around the terminal afferent vessels (portal triad). Zone 1 cells are closest to the source of O_2 and nutrition and are usually the last to be injured and the first to regenerate. More distal zones 2 and 3 are perfused with blood of lesser O_2 content. They are presumably less resistant to toxins and O_2 deprivation.

The biliary tree begins as tiny bile canaliculi typically located in the centrilobular area between hepatocytes, which actually form the limiting walls of the canaliculi. Microvilli extend from the hepatocyte into the canaliculus, and the thin protoplasmic rim of the hepatocyte next to the canaliculus contains many specialized organelles, presumably involved in the formation of bile. As bile is formed, it moves via bile canaliculi from areas around terminal venules (zone 3) toward the portal triad (zone 1). Bile then enters small terminal bile ductules and advances into interlobular bile ducts, which increase in size as they approach the porta hepatis. Intrahepatic bile duct walls are heavily invested with fibrous and elastic tissue and near the hilum contain smooth muscle cells.

Hepatocytes represent approximately 80% of the liver's parenchymal mass. Their function is complex and diverse. They absorb digestive material from the portal venous blood. They store proteins, vitamins, carbohydrates, and lipids and release these compounds into the blood in bound and unbound forms. They excrete bile salts, which facilitate absorption of fat from the intestines, and they synthesize plasma proteins, glucose, cholesterol, fatty acids, and phospholipids. These cells also metabolize, detoxify, and inactivate exogenous and endogenous compounds, including drugs, some poisons, steroids, and most other hormones. They play a role in the immune system as well.

Such a variety of functions requires a complex system of intracellular organelles. These structures have been well documented by ultrastructural methods. Each liver cell contains approximately 800 mitochondria, which occupy about one fifth of the cell volume and are important for oxidative phosphorylation and the oxidation of fatty acids. Lysosomes can be found in the pericanalicular area and perform digestive and catabolic functions on various exogenous substances. It is reasonable to assume that both smooth and rough endoplasmic reticula are involved in almost every hepatocyte function. Hepatic drug-metabolizing activities, as well as conversion of cholesterol to bile acids and certain steps in cholesterol biosynthesis, appear to occur within the endoplasmic reticulum. The Golgi complex is involved in the production of very-low-density lipoproteins (VLDLs), glycoprotein synthesis, albumin secretion, and possibly bile secretion. Other cellular inclusions contain stores of fat droplets and other compounds, including stores of glycogen that first appear in zone 1 but disappear from zone 3. Large, reticuloendothelial Kupffer's cells primarily phagocytize bacteria and other foreign matter from the blood. Other hepatic cell types include endothelial cells, lipocytes, and sinusoidal lining cells.

OVERVIEW OF METABOLIC LIVER FUNCTIONS

Many important biochemical pathways are necessary for general homeostasis, and good reviews exist for this complex topic.[290] This section discusses hemoglobin degradation and glucose, protein, lipoprotein, and cholesterol metabolism.

Hemoglobin Degradation

Because of its complex ultrastructural organization, the liver is capable of synthesizing, metabolizing, and excreting numerous substances.[290] Degradation of heme products to result in the formation of bilirubin is clinically important. When senescent erythrocytes are destroyed by the reticuloendothelial system (i.e., mononuclear phagocytic cells of the spleen, bone marrow, and liver), the released hemoglobin is split into globin and heme. Heme becomes a substrate from which bile pigments are formed. The microsomal enzyme heme oxygenase participates in the formation of biliverdin (as well as endogenous carbon monoxide) (Fig. 73-5), which is reduced to bilirubin and released into the plasma. Free bilirubin combines with plasma albumin and is transported to the liver, apparently the only organ capable of removing it under normal circumstances (Fig. 73-6). Bilirubin is released from the albumin and absorbed by hepatocytes. **Within the liver cell, bilirubin is esterified (conjugated) with monosaccharides, chiefly glucuronic acid, and effectively detoxified. Bilirubin is then excreted into the bile and through the common bile duct into the intestine.** Bacterial enzymes in the distal small intestine and colon convert bilirubin into urobilinogens, which are largely eliminated in the feces. A small portion of the urobilinogens are reabsorbed and undergo enterohepatic circulation and potentially urinary excretion.

Hyperbilirubinemia can result from an overproduction of bilirubin or a defective elimination of bilirubin. Overproduction results in unconjugated hyperbilirubinemia and usually is caused by hemolysis, large hematomas, or ineffective erythropoiesis. Defective elimination typically results from impaired hepatic elimination of conjugated bilirubin and results in conjugated hyperbilirubinemia; frequent causes are cholestatic diseases and biliary obstruction. Any condition that interferes with hepatic uptake or conjugation of bilirubin (e.g., hyperbilirubinemia of newborn, true "breast milk jaundice," Gilbert's syndrome, Crigler-Najjar syndrome) can also result in unconjugated hyperbilirubinemia. Conjugated hyperbilirubinemia is not accompanied by any apparent neurologic symptoms or toxicity, but unconjugated hyperbilirubinemia can result in severe neurologic dysfunction and a fatal encephalopathy termed kernicterus, seen primarily in the newborn.[170,236] Kernicterus is characterized by yellow discoloration of the brain, especially in the basal ganglia, cochlear and cerebellar nuclei, hippocampal formation, and colliculi.

Bilirubin is toxic for a variety of enzymatic processes. This effect occurs at high bilirubin concentrations and can be modified by raising the albumin concentration.[135] Extremely high unconjugated bilirubin levels may play a role in the uncoupling of oxidative phosphorylation in mitochondria. Other methods suggested as explanations for the neurotoxicity of unconjugated hyperbilirubinemia include bilirubin-mediated changes in adenosine triphosphatase (ATPase) and the inhibition of protein synthesis and cellular growth. Membrane function may also be altered by excess bilirubin.[227]

Glucose Metabolism

The liver has a distinct role in the modulation of glucose metabolism. In general, the three "glucose states" are the fed

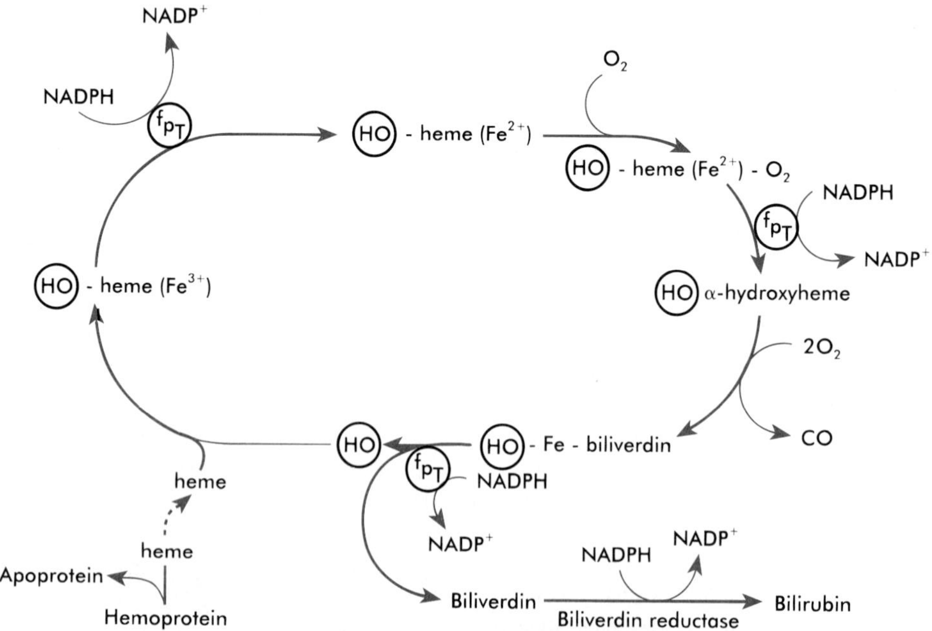

Fig. 73-5. Postulated reaction sequence of heme degradation by microsomal heme oxygenae (*HO*). f_{pt}, NADPHcytochrome *c* reductase. (Modified from Zakim D, Boyer TD, editors: *Hepatology: a textbook of liver disease,* ed 2, Philadelphia, 1990, WB Saunders.)

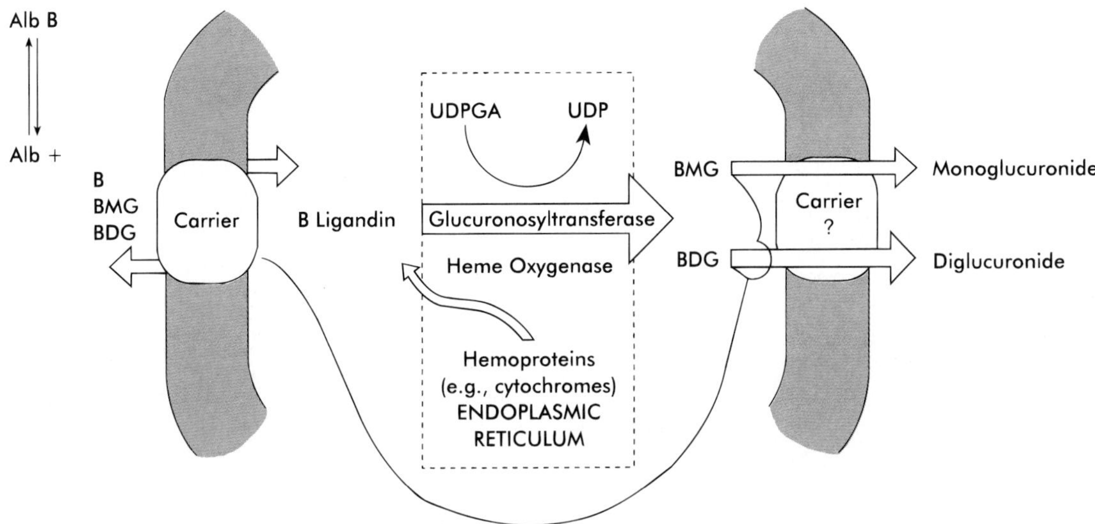

Fig. 73-6. Bilirubin transport and conjugation in hepatocyte. Bilirubin is taken from plasma into hepatocyte at the sinusoidal plasma membrane. Minor fraction is formed in the hepatocyte from breakdown of heme compounds. Inside the liver cell, bilirubin is transferred to the endoplasmic reticulum, where it is conjugated by uricline diphosphate (UDP) glucuronosyltransferase, resulting in formation of bilirubin monoglucuronides and diglucuronide. Conjugated pigments are transported across canalicular membrane and excreted in bile. (From Zakim D, Boyer TD, editors: *Hepatology: a textbook of liver disease,* ed 2, Philadelphia, 1990, WB Saunders.)

state, the postabsorptive state, and the fasted state.[289] The liver's role in this process appears to be controlled partly by the concentration of glucose in the portal vein and ultimately the sinusoids. During the process of attaining the fed state, glucose is distributed directly from the intestine to tissues. Most tissues can store glucose or oxidize it immediately for energy needs. The brain and erythrocytes, however, do not have this capacity and must use glucose immediately. In muscle, glucose can be stored as glycogen, for use later during work. However, muscle glycogen cannot directly return as serum glucose because it lacks the enzyme glucose-6-phosphatase. Within the liver, glucose is used to saturate glycogen stores during a meal, with the remainder used to form fatty acids. These fatty acids are esterified and secreted as VLDLs, which transport the fatty acids to fat cells. Amino acids ingested during a meal are distributed to tissues for protein synthesis (Fig. 73-7).

During the postabsorptive state, the liver returns glucose to the blood rather than storing it, and the fat cells release fatty acids. The liver's released glucose comes from stored glycogen, and is available for central nervous system (CNS), erythrocyte, and muscular use, although the latter has its own glycogen stores for use during work that can be repleted by the glucose released from the liver. During this phase of energy use, oxidation of fatty acids stored as triglycerides in adipocytes increases, and the relative importance of glucose oxidation declines (Fig. 73-8).

After approximately 48 hours in humans, postabsorptive fasting depletes the liver of glycogen stores (Fig. 73-9). Gluconeogenesis must take over to form glucose from various amino acids. Lactate and glycerol can serve as substrates for the synthesis of glucose but are quantitatively less important than protein-derived amino acids. Various enzymes permit the linking of the glycolytic pathway (Fig. 73-10) and the tricarboxylic acid (TCA) pathway (Fig. 73-11 on page 1912), the generation of amino acids, and the removal of ammonia through the urea cycle (Fig. 73-12 on page 1912). This contributes to the negative nitrogen balance seen with fasting. All amino acids, except leucine, can be channelled into glucose production. As ketones increase in concentration late in the course of fasting, the brain is able to use them for fuel.

Because of these mechanisms, hypoglycemia occurs infrequently. However, patients with severe liver disease, especially fulminant hepatitis, may not be able to maintain normal blood glucose levels. Patients with cirrhosis, on the other hand, often have no demonstrable evidence of hypoglycemia, possibly because of glucose production in the medullary regions of the kidney.[145] Interestingly, congestive heart failure (CHF) may be associated with hypoglycemia in patients with severe cirrhosis, possibly from effects on the kidney as well as the liver. Hypoglycemia associated with ethanol ingestion is a common form of acquired hypoglycemia and of special importance to physicians dealing with acute patient care in emergency rooms, intensive care units, and operating rooms. Although this may occur in patients without liver disease and in nonalcoholic patients, such hypoglycemia is much more common in abusers of ethanol. Ethanol inhibits the previously mentioned gluconeogenesis from amino acids, glycerol, and lactate, an effect seen during the fasted state when liver glycogen stores are depleted. Because cirrhotic and alcoholic patients presumably have decreased stores of

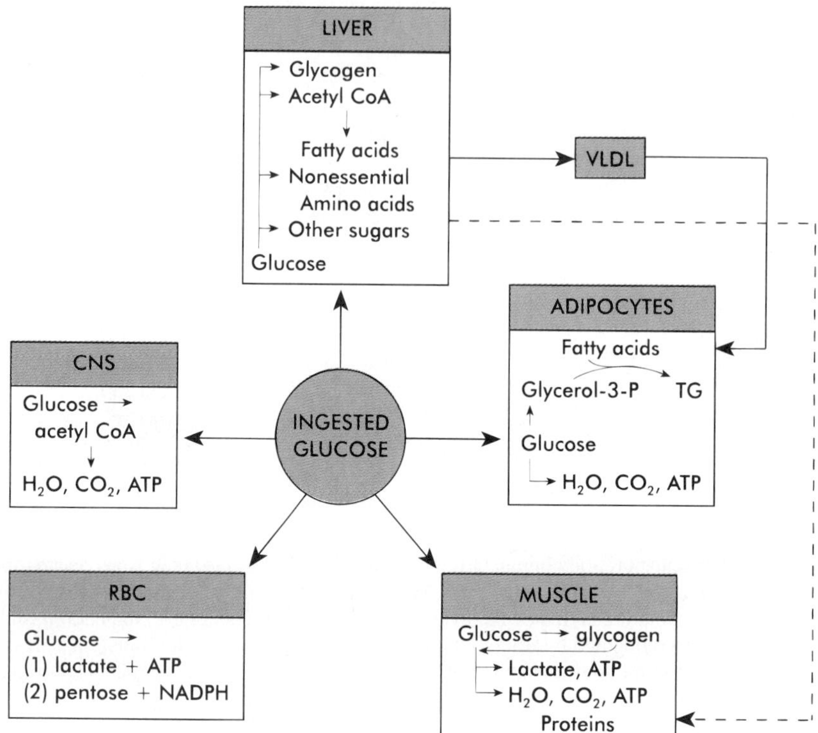

Fig. 73-7. Pattern of supply and use of glucose in fed state. Ingested glucose is shown in the lumen of intestine. This does not show that all absorbed sugar passes into the portal vein and thus into or through the liver. (From Zakim D, Boyer TD, editors: *Hepatology: a textbook of liver disease,* ed 2, Philadelphia, 1990, WB Saunders.)

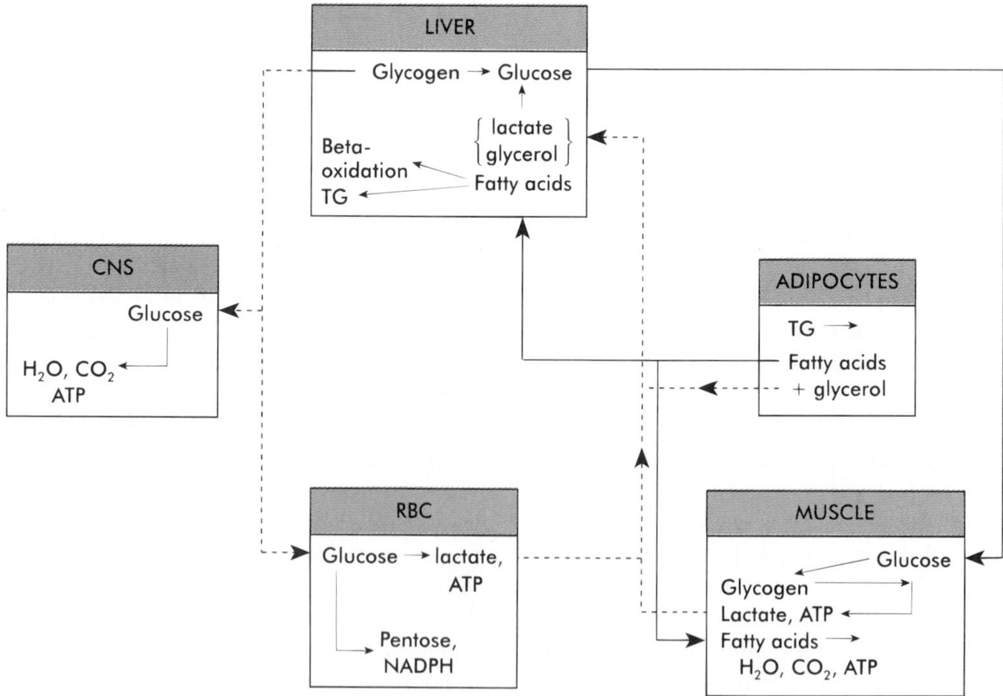

Fig. 73-8. Pattern of supply and use of glucose in the postabsorptive state. Notice the reversal in direction of the supply of carbon atoms (as glucose and fatty acids) between the liver and adipose tissue compared with Fig. 73-7. As opposed to fed state, liver is sole source of glucose in postabsorptive state. (From Zakim D, Boyer TD, editors: *Hepatology: a textbook of liver disease,* ed 2, Philadelphia, 1990, WB Saunders.)

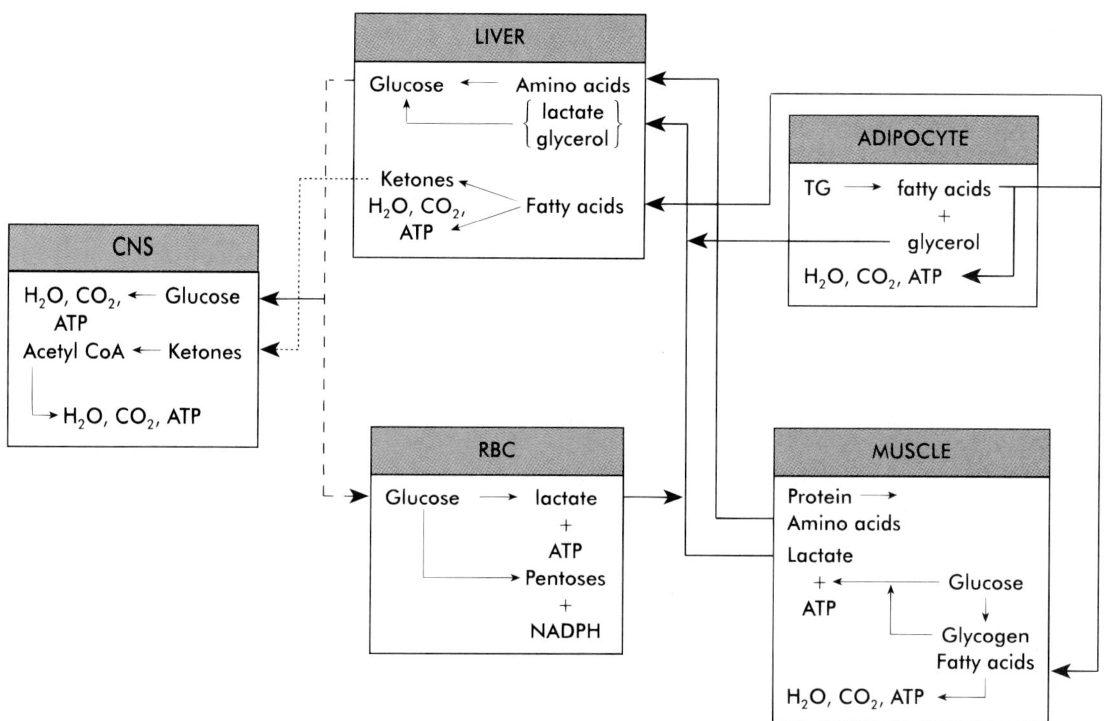

Fig. 73-9. Pattern of supply and use of glucose in the fasted state. Compared with Fig. 73-7, liver glycogen is depleted, amino acids derived from muscle protein are delivered to liver to support synthesis of glucose, and the liver supplies the central nervous system (CNS) with two oxidizable substrates—glucose and ketone bodies. Although not shown, the liver also supplies the cardiac and skeletal muscles. (From Zakim D, Boyer TD, editors: *Hepatology: a textbook of liver disease,* ed 2, Philadelphia, 1990, WB Saunders.)

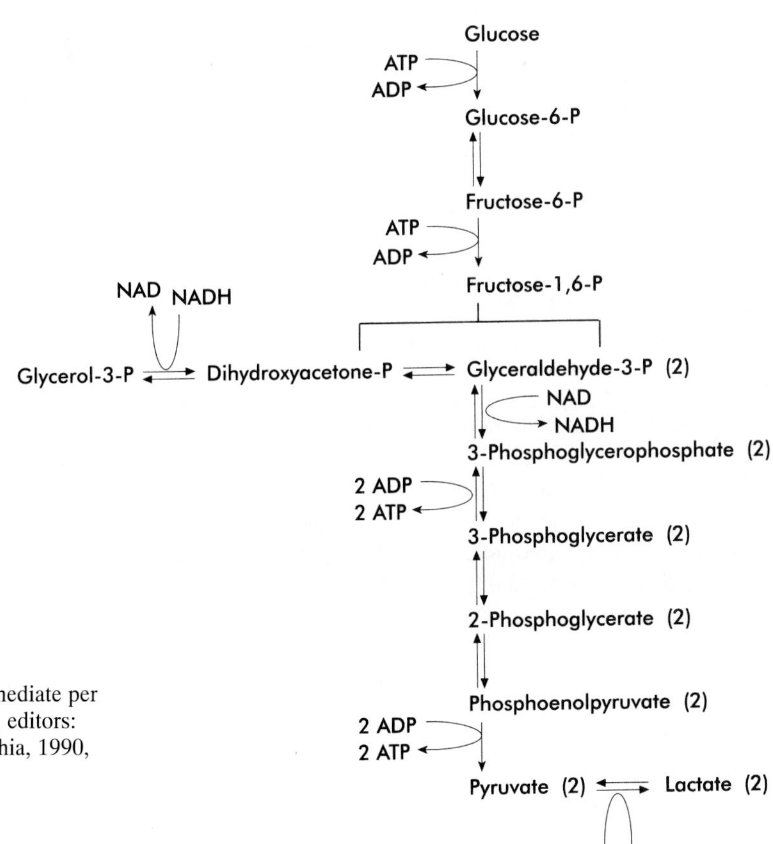

Fig. 73-10. Glycolytic pathway. 2, Two moles of intermediate per mole of glucose consumed. (From Zakim D, Boyer TD, editors: *Hepatology: a textbook of liver disease,* ed 2, Philadelphia, 1990, WB Saunders.)

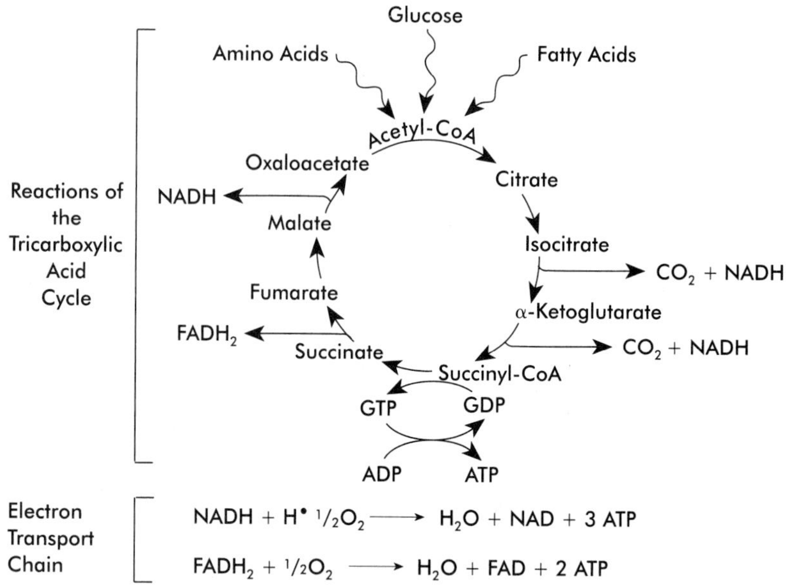

Fig. 73-11. Sequence of reactions in tricarboxylic acid (TCA) cycle and coupling of TCA cycle to synthesis of adenosine triphosphate (ATP). (From Zakim D, Boyer TD, editors: *Hepatology: a textbook of liver disease,* ed 2, Philadelphia, 1990, WB Saunders.)

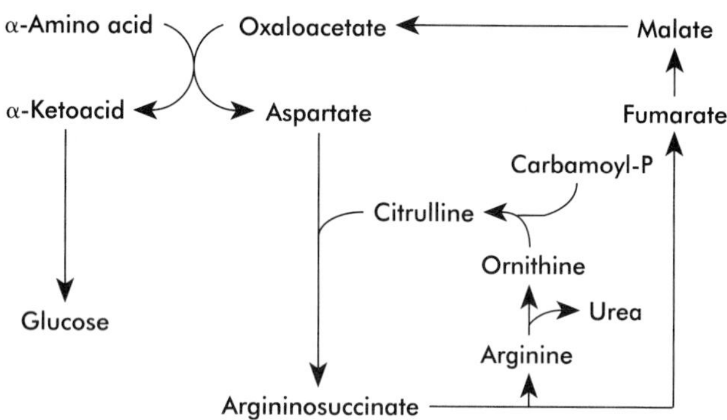

Fig. 73-12. Role of urea cycle in disposing of alpha-amino groups. Amino groups of urea come from carbamoylphosphate and aspartate. (From Zakim D, Boyer TD, editors: *Hepatology: a textbook of liver disease,* ed 2, Philadelphia, 1990, WB Saunders.)

glycogen, they are at risk of this problem after a shorter fast than normal individuals.[198] Glucose can be metabolized by the pentose pathway to form five-carbon sugars necessary in the formation of nucleic acids. This pathway generates NADPH (nicotinamide adenine dinucleotide, reduced), which is used as the reducing agent in the synthesis of fatty acids and steroids and for detoxification of pharmacologic agents. Fructose is also metabolized within the liver via the fructose pathway. Fructokinase is sufficiently active to transiently reduce hepatic concentrations of adenosine triphosphate (ATP) and serum levels of phosphate. Fructose leads to the catabolism of large amounts of adenine nucleotides, increasing the production of uric acid. Fructose can also lead to a greater production of lactate than glucose and in some patients may exacerbate acidosis. Ingested galactose is metabolized after conversion to glucose.

Excess glucose not used by the liver is converted by the liver to fatty acids, which are transported to adipose tissue and stored as triglycerides. During periods of fasting, this process is reversed, and lipolysis frees up fatty acids for metabolism within the liver. Here they are oxidized completely to CO_2 and water in the beta-oxidation cycle and the tricarbolic acid cycle. Acetyl-CoA (Coenzyme A) is derived from glucose (via pyruvate), amino acids, and fatty acids (via the beta-oxidation cycle) but is also a major component of the formation of fatty acids within the hepatocyte cytoplasm.

Protein Metabolism

The liver is responsible for the synthesis of most plasma proteins, with albumin being the major protein secreted. Human albumin is a single polypeptide chain containing 584 amino acids, but it is not glycosylated. Its structure, which allows binding of specific ligands, forms nine double loops stabilized by disulfide bridges.[202] The binding of diverse substances to albumin (e.g., metals, vitamins, amino acids, fatty acids, drugs, peptides, steroid hormones) permits transport of some that might otherwise be poorly soluble in plasma.

Most other plasma proteins secreted by the liver undergo glycosylation, becoming glycoproteins. This process involves the attachment of oligosaccharide units to the amide side chains of asparagine (*n*-linked glycosylation), or to the $^{-}$OH groups of serine or threonine (*o*-linked glycosylation). The glycoproteins are involved in many biologic functions, including hemostasis, protease inhibition, and specialized transport. Table 73-1 lists the major proteins secreted by the liver along with their respective serum concentrations.[61]

The synthesis of plasma proteins entails the complex translation of messenger ribonucleic acid (mRNA) through

Table 73-1 Proteins secreted by the liver

Name	Serum concentration (mg/dl)
Albumin	4500–5000
Fibrinogen	200–450
α_2-macroglobulin	150–420
Haptoglobin	40–180
Hemopexin	50–100
Ceruloplasmin	15–60
Antithrombin III	17–30
Transferrin	3.0–6.5
α_1-antitrypsin	1.3–1.4
C-reactive protein	< 1*
α_1-acid glycoprotein	Trace*
α_1-fetoprotein	Trace

*Rises with inflammation.

sequential phases of protein chain initiation, elongation, and termination. Proteins destined for intracellular function are generally translated by cytoplasmic ribosomes, and those destined for incorporation into membranes or for secretion into plasma are formed on the surface of the endoplasmic reticulum (ER). Various peptide leader segments and signal recognition particles permit recognition of the proteins undergoing synthesis, thus allowing such selective compartmentalization by ultimate intracellular or membrane/secretory function.

Albumin is formed in the Golgi apparatus after a two-step proteolytic cleavage, first of preproalbumin in the ER, then of proalbumin. Albumin has a half-life of approximately 20 days and is thus not a good indicator of liver function in patients with acute hepatic disease. Glycoproteins are formed with oligosaccharides synthesized in the ER and attached to polypeptides in the ER and Golgi apparatus. Glycosylation appears to confer stability to protein molecules and may play a role in the transport of intracellular proteins. Vesicles transport secretory proteins through the hepatocyte to the plasma membrane, where they fuse with the membrane and release their contents into the circulation. This step may depend on calcium.

Various conditions alter protein synthesis by the liver. Ethyl alcohol clearly impairs protein synthesis in *in vitro* studies and protein secretion in both *in vitro* and *in vivo* investigations. This is probably caused by acetaldehyde, the first metabolite of ethanol oxidation. Alpha$_1$-antitrypsin deficiency ensues from a point mutation, leading to a single amino acid substitution. This change results in improper transport and glycosylation of the polypeptide and its accumulation within the hepatocyte. Alcoholic cirrhosis is associated with decreased serum albumin levels, but the size of the exchangeable albumin pool may be normal or even increased, suggesting a normal capacity for synthesis.[121,221,278] Albumin secretory ability may be impaired, however, since biopsy studies have revealed accumulation of protein in the ER and Golgi membranes.[78] Decreased levels of the glycoproteins haptoglobin, alpha$_1$-acid glycoprotein (orosomucoid), and transferrin have also been described in patients with alcoholic cirrhosis.

The decreased albumin seen in liver disease may affect protein binding for many substances, including drugs administered during anesthesia, resulting in increased free or active agents. Because liver disease often impairs metabolism as well, drug toxicity can be potentiated. Narcotics and barbiturates are highly protein (albumin) bound, and a decrease in serum albumin can be associated with an increased incidence of side effects. Similar considerations may at least partially explain the increased susceptibility of patients with severe liver disease to sedatives and tranquilizers. Although a significant proportion of most nondepolarizing muscle relaxants are albumin bound, decreased protein binding does not seem to contribute significantly to the altered function of these muscle relaxants in patients with liver and renal disease.[100]

Lipoprotein and Cholesterol Metabolism

The liver plays a major role in lipoprotein and cholesterol metabolism.[55] Lipids are poorly soluble in plasma and thus require carrier proteins called *apoproteins,* synthesized primarily in the intestine and the liver. The lipoproteins are structured with polar regions facing externally (phospholipids, polar portions of apoprotein) and hydrophobic portions internally (cholesterols, triglycerides). Most lipoproteins are absorbed from the diet and are divided into four classes: (1) chylomicrons; (2) VLDLs; (3) low-density lipoproteins (LDLs); and (4) high-density lipoproteins (HDLs).

Chylomicrons leave the intestine via the mesenteric lymph and generally exist in serum for less than an hour. They bind to endothelial cells in various tissues, where the triglyceride components are hydrolyzed by lipoprotein lipase, releasing free fatty acids for local metabolism or storage. HDL-like substances and chylomicron remnants result from this; cholesterol from the latter is handled by the liver.

VLDLs arise from the intestine as well as the liver and represent the principal lipoprotein secreted by the liver. VLDLs are believed to bind to the same site as the chylomicron and metabolized in much the same way. In humans, most VLDLs are converted to LDLs. Several drugs, including colchicine and tetracycline, alter VLDLs by the liver. LDL metabolism depends on cell membrane receptors, which are present in most tissues but are abundant in the liver, intestine, and adrenal gland. Within these cells, LDLs are metabolized to cholesterol, amino acids, and peptides. LDL serum levels have been associated with atherosclerosis, and several varieties of hypercholesterolemia are associated with reduced receptor numbers or improperly functioning receptors. In these patients, LDLs are handled by some other pathway. LDL metabolism occurs primarily in the liver, whether by receptor-dependent or nondependent pathways. The metabolism of HDLs is less well understood. Although HDL-like material is seen in mesenteric lymph, HDL is probably produced by various tissues, including the liver, and by the metabolism of VLDLs and chylomicrons in serum.

The liver is the most active site of cholesterol biosynthesis, although most cells can synthesize cholesterol at some point in their life cycle. Cholesterol is important in the production of bile salts, steroid hormones, and as a constituent of cell walls. Synthesis begins with acetyl-CoA; passes through mevalonate, squalene, and lanosterol; and finally results in cholesterol. Cholesterol is stored as the esterified form. Cholesterol catabolism leads to the formation of bile salts, which in turn are necessary for cholesterol absorption from the intestine. This represents the major pathway for cholesterol elimination. Cholesterol is also secreted directly into the bile.

PHARMACOKINETICS AND PHARMACODYNAMICS

The liver plays a critical role in the kinetics and dynamics of pharmacologic agents and toxins; several comprehensive reviews of this topic are available.[14,112,223] An extensive discussion is beyond the scope of this chapter, but this section covers important concepts. For many substances the liver serves as the primary site of biotransformation and initiates transfer of unchanged drug into the biliary tract for eventual GI elimination. After oral administration of a drug, the liver may metabolize a substantial portion before it reaches the systemic circulation, thus effectively influencing its bioavailability. In addition, some drugs require biotransformation of inactive forms within the liver to one that is metabolically active (e.g., prednisone, azathioprine).

In general, elimination occurs via excretion of unchanged drug, primarily in the bile or the urine, or through metabolism into one or more metabolites. Excretion as an unchanged drug occurs more often with polar compounds or those ionized at physiologic pH. Metabolic biotransformation generally is necessary for more nonpolar drugs that are not ionized at physiologic pH. Dissemination of drugs within the body is generally termed *distribution,* which occurs simultaneously with elimination. With a constant rate of administration, after four to five half-lives, steady-state conditions arise when distribution and elimination are essentially equal. The volume of distribution (V_d) of a drug is the volume that a known amount of administered drug (d_a) would have to occupy to give the measured serum concentration (d_{sc}):

$$V_d = d_a/d_{sc}$$

A drug with a low serum concentration may have a V_d of hundreds of liters, indicating that the drug is somewhere other than in the plasma or was not measured by the assay. Clearance (CL) is simple in concept but complex and difficult to quantify. It refers to the rate of elimination (RE) by any and all routes relative to the concentration (C) of an agent in any biologic fluid and in general can be described as:

$$CL = RE/C$$

Depending on variables involved, both V_d and CL can lead to estimations that are not physiologic. However, they do serve to illuminate issues concerning the distribution and elimination of pharmacologic agents.

Based on the efficiency of drug removal by the liver, both highly and poorly extracted drugs exist. For efficiently handled drugs, the concentration leaving the liver is very small compared with that entering; the extraction ratio (ER) approaches 1, and clearance is limited by blood flow. However, bioavailability (F) of drugs that are highly extracted by the liver is quite sensitive to the ER:

$$F = 1 - ER$$

Small changes in the ER result in major changes in systemic availability. For example, if the ER decreases from 94% to 88%, approximately a 6% decrease in ER, the availability increases by 100% from 6% to 12%. In addition, for highly extracted drugs, any form of shunting around the liver, whether disease related (intrahepatic and extrahepatic) or surgically created, results in increased availability. Highly extracted drugs also undergo extremely fast, nonrestrictive dissociation from carrier binding sites for efficient extraction to occur. Because of this, highly extracted drugs are less sensitive to changes in carrier protein binding than poorly extracted ones. In addition, when V_d decreases for poorly extracted drugs, reductions in loading doses are required. When V_d is increased, however, as in many liver diseases, an increase in drug loading doses is often not required and could result in toxicity. This is because the increase in V_d in liver disease may be associated with greater concentrations of unbound (i.e., pharmacologically active) drug, which may not be measured in the drug concentration assay.

In general, clearance is more consistently decreased for highly extracted drugs in patients with hepatic disease than for poorly extracted drugs. Liver disease results in a global generalized decrease in the mass of functioning hepatocytes. Remaining liver cells presumably function normally and receive normal blood flow. The blood perfusing areas of nonfunctioning liver cells represents shunt flow, resulting in decreased extraction of highly extracted drugs. The reduced mass of intact liver cells would then have difficulty handling the poorly extracted drugs, which results in their reduced clearance as well. Changes in clearance can serve as an approximate guide for dosing medications. For example, if it is known that the clearance of a drug is decreased by approximately 50% in liver disease, either the dose can be halved or the dose interval can be doubled. For poorly extracted drugs, any condition that decreases carrier binding (albumin, $alpha_1$-acid glycoprotein) results in free drug available for elimination, which increases extraction. For highly extracted drugs, conditions that decrease carrier proteins and increase unbound drug do not increase the already rapid extraction; however, higher active serum levels may result.[14]

Secretion of drugs into the biliary system is not well understood. As mentioned, drugs are either eliminated after some form of metabolic biotransformation or after secretion in an unchanged form into the bile. After reaching the GI tract, the drug can be eliminated in its unchanged form in the feces, reabsorbed, or metabolized with reabsorption and/or elimination. Again, drugs that have polar characteristics and are ionized at physiologic pH are available for biliary excretion, but nonpolar, un-ionized drugs, although they may be secreted into the bile, are then reabsorbed. Large-molecular-weight compounds may also be excreted into the bile. Although bile flow is quite slow (< 1 ml/minute), biliary clearance can be significant for drugs that are actively secreted into the bile.

Drug Therapy in Liver Disease

Although the pharmacokinetics and pharmacodynamics of many drugs have been studied in patients with liver disease, most patients have had either acute hepatitis or cirrhosis. Other liver diseases, such as those associated with cholestasis and chronic passive congestion, are not as well studied. Because of the uncertain capacity of liver function in most patients with liver disease, considerable overlap presumably exists with healthy patients. It is therefore difficult to generalize from "mean" data to the individual patient. One should cautiously approach drug therapy in patients with liver disease, determine serum concentrations when appropriate, and as is the rule in anesthesia practice, titrate dose to effect.

Some specifics should be mentioned. **Drugs with actions in the CNS, such as sedatives, narcotic analgesics, and other psychoactive drugs, are of particular concern in patients with severe liver disease. Even when the pharmacokinetics are only minimally disturbed or even unchanged, excessive sedation or the triggering or exacerbation of hepatic encephalopathy may occur.**[12,150] This susceptibility to increased sedation may be related to the role of gamma-aminobutyric acid (GABA) and GABA receptors in the pathogenesis of hepatic encephalopathy.[232,233]

A substantial decrease occurs in the clearance of benzodiazepines metabolized primarily by oxidative pathways (e.g., diazepam, midazolam), with a significant increase in half-life. The shorter half-life and brief hypnotic effects of midazolam have resulted in its wide use, but prolonged sedation and delayed elimination can occur in patients with cirrhosis.[168] The pharmacodynamics of other benzodiazepines eliminated by glucuronidation (e.g., lorazepam) are not as greatly altered by liver disease, and dosage adjustments may not be required.[14]

Meperidine clearance is substantially reduced in liver disease, with a greatly prolonged half-life.[139,188,204] The dose should be decreased and the time to achieve steady-state levels increased. Morphine metabolism is fairly normal in patients with stable cirrhotic disease, probably because its disposition is via glucuronidation.[201] End-stage liver disease, however, is associated with decreased metabolism and an increased cerebral sensitivity. Fentanyl has a high volume of distribution, probably because of its high lipid solubility. Both clearance and extraction ratios are high. Kinetics are similar in control subjects as in cirrhotic patients before end-stage decompensation, but with severe liver disease, fentanyl dosage must be reduced.[116] Cimetidine may be associated with prolonged fentanyl elimination.

Beta blockers are used to control portal hypertension in cirrhotic patients. These drugs undergo reduced clearance with severe liver disease,[217] and reduced dosage is required. Lidocaine metabolism is greatly impaired as well.[263,282] Diuretics are frequently used in patients with hepatic failure to treat fluid retention. However, natriuretic efficacy is reduced, and overzealous use may result in hypokalemia and intravascular volume depletion which may precipitate hepatic encephalopathy.

Histamine$_2$- (H_2-) receptor antagonists are widely used in cirrhotic patients for treatment of gastritis, GI hemorrhage, and peptic ulcer disease. Cimetidine clearance is reduced in patients with ascites, hypoproteinemia, and encephalopathy, and dosage may need to be reduced by as much as 50%.[268,293] Elimination may also be impaired by the renal dysfunction typically seen in hepatic decompensation. Because of this, other agents (e.g., sucralfate) may need to be substituted for cimetidine. Ranitidine kinetics appear to be similar to those of cimetidine.[288]

Patients with hepatic failure are resistant to both *d*-tubocurarine and pancuronium because both depend partly on biliary excretion for elimination. Because of an increased V_d, a larger dose may be required to achieve a given level of neuromuscular blockade. Once established, however, subsequent doses are smaller and blockade should last longer because elimination is delayed. The usefulness of vecuronium in liver disease may not be as limited as one might predict from its dependence on biliary excretion. A dose-dependent phenomenon may exist; that is, smaller doses may be eliminated adequately.[5,154,155] Because of its unusual mode of degradation, atracurium should not lead to prolonged blockade in patients with end-stage liver disease. This is confirmed by clinical studies,[271] and some would suggest atracurium as the neuromuscular blocking drug of choice in patients with liver disease. Both vecuronium and atracurium do have a somewhat slower onset of action in liver disease, possibly because of an increased V_d. Patients with cholestatic diseases also tend to have a decreased clearance of vecuronium and pancuronium, probably because increased plasma bile salts reduce their hepatic uptake. Succinylcholine biodegradation requires pseudocholinesterase, which is synthesized by the liver. Pseudocholinesterase levels are decreased in patients with liver disease but generally are not low enough to result in a significantly prolonged succinylcholine apnea.

The effects of inhalational anesthetics on the liver are discussed elsewhere (see Chapters 19 and 51). Briefly, the newer halogenated anesthetic agents are reasonably well tolerated by patients with liver disease. Experimentally, liver blood flow is preserved best with isoflurane.[95,104] The use of inhalational anesthetics permits the omission or reduced dosage of many "fixed" intravenous (IV) drugs, thereby decreasing their contribution to intraoperative complications (e.g., hemorrhage, hypotension) as well as their inherent effects on postoperative speed of emergence from anesthesia. Because halogenated agents are mainly eliminated via the lungs, biotransformation by the liver plays a minor role (except for halothane) in this process. It remains to be seen what place the experimental agents desflurane and sevoflurane will have in the patient with liver disease.

CLINICAL LIVER DISEASE

Most patients with hepatic disease either have acute or chronic disease affecting the hepatic parenchyma or have disease-producing cholestasis. The manifestations of diseases within these categories are sufficiently similar that they provide a convenient forum for discussing the major issues in patients with moderate-to-severe liver dysfunction. Anesthetic considerations are discussed where appropriate.

Parenchymal Liver Disease

Parenchymal liver disease has both acute and chronic varieties, as well as a large middle spectrum, and has many etiologies. Whether caused by viral infection (hepatitis types A, B, and C [i.e., non-A, non-B]; delta-hepatitis; others), drugs (e.g., acetaminophen, halothane), toxins (e.g., ethyl alcohol), inborn errors of metabolism (e.g., Wilson's disease), or immunologic disease, manifestations may be similar. These conditions share variably progressive changes in liver architecture and biochemical function. Eventually the metabolic reserve of the liver is compromised, either by the magnitude of decline in number of hepatocytes or by some concomitant process, such as infection and fever, dietary indiscretion, or GI hemorrhage. At this time, the classic features of liver disease become more obvious: jaundice, hypoalbuminemia, portal hypertension with bleeding varices, and abnormalities of the cardiovascular, renal, central nervous system (CNS), and coagulation systems. Significant ascites may develop. Child's criteria[49] for the estimation of the influence of liver disease on surgical outcome were developed with these concerns in mind.

Acute Liver Disease

Acute liver disease occurs quite often. Usually the patient has no previously suspected liver malfunction or metabolic condition with an hepatic manifestation. Determining the diagnosis is sometimes difficult. Although some causes of acute hepatic dysfunction are characteristically short-lived and even asymptomatic (e.g., hepatitis A and B), a certain percentage (e.g., hepatitis B and C) progress to variable degrees of chronic liver disease. Historically, operation in patients with acute hepatitis has carried a high mortality.[120]

Fulminant hepatic failure

A subset of patients with acute hepatic injury develop fulminant hepatic failure (FHF). This catastrophic process results from massive destruction of hepatocytes by a variety of etiologic agents (Box 73-1). The diagnosis of FHF requires the presence of an acute encephalopathy, which some authorities believe should occur within 8 weeks of the onset of the hepatic disease for the diagnosis to apply.[266] This encephalopathy is often associated with cerebral edema. Because of the magnitude of liver impairment, metabolic derangements are severe. A serious coagulopathy develops, related both to decreased synthesis of normal clotting proteins and to thrombocytopenia and altered platelet function. GI hemorrhage often occurs,[92] and intracranial bleeding may also develop. Although hypotension (< 80 mm Hg) occurs frequently in patients with FHF, the etiology is often elusive. One series discovered a cause (hemorrhage, infection, cardiac or respiratory abnormality, extracorporeal perfusion, preterminal state) in only 40% of reported patients.[264] A high cardiac output and low systemic vascular resistance (SVR) resemble those of patients with more chronic end-stage liver disease.[24]

BOX 73-1
MAJOR CAUSES OF FULMINANT HEPATIC FAILURE

Viral infection
- Hepatitis A
- Hepatitis B
- Delta hepatitis
- Hepatitis C (non-A, non-B)

Drugs, chemicals, poisons
- Acetaminophen
- Ethyl alcohol
- Halothane
- Phosphorus
- *Amanita phalloides*

Miscellaneous
- Acute fatty liver of pregnancy
- Reye's syndrome
- Wilson's disease

Hypoxemia frequently occurs in FHF. It may be accompanied by lactic acidosis, and it may occur with no other evidence of pulmonary insult (e.g., pneumonia, atelectasis, pulmonary edema).[22,23] Intrapulmonary shunting is found in these patients, along with a dilated pulmonary vascular bed.[265,280] Pulmonary edema affects as many as 30% of patients with FHF. However, this edema is not believed to be related to left ventricular dysfunction (normal filling pressures), renal dysfunction, or hypoalbuminemia, but may be related to cerebral edema. Electrolyte and acid-base disturbances usually accompany the renal failure that occurs in 30% to 75% of patients with FHF.[194] Most patients initially have only functional renal impairment, which should resolve when the hepatic process improves.[216] Because urea synthesis in FHF may be greatly depressed, serum creatinine and urinary output become better indices of renal function than blood urea nitrogen (BUN).[231,245]

Hypoglycemia (< 40 mg/dl) occurs in approximately 40% of patients with FHF. It may develop rapidly, and care providers should maintain a high index of suspicion. Suspected etiologies include impaired release from the destroyed hepatocytes, impaired gluconeogenesis, and the impaired catabolism of insulin, which can be elevated in patients with FHF.[213,225]

Treatment for patients with FHF involves intense supportive care. As their systems fail, they should be maintained as long as justifiable. However, we have only a rudimentary understanding of the relative importance of the various biochemical disturbances of FHF. To date, no temporary hepatic support devices (e.g., charcoal hemoperfusion) have withstood proper scrutiny. Cerebral edema should be aggressively diagnosed and treated. When massive hepatic necrosis is discovered, the patient should be transferred to a center with the facilities to manage both the predictable encephalopathy and the possible liver transplantation.

Chronic Parenchymal Disease (Cirrhosis)

Chronic parenchymal disease results from various conditions (Box 73-2), including those listed for FHF (except hepatitis A). Although this list is not complete, it represents the more common causes of chronic hepatic impairment. The largest affected groups, however, are those patients with disease caused by viral infection and alcohol consumption.

Cirrhosis is the final common pathologic lesion in various types of liver inury. Classification solely by etiology or histologic morphology, however, is not adequate, because a given hepatic insult may produce several histologic patterns, and a given pattern of injury can be caused by a variety of insults. In general, as liver cells die, extensive connective tissue deposition, fibrosis, and distortion of intravascular channels occur. In addition, the liver's repair work produces areas of regenerating nodules of hepatocellular tissue. These pathologic changes are considered essentially irreversible. As this process evolves with repeated insults to the liver, several sequelae occur. Increased resistance to blood flow through the portal system is one of the factors producing portal hypertension. In the patient with abnormal albumin distribution and kinetics and altered renal function, ascites may develop. Systemic and organ-specific hemodynamic changes occur. Other important sequelae include impaired oxygenation, altered nervous system function, and a coagulopathy.

BOX 73-2
MAJOR CAUSES OF CHRONIC PARENCHYMAL LIVER DISEASE

- Viral infection
  - Chronic active and persistent hepatitis
    - Hepatitis B
    - Hepatitis C (non-A, non-B)
    - Δ hepatitis
  - Drugs, chemicals, toxins
    - Ethyl alcohol
  - Inborn errors of metabolism
    - Wilson's disease
    - Other carbohydrate, protein, lipid, etc. errors
  - Miscellaneous
    - Hemochromatosis
    - α_1-antitrypsin deficiency
    - Cystic fibrosis

Portal Hypertension

The portal vein receives blood from the superior mesenteric vein (small bowel, right colon), inferior mesenteric vein (transverse and left colon, rectum), splenic vein, as well as from the left gastric (i.e., coronary), gastroepiploic, and pancreatic veins. Portal blood enters the liver via right and left branches and mixes with arterial blood either in the portal venules or at the sinusoids. Blood from the sinusoids enters the hepatic veins, which join the IVC just below the diaphragm. No valves exist in the portal system, and normally, resistance to flow is quite low, even with changes in blood flow. Because of pores and microvilli at the sinusoidal endothelial membrane, free passage of proteins into tissue fluid occurs at low venous pressures (e.g., < 2 mm Hg). Above 10 mm Hg, no permeability barrier exists to the movement of large amounts of fluid and protein into the extracellular space (Disse's space).[1,110,238] This contrasts with the usual Starling forces that operate to control fluid shifts between the intracellular and extracellular spaces in other tissue beds.

Normal portal venous pressure is 5 to 10 mm Hg (7 to 14 cm H_2O). A wedge hepatic venous pressure or a direct portal venous pressure more than 5 mm Hg greater than IVC pressure, a splenic pressure greater than 15 mm Hg, or a portal venous pressure measured at operation of greater than 22 mm Hg (30 cm H_2O) indicates the presence of portal hypertension.

As portal hypertension evolves, various portal system collaterals can develop. Many are not clinically obvious. However, esophageal variceal bleeding and its treatment represent a significant medical challenge in the management of cirrhotic patients. Varices may also develop in adhesions from prior abdominal surgical procedures and around the stoma of ileostomies or colostomies created after resection of inflammatory bowel disease. These may lead to GI hemorrhage, as well as increased bleeding at subsequent surgical procedures.

Splenomegaly is frequently encountered in patients with portal hypertension, but a poor correlation exists between portal venous pressure and the spleen's actual size.[274] Evidence of hypersplenism may develop (e.g., thrombocytopenia), but this usually does not create clinical problems unless the patient requires a surgical procedure.

Although increased portal venous inflow may contribute to portal hypertension in some diseases or in some patients, it is more likely that portal hypertension develops mainly in response to increased vascular resistance, according to the so called backward theory. In alcoholic patients, the increased resistance appears to be primarily at the sinusoidal level. Patients with other diseases have either a presinusoidal site of increased resistance (e.g., primary biliary cirrhosis, Wilson's disease, chronic active hepatitis) or resistance increased at a postsinusoidal site (e.g., hepatic vein thrombosis, constrictive pericarditis). Resistance in portocaval collaterals also determines whether portal blood continues to flow through the liver or becomes *hepatofugal,* that is, away from the liver through the collaterals. Not all clinical and experimental observations fit the backward theory of portal hypertension. For example, in experimental animals, restriction of transhepatic portal flow does not always produce portal hypertension comparable with that encountered clinically and does not produce bleeding from esophageal varices. In addition, acute portal hypertension, induced by specific narrowing of the portal vein, is accompanied by substantially decreased portal venous O_2 saturation, increased arteriomesenteric-venous O_2 content difference, increased mesenteric vascular resistance, and decreased mesenteric arterial flow. On the contrary, completely opposite changes are observed in patients with cirrhosis and portal hypertension.

To explain the clinical and physiologic features in patients with cirrhosis that do not fit the backward theory, a forward theory has been proposed.[284] This theory suggests that certain humoral factors (e.g., glucagon, other vasodilating compounds) lead to vasodilatation and formation of arteriovenous (AV) fistulas in the intestine and spleen, which result in a hyperdynamic state with both increased splanchnic blood flow and increased cardiac output. However, portal blood flow is substantially decreased because of portocaval shunting, whereas hepatic arterial blood flow is maintained or even increased.

Ascites

Ascites is one of the primary manifestations of advanced cirrhosis and portal hypertension and portends a poor prognosis. It is associated with altered renal function but is more directly caused by the altered fluid dynamics of portal hypertension. As mentioned earlier, the hepatic sinusoids are lined by an endothelial layer with pores that are not covered by a basement membrane. Because of the normally low sinusoidal pressures, however, a favorable oncotic pressure gradient of 4 to 8 mm Hg (plasma/lymph protein concentration ratio of 1.1:1.4) is maintained.[106] As portal pressure increases, the hepatic control of protein loss into the interstitium is compromised, and the protein content of both the hepatic interstitial fluid and the hepatic lymph flow increases. Thus, the osmotic barrier to interstitial fluid transudation is overcome by the high sinusoidal pressure. Because this increased interstitial fluid and lymph can overwhelm the lymphatic system's ability to return protein to the vascular compartment,[285] ascites results.

Over time, the sinusoid undergoes "capillarization," which decreases the amount of protein that actually enters the lymph and partially restores the osmotic gradient but does not prevent the formation of ascites. Because of this, hepatic lymph in cirrhotic patients contains only approximately 60% of the protein in plasma.[235] Intestinal or splanchnic lymph also contributes to ascites formation but contains much less protein (18% of plasma). The percentage of ascites formed by hepatic or splanchnic lymph is undetermined, but the protein content of ascites is less than 50% that of plasma.[34]

The amount of ascites that accumulates results from an equilibrium between the rate of formation and the rate of absorption. Experimentally, increased intraperitoneal pressure decreases the rate of formation and increases the rate of absorption of ascitic fluid.[295] In humans, the rate of ascites formation is greatest just after paracentesis, when the intraperitoneal pressure is decreased, suggesting similar dynamics.[243]

The treatment of patients with ascites has implications for the anesthesiologist. Sodium and water restriction, diuretic therapy, and abdominal paracentesis may promote intravascular volume depletion. Although large-volume paracentesis (approximately 5 l) leads to an increase in cardiac output immediately after the procedure as well as 24 hours later, decreases in central venous pressure (CVP), pulmonary capillary wedge pressure (PCWP), and creatinine clearance are still measurable at 24 hours. This suggests that patients become hypovolemic as the ascitic fluid reaccumulates, but most tolerate this well.[115,140,251] Interestingly, the decrease in CVP may not be seen in patients with clinical edema, suggesting that the edema fluid is in direct equilibrium with plasma. Infusion of albumin while performing paracentesis has become important in treating ascites rather than using diuretics alone.[103,209]

Elective Operation and Anesthesia in Patients with Newly Suspected Liver Disease

Conclusions about anesthesia and surgical procedures in the setting of abnormal liver function tests are uncertain. Studies of postoperative problems have been done by gastroenterologists, surgeons, and anesthesiologists. Almost invariably, they indicate an increase in both postoperative morbidity and mortality over patients without preoperative evidence of liver dysfunction. Most of these studies, however, did not consider in the presence or absence of comorbid disease.

Operation during acute viral hepatitis had been reported to lead to 9.5% mortality and 11.9% morbidity.[120] When liver disease was present but either not suspected or ignored prior to operation, there was 4% to 31% mortality and 25% to 61% morbidity; one study has noted that all patients with acute viral or alcoholic hepatitis died postoperatively.[128,207] In nonelective abdominal procedures in cirrhotics with ascites, there was 20% mortality and 47% morbidity in patients with bilirubin > 3.5, PT > 2 sec beyond control, and high blood loss.[164] Although we may have problems with the age of some of these reports or quibble over the type of operation and the handling of the resulting data, such studies suggest that **operation in those with liver disease carries risks well beyond those of otherwise normal patients.**

Liver disease represents a hard-to-define continuum ranging from patients with acute disease, either self-limiting or fulminant, to those with disease that will become chronic, or has already become chronic, symptomatic or not. In otherwise healthy ASA 1 surgical patients, 11 of every 7620 (1 of every 700) had clearly abnormal liver function tests (defined as results more than twice the upper limits of normal) and had their procedures cancelled. All had definitive liver disease diagnosed and three subsequently became jaundiced.[237] However, we are more often presented with unsuspected abnormal liver function tests that are less clearly significantly abnormal, and we seldom know whether it is early or late in a disease process or whether we are simply observing laboratory error. **Conventional wisdom, based on some admittedly older studies, would be to delay elective operation until resolution or better definition of the etiology of newly recognized liver dysfunction.** There may also be differences between the risks for patients with acute hepatic disease and those with chronic disease. Although morbidity and mortality in this population of patients in the 1990s may actually be lower than in the past, due to newer surgical procedures (e.g., laparoscopy), better perioperative nutrition, newer drugs, and better understanding of the actions of drugs on splanchnic and hepatic blood flow, prudence still dictates considerable respect for the potential for perioperative morbidity and mortality.

When the considered decision of the patient, surgeon, and anesthesiologist is that "elective" operation and anesthesia is to proceed, the anesthesiologist needs to keep in mind what is known about the effects of operation and anesthesia on splanchnic and hepatic circulations, and hepatic function. **All general anesthesia causes a dose-related reduction in liver blood flow to some extent, with halothane producing a greater decrease than isoflurane.**[97,104] **Minor peripheral operations generally have less effect on liver blood flow than more major procedures such as laparotomy, which is accompanied by a reduction in portal blood flow and an increase in hepatic arterial blood flow.**[29,93,177] During laparotomy, however, isoflurane tends to return liver blood flow toward normal.[19,95,97] Acidosis, whether metabolic or respiratory, increases intrahepatic portal venular resistance, and may increase shunting of hepatic blood away from hepatocytes, resulting in insufficient delivery of O_2 to hepatocytes. Moderate hypocapnia does not deteriorate hepatic circulation and function to a significant extent.[89,94] PEEP (positive end-expiratory pressure) is associated with a reduction in cardiac output and both hepatic arterial and portal venous flow.[37] **Spinal anesthesia (without operation) reduces liver blood flow if arterial pressure is allowed to decrease, but has limited effects when fluid support is administered to maintain systemic pressure.**[109] In a small series of patients with mild alcoholic hepatitis, there was no difference in outcome between patients given either an enflurane or narcotic-based general anesthetic or a spinal anesthetic for peripheral orthopedic, ear-nose-throat, plastic, and general surgery procedures.[296] However, both halothane general anesthesia and bupivacaine spinal anesthesia for knee arthrotomy induced similar increases in hepatic microsomal enzyme activity in healthy patients.[165] Additionally, drugs used by patients, as well as by anesthesiologists, affect liver blood flow. Cimetidine reduces blood flow by 25% to 33%,[77] and this disturbs the clearance of propranolol and lidocaine.[76] Ranitidine also decreases hepatic blood flow but has much less effect on microsomal oxidase hepatic drug elimination.[292] As newer pharmaceuticals and anesthetics are developed, we need to periodically update our knowlege in this area.

HEMODYNAMIC CHANGES IN LIVER DISEASE

Both the arterial and the venous systems are greatly affected by severe liver disease, and changes in cardiac function are prominent. Intravascular volume, although generally believed to be increased, is influenced by changes in oncotic pressure and renal function but may not be increased in proportion to the generalized vasodilatation. As much as 60% to 80% of portal blood may be systemically shunted away from the liver.[114] An incompletely understood, complex mix of associations drives these interactions among the various organs and vascular beds. In addition, sympathetic nervous system modulation is abnormal,[291] and blood flow through many vascular beds is altered (Box 73-3).

Cardiovascular Function

At least 50% to 80% of patients with chronic liver disease have a significantly increased cardiac index.[144,187,200] This hyperdynamic state includes a low systemic vascular resistance (SVR), normal-to-low mean arterial pressure,

BOX 73-3
HEMODYNAMIC CHANGES IN CIRRHOSIS

↓ Systemic vascular resistance from peripheral vasodilation and arteriovenous shunting
↑ Blood volume
↑ Cardiac output
Arterial pressure, filling pressures, and heart rate maintained until end-stage disease
Evidence suggesting cardiomyopathy (e.g., blunted response to catecholamines)
↓ Arteriovenous O_2 content difference and ↑ venous O_2 content
↓ Response to catecholamines
↑ Pulmonary, splanchnic, muscle, and skin blood flow
↓ Portal flow to liver; normal to ↑ hepatic arterial flow
Normal to ↓ renal blood flow
↓ Albumin and oncortic pressure

normal to increased heart rate, and increased blood volume. Left ventricular and left atrial dimensions can be increased, coincident with increased systolic ventricular performance.[163] Because the myocardial response to the increased concentrations of norepinephrine seen in patients with liver disease appears blunted, an element of cardiomyopathy probably exists as well.[124] Stimuli for the increased norepinephrine production include a decreased "effective" blood volume[190] and possibly the degree of portal hypertension (i.e., via an hepatic baroreceptor).[125,143]

Although arterial desaturation may exist, peripheral blood flow is usually increased to a degree associated with normal or increased O_2 delivery. The O_2 tension and saturation of peripheral and mixed venous blood are increased, with narrowing of the arteriovenous (AV) O_2 content difference. However, this presumably represents the widespread (e.g., in splanchnic organs, lungs, skin) presence of AV fistulas rather than supranormal O_2 delivery at the tissue level. Tissue O_2 delivery may not meet demands during periods of stress, despite an increased cardiac output.[182,183]

A variety of intrahepatic shunts exist in cirrhosis.[205] Combined with the extrahepatic "preportal" shunts seen with portal hypertension, considerable opportunity exists for substances normally metabolized by the liver to bypass normal degradation and thereby reach the systemic circulation. It is believed that serum concentrations of various circulating vasodilator substances are maintained or increased in this way.[18] This at least partially explains both the decrease in SVR and the poor response of cirrhotic patients to vasopressor drugs, including angiotensin II.[62,151] Prostaglandins may also be involved in this resistance to pressor compounds.[297] Portal obstruction alone, with preserved liver function, contributes to portal hypertension, portasystemic shunting, and the hyperdynamic cardiovascular function characteristic of patients with cirrhosis.[156]

Glucagon concentrations are increased in cirrhotic patients, probably secondary to increased pancreatic secretion and to decreased hepatic metabolism.[173] In addition to glucagon's hemodynamic effects on the heart (positive inotropic) and renal vasculature (stimulation of renin secretion through "effective" hypovolemia[32]), glucagon appears to cause a considerable reduction in splanchnic arteriolar resistance. This results in increased portal blood flow and increased portal pressure, thus contributing to the portocollateral shunt flow[17,18,247] and the decreased vascular responsiveness to infused catecholamines and vasopressors.[30,214] Other substances (e.g., ferritin, vasoactive intestinal polypeptide) may also be responsible for peripheral vasodilation, decreased SVR, and increased AV shunting.

Cardiac output is not invariably increased in patients with cirrhosis. In patients with massive ascites, cardiac output may even be normal before paracentesis and only clearly increased after ascites removal. Some experts suggest that the abdominal pressure is transmitted to the chest, decreasing the transmural filling pressures and increasing the mean right atrial pressure, thus resulting in decreased venous return. Cardiac output and ventricular stroke work increase dramatically, and right atrial pressure decreases as volume is removed.[115]

Renal Circulation

Renal blood flow and function can be normal in the early stages of chronic liver disease. A decrease in renal cortical blood flow, however, is probably one of the first signs of impaired renal function.[73,138] A distribution of blood flow away from cortical nephrons may partially explain the sodium retention characteristic of cirrhotic patients. In advanced stages of liver disease with edema and massive ascites, patients have variable degrees of reduced renal blood flow. Severe renal hypoperfusion plays an important role in the pathogenesis of the hepatorenal syndrome, which sometimes complicates cirrhosis. This decrease in renal blood flow, especially cortical blood flow, is believed to result from increased renal vascular resistance, despite a relatively high cardiac output and low total SVR. It occurs in the setting of a marked stimulation of several renal vasoconstrictors such as the renin-angiotensin-aldosterone system, the sympathetic nervous system, and antidiuretic hormone.[9] Thus, although many other organs and tissues are hyperperfused (e.g., preportal organs and tissues, skin, lungs, muscles), the kidneys are underperfused. This increase in renal vascular resistance is caused by increased resistance in afferent, more than efferent, arterioles.

Hepatic Circulation

Portal hypertension is the main feature of the abnormal splanchnic circulation seen in cirrhotic patients. As mentioned earlier, portal pressure is a function of one or more of three factors: (1) flow into the portal system; (2) resistance to portal flow; and (3) resistance in portacaval collaterals. The splanchnic circulation is affected by certain factors (e.g., glucagon, bile acids, other vasodilating compounds[18]) that lead to vasodilatation and formation of AV fistulas in the intestine and the spleen. This results in a hyperdynamic state, with increased splanchnic blood flow and increased cardiac output. Regarding the overall hepatic blood flow, portal blood flow is substantially decreased, whereas hepatic arterial blood flow is maintained or even increased. Portal flow may actually be reversed, either in the main portal vein or in the feeding veins.[39,90] In most cirrhotic livers, however, hepatic O_2 supply is maintained; only total hepatic blood flow is decreased. This has pharmacokinetic significance: Compounds and drugs that have a high hepatic clearance will be eliminated more slowly than those in normal patients.

RENAL FUNCTION IN PATIENTS WITH LIVER DISEASE

Renal failure may occur in 50% to 75% of patients dying of cirrhosis[66] and potentially complicates anesthesia management during surgery for patients with severe liver disease. Various interrelated changes in renal function and water and electrolyte handling accompany declining liver function. A comprehensive review of this topic is beyond the scope of this chapter but is available in other resources.[65]

Patients with end-stage liver disease who have edema and ascites (e.g., Läennec's cirrhosis) share an abnormal handling of water. Traditionally, ascites and edema have been believed to result from an alteration of Starling forces (decreased colloid oncotic pressure, increased portal pressure) leading to ascites transudation and decreased plasma volume. The decreased plasma volume serves as an afferent signal for sodium and water retention (underfill theory). Because this theory does not acknowledge that sodium retention is known to precede ascites formation, other explanations have been given.

Others have proposed that edema and ascites formation in the setting of decreased oncotic pressure and increased portal pressure are fundamentally the result of a primary renal defect that promotes sodium and water retention (overflow theory). However, head-out-of-water immersion studies (which produce an increase in central volume) performed in cirrhotic patients strongly suggest that "underfill" better conceptualizes the problem. In these patients, immersion leads to a marked natriuresis and kaliuresis, as well as a significant increase in creatinine clearance. Plasma aldosterone is often elevated in patients with cirrhosis, attributable both to increased adrenal secretion and to decreased hepatic degradation. Although this may contribute to sodium retention, water immersion studies again suggest that a decreased effective plasma volume is a primary condition associated with the formation of edema and ascites.[72] Increased renal prostaglandins appear to be related to the diuresis, natriuresis, and improved creatinine clearance seen in cirrhotic patients during water immersion.[70,71] Natriuretic factors, estrogens and prolactin, kallikreins, and vasoactive intestinal peptides have all been studied in the cirrhotic population with variable results (Table 73-2). In addition, many believe that sympathetic activity, as measured by norepinephrine, is increased, but the effect on sodium and water retention is inconclusive.[69]

Table 73-2 Factors contributing to edema and ascites

Factor	Concentration in cirrhosis	Effect on sodium excretion
Effective plasma volume	↓↓	↓↓
Aldosterone	N to ↑	↓
Oncotic pressure	↓	↓
Norepinephrine	N to ↑	?
Renal prostaglandins	↑	↑
Natriuretic factor	N to ↑	?
Kallikrein system	↓ to ↑	?
Estrogens	N to ↑	↓
Prolactin	? ↑	? ↓
Vasoactive intestinal peptides	↑	? ↓

↓—Decreased; ↓↓—extremely decreased; ↑—increased; N—no change.

The "peripheral arterial vasodilation hypothesis[240]" looks at issues that are not adequately explained by either the "underfill" or "overflow" models. According to this theory, splanchnic arterioloar vasodilation secondary to portal hypertension is the initial event, and baroreceptor-mediated activation of the renin-angiotensin-aldosterone system, the sympathetic nervous system and antidiuretic hormone form an intermediate step (not because circulating blood volume is decreased but because the arterial vascular compartment is disproportionally enlarged), with resultant renal sodium and water retention. This becomes a "revised underfill theory."

Most patients with decompensated cirrhosis demonstrate a moderately impaired renal concentrating ability. However, most patients with compensated cirrhosis can excrete water without significant limitation. In general, patients with cirrhosis excrete a dilute urine in response to water loading, mainly because of lower rates of sodium and urea excretion. A general correlation exists between a patient's clinical status and his or her relative impairment of diluting ability.

Dilutional hyponatremia often results from this impaired handling of water in liver disease, regardless of the patient's "volume status," when water intake is in excess of the ability to excrete it. Thiazide diuretics and aldosterone inhibitors such as spironolactone may contribute to the decreased sodium concentration. In lieu of other medical considerations, water restriction is the treatment for this process. Antidiuretic hormone (ADH), catecholamines, and prostaglandins may also play a role in this impaired water excretion.

Neurotransmitter amino acid transport systems in the brain and spinal cord appear to require adequate sodium (Na^+) ions for proper function; loss of these ions during hyponatremia may at least partially explain the encephalopathy seen in patients with severe liver disease.[87,88] A longstanding association exists between hyponatremia and central pontine myelinolysis (CPM), especially in alcoholic patients with liver disease. Rapid correction of symptomatic hyponatremia to mildly hyponatremic concentrations is no longer believed to be the etiology of this condition.[10,11,38,192] However, overcorrection to a hypernatremic state (> 150 mEq/l) has recently been suggested as contributing to CPM development.[11] In general, severe brain damage during hyponatremia has been associated with: (1) the occurrence of hypoxia, usually from respiratory arrest; (2) correction of sodium to > 135 mEq/L in the first 48 hours; (3) increasing serum sodium by > 25 mmol in the first 24 hours; (4) hypernatremia (> 145 mEq/l) in liver disease patients treated with lactulose (especially if it develops over < 48 hours); (5) associated medical conditions (e.g., cirrhosis, metastatic cancer) that alters the blood–brain barrier; and (6) delay in institution of therapy.[6] **The mortality for patients with severe liver disease, hyponatremia of < 120 mEq/l, and CNS symptoms is more than 60%.** Recently, others have suggested that treatment for acute hyponatremia should be more aggressive than that for chronic hyponatremia. Acute hyponatremia is defined as a decrease exceeding 0.5 mmol/l/hour or as occurring over 2 to 3 days when large amounts of fluids, especially hypotonic, have been administered. This form of hyponatremia can be treated with more than 1 mmol/l/hour to achieve mildly hyponatremic levels.[52]

Hypokalemia often accompanies the hyponatremia. Potassium loss occurs because of: (1) loss of lean body mass and replacement with ascites; (2) increased urinary loss secondary to the use of diuretics; and (3) GI losses from emesis and diarrhea.[6] Replacing potassium does not improve the ability to correct the decreased serum sodium.

Hypernatremia is also seen in patients with severe liver disease. As many as 35% of patients receiving loop diuretics with encephalopathy or those taking lactulose develop this condition.[189,273,279] As in other disease states, hypernatremia develops from an excessive loss of free water or an excessive gain in sodium. The sodium gain usually results from the administration of hypertonic sodium-containing solutions such as hypertonic NaCl or $NaHCO_3$. The free water loss is often the result of inadequately monitored lactulose administration. The metabolism of lactulose acidifies intestinal contents, which draws ammonia intraluminally, where it is converted to the ammonia ion. Because the metabolic products of lactulose create an osmotic gradient, drawing water into the intestine, diarrhea may result. Sodium can be reabsorbed in the ileum and colon, but the water is lost. Insensible water losses from tachypnea and fever, inadequate intake related to encephalopathy, and abnormal losses associated with diuretic therapy may also contribute. Severe hypernatremia may lead to loss of brain volume and subsequent intracranial bleeding, with a mortality greater than 80% in cirrhotic patients. Treatment includes correction of the shock state with colloid to stabilize hemodynamics, correction of the fluid deficit over approximately 48 hours, decreasing osmolarity by only 1 to 2 mOsm/l/hour, and frequent monitoring of electrolytes.

Hepatorenal Syndrome

A spectum of relatively acute azotemic syndromes can affect the patient with hepatic disease. The progressive oliguric renal failure complicating advanced liver disease is termed *hepatorenal syndrome* (HRS) when clinical, laboratory, and anatomic evidence do not suggest another known cause for the renal failure. The conditions most often confused with HRS are prerenal azotemia and acute tubular necrosis (ATN). In addition, in the patient with severe liver disease, bilirubin metabolites can interfere with the measurement of creatinine and artifactually decrease the serum values.[119] This may mask a rising creatinine level or, alternatively, suggest improved renal function. Other characteristics included in the differential evaluation of the liver disease patient with oliguria are listed in Table 73-3.

A consistent finding in HRS is a urinary sodium concentration of < 10 mEq/l, but this is a feature of prerenal failure as well. Some patients develop what is believed to be HRS but have a much higher urinary sodium (20 to 30 mEq/l); some of these conditions may progress to ATN. Patients with HRS retain their concentrating ability, as do patients with prerenal azotemia.

Table 73-3 Hepatorenal syndrome — International Ascites Club Diagnostic Criteria

Major Criteria

- Chronic or acute liver disease with advanced hepatic failure and portal hypertension
- Low GFR (i.e., serum creatinine > 1.5 mg/dl or 24 hr) (creat. clearance < 40 ml/min)
- Absence of shock or ongoing bacterial infection
- Absence of current or recent treatment with nephrotoxic drugs
- Absence of GI fluid losses (repeated emesis or intense diarrhea) or renal fluid losses (weight loss > 500 g/day for several days in patients with ascites without peripheral edema or 1000 g/d in patients with peripheral edema)
- No sustained improvement in renal function (decrease in serum creatinine to ≤ 1.5 mg/dl or increase in creatinine clearance to ≥ 40 ml/min) following diuretic withdrawal and expansion of plasma volume with 1.5 l of isotonic saline
- Proteinuria < 500 mg/dl and no ultrasonographic evidence of obstructive uropathy or parenchymal renal disease

Additional criteria

- Urine volume < 500 ml/d
- Urine sodium < 10 mEq/l
- Urine osmolality greater than plasma osmolality
- Urine erythroctye < 50/hi power field
- Serum Na concentration < 130 mEq/l

GFR—glomerular filtration rate; GI—gastrointestinal.

The specific cause of HRS is not known; however, it is strongly suspected to be a functional rather than a pathologic derangement. Fluid restriction and excessive diuretic therapy may serve to initiate HRS in the patient with severe renal dysfunction; pathologic changes are minimal and inconsistent. In addition, the continued ability to concentrate and reabsorb sodium implies a persistence of renal tubular functional integrity. When kidneys from HRS patients have been transplanted, function has returned. Patients with HRS who undergo successful liver transplantation have also had return of renal function.

Studies have documented decreased mean renal blood flow and reduced cortical blood flow in patients with HRS,[68] which are not seen in other varieties of renal failure. Such selective renal hypoperfusion is a unique feature of this process. Decreased "effective" blood volume and SVR, as well as the augmented sympathetic nervous system activity seen in severe cirrhosis, presumably contribute to these renal perfusion abnormalities. Alterations in the renin-angiotensin system,[41] prostaglandins,[8] thromboxanes,[215,298] and the kallikrein system probably have a role in the pathogenesis of HRS as well.

Treatment of patients with HRS first requires differentiation from more readily treatable conditions, because the onset of oliguria should *not* directly imply the presence of HRS. One must especially look for prerenal failure, because it should be reversible when treated appropriately. Therapy is often supportive and may require the measurement of filling pressures during volume challenges. Attempts should be made to treat severe anemia and metabolic abnormalities such as acidosis and encephalopathy. Enhancing renal perfusion and promoting decreased sodium reabsorption (e.g., with dopamine) may have a place in the management of patients with HRS. Dialysis may be effective in the treatment of acute hepatic disease and HRS. Portocaval shunts, continuous AV ultrafiltration, and peritoneovenous shunts have all been reported as leading to improved renal function. Finally, successful orthotopic liver transplantation should lead to reversal of true HRS.[67]

Recently HRS has been divided into two clinical forms: (1) Type 1 is characterized by rapid reduction in renal function over 2 weeks or less; and (2) Type 2—renal failure without a rapidly progressive course.[9] The recently published International Ascites Club Diagnostic Criteria for the HRS are listed in Table 73-3.[9] These criteria reflect the difficulty in arriving at this diagnosis with certainty.

Often, operation in this group of patients is not elective, and ample time to improve the patient's condition may not be available. One hopes that patients with severe hypo- or hypernatremia or hypo- or hyperkalemia will have time for their electrolytes and volume to be reversed toward normal values. Principles used in the intensive care unit for the management of the patient with electrolyte abnormalities should also apply to the care of the patient in the operating room. Wide swings in electrolytes and osmolarity should be avoided, if possible, by appropriate use of replacement solutions with the proper composition. Appropriate laboratory evaluations should be conducted frequently. Volume management may need to be guided by information obtained from central venous or pulmonary artery (PA) catheters. Intensive care observation and dialysis may be needed postoperatively.

COAGULATION AND LIVER DYSFUNCTION

For coagulation to occur properly, three essential elements of a diverse system must work together: (1) the vascular injury or tissue reactions; (2) the clotting cascade (intrinsic and extrinsic) reactions; and (3) the clot-limiting reactions (Box 73-4). All are necessary; none is sufficient by itself in sustaining normal hemostasis. The liver, by virtue of the many coagulation factors it synthesizes, is intimately involved with each of these components of coagulation. Hepatocellular diseases and diseases affecting liver function lead to alterations in these coagulation systems, which are measurable by laboratory means if not by clinical assessment. Patients with severe liver disease generally have profound life-threatening disturbances of the coagulation process. A brief review of normal coagulation is useful when discussing this topic.

BOX 73-4
ESSENTIAL ELEMENTS IN COAGULATION

Vascular injury/tissure reactions
Clotting cascade reactions
  Intrinsic
  Extrinsic
Clot-limiting reactions

Normal Coagulation[81]

Tissue injury initiates coagulation with the attraction of platelets to endothelial and subendothelial collagen. The platelets then undergo a "release reaction" whereby various substances are extruded to the platelet surface as it swells, becomes sticky, and develops fibrinogen receptors. Fibrinogen then binds to these receptors, at first reversibly and then irreversibly, and ultimately large platelet aggregates plug the site of injury. Several platelet enzymes, including membrane phospholipases, cyclo-oxygenases, and thromboxane, enhance aggregation and constrict the bleeding vessel. Additionally, a large protein—*factor VIII:von Willebrand factor* (factor VIII:VWF; distinct from factor VIII coagulant activity, factor VIII:C)—binds the platelet aggregates to the subendothelial collagen, which is necessary for further stabilization of the plug.

This mechanism is adequate for initial control of bleeding, but ultimate hemostasis requires the involvement of the clotting cascade to ensure ultimate stability of the clot. This cascade proceeds by two pathways to the conversion of *prothrombin* to thrombin, which then cleaves *fibrinogen* to fibrin.

The intrinsic system also begins with activation by the vascular injury. Factor XII (Hageman) binds to the exposed endothelium and is cleaved to an activated form (XIIA) through the actions of *kallikrein* and high-molecular weight kinogen (HMWK). XIIA then activates factor XI to form XIA at the surface of platelets in the developing clot, also facilitated by HMWK. XIA activates factor IX (prothrombin complex [PTc], or Christmas factor) to IXA, requiring calcium. IXA then serves, in the presence of calcium and a cofactor, factor VIII:C, (the antihemophilic factor), to cleave factor X to XA. At the platelet surface, phospholipid (*platelet factor 3* [PF3]) membrane, XA, in the presence of factor V and calcium, cleaves *prothrombin* (factor II) to form *thrombin* (factor IIA), which is available to cleave fibrin from fibrinogen.

The extrinsic system involves the activation of circulating

factor VII by tissue factor, which is released by injured vascular endothelial cells, as well as injured cells of other tissues (e.g., lung, brain, uterus). Once activated, VIIA cleaves factor X in a manner similar to IXA (i.e., intrinsic system), forming XA. It is now known that VII can also be activated by other activated clotting factors, making the intrinsic system complex and not readily summarized. Because these activated factors are from the extrinsic system, distinctions between the systems have become somewhat obscured, but they remain independent. Patients with a deficiency of one system and not the other will have a bleeding tendency. Both systems are needed for optimal activation of factor X and the cleaving of prothrombin to form *thrombin* that ensues.

Thrombin, formed either via the intrinsic or extrinsic pathway, reacts with *fibrinogen* to form *fibrin.*

Fibrin polymerizes with itself first by hydrogen bonds and then covalently through the action of factor XIII (fibrin-stabilizing factor). A fibrin mesh forms around the platelet aggregate, yielding a well-anchored hemostatic plug.

To keep the coagulation process under control, a complex system of reactions exists to *limit* the formation of clot to the area of endothelial injury. As blood flow returns to the injured vessel, clotting factors are diluted, and therefore growth of the clot is inhibited. However, a fibrinolytic system of specific factors to limit clot size is set into motion by the same stimuli that initiate the clotting process.

Plasminogen circulates in the plasma. When activated at the surface of a developing thrombus by *tissue plasminogen activator* ([TPA], released by vascular endothelium), plasmin is formed, and the major fibrinolytic process is activated. Endothelial injury therefore is central to the initiation of both clotting and limiting activities.

Plasmin digests both *fibrinogen* and fibrin but cleaves *fibrinogen* at a site other than that used by *thrombin* to convert fibrinogen to *fibrin.* During these reactions, plasmin splits off small fragments, leaving behind degraded fibrinogen remnants that produce ineffective clot when they react with *thrombin.* As the process continues, these remnants become smaller and no longer engage *thrombin* but can become assimilated within the *fibrin* polymers, producing a weaker enmeshment. This system of limiting and weakening the thrombin-mediated formation of *fibrin* is important for the maintenance of small vessel patency following vascular injury. Inhibitors of the *plasminogen-plasmin* inhibiting system also exist. One of these, alpha$_2$-*antiplasmin,* is responsible for an extremely rapid inactivation of circulating *plasmin* and a slower inactivation of *plasmin* bound to fibrin.

In addition to fibrinolysis, other inhibitors of coagulation are present. *Antithrombin III* (AT III) is the most important of these. It complexes with *thrombin, XIIA, XIA, IXA,* and XA, resulting in inactive form.[45,50,142,249] Heparinlike substances released by vascular endothelial cells enhance this inhibition by approximately one-thousandfold. These inactivated complexes are cleared by the liver.

Activated *Protein C* modulates coagulation by inhibiting factors V and VIII. It is activated by *thrombin* in reactions that are enhanced by *thrombomodulin* (a constituent of the endothelial cell membrane) and another circulating factor, *protein S.*

Congenital deficiencies of either AT III or *Protein C* result in a thrombotic state. A *Protein C inhibitor* is also normally present—a deficiency of which leads to a bleeding tendency (see Chapter 19 for laboratory evaluation of liver function).

Coagulation Process in Liver Disease[81]

With the possible exception of *factor VIII,*[283] the liver produces the majority of both procoagulant and inhibitor factors. As such, deficiencies of these factors parallel the depressed protein synthesis of liver disease, as reflected by decreased serum albumin concentrations.[107,196,270]

Six factors are known to require carboxylation after release from the liver for proper function. Vitamin K is necessary for this process to occur (Box 73-5). When it is deficient, these vitamin K–dependent factors are no longer able to bind calcium or adhere to lipids correctly, resulting in a coagulopathy.[4] Extrahepatic or intrahepatic cholestasis, malabsorption, dietary deficiency (often associated with antibiotic use), biliary fistulas, and cholestyramine use typically result in vitamin K deficiency because of poor intake and/or absorption. Parenteral therapy (3 mg of vitamin K$_1$ in the adult) should correct this deficiency if caused by the conditions similar to those mentioned. However, because carboxylation may be impaired in patients with severe liver disease, vitamin K, even if deficient, would not be expected to be of much value to these patients.

Most of the important factors involved in coagulation are primarily or exclusively formed by the liver (Box 73-6). Therefore, most can be shown to be decreased during the course of chronic liver disease. However, the course of chronic liver disease is quite variable, and the laboratory and clinical manifestations of coagulopathy vary greatly as well. Severe cirrhosis leads to marked abnormalities that contribute to morbidity and mortality, whereas acute viral disease may cause only mild coagulation disturbances. Fulminant hepatic failure usually encompasses profound changes in the coagulation mechanisms. Patients with cholestatic diseases, however, often have increased factor levels, believed to represent stimulated protein production in these disorders.[44]

BOX 73-5
VITAMIN K-DEPENDENT FACTORS

II (Prothrombin)
VII
IX (Christmas factor)
X
Protein C
Protein S

BOX 73-6
FACTORS TOTALLY OR PARTIALLY SYNTHESIZED BY THE LIVER

Procoagulants	Inhibitors
Vitamin K-dependent factors	Antithrombin-III
XII	Protein C
XI	Protein S
IX	α_2-antitrypsin
VIII	
Fibrinogen	
XIII	

An underproduction of the procoagulant factors reflects the underlying derangements of protein synthesis seen in liver disease.[107] Severe liver disease appears to produce a deficiency in vitamin K–dependent factors (when vitamin K is not deficient) that is more severe than decreases in other factors. Factor V is not only decreased in severe liver disease but is also sensitive to degradation by plasmin and consumption by thrombin formation, as in disseminated intravascular coagulation (DIC). Intrinsic system factors XII, XI, HMWK, and prekallikrein are generally believed to be decreased in liver disease.[56,212] Factor VIII is produced at both hepatic and nonhepatic sites. Factor VIII:C is normally elevated in both acute and chronic liver disease and decreases only in the most severe forms of fulminant disease or during DIC. Regarded as an "acute phase reactant" by many experts, the reasons for the elevated levels with VIII:C are not understood. Factor XIII is only partially formed in the liver; concentrations are decreased in liver disease, but clinically significant problems are rarely noted.[171]

Fibrinogen concentrations are normal to increased in patients with acute and chronic liver disease, cholestatic disease, and primary and metastatic liver tumors. As an "acute phase reactant" analogous to factor VIII, fibrinogen is selectively produced either by the liver or at extrahepatic sites. Concentrations may fall below 100 mg/dl when liver function is extremely poor, indicating a poor prognosis.[63] Significant DIC or fibrinolysis will also lower fibrinogen levels. Abnormal fibrinogen (i.e., dysfibrinogenemia) is produced in a variety of liver diseases, including cirrhosis.[85]

Inhibitor proteins also may be decreased in patients with liver disease. AT III levels are quite decreased in cirrhosis,[239] viral and fulminant hepatitis,[33,230] fatty liver of pregnancy,[186] and hepatoma[7] but only moderately decreased in milder cases of hepatitis. In general, AT III concentrations are decreased out of proportion to the degree of liver dysfunction and are especially low in patients with a positive hepatitis B surface antigenemia or with ascites.[46,142] Thrombosis, however, is not a clinical problem, probably because of the concomitant decrease in procoagulants. AT III levels are normal or increased in cholestatic diseases.[111,118]

Protein C—the inhibitor of factors VA and VIIIA—can be normal in cholestatic disease and acute alcoholic hepatitis but is generally decreased in cirrhosis, viral and chronic active hepatitis, and in the late stages of primary biliary cirrhosis.[137,250] Alpha$_2$-antitrypsin, an inhibitor of plasmin, is also decreased in patients with cirrhosis and fulminant hepatitis.[141]

Fibrinolysis and disseminated intravascular coagulation

Arriving at the diagnosis of fibrinolysis versus DIC in the patient with liver disease is a formidable task. The overuse of various factors characteristic of fibrinolysis (increased activity of plasmin) and DIC (increased activity of procoagulants *and* inhibitors) must be seen in the light of the underproduction of factors in most liver diseases.

It has been known for many decades that the clotted blood from a cirrhotic patient readily liquifies.[105] It is now known that TPA levels are elevated in cirrhotic patients, probably from inadequate clearance by the diseased liver.[113] This leads to decreased plasminogen levels because of enhanced conversion of plasminogen to plasmin and exaggerated fibrin degradation. In addition, decreased production of inhibitors of fibrinolysis (e.g., alpha$_2$-antitrypsin) contributes to this fibrinolytic condition. The increased concentrations of plasmin lead to a consumption of fibrin and to a lesser extent fibrinogen and attendant increases in serum levels of fibrin degradation products.

Disseminated intravascular coagulation is a state in which the coagulation system becomes "turned on" by poorly understood stimuli, leading to decreased factor concentrations but increased thrombin levels. The increased thrombin activity requires a secondary increase in the fibrinolytic system to control the coagulation. Factors and platelets are consumed in this process. When formation and removal are nearly equal, a "balanced" consumption exists that can be missed by standard laboratory tests. If the process initiating the DIC leads to a more aggressive activation of the coagulation system, true "consumption" of factors and platelets ensues, with prolongation of laboratory measurements and thrombocytopenia. Factor VIII:C, which should be increased in liver disease but decreased in severe DIC, may be the only clue to the proper diagnosis.

Therefore, excessive fibrinolysis can be a primary event, as often seen in liver disease, or a secondary response to increased factor activation and thrombin generation, as seen in DIC. Many studies have failed to clarify the role of DIC in the coagulation abnormalities of patients with severe liver disease, and an element of both may exist simultaneously in many patients. Newer tests may better discriminate between the conflicting and complementary elements of liver disease and DIC.[43] During liver transplantation, primary fibrinolysis is recognized as a significant problem.[31]

Invasive Procedures and Surgery in Patients with Coagulopathy

Patients with liver disease come to the operating room and procedure suites for a variety of diagnostic and therapeutic procedures. Although excessive bleeding can occur spontaneously in these patients, it is more likely to accompany some hemostatis stress, such as variceal tears and invasive and surgical procedures. Most experts would recommend that **the prothrombin time (PT) should be corrected to within 2 seconds of control values by the infusion of fresh frozen plasma (FFP), which contains normal procoagulant and inhibitor coagulation proteins.** The desired effect may not result, however, with 20 ml/kg or less of FFP.[129,254] The effect also may be limited by intravascular volume overload considerations, as in patients with concomitant renal failure. Plasmapheresis before FFP administration may lessen this problem. **The therapeutic effects of FFP administration are limited by the half-lives of its constituent factors, especially factor VII (half-life of 4 to 8 hours). Within 24 hours after correction, the PT will have returned to the pretreatment baseline values.**

Platelets should be administered to achieve counts greater than 100,000/ml. Because one transfused platelet unit raises the count by only about 10,000/ml, and because platelets will continue to be used and diluted by surgical injury and blood replacement, multiple units may be required intraoperatively and in the early postoperative period. Many experts administer the platelets after the patient arrives in the operating room to achieve maximal benefit.

Vitamin K therapy is often administered before surgery in patients with liver disease and a demonstrated coagulopathy. Many experts believe that a degree of malabsorption, coincident with the severe hepatocellular disease, may be responsible for a part of the coagulation abnormality. Positive results with vitamin K should be seen within 24 hours, if they are to occur.

During extended procedures, the possibility of exaggerated fibrinolysis may arise. If a thromboelastograph is available, this test may help detect the process. Epsilon-aminocaproic therapy may be effective for patients with this abnormality.[86]

THE NERVOUS SYSTEM IN LIVER DISEASE

The neurologic aspects of severe liver disease have been recognized at least since the time of Hippocrates, who wrote, "Those . . . mad . . . from bile are vociferous, malignant and will not be quiet."[127] Many authors and physicians described variations of the symptoms and their musings as to etiologies over the ensuing centuries.[234] Although much more is known today, disagreement over both etiology and treatment still exists.

It is agreed that uncomplicated hepatic encephalopathy is a reversible functional change in the patient's level of consciousness that can vary from lethargy and confusion (hepatic encephalopathy) to stupor and coma (hepatic coma). Encephalopathy occurs often in patients with severe liver disease, but one must remember that other diseases can mimic hepatic encephalopathy. Some of these conditions are not reversible without specific medical or surgical therapy (Box 73-7). Because of the relatively acute nature of FHF, physical findings may be more or less limited to the nervous system. However, for the cirrhotic patient, physical findings include the stigmata of chronic liver disease. Encephalopathic symptoms range from personality changes, to alterations in speech characteristics, to mental confusion, and ultimately to coma. Depending on the patient's place in this continuum, tremor, rigidity, hyperactive reflexes, extensor plantar reflexes, decerebrate posturing, or flaccidity may be seen (Table 73-4). These symptoms should regress with successful therapy.[161,184] Patients who die while exhibiting hepatic encephalopathy usually demonstrate minor pathologic changes (Alzheimer's type II astrocyte proliferation[191]). Only a few patients develop hepatocerebral degeneration, which involves cellular destruction in the gray matter and basal ganglia and leads to athetosis, dementia, and dystonia.[80]

A characteristic physical finding is asterixis, or liver "flap." When the patient is asked to extend the upper extremities with the wrists dorsiflexed, the hand will fall forward after a short time (up to 30 seconds), followed by a quick return to the dorsiflexed position. This occurs because of brief periods of electrical silence in the muscles tested.[153]

Some patients with severe liver disease develop spinal cord symptoms because of a transverse myelopathy. This is demonstrated by gait disturbances and eventually loss of bladder control but does not include sensory changes (which should be present if symptoms are caused by an alcoholic neuropathy). The primary pathologic finding is demyelination of the corticospinal tracts, but axonal degeneration may be seen in the cerebellar tracts and dorsal columns as well.[91] Central pontine myelinolysis (CPM) has been associated both with rapid correction and overcorrection of hyponatremia.[11]

Laboratory findings during hepatic encephalopathy include abnormalities of synthetic function seen in patients with severe liver disease. Hyponatremia may contribute to or mimic encephalopathic symptoms.

Respiratory alkalosis may be present in the early stages, probably as some poorly understood response to increased nitrogenous compounds[134] or electrolyte disturbances.[277] This is a complex process involving alterations of both cerebrospinal fluid (CSF) and arterial pH, and artificial correc-

BOX 73-7
CONDITIONS THAT MIMIC HEPATIC ENCEPHALOPATHY

Subdural hematoma
Intracranial hemorrhage
Hypoglycemia
Hyponatremia
Hypernatremia
Meningitis, including tuberculosis

Table 73-4 Classification system for hepatic encephalopathy

Level of encephalopathy	Level of consciousness	Intellectual function	Neurologic findings
0	Normal	Normal	None
1	Trivial lack of awareness	Short attention span	Slight tremor
	Personality change	Easy forgetfulness	Poor coordination
	Day-night reversal		Asterixis
2	Lethargic	Loss of orientation	Asterixis
	Inappropriate behavior		Abnormal reflexes
3	Asleep but arousable	Loss of ability to calculate	Asterixis
	Confused when awake	Loss of meaningful communication	Abnormal reflexes
4	Unarousable	Absent	Babinski response
			Decerebrate
			Pupillary responses preserved

Modified from Zakim D, Boyer TB, editors: *Hepatology: A textbook of liver disease,* ed 2, Philadelphia, 1990, WB Saunders.

tion has been associated with a more rapid decline in neurologic status.[206] Late in the course of encephalopathy, respiratory acidosis may develop.[208] Increased ammonia levels, although often noted, are of disputed value as an aid to clinical management. Infusion of ammonia in animals can cause severe cerebral symptoms. Such an infusion in patients with liver disease or portosystemic shunts leads to symptoms similar to imminent hepatic coma.[175] In addition, increased ammonia is a feature of several diseases with neurologic sequelae, including Reye's syndrome and urea cycle enzyme deficiencies. Unfortunately, arterial ammonia concentrations can be normal in the encephalopathic patient,[82] and fasting venous levels have not been shown to correlate well with the stage of encephalopathy.[255]

The physical and biochemical changes of hepatic encephalopathy have led to several theories concerning the pathophysiology of this complex condition (Box 73-8). One theory suggests that encephalopathy represents the synergistic effects of several substances normally metabolized by the liver.[294] Another, the Octopamine/False Neurotransmitter Theory, has not been documented.[59,130] Currently, the GABA-ergic Neurotransmitter Theory holds some promise. According to this hypothesis, the GABA receptor/chloride channel is reversibly altered during hepatic encephalopathy, which permits inhibitory (i.e., sedation, coma) processes to dominate. Interestingly, some GABA receptors are physically associated with benzodiazepine receptors, and the density of benzodiazepine receptors is increased in patients with hepatic encephalopathy. This may explain the sensitivity of patients with hepatic disease to sedative/hypnotic medications. Experimentally, benzodiazepine antagonists have been shown to quickly antagonize hepatic coma.[79,226,242] This is an interesting area of research not only for the treatment of hepatic coma, but also for an understanding of brain neurochemistry. Whether caused by an accumulation of inhibitory neurotransmitter substances to altered nerotransmission, or to the failure to synthesize some substance(s) necessary for cerebral function (other than glucose), hepatic encephalopathy is an enigmatic process.

BOX 73-8
THEORIES OF HEPATIC ENCEPHALOPATHY

Synergistic theory
False neurotransmitter theory
GABA-ergic theory

FULMINANT HEPATIC FAILURE

The encephalopathy of FHF is considerably more ominous than that of chronic liver disease and is accompanied by an extraordinary variety of clinical and metabolic changes. Because of the acute nature of FHF, the physical findings of more chronic liver disease, except for jaundice, are often absent, at least initially. Early in the course of FHF, encephalopathy, behavioral changes, and slowed mentation result from bilateral forebrain dysfunction. Behavioral changes can be manifest by simple personality changes, but psychotic-like behavior may also occur. Brain stem impairment can occur later, with loss of consciousness. Delirium may develop during both the evolution and resolution phases of the encephalopathic process. Seizures may also arise but are not characteristic.

Unfortunately, cerebral edema occurs and is a striking finding at autopsy of patients with FHF.[92,272] **Signs of increased intracranial pressure (ICP) may be present in as many as 80% of patients with FHF.[64,102] Increased ICP is considered a specific neurologic complication of acute liver failure that is quite distinct from the hepatic encephalopathy seen in chronic liver disease and in preterminal hypoxic events.[20]** Although the precise cause has remained elusive, postulated mechanisms for cerebral edema include disruption of the blood–brain barrier (BBB), altered osmoregulation, and interstitial expansion of the extracellular space. Any or all of these may be contributing to the cerebral edema in patients with FHF. Cerebral edema is not a requirement for the diagnosis of FHF or hepatic encephalopathy, but it is a major factor in the death of patients with FHF. Over the past 20 years, 65% to 94% of patients with FHF in stage IV coma have died.[16,193,210] Although survival with medical therapy alone has improved during this period, mortality is still extremely high.

Liver transplantation, including auxiliary liver transplantation (in which a portion of the native liver is left in place to recover[48]) has emerged as definitive treatment for patients who have FHF with encephalopathy. The intensive therapy required while awaiting a donor liver has led many centers to monitor ICP once stage III encephalopathy has developed.[47,157] In addition to changes in ICP during routine intensive care, predictable rises occur with vascular clamping and unclamping during the transplantation procedure itself. Such monitoring potentially allows for rational treatment of increased ICP when it becomes significant, whether with osmotic agents, diuretics, or pharmacologic coma.

Anesthetic Considerations in Patients with Hepatic Encephalopathy

Unfortunately, some patients who are encephalopathic or who have a history of recent or recurrent encephalopathy require various types of surgical intervention. After a thorough neurologic evaluation, one hopes sufficient time exists to at least partially correct electrolyte abnormalities, realizing that overzealous treatment of hyponatremia and hypernatremia are both associated with the potential for permanent neurologic damage (i.e., CPM). Hypoglycemia, if present, should be corrected. Conditions capable of inciting or exacerbating encephalopathy should be sought and therapy initiated, if not completed (Box 73-9). Patients with hepatic coma, especially those with FHF, may have increased ICP. In these patients, one should consider monitoring ICP expectantly, especially during operation.[157] At the very least, anesthetic management should apply those considerations useful in patients with abnormal intracranial compliance. Ideally, patients with encephalopathy or hepatic coma should have these conditions normalized. This may not be possible, or the surgical procedure may be intended to ultimately reverse the problem (e.g., liver transplantation).

BOX 73-9
INCITING AND CONTRIBUTING FACTORS IN HEPATIC ENCEPHALOPATHY

Decreased or increased sodium
Decreased phosphate
Hypoglycemia
Infection
Constipation
Gastrointestinal bleeding
Hypovolemia

PULMONARY FUNCTION IN LIVER DISEASE: HEPATOPULMONARY SYNDROME

A limiting factor for both the well-being of patients with severe liver disease and their evaluation before surgical procedures is altered dynamics of oxygenation. Evidence of this defect is present before significant hypoxemia actually develops,[137] and changes can be seen in patients with both acute and chronic liver disease.[280] **As many as 12% to 28% of patients with cirrhosis demonstrate moderate hypoxemia, with an arterial O_2 tension ($Pa{O_2}$) < 70 mm Hg. A smaller percentage have severe hypoxemia with a $Pa{O_2}$ < 50 mm Hg. This hepatopulmonary syndrome**[3,147,148,244] has multiple etiologies (Box 73-10). Symptoms and signs are often dyspnea, dusky lips and fingertips, and clubbing of the digits and may include a worsening of dyspnea when the patient assumes the seated or standing position (platypnea), which results from worsened oxygenation in the upright position (orthodeoxia). Anesthesiologists are becoming increasingly involved with more aggressive surgical procedures in this group of patients.

Patients with chronic liver disease are at risk for the same conditions that injure lung tissue in persons without liver disease. Many patients have an element of chronic lung disease, especially bronchitis and the emphysematous changes that occur with long-term smoking. The recurrent minor and major pulmonary infections increase the considerable potential for hypoxemia.

Liver disease itself, however, induces several changes that alter normal gas exchange. Ascites may severely restrict

BOX 73-10
CAUSES OF HYPOXEMIA IN SEVERE LIVER DISEASE

Chronic lung disease

Acute exacerbations
Changes seen with liver disease
Ventilation-perfusion mismatching
  Premature airway closure
  Pulmonary emboli
  Dilated pulmonary vessels
  Diffusion-perfusion deficit
Impaired hypoxic pulmonary vasoconstriction
Diaphragm dysfunction with ascites
Pleural effusion
Pulmonary edema
Pulmonary complications of specific liver diseases
  (e.g., primary billiary cirrhosis, $alpha_1$-antitrypsin deficiency)
True arteriovenous shunting

diaphragmatic excursion. Pleural effusions are seen in 5% to 10% of these patients and are probably caused by small (< 5 mm) diaphragmatic defects through which ascitic fluid can pass, but they may occur with or without clinical evidence of ascites. High diaphragms and pleural effusions may lead to atelectasis and ventilation/perfusion mismatching.

True arteriovenous communications may also be present but generally are not believed to represent a major contributor to hypoxemia in most patients with liver disease. Abnormalities resembling cutaneous spider nevi have been reported on the pleural surface, as well as precapillary AV communications within the lung parenchyma.[21,224] These "true shunts" result in decreased Pa_{O_2} and as such do not respond to increased inspired O_2. Patients with cutaneous spider nevi may be a subgroup at increased risk for hypoxemia.[218]

Two clinical techniques suggest a different mechanism for the hypoxemia of liver disease. Both contrast-enhanced two-dimensional echocardiography (CE2DE)[126,149,248] and technetium-99-labeled macroaggregated albumin (^{99}Tc-MAA) scans[98] shed some light on this problem. Both involve injection of substances with diameters larger than those of the normal pulmonary capillary bed. When the substance shows up in the left side of the heart within several beats of injection (CE2DE) or over the brain or kidneys (^{99}Tc-MAA), either intrapulmonary or intracardiac shunts exist or the vessels are abnormally dilated. Because oxygenation in patients with severe liver disease may improve with the administration of 100% O_2, any "shunting" must not be from shunts in the true sense of the word. Because precapillary dilatations of pulmonary vessels have long been described in severe liver disease,[21] all this information suggests that dilated pulmonary vessels contribute to a diffusion/perfusion defect. Those dilatations near gas exchange units would be available to improve oxygenation when increased inspired O_2 is provided.

Others have used the multiple inert gases elimination technique (MIGET). They suggest that a state of diminished or blunted hypoxic pulmonary vasoconstriction exists that is responsible for the dilated vascular bed, low pulmonary vascular tone, and subsequent ventilation-perfusion mismatching and hypoxemia.[218,269] Presumably, either a dilating substance is not metabolized by the diseased liver, or some vasoconstrictor substance is inhibited or absent. Several such dilator substances have been proposed, including vasoactive intestinal peptide, glucagon, and atrial natriuretic factor, as well as deficient vasoconstrictors.[148]

Several liver disorders are associated with specific lung diseases. These include the association of primary biliary cirrhosis with lymphocytic interstitial pneumonitis and the ultimate development of severe emphysematous changes in patients with alpha$_1$-antitrypsin deficiency.[147]

Therapy for this vexing clinical problem is not simple. Besides treating intercurrent infections and bronchospasm, if present, or the administration of O_2 to those who seem to respond, other therapy has been limited. Almitrine bismesylate has been reported to improve ventilation/perfusion inequalities[146] but is not available in the United States. A somatostatin analog, octreotide (Sandostatin), has been associated with rapid improvement in oxygenation, possibly through antagonism of neuropeptides that induce pulmonary vasodilation.[148] Emerging evidence suggests that many of the changes resulting in hypoxemia are functional, because the number of patients with hypoxemia who successfully undergo liver transplantation with subsequent resolution of their hypoxemia is increasing.[74,75,260] Therefore, hypoxemia is currently listed as only a relative contraindication to liver transplantation. NO may have a therapeutic role in those patients with pulmonary hypertension.

CHOLESTATIC DISEASE

Severe parenchymal disease can include prominent elements of cholestasis, that is, abnormal excretion of bilirubin, cholesterol, and bile acids. However, certain diseases can present initially as a progressive disturbance of biliary drainage, with symptoms primarily being pruritus, jaundice, and malabsorption of fat-soluble vitamins.

Primary biliary cirrhosis (PBC) is a chronic progressive cholestatic disease caused by an inflammatory destruction of intrahepatic bile ducts and by periportal hepatitis with piecemeal necrosis of hepatocytes, which eventually results in cirrhosis and portal hypertension. Although middle-aged women are affected 9 to 10 times more often than men, other age groups are affected.[50] Symptoms are often pruritus, jaundice, and fatigue,[246] and initial laboratory evaluation reveals abnormal function of a cholestatic rather than a hepatocellular nature. Bile acids are elevated in all patients and are presumably toxic to the liver and other organs because they can damage cell membranes. Although associated with several autoimmune diseases (e.g., scleroderma, Sjögren's syndrome, thyroiditis, CREST syndrome [calcinosis cutis, Raynaud's phenomenon, esophageal dysfunction, sclerodactyly, telangiectasia]), positive tests of various autoantibodies—including the antimitochondrial M_2—do not seem to be related to pathogenetic mechanisms responsible for PBC.[117,169] Eventually, PBC results in progressive destruction of portal and periportal tissue. Sufficient scarring and fibrosis result in cirrhosis. Treatment for patients with PBC may include symptomatic therapy, as well as immunosuppression based on the histologic stage of disease.[169] The clinical course is complicated by steatorrhea and the malabsorption of lipid-soluble vitamins (e.g., A, D, K). As cirrhosis evolves, its manifestations, including portal hypertension and end-stage liver disease, will develop in most patients.

Primary sclerosing cholangitis is another major cholestatic disease distinguished by a progressive inflammatory sclerosis and obliteration of the extrahepatic bile ducts, with or without involvement of the intrahepatic ducts. Although it may be an isolated process, inflammatory bowel disease occurs in 50% to 75% of patients, with most having ulcerative colitis. In addition, an association exists with other diseases, including thyroiditis,[13] mediastinal fibrosis,[122] bronchiectasis,[199] and Sjögren's syndrome.[181] Papillary stenosis and sclerosing cholangitis are also complications of AIDS (acquired immunodeficiency syndrome), possibly in association with cytomegalovirus and *Cryptosporidia* infection.[108] Initial signs and symptoms of primary sclerosing cholangitis are chronic or intermittent biliary obstruction with pruritus and jaundice, but cirrhosis, with portal hypertension and liver failure, eventually develops. Until the advent of liver transplantation, therapy was limited to the control of symptoms, treatment of infections, and replacement of nutrients lost with cholestasis.

INBORN ERRORS OF METABOLISM

Several infrequently occurring diseases have clinical manifestations secondary to inborn errors of hepatic metabolism; Box 73-11 provides a partial list. Patients with such metabolic diseases may have grossly normal liver histology. Some endogenous chemical is not produced, is produced in excess, or is abnormal, or an ingested substance is metabolized in an aberrant fashion. Of special importance to anesthesiologists is *acute intermittent porphyria,* the most serious form of the "hepatic" porphyrias. As a result of an inborn error of porphyrin metabolism, excessive amounts of porphobilinogen accumulate, resulting in abdominal pain and variable neurologic deficits, including demyelination; autonomic, cranial nerve, and cerebellar dysfunction; and bulbar paralysis. Barbiturates, benzodiazepines, phenytoin, ketamine, and etomidate are among the drugs reported to trigger this condition.

OPERATIONS ON THE LIVER

Several surgical procedures are performed only on patients with liver disease. These patients are often extremely ill, and the procedures are demanding. The following sections discuss hepatic resection, procedures for portal hypertension and ascites, and orthotopic liver transplantation.

Hepatic Resection

In the Western world, most patients who undergo some degree of hepatic resection have essentially normal liver function.[84,259] Most have a primary liver tumor or a metastasis from a GI cancer (Box 73-12). Some have more than one lesion that is deemed resectable, either from the preoperative evaluation or after discovery at laparotomy. Another large group of patients who may require some degree of hepatic surgery are those with traumatic abdominal injury; often the liver insult is part of multisystem trauma. Patients with extensive malignant disease who are not candidates for resection often have a chemotherapy infusion pump inserted before the conclusion of the operation.

Preoperative assessment involves attempts to obtain a tis-

BOX 73-11
INBORN ERRORS AFFECTING THE LIVER

- Carbohydrate metabolism
  - Galactosemia
  - Glycogen storage diseases
  - Fructose intolerance
- Protein metabolism
  - Tyrosinemia
- Copper metabolism
  - Wilson's disease
- Lipid metabolism
  - Gaucher's disease
  - Niemann-Pick disease
- Bile acid metabolism
  - Byler's disease
  - Zellweger's syndrome
- Porphyrin metabolism

BOX 73-12
POTENTIALLY RESECTABLE HEPATIC LESIONS

Benign

- Hemangioma
- Focal nodular hyperplasia
- Liver cell adenoma

Malignant

- Metastatic
  - From possibly widespread metastasis
    - Lung
    - Breast
    - Esophagus
    - Stomach
    - Pancreas
    - Upper gastrointestinal tract
    - Melanoma
  - From possibly "hepatic only" metastasis
    - Colon
    - Rectum
    - Pancreatic islet cell
    - Carcinoid
    - Gastrointestinal sarcoma
- Primary hepatic
  - Hepatocellular
  - Cholangiocarcinoma
  - Hepatoblastoma
  - Angiosarcoma
  - Lymphoma
- Local extension into liver
  - Gallbladder and extrahepatic bile ducts
  - Colon
  - Stomach
  - Duodenum
  - Adrenal gland

sue diagnosis and to look for metastases or a primary tumor, as appropriate. Some lesions, such as suspected hemangiomas, hydatid cysts, and highly vascularized tumors, are dangerous to percutaneous biopsy. Ultrasound should distinguish cystic from solid lesions. The results of computed tomography (CT) and magnetic resonance imaging (MRI) scans can better determine the size and number of masses, as well as the potential for involvement of major vascular structures, such as the IVC, portal venous system, and major arteries. Often, however, the results of these tests are not completely definitive, and final decisions about the extent of disease and appropriate procedures are not possible until a thorough evaluation has been conducted at laparotomy. The necessity for preoperative arteriography is debated, but knowledge of an aberrant vascular supply is usually helpful, especially if drug infusion devices are placed.

The initial incision for hepatic resection procedures is usually right subcostal. Following this, a major portion of the operation involves extensive evaluation of the nonhepatic abdominal contents for evidence of additional lesions, as well as a thorough examination of the liver for disease not recognized preoperatively. This can entail the use of intraoperative ultrasound. For large or inaccessible right-sided lesions, the incision may need to be extended into the right chest. Occasionally, the sternum may be partially divided for similar considerations. During the process of assessing the liver, many ligamentous attachments are severed. After a decision to proceed with a resection, additional mobilization may still be required. At some point, the hilar vessels are usually completely dissected free for eventual hemorrhage control or ligation if necessary.

The goal of curative resections is to completely remove the tumor. This generally means that a 1- to 2-cm margin is desired. Wedge resections are usually possible for small lesions located peripherally along the free edges of the liver. Sometimes concern for viability of remaining tissue demands a more formalized lobectomy than a wedge resection. No avascular planes exist for dissection in liver resection. Although the portal triad vessels branch together and become the basis for dividing the liver into segments and lobes, the hepatic veins cross these planes at right angles. As dissection proceeds with blunt instruments or with the ultrasonic dissector (e.g., Cavitron®), numerous vessels are encountered. If these vessels tear or bleed before ligation with suture or clips, they may retract into the liver parenchyma and continue to bleed. Manual pressure on the liver tissue usually controls this bleeding.

Several clues should alert the anesthesiologist to more extensive operation and the potential for more extensive bleeding. A lobectomy is usually associated with more bleeding than a wedge resection, although large wedge resections violate the planes just referred to and can have considerable blood loss. Although eight segments in the liver are described[28] (see Fig. 73-1), major liver resection is usually divided into wedge, lobe, right or left extended lobectomy, and left lateral segmentectomy (Figs. 73-13 and 73-14). The extended right lobectomy (called a trisegmentectomy if dissection proceeds as far as the sulcus of the falciform ligament)[256] is a major resection with potential for significant bleeding. A left trisegmentectomy, which includes resection of the left hepatic lobe and an anterior segment of the right lobe near the right hepatic vein, has been termed an "anatomic fantasy"[259] and generally leads to significant intraoperative blood loss. Tumor near major vessels always presents the potential for sudden catastrophic blood loss. Some surgeons routinely (and others in emergencies)

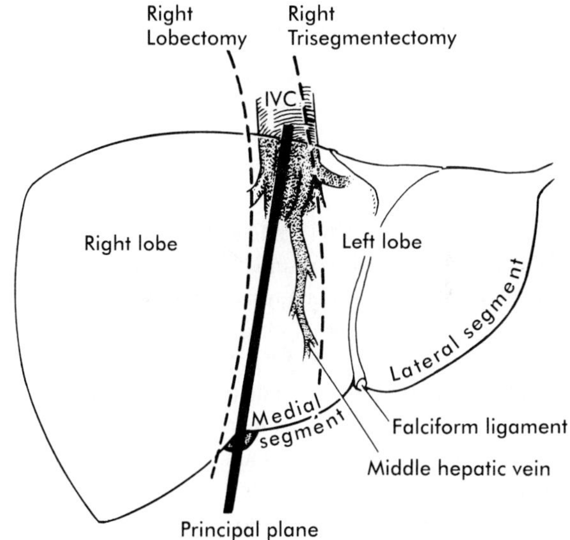

Fig. 73-13. Definition of formal right hepatic resections. (From McDermott WV, editor: *Surgery of the liver,* Boston, 1989, Blackwell Scientific.)

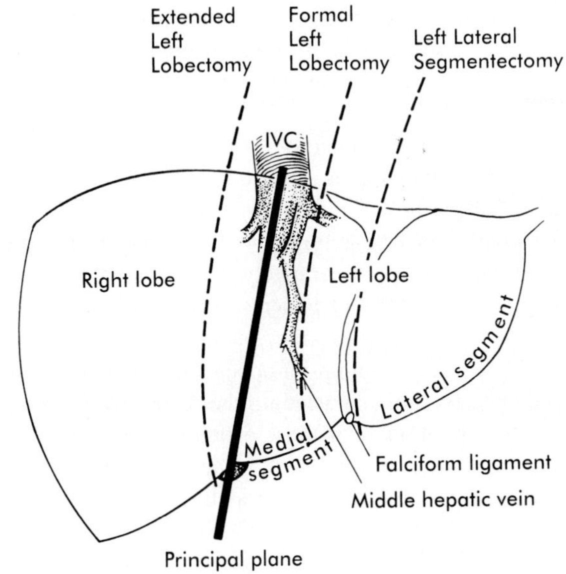

Fig. 73-14. Definition of formal left hepatic resections. Note that the plan of dissection for the extended left is anterior to the right hepatic vein. (From McDermott WV, editor: *Surgery of the liver,* Boston, 1989, Blackwell Scientific.)

clamp the inflow vessels in the hilar area (Pringle maneuver) to control bleeding. Occasionally, the hepatic veins or the suprahepatic IVC is clamped to gain control of hemorrhaging. Either of these tactics leads to warm ischemia. Clamping of the suprahepatic IVC has serious hemodynamic effects in patients without major shunting from portal hypertension. If tumor extends into the diaphragmatic tissue, it may be removed with portions of the diaphragm. This defect is then closed primarily or with prosthetic material.

Anesthetic considerations

In planning the anesthetic management for patients undergoing hepatic resections, one must anticipate the planned procedure. The anesthesiologist should query the surgeon about the likelihood of any resection at all. When evidence suggests that a resection may not be possible, it may be reasonable to postpone invasive monitoring until a definite decision has been made. Time must then be allocated intraoperatively to place an arterial cannula, central venous access, and large-bore transfusion cannulae. Because significant bleeding can occasionally occur if a major vessel is torn during the evaluation phase, many anesthesiologists prefer to establish vascular access before or shortly after the induction of anesthesia. Even if the patient's preoperative liver function is entirely normal, one should anticipate that liver function will be impaired postoperatively, either from loss of hepatocellular mass or from the direct trauma of surgical manipulation.

Intraoperatively, medication doses should be titrated to desired effect, both for narcotics and muscle relaxants. Extremes of CO_2 tension (Pco_2) should be avoided. Hypocapnia appears to lower hepatic arterial blood flow during abdominal surgery, whereas hypercapnia is associated with increased portal and total hepatic blood flow and appears to depress both hepatic function and hepatic oxygen uptake.[89,94] **Isoflurane is often recommended for liver operations because it is associated with better maintenance of liver blood flow.**[95,104]

Patients usually undergo traction on their upper abdomens and diaphragms for extended periods. Most patients, except those undergoing very limited procedures (e.g., small wedge resection) should be managed in an intensive care unit postoperatively. Even with this management, more than 90% of patients develop some pulmonary complication (e.g., pleural effusion, atelectasis, pneumonia).[252] For patients with prior upper-abdominal operation or portal hypertension, the bleeding should be anticipated to be more than "routine." For those patients with some element of cardiac disease or for elderly patients, in whom the perioperative stress of this surgery may uncover coronary artery disease (CAD), additional monitoring (e.g., PA catheter) may be warranted. Also, if the operation is extensive, the blood sugar should be monitored to detect the infrequent patient who will develop intraoperative hypoglycemia. If the right chest is entered, the surgeon may ask for a brief increase in inflation pressures during evacuation of air from the pleural space before closing the chest wound. Such maneuvers can greatly decrease venous return and should be done cautiously.[25,241] As in other abdominal procedures, the patient must be kept warm; using adequate fluid and blood warmers and warming blankets and raising the temperature in the operating room are all beneficial.

Procedures for Portal Hypertension and Ascites

Most chronic diseases affecting the liver eventually result in sufficient destruction of tissue and fibrotic changes that obstruction to venous flow through the liver develops. Portal hypertension results, with an array of collateral channels around the liver, often with repeated episodes of esophageal variceal bleeding and production of ascites. Variceal hemorrhage is often life threatening. In addition to transfusion and optimal replacement of coagulation factors and platelets, several types of surgical therapy have evolved (Box 73-13). Patients undergoing these procedures are often extremely ill, and morbidity and mortality can be great; for any given patient, controversy may arise as to the correct procedure or whether any procedure is indicated.

The nonshunting procedures include transesophageal sclerotherapy, percutaneous embolization of variceal vessels, some form of surgical ligation of varices, and portal-azygos disconnection procedures.

Transesophageal sclerotherapy is currently considered the treatment of choice for acutely bleeding varices and can be performed using either a flexible fiberoptic scope or a rigid esophagoscope. Because the procedure often requires only mild sedation (in adults), the fiberoptic approach is

BOX 73-13
PROCEDURES FOR PORTAL HYPERTENSION AND ASCITES

Nonshunting procedures

- Esophageal sclerotherapy
- Percutaneous varicieal embolization
- Surgical variceal ligation
- Portal-azygos disconnection

Vascular shunting procedures

- Nonselective
  - Portocaval
    - End-to-side
    - Side-to-side
  - Mesocaval
  - Proximal splenorenal
- Selective
  - Distal splenorenal
- Mesonatrial

Intrahepatic shunts (TIPS)

Peritoneovenous shunts

more often used and may last less than 1 hour. The agents used for sclerotherapy are usually sodium morrhuate, ethanolamine, or polidocanol. These chemicals are "inflammatory, vasoconstrictive, thrombogenic, protein-precipitating lipid liquids that induce tissue necrosis."[53] Sclerotherapy involves injection of one of these agents either directly into the varix or into the perivariceal area. The surgeon's visibility is often impaired by active bleeding, despite the local or systemic vasopressin often administered to patients who are actively bleeding. If injected systemically, these compounds can produce: (1) decreased mean arterial pressure; (2) decreased cardiac output; (3) decreased hepatic blood flow (probably secondary to 1 and 2);[42] and (4) acute respiratory failure.[180]

Acute and chronic complications of sclerotherapy can be severe. They include bleeding, esophageal rupture, pneumothorax, chest pain, mediastinitis, esophageal stricture, small pleural effusions, and adult respiratory distress syndrome (ARDS). The overall mortality associated with injection sclerotherapy is approximately 10%, relatively modest considering the seriousness of the underlying disease.[83] The mortality rate for esophageal rupture, which occurs in approximately 9% of patients, is greater.[262] Some centers regard sclerotherapy as inferior to emergency portacaval shunting, although the latter procedure is considerably more invasive.[197] In addition, patients who have had a previous sclerotherapy should be considered as having an abnormal gastroesophageal junction.[101] Occasionally, embolization of varices, collaterals, and feeding veins is undertaken via transhepatic catheterization of the portal vein and its branches as a temporary measure to control hemorrhaging.

Open transesophageal variceal ligation and various esophagogastric transection/reanastomosis procedures for the same purpose are considerably more invasive, nonshunting procedures for decompression of the portal system. Only an open approach to the stomach, however, addresses gastric varices. Operative mortality for the transesophageal variceal ligation procedure is considerable, and some form of elective shunt is usually performed at a later date. Various esophagogastric devascularization procedures have been described (under general heading of "Sugiura procedure"),[261] which can include splenectomy, extensive ligation of veins around the distal esophagus and upper stomach, and ligation of the hepatic, left gastric, and splenic arteries. These procedures are difficult to evaluate and are performed primarily in Japan. Long-term patient survival has been low. In the United States, variceal ligation has been associated with considerable mortality and a high recurrence of variceal bleeding.

Various portosystemic shunts have been performed in an effort to decompress the splanchnic-portal venous system. Considerations that may result in choosing one shunt over another include emergency versus elective surgery, the patient's size and age, and individual anatomic necessities. Liver blood flow is also affected by the nature of the shunt.

Nonselective or "total" shunts, such as the end-to-side portocaval shunt (Fig. 73-15), essentially deprive the liver of splanchnic flow and may produce encephalopathy even in normal patients. In patients with longstanding portal hypertension, side-to-side portocaval, proximal splenorenal (with splenectomy), mesocaval, and portorenal shunts have the potential to be functionally total (i.e., because of reversed flow). Whether or not they are "total" depends on the relative inflow pressures, intrahepatic and intravascular resistances, shunts between the hepatic arterial system and the portal system (e.g., at the sinusoidal level), and any collaterals present.

A selective shunt (Fig. 73-16), in contrast, does not deprive the liver of splanchnic/portal flow because only the coronary (gastric) and the splenic veins are diverted. However, even these shunts may become nonselective with time.[167] Because intraoperatively measured preshunt and postshunt portal pressures may not reliably characterize measured flows,[258] operative assessment of flow is the better standard. In general, the hemodynamic effects of opening a portosystemic shunt are moderate at best and include a mild, very temporary increase in CVP and cardiac output and imperceptible changes in systemic pressure. The anesthesiologist can assist the surgical team in measuring the necessary pressures during shunt operations; a recording system that permits well-calibrated paper recording is preferred.

Patients with the Budd-Chiari syndrome have partial or total thrombosis of the hepatic veins that may extend into the upper IVC. They may be seen subacutely (several weeks to several months) or less often after a more chronic course.[179] The obstruction to venous flow can lead to necrosis of hepatocytes secondary to the marked increase in sinusoidal pressure and to decreased hepatic arterial and portal blood flow. A variety of shunts have been performed for patients with this condition, but the most successful appear to be side-to-side portocaval shunts and both mesocaval "H" grafts and "C" shunts. The success of any shunt depends on a patent IVC permitting flow to reach the right atrium, as well as the portal-to-systemic pressure gradient driving that flow. If the liver is so congested that the caudate lobe enlarges and compresses the IVC, or if the thrombotic process extends into the IVC and blocks venous return, these procedures do not help because collaterals around the obstructed IVC are inadequate to decompress the system. Patients with obstruction of the IVC have been treated with a mesoatrial shunt. A long synthetic graft is extended from the superior mesenteric vein into the chest for anastomosis with the right atrium. Appropriate pressure gradients and myocardial contraction facilitate flow. Results of this procedure appear promising.[228]

Of interest to the anesthesiologist are the hemodynamic changes associated with the acute opening of the mesoatrial shunt. **Patients with Budd-Chiari syndrome usually have a normal cardiac index and SVR before operation and do not manifest the hyperdynamic, low-resistance state of chronic cirrhosis. On opening the mesoatrial shunt, the cardiac index increases by approximately 50%, and**

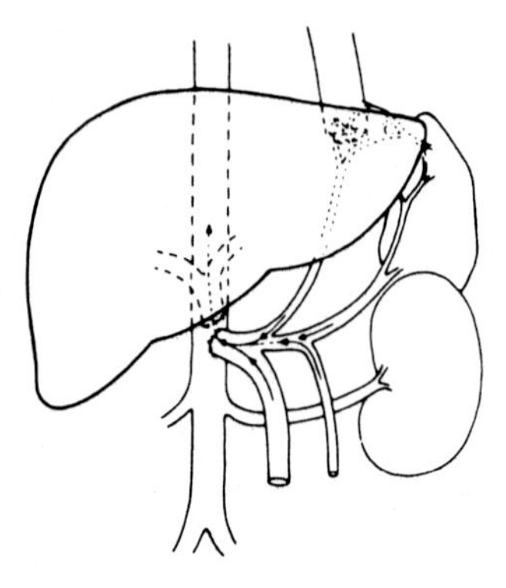

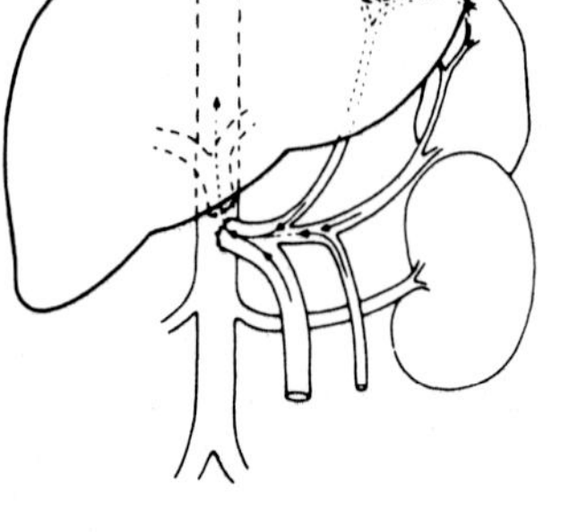

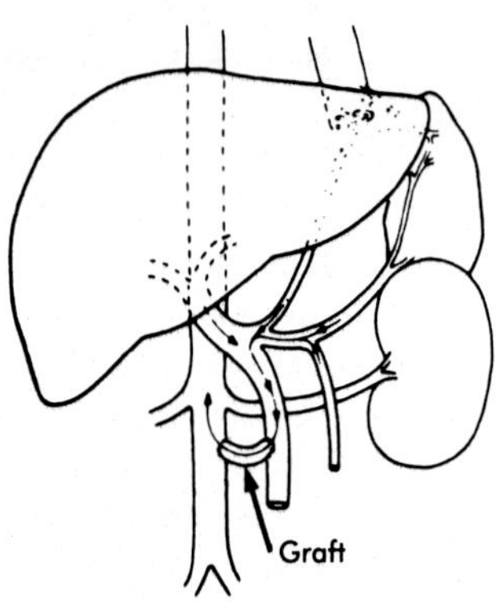

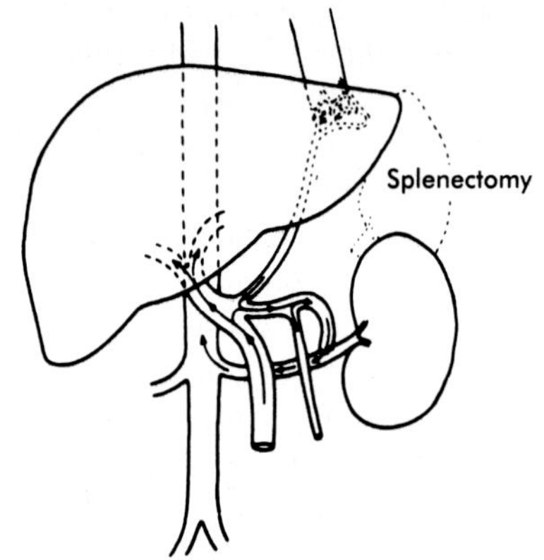

Fig. 73-15. Four types of nonselective portosystemic vascular shunts. Arrows indicate the direction of blood flow. (From Conn HO: In Schaffner F, et al, editors: *The liver and its diseases,* New York, 1974, Intercontinental Medical.)

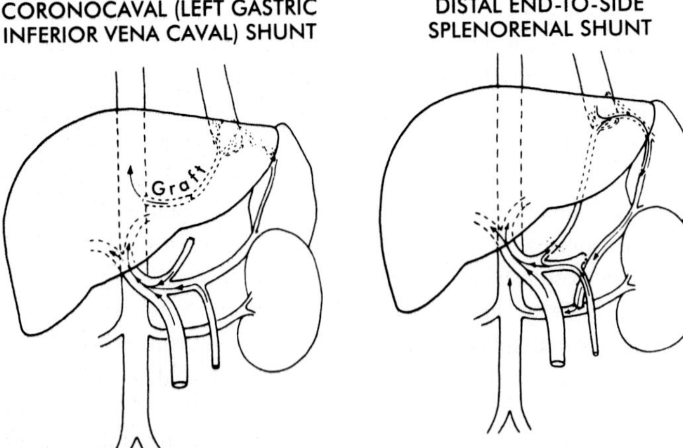

Fig. 73-16. Selective portosystemic vascular shunts. Arrows indicate portal and systemic flows after selective shunting. (From Conn HO: In Schaffner F, et al, editors: *The liver and its diseases,* New York, 1974, Intercontinental Medical.)

the SVR decreases by approximately 40%. Both right atrial and PCWP increase promptly by approximately 5 mm Hg. Shunting therefore appears to alter hemodynamics in the direction of those seen in patients with chronic liver disease and cirrhosis. This is postulated to result both from the volume effects of the shunt and the release into the general circulation of a vasodilator substance.[15]

The transjugular intrahepatic portosystemic shunt (TIPS) is an artificial fistula between branches of the portal vein and the systemic circulation, created by a stent placed in the substance of the liver. This is usually undertaken via the jugular vein, but can also be performed by other approaches (e.g., transfemoral vein). The TIPS diverts flow from the portal system to the systemic and leads to a significant decrease in the portosystemic gradient (e.g., mean 20 → 10 mm Hg[54,267]). It is technically successful in approximately 90% of patients. There is usually a significant decrease in ascites, and there is potential for improvement in renal function as well. An encephalopathy can develop, as in other forms of portosystemic shunting, but is usually mild and easily treated. TIPS is indicated for the management of variceal bleeding and intractable ascites.

Although a seemingly simple procedure, use of TIPS is very challenging and should only be performed in centers with the proper radiographic equipment and capable of responding quickly to untoward events.[123] Complications include early and late hemorrhage, liver capsule perforation, hemolysis,[229] and the side effects of large volumes of contrast material. Although it is often performed with sedation, general anesthesia may be required. Close hemodynamic monitoring is needed. In general, with opening of the shunt in spontaneously breathing sedated patients, there is a significant decrease in the portoatrial pressure gradient and in the SVR, and a significant increase in cardiac index, pulmonary vascular resistance, and mean PA pressure. This increase in pulmonary pressures is sustained.[267] Because TIPS allows a "nonsurgical" treatment in patients who are often quite unstable, this procedure is becoming increasingly used either as a backup to sclerotherapy or as primary therapy. It is favored for patients who will subsequently require liver transplantation,[174] in order to avoid the adhesions following an open procedure.

Peritoneovenous shunting is used to treat patients with intractable ascites. There are two basic types: the LeVeen[159] and Denver[222] shunts. Both have a pressure-sensitive valve with an opening pressure of 3 to 5 cm H_2O that permits one-way flow of ascitic fluid. The Denver shunt also has a small pumping chamber designed to allow the patient to pump/flush the tubing and pressure chamber. No particulate or bacterial filter exists in either shunt. Insertion may be performed in extremely ill patients and is often performed under monitored anesthesia care. An incision is made for tunnelling the catheter into the peritoneal cavity at the distal end and into a neck vein at the proximal end. The catheter's proximal tip rests at the right atrium. The hemodynamic effects seen acutely with the opening of these shunts range from minor increases in the CVP and mean arterial pressures to intravascular fluid overload. Other complications of peritoneovenous shunting include thrombosis and failure of the shunt, peritonitis with generalized septicemia, endotoxemia, central venous thrombosis and embolism, and a post-shunt coagulopathy similar to DIC.

Anesthetic management of patients undergoing these procedures can be complicated by this coagulopathy. When blood is instilled into the peritoneal cavity, it clots because of soluble collagen procoagulants in peritoneal fluid, a process that consumes platelets and fibrinogen. Subsequently, the clots are lysed by TPA. Similar events presumably occur when ascitic fluid reaches the general circulation. This may result in a DIC-like state with a prolonged PT and PTT, increased concentration of fibrin degradation products, and a fall in platelet count and fibrinogen levels. Treatment is facilitated by replacement of factors (FFP), platelets, epsilon-aminocaproic acid (Amicar®, Lederle, Wayne, NJ), and fibrinogen.[160]

Liver Transplantation

Orthotopic liver transplantation has become the final common hope for a large group of patients with various end-stage acute and chronic liver diseases, as well as with metabolic diseases and hepatic malignancies (Box 73-14). Most manifest the profound disturbances in synthetic and degradative functions common to patients with severe liver disease or the deficiency associated with a metabolic disease.

With the introduction of cyclosporin A (Sandoz Pharmaceuticals, Hanover, NJ) in 1979 and the subsequent use of monoclonal antibody against certain T cells (OKT3®, Ortho Pharmaceuticals, Raritan, NJ), **5-year survival rates after liver transplantation range from 55% to 85%, as compared with medical therapy alone, which results in a 0% to 30% survival rate.**[60,131,136,281] Newer antilymphocyte therapy, such as the Macrolide FK506 (Fujisawa Pharmaceutical, Osaka, Japan), continues to extend patient survival.

The anesthesiologist has a vital role in the pretransplant evaluation process. In addition to acquainting the patient and family with the issues and risks involved in the surgical procedures, the pretransplant consultation permits evaluation of those aspects of the patient's illness that may affect intraoperative course and stability. If the patient is encephalopathic, is increased ICP suspected (especially important in FHF), and is it being measured? If renal dysfunction or electrolyte abnormalities are present, has management been effective? What is known of the patient's cardiovascular dysfunction—is it hyperdynamic?[144,187] (Ischemic heart disease should impose a significant risk of perioperative myocardial infarction [MI].) Is there any reason to suspect pulmonary hypertension, which is six to seven times more prevalent in cirrhotic patients than in the general population[176] and may be associated with increased perioperative mortality?[133] Has dyspnea or hypoxia been a feature of the patient's clinical course? How severe is the synthetic defect as measured by the coagulation tests? Is thrombocytopenia present? Are other organs planned to accompany the liver transplant (e.g., liver-kidney, liver-heart-lung)? Is a major vascular procedure planned (e.g., portal venous thrombosis requiring portal vein reconstruction)?[158] Has the patient undergone major abdominal operation in the past? (If yes, bleeding will be predictably increased during the transplant procedure.[58]) Has testing for HIV been completed?

BOX 73-14
INDICATIONS FOR LIVER TRANSPLANTATION

Fulminant hepatic failure

- Viral hepatitis (e.g., A, B, delta)
- Drug induced
- Metabolic
  - Wilson's disease
  - Reye's syndrome
  - Organic acidurias
  - Other

End-stage chronic liver disease

- Predominantly hepatocellular disease
  - Alcoholic liver disease
  - Chronic viral liver disease
  - Idiopathic autoimmune liver disease
  - Chronic drug-induced liver disease
- Predominantly cholestatic disease
  - Primary biliary cirrhosis
  - Primary sclerosing cholangitis
  - Biliary atresia
  - Familial cholestatic syndromes
- Predominantly vascular disease
  - Budd-Chiari syndrome
  - Venoocclusive disease
- Polycystic disease

Nonresectable hepatic malignancies

- Hepatocellular carcinoma
- Cholangiocarcinoma
- Carcinoid
- Other

Metabolic liver disease

- α_1-antitrypsin deficiency
- Wilson's disease
- Hemochromatosis
- Glycogen storage diseases, types I and IV
- Homozygous type II hyperlipoproteinemia
- Urea cycle deficiences
- Others

Modified from Maddrey WC, Van Thiel DH: Liver transplantation: An overview, *Hepatology*, 8:948, 1988.

It is often difficult for hepatologists to determine precisely when a patient should enter the transplantation process. Although imprecise information is available for judging the rate of progression of a given disease in an individual patient, general criteria for the timing of transplantation have been established (Box 73-15). Despite these criteria, many patients die during the evaluation period or while awaiting transplantation,[99] often because of severe infection or hemorrhaging. Because patient outcome has improved dramatically over the past decade, it is no longer adequate to transplant solely those candidates on life support in intensive care units.[257] Both absolute and relative contraindications to liver transplantation have evolved as experience has been gained in various centers (Box 73-16).

All transplantation operations involve issues of multisystem illness in the recipient, donor organ selection, duration and quality of preservation of the donor organ, the timing and physiologic effects of immunosuppressive drugs, and both the physiologic and "reperfusion injury" effects that occur when blood flow is restored to the transplanted organ. Liver transplantation also is overshadowed by the hemodynamic state during the anhepatic phase (whether or not venovenous bypass is used), by the potential for hemodynamic

BOX 73-15
GENERAL CRITERIA FOR LIVER TRANSPLANTATION

Acute liver failure

- Bilirubin > 10–20 mg/dl and increasing
- Prothrombin time > 10 seconds above control and increasing
- Progressive encephalopathy of at least grade 3
- Metabolic acidosis
- Rapid loss of liver mass, as documented by imaging

Chronic liver disease

- Cholestatic liver disease
  - Bilirubin > 10–15 mg/dl
  - Intractable pruritus
  - Intractable bone disease
- Hepatocellular liver disease
  - Albumin < 2.5 mg/dl
  - Hepatic encephalopathy
  - Prothrombin time > 5 seconds above control
- Factors common to both categories
  - Hepatorenal syndrome
  - Recurrent severe infections (biliary sepsis, septicemia, spontaneous bacterial peritonitis)
- Intractable ascites
- Development of hepatocellular carcinoma
  - Social and vocational invalidism

Modified from Maddrey WC, Van Thiel DH: Liver transplantation: an overview, *Hepatology* 8:948, 1988; and Starzyl TE, Demetris AJ, Van Thiel D: Liver transplantation, *N Engl J Med* 321:1014, 1989.

BOX 73-16
CONTRAINDICATIONS TO LIVER TRANSPLANTATION

Absolute contraindications

- Sepsis outside hepatobiliary tree
- Metastatic hepatobiliary malignancy
- Advanced cardiopulmonary disease
- AIDS

Relative contraindications

- Advanced chronic renal failure
- Age > 60 years
- Portal vein thrombosis
- Cholangiocarcinoma
- Hypoxemia with intrapulmonary right-to-left shunts
- Hepatitis: HBsAg and HBeAg positivity
- Prior portocaval shunting procedure
- Prior complex hepatobiliary surgery
- Active alcohol and/or drug abuse
- HIV positivity without clinical AIDS
- Advanced malnutrition

Modified from Maddrey WC, Van Thiel DH: Liver transplantation: an overview, *Hepatology* 8:948, 1988.

collapse with the reperfusion of the engrafted liver, and by coagulation defects, which are usually present preoperatively and worsen during surgery. In addition, any preexisting neurologic or renal impairment will usually not improve during the surgical procedure.

Surgical aspects

The liver transplantation process can be divided into four phases:

Stage 0—Before the incision; largely the domain of the anesthesiologist
Stage 1—Before removal of the diseased liver
Stage 2—Anhepatic phase
Stage 3—Neohepatic phase

During stage 0, the patient is prepared for operation with appropriate monitoring and pharmacologic and hemostatic therapy, and anesthesia is induced. Percutaneous access catheters for venovenous bypass (VVB) return can be placed by the anesthesia team as well.[195] During stage 1, the liver is mobilized and appropriate vessels prepared for eventual anastomosis to the new liver. The recipient's femoral, portal (if used), and axillary (if not placed percutaneously by the anesthesia team) veins are also prepared for cannulation for VVB, if it is to be used. The donor organ is prepared for transplantation at the "back table." This stage may last 4 to 6 hours.

During stage 2, the donor organ is engrafted into the recipient. Generally the portal circulation is established first, followed by the arterial supply. However, some centers reestablish both circulations together, when possible, in the belief that the regional microperfusion, warm ischemia time that would occur during the arterial anastomosis is prevented. Before reperfusion, the increased potassium preservation solution (University of Wisconsin [UW] solution) is flushed from the liver. Stage 2 generally lasts 1 to 2 hours. During stage 3, the VVB is discontinued, the hepatic artery is anastomosed (if not done together with the portal vein), and biliary drainage, either through a direct bile duct anastomosis or via a Roux-en-Y loop, is reestablished. General operative evaluation is also performed to check for bleeding, continued adequacy of liver perfusion, and evidence of graft function. Fibrinolysis frequently occurs during this phase and requires aggressive coagulation management. Stage 3 generally lasts 3 to 4 hours.

Anesthetic considerations. Unlike most elective operations for patients with significant multisystem dysfunction, very few of the abnormalities present in the liver transplant patient will have been "corrected" before the procedure. Because of the potential for significant hemodynamic fluctuation during operation, most centers measure cardiac output and filling pressures, usually with a PA thermodilution catheter (standard, mixed venous O_2, or right-sided heart ejection fraction). Some centers are using transesophageal echocardiography as well. At least one arterial catheter is placed in a site that will not be disturbed by cannulae for the VVB. Large-bore infusion catheters are necessary. Most centers have developed or purchased a rapid-infusion device with a reservoir capacity. Some centers monitor the IVC pressure to detect increases secondary to surgical retraction, which can cause hypotension from venous obstruction; such an increase suggests mechanical rather than volume or pharmacologic therapy. Knowledge of the IVC pressure may also allow assessment of venous pressure gradients after anastomosis of the donor liver.[178]

When planning anesthesia induction, one should remember the potential for an incompetent gastroesophageal junction because of prior sclerotherapy, for increased abdominal pressure secondary to ascites, and for an uncertain volume status in many patients.

Fluid and blood product management during liver transplantation varies from aggressive replacement of deficits and losses to restricted fluids and blood product administration.[162,219,253] The latter is only possible when acceptable hemodynamics ensue. Evidence in the surgical and critical care literature shows that excessive use of fluids and blood products portends a more protracted postoperative course.[166]

Except for patients with liver cancer, who usually have essentially normal liver function, coagulation abnormalities are almost always present (Table 73-5). Most centers use standard laboratory coagulation measurements plus an *in vitro* assessment of coagulation with either the thrombelastograph or the Sonoclot® device. These machines are particularly useful for the detection and treatment of platelet dysfunction and fibrinolysis.[132] Treatment of coagulation abnormalities should be aggressive and begin before the in-

Table 73-5 Coagulation abnormalities in liver transplant recipients

Group	aPTT	PT	Platelet	FIB	FSP	ELT	AT III	TT
PNC	79	95	90	40	25	20	95	85
SC	75	25	63	0	0	0	50	63
PBC	38	25	38	0	13	0	25	56
CA	10	0	0	0	0	0	22	55
Misc	80	80	70	50	11	33	90	80

Numbers represent percent abnormal in each category. PNC—Postnecrotic cirrhosis; SC—sclerosing cholangitis; PBC—primary biliary cirrhosis; CA—carcinoma; Misc—miscellaneous hepatocellular disease; aPTT—activated partial thromboplastin time; PT—prothrombin time; FIB—fibrinogen; FSP—fibrin split products; ELT—euglobulin lysistime (a measure of fibrinolysis); AT III—antithrombin III; TT—thrombin time.

Modified from Bontempo F, Lewis J, Ragni M, et al: The preoperative coagulation pattern in liver transplant patients. In Winter PM, Kang YG, editors: *Hepatic transplantation: Anesthetic and perioperative management,* New York, 1986, Praeger.

cision, if necessary, despite the theoretic potential for VVB tubing surfaces to activate clotting factors. Platelet dysfunction has been successfully treated with DDAVP (1-deamino-8-*d*-arginine vasopressin; desmopressin).[2,40] Fibrinolysis has been treated with epsilon-aminocaproic acid (Amicar).[132]

Aprotinin can also be effective in treating fibrinolysis.[51,57,172] **Metabolic acidosis, hyperkalemia, hypothermia, and hypocalcemia frequently occur in the latter stages of liver transplantation and may act in concert to decrease coagulation.** Manipulation of coagulation is becoming an exciting aspect of the anesthetic management of liver transplant patients and will undoubtedly have importance in other surgical and intensive care settings.

Reperfusion of the new liver is a uniquely unstable period; as many as 30% of transplanted patients will have hypotension, occasionally accompanied by bradycardia and often difficult to treat. Many factors (Box 73-17) may play a role. Both hypovolemia and transient "hypervolemia" caused by splanchnic and lower body volume unloading with reperfusion have been implicated. Cardiac dysfunction may result from a residual bolus of high-potassium preservative solution reaching the heart, suspected "myocardial depressant factors," hypocalcemia, or a transient bolus of low-temperature flush solution. Emboli (air or thrombus), acute pulmonary hypertension, and decreased SVR from poorly described vasodilator substances may also play a role. If the hypotension is of sufficient severity and duration, myocardial ischemia may become a dominant problem. Hypotension at other times during the surgical procedure may be caused by hemorrhage, retraction of the liver obstructing venous return, low SVR, hypocalcemia (acutely associated with massive transfusion), metabolic acidosis and hyperkalemia, and medication administration (e.g., OKT3, IV hepatitis B immune globulin, anesthetics).

Most centers use devices to adequately warm and rapidly administer blood products and fluids. Although such devices are essential during major hemorrhaging, the ability to administer blood at a fast rate generally results in symptomatic hypocalcemia, requiring frequent bolus infusions of calcium. Some centers use cell-saving devices, when appropriate, to limit blood product administration. Some patients may have unrecognized bacterial peritonitis or biliary infection at the time of transplantation; autotransfused blood may not be bacteria free in this setting. Blood replacement therapy is aimed at keeping the hematocrit at approximately 25% to 30%. Hematocrits above 35% are associated with an increased incidence of postoperative hepatic artery thrombosis.

BOX 73-17
SUGGESTED ETIOLOGIES FOR HEMODYNAMIC INSTABILITY WITH LIVER REPERFUSION

- Hypovolemia
  - Inadequate venous return
  - Hemorrhage
- Cardiac dysfunction
  - Transient hyperkalemia
  - Hypothermic fluid bolus
  - Hypocalcemia with rapid transfusion
  - Metabolic acidosis
  - Emboli (air, thrombus)
  - "Myocardial depressant factors"
  - Myocardial ischemia
- Transient hypervolemia
  - Release of splanchnic and lower body venous blood volume
- Lowered systemic vascular resistance
  - ? Vasodilator substances

Venovenous bypass is used during hepatic transplantation to maintain volume loading for the right ventricle, to relieve splanchnic and systemic abdominal venous congestion, and it is hoped, to improve renal function during stage 2 of the transplant procedure. Cardiac output decreases somewhat during this procedure, because the bypass system may not be able to achieve flows comparable to the excluded vascular tree because circuit resistance is greater than in the native vessels. This is generally not a problem, but in patients with limited portal collaterals, interruption of VVB flow by kinking, for example, may not be well tolerated. Flows in the femoral and portal limb (if used) need not be equal and may vary considerably during the procedure. If air or thrombus is seen in the VVB tubing, the bypass should be abruptly discontinued, and the hemodynamic consequences of limited or absent VVB will become obvious. This may require volume loading and pressor support. Not all transplant centers agree that VVB is essential for the overall magement of OLT patients, and in fact, most pediatric patients are managed without it.

Several special situations are worthy of note. **Patients with acute fulminant hepatitis are at special risk of preoperative hypoglycemia, which persists into the operative period. Also, many of these patients have altered intracranial compliance and increased ICP.** Most centers begin assessing this condition with invasive monitoring when the patient reaches stage III hepatic coma.[276] Intraoperatively, increases in ICP can occur with IVC cross-clamping and with reperfusion of the new liver.[35,157] Patients with hepatitis B viral disease are a unique subset of infected patients. During the anhepatic phase of surgery, one presumes that the primary residence of hepatitis B virus has been removed. Centers are currently examining whether interferon, hepatitis B immune globulin, and hepatitis B vaccine have any modulating effect on development of hepatitis B seropositivity or on hepatitis after transplantation. Preliminary results seem encouraging,[104,220,275] recognizing that the hepatitis B virus has been located in various tissues other than the liver.

"Renal" dose dopamine is used at some centers in an effort to maintain or improve urinary output and "protect" the kidneys.[203] Positioning during liver transplantation usually requires that hefty retractors are placed either above or below extended arms. Careful placement of the patient on the table and padding of the upper arm should prevent nerve damage.[36] Temperature conservation and pressure sores are also a major concern during this lengthy procedure. Many centers wrap the patient in both foam padding and some form of thermal covering to address both problems simultaneously. When VVB is used, a predictable temperature loss occurs as blood circulates through tubing in a "cold" operating room.

Anesthetic drug administration during liver transplantation is not as complicated as one might believe. Contradictory considerations, however, do arise. Although decreased hepatic synthetic and degradative functions should dictate lower dosage of many medications, an increased volume of distribution secondary to the renal dysfunction and altered oncotic pressure suggest that more drug might be required. Because anesthesia induction requires appropriate brain concentrations of the drug used for a short period, these considerations are not important for induction purposes. Essentially, normal doses of the standard induction drugs (minus the patient's weight attributable to ascites) are acceptable. Narcotics, inhalational agents, and nondepolarizing muscle relaxants are used for the maintenance of anesthesia and should be titrated to effect, which virtually eliminates the need to consciously consider such variables as volumes of distribution and oncotic pressure. However, because of these latter concerns, IV drugs may continue to be excreted for a considerable time postoperatively and may contribute to postoperative CNS and neuromuscular depression. Of the inhalational anesthetics, isoflurane has been experimentally associated with the best preservation of hepatic blood flow.[19,95,97]

After anastomosis and perfusion, one should remember that the new liver is denervated and that the ability to autoregulate blood flow is limited to humoral (e.g., catecholamines) and metabolic means. Maintenance of perfusion pressure by pharmacologic intervention may be required during this time. The massive volumes of crystalloid and blood products that may be required during some transplant procedures, especially in the patient with depressed renal function, may lead to alterations in electrolyte balance. CPM can be associated with overcorrection of serum sodium levels (see earlier discussion).[287]

Despite the difficulties just mentioned, many patients may be ready to resume spontaneous ventilation within the first 24 hours postoperatively. The transplant patient will face many obstacles until recovery is complete, including the potential for severe infections, rejection episodes, nutritional inadequacy, continued metabolic illness, and repeated surgical events. In this light, the improvements in outcome over the last decade are all the more rewarding.

KEY POINTS

- The hepatic artery is richly invested with smooth muscle capable of altering arterial flow. The portal vessels have less myogenic control, which results in more passive changes in portal blood flow.
- Approximately 25% of the cardiac output courses through the liver, which represents a blood flow of approximately 100 ml/100 g of tissue. The hepatic artery distributes approximately 25% of total liver blood flow and supplies approximately 45% to 50% of hepatic oxygen (O_2).
- Regulation of the hepatic arteriolar tone is mainly achieved by local and intrinsic mechanisms that adjust hepatic arterial flow to compensate for changes in portal blood flow. This buffer response results in an increase in hepatic arterial flow when portal flow decreases.[96,152]
- Within the liver cell, bilirubin is esterified (conjugated) with monosaccharides, chiefly glucuronic acid, and effectively detoxified. Bilirubin is then excreted into the bile and through the common bile duct into the intestine.

- Hyperbilirubinemia can result from an overproduction of bilirubin or a defective elimination of bilirubin.
- Bilirubin is toxic for a variety of enzymatic processes.
- The decreased albumin seen in liver disease may affect protein binding for many substances, including drugs administered during anesthesia, resulting in increased free or active agents. Because liver disease often impairs metabolism as well, drug toxicity can be potentiated. Narcotics and barbiturates are highly protein (albumin) bound, and a decrease in serum albumin can be associated with an increased incidence of side effects.
- In general, clearance is more consistently decreased for highly extracted drugs in patients with hepatic disease than for poorly extracted drugs.
- Drugs with actions in the CNS, such as sedatives, narcotic analgesics, and other psychoactive drugs, are of particular concern in patients with severe liver disease. Even when the pharmacokinetics are only minimally disturbed or even unchanged, excessive sedation or the triggering or exacerbation of hepatic encephalopathy may occur.[12,150]
- Patients with hepatic failure are resistant to both d-tubocurarine and pancuronium, because both partly depend on bilary excretion for elimination.
- Normal portal venous pressure is 5 to 10 mm Hg (7 to 14 cm H_2O). A wedge hepatic venous pressure or a direct portal venous pressure more than 5 mm Hg greater than IVC pressure, a splenic pressure greater than 15 mm Hg, or a portal venous pressure measured at surgery of greater than 22 mm Hg (30 cm H_2O) indicates the presence of portal hypertension.
- Operation in patients with liver disease carries risks well beyond those of otherwise normal patients.
- Conventional wisdom, based on some older studies, would be to delay elective surgery until resolution or better definition of the etiology of newly recognized liver dysfunction.
- All general anesthesia causes a dose-related reduction in liver blood flow to some extent, with halothane producing a greater decrease than isoflurane.[97,104] Minor peripheral surgeries in general have less effect on liver blood flow than more complex procedures such as laparotomy, which is accompanied by a reduction in portal blood flow and an increase in hepatic arterial blood flow.[29,93,177]
- Spinal anesthesia (without operation) reduces liver blood flow if arterial pressure is allowed to decrease, but has limited effects when fluid support is administered to maintain systemic pressure.[109]
- At least 50% to 80% of patients with chronic liver disease have a significantly increased cardiac index.[144,187,200]
- Portal hypertension is the main feature of the abnormal splanchnic circulation seen in cirrhotic patients.
- Renal failure may occur in 50% to 75% of patients dying of cirrhosis.[66]
- The mortality is more than 60% for patients with severe liver disease, hyponatremia of < 120 mEq/l, and CNS symptoms.
- With the possible exception of *factor VIII,*[283] the liver produces the majority of both procoagulant and inhibitor factors. As such, deficiencies of these factors parallel the depressed protein synthesis of liver disease, as reflected by decreased serum albumin concentrations.[107,196,270]
- The PT should be corrected to within 2 seconds of control values by the infusion of FFP, which contains normal procoagulant and inhibitor coagulation proteins.
- The therapeutic effects of FFP administration are limited by the half-lives of its constituent factors, especially factor VII (half-life of 4 to 8 hours). Within 24 hours after correction, the PT will have returned to the pretreatment baseline values.
- Signs of increased ICP may be present in as many as 80% of patients with FHF.[64,102] Increased ICP is considered a specific neurologic complication of acute liver failure that is quite distinct from the hepatic encephalopathy seen in chronic liver disease and in preterminal hypoxic events.[20]
- As many as 12% to 28% of patients with cirrhosis demonstrate moderate hypoxemia, with an arterial O_2 tension (Pao_2) < 70 mm Hg. A smaller percentage have severe hypoxemia with a $Pao_2 < 50$ mm Hg. This is known as hepatopulmonary syndrome.[3,147,148,244]
- Isoflurane is often recommended for liver operation because it is associated with better maintenance of liver blood flow.[89,94]
- Patients with Budd-Chiari syndrome usually have a normal cardiac index and SVR before operation and do not manifest the hyperdynamic, low-resistance state of chronic cirrhosis. On opening the mesoatrial shunt, the cardiac index increases by approximately 50%, and the SVR decreases by approximately 40%. Both right atrial pressure and PCWP increase promptly by approximately 5 mm Hg.
- Orthotopic liver transplantation has become the final common hope for a large group of patients with various end-stage acute and chronic liver diseases, as well as those with metabolic diseases and hepatic malignancies.
- Five-year survival rates after liver transplantation range from 55% to 85%, as compared with medical therapy alone, which results in a 0% to 30% survival rate.[60,131,136,281]
- Fluid and blood product management during liver transplantation varies from aggressive replacement of deficits and losses to restricted fluids and blood product administration.[162,219,253]
- Metabolic acidosis, hyperkalemia, hypothermia, and hypocalcemia frequently occur in the latter stages of liver transplantation and may act in concert to decrease coagulation.
- Reperfusion of the new liver is a uniquely unstable pe-

riod, because as many as 30% of transplanted patients will have hypotension, occasionally accompanied by bradycardia and often difficult to treat.

- VVB is used during hepatic transplantation to maintain volume loading for the right ventricle, to relieve splanchnic and systemic abdominal venous congestion, and it is hoped, to improve renal function during stage 2 of the transplant procedure.
- Patients with acute fulminant hepatitis are at special risk of preoperative hypoglycemia, which persists into the operative period. Also, many of these patients have altered intracranial compliance and increased ICP.

KEY REFERENCES

Arroyo V, Ginès P, Gerbes AL, et al: Definition and diagnostic criteria of refractory ascites and hepatorenal syndrome in cirrhosis, *Hepatology* 23:164–176, 1996.

Bakti G, Fisch H, Karlaganis G, et al: Mechanisms of the excessive sedative response of cirrhotics to benzodiazepines: Model experiments with triazolam, *Hepatology* 7:629, 1987.

Bass NM, Williams RL: Hepatic function and pharmacokinetics. In Zakim D, Boyer TD, editors: *Hepatology: A textbook of liver disease,* ed 2, Philadelphia, 1990, WB Saunders.

Beattie C, Sitzmann JV, Cameron JL: Mesoatrial shunt hemodynamics, *Surgery* 104:1, 1988.

Benoit JN, Granger DN: Splanchnic hemodynamics in chronic portal hypertension, *Semin Liver Dis* 6:287, 1896.

Brajbord D, Ramsay M, Paulsen A, et al: A prospective analysis of upper extremity neuropathy following hepatic transplantation, *Anesth Analg* 68:766, 1989.

Carr JM: Disseminated intravascular coagulation in cirrhosis, *Hepatology* 10:103, 1989.

Epstein M, editor: *The kidney in liver disease,* ed 3, Baltimore, 1988, Williams & Wilkins.

Fiore L, Levine J, Deykin D: Alterations of hemostasis in patients with liver disease. In Zakim D, Boyer TD, editors: *Hepatology: A textbook of liver disease,* ed 2, Philadelphia, 1990, WB Saunders.

Fraser CL, Arieff AI: Hepatic encephalopathy, *N Engl J Med* 313:865, 1985.

Gelman S: Carbon dioxide and hepatic circulation, *Anesth Analg* 69:149, 1989.

Gelman S, Dillard E, Bradley E: Hepatic circulation during surgical stress and anesthesia with halothane, isoflurane or fentanyl, *Anesth Analg* 66:936, 1987.

Gelman S, Ernst E: Role of pH, Pco_2 and O_2 content of portal blood in hepatic circulatory autoregulation, *Am J Physiol* 233:E255, 1977.

Goldfarb G, Debaene B, Ange E, et al: Hepatic blood flow in humans during isoflurane-N_2O and halothane-N_2O anesthesia, *Anesth Analg* 71:349, 1990.

Groothuis GMM, Meijer DKF: Drug traffic in the hepatobiliary system, *J Hepatol* 24:(suppl 1) 3–28, 1996.

Kowalski HJ, Abelmann WH: The cardiac output at rest in Laennec's cirrhosis, *J Clin Invest* 32:1025, 1953.

Krowka MJ, Cortese DA: Hepatopulmonary syndrome: An evolving perspective in the era of liver transplantation, *Hepatology* 11:138, 1990.

Laidlaw J, Read A, Sherlock S: Morphine tolerance in hepatic cirrhosis, *Gastroenterology* 40:389, 1961.

LeRoux P, Elliott J, Perkins J, et al: Intracranial pressure monitoring in fulminant hepatic failure and liver transplantation, *Lancet* 335:1291, 1990.

Lewis BS, Tur-Kaspa R, Lewis N, et al: Left ventricular function in liver cirrhosis: an enchocardiographic study, *Isr J Med Sci* 16:489, 1980.

Murray JF, Dawson AM, Sherlock S: Circulatory changes in chronic liver disease, *Am J Med* 24:358, 1958.

Neal E, Meffin P, Gregory P, et al: Enhanced bioavailability and decreased clearance of analgesics in patients with cirrhosis, *Gastroenterology* 77:96, 1979.

Rakela J, Lange S, Ludwig J, et al: Fulminant hepatitis: Mayo Clinic experience with 34 cases, *Mayo Clin Proc* 60:289, 1985.

Rowland M, Tozer TN: *Clinical pharmakokinetics,* ed 2, Philadelphia, 1989, Lea & Febiger.

Schafer D, Jones E: Hepatic encephalopathy and the gamma aminobutyric acid neurotransmitter system, *Lancet* 1:18, 1982.

Schafer DF, Jones EA: Hepatic encephalopathy. In Zakim D, Boyer TD, editors: *Hepatology: A textbook of liver disease,* ed 2, Philadelphia, 1990, WB Saunders.

Zakim D, Boyer TD, editors: *Hepatology: A textbook of liver disease,* ed 2, vol 1, Philadelphia, 1990, WB Saunders.

REFERENCES

1. Ackroyd F, Mito M, McDermott W: Autonomic vasomotor controls in hepatic blood flow, *Am J Surg* 112:356, 1966.
2. Agnelli G, Berrettini M, De Cunto M, et al: Desmopressin-induced improvement of abnormal coagulation in chronic liver disease, *Lancet* 1:645, 1983.
3. Agustí AGN, Roca J, Bosch J, et al: The lung in patients with cirrhosis, *J Hepatol* 10:251, 1990.
4. Ansell JE, Kumar R, Deykin D: The spectrum of vitamin K deficiency, *JAMA* 237: 40, 1977.
5. Arden J, Lynam D, Castagnoli K, et al: Vercuronium and alcoholic liver disease: A pharmacokinetic and pharmacodynamic analysis, *Anesthesiology* 68:771, 1988.
6. Arieff A, Papadakis MA: Hyponatremia and hypernatremia in liver disease. In Epstein M, editor: *The kidney in liver disease,* Baltimore, 1988, Williams & Wilkins.
7. Arnman R, Gyzander E, Hedner U, et al: Natural protease inhibitors to fibrinolysis in liver diseases, *Hepatogastroenterology* 27:254, 1980.
8. Arroyo V, Ginés P: Prostaglandins and the treatment of hepatorenal syndrome in cirrhosis, *J Hepatol* 11:142, 1990.
9. Arroyo V, Ginés P, Gerbes AL, et al: Definition and diagnostic criteria of refractor ascites and hepatorenal syndrome in cirrhosis, *Hepatology* 23:164–176, 1996.
10. Ayus JC, Krothapalli RK, Arieff AI: Changing concepts in treatment of severe symptomatic hyponatremia: Rapid correction and possible relation to central pontine myelinolysis, *Am J Med* 78:897, 1985.
11. Ayus JC, Krothapalli R, Arieff AI: Treatment of symptomatic hyponatremia and relationship to brain damage: Prospective study, *N Engl J Med* 317:1190, 1987.
12. Bakti G, Fisch H, Karlaganis G, et al: Mechanisms of the excessive sedative response of cirrhotics to benzodiazepines: Model experiments with triazolam, *Hepatology* 7:629, 1987.
13. Bartholomew S, Cain J, Woolner L, et al: Sclerosing cholangitis: Its possible association with Riedel's struma and fibrous retroperitonitis—report of two cases, *N Engl J Med* 269:8, 1963.
14. Bass NM, Williams RL: Hepatic function and pharmacokinetics. In Zakim D, Boyer TD, editors: *Hepatology: A textbook of liver disease,* ed 2, Philadelphia, 1990, WB Saunders.
15. Beattie C, Sitzmann JV, Cameron JL: Mesoatrial shunt hemodynamics, *Surgery* 104:1, 1988.
16. Benhamou J, Rueff B, Sicot C: Severe hepatic failure: A critical study of current therapy. In Orlandi F, Jezequel A, editors: *Liver and drugs,* New York, 1972, Academic.
17. Benoit JN, Barrowman JA, Harper SL, et al: Role of humoral factors in the intestinal hyperemia associated with chronic portal hypertension, *Am J Physiol* 247:G486, 1984.
18. Benoit JN, Granger DN: Splanchnic hemodynamics in chronic portal hypertension, *Semin Liver Dis* 6:287, 1986.
19. Benumof J, Bookstein J, Saidman L, et al: Diminished hepatic arterial blood flow during halothane administration, *Anesthesiology* 45:545, 1976.
20. Berk P, Popper H: Fulminant hepatic failure, Annotated abstracts of a workshop held at the National Institutes of Health, 1977, *Am J Gastroenterol* 69:349, 1978.
21. Berthelot P, Walker JG, Sherlock S, et al: Arterial changes in the lungs in cirrhosis of the liver—lung spider nevi, *N Engl J Med* 274:291, 1966.
22. Bihari D, Gimson A, Lindridge J, et al: Lactic acidosis in fulminant hepatic failure: Some aspects of pathogenesis and prognosis, *J Hepatol* 1:405, 1985.
23. Bihari D, Gimson A, Waterson M, et al: Tissue hypoxia during fulminant hepatic failure, *Crit Care Med* 13:1034, 1985.
24. Bihari D, Gimson A, Williams R: Cardiovascular, pulmonary and renal complications of fulminant hepatic failure, *Semin Liver Dis* 6(2):119, 1986.
25. Biondi JW, Schulman DS, Soufer R, et al: The effect of incremental positive end-expiratory pressure on right ventricular hemodynamics and ejection fraction, *Anesth Analg* 67:144, 1988.
26. Bioulac-Sage P, Lafon M, Saric J, et al: Nerves and perisinusoidal cells in human liver, *J Hepatol* 10:105, 1990.
27. Bismuth H: Surgical anatomy and anatomical surgery of the liver, *World J Surg* 6:3, 1982.
28. Bismuth H, Houssin D, Castaing D: Major and minor segmentectomies in liver surgery, *World J Surg* 6:10, 1982.
29. Bohrer SL, Rogers EL, Koehler RC, Traystman RJ: Effect of hypovolemic hypotension and laparotomy on splanchnic and hepatic arterial blood flow in dogs, *Curr Surg* 38:325–328, 1981.
30. Bomzon A, Blendis LM: Vascular reactivity in experimental portal hypertension, *Am J Physiol* 252:G158, 1987.
31. Bontempo FA: Primary or secondary fibrinolysis? First Symposium of the International Society for Perioperative Care in Liver Transplantation, Pittsburgh, 1990.
32. Bosch J, Ginés P, Arroyo V, et al: Hepatic and systemic hemodynamics and the neurohumoral systems in cirrhosis. In Epstein M, editor: *The kidney in liver disease,* Baltimore, 1988, Williams & Wilkins.
33. Boyadjian H: Changes in antithrombin III activity in the various clinical forms of viral hepatitis, *Folia Med* 23:11, 1981.
34. Boyer T, Kahn A, Reynolds T: Diagnostic value of ascitic fluid LDH, protein, and WBC levels, *Arch Intern Med* 138:103, 1978.
35. Brajbord D, Parks R, Ramsay M, et al: Management of acute elevation of intracranial pressure during hepatic transplantation, *Anesthesiology* 70:139, 1989.
36. Brajbord D, Ramsay M, Paulsen A, et al: A prospective analysis of upper extremity neuropathy following hepatic transplantation, *Anesth Analg* 68:766, 1989.
37. Brienza N, Revelly J-P, Ayuse T, Robotham JL: Effects of PEEP on Liver arterial and venous blood flows, *Am J Respir Crit Care Med* 152:504–510, 1995.
38. Burcar PJ, Norenberg MD, Yarnell PR: Hyponatremia and central pontine myelinolysis, *Neurology* 27:223, 1977.
39. Burns P, Taylor K, Blei A: Doppler Flowmetry and portal hypertension, *Gastroenterology* 92:824, 1987.
40. Burroughs A, Matthews K, Qadiri M, et al: Desmopressin and bleeding time in patients with cirrhosis, *Br Med J* 291:1377, 1985.
41. Cade R, Wagemaker H, Vogel S, et al: Hepatorenal syndrome: Studies of the effect of vascular volume and intraperitoneal pressure on renal and hepatic function, *Am J Med* 82:427, 1987.
42. Camara DS, Caruana JA, Chung RS, et al: The hemodynamic effects of the sclerosant sodium morrhuate in dogs, *Surg Gynecol Obstet* 161:327, 1985.
43. Carr JM: Disseminated intravascular coagulation in cirrhosis, *Hepatology* 10:103, 1989.
44. Cederblad G, Korsan-Bengtsen K, Olsson R: Observations of increased levels of blood coagulation factors and other plasma proteins in cholestatic liver disease, *Scand J Gastroenterol* 11:391, 1976.
45. Chan TK, Chan V: Antithrombin III, the major modulator of intravascular coagulation, is synthesized in human endothelial cells, *Thromb Haemost* 46:504, 1981.
46. Chan V, Lai CL, Chan TK: Metabolism of antithrombin III in cirrhosis and cancer of the liver, *Clin Sci* 60:681, 1981.
47. Chapin J, University of Nebraska; Wiesner R, Mayo Clinic: 1991, Personal communication.
48. Chenard-Neu M-P, Boudjema K, Bernuau J, et al: Auxiliary liver transplantation: Regeneration of the native liver and outcome in 30 patients with fulminant hepatic failure—a multicenter European study, *Hepatology* 23:1119–1127, 1996.
49. Child CG, editor: *The liver and portal hypertension,* Philadelphia, 1965, WB Saunders.
50. Christensen E, Crowe J, Doniach D, et al: Clinical pattern and course of disease in primary biliary cirrhosis based on an analysis of 236 patients, *Gastroenterology* 78:236, 1980.
51. Christophe J, Rouget C, Roullier M, et al: Use of ATIII concentrate during liver transplantation, First Symposium for the International Society for Perioperative Care in Liver Transplantation (abstract). Pittsburgh, 1990.
52. Cluitmans FHM, Meinders AE: Management of severe hyponatremia: Rapid or slow correction? *Am J Med* 88:161, 1990.
53. Conn HO: Complications of portal hypertension. In Gitnick G, editor: *Current hepatology,* Chicago, 1985, Mosby–Year Book.
54. Conn HO: Transjugular intrahepatic portal-systemic shunts: The state of the art, *Hepatology* 17:148–158, 1993.

55. Cooper AD: Hepatic lipoprotein and cholesterol metabolism. In Zakim D, Boyer TD, editors: *Hepatology: A textbook of liver disease,* ed 2, Philadelphia, 1990, WB Saunders.
56. Cordova C, Musca A, Violi F, et al: Prekallikrein behaviour in chronic active hepatitis and in cirrhotic patients, *Haemostasis* 14:218, 1984.
57. Cottam S, Hunt B, Segal B, et al: Aprotinin inhibits tissue-plasminogen activator mediated fibrinolysis during orthotopic liver transplantation, First Symposium of the International Society for Perioperative Care in Liver Transplantation, Pittsburgh, 1990.
58. Cuervas-Mons V, Rimola A, Van Thiel D, et al: Does previous abdominal surgery alter the outcome of pediatric patients subjected to orthotopic liver transplantation? *Gastroenterology* 90:853, 1986.
59. Cuilleret G, Pomier-Layrargues G, Pons F, et al: Changes in brain catecholamine levels in human cirrhotic hepatic encephalopathy, *Gut* 21:565, 1980.
60. Darby H, Selden C, Hodgson HJ: Prolonged survival of cyclosporin treated allogeneic hepatocellular implants, *Transplantation* 42:325, 1986.
61. Donohue T, Jennett R, Tuma D, et al: Synthesis and secretion of plasma proteins by the liver. In Zakim D, Boyer D, editors: *Hepatology: A textbook of liver disease,* ed 2, Philadelphia, 1990, WB Saunders.
62. Douglas WW: Polypeptides—angiotensin, plasma kinins, and others. In Gilman AG, Goodman LS, Rall TW, et al, editors: *The pharmacological basis of therapeutics,* ed 7, New York, 1985, Macmillan.
63. Dymock IW, Tucker JS, Woolf IL, et al: Coagulation studies as a prognostic index in acute liver failure, *Br J Haematol* 29:385, 1975.
64. Ede R, Gimson A, Bihari D, et al: Controlled hyperventilation in the prevention of cerebral oedema in fulminant hepatic failure, *J Hepatol* 2:43, 1986.
65. Epstein M, editor: *The kidney in liver disease,* ed 3, Baltimore, 1988, Williams & Wilkins.
66. Epstein M: Renal sodium handling. In Epstein M, editor: *The kidney in liver disease,* ed 3, Baltimore, 1988, Williams & Wilkins.
67. Epstein M: Functional renal abnormalities in cirrhosis: Pathophysiology and management. In Zakim D, Boyer TD, editors: *Hepatology: A textbook of liver disease,* ed 2, Philadelphia, 1990, WB Saunders.
68. Epstein M, Berk DP, Hollenberg NK, et al: Renal failure in the patient with cirrhosis: The role of active vasoconstriction, *Am J Med* 49:175, 1970.
69. Epstein M, Larios O, Johnson G: Effects of water immersion on plasma catecholamines in decompensated cirrhosis: implications for deranged sodium and water homeostatis, *Miner Electrolyte Metab* 11:25, 1985.
70. Epstein M, Lifschitz M, Hoffman DS: Relationship between renal prostaglandin E and renal sodium handling during water immersion in normal man, *Circ Res* 45:71, 1979.
71. Epstein M, Lifschitz M, Ramachandran M: Characterization of renal PGE responsiveness in decompensated cirrhosis: Implications for renal sodium handling, *Clin Sci* 63:555, 1982.
72. Epstein M, Pins DS, Schneider N, et al: Determinants of deranged sodium and water homeostasis in decompensated cirrhosis, *J Lab Clin Med* 87:822, 1976.
73. Epstein M, Schneider NS, Befeler B: Relationship of systemic and intrarenal hemodynamics in cirrhosis, *J Lab Clin Med* 89:1175, 1977.
74. Eriksson L, Söderman C, Ericzon B, et al: Normalization of ventilation/perfusion relationships after liver transplantation in patients with decompensated cirrhosis: evidence for a hepatopulmonary syndrome, *Hepatology* 12:1350, 1990.
75. Eriksson LS, Söderman C, Wahren J, et al: Is hypoxemia of cirrhotic patients due to a functional 'hepato-pulmonal' syndrome? *J Hepatol* 7:S29, 1988.
76. Feely J, Wilkinson GR, McAllister CB, et al: Increased toxicity and reduced clearance of lidocaine by cimetidine, *Ann Intern Med* 96:592, 1982.
77. Feely J, Wilkinson GR, Wood AJJ: Reduction of liver blood flow and propranolol metabolism by cimetidine, *N Engl J Med* 304:692, 1981.
78. Feldman G, Maurice M: Morphological findings of liver protein synthesis and secretion. In Popper H, Bianchi L, Reuther W, editors: *Membrane alterations as a basis of liver injury,* Baltimore, 1977, University Park.
79. Ferenci P, Grimm G, Gangl A: Successful long-time treatment of chronic hepatic encephalopathy with a benzodiazepine antagonist, *Hepatology* 7:1064, 1987.
80. Finlayson MH, Superville B: Distribution of cerebral lesions in acquired hepatocerebral degeneration, *Brain* 104:79, 1981.
81. Fiore L, Levine J, Deykin D: Alterations of hemostasis in patients with liver disease. In Zakim D, Boyer TD, editors: *Hepatology: A textbook of liver disease,* ed 2, Philadelphia, 1990, WB Saunders.
82. Fisher CJ, Faloon WW: Blood ammonia levels in hepatic cirrhosis: Their control by the oral administration of neomycin, *N Engl J Med* 256:1030, 1957.
83. Fleig WE, Stange EF, Ruettenauer K, et al: Emergency endoscopic sclerotherapy for bleeding esophageal varices: A prospective study in patients not responding to balloon tamponade, *Gastrointest Endosc* 29:8, 1983.
84. Foster JH: Liver resection techniques, *Surg Clin North Am* 69:235, 1989.
85. Francis J, Armstrong DJ: Acquired dysfibrinogenemia in liver disease, *J Clin Pathol* 35:667, 1982.
86. Francis RB, Feinstein DI: Clinical significance of accelerated fibrinolysis in liver disease, *Haemostasis* 14:460, 1984.
87. Fraser CL, Arieff AI: Fluid and electrolyte disorders and the central nervous system. In Maxwell MH, Kleeman CR, Narins RG, editors: *Disorders of fluid and electrolyte metabolism,* ed 4, New York, McGraw-Hill.
88. Fraser CL, Arieff AI: Hepatic encephalopathy, *N Engl J Med* 313:865, 1985.
89. Fujita Y, Sakai T, Ohsumi A, et al: Effects of hypocapnia and hypercapnia on splanchnic circulation and hepatic function in the beagle, *Anesth Analg* 69:152, 1989.
90. Gaiani S, Bolondi L, Bassi S, et al: Prevalence of spontaneous hepatofugal portal flow in liver cirrhosis: Clinical and endoscopic correlation in 228 patients, *Gastroenterology* 100:160, 1991.
91. Gauthier G, Wildi E: L'encéphalomyélopathie porto-systémic, *Rev Neurol (Paris)* 131:319, 1975.
92. Gazzard B, Portmann B, Murray-Lyon, et al: Causes of death in fulminant hepatic failure and relationship to quantitative histological assessments of parenchymal damage, *Q J Med* 44:615, 1975.
93. Gelman S: Disturbances in hepatic blood flow during anesthesia and surgery, *Arch Surg* 111:881–883, 1976.
94. Gelman S: Carbon dioxide and hepatic circulation, *Anesth Analg* 69:149, 1989.
95. Gelman S, Dillard E, Bradley E: Hepatic circulation during surgical stress and anesthesia with halothane, isoflurane, or fentanyl, *Anesth Analg* 66:936, 1987.
96. Gelman S, Ernst E: Role of pH, Pco_2 and O_2 content of portal blood in hepatic circulatory autoregulation, *Am J Physiol* 233:E255, 1977.
97. Gelman S, Fowler K, Smith L: Liver circulation and function during isoflurane and halothane anesthesia, *Anesthesiology* 61:726, 1984.
98. Genovesi MG, Tierney DF, Taplan GV, et al: An intravenous radionuclide method to evaluate hypoxemia caused by abnormal alveolar vessels: limitations of conventional techniques, *Am Rev Respir Dis* 114:59, 1976.
99. Ghent CN: The liver transplant candidate: assessment and followup. In Maddrey WC, editor: *Transplantation of the liver,* New York, 1988, Elsevier.
100. Ghonheim M, Kramer S, Bannow R, et al: Binding of d-tubocurarine to plasma protein in normal man and in patients with hepatic or renal disease, *Anesthesiology* 39:410, 1973.
101. Gibbs C, Schwartz D, Wynne J, et al: Antacid pulmonary aspiration in the dog, *Anesthesiology* 51:380, 1979.
102. Gimson A, Braude S, Mellon P, et al: Earlier charcoal haemoperfusion in fulminant hepatic failure, *Lancet* 2:681, 1982.
103. Gines P, Arroyo V, Quintero E, et al: Comparison of paracentesis and diuretics in the treatment of cirrhotics with tense ascites, *Gastroenterology* 93:234, 287.
104. Goldfarb G, Debaene B, Ang E, et al: Hepatic blood flow in humans during isoflurane-N_2O and halothane-N_2O anesthesia, *Anesth Analg* 71:349, 1990.
105. Goodpasture EW: Fibrinolysis in chronic hepatic insufficiency, *Bull Johns Hopkins Hosp* 25:330, 1914.
106. Granger D, Miller T, Allen R, et al: Permselectivity of cat liver blood-lymph barrier to endogenous macromolecules, *Gastroenterology* 77:103, 1979.
107. Green G, Poller L, Thompson JM, et al: Factor VII as a marker of hepatocellular synthetic function in liver disease, *J Clin Pathol* 29:971, 1976.
108. Greenberger N, Isselbacher K: Diseases of the gallbladder and bile ducts. In Wilson J, Braunwald E, Isselbacher K, et al, editors:

Principles of internal medicine, ed 12, New York, 1991, McGraw-Hill.

109. Greene NM, Brull SJ: Hepatic function. In Greene NM, Brull SJ, editors: *Physiology of spinal anesthesia,* ed 4, Baltimore, 1993, Williams & Wilkins.
110. Greenway C, Stark R: Hepatic vascular bed, *Physiol Rev* 51:23, 1971.
111. Griffin JH, Mosher DF, Zimmerman TS, et al: Protein C, an antithrombotic protein, is reduced in hospitalized patients with intravascular coagulation, *Blood* 60:261, 1982.
112. Groothuis GMM, Meijer DKF: Drug traffic in the hepatobiliary system, *J Hepatol* 24:(sup 1)3–28, 1996.
113. Grossi CE, Rousselot LM, Panke WF: Coagulation defects in patients with cirrhosis of the liver undergoing porta-systemic shunts, *Am J Surg* 104:512, 1962.
114. Groszmann RJ, Kotelanski B, Cohn JN, et al: Quantitation of portasystemic shunting from the splenic and mesenteric beds in alcoholic liver disease, *Am J Med* 53:715, 1972.
115. Guazzi M, Polese A, Magrini F, et al: Negative influences of ascites on the cardiac function of cirrhotic patients, *Am J Med* 59:165, 1975.
116. Haberer J, Schoeffler P, Couderc E, et al: Fentanyl pharmacokinetics in anaesthetized patients with cirrhosis, *Br J Anaesth* 54:1267, 1982.
117. Hadziyannis S, Scheuer P, Feizi T, et al: Immunological and histological studies in primary biliary cirrhosis, *J Clin Pathol* 23:95, 1970.
118. Hallen A, Nilsson IM: Coagulation studies in liver disease, *Thromb Haemost* 11:51, 1964.
119. Halstead AC, Nanji AA: Artifactual lowering of serum creatinine in the presence of hyperbilirubinemia—a method dependent artifact, *JAMA* 251:38, 1984.
120. Harville D, Summerskill W: Surgery in acute hepatitis: causes and effects, *JAMA* 184:257, 1963.
121. Hasch E, Jarnum S, Tygstrup N: Albumin synthesis rate as a measure of liver function in patients with cirrhosis, *Arch Intern Med* 182:38, 1967.
122. Hawk WA, Hazard J: Sclerosing retroperitonitis and sclerosing mediastinitis, *Am J Clin Pathol* 32:321, 1959.
123. Hebbard GS, Jones R, Fitt G, et al: Transjugular intrahepatic portal-systemic shunts (TIPS)—initial experience and clinical outcome, *Aust NZ J Med* 24:141–148, 1994.
124. Henriksen JH, Christensen NJH, Ring-Larsen H: Noradrenaline and adrenaline concentrations in various vascular beds in patients with cirrhosis: relation to hemodynamics, *Clin Physiol* 1:293, 1981.
125. Henriksen JH, Ring-Larsen H, Christensen NJ: Circulating noradrenaline and central haemodynamics in patients with cirrhosis, *Scand J Gastroenterol* 20:1185, 1985.
126. Hind CRK, Wong CM: Detection of pulmonary arteriovenous fistulae in patients with cirrhosis by contrast two dimensional echocardiography, *Gut* 22:1042, 1981.
127. Hippocrates: *The genuine works of Hippocrates,* New York, 1929, W Wood (translated by F Adams).
128. Jackson FC, Christophersen EB, Peternel WW, Kirimli B: Preoperative management of patients with liver disease, *Surg Clin North Am* 48:907–930, 1968.
129. Jagathambal K, Grunwald HW, Rosner F: Evaluation and management of the bleeding patient, *Med Clin North Am* 65:133, 1981.
130. James JH, Siparo V, Jeppsson B, et al: Hyperammonemia, plasma amino acid imbalance and blood-brain amino acid transport: A unified theory of portal-systemic encephalopathy, *Lancet* 2:772, 1979.
131. Jenkins RL: Liver transplantation in the adult, *Transplant Rev* 1:1, 1987.
132. Kang YG: Monitoring and treatment of coagulation. In Winter PM, Kang YG, editors: *Hepatic transplantation: Anesthetic and perioperative management,* New York, 1986, Praeger.
133. Kang YG: 1991, Personal experience and communication.
134. Karetzky MS, Mithoefer JC: The cause of hyperventilation and arterial hypoxia in patients with cirrhosis of the liver, *Am J Med Sci* 254:797, 1967.
135. Karp WB: Biochemical alterations in neonatal hyperbilirubinemia and bilirubin encephalopathy: a review, *Pediatrics* 64:361, 1979.
136. Keating JJ, Johnson RD, Johnson PJ, et al: Clinical course of cirrhosis in young adults and therapeutic potential of liver transplantation, *Gut* 26:1359, 1985.
137. Kelley DA, O'Brien JO, Hutten RA, et al: The effect of liver disease on factors V, VII and protein C, *Br J Haematol* 61:541, 1985.
138. Kew MC, Varma RR, Williams HS, et al: Renal and intrarenal bloodflow in cirrhosis of the liver, *Lancet* 2:504, 1971.
139. Klotz U, McHorse T, Wilkinson G, et al: The effects of cirrhosis in the disposition and elimination of meperidine in man, *Clin Pharmacol Ther* 16:667, 1974.
140. Knauer C, Lowe H: Hemodynamics in the cirrhotic patient during paracentesis, *N Engl J Med* 276:491, 1967.
141. Knott E, Drijfhout HR, Tencate JW, et al: Alpha 2-plasmin metabolism in patients with liver cirrhosis, *J Lab Clin Med* 105:353, 1985.
142. Knott E, Tencate JW, Drijfhout HR, et al: Antithrombin III metabolism in patients with liver disease, *J Clin Pathol* 37:523, 1984.
143. Kostreva DR, Castañer A, and Kampine JP: Reflex effects of hepatic baroreceptors on renal and cardiac sympathetic nerve activity, *Am J Physiol* 238:R390, 1980.
144. Kowalski HJ, Abelmann WH: The cardiac output at rest in Laennec's cirrhosis, *J Clin Invest* 32:1025, 1953.
145. Krebs HA, Bennett DAH, DeGasquet P, et al: Renal gluconeogenesis: the effect of diet on the gluconeogenic capacity of rat-kidney-cortex slices, *Biochem J* 31(86):22, 1963.
146. Krowka MJ, Cortese DA: Severe hypoxemia associated with liver disease: Mayo Clinic experience of experimental use of almitrine bismesylate, *Mayo Clin Proc* 62:164, 1987.
147. Krowka MJ, Cortese DA: Pulmonary aspects of liver disease and liver transplantation, *Clin Chest Med* 10:593, 1989.
148. Krowka MJ, Cortese DA: Hepatopulmonary syndrome: an evolving perspective in the era of liver transplantation, *Hepatology* 11:138, 1990.
149. Krowka MJ, Tajik AJ, Dickson ER, et al: Intrapulmonary vascular dilatations (IVPD) in liver transplant candidates: screening by two-dimensional contrast enhanced echocardiography, *Chest* 96:164S, 1989.
150. Laidlaw J, Read A, Sherlock S: Morphine tolerance in hepatic cirrhosis, *Gastroenterology* 40:389, 1961.
151. Laragh JH, Cannon PJ, Bentzel CJ, et al: Angiotensin II, norepinephrine, and the renal transport of electrolytes and water in normal man and in cirrhosis with ascites, *J Clin Invest* 42:1179, 1963.
152. Lautt WW: Mechanism and role on intrinsic regulation of hepatic arterial blood flow: hepatic buffer response, *Am J Physiol* 249:G549, 1985.
153. Leavitt S, Tyler HR: Studies in asterixis, *Arch Neurol* 10:360, 1964.
154. LeBrault C, Berger J, D'Hollander A, et al: Pharmacokinetics and pharmacodynamics of vecuronium (ORG NC45) in patients with cirrhosis, *Anesthesiology* 62:601, 1985.
155. LeBrault C, Duvaldstein P, Henzel D, et al: Pharmacokinetics and pharmacodynamics of vecuronium in patients with cholestasis, *Br J Anaesth* 58:983, 1986.
156. LeBrec D, Bataille C, Bercoff E, et al: Hemodynamic changes in patients with portal venous obstruction, *Hepatology* 3:550, 1983.
157. LeRoux P, Elliott J, Perkins J, et al: Intracranial pressure monitoring in fulminant hepatic failure and liver transplantation, *Lancet* 335:1291, 1990.
158. LeRut J, Tzakin AG, Bron K, et al: Complications of venous reconstruction in human orthotopic liver transplantation, *Ann Surg* 205:404, 1987.
159. LeVeen HH, Christoudias G, Moon IP, et al: Peritoneo-venous shunting for ascites, *Ann Surg* 180:580, 1974.
160. LeVeen HH, Moon IP, Ahmed N, et al: Coagulopathy postperitoneovenous shunt, *Ann Surg* 205:305, 1987.
161. Levy DE, Bates D, Caronna JJ, et al: Prognosis in nontraumatic coma, *Ann Intern Med* 94:293, 1981.
162. Lewandowski K, Hopfe T, Rossaint R, et al: Restrictive transfusion of blood products in 75 orthotopic liver transplantations, First Symposium of the International Society for Perioperative Care in Liver Transplantation, Pittsburgh, 1990.
163. Lewis BS, Tur-Kaspa R, Lewis N, et al: Left ventricular function in liver cirrhosis: an echocardiographic study, *Isr J Med Sci* 16:489, 1980.
164. Lindenmuth WW, Eisenberg MM: The surgical risk in cirrhosis of the liver, *Arch Surg* 86:235–242, 1963.
165. Loft S, Boel J, Kyst A, et al: Increased hepatic microsomal enzyme activity after surgery under halothane or spinal anesthesia, *Anesthesiology* 62:11–16, 1985.
166. Lowell JA, Schifferdecker C, Driscoll DF, et al: Postoperative fluid overload: not a benign problem, *Crit Care Med* 18:728, 1990.

167. Malt RA: Elective portasystemic shunts. In McDermott WV, editor: *Surgery of the liver,* Boston, 1989, Blackwell Scientific.
168. MacGilchrist A, Birnie G, Cook A, et al: Pharmacokinetics and pharmacodynamics of intravenous midazolam in patients with severe alcoholic cirrhosis, *Gut* 27:190, 1986.
169. MacKay I, Gershwin ME: Primary biliary cirrhosis: current knowledge, perspectives, and future directions, *Semin Liver Dis* 9:149, 1989.
170. Maisels MJ: Neonatal jaunice. In Avery GB, editor: Neonatology—pathophysiology and management of the newborn, ed 2, Philadephia, 1981, JB Lippincott.
171. Mandel EE, Gerhold WM: Plasma fibrin-stabilizing factor: acquired deficiency in various disorders, *Am J Clin Pathol* 52:547, 1969.
172. Marcel RJ, Stegall WC, Suit CT, et al: Continuous small-dose aprotinin controls fibrinolysis during orthotopic liver transplantation, *Anesth Analg* 82:1122–1125, 1996.
173. Marco J, Diego J, Villaneuva ML, et al: Elevated plasma glucagon levels in cirrhosis of the liver, *N Engl J Med* 289:1107, 1973.
174. Menegaux F, Baker E, Keeffe EB, et al: Impact of transjugular intrahepatic portosystemic shunt on orthotopic liver transplantation, *World J Surg* 866–871, 1994.
175. McDermott WV, Adams RD: Episodic stupor associated with an ECK fistula in man with particular reference to ammonia metabolism, *J Clin Invest* 33:1, 1954.
176. McDonnell PJ, Toye PA, Hutchens GM: Primary pulmonary hypertension and cirrhosis: are they related? *Am Rev Respir Dis* 127:437, 1983.
177. McNeill JR, Pang CC: Effect of pentobarbital anesthesia and surgery on the control of arterial pressure and mesenteric resistance in cats. Role of vasopressin and angiotensin, *Can J Physiol Pharmacol* 60:363–368, 1982.
178. Merritt WT, Beattie C, Peck R, et al: Vena caval pressure gradients during liver transplantation, *Transplantation* 50:336, 1990.
179. Mitchell MC, Boitnott JK, Kaufman S, et al: Budd-Chiari syndrome: etiology, diagnosis and management, *Medicine* 61:199, 1982.
180. Monroe P, Morrow CR, Miller E, et al: Acute respiratory failure after sodium morrhuate esophageal sclerotherapy, *Gastroenterology* 85:693, 1983.
181. Montefuso P, Geiss A, Bronzo, et al: Sclerosing cholangitis, chronic pancreatitis, and Sjögren's syndrome: a syndrome complex, *Am J Surg* 147:822, 1984.
182. Moreau R, Lee SS, Hadengue A, et al: Relationship between oxygen transport and oxygen uptake in patients with cirrhosis: effects of vasoactive drugs, *Hepatology* 9:427, 1989.
183. Moreau R, Lee SS, Soupison T, et al: Abnormal tissue oxygenation in patients with cirrhosis and liver failure, *J Hepatol* 7:98, 1988.
184. Morgan MY, Hawley KE: Lacitol vs. lactulose in the treatment of acute hepatic encephalopathy in cirrhotic patients: a double-blind, randomized trial, *Hepatology* 7:1278, 1987.
185. Mortality patterns—United States, 1987, *MMWR* 39:193, 1990.
186. Mosvold J, Abildgaard U, Jenssen H, et al: Low antithrombin III in acute hepatic failure at term, *Scand J Haematol* 29:48, 1982.
187. Murray JF, Dawson AM, Sherlock S: Circulatory changes in chronic liver disease, *Am J Med* 24:358, 1958.
188. Neal E, Meffin P, Gregory P, et al: Enhanced bioavailability and decreased clearance of analgesics in patients with cirrhosis, *Gastroenterology* 77:96, 1979.
189. Nelson DC, McGrew WRG, Hoyumpa AM: Hypernatremia and lactulose therapy, *JAMA* 249:1295, 1983.
190. Nicholls KM, Shapiro MD, Van Putten VJ, et al: Elevated plasma norepinephrine concentrations in decompensated cirrhosis: association with increased secretion rates, normal clearance rates, and suppressibility by central blood volume expansion, *Circ Res* 56:457, 1985.
191. Norenberg MD: The astrocyte in liver disease, *Adv Cell Neurobiol* 2:303, 1981.
192. Norenberg MD, Leslie KO, Robertson AS: Association between rise in serum sodium and central pontine myelinolysis, *Ann Neurol* 1:128, 1982.
193. O'Grady J, Gimson A, O'Brien C, et al: Controlled trials of charcoal hemoperfusion and prognostic factors in fulminant hepatic failure, *Gastroenterology* 94:1186, 1988.
194. O'Grady J, Williams R: Management of acute liver failure, *Schweiz Med Wochenschr* 116:541, 1986.
195. Oken AC, Frank SM, Merritt WT, et al: A new percutaneous technique for establishing venous bypass access in orthotopic liver transplantation, *J Cardiothoracic Anesth* 8:58–60, 1994.
196. Orlando M: Factor VII in liver cirrhosis, *Haemostasis* 11:73, 1982.
197. Orloff MJ, Krims P: Effect of endoscopic sclerotherapy on rebleeding and survival of cirrhotic patients with bleeding esophageal varices (abstract), *Gastroenterology* 90: 1574, 1986.
198. Owen OE, Patel MS, Block BSB, et al: Gluconeogenesis in normal, cirrhotic and diabetic humans. In Hanson RW, Mehlman MA, editors: *Glyconeogenesis: its regulation in mammalian species,* New York, 1976, John Wiley-Interscience.
199. Pang JA, Vicary F: Carcinoma of the colon, sclerosing cholangitis, pericholangitis, and bronchiectasis in a patient with chronic ulcerative colitis, *J Clin Gastroenterol* 6:361, 1984.
200. Park SC, Beerman LB, Gartner JC, et al: Echocardiographic findings before and after liver transplantation, *Am J Cardiol* 55:1373, 1985.
201. Patwardhan R, Johnson R, Hoyumpa A, et al: Normal metabolism of morphine in cirrhosis, *Gastroenterology* 81:1006, 1981.
202. Peters T: Serum albumin. In Anfinsen C, Edsall J, Richards F, editors: *Advances in protein chemistry,* vol 37, New York, 1985, Academic.
203. Polson R, Park G, Lindop M, et al: The prevention of renal impairment in patients undergoing orthotopic liver grafting by infusion of low dose dopamine, *Anesthesiology* 42:15, 1987.
204. Pond S, Tong T, Benowitz N, et al: Enhanced bioavailability of pethidine and pentazocine in patients with cirrhosis of the liver, *Aust NZ J Med* 10:515, 1980.
205. Popper H, Elias H, Petty DE: Vascular pattern in the cirrhotic liver, *Am J Clin Pathol* 22:717, 1952.
206. Posner JB, Plum F: The toxic effects of carbon dioxide and acetazolamide in hepatic encephalopathy, *J Clin Invest* 39:1246, 1960.
207. Powell-Jackson P, Greenway B, Williams R: Adverse effects of exploratory laparotomy in patients with unsuspected liver disease, *Br J Surg* 69:449–451, 1982.
208. Prytz H, Thomsen AC: Acid-base status in liver cirrhosis: disturbances in stable, terminal and porta-caval shunted patients, *Scand J Gastroenterol* 11:249, 1976.
209. Quintero E, Gines P, Arroyo V, et al: Paracentesis versus diuretics in the treatment of cirrhotics with tense ascites, *Lancet* 1:611, 1985.
210. Rakela J, Lange S, Ludwig J, et al: Fulminant hepatitis: Mayo Clinic experience with 34 cases, *Mayo Clin Proc* 60:289, 292, 1985.
211. Rappaport AM, Borowy ZJ, Lougheed WM, et al: Subdivision of hexagonal liver lobules into a structural and functional unit: role in hepatic physiology and pathology, *Anat Rec* 119:11, 1954.
212. Ratnoff OD: The hemostatic defects of liver disease. In Ofston D, Bennett B, editors: *Biochemistry, physiology, and pathology,* London, 1977, John Wiley & Sons.
213. Record C, Chase R, Alberts K, et al: Disturbances in glucose metabolism in patients with liver damage due to paracetamol overdose, *Clin Sci Mol Med* 49:473, 1975.
214. Richardson PDI, Withrington PG: The inhibition by glucagon of the vasoconstrictor actions of noradrenaline, angiotensin and vasopressin on the hepatic arterial vascular bed of the dog, *Br J Pharmacol* 57:93, 1976.
215. Rimola A, Gines P, Arroyo V, et al: Urinary excretion of 6-keto-prostaglandin F1 alpha, thromboxane B2 and prostaglandin E2 in cirrhosis with ascites: relationship to functional renal failure (hepatorenal syndrome), *J Hepatol* 3:111, 1986.
216. Ring-Larsen H, Palazzo J: Renal failure in fulminant hepatic failure and terminal cirrhosis: a comparison between incidence, types and prognosis, *Gut* 22:585, 1981.
217. Rocher I, Decourt S, Leneveu A, et al: Hemodynamic and pharmacokinetic study of propranolol and atenolol in cirrhosis patients, *Int J Clin Pharmacol Ther Toxicol* 23:406, 1985.
218. Rodriquez-Rosin R, Roca J, Agusti A, et al: Gas exchange and pulmonary vascular reactivity in patients with liver cirrhosis, *Am Rev Respir Dis* 135:1085, 1987.
219. Rossaint R, Slama K, Jaeger M, et al: Fluid restriction and early extubation for successful liver transplantation, *Transplant Proc* 22:1533, 1990.
220. Rossi G, Grendele M, Colledan M, et al: Prevention of hepatitis B virus reinfection after liver transplantation, First Symposium of the Society for Perioperative Care in Liver Transplantation (abstract), Pittsburgh, 1990.

221. Rothschild M, Oratz M, Zimmon D, et al: Albumin synthesis in cirrhotic subjects with ascites studies with carbonate-^{14}C, *J Clin Invest* 48:344, 1969.
222. Roussel JGJ, Kroon BBR, Hart GAM: The Denver type for peritoneovenous shunting of malignant ascites, *Surg Gynecol Obstet* 162:235, 1986.
223. Rowland M, Tozer TN: *Clinical pharmakokinetics,* ed 2, Philadelphia, 1989, Lea & Febiger.
224. Rydell R, Hoffbauer FW: Multiple pulmonary arteriovenous fistulas in juvenile cirrhosis, *Am J Med* 21:450, 1956.
225. Samson R, Trey C, Timme A, et al: Fulminating hepatitis with recurrent hypoglycemia and hemorrhage, *Gastroenterology* 53:291, 1967.
226. Samson Y, Bernuau J, Pappata S, et al: Cerebral uptake of benzodiazepine measured by positron emission tomography in hepatic encephalopathy, *N Engl J Med* 316:414, 1987.
227. Sanchez E, Tephly TR: Activation of hepatic microsomal glucuronyl transferase by bilirubin, *Life Sci* 13:1483, 1973.
228. Sanfey H, Boitnott JK, Cameron JL: Surgical management of patients with the Budd-Chiari syndrome, *World J Surg* 8:706, 1984.
229. Sanyal AJ, Freedman AM, Purdum PP, et al: The hematologic consequences of transjugular intrahepatic protosystemic shunts, *Hepatology* 23:32–39, 1996.
230. Sato S, Murakami A, Yoshida T, et al: Usefulness of antithrombin III and alpha 2-antiplasmin inhibitor in early differentiation of fulminant hepatitis and severe form of acute hepatitis, *Gastroenterol Jpn* 18:128, 1983.
231. Schafer D: Fulminant hepatic failure. In Thomas H, Jones E, editors: *Recent advances in hepatology,* vol 2, Edinburgh, 1986, Churchill-Livingstone.
232. Schafer D: Hepatic coma: studies on the target organ, *Gastroenterology* 93:1131, 1987.
233. Schafer D, Jones E: Hepatic encephalopathy and the gamma-aminobutyric acid neurotransmitter system, *Lancet* 1:18, 1982.
234. Schafer DF, Jones EA: Hepatic encephalopathy. In Zakim D, Boyer TD, editors: *Hepatology: A textbook of liver disease,* ed 2, Philadelphia, 1990, WB Saunders.
235. Schaffner F, Popper H: Capillarization of hepatic sinusoids, *Gastroenterology* 44:239, 1963.
236. Scheidt PC, Mellits ED, Hardy JB, et al: Toxicity to bilirubin in neonates: infant development during first year in relation to maximum neonatal serum bilirubin concentration, *J Pediatr* 91:292, 1977.
237. Schemel WH: Unexpected hepatic dysfunction found by multiple laboratory screening, *Anesth Analg* 55:810–812, 1976.
238. Schenk W, McDonald J, McDonald K, et al: Direct measurement of hepatic blood flow in surgical patients with related observations on hepatic flow dynamics in experimental animals, *Ann Surg* 156:463, 1962.
239. Schipper HG, Tencate JW: Antithrombin III transfusion in patients with hepatic cirrhosis, *Br J Haematol* 52:25, 1982.
240. Schrier R, Arroyo V, Bernardi M, et al: Peripheral arteriolar vasodilation hypothesis: A proposal for the initiation of renal sodium and water retention in cirrhosis, *Hepatology* 8:1151, 1988.
241. Schulman DS, Biondi JW, Matthay RA, et al: Effect of positive end-expiratory pressure on right ventricular performance: importance of baseline right ventricular function, *Am J Med* 84:57, 1988.
242. Scollo-LaVizzari G, Steinmann E: Reversal of hepatic coma by benzodiazepine antagonist (Ro 15-1788), *Lancet* i:1324, 1985.
243. Shear L, Ching S, Gabuzda G: Compartmentalization of ascites and edema in patients with hepatic cirrhosis, *N Engl J Med* 282:1391, 1970.
244. Sherlock S: *Disorders of the liver and biliary system,* ed 2, Oxford, 1989, Blackwell Scientific.
245. Sherlock S, Parbhoo S: The management of acute hepatic failure, *Postgrad Med J* 47:493, 1971.
246. Sherlock S, Scheuer P: The presentation and diagnosis of 100 patients with primary biliary cirrhosis, *N Engl J Med* 289:674, 1973.
247. Sherwin R, Joshe P, Hendler R, et al: Hyperglucagonemia in Laennec's cirrhosis, *N Engl J Med* 290:239, 1974.
248. Shub C, Tajik AJ, Seward JB, et al: Detecting intrapulmonary right to left shunting with contrast echocardiography: observations in a patient with diffuse pulmonary arteriovenous fistulas, *Mayo Clin Proc* 51:81, 1976.
249. Sie P, Letrenne E, Caranobe C, et al: Factor II related antigen and antithrombin III levels as indicators of liver failure in consumption coagulopathy, *Thromb Haemost* 47:218, 1982.
250. Silvani V, Mannucci PM, D'Angelo A, et al: The significance of protein C antigen in acute and chronic liver and biliary disease, *Am J Clin Pathol* 84:454, 1985.
251. Simon D, McCain J, Bonkovsky H, et al: Effects of therapeutic paracentesis on systemic and hepatic hemodynamics and on renal and hormonal function, *Hepatology* 7:423, 1987.
252. Sitzman J: 1991, Personal communication.
253. Slama K-J, Rossaint R, Jaeger M, et al: O_2 delivery during anesthesia for liver transplantation using a regimen of fluid restriction, *Transplant Proc* 22:1565, 1990.
254. Spector I, Corn M, Tictin HE: Effect of plasma transfusions on the prothrombin time and clotting factors in liver disease, *N Engl J Med* 275:1032, 1966.
255. Stahl J: Studies of the blood ammonia in liver disease, *Ann Intern Med* 58:1, 1963.
256. Starzl TE, Bell RH, Beart RW, et al: Hepatic trisegmentectomy and other liver resections, *Surg Gynecol Obstet* 141:429, 1975, 1991.
257. Starzl TE, Demetris AJ, Van Thiel D: Liver transplantation. Part I, *N Engl J Med* 321:1014, 1989.
258. Steegmuller KW, Marklin H-M, Hollis HW: Intraoperative hemodynamic investigations during portacaval shunt, *Arch Surg* 119:269, 1984.
259. Steele G: Technique of hepatic lobectomy. Trisegmentectomy, and a variety of hepatic wedge resections. In McDermott WV, editor: *Surgery of the liver,* Boston, 1989, Blackwell Scientific.
260. Stoller JK, Moodie D, Schiavone WA, et al: Reduction of intrapulmonary shunt and resolution of digital clubbing associated with primary biliary cirrhosis after liver transplantation, *Hepatology* 11:54, 1990.
261. Sugiura M, Futagawa S: Further evaluation of the Sugiura procedure in the treatment of esophageal varices, *Arch Surg* 112:1317, 1977.
262. Terblanche J, Yaleoob E, Bornman P: Acute bleeding varices: a five-year prospective evaluation of tamponade and sclerotherapy, *Ann Surg* 194:521, 1981.
263. Thompson P, Melmon K, Richardson J, et al: Lidocaine pharmacokinetics in advanced heart failure, liver disease, and renal failure in humans, *Ann Intern Med* 78:499, 1973.
264. Trewby P, Williams R: Pathophysiology of hypotension in patients with fulminant hepatic failure, *Gut* 18:1021, 1977.
265. Trewby P, Williams R, Williams A, et al: Intra-pulmonary vascular shunts in fulminant hepatic failure, *Digestion* 14:466, 1976.
266. Trey C, Davidson CS: The management of fulminant hepatic failure. In Popper H, Schaffner F, editors: *Progress in liver diseases,* New York, 1970, Grune & Stratton.
267. Van der Linden P, Le Moine O, Ghysels M, et al: Pulmonary hypertension after transjugula intrahepatic portosystemic shunt: effects on right ventricular function, *Hepatology* 23:982–987, 1996.
268. Villeneuve J-P, Fortunet-Fouin H, Arsene D: Cimetidine kinetics and dynamics in patients with severe liver disease, *Hepatology* 3:923, 1983.
269. Wagner PD, Naumann PF, Laravuso RB: Simultaneous measurement of eight foreign gases in blood by gas chromatography, *J Appl Physiol* 36:600, 1974.
270. Walker IR: Factors XI and XII are low in patients with liver disease, *Dig Dis Sci* 28:967, 1983.
271. Ward S, Neal E: Pharmacokinetics of atracurium in hepatic failure, *Br J Anaesth* 55:1169, 1983.
272. Ware AJ, D'Agostino AN, Combes B: Cerebral edema: a major complication of massive hepatic necrosis, *Gastroenterology* 61:877, 1971.
273. Warren SE, Mitas JA, Swerdin AHR: Hypernatremia in hepatic failure, *JAMA* 243:1257, 1980.
274. Westaby S, Wilkinson S, Williams R: Spleen size and portal hypertension in cirrhosis, *Digestion* 17:63, 1978.
275. Wiesner R, Mayo Clinic: 1991, Personal communication.
276. Wiesner RH: Acute fulminant hepatitis, First Symposium of the International Society for Perioperative Care in Liver Transplantation, Pittsburgh, 1990.
277. Wilder CE, Morrison RS, Tyler JM: Relationship between serum sodium and hyperventilation in cirrhosis, *Am Rev Respir Dis* 96:971, 1967.
278. Wilkinson P, Mendenhall C: Serum albumin turnover in normal subjects and patients with cirrhosis measured by I^{131}-labeled human albumin, *Clin Sci* 34:1, 1968.

279. Wilkinson SP, Blendis LM, Williams R: Frequency and type of renal and electrolyte disorders in fulminant hepatic failure, *Br Med J* 1:186, 1974.
280. Williams A, Trewby P, Williams R, et al: Structural alterations to the pulmonary circulation in fulminant hepatic failure, *Thorax* 34:447, 1979.
281. Williams R, Blackburn A, Neuberger J, et al: Long-term use of cyclosporin in liver grafting, *Q J Med* 57:897, 1985.
282. Williams R, Blaschke T, Meffin P, et al: Influence of viral hepatitis on the disposition of two compounds with high hepatic clearance: lidocaine and indocyanine green, *Clin Pharmacol Ther* 20:290, 1976.
283. Wion KL, Kelly D, Summerfield JA, et al: Distribution of factor VIII mRNA and antigen in human liver and other tissues, *Nature* 317:726, 1985.
284. Witte C, Witte M: Splanchnic circulatory and tissue fluid dynamics in portal hypertension, *Fed Proc* 42:287, 1986.
285. Witte M, Witte C, Dumont A: Estimated net transcapillary water and protein flux in the liver and intestines of patients with portal hypertension from hepatic cirrhosis, *Gastroenterology* 80:265, 1980.
286. Wright TL, Boyer TD: Diagnosis and management of cirrhotic ascites. In Zakim D, Boyer TD, editors: *Hepatology: A textbook of liver disease,* ed 2, Philadelphia, 1990, WB Saunders.
287. Wszolek Z, McComb R, Pfeiffer R, et al: Pontine and extrapontine myelinolysis following liver transplantation, *Transplantation* 48:1006, 1989.
288. Young C, Daneshmend T, Roberts C: Effects of cirrhosis and ageing on the elimination and bioavailability of ranitidine, *Gut* 23:819, 1982.
289. Zakim D: Metabolism of glucose and fatty acids by the liver. In Zakim D, Boyer TD, editors: *Hepatology: A textbook of liver disease,* ed 2, Philadelphia, 1990, WB Saunders.
290. Zakim D, Boyer TD, editors: *Hepatology: a textbook of liver disease,* ed 2, volume 1, Philadelphia, 1990, WB Saunders.
291. Zambraski EJ, DiBona GF: Sympathetic nervous system activity in hepatic cirrhosis. In Epstein M, editor: *The kidney in liver disease,* ed 3, Baltimore, 1988, Williams & Wilkins.
292. Zeldis JP, Friedman LS, Isselbacher KJ: Ranitidine: a new H_2-receptor antagonist, *N Engl J Med* 309:1368, 1983.
293. Ziemniak J, Bernhard J, Schentag J: Hepatic encephalopathy and altered cimetidine kinetics, *Clin Pharmacol Ther* 34:375, 1983.
294. Zieve L, Doizaki WM: Brain and blood methanethiol and ammonia concentrations in experimental hepatic coma and coma due to injections of various combinations of these substances, *Gastroenterology* 79:1070, 1980.
295. Zink J, Greenway C: Intraperitoneal pressure in formation and reabsorption of ascites in cats, *Am J Physiol* 233:H185, 1977.
296. Zinn SE, Fairley HB, Glenn JD: Liver function in patients with mild alcoholic hepatitis after enflurane, nitrous oxide-narcotic, and spinal anesthesia, *Anesth Analg* 64:87–90, 1985.
297. Zipser RD, Hoefs JC, Speckart PF, et al: Prostaglandins: modulators of renal function and pressor resistance in chronic liver disease, *J Clin Endocrinol Metab* 48:895, 1979.
298. Zipser RD, Radvan GH, Kronborg KJ, et al: Urinary thromboxane B_2 and prostaglandin E_2 in the hepatorenal syndrome: evidence for increased vasoconstrictor and decreased vasodilator factors, *Gastroenterology* 84:697, 1983.

CHAPTER 74

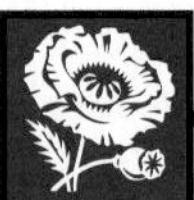

Anesthesia for Endocrine Surgery

ROSE CHRISTOPHERSON
WINSTON C. V. PARRIS

NEOPLASMS SECRETING VASOACTIVE SUBSTANCES

Pheochromocytoma

Pathophysiology

Pheochromocytoma is a catecholamine secreting tumor of the adrenal medulla. **Most pheochromocytomas secrete both epinephrine and norepinephrine, with a larger-than-normal proportion of the secretion as norepinephrine.** Pheochromocytomas are usually solitary tumors, occurring most commonly in the right adrenal, but they are bilateral in 10% of adults and 25% of children. Extra-adrenal origins in the paravertebral sympathetic nerves occur in 10% of cases. Almost all of these are intra-abdominal. Rarely, tumors occur in the neck, thorax, or urinary bladder.

Pheochromocytoma can occur in association with other diseases. Multiple endocrine neoplasia (MEN) type IIA includes pheochromocytoma, medullary carcinoma of the thyroid, and parathyroid hyperplasia; MEN type IIB includes pheochromocytoma, medullary carcinoma of the thyroid, and neuromas of the oral mucosa. Both von Recklinghausen's neurofibromatosis and von Hippel-Lindau disease may be associated with pheochromocytoma. When pheochromocytoma occurs as part of a familial syndrome, it is usually bilateral.

Pheochromocytomas occur most often in early to mid-adulthood. They are associated with paroxysms of hypertension severe enough to place patients at risk for cerebral hemorrhage, myocardial infarction (MI), dysrhythmia, and congestive heart failure (CHF). Paroxysms may be associated with physical stress on the tumor (e.g., pressure on the abdomen.) **Symptoms of pheochromocytoma include sweating, headache, palpitations, and tremor.** On physical examination, patients often have orthostatic hypotension, probably caused by reduced blood volume. Most patients with pheochromocytoma are hypertensive between attacks, although 10% are normotensive. Sequelae of chronic hypertension may be present.

Diagnosis is usually confirmed by measurement of urinary vanillylmandelic acid (VMA), metanephrine, and unconjugated catecholamines over a 24-hour period. Because of the paroxysmal nature of the disease, a failure to find elevated VMA on a single 24-hour urine collection does not rule out pheochromocytoma. In some cases, although VMA is not greatly increased, the ratio of norepinephrine to epinephrine is increased, and the diagnosis can be made on this basis. Urinary metanephrines are less reliably increased than VMA with pheochromocytoma.[19] See Chapter 17 for further discussion of diagnosis of pheochromocytoma.

Patient preparation

Preoperative preparation of the patient with pheochromocytoma is discussed in detail in Chapter 17. It consists of alpha blockade with phenoxybenzamine, phentolamine, and/or prazosin, and volume expansion. The choice of the pure $alpha_1$ blocker, prazosin, versus the $alpha_1$ and $alpha_2$ blockers, phenoxybenzamine and phentolamine, depends on the patient's symptoms and the pattern of catecholamine secretion. When $alpha_2$ presynaptic inhibitory neurons are blocked, feedback inhibition of norepinephrine release is lost. This can result in tachycardia, dysrhythmias, increased contractility, and cardiac ischemia caused by loss of feedback inhibition of cardiac $alpha_2$ receptors. Blockade of $alpha_1$ receptors only with prazosin can result in profound hypotension following the first dose. Because feedback inhibition of norepinephrine release is left intact, there is no release of norepinephrine in response to the decrease in blood pressure because of $alpha_1$ blockade.[14] Beta blockade may be added to alpha blockade for patients with severe tachydysrhythmias; however, beta blockade in patients who are not well alpha blocked may result in severe hypertension. It may take up to 2 weeks to establish appropriate adrenergic blockade and volume expansion preoperatively. It may be wise to withhold long-acting oral alpha and beta blockers the morning of surgery, so that patients are only partially blocked with these agents by the time the tumor is removed.[14]

Premedication with diazepam and promethazine appears to be safe; however, it does not prevent hypertension on arrival in the operating room.[13] Droperidol has been used; however, transient hypertension has also been reported in association with administration of droperidol to patients with pheocromocytoma.[14]

Monitoring

Monitoring requirements for intraoperative management may vary depending on the severity of the disease. Intra-arterial catheters are useful in all patients, because of the large changes in blood pressure that may be expected. Central venous access is necessary in all patients, both to confirm adequacy of intravascular volume and to administer multiple vasoactive drugs as required.

Patients with myocardial dysfunction caused by increased catecholamines may require monitoring with a pulmonary artery (PA) catheter. Indeed, a PA catheter may be useful in nearly all patients for the measurement of cardiac output and calculation of systemic vascular resistance (SVR). A decreased SVR is consistent with effective alpha blockade. The SVR has been used to determine whether a patient has a sufficient alpha blockade to tolerate beta blockade.[24] It is wise to insert these invasive monitors prior to induction (if not even further in advance of operation), to manage volume status and alpha and beta blockade. Cardiovascular instability can occur during the insertion of any of these monitors, because of the neurohumoral effects of the underlying disease.

Cardiovascular drugs

Phentolamine, nitroprusside (SNP), and beta blockers should be available. Nonetheless, very large doses of SNP are sometimes required to control hypertension. It is then useful to infuse phentolamine for basal control, using SNP for rapid changes and fine control. Use of nitroglycerin has been reported[14]; but it reduces preload, so it should be considered only when adequate volume status has been confirmed by central venous or pulmonary artery wedge pressure. Magnesium sulfate ($MgSO_4$) has been used as a sole agent or supplemented by SNP and phentolamine with good results.[15] Esmolol has been used successfully by intravenous bolus and by infusion at standard doses.[24] Short-acting agents are preferable, because serum catecholamines decrease quickly to normal after excision of the tumor. Large doses of long-acting alpha and beta blockade may then exacerbate hypotension. For a summary of reported adverse drug reactions in patients with pheochromocytoma see Table 74-1. Resection of a pheochromocytoma can be accompanied by significant blood loss, therefore adequate venous access and blood products must be available for continued volume resuscitation.

Anesthetic management

A number of anesthetic regimens have been used successfully. Although adverse reactions have been reported with many drugs (Table 74-1), those same drugs have been used safely in selected patients. Midazolam has been used to sedate patients without adverse consequences. **Drugs associated with histamine release, including morphine, curare, and atracurium, probably should not be used, because histamine provokes release of catecholamines from chromaffin granules.** Probably the safest muscle relaxant for patients with pheochromocytoma is vecuronium, which causes no histamine or catecholamine release and is not associated with significant heart rate or blood pressure changes in intubating doses. Etomidate may be an attractive induction agent, because it does not cause histamine release or hypotension. Fentanyl or alfentanil are good choices for induction and maintenance narcotics because they do not cause histamine release.[14] Because hypertension occurs frequently at the time of laryngoscopy,[4] it is wise to administer one of these narcotics to blunt this response. If the tumor has been successfully resected, longer-acting narcotics (e.g., morphine) may be used postoperatively, because histamine release should no longer cause release of abnormally large amounts of catecholamines.

Nitrous oxide and enflurane can be used for maintenance of anesthesia.[15] Halothane and isoflurane are probably less attractive agents for maintenance because of their tendencies to sensitize the heart to catecholamine-induced dysrhythmias and to exacerbate tachycardia, respectively.

It may be necessary to support the blood pressure with phenylephrine after ligation of veins draining the tumor. A patient who was treated primarily with a long-acting beta blocker required an epinephrine infusion to support the blood pressure for 24 hours postoperatively.[15]

Carcinoid Tumors and Carcinoid Syndrome

Pathophysiology

Carcinoid tumors arise from endocrine argentaffin or Kulchitsky cells in the lung, small intestine, bronchi, or ovaries. These cells are involved in amine precursor uptake and decarboxylation (APUD). The intestinal tumors are

Table 74-1 Adverse reactions to drugs in patients with pheochromocytoma

Drug	Reaction
Beta blockers[4]	Hypertension in patients with inadequate alpha blockade
Prazosin[14]	Hypotension on first dose due to negative feedback from unblocked presynaptic $alpha_2$ receptors
Droperidol[4,14]	Transient hypertension
Succinylcholine[4,14]	Hypertension, possibly due to fasciculations causing pressure on tumor; dysrhythmias; catecholamine release due to cholinergic agonism
Pancuronium[4,14]	Hypertension; indirect sympathomimetic agent causing increased catecholamines
Halothane[4,14]	Sensitization of heart to catecholamine-induced dysrhythmias
Phenoxybenzamine[14] Phentolamine[14]	Tachycardia and cardiac ischemia due to blockade of cardiac presynaptic $alpha_2$ inhibitory receptors
Morphine[14]	Histamine release from chromaffin granules
Tubocurarine[14]	Histamine release, one fatality
Atracurium[14]	Histamine release
Atropine[14]	Potentiates catecholamine-induced tachycardia

found most often in the appendix and ileum. In either location, they secrete serotonin. Carcinoid tumors may also secrete insulin, adrenocorticotrophic hormone, melanocyte-stimulating hormone, gastrin, glucagon, bradykinin, substance P, histamine, prostaglandins, vasoactive intestinal peptide, calcitonin, or numerous other substances.[17]

Carcinoid syndrome occurs rarely. Carcinoid tumors of the gut can produce carcinoid syndrome only if they are metastatic to the liver. Bronchial and other carcinoid tumors outside the gut, in which endocrine secretions are not immediately cleared by the liver, can produce carcinoid syndrome without metastasis. Overall, only approximately 5% of patients with carcinoid tumors have the symptoms of carcinoid syndrome. **The symptoms of carcinoid syndrome include flushing, diarrhea, anxiety, wheezing, tachycardia, salivation, lacrimation, hyperthermia, and facial edema.** Endocardial and valvular fibrosis occur downstream of the tumor, that is, in the right side of the heart in intestinal tumors, and in the left side of the heart in bronchial tumors. Typically, valvular disease is a combination of pulmonary stenosis and tricuspid insufficiency, possibly with right heart failure, in patients with extrapulmonary tumors.[17]

Preoperative management

Because of the large number of vasoactive substances that are secreted by carcinoid tumors, anesthetic management is challenging. Bouts of hypertension, tachycardia, hypotension, and bronchospasm have been reported in response to histamine release, exogenous or endogenous catecholamines, and physical stimuli such as preoperative abdominal scrubbing or succinylcholine-induced fasciculations.[17] Pretreatment of these patients with a number of medications, including somatostatin, its long-acting analog octreotide,[17,28] H1 and H2 blockers,[13,17] and methylprednisolone, which blocks prostaglandin synthesis,[28] is advisable.

Patients with any signs or symptoms suggestive of right-sided heart failure or valvular lesions should have a preoperative diagnostic workup sufficient to characterize valvular lesions and cardiac function.

Monitoring

Invasive hemodynamic monitoring with an intra-arterial catheter is appropriate for any patients with carcinoid syndrome, because they are prone to both severe hypertension and severe hypotension. If insertion of an intra-arterial catheter is delayed until a carcinoid crisis occurs, it may be difficult to cannulate the artery because of severe vasospasm.[21] Central venous access should be obtained, both to assess volume status and to administer drugs. Patients with carcinoid syndrome often have diarrhea and may be dehydrated. Patients with valvular lesions or failure of the right side of the heart may benefit from a PA catheter for monitoring and diagnosis of cardiovascular changes. It may not be easy to position the catheter, however, in the presence of tricuspid regurgitation and pulmonary stenosis. In one series of patients with carcinoid syndrome, all were monitored with a PA catheter, and no difficulty with proper placement was noted. The prevalence and severity of valvular lesions were also not reported in this series.[36]

Anesthesia

The goal should be to maintain the patient as stable and stress free as possible. All drugs that cause histamine release, as well as catecholamines and drugs that cause release of endogenous catecholamines, should be avoided. Patients with carcinoid syndrome reputedly awaken slowly,[36] so extubation at the end of the case should not be a primary goal. Facilities for postoperative ventilation should be available. Induction with droperidol 0.15 mg/kg, fentanyl 15 μg/kg, pancuronium, and topical lidocaine, with maintenance of 65% NO, fentanyl 500 μg/hr, and pancuronium as needed, has resulted in a stable course.[36] Another stable anesthetic resulted from induction with fentanyl 250 μg, etomidate 10 mg, and vecuronium 6 mg, with maintenance provided by isoflurane and N_2O.[32]

Systemic Mastocytosis

Pathophysiology

Systemic mastocytosis is a clinical syndrome characterized by the abnormal proliferation of mast cells. It is manifested by dizziness, flushing, palpitations, pruritis, dermographia, nausea, vomiting, diarrhea, hypotension, syncope, and in some cases cardiovascular collapse. The syndrome tends to involve the reticuloendothelial system, especially the spleen, liver, and bone marrow, but it may involve all the tissues of the body with the possible exception of the central nervous system (CNS).

Patients with systemic mastocytosis have proliferating mast cells that contain large metachromatic granules which secrete large quantities of histamine, heparin, serotonin, substance P, and hyaluronic acid. Most of the symptoms are related to these substances. The etiology of the disease may be multifactorial. The natural course of the disease is variable. In childhood, a cutaneous form called *urticaria pigmentosa* occurs. It is not usually associated with systemic symptoms or cardiovascular collapse. It regresses spontaneously in approximately 50% of patients. If it continues into adulthood, however, subsequent regression is rare.

Acute exacerbations of systemic mastocytosis do not respond to H1 and H2 blockers. Patients having acute exacerbations overproduce prostaglandin D2 (PGD2), which is a potent peripheral vasodilator.[41] When combined with antihistaminic drugs, aspirin, and other nonsteroidal anti-inflammatory drugs (which inhibit prostaglandin synthesis) may both prevent exacerbations and control symptoms during ongoing attacks Epinephrine in small doses has been shown to be very effective in controlling the symptoms of systemic mastocytosis. It occupies beta receptors on mast cells, causing inhibition of prostaglandin and histamine release.[40]

Mast cell activators include most narcotic analgesics, some radiologic contrast media, ethyl alcohol, many muscle relaxants, preservatives in some medications, some antibiotics, nonsteroidal anti-inflammatory agents (for some patients), alpha adrenergic agonists, cholinergic receptor agonists, ester-linked local anesthetics, thiobarbituates, dextran, decamethonium, and thiamine. Some foods may also cause exacerbations of mastocytosis.

Preoperative management

Most patients with systemic mastocytosis who present for elective surgery are well-controlled with a number of medications including H1 and H2 blockers, somatostatin, and nonsteroidal anti-inflammatory drugs. Patients whose disease is well controlled should receive their regularly scheduled medications on the day of operation. It is prudent to postpone operation in patients scheduled for elective procedures if there is a clinical suspicion of undiagnosed systemic mastocytosis.

Preoperative laboratory tests should include serum PGD2 and histamine, urine PGD2 metabolites, prostaglandin F2 alpha, and 5-HIAA, as well as routine tests indicated for the type of surgery.

Intradermal skin tests should be performed prior to operation for all agents that may be administered during anesthesia. Preservative-free normal saline may be used as a control. 0.1 ml of each agent is injected intradermally. The test is positive if an area of hyperemia greater than 1 cm or induration greater than 1 mm occurs.

Monitoring

The use of invasive hemodynamic monitoring, especially an intra-arterial catheter, must be weighed against the stress that may accompany vascular cannulation, and the need to give sedation or local anesthesia for insertion of catheters. It may be advisable to induce anesthesia before invasive monitors are inserted. Depending upon the severity of the disease and the type of operation, PA catheterization may be necessary.

Anesthesia

Choice of anesthesia may include local anesthesia, with sedation, for minor surgery. Nonetheless, the patient should be protected from emotional stress, loud noises, and hypothermia, and skin tests are required for all drugs that may be used.

Just before general anesthesia, diphenhydramine 25 mg should be administered intravenously as prophylaxis against histamine release. A second dose should be given prior to endotracheal (ET) intubation. Induction using an inhalation technique is advisable. Inhalational agents, especially ether-linked halogenated compounds, have been shown in animal studies to inhibit degranulation of mast cells.[39] We recommend the use of isoflurane with N_2O, if there is no other contraindication. More recently introduced inhalational agents (desflurane, seroflurane) have not yet been tested in these patients. IV fluids should be administered generously (500 to 1000 ml) during induction to compensate for anesthesia-induced vasodilation. Noise and other sensory stimuli should be controlled during induction, because these may stimulate degranulation of mast cells. Several serious cardiovascular events have occurred during anesthesia induction associated with loud noise.

If possible, the trachea should be intubated without aid of a muscle relaxant. If relaxants are required, vecuronium or pancuronium should be relatively safe. Succinylcholine has been used, usually without complications, but there have been a few reports of major cardiovascular problems following its administration. Newer muscle relaxants have not yet been tested in this population of patients.

Anesthesia may be maintained with O_2, isoflurane, and NO. Isoflurane may protect the patient by inhibiting mast cell degranulation.[39] Thus, this phase of anesthesia is usually uneventful. Joints and bony prominences should be protected from pressure, because continued pressure may cause hemarthroses or ecchymosis due to heparin released by mast cells. Extremes of temperature may provoke exacerbation of mastocytosis, therefore, temperature control in the operating room is important.

If an acute exacerbation of mastocytosis occurs intraoperatively, it should be treated first with a small bolus of epinephrine, 0.5 μg/kg. This should be followed, if needed, by an epinephrine infusion of 1-3 μg/kg/minute. This is the mainstay of management of complications of systemic mastocytosis.[40] Any drugs, anesthetic agents, or interventions suspected of causing the exacerbation should be stopped. O_2 concentration should be increased; appropriate supportive care such as IV fluids should be administered. Serum histamine and urine and serum samples for PGD2 and prostaglandin F2 alpha should be obtained.

Awakening patients from anesthesia can reintroduce stresses they may have been prevented by deeper levels of anesthesia during operation. Muscle relaxants may be reversed in the usual manner. If patients have not received a muscle relaxant, the trachea should be extubated during deep anesthesia to avoid possible laryngospasm and subsequent requirement for muscle relaxant. Noise levels and other sensory stimuli must be eliminated. Emotional or physical stress can cause an exacerbation, thus leaving the trachea intubated is not without risk.

THYROIDECTOMY

Anatomy

The thyroid gland consists of two lateral lobes connected by an isthmus, which crosses the trachea inferior to the thyroid cartilage at approximately the second to fourth tracheal rings. As the thyroid enlarges, it can extend retrosternally. It may displace and occasionally impair the function of the recurrent laryngeal nerve, which lies in a groove between and just lateral to the trachea and esophagus. The recurrent laryngeal nerve courses through the thyroid fascia or between branches of arteries supplying the thyroid in 25% of patients.[16] The thyroid can displace the carotid sheath. It can extend posterior to the trachea and larynx and it can enlarge greatly on one or both sides of the airway, causing deviation and/or compression of airway structures. Thyroid carcinoma can also invade any of these structures.

Anatomic abnormalities remote from the site of operation occur in association with thyroid disease. Patients with hyperthyroidism or a history of hyperthyroidism may have exophthalmos, placing them at increased risk for perioperative corneal abrasions. Patients with congenital hypothyroidism may have greatly enlarged tongues, making both ventilation and intubation difficult.

Pathophysiology

The thyroid gland produces thyroxine (T4) and a small amount of triiodothyronine (T3). T4 is cleaved in the peripheral tissues to T3, which is the more potent thyroid hormone. For a discussion of normal ranges of these hormones, diagnosis, and preoperative treatment of hypothyroidism and hyperthyroidism, see Chapter 17.

Congenital absence of thyroid hormones results in cretinism, a combination of mental retardation, dwarfism, and coarsened facial features. Fortunately, this condition is now rare. **Adult onset hypothyroidism results in gradual onset of mental slowness; reduced basal metabolic rate (BMR) with associated obesity, hypothermia, cold intolerance, fatigue, dry skin, constipation, hoarseness, edema, and goiter. In severe cases, there may be a reduction in cardiac function caused by cardiomyopathy and bradycardia.** The diagnosis is often delayed, because patients tend not to complain of these symptoms, because their mental function slows. Thus adult onset hypothyroidism, or myxedema, is relatively common. Myxedema can and in most cases should be treated with thyroid hormone replacement. This treatment, however, may cause tachycardia and increased myocardial oxygen demand. Therefore, in patients with known or suspected coronary artery disease (CAD), appropriate monitoring should be considered as thyroid hormone replacement is administered. Patients with cardiomyopathy or bradycardia caused by myxedema but who do not have CAD should benefit from thyroid hormone replacement.

Hyperthyroidism occurs most commonly in women 20 to 40 years of age and may be caused by autoimmune mechanisms. Patients may have an increased sensitivity to catecholamines. Exophthalmos is common, requiring special attention to eye protection. Patients usually have goiters, which may compromise their airways directly or through dysfunction of the recurrent laryngeal nerve.

The most common form of thyrotoxicosis is Graves' disease. It often goes into long periods of remission; therefore it is usually treated with antithyroid drugs or radioactive iodine rather than operation. Patients with Graves' disease may have severe ophthalmopathy, which usually resolves with attainment of euthyroid condition. Toxic nodular goiter involves hyperfunction of one or many thyroid nodules. Spontaneous remission is rare. Radioactive iodine or operation are the usual treatments. Silent thyroiditis is a condition of periods of thyrotoxicosis interspersed with euthyroidism. It is self-limited, but biopsy of the gland may be required for diagnosis.[10] Chronic lymphoid (Hashimoto's) thyroiditis is difficult to diagnose without a biopsy, but this form of euthyroid goiter responds to the same treatment as other types of benign nontoxic thyroid enlargement, and biopsy may not be necessary. Subacute thyroiditis can appear with thyrotoxicosis and may require biopsy for diagnosis. Acute thyroiditis is caused by bacterial infection and is essentially an abscess. Patients almost always are euthyroid. Incision and drainage are often necessary.[16]

Monitoring

For a simple thyroidectomy in an otherwise healthy patient, noninvasive monitoring with electrocardiogram, sphygmomanometer, end-tidal capnometer, pulse oximeter, and thermometer is sufficient. There should be a low threshold, however, for invasive blood pressure monitoring with an intra-arterial catheter in patients who have large tumors that will require dissection near the carotid arteries. Such dissection can stimulate reflexes that result in bradycardia and hypotension. Straightforward thyroidectomy should be a relatively brief procedure with no hidden blood loss and no major fluid shifts; therefore a urinary catheter should not be necessary. The thyroid gland is very vascular, and uncontrolled bleeding can occur if vessels are cut before ligation.

In cases where the thyroid is very large, the surgeon may retract the larynx during dissection. This can cause intermittent ball-valve obstruction of the ET tube with impaired expiratory flow, which can result in a rising intrathoracic pressure and reduced venous return with each positive pressure breath. This situation can be detected quickly by direct intra-arterial pressure monitoring. It can be treated by less vigorous retraction (if possible), or by making the patient apneic for brief periods of retraction.

Patients with cardiomyopathies, CHF, or severe CAD may need central venous or PA catheters to monitor the effects of anesthesia on cardiovascular function. Such monitoring is not required for the operation itself, which usually involves no significant fluid shifts and little blood loss.

Airway

Large goiters may make tracheal intubation difficult. The extent of the goiter and its displacement or impingement on the airway can be evaluated by physical examination and by computed tomography (CT) or magnetic resonance imaging (MRI) scan. Recurrent laryngeal nerve function should be evaluated preoperatively by mirror or fiberoptic examination of the vocal cords. The enlarged thyroid may impinge on a recurrent laryngeal nerve, causing vocal cord paralysis. When paralysis is unilateral, it causes hoarseness but no compromise to respiration.[16] Usually the trachea can be intubated in the conventional way, using oral laryngoscopy after induction of general anesthesia and paralysis. Short-acting relaxants should be used, however, because occasionally oral intubation may be difficult or impossible. Alternatives include blind nasal intubation, fiberoptic oral or nasal intubation, or a laryngeal mask airway (although the latter is not generally recommended for the operation itself, because direct access to the oral cavity is limited by the sterile surgical field).

Unilateral damage to the recurrent laryngeal nerve may occur in 1% to 3% of thyroidectomies. Bilateral nerve damage is much more rare. Loss of recurrent laryngeal nerve function may be caused by blunt surgical trauma, inadvertent ligation of the nerve, or sectioning of the nerve. The involved cord is first flaccid, then spastic. Function usually returns within 3 to 9 months. Occasionally, when the nerve has been ligated, removal of the ligature may restore function. Therefore reexploration of the wound may be indicated if new vocal cord paralysis is discovered postoperatively.[16]

There are a number of possible causes of postoperative respiratory distress, including bilateral vocal cord paralysis, hemorrhage, and laryngeal edema. Tracheomalacia may occur after surgery for carcinoma. In the past, we performed laryngoscopic examination postoperatively to determine whether vocal cord paralysis was present. However, the probability of bilateral cord paralysis is extremely low. Therefore, we no longer perform this examination. The surgeon may request postoperative laryngoscopy during spontaneous ventilation if bilateral vocal cord damage is suspected. In that case, the trachea can be extubated during deep anesthesia, and laryngoscopy can be performed at the time of extubation. A paralyzed cord does not move, lies in midposition, and is at a slightly lower level in the larynx than the opposite cord.[7]

Reintubation for unilateral vocal cord paralysis is not indicated if this is the patient's only problem. Edema of the false cords is often found within 24 hours of operation, probably caused by external trauma to the larynx and temporary reduction in venous or lymphatic drainage. Unilateral vocal cord paralysis may exacerbate airway compromise because of edema during the postoperative period. It is reasonable to extubate the trachea in patients with unilateral cord paralysis if they can be observed closely for a number of hours postoperatively. Bilateral vocal cord paralysis requires continued endotracheal intubation until full recovery, and until a plan of action for chronic care is devised.

Postoperative hemorrhage is the most acute airway complication of thyroidectomy. The immediate surgical treatment is reopening of the wound and removal of the hematoma.[16] It may be necessary for the anesthesiologist to immediately reintubate the trachea, because even small amounts of bleeding in the area of the thyroid gland can cause significant, rapid obstruction of the airway. If reintubation is delayed, it may become much more difficult because of local swelling and tracheal deviation.

Induction

The main consideration in choosing induction agents for patients undergoing thyroidectomy involves an analysis of specific airway abnormalities. In general, short-acting agents are desirable because, if the trachea cannot be intubated using oral laryngoscopy, then spontaneous ventilation will resume promptly. Airways that are compromised or displaced by goiter or even thyroid cancer are unlikely to collapse; therefore induction with inhalational agents while maintaining spontaneous ventilation is acceptable. Long-acting neuromuscular blockade at the time of induction is unadvisable because tracheal intubation will be difficult, even in some patients with small goiters.

Positioning

After induction and intubation, the patient should be positioned with padding under his/her shoulders to extend the neck. Alternatively, an inflatable bag may be placed under the patient's shoulders. This may be inflated intraoperatively to extend the neck, then deflated to facilitate closure. The head of the table should be elevated slightly to facilitate venous return. The knees and hips may be flexed slightly, to maintain venous drainage, but the legs should remain slightly lower than the surgical site. The elbows should be padded and the arms tucked at the sides.

The head should be positioned symmetrically on a head ring. Optimal surgical exposure requires significant neck extension. Overextension that allows the weight of the head to hang on the spine may cause severe postoperative neck pain, vertebral artery compression, and if combined with sufficient pressure exerted at the surgical site, even dislocation or fracture of the spine. The anesthetist should verify that most of the weight of the head is actually supported by the head ring and operating table and not by the cervical spine. The patient may be positioned so that the hinge between the head and back sections of the operating table is under the first or second thoracic vertebra. This allows neck extension to be increased intraoperatively if necessary. This manipulation has not proven necessary when an inflatable bag has been used under the shoulders. If neck extension is increased intraoperatively by any manipulation, the anesthetist must reconfirm that the table and head ring continue to bear the weight of the head. Special attention must be paid to eye protection for patients with exophthalmos.

Maintenance

The two greatest stimuli, after laryngoscopy, are skin incision and manipulation of the larynx that causes contact with the ET tube. Injection of a long-acting local anesthetic at the surgical site reduces both response to incision and the need for postoperative narcotics. Stimulation of the airway mucosa can be blunted by IV lidocaine, either given in 20- to 40-mg boluses as needed or as a continuous infusion. Maintenance of general anesthesia for thyroidectomy can be difficult, because most of the operation is not stimulating and hypotension may occur. Patients often do not tolerate deep anesthesia because of the lack of stimulation; then when the airway mucosa is stimulated, they exhibit both motor (coughing) and cardiovascular responses (hypertension, tachycardia).

Because IV lidocaine has relatively little effect on blood pressure and heart rate, yet it blunts airway reactivity, it is a useful adjunct. Some surgeons may wish to stimulate the recurrent laryngeal nerve to confirm its identity, but most are satisfied with anatomic identification. Paralysis with a nondepolarizing muscle relaxant makes the maintenance of a light anesthetic plane possible. Nitrous oxide is not contraindicated in thyroid surgery. Isoflurane reportedly does not cause increases in T4 outside the normal range,[26] whereas both ether and halothane do.[25] These considerations, while of theoretical interest, should not be of practical importance in patients who have been properly prepared preoperatively and are euthyroid.

PARATHYROIDECTOMY

Pathophysiology

Since the advent of automated clinical chemistry screening tests, the prevalence of primary hyperparathyroidism has been discovered to be 0.1% to 0.2%. The majority of patients who have hyperparathyroidism are asymptomatic patients with increased serum calcium levels. The diagnosis is made when the parathyroid hormone (PTH) level is also increased. The peak incidence of primary hyperparathyroidism is in the sixth and seventh decade; it is more common in women than in men. Most patients (80% to 85%) have a single parathyroid adenoma. Less commonly, all four glands may be hyperplastic; this may be idiopathic or it may occur in conjunction with MEN type I or II. Fewer than 1% of patients with primary hyperparathyroidism have parathyroid carcinoma.[16]

The relation of hypercalcemia to parathyroid hormone and vitamin D metabolism is discussed in detail in Chapter 17. Patients with mildly increased serum calcium are frequently asymptomatic or have nonspecific symptoms, including poor appetite, depression, weakness, and joint pain. Hypertension may be present, due either to renal damage or to mechanisms involving renin or hypercalcemia.[16] There is controversy regarding whether or not these patients should undergo parathyroidectomy.[3,16,18]

Hyperparathyroidism was originally described as a "disease of bones and stones," because the disease was diagnosed only when it had reached an advanced stage with evidence of demineralization of bone and formation of renal calculi. Hyperparathyroidism causes increased excretion of phosphate and a more alkaline urine than normal, as well as increased calcium excretion. This leads to formation of renal calculi, nephrocalcinosis, and in severe cases, polyuria and polydipsia.

Chronic severe hyperparathyroidism can lead to hypercalcemic crisis, with serum calcium values of 16 mg/dl or greater. This occurs in patients with longstanding renal failure, who then develop anorexia, vomiting, polyuria, and muscle weakness. They may progress to lethargy, confusion, severe weakness, and coma. The QT interval of the ECG becomes very short when serum calcim is increased markedly. Medical therapy should begin with rehydration using normal saline at a rate of 250 to 300 ml/hr. Once adequate volume status is achieved, a loop diuretic, such as furosemide, should be administered to increase calcium excretion. Thiazide diuretics should not be administered, because they tend to reduce renal excretion of calcium. Patients requiring this treatment may also require monitoring of central venous or PA pressure, because they are at risk both for fluid overload and exacerbation of dehydration.

Patients who are having a hypercalcemic crisis caused by hyperparathyroidism should undergo parathyroidectomy as soon as possible after restoration of intravascular volume and calcium diuresis, because prolonged medical therapy is associated with mortality.[16] Thus significantly hypercalcemic patients may occasionally present for relatively urgent surgery. Severely hypercalcemic patients are very sensitive to digitalis and can develop toxicity at relatively low serum digitalis values.[16]

Anatomy

There are usually four parathyroid glands; however, in an autopsy study, only three glands were found in 13% of subjects, and five glands were found in 6%.[16] The superior parathyroid glands develop along with the thyroid from the fourth branchial pouch, and because they migrate very little during development, they are found in association with the superior thyroid artery behind the upper pole of the thyroid. The inferior parathyroid glands are more variable because they develop with the thymus from the third branchial pouch, then migrate to a lower position. They are usually found behind the lower pole of the thyroid gland, in association with the inferior thyroid artery, but they may be found anywhere from just below the mandible to the pericardium.[16]

Surgical approach

As noninvasive imaging technology improves, the surgical approach to parathyroidectomy is likely to change. Currently, there is no noninvasive imaging technique reliable enough to consider it unnecessary to explore both sides of the neck. Sampling of neck veins for different levels of parathyroid hormone does not always give a clear location of the adenoma(s). Although arteriography can be useful, it has also been associated with several cases of hemi- and quadriplegia.[16] The safest way to locate the parathyroid adenoma is to identify all parathyroid glands intraoperatively on both sides of the neck. If one gland is enlarged, it is removed, and a biopsy is also taken from a normal gland. Pathologic confirmation of the identity of the adenoma and of normal parathyroid tissue is obtained. If all the glands are hyperplastic, a subtotal parathyroidectomy is performed, removing all but one gland or part of one gland. The surgeon's goal is to identify the adenomatous or hyperplastic gland and remove it on the first operation, leaving some normal tissue behind, because re-explorations are more likely to be associated with complications. The recurrent laryngeal nerve is used as a landmark for locating the parathyroid glands; therefore the surgeon tends to identify it early in the dissection.[16] As in thyroidectomy, the recurrent laryngeal nerve can be damaged during dissection, and this is more likely to occur during re-exploration, when the nerve may be hidden in scar tissue.

Despite the generally accepted policy of exploring both sides of the neck, good results have been reported from unilateral neck explorations under local anesthesia in high-risk patients. A combination of ultrasound, thallium subtraction scanning, and CT scanning was used to localize the tumors, then the exploration was performed using an incision over the sternocleidomastoid rather than the usual low cervical incision and bilateral dissection. Two of the 29 patients in the series had hyperplasia in all four glands; therefore, they required second operations.[30] As diagnostic imaging improves, this approach may become more common.

Anesthetic management

The anesthetic management for parathyroidectomy is similar to that for thyroidectomy. In both cases, the surgery is not a major physiologic trespass: blood loss is minimal and fluid shifts are not common. No invasive hemodynamic monitoring is required based on the surgical procedure, although such monitoring may be required in occasional cases because of concomitant medical problems.

Because parathyroid adenomas are almost always small, they do not cause deviation or compression of the airway. No unusual precautions need to be taken when preparing to intubate the trachea. Any hypnotic and barbiturate may be used. The choice of long- versus short-acting muscle relaxant should be made based on the surgeon's desire to test the function of the recurrent laryngeal nerve; however, it is usually not necessary to test the nerve to identify it. One severely hypercalcemic parathyroid patient had an accelerated rate of metabolism of atracurium but problems with neuromuscular blockers are not common.[2] Positioning for parathyroidectomy is similar to that for thyroidectomy and is described in that section of this chapter.

Anesthetic maintenance may require frequent changes in depth of anesthesia, because the procedure alternates between neck exploration and the wait for biopsy results. The operation is not very stimulating, except for skin incision and any stimulation of the laryngeal and tracheal mucosa as glottic structures are moved against the ET tube. Because the recurrent laryngeal nerve can be damaged intraoperatively, it may be appropriate to examine the vocal cords after extubation in the operating room. This is discussed in detail in the section on airway management for thyroidectomy.

Postoperative complications

Postoperative complications include hemorrhage, hematoma, and damage to the recurrent laryngeal nerve. These occur rarely. Obviously, a large hematoma could cause airway obstruction, which could be relieved by reintubation or drainage of the hematoma. Recurrent laryngeal nerve damage must be bilateral to cause airway compromise, and this is extremely rare in first operations on either the thyroid or parathyroid.

Hypoparathyroidism can occur transiently after excision of the adenoma(s). It is most common in patients with underlying renal disease, who tend to lose calcium, or patients with bone disease, who may absorb large amounts of calcium into their bones as the parathyroid hormone level decreases. The serum calcium tends to be least on the second or third postoperative day. Serum calcium should be measured every 12 hours for several days. **Hypocalcemic patients experience an increase in neuromuscular excitability, which can develop into tetany, carpopedal spasm, and laryngeal stridor.** This can be fatal. The QT interval is prolonged in hypocalcemic patients. The treatment for hypocalcemia in the first few postoperative days is IV calcium gluconate, 1 to 2 g over 8 hours. Usually, the hypoparathyroidism is transient. For more persistent hypocalcemia, patients are given oral calcium supplements.

DIABETES

Associated Diseases

A number of disease conditions are associated with diabetes (Box 74-1). These diseases increase the probability both that

BOX 74-1
COMPLICATIONS OF DIABETES MELLITUS

Macrovascular disease
- Coronary atherosclerosis
- Peripheral vascular disease

Microvascular disease
- Nephropathy
- Retinopathy

Neuropathy
- Distal polyneuropathies
- Neuromuscular disease
- Acute mononeuropathy
- Autonomic neuropathy
  - Gastrointestinal
  - Genitourinary
  - Cardiovascular

Dermopathy

a diabetic patient will require operation and that perioperative morbidity will be increased. The prevalence of diabetes depends on the definition used for diagnosis. It is approximately 1% overall in the U.S. with approximately 25% of diabetics insulin dependent (type 1) and the remainder non-insulin dependent (type 2).[8] **The perioperative mortality of diabetic patients has been reported as 3.7% to 13.2%.**[12] Perioperative morbidity and mortality often result from concomitant diseases.

Atherosclerotic vascular disease occurs 2.5 times more frequently in people with diabetes than in the general population. CAD and CHF are the cause of death of more than 70% of patients with diabetes.[9] CAD is especially insidious in these patients, because it may be asymptomatic or have atypical symptomatology, including epigastric distress, neck or bilateral shoulder pain, or symptoms of CHF. CAD may also occur in patients with type I diabetes as early as the late teens.[9] It often involves distal and proximal stenoses and therefore may not be treatable with angioplasty or coronary artery bypass grafting. Cardiomyopathy may be seen in patients with angiographically normal coronary arteries, probably caused by microvascular disease.[8] The anesthesiologist caring for a diabetic surgical patient must assess, monitor, and treat any cardiac disease that may be present.

Diabetic patients compose approximately one fourth to one third of all patients with peripheral vascular disease. They frequently require lower extremity bypass grafting. Because they often have distal disease that is not amenable to grafting, they frequently also require amputation. CAD is common in patients with peripheral vascular disease; therefore, diabetic patients require especially careful cardiovascular assessment, monitoring, and treatment.

Diabetic microvascular disease includes nephropathy and retinopathy, both of which begin to appear approximately 15 years after the diagnosis of type I diabetes. Nephropathy is first apparent as albuminuria, which progresses to azotemia over approximately 10 years.[9] Renal insufficiency with associated hypertension tends to exacerbate all vascular complications of diabetes. Diabetic patients have difficulties with hemodialysis because of their metabolic instability and atherosclerosis. They are frequent recipients of renal transplants. With increasing frequency, renal transplants have been accompanied by transplantation of pancreatic tissue. This can be curative for the diabetes.[8] **Out of 60 diabetic patients evaluated before renal transplantation with thallium stress tests and/or cardiac catheterization, 23 (38%) were found to have significant CAD.**[29]

Retinopathy is present in at least 50% of patients with poorly controlled diabetes after 15 years; more than 90% of patients who have had diabetes for 30 years also have retinopathy.[8] Diabetic retinopathy is the leading cause of blindness in Europe and North America.[23] It leads ultimately to proliferative retinopathy and retinal detachment.

In addition to retinopathy, diabetic patients tend to develop cataracts. This is probably caused by the production of sorbitol in the lens during hyperglycemic states. The sorbitol accumulates and may cause cataracts because of its osmotic effect.[23] Euglycemia does not prevent the formation of cataracts in diabetics.[9] Thus diabetic patients require ophthalmologic surgery for a number of conditions.

Diabetic neuropathy often occurs early in the course of the disease. It has multifactorial causes and tends to respond better to maintenance of euglycemia than the other complications of diabetes. Acute onset of neuropathies can be caused by infarction due to blockage of one or more of the vasa nervorum that supply the nerves. Gradual, progressive neuropathy is probably caused by the collection of excess sorbitol in the Schwann cells.[9] Neuropathies can involve virtually any nerve. **Most commonly, diabetic patients develop distal polyneuropathies, which are symmetric and begin at the feet.**

Neuropathies affecting the autonomic nervous system are of most concern to the anesthesiologists. Gastroparesis is relatively common and treatable by administering metoclopramide as a premedication. The use of cricoid pressure during induction of anesthesia is also advisable for these patients.

Cardiovascular neuropathy is relatively common in diabetic patients. Symptoms of orthostatic hypotension should be sought during the preoperative workup. A decrease in blood pressure of 25 mm Hg systolic or 10 mm Hg diastolic on standing without a compensatory increase in heart rate is diagnostic.[9] Alternatively, a Valsalva maneuver can be performed by having the patient raise their intrathoracic pressure to 40 mm Hg for 15 seconds, while being monitored by ECG. Normally the heart rate increases during Valsalva. The normal ratio of the longest interval between beats after release to the shortest interval during Valsalva is at least 1.2. A ratio of less than 1.1 is evidence of autonomic neuropathy.[8]

This test is easy to perform in the operating room, because an airway pressure gauge and ECG are readily available.

Vagal neuropathy generally develops before deficits in the sympathetic nervous system. Upon induction of general anesthesia, these patients may become hypotensive; therefore, a relatively slow induction with careful attention to the patient's volume status is advisable. In a study of diabetic and nondiabetic patients undergoing ophthalmologic surgery under general anesthesia, 35% of the diabetic patients became hypotensive (systolic blood pressure < 90 mm Hg) and required a pressor. This was significantly different from control patients and was common in patients with other evidence of neuropathy. Because some patients with evidence of cardiac, vascular, or renal disease were excluded and because the operation itself did not present a great stress, the likelihood of other diabetics becoming hypotensive and requiring a pressor is probably greater than 35%. Most episodes of hypotension occurred in the period after laryngoscopy and before incision.[5]

Regional anesthesia in diabetic patients also involves risk. They may experience partial sympathectomy from their disease; therefore, the sympathectomy associated with a spinal or epidural anesthesia should not change their hemodynamics greatly. Because of their neuropathy, sympathetic blockade may extend several segments above sensory blockade. They may therefore be prone to bradycardia and hypotension at levels of sensory blockade not usually associated with either sympathectomy or blockade of the cardiac accelerator nerves. Lesser regional anesthetics (e.g., axillary or retrobulbar block) cause much less vasodilation and therefore should be associated with less hypotension.

Life-threatening bradycardia and hypotension have been reported in diabetic patients undergoing general anesthesia. One patient who had renal failure, peripheral neuropathy, retinopathy, peripheral vascular disease, and symptoms of autonomic dysfunction required an intraperitoneal catheter for dialysis. Shortly after incision, the patient's heart rate decreased from 60 to 38 beats/min, and blood pressure decreased to 50/30 mm Hg. The patient did not respond to a total of 1.2 mg of atropine and 40 mg ephedrine but did respond to cardiac massage and epinephrine. Similar bradycardic episodes occurred twice during the case. MI was ruled out postoperatively. This patient subsequently underwent five procedures under local anesthesia, ankle block, or axillary block, in one case with supplementation of the axillary block with N_2O, uneventfully.[6] Another diabetic patient required a series of surgical procedures because of a foot infection. These were carried out without incident under spinal anesthesia twice and local anesthesia once. The patient then refused spinal anesthesia and received a general anesthetic, which went smoothly until the muscle relaxant was reversed with 3 mg of neostigmine and 0.6 mg of glycopyrrolate. At that time, the heart rate decreased to 42 beats/min, and the blood pressure decreased to 68/40 mm Hg. The patient was unresponsive to 1.2 mg of atropine but responded to epinephrine and cardiac massage. Postoperatively, MI was ruled out.[38] In postoperative testing in both cases, the patients were found to have severe autonomic neuropathies. The fact that atropine was ineffective in both cases is probably important. Where there is a severe parasympathetic neuropathy, there is very little cholinergic tone. Therefore, a drug that blocks the cholinergic stimulus to the heart is unlikely to be effective. **The anesthesiologist should be quick to use a direct-acting pressor (e.g., epinephrine) if vagolytic or indirect-acting agents have not been effective in raising blood pressure in diabetic patients.**

Diabetic autonomic neuropathy has respiratory and cardiovascular effects. Of twelve cardiorespiratory arrests in young diabetic patients with severe autonomic neuropathy, five occurred during or shortly after anesthesia. Two patients were under general anesthesia with close cardiovascular monitoring and spontaneous respirations when they became apneic. One of these patients became moderately hypotensive (90/70 mm Hg) with a heart rate of 90, which was unresponsive to atropine. One patient was under epidural anesthesia and became apneic after receiving 100% oxygen. Two patients were found apneic and pulseless during their stay in the recovery room after receiving general anesthesia. All were easily resuscitated.[23]

In summary, diabetic patients may come for a wide variety of operations either related or unrelated to diabetes. Their anesthetic and monitoring plan may need to be modified, especially if they have cardiovascular disease or autonomic insufficiency. They may be at increased risk for cardiac or respiratory arrest either intraoperatively or in the immediate postoperative period.

Perioperative Management of Glucose and Insulin

The most serious perioperative morbidity in diabetic patients is related to cardiovascular, renal, neurologic, or respiratory complications, as discussed previously. No regimen for perioperative control of blood glucose should be so complicated that it distracts the anesthesiologist from appropriate attention to these important concerns. There is evidence, however, that blood glucose values above 200 mg/dl are associated with both glycosuria and poor wound healing and strength.[11] Therefore, efforts should be made to keep the blood glucose below 200 mg/dl, while avoiding the more serious complication of perioperative hypoglycemia. The plan for achieving perioperative glucose control should be simple enough to be used during relatively complicated procedures, and it should be consistent within a given hospital, so that errors do not occur as the patient's care is transferred from the preoperative ward to the operating room and then to the postoperative recovery room and the postoperative surgical ward.

Oral hypoglycemic agents should not be given the morning of operation. Long-acting sulfonylureas and metformin, or biguanide, should be stopped 2 to 3 days preoperatively and replaced with shorter-acting agents (e.g., chlorpropamide).[1] Traditionally, patients who require insulin receive half their usual dose of regular insulin, and an IV infusion containing 5% dextrose is started. There is controversy regarding whether or not ultralente insulin should be stopped several days before surgery[1] or continued at the patient's usual dose.[11] The fasting blood sugar should be measured preoperatively in insulin-dependent diabetics.

There is no evidence that subcutaneously administered insulin is inadequate for preoperative or postoperative glucose control.[11] Nonetheless, blood flow to the skin tends to increase under anesthesia; therefore the uptake of subcutaneously administered insulin may be variable during anesthesia. Despite this, an alternative method of intraoperative control is to give 10 units of subcutaneous insulin, then start an infusion of 5% dextrose, which is varied depending upon the patient's blood sugar.[8] Regardless of the method of insulin therapy, it is prudent for the anesthesiologist to measure the blood sugar at regular intervals during operation. A goal of whole blood glucose levels of 120 to 180 mg/dl should be sought.[1] If it is necessary to administer insulin intraoperatively, it should be administered as a continuous IV infusion rather than as an IV bolus. The serum half-life of IV insulin is approximately 5 minutes with a biologic half-life of 20 minutes or less, and a large insulin bolus can put the patient at risk for dysrhythmias caused by intracellular shifts of potassium, phosphorus, and magnesium.[11]

There is controversy regarding whether or not glucose and insulin should be administered as separate infusions[11] or combined in a single infusion.[1] We believe they should be combined in a single infusion to prevent the possibility of insulin overdose caused by blockage of the dextrose infusion or inadvertent flushing of the insulin infusion. We have used 5% dextrose solutions with 0.32 units insulin/g of dextrose (16 units/l), with 20 mEq potassium/l, administered at 100 ml/hour in adults. We start this infusion only if the patient's blood glucose is above 200 mg/dl and stop the infusion on transfer of the patient to the recovery room. This is a simple infusion and it contains a relatively low dose of insulin; if no downward trend in the blood sugar is seen, 1 to 2 additional units of insulin can be added without mixing another infusion. Blood glucose values should be measured hourly while patients are receiving an insulin infusion. Potassium values should be determined at least the first hour after the insulin infusion has been started.

Postoperative glucose management is achieved through blood tests every four hours and administration of regular insulin on a sliding scale. This is appropriate, because blood flow to the skin returns to normal after emergence from anesthesia and because this regulation approximates what the patient will receive on the ward or after discharge home.

In conclusion, the anesthesiologist should choose a system of glucose control simple enough not to cause distraction from the prevention of major cardiovascular, respiratory, renal, or neurologic morbidity. The system should be compatible with the plan used by other clinicians who manage the patient preoperatively and postoperatively. Blood glucose values should be determined frequently while the patient is under anesthesia. Insulin should be administered, if necessary, by continuous infusion, to maintain blood glucose levels at 120 to 180 mg/dl.

KEY POINTS

- Although phentolamine has been used traditionally to control intraoperative blood pressures in patients with pheochromocytoma, we have found nitroprusside to be preferable. Nitroprusside has a rapid onset and short half-life, and it is more familiar to most anesthesiologists.
- Drugs associated with histamine or catecholamine release should be avoided for patients with pheochromocytoma.
- Carcinoid tumors arise from endocrine argentaffin or Kulchitsky cells in the lung, small intestine, bronchi, or ovaries.
- Carcinoid syndrome occurs rarely in those patients with carcinoid tumors. The symptoms include flushing, diarrhea, anxiety, wheezing, tachycardia, salivation, lacrimation, hyperthermia, and facial edema.
- Invasive monitoring with an intra-arterial catheter is appropriate for any patients with carcinoid syndrome, because they are at risk for both hypertension and hypotension. Central venous access is indicated, both to assess volume status and to administer vasoactive drugs.
- All drugs that cause histamine release, as well as catecholamines, should be avoided. Patients with carcinoid syndrome reputedly awaken slowly, so early extubation should not be a primary goal.
- Patients with systemic mastocytosis should be skin tested for every drug they are expected to receive during anesthesia. This implies a simple anesthetic plan using as few drugs as possible.
- Epinephrine is the treatment of choice for intraoperative exacerbations of systemic mastocytosis. It occupies receptors on mast cell membranes and prevents release of histamine. Isoflurane tends to stabilize mast cell membranes, smoothing the intraoperative course for patients with systemic mastocytosis.
- There are a number of possible causes of postoperative respiratory distress after thyroidectomy, including bilateral vocal cord paralysis, hemorrhage, and laryngeal edema. Tracheomalacia may occur after operation for carcinoma.
- The main consideration in choosing induction agents for patients having thyroidectomy is the extent of airway ab-

normality. Long-acting neuromuscular blockade at the time of induction is not advisable.

- Patients who have a hypercalcemic crisis caused by hyperparathyroidism should undergo parathyroidectomy as soon as possible after restoration of intravascular volume and calcium diuresis.
- The anesthetic management for parathyroidectomy is similar to that for thyroidectomy. In both cases, the surgery is not a major physiologic trespass: blood loss is minimal and fluid shifts are uncommon. No invasive hemodynamic monitoring is required based on the surgical procedure itself.
- Hypoparathyroidism can occur transiently after parathyroidectomy. The serum calcium tends to be least on the second or third postoperative day. Hypocalcemic patients experience an increase in neuromuscular excitability, which can develop into tetany, carpopedal spasm, and laryngeal stridor.
- Atherosclerotic vascular disease occurs 2.5 times more frequently in diabetic patients than in the general population.
- Coronary artery disease is especially insidious in patients with diabetes, because it may be asymptomatic or have atypical symptomatology.
- Diabetic patients make up approximately one fourth to one third of all patients with peripheral vascular disease.
- Diabetic microvascular disease includes nephropathy and retinopathy.
- Neuropathies affecting the autonomic nervous system are of great concern to the anesthesiologist. Gastroparesis is relatively common and treatable by administering metoclopramide as a premedication.
- Cardiovascular neuropathy is also common in diabetic patients. Symptoms of orthostatic hypotension should be sought. Vagal neuropathy generally develops before deficits in the sympathetic nervous system. These patients may become hypotensive on induction of general anesthesia. Life-threatening bradycardia and hypotension have been reported in diabetic patients undergoing general anesthesia.
- Diabetic autonomic neuropathy has respiratory and cardiac effects. Perioperative respiratory depression and arrest may occur.
- Management of blood glucose in the perioperative period should be simple enough to allow the anesthesiologist to focus attention on the patient's associated cardiovascular, respiratory, neurologic, and renal diseases. It should be consistent within a given hospital, so that errors are not made as patients are transferred between preoperative, intraoperative, and postoperative care personnel.
- If insulin is given intraoperatively, it should be given by continuous IV infusion rather than IV bolus. The goal of therapy should be a blood glucose value of 120 to 180 mg/dl.

KEY REFERENCES

Alberti KGMM: Diabetes and surgery, *Anesthesiology* 74:209, 1991.

Hirsch IB, McGill JB, Cryer PE, et al: Perioperative management of surgical patients with diabetes mellitus, *Anesthesiology* 74:346, 1991.

Hull CJ: Pheochromocytoma, *Brit J Anaesth* 58:1453, 1986.

Parry T, Perera J, Hammond JE: Anesthesia and gastric carcinoid, *Anesthesia* 41:1265, 1986.

Scott HW, Parris WCV, Sandidge PC, et al: Hazards in the operative management of patients with systemic mastocytosis, *Ann Surg* 197:507–514, 1983.

Sebel PS: Thyroid and parathyroid disease. In Nimmo WS, Smith G, editors: *Anesthesia,* Cambridge, 1990, Blackwell Scientific Publications.

REFERENCES

1. Alberti KGMM: Diabetes and surgery, *Anesthesiology* 74:209, 1991.
2. Al-Mohaya S, Naguib M, Abdelatif M, et al: Abnormal responses to muscle relaxants in a patient with primary hyperparathyroidism, *Anesthesiology* 65:554, 1986.
3. Bilezikian JP: Primary hyperparathyroidism. In Stein JH, editor: *Internal medicine,* ed 3, Boston, 1990, Little, Brown and Co.
4. Braude BM, Leiman BC, Moyes DG: Etomidate infusion for resection of pheochromocytoma, *S Afr Med J* 69:60, 1986.
5. Burgos CG, Ebert TJ, Asiddao C, et al: Increased intraoperative cardiovascular morbidity in diabetics and autonomic neuropathy, *Anesthesiology* 70:591, 1989.
6. Ciccarelli LL, Ford CM, Tsueda K: Autonomic neuropathy in a diabetic patient with renal failure, *Anesthesiology* 64:283, 1986.
7. Ellis H: *Anatomy for anaesthetists,* St. Louis, 1983, Blackwell Scientific Publications.
8. Foster DW: Diabetes Mellitus. In Isselbacher KJ, Braunwald E, Wilson JD, et al, editors: *Harrison's principles of internal medicine,* ed 13, New York, 1994, McGraw-Hill.
9. Garber AJ: Diabetes mellitus. In Stein JH, editor: *Internal medicine,* ed 3, Boston, 1990, Little, Brown and Co.
10. Greer MA: Disorders of the thyroid. In Stein, JH, editor: *Internal medicine,* ed 3, Boston, 1990, Little, Brown and Co.
11. Hirsch IB, McGill JB, Cryer PE, et al: Perioperative management of surgical patients with diabetes mellitus, *Anesthesiology* 74:346, 1991.
12. Horton JN: Anaesthesia and diabetes. In Nimmo WS, Smith G, editors: *Anaesthesia,* Chicago, 1989, Blackwell Scientific Publications.

13. Hughes EW, Hodkinson BP: Carcinoid syndrome: the combined use of ketauseria and octreotide in the management of an acute crisis during anesthesia, *Anaesth Intens Care* 17:367, 1989.
14. Hull CJ: Pheochromocytoma, *Brit J Anaesth* 58:1453, 1986.
15. James MFM: Use of magnesium sulfate in the anaesthetic management of phaeochromocytoma: a review of 17 anaesthetics, *Br J Anaesth* 62:616, 1989.
16. Kaplan EL: Thyroid and parathyroid. In Schwartz SI, editor: *Principles of surgery,* ed 6, New York, 1994, McGraw-Hill.
17. Kaplan LM: Endocrine tumors of the gastrointestinal tract and pancreas. In Isselbacher KJ, Braunwald E, Wilson JD, et al, editors: *Harrison's principles of internal medicine,* ed 13, New York, 1994, McGraw-Hill.
18. Lafferty FW, Hubay CA: Primary hyperparathyroidism: a review of the long-term surgical and non-surgical morbidities as a basis for a rational approach to treatment, *Arch Intern Med* 149:789, 1989.
19. Landsberg L, Young JB: Pheochromocytoma. In Isselbacher KJ, Braunwald E, Wilson JD, et al, editors: *Harrison's principles of internal medicine,* ed 13, New York, 1994, McGraw-Hill.
20. Lightdale CJ: Tumors of the small and large intestine. In Stein JH, editor: *Internal medicine,* ed 3 Boston, 1990, Little, Brown and Co.
21. Marsh HM, Martin JK, Kools LK, et al: Carcinoid crisis during anesthesia: successful treatment with a somatostatin analogue, *Anesthesiology* 66:89, 1987.
22. Martin JT: The head-elevated positions. In Martin JT, editor: *Positioning in anesthesia and surgery,* Philadelphia, 1987, WB Saunders.
23. Merimee TJ: Diabetic retinopathy: a synthesis of perspectives, *N Engl J Med* 322(14):978, 1990.
24. Nicholas E, Deutschman CS, Allo M, et al: Use of esmolol in the intraoperative management of pheochromocytoma, *Anesth Analg* 67:1114, 1988.
25. Oyama T, Shibata S, Matsuki A, et al: Serum endogenous thyroxine levels in man during anaesthesia and surgery, *Brit J Anaesth* 41:103, 1969.
26. Oyama T, Latto P, Holaday DA, et al: Effect of isoflurane anaesthesia and surgery on thyroid function in man, *Can Anaesth Soc J* 22:474, 1975.
27. Page MM, Watkins PY: Cardiorespiratory arrest and diabetic autonomic neuropathy, *Lancet* 1/7/78, p. 14.
28. Parry T, Perera J, Hammond JE: Anesthesia and gastric carcinoid, *Anesthesia* 41:1265, 1986.
29. Philipson JD, Carpenter BJ, Itzkott J, et al: Evaluation of cardiovascular risks for renal transplantation in diabetic patients, *Am J Med* 81:630, 1986.
30. Pyrtek LJ, Belkin M, Bartus S, et al: Parathyroid gland exploration with local anesthesia in elderly and high-risk patients, *Arch Surg* 123:614, 1988.
31. Roizen MF: Anesthetic implications of concurrent diseases. In Miller RD, editor: *Anesthesia,* ed 2, New York, 1986, Churchill-Livingstone.
32. Roy RC, Carter RF, Wright PD: Somatostain, anaesthesia, and the carcinoid syndrome, *Anaesthesia* 42:627, 1987.
33. Sebel PS: Thyroid and parathyroid disease. In Nimmo WS, Smith G, editors: *Anesthesia,* Cambridge, 1989, Blackwell Scientific Publications.
34. Shaw JM: Genetic aspects of urticaria pigmentosa, *Arch Dermatol* 97:137–138, 1968.
35. Snider D, King L: Diabetes and other endocrine disorders. In Breslow MJ, Miller CF, Rogers MC, editors: *Perioperative management,* St Louis, 1990, Mosby–Year Book.
36. Tornebrandt K, Nobin A, Ericsson M, et al: Circulation, respiration, and serotonin levels in carcinoid patients during neurolept anaesthesia, *Anesthesia* 38:957, 1983.
37. Townsend CM, Thomson JC: Small intestine. In Schwartz SI, editor: *Principles of surgery,* ed 5, New York, 1989, McGraw-Hill.
38. Triantafillon AN, Tsueda K, Berg J, et al: Refractory bradycardia after reversal of muscle relaxant in a diabetic with vagal neuropathy, *Anesth Analg* 65:1237, 1986.
39. Tsunoo M, Kimura F, Nakamura T, et al: Mast cell disruptive effect of local anesthetics and its prevention with special reference to the effect of aliphatic anesthetics, *Nippon Ida Diag Z* 36:195–198, 1969.
40. Turk J, Oates JA, Roberts LJ II: Intervention with epinephrine in hypotension associated with mastocytosis, *J Allerg Clin Immunol* 71:189–192, 1983.
41. Wasserman MA, DuCharme DW, Griffin RL, et al: Bronchopulmonary and cardiovascular effects of prostaglandin D2 in the dog, *Prostaglandin* 13:255–269, 1972.

CHAPTER 75

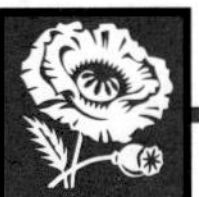

Anesthetic Considerations for Genitourinary and Renal Surgery

MAGED S. MIKHAIL
DURAIYAH THANGATHURAI

Anesthesia for patients undergoing urologic procedures involves the application of a variety of anesthetic techniques in those of all age groups. These procedures vary from relatively minor procedures, such as diagnostic cystoscopy, to extensive and often complicated cancer operations that may involve considerable blood loss. Anesthesiologists should possess a basic understanding of common urologic procedures and their anesthetic requirements. Urologists regularly use patient positions other than the supine position, therefore familiarity with these positions and their potential adverse effects also is necessary.

ANATOMIC CONSIDERATIONS

Kidneys

The kidneys lie retroperitoneally in the abdomen between the T12 and L4 vertebrae. In most patients, each kidney is supplied by a single renal artery that originates from the aorta just below the superior mesenteric artery. The right renal artery passes behind the inferior vena cava. **Compression or retraction of the inferior vena cava during renal surgery can result in systemic arterial hypotension due to decreased venous return.** The single renal vein that usually drains each kidney lies anterior to the ipsilateral renal artery. The left renal vein crosses anterior to the aorta before it joins the inferior vena cava. Because of the proximity of these large blood vessels, renal surgery can be associated with considerable blood loss.

Renal innervation (Fig. 75-1) consists primarily of sympathetic and afferent fibers. The renal neural plexus is an extension of the celiac plexus, but it also receives fibers from the lesser or lowest splanchnic nerves and from the vagus nerves. Sympathetic fibers from T10 to L1 pass into the kidneys along the renal arteries and are predominantly vaso-

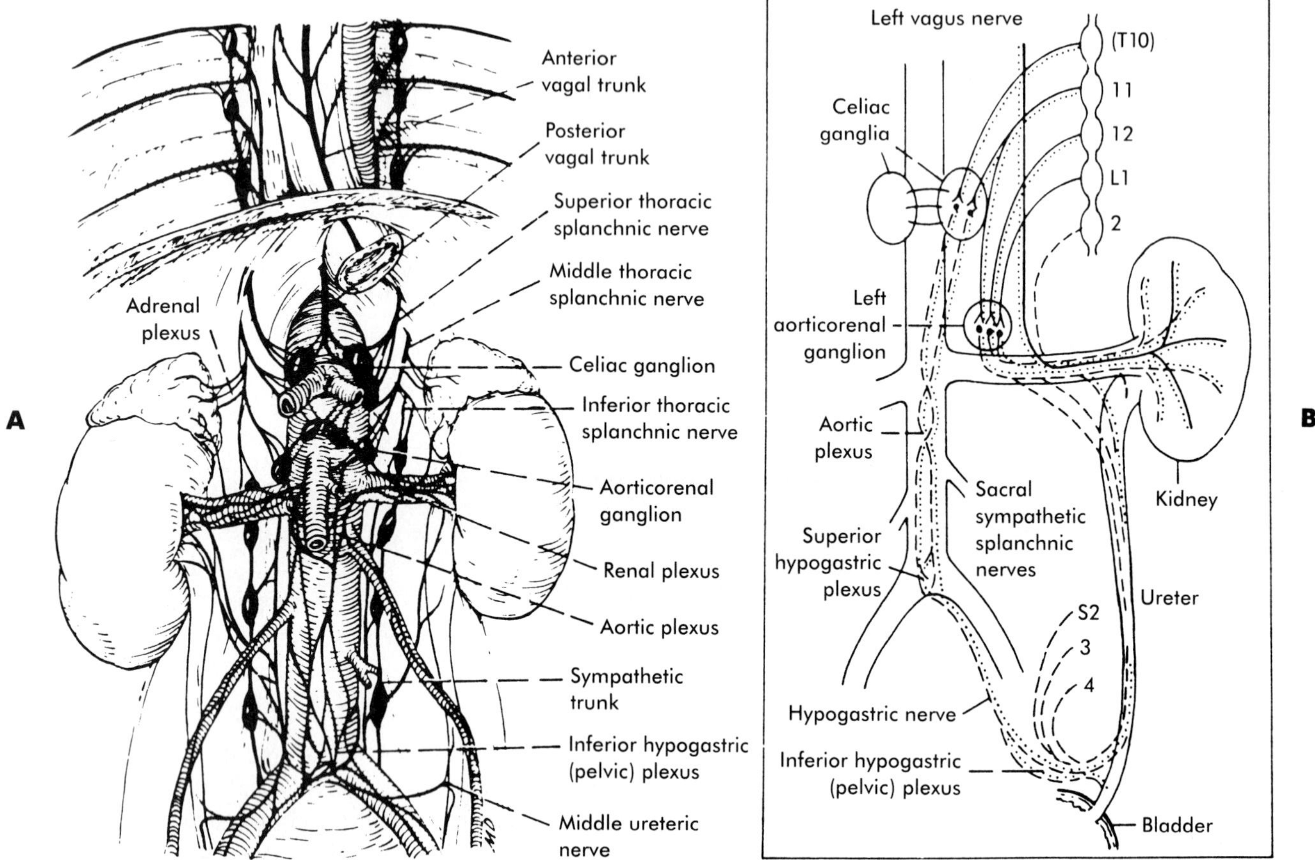

Fig. 75-1. A, Gross anatomy and innervation of the kidneys. **B,** Schematic illustration of the autonomic and sensory nerve pathways. (Modified and reproduced, with permission, from Bonica JJ: *Management of pain*, Philadelphia, 1990, Lea & Febiger.)

constrictor in function.[26] Surgical dissection near the aorta can produce reflex vasoconstriction of renal vessels, which may contribute to perioperative renal dysfunction.

Effective surgical anesthesia of the kidneys requires somatic blockade of the T8 to L3 spinal nerve roots to anesthetize the overlying muscles and skin. Some patients may still perceive pain via afferent fibers that travel in the vagus nerve.[22]

Ureters

The ureter is a continuation of the lower renal pelvis. It descends along the psoas muscle in the retroperitoneum. At the pelvic brim, the ureters cross anterior to the bifurcation of the common iliac arteries before they pass into the posterolateral wall of the base of the bladder. The ureters receive their blood supply from multiple blood vessels adjacent to their path. The long path of the ureters makes them vulnerable to injury or transection during retroperitoneal surgery.

A microscopic ureteric nerve plexus exists along the entire path of the ureters. It is derived from the renal, hypogastric, and pelvic plexuses (Fig. 75-1) and contains many afferent visceral pain fibers.[12] Afferent fibers travel with sympathetic (T10–L2) and parasympathetic fibers of the pelvic splanchnic nerves (S2–S4) into the spinal cord. Regional anesthesia with a T10 sensory level usually produces adequate anesthesia of the ureters.

Bladder

The bladder lies between the pubic bone and the rectum and is covered superiorly by peritoneum. Its arterial supply is derived from the internal iliac (hypogastric) arteries, consisting of two to three superior vesical arteries (branches of the umbilical artery), an inferior vesical artery, which has a variable origin from the internal iliac artery, and branches of the obturator, inferior gluteal, and in women, vaginal and uterine arteries.[197] Venous drainage of the bladder does not follow the same path as arterial inflow but converges at the bladder neck to form an extensive vesical plexus. This venous plexus drains into the internal iliac veins after it is joined by the prostatic venous plexus and the deep dorsal vein of the penis (in men) near the inferior vesical arteries. **The confluence of all these vessels in the lateral, inferior, and posterior aspects of the bladder, together with anatomic variations, greatly increases the risk of major hemorrhage during operations in this area.**

A vesical neural plexus is located on each side of the

bladder between it and the lateral pelvic wall. This plexus, which is a continuation of the inferior hypogastric (pelvic) plexus, contains afferent, sympathetic, and parasympathetic fibers (Fig. 75-2). Sympathetic fibers are derived from lumbar splanchnic nerves (T11–L2 spinal levels), whereas parasympathetic fibers reach the bladder via the pudendal nerve (S2–S4). Afferent fibers, which carry most visceral sensation, travel with the parasympathetic fibers.[73] Sacral parasympathetic outflow produces contraction of bladder wall and inhibition of the involuntary (internal) urinary sphincter. Stimulation of sympathetic nerves relaxes the smooth muscle of the urinary bladder and contracts the internal urinary sphincter. The pudendal nerve controls the external urinary sphincter, allowing volitional emptying of the bladder.

Prostate

The prostate is a pear-shaped organ that surrounds a segment of the male urethra beneath the bladder. It is enclosed by a thick fibrous capsule that contains its blood supply and innervation along its posterolateral aspects. The gland also receives an additional blood supply at its junction with the bladder. Both blood supplies are primarily derived from the inferior vesical arteries. The prostate's rich venous plexus communicates with the vesical plexus and the dorsal vein of the penis (see previous) and can be responsible for extensive intraoperative hemorrhage during retropubic prostatectomy.[206]

The prostatic nerve plexus is a continuation of the vesical plexus. Innervation is primarily sympathetic and derived from the hypogastric plexus (T11–L2). Most afferent fibers travel along the pelvic splanchnic nerves (parasympathetic fibers) to enter the spinal cord at S2–S4 (Fig. 75-2).

Urethra

Innervation of the urethra is similar to the prostate. Additional innervation may be provided by the deep perineal branches of the pudendal nerve (S2–S4) and the pudendal branch of the posterior femoral cutaneous nerve (S1–S3).

Testis

The testis' blood supply and innervation are related to their embryologic origin near the kidneys. The testicular arteries originate directly from the aorta just below the renal arteries. The testicular venous plexus ascends all the way up to

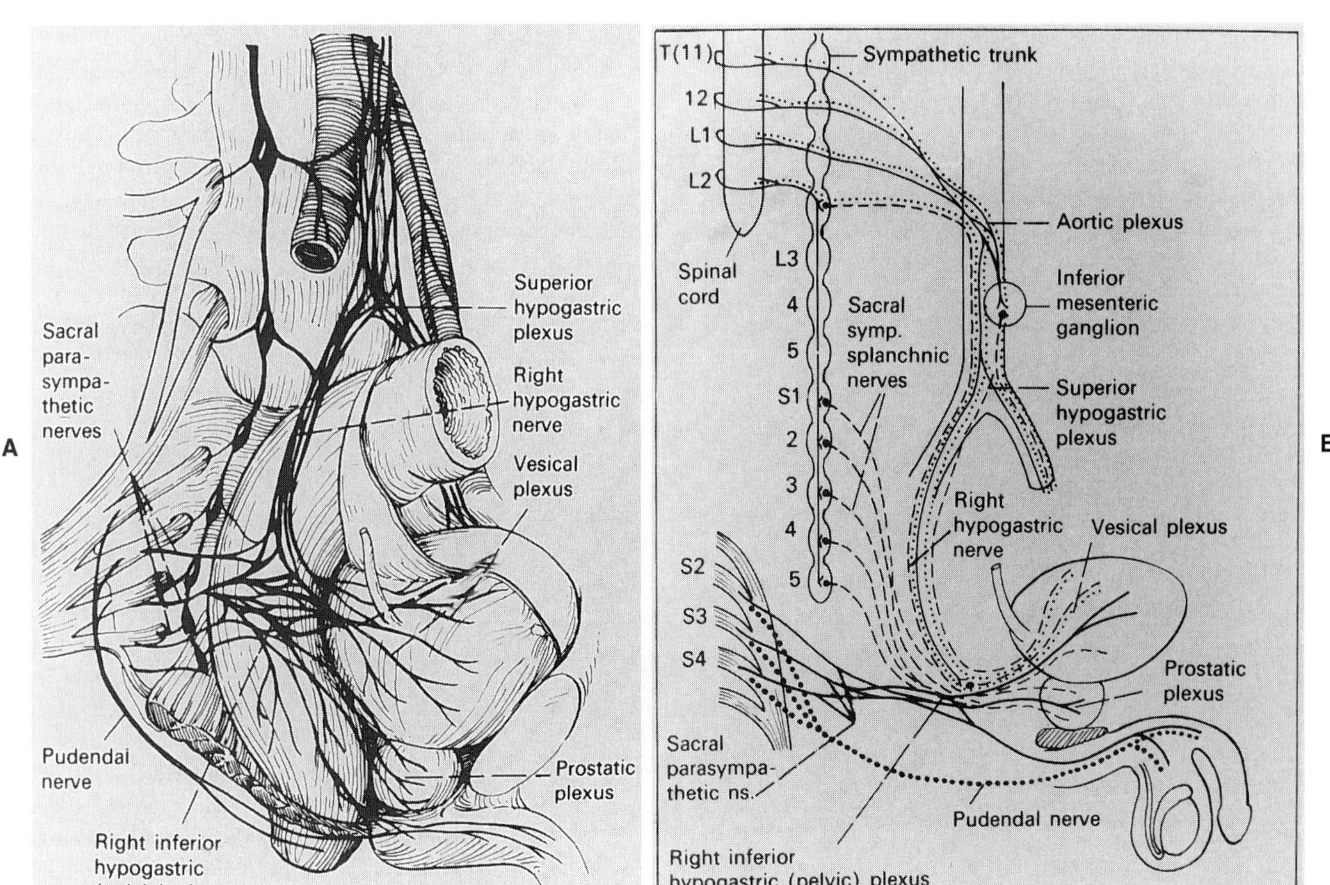

Fig. 75-2. A, Gross anatomy and innervation of the bladder and prostate. **B,** Schematic illustration of the autonomic and sensory nerve pathways. (Modified and reproduced, with permission, from Bonica JJ: *Management of pain*, Philadelphia, 1990, Lea & Febiger.)

drain directly into the vena cava on the right side and into the left renal vein on the left side.

The testicular nerve plexus originates from the aortic plexus at the level of the arterial supply and follows the arteries down into the scrotum. In contrast, the nerve supply to the epididymis and ductus deferens originates from the superior hypogastric and pelvic plexuses. Testicular anesthesia therefore requires regional anesthesia to at least a T10 sensory level.

Male Genitalia

Sensory innervation of the anterior scrotum in men is provided by the ilioinguinal nerve (T12–L2) and the genital branch of the genitofemoral nerve (L1–L2). The posterior scrotum is innervated by the medial and lateral scrotal branches of the perineal nerve and by the perineal branch of the posterior femoral cutaneous nerve (S1–S3). The perineal nerve is a terminal branch of the pudendal nerve (S2–S4).

The innervation of the root of the penis is provided by the ilioinguinal nerve, but the body and glans are innervated by the paired dorsal nerves of the penis, which are continuations of the pudendal nerves (Fig. 75-3).

Parasympathetic (S2–S4) and sympathetic (L1–L2) innervation reach the penis via the prostatic plexus. Afferent impulses from the pudendal nerve or psychic stimulation can cause parasympathetic-mediated arteriolar dilation, leading to engorgement of cavernous tissue and erection. In contrast, sympathetic-mediated vasoconstriction inhibits erection.

Female Genitalia

The posterior labia majora, labia minora, and vestibule are supplied by the posterior labial nerves, which are branches of the pudendal nerves. The mons pubis and anterior portion of the labia are supplied by the anterior labial nerves, which are branches of the ilioinguinal and genitofemoral nerves. The clitoris is supplied by the dorsal nerve of the clitoris, which is a terminal branch of the pudendal nerve.

COMMONLY USED PATIENT POSITIONS

Lithotomy

The lithotomy position (Fig. 75-4) is frequently used for patients undergoing urologic procedures, including cystoscopy and transurethral resection of the prostate. The patient is placed in the supine position and the legs are elevated such that the hips and knees are flexed; two posts with ankle straps or special leg holders are used to maintain the position. At least two people are needed to safely move the patient's legs simultaneously up or down. If strap supports are used the legs should be padded and allowed to hang freely. Extreme lithotomy (Fig. 75-5) often is used for perineal prostatectomy.

Lithotomy position can have important physiologic consequences, including decreased vital capacity,[36] lung volume, and lung compliance.[16] A small decrease in functional residual capacity (FRC) may result in hypoxemia, especially in obese patients. This effect may be accentuated by an extreme (> 30°) head-down (Trendelenburg) position.[179] Passive elevation of the legs increases venous return acutely and may exacerbate borderline congestive heart failure. Mean blood pressure may increase, but cardiac output often does not change significantly.[164] Conversely, rapid lowering of the legs can suddenly decrease venous return and produce

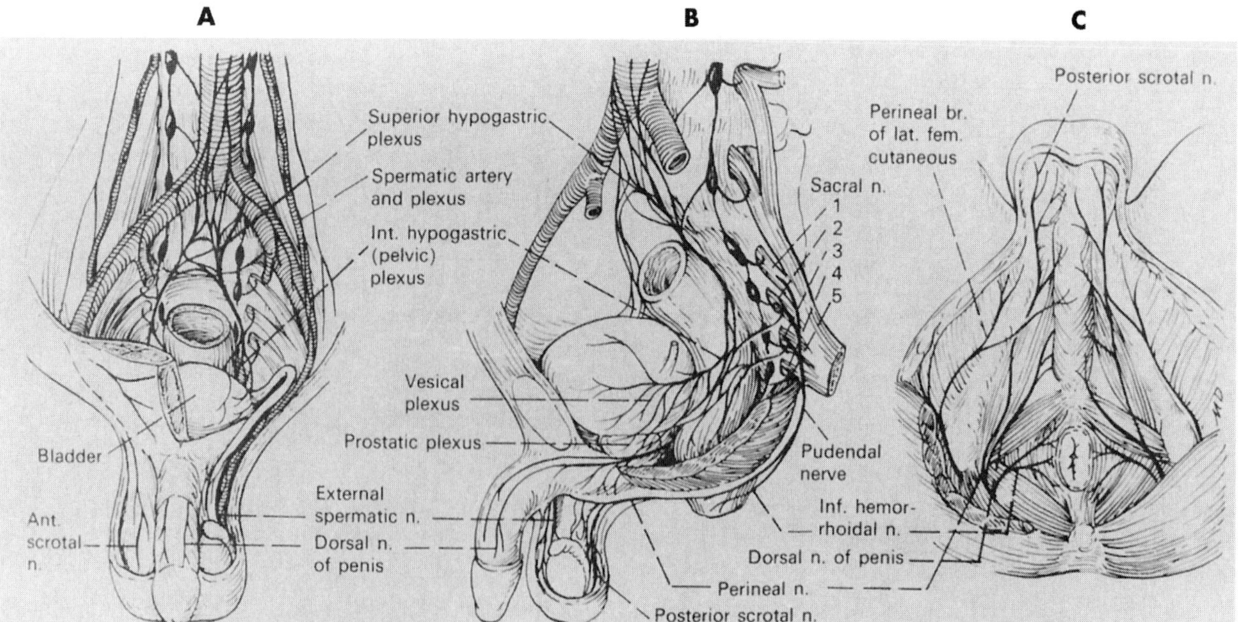

Fig. 75-3. Gross anatomy and innervation of the male genitalia. **A,** Anterior view. **B,** Sagittal view. **C,** Perineal view. (Modified and reproduced, with permission, from Bonica JJ: *Management of pain*, Philadelphia, 1990, Lea & Febiger.)

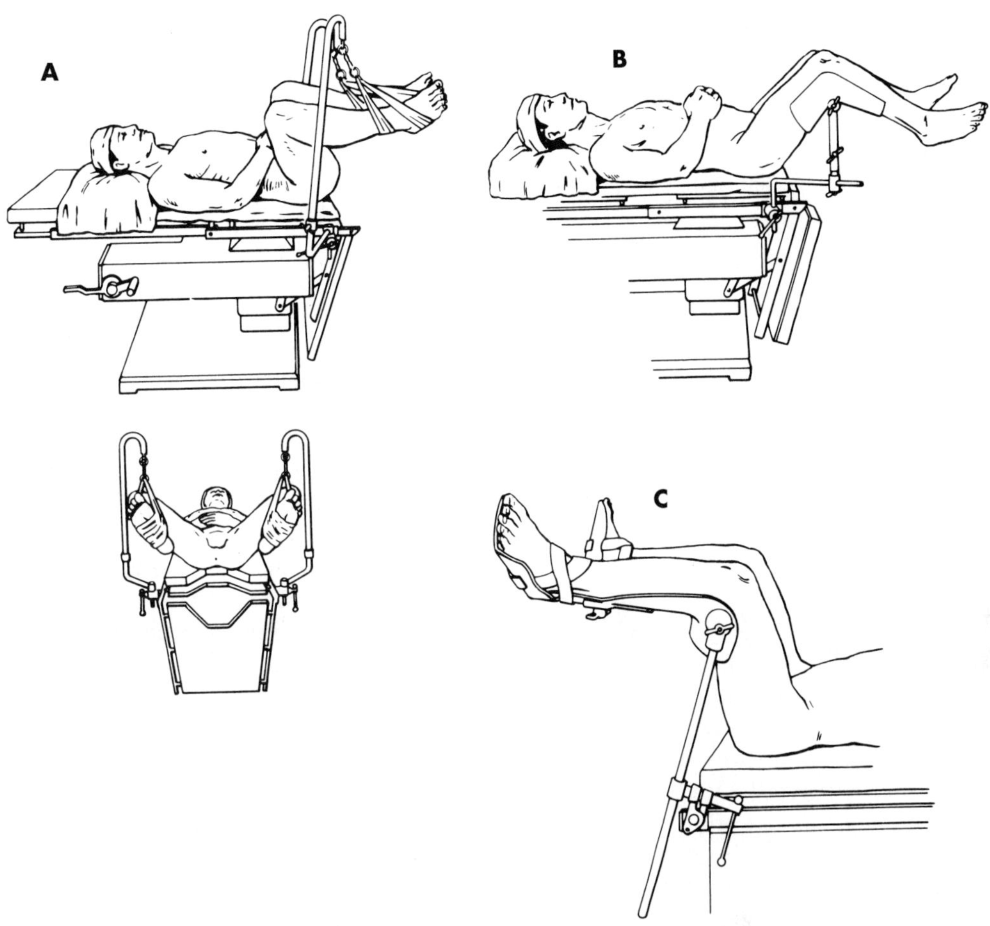

Fig. 75-4. The lithotomy position. **A,** Strap stirrups. **B,** Bier-Hoff stirrups. **C,** Allen stirrups. (Modified and reproduced, with permission, from Martin JT: *Positioning in anesthesia,* Philadelphia, 1988, WB Saunders.)

arterial hypotension, especially in hypovolemic patients.[121] Vasodilation from either general or regional anesthesia can exacerbate the latter effect. Arterial blood pressure should therefore always be measured immediately after the legs are lowered, and if found to be unacceptably low, the legs should be raised again.

Failure to properly position patients can result in several iatrogenic injuries.[16] **Risk factors associated with postoperative motor neuropathy include lithotomy duration of more than 4 hours, body mass index less than 20 kg/m², and a recent smoking history.**[210] **Injury to the common peroneal nerve, resulting in loss of dorsiflexion of the foot, occurs when the lateral thigh rests on the strap support because the nerve is compressed as it winds laterally around the head of the fibula.**[180] In contrast, when the legs are allowed to rest on medially placed strap supports, compression of the saphenous nerve can result in numbness along the medial calf.[29] Excessive flexion of the thigh can injure the obturator or femoral nerves.[201] Extreme hip flexion also may stretch the sciatic nerve. Prolonged lithotomy and the extreme lithotomy position have been rarely associated with a compartment syndrome and rhabdomyolysis.[4,79,125] As the foot of the operating room table is lowered, the hands or fingers can get caught in the gap between the lower and middle sections of the table.[47] The incidence of back pain after lithotomy position may be as high as 37%,[32] although the most common neurologic injury in urologic patients may be to the nerves of the brachial plexus.[16]

Trendelenburg

The supine head-down position, also called Trendelenburg position, may be used to displace cephalad the abdominal organs from the pelvis or to allow better access to the perineum.

The most important respiratory effects of this position are limitation of diaphragmatic motion and decreased lung volume.[16] This position predisposes to reductions in FRC and promotes atelectasis.[179] The degree of impairment is likely related to the angle of tilt from the horizon. Although secretions may tend to pool in the pharynx, Trendelenburg position does not appear to increase the risk of clinically significant pulmonary aspiration in patients without a history of gastroesophageal reflux.[53] Endotracheal tubes may migrate into an endobronchial position because the position of the carina may shift upward.[93]

Although the Trendelenburg position may lower venous pressure and thus, at least theoretically, reduce venous bleeding during pelvic surgery, even 10° of head-down tilt has been associated with venous air embolism.[150] Although increased venous return to the heart may be expected to increase arterial blood pressure or cardiac output, investigators have failed to show a beneficial effect of the head-down position on blood pressure or cardiac output.[164,177] Steep Trendelenburg position may increase venous return and pulmonary blood flow sufficiently to promote respiratory distress in patients with impaired ventricular function.[172]

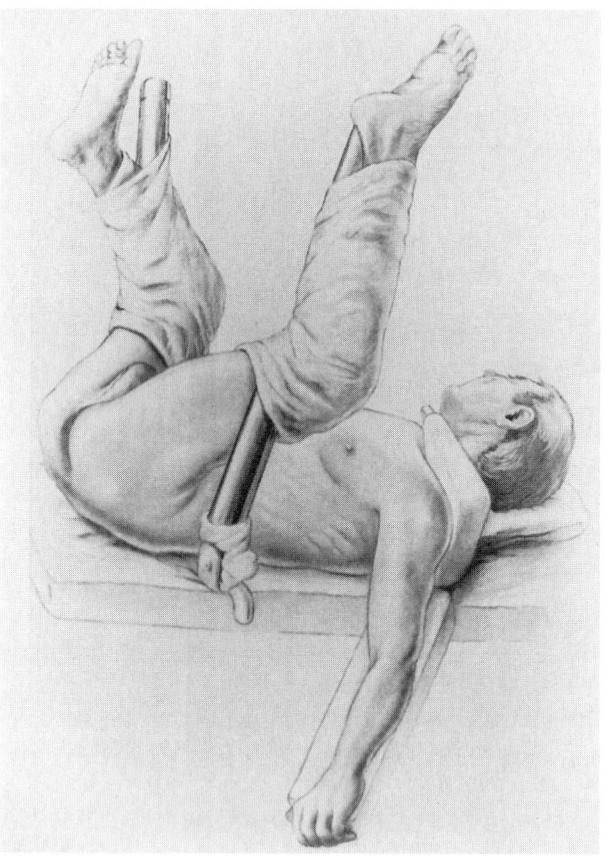

Fig. 75-5. Extreme lithotomy position is used for perineal surgery. (Modified and reproduced, with permission, from Skinner DG, Lieskovsky G: *Diagnosis and management of genitourinary cancer,* Philadelphia, 1988, WB Saunders.)

Extreme head-down position produces venous pooling in the upper half of the body.[214] Increases in central venous pressure and intracranial pressure can promote cerebral edema and reduce cerebral blood flow (especially when associated with a low systemic arterial blood pressure). Cerebral hemorrhage has been reported in patients after prolonged Trendelenburg position.[154] The Trendelenburg position also has been implicated as a factor in postoperative alopecia.[2]

As with the lithotomy position, the most common nerve injury associated with Trendelenburg position is brachial plexus injury.[16] The latter is more likely to occur when the arm is hyperabducted or hyperextended on an arm board or with the use of shoulder braces. The use of muscle relaxants, especially with steep Trendelenburg position (> 30°) together with lithotomy position may increase the incidence of postoperative neuropathy.

Kidney Rest

This position, also called *lateral flexed position,* is used to obtain good surgical exposure of the kidney or ureter on one side. The patient is placed in lateral position with the dependent leg flexed and the other leg extended (Fig. 75-6). A roll is placed under the dependent upper chest to prevent pressure on the brachial plexus in the axilla. The operating table is then extended to achieve maximal separation between the iliac crest and the costal margin on the operative side. Finally, the kidney rest, which is located in the groove where the table bends, is elevated to raise the nondependent iliac crest higher and further enhance surgical exposure.

This position often is associated with serious adverse respiratory and circulatory effects. FRC is reduced in the dependent lung but may increase in the nondependent lung.[124]

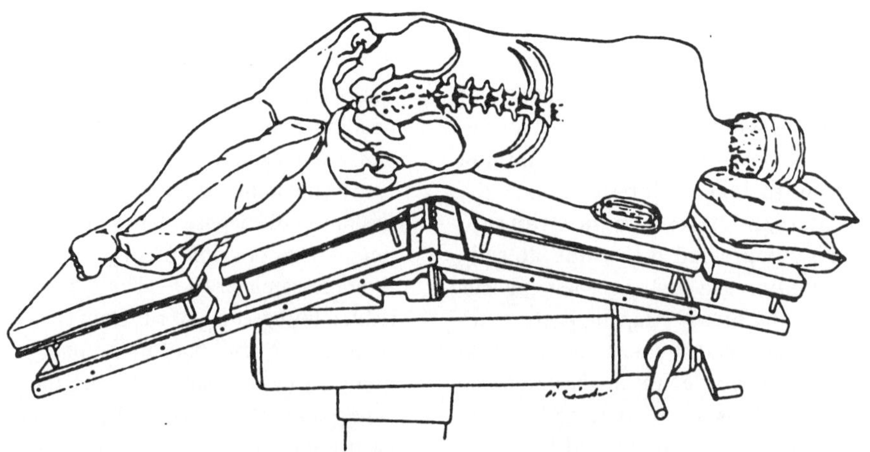

Fig. 75-6. The kidney rest position, also called *lateral flexed position,* often is used for renal surgery. (Modified and reproduced, with permission, from Martin JT: *Positioning in anesthesia and surgery,* Philadelphia, 1987, WB Saunders.)

In the anesthetized patient receiving controlled ventilation, ventilation to perfusion mismatching occurs because the dependent lung receives greater blood flow than the nondependent lung, whereas the nondependent lung receives greater ventilation.[216] This condition promotes atelectasis in the dependent lung and favors hypoxemia.[45] Pansard et al.[157] have noted that the arterial-to-end-tidal gradient for CO_2 progressively increases during general anesthesia in this position. Elevation of the kidney rest can dramatically decrease venous return to the heart by compressing the inferior vena cava.[128] Venous pooling in the legs also decreases venous return and aggravates any arterial hypotension.

Hyperextended Supine

This position, also called hyperlordosis, is used by many surgeons to facilitate exposure of the pelvis during retropubic prostatectomy and cystectomy (Fig. 75-7). The patient is positioned supine with the iliac crest over the break in the operating table. The table then is extended such that the distance between the iliac crest and the costal margin increases maximally without putting excessive strain on the patient's back. Finally, the table is tilted head-down to make the operative field horizontal. A variation of this position includes the frog-leg position, where the knees are flexed and the hips are abducted and externally rotated (Fig. 75-8).

Another variation of this position is used for thoracoabdominal incisions (Fig. 75-9). The patient is positioned close to the edge of the table on the operative side with the iliac crest positioned over break in the table. The leg on the nonoperative side is flexed 30°, and the knee is flexed 90°. The leg on the operative side remains straight. The shoulder on the ipsilateral side is elevated 30° with a roll to allow that arm to come across the chest into an adjustable arm rest ("airplane"). The other arm is extended on an arm board. The table finally is hyperextended and placed in the head-down position to make the operative field horizontal.

Although the adverse effects of this position have not been studied, its physiologic consequences appear to be similar to the Trendelenburg position. The potential for neurologic injuries and back injury exists because of complex nature of the position. Careful positioning and generous padding of the arms and legs are warranted. Positioning the pelvis above the heart may predispose to venous air embolism.[6,162]

Prone

The prone position may be used for percutaneous extraction of renal calculi. After induction of general anesthesia, the patient is turned prone as a single unit (requiring at least four people). Turning the patient into the prone position is a critical period because monitor disconnections are hard to avoid and because hypotension frequently occurs as a result of blunted postural sympathetic reflexes. Care should be taken to maintain the neck in a neutral position. In the prone position, the head may be turned to the side (not exceeding the patient's normal range of motion) or may remain face down in a specially designed cushioned head holder. Extreme caution is necessary to avoid retinal ischemia from pressure on either globe or pressure necrosis of the nose, ears, forehead, breasts (women), or genitalia (men). The chest should rest on parallel rolls (usually foam or towels) to facilitate ventilation. The arms should be at the patient's sides in a comfortable position with the elbows flexed, avoiding excessive abduction at the shoulder.

Vital capacity and tidal volume decrease in patients in the prone position.[14] This reduction appears to be a result of restriction of thoracic excursion by the patient's weight. Abdominal contents also may be displaced cephalad and interfere with diaphragmatic movement. Pulmonary blood flow appears to be preserved.[107] Intrapulmonary shunting generally does not increase in patients in the prone position.[190] When abdominal compression is avoided, some investigators report an increase in FRC with improvement of ventilation to perfusion matching[163] and an increase in arterial oxygen tension when anesthetized patients are turned into the prone position.[160]

The hemodynamic effects of the prone position are primarily a decrease in venous return[47] that may be compensated by an increase in systemic vascular resistance. Abdominal compression, especially in obese patients, can impede venous return. In contrast, Eggers et al.[61] report little change in cardiac index or stroke volume when patients are turned from the supine to prone position.

Brachial plexus injury also accounts for the majority of

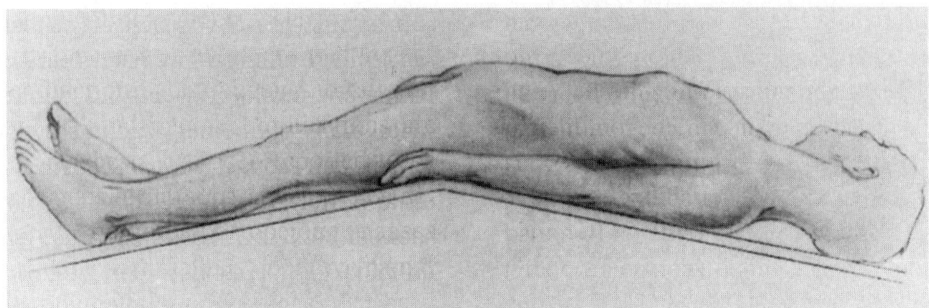

Fig. 75-7. The hyperextended supine position is used to facilitate exposure of the pelvis during retropubic prostatectomy and cystectomy. (Modified and reproduced, with permission, from Skinner DG, Lieskovsky G: *Diagnosis and management of genitourinary cancer,* Philadelphia, 1988, WB Saunders.)

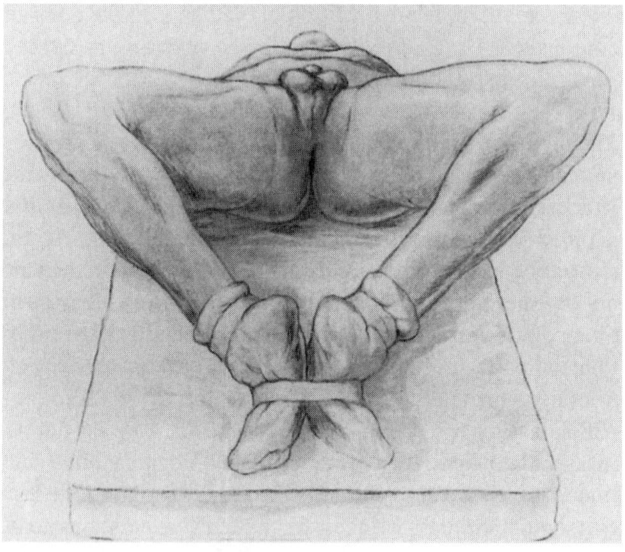

Fig. 75-8. The frog-leg position is a variation of the hyperextended supine position where the knees are flexed and the hips are abducted and externally rotated. (Modified and reproduced, with permission, from Skinner DG, Lieskovsky G: *Diagnosis and management of genitourinary cancer,* Philadelphia, 1988, WB Saunders.)

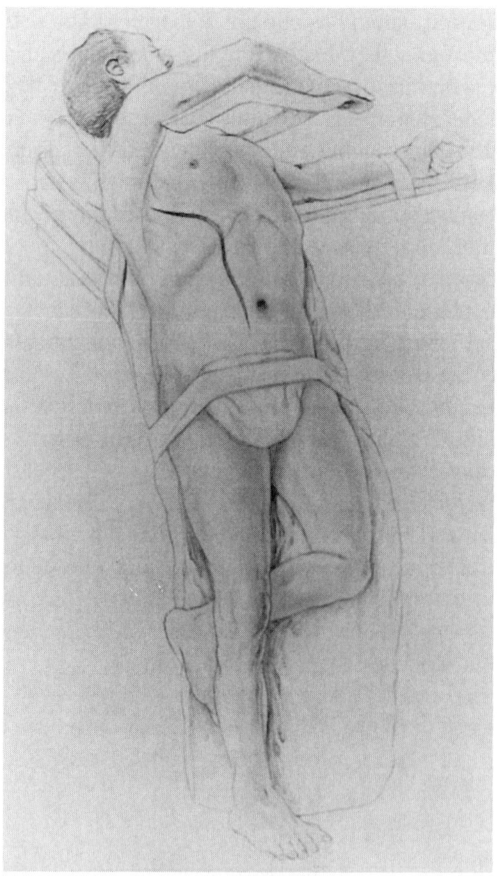

Fig. 75-9. This modification of the hyperextended supine position often is used for thoracoabdominal operations. (Modified and reproduced, with permission, from Skinner DG, Lieskovsky G: *Diagnosis and management of genitourinary cancer,* Philadelphia, 1988, WB Saunders.)

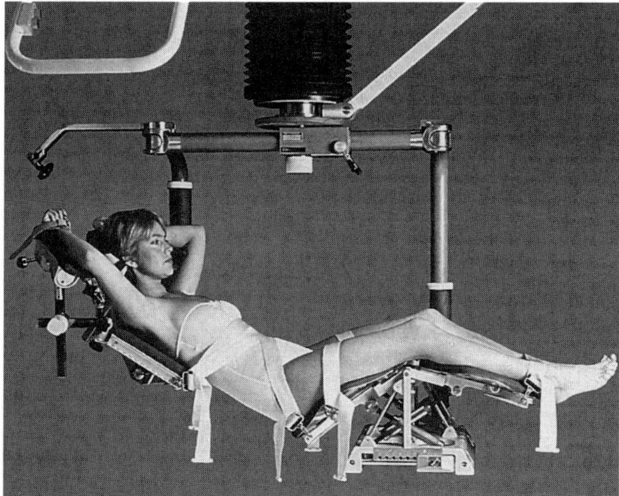

Fig. 75-10. The sitting position is used for water bath lithotripsy. (Reproduced with permission of Dornier Medical Systems, Inc., Kennesaw, GA.)

postoperative neuropathies after being in the prone position.[16] Extending the arm over the head can compress the brachial plexus against the first rib and clavicle. External rotation of the arm can cause the humeral head to stretch the brachial plexus. Abduction of the arm and turning the head to the contralateral side stretch cervical nerve roots.

Other nerve injuries may involve the facial, lateral femoral cutaneous, femoral, and posterior tibial nerves.[183] Branches of the facial nerve may be compressed by excessive pressure on a head rest. Uneven pressure or misplacement of supports under the patient may compress the lateral femoral cutaneous nerve against the iliac spines or the femoral nerve. Excessive pressure on the eye in the patient in the prone position leads to blindness as a result of thrombosis of the retinal artery.[16]

Sitting

The sitting position may be used for water bath lithotripsy (Fig. 75-10). Postural hypotension readily occurs in this position during anesthesia because both general and regional anesthesia blunt or abolish normal compensatory sympathetic reflexes.[45] Systemic arterial hypotension is accentuated by volume depletion. Although functional residual capacity may initially increase,[57] a decrease is typically seen following immersion in water (below).

Careful positioning of the patient helps avoid nerve injuries. Pressure points such as the elbows and ischial spines should be protected with padding.

EXTRACORPOREAL SHOCK WAVE LITHOTRIPSY

Preoperative considerations

Patients with renal or ureteral calculi in the upper two thirds of the ureters (above the iliac crest) frequently undergo extracorporeal shock wave lithotripsy (ESWL). This procedure disrupts kidney stones by focusing high-energy shock waves at them. With older units (Dornier HM3), the patient is placed in a hydraulic chair and immersed in a heated water bath; the patient is then positioned with the aid of two image intensifiers, such that the stone lies in the second focus of an elliptical reflector, whereas the source of the shock waves (spark gap) is in the first focus (Fig. 75-11). Newer units (Siemens Lithostar and Dornier MFL 5000) use a small amount of mineral oil on the skin to acoustically couple the patient to the energy source and therefore do not require a water bath; the shock waves are transmitted by a water-filled casing, which comes in contact with the patient via a plastic membrane.[161] Either radiography or ultrasound examination is used to localize the stone.

Shock waves may be generated electromagnetically, from piezoelectric crystals, or by discharging an underwater capacitor beneath the patient in the first focus of the elliptical reflector. Unlike ultrasound waves, which are used for diagnostic imaging, acoustic shock waves are unharmonic and have nonlinear characteristics. Because most tissues have the same acoustic density as water, shock waves travel through the body without damaging tissues. The change in acoustic impedance at the tissue–stone interface creates cavitational forces on the stone at the entry and exit sites; energy absorption produces stress, shear, and tear forces that promote fragmentation.[189]

The goal of the procedure is to fragment the stone sufficiently to allow its passage down the urinary tract. Some stones, like calcium oxalate dihydrate, usually fragment easily, whereas others such as cystine and calcium oxalate monohydrate may be recalcitrant to fragmentation.[189] Ureteral stents may be placed cystoscopically before the lithotripsy to facilitate passage of stone fragments. Tissue damage can occur if the shock waves are inadvertently focused at air–tissue interfaces such as in the lung and intestine.[130] Children may be more likely to suffer lung damage. Contraindications include inability to position the patient with the lungs and intestines clear of the direct path of shock waves, urinary obstruction below the stone, untreated infection which could result in sepsis, a bleeding diathesis, aortic aneurysm, cardiac pacemaker, orthopedic implant in the lumbar region, pregnancy, morbid obesity, and spinal hemangioma.[215] The presence of an aortic aneurysm, cardiac pacemaker, or orthopedic prosthetic device is currently considered only a relative contraindication in most centers. Ecchymosis, bruising, or blistering of the skin over the treatment site, subcapsular hemorrhage, and intrarenal hematomas are not uncommon.[108] Perinephric hematomas may occasionally be responsible for a dramatic decrease in hematocrit or arterial hypotension postoperatively.[188] Strohmaier et al.[191,192] recently reported that administration of calcium channel blockers before ESWL has a protective effect on renal tubular cells.

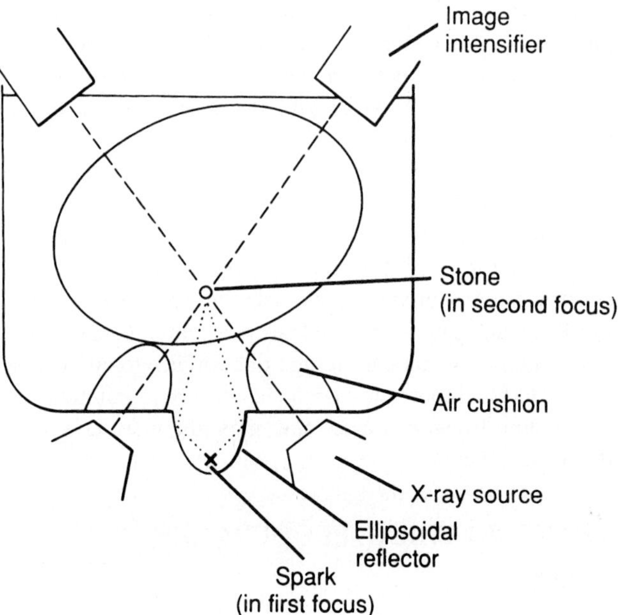

Fig. 75-11. Schematic of a spark gap lithotriptor. The source of the shock waves (spark gap) lies in the first focus of an elliptical reflector, whereas the patient is positioned with the aid of two image intensifiers such that the stone lies in the second focus. (Modified and reproduced, with permission, from Morgan GE, Mikhail MS: *Clinical anesthesiology,* ed 2, Stamford, 1996, Appleton & Lange.)

Anesthetic management

Patients with a history of cardiac arrhythmias and those with a pacemaker may be at increased risk of developing arrhythmias during the procedure.[189,207] Shock waves can occasionally inhibit, reprogram, or damage the internal components of some pacemakers.[63] Patients with cardiac pacemakers generally can undergo lithotripsy safely, providing the pacemaker is not in the direct path of the shock wave. A magnet or reprogramming machine and pharmacologic agents to support heart rate and rhythm (such as epinephrine and isoproterenol) should be immediately available.[58,72,118] Synchronization of the shock waves with the R wave from electrocardiography (ECG) decreases the incidence of arrhythmias. Shock waves typically are timed to be 20 ms after the R wave to correspond to the ventricular refractory period. Greenstein et al.[78] studied the incidence of cardiac arrhythmias during nonsynchronized ESWL treatments and concluded that nonsynchronized shocks can be safely administered to most patients.

Effects of immersion. Immersion into a heated water bath can transiently produce hypotension as a result of vasodilation. **The hydrostatic pressure of the water on the legs and abdomen redistributes blood into the chest and subsequently increases arterial blood pressure to normal level.[19] This sudden increase in venous return increases central venous and pulmonary artery pressures and can precipitate congestive heart failure in patients with limited cardiac reserve. Behnia et al.[20] reported that cardiac output generally decreases, whereas systemic vascular**

resistance increases after immersion. Moreover, the increase in intrathoracic blood volume reduces FRC by 30% to 60% and can predispose patients to hypoxemia.[31]

Choice of anesthesia. Pain during lithotripsy results from dissipation of energy at the skin where the shock waves enter the body and at tissues near the stone. Topical anesthesia at the skin alone does not eliminate the pain.[23] The pain generally is greatest at the skin interface and proportionate to the intensity of the shock waves.[63] Water bath lithotripsy typically uses 1500 to 2000 relatively high-intensity shock waves (18 to 22 kV), for which patients typically require either regional or general anesthesia. A few selected patients may tolerate the procedure with local anesthetic infiltration of the skin together with intravenous (IV) heavy sedation,[123] but an increased number of low-intensity shock waves (14 to 16 kV) sessions are required.[158] Studies comparing general versus regional anesthesia fail to show any differences in morbidity or mortality rates.[109] An alternative technique uses intercostal blocks combined with local skin infiltration.[129]

Newer lithotripsy units couple the shock waves directly to the skin and use 2000 to 3000 low-intensity shock waves (10 to 18 kV), which most patients tolerate with only light sedation.[114,143,196] Most sedation techniques use various combinations of midazolam, propofol, and an opioid. Some investigators have reported good success and less drug consumption with patient-controlled analgesia using alfentanil.[117] Modification of older water bath lithotriptors (HM3) such that the shock waves are distributed over a greater area of skin interface also allows patients to undergo the procedure without the need for regional or general anesthesia.[9] Use of a topical anesthetic in the form of EMLA cream does not reduce analgesic requirements.[136,144]

Regional anesthesia. Regional anesthesia greatly facilitates positioning and monitoring of patients during water bath lithotripsy. Epidural anesthesia is preferred more than spinal anesthesia because of the potential for a postdural puncture headache with the latter (especially in patients in the upright position) and less control over the sensory level.[59] Spinal anesthesia has been associated with a high (up to 45%) incidence of postdural puncture headache.[171]

Continuous epidural anesthesia with a T6 sensory level provides adequate anesthesia because renal innervation is derived from T10 to L1. Light sedation also is generally desirable. Cook et al.[44] found that the addition of epidural fentanyl did not dramatically improve the intensity of the anesthesia but improved postoperative analgesia. As little air as possible should be used during placement of the catheter because large amounts of air in the epidural space could theoretically dissipate shock waves and promote injury to spinal neural tissue.[54] Korbon et al.[116] reported a decrease in the compliance of the epidural space in patients with repeat epidural anesthesia for serial lithotripsies; this unconfirmed report suggests that dural puncture may be more likely during subsequent attempts at epidural anesthesia. Supplemental oxygen by face mask or nasal cannula is given to avoid hypoxemia. Intravascular volume expansion with 1000 to 1500 ml of lactated Ringer's injection helps prevent severe postural hypotension after epidural activation, positioning in the hydraulic chair, and immersion in the warm bath. Fluid therapy typically is generous during the procedure to maintain brisk urinary flow and flush stone debris and blood clots. A small dose of furosemide (10 to 20 mg) also may be desirable in patients with poor cardiac reserve.

A major disadvantage of regional anesthesia is the inability to control diaphragmatic movement. Excessive diaphragmatic excursion during spontaneous ventilation in some patients can move the stone in and out of the wave focus and may prolong the procedure. Cooperative patients may be asked to breathe with a more rapid and shallow respiratory pattern. Bradycardia (e.g., from high sympathetic blockade) also prolongs the procedure if the shock waves are coupled to the ECG.

General anesthesia. General endotracheal anesthesia is preferred by many patients and some urologists because it allows control of diaphragmatic excursion. General anesthesia for water bath lithotripsy is complicated by the inherent risks of placing an unconscious supine patient into a chair, elevating and lowering the chair into the water bath, and then reversing the sequence at the end. Light general anesthesia with muscle paralysis generally is preferred to avoid excessive hypotension. Muscle paralysis assures immobility of the patient, avoids the need for deep anesthesia, and provides control over diaphragmatic movement. Use of high-frequency jet ventilation instead of conventional ventilation does not appear to decrease the number of shocks required or radiation exposure during fluoroscopy[219] and generally has been unsatisfactory.[21] IV fluid loading with 1000 ml of lactated Ringer's injection generally is advisable before moving patients upright into the hydraulic chair to prevent postural hypotension.

Monitoring. Water immersion complicates routine monitoring. ECG pads should be protected with water-proof dressings before immersion. Close ECG monitoring is indicated because even R wave-triggered shocks can induce supraventricular or ventricular arrhythmias.[207] The decrease in FRC with immersion mandates close monitoring of oxygen saturation in patients at high risk for developing hypoxemia. Body temperature should be closely monitored after immersion because hypo- and hyperthermia have been described.[97,131]

TRANSURETHRAL PROCEDURES

Cystoscopy

Preoperative considerations

Cystoscopy is one of the most commonly performed urologic procedures. It usually is performed on an outpatient basis. The most common indications include hematuria, recurrent urinary infections, and urinary obstruction. The urologist may use either a rigid or flexible endoscope. Bladder biopsies, removal of bladder and prostatic tumors, extraction of renal stones, retrograde pyelography, and placement or manipulation of ureteral catheters generally are performed with rigid cystoscopy. Transurethral resection of the prostate is discussed separately in the following section.

Anesthetic management

Obturator reflex. Stimulation of the obturator nerve by electrocautery current through the lateral bladder wall produces external rotation and adduction of the thigh. The resulting muscle contractions can produce musculoskeletal injury or cause the surgeon to perforate the bladder with the cystoscope. **Regional anesthesia does not abolish the obturator reflex unless obturator nerve blocks also are performed.**[70] **The muscle contractions are reliably blocked only by muscle paralysis during general anesthesia.**

Autonomic hyperreflexia. Patients with spinal cord injuries often undergo repeat cystoscopies, especially for stone manipulations. **When the cord lesion is above T6–T7, autonomic hyperreflexia may be encountered during the procedure. This disorder is characterized by paroxysms of generalized sympathetic hyperactivity in response to stimulation below the cord lesion.**[10] **The most typical presentation is sudden hypertension and bradycardia.** Below the lesion, the patient displays pallor, pilomotor erection with somatic and viseral muscle contraction, and increased spasticity. Above the lesion, there often is flushing of the face and neck, congestion of mucous membranes, sweating, and mydriasis. Attacks generally are self-limited but can be life-threatening. Severe, sustained hypertension can lead to hypertensive encephalopathy, stroke, arrhythmias, myocardial ischemia, and death.

Choice of anesthesia. The choice of anesthetic technique for cystoscopy varies with age, gender, and medical condition and with the purpose of the procedure. Children typically require general anesthesia. In contrast, topical anesthesia is adequate for diagnostic studies in most women because of their short urethra. Most young male patients require regional or general anesthesia even for diagnostic studies. Operative cystoscopies involving biopsies, cauterization, or manipulation of ureteral catheters are performed during regional or general anesthesia. General anesthesia with muscle paralysis may be preferable when extensive cauterization is anticipated in the area of the obturator nerve (see previous).

Patients with a high spinal cord lesion or a history of autonomic hyperreflexia require special consideration. Regional and general anesthesia are used. Although spinal and epidural anesthesia can effectively block autonomic hyperreflexia,[199] they often are technically difficult because of spinal deformities; moreover, anesthetic level often is difficult to ascertain. There is no evidence that regional anesthesia worsens neurologic function postoperatively.[10] General anesthesia is complicated by the problem that light anesthesia can lead to hyperreflexia, whereas deep anesthesia readily produces arterial hypotension. Topical anesthesia generally is not successful in preventing hyperreflexia.

Topical anesthesia. Flexible cystoscopy can be performed in most patients with topical (viscous) and intravesical lidocaine.[99] Patients tolerate the procedure well, providing the surgeon does not overdistend the bladder. Diagnostic rigid cystoscopy with topical anesthesia of the urethra also can be carried out in most women and in many cooperative elderly male patients. IV sedation with a benzodiazepine, opioid, or propofol usually is desirable when a rigid cystoscope is used.

General anesthesia. General anesthesia is used for most patients because of the short duration (10 to 20 minutes) and outpatient setting of the procedure. Moreover, most patients are apprehensive about the procedure and prefer to be asleep. Light general anesthesia using thiopental or propofol with nitrous oxide and a halogenated agent is most commonly selected. Airway management typically involves either a conventional or laryngeal mask. Endotracheal intubation may be advisable in morbidly obese patients. Oxygen saturation should be closely monitored whenever patients with marginal pulmonary reserve are placed in the lithotomy or Trendelenburg position. Succinylcholine should be avoided in patients with spinal cord lesions.[200]

Regional anesthesia. Epidural and spinal blocks with a T10 sensory level provide satisfactory anesthesia for cystoscopic procedures. Most clinicians prefer regional anesthesia, especially for procedures lasting more than 30 minutes in elderly and high-risk patients. Satisfactory sensory blockade may require 15 to 20 minutes for epidural anesthesia compared with 5 to 10 minutes for spinal anesthesia. If spinal anesthesia is chosen, hyperbaric bupivicaine (10 to 12 mg) or tetracaine (8 to 10 mg) usually provides an adequate sensory level for most patients undergoing cystoscopies. Studies fail to demonstrate that immediate elevation of the legs after intrathecal injection of a hyperbaric anesthetic solution increases the level of anesthesia or the incidence of severe hypotension.[168] Further, Trendelenburg position does not always increase the cephalad spread of hyperbaric local anesthetic during spinal anesthesia.[178] The site of injection appears to influence cephalad spread. Tuominen et al.[202] reported the sensory level to be several dermatomes higher when intrathecal injections were made at L2–L3 compared with injections at L4–L5.

Transurethral Resection of the Prostate

Preoperative considerations

Obstructive uropathy resulting from prostatic enlargement is one of the most commonly observed problems in men aged more than 60 years. If not recognized and managed promptly, it can result in hydronephrosis, uremia, and irreversible kidney damage. The most common cause of obstruction is benign adenomatous hyperplasia of the prostate. Many patients eventually opt for surgical relief because conservative treatment often is unsuccessful in relieving symptoms. One of four surgical procedures may be selected to remove hyperplastic prostatic tissue, including suprapubic (transvesical) prostatectomy, perineal prostatectomy, retropubic prostatectomy, and transurethral resection of the prostate (TURP). Although morbidity and mortality rates may be somewhat comparable between operations,[51] the transurethral approach is nearly always selected for patients with prostate glands weighing less than 60 g.[149] The mortality rate for patients undergoing TURP is about 0.2%.[139] Suprapubic prostatectomy usually is chosen for patients with prostate glands exceeding 60 g. Alternative management includes transurethral incision of the prostate, laser prostatectomy, balloon dilation, microwave hyperthermia, and high-intensity ultrasound. Most of these procedures require either light general anesthesia or IV sedation.

Carcinomatous enlargement of the prostate also frequently causes urinary obstruction in elderly men. Patients with advanced prostatic carcinoma may present for transurethral resections to relieve symptomatic urinary obstruction as an adjunct to hormonal therapy. Curative surgery for prostatic carcinoma requires radical retropubic prostatectomy.

Patients undergoing prostate surgery have a relatively high (up to 60%) prevalence of cardiovascular, pulmonary, or renal disease.[139] They should be carefully evaluated for coexistent cardiac and pulmonary disease and for renal dysfunction. **Myocardial infarction, pulmonary edema, and renal failure are common causes of perioperative morbidity and mortality. Sepsis has also recently emerged as a major cause of mortality.**[139] Blood should be crossmatched for anemic patients and for patients with large glands (>30 to 40 g) because prostatic bleeding can be difficult to control through the cystoscope. A type and screen is adequate for most other patients.

Anesthetic management

Transurethral resection of the prostate enlarges the urinary channel between the urethra and bladder. The procedure usually is performed by passing a loop through a special cystoscope, called a *resectoscope.* The median and lateral lobes of the prostate tissue are cut by applying a cutting electrocautery current to the loop. Distention of the bladder with intermittent or continuous irrigation with fluid is required to keep blood and tissue from obstructing the view.

TURP can be associated with serious complications because of the characteristics of the prostate and because of the large amounts of irrigation fluid often used (Table 75-1).[139]

TURP syndrome. The procedure often opens the extensive network of venous sinuses in the prostate, potentially allowing systemic absorption of the irrigating fluid. Electrolyte solutions are not used for irrigation because they disperse the electrocautery current. Use of water provides excellent visibility because its hypotonicity lyses any erythrocytes, but it can readily result in acute water intoxication. Water irrigation generally is restricted for cystoscopy and resection of bladder tumors. Near-isotonic nonelectrolyte irrigating solutions, such as glycine 1.5% (230 mOsm/l) or Cytal, a mixture of sorbitol 2.7% and mannitol 0.54% (195 mOsm/l), are most commonly used during TURP. Less common solutions include mannitol, 3%, sorbitol, 3.3%, dextrose, 2.5% to 4%, and urea, 1%.

Table 75-1 Complications associated with TURP

Complication	Incidence (%)
Bleeding requiring transfusion	2.5
TURP syndrome	2
Cardiac arrhythmia	1.1
Bladder perforation	0.9

Data from Mebust WK, Holtgrewe HL, Cockett ATK, et al: Transurethral prostatectomy — immediate and postoperative complications: a cooperative study of 13 participating institutions evaluating 3885 patients, *J Urol* 141:243; 1989.

The absorption of large amounts of fluid (> 2 to 3 l) can produce a constellation of symptoms and signs commonly referred to as the TURP syndrome.[105,133,140] **This potentially fatal syndrome presents during or immediately after the procedure. Its manifestations are primarily circulatory fluid overload, water intoxication, and occasionally toxicity from the solute in the irrigating fluid.**

A fair amount of water absorption can occur because all irrigating fluids are hypotonic. Subclinical hemolysis occurs even with glycine solutions.[17] Absorption of irrigation fluid depends on the duration of the resection and on the height (pressure) of the irrigation fluid. The syndrome has been reported to present after only 15 minutes of resection.[102] Most resections last about 45 to 60 minutes. An average of 10 to 30 ml/min of the irrigating fluid is absorbed during TURP.[81]

Absorption of a large amount of irrigation fluid can produce signs of pulmonary congestion or florid pulmonary edema in patients with limited cardiac reserve. The hypotonicity of these fluids also readily produces acute hyponatremia and hypoosmolality, which may lead to serious neurologic manifestations. Increased circulating levels of vasopressin (ADH) may be contributory.[82,83] Some clinicians routinely administer furosemide to reduce the risk of clot retention and to promote diuresis and possibly prevent TURP syndrome.[52] A progressive increase in blood pressure may be an early clue of water absorption and hypervolemia when central venous or pulmonary artery pressure measurements are not available. Cardiac manifestations include arrhythmias, hypotension, and pulmonary edema.[1] ECG changes, such as widening of the QRS complex and ST segment elevation, may occur at levels of less than 115 mEq/l.

Central nervous system (CNS) symptoms related to hyponatremia include restlessness, headache, irritability, confusion, blindness, coma, and seizures. Symptoms are more readily diagnosed intraoperatively in patients receiving regional anesthesia. They present on emergence in patients undergoing TURP with general anesthesia. Serial measurements of serum sodium may be helpful in detecting major fluid absorption and alerting the anesthetist to potential CNS and cardiac complications. Neurologic symptoms generally are not present until serum sodium levels decrease below 120 mEq/l. Lower sodium levels have been associated with coma.[94] Marked hypotonicity in plasma ([Na+] < 100 mEq/l) also can result in intravascular hemolysis.

Toxicity also may occur in some patients from absorption of the solute in the irrigation fluid. Marked hyperglycinemia has been reported to result in CNS toxicity and circulatory depression in patients receiving more than 1 l of glycine solutions. Nausea, malaise, vomiting, confusion, stupor, and coma have been associated with hyperglycinemia. Plasma glycine levels in excess of 1000 mg/l have been reported (normal, 13 to 17 mg/l).[156] Glycine, which is known to be an inhibitory neurotransmitter in the CNS, also has been implicated in rare instances of transient blindness after TURP.[48,156,166] Use of glycine solutions appears to prolong visual evoked potentials, but the correlation between latency and serum glycine concentration is poor; glycine metabolites may therefore be responsible.[37,86] **Hyperammonemia with marked CNS toxicity also has been described and is presumably from the metabolic degradation of glycine.**[98,165] Blood ammonia levels can exceed 500 μmol/l (normal, 5 to 50 μmol/l).[98] Large amounts of sorbitol or dextrose solutions could exacerbate hyperglycemia in diabetic patients. Absorption of large amounts of a mannitol solution can produce fluid overload as a result of acute intravascular volume expansion.

Successful management of the TURP syndrome is directed at early recognition and is based on the severity of symptoms. Hypoxemia and hypoperfusion should be avoided while the absorbed water is eliminated. The majority of patients can be treated with oxygen therapy, fluid restriction, and a loop diuretic. Severely symptomatic hyponatremia producing seizures or coma should be managed with hypertonic saline. The amount of hypertonic saline solution (usually 3%) is based on the patient's serum sodium concentration, and the rate should not be faster than 100 ml/h so that circulatory fluid overload is not exacerbated. Midazolam (2 to 4 mg), diazepam (3 to 5 mg), or thiopental (50 to 100 mg) can be used to terminate seizure activity. Phenytoin, 10 to 20 mg/kg IV (no faster than 50 mg/min), also may be advisable to provide more sustained anticonvulsant activity. Endotracheal intubation should be undertaken in obtunded patients to prevent aspiration until the mental status normalizes.

Hypothermia. Large volumes of irrigating fluids at room temperature are a potential source of heat loss for the patient.[8,89] To prevent hypothermia, irrigating solutions can be warmed to body temperature before they are used. Shivering may dislodge clots and promote postoperative bleeding. Anesthetic techniques do not appear to significantly differ in their effects on heat loss.[187]

Bladder perforation. Bladder perforation is estimated to occur in 1% of patients undergoing TURP.[139] Overdistention of the bladder with irrigation or penetration of the resectoscope through the bladder wall can be responsible. Most perforations are extraperitoneal and usually are associated with poor return of the irrigating fluid.[110] Alert patients may complain of nausea, diaphoresis, and retropubic, lower abdominal, or periumbilical pain. **Large extraperitoneal and most intraperitoneal perforations present as sudden unexplained hypotension with generalized abdominal pain. General anesthesia or heavy sedation can mask perforation, although perforation should be suspected after sudden hypo- or hypertension, especially when associated with reflex bradycardia.**

Bleeding and coagulopathy. Intraoperative bleeding necessitates transfusion in about 2.5% of patients undergoing TURP; an additional 3.7% eventually require transfusion postoperatively.[139] Factors associated with transfusion include a prostate gland weighing more than 35 to 45 g or a resection greater than 90-minutes duration.[139,184] Intraoperative blood loss is reported to be approximately 3 to 5 ml per minute of resection.[90] Studies on the relationship between the type of anesthesia and blood loss are conflicting. Some studies report a major reduction in blood loss with epidural anesthesia compared with general anesthesia.[3,126,127] Others could not demonstrate any differences in bleeding between epidural and general anesthesia[152] or between spinal and general anesthesia.[137,184] Blood loss was similar during general anesthesia whether spontaneous or mechanical ventilation was used.[137,152] Using warmed irrigating fluids had no effect on blood loss.[91]

Disseminated intravascular coagulation (DIC) has been reported after TURP and generally is thought to be a result of the release of thromboplastins from the prostate into the circulation during surgery.[68,90] As many as 6% of patients may develop subclinical intravascular coagulopathies.[184] Dilutional thrombocytopenia caused by absorption of irrigation fluid may contribute to bleeding. Patients with metastatic carcinoma of the prostate have been reported to develop primary fibrinolysis; tumor secretion of fibrinolytic enzymes (fibrinolysins) is likely responsible in such instances. Coagulopathy usually manifests as diffuse uncontrollable bleeding but should be confirmed by laboratory tests. Primary fibrinolysis should be managed with ϵ-aminocaproic acid (Amicar), 5 g, followed by 1 g/hour IV. The management of DIC in this setting is complicated and should be undertaken in consultation with a hematologist because heparin therapy may be indicated in addition to replacement of clotting factors and platelets.

Septicemia and other complications. The prostate often harbors chronic infection. Extensive manipulation or surgery frequently produces transient bacteremia. Preoperative prophylactic antibiotic therapy decreases the likelihood of major bacteremic and septic episodes after TURP.[88]

Fatal massive air embolism has been described at the end of TURP when air is introduced into the bladder.[203] The air presumably entered the circulation via opened prostatic veins.

Choice of anesthesia. Dobson et al.[56] studied hemodynamics changes in patients receiving spinal anesthesia and compared them with those in patients having general anesthesia. They found major changes only after induction. Mean arterial pressure decreased similarly with both techniques, but general anesthesia also was associated with significant reductions in cardiac output. The incidence of perioperative myocardial ischemia appears to be similar.[60] Moreover, both techniques appear to have a similar mortality rate.[100] Spinal anesthesia is most commonly used in the United States.[139]

Studies comparing cognitive function in patients receiving regional anesthesia with those having general anesthesia have found no differences in short-term and long-term cognitive scores.[13,40,74,80,153] Although most studies show a decline in cognitive function in the first few hours or days after surgery, nearly all patients eventually had full recovery. Nilsson and Hahn[153] have suggested that the amount of fluid absorption is the most important factor that correlates with changes in mental status. Studies evaluating the influence of preoperative mental function on postoperative cognitive impairment are inconsistent.[80,181] When compared with general anesthesia, regional anesthesia in some studies appears to decrease surgical blood loss[3,126,127] and may reduce the incidence of postoperative venous thrombosis.[95] Whelan et al.[213] reported that patients undergoing TURP during general anesthesia had a transient decrease in immunocompetence, whereas those receiving spinal anesthesia did not; although interesting, the clinical importance of this study remains unclear. Regional anesthesia may be less likely to mask symptoms and signs of TURP syndrome or bladder perforation.

The possibility of vertebral metastasis should be considered in patients with carcinoma, especially in those with back pain. Metastatic disease to the lumbar spine generally is considered a relative contraindication to regional anesthesia.[148] Minor, transient low frequency hearing loss may be common after spinal anesthesia and is reported to occur even with 26-gauge needles.[208,209] The incidence of postdural puncture headache appears to be low after TURP, possibly because of the older age and male gender of this group of patients.

Either spinal or epidural anesthesia with a T10 sensory level can provide excellent anesthesia for those undergoing TURP. Hyperbaric tetracaine, 8 to 10 mg, or bupivicaine, 10 to 12 mg, is most commonly used. Addition of epinephrine, 0.2 mg, prolongs and enhances the effectiveness of the block, especially with lower doses of local anesthetic.[35] Preoperative, oral clonidine, 0.15 mg, also can prolong tetracaine spinal anesthesia.[155] Lower sensory levels may be adequate if bladder pressure is kept low (< 15 mm Hg).[18] Addition of 0.1 or 0.2 mg of morphine to the intrathecal local anesthetic also provides sustained postoperative analgesia;[111] higher dosages increase the incidence of nausea and vomiting. Intrathecal meperidine, 0.5 to 1.0 mg/kg, alone can provide intraoperative anesthesia and postoperative analgesia of shorter duration.[76,119]

Transurethral injection of local anesthetics into the prostate allows TURP without regional or general anesthesia in selected patients.[25] This technique may facilitate TURP in the outpatient setting.[138]

Monitoring. Mental status is the best monitor for detecting early signs of the TURP syndrome and bladder perforation. Addition of ethanol to the irrigation fluid in conjunction with expired breath analysis for ethanol can allow quantification of the absorption of irrigating fluid;[84,85,101,186] unfortunately, this technique is largely a research tool. A decrease in arterial oxygen saturation may be a relatively late sign of fluid overload. Close temperature monitoring is advisable during long resections to detect hypothermia. Blood loss is especially difficult to assess because of the use of large volumes of irrigating solutions, so clinical signs of hypovolemia should be relied on. Blood loss may be estimated based on the duration of the resection.[90] Transient, postoperative decreases in hematocrit reflect blood loss and hemodilution from absorption of irrigation fluid.

Several investigators have reported a disturbingly high rate (18%) of intraoperative myocardial ischemia in patients undergoing TURP.[60,96] Patients with a history of ischemic heart disease should be monitored closely in the intra- and postoperative periods. Edwards et al.[60] emphasized that not only are these patients at high risk for ischemia but that the incidence and duration of ischemic episodes were highest after surgery.

MAJOR CANCER SURGERY

Urologic tumors account for a large percentage of all malignancies in the United States. Adenocarcinoma of the prostate is the most common malignancy in men and the second most common cause of cancer deaths in men aged more than 55 years. Bladder, renal, and testicular cancers, although less common, are neoplasms for which curative and palliative surgery plays an important role in management. Anesthesiologists may increasingly encounter patients undergoing operations for these tumors because of a steady increase in average life expectancy (these malignancies generally affect older individuals) and because of an increase in the incidence of some of these malignancies.

Surgery for Prostate Cancer

Preoperative considerations

Prostate cancer is a disease of aging, rarely occurring before age 40 years and reaching a peak incidence at age 80 years. The incidence of adenocarcinoma of the prostate is estimated to be 75% in patients aged more than 75 years.[149] Management varies from surveillance to aggressive surgical therapy because of the tumor's spectrum of clinical behavior. Important variables that influence management include the grade and stage of the malignancy, patient age, and the presence of other medical illnesses. Patients may come to the operating room for pelvic lymph node dissection to stage the cancer, radical prostatectomy, salvage prostatectomy or cystoprostatectomy (after failure of radiation therapy), or bilateral orchiectomy for hormonal therapy.

Anesthetic management

Pelvic lymph node dissection. Staging of prostate cancer is traditionally based on clinical (rectal) examination and a computed tomography (CT) or magnetic resonance imaging (MRI) scan to detect lymph node involvement and a bone scan. Transrectal ultrasound examination also is currently heavily relied on for biopsies and evaluating tumor size and possible extracapsular extension. Pelvic lymph node dissection has increasingly been advocated in recent years to more accurately stage the cancer. This has been in large part a result of development of a laparoscopic technique. Many urologists believe that the combination of a preoperative prostate-specific antigen (PSA) level with the Gleason score of the biopsy provide sufficient information in most patients to avoid the need for a staging lymph node dissection.[149]

Laparoscopic pelvic lymph node dissection (LPLND) differs from most other laparoscopic procedures in that: (1) the patient is placed in steep Trendelenburg position and rotated from side to side for surgical exposure, (2) greater CO_2 absorption can potentially take place because the retroperitoneum is entered, and (3) the copious fluid used to irrigate clots from the pelvic fossa can produce hypothermia.[211] The procedure is carried out during general endotracheal anesthesia because of its duration, steep Trendelenburg position, necessity for abdominal distention, and desirability of being able to increase the patient's minute ventilation. Most clinicians avoid nitrous oxide to prevent bowel distention and expansion of residual intra-abdominal gas.

Radical retropubic prostatectomy. Radical retropubic prostatectomy typically is performed in conjunction with pelvic lymph node dissection through a lower, midline, abdominal incision. The operation is used for localized prostatic cancer or occasionally as a salvage procedure after radiation.[38] It involves *en bloc* removal of the entire prostate gland, the seminal vesicles, ejaculatory ducts, and part of the bladder neck. Although the prostate is always approached anteriorly, the dissection may proceed either from the urethra upward (Campbell) or from the bladder downward (Walsh); the latter technique more often is chosen for preservation of sexual function ("nerve-sparing" prostatectomy). After the prostatectomy, the remaining bladder neck is anastomosed directly to the urethra over an indwelling urinary catheter. The surgeon may ask for IV administration of indigo carmine for visualization of the ureters. This agent can be associated with either hyper- or hypotension.[104,176] If sexual function cannot be preserved, a first stage penile prosthesis (reservoir) often is placed. Radical retropubic prostatectomies are often associated with major operative blood loss. Direct arterial pressure monitoring is advisable in most patients. Some authors also advocate routine use of central venous pressure monitoring.[145] Albin et al.[6] suggest the use of a precordial Doppler because of the potential for venous air embolism.[162]

Blood loss appears to vary considerably from center to center; values less than 500 ml are not uncommon, but some institutions report average blood losses in excess of 1500 ml.[174] **Anatomic factors that may affect blood loss include positioning, pelvic anatomy, and size of the prostate; surgical factors may include operative technique, early ligation of the dorsal vein of the penis plexus, and temporary clamping of the hypogastric artery. Blood loss appears to be similar in patients receiving general anesthesia and those having regional anesthesia.**[174] Controlled hypotension also may play a role in reducing operative blood loss. There is value of preoperative autologous blood donation for reducing allogenic transfusions, but this value has been questioned as a cost-effective strategy.[75,145,217] Hemodilution may be an effective but less costly strategy.[151]

Retropubic prostatectomy can be performed during general, epidural, or spinal anesthesia. Postoperative morbidity appears to be similar in patients receiving epidural and general anesthesia.[173] Regional anesthesia requires a T6 sensory level, but because the hyperextended supine position is typically used, patients often do not tolerate regional anesthesia without heavy sedation. Moreover, the combination of prolonged Trendelenburg with administration of large amounts of IV fluids can produce edema of the upper airway, which may complicate anesthetic management should endotracheal intubation become necessary.

Use of epidural opioids for postoperative analgesia does not appear to be clearly superior to IV patient-controlled analgesia (PCA).[7,122,175] Shir et al.[175] reported that epidural anesthesia may have a preemptive analgesic effect because it decreases postoperative pain requirements, although they could not demonstrate this effect in patients receiving epidural and general anesthesia. More recently, Liu et al.[122] found no differences in pain relief or recovery between patients receiving hydromorphone either epidurally or by IV PCA; the latter group of patients did require less hydromorphone. Use of ketorolac as an adjuvant to epidural fentanyl analgesia has been shown to decrease fentanyl requirements, improve analgesia, and promote earlier return of bowel function without increasing transfusion requirements.[77] The same effect may be expected with IV opioids administered by PCA.

Extensive dissection near the pelvic veins likely increases the risk of thromboembolic complications. Hendolin et al.[95] have suggested that epidural anesthesia reduces the incidence of postoperative deep vein thrombosis after open prostatectomy, but many surgeons routinely use warfarin postoperatively to reduce the incidence of postoperative thrombophlebitis and pulmonary embolism. Prophylactic minidose heparin has been reported to increase operative blood loss and transfusion requirements,[24] whereas sequential pneumatic (leg) compression devices appear to delay but not reduce deep vein thrombosis.[41] The beneficial antithrombotic effect of epidural anesthesia is likely lost with warfarin therapy. Moreover, postoperative anticoagulation may increase the risk of epidural hematoma.

Other surgical complications include hemorrhage, injury to the obturator nerve, ureter, and rectum, and urinary incontinence and impotence.[11]

Radical perineal prostatectomy. Unlike the retropubic approach, this approach for radical prostatectomy does not allow simultaneous lymph node dissection. Pelvic lymph node dissection should be carried out separately first. The procedure also does not easily allow preservation of the pelvic nerve plexus and thus sexual function. Claims that the transperineal approach is associated with less blood loss may be unfounded.

Anesthetic management is complicated by the extreme (exaggerated) lithotomy position. Careful positioning is required to decrease the likelihood of musculoskeletal or neurologic injuries. Patients typically require general endotracheal anesthesia because of this position, which is uncomfortable and interferes with diaphragmatic excursion. The procedure can be associated with considerable blood loss (> 2.0 l). Two large-bore IV catheters and direct arterial pressure monitoring generally are indicated.

Bilateral orchiectomy. This procedure usually is performed for local control of the tumor in patients with metastatic adenocarcinoma of the prostate. It effectively ablates production of androgens from the testicles. The procedure is relatively short (20 to 45 minutes) and is performed through a single midline scrotal incision. Although bilateral orchiectomy can be performed under local anesthesia, most patients and many clinicians prefer general anesthesia. Regional anesthesia also may be appropriate if metastatic disease of the lumbar spine can be excluded.

Surgery for Bladder Cancer and Urinary Diversion

Preoperative considerations

Bladder cancer is the second most common malignancy of the genitourinary tract. Its incidence is highest in elderly patients (average age, 65 years) with a 3:1 male-to-female ratio. Transitional cell carcinoma is most common. The association of cigarette smoking with carcinoma of the bladder contributes to coexistent coronary artery and chronic obstructive pulmonary disease in many of these patients. Impaired renal function may be age-related or a result of urinary tract obstruction. Staging includes cystoscopy and CT or MRI scans. Intravesical chemotherapy may be used for superficial tumors, whereas transurethral resection may be carried out for single low grade noninvasive tumors. Preoperative radiation may be administered to some patients to reduce tumor size before radical cystectomy.

Anesthetic management

Radical cystectomy. Radical cystectomy is a major operation that is commonly associated with considerable blood loss.[167] The procedure is performed through a large midline incision that extends from the pubis to xyphoid. All anterior pelvic organs, including the bladder, prostate, and seminal vesicles, are removed in men; part of the urethra also may be taken. The resection in women includes the uterus, cervix, ovaries, part of the urethra, and the anterior vaginal vault. Pelvic node dissection also is performed bilaterally. After cystectomy, urinary diversion is undertaken.

Radical resection of these cancers typically requires 3 to 4 hours and frequently necessitates blood transfusion. General endotracheal anesthesia with a muscle relaxant provides optimal operating conditions. Controlled hypotensive anesthesia may reduce intraoperative blood loss and transfusion requirements.[5] Supplementation of general anesthesia with spinal or continuous epidural anesthesia can facilitate the induced hypotension and decreases general anesthetic requirements. Moreover, an epidural catheter provides a highly effective route for postoperative analgesia. A major drawback in the use of regional anesthesia is hyperperistalsis, which often produces a small contracted bowel (to be discussed).

Close monitoring of intravascular volume and blood loss is essential during these procedures. Direct intra-arterial pressure monitoring is indicated in all patients. Multiple large-bore IV catheters are desirable in case rapid transfusion becomes necessary. Central venous pressure monitoring is advisable in patients with limited cardiac reserve, whereas pulmonary artery pressure monitoring is indicated for those with a history of ventricular dysfunction. Urinary output should be monitored continuously and correlated with the progress of the operation because the urinary path is interrupted at an early point during most of these procedures.

Urinary diversion. Urinary diversion is most commonly performed immediately after radical cystectomy. Several procedures are currently used, but all entail implanting the ureters into a segment of bowel. The bowel segment is either left *in situ,* such as in ureterosigmoidostomy (uncommon), or divided with its mesenteric blood supply intact and attached to a cutaneous stoma or urethra. Depending on the type of procedure, the isolated bowel can function either as a conduit (ileal conduit) or be reconstructed to form a continent reservoir (such as a Kock pouch). Conduits may be formed from ileum, jejunum, or colon. Continent urinary diversions include ureterosigmoidostomy and small bowel (Kock, Camey), large bowel (Indiana), and gastric reservoirs.

Good anesthetic management depends on keeping the patient well hydrated and on maintaining a brisk urinary output. If the procedure follows a radical cystectomy, central venous pressure monitoring often is used to guide IV fluid administration. The point at which the ureters are divided should be noted to prevent overzealous fluid administration in response to an abrupt decrease in urine output. When regional anesthesia is used as part of the anesthetic technique, unopposed parasympathetic activity as a result of sympathetic blockade can result in a contracted, hyperactive bowel that makes construction of a continent ileal reservoir technically difficult. The use of a large dose of anticholinergic (glycopyrrolate, 1 mg) or papaverine (50–100 mg as a slow IV infusion over 2 or 3 hours) often alleviates this problem.[132]

Prolonged contact of urine with bowel mucosa may

allow sufficient exchange of ions across the bowel to produce metabolic disturbances. Hyponatremic, hypochloremic, or hyperkalemic metabolic acidosis can occur after jejunal conduits. In contrast, colonic and ileal conduits can be associated with hyperchloremic metabolic acidosis. Hyponatremic metabolic alkalosis has been described when gastric mucosa is used.

Surgery for Testicular Cancer

Preoperative considerations

Ninety-five percent of all testicular tumors are germ cell tumors; they are commonly classified either as seminomas or nonseminomas. The latter includes embryonal teratoma, choriocarcinoma, and mixed tumors. The initial management for all these tumors is radical (inguinal) orchiectomy. Subsequent management depends on tumor histology.

Seminomas are very radiosensitive and are managed with retroperitoneal radiotherapy because (with the exception of choriocarcinoma) malignant testicular tumors usually spread lymphatically. Chemotherapy is used for patients who relapse after radiation. Patients with large bulky seminomas or those with increased alpha-fetoprotein levels (usually associated with nonseminomas) are treated primarily with chemotherapy. Chemotherapeutic regimens commonly used include cisplatin, vincristine, and bleomycin; vinblastine, cyclophosphamide, dactinomycin, bleomycin, and cisplatin; and cisplatin and etoposide. Retroperitoneal lymph node dissection (RPLND) is undertaken only for patients with residual tumor after chemotherapy.

In contrast, RPLND plays a more prominent role in the treatment of patients with nonseminomatous germ cell tumors. Low stage disease is managed with RPLND or, in some patients, with surveillance. High stage disease usually is managed with chemotherapy followed by RPLND.

Patients undergoing RPLND for testicular cancer are typically aged 15 to 35 years but often are at increased risk of morbidity from the residual effects of preoperative chemotherapy. In addition to bone marrow suppression, specific organ toxicity may be encountered, such as renal impairment after cisplatin, pulmonary fibrosis after bleomycin, and neuropathy after vincristine.

Anesthetic management

Radical orchiectomy. All malignant testicular tumors are removed via inguinal orchiectomy. The procedure may be carried out with regional or general anesthesia; most patients prefer the latter. Anesthetic management may be complicated by reflex bradycardia from traction on the spermatic cord.

Retroperitoneal lymph node dissection. This operation usually is performed for staging and management of nonseminomatous testicular cancers. A thoracoabdominal incision extending from the posterior axillary line over the eighth to tenth ribs to a paramedian line halfway between the xiphoid and the umbilicus is most commonly used to gain access to the retroperitoneum. Alternatively, a midline transabdominal approach may be chosen. All lymph node tissue between the ureters from the renal vessels to the iliac bifurcation is removed. With the standard RPLND, all sympathetic fibers are disrupted, resulting in loss of normal ejaculation and infertility. A modified technique may be used in some patients to preserve fertility; the dissection below the level of the inferior mesenteric artery is limited to only nodal tissue on the ipsilateral side of the tumor.

Patients receiving bleomycin preoperatively appear to be at increased risk of developing postoperative pulmonary insufficiency.[134,205] **Although somewhat controversial, use of high inspired oxygen concentrations has been associated with the development of adult respiratory distress syndrome (ARDS) postoperatively.** Excessive IV fluid administration also may be contributory. Anesthetic management requires use of the lowest inspired concentration of oxygen compatible with an acceptable hemoglobin oxygen saturation (> 90%). Positive end-expiratory pressure (PEEP), 5 to 10 cm H_2O, may optimize oxygenation. Some clinicians also prefer to use an air–oxygen mixture because nitrous oxide has been associated with bone marrow suppression.

Evaporative and redistributive fluid losses ("third spacing") are considered a result of the large wound and extensive surgical dissection. Fluid replacement should be sufficient to maintain an adequate urinary output (> 0.5 ml/kg/h); the combined use of colloid and crystalloid solutions in a ratio of 1:2 or 1:3 may be more effective in preserving urinary output than crystalloid alone. Mannitol (0.25 to 0.5 g/kg) usually is given before dissection near the renal arteries. Mannitol is thought to prevent ischemic renal injury from surgically induced spasm of the renal arteries by preserving renal blood and tubular flow.

The postoperative pain associated with thoracoabdominal incisions often is severe and typically associated with considerable splinting of respirations. Aggressive postoperative analgesia is necessary to avoid atelectasis. Continuous epidural analgesia, interpleural analgesia, and intercostal nerve blocks can facilitate management. Because ligation of intercostal arteries during left-sided dissections has rarely resulted in paraplegia, it may be prudent to document normal motor function postoperatively before institution of epidural anesthesia. These vessels feed the arteria radicularis magna (artery of Adamkiewicz), which supplies most of the arterial blood flow to the lower half of the spinal cord. The arteria radicularis magna originates on the left side in most patients. The unilateral sympathectomy after modified RPLND usually results in the ipsilateral leg being warmer than the contralateral one.

Surgery for Renal Cancers

Preoperative considerations

Radical nephrectomy is most commonly performed for adenocarcinoma of the kidney (renal cell carcinoma or hypernephroma). The tumor has a male-to-female ratio of 2:1 and a peak incidence in the fifth and sixth decades of life. The classic triad of hematuria, flank pain, and palpable mass occurs only in 10% of patients. It often is termed *the internist's tumor* because of a frequent association with paraneoplastic syndromes, such as erythrocytosis, hypercalcemia, hypertension, and nonmetastatic hepatic dysfunction.

Surgery typically is performed for carcinomas confined to the kidneys. **In approximately 5% to 10% of patients, the tumor extends into the renal vein and inferior vena cava as a thrombus. A tumor thrombus complicates but does not necessarily preclude surgery (to be discussed).** Staging includes CT or MRI scans and often an arteriogram and venogram. Preoperative arterial embolization may reduce operative blood loss.

Preoperative evaluation should focus on defining the degree of renal impairment and on searching for the presence of associated systemic diseases. Preexisting renal impairment depends on tumor size in the affected kidney and on underlying systemic disorders, such as hypertension and diabetes. Smoking is a well-established risk factor for renal adenocarcinoma; not surprisingly, patients have a high incidence of underlying coronary artery and chronic obstructive lung disease. Although some patients present with erythrocytosis, the majority of patients are anemic. Preoperative blood transfusion may be advisable to increase hemoglobin concentration more than 10 g/dl when a large tumor is to be resected.

Anesthetic management

Radical nephrectomy. An anterior subcostal (unilateral chevron), flank, midline, or thoracoabdominal incision may be used. Many surgeons prefer the thoracoabdominal approach for large tumors and for when a thrombus is present. The kidney rest position is used for a flank incision, whereas variations of the hyperextended supine position are used for other incisions. The renal artery and vein are ligated, and the kidney, adrenal, and perinephric fat are removed *en bloc* with the surrounding (Gerota's) fascia. Lymphadenectomy also is usually carried out.

General endotracheal anesthesia is used for this procedure. Extensive blood loss frequently is encountered because these tumors are very vascular and often very large at presentation. As with RPLND, retraction of the inferior vena cava may be associated with transient arterial hypotension. Direct arterial pressure monitoring is indicated in most patients. Central venous cannulation generally is advisable for venous pressure monitoring and for rapid transfusion when necessary. Pulmonary artery catheterization is indicated for patients with a history of cardiac dysfunction. Controlled hypotension to reduced blood loss is a two-edged sword because of its potential to impair renal function. Reflex renal vasoconstriction in the unaffected kidney also can induce intra- and postoperative renal dysfunction. Administration of mannitol before the dissection generally is advisable.

A pneumothorax can develop after the flank approach if the pleura is entered; this complication should be excluded by a postoperative chest radiograph. A chest tube is routinely placed only after the thoracoabdominal approach.

Radical nephrectomy with excision of a vena cava thrombus. In some medical centers, complicated resections of tumors with a thrombus growing into the inferior vena cava are successfully performed. The tumor thrombus may extend only into the inferior vena cava but below the liver (level I), up to the liver but below the diaphragm (level II), or above the diaphragm into the right atrium (level III). The rationale for surgery is that these patients generally have a very short life expectancy without surgery. Moreover, surgery can dramatically prolong life and improve the quality of life in selected patients. Metastases may regress in some patients after resection of the primary tumor. A ventilation-to-perfusion scan may be used to detect tumor embolization preoperatively.

The thoracoabdominal approach almost always is used. The presence of a large thrombus, especially level II or III thrombus, greatly complicates anesthetic management. Invasive pressure monitoring and multiple large-bore IV catheters therefore are necessary. Central venous pressure typically is high and likely reflects the degree of venous obstruction by the thrombus. The presence of a level III (and possibly level II) thrombus contraindicates flotation of a pulmonary artery catheter, which can dislodge and embolize thrombus fragments. A low-lying central venous catheter may be equally detrimental, especially on the right side. Use of transesophageal echocardiography has been suggested.[193]

Operative blood loss averages 10 to 20 U of packed erythrocytes but can exceed 50 U. Obstruction of the inferior vena cava dilates venous collaterals from the lower body that traverse the abdominal wall, retroperitoneum, and the epidural space. Transfusion of platelets, fresh frozen plasma, and cyroprecipitate often is necessary. Problems associated with massive blood transfusion are to be expected.

Patients also are at serious risk for potentially catastrophic pulmonary embolization of the tumor. **Tumor embolization may be heralded by sudden supraventricular arrhythmias, arterial desaturation, or profound systemic hypotension.** When the tumor occupies more than 40% of the right atrium, cardiopulmonary bypass with or without hypothermic circulatory arrest may be indicated.[212] The latter greatly increases operative blood loss.

KIDNEY TRANSPLANTATION

Preoperative considerations

The success of renal transplantation has largely been a result of recent advances in immunosuppressive therapy. The procedure has greatly improved the quality of life and lowered the morbidity and mortality rates of patients with end-stage renal disease (ESRD).[66] Early renal transplantation in small children with ESRD improves growth and development.[103] Moreover, the procedure has proved to be cost-effective.[62] Common indications for transplantation, in decreasing frequency, include diabetic nephropathy, hypertensive kidney disease, glomerulonephritis, and polycystic kidney disease.

With present immunosuppressive regimens, cadaveric

transplantations have achieved almost the same 3-year graft survival rates (80% to 90%) as living-related donor grafts (90%). Additionally, restrictions on candidates for renal transplantation have gradually decreased such that active infection or cancer are the only remaining absolute contraindications. Advanced age (> 60 years) and severe cardiovascular disease now are considered only relative contraindications. Although the role of HLA tissue matching in living-related renal transplantations is well established, its importance in cadaveric transplantation is more controversial.[28]

Preoperative evaluation. Preoperative optimization of the patient's medical condition with dialysis is mandatory. Current organ preservation techniques allow ample time (24 to 48 hours) for preoperative dialysis of cadaveric recipients. Living-related transplantations are performed electively with the donor and recipient anesthetized simultaneously in separate operating rooms.

Patients often have multiple metabolic abnormalities, which can be corrected with dialysis. The inability to excrete potassium makes hyperkalemia a serious problem. **The recipient's serum potassium concentration should be lower than 5.5 meq/l before surgery to avoid intraoperative arrhythmias or myocardial depression.** Hyperphosphatemia, hypermagnesemia, metabolic acidosis, and hypocalcemia also are common. Hyponatremia usually reflects excessive water intake. Excessive sodium manifests as peripheral edema, congestive heart failure, and hypertension.

Congestive heart failure may be present as a result of inadequate fluid removal during dialysis. Pulmonary congestion can be managed with digoxin, nitrates, angiotensin-converting enzyme (ACE) inhibitors, or diuretics if the patient still forms urine. Patients frequently have underlying hypertensive heart disease or coronary artery disease. Because diabetes is a common cause of ESRD, accelerated atherosclerosis often is also present. Preoperative coronary angiography may be considered in diabetic patients and in those with a history suggestive of coronary artery disease. Echocardiography, especially with dobutamine, may be helpful in identifying patients at risk for perioperative cardiac complications. Significant pleural and pericardial effusions are unusual in well-dialyzed patients but, if present, can further compromise pulmonary and cardiac function.

Systemic arterial hypertension is common in patients with ESRD. Salt and water retention caused by inadequate dialysis often is contributory. Antihypertensive medications may include ACE inhibitors, calcium channel blockers, or beta-adrenergic blockers. Antihypertensive medications generally should be continued on schedule up to the time of surgery.

Low erythropoietin production by the kidney, nutritional deficiencies, and bone marrow depression frequently results in hemoglobin levels of 6 to 8 g. The half-life of erythrocytes is decreased in uremic patients; the mechanical trauma associated with hemodialysis is contributory. Increased cardiac output, increased levels of 2,3-diphosphoglycerate (2,3-DPG), and a shift of the oxyhemoglobin dissociation curve to the right resulting from metabolic acidosis are likely compensatory mechanisms in these patients. Chronic erythropoietin administration effectively reduces the severity of the anemia (hemoglobin levels, > 10 g). Although early studies report that preoperative erythrocyte transfusions improved graft survival in cadaveric renal transplantation, the beneficial effect of this practice appears to have been lost in the cyclosporine era.[141]

Platelet dysfunction is commonly observed in uremic patients. Dialysis frequently restores platelet function to normal. Coagulation factor defects also may be present in patients with associated liver dysfunction. Platelet count, bleeding time, prothrombin time (PT), and partial thromboplastin time (PTT) generally should be checked preoperatively.

Immunosuppression as a result of chronic uremia makes patients with ESRD susceptible to infection. Many patients are chronic carriers of hepatitis B and C viruses; the care of these patients therefore may entail increased risk to health care workers.

Peripheral neuropathy is common in those with long-standing ESRD. The neuropathy typically involves the distal lower extremities and may initially only be a sensory defect. Improvement commonly follows dialysis. Anorexia, nausea, and vomiting may result from peptic ulcer disease and inadequate dialysis.

Anesthetic management

The operation usually is carried out through a curvilinear lower quadrant incision. The donor kidney is placed extraperitoneally into the iliac fossa, and the renal vessels are anastomosed to the iliac vessels; the ureter is attached directly into bladder. In small patients (< 20 kg), the kidney is placed intraperitoneally and anastomosed to the aorta and the inferior vena cava. Nephrectomy is performed only in the presence of intractable hypertension or chronic infection. Immunosuppression is started on the day of surgery with combinations of corticosteroids, cyclosporine, and azathioprine. Some centers avoid cyclosporine in the first few days and instead use antithymocyte globulin or monoclonal antibodies directed against specific subsets of T lymphocytes. A calcium channel blocker also may simultaneously be administered to lessen the likelihood of cyclosporine-induced renal toxicity.[218]

Choice of anesthesia. Patients with severe diabetes often exhibit marked autonomic dysfunction that can result in accentuation of bradycardia and hypotension or marked hypertension, regardless of anesthetic technique.[113] Although spinal and epidural anesthesia have been successfully used,[120] most transplantations are done during general anesthesia.[92] Contraindications to spinal or epidural anesthesia include coagulopathy, systemic or local infection at the block site, or patient refusal. Regional anesthesia may be considered in the rare patient who is not optimally prepared for general anesthesia.

All general anesthetic agents and techniques have been

used in the anesthetic treatment of patients with ESRD. A rapid-sequence induction is recommended by some authors because dialysis may prolong gastric emptying.[218] Patients may not tolerate profound depths of anesthesia with halogenated agents because of hypotension. Relative hypovolemia from recent hemodialysis often is contributory. Although the pharmacokinetics of most induction agents is not appreciably altered by renal failure,[33,112,146] the induction dose of thiopental or propofol generally should be reduced to avoid excessive hypotension. Decreased protein binding of thiopental as a result of hypoalbuminemia increases the free drug; metabolic acidosis also likely increases the fraction of unionized thiopental. Some clinicians prefer etomidate for induction. The use of IV lidocaine or opioids for attenuation of the hypertension associated with laryngoscopy is important because many patients display marked hypertension after endotracheal intubation.

All volatile agents, including methoxyflurane and enflurane, have been used without any apparent detrimental effect on graft function;[182] nonetheless, these two agents are probably best avoided. Sevoflurane should likewise be avoided because of its potential to increase serum fluoride levels, even though no renal toxicity has been documented.[42,69]

Most neuromuscular blocking drugs are renally excreted and therefore have reduced clearance and increased duration of action in these patients.[182] The response to succinylcholine generally is unaffected by ESRD in patients with a normal serum potassium.[115,142] Although decreased levels of pseudocholinestase are described in patients on dialysis,[198] little if any prolongation is observed clinically. Of all the nondepolarizing agents available, only atracurium and cisatracurium clearly are not prolonged,[65] although accumulation of the metabolite laudanosine has been reported with use of atracurium.[204] The prolongation of mivacurium also is not clinically significant.[43] The duration of action for rocuronium and vecuronium is moderately prolonged, but these agents are commonly used.[46,64,194] Elimination of all other nondepolarizing muscle relaxants heavily depends on normal renal function. These agents should not be used in case the renal transplant does not immediately function properly. Regardless of the relaxant selected, use of a nerve stimulator is critical to avoid residual paralysis. Fortunately, the half-lives of neostigmine, pyridostigmine, and edrophonium and of anticholinergic agents are prolonged in patients with ESRD so that "recurarization" is not likely.[49,50,147]

Morphine clearance is reduced in patients with renal failure.[15,169] Its effect also is likely prolonged because of increased levels of its metabolites, especially morphine-6-glucuronide.[55,159] Large doses of meperidine should be avoided because of the accumulation of the potentially epileptogenic metabolite, normeperidine, in patients with renal failure.[195] Fentanyl, alfentanil, and sufentanil pharmacokinetics are not dramatically altered in patients with renal failure.[27,39,71,135,170]

Monitoring. Direct arterial pressure monitoring is desirable in most patients to detect potentially wide swings in blood pressure[67] and to allow measurement of blood gases, serum electrolytes, and glucose. Central venous pressure monitoring also is very useful in ensuring adequate hydration and avoiding fluid overload. Normal saline or half-normal saline solutions are commonly used because lactated Ringer's solution contains potassium. A urinary catheter is placed preoperatively. A brisk urine flow after the arterial anastomosis generally indicates good graft function. The diuresis that follows may resemble nonoliguric renal failure. If the graft ischemic time was prolonged, an oliguric phase may precede the diuretic phase, in which case fluid therapy should be adjusted appropriately. The judicious use of furosemide (40 to 100 mg) or mannitol (0.25 to 0.5 g/kg) may be indicated in such patients. Some centers routinely use an IV, low-dose dopamine infusion (3 μg/kg/min), but Kadieva et al.[106] could not clearly demonstrate a beneficial effect in most patients. Hyperkalemia has been reported after release of the vascular clamp after completion of the arterial anastomosis. Release of potassium contained in the preservative solution (usually University of Wisconsin solution) has been implicated in those patients. Serum electrolyte concentrations should be monitored closely after completion of the anastomosis. Hyperkalemia may be suspected from peaking of the T wave on the ECG. Most patients generally can be extubated immediately after the procedure.

PEDIATRIC UROLOGIC PROCEDURES

Preoperative considerations

Common pediatric urologic procedures in most anesthetic practices include circumcision, urethral meatotomy, and orchiopexy. Depending on the age of the patient, these procedures may be performed with local, regional, light general anesthesia, or more frequently with a combination thereof. Occasionally, more complex procedures such as resection of a Wilms' tumor or neuroblastoma are encountered. These more complicated operations frequently result in major blood loss and usually require general anesthesia with invasive monitoring.

Anesthetic management

Circumcision. Local anesthesia usually is used for circumcisions in the neonatal period, whereas general anesthesia is used in older boys. Concomitant use of caudal anesthesia (bupivacaine up to 3 mg/kg) permits light general anesthesia and provides excellent postoperative analgesia. Use of caudal anesthesia does not appear to delay discharge of the ambulatory pediatric patient.[34] A penile block (Fig. 75-12) may alternately be used for postoperative analgesia.[30] The penile block is performed by injecting local anesthetic (1 to 4 ml of 0.5% bupivacaine without epinephrine) in the area of the dorsal nerves of the penis close to the pubic bone. Epinephrine-containing solutions are not used because they could compromise penile blood flow.

Orchiopexy. Patients with an undescended testicle generally require full general anesthesia because of the often intense stimulus of traction on the spermatic cord. Reflex

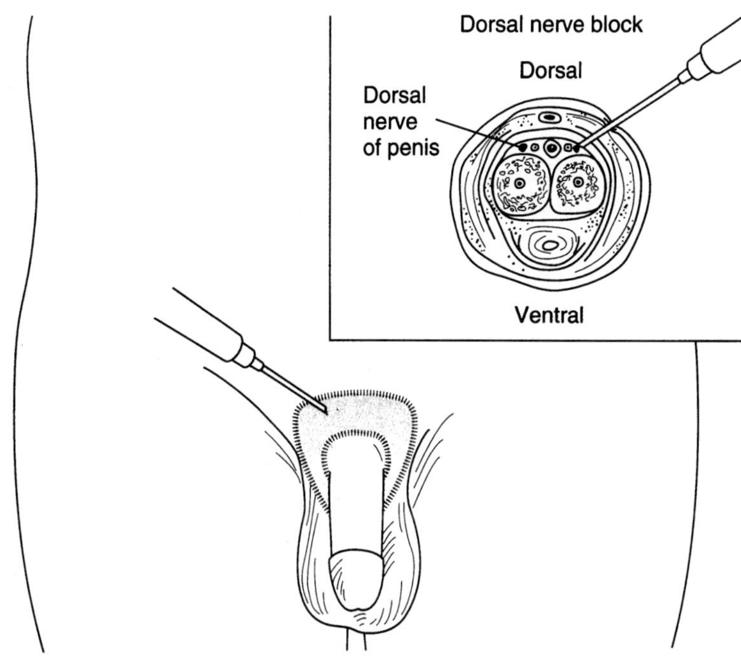

Fig. 75-12. Ring block of the penis. (Modified and reproduced, with permission, from Morgan GE, Mikhail MS: *Clinical anesthesiology,* ed 2, Stamford, 1996, Appleton & Lange.)

bradycardia should be managed aggressively with atropine. The procedure typically is carried out using an inguinal incision and often involves repair of a coexisting inguinal hernia; abdominal exploration may be necessary to locate the testicle in some patients. The concomitant use of caudal anesthesia permits reduction in the depth of general anesthesia required and provides good postoperative analgesia. Inguinal or iliohypogastric nerve block also provides equivalent postoperative pain relief.[87]

Surgical detorsion of the spermatic cord. Torsion of the spermatic cord (testicle) is typically encountered in adolescent boys. Emergency surgery is indicated within 3 or 4 hours to relieve the torsion and prevent residual testicular atrophy. The diagnosis usually is confirmed by color Doppler ultrasonography or a scintillation scan. Patients typically have a full stomach. General or regional anesthesia may be used in young adults, but most children require general anesthesia. Combined caudal anesthesia with light general anesthesia often is used.

Resecetion of Wilms' tumor. Wilms' tumor, or nephroblastoma, is the most common abdominal neoplasm in children. It has a peak incidence between the ages of 3 and 4 years. Up to 15% of patients have other congenital anomalies. They usually present with a palpable abdominal mass on physical examination. Hypertension is present in 25% to 60% of patients and may be related to elevated renin levels or compression of the renal arteries. Pulmonary metastases are common at the time of diagnosis. The tumor, which may invade the vena cava, is radiosensitive and chemosensitive. Chemotherapy usually is preferred to minimize the risk of growth impairment and organ toxicity and is given before surgery. Chemotherapeutic agents may include actinomycin-D, vincristine, doxorubicin, cyclophosphamide, and cisplatin. Radiation therapy may be given postoperatively in patients with extensive disease.

Anesthetic management of these patients may be complicated by abdominal distention that is associated with bowel obstruction and pulmonary compromise. Patients should be treated as having a full stomach. Oxygen saturation should be monitored carefully; desaturation occurs readily because of the abdominal distention, pulmonary metastases, or surgical retraction.[185] The vascularity of this tumor predisposes to major intraoperative bleeding. Patients therefore are best treated with general anesthesia, intra-arterial, and possibly central venous pressure monitoring. Multiple large-bore IV catheters should be placed in anticipation of the need for blood replacement. Further, catheters should be above the diaphragm because the inferior vena cava may be clamped.

Resection of neuroblastoma. This relatively rare tumor originates from neural crest cells either from the adrenal or postganglionic adrenergic cells of the sympathetic nervous system. Although the majority of neuroblastomas are intra-abdominal, 20% are intrathoracic, usually in the posterior mediastinum; they therefore rarely compromise the airway.[185] Intra-abdominal tumors often involve the kidneys. Most neuroblastomas secrete catecholamines, but only 20% of patients have hypertension. Spinal cord involvement may result in gait impairment and bowel and bladder dysfunction.

Anesthetic management depends on the location of the tumor. Management of abdominal neuroblastomas is similar to that of Wilms' tumor. Unlike pheochromocytomas, problems with intraoperative hypertension are not common.

KEY POINTS

- A variety of patient positions are commonly used in urologic procedures; these positions include lithotomy, Trendelenburg, extreme lithotomy, kidney rest position, hyperextended supine position, prone, and sitting. These positions often are associated with major alterations in cardiopulmonary physiology. Moreover, improper positioning can lead to iatrogenic injuries, the most common being brachial injury. Risk factors associated with postoperative motor neuropathy of the lower extremities include lithotomy duration of more than 4 hours, body mass index less than 20 kg/m^2 and a recent smoking history.
- Older extracorporeal shock wave lithotripsy (ESWL) units use high-intensity shock waves; patients usually require general or epidural anesthesia with a T6 sensory level. These units require that the patient be immersed in a sitting position into a water bath. Immersion increases venous return but decreases functional residual capacity. Studies comparing the use of general anesthesia and regional anesthesia indicate no difference in morbidity rates.
- ESWL with newer units uses a higher number of less painful, low-intensity shock waves without immersion; most patients require only light sedation.
- Diagnostic or operative cystoscopy usually is performed with either general or spinal anesthesia (T10 sensory level). Diagnostic cystoscopy often can be performed with topical anesthesia and light sedation, especially in women. Electrocautery in the lateral bladder wall can stimulate the obturator nerve, resulting in external rotation and adduction of the thigh; the obturator reflex is only abolished by muscle paralysis during general anesthesia.
- Transurethral resection of the prostate (TURP) can be associated with a variety of complications, including the TURP syndrome, bladder perforation, hemorrhage, coagulopathy, hypothermia, and septicemia.
- The TURP syndrome follows absorption of large amounts (> 2 to 3 l) of irrigating fluid. The syndrome presents during or immediately after surgery as headache, restlessness, confusion, blindness, coma, cyanosis, dyspnea, arrhythmias, hypotension, or seizures. Manifestations reflect circulatory fluid overload, water intoxication, and occasionally toxicity from the solute (usually glycine) in the irrigating solution. Fluid absorption primarily depends on the hydrostatic pressure (height of the fluid bag) and the duration of the resection. An average of 10 to 30 ml/min of fluid is absorbed. Hyperglycinemia and hyperammonemia are described in patients with TURP syndrome. Symptoms can be more readily diagnosed in patients receiving regional anesthesia.
- Spinal anesthesia is most commonly used for TURP, but studies show little or no difference in morbidity or mortality rates between general and regional anesthesia. Some investigators report up to an 18% incidence of perioperative myocardial ischemia in patients undergoing TURP. The latter may reflect the relatively high incidence of cardiovascular disease in these patients.
- Radical surgery for urologic malignancies can be associated with considerable blood loss. Direct intra-arterial blood pressure monitoring and multiple large bore venous cannulae generally are advisable. Controlled hypotension may reduce intraoperative bleeding and transfusion requirements. The value of preoperative autologous blood donation has been questioned as a cost-effective strategy for radical prostatectomy. Postoperative analgesia with epidural opioids does not appear to be clearly superior to IV opioids via patient-controlled analgesia after radical prostatectomy.
- Patients with testicular malignancies and undergoing retroperitoneal lymph node dissections may be at increased risk of postoperative morbidity from the residual effects of preoperative chemotherapy, especially bleomycin. Prophylactic infusion of mannitol before surgical dissection may reduce perioperative renal dysfunction. Although controversial, the inspired oxygen concentration should be kept to the minimum level compatible with adequate oxygenation to reduce the incidence of postoperative respiratory failure in patients who have received bleomycin.
- The medical condition of patients undergoing renal transplantation should be optimized with preoperative dialysis. Nearly all anesthetic agents and techniques have been used for renal transplantation. Most transplantations are performed during general anesthesia. Patients with end-stage renal disease, especially those with diabetes, often exhibit marked autonomic dysfunction. Exaggerated hypotension after induction and hypertension after endotracheal intubation are common. Relative hypovolemia after hemodialysis may be contributory. Direct arterial pressure monitoring is therefore usually desirable; central venous pressure monitoring also is very useful in ensuring adequate hydration and avoiding fluid overload. Hyperkalemia can occur after release of the vascular clamp after completion of the arterial anastomosis and is a result of release of potassium contained in the preservative solution.
- Common urologic procedures in children include circumcision, urethral meatotomy, and orchiopexy. Depending on the age of the patient, they may be performed with local, regional, light general anesthesia, or a combination thereof. Complex procedures, such resection of a Wilms' tumor or neuroblastoma, are less common but result in major blood loss and require general anesthesia with invasive monitoring.

KEY REFERENCES

Battillo JA, Hendler MA: Effects of patient positioning during anesthesia. In Lebowitz RW, editor: *Anesthesia for urological surgery, Int Anesth Clin* 31:67, 1993.

Dobson PM, Caldicott LD, Gerrish SP, et al: Changes in hemodynamic variables during transurethral resection of the prostate: comparison of general and spinal anaesthesia, *Br J Anaesth* 72:267, 1994.

Eide TR: Anesthetic considerations for extracorporeal shock wave lithotripsy. In Lebowitz RW, editor: *Anesthesia for urological surgery, Int Anesth Clin* 31:47, 1993.

Jensen V: The TURP syndrome, *Can J Anaesth* 38:90, 1991.

Kirvela M, Scheinin M, Lindgren L: Haemodynamic and catecholamine responses to induction of anaesthesia and tracheal intubation in diabetic and non-diabetic uraemic patients, *Br J Anaesth* 74:60, 1995.

Liu S, Carpenter RL, Mulroy MF, et al: Intravenous versus epidural administration of hydromorphone: effects on analgesia and recovery after radical retropubic prostatectomy, *Anesthesiology* 82:682, 1995.

Mathes DD: Bleomycin and hyperoxia exposure in the operating room, *Anesth Analg* 81:624, 1995.

Mebust WK, Holtgrewe HL, Cockett ATK, et al: Transurethral prostatectomy—immediate and postoperative complications: a cooperative study of 13 participating institutions evaluating 3885 patients, *J Urol* 141:243, 1989.

Monk TG, Boure B, White P, et al: Comparison of intravenous sedative-analgesic techniques for outpatient immersion lithotripsy, *Anesth Analg* 72:616, 1991.

Shir Y, Frank SM, Brendler, et al: Postoperative morbidity is similar in patients anesthetized with epidural and general anesthesia for radical prostatectomy, *Urology* 44:232, 1994.

Shir Y, Raja SN, Frank SM: The effect of epidural versus general anesthesia on postoperative pain and analgesic requirements in patients undergoing radical prostatectomy, *Anesthesiology* 80:49, 1994.

Smith CE, Hunter JM: Anesthesia for renal transplantation: relaxants and volatiles, *Int Anesth Clin* 33:69, 1995.

Warner MA, Martin JT, Schroeder DR, et al: Lower-extremity motor neuropathy associated with surgery performed on patients in a lithotomy position, *Anesthesiology* 81:6, 1994.

Yamada AH, Lieskovsky G, Skinner DG, et al: Impact of autologous blood transfusion on patients undergoing radical prostatectomy using hypotensive anesthesia, *J Urol* 149:73, 1993.

Yao FS: Anesthesia for renal transplantation. In Malhorta V, editor: *Anesthesia for renal and genito-urologic surgery,* New York, 1996, McGraw-Hill.

REFERENCES

1. Aasheim GM: Hyponatremia during transurethral surgery, *Can J Anaesth* 20:274, 1973.
2. Abel RR, Lewis GM: Postoperative alopecia, *Arch Dermatol* 81:72, 1960.
3. Abrams PH, Shah PJR, Bryning K, et al: Blood loss during transurethral resection of the prostate, *Anaesthesia* 37:71, 1982.
4. Adler LM, Loughlin JS, Morin CJ, et al: Bilateral compartment syndrome after a long gynecologic operation in the lithotomy position, *Am J Obstet Gynecol* 162: 1271, 1990.
5. Ahlering TE, Henderson JB, Skinner DG: Controlled hypotensive anesthesia to reduce blood loss in radical cystectomy for bladder cancer, *J Urol* 129:953, 1983.
6. Albin MS, Ritter RR, Reinhart R, et al: Venous air embolism during radical retropubic prostatectomy, *Anesth Analg* 74:151, 1992.
7. Allaire PH, Messick JM, Oesterling JE, et al: A prospective randomized comparison of epidural infusion of fentanyl and intravenous administration of morphine by patient-controlled analgesia after radical prostatectomy, *Mayo Clin Proc* 67:1031, 1992.
8. Allen TD: Body temperature changes during prostatic resection as related to the temperature of the irrigating solution, *J Urol* 110:433, 1973.
9. Allman DB, Richlin DM, Ruttenberg M, et al: Analgesia in anesthesia-free extracorporeal shock wave lithotripsy: a standard protocol, *J Urol* 59:533, 1991.
10. Amzallag M: Autonomic hyperreflexia. In Lebowitz RW, editor: *Anesthesia for urological surgery, Int Anesth Clin* 31:57, 1993.
11. Andriole GL, Smith DS, Rao G, et al: Early complications of contemporary anatomical radical retropubic prostatectomy, *J Urol* 152:1858, 1994.
12. Ansell JS, Gee WF: Diseases of the kidney and ureter. In Bonica JJ, editor: *The management of pain,* Philadelphia, 1990, Lea & Febiger.
13. Asbjorn J, Jakobsen BW, Pilegaard HK, et al: Mental function in elderly men after surgery during epidural analgesia, *Acta Anaesthesiol Scand* 33:369, 1989.
14. Attinger EO, Herschfus JA, Segal M: The mechanics of breathing in different body positions: II: In cardiopulmonary disease, *J Clin Invest* 35:912, 1956.
15. Ball M, Moore RA, Fischer A, et al: Renal failure and the use of morphine in the intensive care, *Lancet* 784 1985.
16. Battillo JA, Hendler MA: Effects of patient positioning during anesthesia. In Lebowitz RW, editor: *Anesthesia for urological surgery, Int Anesth Clin* 31:67, 1993.
17. Beal JL, Freysz M, Berthelon G, et al: Consequences of fluid absorption during transurethral resection of the prostate using distilled water or glycine 1.5 per cent, *Can J Anaesth* 36:278, 1989.
18. Beers RA, Kane PB, Nsouli I, et al: Does a mid-lumbar block level provide adequate anaesthesia for transurethral prostatectomy? *Can J Anaesth* 41:807, 1994.
19. Begin R, Epstein M, Sackner MA, et al: Effects of immersion to the neck on pulmonary circulation and tissue volume, *J Appl Physiol* 40:293, 1976.
20. Behnia R, Shanks CA, Ovassapian O, et al: Hemodynamic responses associated with lithotripsy, *Anesth Analg* 66:354, 1987.
21. Berger JJ, Boysen PG, Gravenstein J, et al: Failure of high frequency jet ventilation to ventilate patients adequately during extracorporeal shock wave lithotripsy, *Anesth Analg* 66:262, 1987.

22. Bernstein S: Regional anesthesia for urological surgery. In Lebowitz RW, editor: *Anesthesia for urological surgery, Int Anesth Clin* 31:57, 1993.
23. Bierkens AF, Maes RM, Hendrikx AJM, et al: The use of local anesthesia in second generation extracorporeal shock wave lithotripsy: eutectic mixture of local anesthetics, *J Urol* 146:287, 1991.
24. Bigg EW, Catalona WJ: Prophylactic minidose heparin in patients undergoing radical retropubic prostatectomy, *Urology* 34:309, 1992.
25. Birch BR, Gelister JS, Parker CJ, et al: Transurethral resection of prostate under sedation and local anesthesia (sedoanalgesia). Experience in 100 patients, *Urology* 38:113, 1991.
26. Bonica JJ: Applied anatomy relevant to pain. In Bonica JJ, editor: *The management of pain,* Philadelphia, 1990, Lea & Febiger.
27. Bower S, Sear JW: Disposition of alfentanil in patients receiving a renal transplant, *J Pharm Pharmacol* 41:654, 1989.
28. Bretan PN, Burke EC: Renal transplantation. In Tanagho EA, McAninch JW, editors: *General urology,* ed 14, Norwalk, 1995, Appleton & Lange.
29. Britt BA, Gordon RA: Peripheral nerve injuries associated with anesthesia, *Can Anaesth Soc J* 11:514, 1964.
30. Broadman LM, Hannallah RS, Belmar AB et al: Post-circumcision pain—a prospective evaluation of subcutaneous ring block of the penis, *Anesthesiology* 67:399, 1987.
31. Bromage PR, Bonsu AK, el Faqih SR, et al: Influence of Dornier HM3 system on respiration during extracorporeal shock wave lithotripsy, *Anesth Analg* 68:363, 1989.
32. Brown EM, Elman DS: Postoperative backache, *Anesth Analg* 40:683, 1961.
33. Burch PG, Stanski DR: Decreased protein binding and thiopental kinetics, *Clin Pharmacol Ther* 32:212, 1982.
34. Burns AM, Shelly MP, Dewar AK: Caudal analgesia for pediatric day care surgery: assessment of motor function prior to discharge, *J Clin Anesth* 2:27, 1990.
35. Carpenter RL, Smith HS, Bridenbaugh LD: Epinephrine increases the effectiveness of tetracaine spinal anesthesia, *Anesthesiology* 71:33, 1989.
36. Case EH, Stiles JA: Effects of various surgical positions on vital capacity, *Anesthesiology* 7:29, 1946.
37. Casey WF, Hannon V, Cunningham A, et al: Visual evoked potentials and changes in serum glycine concentration during transurethral resection of the prostate, *Br J Anaesth* 60:525, 1988.
38. Catalona WJ: Surgical management of prostatic cancer: contemporary results with anatomic radical prostatectomy, *Cancer* 75:1903, 1995.
39. Chauvin M, Lebrault C, Levron JC, et al: Pharmacokinetics of alfentanil in chronic renal failure, *Anesth Analg* 66:53, 1987.
40. Chung FF, Chung A, Meier RH, et al: Comparison of perioperative mental function after general anaesthesia and spinal anaesthesia with intravenous sedation, *Can J Anaesth* 36:382, 1989.
41. Cisek LJ, Walsh PC: Thromboembolic complications following radical retropubic prostatectomy. Influence of external sequential pneumatic compression devices, *Urology* 42:406, 1993.
42. Conzen PF, Nuscheler M, Melotte A, et al: Renal function and serum fluoride concentrations in patients with stable renal insufficiency after anaesthesia with sevoflurane or enflurane, *Anesth Analg* 81:569, 1995.
43. Cook DR, Freeman JA, Lai AA, et al: Pharmacokinetics of mivacurium in normal patients and in those with hepatic or renal failure, *Br J Anaesth* 69:580, 1992.
44. Cook RJ, Neerhut R, Thomas DG: Does combined epidural lignocaine and fentanyl provide better anaesthesia for ESWL than lignocaine alone? *Anaesth Intensive Care* 19:357, 1991.
45. Coonan TJ, Hope CE: Cardio-respiratory effects of changes in body position, *Can Anaesth Soc J* 30:424, 1983.
46. Cooper RA, Maddineni VR, Mirakhur RK, et al: Time course of neuromuscular effects and pharmacokinetics of rocuronium bromide (Org 9426) during isoflurane anaesthesia in patients with and without renal failure, *Br J Anaesth* 71:222, 1993.
47. Courington FW, Little DM Jr: The role of posture in anesthesia, *Clin Anesth* 3:24, 1968.
48. Creel DJ, Wang JML, Wong KC: Transient blindness associated with transurethral resection of the prostate, *Arch Ophthalmol* 105:1537, 1987.
49. Cronnelly R, Stanski DR, Miller RD, et al: Pyridostigmine kinetics with and without renal function, *Clin Pharmacol Ther* 28:78, 1980.
50. Cronnelly R, Stanski DR, Miller RD, et al: Renal function and the pharmacokinetics of neostigmine in anesthetized man, *Anesthesiology* 51:222, 1979.
51. Crowley AR, Horowitz M, Chan E, et al: Transurethral resection of the prostate versus open prostatectomy: long term mortality comparison, *J Urol* 153:695, 1995
52. Crowley, K, Clarkson K, Hannon V, et al: Diuretrics after transurethral prostatectomy: a double-blind controlled trial comparing frusemide and mannitol, *Br J Anaesth* 65:337, 1990.
53. Culver GA, Makel HP, Beecher HK: Frequency of aspiration of gastric contents by lungs during anesthesia, *Ann Surg* 133:289, 1951.
54. Deam RK, Scott DA: Neurological damage resulting from extracorporeal shock wave lithotripsy when air is used to locate the epidural space, *Anaesth Intensive Care* 21:455, 1993.
55. Dhonneur G, et al: Plasma and cerebrospinal fluid concentrations of morphine and morphine glucuronides after oral morphine. The influence of renal failure, *Anesthesiology* 81:87–93, 1994.
56. Dobson PM, Caldicott LD, Gerrish SP, et al: Changes in hemodynamic variables during transurethral resection of the prostate: comparison of general and spinal anaesthesia, *Br J Anaesth* 72:267, 1994.
57. Don HF: The measurement of trapped gas in the lungs at functional residual capacity and the effects of posture, *Anesthesiology* 35:582, 1971.
58. Drach GW, Weber C, Donovan JM: Treatment of pacemaker patients with extracorporeal shock wave lithotripsy: experience from 2 continents, *J Urol* 143:895, 1990.
59. Duvall JO, Griffith DP: Epidural anesthesia for extracorporeal shock wave lithotripsy, *Anesth Analg* 64:544, 1985.
60. Edwards ND, Callaghan LC, White T, et al: Perioperative myocardial ischaemia in patients undergoing transurethral surgery: a pilot study comparing general with spinal anaesthesia, *Br J Anaesth* 74:368, 1995.
61. Eggers GWN, de Groot WJ, Tanner CR, et al: Hemodynamic changes associated with various surgical positions, *JAMA* 185:1, 1963.
62. Eggers PW: Effect of transplantation on the Medicare end-stage renal disease program, *N Eng J Med* 318:223, 1988.
63. Eide TR: Anesthetic considerations for extracorporeal shock wave lithotripsy. In Lebowitz RW, editor: *Anesthesia for urological surgery, Int Anesth Clin* 31:47, 1993.
64. Fahey MR, Morris RB, Miller RD, et al: Pharmacokinetics of ORG NC45 (Norcuron) in patients with and without renal failure, *Br J Anaesth* 53:1049, 1981.
65. Fahey MR, Rupp SM, Fisher DM, et al: The pharmacokinetics and pharmacodynamics of atracurium in patients with and without renal failure, *Anesthesiology* 61:699, 1984.
66. Flechner SM: Current status of renal transplantation. Patient selection, results, and immunosuppression, *Urol Clin North Am* 21:265, 1994.
67. Freilich JD, Waterman PM, Rosenthal JT: Acute hemodynamic changes during renal transplantation, *Anesth Analg* 63:158, 1984.
68. Friedman NJ, Silvija Hoag M, Robinson AJ, et al: Hemorrhagic syndrome following transurtheral prostatic resection for benign adenoma, *Arch Intern Med* 124:341, 1969.
69. Frink EJ, Ghantous H, Malan TP, et al: Plasma inorganic fluoride with sevoflurane anesthesia: correlation with indices of hepatic and renal function, *Anesth Analg* 74:231, 1992.
70. Fujita Y, Kimura K, Furukawa Y, et al: Plasma concentrations of lignocaine after obturator nerve block combined with spinal anaesthesia in patients undergoing transurethral resection procedures, *Br J Anaesth* 68:596, 1992.
71. Fyman PN, Reynolds JR, Moser F, et al: Pharmacokinetics of sufentanil in patients undergoing renal transplantation, *Can J Anaesth* 35:312, 1988.
72. Garza J, Tansey M, Florio J: The effect of extracorporeal shock wave lithotripsy on implantable cardiac pacemakers, *PACE* 10:675, 1987.
73. Gee WF, Ansell JS: Pelvic and perineal pain of urologic origin. In Bonica JJ, editor: *The management of pain,* Philadelphia, 1990, Lea & Febiger.
74. Ghoneim MM, Hinrichs JV, O'Hara MW, et al: Comparison of psychologic and cognitive functions after general or regional anesthesia, *Anesthesiology* 69:507, 1988.
75. Goodnough LT, Grishaber JE, Birkmeyer JD, et al: Efficacy and cost effectiveness of autologous blood predeposit in patients undergoing radical prostatectomy, *Urology* 44:226, 1994.

76. Grace D, Fee JP: Anaesthesia and adverse effects after intrathecal pethidine hydrochloride for urological surgery, *Anaesthesia* 50:1036, 1995.
77. Grass JA, Sakima NT, Valley M, et al: Assessment of ketorolac as an adjuvant to fentanyl patient-controlled epidural anesthesia after radical prostatectomy, *Anesthesiology* 78:642, 1993.
78. Greenstein A, Kaver I, Lechtman V, et al: Cardiac arrhythmias during nonsynchronized extracorporeal shock wave lithotripsy, *J Urol* 154:1321, 1995.
79. Guzzi LM, Mills LM, Greenman P: Rhabdomyolysis, acute renal failure, and the exaggerated lithotomy position, *Anesth Analg* 77:635, 1993.
80. Haan J, van Kleef JW, Bloem BR, et al: Cognitive function after spinal or general anesthesia for transurethral prostatectomy in elderly men, *J Am Geriatr Soc* 39:596, 1991.
81. Hagstrom RS, Dennise SA, Rowland HS, et al: Studies on fluid absorption during transurethral prostatic resection, *J Urol* 73: 852, 1955.
82. Hahn RG, Rundgren M: Vasopressin and amino acid concentrations in serum following absorption of irrigating fluid containing glycine and ethanol, *Br J Anaesth* 63:337, 1989.
83. Hahn RG, Rundgren M: Vasopressin responses during transurethral resection of the prostate, *Br J Anaesth* 63:330, 1989.
84. Hahn RG: Early detection of the TURP syndrome by marking the irrigating fluid with 1% ethanol, *Acta Anaesthesiol Scand* 33:146, 1989.
85. Hahn RG: Ethanol monitoring of irrigating fluid absorption, *Eur J Anaesth* 13:102, 1996.
86. Hahn RG: Serum amino acid patterns and toxicity symptoms following the absorption of irrigant containing glycine in transurethral prostatic surgery, *Acta Anaesth Scand* 32:493, 1988.
87. Hannallah RS, Broadman LM, Belman AB, et al: Comparison of caudal and ilioinguinal/iliohypogastric nerve blocks for control of postorchiopexy pain in pediatric ambulatory surgery, *Anesthesiology* 66: 832, 1987.
88. Hargreave TB, Botto H, Rikken GH, et al: European collaborative study of antibiotic prophylaxis for transurethral resection of the prostate, *Eur Urol* 23:437, 1993.
89. Harioka T, Murakawa M, Noda J, et al: Effect of continuously warmed irrigating solution during transurethral resection, *Anaesth Intensive Care* 16:324, 1988.
90. Hatch PD: Surgical and anaesthetic considerations in transurethral resection of the prostate, *Anaesth Intensive Care* 15:203, 1987.
91. Heathcote PS, Dyer PM: The effect of warm irrigation on blood loss during transurethral prostatectomy under spinal anaesthesia, *Br J Urol* 58:669, 1986.
92. Heino A, Orko R, Rosenberg PH: Anaesthesiological complications in renal transplantation: a retrospective study of 500 transplantations, *Acta Anaesthol Scand* 30:574, 1986.
93. Heinonen J, Takki S, Tammisto T. Effect of the Trendelenburg tilt and other procedures on the position of endotracheal tubes, *Lancet* 1:850, 1969.
94. Henderson DJ, Middleton RG: Coma from hyponatremia following transurethral resection of the prostate, *Urology* 15:267, 1980.
95. Hendolin H, Mattila MAK, Poikolainen E: The effect of lumbar epidural analgesia on the development of deep vein thrombosis of the legs after open prostatectomy, *Acta Chir Scand* 147:425, 1981.
96. Heyns CF, Ritttoo D, Sutherland GR, et al: Intra-operative myocardial ischaemia detected by biplane transoesophageal echocardiography during transurethral prostatectomy, *Br J Urol* 71:716, 1993.
97. Higgens TL, Miller EV, Roberts J: Accidental hypothermia as a complication of extracorporeal shock wave lithotripsy under general anesthesia, *Anesth Analg* 66:389, 1987.
98. Hoekstra PT, Kahnoski R, McCamish MA, et al: Transurethral prostatic resection syndrome—a new perspective: encephalopathy with associated hyperammonemia, *J Urol* 130:704, 1983.
99. Holmang S, Aldenborg F, Hedelin H: Extirpation and fulguration of multiple superficial bladder tumour recurrences under intravesical lignocaine anaesthesia, *Br J Urol* 73:177, 1994.
100. Hosking MP, Lobdell CM, Warner MA, et al: Anaesthesia for patients over 90 years of age: outcomes after regional and general anaesthetic techniques for two common surgical procedures, *Anaesthesia* 44:142, 1989.
101. Hulten J, Samra VJ, Hyertberg H, et al: Monitoring of irrigating fluid absorption during transurethral prostatectomy. A study in anesthetized patients using a 1% ethanol tag solution, *Anaesthesia* 46:349, 1991.
102. Hurlbert BJ, Windgard DW: Water intoxication after fifteen minutes of transurethral resection of the prostate, *Anesthesiology* 50:355, 1979.
103. Inglefinger J, Grupe W, Harmon W, et al: Growth acceleration following renal transplantation in children less than 7 years of age, *Pediatrics* 68:255, 1981.
104. Jeffords DL, Lange PH, DeWolf WC: Severe hypertensive reaction to indigo carmine, *Urology* 9:180, 1977.
105. Jensen V: The TURP syndrome, *Can J Anaesth* 38:90, 1991.
106. Kadieva VS, Friedman L, Margolius LP, et al: The effect of dopamine on graft function in patients undergoing renal transplantation, *Anesth Analg* 76:362, 1993.
107. Kaneko K, Milic-Emili J, Dolovich MB, et al: Regional distribution of ventilation and perfusion as a function of body position, *J Appl Physiol* 21:767, 1966.
108. Kaude JV, Williams CM, Millner MR, et al: Renal morphology and function immediately after extracorporteal shock wave lithotripsy, *AJR AMJ Roentgenol* 145:305, 1985.
109. Kelly RE, Binion M, Malhotra V, et al: Pulmonary function after extracorporeal shock wave lithotripsy—a comparison of general and regional anaesthesia, *Can J Anaesth* 36:137, 1989.
110. Kenyon HR: Perforations in transurethral operations: technique for immediate diagnosis and management of extravasations, *JAMA* 142:798, 1950.
111. Kirson LE, Goldman JM, Slover RB: Low-dose intrathecal morphine for postoperative pain control in patients undergoing transurethral resection of the prostate, *Anesthesiology* 71:192, 1989.
112. Kirvela M, Olkkola KT, Rosenberg PH, et al: Pharmacokinectics of propofol and haemodynamic changes during induction of anaesthesia in uraemic patients, *Br J Anaesth* 68:178, 1992.
113. Kirvela M, Scheinin M, Lindgren L: Haemodynamic and catecholamine responses to induction of anaesthesia and tracheal intubation in diabetic and non-diabetic uraemic patients, *Br J Anaesth* 74:60, 1995.
114. Knudsen F, Jorgensen S, Bonde J, et al: Anesthesia and complications of extracorporeal shock wave lithotripsy of urinary calculi, *J Urol* 148:1030, 1992.
115. Koide M, Waud BE: Serum potassium concentrations after succinylcholine in patients with renal failure, *Anesthesiology* 36:142, 1972.
116. Korbon GA, Lunch C, Arnold WP, et al: Repeated epidural anesthesia for extracorporeal shock wave lithotripsy unreliable, *Anesth Analg* 66:669, 1987.
117. Kortis HI, Amory DW, Wagner BK, et al: Use of patient-controlled analgesia with alfentanil for extracorporeal shock wave lithotripsy, *J Clin Anesth* 7:205, 1995.
118. Langberg J, Abber J, Thuroff JW, et al: The effects of extracorporeal shock wave lithotripsy on pacemaker function, *Pacing Clin Electrophysiol* 10:1142, 1987.
119. Lewis RP, Spiers SP, McLaren IM, et al: Pethidine as a spinal anaesthetic agent—a comparison with plain bupivacaine in patients undergoing transurethral resection of the prostate, *Eur J Anaesthesiol* 9:105, 1992.
120. Linke CL, Merin RG: A regional anesthetic approach for renal transplantation, *Anesth Analg* 55:69, 1976.
121. Little DM Jr: Posture and anesthesia, *Can Anaesth Soc J* 7:2, 1960.
122. Liu S, Carpenter RL, Mulroy MF, et al: Intravenous versus epidural administration of hydromorphone: effects on analgesia and recovery after radical retropubic prostatectomy, *Anesthesiology* 82:682, 1995.
123. Loening S, Karamolowsky EV, Willoughby B: Use of local anesthesia for extracorporeal shock wave lithotripsy, *J Urol* 137: 626, 1987.
124. Lumb AB, Nunn JF: Respiratory function and rib cage contribution to ventilation in body positions commonly used during anesthesia, *Anesth Analg* 73:422, 1991.
125. Lydon JC, Spielman FJ: Bilateral compartment syndrome following prolonged surgery in the lithotomy position, *Anesthesiology* 60:236, 1984.
126. Mackenzie AR: Influence of anaesthesia on blood loss in transurethral prostatectomy, *Scot Med J* 35:14, 1990.
127. Madsen RE, Madsen PO: Influence of anaesthesia form on blood loss in transurethral prostatectomy, *Anesth Analg* 46:330, 1967.
128. Malatinsky J, Kadlic T: Inferior venal caval occlusion in the left lateral position: a case report, *Br J Anaesth* 46:165, 1974.

129. Malhotra V, Long CW, Meister MJ: Intercostal blocks with local infiltration anesthesia for extracorporeal shock wave lithotripsy, *Anesth Analg* 66:85, 1987.
130. Malhotra V, Rosen RJ, Slepian RL: Life threatening hypoxemia in an adult due to shock wave induced pulmonary contusion, *Anesthesiology* 75:529, 1991.
131. Malhotra V: Hyperthermia and hypothermia as complication of extracorporeal shock wave lithotripsy, *Anesthesiology* 67:448, 1987.
132. Malkowicz SB, Avon MR, Thangathurai D, et al: Intravenous papaverine in constructing continent urinary reservoir, *Urology* 33:431, 1989.
133. Marx GF, Orkin LR: Complications associated with transurethral surgery, *Anesthesiology* 23:802, 1962.
134. Mathes DD: Bleomycin and hyperoxia exposure in the operating room. *Anesth Analg* 81:624, 1995.
135. McClain DA, Hug CC Jr: Intravenous fentanyl kinetics, *Clin Pharmacol Ther* 28: 106, 1980.
136. McDonald PF, Berry AM: Topical anaesthesia for extracorporeal shock wave lithotripsy, *Br J Anaesth* 69:399, 1992.
137. McGowan SW, Smith GFN: Anaesthesia for transurethral prostatectomy, *Anaesthesia* 35:847, 1980.
138. McLaughlin MG, Kinahan TJ: Transurethral resection of the prostate in the outpatient setting, *J Urol* 143:951, 1990.
139. Mebust WK, Holtgrewe HL, Cockett ATK, et al: Transurethral prostatectomy—immediate and postoperative complications: a cooperative study of 13 participating institutions evaluating 3885 patients, *J Urol* 141:243, 1989.
140. Mebust WK: Transurethral prostatectomy, *Urol Clin North Am* 17:575, 1990.
141. Melzer JS, Salvatierra O: The blood transfusion effect in cadaveric donor transplantation; the University of California, San Francisco experience, *Transpl Immunol Lett* 4:6, 1987.
142. Miller RD, Way WL, Hamilton WK, et al: Succinylcholine induced hyperkalemia in patients with renal failure? *Anesthesiology* 36:138, 1972.
143. Monk TG, Boure B, White P, et al: Comparison of intravenous sedative–analgesic techniques for outpatient immersion lithotripsy, *Anesth Analg* 72:616, 1991.
144. Monk TG, Ding Y, White PF, et al: Effect of topical eutectic mixture of local anesthetics on pain response and analgesic requirement during lithotripsy procedures, *Anesth Analg* 79:506, 1994.
145. Monk TG: Cancer of the prostate and radical prostatectomy. In Malhorta V, editor: *Anesthesia for renal and genito-urologic surgery,* New York, 1996, McGraw-Hill.
146. Morcos WE, Payne JP: The induction of anaesthesia with propofol (Diprivan) compared in normal and renal failure patients, *Postgrad Med J* 61:62, 1985.
147. Morris RB, Cronnelly R, Stanski DR, et al: Pharmacokinetics of edrophonium in anephric and renal transplant patients, *Br J Anaesth* 53:1311, 1981.
148. Mutoh S, Aikou I, Ueda S: Spinal coning after lumbar puncture in prostate cancer with asymptomatic vertebral metastasis: a case report, *J Urol* 145:834, 1991.
149. Narayan P: Neoplasms of the prostate gland. In Tanagho EA, McAninch JW, editors: *General urology,* ed 14, Norwalk, 1995, Appleton & Lange.
150. Naulty JS, Meisel LB, Datta, et al: Air embolism during radical hysterectomy, *Anesthesiology* 57:420, 1982.
151. Ness PM, Bourke DL, Walsh PC: Randomized trial of perioperative hemodilution versus transfusion of preoperatively deposited autologous blood in elective surgery, *Transfusion* 32:226, 1992.
152. Nielsen KK, Andersen K, Asbjorn J, et al: Blood loss in transurethral prostatectomy: epidural versus general anaesthesia, *Int Urol Nephrol* 19:287, 1987.
153. Nilsson A, Hahn RG: Mental status after transurethral resection of the prostate, *Eur Urol* 26:1, 1994.
154. Oliver SB, Cucchiara RF, Warner MA, et al: Unexpected focal neurologic deficit on emergence from anesthesia: a report on three cases, *Anesthesiology* 67:823, 1987.
155. Ota K, Namiki A, Iwasaki H, et al: Dosing interval for prolongation of tetracaine spinal anesthesia by oral clonidine in humans, *Anesth Analg* 79:1117, 1994.
156. Ovassapian A, Joshi CW, Brunner EA: Visual disturbances: an unusual symptom of transurethral prostatic resection reaction, *Anesthesiology* 57:332, 1982.
157. Pansard JL, Cholley B, Devilliers C, et al: Variation in arterial to end-tidal CO2 tension differences during anesthesia in the "kidney rest" lateral decubitus position, *Anesth Analg* 75:506, 1992.
158. Pettersson B, Tiselius HG, Andersson A, et al: Evaluation of extracorporeal shock wave lithotripsy without anesthesia using a Dornier HM3 lithotriptor without technical modifications, *J Urol* 142:1189, 1989.
159. Portenoy RK, Foley KM, Stulman J, et al: Plasma morphine and morphine-6-glucuronide during chronic morphine therapy for cancer pain: plasma profiles, steady-state concentrations and the consequences of renal failure, *Pain* 57:13, 1991.
160. Posner A, Brody D, Ravin M: Effect of prone position with constant volume ventilation on PaO2 in man, *Anesth Analg* 44:435, 1965.
161. Rassweiler J, Henkel TO, Kohrmann KU, et al: Lithotripter technology: present and future, *J Endourology* 6:1, 1992.
162. Razvi HA, Chin JL, Bhandari R: Fatal air embolism during radical retropubic prostatectomy, *J Urol* 151:433, 1994.
163. Rehder K, Knopp TJ, Sessler AD: Regional intrapulmonary gas distribution in awake and anesthetized-paralyzed prone man, *J Appl Physiol* 45:528, 1978.
164. Reich DL, Konstadt SN, Hubbard M, et al: Do Trendelenburg and passive leg raising improve cardiac performance? *Anesth Analg* 67:S184, 1988.
165. Roesch R, Stoelling RK, Lingman JE, et al: Ammonia toxicity resulting from glycine absorption during a transurethral resection of the prostate, *Anesthesiology* 58:577, 1983.
166. Russell D: Painless loss of vision after transurethral resection of the prostate, *Anaesthesia* 45:218, 1990.
167. Ryan DW: Anesthesia for cystectomy, *Anaesthesia* 37:557, 1982.
168. Schmidt KA, Snyder SA: Effect of horizontal lithotomy position on hyperbaric tetracaine spinal anesthesia, *Anesth Analg* 67:894, 1988.
169. Sear J, Moore A, Hunniset A, et al: Morphine kinetics and kidney transplantation: morphine removal is influenced by renal ischemia, *Anesth Analg* 64:1065, 1985.
170. Sear JW: Sufentanil disposition in patients undergoing renal transplantation: influence of choice of kinetic model, *Br J Anaesth* 63:60, 1989.
171. Sengupta P: Prevention of postdural puncture headache after spinal anaesthesia for extracorporeal shock-wave lithotripsy. An assessment of prophylactic epidural blood patching, *Anaesthesia* 44:54, 1989.
172. Sharp JT: The effect of body position change on lung compliance in normal patients and in patients with congestive heart failure, *J Clin Invest* 35:659, 1959.
173. Shir Y, Frank SM, Brendler, et al: Postoperative morbidity is similar in patients anesthetized with epidural and general anesthesia for radical prostatectomy, *Urology* 44:232, 1994.
174. Shir Y, Raja SN, Frank SM, et al: Intraoperative blood loss during radical retropubic prostatectomy: epidural versus general anesthesia, *Urology* 45:993, 1995.
175. Shir Y, Raja SN, Frank SM: The effect of epidural versus general anesthesia on postoperative pain and analgesic requirements in patients undergoing radical prostatectomy, *Anesthesiology* 80:49, 1994.
176. Shir Y, Raja SR: Indigo carmine-induced severe hypotension in patients undergoing radical prostatectomy, *Anesthesiology* 79: 378, 1993.
177. Sibbald WJ, Patterson NA, Holliday RL, et al: The Trendelenburg position: hemodynamic effects in hypotensive and normotensive patients, *Crit Care Med* 7:218, 1979.
178. Sinclair CJ, Scott DB, Edstrom HH: Effect of the Trendelenburg position on spinal anesthesia with hyperbaric bupivacaine, *Br J Anaesth* 54:497, 1982.
179. Slocum HC, Hoeflich EA, Allen CR: Circulatory and respiratory distress from extreme positions on the operating table, *Surg Gynecol Obstet* 84:1065, 1947.
180. Slocum HC, O'Neal KC, Allen CR: Neurovascular complications from malposition on the operating table, *Surg Gynecol Obstet* 86:729, 1948.
181. Smith C, Carter M, Sebel P, et al: Mental function after general anaesthesia for transurethral procedures, *Br J Anaesth* 67:262, 1991.
182. Smith CE, Hunter JM: Anesthesia for renal transplantation: relaxants and volatiles, *Int Anesthesiol Clin* 33:69, 1995.
183. Smith RN, Gramling ZW, Volpitto PP: Problems related to the prone position for surgical operation, *Anesthesiology* 22:189, 1961.
184. Smyth R, Cheng D, Asokumar B, et al: Coagulopathies in patients after transurethral resection of the prostate: spinal versus general anesthesia, *Anesth Analg* 81:680, 1995.

185. Spear RM, Deshpande, Davis PJ: Anesthesia for general, urologic, and plastic surgery. In *Smith's anesthesia for infants and children,* ed 5. St. Louis, 1990, CV Mosby.
186. Stalberg HP, Hahn RG, Jones AW: Ethanol monitoring of transurethral prostatic resection during inhaled anesthesia, *Anesth Analg* 75:983, 1992.
187. Stjerstrom H, Henneberg S, Eklund A, et al: Thermal balance during transurethral resection of the prostate: a comparison of general anaesthesia and epidural analgesia, *Acta Anaesthesiol Scand* 29:743, 1985.
188. Stoller ML, Litt L, Salazar RG: Severe hemorrhage after extracorporeal shock-wave lithtripsy, *Ann Intern Med* 111:612, 1989.
189. Stoller ML: Extracorporeal shock wave lithotripsy. In Tanagho EA, McAninch JW, editors: *General urology,* ed 14, Norwalk, 1995, Appleton & Lange.
190. Stone JG, Khambatta HJ: Pulmonary shunts in the prone position, *Anaesthesia* 33:512, 1978.
191. Strohmaier WL, Bichler KH, Koch J, et al: Protective effect of verapamil on shock wave induced renal tubular dysfunction, *J Urol* 150:27, 1993.
192. Strohmaier WL, Koch J, Balk N, et al: Limitation of shock-wave-induced renal tubular dysfunction by nifedipine, *Eur Urol* 25:99, 1994.
193. Swenson JD, Hullander RM, Nolan JF, et al: Renal cell carcinoma in the inferior vena cava demonstrated by transesophageal echocardiography, *J Cardiothorac Vasc Anesth* 7:335, 1993.
194. Szenohradszky J, Fisher DM, Segredo V, et al: Pharmacokinetics of rocuronium bromide (ORG 9426) in patients with normal renal function or patients undergoing cadaver renal transplantation, *Anesthesiology* 77:899, 1992.
195. Szeto HH, Inturrisi CE, Houde R, et al: Accumulation of normeperidine, an active metabolite of meperidine, in patients with renal failure or cancer, *Ann Intern Med* 86:738, 1977.
196. Tailly GG: Experience with the Dornier HM4 and MPL9000 lithotriptors in urinary stone treatment, *J Urol* 144:622, 1991.
197. Tanagho EA: Anatomy of the genitourinary tract. In Tanagho EA, McAninch JW, editors: *General urology,* ed 14, Norwalk, 1995, Appleton & Lange.
198. Thomas JL, Holmes JH: Effect of hemodialysis on plasma cholinesterase, *Anesth Analg* 49:323, 1970.
199. Thorn-Alquist A: Prevention of hypertensive crises in patients with high spinal lesions during cystoscopy and lithotripsy, *Acta Anaesthesiol Scand* 57:79, 1975.
200. Tobey RE: Paraplegia, succinylcholine and cardiac arrest, *Anesthesiology* 32:259, 1970.
201. Tondare AS, Nadkarni AV, Sathe CH, et al: Femoral neuropathy: a complication of lithotomy position under spinal anesthesia, *Can Anaesth Soc J* 30:84, 1983.
202. Touminen M, Taivainen T, Rosenberg PH: Spread of spinal anaesthesia with plain 0.5% bupivacaine: influence of the vertebral interspace used for injection, *Br J Anaesth* 62:358, 1989.
203. Vacanti CA, Lodhia KL: Fatal massive air embolism during transurethral resection of the prostate, *Anesthesiology* 74:186, 1991.
204. Vandenbrom RH, Wierda JM, Agoston S: Pharmacokinetics and neuromuscular blocking effects of atracurium besylate and two of its metabolites in patients with normal and impaired renal function, *Clin Pharmacokinet* 19:230, 1990.
205. Waid-Jones MI, Coursin DB: Perioperative considerations for patients treated with bleomycin, *Chest* 99:993, 1991.
206. Walsh PC: Technique of radical retropubic prostatectomy with preservation of sexual function—an anatomic approach, In Skinner DG, Lieskovsky G, editors: *Genitourinary cancer,* Philadelphia, 1988, WB Saunders.
207. Walts LF, Atlee JL: Supraventricular tachycardia associated with extracorporeal shock wave lithotripsy, *Anesthesiology* 65:521, 1986.
208. Wang LP, Fog J, Bove M: Transient hearing loss following spinal anaesthesia, *Anaesthesia* 42:1268, 1987.
209. Wang LP, Magnusson M, Lundberg J, et al: Auditory function after spinal anesthesia, *Reg Anesth* 18:162, 1993.
210. Warner MA, Martin JT, Schroeder DR, et al: Lower-extremity motor neuropathy associated with surgery performed on patients in a lithotomy position, *Anesthesiology* 81:6, 1994.
211. Weingram J: Laparoscopic and laser surgery. In Malhorta V, editor: *Anesthesia for renal and genito-urologic surgery,* New York, 1996, McGraw-Hill.
212. Welch M, Bazaral MG, Schmidt R, et al: Anesthetic management for surgical removal of renal carcinoma with caval or atrial tumor thrombus using deep hypothermic circulatory arrest, *J Cardiothorac Anesth* 3:580, 1989.
213. Whelan P, Morris PJ: Immunological responsiveness after transurethral resection of the prostate: general versus spinal anesthesia, *Clin Exp Immunol* 48:661, 1982.
214. Wilcox S, Vandam LD: Alas, poor Trendelenburg and his position! A critique of its uses and effectiveness, *Anesth Analg* 67:574, 1988.
215. Wilson WT, Preminger GM: Extracorporeal shock wave lithotripsy: an update, *Urol Clin North Am* 17:231, 1990.
216. Wulff KE, Aulin I: The regional lung function in the lateral decubitus position during anesthesia and surgery, *Acta Anaesth Scand* 16:195, 1972.
217. Yamada AH, Lieskovsky G, Skinner DG, et al: Impact of autologous blood transfusion on patients undergoing radical prostatectomy using hypotensive anesthesia, *J Urol* 149:73, 1993.
218. Yao FS: Anesthesia for renal transplantation. In Malhorta V, editor: *Anesthesia for renal and genito-urologic surgery,* New York, 1996, McGraw-Hill.
219. Zeitlin GL, Roth R: Effects of three anesthetic techniques on the success of extracorporeal shock wave lithotripsy in nephrolithiasis, *Anesthesiology* 68:272, 1988.

CHAPTER 76

Anesthesia for Obstetrics

BETH GLOSTEN

The pregnant patient presents unique issues to the anesthesia provider. Pregnancy itself alters maternal physiology and influences the potential complications and responses to anesthetics for pain relief during labor or cesarean delivery. The anesthetic techniques and agents should not only be effective, but have minimal effect on maternal and fetal well-being. The presence of certain medical conditions in either mother or fetus or obstetric complications further complicate anesthetic management. This chapter will review the important physiologic features of pregnancy and anesthetic care for both normal and high-risk pregnant patients.

PHYSIOLOGIC CHANGES DURING PREGNANCY

Pregnancy, labor, and delivery are associated with profound physiologic changes involving all organ systems. These changes should be recognized by the anesthesia provider.

Cardiovascular Changes

The cardiovascular system undergoes major alterations to meet increased demands of pregnancy[138,156,195,237] (Table 76-1). Maternal blood volume increases throughout pregnancy, the maximum rates of increase occurring during the

Table 76-1 Changes in the cardiovascular system

Variable	Direction of change	Average change (%)
Blood volume	↑	+35
Plasma volume	↑	+45
Red blood cell volume	↑	+20
Cardiac output	↑	+40
Stroke volume	↑	+30
Heart rate	↑	+15
Femoral (uterine) venous pressure	↑	+15 mm Hg
Total peripheral resistance	↓	−15
Mean arterial blood pressure	↓	−15 mm Hg
Systolic blood pressure	↓	−0–15 mm Hg
Diastolic blood pressure	↓	−10–20 mm Hg
Central venous pressure	No change	

From Cheek TG, Gutche B: Maternal physiologic alterations during pregnancy. In Shnider SM, Levinson, G, editors: *Anesthesia for obstetrics,* ed 2, Baltimore, 1987, Williams & Wilkins.

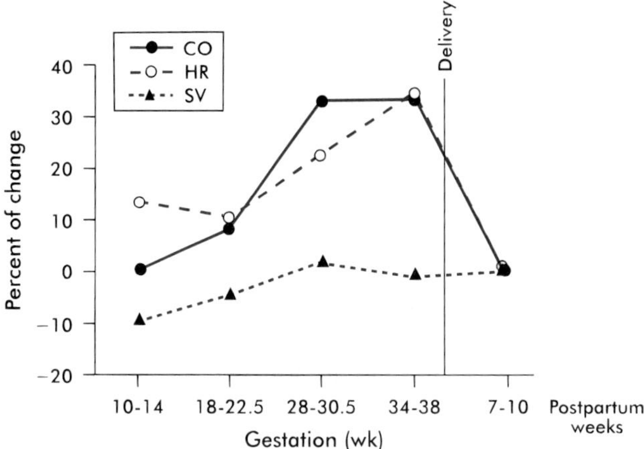

Fig. 76-1. Percent changes in cardiac output (CO), heart rate (HR), and stroke volume (SV) during gestation with the postpartum period used as a control. (From Mashini IS, Albazzaz SJ, Fadd HE: Serial noninvasive evaluation of cardiovascular hemodynamics during pregnancy, *Am J Obstet Gynecol* 156:1208, 1987.)

second trimester.[237] Although blood volume increases by 35%, plasma volume and erythrocyte volume increases by 45% and 20%, respectively. As a result, hematocrit decreases from hemodilution. The increased blood volume is well tolerated by healthy pregnant women. Patients with cardiac disease (e.g., mitral stenosis) may become symptomatic as pregnancy progresses until cardiac function cannot meet the demands of pregnancy.

Cardiac output increases approximately 30% to 40% during the first trimester, with a second smaller increase during the second trimester due to increases in heart rate, and greater increases in stroke volume (Table 76-1 and Fig. 76-1).[36,156,237] During labor, cardiac output is further increased both from the sympathetic stimulation of pain, as well as the episodic autotransfusion of blood into the central circulation from the contracting uterus. It is estimated that with each uterine contraction, 300 to 500 ml enters the maternal system.[105] This autotransfusion can increase cardiac output and central blood volume by 10% to 25 % above prelabor values.[236] The greatest increase in cardiac output occurs immediately after delivery when cardiac output can be up to 80% above prelabor values.[99] This again is attributed to autotransfusion from the contracted uterus. Prepregnancy cardiac output levels are generally regained several weeks postpartum, and the normal nonpregnant blood volume is reached by about 2 weeks postpartum.[195] Fig. 76-1 describes the peripartum changes in cardiac output, heart rate, and stroke volume.

Measurement of cardiac output after the twenty-eighth week gestation depends on patient position. Lees[137] and Kerr[130] demonstrated that early reports of decreased cardiac output in the third trimester were due to obstruction of the inferior vena cava (IVC) by the gravid uterus resulting in decreased venous return. Caval compression leads to the development of collateral routes for venous return (intervertebral, epidural, azygous venous systems). Some pregnant women at term will be symptomatic from this decreased venous return and display the "supine hypotensive syndrome" with hypotension, tachycardia, and diaphoresis when lying supine. Manual displacement of the uterus by placing the patient in the semi- or full lateral position with a wedge under the left hip will prevent aortocaval compression. Proper patient positioning is extremely important during the administration of anesthesia. Anesthetic-induced decreased venous tone in the lower extremities will exacerbate decreased venous return. With the supine position and caval compression, the resulting decreased cardiac output and increased venous pooling can impair uterine blood flow and fetal well-being.

Despite increases in cardiac output and blood volume, blood pressure is not elevated during normal pregnancy resulting in a decrease in peripheral vascular resistance. These changes in vascular tone are apparently mediated by changes in prostaglandin and prostacyclin levels, resulting in alterations in blood flow distribution that improve O_2 delivery to the uterus.[253]

Hematologic Changes

Plasma volume increases to a greater extent than does erythrocyte volume, resulting in the relative anemia of pregnancy, with the normal hemoglobin in the range of 12 g/dl.[237] Although blood viscosity decreases, the pregnant woman becomes hypercoagulable because of increases in platelets and certain coagulation factors (Table 76-2).

Table 76-2 Coagulation factors and inhibitors during normal pregnancy

Factor	Nonpregnant (%)	Late pregnancy (%)
Factor I (fibrinogen)	200–450 mg/dl	400–650 mg/dl
Factor II (prothrombin)	75–125	100–125
Factor V	75–125	100–150
Factor VII	75–125	150–250
Factor VIII	75–150	200–500
Factor IX	75–125	100–150
Factor X	75–125	150–250
Factor XI	75–125	50–100
Factor XII	75–125	100–200
Factor XIII	75–125	35–75
Antithrombin III	85–110	75–100
Antifactor Xa	85–110	75–100
Platelets		Slight ↑
Fibrinolysis		Slight ↓

From Cheek TG, Gutche B: Maternal physiologic alterations during pregnancy. In Shnider SM, Levinson G, editors: *Anesthesia for obstetrics,* ed 2, Baltimore, 1987, Williams & Wilkins.

Table 76-3 Maternal respiratory alterations at term

Variable	Change	Change (%)
Respiratory parameters		
Minute ventilation	↑↑↑↑	+50
Alveolar ventilation	↑↑↑↑↑	+70
Tidal volume	↑↑↑	+40
Respiratory rate	↑	+15
Closing volume	±↓	0
Airway resistance	↓↓	−36
Vital capacity	±	0
Inspiratory lung capacity	±	0
Functional residual capacity	↓↓	−20
Total lung capacity	±	0
Expiratory reserve volume	↓↓	−20
Residual volume	↓↓	−20
Oxygen consumption	↑↑	+20
Blood gas values		
Arterial pH	±	0
Arterial P_{CO_2}	↓	−10 mm Hg
Arterial P_{O_2}	↑	+10 mm Hg
Serum HCO_3^-	↓	−4 mEq

Modified from Skaredoff MN, Ostheimer GW: Physiologic changes during pregnancy: effects of major regional anesthesia, *Reg Anesth* 6:28, 1981.

Gastrointestinal Changes

Increased levels of progesterone result in delayed gastric emptying and decreased esophageal mobility.[101] This, in combination with displacement of the stomach by the gravid uterus, can result in gastroesophageal reflux and puts the patient at risk for aspiration during general anesthesia.[205] Generally, every parturient is managed as a patient with a full stomach after the first trimester.

Hepatic Changes

Levels of hepatic enzymes such as alkaline phosphatase serum glutamic-oxaloacetic transaminase (SGOT), lactic dehydrogenase (LDH), and cholesterol increase during pregnancy.[163] Bilirubin is unchanged, and albumin decreases, although the total protein concentration increases. Decreased plasma protein concentrations result in a lessening of plasma oncotic pressure during pregnancy. Plasma cholinesterase levels are decreased; however, there is no clinically significant prolongation of the action of succinylcholine or ester-type local anesthetics in the dosages generally given.[25]

Respiratory Changes

Oxygen demand increases during pregnancy. O_2 content decreases slightly because of the lesser hematocrit. O_2 delivery increases because of increases in cardiac output and a shift to the right in the maternal oxyhemoglobin dissociation P_{50}.[126] Respiratory changes also result in increases in O_2 supply (Table 76-3).[224] Although functional residual capacity (FRC) is decreased due to cephalad displacement of the diaphragm by the gravid uterus, the thoracic anteroposterior diameter enlarges.[196] Minute ventilation at term is double that in the nonpregnant patient. Increased minute ventilation results in a decrease in arterial P_{CO_2}, but arterial pH is normalized by a decrease in serum bicarbonate.[196]

As pregnancy progresses, the contribution of abdominal breathing is decreased and the parturient may have airway closure during normal tidal ventilation.[24] This, in combination with the decrease in FRC and increase in O_2 consumption, makes the pregnant patient (particularly if obese) prone to atelectasis and the development of an increased alveolar-arterial O_2 gradient when in the supine position. Hypoxemia may then develop during somnolence associated with administration of parenteral analgesics or during apnea associated with the induction of general anesthesia.

Renal Changes

Progesterone causes the renal pelvis and ureters to dilate. Increases in intravascular volume and aldosterone levels cause an increase in renal plasma flow and glomerular filtration rate.[75] Therefore, blood urea nitrogen and serum creatinine are decreased. Glycosuria is common because of both hormonal changes and the increased glucose load presented to the renal tubules.

Skin and Mucous Membrane Changes

Mucous membranes become extremely fragile during the third trimester of pregnancy. This likely reflects blood vessel engorgement from the increased plasma volume. Manipulation of the nasal passages is best avoided

to prevent severe nosebleeds. Difficult laryngoscopy can lead to easy bleeding, increasing the problems.

Increased extracellular fluid can result in dependent edema. The upper airway and vocal cords can also become edematous. Airway edema likely contributes to difficulties with tracheal intubation. Smaller diameter endotracheal (ET) tubes (6.0 to 7.0 mm) are usually necessary.

Nervous System Changes

Pregnancy is associated with a decrease in local anesthetic dose requirements (Table 76-4). Pregnant women need approximately 25% less local anesthetic for regional anesthesia than nonpregnant women.[29] Both anatomic and hormonal effects may be responsible. Distention of the epidural veins may decrease the size of the epidural space and facilitate spread of epidural local anesthetic. Exaggerated lumbar lordosis may enhance cephalad spread of spinal local anesthetics. Further, hormonal changes of pregnancy may alter nerve response to local anesthetics. Isolated nerves from pregnant rabbits or from rabbits chronically treated with progesterone are significantly more sensitive to bupivacaine-induced conduction blockade than nerves from nonpregnant animals.[70]

Pregnancy also decreases the requirement for inhalational agents by 25% to 40% in animals[186] and by approximately 28% in humans in the first trimester of pregnancy.[93] This effect is diminished by about the third postpartum day.[42] Increased plasma and central nervous system (CNS) progesterone levels may be responsible. In animals, high plasma levels of progesterone are inversely correlated with the minimal anesthetic concentration (MAC) for halothane.[71]

Musculoskeletal Changes

The hormone relaxin is produced by the placenta and causes ligamentous relaxation.[129] Lumbar lordosis is increased by center of gravity changes due to the presence of the gravid uterus. These changes result in a high percentage of parturients reporting back pain and sciatic symptoms. Regional anesthesia does not increase the incidence of postpartum back symptoms.[169]

UTERINE BLOOD FLOW

Uterine blood vessels are normally maximally dilated, and therefore uterine blood flow is directly related to perfusion pressure as described by the following equation:

$$\text{Uterine blood flow} = \frac{\text{Maternal mean arterial pressure} - \text{Venous pressure}}{\text{Uterine vascular resistance}}$$

Thus any factor increasing uterine vascular resistance, decreasing maternal arterial pressure, or increasing uterine venous pressure can reduce uterine blood flow and impair O_2 delivery to the fetus (Table 76-5).

During regional anesthesia, maternal hypotension should be avoided. Regional anesthesia uncomplicated by hypotension is not associated with decreases in intervillous blood flow.[121,123] Hypotension is prevented by prehydration with intravenous (IV) fluids and proper positioning of the patient with uterine displacement. If hypotension occurs, it is treated promptly. Vasopressors with predominant alpha-adrenergic activity have been shown in animals to increase uterine vascular resistance and decrease uterine blood flow.[81] **Ephedrine, which acts on both alpha and beta receptors, has been shown to maintain uterine blood flow and has classically been the vasopressor of choice to treat hypotension stemming from regional anesthesia in the obstetric patient.** Recent studies in healthy, well-hydrated women undergoing epidural or spinal anesthesia for cesarean section have shown that the use of the alpha-agent phenylephrine to treat hypotension does not cause fetal acidosis.[171,198] Thus in conditions in which the tachycardia caused by ephedrine would be detrimental (i.e., patients with preexisting tachycardia or certain cardiac lesions), phenylephrine can be considered as an antihypotensive agent although there are no current reports of its use in the high-risk parturient.

An increase in intensity or duration of uterine contractions will decrease blood flow through the placenta. If the uterus is excessively stimulated by oxytocin, placental blood flow can be severely compromised and fetal distress can

Table 76-4 Anesthetic requirements during pregnancy

Variable	Change	Change (%)
Inhalational agents	↓ MAC	−25–40
Local anesthetics		
Epidural agents	↓ Dose	−20–30
Spinal agents	↓ Dose	−20–30

Table 76-5 Factors decreasing uterine blood flow

Factor	Etiology
Decreased maternal arterial pressure	Hypovolemia (abruptio placenta, placenta previa)
	Sympathetic block from regional anesthesia
	Aortocaval compression; supine hypotensive syndrome
Increased uterine venous pressure	Caval compression; supine hypotensive syndrome
Increased uterine vascular resistance	Hypertension
	Preeclampsia
	Alpha agonists
	Uterine contractions
	Uterine hyperstimulation with oxytocin
	Abruptio placenta
	High concentrations of local anesthetics

occur. High concentrations of local anesthetics have been shown to increase uterine vascular resistance. These levels are not achieved after epidural anesthesia. In the gravid ewe, concentrations of local anesthetics in the range found after paracervical block, where the anesthetic is injected close to the uterine arteries, have been associated with a 25% decrease in uterine blood flow.[85]

UPTAKE, DISTRIBUTION, AND METABOLISM OF DRUGS IN THE FETUS AND NEWBORN

A portion of all drugs administered to the mother will pass to the fetus.[168,252] **The amount transferred to the fetus is classically described by the ratio of the concentration of drug in the umbilical vein with that in the maternal vein (UV/MV ratio) at the time of delivery.** The factors that will ultimately determine the fetal or newborn drug concentration and effect on the newborn are listed in Box 76-1.

Maternal Drug Concentration

The maternal concentration of free drug that ultimately determines the placental transfer depends on several factors:

- *Site of administration.* Peak blood levels of drugs are highest in areas of dense vascularity. For the various anesthetic techniques used in obstetrics, peak blood levels from highest to lowest are as follows:

intravenous → paracervical block → caudal epidural → lumbar epidural → intramuscular (IM) injection → subarachnoid block.

To some extent, peak blood levels of local anesthetics can be decreased by the addition of epinephrine.

BOX 76-1
FACTORS AFFECTING UPTAKE DISTRIBUTION, AND METABOLISM OF DRUGS IN THE FETUS AND NEWBORN

Maternal drug concentration
- Site of administration
- Total dosage
- Maternal protein binding
- Maternal clearance and metabolism
- Maternal blood pH

Placental transfer
- Diffusion constant
- Placental factors (area, distance, metabolism)

Fetal drug concentration
- Fetal circulation
- Fetal pH
- Fetal protein binding
- Fetal metabolism
- Tissue binding

- *Total dosage.* The amount of drug crossing the placenta will obviously increase with increased amounts of maternally administered drug. A diffusable drug given by IV bolus produces a maternal arterial concentration that rapidly declines as the drug is redistributed about the body. The umbilical venous concentration may exceed maternal arterial concentration (Fig. 76-2).[220]
- *Maternal protein binding.* An equilibrium state is established between the protein bound portion and unbound portion of the drug. Only the unbound fraction is available for placental transfer. The rate of placental diffusion is believed to be inversely correlated with the protein binding capacity of maternal blood for the specific agent (Table 76-6).[57]

Protein binding is a dynamic process, and as the "free" drug concentration decreases because of redistribution and placental transfer, more drug enters the free-drug compartment from the bound portion. Thus the importance of protein binding in placental transfer is probably limited.

- *Clearance and metabolism.* Maternal metabolism will remove the drug from the circulation and make it un-

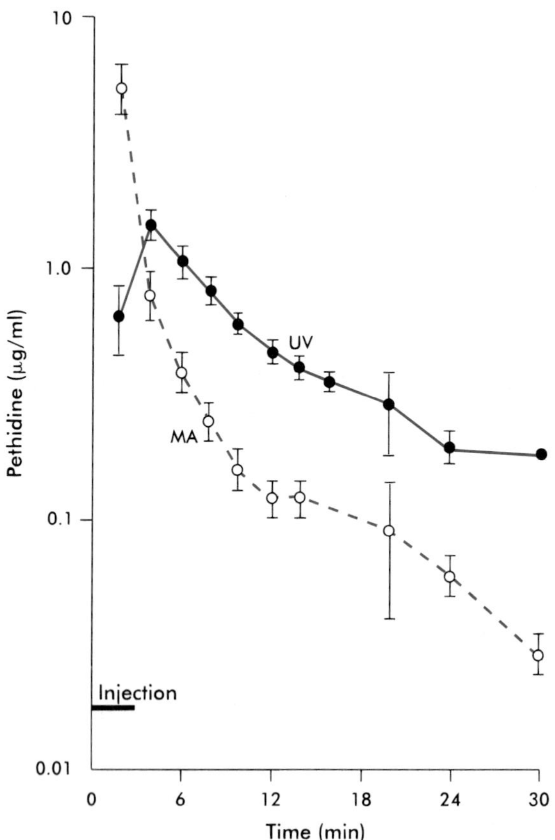

Fig. 76-2. Pethidine (meperidine) concentrations in maternal artery (MA) and umbilical vein (UV) in ewes and lambs following 1.5 mg/kg given intravenously to the mother. (From Shier RW, Sprague AD, Dilts PV: Placental transfer of meperidine HCl. Part II, *Am J Obstet Gynecol* 115:556, 1973.)

Table 76-6 Relationship between plasma protein binding capacity and umbilical vein/maternal blood (UV/M) ratio of various local anesthetic agents

Agent	Protein binding capacity (%)	Maternal arterial or venous blood levels (μg/ml)	Umbilical vein levels (μg/ml)	UV/M ratio
Prilocaine	55	1.03–1.5	1.07–1.5	1.0–1.18
Lidocaine	64	1.23–3.5	0.8–1.8	0.52–0.69
Mepivacaine	77	2.91–6.9	1.9–4.9	0.69–0.71
Bupivacaine	95	0.26	0.08–0.11	0.31–0.44
Etidocaine	94	0.25–1.3	0.07–0.45	0.14–0.35

From Covino BG, Vasallo HG: *Local anesthetics, mechanisms of action and clinical use,* New York, 1976, Grune & Stratton.

available for placental transfer. In some cases, the metabolites themselves can transfer across the placenta and affect the fetus (such as the normeperidine metabolite of meperidine).

- *Maternal pH.* Only the more lipid soluble unionized form of acid or base molecules will freely equilibrate across the placenta. Because fetal pH is slightly less than the maternal pH, bases (e.g., local anesthetics) will be more ionized in the fetus and be less likely to cross the placenta back into the maternal circulation.

Placental Transfer

The placenta is a highly vascular organ whose function is to bring maternal and fetal circulations into close proximity for purposes of gas and nutrient exchange. As such, maternally administered medications may cross to the fetus. Various factors govern drug transfer across the intervillous space. These factors are summarized in the following equation:

$$Q/t = \frac{KA(Cm - Cf)}{D}$$

Where Q/t = amount of drug diffused/unit time (rate of transfer); K = diffusion coefficient of drug; A = surface area of placental membrane; D = thickness of placental membrane; and (Cm − Cf) = diffusion gradient (maternal drug concentration minus fetal drug concentration).

Diffusion coefficient

This value is constant for each agent and depends on characteristics such as molecular weight and lipid solubility. Drugs with molecular weights of greater than 1000 dalton (such as insulin and heparin) cannot cross the placenta by simple diffusion. Most anesthetic agents can freely transfer across the placenta.

Placental factors

The distance over which diffusion should occur is related to the maturity of the chorionic villi. At term the average distance across the mature villi is approximately 2 mm. Certain diseases of pregnancy, such as chronic hypertension and preeclampsia, increase the diffusion distance. Metabolism of drugs in the placenta itself has little clinical significance.

Fetal Drug Concentration

Fetal circulation

The fetal circulation plays an important role in the pattern of drug distribution (Fig. 76-3).[212] All drugs enter the fetal circulation from the placenta through the umbilical vein. From the umbilical vein about 40% to 60% of the blood passes through the fetal liver; the rest bypasses the liver through the ductus venosus and enters the heart through the IVC. This first pass perfusion through the liver is a buffer against attainment of high fetal drug levels. The drug concentration initially seen by the fetal heart and brain is much less than the umbilical vein concentration because of the first pass effect through the fetal liver and progressive dilution by blood returning to the heart from other parts of the fetal circulation. Asphyxia produces fetal catecholamine release, which increases the percentage of blood flow through the ductus venosus. A greater proportion of umbilical venous flow is shunted directly to the heart, and delivery of anesthetic to the heart and brain is greater.

Fetal pH

Drugs such as local anesthetics are weak bases that are in equilibrium between ionized and un-ionized forms. The fetal pH is less than the maternal pH, therefore the local anesthetic that diffuses across the placenta will be "trapped" in the fetus as the ionized acid to a certain extent (i.e., local anesthetic will preferentially cross as fetal pH becomes more acidic). This trapping of local anesthetic with fetal acidosis was reported in human infants by Brown;[31] in his series, the infants with the lowest pH had systemic levels of local anesthetic that actually exceeded maternal levels. For this reason, in cases of fetal distress, 2-chloroprocaine, which has the shortest systemic half-life, is the suggested agent if epidural anesthesia is to be done.

Fetal tissue and protein binding

The total amount of plasma protein binding sites is less in the fetus, which leads to an increase in the unbound fraction present in the fetal circulation. On the other hand, uptake of drug by the fetal tissues tends to decrease fetal drug concentra-

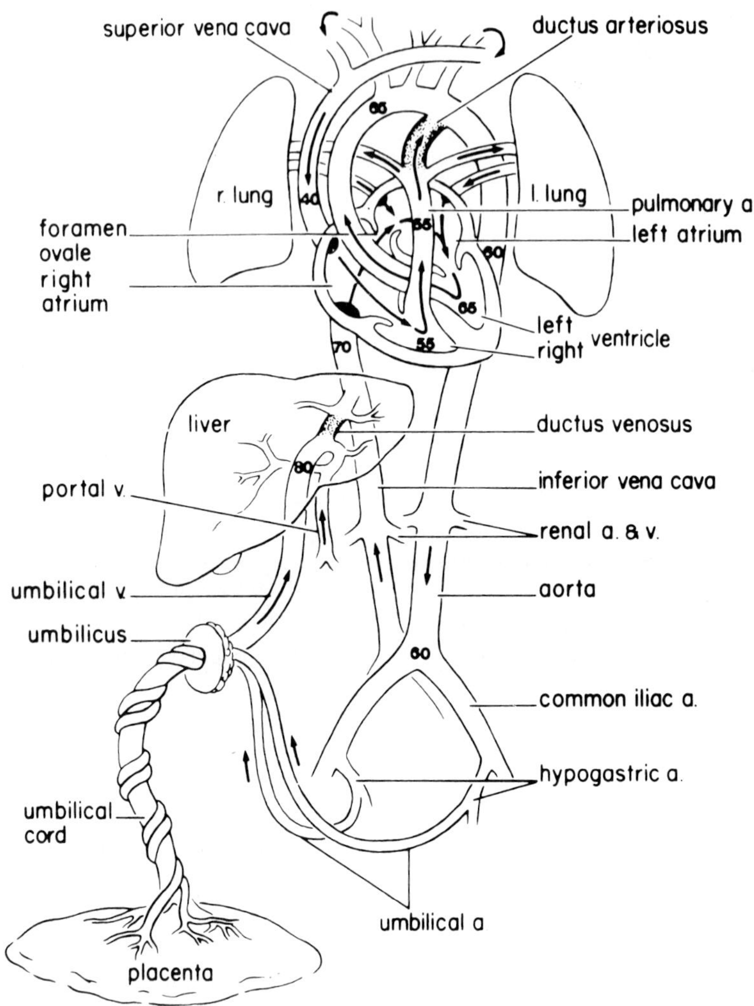

Fig. 76-3. The fetal circulation. Arrows indicate the direction of blood flow, and the numbers represent approximate values of the percent saturation of the blood with oxygen *in utero.* Note that the umbilical venous blood can bypass the liver via the ductus venosus, and that relatively well oxygenated blood entering the right atrium via the inferior vena cava can enter the left atrium via the foramen ovale. Relatively deoxygenated blood from the upper body enters the right ventricle and flows into the aorta via the ductus arteriosus to return to the placenta via the umbilical artery. (From Parer JT: *Handbook of fetal heart rate monitoring,* Philadelphia, 1983, WB Saunders.)

tion. Tissue binding in a specific target organ in the fetus is governed by factors including tissue blood flow, arterial to venous drug concentration gradient, and lipid solubility of the drug.

Fetal metabolism

The metabolic pathways in the fetus and newborn may not be completely mature. While *in utero,* the fetus can rely on maternal metabolism for drug clearance. After birth, the half-lives of many drugs, including local anesthetics, are prolonged in the newborn compared with the adult.[223]

EFFECTS OF MATERNALLY ADMINISTERED AGENTS ON THE FETUS AND NEWBORN

Methods of Evaluation

There has been great concern about the effects of medication given during labor and delivery on infant outcome. Various agents have resulted in a wide array of effects ranging from changes in the pattern of the fetal heart rate to subtle changes in neonatal tone to more severe neonatal depression. Several neuro/psychologic have been described in attempts to determine the effects of maternally administered drugs on the neonate. This section will describe the most common methods of evaluating drug effects in the neonate. The evidence describing both physiologic and neurobehavioral side effects for specific drugs used by the anesthesia provider will be reviewed.

Several types of neonatal evaluation have become popular (Box 76-2). Some investigators have relied on laboratory evidence of fetal well-being as demonstrated by umbilical artery and vein acid base values at the time of delivery. The traditional method for evaluating neonatal condition at birth has been with the APGAR scoring system.[13] The score evaluates heart rate, respiratory effort, muscle tone, reflex irritability, and color at 1 and 5 minutes of life with a maximum score of

10 (Table 76-7). This method may be insensitive to subtle or delayed effects of anesthetic agents. Infants may show alterations in neurologic or behavioral function despite a normal APGAR score. For this reason, tests of neurobehavioral function have been developed to study anesthetic effects. In general these tests evaluate the neonate's muscle tone, ability to alter his/her state of arousal, ability to suppress meaningless stimuli, and reflex motor responses. The Brazelton Neonatal Behavioral Assessment Scale (NBAS) is the most complete and is considered the gold standard for neurobehavioral examinations.[27] It is infrequently used because of the time and training required to administer it. In 1974, Scanlon developed the Early Neonatal Neurobehavioral Scale (ENNS);[217] an easier-to-perform, less complicated, and shorter examination, which uses modified and selected items from the Brazelton examination. This test has been used extensively to evaluate the effects of anesthetic drugs. In 1979, Amiel-Tison devised the Neurologic and Adaptive Capacity Score (NACS).[12] This test is shorter than previous examinations, and some investigators believe it may not be complete enough to detect subtle effects.[235] **It should be remembered that there are no valid long-term studies to determine if the findings on *any* of these examinations have a significant correlation with later mental and neurologic development of the newborn.**

Neonatal Effects of Specific Agents

Tranquilizers

Benzodiazepines are used uncommonly in obstetrics because the amnestic effects are usually undesirable to the mothers. Maternal doses of diazepam greater than 10 mg have been associated with neonatal hypotonia, hypothermia, and respiratory depression.[59] Metabolites can be present in the neonate for up to 8 days.

BOX 76-2
METHODS OF EVALUATING THE NEONATE FOR EFFECTS OF MATERNALLY ADMINISTERED DRUGS

Fetal acid base status
Time to onset of sustained respiration
APGAR score
Neurobehavioral examinations
- Brazelton (NBAS)
- Scanlon (ENNS)
- Amiel-Tison (NACS)

Opioids

Opioids remain the most commonly used agents for obstetric pain relief. Meperidine is the opioid used most frequently. Maternally administered meperidine may produce neonatal depression that is related to total dose and to the time interval between administration and delivery. Maximal depression occurs with delivery within 1 to 3 hours after IM injection; less depression was seen if meperidine was given within 1 hour or more than 3 hours after delivery.[222] This is likely due to the accumulation of meperidine in the fetus because of slower elimination by the fetus and the presence of the active metabolite of meperidine (normeperidine).[175]

Morphine is used only during very early labor in obstetrics because in equianalgesic doses morphine produces more respiratory depression of the newborn than does meperidine.[251]

No significant abnormalities have been demonstrated in infants of mothers receiving up to 1 μg/kg of IV fentanyl before cesarean section.[79] Rayburn used 50 to 100 μg bolus doses of fentanyl every hour as needed for labor analgesia (range 50 to 600 μg, total) and found no effect on APGAR or neurobehavior scores in the neonates.[201]

Butorphanol (Stadol) and nalbuphine (Nubain) are two agonist-antagonist opioids. These agents are popular because of a purported ceiling effect on respiratory depression. Butorphanol in doses of 1 or 2 mg IV or IM has been shown to be safe for the neonate.[150] IV nalbuphine given during labor in total doses ranging from 3 mg to 42 mg has not been associated with neonatal side effects.[86]

Epidural and subarachnoid opioids are used more frequently in obstetrics. The small doses of intrathecal fentanyl or morphine used in obstetrics have not been demonstrated to have adverse neonatal effects.[19,115] **Similarly, the use of epidural fentanyl or sufentanil for analgesia during labor or cesarean delivery has not been demonstrated to have adverse neonatal effects.**[52,194,214,245]

Anesthetic induction agents

Thiopental and thiamylal rapidly cross the placenta (Table 76-8). The newborn is relatively unaffected by the usual in-

Table 76-7 APGAR score

Evaluation	Score 0	1	2
Heart rate	Absent	< 100 beats/min	> 100 beats/min
Respiratory effort	Absent	Slow, irregular	Strong cry
Tone	Flaccid	Some extremity flexion	Strong flexion
Reflex irritability to stimulus	No response	Grimace	Cry
Color	Blue	Blue extremities only	Pink

duction doses of these drugs (4 to 6 mg/kg) because of the first pass effect through the fetal liver and progressive dilution of the drug in the fetal circulation before reaching the brain.[82] Maternal redistribution also lessens placental passage. Repeated maternal doses of thiopental will result in neonatal depression. **No differences in neonatal outcome after elective cesarean delivery have been reported when comparing regional anesthesia with general anesthesia with thiopental, N_2O, and low concentrations of inhaled agent.**[255]

Ketamine used in doses of less than 1.5 mg/kg for induction of general anesthesia for cesarean delivery is not associated with neonatal depression.[118] Etomidate, 0.3 mg/kg is equivalent to thiopental in terms of neonatal outcome. Administration of 2.0 to 2.5 mg/kg of propofol is also similar to thiopental. If propofol is used to maintain anesthesia prior to delivery, if the induction of anesthesia to delivery interval is prolonged (>14 minutes), neonatal depression may occur.

Inhalation agents

Inhaled agents such as N_2O have been shown to rapidly cross the placenta and equilibrate after about 15 minutes of anesthesia.[155] During general anesthesia concentrations of 50% N_2O have not been shown to significantly depress the neonate unless the induction to delivery interval is abnormally prolonged. The addition of 0.5% halothane, 0.75% isoflurane, or 1% enflurane has not been associated with abnormalities in neurobehavioral examinations.[248] In all cases involving general anesthesia with potent inhaled agents, the time from induction of anesthesia to delivery of the infant should be minimized because after intervals of greater than 15 minutes, concentrations of N_2O in maternal and fetal circulations equilibrate and neonatal depression can result because of anesthetic effect and diffusion hypoxia.[155]

Muscle relaxants

Muscle relaxants are highly ionized agents with low lipid solubility; placental transfer is minimal (Table 76-8).

Local anesthetics

The direct effect of local anesthetics on the neonate is related to the concentration of drug that reaches the fetus via the umbilical vein. If the fetus becomes acidotic, ion trapping of the local anesthetic can occur, increasing the UV/MV ratio.[31] The plasma levels of local anesthetic seen after spinal anesthesia would be far too low to expect any direct drug effects on the neonate. Greater systemic concentrations of local anesthetics are reached after epidural, pudendal, paracervical, and caudal techniques.

If the fetal concentration of local anesthetic exceeds the toxic range, the syndrome of local anesthetic intoxication can occur, manifested as apnea, bradycardia, and convulsions in the first few minutes after birth.[83] In sheep, the doses of local anesthetic required to produce convulsions in the fetal lamb are much greater than in the adult ewe.[232] This greater threshold may be due to the greater volume of distribution in the neonate.

Table 76-8 Placental passage of commonly used anesthetic medications

Drug	Umbilical vein/ maternal vein ratio
Thiopental	1.08 (range 0.5–1.5)
Ketamine	0.54 (range 0.4–0.7)
Propofol	0.7
Etomidate	0.5
Pancuronium	0.19
Vecuronium	0.11
Morphine	0.92
Meperidine	0.81, may exceed 1.0 after 2–3 hours
Fentanyl	0.57
Sufentanil	0.2 (in sheep; levels too low to measure in humans)
Butorphanol	0.84
Nalbuphine	0.97

Data from references 62, 63, 96, 106, 146, 172, 242.

There has been considerable investigation as to the direct effects of local anesthetic on the neonate in the concentrations generally seen after epidural anesthesia. Early studies reported poorer neurobehavioral scores in infants of mothers receiving epidurals with lidocaine or mepivacaine than in infants of mothers who did not receive epidural anesthesia.[217] Although this study resulted in great concern over the use of epidural lidocaine in obstetrics, it was later criticized because of inadequate control groups and combinations of medications used in the study group. Later better controlled studies have not demonstrated significant neonatal effects of lidocaine, bupivacaine, or 2-chloroprocaine in the doses normally used for epidural anesthesia.[2,68] Preliminary clinical studies evaluating the maternal and neonatal effects of epidural ropivacaine (a newly developed amide local anesthetic) for cesarean delivery anesthesia suggest that it is equivalent to bupivacaine in terms of neonatal neurobehaviour.

Miscellaneous medications

Atropine can cross the placenta and has been associated with decreased fetal heart rate variability[1,104] which could mask signs of fetal distress. Glycopyrrolate, a quarternary compound does not cross the placenta to any great extent.[1] Metoclopramide and cimetidine have been used before cesarean delivery to accelerate gastric emptying and decrease gastric acidity; no adverse effects of these agents have been reported.[110]

DETERMINATION OF FETAL WELL-BEING

There are numerous methods available to evaluate fetal well-being (Table 76-9). The anesthesia provider needs to be familiar with the commonly used techniques so that fetal

Table 76-9 Techniques to assess fetal well-being

Fetal heart rate monitoring—heart rate, variability, periodic changes
Nonstress test and contraction stress test
Fetal scalp blood sampling and scalp stimulation test
The biophysical profile:

	Normal (2 points)	Abnormal (0 points)
Fetal breathing movements	1 episode > 30 sec in 30 min	Absent or less than normal
Feta body movements	> 3 body/limb movements in 30 min	< 2 movements in 30 min
Fetal tone	> 1 active extension plus flexion of limb, trunk	Absent or less than normal
Fetal heart rate reactivity	> 2 accelerations of > 15 beats per minute for > 15 seconds, with fetal movement, in 20 minutes	Absent or less than normal
Amniotic fluid	> 1 pocket, > 1 cm in perpendicular planes	Absent or less than normal

Data from Manning FA, et al: *Am J Obstet Gynecol* 136:787, 1980.

status can be assessed before undertaking anesthetic care of the mother and a worrisome fetal status can be recognized.

Fetal Heart Rate Monitoring

Fetal heart rate (FHR) can be monitored externally using ultrasound or internally via a fetal scalp electrode.[87] Although assessment of FHR patterns is useful to confirm fetal well-being both before and during labor, its use in recognizing fetal compromise is less clear. That is, a normal FHR pattern indicates the presence of a normal, well-oxygenated fetus, whereas an abnormal FHR pattern may indicate the presence of fetal compromise.[48] The most important components of FHR monitoring are rate, beat-to-beat variability, and pattern.

Rate

Under normal conditions at term, the FHR is modulated by parasympathetic and sympathetic nerves and ranges between 120 and 160 beats/min. **Responses to hypoxia depend on the nature of the insult. In the absence of active labor, the fetus compensates for slowly developing asphyxia with an increase in heart rate.** Acute profound hypoxia causes slowing of the fetal heart. The presence of a maternal fever can cause fetal tachycardia.

Beat-to-beat variability

Beat-to-beat variability is an important component of the normal FHR tracing and is the best indicator of fetal well-being and reflects a normally functioning, well-oxygenated CNS. Short-term variability represents a beat-to-beat difference of 2 to 3 beats; this is superimposed on a pattern of long-term variability of fluctuations of 5 to 20 beats/min. Various medications such as atropine and opioids administered maternally can diminish variability. Loss of beat-to-beat variability in the absence of medication is a sign of fetal CNS depression secondary to hypoxia.

Fetal heart rate pattern

Patterns of periodic decelerations of the FHR in association with uterine contractions (UC) as measured by a tocodynamometer are used to monitor fetal status. Three types of decelerations are described (Fig. 76-4).[43]

Early deceleration patterns begin with the onset of the UC, rarely drop below 110 beats/min, and usually return to baseline at the same time as the uterine pressure curve. This pattern is probably of vagal origin due to head compression and does not indicate fetal asphyxia.

Late decelerations are recurrent decelerations that begin 20 seconds or more after the onset of the UC. Duration and intensity of each is generally proportional to that of the accompanying UC. Late decelerations indicate uteroplacental insufficiency. **Late decelerations associated with normal FHR variability are probably the result of hypoxia-induced stimulation of fetal chemoreceptors which causes a vagal discharge. In contrast, late decelerations accompanied by diminished or absent variability are more ominous and represent severe or prolonged O_2 deprivation causing direct fetal myocardial hypoxic depression.**

Variable decelerations are so named because they are variable in configuration and bear no consistent temporal relationship to the onset of the contraction. This results in a bradycardia in which onset is probably vagally mediated. Repetitive cord compression can lead to hypoxemia, loss of FHR variability, and direct myocardial depression.

The anesthesia provider should be aware of the FHR pattern before administering or reinforcing any anesthetic. Should an FHR pattern of concern appear, the anesthesia provider should help to improve the uterine environment by administering supplemental O_2 to the mother, altering maternal position to maximize uterine blood flow, and correct any maternal hypotension.

Stress Testing

FHR monitoring is used before labor to assess fetal well-being. A nonstress test involves external fetal monitoring for approximately 20 minutes. A negative (normal) nonstress test involves observing two accelerations of the fetal heart rate of 10 beats per minute which last for 10 seconds. A nonreactive nonstress test may trigger further fetal evaluation with a contraction stress test. During UC, uterine blood flow and therefore fetal O_2 delivery decrease. With placental insufficiency, this may result in fetal hypoxia and abnormality in FHR patterns. Oxytocin is used to stimulate contractions. A positive (abnormal) contraction stress test consists of per-

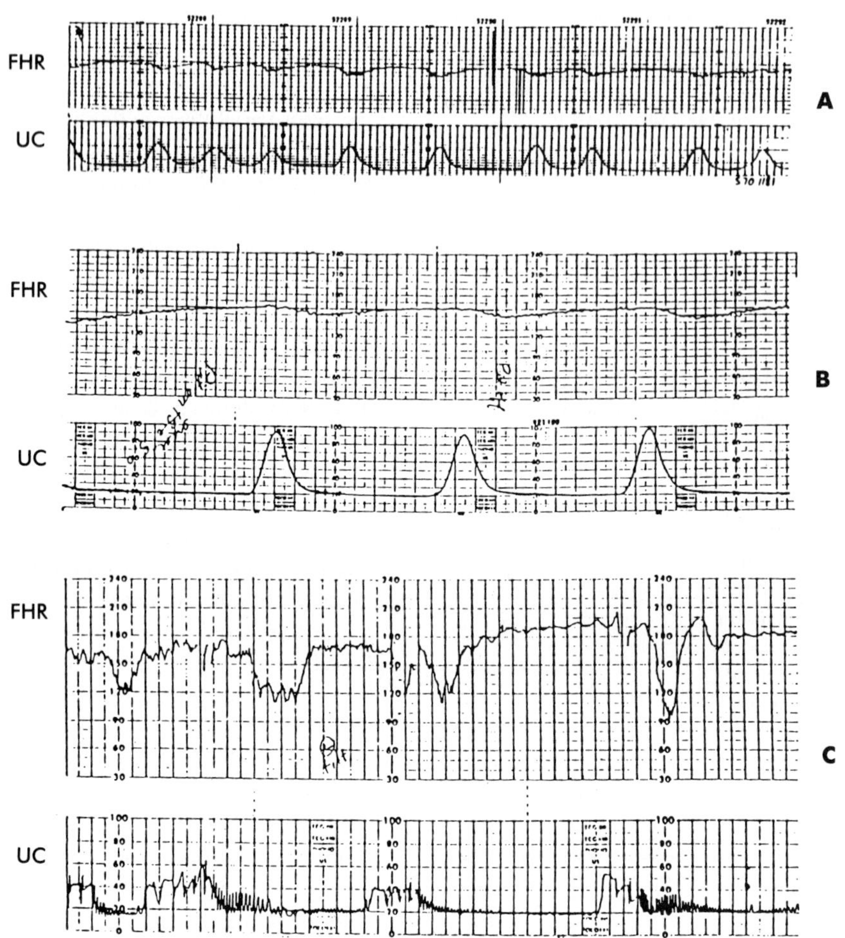

Fig. 76-4. Examples of periodic changes of fetal heart rate. **A,** Early decelerations. **B,** Late decelerations. **C,** Variable decelerations. (From Chestnut DH: Fetal distress. In James FM, Wheeler AS, Dewan DM, editors: *Obstetric anesthesia: the complicated patient,* Philadelphia, 1988, FA Davis.)

sistent late decelerations and requires further evaluation and possible emergency or urgent delivery.

Fetal Biophysical Profile

The biophysical profile is an ultrasound examination of the fetus. The fetus receives a score based on the results of a nonstress test, body muscle tone, amniotic fluid volume, breathing movements, and body movements (Table 76-9).[152] A poor score (4 or less) indicates abnormalities in fetal status, suggests the fetus is a risk for asphyxia and may prompt a decision to deliver the fetus.

Fetal Scalp Sampling

Abnormalities in the FHR pattern during labor may cause the obstetrician to be concerned about the fetal status and perform fetal capillary blood sampling to further evaluate fetal well-being. This procedure can only be performed on women with a dilated cervix and ruptured membranes. Fetal capillary blood pH values have been shown to correlate well with fetal umbilical blood gas values and APGAR score.[53] Values less than 7.20 (severe acidosis) indicate significant asphyxia and generally require immediate delivery of the infant. Values from 7.20 to 7.24 are intermediate and require close monitoring and possibly repeat sampling. The less invasive "scalp stimulation test" (tactile stimulation of the fetal scalp) has also been used to assess fetal well-being. An increase in FHR by 15 beats per minute lasting 10 seconds after scalp stimulation correlates with a fetal scalp pH of greater than 7.20.[48]

ANESTHESIA FOR VAGINAL DELIVERY

During the first stage of labor (defined as the onset of regular uterine contractions which results in progressive thinning and dilation of the uterine cervix), pain results from stretching of the uterus and cervix. Pain sensations are carried by visceral afferents entering the spinal cord at the T10 to L1 levels. This pain is often described as dull, aching, or cramping, and is poorly localized. Pain is mediated by "high threshold" nociceptors; although an intense stimulus is necessary to trigger these fibers, once they are activated, the threshold for stimulation is reduced. This may contribute to the increased pain reported during a long labor. Other factors influencing the pain response include use of oxytocin, parity, and participation in childbirth preparation classes. During the second stage of labor (defined as the time from complete cervical dilation to delivery of the fetus) as the fetal head descends into the birth canal the lower lumbar and sacral dermatomes are involved (mainly S2, S3, S4) in pain transmission. In this stage, pain increases and becomes more somatic in nature (sharp and well localized). A variety of techniques are available for pain relief during labor and vaginal delivery (Box 76-3).

Psychologic Techniques

The most commonly used method of psychoprophylaxis is that of Lamaze, which teaches the use of specific breathing patterns during contractions.[135] The preparative classes generally allow the parturient to be well informed about the process of labor and delivery, to help allay anxiety. A potential problem with this method is that if incorrectly performed, excessive maternal hyperventilation will result. A sharp decrease in maternal P_{CO_2} will cause uterine vasoconstriction and may compromise O_2 delivery to the fetus.[142,176] A second concern is that the parturient must not be influenced to feel that she has "failed" if psychoprophylaxis alone is inadequate for the pain of labor and delivery. She should be informed that other methods of obstetric pain relief will be available as needed and when requested.

Systemic Medication

Opioids

Direct effects of opioids on the fetus have been discussed previously; maternal side effects include potential respiratory depression, pruritus, nausea, and vomiting. Side effects can be minimized if these drugs are administered properly. The advantage of systemic opioids for labor analgesia is their ease of administration, and they remain the most commonly used means of treating labor pain (Table 76-10).[102] The main disadvantage is that analgesia is imperfect. Because the pain of labor is episodic, administering a dose of opioid sufficient to eliminate all UC pain would result in significant maternal somnolence and respiratory depression in between UCs (not to mention the potential for newborn depression). Therefore, much lesser doses are used. A realistic goal for the use of systemic opioids for labor analgesia is to "take the edge off" labor pain.

Meperidine is currently the most commonly used opioid for labor analgesia. It is given in dosages of 10 to 50 mg IV or 50 to 100 mg IM with a duration of pain relief of 2 to 4 hours. As previously described, if meperidine is administered IM less than 1 hour or more than 3 hours before delivery, neonatal respiratory depression is minimized.[175,222,251] The possibility of accumulation of normeperidine in the fetus should be remembered.[134]

Morphine has been used extensively for pain relief during labor. Dosages of 5 to 10 mg IM or 2 to 3 mg IV provide analgesia lasting 2 to 4 hours. Morphine use has lost its popularity since the development of meperidine. Further, when equianalgesic doses of morphine and meperidine were compared, morphine resulted in a relatively greater amount of neonatal depression.[251] Morphine is usually used only in very early labor.

Fentanyl has been used for labor analgesia. In bolus doses of 25 to 100 μg, it has a rapid onset of analgesia with few side effects.[201] Administration via patient-controlled analgesia (PCA) has been described with success.[208]

Nalbuphine (Nubain) and butorphanol (Stadol) are used for analgesia during labor, perhaps to take advantage of the reported ceiling of respiratory depression with these drugs.[125,207] Butorphanol is administered in dosages of 1 to 2 mg IM or IV and is effective in reducing labor pain without significant side effects.[197] Nalbuphine given in 3-mg doses during labor has been shown to be comparable with meperidine in terms of pain relief.[86]

Tranquilizers

Tranquilizers, such as the benzodiazepines and phenothiazines, are occasionally used to relieve anxiety during labor and delivery. The benzodiazepines are used rarely, because

BOX 76-3
ANALGESIC TECHNIQUES FOR LABOR AND VAGINAL DELIVERY

- Psychologic techniques
- Systemic medications
  - Opioids
  - Tranquilizers
  - Barbiturates
  - Patient-controlled opioid analgesia
- Inhalational analgesia (NO_2)
- Regional analgesia
  - Paracervical block (first stage of labor only)
  - Pudendal block (second stage of labor only)
  - Spinal analgesia (opioids +/− local anesthetics)
  - Lumbar epidural analgesia
  - Caudal analgesia

Table 76-10 Distribution of labor analgesic techniques in the United States in 1992

Technique	Patents (%)
None	22
Systemic medication	54
Epidural	29
Spinal	4

Data from Hawkins JL, et al: *Anesthesiology* 81:A1128, 1994.

many women do not desire amnesia of their labor and delivery experience. Phenothiazines may be combined with opioids to increase sedation and decrease the opioid side effects. Hydroxyzine (Vistaril) in doses of 50 to 100 mg IM and promethazine (Phenergan) in doses of 25 to 50 mg IM or 15 to 25 mg IV have been used to enhance analgesia without significant neonatal side effects.[33,34] Phenothiazines such as promazine (Sparine), chloropromazine (Thorazine), and prochlorperazine (Compazine) are generally not used in obstetrics because their greater alpha-adrenergic blocking actions could potentially produce hypotension.

Barbiturates

Barbiturates, such as secobarbital (Seconal) and pentobarbital (Nembutal), are no longer popular for use during labor because of demonstration of protracted effects on the newborn.[26] Further, the antianalgesic effect of barbiturates make their use during labor pain irrational.

Patient-controlled intravenous analgesia

Classically, systemic agents have been administered IM or IV during labor on a schedule determined by the obstetrician. With the recent development of PCA, another modality is available for drug administration during labor. Several studies have reported the successful use of PCA with meperidine, nalbuphine, and fentanyl during labor.[86,191,208,219] More work is needed to define proper dosing parameters and lockout intervals so that pain relief can be optimized with minimal side effects.

Inhalation Analgesia

Because of concerns about loss of airway reflexes and aspiration, inhalational analgesia using potent inhaled agents is rarely used for vaginal delivery. A mixture of 50% N_2O and 50% O_2 (Entonox) is available for self-administration during labor.[116] Those who advocate its use feel that it provides amnesia and analgesia, but if self-administered, will not cause unconsciousness and loss of airway reflexes. The analgesic efficacy is questionable.[116]

In rare instances, general anesthesia may be required for vaginal delivery, as in the instance of acute fetal distress requiring forceps delivery without time for administration of a regional anesthetic. Usual precautions (e.g., prophylaxis against pulmonary aspiration of gastric contents, airway evaluation) should be taken. General anesthesia may also be used to provide uterine relaxation for intrauterine manipulation (such as internal podalic version).

Regional Anesthesia

Regional anesthetic techniques provide excellent pain relief for labor and delivery without the sedative effects of systemic medications. Administration of major regional analgesia for labor should follow a preanesthetic evaluation (including medical, obstetric, and fetal issues), obtaining informed consent, establishing adequate IV access, prehydration with 500 to 1000 ml of balanced salt solution, and having emergency airway and resuscitation equipment available.

Epidural anesthesia

Epidural anesthesia is the most effective form of regional analgesia used for labor and delivery.[188] The placement of an epidural catheter provides the ability to titrate the anesthetics given, and anesthesia can be maintained over an extended period of time. The sensory level and density of the block can be altered as the obstetric situation dictates. Epidural analgesia has some potential physiologic benefits. By reducing pain, maternal catecholamine levels are reduced,[221] intervillous blood flow is improved (when hypotension is avoided), uterine activity may improve,[136] and the hyperventilation triggered by painful contractions is eliminated. Epidural (and spinal) anesthesia is considered contraindicated in a few circumstances (Box 76-4). Other problems that might preclude regional anesthesia include preexisting neurologic disease, previous back surgery, maternal systemic infection, mild isolated abnormalities of tests of coagulation. These conditions should be evaluated on an individual basis. Box 76-5 describes a technique for epidural anesthesia.

Choice of drugs for epidural anesthesia

The agent chosen for epidural anesthesia for vaginal delivery should provide effective analgesia with minimal hypotension and skeletal muscle relaxation. Both epidural opioids and local anesthetics are used for epidural analgesia in the laboring patient.

Use of epidural opioids alone has proved to be effective usually only for the pain of early labor. Three to 5 mg of morphine suffers from a long latency, lack of efficacy in the late first and second stages of labor, and high incidence of side effects (e.g., nausea, vomiting, pruritus).[114] Therefore, it is uncommonly used for labor analgesia. Fentanyl (50 to 100 μg),[38] sufentanil (5 to 10 μg)[229] and meperidine (25 to 50 mg)[18] provide analgesia during early labor for 1 to 2 hours.

Local anesthetics are the mainstay of effective labor analgesia. Bupivacaine (0.125% to 0.25%) is the most commonly used local anesthetic for labor analgesia be-

BOX 76-4
CONTRAINDICATIONS TO REGIONAL ANALGESIA OR ANESTHESIA IN THE PARTURIENT

Uncorrectable maternal hypovolemia
Overt maternal coagulopathy
Infection in the skin at the site of needle placement
Patient refusal
Presence of a mass lesion causing increased intracranial pressure

cause of its relatively long duration of action, lack of tachyphylaxis, and minimal motor block when dilute solutions are administered. Lidocaine (0.75% to 1.0%) is also effective, but may be less so than bupivacaine.[167] Although it has a rapid onset of action, 2-chloroprocaine (2%) is used less often for labor analgesia because of its short duration and possible interference with subsequent epidural injections of bupivacaine and opioids.[54,97] Finally, ropivacaine, a new amide local anesthetic (which at the time of this writing was undergoing preliminary investigation in preparation for approval for use by the FDA) appears to be similar in clinical effects to bupivacaine with animal studies demonstrating less cardiotoxicity.[216] Epinephrine (1/800,000 to 1/200,000 concentrations) may be added to local anesthetics for labor analgesia; use of this drug is often avoided because of concerns that absorbed epinephrine may act as a tocolytic and because it may increase motor block.

Combining epidural opioids with local anesthetics is the most common technique used for labor analgesia. By taking advantage of the different mechanisms of analgesia offered by the two agents, effective analgesia for all stages of labor results with minimal motor block. Fentanyl, 50 to 100 μg added to bupivacaine 0.25% hastens the onset and increases the duration of analgesia.[52,124] Administration of 10 to 30 μg of sufentanil also enhances bupivacaine analgesia,[243] but caution should be used administering this drug, because 30 μg of IV sufentanil can cause important maternal respiratory depression. Administration of 25 mg of meperidine also improves bupivacaine analgesia.[32]

After establishing an epidural block (Box 76-5), analgesia for labor is nicely maintained with a continuous infusion of dilute local anesthetic with or without addition opioid.[109,143] For example, bupivacaine, 0.0625% plus 1–2 μg/ml of fentanyl (8–15 ml/hr) provides effective analgesia with minimal motor block.[39,45] Potential benefits of this technique include maintenance of a stable analgesic level, the need for fewer bolus injections, and improved patient satisfaction. Examples of recipes for continuous infusion solutions appear in Table 76-11. When using an infusion technique, is it essential to monitor the patient and record vital signs at specified intervals to ensure that the patient is stable and that the sensory level is not rising or receding. The regimens presented in the Table 76-11 are by no means the only ones that have been successful.

For spontaneous or forceps assisted vaginal delivery, an epidural catheter used for labor analgesia can be reinforced, if necessary, with 1- to 3.5-ml bolus doses of 1% to 2% lidocaine or 2% to 3% 2-chloroprocaine to achieve sacral anesthesia.

BOX 76-5
A TECHNIQUE FOR ADMINISTERING EPIDURAL ANALGESIA FOR LABOR

- Preoperative evaluation including medical, obstetric, anesthetic, and fetal issues
- Informed consent
- Prehydration with 500 to 1000 ml of non–dextrose-containing crystalloid solution
- Maternal monitors—blood pressure, heart rate; fetal monitoring continued whenever possible
- Resuscitation equipment available
- Supplemental O_2 is administered to the mother
- Lateral position (perhaps more comfortable) or sitting position (obese patients)
- Sterile prep and drape of lumbar interspace
- Identification of epidural space with loss of resistance to air or saline
- Placement of an epidural catheter approximately 3 cm (single orifice) or 5 cm (multiple orifice) into space
- Aspiration of the catheter evaluating for intravascular or intrathecal placement
- Test the catheter for intravascular placement (e.g., 3 ml 0.25% bupivacaine plus 1/200,000 epinephrine, 1 to 2 ml of air) and intrathecal placement (3 ml 0.25% bupivacaine or 1.5% lidocaine)
- Secure the catheter and position the mother with uterine displacement
- Inject induction dose of local anesthetic (such as 5 to 10 ml 0.125% to 0.25% bupivacaine +/− fentanyl 50 μg)
- Monitor maternal blood pressure every 1 to 2 minutes for approximately 15 minutes; treat any hypotension (systolic blood pressure < 100 mm Hg or > 20% to 30% fall) with positioning oxygen, IV fluids, and ephedrine; be sure to monitor fetal heart rate
- Check for evidence of bilateral analgesic level (usually T10 level necessary) and analgesic efficacy. Institute a continuous infusion of 0.0625% bupivacaine containing fentanyl, 2 μg/ml

Complications

Hypotension can occur after induction of epidural anesthesia secondary to sympathetic block. It is usually defined as a decrease in systolic blood pressure to less than 100 mm Hg or more than 20% to 30%, and is prevented by IV hydration

Table 76-11 Continuous infusion protocols

Drug	Concentration	Infusion rate (ml/hr)
Plain bupivacaine	0.125%	8–15
Bupivacaine plus fentanyl	0.0625% 1–2 μg/ml	8–15
Bupivacaine plus sufentanil	0.0625% 0.2–0.3 μg/ml	8–15

Modified from Naulty JS: Continuous infusions of local anesthetics and narcotics for epidural anesthesia in the management of labor, *Intern Anesth Clin* 28:17, 1990.

with non–dextrose-containing crystalloid solutions and proper maternal positioning with uterine displacement. Hypotension is treated with fluid infusion and 5- to 10-mg doses of ephedrine.

The method used to test for proper location of the epidural catheter in the obstetric patient is controversial. For IV testing, the epinephrine test dose (15 μg) may be problematic. In animals, IV epinephrine decreases intervillous blood flow in a dose-related manner.[47] The possible deleterious effects of epinephrine on uterine blood flow should be considered, although at the low concentrations used, the effects are probably small. Further, the effects are transient. There may be difficulty in using maternal heart rate changes to identify intravascular injections. Laboring patients may show a 20% to 30% increase in heart rate with contractions.[141] Proper timing of the test dose may improve reliability. Other IV test doses include 1 to 2 ml of air (listening for evidence of IV air by placing a doppler over the maternal precordium),[140] and subjective symptoms of local anesthetics. The main goal is to avoid local anesthetic toxicity from IV injection. This is achieved primarily by fractionating the dose of local anesthetic.

Because the total dose of local anesthetic administered during epidural anesthesia is significant, the potential for a systemic toxic reaction exists. This can occur when local anesthetic is either injected inadvertently into a blood vessel or if the total dose of anesthetic injected into the epidural space is so large that intravascular absorption results in toxic systemic levels (unusual following epidural analgesia for labor, but possible during epidural anesthesia for cesarean delivery). The signs and symptoms of overdose are related to the systemic concentration.[239] Patients usually will complain initially of lightheadedness, tinnitus, and circumoral numbness. Later symptoms include frank convulsions and dysrhythmias. If a toxic reaction occurs, supportive therapy is used to prevent maternal and fetal hypoxia.[154,225] The mother's airway needs to be supported; this may require ET intubation if loss of consciousness persists for more than a few seconds. In general, seizures are short and self-limited; a small dose of IV diazepam or an ultra–short-acting barbiturate may occasionally be required to stop convulsions. Hypotension is treated with fluids and vasopressors. If monitoring reveals that the fetus is in distress that is not relieved by these supportive measures, emergency delivery may be required.

Identification of subarachnoid catheter placement is achieved by administering a small dose of local anesthetic (such as 3 ml of 0.25% bupivacaine or 1.5% to 2% lidocaine) and testing the patient for any evidence of block after 3 to 5 minutes.

Testing the epidural catheter for proper placement should be done any time a bolus dose of local anesthetic is administered (e.g., a reinforcing dose during labor, for vaginal delivery, or extending a block for cesarean delivery). Epidural catheters can migrate over time or during patient movement, and this should be detected.

Sometimes epidural analgesia fails to provide perfect labor analgesia either because no block is achieved or it is asymmetric or patchy. If a patient with a previously functioning epidural complains of pain, reasons may include failure of the epidural catheter, an inadequate dose of anesthetic, a change in labor pain (rapid progression to advanced first stage of labor), or abnormal presentation of the fetus.

The incidence of accidental dural puncture during performance of epidural anesthesia is approximately 1% to 2% and likely depends upon operator experience. Approximately 60% to 75% of these patients will ultimately develop postdural puncture headache and the many of these patients will require treatment.

The incidence of persistent neurologic symptoms after epidural anesthesia is extremely rare. In a review of over 32,000 cases of lumbar and caudal epidurals, the incidence of permanent sequelae was only 0.02%.[73]

Concern exists about the potential effects of epidural anesthesia on labor. Many retrospective and uncontrolled studies reported an association between use of epidural anesthesia and longer first and second stages of labor as well as increased need for operative or instrumental delivery. The importance of selection bias is important when interpreting these results—the patients with long labors, large babies, extreme pain, and other risk factors for operative delivery are patients who are most likely to request epidural analgesia.[254] Epidural anesthesia is usually requested only after labor is well established. The overall effect of epidural anesthesia on the first stage of labor is minimal.[230] The second stage of labor has been reported to be slightly prolonged by regional anesthesia.[119] The potential for instrumental delivery can be minimized by the use of smaller concentrations of anesthetic and effective coaching.[45,158] The influence of epidural analgesia on the need for Cesarean delivery is also controversial, with some experts claiming an effect when epidural analgesia is established in early labor (< 5 cm cervical dilation)[233] while other experts did not find such an effect.[44,46]

Caudal anesthesia

Caudal anesthesia involves the injection of 15 to 25 ml of local anesthetic through the sacral hiatus into the caudal canal, which is the most distant segment of the epidural space. Caudal block was initially quite popular for obstetric anesthesia,[76] but it is now used infrequently for several reasons. Because the local anesthetic is injected at the sacral hiatus, it may be difficult to provide a level of anesthesia much greater than T10 should this be needed. Because the extent of caudal anesthesia is largely volume related, large doses of local anesthetic may be required, increasing the risk of a systemic toxic reaction. Because of the close proximity of the fetal presenting part to the coccyx, unintentional injection into the fetal head is a possible complication. Finally, a caudal block produces good sacral analgesia—but early in labor, selective block of T10 to L1 segments is the goal.

Spinal anesthesia

Spinal analgesia/anesthesia may be administered to laboring patients under some circumstances: (1) intrathecal opioids

+/− small doses of local anesthetics may be used for labor analgesia; (2) on occasion, if placement of an epidural is complicated by dural puncture, the epidural catheter can be threaded into the intrathecal space to provide continuous spinal analgesia; and (3) a low level of spinal anesthesia can be administered for vaginal delivery, particularly if outlet forceps, vacuum extraction, or extensive episiotomy repair is required. This technique of "saddle block" anesthesia is performed by administering 30 to 50 mg of hyperbaric lidocaine or 7.5 mg of hyperbaric bupivacaine. This dose of anesthetic will usually result in approximately a T10 sensory level.

Morphine was the first intrathecal opioid used for labor analgesia. Doses of 0.5 to 2 mg were used initially. Problems included long latency, inadequate analgesia in the late first and second stages of labor, and a high incidence of pruritus, nausea, and vomiting (Table 76-12).[3] The long latency can be overcome by combining it with 10 to 25 μg of fentanyl.[139] Side effects are still problematic (even with the 0.25-mg dose) and limit the use of morphine in laboring women. If used, morphine potentiates the efficacy of subsequently administered epidural bupivacaine—very dilute solutions (0.0625%) are effective.[8] Other intrathecal opioids offer effective pain relief during labor. Fentanyl (10 to 25 μg) and sufentanil (10 μg) both provide a rapid onset of analgesia lasting 1 to 2 hours (Table 76-12).[182] Administration of either spinal fentanyl or sufentanil can be accompanied by a decrease in maternal blood pressure.[51] The most likely etiology is pain relief, but it is prudent to monitor maternal blood pressure and FHR and have appropriate IV access before administering these drugs. Intrathecal meperidine (10 to 20 mg) has unique effects.[112] Because of its local anesthetic action, meperidine produces a much denser block than other opioids. It has been successfully used for labor analgesia in the late first and second stages of labor (Table 76-12). The anesthesia provider should watch for evidence of sympathetic block and hypotension. Another option for analgesia late in labor is a combination of intrathecal fentanyl or sufentanil with a small dose of bupivacaine (2.5 mg).[5]

Spinal opioids can be administered either as a single injection, via a continuous spinal catheter (seldom used, as noted previously), or by using the combined spinal-epidural technique. The latter procedure involves identification of the epidural space, placement of a long spinal needle through the epidural needle, piercing the dura, injecting the spinal drug, removing the spinal needle, and then threading an epidural catheter for use later in labor.[182] Either extra-long spinal needles or manufactured combined spinal-epidural kits can be used.

Table 76-12 Intrathecal opioids for labor analgesia

Opioid	Dose	Duration (hr)	Comments
Morphine	0.25 mg	1–4	Long latency High incidence of side effects
Fentanyl	10–25 μg	0.5–1.5	Rapid onset
Sufentanil	10 μg	1.0–2.0	Rapid onset
Meperidine	10–20 mg	1.0–3.0	Local anesthetic effect

Data from Norris MC, Arkoosh VA: *Intern Anesth Clin* 32:69, 1994; Ross BK. in Chestnut D, editor: *Obstetric anesthesia: Principles and practice.* St. Louis, 1994, Mosby–Year Book.

Complications

Hypotension is a common complication of spinal anesthesia with local anesthetics because of the combination of sympathetic vasomotor blockade and compression of the aorta by the gravid uterus. Reduction in maternal blood pressure requires prompt correction with fluid and vasopressor therapy to ensure fetal well-being. Even brief periods of hypotension (2 to 3 minutes) have been associated with mild neonatal acidosis.[55]

Nausea and vomiting in the patient are not infrequent after spinal anesthesia. The mechanism probably involves systemic hypotension decreasing cerebral blood flow. The incidence of nausea and vomiting is significantly reduced with prompt treatment of decreased baseline blood pressure with ephedrine.[64]

The incidence of postdural puncture headache in the obstetric patient using the 26-gauge Quincke needle ranges from 1% to 10% in various studies.[98] Recent evidence suggests that inserting the spinal needle parallel to the dural fibers may reduce the incidence of headache.[166] Headache incidence also is reduced with use of a 27-gauge needle, although the failure rate may be greater. Recent reports indicate that use of 24- or 25-gauge spinal needles with a conical tip (such as the Whitacre or Sprotte needle) result in lesser headache incidence than when the 25- or 26-gauge cutting-edge Quincke needle is used.[98]

Postdural puncture headache will usually present as positional symptoms during the first or second postpartum day. Treatment consists initially of hydration and oral analgesics. Recent studies suggest that oral caffeine tablets (300 mg) may be effective.[35] If the headache does not improve over 24 hours or delays discharge from the hospital, an epidural blood patch can be performed. In this technique, 10 to 20 ml of autologous blood are injected in a sterile manner into the epidural space at the site of the dural puncture. The success rate for this procedure is greater than 90%.[4]

The incidence of neurologic complications following spinal anesthesia is extremely small. In a prospective review of over 10,000 patients receiving spinal anesthesia with lidocaine, only two patients had nerve root problems believed to be due to spinal anesthesia.[190]

Total spinal anesthesia occurs with unexpectedly high subarachnoid spread of local anesthetic. If loss of control of the airway occurs, the parturient should be oxygenated, usually via an ET tube. Fluids and ephedrine will be necessary to maintain blood pressure. The FHR should be monitored.

Paracervical block

Paracervical block is a fairly simple technique for pain relief during the first stage of labor. Local anesthetic is injected lateral to the cervix at the fornix of the vagina so that pain impulses from the uterus and cervix during the first stage of labor are blocked (Fig. 76-5). This technique is no longer commonly used because it is associated with a high incidence of fetal bradycardia occurring within several minutes of the block. This may be due to the close proximity of the uterine vessels to the area in which the local anesthetic is injected, resulting in uterine artery vasoconstriction and high levels of local anesthetic in the fetal circulation.[15]

Pudendal block

Pudendal nerve block provides anesthesia for outlet forceps and episiotomy repair. The pudendal nerve originates from sacral roots 2 through 4 and supplies the lower part of the vaginal canal and perineum. The pudendal nerve is blocked with 5 to 10 ml of local anesthetic at the attachment of the ischial spine and the sacrospinous ligament. Usually a transvaginal approach is used. Frequent aspiration is required to avoid intravascular injection into the pudendal vessels. This block is generally performed by the obstetrician. Maternal and neonatal blood levels of local anesthetic after pudendal block have been found to be similar to those seen after epidural anesthesia.[164]

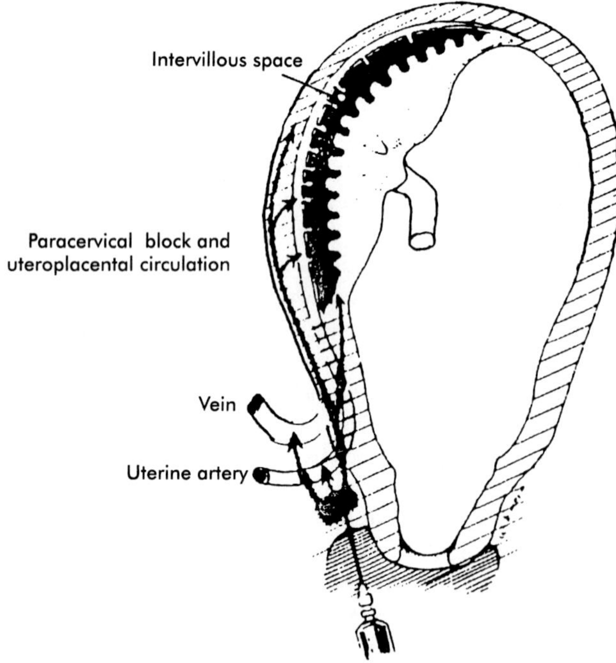

Fig. 76-5. Diagram of paracervical area in relation to uteroplacental circulation. (From Asling JH, Shnider SM, Margolis AJ, et al: Paracervical block anesthesia in obstetrics. II. Etiology of fetal bradycardia following paracervical block anesthesia, *Am J Obstet Gynecol* 107:626, 1970.)

ANESTHESIA FOR CESAREAN DELIVERY

In recent years, the frequency of cesarean section has increased markedly so that its present use in the United States is approximately 20% depending on geographic region and population characteristics.[228] With proper technical skills and an understanding of maternal and fetal physiology, spinal or epidural anesthesia can be used successfully. With cases in which regional anesthesia is contraindicated, an awareness of the risks involved and their appropriate management makes general anesthesia an acceptable alternative. The distribution of anesthetic techniques for cesarean delivery in the United States is presented in Table 76-13.[102]

Spinal Anesthesia

The advantages and disadvantages of spinal anesthesia are outlined in Box 76-6. A technique of administration of spinal anesthesia in the parturient is described in detail in Box 76-7. When administering spinal anesthesia for ce-

Table 76-13 Anesthesia for cesarean delivery in the United States in 1992

Anesthetic	Patients (%)
Spinal	40
Epidural	44
General	17

Data from Hawkins JL, et al: *Anesthesiology* 81:A1128, 1994.

BOX 76-6
ADVANTAGES AND DISADVANTAGES TO SPINAL ANESTHESIA FOR CESAREAN DELIVERY

Advantages

- Rapid onset of block
- Simple technique
- Small amount of drug required
- Reliable (less failure rate than epidural)
- Mother is awake
- Able to use intrathecal opioids for postoperative analgesia

Disadvantages

- Rapid onset of hypotension
- Single-injection technique—limited duration of anesthesia

BOX 76-7
A TECHNIQUE FOR ADMINISTERING SPINAL ANESTHESIA FOR CESAREAN DELIVERY

- Ensure adequate IV access
- Administer 30 ml of clear, nonparticulate antacid
- Prehydrate with 1.5 to 2.0 l non–dextrose-containing IV fluids
- Maternal monitors applied and supplemental O_2 given
- Position in right lateral decubitus position (or sitting)
- Locate subarachnoid space with 24- or 25-gauge conical tip spinal needle
- Inject 1.6 ml 0.75% hyperbaric bupivacaine (12 mg) +0.2 mg epinephrine +/−0.2 mg preservative-free morphine
- Place patient supine with left uterine displacement
- Monitor blood pressure every minute for 15 to 20 minutes, treat hypotension aggressively
- Check block level frequently. A T4 block level is usually necessary. If too low, tilt patient's head down. If too high, do not place patient in the head-up position (this risks sever hypotension from venous pooling)
- Elevate the legs to maintain venous return, and communicate with the patient continuously to assess adequacy of airway protection

sarean delivery, at least 1500 to 2000 ml of a balanced salt solution should be administered acutely to counteract the hypotension that often accompanies the rapid onset of high sympathetic block. A sensory level of at least the T4 dermatome is necessary for adequate anesthesia. This level is achieved in the pregnant patient with doses of local anesthetic below those required in nonpregnant patients. Hyperbaric bupivacaine is becoming the agent most commonly used for cesarean section. However, the spread of spinal hyperbaric bupivacaine in the parturient cannot be predicted by patient factors, such as height or weight.[180,181] Although increasing the dose from 12 to 15 mg will on average increase the height of spinal block, it is not possible to predict the extent of block in a given patient (Fig. 76-6). A reasonable dose is approximately 12 mg of hyperbaric bupivacaine—the patient should be observed for development of an inadequate block, which might be improved with a head-down tilt, as well as a block that is too high. The addition of 0.2 mg of epinephrine has been shown to improve the quality of bupivacaine spinal anesthesia for cesarean delivery.[9] The addition of intrathecal opioids also enhances the quality of perioperative analgesia. The addition of a small dose of morphine (0.2 mg) results in postoperative analgesia lasting up to 24 hours.[7] Adding fentanyl in doses of 6.25 to 12.5 μg may also improve intraoperative analgesia.[115]

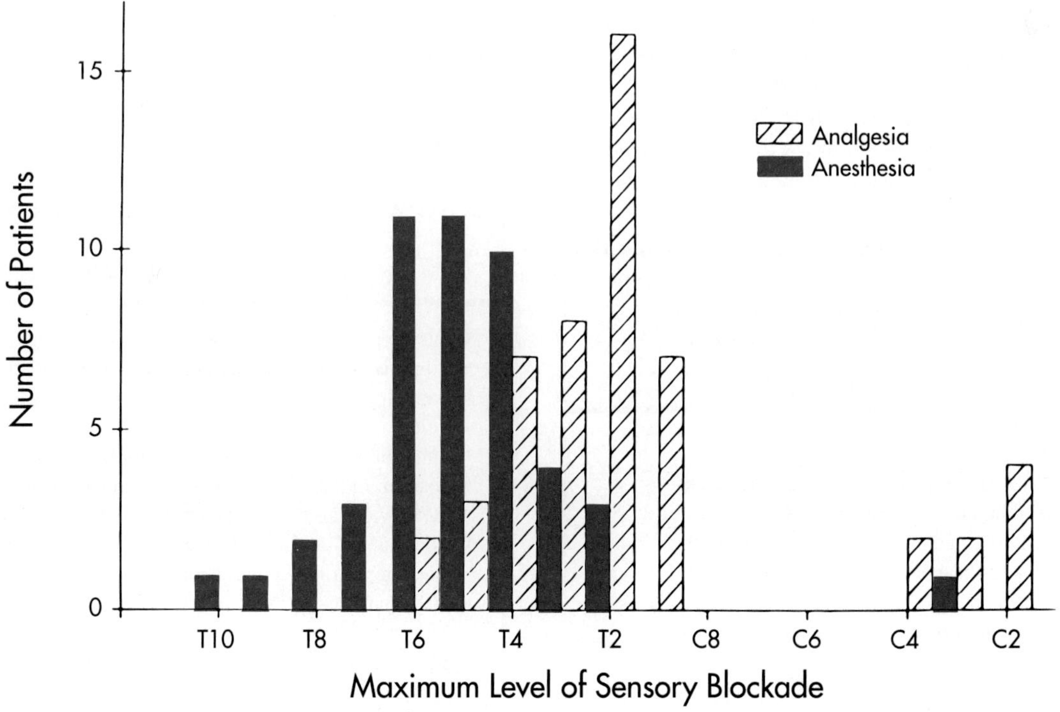

Fig. 76-6. The maximum cephalad extent of analgesia to pin prick and anesthesia to light touch in 52 term parturients following subarachnoid injection of 15 mg hyperbaric bupivacaine. (From Norris MC: Patient variables and the subarachnoid spread of hyperbaric bupivacaine in the term parturient, *Anesthesiology* 72:478–482, 1990.)

The complications of spinal anesthesia have been described earlier and include a relatively high incidence of hypotension, intrapartum nausea and vomiting, and risk of postdural puncture headache.

Epidural Anesthesia

The advantages and disadvantages of epidural anesthesia for cesarean delivery are listed in Box 76-8. Disadvantages of this technique include the need for large amounts of local anesthetic agent and the slower onset of sensory anesthesia.[204] **Advantages include the slower onset of sympathetic block which promotes hemodynamic stability (useful in patients with hypertension or other cardiac disease).** The flexibility of epidural anesthesia is also a benefit; a catheter used for labor analgesia can be used for surgery, and if surgical complications prolong operative time, the anesthetic block can be reinforced to maintain a suitable block. A technique of administering epidural anesthesia for cesarean delivery is described in detail in Box 76-9.

The most commonly used agents for epidural anesthesia for cesarean delivery are 2% lidocaine +/− epinephrine 1:200,000 or 3% 2-chloroprocaine. In general, 15 to 30 ml of either of these agents will provide a sensory level to T4 (Table 76-14). Bupivacaine, 0.5%, is also a suitable epidural anesthetic for cesarean delivery. It is used less often because of its slower onset of block. The relatively rapid onset of 2-chloroprocaine makes it the agent of choice when the sensory level needs to be raised rapidly for an emergency cesarean delivery. The rapid maternal and fetal metabolism of this agent avoids accumulation in the fetus and makes this a good agent to use when fetal acidosis is present.[189] For the routine, nonurgent cesarean section, 2% lidocaine with epinephrine is preferred because of its longer duration of action, requiring fewer reinforcements, and absence of interference with epidural opioids. Ropivacaine has also been evaluated for cesarean delivery anesthesia and its effects are comparable with those of bupivacaine.[67]

Adding epinephrine to lidocaine will enhance analgesia and increase the duration of the block. The effect of added epinephrine on maternal systemic absorption of lidocaine is controversial with some reports indicating less absorption[157,184] and some showing an unimportant effect.[30]

There has been concern about the addition of epinephrine in obstetrics because of possible detrimental effects on uterine blood flow. Although some animal studies have reported a transient decrease in uterine blood flow after the administration of small IV doses of epinephrine, the amount of epinephrine that would be absorbed from the epidural space during anesthesia for cesarean section probably does not have significant clinical effects on uterine blood flow.[11]

General Anesthesia

Although general anesthesia provides a rapid induction of anesthesia without hypotension, the risks of airway manage-

BOX 76-8
ADVANTAGES AND DISADVANTAGES TO EPIDURAL ANESTHESIA FOR CESAREAN DELIVERY

Advantages

- Slower onset of sympathetic block provides less hypotension and improved hemodynamic stability
- Use of a catheter technique allows prolongation of surgical anesthesia
- Mother is awake
- Able to use epidural opioids for postoperative analgesia

Disadvantages

- Slow onset of surgical anesthesia
- Requires large dose of local anesthetics
- Greater failure rate than spinal anesthesia

Table 76-14 Local anesthetics for epidural anesthesia for cesarean section

	3% 2-chloroprocaine	2% Lidocaine with epinephrine
Dose	15–25 ml	15–25 ml
Onset of action	3–5 min	5–15 min
Duration of action	40–50 min	60–75 min

BOX 76-9
A TECHNIQUE FOR ADMINISTERING EPIDURAL ANESTHESIA FOR CESAREAN DELIVERY

- Ensure adequate IV access
- Administer 30 ml of clear, nonparticulate antacid
- Prehydrate with 1.5 to 2.0 l non–dextrose-containing IV fluids
- Maternal monitors applied and supplemental O_2 given
- Position in lateral decubitus position (or sitting)
- Identify epidural space and place epidural catheter
- Administer a test to check for intravascular or intrathecal placement of the epidural catheter
- Place patient supine with left uterine displacement
- Administer 5-ml increments of 2% lidocaine +/− epinephrine 1:200,000 to obtain a T4 sensory level
- A total dose of 20 to 30 ml is usually necessary; also inject 50 μg epidural fentanyl
- Monitor blood pressure every minute for 15 to 20 minutes and treat hypotension aggressively

ment problems and maternal aspiration restrict its use to circumstances where regional anesthesia is not feasible. Examples include the patient with fetal distress requiring emergency cesarean delivery and the patient with hemodynamic instability from obstetric hemorrhage. The advantages and disadvantages to general anesthesia for cesarean delivery are listed in Box 76-10. A technique for administering general anesthesia to the parturient is described in Box 76-11.

The importance of proper airway evaluation of the patient presenting for cesarean delivery cannot be overemphasized. The inability to intubate and oxygenate the mother is a leading cause of anesthesia related maternal mortality.[80,159,174] Factors which increase the likelihood of a difficult intubation in obstetrics include increasing Mallampati airway classification, receding mandible, short neck, and protruding maxillary incisors.[206] If a difficult airway is anticipated, the anesthesia provider should inform the obstetrician that a rapid induction of general anesthesia could be risky for the mother. In these cases, an epidural block should be established during labor, with assurance of its effectiveness. The block can be extended should cesarean delivery be necessary. **Unfortunately, not all cases of airway difficulties can be predicted from a preoperative airway examination.** Management of the patient will depend upon the ability to maintain an adequate mask airway and the reason for cesarean delivery (i.e., fetal distress or not). Principles to follow when faced with a difficult airway in the obstetric patient are presented in Box 76-12. An algorithm for management of the difficult airway in the obstetric patient should be understood by all team members and followed. Fig. 76-7 presents such an algorithm. The more complex the algorithm, the less use it may have in a true crisis management situation.

Several maneuvers are carried out to limit the chance of pulmonary acid aspiration during general anesthesia. Clear, nonparticulate oral antacids are given before induction of anesthesia to increase gastric pH.[92] **H_2 blockers may also help increase gastric pH; 50 mg of IV ranitidine is effective by 30 minutes after administration.**[211] **Metoclopramide may also facilitate gastric emptying and increase tone in the lower esophageal sphincter.**[133] **Finally, a rapid sequence induction of anesthesia with cricoid pressure is performed.**

Preoxygenation with 100% O_2 is essential before induction of anesthesia because pregnancy-related decreased functional residual capacity (FRC) and increased O_2 consumption can result in rapid O_2 desaturation during intubation.[14] In an acute emergency, four deep breaths of 100% O_2 will provide reasonable preoxygenation.[183]

Nitrous oxide can be initially administered at a concentration of 50% to provide the fetus with a high O_2 concentration and should then be increased to 70% after delivery of the infant. Isoflurane or enflurane is used before delivery of the infant at doses generally 25% to 40% less than the dose required in the nonpregnant patient.[186] After delivery, these agents are decreased to avoid any uterine relaxation they may produce.[177]

Newborn depression after *in utero* exposure to general

BOX 76-10
ADVANTAGES AND DISADVANTAGES TO GENERAL ANESTHESIA FOR CESAREAN DELIVERY

Advantages

- Rapid onset
- Low rate of failure
- Able to administer a high FIO_2
- Control of the maternal airway

Disadvantages

- Risk of difficult intubation
- Risk of aspiration
- Risk of hypoxia during apnea
- Neonatal depression from placental passage of anesthetics
- Maternal awareness
- Decreased uterine tone from potent inhaled anesthetics

BOX 76-11
A TECHNIQUE FOR ADMINISTERING GENERAL ANESTHESIA FOR CESAREAN DELIVERY

- Ensure adequate IV access
- Administer 30 ml of clear, nonparticulate antacid
- Position with left uterine displacement
- Maternal monitors include ECG, blood pressure, pulse oximeter, end-tidal CO_2
- Preoxygenate
- Surgeons prep and drape the abdomen
- A rapid-sequence induction of anesthesia is performed with 4 to 6 mg/kg of thiopental or 1.0 to 1.5 mg/kg of ketamine followed by 1 to 1.5 mg/kg of succinylcholine. Apply cricoid pressure and intubate the trachea after skeletal muscle relaxation. Confirm proper ET intubation with capnography
- Maintain anesthesia prior to delivery with 50% NO_2 in O_2 and 0.5 MAC isoflurane
- Avoid maternal hyperventilation
- After delivery, anesthesia is deepened with 70% NO_2 in O_2 and IV opioids and benzodiazepines. The isoflurane is reduced or discontinued if uterine atony is noted. Skeletal muscle relaxation is maintained with small doses of vecuronium or atracurium

BOX 76-12
PRINCIPLES OF MANAGING THE DIFFICULT AIRWAY IN THE OBSTETRIC PATIENT

- Try to predict airway problems in advance with a thorough preoperative evaluation
- In patients with likely difficult airways, perform a regional anesthetic or an awake intubation
- If an unpredicted difficult airway occurs:
  - Avoid repeated attempts at laryngoscopy—this will only increase airway edema and intubation difficulties
  - Try something different with each intubation attempt—a different laryngoscope, patient head position, etc.
  - Avoid repeated doses of succinylcholine—allow spontaneous ventilation to return
  - Maintain cricoid pressure throughout
  - Monitor O_2 saturation
  - If mask ventilation and oxygenation is possible, consider why the cesarean is being performed. If it is for severe fetal distress, general anesthesia can then be maintained by mask with cricoid pressure. Use a high FIO_2. The laryngeal mask airway has been suggested for use in this situation.[23]
  - If mask ventilation and oxygenation is possible but the reason for the cesarean delivery is not severe fetal distress, awaken the mother and proceed with an awake intubation or regional anesthetic.
  - If mask ventilation and oxygenation are not possible, do whatever is necessary to oxygenate the mother, regardless of the reason for cesarean delivery. Means to oxygenate the mother might include the laryngeal mask airway, the Combitube, transtracheal jet ventilation, or cricothyroidotomy. Allow the mother to awaken and proceed with an awake intubation or regional anesthetic.

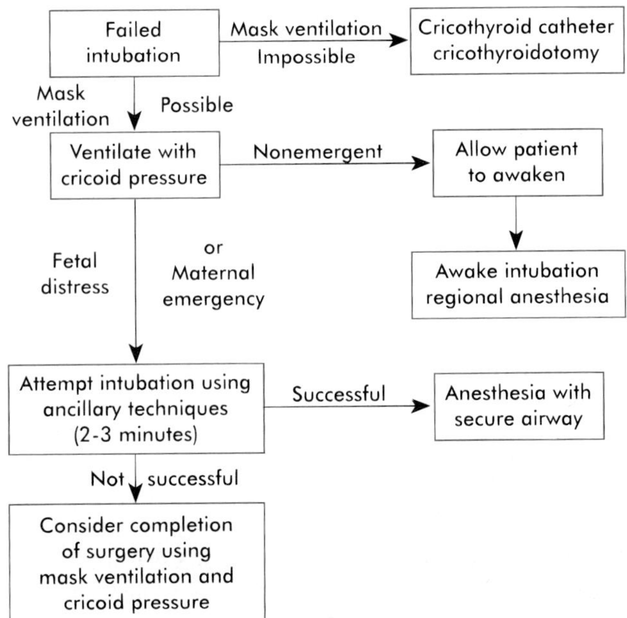

Fig. 76-7. Sample protocol for failed intubation. (From Malan TP, Johnson MD: The difficult airway in obstetric anesthesia: techniques for airway management and the role of regional anesthesia, *J Clin Anesth* 1:104, 1988.)

anesthetics is a concern. A comparison of neonatal condition after elective cesarean delivery with general anesthesia versus epidural anesthesia did not demonstrate significant differences.[117] Another retrospective report found use of general anesthesia to be associated with lesser APGAR scores and greater need for supplemental O_2 in the newborn.[185] Selection bias likely influenced these results; general anesthesia was administered in circumstances of preexisting fetal compromise which influenced neonatal care. Nonetheless, efforts should be made to minimize fetal exposure to anesthetics. Limiting the time between induction of anesthesia and delivery will help limit neonatal depression. N_2O will equilibrate across the placenta after approximately 15 minutes.[155] Anesthetic-related neonatal depression is unlikely when infants are delivered within 10 minutes of induction when 50% N_2O and a small dose of a volatile agent are used.[248] The time from uterine incision to delivery of the infant can also influence neonatal condition. A uterine incision to delivery interval of greater than 180 seconds was associated with lesser APGAR scores and fetal acidosis during either general anesthesia or spinal anesthesia.[72]

With efforts to minimize neonatal depression, adequate maternal anesthesia should not be sacrificed. Awareness and recall may occur during general anesthesia for cesarean delivery.[131] The use of low concentrations of potent volatile anesthetic agents has significantly decreased the incidence of awareness.[248] Patients should be queried about intraoperative recall after general anesthesia for cesarean delivery.

Postoperative Pain Relief

Various modalities of pain management following cesarean section are available. Obstetric patients usually want to receive as little sedative medication as possible, particularly if nursing. Subarachnoid opioids can be added to the local anesthetic used for spinal anesthesia for cesarean section. Intrathecal morphine (0.25 mg) and epidural morphine (3 to 4 mg) provide prolonged postoperative analgesia (12 to 20 hrs).[41] Appropriate patient monitoring following injection of intrathecal or epidural morphine is somewhat controversial. Because of the risk of delayed respiratory depression, hourly nursing checks of the patient's level of sedation and respiratory rate, for approximately 24 hours after drug administration, has been described as a reasonable practice.[202,203] IV PCA is another well-accepted form of postoperative analgesia.[100]

MANAGEMENT OF ANESTHESIA FOR THE HIGH-RISK PARTURIENT

Parturients with conditions that may compromise the well-being of mother and fetus are classified as "high risk." Anesthetic decisions should be based on understanding the pathophysiology of each condition so that specific problems can be anticipated and properly managed. Either maternal or fetal problems can result in a "high-risk" pregnancy. Maternal conditions may be related to complications of pregnancy or may be secondary to pre-existing maternal medical problems.

Maternal Obstetric Complications

Maternal complications associated specifically with pregnancy include obstetric hemorrhage and pregnancy-induced hypertension.

Antepartum hemorrhage

Severe bleeding during the antepartum period is usually associated with placental abnormalities such as placenta previa or abruptio placenta, and rarely, with uterine rupture (Table 76-15).

Placenta previa involves abnormal implantation of the placenta in the lower uterine segment and usually presents with painless vaginal bleeding. The significance of the previa depends upon the specific location of the placenta (Fig. 76-8). In severe cases, the placenta obstructs descent of the fetal presenting part, and hemorrhage can occur as the uterus contracts and the cervix dilates. Placenta previa occurs in up to 1% of third-trimester pregnancies and is associated with a maternal mortality of approximately 1%.[4,60] Risk factors include prior uterine surgery, prior placenta previa, and advanced maternal age.

Obstetric management depends on the degree of previa, amount of bleeding, and maturity of the fetus. Usually the degree of previa can be defined by ultrasound; if this is unavailable, the obstetrician may perform a vaginal examination using a "double set-up" wherein everything is ready to immediately perform caesarian section. During the vaginal examination, bleeding may become profuse, and the anesthesia provider should be prepared to rapidly induce general anesthesia for an emergency cesarean delivery. Otherwise, vaginal examinations are avoided.

If bleeding is minimal and the fetus is premature, the obstetrician may admit and monitor the parturient. Any UCs may be suppressed with tocolytic agents. In these cases, bleeding may occur at any time; the anesthesia provider should evaluate the patient and be familiar with the medical and obstetric history. Large-bore IV access should be available.

If hemorrhage from placenta previa occurs requiring emergency delivery, general anesthesia is indicated. Administration of 1 mg/kg of ketamine, or 0.3 mg/kg of etomidate are appropriate induction agents. If bleeding is absent or minimal and the patient presents for nonurgent cesarean delivery, a regional anesthetic may be used. The anesthesia provider should be prepared for excessive blood loss because the obstetrician may need to cut through the placenta during surgery, and the lower uterine segment may contract poorly after delivery of the placenta.

The incidence of placenta previa is greater in subsequent pregnancies. Further, if a patient presents with a placenta previa after a prior cesarean delivery, be aware of the risk of placenta accreta.[49] This is a condition in which the placenta invades the uterine wall. As such, the placenta cannot be easily removed from the uterus, and massive bleeding can occur requiring emergency gravid hysterectomy.

Abruptio placenta occurs in approximately 1% of pregnancies and involves premature separation of a normally implanted placenta. This condition usually presents as painful vaginal bleeding with frequent uterine contractions and/or a rigid uterus.[95] Of concern is that it may be difficult to estimate the amount of bleeding because hemorrhage can be concealed behind the separated placenta.

Table 76-15 Antepartum hemorrhage

	Placenta previa	Abruptio placentae	Uterine rupture
Incidence	0.1%–1.0%	0.2%–2.4%	0.08%–0.1%
Presenting symptoms	Painless vaginal bleeding	Painful vaginal bleeding; abnormalities in FHR; irritable uterus	Pain with or without vaginal bleeding; abnormalities in FHR; irritable uterus
Predisposing condition	Previous pregnancy with placenta previa	Hypertension, uterine abnormalities, history of cocaine abuse	Previous uterine surgery, prolonged intrauterine manipulation
Associated complications	Potential for massive blood loss	Potential for massive blood loss; blood loss may be concealed; DIC; renal failure	Potential for massive blood loss

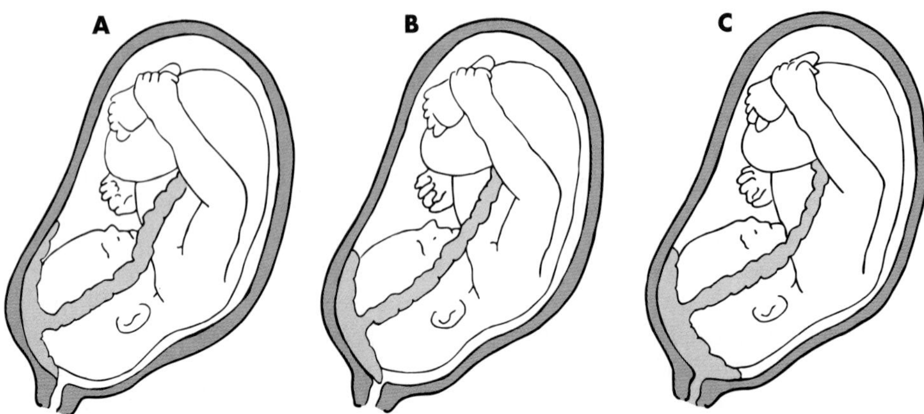

Fig. 76-8. Various forms of placenta previa. **A,** Marginal previa. **B,** Moderate previa. **C,** Complete previa.

Abruptio placenta can significantly affect fetal well-being both from maternal hemorrhage and decreased maternal cardiac output, and from loss of placental surface area for gas exchange. Risk factors include chronic hypertension, multiparity, advanced maternal age, cocaine use, trauma, and prior history.

Approximately 10% of cases of abruptio placenta may be complicated by disseminated intravascular coagulation (DIC), particularly in cases of chronic abruption where the systemic circulation may be showered with elements of the expanding hematoma or fetal demise. In these cases, patients may present with abnormal clotting studies and thrombocytopenia. If DIC occurs, fibrin and myoglobin may be present in the glomeruli resulting in some degree of acute renal failure.[148]

If the abruption is small, vaginal delivery can be attempted. Regional anesthesia can be used if maternal volume status and clotting studies are normal. In a severe abruption with acute fetal distress, emergency cesarean delivery should be performed under general anesthesia. Massive and rapid blood transfusion may be required. In a severe abruption, neonatal hypovolemia may complicate resuscitation.

Uterine rupture is a devastating event that can result in both maternal and fetal mortality. Predisposing conditions include previous uterine surgery (especially with a classical uterine incision) prolonged difficult labor, or uterine manipulation.[160] **Uterine rupture may present as maternal hemodynamic instability, fetal distress, or uterine irritability.** This is a catastrophic event that requires immediate cesarean delivery under general anesthesia, possible obstetric hysterectomy, and full active resuscitation of both mother and infant.

True uterine rupture is distinctly different from uterine scar dehiscence; a condition in which separation of a prior uterine incision occurs. This can happen in patients undergoing vaginal birth after cesarean delivery (VBAC), but is not usually associated with the hemorrhage and maternal and fetal instability typical of a true uterine rupture. When VBAC was first proposed, there was concern that performing regional anesthesia in these patients would mask maternal signs of uterine rupture (pain). Pain is not the usual presenting symptom of a uterine rupture, and there is now substantial experience demonstrating that epidural anesthesia for vaginal delivery can be safely performed in patients who have previously undergone cesarean delivery (and may actually improve a patient's acceptance of VBAC over repeat cesarean).[37,238] Continuous electronic monitoring of uterine activity and FHR is prudent in these cases. If the trial of vaginal delivery fails, the epidural block may be extended to a surgical level for cesarean delivery.

Postpartum hemorrhage

The most common causes of postpartum hemorrhage include lacerations, retained placenta, uterine atony, and uterine inversion.

Cervical and vaginal lacerations may be difficult for the obstetrician to identify and may result in prolonged bleeding. Epidural anesthesia, if present for delivery, is generally adequate for repair of these lesions. Occasionally, a saddle block may be required. Be aware that blood loss is difficult to estimate after vaginal delivery; carefully assess maternal hemodynamic status before preceding with an anesthetic. Sedation (such as IV ketamine, 10-mg increments or fentanyl 25-μg increments) may be a reasonable option in circumstances of hypovolemia. Rarely, general anesthesia is necessary in these cases.

Retained placenta occurs in about 1% of all vaginal deliveries. The placenta that has failed to separate causes continued bleeding from the intervillous spaces. Usually, manual exploration of the uterus is required. Regional anesthesia will provide patient comfort. Caution should be used inducing regional anesthesia if maternal hemorrhaging has been significant. IV analgesia is another option (see previous paragraph). In some cases uterine relaxation may be needed. Case reports indicate that small doses of IV nitroglycerin (50 to 100 μg) successfully relax the uterus for removal of the placenta. However, controlled trials of the uterine-relaxing effect of nitroglycerin are lacking. General anesthesia is another option for providing uterine relaxation. Studies on human uterine muscle have shown that all the potent inhaled anesthetics cause dose-dependent uterine muscle relaxation.[177] The dose necessary to achieve a rapid clinical effect is usually greater than 1 MAC. Therefore, intubation is mandatory and precautions should be taken to prevent aspiration as described in the section on general anesthesia for cesarean delivery.

Uterine atony occurs when the myometrium fails to adequately contract after delivery. This is first treated with uterine massage and oxytocin infusion (20 to 40 units/l of IV fluids), and evaluating that the placenta has been completely delivered. Oxytocin should not be given as a bolus dose, as it may cause hypotension.[226] If these measures fail to produce uterine muscle contraction, the 15-methyl analog of prostaglandin F2 alpha, namely 250 μg of carboprost tromethamine (Hemabate), can be given IM. This drug is a potent uterotonic agent;[103] side effects include bronchospasm in asthmatic patients,[84] gastric hypermotility, and occasionally hypertension. Alternatively, the ergot alkaloids methylergonovine maleate or ergonovine maleate (Methergin or Ergotrate) can be given. The dose is 0.2 mg IM. These drugs are alpha agonists and should be avoided in hypertensive patients. Patients who have recently received vasopressors are also at risk for hypertension following administration of these drugs.[226]

Uterine inversion is a rare but potentially devastating complication that occurs when the uterine fundus is inverted through the cervix into the vagina. The incidence is about 1 in 6000 deliveries, and predisposing factors include retained placenta, prolonged labor, and precipitous delivery.[250] Acute inversion results in symptoms of hemorrhage and shock, and the anesthesia provider should quickly induce uterine muscle relaxation. This can be accomplished with volatile anesthetics; the use of IV nitroglycerin in this setting has also been described.

Hypertensive disorders of pregnancy

Pregnancy-induced hypertension occurs with an overall incidence of 3% to 7% and is one of the major cause of maternal morbidity and mortality.[108] The American College of Obstetrics and Gynecology has classified hypertension during pregnancy into four groups:

- Preeclampsia-eclampsia
- Chronic hypertension
- Chronic hypertension with superimposed preeclampsia
- Gestational hypertension

Despite multiple attempts over decades to define its origin, the etiology of preeclampsia remains unknown. The clinical diagnosis is made in the presence of at least two of the following clinical findings:

Hypertension. Systolic blood pressure of at least 140 mm Hg or greater than 30 mm Hg above prepartum levels, or diastolic blood pressure of at least 90 mm Hg or 15 mm Hg above normal; this change should be seen with two blood pressure measurements taken at least 6 hours apart.

Generalized edema

Proteinuria. Greater than 300 mg protein in a 24-hour collection.

These symptoms should occur after the twentieth week of gestation. A patient has severe preeclampsia if blood pressure is geater than 160/100, proteinuria greater than 5 grams/24 hrs, oliguria, cerebral or visual disturbances, pulmonary edema, epigastric pain (presumably due to hepatic involvement), impaired liver function, thrombocytopenia, hepatic rupture, or HELLP (hemolysis, elevated liver enzymes, low platelets) syndrome are present. If a convulsion occurs, the patient has eclampsia.

The pathophysiology of preeclampsia-eclampsia is unclear; recent studies show that there may be an imbalance in the production of the prostaglandins thromboxane and prostacyclin.[247] There is a significant increase in the thromboxane/prostacyclin ratio in preeclamptic patients. Thromboxane and prostacyclin have two distinctly separate clinical effects (Box 76-13). The relative increase in thromboxane leads to vasoconstriction and decreased uteroplacental blood flow.[247] This reduced perfusion causes release of some factor which activates endothelial cells resulting in increased sensitivity to vasopressors and activation of the coagulation cascade. Endothelial damage could be the inciting event leading to the imbalance in thromboxane and prostacyclin. A second theory proposes that immunologic rejection of fetal tissues results in placental vasculitis and ischemia; placental ischemia causes renin release and widespread vasoconstriction.

Preeclampsia should be recognized as a multisystem disease characterized by inadequate organ perfusion due to widespread vasoconstriction. There is relative intravascular volume depletion but increased extravascular sodium and water retention (edema). Preeclampsia can result in thrombocytopenia, abnormal clotting studies, abnormalities in renal function, and elevation of liver enzymes. Rarely, hepatic rupture can occur. The hemo-

BOX 76-13
PROSTAGLANDIN IMBALANCE IN PREECLAMPSIA

Effects of thromboxane (increased)

↑ Vasoconstriction
↑ Platelet aggregation
↑ Uterine activity
↓ Uteroplacental blood flow

Effects of prostacyclin (decreased)

↓ Vasoconstriction
↓ Platelet aggregation
↓ Uterine activity
↑ Uteroplacental blood flow

dynamic characteristics of patients with preeclampsia are diverse.[40] Many patients will have relatively low pulmonary capillary wedge pressures (PCWP) and high cardiac output.[149] As disease severity increases, systemic vascular resistance (SVR) increases and cardiac output decreases. Serum protein content and colloid osmotic pressure are less in preeclamptic than normal pregnant patients.[256] The laryngeal edema of normal pregnancy can be aggravated to the point of airway obstruction. Pulmonary edema may develop from either cardiac failure, low oncotic pressure, or increased capillary permeability. Cerebral edema and hemorrhage can occur; cerebral hemorrhage is the leading cause of death in these patients.[108] Intravascular hypovolemia and vasoconstriction lead to impaired placental blood flow. The fetus is at risk for intrauterine growth retardation, premature delivery, and perinatal mortality.[144]

Management of these patients involves maximizing organ perfusion, optimizing placental blood flow, and preventing complications.

Magnesium is administered parenterally to prevent seizures.[147] Its mechanism is either by decreasing excitability of the muscle membrane or by improving cerebral blood flow from vasodilation. The patient is given a loading dose of 4 g over approximately 10 minutes and then placed on a continuous infusion of 1 to 2 g/hr to maintain a blood level of 4 to 8 mEq/l. Magnesium renders a patient more sensitive to the effects of nondepolarizing muscle relaxants by reducing the excitability of the muscle membrane, decreasing acetylcholine release and decreasing the sensitivity of the endplate to acetylcholine.[91] Magnesium also acts as a mild vasodilator and can reduce blood pressure, particularly after administration of a loading dose.[56]

Antihypertensive drugs are used to control blood pressure. Hydralazine is a commonly used antihypertensive agent in obstetrics.[107] It is usually given in 5-mg increments IV. Recently labetalol in 5 to 10 mg increments up to 1 mg/kg has been used in patients with preeclampsia, and has been shown to successfully reduce maternal blood pressure without reducing placental blood flow.[122] In a hypertensive crisis, continuous arterial blood pressure monitoring with an arterial line may be necessary to guide therapy.

The use of continuous lumbar epidural analgesia in these patients has significant advantages, provided it is done with care. If the patient is gently hydrated, blood pressure kept within 10% to 20% of baseline, and hypotension avoided, epidural anesthesia does not adversely affect uterine blood flow and in fact may lead to a significant improvement in uterine perfusion.[179] These patients are at risk for uteroplacental insufficiency and may demonstrate fetal distress, requiring urgent cesarean delivery. In these cases, the epidural catheter can be used to raise the level of sensory anesthesia and avoid the risks of ET intubation in these patients, which might be difficult because of laryngeal edema.

Before administering epidural anesthesia, medical management should be optimized. Blood pressure should be controlled (diastolic blood pressure between 90 and 100 mm Hg) with IV hydralazine or labetalol. How the disease is affecting each organ system should allow therapies to be rational. Invasive arterial and/or central venous pressure (CVP) monitoring can be instituted if severe hypertension or unclear volume status exist. Prehydration can be empiric, such as 250 to 500 ml crystalloid, or as guided by the CVP (with the goal of increasing CVP by 2 to 3 cm H_2O). If the patient suffers from pulmonary edema, refractory hypertension, or oliguria in the face of a normal CVP, a pulmonary artery catheter may be indicated to assist fluid management and guide antihypertensive therapy.

Preeclampsia may be complicated by abnormalities in blood coagulation. Patients with HELLP syndrome are likely to have a coagulopathy (low platelets and abnormal clotting studies). Other patients with preeclampsia may have thrombocytopenia and abnormal platelet function.[128] The level of platelet count below which the risk of bleeding is high and regional anesthesia should be avoided is unknown. A conservative stance is to require a platelet count of greater than 100,000 mm^3 before administering an epidural anesthetic. Which is the best test for evaluating platelet function is unclear. Further, retrospective studies indicate that epidural anesthesia has safely been administered to parturients with thrombocytopenia (unknown at the time of anesthesia) without problems.[200] Despite this, it is reasonable to avoid regional anesthesia in patients with an obvious coagulopathy. In patients with isolated thrombocytopenia without evidence of abnormal bleeding, each case should be considered individually considering the risks and benefits of epidural anesthesia. Although some have advocated use of the bleeding time to clarify a patient's coagulation status, the utility of this test in predicting bleeding has not been confirmed.

If cesarean delivery is required, epidural anesthesia can be used and has advantages in the preeclamptic patient. Overvigorous maternal hydration should be avoided to prevent pulmonary and cerebral edema. On the other hand, abrupt hypotension should be avoided to prevent fetal compromise. Moderate hydration (500 to 1000 ml crystalloid), vigilance and relatively slow establishment of an epidural block will allow treatment of blood pressure changes. As the block progresses cephalad, IV fluid and ephedrine therapy can be given to preserve a normal blood pressure. Small doses of ephedrine (2.5 mg) are given, because these patients can have an exaggerated response to vasopressors. Because spinal anesthesia may be associated with a rapid sympathetic block, it is used less often in the severely hypertensive patient.

If coagulopathy exists or an emergency cesarean delivery is required in the patient without an epidural catheter, general anesthesia may be needed. Inducing general anesthesia in these patients can be hazardous because of the potential for airway bleeding and edema and difficult intubation. Severe maternal hypertension with laryngoscopy and intubation can also occur.[111] Before induction of general anesthesia, the blood pressure can be treated with hydralazine or labetalol. If an arterial line is in place, nitroprusside can also be used to control the hypertensive response to laryngoscopy. A monitor of neuromuscular function should be employed to assist dosing the patient with muscle relaxants in the face of magnesium sulfate therapy.

Preexisting Medical Problems

Preexisting medical problems in the parturient may require alterations in obstetric and anesthetic management.

Diabetes mellitus

Diabetes mellitus is one of the most common medical problems in pregnancy. This disorder ranges from gestational diabetes (glucose intolerance diagnosed during pregnancy) to the more severe, insulin-dependent forms involving complications of other organ systems.

During the second half of pregnancy, maternal levels of glucose may be greater because of the anti-insulin effects of human placental lactogen, progesterone, and cortisol.[151] In diabetic women, the physiologic changes of insulin resistance and ketogenesis increase metabolic disturbances and make them more prone to hyperglycemia and ketoacidosis.

Morbidity and mortality are much greater in the diabetic parturient and fetus.[69,89] **The associated vascular disease can result in major cardiac, renal, or CNS complications.** Diabetic ketoacidosis is a major cause of perinatal mortality, with a fetal death rate as high as 90%. Infants of diabetic mothers have an increased risk of major congenital anomalies (particularly cardiac), fetal distress, intrauterine fetal demise, prematurity, and neonatal hypoglycemia.[88]

Insulin therapy during pregnancy is used to maintain the parturient in tight control because poor metabolic control seems to be related to a greater incidence of neonatal abnormalities.[88] Fetal monitoring with nonstress tests is essential during the end of the third trimester to detect fetal problems and prevent intrauterine fetal demise.

During labor and delivery, the blood glucose level should be maintained at less than 120 mg/dl to prevent rebound neonatal hypoglycemia. This is best accomplished by continuous low-dose IV infusion of insulin. Monitor blood glucose frequently and administer supplemental insulin or glucose as needed.

Uteroplacental blood flow has been shown to be compromised even in cases of mild gestational diabetes.[120] Therefore, the fetus of the diabetic mother is at increased risk for hypoxia and fetal distress.

Anesthetic management should attempt to optimize uteroplacental blood flow. Lumbar epidural block has been shown to provide excellent pain relief on these patients without adverse fetal effects.[66] If cesarean delivery is required, epidural or spinal anesthesia can be used. Although there have been concerns that spinal anesthesia in these patients results in more acidotic infants, later studies in diabetic parturients in which hypotension was promptly treated have not shown fetal acidosis after spinal anesthesia for cesarean delivery.[65,66] Of note is that in diabetics, as in all patients, acute hydration should be provided with a dextrose-free solution to prevent maternal and neonatal hyperglycemia, which can cause neonatal acidosis and rebound hypoglycemia.

Cardiac disorders

Anesthesia for the pregnant patient with heart disease requires knowledge of the pathophysiology of the specific lesion and an understanding of the physiologic impact of pregnancy on that lesion. Consultation with the patient's cardiologist is essential so that the patient's physiology is clearly understood and plans made for appropriate hemodynamic monitoring of each patient (e.g., arterial line, central venous, or pulmonary artery catheter). Recall that the pain and work of labor poses significant increases in cardiac work that may be poorly tolerated by the patient with borderline cardiac function. Further, the time of greatest physiologic stress for many cardiac patients is the immediate postpartum period. Be prepared to prevent the stress of pain during labor, minimize the hemodynamic effects of labor and continue monitoring these patients after delivery. Only very general guidelines will be presented for management of the patient with various cardiac lesions. The reader is referred to more comprehensive textbooks of obstetric anesthesia for in-depth consideration of the various cardiac lesions.

The most common acquired cardiac lesion presenting during pregnancy is mitral stenosis, generally secondary to rheumatic heart disease.[50] The increased cardiac output in response to pain during labor and delivery can be attenuated by lumbar epidural analgesia. Pulmonary artery pressure monitoring is often necessary to avoid sudden changes in left atrial pressure. Phenylephrine is preferred as a vasopressor as tachycardia is not well tolerated.

Pregnancy is typically well-tolerated in patients with mitral insufficiency. The increased heart rate and decreased SVR of pregnancy enhances forward cardiac output; left ventricular failure and pulmonary congestion can occur. Also, the patient is at risk of developing atrial fibrillation because of the dilated left atrium.[153] Lumbar epidural anesthesia is recommended to provide some degree of afterload reduction and prevent large increases in SVR. Bradycardia should be avoided, and ephedrine is the vasopressor of choice.

Mitral valve prolapse occurs in 5% to 10% of childbearing-age women. The great majority of patients are asymptomatic and require no special consideration other than perhaps antibiotic prophylaxis. Symptomatic patients are managed as patients with mitral insufficiency.

With aortic insufficiency, left ventricular volume overload can result in left ventricular failure and pulmonary edema. In these patients, epidural anesthesia is recommended for labor and delivery to decrease SVR. Bradycardia is poorly tolerated, and ephedrine is the preferred vasopressor.

Patients with significant aortic stenosis may not be able to respond to the increased demands of pregnancy.

Pulmonary artery catheter monitoring may help avoid acute decreases in filling pressure, blood pressure, cardiac output and coronary filling, but PA catheter placement in patients with ventricular hypertrophy can have increased risk of ventricular fibrillation. Sudden increases in filling pressure may result in left ventricular failure. Tachycardia should be avoided. If regional anesthesia is to be given, a continuous technique with gradual onset and the lowest level of sensory analgesia possible should be administered to minimize sympathetic block. Epidural opioids alone can be given to avoid the sympathetic block produced by local anesthetics. This will provide adequate analgesia for at least the first stage of labor and either a caudal catheter, pudendal block, or local infiltration can be used for delivery. Epidural anesthesia for cesarean delivery has been used, but should be administered slowly with appropriate hemodynamic monitors to preserve preload and blood pressure.[78] General anesthesia should avoid tachycardia.

With development of improved pediatric surgical techniques, most women with congenital heart disease will have had successful corrective procedures early in childhood and no special anesthetic considerations are required. The most common such conditions are patent ductus arteriosus, atrial septal defect, and ventricular septal defect. Should a defect remain, it usually results in a left-to-right shunt. In these cases, increases in SVR and marked increases in heart rate should be avoided. Large increases in left-to-right shunting may result in right ventricular failure. Avoid air bubbles in IV lines (periodic right-to-left shunting may occur). Epidural anesthesia can be used for labor and delivery. For cesarean delivery, either regional or general anesthesia can be used. Central monitoring may be necessary in patients with large shunts leading to right ventricular failure.

Patients with cyanotic congenital heart disease may tolerate pregnancy poorly. These conditions are characterized by a right-to-left shunt and include unrepaired tetralogy of Fallot, Eisenmenger's syndrome, and pulmonary hypertension. Air bubbles should be cleared from IV lines. Hemodynamic changes that increase right-to-left shunting will increase cyanosis and are devastating to these patients. Avoid increased pulmonary vascular resistance (pain, hypoxia, hypercarbia, acidosis). Administer supplemental O_2. Decreases in both SVR and preload should be avoided. The decreases in SVR associated with regional anesthesia may not be tolerated. Systemic or neuraxial opioids, or very dilute local anesthetics in small doses can be used for labor and delivery.[192,193] General anesthesia may be required for cesarean delivery, although epidural anesthesia has been described.[227]

Respiratory disorders

Asthma is the most common respiratory disorder seen in the parturient. The effect of pregnancy on the course of the disease is unpredictable; in general, patients with more severe disease will experience a deterioration during pregnancy.[253]

The main goal of treatment during pregnancy is to avoid asthmatic attacks that may compromise O_2 delivery to the fetus. Drug therapy is continued. Should an asthmatic attack occur during pregnancy, treatment is started with supplemental O_2, inhaled bronchodilators, subcutaneous beta-sympathomimetics, and steroids, if necessary.

Asthma medications should be continued during the peripartum period. Epidural anesthesia is recommended for labor and delivery. Should the patient require an emergency procedure, the epidural block can be extended. This will avoid the need for general anesthesia in the patient and the risk of severe bronchoconstriction. If general anesthesia is needed, ketamine is a reasonable induction agent because of its bronchodilating effect. Adequate anesthesia should be maintained with N_2O and a volatile agent to aid in maintaining bronchodilation.

Cigarette smoking often complicates pregnancy. Associated problems with maternal cigarette use include fetal intrauterine growth retardation, and maternal obstetric bleeding.[165] The reason for the bleeding risk is believed to be abnormalities of placental vascular structure which develop in response to decreased oxygen delivery.

Neurologic disorders

Controversy surrounds the choice of anesthesia for the obstetric patient with preexisting disease of the nervous system. If the patient's neurologic condition changes postoperatively, the cause may be unclear and the anesthetic technique or drug may be blamed. To develop a rational anesthetic plan, an understanding of the patient's neurologic and general medical condition is needed. Unfortunately, the anesthetic literature available on most of these conditions is limited.

Chronic back problems

Ligamentous strain from the lumbar lordosis of pregnancy results in up to 50% of pregnant women reporting back pain, often associated with symptoms of pain radiating down the legs. Parturients may also present with a history of intervertebral disk disease. There is no evidence that regional anesthesia will exacerbate these problems.[28] Postpartum back pain can be minimized by assuring proper patient position during labor and delivery to avoid excessive strain.

In patients with previous back surgery for disc disease or scoliosis, performing regional anesthesia may be difficult because of altered anatomy or adhesions. In many cases, epidural anesthesia can be performed successfully. However, the patient should be aware that the epidural block may be patchy and inadequate because of alterations in the epidural space from previous surgery. The possibility of unintentional dural puncture may be increased. For cesarean delivery, spinal anesthesia may be easier to perform with more predictable results.

Multiple sclerosis

Multiple sclerosis causes neurologic disability in young and middle-aged adults with a frequency of 0.5/1000. The disease is characterized by random and multiple sites of demyelination in the brain and spinal cord and does not affect the peripheral nervous system. The course consists of waxing and waning symptoms at unpredictable time intervals over years. The relapse rate during the first 3 months postpartum is about three times more common than in the nonpregnant state. Several studies have implicated spinal anesthesia in the exacerbation of multiple sclerosis during the postoperative period in the nonobstetric patient.[17] The numbers of actual relapses reported in these studies are very small and the relationship of the relapses to the anesthetic technique is unclear because other conditions in the postoperative period may also predispose to relapse. Later studies in both obstetric and nonobstetric patients have reported the use of both spinal and epidural anesthesia in these patients without neurologic complications.[16] The patient should be informed that there is an increased incidence of relapse in the postpartum period, regardless of the use of anesthesia.

Viral disease

There has been concern that performing regional anesthesia in a patient who has a history of herpes might risk contaminating the patient's cerebrospinal fluid (CSF) with herpes virus particles and cause meningitis. The patient is viremic only during the primary infection. During recurrent episodes, even when vesicles are present, the patient is *not* viremic and spinal or epidural anesthesia *can* be administered.[199] Opinions vary regarding the use of regional anesthesia in the patient with a past history of polio. Case reports of recrudescence of symptoms after spinal anesthesia exist. Epidural anesthesia has been used successfully for labor and delivery or cesarean delivery without postpartum complications.[58]

Spinal cord injury

Regional anesthesia can be extremely beneficial to the obstetric patient with spinal cord injury. If the lesion is below the level of T10, patients will experience labor pain. For patients with spinal cord injuries above the level of T6, autonomic hyperreflexia may occur. This sympathetic response can be elicited by cutaneous or visceral stimulation below the level of spinal cord transection; patients exhibit severe hypertension, headache, and flushing above and blanching below the level of the lesion. This can be triggered by UCs during labor.[6] Regional anesthesia is an excellent choice for preventing autonomic hyperreflexia.[127,249] Usually only a low concentration of local anesthetic agent or opioid is required. If epidural anesthesia alone does not completely prevent or control the hypertension, IV agents such as hydralazine, trimethaphan, or nitroprusside have been used successfully.

Cerebrovascular accidents

Cerebral hemorrhage can be seen in association with aneurysms, arteriovenous malformations, and preeclampsia or eclampsia. Hypertension should be treated aggressively and abrupt changes in blood pressure avoided. For the parturient with a history of a cerebrovascular accident, epidural anesthesia is a good choice for labor and vaginal or cesarean delivery, provided intracranial pressure is not elevated. If general anesthesia is required, the hypertensive response to intubation should be attenuated with IV lidocaine, antihypertensive medications such as labetalol, trimethaphan, or sodium nitroprusside, and adequate doses of anesthetic induction agents.

Obesity

The obese parturient presents physiologic and technical challenges to the obstetrician and anesthesia provider.[94] Obesity is defined as body weight greater than 120% of ideal body weight; morbid obesity is defined as twice normal body weight or a body mass index greater than 30, where body mass index = $wt(kg)/(ht(m))^2$. The obese parturient has a greater incidence of pregnancy complications including hypertension, diabetes, breech presentation, macrosomic infants, and need for cesarean delivery.[90,113] The decrease in functional residual capacity normally seen in pregnancy is worsened by obesity causing ventilation/perfusion mismatch and airway closure, particularly in the supine position.[24] Pregnancy increases the cardiovascular demands of a system already stressed by obesity. The supine position can result in severe supine hypotensive syndrome. Gastric volumes are increased, emptying is delayed, and patients are at risk for regurgitation.[241] Inducing general anesthesia for cesarean section can be hazardous due to airway difficulties, hypoxia, and regurgitation.[113] Obesity is a risk factor for increased anesthesia-related maternal mortality.[80,159]

Induction of a continuous regional anesthetic technique in obese patients is recommended as early in labor as possible. Regional anesthesia may be technically difficult and repeated attempts necessary.[113] Having a tested epidural catheter in place will limit the need for general anesthesia should emergency cesarean delivery be required. Single-shot spinal anesthesia is not preferred in these patients for several reasons; first, the level of anesthetic block is unpredictable and may be greater than anticipated; second, hypotension may be quite severe and difficult to manage; and third, surgery times are often prolonged and the block may wear off before surgery is completed. Continuous spinal anesthesia has been used with success in the morbidly obese parturient.

Postoperatively, the obese patient should be observed for adequate respiratory function. Early ambulation should be encouraged to avoid pulmonary atelectasis and deep venous thrombosis.

Maternal substance abuse and addiction

Maternal addiction is seen with distressing frequency. The most commonly abused substances are alcohol, opioids, and cocaine. IV drug use and venous thrombosis may lead to difficulties with IV access. Mothers with a history of opioid abuse may experience withdrawal symptoms if opioids are not given during hospitalization. Withdrawal symptoms may also be precipitated if these women receive opioid agonist-antagonist agents such as butorphanol. The response to neuraxial opioids is unpredictable; postoperative pain relief can be difficult to manage and is more easily accomplished with PCA.

Cocaine is a potent vasoconstrictor that has been shown in animal studies to significantly decrease uterine blood flow.[170] Parturients with a history of cocaine abuse can present with hypertension, tachycardia, other cardiac arrhythmia, seizure, cerebrovascular accident, myocardial infarction, or pulmonary edema. Acute cocaine intoxication may be difficult to distinguish from preeclampsia. Cocaine use during pregnancy is associated with a greater incidence of premature rupture of membranes, preterm delivery, and abruptio placenta.[10,178] If cocaine abuse has occurred in proximity to the onset of labor, significant hypertension and tachycardia will require treatment with IV labetalol. Relative volume-depletion may result in significant hypotension during the induction of regional anesthesia, and the response to ephedrine may be unpredictable. Significant hypertension can occur during laryngoscopy and intubation during the induction of general anesthesia. The infants of drug-addicted mothers will frequently need to be treated for withdrawal.

Fetal Conditions Complicating Pregnancy

Fetal conditions complicating pregnancy include prematurity, postmaturity, multiple gestations, abnormal presentations, and cord prolapse.

Prematurity

Preterm delivery occurs in up to 10% of all births and is defined as delivery at 36 weeks of gestation or less. Prematurity is the major cause of neonatal mortality.[213] Although advances in neonatal care have improved outcome, these infants are still at risk for pulmonary complications secondary to respiratory distress syndrome and CNS complications from intracranial hemorrhage.

To prevent these complications, various tocolytic agents are employed when preterm labor occurs. These tocolytic agents have a variety of maternal and fetal side effects that the anesthesia provider should be familiar with (Table 76-16).[226]

Table 76-16 Side effects of tocolytics

Drug	Maternal effects	Fetal effects
Beta-adrenergic agents	↓ BP ↑ HR CHF Dysrhythmias Pulmonary edema Headache ↑ Glucose ↓ Potassium	↑ HR ↑ Glucose
Magnesium sulfate	Pulmonary edema Drowsiness ↑ Sensitivity to muscle relaxants	Hypotonia
Calcium channel blockers	↓ BP ↓ Cardiac conduction	

Beta-adrenergic drugs such as ritodrine and terbutaline are used for tocolysis. These agents act by direct stimulation of the beta-adrenergic receptors present in uterine smooth muscle, resulting in increased intracellular cyclic adenosine monophosphate (cAMP) and uterine relaxation. Ritodrine is the only beta-mimetic currently approved for tocolysis by the FDA, but terbutaline is more commonly used because it is available as both oral and IV preparations and is less expensive. The beta-adrenergic drugs have significant side effects. Most experience tachycardia (from either a direct $beta_1$ effect or in responses to the $beta_2$ mediated vasodilation). Chest pain can complicate administration of these drugs. Pulmonary edema can also occur; the etiology is probably multifactorial, and includes cardiogenic and noncardiogenic reasons.[21,22] Patients receiving beta-adrenergic therapy are at risk for fluid overload and cardiogenic pulmonary edema due to stimulated antidiuretic hormone activity from beta-adrenergic agonist.[218] Further, preterm labor is often precipitated by an infectious process which will predispose to increased capillary permeability and noncardiogenic pulmonary edema. Risk factors for pulmonary edema while receiving beta-adrenergic agonists for tocolytic therapy include anemia, preexisting cardiac disease, multiple gestation, excessive hydration, tachycardia, prolonged tocolytic therapy, and associated infection (chorioamnionitis).

Magnesium sulfate has been shown to reduce uterine contractility and has been used as a tocolytic, particularly in cases where beta-mimetics alone have not been successful or are contraindicated.[240] Serum magnesium levels are maintained between 5.0 and 7.0 mg/100 ml.

If tocolysis fails, the anesthesia provider may be required to administer an anesthetic for labor and delivery to a patient who has recently been treated with one of these agents. The respiratory status of patients on beta-mimetic therapy should be closely monitored. Hydration before regional anesthesia should be modest. Neosynephrine may be the preferred vasopressor. If patients receiving magnesium sulfate require general anesthesia, careful neuromuscular blockade monitoring is required, as previously discussed. In addition, uterine atony may occur after delivery.

The method of delivery of the preterm fetus is controversial. Recent studies indicate that cesarean delivery of these infants may not decrease morbidity.[20] Obstetricians may elect to deliver the premature breech infant by cesarean delivery. The breech is smaller than the head in the preterm infant; vaginal delivery may risk entrapment of the fetal head behind an incompletely dilated cervix. In **selecting an anesthetic, the anesthesia provider should be aware that the**

preterm fetus is particularly susceptible to maternally administered drugs. The preterm fetus has immature enzyme systems available for drug metabolism, an incomplete blood–brain barrier, and less protein available for drug binding. The preterm fetus is capable of metabolizing both ester- and amide-type local anesthetics and is in fact somewhat less sensitive to the CNS toxicity of lidocaine than is the full-term fetus.[232] After delivery, the preterm infant may require aggressive resuscitation and appropriate personnel should be available.

Postmaturity

The postmature fetus is at risk for uteroplacental insufficiency, meconium aspiration, and fetal distress. The efficacy of the placenta declines with postmaturity, and it may not be capable of maintaining adequate gas exchange. The anesthesia provider should evaluate these patients as concerns of fetal well-being may trigger urgent or emergent cesarean delivery.

Multiple gestations

The parturient with **multiple gestation** will frequently present with premature labor and/or breech presentation. If time permits, induction of an epidural anesthetic will provide excellent anesthesia for vaginal delivery. During attempted vaginal delivery of a multiple gestation, the sensory level of epidural analgesia should be maintained at about T6 so that if problems aincrease during attempted delivery of the second infant, the epidural can be used to provide anesthesia for emergency cesarean delivery. If cesarean section is not urgent, either epidural or spinal anesthesia can be used; the larger uterus will predispose these patients to severe supine hypotensive syndrome. The full lateral position may be necessary to avoid caval compression. Overdistention of the uterus is a risk for uterine atony and postpartum hemorrhage. Adequate personnel should be available for resuscitation of more than one infant.

Abnormal presentations

Normally, the presenting part of the fetus is the head with the occiput facing anteriorly. **As the fetus descends, the occiput may not properly rotate into the anterior position and the fetal head will present facing posteriorly.** In this situation, it is more difficult for the head to descend through the pelvis. Labor may be difficult and prolonged, and the patient may experience severe back pain. Forceps rotation may be necessary. Cesarean delivery may be necessary if attempts at vaginal delivery fail. Epidural anesthesia is a good choice in these cases because it provides segmental analgesia during labor and can be extended should forceps be required.

With breech presentation, either the fetal buttocks or lower extremities are the presenting parts. This presentation is more common in the premature fetus.[173] The obstetrician may attempt to externally rotate the fetus. If vaginal delivery of a breech infant is attempted, epidural anesthesia is recommended to allow optimal perineal muscle relaxation for delivery of the head. Because vaginal breech deliveries are associated with increased neonatal morbidity,[173] the obstetrician may decide to perform a cesarean delivery. Either spinal or epidural anesthesia can be used. During either vaginal or cesarean delivery of a breech infant, there may be difficulty extracting the head of the infant. The anesthesia provider should be prepared to provide uterine muscle relaxation.

Cord prolapse is seen more commonly with breech presentations because the lower uterus is not filled by the fetal head and there is an opportunity for the cord to become the presenting part. As such, the cord is compressed, the fetal blood supply is cut off, and emergency cesarean delivery is needed.

NEONATAL RESUSCITATION

There is a complex adaptation from intrauterine to extrauterine life that the newborn should accomplish at birth. Hypoxia, hypercarbia, and cold are among the stimuli that will initiate breathing. Because the fetal lung is gas-free, the inspiratory pressure that the infant needs to initially expand the lung can be as high as 70 cm H_2O.[246] Later breaths require less inspiratory pressure. The onset of regular breathing should occur within the first 30 seconds of life, and the newborn respiratory rate is about 30 to 40 breaths/min.

The fetal circulation has been discussed in an earlier section. Adaptation of the circulatory system to extrauterine life requires closure of the right-to-left shunts that exist between the right and left atria through the foramen ovale and between the PA and the aorta through the ductus arteriosus.[212] Normal values for blood gases *in utero* and in the first hours of life are listed in Table 76-17.[132] The normal newborn heart rate should be about 120 beats/min. Normal newborn blood pressure varies with gestational age. In the full-term infant, the systolic blood pressure should be 60 to 70 mm Hg. **The neonate is unable to maintain body temperature by shivering and uses nonshivering thermogenesis to break down brown fat and maintain body temperature.**[61] **Thus, a huge increase in O_2 consumption will occur if the newborn is inadequately warmed.**

Table 76-17 Blood gas values in the fetus and newborn

	Umbilical vein	Umbilical vein	Neonatal artery	
	Values *in utero*		60 min	24 hr
pH	7.30–7.35	7.28–7.32	7.30–7.36	7.33–7.40
Pco_2 (mm Hg)	32–42	42–52	32–40	30–36
Po_2 (mm Hg)	30–42	15–25	50–70	65–85

Understanding these physiologic adaptations will allow those responsible for neonatal resuscitation to best direct their efforts. Infants likely to need resuscitation can often be identified before delivery. Abnormalities in FHR pattern or fetal scalp pH values can indicate an initially depressed neonate. A history of obstetric hemorrhage, preeclampsia, or other high-risk conditions can also identify an infant that will need resuscitation.

Neonatal resuscitation equipment should be readily available for use in the delivery room. A list of suggested equipment is given in Box 76-14.

There are some anatomic differences to remember when managing the neonatal airway. The head is relatively large with a prominent occiput, the neck is short, and the tongue is relatively large. The cricoid cartilage is the narrowest part of the airway. The chest is relatively small, and it may be difficult to distinguish an ET from an esophageal intubation just by listening to breath sounds.

The APGAR score described previously is initially used to identify infants in need of resuscitation. The following standards for neonatal resuscitation based on the APGAR score were recommended by the American Heart Association. The infant with an APGAR score of 7 to 10 is healthy, cries shortly after delivery, maintains tone and color, and has a heart rate of greater than 100 beats/min. These infants require only routine delivery room care. The infant should be dried and placed under a radiant warmer. Secretions in the mouth and nose should be suctioned gently with a bulb syringe; remember that vigorous suctioning in the first 5 minutes after birth can result in bradycardia by producing a vagal response.

The infant with an APGAR score of 4 to 6 is depressed and may not breathe immediately. The airway should be cleared with a bulb syringe and the infant stimulated. If the infant does not breathe immediately and the heart rate is less than 100 beats/min, ventilation with a bag and mask should be initiated. Adequacy of ventilation can be assessed by watching chest movement and palpating the umbilical cord for heart rate. Usually the heart rate increases rapidly when ventilation is successful. Long, positive pressure inflations are better than fast, short inflations because high opening pressures may be needed, as previously discussed. A rate of about 60 breaths/min is used.

The infant with an APGAR score of 0 to 3 is flaccid, apneic, pale, and unresponsive. Immediate ventilation with 100% O_2 should be initiated and the infant should be intubated.

When the heart rate persists at less than 100 beats/min despite adequate ventilation, closed chest cardiac massage is begun. Two thumbs are placed on the middle third of the sternum to avoid potential damage to abdominal organs. The sternum is compressed 1 inch at a rate of 120 compressions/min. Compressions are always accompanied by positive pressure ventilation at a rate of 60/min.

If the heart rate is still low, drug therapy should be started (Table 76-18). The umbilical vein is identified as the thin-walled structure in the center of the umbilical cord (the two umbilical arteries are thicker-walled structures on either side of the vein). A 5-French catheter can be used to catheterize the umbilical vein after flushing with heparinized saline. It is inserted just to the point where blood return is obtained. Once the catheter is in place, drugs can be administered.

The AHA now suggests that atropine and calcium are not useful in the acute phase of neonatal resuscitation. Sodium bicarbonate in a dose of 1 to 2 mg/kg may be useful in prolonged arrests, but its use is now discouraged in brief arrests because of the association between acute sodium loads and the incidence of cerebral intraventricular hemorrhage. Epinephrine will improve perfusion pressure, contractility, and heart rate. Epinephrine can be given IV or via the ET tube in a dose of 0.01 to 0.03 mg/kg, which is 0.1 to 0.3 ml/kg of a 1:10,000 solution. This is given if heart rate is less than 80 despite adequate ventilation and cardiac compression.

Volume expanders are indicated if evidence of fetal/maternal bleeding is present. Ten ml/kg of 5% albumin or emergency release O-negative blood can be given.

BOX 76-14
NEONATAL RESUSCITATION EQUIPMENT

- Warming table with radiant heater
- Warm blankets
- Bulb syringe
- Source of O_2
- Suction
- Laryngoscopes—Miller 0 for premature infants, Miller 1 for full-term infants
- Face masks
- Endotracheal tubes:
  - 2.5 for infant < 29 weeks
  - 3.0 for infant 39–38 weeks
  - 3.1 for full-term infant
- Plastic meconium aspirators that connect to wall suction
- Monitors—ECG, blood pressure, pulse oximeter
- Medications

Table 76-18 Drug therapy during neonatal resuscitation

Drug	Concentration	Dose
Epinephrine	1:10,000	0.01–0.03 mg/kg
Sodium bicarbonate	0.5 mEq/ml	1–2 mEq/kg
Volume expander		
5% albumin		10 ml/kg
O^- blood		10 ml/kg
Naloxone	0.02 mg/ml	0.01 mg/kg

If depression due to opioids is suspected, naloxone can be given IV or IM in a dose of 0.01 mg/kg of a neonatal solution. The neonatal solution contains 0.02 mg/ml. Therefore, 2 ml IM are given to a full-term infant. The duration of opioids can exceed that of the naloxone, and that naloxone can induce a withdrawal reaction in an infant of a opioid-addicted mother.

There are numerous specific etiologies that can cause symptoms of respiratory distress and cyanosis in the newborn. The management of meconium aspiration will be discussed because this is one of the most common situations that occur in the delivery room.

Infants who aspirate meconium *in utero* can have severe parenchymal disease and respiratory distress, and aggressive airway management in the delivery room is essential in reducing morbidity.[234] Meconium passage occurs in about 9% of all live births and reflects release of the anal sphincter in response to asphyxia. Fetuses at risk include those who are postmature or who have suffered peripartum asphyxia. Fifty percent of infants who have meconium-stained amniotic fluid will have meconium in the trachea. Inhalation of meconium results in development of a chemical pneumonitis and plugging of the airways with air trapping and ventilation-perfusion mismatch. Earlier studies showed that immediate laryngoscopy and direct tracheal suctioning significantly reduced neonatal mortality.[234] Later studies have generated controversy, by contending that in vigorous infants born with thinly meconium-stained amniotic fluid, immediate tracheal suctioning may not be necessary.[145] Tracheal suctioning is usually done when thick meconium is present.

ANESTHESIA FOR SURGERY DURING PREGNANCY

The need for nonobstetric surgery may arise during pregnancy. Elective surgery should be delayed until after delivery. If surgery should be performed, some simple principles exist. The fetus is a vulnerable second patient, whose well-being is completely dependent upon the mother to maintain a healthy uterine environment. Supplemental O_2 is usually given to the mother. Prevention of aorto-caval compression, maintenance of normal P_{CO_2}, and normal cardiac output and blood pressure are sound goals. These principles are more important than any specific anesthetic technique.

If the need for surgery arises during the first trimester of pregnancy, concerns of drug-related teratogenicity should be considered. This vulnerable period is day 15 to approximately day 90 of gestation. Maternal physiology is an important determinant of fetal development. For example, hyperglycemia in a diabetic patient is a known teratogen, with such fetuses at risk for cardiac defects. Maternal stress, hypoxia, and hyperthermia are also harmful. With respect to anesthetic agents, although many have been studied for possible teratogenic effects in animals, the application of the results in humans is unclear (e.g., thalidomide, a known teratogen in humans, was not found to be teratogenic in rats). Anesthetic induction agents, potent inhaled agents, and lidocaine appear to be devoid of teratogenic effects. Cocaine, however, does have adverse effects. Diazepam exposure in the first trimester has been reported to be associated with fetal cleft palate; many of the women taking diazepam were being treated for some problem and also used other medications.[215] The implication that diazepam is teratogenic is controversial. Nonetheless, regular users of diazepam (and possibly all benzodiazepines) in the first trimester should consider this report.

The use of N_2O during pregnancy, particularly in the first trimester, has been questioned. N_2O decreases methionine synthetase activity and theoretically could interface with DNA synthesis. Prolonged exposure of pregnant rats to N_2O in early gestation increases the rate of fetal resorption and formation of congenital anomalies. Interestingly, these effects are reduced if the animals also receive a potent inhaled anesthetic.[161] This suggests that perhaps the adverse effects of N_2O seen in rats is mediated by something other than impaired DNA synthesis (such as adrenergic stimulation). **No adverse effect of N_2O has been demonstrated when it has been used as part of a general anesthetic during pregnancy in humans.** Retrospective surveys of humans exposed chronically to low doses of N_2O (such as operating room personnel, dental care providers) suggest that there is an increased risk of spontaneous abortion and anomalies and decreased fertility in these women when compared with those who work in environments uncontaminated by N_2O. These data may be flawed by the lack of control of other work conditions (e.g., level of stress, age of employees), and most important, by recall or response bias,[231] i.e., if a woman exposed to N_2O while working in a dental office had a miscarriage, she might be much more likely to accurately complete a reproductive health questionnaire than someone who knows of no controversies about her workplace and/or who has not had pregnancy problems. Surveys of women undergoing anesthesia and surgery during pregnancy demonstrate an increased risk of fetal loss, intrauterine growth retardation, and premature delivery.[77,162] No difference in the incidence of fetal anomalies has been reported, despite the use of general anesthesia using N_2O. Again, the greatest risk to the unborn fetus is the alteration in uterine environment as a result of the condition leading to surgery, the need for anesthesia and surgery, or uterine contractions occurring after surgery. From the data available, no specific anesthetic technique can be implicated as problematic.

It is reasonable to limit drug exposure when planning an anesthetic for surgery during pregnancy. Regional anesthetic techniques, when appropriate, can achieve this goal. Minimal anesthetic can be used (particularly with spinal anesthesia). Prevention and treatment of hypotension is key to successful management. When regional anesthesia is not appropriate (because of surgical location or patient preferences), prevention of maternal hypoxia, hypo- or hypercapnia, aspiration prophylaxis, and maintaining normal blood pressure are key goals.

The uterus becomes an intra-abdominal organ after about 12 weeks. After about 18 weeks, it is usually possible to auscultate the FHR using doppler ultrasound. Whenever possible, FHR monitoring should be carried out during surgery. A person dedicated to obtaining and interpreting the FHR tracing should be available. Certainly an intervention such as cesarean delivery would not be undertaken at an early gestational age, but nonreassuring FHR changes could lead to maternal hemodynamic or position changes, or relocation of surgical retractors with the goal to improve uteroplacental function. When the fetus is viable, changes in the FHR monitor might result in operative delivery. Documentation of fetal heart tones before and after surgery should be completed. A tocolytic agent can be administered after surgery to prevent uterine contractions.

ANESTHESIA FOR *IN VITRO* FERTILIZATION

With recent improvements in techniques and success rates, *in vitro* fertilization procedures, or assisted reproductive technologies are becoming more common. Most ovum retrievals are performed using a transvaginal approach with ultrasound guidance. Laparoscopic retrieval is possible but is used less frequently. After fertilization occurs, embryo transfer can be performed transvaginally 48 hours after the initial procedure. Embryo transfer does not require anesthesia. Other procedures include gamete intrafallopian tube transfer (GIFT), in which oocytes and sperm are placed into a fallopian tube under laparoscopic guidance with the patient under general anesthesia—this occurs just after egg harvest, and zygote intrafallopian transfer (ZIFT), in which a zygote (single-cell fertilized egg) is placed laparoscopically into the fallopian tube—this occurs several hours after fertilization.

Controversy exists regarding the risks associated with anesthetics or analgesics administered for assisted reproductive technologies. A review of putative toxic effects of anesthetics and adjuvants administered during egg retrieval suggests that from the available animal (usually mouse) data, high concentrations of O_2, lidocaine (blood concentrations as low as 1 μg/ml), and N_2O might interfere with cell division.[187] Although it is difficult to apply data from animal models directly to humans, in the absence of more relevant information, it is perhaps reasonable to avoid these agents if/when other suitable alternatives exist. Opioids, midazolam, low-dose (0.5%) isoflurane and propofol do not appear to have toxic effects on cell division.

For transvaginal ovum retrieval, IV sedation is often sufficient. Small doses of fentanyl with midazolam or low-dose propofol sedation are effective. Spinal anesthesia may be the preferred regional anesthetic technique: A small dose of either lidocaine or bupivacaine can be given, sacral analgesia is easily obtained, and the larger dose of local anesthetics (particularly lidocaine) needed for epidural anesthesia is avoided.

The best general anesthetic for a laparoscopic procedure is unknown. Human studies are difficult to perform and control because other factors influencing pregnancy outcome (e.g., patient age, reason for infertility, duration of anesthesia, and duration of CO_2 insufflation) may not be controlled. Further, large numbers of patients are needed, because the success rate for the different assisted reproductive techniques is already fairly low (25% to 35%). Rosen et al.[209] found pregnancy success rates to be equivalent in patients undergoing laparoscopic egg retrieval with either an O_2/N_2O/isoflurane anesthetic or an O_2/isoflurane anesthetic. Vincent et al.[244] found success rates for ZIFT patients to be lesser in those who received a propofol/O_2/ N_2O anesthetic compared with an O_2/ N_2O/isoflurane anesthetic. The significance of these results is unclear. Further work is necessary to define optimal anesthetic techniques for *in vitro* fertilization procedures.

SUMMARY

Pregnancy results in dramatic physiologic changes. Anesthesia providers should consider these changes and recognize the vulnerability of the unborn fetus. Management should optimize uteroplacental blood flow. Although systemic opioids are used most commonly for labor analgesia, regional analgesia provides the most effective pain relief during labor. Spinal, epidural, or general anesthesia is appropriate for cesarean delivery depending upon the situation, but general anesthesia is associated with significant risk (e.g., failed intubation, pulmonary aspiration). When pregnancy is complicated by medical problems, the interaction of that medical condition with the stresses of pregnancy should be appreciated.

KEY POINTS

- Pregnancy, labor, and delivery are associated with profound physiologic changes involving all organ systems. These changes require specific consideration by the anesthesia provider and may result in alterations in the anesthetic techniques and drug dosages used in the nonpregnant patient.
- All drugs enter the fetal circulation from the placenta through the umbilical vein. From the umbilical vein, approximately 40% to 60% of the blood passes through the fetal liver; the rest of the blood bypasses the liver through the ductus venosus and enters the heart through the IVC. The first-pass perfusion through the liver is a buffer against attainment of high fetal drug levels.
- Opioids remain the most commonly used agents for obstetric pain relief. Meperidine is the opioid used most frequently. Maternally administered meperidine may produce neonatal depression related to total dose and to the time interval between administration and delivery. Maximal depression occurs with delivery within 1 to 3 hours after IM injection.
- The most important components of FHR monitoring are rate, beat-to-beat variability, and pattern.
- Regional anesthetic techniques provide excellent pain relief for labor and delivery without the sedative effects of systemic medications. Several general principles apply to the use of any regional technique in obstetrics. First, adequate IV access is required. Second, adequate prehydration with 500 to 1000 ml of a balanced salt solution is needed, particularly before administering techniques that may result in sympathetic blockade. Third, equipment should always be available for resuscitation should a complication occur. Several different techniques of regional analgesia for labor are used. Although epidural opioids alone are usually only effective early in labor, local anesthetics combined with opioids work well for much of labor and delivery. Spinal opioids are also effective analgesics during the first stage of labor.
- In recent years, the frequency of cesarean section has increased markedly; the present use in the United States is approximately 20%, depending on geographic region and population characteristics. With proper technical skills and an understanding of maternal and fetal physiology, spinal or epidural anesthesia can be used successfully. With cases in which regional anesthesia is contraindicated, an awareness of the risks involved and their appropriate management makes general anesthesia an acceptable alternative.
- The main risk of general anesthesia in the obstetric patient is failure to secure a patent airway. This has become the leading cause of anesthesia-related maternal mortality. Preoperative evaluation of the airway may help identify patients at risk. However, a difficult airway may not always be predicted. Therefore, a difficult intubation algorithm should be rehearsed.
- Comparison of neonatal condition after cesarean section with general anesthesia or epidural anesthesia has not demonstrated significant differences. The time from uterine incision to delivery of the infant can influence neonatal condition. A uterine incision-to-delivery interval of greater than 180 seconds was associated with lesser APGAR score and fetal acidosis during either general anesthesia or spinal anesthesia.
- Obstetric hemorrhage contributes to maternal mortality. Placenta previa may require emergent cesarean delivery for hemorrhage with aggressive maternal resuscitation. Placenta previa occurring in a patient with prior cesarean delivery may be complicated by placenta accreta. Abruptio placenta can be associated with concealed blood loss, DIC, renal failure, and severe fetal distress or fetal demise.
- Preeclampsia is a multisystem disease that presents with hypertension, proteinuria, and generalized edema and is characterized by organ hypoperfusion. There is widespread peripheral vasoconstriction resulting in intravascular volume depletion and extravascular sodium and water retention. Intravascular volume and protein content are markedly less than in normal pregnancy. The laryngeal edema of normal pregnancy can be aggravated to the point of airway obstruction. Cerebral edema and hemorrhage can occur, cerebral hemorrhage being the leading cause of death in these patients. Regional analgesia or anesthesia is appropriate in preeclamptic patients with normal coagulation. Maintaining hemodynamic stability and good uteroplacental function are priorities.
- Maternal drug addiction also is being seen with increasing frequency. The most commonly abused substances are alcohol, opioids, and cocaine. Mothers with a history of opioid abuse may experience withdrawal symptoms if opioids are not given during labor and delivery; their neonates may also experience withdrawal. Cocaine intoxication can lead to abruptio placenta and severe hypertension.
- Fetal conditions complicating pregnancy include prematurity, postmaturity, multiple gestations, abnormal presentations, and cord prolapse.
- Anesthesia for surgery during pregnancy should optimize the uterine environment by maintaining normal maternal oxygenation, ventilation, and cardiac output. Monitoring of the FHR should be performed whenever feasible.

KEY REFERENCES

Archer GW Jr, Marx GF: Arterial oxygen tension during apnoea in parturient women, *Br J Anaesth* 46:358, 1974.

Chestnut DH, Owen CL, Bates JN, et al: Continuous infusion epidural analgesia during labor: a randomized, double-blind comparison of 0.0625% bupivacaine 0.0002% fentanyl versus 0.125% bupivacaine, *Anesthesiology* 68:754, 1988.

Endler GC, Mariona FG, Sokol RJ, et al: Anesthesia-related maternal mortality in Michigan, 1972 to 1984, *Am J Obstet Gynecol* 159:187, 1988.

Eng M, Berges PU, Ueland K, et al: The effects of methoxamine and ephedrine in normotensive pregnant primates, *Anesthesiology* 35:354, 1971.

Kerr MG, Scott DB, Samuel E: Studies of the inferior vena cava in late pregnancy, *Br Med J* 1:532, 1964.

Lees MM, Taylor SH, Scott DB, et al: A study of cardiac output at rest throughout pregnancy, *J Obstet Gynaecol Br Commonw* 74:319, 1967.

Leighton BL, DeSimone CA, Norris MC, et al: Intrathecal narcotics for labor revisited: the combination of fentanyl and morphine intrathecally provides rapid oset of profound analgesia, *Anesth Analg* 69:122, 1989.

Newsome LR, Bramwell RS, Curling PE: Severe preeclampsia: hemodynamic effects of lumbar epidural anesthesia, *Anesth Analg* 65:31, 1986.

Rocke DA, Murray WB, Rout CC, et al: Relative risk analysis of factors associated with difficult intubation in obstetric anesthesia, *Anesthesiology* 77:67, 1992.

Ueland K, Hansen JM: Maternal cardiovascular dynamics II. Posture and uterine contractions, *Am J Obstet Gynecol* 103:1, 1969.

REFERENCES

1. Abboud T, Raya J, Sadri S, et al: Fetal and maternal cardiovascular effects of atropine and glycopyrrolate, *Anesth Analg* 62:426, 1983.
2. Abboud TK, Khoo SS, Miller F, et al: Maternal, fetal, and neonatal responses after epidural anesthesia with bupivacaine, 2-chloroprocaine, or lidocaine, *Anesth Analg* 61:638, 1982.
3. Abboud TK, Shnider SM, Dailey PA, et al: Intrathecal administration of hyperbaric morphine for the relief of pain in labor, *Br J Anaesth* 56:1351, 1984.
4. Abdul-Karim RW, Chevli RN: Antepartum hemorrhage and shock, *Clin Obstet Gynecol* 19:533, 1976.
5. Abouleish A, Abouleish E, Camann W: Combined spinal-epidural analgesia in advanced labour, *Can J Anaesth* 41:575, 1994.
6. Abouleish E: Hypertension in a paraplegic parturient, *Anesthesiology* 53:348, 1980.
7. Abouleish E, Rawal N, Decreaseon K, et al: Combined intrathecal morphine and bupivacaine for cesarean section, *Anesth Analg* 67:370, 1988.
8. Abouleish E, Rawal N, Shaw J, et al: Intrathecal morphine 0.2 mg versus epidural bupivacaine 0.125% or their combination: Effects on parturients, *Anesthesiology* 74:711, 1991.
9. Abouleish EI: Epinephrine improves the quality of spinal hyperbaric bupivacaine for cesarean section, *Anesth Analg* 66:395, 1987.
10. Acker D, Sachs BP, Tracey KJ, et al: Abruptio placentae associated with cocaine use, *Am J Obstet Gynecol* 146:220, 1983.
11. Albright GA, Jouppila R, Hollmen AI, et al: Epinephrine does not alter human intervillous blood flow during epidural anesthesia, *Anesthesiology* 54:131, 1981.
12. Amiel-Tison C, Barrier G, Shnider SM, et al: A new neurologic and adaptive capacity scoring system for evaluating obstetric medications in full-term newborns, *Anesthesiology* 56:340, 1982.
13. Apgar V: A proposal for a new method of evaluation of the newborn infant, *Anesth Analg* 32:260, 1953.
14. Archer Jr GW, Marx GF: Arterial oxygen tension during apnoea in parturient women, *Br J Anaesth* 46:358, 1974.
15. Asling JH, Shnider SM, Margolis AJ, et al: Paracervical block anesthesia in obstetrics. II. Etiology of fetal bradycardia following paracervical block anesthesia, *Am J Obstet Gynecol* 107:626, 1970.
16. Bader AM, Hunt CO, Datta S, et al: Anesthesia for the obstetric patient with multiple sclerosis, *J Clin Anesth* 1:21, 1988.
17. Bamford C, Sibley W, Laguna J: Anesthesia in multiple sclerosis, *Can J Neurol Sci* 5:41, 1978.
18. Baraka A, Maktabi M, Noueihid R: Epidural meperidine-bupivacaine for obstetric analgesia, *Anesth Analg* 61:652, 1982.
19. Baraka A, Noueihid R, Hajj S: Intrathecal injection of morphine for obstetric analgesia, *Anesthesiology* 54:136, 1981.
20. Barrett JM, Boehm FH, Vaughn WK: The effect of type of delivery on neonatal outcome in singleton infants of birth weight of 1,000 g or less, *JAMA* 250:625, 1983.
21. Benedetti TJ: Maternal complications of parenteral B-sympathomimetic therapy for premature labor, *Am J Obstet Gynecol* 145:1, 1983.
22. Benedetti TJ, Hargrove JC, Rosene KA: Maternal pulmonary edema during premature labor inhibition, *Obstet Gynecol* 59:335, 1982.
23. Benumof JL: Laryngeal mask airway and the ASA difficult airway algorithm, *Anesthesiology* 84:686, 1996.
24. Bevan DR, Holdcroft A, Loh L, et al: Closing volume and pregnancy, *Br Med J* 1:13, 1974.
25. Blitt CD, Petty WC, Alberternst EE, et al: Correlation of plasma cholinesterase activity and duration of action of succinylcholine during pregnancy, *Anesth Analg* 56:78, 1977.
26. Brazelton TB: Effect of prenatal drugs on the behavior of the neonate, *Am J Psychiatry* 126:1261, 1970.
27. Brazelton TB: *Neonatal behavioral assessment scale,* Philadelphia, 1973, JB Lippincott.
28. Breen TW, Ransil BJ, Groves PA, et al: Factors associated with back pain after childbirth, *Anesthesiology* 81:29, 1994.
29. Bromage PR: Continuous lumbar epidural analgesia for obstetrics, *Can Med Assoc J* 85:1136, 1961.
30. Brose WG, Cohen SE: Epidural lidocaine for cesarean section: Effect of varying epinephrine concentration, *Anesthesiology* 69:936, 1988.
31. Brown WU, Bell GC, Alper MH: Acidosis, local anesthetics, and the newborn, *Obstet Gynecol* 48:27, 1976.
32. Brownridge P, Plummer J, Mitchell J, et al: An evaluation of epidural bupivacaine with and without meperidine in labor, *Reg Anesth* 17:15, 1992.
33. Burt RA: The fetal and maternal pharmacology of some of the drugs used for the relief of pain in labor, *Br J Anaesth* 43:824, 1971.
34. Busacca M, Gementi P, Gambini E, et al: Neonatal effects of the administration of meperidine and promethazine to the mother in labor, *J Perinat Med* 10:48, 1982.
35. Camann WR, Murray RS, Mushlin PS, et al: Effects of oral caffeine on postdural puncture headache, *Anesth Analg* 70:181, 1990.

36. Capeless EL, Clapp JF: Cardiovascular changes in early phase of pregnancy, *Am J Obstet Gynecol* 161:1449, 1989.
37. Carlson C, Nybell-Lindahl G, Ingemarsson I: Extradural block in patients who have previously undergone caesarean section, *Br J Anaesth* 52:1980.
38. Carrie LES, O'Sullivan GM, Seegobin R: Epidural fentanyl in labor, *Anesthesia* 36:965, 1981.
39. Celleno D, Capogna G: Epidural fentanyl plus bupivacaine 0.125 percent for labour: analgesic effects, *Can J Anaesth* 35:375, 1988.
40. Chadwick HS, Easterling TR: Anesthetic concerns in the patient with preeclampsia, *Semin Perinatol* 15:397, 1991.
41. Chadwick HS, Ready LB: Intrathecal and epidural morphine sulfate for postcesarean analgesia—A clinical comparison, *Anesthesiology* 68:925, 1988.
42. Chan MT, Gin T: Postpartum changes in the minimum alveolar concentration of isoflurane, *Anesthesiology* 82:1360, 1995.
43. Chesnut DH: Fetal distress. In James FM, Wheeler AS, Dewan DM, editors: *Obstetric anesthesia: The complicated patient,* Philadelphia, 1988, FA Davis.
44. Chestnut DH, McGrath JM, Vincent RD, et al: Does early administration of epidural analgesia affect obstetric outcome in nulliparous women who are in spontaneous labor? *Anesthesiology* 80:1201, 1994.
45. Chestnut DH, Owen CL, Bates JN, et al: Continuous infusion epidural analgesia during labor: a randomized, double-blind comparison of 0.0625% bupivacaine 0.0002% fentanyl versus 0.125% bupivacaine, *Anesthesiology* 68:754, 1988.
46. Chestnut DH, Vincent RD, McGrath JM, et al: Does early administration of epidural analgesia affect obstetric outcome in nulliparous women who are receiving intravenous oxytocin? *Anesthesiology* 80:1193, 1994.
47. Chestnut DH, Weiner CP, Martin JG, et al: Effect of intravenous epinephrine on uterine artery blood flow velocity in the pregnant guinea pig, *Anesthesiology* 65:633, 1986.
48. Clark Sl, Gimovsky ML, Miller FC: The scalp stimulation test: a clinical alternative to fetal scalp blood sampling, *Am J Obstet Gynecol* 148:274, 1984.
49. Clark SL, Koonings PP, Phelan JP: Placenta previa/accreta and prior cesarean section, *Obstet Gynecol* 66:89, 1985.
50. Clark SL, Phelan JP, Greenspoon J, et al: Labor and delivery in the presence of mitral stenosis: central hemodynamic observations, *Am J Obstet Gynecol* 152:984, 1985.
51. Cohen SE, Cherry CM, Holbrook RH, et al: Intrathecal sufentanil for labor analgesia—sensory changes, side effects, and fetal heart rate changes, *Anesth Analg* 77:1155, 1993.
52. Cohen SE, Tan S, Albright GA, et al: Epidural fentanyl//bupivacaine mixtures for obstetric analgesia, *Anesthesiology* 67:403, 1987.
53. Cohen WR, Schifrin BS: Diagnosis and management of fetal distress during labor, *Semin Perinatol* 2:155, 1978.
54. Corke BC, Carlson CG, Dettbarn WD: The influence of 2-chloroprocaine on the subsequent analgesic potency of bupivacaine, *Anesthesiology* 60:25, 1984.
55. Corke BC, Datta S, Ostheimer GW, et al: Influence of hypotension during spinal anesthesia during cesarean section on infant outcome, *Anaesthesia* 37:658, 1982.
56. Cotton DB, Gonik B, Dorman KF: Cardiovascular alterations in severe pregnancy-induced hypertension: Acute effects of intravenous magnesium sulfate, *Am J Obstet Gynecol* 148:162, 1984.
57. Covino BG, Vassallo HG: *Local anesthetics: Mechanisms of action and clinical use,* New York, 1976, Grune and Stratton.
58. Crawford JS, James III FM, Nolte H, et al: Regional analgesia for patients with chronic neurological disease and similar conditions, *Anaesthesia* 35:821, 1981.
59. Cree JE, Meyer J, Hailey DM: Diazepam in labour: its metabolism and effect on the clinical condition and thermogenesis of the newborn, *Br Med J* 1973.
60. Crenshaw C, Jones DE, Parker RT: Placenta previa: a survey of twenty years experience with improved perinatal survival by expectant therapy and cesarean delivery, *Obstet Gynecol Surv* 28:461, 1973.
61. Dahm LS, James LS: Newborn temperature and calculated heat loss in the delivery room, *Pediatrics* 49:504, 1972.
62. Dailey PA, Fisher DM, Shnider SM, et al: Pharmacokinetics, placental transfer, and neonatal effects of vecuronium and pancuronium administered during Cesarean section, *Anesthesiology* 60:469, 1984.
63. Dailland P, Cockshott ID, Lirzin JD, et al: Intravenous propofol during Cesarean section: placental transfer, concentrations in breast milk, and neonatal effects. A preliminary study, *Anesthesiology* 71:827, 1989.
64. Datta S, Alper MH, Ostheimer GW, et al: Method of ephedrine administration and nausea and hypotension during spinal anesthesia for cesarean section, *Anesthesiology* 56:68, 1982.
65. Datta S, Brown Jr WU: Acid-base status in diabetic mothers and their infants following general or spinal anesthesia for cesarean section, *Anesthesiology* 47:272, 1977.
66. Datta S, Brown Jr WU, Ostheimer GW, et al: Epidural anesthesia for cesarean section in diabetic parturients: maternal and neonatal acid-base status and bupivacaine concentration, *Anesth Analg* 60:574, 1981.
67. Datta S, Camann W, Bader A, et al: Clinical effects and maternal and fetal plasma concentratons of epidural ropivacaine versus bupivacaine for cesarean section, *Anesthesiology* 82:1346, 1995.
68. Datta S, Corke BC, Alper MH, et al: Epidural anesthesia for cesarean section: a comparison of bupivacaine, chloroprocaine, and etidocaine, *Anesthesiology* 52:48, 1980.
69. Datta S, Kitzmiller JL: Anesthetic and obstetric management of diabetic pregnant women, *Clin Perinatol* 9:153, 1982.
70. Datta S, Lambert DH, Gregus J, et al: Differential sensitivites of mammalian nerve fibers during pregnancy, *Anesth Analg* 62:1070, 1983.
71. Datta S, Migliozzi RP, Flanagan HL, et al: Chronically administered progesterone decreases halothane requirements in rabbits, *Anesth Analg* 68:46, 1989.
72. Datta S, Ostheimer GW, Weiss JB, et al: Neonatal effect of prolonged anesthetic induction for cesarean section, *Obstet Gynecol* 58:331, 1981.
73. Dawkins CJM: An analysis of the complications of extradural and caudal block, *Anaesthesia* 24:554, 1969.
74. DiGiovanni AJ, Galbert MW, Wahle WM: Epidural injection of autologous blood for postlumbar-puncture headache II. Additional clinical experiences and laboratory investigation, *Anesth Analg* 51:226, 1972.
75. Dignam WJ, Titus P, Assali NS: Renal function in human pregnancy. I. Changes in glomerular filtration rate and renal plasma flow, *Proc Soc Exp Biol Med* 97:512, 1958.
76. Dogu TS: Continuous caudal analgesia and anesthesia for labor and vaginal delivery. A review of 4071 confinements, *Obstet Gynecol* 33:92, 1969.
77. Duncan PG, Pope WD, Cohen MM, et al: Fetal risk of anesthesia and surgery during pregnancy, *Anesthesiology* 64:790, 1986.
78. Easterling TR, Chadwick HS, Otto CM, et al: Aortic stenosis in pregnancy, *Obstet Gynecol* 72:113, 1988.
79. Eisele JH, Wright R, Rogge P: Newborn and maternal fentanyl levels at cesarean section, *Anesth Analg* 61:179, 1982.
80. Endler GC, Mariona FG, Sokol RJ, et al: Anesthesia-related maternal mortality in Michigan, 1972 to 1984, *Am J Obstet Gynecol* 159:187, 1988.
81. Eng M, Berges PU, Ueland K, et al: The effects of methoxamine and ephedrine in normotensive pregnant primates, *Anesthesiology* 35:354, 1971.
82. Finster M, Morishima HO, Mark LC, et al: Tissue thiopental concetntrations in the fetus and newborn, *Anesthesiology* 336: 55, 1972.
83. Finster M, Poppers PJ, Sinclair JC: Accidental intoxication of the fetus with local anesthetic drug during caudal anesthesia, *Am J Obstet Gynecol* 92:922, 1965.
84. Fishburne Jr JI, Brenner WE, Braaksma JT, et al: Cardiovascular and respiratory responses to intravenous infusion of prostaglandin F2α in the pregnant woman, *Am J Obstet Gynecol* 114:765, 1972.
85. Fishburne JI, Greiss FC, Hopkinson R, et al: Responses of the gravid uterine vasculature to arterial levels of local anesthetic agents, *Am J Obstet Gynecol* 133:753, 1979.
86. Frank M, McAteer EJ, Cattermole R, et al: Nalbuphine for obstetric analgesia—a comparison of nalbuphine with pethidine for pain relief in labour when administered by patient-controlled analgesia (PCA), *Anaesthesia* 42:697, 1987.
87. Freeman RK, Caribe TJ: *Fetal heart rate monitoring,* Baltimore, 1989, Williams & Wilkins.
88. Gabbe SG: Congenital malformations in infants of diabetic mothers, *Obstet Gynecol Surv* 32:125, 1977.
89. Gabbe SG, Mestman JH, Freeman RK, et al: Management and outcome of pregnancy in diabtes mellitus, classes B to R, *Am J Obstet Gynecol* 129:723, 1977.
90. Garbaciak JA, Richter M, Miller S, et al:

Maternal weight and pregnancy complications, *Obstet Gynecol* 152:238, 1985.

91. Ghoneim MM, Long JP: The interaction between magnesium and other neuromuscular blocking agents, *Anesthesiology* 32:23, 1970.
92. Gibbs CP, Schwartz DJ, Wynne JW, et al: Antacid pulmonary aspiration in the dog, *Anesthesiology* 51:380, 1979.
93. Gin T, Chan MT: Decreased minimum alveolar concentration of isoflurane in pregnant humans, *Anesthesiology* 80:71, 1994.
94. Glosten B: Obesity and obstetric anesthesia, *Semin Anesthesiol* 11:43, 1992.
95. Gottesfeld KR: Managing the placental abruption, *Contemp Obstet Gynecol* 22:20, 1983.
96. Gregory MA, Davidson DG: Plasma etomidate levels in mother and fetus, *Anaesthesia* 46:716, 1991.
97. Grice SC, Eisenach JC, Dewan DM: Labor analgesia with epidural bupivacaine plus fentanyl: Enhancement with epinephrine and inhibition with 2-chloroprocaine, *Anesthesiology* 72:623, 1990.
98. Halpern S: Postdural puncture headache and spinal needle design, *Anesthesiology* 81:1376, 1994.
99. Hansen JM, Ueland K: The influence of caudal analgesia on cardiovascular dynamics during normal labor and delivery, *Acta Anaesthesiol Scand Suppl* 23:449, 1966.
100. Harrison DM, Sinatra R, Morgese L, et al: Epidural narcotic and patient-controlled analgesia for post-cesarean section pain relief, *Anesthesiology* 68:454, 1988.
101. Hart DM: Heartburn in pregnancy, *J Int Med Res* 1:1, 1978.
102. Hawkins JL, Gibbs CP, Orleans M, et al: Obstetric anesthesia workforce survey—1992 versus 1981 (abstract), *Anesthesiology* 81:A1128, 1994.
103. Hayashi RH, Castillo MS, Noah M: Management of severe postpartum hemorrhage with a prostaglandin F2 alpha analogue, *Obstet Gynecol* 63:806, 1984.
104. Hellman LM, Johnson HL, Tolles WE, et al: Some factors affecting the fetal heart rate, *Am J Obstet Gynecol* 82:1055, 1961.
105. Hendricks CH: Hemodynamics of a uterine contraction, *Am J Obstet Gynecol* 76:968, 1958.
106. Herman NL: The placenta: anatomy, physiology, and transfer of drugs, In Chestnut DH editor: *Obstetric Anesthesia—principles and practice,* New York, 1994, Mosby–Year Book.
107. Hibbard BM, Rosen M: The management of severe pre-eclampsia and eclampsia, *Br J Anaesth* 49:3, 1977.
108. Hibbard LT: Maternal mortality due to acute toxemia, *Obstet Gynecol* 42:263, 1973.
109. Hicks JA, Jenkins JG, Newton MC, et al: Continuous epidural infusion of 0.075% bupivacaine for pain relief in labour, *Anaesthesia* 43:289, 1988.
110. Hodgkinson R, Glassenberg R, Joyce THI, et al: Comparison of cimetidine (Tagamet®) with antacid for safety and effectiveness in reducing gastric acidity before elective cesarean section, *Anesthesiology* 59:86, 1983.
111. Hodgkinson R, Husain FJ, Hayashi RH: Systemic and pulmonary blood pressure during caesarean section in parturients with gestational hypertension, *Can Anaesth Soc J* 27:389, 1980.
112. Honet JE, Arkoosh VA, Norris MC, et al: Comparison among intrathecal fentanyl, meperidine, and sufentanil for labor analgesia, *Anesth Analg* 75:734, 1992.
113. Hood DD, Dewan DM, Kashtan K: Anesthesia outcome in the morbidly obese parturient, *Anesthesiology* 73:A952, 1990.
114. Hughes SC, Rosen MA, Shnider SM, et al: Maternal and neonatal effects of epidural morphine for labor and delivery, *Anesth Analg* 63:319, 1984.
115. Hunt CO, Naulty JS, Bader AM, et al: Perioperative analgesia with subarachnoid fentanyl-bupivacaine for cesarean delivery, *Anesthesiology* 71:535, 1989.
116. Irestedt L: Current status of nitrous oxide for obstetric pain relief, *Acta Anaesthesiol Scand* 38:771, 1994.
117. James FM, Crawford JS, Hopkinson R, et al: A comparison of general anesthesia and lumbar epidural analgesia for elective cesarean section, *Anesth Analg* 56:228, 1977.
118. Janeczko GF, el-Etr AA, Younes S: Low-dose ketamine anesthesia for obstetrical delivery, *Anesth Analg* 53:828, 1974.
119. Johnson WL, Winter WW, Eng M, et al: Effect of pudendal, spinal, and peridural block anesthesia on the second stage of labor, *Am J Obstet Gynecol* 113:166, 1972.
120. Jones CJP, Fox H: Placental changes in gestational diabetes—an ultrastructural study, *Obstet Gynecol* 48:274, 1976.
121. Jouppila P, Jouppila R, Barinoff T, et al: Placental blood flow during caesarean section performed under subarachnoid blockade, *Br J Anaesth* 56:1379, 1984.
122. Jouppila P, Kirkinen P, Koivula A, et al: Labetalol does not alter the placental and fetal blood flow or maternal prostanoids in pre-eclampsia, *Br J Obstet Gynaecol* 93:543, 1986.
123. Jouppila R, Jouppila P, Kuikka J, et al: Placental blood flow during caesarean section under lumbar extradural analgesia, *Br J Anaesth* 50:2275, 1978.
124. Justins DM, Francis D, Houlton PG, et al: A controlled trial of extradural fentanyl in labour, *Br J Anaesth* 54:409, 1982.
125. Kallos T, Caruso FS: Respiratory effects of butorphanol and pethidine, *Anaesthesia* 34:633, 1979.
126. Kamban JR, Handte RE, Brown WR, et al: Effect of pregnancy on oxygen dissociation, *Anesthesiology* 59:A395, 1983.
127. Katz VL, Thorp Jr JM, Cefalo RC: Epidural analgesia and autonomic hyperreflexia: a case report, *Am J Obstet Gynecol* 162:471, 1990.
128. Kelton JG, Hunter DJ, Neame PB: A platelet function defect in preeclampsia, *Obstet Gynecol* 65:107, 1985.
129. Kemp BE, Niall HO: Relaxin, *Vitam Horm* 41:79, 1985.
130. Kerr MG, Scott DB, Samuel E: Studies of the inferior vena cava in late pregnancy, *Br Med J* 1:532, 1964.
131. King H, Ashley S, Brathwaite D, et al: Adequacy of general anesthesia for cesarean section, *Anesth Analg* 77:84, 1993.
132. Koch G, Wendel H: Adjustment of arterial blood gases and acid base balance in the normal newborn infant during the first week of life, *Biol Neonat* 12:136, 1968.
133. Koch-Weser J, Schulze-Delrieu K: Drug therapy—metoclopramide, *N Engl J Med* 305:28, 1981.
134. Kuhnert BR, Linn PL, Kennard MJ, et al: Effects of low doses of meperdine on neonatal behavior, *Anesth Analg* 64:335, 1985.
135. Lamaze F: *Painless childbirth: psychprophylactic method,* London, 1958, Burke.
136. Lederman RP, Legerman E, Work B, et al: Anxiety and epinephrine in multiparous women in labor: Relationship to duration of labor and fetal heart rate pattern, *Am J Obstet Gynecol* 153:870, 1985.
137. Lees MM, Scott DB, Kerr MG, et al: The circulatory effects of recumbent postural change in late pregnancy, *Clin Sci* 32:453, 1967.
138. Lees MM, Taylor SH, Scott DB, et al: A study of cardiac output at rest throughout pregnancy, *J Obstet Gynaecol Br Commonw* 74:319, 1967.
139. Leighton BL, DeSimone CA, Norris MC, et al: Intrathecal narcotics for labor revisited: the combination of fentanyl and morphine intrathecally provides rapid oset of profound analgesia, *Anesth Analg* 69:122, 1989.
140. Leighton BL, Gross JB: Air: an effective indicator of intravenously located epidural catheters, *Anesthesiology* 71:848, 1989.
141. Leighton BL, Norris MC, Sosis M, et al: Limitations of epinephrine as a marker of intravascular injection in laboring women, *Anesthesiology* 66:688, 1987.
142. Levinson G, Shnider SM, deLorimier AA, et al: Effects of maternal hyperventilation on uterine blood flow and fetal oxygenation and acid-base status, *Anesthesiology* 40:340, 1974.
143. Li DF, Rees GAD, Rosen M: Continuous extradural infusion of 0.0625% or 0.125% bupivacaine for pain relief in primigravid labour, *Br J Anaesth* 57:264, 1985.
144. Lin CC, Lindheimer MD, River P, et al: Fetal outcome in hypertensive disorders of pregnancy, *Am J Obstet Gynecol* 142:255, 1982.
145. Linder N, Aranda JV, Tsur M, et al: Need for endotracheal intubation and suction in meconium-stained neonates, *J Pediatr* 112:613, 1988.
146. Little B, Chang T, Chucot L, et al: Study of ketamine as an obstetric anesthetic agent, *Am J Obstet Gynecol* 113:247, 1972.
147. Lucas MJ, Leveno KJ, Cunningham FG: A comparison of magnesium sulfate with phenytoin for the prevention of eclampsia, *N Engl J Med* 333:201, 1995.
148. Lunan CB: The management of abruptio placentae, *J Obstet Gynaecol Br Commonw* 80:120, 1973.
149. Mabie WC, Ratts TE, Sibai BM: The central hemodynamics of severe preeclampsia, *Am J Obstet Gynecol* 161:1443, 1989.
150. Maduska AL, Hajghassemali M: A double-blind comparison of butorphanol and meperdine in labour: maternal pain relief and effect on the newborn, *Can Anaesth Soc J* 25:398, 1978.
151. Malaisse WJ, Malaisse-Lagae F, Picard C, et al: Effects of pregnancy and chorionic growth hormone upon insulin secretion, *Endocrinology* 84:41, 1969.

152. Manning FA, Platt LD, Sipos L: Antepartum fetal evaluation: development of a fetal biophysical profile, *Am J Obstet Gynecol* 136:787, 1980.
153. Marcus FI, Ewy GA, O'Rourke RA, et al: The effect of pregnancy on the murmurs of mitral and aortic regurgitation, *Circulation* 41:795, 1970.
154. Marx GF: Cardiopulmonary resuscitation of late-pregnant women (letter), 56:156, 1982.
155. Marx GF, Joshi CW, Orkin LR: Placental transmission of nitrous oxide, *Anesthesiology* 2:429, 1970.
156. Mashini IS, Albazzaz SJ, Fadel HE, et al: Serial noninvasive evaluation of cardiovascular hemodynamics during pregnancy, *Am J Obstet Gynecol* 156:1208, 1987.
157. Mather LE, Tucker GT, Murphy TM, et al: The effects of adding adrenaline to etidocaine and lignocaine in extradural anaesthesia II: pharmacokinetics, *Br J Anaesth* 48:989, 1976.
158. Matouskova A, Dottori O, Forssman L, et al: An improved method of epidural analgesia with reduced instrumental delivery rate, *Acta Obstet Gynecol Scand* 83:9, 1979.
159. May AE: Editorial—the Confidential Enquiry into Maternal Deaths 1988–1990, *Br J Anaesth* 73:129, 1994.
160. Mayer DC, Spielman FJ: Antepartum and postpartum hemorrhage. In Chestnut DH editor: *Obstetric anesthesia,* St. Louis, 1994, Mosby–Year Book.
161. Mazze RI, Fujinaga M, Rice SA, et al: Reproductive and teratogenic effects of nitrous oxide, halothane, isoflurane, and enflurane in Sprague-Dawley rats, *Anesthesiology* 64:339, 1986.
162. Mazze RI, Kallen B: Reproductive outcome after anesthesia and operation during pregnancy: a registry study of 5405 cases, *Am J Obstet Gynecol* 161:1178, 1989.
163. McNair RD, Jaynes RV: Alterations in liver function during normal pregnancy, *Am J Obstet Gynecol* 80:500, 1960.
164. Merkow AJ, McGuinness GA, Erenberg A, et al: The neonatal neurobehavioral effects of bupivacaine, mepivacaine, and 2-chloroprocaine used for pudendal block, *Anesthesiology* 52:309, 1980.
165. Meyer MB, Tonascia JA: Maternal smoking, pregnancy complications, and perinatal mortality, *Am J Obstet Gynecol* 128: 494, 1977.
166. Mihic DN: Postspinal headache and relationship of needle bevel to longitudinal dural fibers, *Reg Anesth* 10:76, 1985.
167. Milaszkiewicz R, Payne N, Loughnan B, et al: Continuous extradural infusion of lignocaine 0.75% vs bupivacaine 0.125% in primiparae: quality of analgesia and influence on labour, *Anaesthesia* 47:1042, 1992.
168. Mirkin BL: Perinatal pharmacology: placental transfer, fetal localization, and neonatal disposition of drugs, *Anesthesiology* 43:156, 1975.
169. Moir DD, Davidson S: Postpartum complications of forceps delivery performed under epidural and pudenal nerve block, *Br J Anaesth* 44:1197, 1972.
170. Moore TR, Sorg J, Miller L, et al: Hemodynamic effects of intravenous cocaine on the pregnant ewe and fetus, *Am J Obstet Gynecol* 155:883, 1986.
171. Moran DH, Perillo M, LaPorta RF, et al: Phenylephrine in the prevention of hypotension following spinal anesthesia for cesarean delivery, *J Clin Anesth* 3:301, 1991.
172. Morgan DJ, Blackman GL, Paull JD, et al: Pharmacokinetics and plasma binding of thiopental. II: Studies at Cesarean section, *Anesthesiology* 54:474, 1981.
173. Morgan HS, Kane SH: An analysis of 16,327 breech births, *JAMA* 187:262, 1964.
174. Morgan M: Anaesthetic contribution to maternal mortality, *Br J Anaesth* 59:842, 1987.
175. Morrison JC, Whybrew WD, Rosser SI, et al: Metabolites of meperidine in the fetal and maternal serum, *Am J Obstet Gynecol* 126:997, 1976.
176. Motoyama EK, Rivard G, Acheson F, et al: Adverse effect of maternal hyperventilation on the foetus, *Lancet* 1:286, 1966.
177. Munson ES, Embro WJ: Enflurane, isoflurane, and halothane and isolated human uterine muscle, *Anesthesiology* 46:11, 1977.
178. Neerhof MG, MacGregor SN, Retzky SS, et al: Cocaine abuse during pregnancy: peripartum prevalence and perinatal outcome, *Am J Obstet Gynecol* 161:633, 1989.
179. Newsome LR, Bramwell RS, Curling PE: Severe preeclampsia: hemodynamic effects of lumbar epidural anesthesia, *Anesth Analg* 65:31, 1986.
180. Norris MC: Height, weight, and the spread of subarachnoid hyperbaric bupivacaine the the term parturient, *Anesth Analg* 67:555, 1988.
181. Norris MC: Patient variables and the subarachnoid spread of hyperbaric bupivacaine in the term parturient, *Anesthesiology* 72:478, 1990.
182. Norris MC, Arkoosh VA: Spinal opioid analgesia for labor, *Int Anesthesiol Clin* 32:69, 1994.
183. Norris MC, Dewan DM: Preoxygenation for cesarean section: a comparison of two techniques, *Anesthesiology* 62:827, 1985.
184. Ohno H, Watanabe M, Saitoh J, et al: Effect of epinephrine concentration on lidocaine disposition during epidural anesthesia, *Anesthesiology* 68:625, 1988.
185. Ong BY, Cohen MM, Palahniuk RJ: Anesthesia for cesarean section—effects on neonates, *Anesth Analg* 68:270, 1989.
186. Palahniuk RJ, Shnider SM, Eger EI, II: Pregnancy decreases the requirement for inhaled anesthetic agents, *Anesthesiology* 41:82, 1974.
187. Pavlin DJ: Anesthetic implications of advances in surgical technology, *Anesthesiol Clin North Am* 1996, in press.
188. Philipsen T, Jensen N-H: Maternal opinion about analgesia in labour and delivery. A comparison of epidural blockade and intramuscular pethidine, *Eur J Obstet Gynecol Reprod Biol* 34:205, 1990.
189. Philipson EH, Kuhnert BR, Syracuse CD: Fetal acidosis, 2-chloroprocaine, and epidural anesthesia for cesarean section, *Am J Obstet Gynecol* 151:322, 1985.
190. Phillips OC, Ebner H, Nelson AT, et al: Neurologic complications following spinal anesthesia with lidocaine: a prospective review of 10,440 cases, *Anesthesiology* 30:284, 1969.
191. Podlas J, Breland BD: Patient-controlled analgesia with nalbuphine during labor, *Obstet Gynecol* 70:203, 1987.
192. Pollack KL, Chestnut DH, Wenstrom KD: Anesthetic management of a parturient with Eeisenmenger's syndrome, *Anesth Analg* 70:212, 1990.
193. Power KJ, Avery AF: Extradural analgesia in the intrapartum management of a patient with pulmonary hypertension, *Br J Anaesth* 63:116, 1989.
194. Preston PG, Rosen MA, Hughes SC, et al: Epidural anesthesia with fentanyl and lidocaine for cesarean section: maternal effects and neonatal outcome, *Anesthesiology* 68:938, 1988.
195. Pritchard JA: Changes in blood volume during pregnancy and delivery, *Anesthesiology* 26:393, 1965.
196. Prowse CM, Gaensler EA: Respiratory and acid-base changes during pregnancy, *Anesthesiology* 26:381, 1965.
197. Quilligan EJ, Keegan KA, Donahue MJ: Double-blind comparison of intravenously injected butorphanol and meperidine in parturients, *Int J Gynaecol Obstet* 18:363, 1980.
198. Ramanathan S, Grant GJ: Vasopressor therapy for hypotension due to epidural anesthesia for cesarean section, *Acta Anaesthesiol Scand* 32:559, 1988.
199. Ramanathan S, Sheth R, Turndorf H: Anesthesia for cesarean section in patients with genital herpes infections: a retrospective study, *Anesthesiology* 64:807, 1986.
200. Rasmus KT, Rottman RL, Kotelko DM, et al: Unrecognized thrombocytopenia and regional anesthesia in parturients: a retrospective review, *Obstet Gynecol* 73:943, 1989.
201. Rayburn W, Rathke A, Leuschen P, et al: Fetanyl citrate analgesia during labor, *Am J Obstet Gynecol* 161:202, 1989.
202. Ready LB, Loper KA, Nessly M, et al: Postoperative epidural morphine is safe on surgical wards, *Anesthesiology* 75:452, 1991.
203. Ready LB, Oden R, Chadwick HS, et al: Development of an anesthesiology-based postoperative pain management service, *Anesthesiology* 68:100, 1988.
204. Riley ET, Cohen SE, Macario A, et al: Spinal versus epidural anesthesia for cesarean section: a comparison of time efficiency, costs, charges, and complications, *Anesth Analg* 80:709, 1995.
205. Roberts RB, Shirley MA: Reducing the risk of acid aspiration during cesarean section, *Anesth Analg* 53:859, 1974.
206. Rocke DA, Murray WB, Rout CC, et al: Relative risk analysis of factors associated with difficult intubation in obstetric anesthesia, *Anesthesiology* 77:67, 1992.
207. Romagnoli A, Keats AS: Ceiling effect for respiratory depression by nalbuphine, *Clin Pharmacol Ther* 27:478, 1980.
208. Rosaeg OP, Kitts JB, Koren G, et al: Maternal and fetal effects of intravenous patient-controlled fentanyl analgesia during labour in a thrombocytopenic partuient, *Can J Anaesth* 39:277, 1992.
209. Rosen MA, Foizen MF, Eger EI, et al: The effect of nitrous oxide on *in vitro* fertiliza-

tion success rate, *Anesthesiology* 67:42, 1987.

210. Ross BK: Opioid Techniques. In Chestnut D editor: *Obstetric anesthesia—Principles and practices,* New York, 1994, Mosby–Year Book.
211. Rout CC, Rocke DA, Gouws E: Intravenous ranitidine reduces the risk of acid aspiration of gastric contents at emergency cesarean section, *Anesth Analg* 76:156, 1993.
212. Rudolph AM: The changes in the circulation after birth. Their importance in congenital heart disease, *Circulation* 41:343, 1970.
213. Rush RW, Davey DA, Segall ML: The effect of preterm delivery on perinatal mortality, *Br J Obstet Gynaecol* 85:806, 1978.
214. Russell R, Reynolds F: Epidural infusions for nulliparous women in labour, *Anaes–thesia* 48:856, 1993.
215. Safra MJ, Oakley GP: Association between cleft lip with or without cleft palate and prenatal exposure to diazepam, *Lancet* 478, 1975.
216. Santos AC, Arthur GR, Roberts DJ, et al: Effect of ropivacaine and bupivacaine on uterine blood flow in pregnant ewes, *Anesth Analg* 74:62, 1992.
217. Scanlon JW, Brown Jr WJ, Weiss JB, et al: Neurobehavioral responses of newborn infants after maternal epidural anesthesia, *Anesthesiology* 40:121, 1974.
218. Schrier RW, Lieberman R, Ufferman RC: Mechanism of antidiuretic effect of beta adrenergic stimulation, *J Clin Invest* 51:97, 1972.
219. Scott JS: Obstetric analgesia. A consideration of labor pain and a patient-controlled technique for its relief with meperidine, *Am J Obstet Gynecol* 106:959, 1970.
220. Shier RW, Sprague AD, Diltsm PV: Placental transfer of meperidine HCl. Part II, *Am J Obstet Gynecol* 115:556, 1973.
221. Shnider SM, Abboud TK, Artal R, et al: Maternal catetcholamines decrease during labor after lumbar epidural anesthesia, *Am J Obstet Gynecol* 147:13, 1983.
222. Shnider SM, Moya F: Effects of meperidine on the newborn infant, *Am J Obstet Gynecol* 89:1009, 1964.
223. Shnider SM, Way EL: Plasma levels of lidocaine (Xylocaine®) in mother and newborn following obstetrical conduction anesthesia: clinical applications, *Anes–thesiology* 29:951, 1968.
224. Skaredoff MN, Ostheimer GW: Phys–iologic changes during pregnancy: effects of major regional anesthesia, *Reg Anesth* 6:28, 1981.
225. Smith BE, Hehre FW, Hess OW: Convulsions associated with anesthetic agents during labor and delivery, *Anesth Analg* 43:476, 1964.
226. Spielman FJ, Herbert WNP: Maternal cardiovascular effects of drugs that alter uterine activity, *Obstet Gynecol Surv* 43:516, 1988.
227. Spinnato JA, Kraynack BJ, Cooper MW: Eisenmenger's syndrome in pregnancy: epidural anesthesia for elective cesarean section, *N Engl J Med* 304:1215, 1981.
228. Stafford RS: Alternative strategies for controlling rising Cesarean section rates, *JAMA* 263:683, 1990.
229. Steinberg RB, Powell G, Hu X, et al: Epidural sufentanil for analgesia for labor and delivery, *Reg Anesth* 14:225, 1989.
230. Studd JWW, Crawford JS, Duignan NM, et al: The effect of lumbar epidural analgesia on the rate of cervical dilatation and the outcome of labour of spontaneous onset, *Br J Obstet Gynaecol* 87:1015, 1980.
231. Tannenbaum TN, Goldberg RJ: Exposure to anesthetic gases and reproductive outcome, *J Occup Med* 27:659, 1985.
232. Teramo K, Benowitz N, Heymann MA, et al: Gestational differences in lidocaine toxicity in the fetal lamb, *Anesthesiology* 2:133, 1976.
233. Thorp JA, Hu DH, Albin RM, et al: The effect of intrapartum epidural analgesia on nulliparous labor: A randomized, controlled, prospective trial, *Am J Obstet Gynecol* 169:851, 1993.
234. Ting P, Brady JP: Tracheal suction in meconium aspiration, *Am J Obstet Gynecol* 122:767, 1975.
235. Tronick E: A critique of the neonatal Neurologic and Adaptive Capacity Score (NACS), *Anesthesiology* 56:338, 1982.
236. Ueland K, Hansen JM: Maternal cardiovascular dynamics II. Posture and uterine contractions, *Am J Obstet Gynecol* 103:1, 1969.
237. Ueland K: Maternal cardiovascular dynamics. VII. Intrapartum blood volume changes, *Am J Obstet Gynecol* 126:671, 1976.
238. Uppington J: Epidural analgesia and previous caesarean section, *Anesthesia* 38:336, 1983.
239. Usubiaga JE, Wikinski J, Ferrero R, et al: Local anesthetic-induced convulsions in man—an electroencephalographic study, *Anesth Analg* 45:611, 1966.
240. Valenzuela G, Cline S: Use of magnesium sulfate in premature labor that fails to respond to beta-mimetic drugs, *Am J Obstet Gynecol* 143:718, 1982.
241. Vaughan RW, Bauer S, Wise L: Volume and pH of gastric juice in obese patients, *Anesthesiology* 43:686, 1975.
242. Vertommen JD, Marcus MAE, Van Aken H: The effects of intravenous and epidural sufentanil in the chronic maternal-fetal sheep preparation, *Anesth Analg* 80:71, 1995.
243. Vertommen JD, Vandermeulen E, Van Aken H, et al: The effects of the addition of sufentanil to 0.125% bupivacaine on the quality of analgesia during labor and on the incidence of instrumental deliveries, *Anesthesiology* 74:809, 1991.
244. Vincent RD, Syrop CH, Van Voorhis BJ, et al: An evaluation of the effect of anesthetic technique on reproductive success after laparoscopic pronuclear stage transfer, *Anesthesiology* 82:352, 1995.
245. Viscomi CM, Hood DD, Melone PJ, et al: Fetal heart rate variability after epidural fentanyl during labor, *Anesth Analg* 71:679, 1990.
246. Vyas H, Milner AD, Hopkin IE: Intra–thoracic pressure and volume changes during the spontaneous onset of respiration in babies born by cesarean section and by vaginal delivery, *J Pediatr* 99:787, 1981.
247. Walsh SW: Preeclampsia: an imbalance in placental prostacyclin and thromboxane production, *Am J Obstet Gynecol* 152:335, 1985.
248. Warren TM, Datta S, Ostheimer GW, et al: Comparison of the maternal and neonatal effects of halothane, enflurane, and isoflurane for cesarean delivery, *Anesth Analg* 62:516, 1983.
249. Watson DW, Downey GO: Epidural anesthesia for labor and delivery of twins of a paraplegic mother, *Anesthesiology* 52:259, 1980.
250. Watson P, Besch N, Bowes WA: Management of acute and subacute puerperal inversion of the uterus, *Obstet Gynecol* 55:12, 1980.
251. Way WL, Costley EC, Way EL: Respiratory sensitivity of the newborn infant to meperidine and morphine, *Clin Pharmacol Ther* 6:454, 1965.
252. Wheeler AS, Harris EA: The uterus, placenta, and fetus, *Semin Anesthesiol* 1:101, 1982.
253. Williams DA: Asthma and pregnancy, *Acta Allerg* 22:311, 1967.
254. Wuitchik M, Bakal D, Lipshitz J: The clinical significance of pain and cognitive activity in latent labor, *Obstet Gynecol* 73:35, 1989.
255. Zagorzycki MT, Brinkman CR: The effect of general and epidural anesthesia upon neonatal Apgar scores in repeat cesarean section, *Surg Gynecol Obstet* 155:641, 1982.
256. Zinaman M, Rubin J, Lindheimer MD: Serial plasma oncotic pressure levels and echoencephalography during and after delivery in severe pre-eclampsia, *Lancet* 1:1245, 1985.

CHAPTER 77

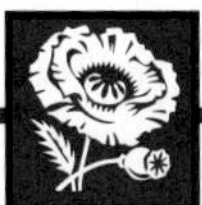

Anesthesia for Gynecologic Surgery

JOSEPH M. GARFIELD
MICHAEL G. MUTO
MARINA D. BIZZARRI-SCHMID

To provide maximum useful information to the reader, we have divided the field of gynecologic surgery into specific areas. One theme stressed throughout the chapter is to include, wherever possible, a description of the surgical anatomy of the region and the basis and rationale for the representative surgical procedures discussed. By providing this background, we communicate a basic understanding of the surgeon's goals and needs and thereby allow anesthesia providers to administer better and more rational anesthetics. We also discuss pertinent physiologic and pharmacologic aspects of anesthetic management, culminating in a discussion of appropriate anesthetic techniques with an emphasis on practical information. We have also included selected references for those interested in pursuing a particular topic in greater depth.

PSYCHOLOGIC OVERVIEW OF GYNECOLOGIC PATIENTS

In administering anesthesia to gynecologic patients, the astute anesthesia caregiver recognizes that gynecologic conditions harbor a strong emotional context. **From the patient's viewpoint, gynecologic problems fall into several principal areas, all of which are capable of inducing fear, anxiety, embarrassment, even guilt: (1) infertility, (2) abortions, both spontaneous and therapeutic, (3) acute and chronic pain, (4) mechanical conditions (i.e., stress and fecal incontinence, draining vesicovaginal and rectovaginal fistulas, uterine prolapse), and (5) potential and actual malignancies.**

Infertility patients may harbor strong feelings of guilt or inadequacy because they are inable to conceive. These patients can be subjected to an escalating series of procedures, including laparoscopy, conservative laparotomy, *in vitro* fertilization, and tubal reconstructions. Some finally conceive, only to suffer miscarriage or ectopic pregnancy. The anesthesia provider must at all times be sensitive to these issues and try to be kind, caring, and supportive.

Patients who suffer a spontaneous or missed abortion, with rare exceptions, undergo a period of intense sadness and mourning for the dead fetus. These patients often undergo surgery attended by local anesthesia with sedation. Comments such as: "Don't worry, you can always become pregnant again," or "This is for the best because the baby was probably defective in some way" must be avoided because they devalue the fetus and relegate it to an interchangeable commodity. Patients who have elective abortions also tend to suffer feelings of guilt. Patients who decide to undergo abortion for such fetal conditions as Down's syndrome or other genetic disease or congenital anomalies experience intense guilt and sadness.

Many patients have surgical procedures for chronic pelvic pain. These patients have often suffered for years and may even be dependent on narcotics. They may appear emotionally brittle. Surgery may represent their final hope for relief. Some of these patients may benefit from psychiatric and pain service consultations before surgery.

Patients with urinary or fecal incontinence are often acutely embarrassed when taken to surgery. These conditions are perceived by patients as unsightly, malodorous, and a reason for others to shun them. Again, anesthesia care must be kind and sensitive.

Patients with potentially malignant breast or pelvic masses are often acutely anxious. These patients fear disfigurement, loss of sexual function and desirability, and face the specters of long-term disability, dependence on others, and eventual death. These issues are real and compelling. Anxiety and fear can have serious physiologic consequences as well, including autonomic dysfunction, dysrhythmias, hypertension, angina, and decreased gastric motility in the perioperative period.

Anesthesia care givers must always ensure that their patients are not exposed or uncovered. This includes their entire perioperative time. Also, patients in gowns often feel cold and are vasoconstricted. Warm blankets will make a patient much more comfortable, less anxious, and will show sensitivity. Edentulous patients are often embarrassed when their dentures are removed and even try to cover their mouths with the bedsheets. When performing invasive procedures in the preoperative holding area, there must be no residue of blood upon completion. This can be upsetting and is easy to avoid.

General Considerations

Gynecologic surgery can be divided into four major categories: transvaginal, perineal, intra-abdominal, and transabdominal (Box 77-1). We have found this schema useful because it is simple to remember yet inclusive and will incorporate new surgical procedures as they are introduced.

Gynecologic patients differ in a number of respects from other surgical patients. Although they are homogeneous relative to their sex, certain genotypic and phenotypic abnormalities involving the X and Y chromosomes can give rise to physical abnormalities including short, stubby stature with webbed neck (Turner's syndrome) and to varying degrees of incomplete masculinization (XY mosaicism).[67] These may present potential airway management and positioning problems. Some of the latter individuals may be mentally retarded or have behavioral abnormalities that may influence selection of anesthetic technique.

BOX 77-1
COMMON GYNECOLOGIC PROCEDURES

Transvaginal

- D&C
- D&E
- Cervical
  - Cone biopsy
  - Cerclage
- Hysteroscopy
- Vaginal reconstruction

Perineal

- Laser fulguration of condylomata
- Hymenotomy
- Marsupialization of Bartholin's cyst
- Anterior-posterior repair
- Vulvectomy
- Stamey urethropexy (urologic)

Intra-abdominal

- Oophorectomy
- Cystectomy
- Salpingectomy
- Salpingostomy
- Myomectomy
- Hysterectomy
- Radical hysterectomy
- Ruptured ectopic pregnancy

Transabdominal

- Laparoscopy
- Pelviscopy

In addition to a kind and sympathetic approach, most patients benefit from preoperative use of intravenous (IV) anxiolytics. The possibility of delayed gastric emptying often indicates an H_2-blocker, metoclopramide, droperidol, and/or an antacid preparation preoperatively to anxious patients and to pregnant patients undergoing abortions.[20]

In addition to identifying and speaking with the patient, reviewing the chart and previous anesthetic records, if available, a discussion with the surgeon before seeing the patient can be of great value in deciding the appropriate anesthetic. In many instances, the surgeon is aware of important information that impacts directly on choice of anesthetic technique but that may not have been entered on the patient's record at the time of the preanesthetic visit. This is particularly important in oncology patients, many of whom have received antineoplastic drugs and may have major decrements in renal, cardiac, and respiratory function. Preoperative preparation of these patients will be discussed in detail in the section on cancer surgery.

During anesthesia and surgery, major problems can include aspiration, hemorrhage, allergic reactions, and cata-

Table 77-1 Medications used in gynecologic surgery

Medication	Uses	Route of administration	Risks
Oxytocin	Induces labor; decreases uterine hypotonicity to reduce hemorrhage postpartum or after abortion; NOTE: oxytocin preparations are synthetic, thus decreasing chance of contamination with antidiuretic hormone	IV infusion; no more than 20 U/1000 ml solution	Uterine hyperactivity; coronary vascoconstriction (if preparation contains antidiuretic hormone [ADH]); hypotension; reflex tachycardia; use with caution with hypovolemic patients or patients with blunted compensatory reflex responses; ADH-like response if given in high doses with risk of water intoxication; should be given in electrolyte-containing solutions, not dextrose in water
Pitressin (vasopressin)	Reduces bleeding during cone biopsy	20 units in 20 ml injected into cervical tissues	Coronary vasospasm; GI smooth muscle stimulation
Ergot derivatives			
Ergonovine	Increases uterine tone	IM/oral	Peripheral vasoconstriction
Methylergonovine	Decreases hemorrhage after abortion; IM—effect within 10 minutes lasts 3 to 6 hours (may be dangerous by IV route)	IM 0.2 mg	Acute hypertension, seizures, cerebrovascular accidents, retinal detachment if given IV; use with *caution* in patients with coronary artery disease, essential hypertension, preeclampsia, atherosclerotic disease; NOTE: nausea and vomiting may reflect a direct central nervous system effect
Prostaglandins			
PGE_2	Increases uterine tone	Intra-amniotic	Nausea; vomiting; bronchospasm; tetanic uterine contractions; hypotension; hypertension
PGF_2	Induces abortion in early pregnancy		
Promit			
Dextran 1	Haptene to prevent anaphylaxis from Dextran 70	IV 20 ml	Almost none

strophic events. A well-running IV infusion is imperative because blood loss can be sudden and profuse. Allergic and toxic reactions to antibiotics as well as to agents and medications specific to gynecologic surgery (Table 77-1) can occur unexpectedly. Catastrophic, life-threatening events, such as a ruptured ectopic pregnancy with severe hypotension or amniotic fluid embolism during dilation and evacuation (D&E), require prompt, aggressive teamwork.

ANESTHETIC MANAGEMENT OF GYNECOLOGIC PATIENTS

Monitors

All patients, including those having attended local anesthesia, must be monitored with an electrocardiogram (ECG), blood pressure cuff, and pulse oximeter. Additional monitors include capnography, a temperature probe, a peripheral nerve stimulator, and a Foley catheter as appropriate. Invasive monitors, such as an arterial catheter, a central venous catheter, or a pulmonary artery (PA) catheter, may be indicated in patients with serious medical problems and/or in patients undergoing radical, prolonged procedures accompanied by extensive fluid shifts and volume replacement.

General Anesthesia

Although general anesthesia can be used for all operative gynecologic procedures, we believe that it must not be used indiscriminately. **We consider general anesthesia best suited for certain specific applications, including: (1) extensive intra-abdominal procedures with the patient in the steep Trendelenburg position for prolonged periods, because the airway is at risk for regurgitation and aspiration as well as glottic and pharyngeal edema; in such cases, a cuffed endotracheal (ET) tube must be inserted; (2) extended laparoscopic and pelviscopic procedures using CO_2 insufflation; (3) patients scheduled for procedures that can be performed with regional anesthesia but for whom regional or local anesthesia is contraindicated or who refuse regional anesthesia; (4) procedures that either require or are best performed with the patient under general anesthesia (i.e., modified radical mastectomy, lumpectomy, and axillary node dissection;**

N.B.: in selected patients, these procedures can be performed using thoracic epidural). General anesthesia is often preferred by patients, especially for day-surgery procedures and may be provided using mask, laryngeal mask airway (LMA) or by ET tube to secure the airway. Many gynecologic operations are very short and performed as outpatient procedures. Thus, deep levels of general anesthesia are required, yet the patient needs to awaken promptly and be soon ready for discharge. General anesthesia by mask or LMA is appropriate in cases in which there are no contraindications, such as a full stomach, obesity, severe anxiety, nausea, vomiting, and emergent surgery. An inhalational induction with the patient breathing spontaneously, bolstered by judicious use of small doses of sodium thiopental or propofol, avoids or minimizes introduction of air into the stomach from positive pressure ventilation. This, in turn, decreases the possibilities of nausea, vomiting, and aspiration. This is an important consideration because patients are often placed in the Trendelenburg position. If a patient receiving a general anesthetic by mask or LMA is placed in the Trendelenburg position, the head of the bed can be somewhat elevated, thereby reducing the possibility of passive regurgitation, yet not compromising most procedures requiring a modest head-down tilt.

Many techniques of general anesthesia are acceptable for gynecologic surgery. As a general rule, anesthesia providers must use those with which they are most comfortable. In lengthy intra-abdominal procedures, N_2O can distend the bowel and compromise surgical access and visibility.[21]

For this reason, we usually use a volatile agent in a mixture of O_2 and air (O_2 only in patients with severe pulmonary disease and shunting, morbid obesity and other such states where arterial desaturation is likely to occur). In grossly obese patients undergoing procedures in the lithotomy position, the functional residual capacity is small in relation to their body size and weight.[47,69] During laryngoscopy, O_2 saturation can plummet if the trachea is not intubated promptly. We try to use regional anesthesia in these patients. If we cannot, we thoroughly preoxygenate the patient before induction to maximize N_2 washout. If there is any suspicion of a difficult airway in such a patient, an awake, sedated nasotracheal or fiber optic intubation must be considered. It can be very useful to have sevoflurane available for such situations, especially where a patient may be difficult to intubate, but relatively easy to ventilate by mask. If laryngoscopy fails, sevoflurane in O_2 can be used to increase depth of anesthesia rapidly, allowing additional attempts.

Regional Anesthesia

Regional anesthesia can be used for much gynecologic surgery, particularly transvaginal and perineal procedures. Regional anesthesia can also be used for abdominal procedures, such as conservative laparotomy, myomectomy, ovarian cystectomy, and hysterectomy. The key to success lies in patient selection and the ability of the surgeon and anesthesia provider to work together. It is important to inquire whether the surgeon thinks that the procedure can be performed within a reasonable period of time (i.e., within 2 hours) without requiring a steep Trendelenburg position and/or extensive exploration and packing of the upper abdomen. If so and the patient is suitable and accepts a regional technique, spinal or epidural anesthesia can be used to advantage.

Specific technique and choice of local anesthetic depends on the magnitude and duration of the operation. The surgical site dictates the level of anesthesia required. When used for intra-abdominal surgery, a level of at least T8 is advised.[9] A level of T4 to T6 can provide satisfactory anesthesia for almost all intra-abdominal gynecologic procedures, especially because few involve the upper abdomen. It is important to warn the patient that she may experience some pressure or pulling. Pretreatment with a narcotic can attenuate this problem. Prophylactic droperidol may prevent the nausea that often results from peritoneal stimulation. IV sedation and supplementary analgesia are important ingredients in regional anesthesia. An excellent block can easily turn into a "failed anesthetic" that requires use of general anesthesia if the patient becomes anxious or develops upper-extremity discomfort from lying on the operating room table for a prolonged period.

Single-Dose Versus Continuous Techniques

Single-dose techniques are indicated for procedures that are either short or of a predictable duration, not to exceed 2 or 3 hours. Conversely, continuous catheter techniques offer control and flexibility, especially when the procedure is of unknown duration; continuous epidural techniques allow postoperative epidural narcotics for pain control.

Spinal Anesthesia

Spinal anesthesia performed with a small-gauge spinal needle is suitable for many procedures. The choice of local anesthetic depends on the operation and whether the patient is an outpatient or an inpatient. Hyperbaric lidocaine in dextrose is excellent for short day-surgery procedures, such as D&C, cone biopsy, and cystoscopy-proctoscopy for staging of cervical cancer patients. It is also excellent for cervical cerclage. Although the latter patients usually stay overnight to be monitored, it is desirable that their anesthetic be as brief as possible. Until recently, 5% lidocaine in 7.5% dextrose, prepared in premixed 2-ml ampules was the most commonly used solution for hyperbaric lidocaine spinal anesthesia. A recent Food and Drug Administration (FDA) directive cautioned against its routine use for single-dose as well as continuous spinal anesthesia due to a number of incidents involving recurrent paresthesias and areas of lower-extremity numbness following its administration.[4] The Anesthesia and Life Support Drug Advisory Committee of the FDA concluded that these adverse effects occurred from maldistribution of the drug during slow injection through a small-bore (25–32 G needle), resulting in drug pooling in localized areas around dependent nerve roots within the subarachnoid space, rather than distribution throughout the cauda equina. This occurrence is similar to that observed with the now discredited spinal microcatheters. In the case of hyperbaric lidocaine spinal, the FDA recommends that if 5% lidocaine in dextrose is to be used, it be diluted 1:1 with either cerebrospinal fluid (CSF) or normal saline solution before subarachnoid injection. Instead, we substitute prepackaged 2-ml ampules of 1.5 % lidocaine solution in 7.5% dextrose (30 mg lidocaine per ampule), for the 5% solution. With the 1.5 % solution, 52.5 (3.5 ml) to 60 mg (4 ml) is appropriate for most cases. Isobaric lidocaine (2% without epinephrine), 50 to 60 mg, can also be used for minor gynecologic procedures, but is more apt to produce a spotty block at sacral nerve roots than a hyperbaric solution.

We discourage use of longer-acting agents (e.g., tetracaine and bupivacaine) in day-surgery patients because they may lead to postoperative problems that preclude same-day discharge. The main disadvantage of spinal anesthesia in day-surgery patients is postdural puncture headache, especially in young women. Good perioperative education and reassurance that help and treatment are available is essential. Whenever possible, either a 25-gauge pencil-point needle, or a 26- or 27-gauge Quincke spinal needle, the latter inserted so that the needle bevel is parallel to the dural fibers, must be used to minimize risk of postdural puncture headache.

Continuous Spinal Anesthesia

This technique, developed in the 1930s, allows for a highly controllable onset of block. It is especially useful in elderly and debilitated patients who may not tolerate sudden hemodynamic changes or high doses of local anesthetics. The classical technique involves insertion of a catheter through a 17-gauge Tuohey or Weiss needle. Because this leaves a sizable hole in the dura after withdrawal of the catheter, we restrict this technique to older patients who are less prone to develop headache. Microcatheters that pass through standard 22- and 26-gauge, 3-inch spinal needles were recently tried. It was believed that these catheters might be used to advantage in younger and middle-aged patients because they carry a lesser risk of postoperative headache, but reports of cauda equina syndrome associated with microcatheters, especially in conjunction with hyperbaric 5% lidocaine in 7.5% dextrose, have led to their abandonment.[4]

Epidural Anesthesia

Continuous epidural anesthesia is especially useful in procedures of uncertain duration, such as vaginal reconstruction, or to provide baseline anesthesia for intra-abdominal procedures. For the latter, a combined epidural-general technique is often used to provide unconsciousness and airway protection during the surgery, with the catheter left in place to allow epidural narcotic/local anesthetic combinations postoperatively. The primary disadvantage of an epidural technique is the time required for a block to become established (i.e., 15 to 25 minutes), which makes it impractical for very short procedures. On occasion, a patient specifically requests an epidural as her sole anesthetic for an intra-abdominal procedure. A continuous epidural works well for hysterectomy, myomectomy, and ovarian cystectomy, provided that steep Trendelenburg position can be avoided or minimized. Advantages are minimal risk of headache, flexibility if the case is prolonged, and the capability for postoperative analgesia. In patients who are adamant about having an epidural instead of a spinal anesthetic for a relatively short procedure, a single-dose technique with a rapidly acting agent (e.g., lidocaine) can be used to advantage.

Caudal Anesthesia

This technique is seldom used in modern gynecologic surgery because it requires relatively high doses of local anesthetic and has an onset of 10 to 20 minutes. For these reasons, most anesthesia providers administer a lidocaine spinal for procedures previously performed with caudal anesthesia (e.g., culdoscopy, hemorrhoidectomy).

Monitored Anesthesia Care

Monitored IV sedation, coupled with a paracervical or intracervical block or local anesthesia, is appropriate for certain procedures, such as D&C, D&E, hymenotomy, and breast biopsy. Some patients may not be good candidates for this type of anesthesia because of surgical considerations (e.g., a high-grade cervical stenosis making insertion of a dilator difficult or a deep breast mass not easily accessible). Other patients may not be suitable candidates for emotional reasons. Sedative and analgesic medications must be given generously before the paracervical or intracervical block is placed, because the block can be somewhat painful. Paracervical tissues are highly vascular. This block can rapidly result in high blood levels of local anesthetic; the patient must be monitored carefully for signs of incipient toxicity.[30]

Ketorolac (Toradol®) is a useful analgesic and anti-inflammatory medication in ambulatory procedures where monitored anesthesia care (MAC) is frequently employed. The usual IV dose is 30 mg, administered as a slow IV bolus. Similar to other nonsteroid anti-inflammatory agents, ketorolac inhibits platelet cyclo-oxygenase. This can result in decreased platelet adhesiveness and increased tendency for bleeding intra- and postoperatively. It is advisable that the drug be administered just prior to closure when hemostatsis has been achieved and it is apparent that no bleeding diathesis exists. Additionally, ketorolac is irritating to the gastric mucous and may not be a good choice in patients with history of ulcer or gastritis.

SURGICAL AND ANESTHETIC CONSIDERATIONS FOR SPECIFIC GYNECOLOGIC PROCEDURES

Perineal and Urologic Surgery

Surgical anatomy

The vulva includes all structures visible externally from the pubis to the perineum and includes the mons pubis, labia

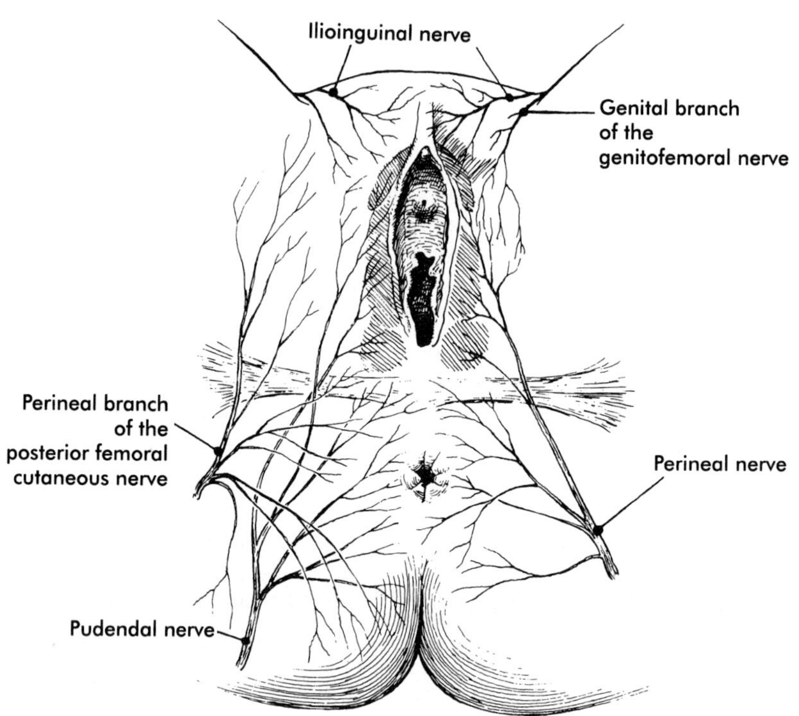

Fig. 77-1. Cutaneous nerves that supply the vulvar and perianal regions in women. (From Wheelas CR: *Atlas of pelvic surgery,* Philadelphia, 1981, Lea & Febiger.)

majora and minora, the clitoris, vestibule, urethra, and the Skene's and Bartholin's glands.

The primary blood supply to the vulva is via the internal pudendal artery, a branch of the internal iliac artery. The nerve supply is via the pudendal nerve that arises from sacral nerve roots 2, 3, and 4 (S2, S3, and S4) (see Fig. 77-8). The pudendal nerve, artery, and accompanying veins pass from the pelvis via the lesser sciatic foramen and along the lateral wall of the ischiorectal fossa. In the area of the ischial tuberosity, the nerve may be readily blocked to achieve anesthesia of the perineum. Pudendal nerve block is used primarily in obstetrics to provide analgesia for vaginal delivery (Fig. 77-1).[70]

The lymphatic drainage of the vulva is predominantly to the superficial inguinal lymph nodes and ultimately to the femoral or deep inguinal and pelvic nodal systems. This is an important avenue in the local spread of vulvar carcinoma and is discussed in the subsection on vulvectomy.

Specific procedures

Minor vulvar procedures. Many minor procedures are performed on the vulva. Although some may be performed with use of attended local anesthesia, most require use of regional or general anesthesia. Patients with extensive preinvasive disease may require multiple vulvar biopsies. Patients presenting with imperforate hymen or a variety of congenital abnormalities of the hymen may require hymenectomy or hymenotomy. The latter patients are usually young and may feel embarrassed about their condition. A brief general anesthetic by mask or LMA is often indicated for this patient population.

Bartholin's gland abscess. Bartholin's gland, a secretory gland located in the labia majora, is a frequent site of abscess formation resulting from the obstruction of its duct (Fig. 77-2).[70] These abscesses rapidly become superinfected and may present as a very painful swollen mass. They are incised and drained, generally with the patient under local anesthesia, in an office or emergency ward setting. With recurrent Bartholin's gland abscess, marsupialization may be required which involves unroofing and suturing the wall of the gland to prevent it from healing closed.

A Bartholin's gland marsupialization is an entirely different procedure from a Bartholin's gland excision. Because of the rich vascular supply of the vulva, attempts at excising Bartholin's glands can be prolonged and entail much greater blood loss than simple marsupialization. The anesthesia provider must know which procedure will be performed. A marsupialization is nicely performed with a hyperbaric lidocaine spinal anesthetic, because these procedures are often done emergently with a likely full stomach. In the case of a Bartholin's gland excision, a longer-acting spinal anesthetic may be needed.

Laser fulguration. Vulvar intraepithelial neoplasia is associated with human papillomavirus (HPV) infections. Recently, there has been a dramatic increase in the prevalence of vulvar intraepithelial neoplasias and decreased age of onset.[74] The CO_2 laser has become popular and effective therapy. Its use has resulted in better cosmetic results and

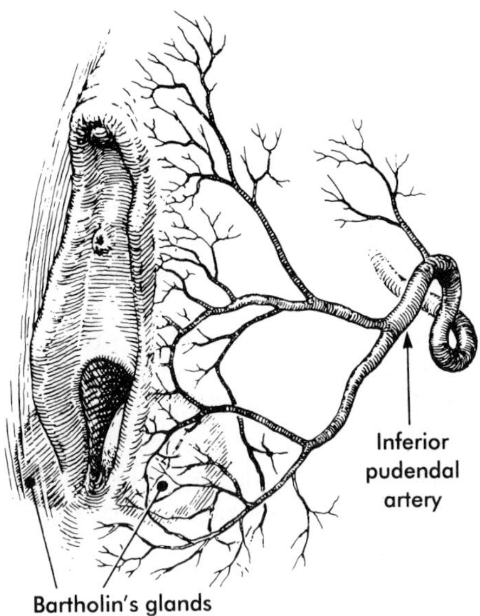

Fig. 77-2. Arterial blood supply to the vulva and Bartholin's glands. (From Wheelas CR: *Atlas of pelvic surgery,* Philadelphia, 1981, Lea & Febiger.)

lesser recurrence rates than those seen with more traditional forms of treatment.[75]

Laser vaporization of vulvar intraepithelial neoplasia is performed in the operating room with the patient receiving general or regional anesthesia and in the lithotomy position. Duration of the procedure depends on extent and distribution of diseased areas. It is frequently performed with the laser colposcope. Operative laser use entails risks both to the patient and operating room staff, including thermal injury from reflecting laser light, ignition of operative drapes resulting in burns, retinal injury, and the theoretic risk of viral inoculation from inhalation of particulates in the laser plume.[56]

Although it is possible to detect human papilloma viral DNA in laser plume, it is unclear whether or not the smoke is infectious.[60,72] Appropriate eye protection and occlusive laser masks for all operating room personnel are important. A properly functioning smoke evacuator devoted to controlling laser plume will greatly reduce exposure.[66]

The primary surgical requirement is that the perineum be immobile during use of the laser. Sudden movements from coughing, straining, or retching can cause the laser beam to strike an unintended area, with serious consequences. If regional anesthesia is used, it is important that a solid motor block be established so that the patient does not move her legs during the procedure. We have found hyperbaric lidocaine to be excellent for procedures up to 90 minutes in length. With addition of epinephrine, 2 hours of satisfactory analgesia and motor block can be achieved yet the block will wear off in time to discharge a day-surgery patient. We have used general anesthesia for these procedures both by mask and with an ET tube. A combination of N_2O (a volatile agent), and adjunctive IV narcotic is reasonable.

All personnel must wear protective eyewear certified for use with the specific type of laser employed. For the patient, at our institution, this regimen includes: (1) eye pads moistened with saline solution placed over both eyes or laser-certified goggles; (2) a special laser-surgical mask, to trap virus-containing particulates if the patient is having regional anesthesia; (3) surgical drapes in place to form a barrier between the laser and the patient's head. These steps usually do not preclude use of a mask, although facial configurations of individual patients may dictate that an LMA or ET tube be used to provide satisfactory eye protection.

Vulvectomy and vulvar trauma. There are three types of vulvectomies: the skinning vulvectomy, the simple vulvectomy, and the radical vulvectomy.

Skinning vulvectomy. Skinning vulvectomy involves the surgical removal of the vulvar skin, generally in areas affected by chronic skin diseases or intraepithelial neoplasias. The skinning vulvectomy may be so extensive that it requires a split-thickness skin graft. These procedures tend to be time consuming because multiple biopsies of margins must be performed to ensure that the disease process for which the vulvectomy is being performed has been eradicated. The need to wait for multiple biopsies prolongs this otherwise straigthforward procedure.

Simple vulvectomy. Simple vulvectomy entails removal of the entire vulva and subcutaneous tissues but not to the depth of the inferior fascia of the urogenital diaphragm. Simple vulvectomies are uncommon and are reserved for serious dermatoses.

Radical vulvectomy. Radical vulvectomy is the traditional procedure for invasive carcinoma of the vulva, and involves removal of all tissue to the inferior fascia of the urogenital diaphragm. There is risk of important blood loss from the region of the vestibular bulbs, pudendal artery, and in the retropubic space of Retzius. Modifications of the radical vulvectomy may be performed for small unilateral or minimally invasive lesions. These include the radical hemivulvectomy and the radical local excision.

Radical vulvectomy is classically accompanied by bilateral inguinal lymphadenectomy. The original description of this operation described the en-bloc resection of inguinal lymph nodes and vulva including intervening skin bridges between the groins and the vulva (Fig. 77-3).[70] This resulted in large defects, frequently requiring grafting to repair. Modification of the radical vulvectomy and inguinal lymphadenectomy involves three separate incisions, one in each groin and the third to encompass the vulva. Two surgical teams may work concurrently as in a combined abdominoperineal resection to shorten operative time. It is uncommon for a vulvectomy to result in extensive blood loss. Dissection of the groin is relatively bloodless. The procedure is performed in proximity to the femoral artery and vein and, therefore, inadvertent injury to these vessels may cause unexpected sudden and extensive blood loss.

Vulvar trauma. **In addition to surgery for neoplasia, major blood loss may be anticipated in cases of vulvar**

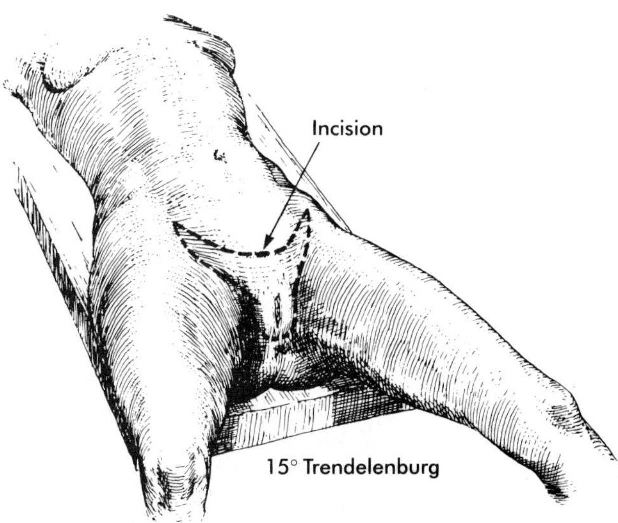

Fig. 77-3. Incision for the classic radical vulvectomy using an en bloc resection. (From Wheelas CR: *Atlas of pelvic surgery,* Philadelphia, 1981, Lea & Febiger.)

trauma. The vulva is highly vascular, particularly in pregnancy. If the vulva is involved in serious impalement injuries and other pelvic trauma, these cases are considered major trauma and often require multiple large-bore IVs, extensive invasive monitoring, and an interdisciplinary approach to surgical management.

Anesthetic management of vulvar and perineal procedures. Regional anesthesia is excellent for all perineal and groin procedures. The type of vulvectomy planned (i.e., skinning versus simple versus radical) allows best planning for anesthesia. We have used continuous epidural and spinal anesthesia for prolonged cases with excellent results. Judicious use of sedatives and an effort by the entire team to refrain from loud and inappropriate comments minimizes patient awareness and anxiety. In most cases, a supplemental general anesthetic is not needed. Although vulvectomy is not usually particularly painful for a prolonged period postoperatively, we usually administer postoperative epidural narcotics if a continuous epidural technique was used.

Urologic and urethral procedures. A variety of surgical procedures are available to correct anatomic alterations that result in stress urinary incontinence in the woman. Weakness of the endopelvic fascia and a loss of pelvic support result in the loss of the posterior urethrovesical angle (Fig. 77-4).[59] This results in decreased function of the anatomic internal urethral sphincter and subsequent loss of urine with cough, sneeze, or strain. Procedures for female stress urinary incontinence are directed toward reestablishing the normal anatomic relationship among urethra, bladder, and pubic symphysis.

Traditional approaches have included retropubic surgery (e.g., Marshall-Marchetti-Krantz or Burch procedure) or the transvaginal Kelly plication. More recently, techniques for transvaginal urethropexy have been introduced. These include the Pereyra and Stamey procedures.[51,64] The goal of these procedures is to provide resuspension of the urethra with reestablishment of the posterior urethrovesical angle by passing permanent sutures from the fascia overlying the pubis to the paraurethral fascia. These procedures are performed with the use of long needles to carry sutures from the vaginal epithelium to the rectus fascia above the pubis. These relatively new operative procedures have dramatically reduced blood loss and operative time of the abdominal operations. From a surgical standpoint, it is paramount, during placement of the paraurethral suture, that the patient not cough or strain. It is also important to avoid breath-holding or coughing in the immediate postoperative period to avoid disrupting the surgical repair. We try to perform these procedures with the patient receiving regional anesthesia whenever possible. Spinal anesthesia provides excellent analgesia combined with profound muscle relaxation and immobility during the procedure. If a general anesthetic must be used, we usually administer a prophylactic antiemetic (e.g., droperidol and/or metoclopramide IV), because postoperative nausea and retching can threaten the integrity of the surgical repair.

Transvaginal Surgery

Surgical anatomy

The vagina is an 8- to 10-cm compliant, plastic, musculomembranous canal that extends from the external genitalia to the uterine cervix (Fig. 77-5).[59] Anteriorly, it is related to the urethra and bladder. Posteriorly, its lower aspect is related to the rectal ampula and perineum, whereas its upper, posterior third is adjacent to the cul-de-sac of Douglas. The primary blood supply to the vagina is derived from the vaginal branches of the uterine artery and the pudendal artery. The lymphatic drainage of the upper third of the vagina is predominately to the parametrial and pelvic lymph nodes, whereas the lower two thirds shares the lymphatic drainage of the vulva, which is predominately to the superficial inguinal lymph nodes. The sensory nerve supply to the vagina arises from S2, S3, and S4 via the pudendal nerve, which can be blocked for episiotomy during vaginal delivery (see Chapter 76). The sympathetic nerve supply arises from the hypogastric plexus (L1-L3), whereas the parasympathetic supply is from sacral segments (see Fig. 77-8).

The vagina offers access to the cervix, endometrial, and peritoneal cavities for such procedures as D&C, D&E, and cervical surgery. New endoscopic techniques including hysteroscopy are becoming more popular. The vagina also offers ready access to the peritoneal cavity. A needle passed posterior to the cervix into the pouch of Douglas allows the surgeon to sample intraperitoneal collections of blood, fluid, or pus (see Fig. 77-5).[59] This procedure, called *culdocentesis,* aids in the diagnosis of hemoperitoneum from ruptured ectopic pregnancy and is often performed in the emergency room.

The uterine cervix (Latin for "neck") enters the vagina at a variable angle through the anterosuperior wall and is com-

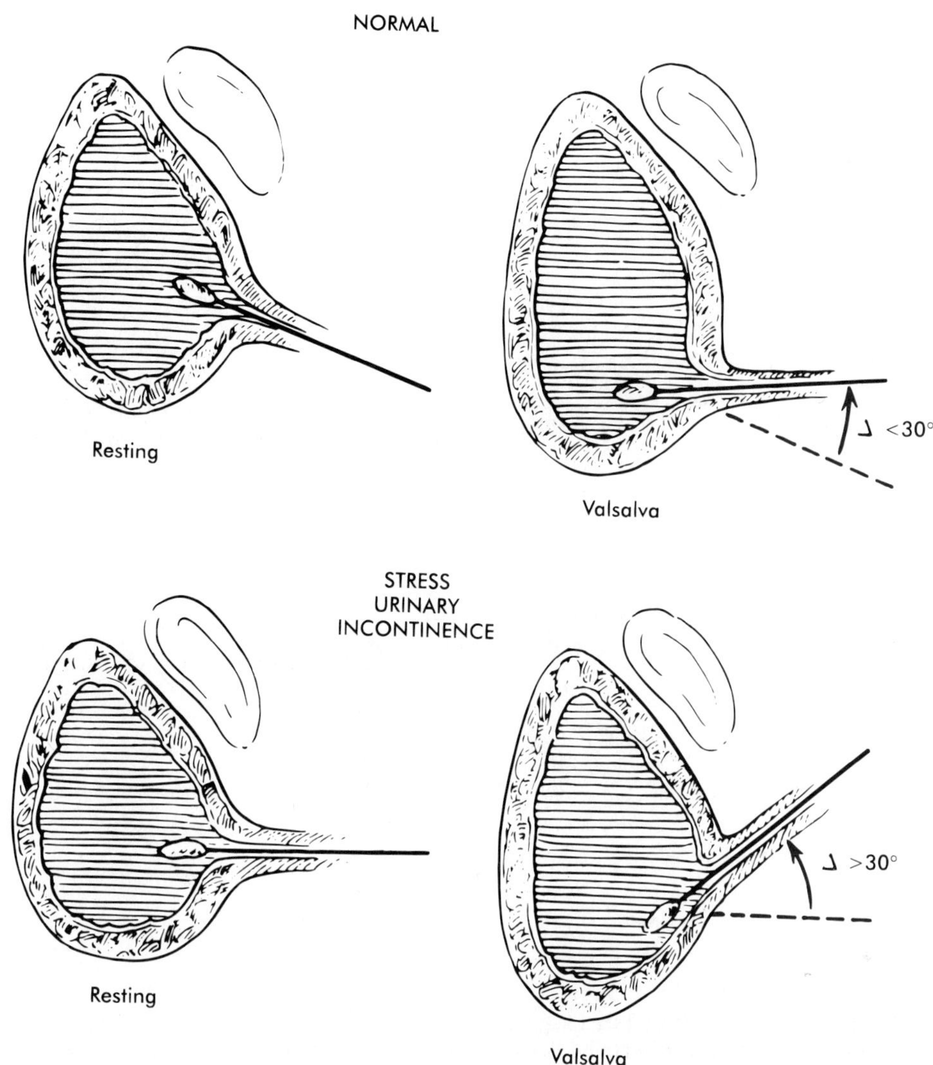

Fig. 77-4. The angle of the posterior urethrovesical junction in a continent and incontinent patient. (From Ryan KJ, Berkowitz R, Barbieri R, editors: *Kistner's gynecology, principles and practice,* ed 5, Littleton, 1990, Year Book Medical.)

posed of myometrial muscle and dense stroma.[25] The cervix is innervated by nerves arising in the hypogastric plexi.[24] The exocervix is poorly supplied by sensory nerves and is relatively insensitive to surgical manipulation. Deeper within the exocervix or along the endocervix the nerve supply is abundant and the region is exquisitely sensitive.[24] The cervical blood supply is derived from the descending branch of the uterine artery. The cervical lymphatic drainage is described in the section on abdominal surgery.

Specific transvaginal procedures

Vaginal plastic procedures. There are a number of vaginal malformations that can be subjected to corrective surgery, including congenital absence of the vagina, failure of appropriate canalization, or failure of fusion of embryonic anlage. These developmental abnormalities lead to the congenital absence of the vagina or a variety of transverse and longitudinal vaginal septa.

Neoplastic processes may involve the vagina. Vaginal intraepithelial neoplasia, referred to as *in situ* dysplastic changes of uncertain malignant potential, may require laser fulguration or excision. Vaginal carcinoma is the rarest of gynecologic malignancies. A more common variant—invasive squamous cell carcinoma—is usually treated primarily with radiotherapy. With regard to anesthetic management, regional or general anesthesia can be used. In selected minor procedures, especially in ill patients, use of attended local anesthesia may be appropriate.

Dilatation and curettage. Dilatation and curettage in which endometrial curettings are obtained for pathologic evaluation, is usually performed to investigate abnormal uterine bleeding. Safe, reliable, and accurate techniques for endometrial biopsies allow the practitioner to obtain a biopsy in an office setting with most patients under paracervical block. Accordingly, patients scheduled for D&C in the operating suite constitute a selected population who may

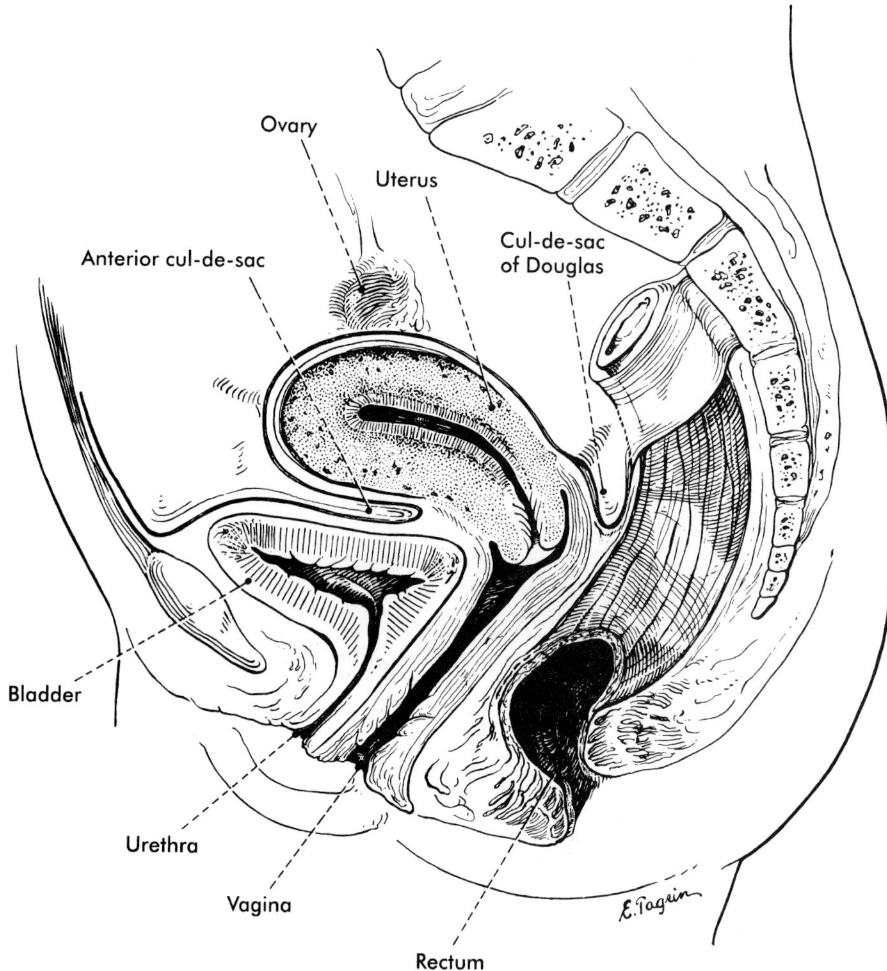

Fig. 77-5. Anatomic relations of the bladder, rectum, and female genital tract in sagittal section. (From Ryan KJ, Berkowitz R, Barbieri R, editors: *Kistner's gynecology, principles and practice,* ed 5, Littleton, 1990, Year Book Medical.)

have serious medical problems, distorted anatomy, or could not tolerate an office biopsy. Some of these patients have become anemic secondary to protracted uterine bleeding. They usually have adapted to their chronically low hematocrits and tolerate spinal and general anesthesia well. Conversely, patients who have had sudden, major uterine bleeding with an abrupt drop in hematocrit to the low 20s may require transfusion before anesthesia, particularly if orthostatic hypotension is present.

A D&C is usually a brief procedure and can be completed in as little as 5 minutes by an experienced gynecologist. The most painful stimulus is from dilation of the cervix, particularly if the patient has cervical stenosis. If general anesthesia is used, a relatively deep level of anesthesia must be present during dilatation to prevent sudden laryngospasm or other manifestations of inadequate anesthetic depth. Spinal anesthesia is excellent for diagnostic D&C. Hyperbaric lidocaine (1.5% lidocaine in 7.5% dextrose, 50 to 60 mg) may be administered with the patient sitting for the lumbar puncture, then gently lowered to the supine position. A T8 to 10 level must be achieved to prevent discomfort during curettage, because the fundus of the uterus is innervated from T10 to L4 (see Fig. 77-8). Use of attended local anesthesia with the surgeon performing a paracervical block, is satisfactory in selected patients, particularly the elderly and frail. It must be remembered that a paracervical block will not relieve the discomfort of uterine curettage, because the fundus of the uterus is separately innervated (see Fig. 77-8),[7] and adjunctive IV narcotic administration may be required. When considering attended local anesthesia for a particular patient, the suitability of the technique must always be discussed beforehand with the surgeon to avoid an unpleasant and unsatisfactory experience.

From a surgical standpoint, the major risk of diagnostic D&C is perforation and subsequent hemorrhage. Although uterine perforations may occur in any anatomic location, they most commonly occur posteriorly or fundally (see Fig. 77-5). When a perforation occurs in the lateral uterine wall, there is a significant risk of injury to the uterine artery and subsequent hemorrhage may ensue. Perforation of the uterus of a premenopausal patient, with its more extensive vascular supply, has greater likelihood of leading to surgical intervention than a perforation in an atrophic postmenopausal uterus. If a perforation is suspected, every attempt is made to localize the exact position of the perforation by gentle probing. Depending on the patient's age and the location of the perforation, the surgeon may wish to observe the patient, proceed to a diagnostic laparoscopy, or proceed directly to laparotomy for surgical repair.

Hysteroscopy. Hysteroscopy is defined as the endoscopic examination of the endocervix and endometrial cavity.[43] Following dilation of the cervical os, a hysteroscope, which may be rigid or flexible, is inserted into the endometrial cavity. The cavity is then distended with either CO_2[3] or liquid distending media to improve visibility and surgical access. The procedure may be performed purely for diagnostic purposes or as a therapeutic procedure. It is important to draw the distinction between diagnostic and operative hysteroscopy because their anesthetic management often differs.

Diagnostic hysteroscopy may be helpful in evaluating patients with unexplained infertility or abnormal uterine bleeding, or for localization of intrauterine contraceptive devices. Hysteroscopes designed for office use are of small caliber and may be either rigid or flexible. These devices may be inserted under paracervical block with minimal cervical dilation. CO_2 is the preferred distention medium for office procedures. Patients brought to the operating room for diagnostic hysteroscopy usually undergo rigid hysteroscopy using glycine distention. These procedures are usually performed as an adjunct to D&C and are brief, employing relatively small volumes of dextran or glycine. Extensive dilation is not required and local anesthesia may suffice.

Operative hysteroscopy is performed for resection of intracavity uterine lesions, such as submucous leimyomas, intrauterine septae, or adhesions. The operative hysteroscope also may be used to visualize and guide endometrial ablations, a conservative therapeutic approach to dysfunctional uterine bleeding in which the endometrial cavity is destroyed by an electrocautery device termed a roller-ball, or by laser, thereby sparing the patient a hysterectomy. Operative hysteroscopes are much larger than diagnostic scopes, and therefore considerable cervical dilation is required to insert the instrument. Resection and hemostasis are accomplished by using a monopolar cutting wire, similar to the instrument used by urologists in the transurethral resection of the prostate. A near iso-osmolar, nonconducting distending medium is required to obtain adequate visualization and exposure during operative procedures. Until recently, 32% dextran (Hyskon®) was the predominant distending medium, but it has been supplanted by glycine at most centers. When using glycine, a frequent and accurate accounting of the volume absorbed (i.e., volume infused minus volume recovered) must be employed to minimize the possibilities of water intoxication, hyponatremia, and ammonia toxicity (see following paragraphs). When resecting intrauterine lesions, some surgeons prefer to place a laparoscope into the abdominal cavity to guard against inadvertent perforation of the myometrium, to further delineate upper genital tract anatomy, to treat concurrent intraperitoneal or adnexal disease or to assess the patency of the fallopian tubes via chromopertubation. Although many surgeons do not routinely use laparoscopy concurrently with operative hysteroscopy, the anesthesia team must be prepared for emergent laparoscopy in the event of a complication.

Table 77-2 Complications of hysteroscopy

Category	Examples
Traumatic and hemorrhagic	Air and carbon dioxide embolism[49,52]; acute hydrothorax
Distention medium hazards	Anaphylaxis Disseminated intravascular coagulation rhabdomyolysis[28]; pulmonary hemorrhage hypervolemia; left ventricular failure electrolyte imbalance; hyponatremia hypothermia; transient blindness
Infection	Uterine and adnexal infection[46]
Electrical and laser damage	Fires; burns; electroshock hazard

It is not necessary for all patients undergoing operative hysteroscopy to have general or regional anesthesia. Some surgeons will perform procedures like endometrial ablation under local anesthesia with sedation. Many patients undergoing endometrial ablation are poor anesthesia risks.

Complications of hysteroscopy. Hysteroscopy is often considered a minor, low-risk procedure. Nonetheless, there are reports of severe complications, including death, in young and healthy patients.[35,38] Brooks has divided the complications of operative hysteroscopy into several major categories, including: (1) traumatic and hemorrhagic; (2) distension medium hazards; (3) infection; and (4) electrical or laser damage.[8] These complications are summarized in Table 77-2.

Anesthesia caregivers must be familiar with the technical aspects of hysteroscopy and especially with the types of distending media, because many complications are specific to the medium used.[28,73] Prompt recognition and treatment of complications are essential. Subtle changes in mental status may be the harbinger of much more serious problems. Standard monitoring, including scrupulous accounting of the quantities of distending medium used and recovered, suffices unless the patient's overall health warrants invasive techniques. Full resuscitative equipment must be immediately available.

The distending solution for hysteroscopy must be nontoxic, nonconductive, isotonic, cause minimal intravascular and intracellular changes, must not crystallize, and must allow for good visibility. Distension media in clinical use include CO_2 gas, low-viscosity fluids (glycine, dextrose, sorbitol/mannitol, and saline) and high-viscosity fluid (dextran-70).

Carbon dioxide[3] is not useful for operative hysteroscopy, because bubbles often obscure the view. When used for diagnostic hysteroscopy, care must be taken to use low flows and low pressure. Only insufflators designed for hysteroscopy (flow rates of 100 to 200 ml/min) must be used to avoid embolism and rupture of the oviducts. CO_2-cooled laser fiber and sapphire tips can produce flow rates of 1000 ml/min and have been associated with several cases of fatal CO_2 embolization.[10,18] This led to a warning issued by the FDA in 1990 not to use gas-cooled laser fibers or tips for intrauterine surgery.[8]

Currently, the most commonly used low-viscosity solution for hysteroscopy is glycine mixed with water to make a 1.5% solution, which is electrolyte-free and somewhat hypo-osmolar (200 mOsm/l). It undergoes oxidative deamination in the liver and kidneys to form ammonia and glyoxylic acid. Glycolylic acid is metabolized to oxalate which may form crystals.[73] Complications from glycine arise as a consequence of its entry into the vascular system. When monitoring the fluid balance with low-viscosity solutions like glycine, it is easy to grossly underestimate the amount of fluid absorbed. Because the irrigating medium often leaks from the cervix around the hysteroscope, the volume of this leakage is not always quantitated and is often overestimated, leading to gross inaccuracies in input-output calculations.[73] When large quantities of glycine enter the circulation, an acute dilutional effect occurs. Although the 1.5% solution used is nearly iso-osmolar, the glycine is metabolized rapidly, with intravascular and intracellular volume changes in response to absorption of large amounts of free water which can seriously alter electrolyte balance. Direct ammonia toxicity can result from glycine metabolism, and CNS toxicity (seizures, mental changes, lethargy) may occur in part from a direct neurotransmitter effect. Glycine functions as an inhibitory neurotransmitter in the brain, increasing conductance of certain ions by binding to ligand-activated ion channels at the postsynaptic membrane.[22]

Glycine is infused into the uterus under pressure and is absorbed by the uterine vessels and peritoneum. Glycine has a intravascular half-life of 85 minutes and is then absorbed intracellularly. Large volumes of solution absorbed in this way can result in excess free water with resultant hypo-osmolar hyponatremia. The "Post-TURP syndrome" is well described in the urology literature and has a "Post-Hysteroscopy syndrome" counterpart. It occurs when large volumes of irrigating fluid are absorbed resulting in hypervolemia, hyponatremia, and decreased osmolarity. The blood–brain barrier is relatively permeable to free water, and cerebral edema may quickly develop. This syndrome is associated with hypertension, bradycardia, mental status changes, nausea, vomiting, headache, agitation, and lethargy. It may progress to seizures, coma, and death if not recognized and treated promptly.

Once the diagnosis is suspected treatment must begin immediately. The procedure must be completed expeditiously. Blood for complete blood count (CBC), serum electrolytes (sodium is the most important) and osmolality must be drawn and sent immediately for testing. Treatment centers upon correcting hyponatremia and hypo-osmolarity. Standard treatment is normal saline and furosemide. Hypertonic saline may result in hypernatremia. Overly rapid correction of the hyponatremia can be harmful. There is controversy as to how rapidly the sodium must be corrected. Central pontine myelinolysis (CPM) has been associated with overly rapid correction. This syndrome is believed to result from brain dessication. Typically, the patient improves initially, then deteriorates neurologically. This deterioration may occur several days later. Patients may develop paresis, mutism, pseudobulbar palsy, behavioral changes, and movement disorders.[73]

Treatment of acute and chronic hyponatremia differ. Hyponatremia is considered chronic if it has persisted for more than 48 hours and must be corrected slowly. Serum sodium must increase by no more than 25 mEq/l over 48 hours. The potential danger of fluid overload requires attention to the amount of fluid infused, recovered and absorbed. Fluid balance (quantity infused − quantity recovered) must be monitored and recorded every 15 minutes. Istre et al.[37] found that glycine deficits of up to 500 ml led to a mean decrease in serum sodium of 2.5 mEq/l; deficits exceeding 500 ml resulted in a mean decrease of 8 mEq/l. These measures are of considerable importance, especially during hysteroscopy under general anesthesia, during which changes in mental status go unmonitored.

High viscosity media present a different set of problems. Dextrans are products of bacterial polymerization of glucose.[73] Dextran-70 has a molecular weight of 70,000 daltons, is imiscible with blood, and is metabolized by the reticuloendothelial system. Hyskon® is a solution of 32% dextran-70 in 10% glucose.

The complications associated with dextran-70 appear the result of allergic reactions or volume overload. Several cases of anaphylactic shock and noncardiogenic pulmonary edema have been reported. Dextran-1 (Promit®) administered 2 minutes before dextran-70 infusion (Hyskon®) has reduced the incidence of anaphylaxis. Dextran-1 acts as a hapten, binding antidextran antibodies and forming low–molecular weight complexes. These are rapidly cleared from the serum, thereby eliminating the high–molecular weight complex that causes the response.[44] Dextran-70 is a potent osmotic agent with an intravascular half-life of several days. The increased osmotic pressure from dextran-70 may cause intravascular volume overload and even pulmonary edema in extreme cases. Each gram of dextran-70 can draw 20 to 27 ml of water into the circulation. Expansion of the intravascular volume can be almost 10 times the volume of dextran absorbed. Treatment ofpulmonary edema from dextran may be challenging, because it may not respond to standard therapy. Dialysis is not effective. Plasmapheresis may be indicated in severe cases. Anaphylaxis must be treated with resuscitative measures to support the airway and circulation. The administration of dextran must, of course, be stopped at the first sign of an adverse event. Disseminated intravascular coagulation (DIC) and other coagulation disorders, oliguria, and renal failure have also been associated with dextran-70. Low–molecular weight dextrans are filtered by the kidney and may precipitate in the renal tubules and cause obstruction. They may cause problems with blood cross-matching, glucose, and bilirubin determination.

We recommend the following measures to improve the safety of hysteroscopy: (1) consider regional anesthesia whenever feasible so that the early behavioral signs of hyponatremia can be detected; (2) conduct frequent and accurate checks of fluid balance to prevent inadvertent fluid overload. With low-viscosity solutions (i.e., glycine, gross overestimates of leakage are often made), which translate into serious underestimates of the quantity absorbed by the patient. Prompt cessation of surgery in the case of fluid overload can avoid major problems.

Dilatation and evacuation. Dilatation and evacuation is the most common procedure used for induced abortion. More than 1 million procedures are performed in the United States on an annual basis. Complication rates from induced abortion are correlated with the week of gestation and the experience of the surgeon.[30,32,53] Most are performed with the patient under attended local anesthesia using a combination of local anesthesia (e.g., paracervical block, with IV sedation and analgesia). Complications include cardiac arrest, seizures, and uterine perforation. With a paracervical block, the patient will report sudden, acute abdominal pain if a uterine perforation occurs. The likelihood of uterine perforation is much greater when this procedure is performed with the patient receiving spinal or general anesthesia because the patient will be unaware of and unable to report the impending event to the surgeon. This is a powerful argument for use of attended local anesthesia whenever possible. Average blood loss from such a procedure is greater when general anesthesia with volatile agents is used, related to uterine relaxation or atony.[14,34] This can be major, especially in an abortion performed after the first trimester, and occurs before uterine tone is regained. Rare surgical complications from D&E include amniotic fluid embolus resulting in sudden cardiopulmonary collapse and profound *disseminated intravascular coagulation* DIC.[31,32,48] DIC is associated with second-trimester abortions, particularly with a long-standing fetal demise. If suspected, a DIC screen must be performed and a hematology consultation obtained.

Paracervical block with IV sedation is the preferred anesthetic for D&E. Some patients insist on general anesthesia. These patients can be often distraught and may have hyperemesis. A full stomach must be assumed. When there is any question regarding emesis or a full stomach, we treat the patient with metoclopramide and insert an ET tube. Once the suction aspiration is begun, the surgeon usually requests that oxytocin be administered IV to increase uterine tone. This causes the uterus to "clamp down" and stop bleeding. Oxytocin must be administered as an infusion (see Table 77-1). In severe cases of uterine atony, 0.2 mg of methylergonovine (Methergine®), can be administered intramuscularly (IM). This drug must not be administered IV except in life-threatening hemorrhagic emergencies, because a catastrophic hypertensive crisis may result. If given IV, injection must be over a 60-sec period and the blood pressure closely monitored. It is best to avoid volatile agents in high concentrations for D&E because their use can contribute to uterine atony.[14,34] Thiopental, N_2O, and a narcotic, with judicious use of a succinylcholine infusion or nondepolarizer ensures adequate anesthesia and muscle relaxation for the procedure.

Complete molar pregnancy. Special attention must be paid to anesthetic management for suction curettage for complete molar pregnancy. A hydatidiform mole is a neoplastic condition resulting from deranged placental growth. Molar pregnancies are associated with vaginal bleeding, resulting in anemia in approximately 50% of cases.[4] Rapid evacuation of large quantities of tissue from an excessively enlarged uterus may result in brisk blood loss which must be anticipated. Patients with molar pregnancies may also present with preeclampsia (27%) and hyperemesis gravidarum (26%) that complicates fluid and electrolyte management.[5] Rare but life-threatening complications of molar pregnancy include hyperthyroidism and pulmonary trophoblastic emboli.[5] Hyperthyroidism occurs in 7% of patients with molar pregnancies. Its cause is unclear but may be related to thyrotropic effects of trophoblastic hormones. If unrecognized, caregivers may be confronted with a full-blown thyroid storm. These patients may require a combination of antithyroid drugs, such as PTU, and treatment with a beta-blocker, (i.e., propranolol and sodium iodide) to combat the manifestations of this condition.[61] Trophoblastic emboli may also occur during molar evacuation, when tissue may enter uterine venous sinuses and eventually the right heart and PA, resulting in varying degrees of respiratory compromise.

Cone biopsy. A cone biopsy is the concentric excision of both exocervical and endocervical stroma of the uterine cervix. The procedure is performed both to aid in the diagnosis of preinvasive or invasive lesions of the cervix and may also be therapeutic, particularly in the case of preinvasive cervical lesions. The cone biopsy is reserved for those cases of preinvasive cervical neoplasia that are present in the endocervical canal or lesions not detected by outpatient biopsy when the patient has had an abnormal Pap smear. Cone biopsy is helpful in establishing the degree or depth of invasive squamous cell carcinoma. The goal is to remove a cone-shaped plug of tissue incorporating two thirds the depth of the endocervix and the entire transformation zone.

The cervix is well vascularized. Accordingly, various surgical approaches have been devised to reduce blood loss. Most gynecologic surgeons place hemostatic sutures in the lateral cervical stroma to ligate descending cervical branches of the uterine artery. Sutures in this location reduce blood flow to the cervix without rendering it ischemic. Dilute solutions of vasopressin (Pitressin®) or epinephrine injected locally can induce local vasospasm and reduce blood loss. Usual dose of vasopressin is 20 units in 20 ml of normal saline solution. Usual dose of epinephrine is 10 to 20 ml of 1% lidocaine with epinephrine in a 1:200,000 ratio. Inadvertent IV injection of these potent vasospastic compounds can have severe consequences. A direct intravascular injection of vasopressin can result in stimulation of gastrointestinal smooth muscle as well as severe vasospasm of the coronary arteries.[33] Most patients who have cone biopsy procedures do not have significant coronary artery disease (CAD), but there is the potential for severe myocardial ischemia if a large amount of vasopressin suddenly enters the bloodstream. Vasopressin may also induce hypertension as the agent is absorbed after injection into the cervical stroma. If severe, a direct-acting vasodilator, such as hydralazine (Apresoline®), may be required. Adrenergic-blocking agents, such as labetalol, are less effective because vasopressin does not act via adrenergic stimulation but rather exerts direct effect on vascular smooth muscle.

Cone biopsy usually takes 30 to 60 minutes, depending on extent of the lesion. Bleeding can be a major problem, especially if the patient is pregnant, although cervical conization is seldom performed in pregnancy. Vasospastic compounds are contraindicated in pregnancy. Approximately one in 10 patients experiences a complication of cervical conization. The majority present with vaginal hemorrhage, usually occurring 7 to 10 days after the procedure. Occasionally, a patient will be taken to the operating room emergently to achieve hemostasis.

Most cone biopsies are performed as day-surgery procedures. We try to use spinal anesthesia whenever possible. If general anesthesia is required, we use the combination of N_2O and a volatile agent. If a patient has a good airway, a mask or LMA can be used with spontaneous or assisted respiration.

Cervical cerclage. Cervical cerclage is a procedure performed to prevent second-trimester pregnancy loss related to an incompetent cervical os. These patients may have suffered several prior miscarriages and are generally between 16 and 21 weeks' gestation. With the patient in the lithotomy position, the surgeon places a circumferential suture around the cervical os. The procedure usually lasts about 30 minutes. We perform this procedure with the patient receiving hyperbaric spinal anesthesia with a modest dose of 1.5% lidocaine in 7.5% dextrose. After IV hydration with 500 to 1000 ml lactated Ringer's solution, we administer the spinal anesthetic with the patient in the sitting position. A level of T12 anesthetizes the cervix and a portion of the fundus, because the latter is occasionally stimulated during this procedure. For most patients, administration of 45 to 55 mg of lidocaine is adequate. Although hypotension seldom occurs, ephedrine is the agent of choice if a vasopressor is needed. We do not administer any adjunctive sedation or narcotic unless absolutely necessary because these patients are highly motivated and prefer not to receive any unnecessary drugs during pregnancy.

If a patient refuses a regional technique and insists on receiving general anesthesia, we administer thiopental and a volatile agent in O_2 along with IV fentanyl if needed.

Because the fetuses of these patients are below the stage of fetal viability, continuous fetal monitoring during the surgical procedure is not routinely performed. These patients are occasionally admitted overnight for observation, because postoperative bleeding, cramping, premature labor, and infection can occur.

Vaginal hysterectomy. Vaginal hysterectomy is used primarily for removal of the uterus and cervix in patients with benign pelvic conditions. The vaginal approach is also used in patients with early stage malignancies of the uterus. The procedure is also performed in patients with loss of pelvic support, with uterine prolapse (i.e., the intussusception of the cervix and uterus into the vaginal canal). Uterine prolapse is a consequence of weakness in the endopelvic fascia, the primary support for the pelvic viscera. Excessive uterine size, prior abdominal surgery, or the suspicion of intrapelvic malignant disease are all contraindications to this procedure.

The procedure requires entry into the anterior and posterior cul-de-sacs to expose the broad ligament containing the uterine artery (Fig. 77-6),[51] using serial placement of ascending hemostatic clamps in paracervical and parametrial tissues, thereby progressively freeing the uterus while achieving hemostasis. Rarely, bleeding from a vascular

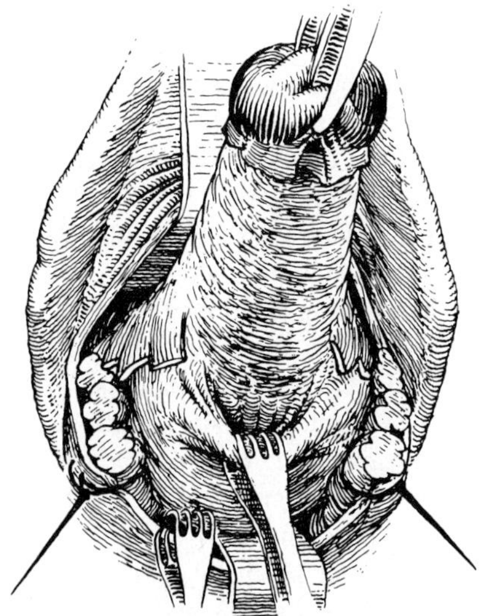

Fig. 77-6. Representation of the later stages of vaginal hysterectomy. The uterosacral ligaments, cardinal ligaments, and uterine arteries have been ligated. With division of the utero-ovarian ligaments, the hysterectomy will be complete. (From Wheelas CR: *Atlas of pelvic surgery,* Philadelphia, 1981, Lea & Febiger.)

pedicle or unsuspected intra-abdominal adhesions requires abandonment of the vaginal approach to complete the procedure abdominally.

The ovaries may be conserved or removed vaginally. In elderly patients, vaginal hysterectomy is frequently performed in association with a repair of a cystocoele or rectocoele.

Vaginal hysterectomy can be managed well with spinal anesthesia. The procedure generally takes 1 to 3 hours; the latter time is usual if hysterectomy is combined with repair of prolapse. We have found a hyperbaric technique with bupivacaine to work well. Epinephrine is added for longer procedures. A T6 to T8 level is needed to block peritoneal sensation when the uterus is placed under traction. On occasion, such traction can initiate a vagal response with severe bradycardia and IV atropine may be needed. If general anesthesia is used, there is usually no need for neuromuscular blockers other than for ET intubation. Because of the length of the procedure and the use of the Trendelenburg position, we tend to insert an ET tube to guard against the possibilities of prolonged facial pressure from a tight-fitting mask and aspiration of gastric contents. Laparascopically-assisted vaginal hysterectomies (LAVH) are frequently performed to simplify the surgery and to decrease blood loss. After induction of general anesthesia, the surgeon inserts the laparoscope, identifies and then divides the ligamentous attachments of most of the uterus along with much of its blood supply. The uterus is then removed vaginally, usually with less blood loss than would otherwise occur. LAVH usually is performed with both arms tucked in at the sides. The operating room team must be certain that both elbows are padded and that the hands and fingers are protected. The blood pressure cuff, IV, and pulse-oximeter sensor must function well with the arms at the sides, because access to these areas will be difficult once the procedure is underway.

Regardless of technique or agents, a large-bore (16-gauge) IV catheter be placed and a blood type and antibody screen be performed preoperatively. On occasion, sudden, uncontrolled hemorrhage occurs during the freeing up of the uterus and the rapid administration of several units of blood may be required.

Intra-abdominal Operations

Surgical anatomy of the pelvis

Anatomic overview. The organs of the true pelvis include the vagina, uterine cervix, uterus, fallopian tube, and ovary with the bladder and rectum in close proximity (see Fig. 77-5). On occasion, after pelvic sepsis and/or tumor invasion, the rectum and bladder form fistulous communications with other pelvic structures (e.g., vesicovaginal and rectovaginal fistulas) that require surgical correction.

The blood supply to the pelvis is largely derived from the internal iliac (hypogastric) artery (Fig. 77-7).[40] The internal iliac artery gives rise to important visceral branches, including the uterine artery, superior, middle, and inferior vesical arteries supplying the urinary bladder, the middle and inferior hemorrhoidal artery, and the vaginal artery. Despite these seemingly discrete, organ-specific vessels, there is a rich and extensive collateral circulation to the pelvic viscera. This is demonstrated by the fact that the internal iliac artery

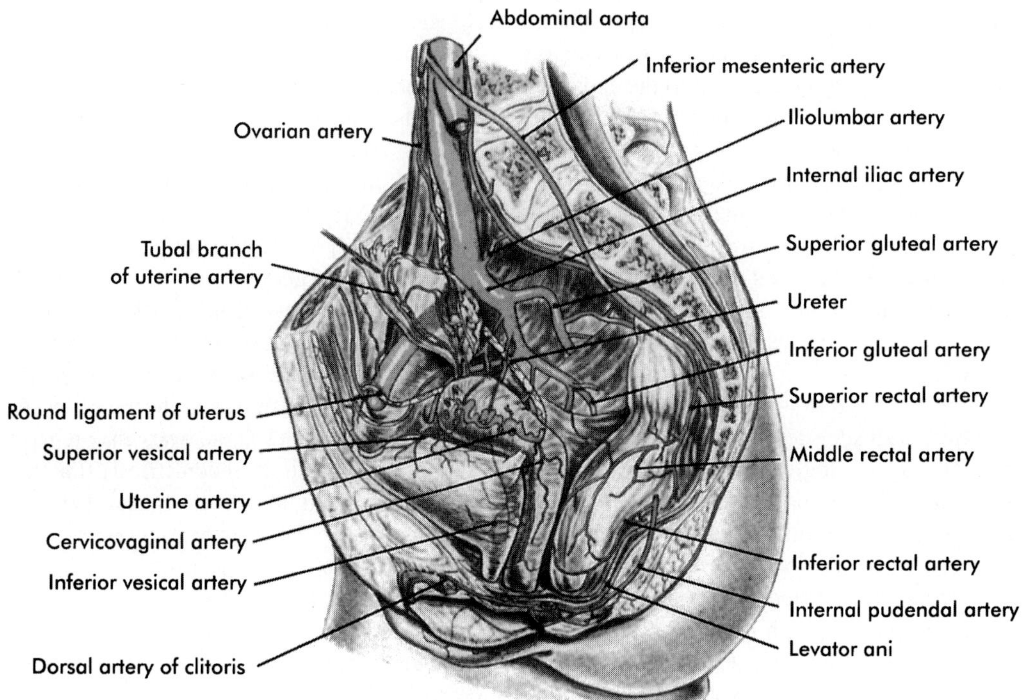

Fig. 77-7. Arterial blood supply to the organs of the female pelvis. (From Langman J, Woerdeman MW: *Atlas of medical anatomy,* Philadelphia, 1978, WB Saunders.)

may be ligated in cases of extensive pelvic dissection or obstetric hemorrhage with no untoward effects. Collateral circulation to the true pelvis arises from the aorta via the ovarian artery, lumbar and vertebral arteries, and the middle sacral artery. There is also collateral supply from branches of the external iliac artery and the femoral artery. A dense venous plexus drains the uterus, vagina, and fallopian tube. These vessels may be engorged in pregnancy and can cause severe bleeding from a ruptured ectopic pregnancy.

The pelvic organs are innervated by both sympathetic and parasympathetic nerves (Fig. 77-8).[7] A majority of the sympathetic fibers enter the hypogastric or presacral plexus. These fibers are derived predominately from the first, second, third, and fourth lumbar nerves (L1 to L4). The presacral plexus brings sympathetic innervation to the uterine fundus, cervix, and vagina. In addition, several important excretory organs, including the rectosigmoid region of the colon, anus, bladder, and urethra, derive their sympathetic innervation from this plexus. Parasympathetic preganglionic fibers arise from the second, third, and fourth sacral nerves (S2 to S4). The sensory nerve supply to the pelvic viscera including the uterus arises from T10 to L4 spinal cord segments. This has important practical implications because uterine pain is usually referred to the lower abdomen or hypogastrium. Pain fibers from the cervix are carried through the uterosacral ligaments to S2, S3, and S4. Pain arising from the cervix is frequently referred to the lumbosacral region and may be confused with lower backstrain, particularly during pregnancy.

The lymphatic drainage of the female reproductive organs is predominately to the pelvic and para-aortic lymph nodes. The uterine cervix drains to paracervical nodes. The most frequently involved node in cervical cancer is the obturator node. Spread may also extend to the external iliac nodal chain. Branches from the fundus of the uterus follow the same path as the uterine cervix (i.e., drainage to the pelvic and para-aortic nodes). The fallopian tube and ovary share common pathways to the pelvic and para-aortic nodes but, in addition, the ovary has lymphatic channels along the ovarian artery and vein that arise from the aorta or vena cava at the first lumbar vertebra. The upper portion of the vagina drains to the pelvic lymph node system. The lower portion, however, drains primarily to the superficial and deep inguinal lymph nodes. The route of lymphatic drainage determines the route of metastases for many gynecologic cancers. Accordingly, these retroperitoneal nodal groups are regarded very seriously and are frequently palpated, biopsied, or radically dissected as part of procedures for malignancies. In performing a hysterectomy for uterine carcinoma, the decision to perform a para-aortic lymph node biopsy is made intraoperatively and is based on gross examination of the total depth of invasion within the myometrial wall and the degree of differentiation of the adenocarcinoma. Para-aortic node biopsy requires an extension of the incision and prolonged operative time with the potential for damage to the great vessels.

Specific intra-abdominal procedures

There are many intra-abdominal gynecologic procedures. These include surgery on the ovary, fallopian tubes, uterus, and cervix. Commonly performed procedures include ovarian cystectomy, oophorectomy, salpingostomy, myomectomy, total abdominal hysterectomy, and to a lesser extent, radical hysterectomy. In addition, there are less common procedures performed for the reconstruction of uterine anomalies. The gynecologic surgeon may approach the pelvis through a variety of transverse or vertical abdominal incisions, and it is important that the anesthesia provider understand their rationale to optimize regional or general anesthesia. Transverse incisions include the Pfannenstiel, the Maylard, and the Cherney incisions. These are all low transverse incisions that offer excellent surgical access to the pelvis while placing the incision in a cosmetic location. They are also strong and not readily disrupted. The Pfannenstiel incision is the most common approach to the uterus for cesarean section. The Maylard and Cherney incisions are modifications of the Pfannenstiel in which the muscle belly or tendon of the rectus abdominis is divided and the superficial epigastric arteries ligated. These latter two incisions offer excellent access to the pelvic side wall and are common approaches for radical hysterectomy.

If access to the upper abdomen is required, as in patients with pelvic masses, this necessitates use of a vertical incision. Vertical approaches include the midline laparotomy and the paramedian incision. These incisions lack the intrinsic strength and structural integrity of a transverse incision. In addition, a large vertical incision intruding into the upper abdomen tends to impede respiration and provoke splinting postoperatively, which can impede recovery and predispose patients to respiratory complications, particularly obese patients.[69] Although it is beyond the scope of this chapter to describe in detail each of the many intra-abdominal surgical operations, representative procedures that most anesthesia providers will encounter will be discussed herein.

Ovarian surgery. Conservative ovarian surgery is performed for a variety of neoplastic and nonneoplastic conditions of the ovary. Benign neoplastic conditions most commonly affecting the ovary include the benign mature cystic teratoma (dermoid cyst) and the simple cystadenoma. In addition, cystic masses in the ovary may represent nonneoplastic processes such as endometriosis (the chocolate cyst) or may arise from infectious causes (see later discussion). Ovarian cystectomies may be performed for these benign processes for conservation of the ovarian stroma. These procedures are generally of short duration and do not entail a great loss of blood. Although most commonly performed with the patient under general anesthesia, simple ovarian cystectomy is well managed with hyperbaric spinal, single-dose, or continuous epidural anesthesia; the latter is preferred if the length of surgery cannot be predicted accurately.

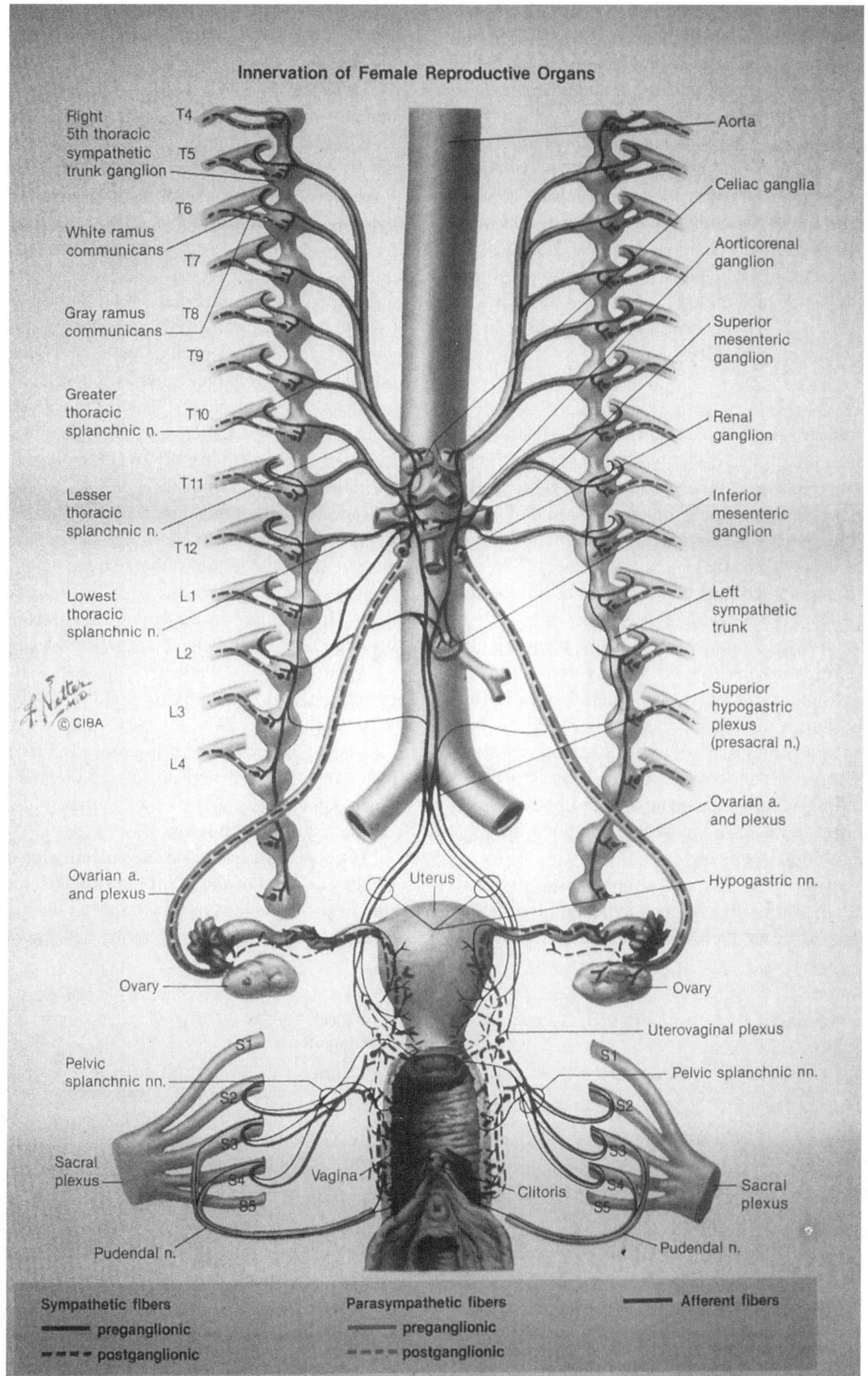

Fig. 77-8. Innervation of female reproductive organs. (From Brass A, editor: *The CIBA collection of illustrations, the nervous system,* vol 1, part 1, West Caldwell, 1984, CIBA.)

Oophorectomy is the removal of an ovary. It may be performed for both benign and malignant processes. These procedures range from straightforward to technically challenging in the presence of inflammation, endometriosis, or metastatic disease and may require extended vertical incisions for adequate exposure. Although regional anesthesia can be used, in uncertain situations it is prudent to inquire beforehand regarding the type and size of incision contemplated, whether upper-abdominal packs will be used, need for a steep Trendelenburg position, and so forth, to determine whether a combined regional-light general anesthesia technique with an ET tube placed for airway protection is indicated. Surgery for ovarian neoplasia is described in the section on gynecologic oncology.

Tubal surgery

Tubal anatomy. The fallopian tubes are paired structures extending from the uterus to the ovary (Fig. 77-9).[40] There are four distinct anatomic subdivisions of the tube: (1) the interstitial; (2) isthmic; (3) ampullary; and (4) infundibular regions. The interstitial portion passes tangentially through the myometrial muscle to the endometrial cavity. The isthmic portion is a narrowed muscular region in the midportion of the tube. The capacious ampullary portion of the tube is the region where fertilization occurs. Finally, the infundibular portion terminating in the fimbria is that portion of the tube most proximal to the ovary. The arterial supply of the fallopian tube is redundant, with branches derived from both uterine and ovarian arteries. The lymphatic drainage follows that of the ovary. The innervation of the tube is complex with both sympathetic and parasympathetic fibers. Sensory nerves terminate in the T10 dermatome and therefore tubal pain may be referred to this region.

A variety of inflammatory and nonneoplastic processes affect the fallopian tube. Benign or malignant neoplasia of the tube is rare. However, there are two disease processes affecting the tube that have important implications for anesthetic management: tubal ectopic pregnancy and tuboovarian abscess.

Tubal ectopic pregnancy. There has been an important increase in the incidence of tubal ectopic pregnancy in the United States. Currently, the overall incidence is approximately 1/100 pregnancies, a much greater figure than in former years. This is predominantly related to a larger population with significant risk factors for ectopic implantation. These include history of pelvic inflammatory disease, intrauterine device (IUD) use, prior tubal reconstruction, failed tubal fulguration, diethylstilbestrol exposure, or prior ectopic gestation.[1] The most common presenting symptoms are nonspecific and include pain and abnormal vaginal bleeding. Physical signs include abdominal tenderness and a palpable pelvic mass.[11] The diagnosis of ectopic pregnancy has been clarified by the development of a highly sensitive radioimmunoassay for the beta subunit of human chorionic gonadotropin. This highly sensitive pregnancy test and new developments in pelvic ultrasonography have improved the early detection of small ectopic pregnancies. Despite these modalities, tubal ectopic pregnancies still can rupture without warning and patients present with acute hemoperitoneum, occasionally of massive proportions, leading to profound hemorrhagic shock, exsanguination, even cardiac arrest. Patients with suspected ectopic tubal gestations are frequently brought urgently to surgery.[45] When the diagnosis is not clear, patients may undergo a diagnostic laparoscopy. With the advent of laparoscopic techniques for resection of ectopic pregnancies, the diagnostic laparoscopy may also be therapeutic (see section on laparoscopy and pelviscopy).

Tubal ectopic gestations are usually located in the ampullary portion of the fallopian tube, because this area is the most capacious and where fertilization most frequently occurs. This region of the tube may be approached

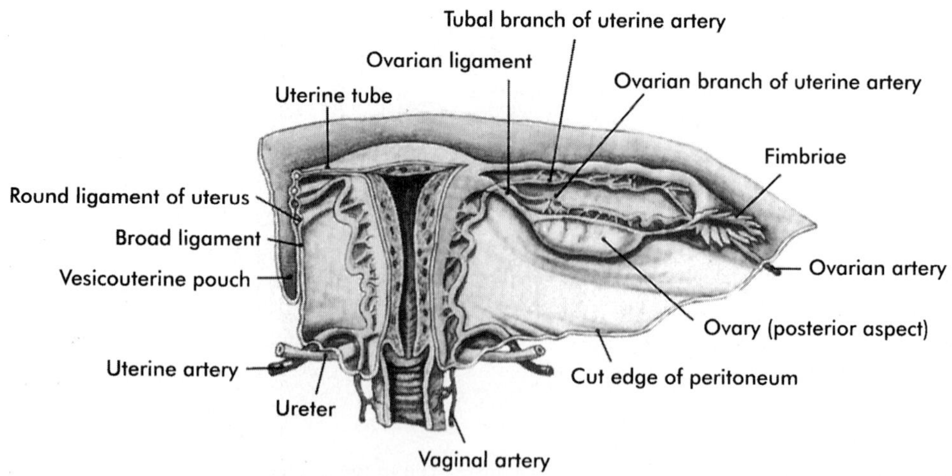

Fig. 77-9. Detailed view of the blood supply to the uterus, fallopian tubes, and ovaries. (From Langman J, Woerdeman MW: *Atlas of medical anatomy,* Philadelphia, 1978, WB Saunders.)

surgically with a variety of conservative procedures, most notably the linear salpingostomy. In this procedure, an incision is made longitudinally in the fallopian tube and the products of conception are allowed to extrude. The procedure may be time consuming because hemostasis at the bed of the implantation site may be difficult to obtain. If sutures alone are not sufficient, a dilute vasopressin solution may be applied or injected into the area.

Fortunately, ectopic gestations lodged in the interstitial portion of the tube are rare. This location demands special note because an ectopic pregnancy implanted here will be surrounded by myometrium within the uterine wall and may achieve significant size before becoming symptomatic. Procedures for extirpation involve a cornual resection (i.e., a resection of the myometrium in the region of the tubal insertion). Ectopic pregnancies in this location may also require a hysterectomy.

Anesthetic management of ruptured ectopic pregnancy with hemoperitoneum is similar to that of a ruptured abdominal aortic aneurysm (AAA) and is centered on rapid fluid resuscitation of the patient, restoration of the circulation, followed by immediate operation. If a patient is brought to surgery in extremis, the airway must be secured, fluids rapidly administered through several large-bore IVs equipped with pressure-infusion devices, and the operation begun immediately. Type-specific or even O-negative blood may be life saving. As in cases of ruptured aortic aneurysm, the operation is the basic resuscitative measure. Fortunately, these patients tend to be young and otherwise healthy. Even in the face of profound blood loss and anemia, they usually do well once volume status is restored and bleeding stopped.

Tubo-ovarian abscess. The tubo-ovarian abscess is a complication of acute salpingitis. Most of these abscesses less than 5 cm in size respond to medical management with broad-spectrum antibiotic therapy. Surgery is reserved for those patients with ruptured tubo-ovarian abscesses, patients with abscesses in excess of 8 cm in size, or in the case of abscesses refractory to drug therapy. A ruptured tubo-ovarian abscess may be accompanied by frank peritonitis and septic shock. A rupture is usually clinically manifested by a pronounced increase in pain and the rapid development of an acute abdomen. Respiratory distress syndrome and coagulopathies may also develop rapidly.

Conservative management for medically unresponsive tubo-ovarian abscess in a stable patient may include percutaneous or laparoscopic drainage. Abscess presently in the pouch of Douglas (cul de sac) may be drained through the vagina. More commonly, however, these abscesses are approached with laparotomy and adenexectomy, either unilateral or bilateral and possible hysterectomy depending upon the extent of the pelvic infection. Unstable patients must be managed in a surgically aggressive manner.

The surgical management of the tubo-ovarian abscess is one of the most difficult and challenging operations in gynecology. There is a great risk of bowel or ureteral injury. Operative times may be protracted and blood loss significant. It is best to be prepared for a difficult case.

Surgical management may include either salpingo-oophorectomy or total abdominal hysterectomy with unilateral or bilateral salpingo-oophorectomy. Regardless of the type of surgery performed, this type of pelvic surgery in patients with acute infection prolongs an already technically difficult procedure. There is a great risk of damage to vital internal organs, including the ureter. If acute pelvic inflammatory disease (PID) is present, the operative time may be lengthened and the probability of significant blood loss is increased.

Myomectomy. Uterine leiomyomas (fibroids) are the most common benign tumor in women. These tumors undergo rapid growth, particularly in the perimenopausal period. Uterine leiomyomas may cause excessive uterine size, menometrorrhagia, pain, ureteral obstruction, and rarely, even lead to first-trimester pregnancy loss. Grossly, these lesions are well circumscribed, nonencapsulated, benign tumors, commonly called *fibroids.* Fibroids may occur in any one of three locations in the uterus: (1) submucosal (within the innermost layer of the uterus); (2) intramural (within the myometrial layer); and (3) subserosal (within the outermost uterine layer). Because of their accessibility, submucous leiomyomas can often be resected hysteroscopically as described in an earlier section on transvaginal surgery, whereas intramural or subserosal locations require pelviscopy or a lapararotomy.

The most common symptoms associated with fibroids are menorrhagia, pelvic pain, or pressure.[1] Large or multiple uterine fibroids can interfere with implantation of the fertilized ovum and the gestational process. Accordingly, the indication for surgical intervention is fibroid-related symptoms in women who wish to retain fertility or to become pregnant. Leuprolide, a drug that mimics the agonistic action of gonadotropin-releasing hormone (GRNH) is sometimes prescribed preoperatively to shrink large fibroids so that they will bleed less. Instead of the cyclic, pulsatile release of GNRH associated with normal menses, leuprolide results in a sustained release of GNRH resulting in a pharmacologically induced menopausal state when the drug is being taken.[68] Accordingly, the patient becomes less anemic at the time of surgery. Leuprolide is not associated with any known interactions with anesthetic agents, sedatives or vasopressors, so it must not interfere with any anesthetic technique in common use.

Approximately 18,000 myomectomies are performed annually in the United States.[36] There are a variety of surgical approaches to the resection of fibroids, depending on their size, number, and location within the uterus. Hemostasis is a major concern during this type of surgery. In this regard, the surgeon and anesthesia provider must be encouraged to work together to have the patient donate at least one, and preferably two, units of autologous blood if the preoperative hematocrit level permits it. This requires advanced planning; donation must ideally take place 4 to 5 weeks before surgery so that two units can be donated with sufficient time for the hematocrit to recover. Too often, the concept of autologous blood donation comes as an afterthought and the patient is too anemic to donate on such short notice. Autologous donation obviates most of the risks of banked blood, and its use must be promoted whenever possible. Techniques to reduce blood loss during myomectomy include the liberal use of electrocautery, the temporary occlusion of the ovarian artery and vein with bulldog vascular clamps, and the placement of a bilateral uterine artery tourniquet to reduce blood flow to the uterus. Some gynecologic surgeons inject vasospastic substances (e.g., vasopressin or epinephrine, 1:200,000 solution) directly into the myometrium surrounding the fibroid.

A myomectomy can range from a straightforward, relatively brief procedure with a 200-ml blood loss to a difficult and prolonged dissection with extensive bleeding. Pedunculated, subserosal fibroids are usually easy to mobilize and resect, whereas intramural fibroids are the most difficult because their blood supply is not discrete and not easily clamped off. After removal of multiple uterine fibroids, the defects may require the surgeon to perform an extensive uterine reconstruction to reestablish normal uterine contours, with the potential for greater additional blood loss. It is important that the anesthesia caregiver know which technique the surgeon will use to remove the fibroids and how hemostasis will be achieved. It should be known beforehand if the surgeon plans to use vascular clamps and tourniquets, because their absence will result in greater blood loss. If vasopressin is used intraoperatively, the anesthesia team must be informed of the dose and time of administration.

Although most myomectomies are performed with the patient under general ET anesthesia, spinal or continuous epidural anesthesia can be used; steep Trendelenburg positioning is seldom required. A regional technique also offers the theoretic advantage of a lesser mean arterial pressure, thereby decreasing overall blood loss.

Uterine reconstructive surgery. A variety of uterine reconstructive procedures are performed for congenital malformations of the uterus that interfere with fertility or gestation. These include procedures performed for the reunification of duplicated uterine horns or uterine septa. These procedures can be managed with general or regional anesthesia.

Abdominal hysterectomy. There are three general types of abdominal hysterectomy. These include: (1) subtotal (supracervical) hysterectomy; (2) total hysterectomy; and (3) radical hysterectomy. The radical hysterectomy is described in detail as part of the section on gynecologic oncology. A subtotal hysterectomy is the removal of part or all of the uterine fundus with preservation of the lower uterine segment or uterine cervix. A total hysterectomy includes removal of both the body of the uterus and, in addition, the uterine cervix. It does not, however, include the removal of the fallopian tubes or ovaries, which are considered separate procedures if performed at the time. Total, rather than subtotal, abdominal hysterectomy is performed whenever possible because removal of the cervix eliminates the possibility of cervical cancer occurring at a later time. Subtotal hysterectomy is a procedure reserved for benign disease in which a lot of distortion of the anatomic relationships of the lower uterine segment, or dense adhesions to the bladder or rectum preclude the surgical removal of the cervix.

The indications for hysterectomy include a variety of benign and malignant diseases. Surgical considerations for removal of the uterus in the presence of malignancy are reviewed in the section on gynecologic oncology. The most common benign conditions for which total hysterectomy is performed include symptomatic uterine fibroids (particularly in postmenopausal women), pelvic pain, and endometriosis. Endometriosis is the ectopic proliferation of endometrial tissue outside the endometrial cavity. This tissue undergoes cyclic changes associated with changes in hormonal status. Endometriosis, particularly when advanced, results in the destruction of normal tissue planes and increased vascularity in the pelvis. Therefore, hysterectomies performed for relief of chronic pelvic pain stemming from endometriosis may be complicated and time consuming. Special note is made of procedures performed either in the presence of acute inflammatory disease (e.g., patients undergoing hysterectomy for PID) or in the presence of endometriosis. These conditions can result in dense adhesions and increased vascularity that can prolong surgery and increase blood loss.

Most hysterectomies are performed with the patient under general ET anesthesia because of the steep Trendelenburg position often required and the propensity for nausea and regurgitation under these conditions. With a gentle surgeon who can operate with little or no Trendelenburg positioning, it is possible (maybe even desirable) to use regional anesthesia. If there is uncertainty regarding duration of the procedure, a long-acting agent or a continuous technique must be strongly considered. A combined technique with an indwelling epidural catheter for postoperative analgesia is excellent for prolonged, major procedures and is discussed further in the section on gynecologic oncology.

Gynecologic Oncology

Gynecologic malignancies have become one of the leading causes of death of women in the United States. In 1988, an estimated 141,000 new cases of gynecologic cancer were diagnosed (this figure includes patients with carcinoma *in situ*), and in 1991, approximately 71,900 new cases of invasive gynecologic malignancies were diagnosed.[55] Many of these patients require extensive and lengthy surgical procedures and undergo, as well, chemotherapeutic regimens with multiple agents, some of which have the potential for major toxic side effects. To deliver optimal anesthetic care to this surgical population, it is essential that anesthesia providers have a good understanding of the relevant disease processes and the medical and surgical interventions they will encounter.

Preoperative assessment

The anesthesia caregiver must have an understanding of the patient's disease, its extent (if known), and the surgical procedure contemplated. It is important to determine if any previous surgical procedures were performed, because the presence of scarring and adhesions may increase the difficulty of dissection, thereby increasing operative time and resulting in greater fluid shifts and blood loss. If the patient has a discrete tumor mass, its size, location, and extent must be known so that appropriate maneuvers can be performed to avoid aortocaval compression and respiratory embarrassment in the relaxed, anesthetized patient in the supine in the Trendelenburg position. Inquiry must include questions about the patient's previous courses of chemotherapy (if any) and the agents, times of treatment, and dosages. These compounds can exert severe toxic effects and disrupt hematopoiesis and myocardial and renal function. Table 77-3 contains a summary of the chemotherapeutic agents commonly used in gynecologic oncology patients. Although most newly diagnosed patients will not have received chemotherapy, many patients having repeat procedures—particularly patients with ovarian cancer—will have had several courses of treatment. As previously mentioned, these drugs are quite toxic and the anesthesia provider must be familiar with their actions and side effects.

Myelosuppressive effects of chemotherapy

Most chemotherapeutic agents used for the treatment of gynecologic malignancies are myelosuppressive. Although the degree and duration of myelosuppression is variable, it occurs at a predictable time interval following a treatment session. Accordingly, it is unusual to plan elective surgery during a chemotherapy nadir when depression of erythrocyte and leukocytes counts are apt to be maximal and bleeding and clotting abnormalities most likely to be manifest. Unfortunately, urgent situations may occur in which surgical intervention during the nadir is unavoidable. Risks of bleeding or infection are real and require support. It is wise to consult with the surgeon and a hematologist when such emergency procedures must be undertaken. In many cases, platelets or fresh frozen plasma (FFP) will be required; it is always prudent to make sure that these components will be available if and when needed.

Physiologic effects of chemotherapy

Certain agents have effects that permanently impair the function of the heart, lungs, and kidneys. Appropriate diagnostic studies and clinical laboratory tests, if indicated, must have been obtained.

Doxorubicin (Adriamycin®) is a drug used in the treatment of both endometrial and ovarian carcinoma and sarcoma.[12] Use of doxorubicin may lead to decreased cardiac function. The patient may remain asymptomatic, but decreased contractility may be seen with serial ECG studies.[41,42] In extreme cases, refractory congestive heart failure (CHF) may develop despite administration of digitalis and other inotropic agents. CHF appears to be a dose-related side effect of doxorubicin therapy. Although reported at cumulative doses as low as 250 mg/M^2, the risk of congestive failure is negligible below cumulative doses of 500 mg/M^2, the usual clinical dose. An ECG estimate of cardiac ejection fraction can be obtained rapidly and provides a reasonably accurate measure of the degree of preoperative cardiac dysfunction.[41,42] The normal value for the ejection fraction is 0.5 to 0.7, whereas a value below 0.4 is considered indicative of severe impairment of left ventricular function.[39] In such patients, especially after doxorubicin therapy, placement of a Swan-Ganz catheter before or after induction of anesthesia can be considered.

Bleomycin (Blenoxane®) is active against squamous cell carcinoma of the cervix and germ cell tumors of the ovary. Bleomycin may cause severe, even fatal pulmonary fibrosis. This toxic manifestation may develop in 5% to 10% of patients receiving bleomycin. Although more common in patients who have received a total cumulative dose of 400 units or who are older than 70 years of age, pulmonary fibrosis has been observed at all dose levels and is consid-

Table 77-3 Chemotherapeutic agents with unique toxicities affecting anesthetic management

Agent	Gynecologic malignancy	Usual dose	System affected	Toxic manifestation	Diagnostic tests
Adriamycin (doxorubicin)	Endometrial carcinoma; ovarian carcinoma	500 mg/M^2	Heart	Myocardial fibrosis; congestive heart failure	Echocardiogram; ejection fraction
Bleomycin (Blenoxane)	Cervical carcinoma; germ cell tumors of the ovary	400 units	Lung	Pulmonary fibrosis	Spirometry; diffusing capacity
cis-Platinum	Endometrial carcinoma; cervical carcinoma	50–75 mg/M^2	Kidney	Renal tubular dysfunction	Creatinine clearance (dose-related)

ered an idiosyncratic reaction to this drug. CO_2 diffusion studies are helpful in quantitating the degree of pulmonary disease.[27]

cis-Platinum (*cis*-dichlorodiamineplatinum) is active against ovarian, endometrial, and cervical carcinoma, and is frequently used by the gynecologic oncologist. *cis*-Platinum can produce renal toxicity, resulting in renal tubular dysfunction. Incidence has been considerably reduced by the routine use of hydration and diuresis before chemotherapy sessions.[12]

Renal toxicity appears to be a dose-related effect with measurable alterations as early as the first dose. Primary manifestations are decreased creatinine clearance and significant electrolyte perturbations, including hypocalcemia, hypomagnesemia, and hypophosphatemia. Serum electrolytes, including serum magnesium, must be checked preoperatively in this population.[12] In addition, *cis*-platinum produces ototoxicity, manifested by tinnitus and hearing loss in the high-frequency range (4000 to 8000 Hz). Peripheral neuropathies, sometimes severe, and myelosupression, manifested by mild-to-moderate leukopenia and thrombocytopenia, occur with this agent.[12]

After obtaining the patient's history, the physical examination is directed toward evaluation of the airway, the cardiopulmonary system, and to those areas potentially affected by previous chemotherapy and radiation therapy. Often ignored until the advent of IV alimentation was the nutritional preparation of the patient for surgery. Studies show an inverse relationship between the serum albumin concentration and incidence of postoperative complications.[63] Serum albumin also serves as a drug carrier for many of the potent medications used in anesthesia, including thiopental and neuromuscular-blocking agents. With the decreased concentrations of serum albumin seen in the elderly and in patients with hepatic or nutritional deficiencies, protein binding decreases and less of these medications may be needed to achieve their desired effects. Acidosis decreases the protein-binding of drugs, particularly highly protein-bound drugs, such as thiopental and digoxin.[65]

Preoperative laboratory studies must be individualized for each patient. A standard chemistry battery to determine hepatic and renal function and electrolyte status in every patient facing a major cancer operation is the practice of some cancer centers. These patients must also have a complete blood count (CBC), and determinations of prothrombin time (PT), partial thromboplastin time (PTT), and bleeding time to identify underlying anemias, continued bone marrow depression, coagulation disorders, and platelet dysfunction that may result in increased bleeding tendencies during surgery. Consultation with the patient's oncologist will assist in further preoperative assessment of the patient's current condition and is helpful in identifying other problems that may require additional preoperative evaluation.

Intraoperative considerations

Many gynecologic oncology patients are quite ill and may require invasive monitoring and even postoperative ventilatory support. Before performing central venous cannulation, a triple-lumen catheter must be considered, because many gynecologic oncology patients require hyperalimentation postoperatively. With good sterile technique, one of the lumens can be reserved for hyperalimentation. The remaining two can be used for central venous pressure (CVP) determinations, fluids, and medications during surgery. Attention to patient temperature, warming fluids, and other appropriate tempearture maintenance techniques must be employed.

Various methods of anesthesia, including general, regional, and combined techniques, have been covered elsewhere in this chapter. We wish to stress several issues. Many patients who undergo debulking procedures have varying degrees of small bowel obstruction from tumor masses must be regarded as having full stomachs and must be managed accordingly. Occasionally, patients come to surgery with huge pelvic tumors, some approaching or even exceeding the size of a full-term uterus. In addition to considering these patients as having full stomachs, it is important to place a wedge directly under the right pelvis in the manner used for obstetric delivery. This serves to displace the uterus or other pelvic mass away from the vena cava, thereby decreasing the possibility of hypotension resulting from caval compression. The anesthesia provider must also remember that surgeons often place packs around the vena cava, and the combination of packing and overzealous retraction can decrease venous return dramatically. If a sudden drop in blood pressure is observed without apparent cause, packs or retractors must be checked and loosened.

Patients with gynecologic malignancies, particularly ovarian cancer, may have a coexistent hypercoagulable state that increases risk of pulmonary thromboembolism. Various regimens are used reduce this risk both intraoperatively and in the postoperative period. These include early ambulation, minidose heparin, dextran, oral anticoagulants, and, recently, the use of external pneumatic compression boots during surgery and the immediate postoperative period.[16] Despite these measures, there is possibility of sudden, unexpected massive pulmonary embolism during surgery. This rare event is catastrophic, requiring prompt diagnosis and treatment if the patient is to survive.[16]

Positioning the patient is also important during these procedures. Major gynecologic intra-abdominal cases are performed in Trendelenburg position with both of the patient's arms extended on armboards, pose a problem for the anesthesia provider. In the steep Trendelenburg position, where gravity tends to outstretch the arms spontaneously, care is taken to keep the patient's arms at an angle less than 90°.[71] If the arms extend beyond this angle for a prolonged period, stretch injury to the brachial plexus may occur. The patient's head must be in a neutral position if possible, because turning it to one side causes the brachial plexus on the contralateral side to be stretched. Combined with an arm abducted to 90° this constitutes a dangerous situation that can result in a serious, prolonged postoperative nerve palsy with major medicolegal ramifications. Pressure against the arm boards by the surgical team must be observed and corrected. Another potential danger is the set of straps used to fasten the arms to the armboard. If applied too tightly at the wrist, they can produce severe nerve compression with postoperative neuropathy, a condition much better avoided than treated.

Representative gynecologic malignancies

Endometrial carcinoma. Endometrial carcinoma is more common among obese, diabetic women in the perimenopausal or postmenopausal age group.[15] The most common presenting symptom is vaginal bleeding resulting from highly vascular and friable neoplastic tissue in the endometrium. For this reason, abnormal bleeding in a perimenopausal or postmenopausal women is a serious event that must be investigated promptly. Fortunately, a diagnosis is readily made by an office endometrial biopsy or by fractional dilatation and curettage in the operating room. Because of its early and obvious manifestation, approximately 85% of patients with endometrial carcinoma present with disease confined to the uterus, which is amenable to surgical therapy.[6,62]

Surgery for endometrial carcinoma usually involves a total abdominal hysterectomy, bilateral salpingo-oophorectomy, and possible para-aortic or pelvic lymph node biopsy. The presence or absence of lymph node metastases has important consequences for both the prognosis and the subsequent therapeutic management of the patient. The likelihood of nodal involvement is related to the stage of the disease, its histologic grade, and the degree to which the tumor has invaded the myometrium.[54] In well-differentiated, superficially invasive lesions, the likelihood of lymph node metastases is so low that the increased operative time and potential morbidity incurred in lymph node biopsy is not warranted. Conversely, poorly differentiated or deeply invasive lesions have a great risk of nodal metastases. This finding, therefore, mandates evaluation of the regional lymph nodes to plan subsequent therapy.[62]

Frequently, the gynecologic surgeon reserves the decision for nodal evaluation until the surgical pathologist performs a gross examination of the excised bivalved uterus to determine the degree of invasion. It is important for the anesthesia provider to be aware of the possibility of para-aortic or pelvic node biopsy and its dependence on the surgical pathologist's report. This procedure extends operative time, requires an extended incision, and carries the potential for major blood loss.

Cervical carcinoma. The widespread use of the Papanicolaou smear (Pap smear) in the evaluation of cytology of the cervix has improved early detection of both preinvasive and invasive cervical carcinoma.[13] Currently, one of every three patients presenting with cervical cancer has her disease confined exclusively to the cervix (early-stage disease). Radiation therapy or surgery are equally effective in treating early-stage cervical carcinoma. The patient and physician, therefore, have an option of two equally effective therapies. The radical (Wertheim) hysterectomy is generally reserved for patients who are young, healthy, and good surgical candidates. Surgery offers preservation of both ovarian and vaginal function.

Clinical staging of invasive carcinoma of the cervix includes an examination with the patient under anesthesia, cystoscopy and proctosigmoidoscopy, a procedure that can be performed satisfactorily with use of single-dose spinal anesthesia. In the case of small central lesions, the gynecologic surgeon frequently schedules the patient for a radical hysterectomy with an initial staging examination, the results of which will determine whether or not the hysterectomy is performed. Occasionally, the staging reveals more extensive disease than appreciated on an outpatient basis, thereby precluding an immediate surgical approach. For this reason, it is imperative that the anesthesia provider confer preoperatively with the gynecologic surgeon regarding the likelihood of progression to radical hysterectomy. This avoids placing invasive monitoring lines and administering large doses of narcotics and neuromuscular-blocking agents in anticipation of a prolonged, radical pelvic dissection when the procedure will be terminated after a brief staging.

The radical (Wertheim) hysterectomy deserves special mention. This procedure, performed to achieve a surgical cure in patients with disease confined to the cervix or uppermost vagina, differs from a total abdominal hysterectomy in several ways. The goal of the radical hysterectomy is to remove the uterus, upper vagina, and all parametrial tissues to the pelvic side wall. As part of this dissection, the ureter, which traverses the parametrial tissues, must be unroofed and moved to a more lateral position. The potential for blood loss in a radical hysterectomy is great. Much of the dissection is performed through highly vascular tissue planes. In addition, the hysterectomy is often accompanied by bilateral pelvic lymphadenectomy. Dissection on or near the great vessels or within the deep pelvic spaces, including the obturator space and in and around the hypogastric vein and venous plexus, bears the potential for major blood loss that is difficult to control. Although major bleeding is rare with this procedure, it is wise to have several units typed, crossmatched, and available within 5 minutes if needed.

In a small number of patients with cervical carcinoma, advanced disease that fails to respond to radiation therapy develops. Sometimes, the local disease becomes so massive that it may spread to the bladder and rectum and cause uremia by compression of the ureters. If the disease is confined to the pelvis without fixation to the pelvic sidewall, pelvic exenteration may offer the only hope of cure. This massive procedure includes a radical hysterectomy, cystectomy with urinary diversion, and proctocolectomy with a permanent colostomy. These patients usually require invasive monitoring and several large-bore IV catheters, because blood loss can be extensive.[50] Major fluid and electrolyte shifts as well as major heat loss can occur. Fluids must be warmed and, if available, a heating mattress must be used. **A combined**

epidural–light general anesthesia technique is often indicated. The epidural component provides sympathetic blockade by its actions at the thoracolumbar sympathetic region. This, in turn, promotes a contracted bowel, which facilitates the dissection and preparation of the ileal conduit for urinary diversion. With general anesthesia, it is prudent to avoid N_2O because its use will distend loops of bowel, particularly the ileal conduit. Low-flow or closed-circuit techniques and the use of passive humidifiers also conserve heat during these long procedures.

Ovarian carcinoma. Ovarian carcinoma is the most lethal of the gynecologic malignancies.[62] Because it is a symptomatically silent tumor, the majority of patients present with advanced and widespread disease. The most common form of ovarian carcinoma is the so-called epithelial tumor that results in abdominal carcinomatosis, ascites and, often, pleural effusions. The goals of the primary surgical procedure are twofold: (1) to establish an accurate surgical stage; and (2) to attempt complete surgical resection of all visible tumor masses, the so-called cytoreductive procedure. The rationale for cytoreductive surgery is to reduce the population of malignant cells to a small fraction, so that those remaining ill be more responsive to chemotherapy.

Patients with advanced ovarian cancer frequently present with a large volume of malignant ascites. Liters of accumulated fluid may reduce diaphragmatic excursion and impair ventilation. Intra-abdominal pressure may also impede venous return. Finally, impaired gastric emptying may result in reflux or regurgitation despite a prolonged fast. Malignant pleural effusions, when present, may further impair ventilation. Preoperative thoracentesis or paracentesis may be necessary on occasion.

Ovarian cancer causes ascites by obstructing the subdiaphragmatic lymphatic channels required for the normal circulation of intraperitoneal fluid.[23] The ascites is a transudate—very different in protein content from the exudative ascites seen in portal hypertension patients. It is unusual for the patient to undergo major fluid shifts with the aspiration of this fluid.

Cytoreductive procedures range considerably in extensiveness. The aggressiveness of the procedure depends on the extent of disease spread, the organ systems involved, and the aggressiveness of the surgeon.[29] Generally, a total abdominal hysterectomy and bilateral salpingo-oophorectomy with omentectomy are performed. In addition, more extensive procedures may include the resection of small or large bowel, a total omentectomy, resection of diaphragmatic or upper-abdominal masses, and splenectomy. These procedures generally involve extensive retroperitoneal dissection, particularly in the pelvis. Bowel resections, bypasses, and colostomies are often required to relieve incipient bowel obstruction from tumor masses. Although the classic radical (Wertheim) hysterectomy is reserved for diseases of the cervix, the procedure may be modified to apply to ovarian cancer.

There is no standard approach to the surgical management of ovarian cancer. The wide range of disease presentation and extent of involvement makes prediction difficult until the abdomen is opened. Accordingly, both the anesthesia and surgical teams must be prepared for many contingencies arising from extensive, protracted dissections, including major blood loss, coagulopathies, significant fluid and electrolyte shifts, and profound heat loss.

Transabdominal Procedures

Laparoscopy and pelviscopy

Laparoscopy is endoscopic examination of the intra-abdominal cavity. It has become one of the most commonly performed procedures in operative gynecology because it allows procedures on the pelvic viscera without opening the abdomen, thereby minimizing hospital stay and morbidity. Although developed as a diagnostic procedure, laparoscopy has evolved to the point that an extensive variety of procedures, including tubal ligations, fulguration of endometriosis, removal of ectopic pregnancies with tubal repair, aspiration and removal of ovarian cysts, and even myomectomies are being performed laparoscopically as day-surgery procedures.

In performing a laparoscopy, after first catheterizing the bladder to ensure that it will be empty, the surgeon inserts a long, hollow needle fitted with a stopcock (Verres needle) periumbilically through the fascial layers and peritoneum. Once in place, the needle is connected to an insufflator, a device that supplies CO_2 until the desired intra-abdominal pressure is attained. For this phase of the procedure, a "manual" as opposed to an "automatic" insufflation mode is used. The manual mode supplies CO_2 at a flow rate of approximately 5 l/min with a pressure limit of 19 mm Hg. During the initial CO_2 insufflation, the surgeon constantly watches the intra-abdominal pressure gauge. In a relaxed patient who is not coughing or otherwise raising intra-abdominal pressure, if the pressure gauge rapidly increases to 19 mm Hg and flow ceases, this usually indicates that the needle is between fascial planes in the muscle layers, rather than in the peritoneal cavity. Under these circumstances, the surgeon withdraws and reinserts the Verres needle.

With a proper intraperitoneal insertion, the intra-abdominal pressure remains well below 19 mm Hg. Generally, 3 l of CO_2, as determined by a gauge on the insufflator, is sufficient to produce the desired degree of intraperitoneal distension. This, in turn, facilitates viewing and minimizes the possibility of puncturing viscera or blood vessels. CO_2 is used because it is nonflammable and absorbed very quickly. This is of paramount importance if the Verres needle inadvertently enters a large vein and causes a massive gas embolus. Recognition and treatment of this complication are discussed in the section on anesthetic management.

After the desired degree of abdominal distention has been attained, the surgeon removes the Verres needle and inserts a trochar. The hollow trochar has a self-sealing opening through which the laparoscope is then passed. Laparoscopes designed exclusively for diagnostic procedures are generally 5 to 7 mm in diameter, whereas those designed for operative laparoscopy may be up to 13 mm in size. The risk of visceral injury with the placement of larger diameter laparoscopes is much greater than with the smaller instruments.

After it is properly placed, the laparoscope is connected to the insufflator, which is usually placed on "automatic" setting, which supplies CO_2 at a flow rate of 200 ml/min as needed to maintain the prevailing intra-abdominal pressure, usually around 12 cm H_2O. If the intra-abdominal pressure increases above the preset level for any reason, gas flow will be interrupted. The insufflation apparatus cannot distinguish between causes of elevated intra-abdominal pressure. Thus it ceases to supply gas if the pressure within the abdomen is high from a valsalva maneuver. This rapidly leads to collapse of the abdomen and poor visualization, and is best prevented by ensuring that good relaxation is present. Once it has been determined that the laparoscope is intraperitoneally placed, a second puncture site is usually made near the bladder for insertion of a cannula to manipulate the uterus and bring desired structures into view. During the laparoscopy, the surgeon usually requests that the patient be placed in the Trendelenburg position so that the upper-abdominal viscera and diaphragm will not impede viewing of the pelvic organs. When the procedure is completed, the laparoscope is removed and the surgeon requests that the patient be returned to the supine position and presses on the abdomen to expel as much CO_2 as possible before removing the trochar and suturing the periumbilical incision. Although it is rapidly taken up and removed by the peritoneal surfaces, residual CO_2 tends to exert pressure on the diaphragm, causing referred pain to the scapulae as the patient awakens. In practice, this pain is self-limited and seldom poses a problem for the patient, particularly when she has been counseled preoperatively to expect this type of temporary discomfort.

Common laparoscopic procedures. There are many indications for laparoscopic examination. These include diagnostic procedures for the evaluation of infertility, for the evaluation of acute or chronic pain, and for the examination of the pelvic mass. In addition, therapeutic laparoscopy may be performed in conjunction with *in vitro* fertilization, reconstructive tubal surgery, and tubal sterilization. Recently, interest has grown in more extensive pelvic operative procedures performed via the operative laparoscope. These include the removal of ectopic pregnancies, ovarian cystectomy, and even myomectomy or salpingo-oophorectomy. Although a complete description of all these procedures is beyond the scope of this chapter, two commonly performed, representative laparoscopic procedures are highlighted in the following sections.

Laparoscopic tubal sterilization. Laparoscopic tubal sterilization procedures have become the most common operation performed in the United States. There are two principal methods for laparoscopic tubal ligation. The most widely performed uses the bipolar electric cautery to coagulate a portion of the fallopian tube. With this device, the surgeon grasps a portion of the tube between the jaws of the cautery forceps that act as positive and negative electrodes. A precisely controlled and localized current can then be applied, which coagulates the tubal segment, thereby occluding it. The inherent safety of the modern bipolar cautery has led to its wide acceptance and greatly reduced the risk of thermal injury and the likelihood of subsequent emergency laparotomy. This method is permanent and difficult to reverse since a portion of the tube is destroyed. A microvascular resection and reanastomosis are needed for reversal. Accordingly, it is used when a woman wishes permanent sterility. Conversely, some women who have had this coagulation procedure later seek to have it reversed. This has prompted the development of techniques that are less destructive. These include the application of Silastic rings or clips that occlude the tube without destroying a large portion of the mesosalpingeal blood supply. Regardless of the technique used, a laparoscopic tubal ligation procedure is brief, usually requiring less than 30 minutes. The procedure is performed with a CO_2 pneumoperitoneum and the patient in a deep Trendelenburg position.

Tubal ectopic pregnancy. **Laparoscopy is frequently used for the diagnosis of tubal ectopic pregnancy and has become a therapeutic modality as well.** The therapeutic resection of ampullary tubal ectopic pregnancies is now an accepted approach to the tubal ectopic pregnancy. It is now common to perform laparoscopy in any patient who has suspected ectopic pregnancy but who does not demonstrate signs and symptoms of rupture (i.e., hemoperitoneum or hypovolemic shock).

Pelviscopic procedures. More extensive surgical procedures have been performed using sophisticated operative laparoscopy equipment. A high patient acceptance, decreased operative time, lesser costs, and the ability to perform many procedures on a day-surgery basis make it likely that the popularity of these procedures will continue to grow. Operative laparoscopy requires the maintenance of a CO_2 pneumoperitoneum for prolonged period of time and the prolonged use of a steep Trendelenburg position. These aspects pose potential hazards for the patient and anesthesia provider and are discussed next.

Anesthetic management. Because laparoscopy and pelviscopy constitutes a major portion of operative gynecology, its anesthetic management is discussed in detail. ***Most laparoscopies, particularly prolonged cases requiring pelviscopic maneuvers, are performed with the patient under general anesthesia.*** CO_2 insufflation is used to distend the abdomen to improve visibility before inserting the laparoscope. The gas tends to impede respiration and cause abdominal discomfort, particularly if the procedure lasts longer than 15 to 20 minutes. Most patients prefer to be asleep for this procedure. Intraperitoneal CO_2 absorption in laparoscopy patients breathing spontaneously during general anesthesia results in a minimal-to-mild respiratory acidosis. This can be compensated with controlled ventilation using greater minute volumes.[2,19] With the combination of intraperitoneal CO_2 and greater minute volumes during controlled ventilation, inspiratory pressures tend to increase, and plateau pressures of 20 to 30 cm H_2O are not uncommon, particularly in obese patients. **The anesthesia provider must observe the inspiratory pressure frequently. If it increases to an unacceptable level during adequate anesthesia and muscle relaxation, the surgeon must release some gas from the abdomen, reduce the degree of Trendelenburg, or both, especially if O_2-saturation decreases concurrently.** Tension pneumothorax related to excessive inspiratory pressures can occur, and must be ruled out when a sudden increase in inspriatory pressure is accompanied by decreasing O_2 saturation. Heat loss during a prolonged laparoscopy or pelviscopy is also common. It is attributable to a combination of factors (i.e., heat transferred to the insufflating gas, heat loss with copious volumes of irrigant), especially when hysteroscopy is performed and heat loss to anesthetic gases in the delivery system. Heat loss can be minimized by instituting corrective measures. These include warming both IV and irrigating solutions, ensuring that irrigating solutions are not allowed to become hot, installing a passive humidifier in the circuit, using low-flow systems and using convective upper-body heating devices.

Regional anesthesia. **With a skilled and gentle surgeon and a properly selected patient, it is possible to use regional (i.e., spinal or epidural) anesthesia or even attended local anesthesia for a diagnostic laparoscopy** or, in exceptional circumstances, laparoscopic tubal ligation. Suitable patients for regional or local anesthesia must be relatively slender, scheduled for a simple diagnostic laparoscopy, and not have undergone prior abdominal surgery that might result in scarring of the abdominal wall, making insertion of the Verres needle and trochar difficult. The patient must be highly motivated to cooperate. When regional or attended local anesthesia is used, all must realize that there will be discomfort from the CO_2, because referred pain pathways to the scapulae are not blocked. This can be minimized with smallest possible amount of CO_2 and minimal degree of head-down tilt. These steps minimize the possibility of respiratory acidosis in an awake, spontaneously ventilating patient. Degree of acidosis is minimal in a brief procedure in a slender patient who has not received large doses of narcotic or lost intercostal function from a high segmental block. It is dangerous to attempt laparoscopy in a spontaneously breathing patient who has preexistent elevated intra-abdominal pressure, a full stomach, is morbidly obese, or suffering from respiratory compromise. Such patients must receive general anesthesia with a controlled airway.

General anesthesia. **General anesthesia is used for the majority of diagnostic and operative laparoscopies. Objectives are to minimize incidence of intraoperative recall and awareness** during this often brief procedure; provide adequate relaxation to avoid risks of perforation of visci and entry into vascular structures; monitor for CO_2 embolus; minimize postoperative grogginess and length of stay, because most of these procedures are performed in day-surgery patients; and minimize postoperative nausea.

Preoperative preparation. Preparation for laparoscopy must begin with the preanesthetic interview. In addition to the standard history and physical examination, the patient must be told to expect transient must er discomfort from the CO_2 insufflation. The possibility of postoperative nausea, which is frequent despite antiemetics, must be mentioned.[26] An adequate IV is important. For routine diagnostic laparoscopies, 18-gauge catheters are usually satisfactory. If a patient has had previous intra-abdominal procedures with adhesions and scarring, an ectopic pregnancy, or if a laparotomy is being considererd, it is wise to consider placing a 16-gauge catheter. After the IV has been placed, we administer a modest dose of midazolam (e.g., 1 to 2 mg IV), in young, healthy patients. This is effective in attenuating short-term state anxiety relative to anesthesia and surgery in this patient population. It also helps reduce incidence of intraoperative awareness. Its relatively short half-life allows rapid postoperative return of cognition. After the patient has been transferred to the operating room, monitors must include a blood pressure cuff, ECG, pulse oximeter, and capnography, particularly to aid in diagnosis of massive air embolism. Depending on the anesthetic technique chosen, a short-acting narcotic, fentanyl, or alfentanil is administered. For routine laparoscopies of 30 minutes or less duration, we usually administer 1.5 μg/kg fentanyl IV 4 to 5 minutes before induction of anesthesia. In addition, we usually administer an IV antiemetic (i.e., 625 mg of droperidol or 4 mg of ondansetron) if the patient has a history of severe nausea with general anesthesia, before induction, especially if the procedure is brief.

Choice of anesthetic agents. There are several general anesthetic techniques available for laparoscopy. These include N_2O and a short-acting narcotic, without use of a volatile agent, and a modified technique in which low concentrations of a volatile agent are added to the basic nitrous-narcotic regimen,[57] and an inhalational technique using a combination of a volatile agent such as desflurane or sevoflurane in O_2 or a mixture of O_2 and compressed air to eliminate bowel distention secondary to N_2O. After preoxygenation, 4 mg/kg of thiopental or 2 mg/kg of propofol is administered for induction of anesthesia, combined with a neuromuscular-blocking agent (see next section) to facilitate intubation of the trachea. While waiting for the neuromuscular blocker to exert its full effect, we administer a volatile agent in O_2 using controlled ventilation. Because the IV induction agent often is redistributed by the time the patient is sufficiently relaxed, the volatile agent helps to ensure that the patient does not experience awareness during laryngoscopy and intubation. It also helps to attenuate undesirable hypertensive responses to ET intubation. After placement and verification of the ET tube, we administer 65% to 70% N_2O in O_2 with a relatively low background concentration of a volatile agent. Addition of a volatile agent decreases the incidence of intraoperative hypertension, allows brief periods of deeper anesthesia, if necessary, and can be eliminated rapidly at the end of the procedure with high flows, thereby promoting rapid emergence. A thiopental, N_2O–narcotic technique can also be effective, particularly with relatively brief procedures. Alfentanil has been advocated for these cases. Using a calibrated infusion pump, a loading dose sufficient to produce an intense, but relatively brief, narcotic effect can be administered, permitting rapid emergence when the infusion is discontinued. We have found the basic N_2O–narcotic technique, supplemented with a short-acting volatile agent, to be quite satisfactory for most diagnostic laparoscopies. It is straightforward, efficacious, and does not require specialized infusion apparatus. For pelviscopies of an anticipated length exceeding 1 hour, we usually avoid N_2O to reduce bowel distention and use a low-flow technique to minimize heat loss. Unfortunately, all of these techniques are associated with a relatively high incidence of postoperative nausea.[26] We usually administer 625 μg of doperidol IV before induction of anesthesia unless contraindicated. In patients especially prone to nausea, 4 mg of ondansetron may be substituted.

Choice of neuromuscular-blocking agents. Choice of neuromuscular-blocking agent depends mainly on the anticipated length of the operation. For brief procedures with anticipated lengths of 20 minutes or less, an inhalational technique without neuromuscular-blocking agents can be used, but sudden coughing, straining, or other patient movement during insertion of a Verres needle of trochar can lead to perforation of an organ or major vessel. A nondepolarizing agent with a short half-life, such as vecuronium or rocuronium, is a good choice for brief laparoscopic procedures. Even though reversal is usually required when these agents are used, they are preferable to succinylcholine infusions, which are more difficult to control, have strong vagotonic effects and carry the potential of overdose and phase-II block. Use of succinylcholine infusions has diminished nearly to the vanishing point in centers.

For most laparoscopic procedures, a nondepolarizing neuromuscular blocker is current practice. After intubation of the trachea with succinylcholine and recovery of twitch, a nondepolarizing agent is administered. Use of succinylcholine can be avoided entirely by using a nondepolarizer initially in a dose sufficient for ET intubation. Provided that a patient has maintained "no-oral-intake" status, has a good airway, and is not at risk for aspiration, this is an excellent technique. After preoxygenation, 4 mg/kg of thiopental is given as an IV bolus injection, followed immediately by an intubating dose of the neuromuscular blocker. Anesthesia is maintained with a volatile agent in O_2 using manual ventilation until the desired degree of relaxation is attained. This technique also minimizes incidence of awareness during ET intubation and eliminates the possibility of postoperative muscle fasciculation pain from succinylcholine. Before attempting extubation, the anesthesia provider must document that reversal is complete by demonstrating that a full train-of-four and sustained tetanus at 100 Hz are present.

Stomach decompression. Before insertion of the Verres needle, the stomach must be decompressed. Manual ventilation before intubation can force air into the stomach, producing gastric dilation and increased probability of perforation by the needle. This can be remedied easily by inserting an orogastric catheter. The patient must not be ventilated when the Verres needle or trochar is inserted. Positive pressure ventilation causes the abdomen to rise and may bring the stomach or other viscera in contact with the needle or trochar during inspiration.

Recognition and management of massive gas embolus. Massive CO_2 embolus during laparoscopy, although rare, is a catastrophic event that is rapidly fatal unless recognized and treated immediately.[17,58] The usual sequence of events is the onset of sudden, severe hypotension and arterial desaturation, often progressing to cardiovascular collapse, occurring shortly after insertion of the Verres needle or laparoscope. One case report describes hypotension and tachycardia in concert with acute, fulminant pulmonary edema 1 to 2 minutes after onset of CO_2 insufflation.[17] With massive embolism, a "mill-wheel" murmur throughout the cardiac cycle may be heard with an esophageal or even precordial stethoscope. This is believed to result from foaming of blood within the right heart and pulmonary outflow tract, precluding sufficient blood flow to the lungs. Capnography may reveal a sudden decrease in expired CO_2 because of an acute increase in "physiologic" dead space. Treatment is largely supportive. CO_2 insufflation must be discontinued immediately. The surgeon may wish to leave the trochar in place if laceration of a large vein is suspected. It may be necessary to place the patient in the left lateral head-down position (Durant's maneuver). This tends to trap gas in the apex of the right ventricle rather than the pulmonary outflow tract and may regenerate forward blood flow. A central venous catheter placed into the right atrium may also help to remove CO_2 gas and foam that may be acting as a mechanical obstruction to cardiac output. Fortunately, CO_2 is highly soluble in blood as compared with air. For this reason, CO_2 rapidly goes into solution in blood vessels and carries a better prognosis than air embolism. If effective cardiac output can be restored, dissolved CO_2 will be rapidly cleared. During a state of cardiovascular compromise or collapse, the patient must be supported with 100% O_2 and vasopressors. If pulmonary edema is present, 5 to 10 cm H_2O positive end-expiratory pressure (PEEP) and use of IV furosemide are efficacious. Unless blood loss is major and uncontrolled, the procedure must be terminated and the patient brought to an intensive care environment for continued observation and supportive therapy. Fortunately, most of these patients can be extubated several hours later and recover fully. The anesthesia care team plays vital roles in recognition and treatment of this potentially fatal complication and almost invariably provides the first diagnosis. Constant awareness can make the difference between death and survival.

KEY POINTS

- Gynecologic surgery can be categorized into four general areas: transvaginal, perineal, intra-abdominal, and trans-abdominal. Despite the multiplicity of gynecologic procedures and the fact that gynecologic cases range from brief procedures requiring 5 to 10 minutes to extensive resections for ovarian and cervical cancer, this simple classification allows us to put any specific procedure into a rational context to plan the appropriate anesthetic.
- The astute anesthesia provider must remember that gynecologic patients often suffer from severe anxiety relating to disorders of the reproductive system, including infertility, sexual dysfunction, and malignancy. Before administering anesthesia to these patients, we must make every effort to gain rapport with their patients and bolster their emotional defenses.
- From the patient's viewpoint, gynecologic problems fall into several principal areas, all of which are capable of inducing fear, anxiety, embarrassment, and guilt. These include infertility; abortions, both spontaneous and therapeutic; acute and chronic pain; mechanical conditions (i.e., stress incontinence, fecal incontinence, draining vesicovaginal and rectovaginal fistulas, uterine prolapse); and potential and actual malignancies.
- All patients, including those having attended local anesthesia, must be monitored with an ECG, blood pressure cuff, and pulse oximeter. Additional monitors include capnography, a temperature probe, a peripheral nerve stimulator, and a Foley catheter as appropriate. Invasive monitors, such as an arterial catheter, a central venous catheter, or a PA catheter, may be indicated in patients with serious medical problems or in patients undergoing radical, prolonged procedures accompanied by extensive fluid shifts and volume replacement.
- Although general anesthesia can be used for all gynecologic operations, we consider it best suited for: (1) extensive intra-abdominal procedures with prolonged periods with the patient in a steep Trendelenburg position when the airway is believed to be at risk for regurgitation, aspiration, and glottic edema; in such cases, a cuffed ET tube must be inserted; (2) extended laparoscopic and pelviscopic procedures using CO_2 insufflation; (3) patients scheduled for procedures that in general can be performed with regional anesthesia but in whom regional or local anesthesia are specifically contraindicated or who refuse regional anesthesia; and (4) procedures that either require or are best performed with the patient under general anesthesia (e.g., modified radical mastectomy, lumpectomy, and axillary node dissection, etc.)
- One important consideration for lengthy intra-abdominal procedures is that N_2O can distend the bowel and compromise the surgeon's access and visibility.
- Regional anesthesia is suitable for most gynecologic surgery, particularly transvaginal and perineal procedures. Regional anesthesia can also be used for abdominal procedures, such as conservative laparotomy, myomectomy, ovarian cystectomy, and hysterectomy. The key to success lies in patient selection and the ability of the surgical and anesthesia teams to work together.
- Spinal anesthesia with a small-gauge spinal needle is suitable for many procedures. The choice of local anesthetic depends on the operation and whether the patient is an outpatient or an inpatient.
- Continuous epidural anesthesia is especially useful in procedures of uncertain duration, such as vaginal reconstruction, or to provide a baseline anesthetic for intra-abdominal procedures.
- Monitored IV sedation, coupled with a paracervical block or local anesthesia, is appropriate for certain procedures such as D&C, D&E, hymenotomy, and breast biopsy.
- Of the minor procedures performed on the vulva, some may be performed with the patient under attended local anesthesia, but most require regional or general anesthesia.
- A Bartholin's gland marsupialization is an entirely different procedure from a Bartholin's gland excision. A Bartholin's gland marsupialization can generally be performed in 15 minutes or less, whereas a formal Bartholin's gland excision is considerably longer.
- Operative laser use entails certain risks, both to the patient and to operating room staff, including thermal injury from reflecting laser light, ignition of operative drapes resulting in burns, retinal injury, and theoretic risk of viral inoculation from inhalation of particulates in the laser plume.
- Regardless of the anesthetic technique, the patient and all members of the surgical team must have eye protection. Personnel must wear goggles or glasses designed for the specific type of laser being used. For the patient, at our institution, this regimen includes: (1) eye pads moistened with saline solution placed over both eyes; (2) placement of goggles over the eye pads; (3) a special laser-surgical mask to trap virus-containing particulates if the patient is having regional anesthesia; (4) surgical drapes in place to form a barrier between the laser and the patient's head.
- A D&C is usually a very brief procedure and can be completed in as little as 5 minutes by an experienced gynecologist. The most painful stimulus is from dilatation of the cervix, particularly if the patient has cervical stenosis. If general anesthesia is used, the anesthesia provider must ensure that a relatively deep level of anesthesia is present during dilatation to prevent sudden laryngospasm or other manifestations of inadequate anesthetic depth. Spinal anesthesia is excellent for diagnostic D&C.

- Attended local anesthesia, with the surgeon performing a paracervical block, is satisfactory in selected patients, particularly the elderly and frail. A paracervical block does not relieve the discomfort of uterine curettage and adjunctive IV narcotic administration may be required.
- Most therapeutic abortions are performed with the patient under attended local anesthesia using a combination of local anesthesia (e.g., paracervical block) with IV sedation and analgesia.
- Special attention must be paid to the anesthetic management of patients undergoing suction curettage for complete molar pregnancy. The rapid evacuation of large quantities of tissue from an excessively enlarged uterus may result in brisk blood loss, which must be anticipated.
- Approximately one in 10 patients experience a complication of cervical conization. The majority present with vaginal hemorrhage, usually 7 to 10 days after the procedure. Occasionally, a patient must be taken to the operating room emergently to obtain hemostasis.
- Hysteroscopy is not an innocuous procedure and has the potential of severe complications. With low-viscosity distention media (i.e., 1.5% glycine), the volume absorbed into the circulation is often grossly underestimated. Glycine can lead to severe dilutional hyponatremia—a syndrome analogous to the "post-TURP syndrome" encountered in men—with mental changes, interstitial pulmonary edema, and toxicity from ammonia, a metabolic product of glycine breakdown.
- General anesthesia is used for the majority of diagnostic and operative laparoscopies. The objectives on which the anesthesia provider must focus are: (1) to minimize the incidence of intraoperative recall and awareness during this often brief procedure; (2) to provide the surgeon with adequate relaxation at all times to avoid the risks of perforation of visci and entry into vascular structures; (3) to monitor for the possibility of CO_2 embolus; (4) to minimize postoperative grogginess and length of stay, because most of these procedures are performed in day-surgery patients; and (5) to minimize postoperative nausea.
- Massive CO_2 embolus during laparoscopy, although rare, is a catastrophic event that is rapidly fatal unless recognized and treated immediately. The usual sequence of events is the onset of sudden, severe hypotension and arterial desaturation, often progressing to cardiovascular collapse, occurring shortly after insertion of the Verres needle or laparoscope. Capnography may reveal a sudden decrease in expired CO_2 on the wave form because of an acute increase in dead space.

KEY REFERENCES

Baratz RA, Karis JH: Blood gas studies during laparoscopy under general anesthesia, *Anesth Analg* 30:463, 1969.

Brownridge P, Cohen SE: Gynecologic procedures suitable for neural blockade. In Cousins MJ, Bridenbaugh PO, editors: *Neural blockade in clinical anesthesia and management of pain*, ed 2, Philadelphia, 1989, JB Lippincott.

Cullen BF, Margolis AJ, Eger EI: The effects of anesthesia and pulmonary ventilation on blood loss during therapeutic abortions, *Anesthesiology* 32:108, 1970.

Drury WL, LaVallee DA, Vacanti CJ: Effects of laparoscopic tubal ligation on arterial blood gases, *Anesth Analg* 50:349, 1971.

Grimes DA, W: Deaths from paracervical anesthesia used for first-trimester abortion, *N Engl J Med* 295:1397, 1976.

Lewis KP: Anesthetic implications in the patient receiving cancer chemotherapy, part 1, *Anesth Rev* 15:35, 1988.

Lewis KP: Anesthetic implications in the patient receiving cancer chemotherapy, part 2, *Anesth Rev* 15:45, 1988.

Powell L, Garfield JM: Anesthetic considerations for gynecologic cancer surgery, *Semin Surg Oncol* 6:194, 1990.

Witz CA, Silverberg KM, Burns WN, et al: Complications associated with the absorption of hysteroscopic fluid media, *Fertil Steril* 60(5):745–756, 1993.

REFERENCES

1. Babknia A, Rock JA, Jones HW: Pregnancy success following abdominal myomectomy for infertility, *Fertil Steril* 30:644, 1978.
2. Baratz RA, Karis JH: Blood gas studies during laparoscopy under general anesthesia, *Anesth Analg* 30:463, 1969.
3. Bartisch EG, Dillon TF: Carbon dioxide hysteroscopy, *Am J Obstet Gynecol* 124: 756, 1976.
4. Bedford RF: 5% lidocaine for spinal anesthesia, *Anesthesiology* 83:33A, 1995.
5. Berkowitz RS, Goldstein DP, DuBeshter B, et al: Management of complete molar pregnancy, *J Reprod Med* 32:634, 1987.
6. Boronow RC, Morrow CP, Creasman WT: Surgical staging and endometrial cancer: clinical pathological findings of a prospective study, *Obstet Gynecol* 63:825, 1984.
7. Brass A, editor: *The CIBA collection of illustrations, the nervous system*, vol 1, part 1, West Caldwell, 1984, CIBA.
8. Brooks PG: Complications of operative hysteroscopy: how safe is it? *Clin Obstet Gynecol* 35(2):256–261, 1992.
9. Brownridge P, Cohen SE: Gynecologic procedures suitable for neural blockade. In Cousins MJ, Bridenbaugh PO, editors:

Neural blockade in clinical anesthesia and management of pain, ed 2, Philadelphia, 1989, JB Lippincott.
10. Brundin J, Thornasson K: Cardiac gas embolism during carbon dioxide hysteroscopy. Risk and management, *Eur J Obstet Reprod Biol* 33(3):241–245, 1989.
11. Burnett LS: Gynecologic causes of the acute abdomen, *Surg Clin North Am* 68:385, 1988.
12. Calabresi P, Chabner BA: Antineoplastic agents. In Gilman AG, Rall TW, Nies AS, et al, editors: *The pharmacological basis of therapeutics,* ed 8, New York, 1985, Pergamon Press.
13. Campodonico I, Escudero P, Suarez E: Carcinoma of the cervix uteri. In Petterson F, Kulstad P, Ludwig H, et al, editors: *Annual report on the results of treatment in gynecologic cancer,* Stockholm, 1985, Tryckeri Balder AB.
14. Cullen BF, Margolis AJ, Eger EI: The effects of anesthesia and pulmonary ventilation on blood loss during therapeutic abortions, *Anesthesiology* 32:108, 1970.
15. Davies JL, Rosenshein NB, Antunes CM: A review of the risk factors for endometrial carcinoma, *Obstet Gynecol Surv* 36:107, 1981.
16. Dehring DJ, Arens JF: Pulmonary thromboembolism: disease recognition and patient management, *Anesthesiology* 73:146, 1990.
17. Desai S, Roaf E, Liu P: Acute pulmonary edema during laparoscopy, *Anesth Analg* 61: 699, 1982.
18. Ditton LN: Presumed carbon dioxide embolism associated with hysteroscopy (letter), *Anaesth Intensive Care* 20(1):123–124, 1992.
19. Drury WL, LaVallee DA, Vacanti CJ: Effects of laparoscopic tubal ligation on arterial blood gases, *Anesth Analg* 50:349, 1971.
20. Duffy BL, Woodhouse PC, Schramm MD, et al: Ranitidine prophylaxis before anaesthesia in early pregnancy, *Anesth Intens Care* 13:29, 1984.
21. Eger EI, Saidman LJ: Hazards of nitrous oxide anesthesia in bowel obstruction and pneumothorax, *Anesthesiology* 26:61, 1965.
22. Erulkar SD: Chemically mediated synaptic transmission: an overview. In Siegel GJ, Agranoff BW, Albers RW, Molinoff PB, editors: *Basic neurochemistry*, ed 5, New York, 1994, Raven Press.
23. Feldman GB, Knapp RC: Lymphatic drainage of the peritoneal cavity and its significance in ovarian cancer, *Am J Obstet Gynecol* 19(7):991–994, 1974.
24. Ferenczy A, Winkler B: Anatomy and histology of the cervix. In Kurman RJ, editor: *Blaustein's pathology of the female genital tract,* ed 3, New York, 1987, Springer-Verlag.
25. Ferenzy A: Anatomy and histology of the cervix. In Blaustein A, editor: *Pathology of the female genital tract,* ed 7, New York, 1982, Springer-Verlag.
26. Garfield JM, Garfield FB, Philip BK, et al: A comparison of clinical and psychological effects of fentanyl and nalbuphine in ambulatory gynecologic patients, *Anesth Analg* 66:1303, 1987.
27. Ginsberg SJ, Comis RL: Pulmonary toxicity of antineoplastic agents, *Semin Oncol* 9:34, 1982.
28. Goldenberg M, Zoiti M, Seidman DS, et al: Transient blood oxygen desaturation, hypercapnia, and coagulopathy after operative hysteroscopy with glycine used as the distending medium. *Am J Obstet Gynecol* 170 (1 Pt 1):25–29, 1994.
29. Griffiths CT, Fuller AF: Intensive surgical and chemotherapeutic management of advanced ovarian cancer, *Surg Clin North Am* 58:131, 1978.
30. Grimes DA, Cates W: Deaths from paracervical anesthesia used for first-trimester abortion, *N Engl J Med* 295:1397, 1976.
31. Grimes DA, Schulz KF, Cates W, et al: Local vs. general anesthesia: which is safer for performing suction curettage abortions? *Am J Obstet Gynecol* 135:1030, 1979.
32. Grimes DA, Schulz KF: Morbidity and mortality from second trimester abortions, *J Reprod Med* 30:505, 1985.
33. Hays RM: Agents affecting the renal conservation of water. In Gilman AG, Rall TW, Nies AS, et al., editors: *The pharmacological basis of therapeutics*, ed 8, New York, 1985, Pergamon Press.
34. Heyman HJ, Barton JJ: Safety of local vs. general anesthesia for second-trimester dilatation and evacuation abortion (letter), *Obstet Gynecol* 68:877, 1986.
35. Howe RS. Third trimester uterine rupture following hysteroscopic uterine perforation, *Obstet Gynecol* 81(5)(Pt 2):827–829, 1993.
36. Hysterectomies in the United States 1965–1984; Vital and Health Statistics Series 13, No 92, Washington, DC, 1987 National Center for Health Statistics.
37. Istre O, Skajaa K, Schjoensby AP, Forman A: Changes in serum electrolytes after transcervical resection of endometrium and submucous fibroids with use of glycine 1.5% for uterine irrigation, *Obstet Gynecol* 80: 218–222, 1992.
38. Jedeikin R, Olsfanger D, Kessler I: Disseminated intravasular coagulopathy and adult respiratory distress syndrome: life-threatening complications of hysteroscopy, *Am J Obstet Gynecol* 162(1):44–45, 1990.
39. Lake CI: Cardiovascular anatomy and physiology. In Barash PG, Cullen BF, Stoelting RK, editors: *Clinical anesthesia,* ed 1, Philadelphia, 1989, JB Lippincott.
40. Langman J, Woerdeman MW: *Atlas of medical anatomy,* Philadephia, 1978, WB Saunders.
41. Lewis KP: Anesthetic implications in the patient receiving cancer chemotherapy, part 1, *Anesth Rev* 15:35, 1988.
42. Lewis KP: Anesthetic implications in the patient receiving cancer chemotherapy, part 2, *Anesth Rev* 15:45, 1988.
43. Lindemann HG: *Atlas derr hysteroskopie,* Stuttgart, 1980, FRG Gustav Fisher.
44. Ljungstrom KG, Renck H, Hedoro H: Hapten inhibition and dextran anaphylaxis, *Anesthesia* 43(9):729, 1988.
45. Lund PR, Sielaff GW, Aiman EJ: *In vitro* fertilization patient presenting in hemorrhagic shock caused by unsuspected heterotopic pregnancy, *Am J Emerg Med* 7:49, 1989.
46. McCausland VM, Fields GA, McCausland AM, et al: Tubovarian abscesses after operative hysteroscopy, *J Reprod Med* 38(3): 198–200, 1993.
47. Mecca RS: Postanesthesia recovery. In Barash PG, Cullen BF, Stoelting RK, editors: *Clinical anesthesia*, ed 1, Philadelphia, 1989, JB Lippincott.
48. Meir PR, Bowes WA: Amniotic fluid embolus-like syndrome presenting in the second trimester of pregnancy, *Obstet Gynecol* 61(suppl):31S, 1983.
49. Oenhaus T, Maurer W: CO_2 embolism during hysteroscopy, *Anaesthetist* 39(4):243–246, 1990.
50. Orr JW, Singleton HM, Soong SJ, et al: Hemodynamic parameters following pelvic exenteration, *Am J Obstet Gynecol* 146:882, 1983.
51. Pereyra AJ, Lebherz TB, Growdon WA: Pubourethral supports in perspective: Modified Pereyra procedure for urinary incontinence, *Obstet Gynecol* 59:643, 1982.
52. Perry PM, Baugham VL: A complication of hysteroscopy air embolism, *Anesthesiology* 73(3):546–547, 1990.
53. Peterson HB, Grimes DA, Cates W, et al: Comparative risk to health from induced abortion at less than 12 weeks gestation performed with local vs. general anesthesia, *Am J Obstet Gynecol* 141:763, 1981.
54. Piver MS, Lele SB, Barlow JJ: Paraaortic lymph node evaluation in stage I endometrial carcinoma, *Obstet Gynecol* 59:97, 1982.
55. Powell L, Garfield JM: Anesthetic considerations for gynecologic cancer surgery, *Semin Surg Oncol* 6:194, 1990.
56. Reid R, Absten GT: Lasers in gynecology, *Lasers Surgery Med* 17: 201–301, 1995.
57. Rising S, Dodgson MS, Steen PA: Isoflurane vs. fentanyl for outpatient laparoscopy, *Acta Anaesthesiol Scand* 29:251, 1985.
58. Root B, Levy MN, Pollack S, et al: Gas embolism death after laparoscopy delayed by "trapping" in portal circulation, *Anesth Analg* 57:232, 1978.
59. Ryan KJ, Berkowitz R, Barbieri R, editors: *Kistner's gynecology, principles and practice,* ed 5, Littleton, 1990, Year Book Medical.
60. Sawchuk WS, Weber PJ, Lowy DR, Dzubow LM: Infectious papilloma virus in the vapor of warts treated with carbon dioxide laser or electrocoagulation; detection and protection, *J Am Acad Dermatol* 21(1): 41–49, 1989.
61. Sieber FE: Evakuation of the Patient with Endocrine Disease and Diabetes Mellitus. In Rogers MC, Tinker JH, Covino BG, Longnecker DE, editors: *Principles and practice of anesthesiology,* ed 1, St. Louis, 1992, Mosby–Year Book.
62. Silverberg E, Lubera JA: Cancer statistics, *Cancer* 38:5, 1988.
63. Smale BF, Mullen JL, Buzby GP, et al: The efficacy of nutritional assessment and support in cancer surgery, *Cancer* 47:2375, 1981.
64. Stamey TA: Endoscopic suspension of the vesicle neck for urinary incontinence, *Surg Obstet Gynecol* 136(4):547, 1973.
65. Swinhoe CF, Reilly CS: Pharmacokinetics of the shocked state, *Anaesth Pharm Rev* 2: 92–102, 1994.
66. The dangers of laser plume, *Health Dev.* 19 (1):4–19, 1990.
67. Tovell HM, Danforth DN: Structural defects of the female reproductive tract. In Danforth D, editor: *Obstetrics and gynecology,* ed 4, Philadelphia, 1982, Harper & Row.
68. *Uterine Leiomyomata.* ACOG Technical Bulletin No. 192, May 1994.
69. Vandam LD, Desai S: Evaluation of the pa-

tient and preoperative preparation. In Barash P, Cullen BF, Stoelting RK, editors: *Clinical anesthesia,* ed 1, Philadephia, 1989, JB Lippincott.

70. Wheelas CR: *Atlas of pelvic surgery,* Philadelphia, 1981, Lea & Febiger.
71. Wilcox S, Vandam LD: Alas, poor Trendelenburg and his position! A critique of its uses and effectiveness, *Anesth Analg* 67: 574, 1988.
72. Wisniewski PM, Warhol MS, Rando RF, et al: Studies on the transmission of viral disease via the carbon dioxide laser plume and ejecta, *J Reprod Med* 35(12):1117–1123, 1990.
73. Witz CA, Silverberg KM, Burns WN, et al: Complications associated with the absorption of hysteroscopic fluid media, *Fertil Steril* 60(5):745–756, 1993.
74. Woodruff JD, Julian C, Puray T: The contemporary challenge of carcinoma *in situ* of the vulva, *Am J Obstet Gynecol* 115:677, 1983.
75. Wright VC, Davies E: Laser surgery for vulvar intraepithelial neoplasia: principles and results, *Am J Obstet Gynecol* 15:374, 1987.

CHAPTER 78

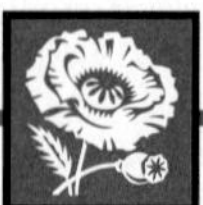

Anesthesia for Surgical Emergencies in Newborns

MYRON YASTER

Except for extraordinary circumstances, all newborns require anesthesia for surgery.[6,15,230] In the past, it was assumed that newborns neither experienced nor perceived painful stimuli to the same degree as adults.[6,164] Most believed that newborns did not have the neurologic substrate necessary for the perception of pain, either because of a lack of myelinization, incomplete pain pathways from the periphery to the cortex, or immaturity of the cerebral cortex. Absolutely no evidence indicates that any of this is true. Newborns respond to noxious stimuli with behavioral, physiologic, metabolic, and hormonal responses suggestive of substantial stress.[5,6,64,138,225]

The neurophysiologic pathways for nociception from the peripheral receptors to the cerebral cortex are developed even in premature infants. Further, the primary pathways of pain transmission involve nonmyelinated C and A delta fibers, so postnatal myelination is not required for most pain perception.[63,148,227,228] Finally, failure to provide anesthesia is associated with an increased incidence of circulatory, respiratory, and metabolic complications in newborns.[7,8] **Thus, most evidence suggests that newborns not only respond to noxious stimuli, but that the failure to provide analgesia and anesthesia significantly increases perioperative morbidity and mortality.**

The newborn differs from the adult and older child in the uptake, distribution, metabolism, and excretion of all drugs.[34,85] Variations in the penetration of drugs into the brain (integrity of the blood–brain barrier) as well as in receptor sensitivity also affect how many drugs react in the newborn.[167,222,242] These differences are extremely important in the anesthetic management of the newborn.

DRUG DISTRIBUTION

How much drug reaches a receptor site depends on the degree of protein binding, tissue volumes, tissue solubility coefficients, and blood flow. In the blood, opioids (fentanyl, morphine), amide local anesthetics (bupivacaine, lidocaine), and muscle relaxants (pancuronium, curare) bind to albumin and other serum proteins, such as alpha$_1$-acid glycoprotein. The unbound or "free" drug is available to cross biologic membranes, bind to receptors, and initiate a pharmacologic effect. Concentrations of both albumin and alpha$_1$-acid glycoprotein are lower in the newborn than at any other stage in life.[34,47,85,127,143] Thus, a greater proportion of active or free drug is available to penetrate the brain, heart, and other viscera. Further, biologic membranes that separate target receptors from the blood vasculature (e.g., the blood–brain barrier) may also be immature at birth and thereby allow agonists with limited lipid solubility (e.g., morphine) to have greater brain permeability. Kupferberg[119] and Way and Way et al.[222] demonstrated that morphine concentrations were two to four times greater in the brains of younger rats than older rats despite equal blood concentrations. On the other hand, decreased protein binding may contribute to the larger apparent volume of distribution of many drugs as well. A large apparent volume of distribution has the effect of diluting the plasma concentrations of parenterally administered drugs and partly explains why some drugs must be given in larger doses (on a mg/kg basis) to achieve a therapeutic effect.

Body composition changes with age. Eighty percent of the newborn's body mass is composed of water (Table 78-1).[102] In the very-low-birth-weight premature infant (<1000 g), total body water can be estimated at 100% (or more) of body weight.[71] This increase in total body water occurs primarily in the extracellular fluid space and also explains the larger apparent volume of distribution of most parenterally administered drugs in the newborn.

Blood flow determines how much drug reaches a target receptor. As in the adult, a high proportion of cardiac output perfuses the newborn's vessel-rich organs, such as the brain, kidney, and intestinal viscera.[53] Very high brain concentrations are achieved following the administration of any lipophilic or inhalational anesthetic agent because the infant's brain receives almost 30% of the entire cardiac output compared with only approximately 15% in the adult. The infant's very small muscle and fat mass provides less uptake of an administered drug and less of a reservoir to lower blood concentrations. Further, the potent vapors are less soluble in neonatal blood than in the adult's blood.[21,123,126,135] **These factors allow higher concentrations of an administered drug (halothane, fentanyl) to be achieved more quickly than might be expected.**

Biotransformation and Elimination

Following administration, the disposition of a drug depends on distribution ($t_{1/2}\alpha$) and elimination. The terminal half-life of elimination ($t_{1/2}\beta$) is directly proportional to the volume of distribution (Vd) and inversely proportional to the total body clearance (Cl) according to the following formula:

$$t_{1/2}\beta = 0.693 \times (Vd/Cl)$$

Thus a prolongation of the $t_{1/2}\beta$ may result from either an increase in a drug's volume of distribution or a decrease in its clearance.

Following redistribution, termination of a drug's effect involves biotransformation, metabolism, and excretion. Many anesthetic agents (e.g., opioids, muscle relaxants, hypnotics) are biotransformed in the liver before excretion. Several of these reactions are catalyzed in the liver by microsomal mixed-function oxidases that require the cytochrome P-450 system, NADPH, and O_2. The cytochrome P-450 system is very immature at birth and does not reach adult levels until 1 or 2 months after birth.[34,83,85] The immaturity of this hepatic enzyme system may explain the prolonged clearance or elimination of some drugs in the first few days to weeks of life.

On the other hand, the P-450 system can be affected by various drugs (e.g., phenobarbital) and substrates and matures regardless of gestational age. Thus, the age from birth, not the duration of gestation, determines how premature and full-term infants metabolize drugs. Greeley and de Bruijn[83] have demonstrated that sufentanil is more rapidly metabolized and eliminated in 2- to 3-week-old infants than in newborns less than a week of age. Elimination may be further prolonged by abnormal or decreased liver blood flow, which may occur following an acute illness or abdominal surgery. Certain conditions that may raise intra-abdominal pressure (e.g., closure of an abdominal wall defect, as with an omphalocele or gastroschisis) may further decrease liver blood flow by shunting blood away from the liver via the still-patent ductus venosus.[136,231,238] Finally, in all newborns, excretion may be reduced compared with the older child or adult, because both glomerular and tubular renal function is reduced in the newborn.

Table 78-1 Composition of body mass in newborn compared with adult

Body compartment	Premature (< 2.5 kg)	Full term (> 2.5 kg)	Adult
Total body water (% body weight)	90–100	70–85	60
Extracellular fluid (% body weight)	40–60	40	20
Intracellular fluid (% body weight)	40	40	40
Blood volume (ml/kg)	90–105	80–95	50–65
Muscle mass (% body weight)	15	20	50
Fat (% body weight)	3	10	15–30

CHOICE OF ANESTHETIC AGENTS

Inhalational Agents

At equipotent doses (minimum alveolar concentration [MAC] median effective dose [ED_{50}]), all the potent inhalational anesthetic agents produce unacceptable hypotension in newborns requiring emergency surgery.[69,70] This depression of blood pressure is caused by both the intrinsic properties of the anesthetic agents and the newborn's myocardium. The newborn attains a higher concentration of halothane (or any of the potent vapors) in the brain and heart than an adult does at the same inspired concentration. If the inspired concentration of an inhaled agent is kept constant, the ratio of the inspired agent (F_I) to its alveolar (F_A) concentration (F_A/F_I) is significantly higher in the newborn compared with the adult because of differences in ventilation and anesthetic uptake. The infant has three to four times the minute ventilation of an older child or adult but the same functional residual capacity (FRC) on an milligrams per kilogram basis (Table 78-2). **Thus inhalational agents rapidly wash in (and wash out) because the time constant of the infant's lung is so greatly reduced compared with that of the adult (0.19 minutes in the infant versus 0.73 minutes in the adult).**[19,42,112,142] Controlled ventilation further exacerbates this.

The uptake of a potent vapor is very rapid in the newborn as well. Because the mass of vessel-rich organs is so small, the uptake of inhalational agents by the tissues is rapid and tissue concentrations saturate quickly. Venous blood returning to the lung arrives at a relatively high anesthetic partial pressure compared with the adult, and this further reduces the F_A/F_I ratio and increases the amount of potent agent in the alveolus.[21,53,54,86,123,172,208] This allows a higher concentration of inhalational agent to be taken up by the blood for delivery to the major organs. End-tidal gas monitoring may help prevent unintentional overdosage.[9,12]

The MAC of halothane or isoflurane is also significantly lower in newborns than in infants 1 to 6 months of age. Further, premature infants have lower MAC requirements than full-term infants.[86,121,124-126,135,211] Thus some of the hypotension associated with the inhalational agents may have occurred because of anesthetic overdose. Nevertheless, even at "true" MAC concentrations, heart rate and blood pressure decrease by 12% and 30%, respectively, in the newborn.[121] This can be partially attenuated by pretreating the infant with an intravenous (IV) anticholinergic such as atropine immediately before induction of anesthesia.[11,69,150,205,244] Atropine requirements in the newborn are higher than in the adult, 0.03 to 0.05 mg/kg versus 0.01 to 0.02 mg/kg, respectively. Additionally, IV doses of atropine less than 0.1 to 0.15 mg may produce paradoxic bradycardia.

The other cause of the extreme hypotension associated with inhalational agents relates to intrinsic properties of the newborn's myocardium. The newborn's myocardium is less compliant than the older child's and the adult's. The newborn has a fixed stroke volume and can increase cardiac output only by increasing heart rate. Also, the newborn's myocardium has decreased contractile mass and a decreased velocity of shortening.[67,209] The negative inotropic and chronotropic effects associated with the inhaled agents are therefore poorly tolerated. Further, the baroreceptor reflexes are blunted or obliterated by these agents as well.[52,84,146,147,194,223] Reflex tachycardia, which is vital in supporting blood pressure and cardiac output, may not occur.

Table 78-2 Respiratory variables in newborn compared with adult

Respiratory variable	Newborn (ml/kg)	Adult (ml/kg)
Tidal volume	7	7
Respiratory rate	30–40	10–15
Dead space volume / Tidal volume	0.3	0.3
Functional residual capacity	20–30	20–30
Vital capacity	50–70	50–70
Alveolar ventilation/FRC	5:1	1.5:1

Fentanyl(s)

Fentanyl and its structurally related relatives, sufentanil and alfentanil, are highly lipophilic drugs that rapidly penetrate all membranes, including the blood–brain barrier. Following an IV bolus, fentanyl is rapidly eliminated from plasma as the result of its extensive uptake by body tissues. The fentanyls are highly bound to alpha$_1$-acid glycoproteins in the plasma, which are reduced in the newborn.[143,200] The fraction of free unbound sufentanil is significantly increased in neonates and children less than 1 year of age (19.5 ± 2.7% and 11.5 ± 1.2%, respectively) compared with older children and adults (8.1 ± 1.4% and 7.8 ± 1.5%, respectively). This correlates to levels of alpha$_1$-acid glycoproteins in the blood.[117,143,144,200]

Fentanyl's pharmacokinetics differ among newborns, children, and adults.[48,73,114,117,143,144,200] The total body clearance of fentanyl is greater in infants 3 to 12 months of age than in children older than 1 year of age or in adults (18.1 ± 1.4, 11.5 ± 4.2, and 10.0 ± 1.7 mL/kg/minute, respectively), and the elimination half-life is longer (233 ± 137, 244 ± 79, and 129 ± 42 minutes, respectively).[117,143,144,200] The prolonged elimination half-life of fentanyl from plasma has important clinical implications. Repeated doses of fentanyl for maintenance of analgetic effects lead to accumulation of fentanyl and its ventilatory depressant effects.[104,105,140] Very large doses (0.05 to 0.10 mg/kg) may be expected to induce long-lasting effects because plasma fentanyl levels will not fall below the threshold level at which spontaneous ventilation occurs during the distribution phases.

In a landmark paper, Robinson and Gregory[183] reported the first use of fentanyl (30 to 50 μg/kg) as the principal anesthetic agent in neonates undergoing ductus ligation surgery. Using heart rate and blood pressure responses as indices of adequate anesthesia, these investigators demonstrated that the combination of fentanyl, O_2, and pancuronium can provide anesthesia with minimal hemodynamic consequences in volume resuscitated neonates.[183] Indeed, the hemodynamic stability associated with fentanyl (and sufentanil) administration in the newborn has been confirmed by several other investigators. In all reported studies, both hypotension and bradycardia are rare, as long as intravascular volume has been restored and a vagolytic agent (either pancuronium or atropine) is administered concomitantly. Further, in a newborn lamb model, fentanyl does not significantly affect heart rate, blood pressure, cardiac output, or the regional distribution of blood flow to the major organs, such as the brain and gastrointestinal (GI) tract, when it was administered in doses of 30 to 3000 μg/kg.[191,232] On the other hand, the safety of "fentanyl" anesthesia may be diminished when other anesthetic agents, such as N_2O, barbiturates, or benzodiazepines, are administered concomitantly.[233,234]

Yaster[229] extended the observations of Robinson and Gregory in a prospective study of premature and full-term infants less than 7 days of age undergoing a variety of thoracic, abdominal, and genitourinary emergency procedures. In this study, fentanyl in doses of 10 to 12.5 μg/kg produced insignificant hemodynamic changes and provided reliable anesthesia for at least 75 minutes.

Several reasons exist for the discrepancies in fentanyl requirements in these studies. Robinson and Gregory studied premature infants varying in age from 1 day to 6 weeks undergoing thoracic surgery. Yaster's patients were younger, with most less than 24 hours old. Analgesic requirements are known to be reduced in the first few days of life. This may be caused by the release of endogenous opioids in response to birth or to fetal and neonatal distress. As mentioned earlier, the blood–brain barrier is immature in the first few days of life, and this may allow more fentanyl to reach the mu receptors within the central nervous system (CNS).[119,222] However, this is more important for less lipid-soluble agonists, such as morphine.[132–134] Alternatively, the increased fraction of free, unbound fentanyl in the newborn may allow more drug to penetrate into the brain.[143] Additionally, fentanyl clearance increases greatly in the first weeks of life, probably as a result of increasing activity of the cytochrome P-450 system and increasing hepatic blood flow following closure of the ductus venosus.[73,95,118] Thus, the increased fentanyl metabolism that occurs in older newborns may increase their anesthetic (fentanyl) requirements. Finally, many patients in Yaster's study underwent abdominal surgery or had significant abdominal pathology such as necrotizing enterocolitis (NEC). Fentanyl clearance and analgetic requirements may be significantly decreased in these patients, particularly if intra-abdominal pressure increases. Increased intra-abdominal pressure ($>$ 15 to 20 mm Hg) greatly reduces liver and splanchnic blood flow and has been documented to occur following closure of abdominal wall defects such as omphalocele or gastroschisis.[118,136,224,231,238] This decreased liver blood flow reduces fentanyl biotransformation and thus anesthetic requirements. Fentanyl dosage may therefore depend on the neonate's postnatal age and on the type of surgery performed, as well as on patient risk factors such as acidosis, hypoxia, and circulatory stability.

The use of fentanyl as a primary anesthetic agent results in the need for postoperative intubation and ventilation, independent of the infant's medical or surgical condition. All opioids produce profound respiratory depression in the newborn.[131] Several studies suggest that the respiratory depression and analgesia produced by mu agonists involve different receptor subtypes. These receptors change in number in an age-related fashion and can be blocked by naloxone. Pasternak et al.[166,167] working with newborn rats, showed that 14-day-old rats are 40 times more sensitive to morphine analgesia than 2-day-old rats. Nevertheless, morphine depresses the respiratory rate in 2-day-old rats to a greater degree than in 14-day-old rats. Thus, the newborn may be particularly sensitive to the respiratory depressant effects of the frequently administered opioids in what may be an age-related receptor phenomenon.

Muscle Relaxants

The structural and functional development of the neuromuscular system is incomplete at birth.[32–35,78,81,82] The newborn has decreased neuromuscular reserve compared with the older child or adult. At a stimulation rate of 20 Hz, many neonates demonstrate tetanic fade, and premature infants demonstrate posttetanic exhaustion. At a higher stimulation rate (50 Hz), all newborns demonstrate posttetanic exhaustion. The ratio of the first and fourth twitches in a train-of-four and the degree of posttetanic facilitation all increase with age. Based on these findings and on clinical criteria, some have suggested that the newborn is sensitive to nondepolarizing muscle relaxants.[32,82]

Several investigators have documented the sensitivity of infants to d-tubocurarine, even if one compensates for the newborn's increased extracellular fluid space and apparent volume of distribution.[62] However, a single dose of curare does not appear to have a longer duration of action in the newborn compared with the adult, because in the neonate, the steady-state plasma concentration associated with a 50% neuromuscular block is only one third that of the adult value.[62] This also means that subsequent doses of curare may lead to a prolonged duration of paralysis.

At appropriate doses, all the nondepolarizing muscle relaxants effectively and rapidly paralyze newborn infants.[43,152] Drug selection is usually based on properties other than neuromuscular blockade. Because pancuronium is a potent vagolytic (cardiac muscarinic blockade), it is the most frequently used agent in the newborn. Unlike in the adult, tachycardia is a desired side effect because the infant responds to a variety of stimuli (e.g., hypoxia, intubation, halothane, and fentanyl administration) with bradycardia. Because the newborn's cardiac output depends on heart rate, bradycardia can potentially be catastrophic. Occasionally, other agents (e.g., atracurium or mivacurium) are selected because end-organ pathology (liver, kidney) may interfere with drug elimination or because duration of paralysis or onset time of paralysis is inappropriate for the surgery performed.[22,60,61,79]

Interestingly, newborns are relatively resistant to succinylcholine, although plasma cholinesterase levels are reduced following birth.[32,33,35,81,82] IV doses of 2 mg/kg, rather than 0.5 to 1 mg/kg, are required for complete paralysis. IV succinylcholine produces many dysrhythmias, including sinus bradycardia, sinus arrest, nodal rhythms, and ventricular ectopy.[91,198] Further, several neonates have developed pulmonary edema and hemorrhage in the absence of upper-airway obstruction following IV use of succinylcholine.[36] Other well-known complications of succinylcholine include malignant hyperthermia, hyperkalemia, myoglobinemia, and increased intraocular and possibly intracranial pressure (ICP). **Because of these effects, increasing numbers of pediatric anesthesiologists are discouraging the routine use of this drug.** Nevertheless, succinylcholine is the most rapid-acting neuromuscular-blocking agent available, and despite the problems associated with its use, no perfect substitute exists for it when "full-stomach" precautions are used or if laryngospasm occurs.[80,122] Thus, my practice is to adhere to the advice of Dr. Dennis Fisher: "Always have it, never use it."

Regional Anesthesia

Continuous epidural analgesia is increasingly being used in the management of acute medical (e.g., cancer, sickle cell vaso-occlusive crisis) and surgical (e.g., trauma, postoperative) pain in older children, because it provides profound pain relief with minimal systemic side effects.[31,213,239] It is now becoming an important tool in the perioperative management of the newborn as well. Epidural anesthesia is used either alone or combined with general inhalational anesthesia in the management of major (e.g., tracheo-esophageal fistula repair, abdominal wall defects, ligation of patent ductus arteriosus) and minor (e.g., inguinal hernia repair, pyloromyotomy) surgical procedures.[19,88,185,203] Other methods, including peripheral nerve blockade have also become common. The penile nerve block in particular is used to provide complete anesthesia and analgesia for neonatal circumcision.[23,45,138] Complications are rare and are related to local anesthetic toxicity caused by either accidental IV administration or by accumulation of excessive amounts of drug administered by either repeated bolus dosing or continuous infusion.[4,14,137,240]

The newborn infant may be at increased risk for local anesthetic toxicity for several reasons. First, young infants ($<$ 3 months of age) have reduced liver blood flow and glomerular function and immature metabolic pathways.[34] Thus, larger fractions of amide local anesthetics are unmetabolized and remain active in the plasma. Clearance is also reduced. With prolonged infusions, the slower clearance of amide local anesthetics will result in higher plasma concentrations than in older children and adults. Second, neonates have lower levels of albumin and alpha$_1$-acid glycoproteins, leading to increased concentrations of unbound drug.[127] The larger volume of distribution at steady state in the neonate may confer some clinical protection by lowering plasma drug levels with bolus administration. Third, the newborn's blood–brain barrier is immature and allows higher concentrations of unbound drugs to enter the CNS.[222] Finally, the ability to detect toxicity in newborn patients is decreased because premonitory signs of CNS irritability, which may precede the onset of dysrhythmias or seizures, may be difficult to recognize because of an inability to communicate. Indeed, the most frequently reported symptoms of minor CNS toxicity—namely "restlessness" and "agitation"—are often misinterpreted as "pain" or "difficulty adjusting to the hospital environment" in young children.

The blood concentration at which lidocaine and bupivacaine toxicity occurs in human newborns is unknown. In adult humans and sheep, minor toxic symptoms, such as agitation, occur at plasma lidocaine concentrations above 5 mg/l, and major symptoms, such as convulsions, are associated with blood lidocaine concentrations of 10 mg/l.[57,156,190] Other factors, such as hypoxia, acidosis, hyponatremia, and hyperkalemia, are known to increase local anesthetic toxicity and lower the threshold at which it occurs.[57,156,190] Clearly, the critically ill, postoperative newborn patient can experience many of these physiologic perturbations.

MONITORING

Critically ill neonates undergoing emergency surgery require as much, if not more, monitoring during anesthesia and surgery than critically ill adults, because the margin of error is so small and because disaster can strike so quickly. Unfortunately, compromises are often made because of the technical difficulty in monitoring small children and because once positioned and draped on the operating room table, observation, palpation, and even auscultation are often difficult, if not impossible to perform. Meticulous attention to detail is absolutely necessary, and one must emphasize that no machine can replace a vigilant anesthesiologist who will evaluate, interpret, and analyze the patient's condition.

Unquestionably the single most important monitor in pediatric anesthesia remains the precordial or esophageal stethoscope. It provides beat-to-beat, breath-by-breath information on the patient's condition. For example, the first indication of cardiovascular deterioration in children may be a change in heart sounds, from brisk and close to muffled and distant. Loss of breath sounds may indicate a mechanical disconnection or an endobronchial intubation well before a mechanical alarm sounds. Despite its importance, this low-technology, inexpensive monitor is rapidly being discarded by anesthesiologists in favor of more glitzy and expensive monitors.

Just slightly less important than the precordial stethoscope is the pulse oximeter.[38,39] This noninvasive, beat-to-beat monitor of O_2 saturation has revolutionized anesthesia monitoring and should be used not only in the operating room but also in the infant's transport to and from the operating room.[153,202,215] **In neonates, the oximeter probe is preferentially placed on the right hand, ear lobe, or on the buccal mucosa.**[107,178]

Newborns can easily shunt venous, desaturated blood across the ductus arteriosus, which causes blood distal to the left subclavian artery to become desaturated.[98,165,189] The right hand (or buccal mucosa) will be perfused with preductal arterial blood, and pulse oximetry will reflect preductal (coronary, cerebral) O_2 saturation. This is important because newborns, particularly premature neonates, are at risk for developing the retinopathy of prematurity (retrolental fibroplasia) if they are exposed to high O_2 concentrations.[16,65] If the sensor is postductal (i.e., on the left hand or on the feet), low arterial O_2 saturations may be measured and too much O_2 may be administered to the patient. On the other hand, one must never compromise O_2 delivery to the neonate's brain to protect the eyes.

The next most important monitor is blood pressure. Newborns, particularly premature newborns less than 1.5 kg, may have normal systolic blood pressures of only 40 mm Hg. Blood pressure measurement and control become major tasks. This is why many pediatric anesthesiologists prefer fentanyl-based anesthetics to inhalational agents when providing anesthesia for newborn surgery. An adequately sized blood pressure cuff, a Doppler ultrasonic transducer, or an automatic blood pressure device is necessary for noninvasive blood pressure determinations in the newborn. However, for most major surgery, continuous invasive intra-arterial monitoring is indicated for the safe delivery of anesthesia. Catheterization of preferably the radial artery is accomplished either percutaneously or by a cutdown. The temporal arteries must be avoided as an intra-arterial site because of the potentially catastrophic brain embolization associated with their use. Alternative catheterization sites include the dorsalis pedis, posterior tibial, and the umbilical arteries. The arterial catheter provides beat-to-beat monitoring and a means to frequently sample for blood gases, hematocrit, and glucose. It is also a very sensitive guide of the patient's intravascular volume status.

It is extremely difficult to judge intravascular volume clinically in the neonate. During abdominal surgery (e.g., NEC), third-space fluid losses may approach 100 to 200 ml/kg. The arterial wave form displayed on a monitor or on a recorder is one of the best signs of early intravascular volume losses (Fig. 78-1). One looks for either a change in the shape of the arterial wave form (decreased area under the curve) or the development of respiratory variation in the wave form. During positive-pressure ventilation, decreased venous return causes a dramatic fall or drift in the arterial wave form with each breath. Typically, this fall occurs when the intravascular volume has been depleted.

In adults, the more frequently used monitors for intravascular volume are either a central venous or a pulmonary artery (PA) catheter. Historically, central venous pressure (CVP) measurements have been considered not only technically difficult to obtain but also useless to interpret. Experiments done in the 1960s during exchange transfusions demonstrated little correlation with blood losses of as much as 20% of the estimated blood volume and CVP as measured by umbilical central venous catheters.[220,221] Unfortunately, these experiments have never been repeated with central venous catheters placed in the internal or external jugular vein and pressure transduced with modern equipment. In my experience the CVP is very useful, particularly in surgery involving major blood or third-space loss, shock, or when intra-abdominal pressure is elevated.[231,238] Further, because these are large-bore catheters securely inserted

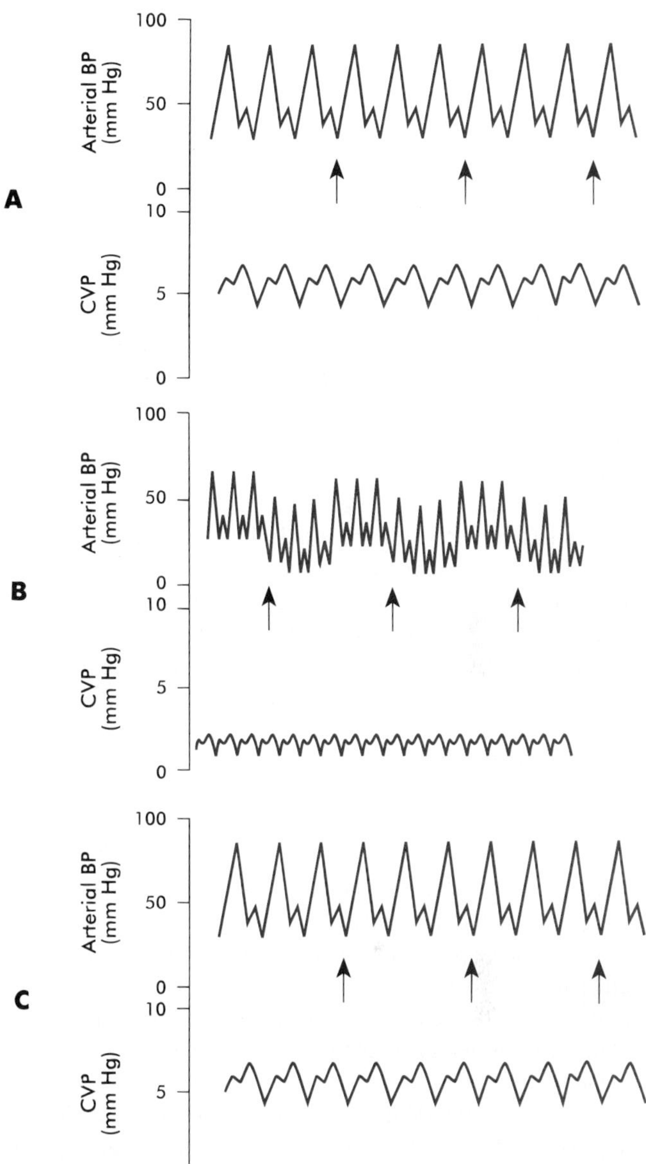

Fig. 78-1. Hypovolemia may be detected on both arterial (BP) and central venous pressure (CVP) wave forms. **A,** Before surgery, systolic blood pressure and CVP average 60 and 6 mm Hg, respectively. With each positive-pressure breath (*arrow*), a small (< 5 mm Hg) fall in blood pressure occurs. **B,** Once the abdomen is opened, each positive-pressure breath produces an exaggerated decrease (> 10 mm Hg) (pulsus paradoxus) and fall in CVP (< 0 to 1 mm Hg) by decreasing venous return. **C,** Following volume resuscitation, the arterial wave form no longer changes with positive-pressure ventilation.

within the vascular tree (usually the internal jugular vein), they supply a reliable means of administering fluids and vasoactive drugs.

One of the mainstays in the assessment of volume status is the measurement of urine output (or lack thereof). Bladder catheterization is easily accomplished using a 5-French feeding tube (not a balloon-tipped Foley catheter). The catheter is secured to the skin with tape and connected to a calibrated urinometer by low-volume tubing. Minimal acceptable urine outputs are 0.5 to 1.0 ml/kg/hour.[194] Unfortunately, in very small children, this small volume of urine may take hours to travel the length of the operating room table to reach the urinometer. Because of this, measurement of urine output during surgery may be of marginal value.

Because neonatal anesthesia is performed with controlled mechanical ventilation, respiratory monitoring is essential. Despite the many technical problems involved in measuring end-tidal CO_2 concentrations through small uncuffed endotracheal (ET) tubes, particularly when using Mapleson circuits, such measurement (together with pulse oximetry) remains a mandatory monitor for the provision of safe anesthesia.[9,10,39,141]

Finally, temperature monitoring is also important. **All newborns are at extraordinarily high risk of becoming cold during transport and in the operating room.** To minimize this risk, many anesthesiologists routinely wrap infants in plastic bags, use overhead warmers and heated water mattresses, turn up the temperature in the operating room, warm IV fluids, and use heated, humidified gases.[17,187,188,195] Temperature is routinely monitored with either a rectal or a nasopharyngeal temperature probe.

FLUIDS

Intraoperative IV fluid therapy provides the infant with maintenance requirements of water, electrolytes, and glucose to replace preoperative deficits and ongoing intraoperative third-space and blood losses.[71,108] Maintenance fluid requirements are calculated based on the assumption that 100 ml of water is required for every 100 calories consumed.[102,129] The newborn's energy (and fluid) requirements are 100 calories (ml)/24 hours in the unanesthetized state, or approximately 4 ml/kg/hour. Under anesthesia, these basal caloric requirements are significantly reduced.[129]

Because most newborns undergoing emergency surgery are in neonatal intensive care units and are receiving IV fluids before surgery, the logical presumption is that preoperative deficits are nonexistent. Unfortunately, this is rarely true.[212] Most newborns have restricted fluid intake in the nursery, despite the presence of a surgical emergency and third-space fluid losses. Further, infants are rarely given solutions containing electrolytes, although the newborn's kidney cannot tolerate a water load and wastes sodium even when overloaded with water. The maximal urine osmolality achievable by the neonatal kidney is only 800 mOsm/l. Unsuspected hypovolemia can be catastrophic when combined with anesthetic drugs.

Surgical trauma, manipulation, or inflammation of the bowel results in internal sequestration of functional extracellular fluids and is often referred to as "third-space" losses. The fluid within the third space acts as sequestered fluid and is nonfunctional in terms of the purpose of extracellular fluid. Replenishment of this interstitial water and salt loss with balanced salt solutions (isotonic crystalloid solutions), such as Ringer's lactate or normal saline, is essential. The magnitude of the third-space loss depends on the site and extent of injury. Abdominal surgery, particularly if extensive bowel pathology is present or surgical manipulation occurs, may require third-space replacement therapy of 10 to 20 ml/kg/hour, whereas peripheral or thoracic surgery may require only 3 to 5 mg/kg/hour.

All blood loss must be replaced with either balanced salt solutions, 5% albumin, or blood. Normally, infants are born with high hematocrits (> 50%), which fall to 30% over the first 3 months of life. Additionally, these erythrocytes are made primarily of hemoglobin F (HbF), which has a greater affinity for O_2 than adult hemoglobin (HbA).[206,207] The partial pressure at which 50% of hemoglobin is saturated (P_{50}) is 19 for HbF versus 27 for HbA. **Because the newborn has limited stores of iron and limited ability to replace lost erythrocytes with new ones, the hematocrit should not be allowed to fall below 35% during surgery.** The allowable erythrocyte loss can be calculated by the following formula:[184]

$$\text{Weight (kg)} \times \text{EBV} \times \frac{\text{Hct}_{\text{start}} - 0.35}{\text{Hct}_{\text{average}}}$$

EBV, estimated blood volume (see Table 78-1) and $\text{Hct}_{\text{average}} = (\text{Hct}_{\text{start}} + 0.35)/2$.

Ideally, blood should be replaced with fresh whole blood, because this mixture contains platelets and clotting factors as well as erythrocytes. Unfortunately, this is rarely, if ever, available. Packed erythrocytes are usually used instead. This blood product typically has a hematocrit of 60% to 70% and has little, if any, factors V and VIII. Large blood losses and massive transfusions (two to three times the EBV) often produce a secondary coagulopathy. This bleeding is usually caused by either dilutional or consumption thrombocytopenia. Platelets can be transfused based on the following formula:[184]

$$\frac{\text{Platelet increment}}{\text{mm}^3} = \frac{30{,}000 \times \text{Number of units}}{\text{EBV(l)}}$$

Fresh frozen plasma (FFP) is rarely necessary and should be given only when a legitimate indication exists. All blood products, including FFP, may be contaminated with viruses. **The newborn should be considered an immunocompromised host. Therefore, one should irradiate any blood product that may contain leukocytes before transfusion because of the possibility of producing a graft-versus-host reaction. Additionally, only CMV negative blood and blood products should be given to the newborn.**

AIRWAY

Understanding the anatomic differences between infants, children, and adults is crucial for successful airway management in the normal child and in the child with a congenital anomaly (see Tables 78-1 and 78-2 and Fig.

78-2).[139,170,180,237] **Infants less than 6 months of age are obligate nose breathers. Anatomic (e.g., choanal atresia), physical (e.g., nasogastric tube), or infectious obstruction of the nasopharynx rapidly causes respiratory distress or failure.**[40,49,171,180,181] The abundant and friable lymphoidal tissue of the nasopharynx also precludes the routine placement of nasopharyngeal airways in this age group when treating upper airway obstruction.

The tongue is relatively large in relation to the mandible in children less than 2 years of age, making visualization of the larynx difficult. The tongue most often obstructs the upper airway when consciousness is lost following the induction of anesthesia. The larynx is also difficult to visualize because it is anterior and more cephalad in the newborn. The larynx is located at the third to fourth cervical vertebrae (C3 to C4) in infants and at C5 to C6 in adults. The vocal cords also differ in their appearance. In infants, vocal cords are 40% ligament and 60% arytenoid cartilage. These ratios are reversed in adults.

The infant's epiglottis is omega-shaped, floppy, and has a 45° angle of entry into the pharyngeal wall. Visualization of the larynx requires lifting the epiglottis directly with an appropriately sized straight laryngoscope blade (0 or 1 Miller blade). The adult's epiglottis, on the other hand, is stiff, flat, and parallel to the tracheal wall. Visualization of the larynx in the adult can be made indirectly by placing the laryngoscope blade in the vallecula (Fig. 78-3).[237]

Finally, the trachea is different as well. **The narrowest part of the airway in children less than 8 to 10 years of age is the cricoid ring. Uncuffed ET tubes are used in this age group to prevent damage to the mucosa underlying this structure.** Further, the infant's trachea may be only 4 to 5 cm in length. This makes endobronchial intubation extremely easy to accomplish even by very experienced practitioners. Proper positioning of the ET tube can be made by auscultation (return of breath sounds after a deliberate right mainstem intubation), palpation of the tip of the ET tube in the sternal notch, inspection of the distal line marker at the level of the vocal cords, or a chest radiograph. Once positioned, the ET tube must be secured with adhesive tape in a way that minimizes the likelihood of dislodgement or acci-

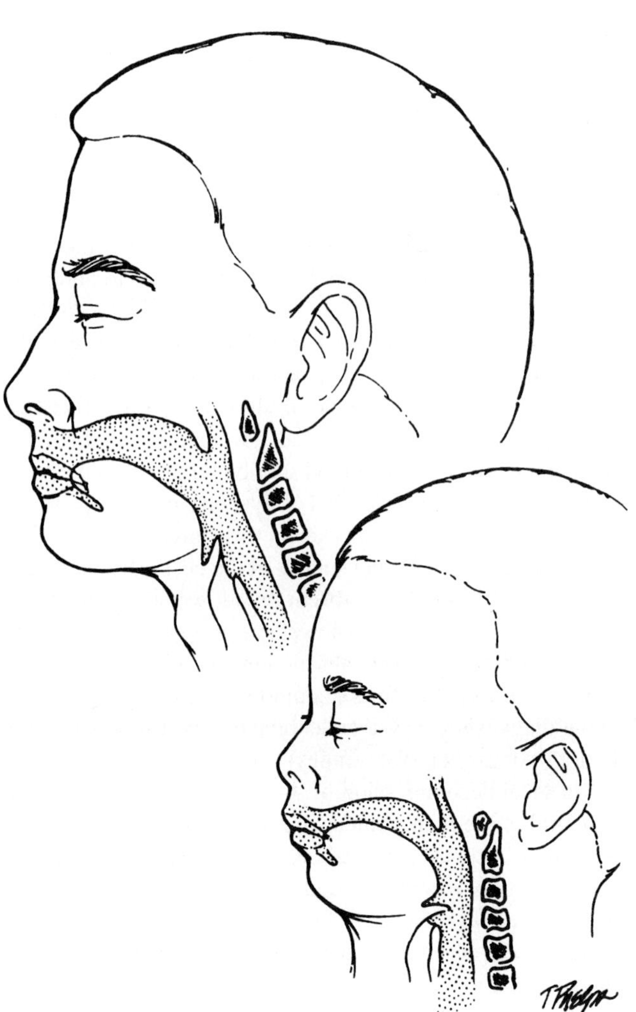

Fig. 78-2. Comparative anatomy of the adult and infant airway.

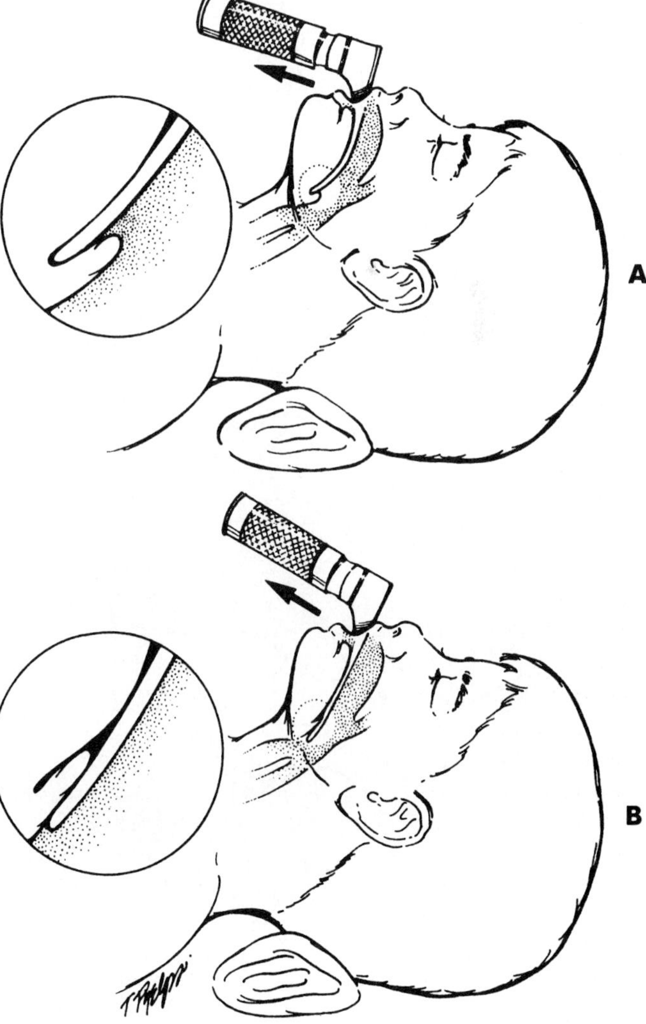

Fig. 78-3. Laryngoscope blades. **A,** A curved (MacIntosh) blade is inserted in the vallecula only. **B,** A straight (Miller) blade is inserted either under epiglottis or above it in the vallecula.

dental extubation. The "fish-mouth" technique, developed by Dr. Lee of the Children's Hospital of Philadelphia, is one preferred technique (Fig. 78-4).

The preferred method for tracheal intubation is controversial. Because of the anatomic considerations previously listed and because the newborn rapidly desaturates following only 15 to 20 seconds of apnea, in the past many anesthesiologists believed it was safer to intubate the newborn "awake." However, recent evidence that awake intubation may cause intraventricular hemorrhage in fragile, premature newborns has counterbalanced this belief.[68,149,169] Further, awake intubations are technically more difficult to accomplish and often result in trauma to the vocal cords, hemorrhage, bradycardia, and desaturation from breath holding. Many clinicians prefer to use a "rapid-sequence" induction in infants requiring full-stomach precautions, that is, infants who are at risk of aspirating their gastric contents (e.g., with intestinal obstruction, NEC) and who have a normal airway on physical examination. After volume resuscitation (10 to 40 ml/kg of Ringer's lactate), preoxygenation, and pretreatment with atropine (0.15 mg), gentle cricoid pressure is applied to occlude the esophagus.[72] If cricoid pressure is applied too vigorously, the position of the larynx may be distorted or the trachea occluded. In hemodynamically stable patients, rapid-sequence IV induction can be accomplished by bolus administration of thiopental (4 to 7 mg/kg), ketamine (2 to 4 mg/kg), or fentanyl (12.5 μg/kg) immediately followed by succinylcholine (2 mg/kg) or pancuronium (0.1 to 0.15 mg/kg). Newborns not requiring full-stomach precautions are in the minority (e.g., those with myelomeningocele, bladder exstrophy), and in these patients anesthesia can be induced by inhalational agents delivered by mask or IV without cricoid pressure.

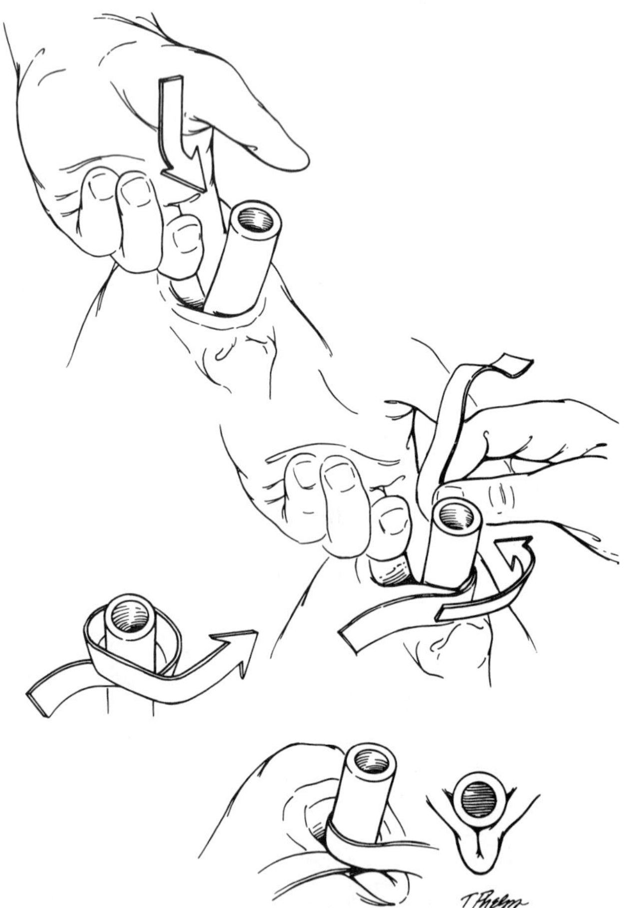

Fig. 78-4. Following preparation of infant's skin with tincture of benzoin or Mastisol, the endotracheal (ET) tube is secured with 1/2-inch adhesive tape using the "fish-mouth technique." Starting at one zygoma, tape is pulled, wrapped around ET tube, and then pulled to opposite zygoma. This technique was developed by Dr. Terry Lee of Children's Hospital of Philadelphia.

SURGICAL EMERGENCIES IN NEWBORNS

It is beyond the scope of this text to discuss the anesthetic management of every surgical emergency that occurs in the first weeks of life. However, by concentrating on those emergencies occurring most frequently, the basic principles provided can be applied to conditions not specifically discussed.

Congenital Diaphragmatic Hernia

The most challenging and frustrating of all neonatal surgical emergencies—congenital diaphragmatic hernia (the herniation of the abdominal viscera into the thorax)—carries a 50% mortality regardless of the method of treatment used. Even early prenatal diagnosis by ultrasound, which now occurs in approximately 20% of patients, has done little, if anything, to affect outcome.[3,92,93,179] The incidence of this devastating problem is reported to be 1 in 2000 to 5000 live births.

Most frequently, the abdominal viscera, including the small bowel and colon, liver, and occasionally the kidney, herniate into the left hemithorax during the first or second trimester and interfere with the development of both the lung parenchyma and its blood supply. Infants born with this anomaly have the classic triad of dyspnea, cyanosis, and apparent dextrocardia. Physical examination reveals a scaphoid abdomen, bowel sounds in the chest, distant or displaced heart sounds, and absent breath sounds in the chest. Chest radiography reveals bowel gas or a gastric tube in the chest, mediastinal shift, absent lung markings, and most ominously, a contralateral pneumothorax. The major differential diagnosis is a cystic adenomatoid malformation of the lung or congenital lobar emphysema.

Surgical decompression of the left hemithorax, although essential in the management of this malformation, does not determine ultimate survival. Rather, outcome depends on the pulmonary vasculature and whether it will respond in an exaggerated, hyperreactive fashion to the stimuli that vasoconstrict and elevate PA pressure.[74,75,155] Histologic studies of the lungs of children born with this anomaly reveal decreased number and size of the bronchi, lung saccules, and alveoli and abnormalities of the pulmonary vascular bed.

The numbers of pulmonary blood vessels are reduced, and the arterial muscularis and media are hypertrophied. **Hyperactive pulmonary artery (PA) vasoconstriction caused by hypoxia, hypercapnia, acidosis, pain, or positive-pressure ventilation can initiate a catastrophic cycle of events in which desaturated blood returning to the lung is preferentially shunted across the still-patent ductus arteriosus and atrial septum into the systemic circulation.** This shunting of blood across the ductus and atrial septum is a return of the circulation to the pattern that existed *in utero* and is referred to as *persistent fetal circulation* (PFC) or *persistent hypertension of the newborn* (PPHN).[27,75,76,165] The goal of anesthetic management is to prevent this catastrophic cascade from occurring by maximizing arterial oxygenation and by preventing pain and metabolic or respiratory acidosis.[25,41,216]

These infants require immediate intubation and decompression of the stomach as soon as the diagnosis is suspected. This is almost always accomplished in the delivery room or in the neonatal intensive care unit before the anesthesiologist's arrival. Medical management is directed at improving oxygenation and increasing pulmonary blood flow. This is accomplished with muscle relaxants (usually pancuronium), analgesics (usually fentanyl, 10 to 50 μg/kg as an initial bolus, followed by a continuous infusion of 3 to 10 μg/kg/hour), mechanical or spontaneous ventilation, using low inflating pressures and pressure support ventilation and correction of acidosis with IV bicarbonate therapy.[154,192,216] Interestingly, this is also the basis of intraoperative anesthetic management as well. Inhalational anesthetic agents are avoided because of their hypotensive and cardiac depressant effects. The importance of inadequate cardiac output in neonates with PFC should not be overlooked. Decreased cardiac output leads to decreased pulmonary perfusion and further hypoxemia. Blood returning to the heart from poorly perfused organs arrives with a lower O_2 content, which potentiates the hypoxemia caused by right-to-left shunting.

Bohn et al.[18,120] have advocated the avoidance of the "mad dash" to the operating room and recommend instead 24 to 48 hours stabilization. Further, these authors and others contend that infants who do not respond to this therapy will fail to survive with surgery or any other therapy, including extracorporeal membrane oxygenation (ECMO).[159,160,226] Bohn et al.[18,120] have also suggested a nomogram to predict the degree of pulmonary hypoplasia in these infants and their chance of survival. They used the preoperative arterial carbon dioxide tension ($Paco_2$) and an index of ventilation, which is determined by the mean airway pressure times the respiratory rate. If the $Paco_2$ could be reduced to less than 40 mm Hg and the ventilatory index was less than 1000, survival was almost universal. On the other hand, if $Paco_2$ and the ventilatory index were greater than 40 and 1000, respectively, death was virtually inevitable. Interestingly, these latter infants were found at autopsy to have less than 10% of the normal number of alveoli *bilaterally*.[18,110,120]

Blood loss is minimal during the surgical repair of this problem in patients who are not on ECMO, and third-space losses can be assumed to average 8 to 10 ml/kg/hour. Aside from routine monitoring, these patients require arterial and central venous catheters. A precordial stethoscope placed in the right axilla may help alert the anesthesiologist to one of the most serious intraoperative catastrophes, development of a contralateral pneumothorax. This is heralded by sudden hypoxia or hypotension. Placement of a chest tube when this occurs may be lifesaving. Some authors have suggested the insertion of a prophylactic chest tube on the contralateral side, because this complication is so catastrophic.

Vasodilator therapy has also been advocated for perioperative control of the elevated PA pressures. Agents suggested for use include isoproterenol, nitroglycerin, tolazoline, adenosine, and adenosine triphosphate (ATP).[113] These are rarely effective because the pulmonary vasodilatation produced is matched by an equal fall in systemic vascular resistance (SVR). On the other hand, inhaled nitric oxide (NO) may be much more useful in the treatment of PA hypertension.[1,106,115,130,197,241,243] NO diffuses across alveolar capillary membranes and stimulates cyclic guanylate cyclase, which increases cyclic GMP. Cyclic GMP is a potent dilator of vascular smooth muscle. Because NO is rapidly metabolized it has a potent local effect and should preferentially dilate only the pulmonary vascular musculature. Finally, the anesthesiologist should anticipate the possibility of a cardiac arrest during this surgery; vasopressors, including dopamine (4 to 10 μg/kg/min) and epinephrine (0.1 to 1.0 μg/kg/min), should always be available for emergency intraoperative administration.[113]

The most recent innovation in the treatment of congenital diaphragmatic hernia is the perioperative use of heart-lung bypass or ECMO.[1,94,106,130,197,241,243] The use of ECMO in the management of congenital diaphragmatic hernia is both controversial and confusing. Infants who either would not survive by the criteria of Bohn et al.[18] or who develop a PFC pattern following surgery (a so-called honeymoon period) may be placed on ECMO to allow the infant's lungs time to develop and restructure. Unfortunately, when to place an infant on ECMO (either before or after surgery), when to perform surgery if the neonate is receiving ECMO, and when to withdraw ECMO support are very parochial decisions that may differ among physicians even within the same institution.[2,109,128,199,214] The usefulness of this very expensive therapeutic modality may remain unknown until controlled multicenter trials are performed.

Omphalocele and Gastroschisis

An *omphalocele* occurs because of the gut's failure to return to the abdominal cavity at the tenth week of gestation.[145] The herniated bowel is covered by the amnion, which protects it from fluid loss, infection, and a chemical, amniotic fluid burn. The apex of the herniated sac is the umbilical cord. *Gastroschisis* results from an intrauterine vascular accident that interrupts the abdominal wall and musculature. The herniated bowel is not covered by any membrane and is "burned" by the amniotic fluid. It is subject to tremendous postnatal evaporative fluid losses as well as infection. In gastroschisis the umbilical cord is found to the side of the herniated bowel.

The optimal method for surgical management of congenital abdominal wall defects remains controversial. Two options exist: primary fascial closure, with or without intraoperative and postoperative muscle paralysis, or a staged repair using either a silicone elastomer pouch or a primary skin closure.[58,177,193,196,210] Primary fascial closure of omphalocele or gastroschisis carries the risk of placing the abdominal contents under pressure, which may produce a reduction in cardiac output, hypotension, bowel ischemia, venous stasis, and postoperative respiratory and renal failure.[77,136,162,231,238] When primary fascial closure cannot be achieved, either because of the large size of the defect or because it critically compromises respiratory or cardiovascular function, the alternative approach is a staged repair using either a silicone elastomer pouch or a skin closure with secondary fascial closure. The staged silicone elastomer repair carries an increased risk of infection as well as the need for multiple anesthetic and surgical procedures. Skin closure with secondary ventral herniorrhaphy incurs the same risks.

Traditional criteria for deciding on which course to choose have been based on the size of the defect, the presence of associated congenital anomalies, or clinical observations of the infant's respiratory rate, pulmonary compliance, blood pressure, skin color, and peripheral perfusion during fascial approximation. Unfortunately, these clinical observations may not be reliable, particularly in paralyzed, anesthetized infants.

Anesthetic management

Infants are intubated and anesthetized with fentanyl (10 to 12.5 μg/kg), pancuronium, and O_2.[229] Aside from routine monitoring, catheters are placed in the right radial artery and the internal jugular vein. Intragastric pressure is measured by a fluid-filled, 12-French oral gastric tube. Yaster et al.[231,238] suggested that successful management of neonates with omphalocele or gastroschisis can be reliably determined by the intraoperative measurement of intragastric and CVP (Fig. 78-5). In this treatment algorithm, primary repair is always attempted. However, if the intragastric pressure rises above 20 mm Hg and the CVP increases by 4 mm Hg or more following closure of the abdominal fascia, the primary repair is abandoned and a staged repair is performed with a silicone elastomer chimney. This algorithm avoids the consequences of acutely elevating intra-abdominal pressure. Following surgery, the patient is taken to the neonatal intensive care unit, still intubated, and placed on controlled mechanical ventilation. Infants treated with a staged repair have their chimneys gradually reduced over 5 to 10 days. CVP and intragastric pressure can be used to guide this therapy as well.

Newborns with abdominal wall defects have significantly increased fluid requirements because of the increase in insensible losses that occur when eviscerated bowel is exposed to the environment.[151] Also, they have extreme third-space losses because of the traumatized, inflamed bowel and adynamic ileus that develops perioperatively. Fluid requirements are even greater in patients with gastroschisis because the herniated viscera lacks a protective covering, resulting in a chemical burn preoperatively.[151]

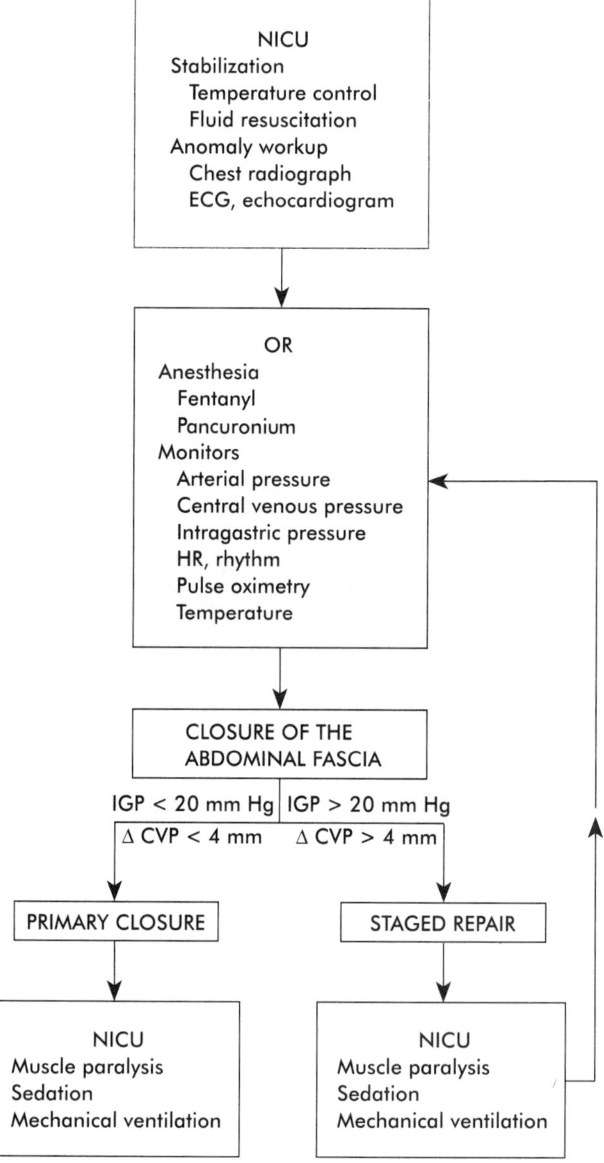

Fig. 78-5. Algorithm for intraoperative and postoperative management of children with congenital abdominal wall defects. Note that one measures actual intragastric pressures and *changes* in central venous pressure.

Intestinal Obstruction and Necrotizing Enterocolitis

Intestinal obstruction is among the most common surgical emergencies in the newborn and is characterized by feeding intolerance, bilious vomiting, and abdominal distension.[46,51,90,112,175] Common sites of obstruction include the duodenum; the jejunum-ileum, particularly the terminal ileum; and the anus. Necrotizing enterocolitis (NEC), on the other hand, is caused by a bacterial invasion of previously injured or ischemic bowel wall. It is characterized by intestinal obstruction, gangrene, perforation, intramural air (*pneumatosis intestinalis*), and peritonitis.* Patients are usually premature and are often septic, hypotensive, thrombocytopenic, and have respiratory failure. Metabolic and respiratory acidosis and electrolyte disturbances also frequently occur.

Duodenal obstruction typically develops within the first hours of life and is extremely common in children with Down's syndrome. An abdominal radiograph reveals the classic "double-bubble" sign, or a dilated, air-filled stomach and proximal duodenum. Because these children have this condition so early in life, usually within the first 12 hours, they are rarely dehydrated or hypochloremic. Small- and large-bowel obstructions typically appear later, usually 2 to 7 days after birth, and are often associated with hemodynamic compromise and metabolic disturbances. Jejunal or ileal atresias are believed to be caused by intrauterine vascular accidents. Meconium ileus is an obstruction of the small bowel caused by inspissated, abnormal meconium and is pathonomic of cystic fibrosis. When this anomaly develops, these infants do not have the lung disease associated with this devastating disease. Malrotations of the bowel also are associated with obstruction and occur often in patients with congenital diaphragmatic hernia and omphalocele or gastroschisis. Infants with Hirschsprung's disease have a functional distal obstruction caused by a lack of ganglia in the rectum and distal colon. Imperforate anus, which should be readily obvious in the delivery room, requires special attention because of the many anomalies associated with it. The *VATER syndrome* (*v*ertebral, *a*nal, *t*racheoesophageal fistula, *e*sophageal atresia, and *r*enal anomalies) carries a 20% incidence of significant congenital heart disease.[37,201] Patients diagnosed with it should have an echocardiogram (ECG) obtained before surgery.

Regardless of the underlying pathology, the major anesthetic challenge in surgical patients with an intestinal obstruction or NEC is maintaining an adequate circulating blood volume and preventing the pulmonary aspiration of gastric contents. Virtually all newborns undergoing emergency abdominal surgery are intravascularly depleted from the massive ongoing third-space losses. Sepsis, bowel manipulation, peritonitis, use of contrast agents, and release of vasoactive peptides significantly deplete the circulating blood volume and extracellular fluid space of water and electrolytes. In patients with NEC, third-space fluid replacement therapy in the perioperative period may exceed 100 to 200 mg/kg/hour. Also, the critically ill septic patient may not be able to tolerate these extreme fluid shifts, and dopamine (4 to 10 μg/kg/min) should be infused to help maintain blood pressure and blood flow. Both arterial pressure and CVP monitors may be required to check intravascular volume in these patients.

All newborns undergoing emergency abdominal surgery may aspirate their abdominal contents at induction of anesthesia. Therefore one must use methods that minimize these risks, such as an awake intubation or a rapid-sequence induction with cricoid pressure. This has been described previously. I prefer to maintain anesthesia with the fentanyl, pancuronium, and O_2 technique for this group of patients, but inhalational agents can also be used as long as N_2O is avoided. N_2O will further distend the bowel and thus complicate fascial closure.

*References 24, 56, 66, 111, 116, 157, 174, 182, 186

Esophageal Atresia and Tracheoesophageal Fistula

Ninety percent of infants born with a tracheoesophageal fistula (TEF) have a blind esophageal pouch and a fistula connecting the distal esophagus and the distal trachea, usually within 1 or 2 cm of the carina.[55,168,176,204] From 30% to 50% of these infants have the associated anomalies of the VATER syndrome (see previous discussion). An investigation of potential cardiac anomalies must therefore be made before surgery. Often suspected prenatally by polyhydramnios, infants have excessive salivation ("mucous mouth"), choking, coughing, aspiration pneumonia, and cyanosis. Attempts at feeding are met with explosive vomiting, and it is impossible to pass an oral or nasogastric tube. A chest radiograph of a coiled oral gastric tube in the cervical esophageal pouch is diagnostic of TEF. Because of the potential for aspiration, contrast media should *not* be instilled to confirm this diagnosis.

The tracheal-to-distal esophageal fistula aerates the GI tract and allows for regurgitation of gastric juice up the fistula into the lung. Thus pulmonary aspiration occurs by two methods. The first involves aspiration of saliva or attempted feedings from the blind esophageal pouch and the second by gastric juice contamination via the fistula tract. If significant aspiration pneumonia occurs, corrective surgery is deferred and a decompressing gastrostomy is placed under local or caudal anesthesia.

As soon as the diagnosis is confirmed, the infant is placed in a head-up position, and the upper pouch is decompressed with a large-bore, sump (Replogle) tube. Following diagnostic workup, the child is transported to the operating room for corrective repair. Routine monitors (see previous discussion) are placed. The precordial stethoscope is placed in the left axilla and carefully secured in place with both a "double-stick" and an "Op-site" dressing. Adequate IV access and a radial artery catheterization complete the preinduction preparation.

Combined technique: epidural plus "light" general anesthesia

Recently, a combined epidural and general anesthesia technique has become the preferred anesthetic method in the management of esophageal atresia and TEF. First proposed by Bosenberg et al.,[19,20] this technique is far superior to the classic technique described in the following section, because it allows the newborn patient to breathe spontaneously throughout the procedure and thereby avoids the potential for gastric dilation. Additionally, the use of continuous epidural analgesia postoperatively provides incomparable analgesia, makes extubation of the trachea relatively easy, and significantly reduces the need for postoperative ventilation.[19,20]

In this technique, paralysis is avoided and the patient breathes spontaneously throughout. Immediately before intubation, the infant is given atropine (0.15 mg IV), and the esophageal pouch is suctioned. The trachea is intubated either without anesthesia, that is, an "awake" intubation, or following an inhalational mask induction using O_2 and halothane only (N_2O is avoided). The tip of the ET tube is placed in midtrachea well above the carina and the fistula. Once the trachea is intubated and the ET tube is secured, the patient is turned to the lateral position and the back is cleaned and prepared with iodine. While the patient continues to breathe just enough halothane to allow immobility during needle insertion, an epidural catheter is placed either at the sacrococcygeal ligament (caudal approach) or at the L3-L4 intervertebral interspace (lumbar approach). It is my preference to use the caudal approach, because it is easier to perform than a lumbar approach and has minimal associated complications (e.g., dural puncture). Although different needles and catheter types and sizes are used, I believe that short (2-inch), large bore needles (17- to 18-gauge), and catheters (19- to 20-gauge) are easiest to place and have the fewest perioperative problems (e.g., inadvertent intravascular placement, kinking at the insertion site, etc.). The epidural catheter is then advanced rostrally to the thorax. Advancing an epidural catheter from a caudal or lumbar approach rostrally to the thorax is quite easy in the neonate because the epidural fat is loose and noncompacted. Local anesthetics, either bupivacaine 0.175 to 0.25% (0.5 to 1 ml/kg) or lidocaine 1% (0.5 ml/kg), are administered through the epidural catheter. One half to two thirds of the initial dose is administered every 60 to 120 minutes as needed.[44,87,88,236] The child continues to breathe halothane and O_2 spontaneously throughout the procedure. Halothane concentrations are adjusted to produce immobility (usually 0.2%–0.4% end-tidal concentrations, or one half of the MAC). Finally, the epidural catheter is left in place at the conclusion of surgery and is used to provide postoperative analgesia using either lidocaine (1 mg/ml, 1 ml/kg/hour) or bupivacaine (1 mg/ml, 0.2 mg/kg/hour).[235]

"Classic approach"

Immediately before intubation, the infant is given atropine (0.15 mg IV), and the esophageal pouch is suctioned. Then, with the infant in a semisitting position, the trachea is intubated when the patient is awake. With the infant spontaneously breathing halothane, the ET tube is positioned by deliberately intubating the right mainstem bronchus and then slowly pulling the tube back until breath sounds are heard in the left axilla and not in the stomach. Isolation of the fistula is possible because in most patients the fistula is approximately 0.5 to 1.0 cm above the carina on the trachea's posterior surface. If the ET tube has a side hole ("Murphy eye"), it should be turned to the left, opposite to its normal orientation, to maximize ventilation of the left lung. Even if the ET tube does not have a side hole, it may be helpful to turn the bevel of the tube 180° so that the curve of the tube faces forward. This reduces ventilation of the fistula and stomach. Once positioned, the ET tube is secured with the fish-mouth technique to avoid displacement of the ET tube down the right mainstem bronchus or, more ominously, into the fistula tract itself (see Fig. 78-4). This is why the precordial stethoscope is securely placed in the left axilla.

Once the ET tube is positioned, anesthetic management is based on the presence or absence of a decompressive gastrostomy and by the preferential flow of gases down the path of least resistance, that is, through the fistula tract into the stomach. Positive-pressure ventilation may allow O_2 and other gases to bypass the lungs and acutely dilate the stomach. This interferes with ventilation and venous return and can lead to cardiopulmonary arrest and gastric rupture. If this occurs, an emergency decompressive gastrostomy may be lifesaving. Unfortunately, although the insertion of a gastrostomy may be lifesaving, it may substitute one problem for another. Airflow resistance through the fistula-stomach-gastrostomy may be so low that ventilation of the lungs becomes impossible. The gastrostomy may need to be intermittently clamped and unclamped or left partially clamped through the procedure. Some experts have advocated the use of a Fogarty catheter, placed either through a bronchoscope or a gastric endoscope, to occlude the fistula tract if this becomes a problem.[59] One must use extreme caution, however, when using a Fogarty catheter passed alongside an ET tube. If it slips out of the fistula tract into the trachea, the catheter can completely occlude the end of the ET tube. Thus, because of these many problems with positive-pressure ventilation, many anesthesiologists recommend an anesthetic technique that employs spontaneous ventilation with halothane. Other experts believe that paralysis is safe because the fistula can be effectively isolated by careful positioning of the ET tube. In my experience using this technique, it is rarely possible to have a spontaneously breathing newborn sufficiently anesthetized to perform surgery without compromising blood pressure and oxygenation.

Regardless of the anesthetic technique that is used, surgery is performed with the patient in the left lateral decubitus position. During the surgical repair the right lung is compressed and packed away, which may result in hypoxemia. Also, the infant may become hypoxemic if the trachea or ET tube is compressed and occluded by the surgeon during ligation of the fistula. Alternatively, the ET tube can become obstructed by blood clots or may migrate into the fistula tract. Thus, to provide a greater margin of safety, I routinely use 100% O_2 during anesthesia, even in premature infants who are at risk for the retinopathy of prematurity.

After ligation of the fistula, a catheter is passed either through the nose or mouth into the blind esophageal pouch to help the surgeon identify the lower end of the esophagus. When the anastomosis of the esophagus is complete, the catheter is removed to a position just above the suture line and is secured in place with waterproof tape. Occasionally, the distal end of the esophagus is too short to reach the proximal pouch. If this occurs, the surgeon may need to exteriorize the upper pouch and place a gastrostomy.

Myelodysplasia

Failure of neural tube closure early in intrauterine development results in a spectrum of abnormalities ranging from spina bifida occulta, a relatively benign process, to myelomeningocele, an abnormality involving vertebral bodies, the spinal cord, and the brain stem.[89,158] The brain stem lesion, the Arnold-Chiari malformation, may be the cause of rather than the effect of the neural tube's failure to close. Ninety percent of infants with myelomeningocele have the Arnold-Chiari malformation, which consists of downward displacement of the brain stem and the cerebellar tonsils through the cervical spinal canal with medullary kinking.[26,158] This, together with obliteration of the foramina of the fourth ventricle, blocks the normal circulation of cerebrospinal fluid (CSF) and leads to progressive hydrocephalus. Associated skeletal anomalies, particularly of the lower extremities, often occur and result in multiple orthopedic procedures as the child grows. Fortunately, the combination of the discovery that maternal folate deficiency is primarily responsible for this defect and better prenatal diagnosis has resulted in a dramatic fall in the number of children born with this defect.

Infants with a meningomyelocele are transported to the operating room in the prone position. The defect is covered with moist, sterile dressings, and great care is taken to avoid contamination and infection. If the meningocele is ruptured, Ringer's lactate is used to replace CSF losses milliliter for milliliter or at an approximate rate of 4 to 6 ml/kg/hour.

The infant must be turned supine for intubation. Positioning is crucial to facilitate this. A foam head ring, or operating room towels folded into a ring, are covered with a sterile drape or towel. The infant is then turned to the supine position with the defect resting in the pocket of the ring. Towels are then placed under the child's back to build up a level platform for intubation (Fig. 78-6). Anesthesia is induced with either inhalational agents (halothane) or IV agents (thiopental, lidocaine). Almost any anesthetic technique is possible for this procedure as long as it allows for rapid extubation following surgery. Succinylcholine does not cause catastrophic hyperkalemia in patients with this defect.[50] **Tracheal intubation may be complicated by significant hydrocephalus. Further, during intubation, the neck should not be excessively flexed, because in patients with Arnold Chiari malformations, this may cause brain stem compression.**[163] Once the trachea is intubated, the ET tube is secured with a fish-mouth technique (see Fig. 78-4), and the child is turned to the prone position for surgery.

A new alternative, proposed by Abajian et al.,[217] is to perform this procedure under spinal anesthesia. In this technique, the patient is not intubated and is positioned prone with facial padding and a small chest roll to elevate the thorax. "Blow-by" O_2 is administered, and a sucrose-tipped pacifier is given to the child to suck on. Using a 26-gauge needle attached to a 1-ml syringe, 0.5 to 0.7 mg/kg of hyperbaric tetracaine (1 ml 10 mg/ml tetracaine mixed with 1 ml of 10% glucose = 5 mg/ml tetracaine) plus epinephrine is injected into the most inferior region of the meningomyelocele sac in an area devoid of neural elements. Because the duration of surgery usually outlasts the duration of spinally administered anesthesia, top-up dosings (0.3 to 0.5 mg/kg) are dripped into the open wound by the surgeon on an as-needed basis.

In my practice, I combine spinal anesthesia with general anesthesia. In the combined technique, I induce general anesthesia, intubate the trachea, turn the patient supine, and then inject tetracaine as previously described. Several min-

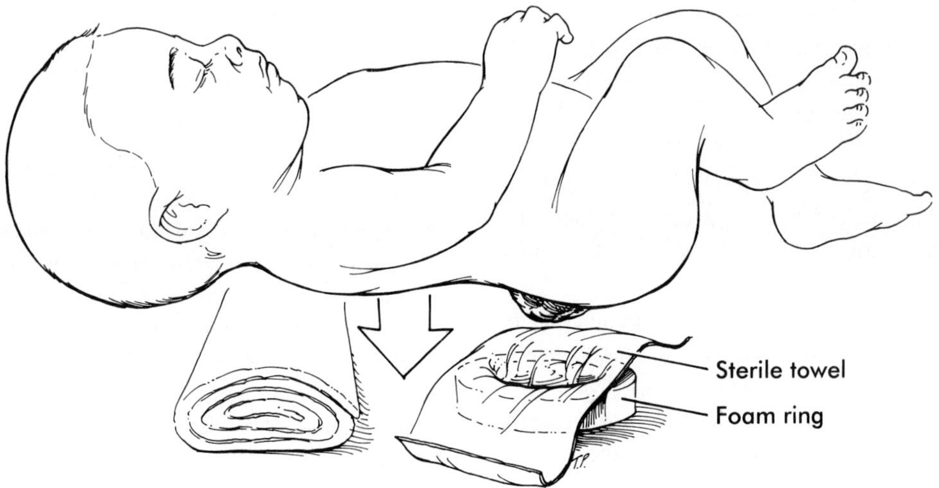

Fig. 78-6. Positioning of newborn with myelomeningocele for ET intubation.

utes later, I lower the concentration of the inspired inhalational anesthetic agent to a level that provides immobility and allows the child to tolerate the ET tube.

The decision to place a ventricular-peritoneal (VP) shunt at the initial surgery or several days later is a surgical one.[26,103,158,173] Some surgeons defer placement of the VP shunt because they think the drain will become infected. Also, because 5% to 10% of these patients do not develop hydrocephalus, some surgeons prefer to wait until the condition develops rather than treating it expectantly.

Patent Ductus Arteriosus

Following birth, the increase in arterial O_2 that occurs by breathing room air results in the closure of the ductus arteriosus.[13,30,76,97,99,142,161,189] In premature infants, this may not occur and often results in a large left-to-right shunt, heart failure, pulmonary edema, and an inability to be weaned from mechanical ventilation. Medical management consists of fluid restriction, diuretic therapy, digoxin, and inhibition of prostaglandin production, usually with parenterally administered indomethacin (0.2 mg/kg).[13,28,29,96,100,101] Indomethacin, a prostaglandin inhibitor, is often successful at pharmacologically closing the ductus within 24 hours of its administration. When indomethacin is not effective, surgical correction becomes essential if the child is to be weaned from mechanical ventilation. Unfortunately, in the smallest of premature infants (less than 1000 g), indomethacin is often unsuccessful because it significantly impairs renal function.

Because these children have been restricted from fluids and are intravascularly volume depleted before surgery, volume expansion with Ringer's lactate is essential to prevent profound hypotension after induction of anesthesia, even when a fentanyl anesthetic is used. Fentanyl (10 to 50 μg/kg) has become the most common anesthetic used.[8,229] N_2O must be avoided, and 100% O_2 is often required to maintain oxyhemoglobin concentrations above 90%, especially once the chest is opened and the lung retracted. **Lung retraction, which is necessary to provide surgical exposure, may result in vagal stimulation, and if the child has not been pretreated with either atropine or pancuronium, bradycardia and hypotension result. During closure of the ductus, hemorrhage and exsanguination may occur if this fragile structure is inadvertently torn by the surgeon.** Thus type and cross-matched blood should always be available before surgery. Also, closure of the ductus is associated with an abrupt rise in diastolic blood pressure, which may contribute to the development of intraventricular hemorrhage in this patient population.[218,219]

Recently, epidural anesthesia has been used to treat postoperative pain in these infants and to reduce intraoperative anesthetic requirements. Both local anesthetics and epidurally administered opioids are effective. Typically, opioids are administered via a caudal approach and local anesthetics via a caudally placed catheter that has been advanced to the thorax.

KEY POINTS

- Except for extraordinary circumstances, all newborns require anesthesia for surgery. Newborns respond to noxious stimuli with behavioral, physiologic, metabolic, and hormonal responses suggestive of substantial stress.
- The newborn differs from the adult and older child in the uptake, distribution, metabolism, and excretion of drugs.
- Concentrations of both albumin and alpha$_1$-acid glycoprotein are lower in the newborn than at any other stage in life. Thus, a greater proportion of active or free drug is available to penetrate the brain, heart, and other viscera.
- At equipotent doses, all the potent inhalational anesthetic agents (e.g., halothane, enflurane, isoflurane) produce unacceptable hypotension in newborns who require emergency surgery.
- Investigators have demonstrated that a combination of fentanyl, O_2, and pancuronium can provide anesthesia in newborns with minimal hemodynamic consequences.
- The use of fentanyl results in the need for postoperative intubation and ventilation, independent of the infant's medical or surgical condition.
- At appropriate doses, all the nondepolarizing muscle relaxants are effective paralytics in the newborn. The selected method is usually based on properties other than neuromuscular blockade.
- Pancuronium is a potent vagolytic and is the most frequently used agent in the newborn.
- Tachycardia is a desired side effect during surgery because the infant responds to a variety of stimuli with bradycardia.
- In neonates, the oximeter probe is preferentially placed in the right hand, earlobe, or on the buccal mucosa.
- An arterial catheter is an extremely sensitive monitor of the infant's intravascular volume status.
- All newborns are at extraordinarily high risk of becoming cold during transport and in the operating room. This risk must be minimized with warmers, heated water mattresses, warm IV fluids, elevated temperature in the operating room, and the use of heated, humidified gases.
- The newborn should be considered an immunocompromised host. Therefore, one should consider irradiating any blood product that may contain leukocytes before transfusion is undertaken.
- Infants less than 6 months of age are obligate nose breathers.

- The preferred method for tracheal intubation in infants for emergency surgery is controversial. Because of anatomic considerations and because the newborn rapidly desaturates following only 15 to 20 seconds of apnea, many anesthesiologists believe it is safer to intubate the newborn "awake." However, other experts now believe that it is safer and easier to intubate the trachea following a "rapid-sequence" induction of anesthesia.
- The goal of anesthetic management in treating congenital diaphragmatic hernia is to maximize arterial oxygenation and prevent pain and metabolic or respiratory acidosis.
- Successful management of neonates with omphalocele or gastroschisis can be reliably determined by the intraoperative measurement of intragastric pressure and CVP.
- The major anesthetic challenge in infants with an intestinal obstruction or NEC is maintaining an adequate circulating blood volume and preventing pulmonary aspiration of gastric contents.
- A combined epidural and general anesthesia technique has become the preferred anesthetic method in the management of esophageal atresia and TEF. This technique allows the newborn patient to breathe spontaneously throughout the procedure and postoperatively makes extubation of the trachea relatively easy.

KEY REFERENCES

Anand KJ, Hickey PR: Halothane-morphine compared with high-dose sufentanil for anesthesia and postoperative analgesia in neonatal cardiac surgery, *N Engl J Med* 326:1–9, 1992.

Anand KJ, Sippell WG, Aynsley-Green A: Randomised trial of fentanyl anaesthesia in preterm babies undergoing surgery: Effects on the stress response, *Lancet* 1:62–66, 1987.

Bissonnette B: Temperature monitoring in pediatric anesthesia, *Int Anesthesiol Clin* 30:63–76, 1992.

Bohn DJ, James I, Filler RM, et al: The relationship between $PaCO_2$ and ventilation parameters in predicting survival in congenital diaphragmatic hernia, *J Pediatr Surg* 19:666–671, 1984.

Bosenberg AT, Bland BA, Schulte-Steinberg O, Downing JW: Thoracic epidural anesthesia via caudal route in infants, *Anesthesiology* 69:265–269, 1988.

Cook DR: Muscle relaxants in infants and children, *Anesth Analg* 60:335, 1981.

Cote CJ, Goldstein EA, Cote MA, et al: A single-blind study of pulse oximetry in children, *Anesthesiology* 68: 184–188, 1988.

Friesen RH, Henry DB: Cardiovascular changes in preterm neonates receiving isoflurane, halothane, fentanyl, and ketamine, *Anesthesiology* 64:238, 1986.

Goudsouzian NG, Standaert FG: The infant and the myoneural junction, *Anesth Analg* 65:1208, 1986.

Greeley WJ, de Bruijn NP: Changes in sufentanil pharmacokinetics within the neonatal period, *Anesth Analg* 67:86, 1988.

Gregory GA: The baroresponses of preterm infants during halothane anaesthesia, *Can Anaesth Soc J* 29:105, 1982.

Hertzka RE, Gauntlett IS, Fisher DM, et al: Fentanyl-induced ventilatory depression: Effects of age, *Anesthesiology* 70:213, 1989.

LeDez KM, Lerman J: The minimum alveolar concentration (MAC) of isoflurane in preterm neonates, *Anesthesiology* 67:301–307, 1987.

Lindahl SG: Energy expenditure and fluid and electrolyte requirements in anesthetized infants and children, *Anesthesiology* 69:377, 1988.

O'Rourke PP, Crone RK, Vacanti JP, et al: Extracorporeal membrane oxygenation and conventional medical therapy in neonates with persistent pulmonary hypertension of the newborn: a prospective randomized study, *Pediatrics* 84: 957, 1989.

Robinson S, Gregory GA: Fentanyl-air-oxygen anesthesia for patent ductus arteriosus in preterm infants, *Anesth Analg* 60:331, 1981.

Truog RD, Schena JA, Hershenson MB, et al: Repair of congenital diaphragmatic hernia during extracorporeal membrane oxygenation, *Anesthesiology* 72:750–753, 1990.

Yaster M: The dose response of fentanyl in neonatal anesthesia, *Anesthesiology* 66:433, 1987.

Yaster M, Buck JR, Dudgeon DL, et al: Hemodynamic effects of primary closure of omphalocele/gastroschisis in human newborns, *Anesthesiology* 69:84, 1988.

REFERENCES

1. Abman SH, Kinsella JP: Inhaled nitric oxide for persistent pulmonary hypertension of the newborn: the physiology matters! *Pediatrics* 96:1153–1155, 1995.
2. Adolph V, Flageole H, Perreault T, et al: Repair of congenital diaphragmatic hernia after weaning from extracorporeal membrane oxygenation, *J Pediatr Surg* 30:349–352, 1995.
3. Adzick NS, Vacanti JP, Lillehei CW, et al: Fetal diaphragmatic hernia: ultrasound diagnosis and clinical outcome in 38 cases, *J Pediatr Surg* 24:654–657, 1989.
4. Agarwal R, Gutlove DP, Lockhart CH: Seizures occurring in pediatric patients re-

ceiving continuous infusion of bupivacaine, *Anesth Analg* 75:284–286, 1992.
5. Anand KJ, Carr DB: The neuroanatomy, neurophysiology, and neurochemistry of pain, stress, and analgesia in newborns and children, *Pediatr Clin North Am* 36:795–822, 1989.
6. Anand KJ, Hickey PR: Pain and its effects in the human neonate and fetus, *N Engl J Med* 317:1321–1329, 1987.
7. Anand KJ, Hickey PR: Halothane-morphine compared with high-dose sufentanil for anesthesia and postoperative analgesia in neonatal cardiac surgery, *N Engl J Med* 326:1–9, 1992.
8. Anand KJ, Sippell WG, Aynsley-Green A: Randomised trial of fentanyl anaesthesia in preterm babies undergoing surgery: effects on the stress response, *Lancet* 1:62–66, 1987.
9. Badgwell JM: Respiratory gas monitoring in the pediatric patient, *Int Anesthesiol Clin* 30:131–146, 1992.
10. Badgwell JM, Heavner JE: End-tidal carbon dioxide pressure in neonates and infants measured by aspiration and flow-through capnography, *J Clin Monit* 7:285–288, 1991.
11. Badgwell JM, Heavner JE, Cooper MW, Cockings E: The cardiovascular effects of anticholinergic agents administered during halothane anaesthesia in children, *Acta Anaesthesiol Scand* 32:383–387, 1988.
12. Badgwell JM, McLeod ME, Lerman J, Creighton RE: End-tidal PCO_2 measurements sampled at the distal and proximal ends of the ET tube in infants and children, *Anesth Analg* 66:959–964, 1987.
13. Barst RJ, Gersony WM: The pharmacological treatment of patent ductus arteriosus. A review of the evidence, *Drugs* 38:249–266, 1989.
14. Berde CB: Convulsions associated with pediatric regional anesthesia, *Anesth Analg* 75:164–166, 1992.
15. Berry FA, Gregory GA: Do premature infants require anesthesia for surgery? editorial, *Anesthesiology* 67:291–293, 1987.
16. Betts EK, Downes JJ, Schaffer DB, Johns R: Retrolental fibroplasia and oxygen administration during general anesthesia, *Anesthesiology* 47:518–520, 1977.
17. Bissonnette B: Temperature monitoring in pediatric anesthesia, *Int Anesthesiol Clin* 30:63–76, 1992.
18. Bohn DJ, James I, Filler RM, et al: The relationship between $PaCO_2$ and ventilation parameters in predicting survival in congenital diaphragmatic hernia, *J Pediatr Surg* 19:666–671, 1984.
19. Bosenberg AT, Bland BA, Schulte-Steinberg O, Downing JW: Thoracic epidural anesthesia via caudal route in infants, *Anesthesiology* 69:265–269, 1988.
20. Bosenberg AT, Hadley GP, Murray WB: Epidural analgesia reduces postoperative ventilation requirements following esophageal atresia repair, *J Pain Symp Manage* 6:209, 1991.
21. Brandom BW, Brandom RB, Cook DR: Uptake and distribution of halothane in infants: in vivo measurements and computer simulations, *Anesth Analg* 62:404–410, 1983.
22. Brandom BW, Woelfel SK, Cook DR, et al: Clinical pharmacology of atracurium in infants, *Anesth Analg* 63:309–312, 1984.
23. Broadman LM, Hannallah RS, Belman AB, et al: Post-circumcision analgesia—a prospective evaluation of subcutaneous ring block of the penis, *Anesthesiology* 67: 399–402, 1987.
24. Buras R, Guzzetta P, Avery G, Naulty C: Acidosis and hepatic portal venous gas: indications for surgery in necrotizing enterocolitis, *Pediatrics* 78:273–277, 1986.
25. Burrows FA, Klinck JR, Rabinovitch M, Bohn DJ: Pulmonary hypertension in children: perioperative management, *Can Anaesth Soc J* 33:606–628, 1986.
26. Charney EB, Rorke LB, Sutton LN, Schut L: Management of Chiari II complications in infants with myelomeningocele, *J Pediatr* 111:364–371, 1987.
27. Clyman RI, Mauray F, Heymann MA, Roman C: Influence of increased pulmonary vascular pressures on the closure of the ductus arteriosus in newborn lambs, *Pediatr Res* 25:136–142, 1989.
28. Clyman RI, Mauray F, Roman C, et al: Circulating prostaglandin E2 concentrations and patent ductus arteriosus in fetal and neonatal lambs, *J Pediatr* 97:455–461, 1980.
29. Clyman RI, Mauray F, Rudolph AM, Heymann MA: Age-dependent sensitivity of the lamb ductus arteriosus to indomethacin and prostaglandins, *J Pediatr* 96:94–98, 1980.
30. Clyman RI, Mauray F, Wong L, et al: The developmental response of the ductus arteriosus to oxygen, *Biol Neonate* 34:177–181, 1978.
31. Cohen DE: Management of postoperative pain in children. In Schechter NL, Berde CB, Yaster M, editors. *Pain in infants, children, and adolescents,* Baltimore, 1993, Williams & Wilkins.
32. Cook DR: Muscle relaxants in infants and children, *Anesth Analg* 60:335–343, 1981.
33. Cook DR: Newborn anaesthesia: pharmacological considerations, *Can Anaesth Soc J* 33:S38–42, 1986.
34. Cook DR, Davis PJ, Lerman J: Pharmacology of pediatric anesthesia. In Motoyama EK, Davis PJ, editors. *Smith's anesthesia for infants and children,* St. Louis, 1996, Mosby–Year Book.
35. Cook DR, Fischer CG: Characteristics of succinylcholine neuromuscular blockage in neonates, *Anesth Analg* 57:63–66, 1978.
36. Cook DR, Westman HR, Rosenfeld L, Hendershot RJ: Pulmonary edema in infants: possible association with intramuscular succinylcholine, *Anesth Analg* 60: 220–223, 1981.
37. Corsello G, Maresi E, Corrao AM, et al: VATER/VACTERL association: clinical variability and expanding phenotype including laryngeal stenosis, *Am J Med Genet* 44:813–815, 1992.
38. Cote CJ, Goldstein EA, Cote MA, et al: A single-blind study of pulse oximetry in children, *Anesthesiology* 68:184–188, 1988.
39. Cote CJ, Rolf N, Liu LM, et al: A single-blind study of combined pulse oximetry and capnography in children, *Anesthesiology* 74:980–987, 1991.
40. Cotton RT, Richardson MA: Congenital laryngeal anomalies, *Otolaryngol Clin North Am* 14:203–218, 1981.
41. Crone RK, Sorensen GK, Orr RJ: Anaesthesia for the neonate, *Can J Anaesth* 38:R105–125, 1991.
42. Crumrine RS, Yodlowski EH: Assessment of neuromuscular function in infants, *Anesthesiology* 54:29–32, 1981.
43. Cunliffe M, Lucero VM, McLeod ME, et al: Neuromuscular blockade for rapid tracheal intubation in children: comparison of succinylcholine and pancuronium, *Can Anaesth Soc J* 33:760–764, 1986.
44. Dalens B: Regional anesthesia in children, *Anesth Analg* 68:654–672, 1989.
45. Dalens B, Vanneuville G, Dechelotte P: Penile block via the subpubic space in 100 children, *Anesth Analg* 69:41–45, 1989.
46. Davenport M: ABC of general surgery in children. Surgically correctable causes of vomiting in infancy, *Br Med J* 312:236–239, 1996.
47. Davis PJ, Cook DR: Clinical pharmacokinetics of the newer IV anaesthetic agents, *Clin Pharmacokinet* 11:18–35, 1986.
48. Davis PJ, Killian A, Stiller RL, et al: Pharmacokinetics of alfentanil in newborn premature infants and older children, *Dev Pharmacol Ther* 13:21–27, 1989.
49. Derkay CS, Grundfast KM: Airway compromise from nasal obstruction in neonates and infants, *Int J Pediatr Otorhinolaryngol* 19:241–249, 1990.
50. Dierdorf SF, McNiece WL, Rao CC, et al: Failure of succinylcholine to alter plasma potassium in children with myelomeningocoele, *Anesthesiology* 64:272–273, 1986.
51. Dillon PW, Cilley RE: Newborn surgical emergencies. Gastrointestinal anomalies, abdominal wall defects, *Pediatr Clin North Am* 40:1289–1314, 1993.
52. Duncan PG, Gregory GA, Wade JG: The effect of nitrous oxide on baroreceptor function in newborn and adult rabbits, *Can Anaesth Soc J* 28:339–341, 1981.
53. Eger EI, II: *Anesthetic uptake and action,* Baltimore, 1974, Williams & Wilkins.
54. Eger EI, II, Saidman LJ, Brandstater B: Minimum alveolar anesthetic concentration: a standard of anesthetic potency, *Anesthesiology* 26:756–763, 1965.
55. Engum SA, Grosfeld JL, West KW, et al: Analysis of morbidity and mortality in 227 cases of esophageal atresia and/or tracheoesophageal fistula over two decades, *Arch Surg* 130:502–508, 1995.
56. Faix RG, Adams JT: Neonatal necrotizing enterocolitis: current concepts and controversies, *Adv Pediatr Infect Dis* 9:1–36, 1994.
57. Feldman HS, Arthur GR, Covino BG: Comparative systemic toxicity of convulsant and supraconvulsant doses of IV ropivacaine, bupivacaine, and lidocaine in the conscious dog, *Anesth Analg* 69:794–801, 1989.
58. Filston HC: Gastroschisis—primary fascial closure. The goal for optimal management, *Ann Surg* 197:260–264, 1983.
59. Filston HC, Chitwood WR, Jr., et al: The Fogarty balloon catheter as an aid to management of the infant with esophageal atresia and tracheoesophageal fistula compli-

cated by severe RDS or pneumonia, *J Pediatr Surg* 17:149–151, 1982.

60. Fisher DM, Canfell PC, Fahey MR, et al: Elimination of atracurium in humans: contribution of Hofmann elimination and ester hydrolysis versus organ-based elimination, *Anesthesiology* 65:6–12, 1986.
61. Fisher DM, Canfell PC, Spellman MJ, Miller RD: Pharmacokinetics and pharmacodynamics of atracurium in infants and children, *Anesthesiology* 73:33–37, 1990.
62. Fisher DM, O'Keeffe C, Stanski DR, et al: Pharmacokinetics and pharmacodynamics of d-tubocurarine in infants, children, and adults, *Anesthesiology* 57:203–208, 1982.
63. Fitzgerald M: Neurobiology of fetal and neonatal pain. In Wall PD, Melzack R, editors: *Textbook of pain,* Edinburgh 1994, Churchill Livingstone.
64. Fitzgerald M, Anand KJ: Developmental neuroanatomy and neurophysiology of pain. In Schechter NL, Berde CB, Yaster M, editors: *Pain in infants, children, and adolescents.* Baltimore, 1993, Williams & Wilkins.
65. Flynn JT: Oxygen and retrolental fibroplasia: update and challenge, *Anesthesiology* 60:397–399, 1984.
66. Foglia RP: Necrotizing enterocolitis, *Curr Probl Surg* 32:757–823, 1995.
67. Friedman WF, George BL: Treatment of congestive heart failure by altering loading conditions of the heart, *J Pediatr* 106:697–706, 1985.
68. Friesen RH, Honda AT, Thieme RE: Changes in anterior fontanel pressure in preterm neonates during tracheal intubation, *Anesth Analg* 66:874-878, 1987.
69. Friesen RH, Lichtor JL: Cardiovascular depression during halothane anesthesia in infants: study of three induction techniques, *Anesth Analg* 61:42–45, 1982.
70. Friesen RH, Lichtor JL: Cardiovascular effects of inhalation induction with isoflurane in infants, *Anesth Analg* 62:411–414, 1983.
71. Furman EB, Roman DG, Lemmer LA, et al: Specific therapy in water, electrolyte and blood-volume replacement during pediatric surgery, *Anesthesiology* 42:187–193, 1975.
72. Gambee AM, Hertzka RE, Fisher DM: Preoxygenation techniques: comparison of three minutes and four breaths, *Anesth Analg* 66:468–470, 1987.
73. Gauntlett IS, Fisher DM, Hertzka RE, et al: Pharmacokinetics of fentanyl in neonatal humans and lambs: effects of age, *Anesthesiology* 69:683–687, 1988.
74. Geggel RL, Murphy JD, Langleben D, et al: Congenital diaphragmatic hernia: arterial structural changes and persistent pulmonary hypertension after surgical repair, *J Pediatr* 107:457–464, 1985.
75. Geggel RL, Reid LM: The structural basis of PPHN, *Clin Perinatol* 11:525–549, 1984.
76. Gersony WM: Patent ductus arteriosus in the neonate, *Pediatr Clin North Am* 33: 545–560, 1986.
77. Goldstein B, Herrin JT, Todres ID: Increased intraabdominal pressure and anuria in the newborn, *J Pediatr Surg* 26:749–750, 1991.
78. Goudsouzian NG: Muscle relaxants in infants and children, *Can Anaesth Soc J* 32: S27–31, 1985.
79. Goudsouzian NG: Atracurium infusion in infants, *Anesthesiology* 68:267–269, 1988.
80. Goudsouzian NG: Recent changes in the package insert for succinylcholine chloride: should this drug be contraindicated for routine use in children and adolescents? (Summary of the discussions of the anesthetic and life support drug advisory meeting of the Food and Drug Administration, FDA building, Rockville, June 9, 1994), *Anesth Analg* 80:207–208, 1995.
81. Goudsouzian NG, Liu LM: The neuromuscular response of infants to a continuous infusion of succinylcholine, *Anesthesiology* 60:97–101, 1984.
82. Goudsouzian NG, Standaert FG: The infant and the myoneural junction, *Anesth Analg* 65:1208–1217, 1986.
83. Greeley WJ, de Bruijn NP: Changes in sufentanil pharmacokinetics within the neonatal period, *Anesth Analg* 67:86–90, 1988.
84. Gregory GA: The baroresponses of preterm infants during halothane anaesthesia, *Can Anaesth Soc J* 29:105–107, 1982.
85. Gregory GA: Pharmacology. In Gregory GA, editor. *Pediatric anesthesia,* New York 1994, Churchill Livingstone.
86. Gregory GA, Eger EI, II, Munson ES: The relationship between age and halothane requirement in man, *Anesthesiology* 30:488–491, 1969.
87. Gunter JB, Dunn CM, Bennie JB, et al: Optimum concentration of bupivacaine for combined caudal—general anesthesia in children, *Anesthesiology* 75:57–61, 1991.
88. Gunter JB, Watcha MF, Forestner JE, et al: Caudal epidural anesthesia in conscious premature and high-risk infants, *J Pediatr Surg* 26:9–14, 1991.
89. Hahn YS: Open myelomeningocele, *Neurosurg Clin North Am* 6:231–241, 1995.
90. Haller JA, Jr., Tepas JJ, Pickard LR, Shermeta DW: Intestinal atresia. Current concepts of pathogenesis, pathophysiology, and operative management, *Am Surg* 49: 385–391, 1983.
91. Hannallah RS, Oh TH, McGill WA, Epstein BS: Changes in heart rate and rhythm after intramuscular succinylcholine with or without atropine in anesthetized children, *Anesth Analg* 65:1329–1332, 1986.
92. Harrison MR, Adzick NS, Estes JM, Howell LJ: A prospective study of the outcome for fetuses with diaphragmatic hernia, *JAMA* 271:382–384, 1994.
93. Harrison MR, Adzick NS, Flake AW: Congenital diaphragmatic hernia: an unsolved problem, *Semin Pediatr Surg* 2: 109–112, 1993.
94. Heiss K, Manning P, Oldham KT, et al: Reversal of mortality for congenital diaphragmatic hernia with ECMO, *Ann Surg* 209:225–230, 1989.
95. Hertzka RE, Gauntlett IS, Fisher DM, Spellman MJ: Fentanyl-induced ventilatory depression: Effects of age, *Anesthesiology* 70:213–218, 1989.
96. Heymann MA, Berman W, Jr., Rudolph AM, Whitman V: Dilatation of the ductus arteriosus by prostaglandin E1 in aortic arch abnormalities, *Circulation* 59:169–173, 1979.
97. Heymann MA, Iwamoto HS, Rudolph AM: Factors affecting changes in the neonatal systemic circulation, *Ann Rev Physiol* 43: 371–383, 1981.
98. Heymann MA, Rudolph AM: Effects of congenital heart disease on fetal and neonatal circulations, *Prog Cardiovasc Dis* 15:115–143, 1972.
99. Heymann MA, Rudolph AM: Control of the ductus arteriosus, *Physiol Rev* 55:62–78, 1975.
100. Heymann MA, Rudolph AM: Effects of prostaglandins and blockers of prostaglandin synthesis on the ductus arteriosus: animal and human studies, *Adv Prosta Thromb Res* 4:363–372, 1978.
101. Heymann MA, Rudolph AM, Silverman NH: Closure of the ductus arteriosus in premature infants by inhibition of prostaglandin synthesis, *N Engl J Med* 295: 530–533, 1976.
102. Hom XB: Fluids and Electrolytes. In Barone MA, editor: *The Harriet Lane handbook,* St. Louis 1996, Mosby–Year Book.
103. Hubballah MY, Hoffman HJ: Early repair of myelomeningocele and simultaneous insertion of ventriculoperitoneal shunt: technique and results, *Neurosurgery* 20:21–23, 1987.
104. Hug CC, Jr., Murphy MR: Fentanyl disposition in cerebrospinal fluid and plasma and its relationship to ventilatory depression in the dog, *Anesthesiology* 50:342–349, 1979.
105. Hug CC, Jr., Murphy MR: Tissue redistribution of fentanyl and termination of its effects in rats, *Anesthesiology* 55:369–375, 1981.
106. Ivy DD, Wiggins JW, Badesch DB, et al: Nitric oxide and prostacyclin treatment of an infant with primary pulmonary hypertension, *Am J Cardiol* 74:414–416, 1994.
107. Jobes DR, Nicolson SC: Monitoring of arterial hemoglobin oxygen saturation using a tongue sensor, *Anesth Analg* 67:186–188, 1988.
108. John E, Klavdianou M, Vidyasagar D: Electrolyte problems in neonatal surgical patients, *Clin Perinatol* 16:219–232, 1989.
109. Johnston PW, Bashner B, Liberman R, et al: Clinical use of extracorporeal membrane oxygenation in the treatment of persistent pulmonary hypertension following surgical repair of congenital diaphragmatic hernia, *J Pediatr Surg* 23:908–912, 1988.
110. Johnston PW, Liberman R, Gangitano E, Vogt J: Ventilation parameters and arterial blood gases as a prediction of hypoplasia in congenital diaphragmatic hernia, *J Pediatr Surg* 25:496–499, 1990.
111. Kanto WP, Jr., Hunter JE, Stoll BJ: Recognition and medical management of necrotizing enterocolitis, *Clin Perinatol* 21: 335–346, 1994.
112. Kays DW: Surgical conditions of the neonatal intestinal tract, *Clin Perinatol* 23: 353–375, 1996.
113. Keeley SR, Bohn DJ: The use of inotropic and afterload-reducing agents in neonates, *Clin Perinatol* 15:467–489, 1988.
114. Killian A, Davis PJ, Stiller RL, et al:

Influence of gestational age on pharmacokinetics of alfentanil in neonates, *Dev Pharmacol Ther* 15:82–85, 1990.

115. Kinsella JP, Neish SR, Ivy DD, et al: Clinical responses to prolonged treatment of persistent pulmonary hypertension of the newborn with low doses of inhaled nitric oxide, *J Pediatr* 123:103–108, 1993.
116. Kliegman RM: Models of the pathogenesis of necrotizing enterocolitis, *J Pediatr* 117:S2–5, 1990.
117. Koehntop DE, Rodman JH, Brundage DM, et al: Pharmacokinetics of fentanyl in neonates, *Anesth Analg* 65:227–232, 1986.
118. Kuhls E, Gauntlett IS, Lau M, et al: Effect of increased intra-abdominal pressure on hepatic extraction and clearance of fentanyl in neonatal lambs, *J Pharmacol Exp Ther* 274:115–119, 1995.
119. Kupferberg HJ, Way EL: Pharmacologic basis for the increased sensitivity of the newborn rat to morphine, *J Pharmacol Exp Ther* 141:105–109, 1963.
120. Langer JC, Filler RM, Bohn DJ, et al: Timing of surgery for congenital diaphragmatic hernia: is emergency operation necessary? *J Pediatr Surg* 23:731–734, 1988.
121. LeDez KM, Lerman J: The minimum alveolar concentration (MAC) of isoflurane in preterm neonates, *Anesthesiology* 67:301–307, 1987.
122. Lerman J, Berdock SE, Bissonnette B, et al: Succinylcholine warning, *Can J Anaesth* 41:165, 1994.
123. Lerman J, Gregory GA, Willis MM, Eger EI, II: Age and solubility of volatile anesthetics in blood, *Anesthesiology* 61:139–143, 1984.
124. Lerman J, Oyston JP, Gallagher TM, et al: The minimum alveolar concentration (MAC) and hemodynamic effects of halothane, isoflurane, and sevoflurane in newborn swine, *Anesthesiology* 73:717–721, 1990.
125. Lerman J, Robinson S, Willis MM, Gregory GA: Anesthetic requirements for halothane in young children 0-1 month and 1-6 months of age, *Anesthesiology* 59: 421–424, 1983.
126. Lerman J, Schmitt-Bantel BI, Gregory GA, et al: Effect of age on the solubility of volatile anesthetics in human tissues, *Anesthesiology* 65:307–311, 1986.
127. Lerman J, Strong HA, LeDez KM, et al: Effects of age on the serum concentration of alpha 1-acid glycoprotein and the binding of lidocaine in pediatric patients, *Clin Pharmacol Ther* 46:219–225, 1989.
128. Levy FH, O'Rourke PP, Crone RK: Extracorporeal membrane oxygenation, *Anesth Analg* 75:1053–1062, 1992.
129. Lindahl SG: Energy expenditure and fluid and electrolyte requirements in anesthetized infants and children, *Anesthesiology* 69:377–382, 1988.
130. Lonnqvist PA, Winberg P, Lundell B, et al: Inhaled nitric oxide in neonates and children with pulmonary hypertension, *Acta Paediatr* 83:1132–1136, 1994.
131. Lynn AM, McRorie TI, Slattery JT, et al: Pharmacokinetics and pharmacodynamics of morphine in infant monkeys, *Dev Pharmacol Ther* 16:41–47, 1991.
132. Lynn AM, McRorie TI, Slattery JT, et al: Age-dependent morphine partitioning between plasma and cerebrospinal fluid in monkeys, *Dev Pharmacol Ther* 17:200–204, 1991.
133. Lynn AM, Nespeca MK, Opheim KE, Slattery JT: Respiratory effects of IV morphine infusions in neonates, infants, and children after cardiac surgery, *Anesth Analg* 77:695–701, 1993.
134. Lynn AM, Slattery JT: Morphine pharmacokinetics in early infancy, *Anesthesiology* 66:136–139, 1987.
135. Malviya S, Lerman J: The blood/gas solubilities of sevoflurane, isoflurane, halothane, and serum constituent concentrations in neonates and adults, *Anesthesiology* 72:793–796, 1990.
136. Masey SA, Koehler RC, Buck JR, et al: Effect of abdominal distension on central and regional hemodynamics in neonatal lambs, *Pediatr Res* 19:1244–1249, 1985.
137. Maxwell LG, Martin LD, Yaster M: Bupivacaine-induced cardiac toxicity in neonates: successful treatment with IV phenytoin, *Anesthesiology* 80:682–686, 1994.
138. Maxwell LG, Yaster M, Wetzel RC, Niebyl JR: Penile nerve block for newborn circumcision, *Obstet Gynecol* 70:415–419, 1987.
139. Maze A, Bloch E: Stridor in pediatric patients, *Anesthesiology* 50:132–145, 1979.
140. McClain DA, Hug CC, Jr: Intravenous fentanyl kinetics, *Clin Pharmacol Ther* 28: 106–114, 1980.
141. McEvedy BA, McLeod ME, Mulera M, et al: End-tidal, transcutaneous, and arterial pCO2 measurements in critically ill neonates: a comparative study, *Anesthesiology* 69:112–116, 1988.
142. McMurphy DM, Heymann MA, Rudolph AM, Melmon KL: Developmental changes in constriction of the ductus arteriosus: responses to oxygen and vasoactive agents in the isolated ductus arteriosus of the fetal lamb, *Pediatr Res* 6:231–238, 1972.
143. Meistelman C, Benhamou D, Barre J, et al: Effects of age on plasma protein binding of sufentanil, *Anesthesiology* 72:470–473, 1990.
144. Meistelman C, Saint-Maurice C, Lepaul M, et al: A comparison of alfentanil pharmacokinetics in children and adults, *Anesthesiology* 66:13–16, 1987.
145. Meller JL, Reyes HM, Loeff DS: Gastroschisis and omphalocele, *Clin Perinatol* 16:113–122, 1989.
146. Merrill DC, McWeeny OJ, Segar JL, Robillard JE: Impairment of cardiopulmonary baroreflexes during the newborn period, *Am J Physiol* 268:H1343–1351, 1995.
147. Merrill DC, Segar JL, McWeeny OJ, et al: Cardiopulmonary and arterial baroreflex responses to acute volume expansion during fetal and postnatal development, *Am J Physiol* 267:H1467–1475, 1994.
148. Meyer RA, Campbell JN, Raja SN: Peripheral neural mechanisms of nociception. In Wall PD, Melzack R, editors: *Textbook of pain,* Edinburgh, 1994, Churchill Livingstone.
149. Millar C, Bissonnette B: Awake intubation increases intracranial pressure without affecting cerebral blood flow velocity in infants, *Can J Anaesth* 41:281–287, 1994.
150. Miller BR, Friesen RH: Oral atropine premedication in infants attenuates cardiovascular depression during halothane anesthesia, *Anesth Analg* 67:180–185, 1988.
151. Mollitt DL, Ballantine TV, Grosfeld JL, Quinter P: A critical assessment of fluid requirements in gastroschisis, *J Pediatr Surg* 13:217–219, 1978.
152. Montgomery CJ, Steward DJ: A comparative evaluation of intubating doses of atracurium, d-tubocurarine, pancuronium and vecuronium in children, *Can J Anaesth* 35:36–40, 1988.
153. Motoyama EK, Glazener CH: Hypoxemia after general anesthesia in children, *Anesth Analg* 65:267–272, 1986.
154. Nakayama DK, Motoyama EK, Evans R, Hannakan C: Relation between arterial hypoxemia and plasma eicosanoids in neonates with congenital diaphragmatic hernia, *J Surg Res* 53:615–620, 1992.
155. Nakayama DK, Mutich R, Motoyama EK: Pulmonary dysfunction in surgical conditions of the newborn infant, *Crit Care Med* 19:926–933, 1991.
156. Nancarrow C, Rutten AJ, Runciman WB, et al: Myocardial and cerebral drug concentrations and the mechanisms of death after fatal IV doses of lidocaine, bupivacaine, and ropivacaine in the sheep, *Anesth Analg* 69:276–283, 1989.
157. Neu J: Necrotizing enterocolitis: the search for a unifying pathogenic theory leading to prevention, *Pediatr Clin North Am* 43:409–432, 1996.
158. Noetzel MJ: Myelomeningocele: current concepts of management, *Clin Perinatol* 16:311–329, 1989.
159. O'Rourke PP, Crone RK, Vacanti JP, et al: Extracorporeal membrane oxygenation and conventional medical therapy in neonates with persistent pulmonary hypertension of the newborn: a prospective randomized study, *Pediatrics* 84:957–963, 1989.
160. O'Rourke PP, Lillehei CW, Crone RK, Vacanti JP: The effect of extracorporeal membrane oxygenation on the survival of neonates with high-risk congenital diaphragmatic hernia: 45 cases from a single institution, *J Pediatr Surg* 26:147–152, 1991.
161. Oberhansli-Weiss I, Heymann MA, Rudolph AM, Melmon KL: The pattern and mechanisms of response to oxygen by the ductus arteriosus and umbilical artery, *Pediatr Res* 6:693–700, 1972.
162. Oldham KT, Coran AG, Drongowski RA, et al: The development of necrotizing enterocolitis following repair of gastroschisis: a surprisingly high incidence, *J Pediatr Surg* 23:945–949, 1988.
163. Oren J, Kelly DH, Todres ID, Shannon DC: Respiratory complications in patients with myelodysplasia and Arnold- Chiari malformation, *Am J Dis Child* 140:221–224, 1986.
164. Owens ME: Pain in infancy: conceptual and methodological issues, *Pain* 20:213–230, 1984.
165. Pang LM, Mellins RB: Neonatal cardiorespiratory physiology, *Anesthesiology* 43: 171–196, 1975.

166. Pasternak GW, Wood PJ: Multiple mu opiate receptors, *Life Sci* 38:1889–1898, 1986.
167. Pasternak GW, Zhang A, Tecott L: Developmental differences between high and low affinity opiate binding sites: their relationship to analgesia and respiratory depression, *Life Sci* 27:1185–1190, 1980.
168. Poenaru D, Laberge JM, Neilson IR, Guttman FM: A new prognostic classification for esophageal atresia, *Surgery* 113: 426-432, 1993.
169. Pokela ML, Koivisto M: Physiological changes, plasma beta-endorphin and cortisol responses to tracheal intubation in neonates, *Acta Paediatr* 83:151–156, 1994.
170. Pransky SM: Evaluation of the compromised neonatal airway, *Pediatr Clin North Am* 36:1571–1582, 1989.
171. Pransky SM, Grundfast KM: Differentiating upper from lower airway compromise in neonates, *Ann Otol Rhinol Laryngol* 94:509–515, 1985.
172. Quasha AL, Eger EI, II, Tinker JH: Determination and applications of MAC, *Anesthesiology* 53:315–334, 1980.
173. Rekate HL: To shunt or not to shunt: hydrocephalus and dysraphism, *Clin Neurosurg* 32:593–607, 1985.
174. Rescorla FJ: Surgical management of pediatric necrotizing enterocolitis, *Curr Opin Pediatr* 7:335–341, 1995.
175. Reyes HM, Meller JL, Loeff D: Neonatal intestinal obstruction, *Clin Perinatol* 16: 85–96, 1989.
176. Reyes HM, Meller JL, Loeff D: Management of esophageal atresia and tracheoesophageal fistula, *Clin Perinatol* 16:79–84, 1989.
177. Reyes HM, Wright JK: Primary closure of gastroschisis. Evaluation of results and technique, *Surg Ann* 11:85–97, 1979.
178. Reynolds LM, Nicolson SC, Steven JM, et al: Influence of sensor site location on pulse oximetry kinetics in children, *Anesth Analg* 76:751–754, 1993.
179. Rice HE, Adzick NS: Prenatal diagnosis: essentials for the pediatric surgeon, *Semin Pediatr Surg* 2:84–91, 1993.
180. Richardson MA, Cotton RT: Anatomic abnormalities of the pediatric airway, *Pediatr Clin North Am* 31:821–834, 1984.
181. Richardson MA, Osguthorpe JD: Surgical management of choanal atresia, *Laryngoscope* 98:915–918, 1988.
182. Ricketts RR: Surgical treatment of necrotizing enterocolitis and the short bowel syndrome, *Clin Perinatol* 21:365–387, 1994.
183. Robinson S, Gregory GA: Fentanyl-air-oxygen anesthesia for ligation of patent ductus arteriosus in preterm infants, *Anesth Analg* 60:331–334, 1981.
184. Rockcress BD: Hematology. In Barone MA, editor: *The Harriet Lane handbook*, St. Louis 1996, Mosby–Year Book.
185. Rosen KR, Rosen DA: Caudal epidural morphine for control of pain following open heart surgery in children, *Anesthesiology* 70:418–421, 1989.
186. Rowe MI, Reblock KK, Kurkchubasche AG, Healey PJ: Necrotizing enterocolitis in the extremely low birth weight infant, *J Pediatr Surg* 29:987–990, 1994.
187. Rowe MI, Taylor M: Transepidermal water loss in the infant surgical patient, *J Pediatr Surg* 16:878–881, 1981.
188. Rowe MI, Taylor M, Sheehan K: Prevention of water and heat losses from the exposed intestine, *J Pediatr Surg* 17:608–610, 1982.
189. Rudolph AM, Heymann MA: The fetal circulation, *Ann Rev Med* 19:195–206, 1968.
190. Rutten AJ, Nancarrow C, Mather LE, et al: Hemodynamic and central nervous system effects of IV bolus doses of lidocaine, bupivacaine, and ropivacaine in sheep, *Anesth Analg* 69:291–299, 1989.
191. Schieber RA, Stiller RL, Cook DR: Cardiovascular and pharmacodynamic effects of high-dose fentanyl in newborn piglets, *Anesthesiology* 63:166–171, 1985.
192. Schreiber MD, Heymann MA, Soifer SJ: Increased arterial pH, not decreased PaCO2, attenuates hypoxia-induced pulmonary vasoconstriction in newborn lambs, *Pediatr Res* 20:113–117, 1986.
193. Schwartz MZ, Tyson KR, Milliorn K, Lobe TE: Staged reduction using a Silastic sac is the treatment of choice for large congenital abdominal wall defects, *J Pediatr Surg* 18: 713–719, 1983.
194. Segar JL, Hajduczok G, Smith BA, et al: Ontogeny of baroreflex control of renal sympathetic nerve activity and heart rate, *Am J Physiol* 263:H1819–826, 1992.
195. Sessler DI: Temperature regulation. In Gregory GA, editor: *Pediatric anesthesia*, New York 1994, Churchill Livingstone.
196. Shaul DB, Schwartz MZ, Marr CC, Tyson KR: Primary repair without routine gastrostomy is the treatment of choice for neonates with esophageal atresia and tracheoesophageal fistula, *Arch Surg* 124: 1188–1190, 1989.
197. Shaul PW: Nitric oxide in the developing lung, *Adv Pediatr* 42:367–414, 1995.
198. Shorten GD, Bissonnette B, Hartley E, et al: It is not necessary to administer more than 10 micrograms.kg-1 of atropine to older children before succinylcholine. *Can J Anaesth* 42:8–11, 1995.
199. Sigalet DL, Tierney A, Adolph V, et al: Timing of repair of congenital diaphragmatic hernia requiring extracorporeal membrane oxygenation support, *J Pediatr Surg* 30:1183–1187, 1995.
200. Singleton MA, Rosen JI, Fisher DM: Plasma concentrations of fentanyl in infants, children and adults, *Can J Anaesth* 34:152–155, 1987.
201. Smith DW: *Recognizable patterns of human malformation*, Philadelphia, 1982, WB Saunders.
202. Soliman IE, Patel RI, Ehrenpreis MB, Hannallah RS: Recovery scores do not correlate with postoperative hypoxemia in children, *Anesth Analg* 67:53–56, 1988.
203. Spear RM, Deshpande JK, Maxwell LG: Caudal anesthesia in the awake, high-risk infant, *Anesthesiology* 69:407–409, 1988.
204. Srikanth MS, Ford EG, Stanley P, Mahour GH: Communicating bronchopulmonary foregut malformations: classification and embryogenesis, *J Pediatr Surg* 27:732–736, 1992.
205. Steward DJ: Anticholinergic premedication for infants and children, *Can Anaesth Soc J* 30:325–328, 1983.
206. Stockman JA, III: Anemia of prematurity. Current concepts in the issue of when to transfuse, *Pediatr Clin North Am* 33: 111–128, 1986.
207. Stockman JA, III, Graeber JE, Clark DA, et al: Anemia of prematurity: determinants of the erythropoietin response, *J Pediatr* 105: 786–792, 1984.
208. Stoelting RK, Eger EI, II: The effects of ventilation and anesthetic solubility on recovery from anesthesia: an *in vivo* and analog analysis before and after equilibrium, *Anesthesiology* 30:290–296, 1969.
209. Strafford MA: Cardiovascular physiology. In Motoyama EK, Davis PJ, editors: *Smith's anesthesia for infants and children*, St. Louis 1996, Mosby–Year Book.
210. Stringel G, Filler RM: Prognostic factors in omphalocele and gastroschisis, *J Pediatr Surg* 14:515–519, 1979.
211. Taylor RH, Lerman J: Minimum alveolar concentration of desflurane and hemodynamic responses in neonates, infants, and children, *Anesthesiology* 75:975–979, 1991.
212. Tepas JJ, III, Mollitt DL, String DL, Pieper P: Error in fluid and calorie calculation in the surgical neonate, *J Pediatr Surg* 26: 132–134, 1991.
213. Tobias JD, Oakes L, Rao B: Continuous epidural anesthesia for postoperative analgesia in the pediatric oncology patient, *Am J Pediatr Hematol Oncol* 14:216–221, 1992.
214. Truog RD, Schena JA, Hershenson MB, et al: Repair of congenital diaphragmatic hernia during extracorporeal membrane oxygenation, *Anesthesiology* 72:750–753, 1990.
215. Tyler IL, Tantisira B, Winter PM, Motoyama EK: Continuous monitoring of arterial oxygen saturation with pulse oximetry during transfer to the recovery room, *Anesth Analg* 64:1108–1112, 1985.
216. Vacanti JP, Crone RK, Murphy JD, ed al: The pulmonary hemodynamic response to perioperative anesthesia in the treatment of high-risk infants with congenital diaphragmatic hernia, *J Pediatr Surg* 19:672–679, 1984.
217. Viscomi CM, Abajian JC, Wald SL, et al: Spinal anesthesia for repair of meningomyelocele in neonates, *Anesth Analg* 81:492–495, 1995.
218. Volpe JJ: Intraventricular hemorrhage and brain injury in the premature infant, Diagnosis, prognosis, and prevention, *Clin Perinatol* 16:387–411, 1989.
219. Volpe JJ: Intraventricular hemorrhage in the premature infant—current concepts. Part II, *Ann Neurol* 25:109–116, 1989.
220. Wallgren G, Hanson JS, Lind J: Quantitative studies of the human neonatal circulation. 3. Observations on the newborn infants central circulatory responses to moderate hypovolemia, *Acta Paediatr Scand* Suppl 179:45, 1967.
221. Wallgren G, Lind J: Quantitative studies of the human neonatal circulation. IV. Observations on the newborn infants peripheral circulation and plasma expansion during moderate hypovolemia, *Acta Paediatr Scand* Suppl 179:57, 1967.
222. Way WL, Costley EC, Way EL: Respiratory senstivity of the newborn infant to meperidine and morphine (abstract). *Clin Pharmacol Ther* 6:454–461, 1965.
223. Wear R, Robinson S, Gregory GA: The effect of halothane on the baroresponse of

adult and baby rabbits, *Anesthesiology* 56:188–191, 1982.

224. Wesley JR, Drongowski R, Coran AG: Intragastric pressure measurement: a guide for reduction and closure of the silastic chimney in omphalocele and gastroschisis, *J Pediatr Surg* 16:264-270, 1981.
225. Williamson PS, Evans ND: Neonatal cortisol response to circumcision with anesthesia, *Clin Pediatr* 25:412–415, 1986.
226. Wilson JM, Lund DP, Lillehei CW, et al: Delayed repair and preoperative ECMO does not improve survival in high-risk congenital diaphragmatic hernia, *J Pediatr Surg* 27:368–372, 1992.
227. Wilson PR, Lamer TJ: *Pain mechanisms: Anatomy and physiology.* In Raj PP, editor: *Practical management of pain,* St. Louis, 1992, Mosby–Year Book.
228. Woolf CJ: The dorsal horn: state-dependent sensory processing and the generation of pain. In Wall PD, Melzack R, editors: *Textbook of pain,* Edinburgh, 1994, Churchill Livingstone.
229. Yaster M: The dose response of fentanyl in neonatal anesthesia, *Anesthesiology* 66: 433–435, 1987.
230. Yaster M: Analgesia and anesthesia in neonates, *J Pediatr* 111:394–396, 1987.
231. Yaster M, Buck JR, Dudgeon DL, et al: Hemodynamic effects of primary closure of omphalocele/gastroschisis in human newborns, *Anesthesiology* 69:84–88, 1988.
232. Yaster M, Koehler RC, Traystman RJ: Effects of fentanyl on peripheral and cerebral hemodynamics in neonatal lambs, *Anesthesiology* 66:524–530, 1987.
233. Yaster M, Koehler RC, Traystman RJ: Interaction of fentanyl and pentobarbital on peripheral and cerebral hemodynamics in newborn lambs, *Anesthesiology* 70:461–469, 1989.
234. Yaster M, Koehler RC, Traystman RJ: Interaction of fentanyl and nitrous oxide on peripheral and cerebral hemodynamics in newborn lambs, *Anesthesiology* 80:364–371, 1994.
235. Yaster M, Kost-Byerly S, Lenox WC, et al: Continuous lidocaine epidural analgesia in postoperative neonates, *Anesthesiology* 1997; in press.
236. Yaster M, Maxwell LG: Pediatric regional anesthesia, *Anesthesiology* 70:324–338, 1989.
237. Yaster M, Maxwell LG: Airway management. In Nichols DG, Yaster M, Lappe DG, Haller JAJ, editors: *Golden hour: The handbook of advanced pediatric life support,* St. Louis, 1996, Mosby–Year Book.
238. Yaster M, Scherer TL, Stone MM, et al: Prediction of successful primary closure of congenital abdominal wall defects using intraoperative measurements, *J Pediatr Surg* 24:1217–1220, 1989.
239. Yaster M, Tobin JR, Billett C, et al: Epidural analgesia in the management of severe vaso-occlusive sickle cell crisis, *Pediatrics* 93:310–315, 1994.
240. Yaster M, Tobin JR, Fisher QA, Maxwell LG: Local anesthetics in the management of acute pain in children, *J Pediatr* 124:165–176, 1994.
241. Zapol WM, Rimar S, Gillis N, et al: Nitric oxide and the lung, *Am J Respir Crit Care Med* 149:1375–1380, 1994.
242. Zhang AZ, Pasternak GW: Ontogeny of opioid pharmacology and receptors: high and low affinity site differences, *Eur J Pharmacol* 73:29–40, 1981.
243. Ziegler JW, Ivy DD, Kinsella JP, Abman SH: The role of nitric oxide, endothelin, and prostaglandins in the transition of the pulmonary circulation, *Clin Perinatol* 22: 387–403, 1995.
244. Zimmerman G, Steward DJ: Bradycardia delays the onset of action of IV atropine in infants, *Anesthesiology* 65:320–322, 1986.

CHAPTER 79

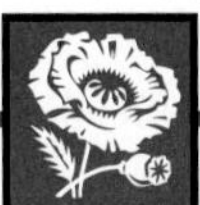

Anesthesia for Children

RANDALL C. WETZEL
LYNNE G. MAXWELL

The intraoperative management of children depends on a thorough understanding of their physiologic and psychologic needs, as detailed in Chapter 25. In addition, familiarity with techniques and equipment specifically designed to provide anesthesia in children is essential. A third critical area is a thorough knowledge of how developmental changes alter the pharmacology of drugs used during anesthesia for children. Meticulous attention to thermoregulation, monitoring, and fluid management is essential to the anesthetic management of children. Finally, specific knowledge regarding pediatric surgical procedures is necessary.

EQUIPMENT

Pediatric Breathing Circuits

To understand pediatric breathing circuits, one should review their developmental history. Mask anesthesia and open anesthetics were used frequently in the early years of anesthesia; however, the development of increasingly complex procedures and the addition of endotracheal (ET) intubation led to several modifications. Understanding how and why these modifications occurred and their effects facilitate the physician's understanding of modern pediatric breathing circuits. One procedure that significantly impacted the development of pediatric circuits was cleft palate repair.

In 1937, Philip Ayre[5] introduced the T-piece technique. This provided flow-by fresh gas to the ET tube and a low dead-space, simple, lightweight, low-resistance, safe system for infants and small children. Ayre noted that the addition of reservoir tubing to the expiratory limb of the T-piece decreased some of the variability in depth of anesthesia by allowing rebreathing of the anesthetic vapor. Rebreathing was proportionate to gas flow and the length of the reservoir tubing. Jackson Rees,[135] working at the Alder Hey Children's

Hospital in Liverpool, England, modified the Ayre's T-piece by adding an open-ended reservoir bag to the expiratory limb (Fig. 79-1). Rees' modification of Ayre's T-piece in 1950 made the length of the expiratory limb irrelevant and allowed the anesthesiologist to provide assisted and controlled ventilation by controlling gas flow out of the reservoir bag and by pressurizing the expiratory limb. Since then, there have been many modifications. These modifications basically consist of adding an expiratory pressure release valve (PRV), varying the volume of the expiratory limb, and changing the site of fresh gas inflow into the circuit. In 1954, Mapleson[101] classified these various arrangements into the Mapleson system of breathing circuits from A to F (Fig. 79-1).

The relative positioning of the expiratory limb, fresh gas flow, reservoir bag, and PRV determines the functional characteristics of each Mapleson circuit. The only fully open circuit is the Ayre's T-piece, where no rebreathing of anesthetic vapor occurs. As soon as an expiratory limb (which provides a reservoir) is added, some degree of rebreathing of expired gas occurs, and the circuit is semiclosed. Whenever the patient's inspiratory flow exceeds that provided by the fresh gas flow, gas is inspired (rebreathed) from the reservoir limb. Understanding these points is essential to the understanding of circuit performance during spontaneous and controlled ventilation for each type of circuit. The advantage of the semiclosed circuits compared with the circle system is that valves and CO_2 rebreathing canisters are eliminated, thus giving minimal resistance to inspiration and not increasing the child's work of breathing. The potential disadvantage is that, to some degree, rebreathing occurs in all these circuits. Rebreathing, however, is not necessarily undesirable. Some degree of rebreathing from the expiratory limb allows conservation of heat, humidification, and anesthetic vapor. In addition, this tends to smooth out anesthetic depth by decreasing the variability of inspired anesthetic concentration. **The major factor that determines the degree of rebreathing, and thus arterial CO_2 tension ($Paco_2$), is the fresh gas flow. The other factor that determines rebreathing in these circuits is whether the patient is breathing spontaneously or is mechanically ventilated.** A brief analysis for each breathing system follows.

The Mapleson A system is the only circuit that has the

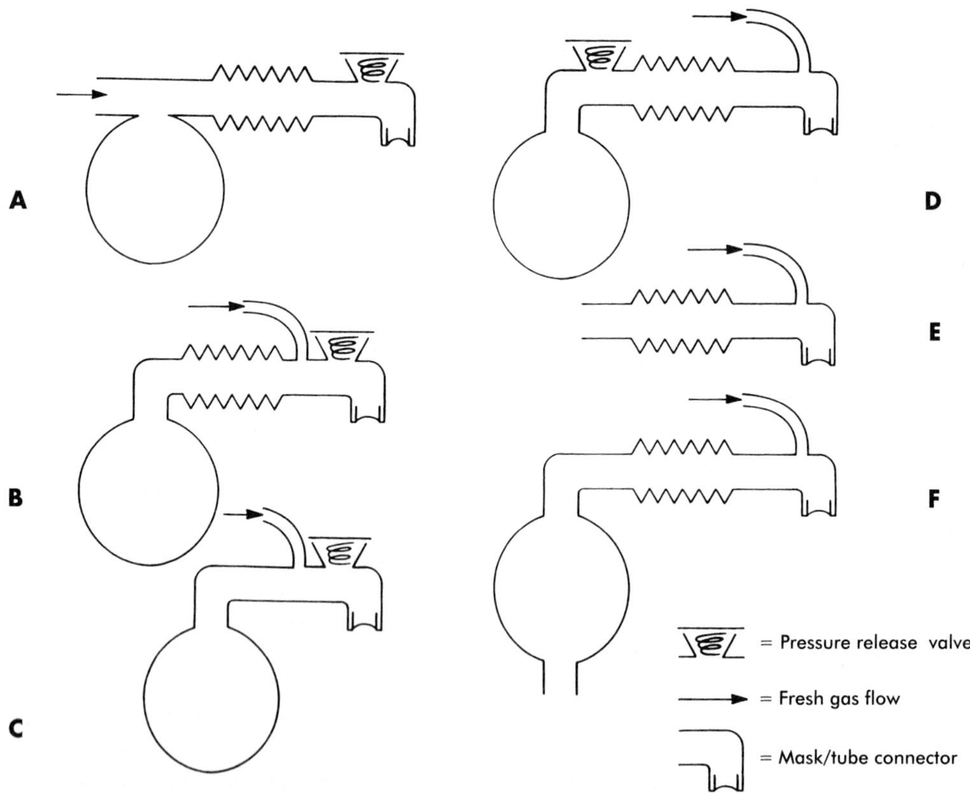

Fig. 79-1. A–F, Mapleson classification of pediatric breathing circuits. **D,** Bain. **E,** Ayre's T-piece. **F,** Jackson Rees. Configuration of fresh gas flow, patient connector, reservoir bag, and pressure release valve (PRV) determines this classification. Specific attention should focus on placement of PRV and fresh gas flow, because these factors most significantly affect these circuits' characteristics.

fresh gas flow located distally near the reservoir bag in the expiratory limb. The pressure PRV is near the patient. This circuit provides the least amount of rebreathing during spontaneous ventilation (i.e. it is the most efficient). In effect, the expiratory and inspiratory limbs are the same. Rebreathing depends on the resistance in the PRV. During spontaneous inspiration with the PRV fully open, fresh gas flows into the patient. During expiration, expired gas flows out of the PRV, whereas all of the reservoir gas is fresh. This situation is dramatically reversed during mechanical ventilation. When the PRV is closed to allow positive pressure in the system, fresh gas flows toward the patient with compression of the reservoir bag. During expiration, expiratory gas fills the reservoir limb. During the next positive-pressure breath, expired gas is pushed toward the patient. To prevent rebreathing and respiratory acidosis with this circuit, very large fresh gas flows are required and the PRV must be partially open. Another disadvantage is that the PRV is near the patient, away from the anesthesiologist, and therefore is difficult to access. Scavenging of expired vapors from the PRV is also difficult. This circuit, although appropriate for spontaneous breathing during induction, is of little value in today's operating rooms.

In the Mapleson B circuit, the fresh gas flow is proximal to the patient. The expiratory and reservoir limbs are not the source of fresh gas flow as in the A circuit. The PRV is also close to the patient. The B circuit's bulky arrangement near the ET tube makes securing the endotracheal tube difficult, and may contribute to its dislodgement. In addition, the B circuit is less efficient during spontaneous ventilation than the Mapleson A circuit, but still allows significant rebreathing during controlled positive-pressure ventilation. The B circuit is infrequently used.

The Mapleson C circuit has a very short expiratory limb with a reservoir bag. Because of its size, this is the basic design for resuscitator bags used for transporting patients. Rebreathing during controlled ventilation is considerably less than with a Mapleson A circuit because of the short expiratory limb. The C circuit has little application for providing anesthesia in the operating room because the anesthesiologist must be quite close to the patient.

In the Mapleson D system, the fresh gas flow is near the ET tube or mask connector, and the PRV is distally located on the expiratory limb. This is quite similar to the Rees modification of the Ayre T piece, and considerations for both circuits are the same. During spontaneous breathing, the fresh gas flow is directed toward the patient, and any overflow passes along the expiratory limb. During expiration, expired gas is directed down the expiratory limb toward the PRV and is diluted by fresh gas inflow. If fresh gas flow is sufficiently high to completely fill the expiratory limb with fresh gas, or when the fresh gas volume in the expiratory limb equals or exceeds the tidal volume, no rebreathing of expired gas can occur during inspiration. During controlled ventilation, the expiratory limb is pressurized by occlusion. Fresh gas and some expiratory gas flow toward the patient. The greater the fresh gas flow, the less rebreathing occurs. Thus one can see that the patient's $Paco_2$ during controlled positive-pressure ventilation depends mainly on the fresh gas flow. **During spontaneous breathing, the Mapleson D circuit requires higher fresh gas flow than the Mapleson A circuit to ensure no rebreathing; however, this is the most efficient circuit for CO_2 clearance during positive-pressure ventilation.**

A Mapleson D circuit becomes a Bain circuit if the fresh gas flow is made coaxial in the expiratory limb.[1] Although these flows are still entirely functionally separated from each other (compared with Mapleson A), they now physically occupy the same space, thus allowing a more convenient circuit, which has achieved some popularity in adult applications. An internal disconnection of the fresh gas conduit, which may be difficult to detect, would convert the system to a Mapleson A circuit and lead to marked rebreathing. This has tended to decrease the popularity of these coaxial systems in the United States.

The patient's respiratory pattern, whether controlled or spontaneous, has a significant impact on the composition of gas in the expiratory limb. The important factors are respiratory rate, patient peak inspiratory flow rate, and tidal volume. Nevertheless, the circuit's fresh gas flow is the most critical determinant of rebreathing. In general, when the average minute ventilation is 100 ml/kg, an adequate fresh gas flow in a Mapleson D circuit is 250 ml/kg to ensure adequate CO_2 clearance. If more CO_2 clearance is required, flows can be increased. It is generally recommended to maintain flow through a Mapleson D circuit at no less than 3 l/min, regardless of the child's age and weight. The length of expiratory limb in the Mapleson D circuit is irrelevant, whether it is 2 or 20 feet long. The degree of CO_2 rebreathing still depends on fresh gas flow, because this flow washes out the proximal segment of the expiratory limb and decreases the amount of expired gas and CO_2 rebreathed by the patient. For example, if the fresh gas flow is 6 l/min (100 ml/sec) and if expiration has ceased for 1 second and the tidal volume is less than 100 ml, the patient will entrain no CO_2 during controlled ventilation. During spontaneous ventilation a similar situation occurs, but fresh gas flow can be even lower, because the reservoir effect of the expiratory limb is decreased by the effect of continuous fresh gas flow during a spontaneous inspiration.

The Ayre T piece and subsequent modifications were designed primarily to allow children, especially young infants, to breathe spontaneously with little resistance. The tremendous advantage that these systems provide in spontaneously breathing children is lost when the child is paralyzed and ventilation is controlled. In addition, the use of newer, low-resistance valves with high gas flows generally facilitates children's ease of breathing, even through adult circle systems.

The major practical advantages of the Mapleson sys-

tems are that they are lightweight, easy to use, generally take up less space than the standard circle systems, and provide warming and humidification of the inspired gas.

Circle Systems

Circle systems are standard anesthesia equipment in the United States. Most modern circle systems, with large respiratory tubing and lightweight unidirectional valve systems, with sufficiently high fresh gas flows, are adequate for children weighing more than 10 kg. More cautious monitoring is necessary with the use of adult circle systems in children than in adults for two reasons:

- The impact of sticky or jammed unidirectional valves is much greater because a child is less able to overcome their resistance. Because of the large ratio of circuit volume-to-tidal volume, the effect of a floating unidirectional valve on the degree of CO_2 rebreathing is significant.
- The compressible volume in these circuits may be close to or even greater than the child's tidal volume, thus making the adjustment of mechanical ventilation difficult.

These problems usually can be detected easily by using capnometry during anesthesia.

Specifically designed pediatric circle systems come in many forms. Modification of fresh gas flow, as in the Ohio circuit, or variation in the location and size of the CO_2 canister are two modifications available. Neither of these modifications is widely used, however, because they require significant changes in the current adult anesthesia configuration. Other alternatives are to decrease the circuit volumes by using smaller pediatric respiratory tubing and small-volume CO_2 rebreathing canisters. These provide some potential benefit; however, the difficulty of using unidirectional valves in any pediatric circuit must always be considered in children less than 10 kg, if they are to breathe spontaneously. The use of low-volume circuits with decreased compressible volume during mechanical ventilation does not eliminate these problems.

Masks

For all anesthetic circuits, fresh gas flow or circle flow should be as close to the patient's airway as possible to decrease the amount of dead space. Therefore, pediatric masks have been designed to have low intrinsic volume and rapid washout. The Rendall-Baker-Soucek masks have time-honored use, good configuration to children's faces, and low volumes. Many modifications in mask design have been used in an attempt to entice the child to willingly accept the anesthetic mask. Clear, soft-plastic masks apparently are more acceptable to children than hard, black rubber masks. Thus, the development of newer masks (Fig. 79-2) has ensured more comfort and acceptability by children. A pneumatic perimeter cuff allows a more reliable seal and fit to a wider variety of facial contours. In addition, the clear mask allows the anesthesiologist to determine lip color and observe for secretions and vomitus. It is also reassuring to see condensation

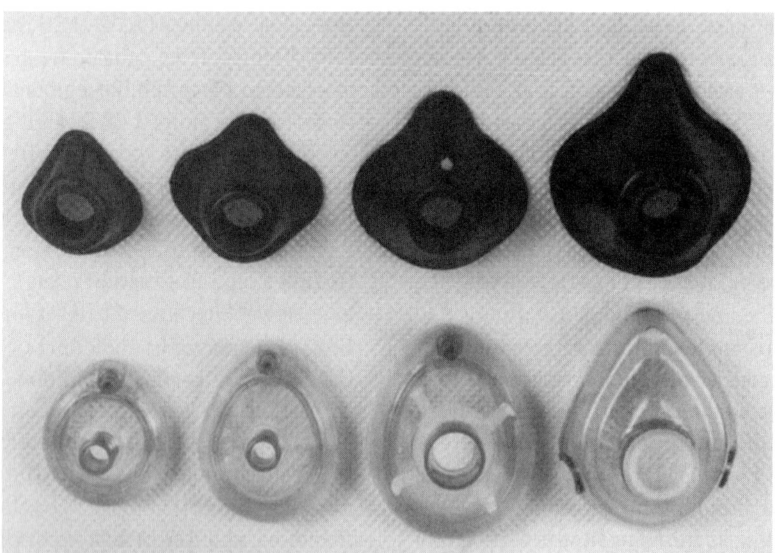

Fig. 79-2. Pediatric anesthesia masks. *Top,* Rendall-Baker-Soucek masks. The pliable outer rim and low intrinsic volume make these ideal for pediatric patients. These masks also come in clear plastic, which is frequently less threatening to infants and children. *Bottom,* Newer design of clear plastic mask, with inflatable or pliable rims to ensure a good seal with children's faces. These clear masks allow anesthesiologists to evaluate patient's airway, check for secretions and vomitus, see fogging of mask, and observe the color of patient's lips.

demonstrating unobstructed breathing. The extra cost of these masks may be justified by these advantages.

Airways

Oral airways come in a variety of sizes appropriate for the smallest premature infant (Fig. 79-3). The purpose of an oral airway is to elevate the tongue from the posterior pharyngeal wall and ensure a patent pharyngeal airway. The use of an overly large airway must be assiduously avoided because placement of the distal end of the airway in the vallecula with posteroinferior dislocation of the epiglottis may lead to airway obstruction. In addition, airway placement down the esophagus with anterior displacement can also cause airway obstruction and increase the resistance to inspiration. The best way to determine the appropriate size for a child is to externally place the airway on the child's face. With the flange at the lips, the distal end of the airway should reach the angle of the mandible. Not only large airways may cause difficulty; small airways also may lead to obstruction by pushing the tongue further back.

Nasal airways also come in various sizes. The anesthesiologist should remember that the purpose of the nasal airway is the same as that of an oral airway—to maintain a patent pharyngeal airway. Therefore, nasal airways should be sufficiently long to ensure this. Again, external examination is suggested: With the flange at the nares, the distal end should reach to the angle of the mandible.

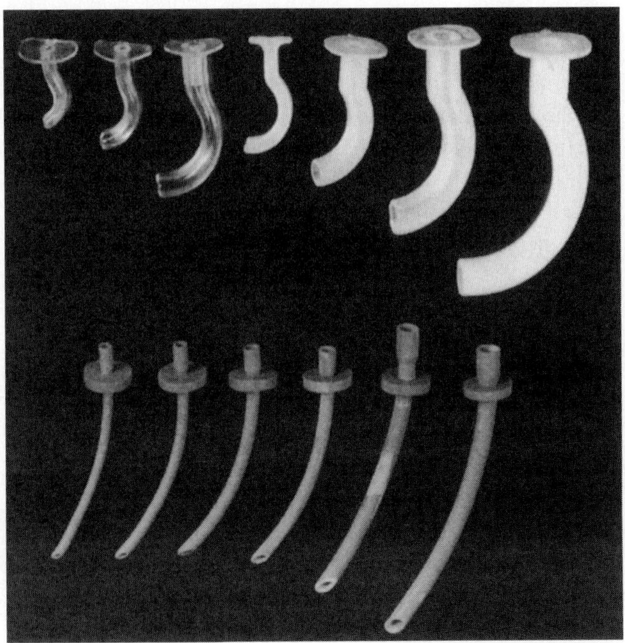

Fig. 79-3. Pediatric oral and nasal airways. *Top,* Oral airways are 000, 00, 0, 40, 50, 70, and 90 mm in length (left to right). *Bottom,* Nasal airways of Rusch type. Movable ring allows depth adjustment so that distal end of nasal airway can be placed in the appropriate location.

Endotracheal Intubation

In the past 30 years, great advances have been made in medical understanding of the requirements of pediatric ET tubes. The composition and design of ET tubes have become largely uniform. The former use of tapered tubes (Cole) made of red rubber or of tubes with high-pressure cuffs, inserted into children with little understanding of laryngeal size and anatomy, led to a high incidence of subglottic stenosis and postoperative laryngeal complications. Several factors are now recognized as important in the skeleton of ET tubes.[21,87]

Most ET tubes today are made of polyvinylchloride, although silastic ET tubes are also becoming more popular. All are implant tested to ensure low irritability to the tracheal mucosa, which only refers to their chemical composition. The tube also should be nontapering and have a uniform external diameter. Ideally, one should be able to tell the size, design, and depth of insertion of the ET tube when it is in place. The only major drawback of PVC tubes is that they are flammable and thus, not indicated for use in laser surgery unless they are suitably wrapped with reflective tape. Another approach is to use graphite-impregnated tubes (Xomed) with decreased flammability. Red rubber tubes are less flammable; however, they should still be wrapped with reflective tape. They may have a high-pressure cuff, which should not be inflated.

The selection of cuffed or uncuffed tubes is also impacted by history. When high-pressure cuffs were used, a high incidence of tracheal injury occurred in small children. This led to the recommendation that cuffed tubes should not be used at all in young children. With new low-pressure, high-compliance cuffs, this is a less stringent requirement; if ventilation and airway protection cannot otherwise be ensured, a cuffed tube may be indicated in even small children. However, for routine anesthesia, the general practice is to use an uncuffed tube in children under 8 years of age. The reason is that a larger internal diameter is possible with uncuffed tubes, with less impingement on the tracheal mucosa.

The selection of ET tube size (i.e., internal diameter) depends on many factors. For airway management, a large ET tube that allows access for suctioning airway secretions to decrease the likelihood of tube obstruction is optimal. In addition, because resistance is inversely proportional to the fourth power of the radius, a larger tube is desirable for airway control. The overwhelming consideration, however, is the potential for tracheal injury.[11] **One must remember that an ET tube may readily pass through the cords but still impinge on the narrowest part of the child's airway—the subglottic area at the cricoid ring. Tracheal injury occurs most frequently at this site.**[76] Many factors are involved.[153] Mucosal injury occurs with any ET tube, generally within minutes of being placed. Ischemia appears to be an aggravating factor, and if lateral pressure from the ET tube excludes capillary flow in the submucosal area, serious injury can be expected.

Thus ensuring the presence of an adequate air leak

around the ET tube clearly is a crucial factor in ET tube maintenance.[11,46,163] The air leak test around an ET tube is performed by slowly increasing airway pressure while noting the airway pressure at which an audible leak begins between the ET tube and the glottis. The safe range is generally considered to be 10 to 30 cm H_2O. The ideal range is 15 to 20 cm H_2O airway pressure. The anesthesiologist should clearly understand that if a tube has a leak at 10 cm H_2O, it may be difficult to ventilate a patient who requires 20 cm H_2O for adequate lung inflation and atelectasis may result. Thus, a higher leak pressure may be desirable in patients who have decreased lung compliance, such as those who may be in the prone position during surgery. In children who are breathing spontaneously, the leak level is only relevant as an indicator of appropriate tube fit. Because laryngeal size varies greatly, following every intubation, a leak test should be routinely performed. If the tube is to be left in for a prolonged time (hours), changing the tube with no leak at 30 cm H_2O is good practice because the incidence of trauma with reintubation is probably less than with prolonged ischemia to the subglottic region.

Other factors also play a role in the etiology of permanent tracheal injury and subglottic stenosis including: infection, hemodynamic instability, patient movement, seizure activity, the piston movement of the tube caused by the ventilator, and the difficulty and frequency of reintubation.[79,129,153,160,165] The anesthesiologist should distinguish between placing an ET tube for elective surgery in healthy patients with normal lungs and in those who have decreased lung compliance or increased secretions, or those who will require prolonged intubation in a pediatric intensive care unit. Ideally, an adequate leak will be provided around a tube that is large enough to minimize airway resistance and allow suctioning and removal of secretions. Compulsive respiratory therapy should minimize postextubation complications. In the operating room, where the patient may have controlled ventilation throughout surgery and secretions are not a problem, anesthesiologists tend to choose smaller tubes, thus decreasing the incidence of airway injury. Balancing the potential risks and benefits requires that the appropriate-sized ET tube be assessed for each individual child's needs.

Because children's anatomy varies greatly, formulas and tabulated recommendations for determining tube size only serve as guidelines. A cursory look at the literature demonstrates the wide variability in recommended tube sizes. These recommendations are not as important as selecting the appropriate tube for the individual patient. A recommended tube with no leak is too large, regardless of the recommendation, just as a recommended tube with a leak at 2 cm H_2O airway pressure is too small. It is advisable to post guidelines in areas where children are anesthetized to provide suggestions for appropriate ET tube size.

Two suggested practical guidelines for determining the appropriate-sized ET tube in children are: (1) comparing the external ET tube diameter to the width of the child's fifth finger at the distal interphalangeal joint; and (2) comparing the diameter of the nares. Neither of these methods has been rigorously evaluated, but they are frequently used. A tube should pass easily into the child's trachea. Whenever a child is intubated in the operating room, appropriate-sized suction catheters must be available. Tube sizes are generally stated in internal diameter and suction catheters in French size. Table 79-1 shows appropriate suction catheters for corresponding ET tubes.

Table 79-1 Sizes of endotracheal tubes and suction catheters suggested for infants and children

Age	Internal tube diameter (mm)	Tube length (oral)* (mm)	Suction catheter (French)
Premature	2.5–3.0	8–9	6
0–6 mo	3.0–3.5	10–11	6
6–12 mo	3.5–4.0	12	8
1–2 yr	4.0	13	8
2–4 yr	4.5	14	8
4–6 yr	5.0	15	10
6–8 yr	5.5	16	10
8–10 yr	6.0–6.5 (optional cuff)	17	10–12
10–12 yr	7.5–8.0 (optional cuff)	18	12
> 12 yr	7.5–8.0 (cuffed)	19–22	12

*Teeth or alveolar ridge to midtrachea.

Laryngoscopes

Many laryngoscopic blades have been specifically designed for various pediatric anesthetic applications. The standard MacIntosh blade is manufactured in a small size. Small Miller blades are also available for neonates and small infants. The anteriorly placed, cephalad location of the larynx in the neonate and infant has led many authors to suggest that the ideal blade is a Miller 0 or 1 blade. This blade is placed in the vallecula and used to elevate the epiglottis for intubation in babies. For children older than 1 year of age, a MacIntosh 1 or 2 blade is frequently adequate and usually can provide good visualization. The selection of a straight versus a curved blade is the anesthesiologist's choice, and he or she should be familiar with the use of both blades. When selecting the appropriate blade, it is essential to remember the details of the child's airway (Fig. 79-4).

It cannot be too strongly emphasized that positioning of the child's head during intubation is critical. The position of the head required to align the airway axes for intubation when using a Miller blade is quite different from when using the MacIntosh blade. Considerable extension is required when using a Miller blade, whereas with the MacIntosh the head should be elevated in the classic sniffing position. Failure to correctly position the head is

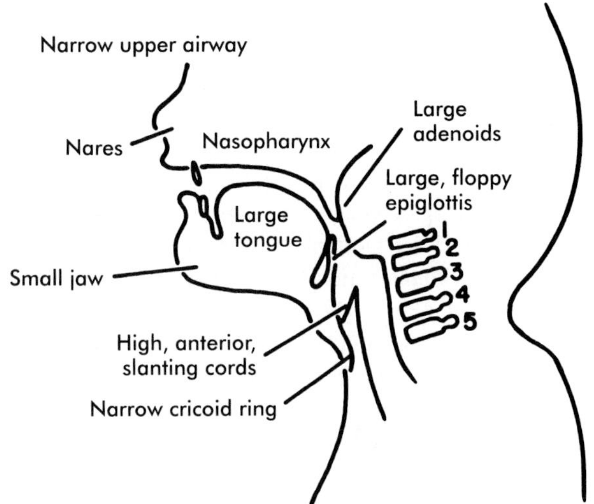

Fig. 79-4. Pediatric airway showing areas different from the adult airway. Familiarity with configuration of infant's and child's airway dictates selection of laryngoscope blades. (From Wetzel RC: Anesthesia for pediatric trauma. In Stene JK, editor: *Trauma anesthesia,* Baltimore, 1991, Williams & Wilkins.)

probably the most common cause of difficulty during intubation with either a straight or a curved blade. Wider straight blades (e.g., the Robertshaw, Flagg, and Wis-Hipple blades) allow the child's relatively large tongue to be removed from the field of view. An interesting modification of the Miller blade is the addition of a channel to provide O_2 flow. The use of this blade could be important in preventing desaturation during intubation because children have a relatively decreased O_2 reserve and higher O_2 consumption.

THE DIFFICULT AIRWAY

It is important to distinguish patients with a "difficult airway" from those who are "difficult to intubate." Children who have choanal atresia may have an obstructed airway that causes problems with mask airway management until the obstruction is relieved with an oral airway; however, these children should not be difficult to intubate unless other associated anomalies are present. Children with enlarged tonsils and adenoids causing sleep apnea predictably have obstructed nasal and oral airways on anesthesia induction. Thus the anesthesiologist should be prepared to use positive end-expiratory pressure (PEEP) or an oral airway during mask induction or preferably to perform an IV induction with placement of an oral airway before paralysis. These patients may require assistance with ventilation but should not present problems with intubation.

Before induction of anesthesia, the patient's head, neck, and airway anatomy should be meticulously assessed to identify patients in whom visualization of the larynx may be difficult. Examination of the head should include assessment of mouth opening, maxillary and especially mandibular size, and tongue size, both absolute and in relation to mandibular size. In addition to congenital abnormalities (see Table 25-7) mouth opening may be limited because of diseases such as juvenile rheumatoid arthritis or in patients who have received irradiation of tumors of the head and neck. Especially in children, careful examination of the teeth is necessary to detect and document preexisting loose or damaged teeth. The ability to visualize the uvula and tonsillar fossae has been predictive of unimpaired visualization of the larynx in adults, but this has never been documented in children and probably has no relation to the ability to visualize the larynx in neonates. Neck examination should be directed at mobility of the cervical spine, which may be limited in patients with the conditions listed in Table 25-7. Children with certain dwarfing syndromes and those with Down syndrome may have atlantoaxial instability from odontoid hypoplasia or laxity of the atlantoaxial ligament. These children may not have difficulty with intubation because of this cervical spine abnormality, but preoperative magnetic resonance imaging (MRI) or computed tomography (CT) scans may be indicated if any neurologic signs of spinal cord compression exist to avoid further damage to the spinal cord during positioning for intubation. The position of the larynx with respect to the midline and the base of the tongue should be determined.

When examination of the patient reveals clear evidence of an anticipated difficulty with airway management or difficult intubation, the anesthesiologist should share this information with the surgeon, who in rare cases might be asked to establish an emergency surgical airway. Therefore, the surgeon should be present at induction, and if the patient has epiglottitis, the surgeon should be prepared with a tracheostomy set. The parents should be informed of the increased risk to the child. Discussion should occur preoperatively regarding the tracheostomy to determine whether elective surgery should be cancelled and the patient awakened if an airway cannot be established.

Patients with anticipated difficult intubation should be premedicated with atropine or glycopyrrolate. These drugs may be administered orally (0.05 ml/kg) and are much more effective in drying secretions when administered in advance than IV in the operating room. Atropine (0.02 mg/kg), however, should again be administered IV in the induction room to prevent reflex bradycardia from laryngoscopy, because the vagolytic effect of an orally administered dose is unreliable and short-lived. Because of the risk of gastric distension associated with management of the difficult airway, some authors have recommended the preoperative administration of a H_2-receptor antagonist and metoclopramide in these patients to decrease the impact of aspiration of gastric contents.[65,136] **In most patients with anticipated difficult airway management, sedative premedication should not be administered before their arrival in the operating room.**

The techniques for securing the airway in the patient with anticipated difficult intubation include intubation under direct visualization (laryngoscopy), either after mask induction or with the patient "awake" (actually sedated). Oral or nasal intubation may also be accomplished "blindly" usually with the patient awake or sedated. Finally, intubation may be accomplished with the child awake (sedated) or after mask intubation with the aid of the fiberoptic bronchoscope. A brief discussion of these techniques follows.

Awake, unsedated intubation during direct laryngoscopy is possible only in neonates or in very debilitated older children. In patients weighing less than 10 kg, using the Miller 1 blade with the attached O_2 channel (oxyscope) may allow for a longer laryngoscopy. However, if the patient holds his or her breath during laryngoscopy, as often occurs, the O_2 flow may not help maintain oxygenation. In patients in whom the ability to visualize the larynx is questionable (Treacher-Collins, Pierre-Robin, Goldenhar) an "awake look" before inhalation induction may be reassuring or may lead to a decision to proceed to a fiberoptically aided technique. All patients with difficult airways should have an IV line started before sedation, laryngoscopy, or inhalational induction. In patients with no known spontaneous airway obstruction, in whom the main concern is laryngeal visualization, sedation before starting the IV line may be provided with rectal midazolam (1 mg/kg) or intramuscular (IM) ketamine (2 to 3 mg/kg). In vigorous patients, after the administration of IV atropine, as noted earlier, further sedation may be titrated to effect. Further sedation is best performed with midazolam or ketamine, avoiding narcotics to preserve spontaneous ventilation. During this period, the nose and mouth may be anesthetized with topical lidocaine (plus 0.25% Neo-Synephrine® for the nose) in preparation for possible oral or nasal airway placement.

Cautious inhalational induction can then be performed. If airway obstruction occurs with mild anesthesia, the prior topicalization of the nose and mouth may allow early placement of nasal or oral airways without stimulation of airway reflexes. If one is fairly confident of the ability to maintain airway patency with spontaneous ventilation, the IV line may be deferred until after the inhalational induction is begun, but it should be started as quickly as possible to provide a route for drug and fluid administration should hypotension, bradycardia, or airway obstruction occur during deepening anesthesia. If the concern is mainly for laryngeal visualization and not airway obstruction, inhalational induction can by performed in a routine fashion, starting with a 70/30 mixture of N_2O and O_2, using high flows. Halothane is added after 2 minutes of the patient breathing the N_2O/O_2 mixture and increased by 0.5% every 30 seconds up to a final concentration of 3% to 4%. The increase in halothane concentration is slowed if coughing or breath holding occurs. If concern exists about a high probability of airway obstruction during induction, such as in patients with epiglottitis, the induction is performed without N_2O (i.e., 100% O_2) from the outset. Performing the induction without N_2O greatly prolongs the time required to achieve an adequate depth of anesthesia. The use of a Mapleson D or other semi-closed valveless circuit with high flows allows more rapid change in the inspired anesthetic concentration than use of a circle system. This is true during induction and also will hasten the patient's emergence from anesthesia if the decision is made not to proceed with intubation.

During inhalational induction, the anesthesiologist should pay careful attention to breath sounds heard through the precordial stethoscope and to a respiratory pattern indicative of obstruction (rocking motion). The mask should be kept in good contact with the patient's face so that the patient's tidal volume can be determined by watching the feeling the reservoir bag. If airway obstruction occurs early in induction and the oropharynx has not been topicalized, placement of an oral airway might trigger airway reflexes that could lead to further coughing, breath holding, or laryngospasm. **The initial response to airway obstruction should be to cease increasing the halothane concentration, improving the patient's jaw lift, and closing the popoff valve of the circuit to deliver 10 cm H_2O of PEEP to the airway.** This level of PEEP will gently distend the soft tissues causing the airway obstruction, and the improved ventilation will allow further deepening of anesthetic level. When the lash reflex is lost, the N_2O is discontinued and the child maintained on 100% O_2 for at least 5 minutes in preparation for laryngoscopy. It is essential that spontaneous ventilation be maintained and the plane of anesthesia be sufficiently deep before laryngoscopy. The IV administration of lidocaine (1 to 1.5 mg/kg) 1 minute before laryngoscopy will deepen the plane of anesthesia and protect against undesired airway reflexes without depressing spontaneous ventilation. During this process, assisted ventilation may be necessary to prevent hypoventilation, but this effort should not be so vigorous as to eliminate spontaneous respiratory effort.

Once the patient is sufficiently anesthetized, as evidenced by the lack of response to stimulation, conjugate gaze, and a reduction in blood pressure by at least 20%, laryngoscopy is attempted. If laryngoscopy causes breath holding, tachycardia, or cough, the attempt is terminated and the patient further anesthetized. A wide range of laryngoscope blades should be available for patients whose larynx is expected to be difficult to visualize. Visualization of the larynx in patients with large tongues or soft tissue masses (e.g., cystic hygroma) may be enhanced by the use of a ear-nose-throat (ENT) laryngoscope. These are anterior commissure scopes that allow visualization of the larynx through a tubular configuration that excludes soft tissue from the line of sight. These laryngoscopes are not battery operated and require a separate light source. The availability of these scopes may be lifesaving or may prevent the need for tracheostomy in children with an "anterior" larynx (i.e., anterior to the line of sight). If the solid tubular laryngoscope is chosen, a long alligator clamp is used to immobilize the ET tube, from which the 15-mm connector has been removed to allow the laryngoscope to be withdrawn without dislodging the tube. Another laryngoscope that may expedite intubation in patients with small mouths or anterior larynges is the Bullard laryngoscope (American ACMI, Stamford, CT), in which the larynx is visualized "around the corner" through the use of a fiberoptic scope.

A fiberoptic bronchoscope may be used nasally or orally in the sedated infant or child to assist difficult intubation if the ability to visualize the larynx by direct laryngoscopy is doubtful (e.g., because the mouth does not open) or mask induction is contraindicated (e.g., because of malignant hyperthermia susceptibility, full stomach) and if the child is large enough to be intubated with a tube that will fit over a bronchoscope (5.0 for Olympus LF-1 and 3.5 for Olympus PF-27M [Olympus Corp., Lake Success, NY]).[47,91,162] The smaller bronchoscopes lack a suction channel and are more difficult to use. These instruments require prior experience with normal and adult airways before management of difficult pediatric airways is attempted.

"Blind" nasal intubation is more difficult in infants and small children than in adults because of the more anterior position of the larynx, and therefore, the greater curve that the tube must make in the pharynx. Sylets and light wands have been used to improve the success of this method. The light wand may also be used in a blind, oral fashion.[41] The hazard of blind methods is that the airway may be traumatized in an unsuccessful attempt, making subsequent attempts more difficult or compromising the patient's ability to ventilate. The nasal approach should be avoided in patients with coagulopathy and in those with head or facial trauma.

Most important, in patients with both anticipated and unanticipated difficulties in airway management, the anesthesiologist must document in the patient's chart and in the anesthetic record the anatomic abnormality that led to the difficulty and what methods were used, both unsuccessful and successful, to achieve intubation. The patient's parents must be informed so that they may tell any future anesthesiologist of the problems. This is especially important when the problem is not obvious on examination. The anesthesiologist also might suggest that these patients wear a Medic-Alert® bracelet.

INHALATIONAL ANESTHESIA

When considering inhalational anesthesia in children, one should remember two statements by Snow in the middle nineteenth century[145]: (1) "In children, the breathing and circulation are more rapid than in adults, and children and youths are put sooner and more easily under the influence of ether;" and (2) "Children recover from the effects of chloroform more rapidly on account of their circulation and respiration." Although we have a much more sophisticated understanding of these concepts today, the basic reality remains unchanged nearly 150 years later.

In addition to the factors mentioned in Chapter 25 that affect the distribution of IV agents, additional factors affect the uptake and distribution of the inhalational anesthetics. The rapid rise of the alveolar concentration of inhalational anesthetic, as measured by the ratio of alveolar to inspired fractional concentration (F_A/F_I) depends on many factors, especially alveolar ventilation (V_A), cardiac output (Q), and the distribution of Q to vessel-rich and vessel-poor groups. All these factors show characteristic developmental changes throughout life.[145] In general, the uptake of inhalational anesthetics occurs more rapidly in children than in adults, as has clearly been shown for N_2O and halothane (Fig. 79-5).

Although total tidal volume on a per kilogram basis (approximately 5 to 7 mg/kg) is relatively constant throughout life, the relationship of alveolar ventilation to functional residual capacity (V_A/FRC) changes dramatically. In infants this ratio is approximately 5:1, whereas in adults it approaches 1.5:1. Thus washout of the FRC would be expected to occur more quickly in infants. This is because FRC (ml/kg) is less in children than in young adults; this is also responsible for the rapid development of hypoxia during apnea in neonates. Thus, if this were the only factor involved, one would expect the alveolar concentration of anesthetic to rise much more rapidly in infants compared with adults and lead to more rapid induction.

Blood-gas partition coefficients also change with age.[96] Differences in plasma protein fraction, blood cell mass, and even hemoglobin type (fetal versus adult) may account for the generally lower blood-gas partition coefficients in younger patients. This tends to cause a more rapid rise in the alveolar concentration of inhalational anesthetic agents. The impact of cardiac output is also of interest. The much higher (per kilogram) cardiac output seen in infants compared with adults (almost two to three times as high) tends to decrease the rate of rise of alveolar concentration of anesthetic gas. The impact of this on uptake and distribution is somewhat offset by the relatively higher distribution of cardiac output to the vessel-rich groups and different blood-tissue partition coefficients in neonates. It has also been shown that the tis-

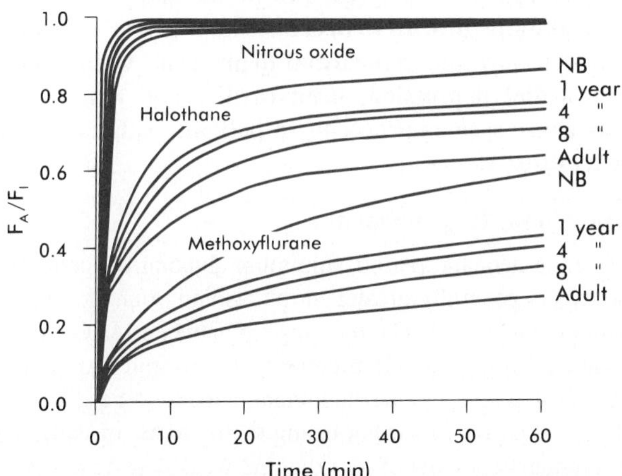

Fig. 79-5. Age dependency of increase in alveolar to inspired fractional concentration (F_A/F_I) with time. Note that for all anesthetics, the newborn's F_A rises more rapidly for a given F_I of anesthetic vapor than that of the adult. (From Eger EI: *Anesthetic uptake and action,* Baltimore, 1974, Williams & Wilkins.)

sue concentration of inhalational anesthetic agents also rises much more rapidly in younger patients. The general effect is that for a given F_1 of anesthetic, tissue concentrations are generally higher in infants than adults. **In summary, all these factors appear to enhance the rapidity of inhalational induction in children compared with adults.**

The effect of intracardiac shunts on the uptake and distribution of anesthetic agents has been of interest to pediatric anesthesiologists since the advent of cardiac surgery. By understanding the impact of intracardiac shunting, insights into the process of uptake and distribution are available; however, the clinical impact of intracardiac shunts is relatively minor. The effect of a right-to-left intracardiac shunt, which relatively decreases pulmonary blood flow in relation to systemic blood flow, is generally to slow the rate of induction. Although in a right-to-left shunt the F_A/F_1 ratio rises more rapidly, arterial blood bypassing the lungs tends to cause a slower rise in arterial concentration and therefore a slower induction. In contrast, the effect of a left-to-right shunt depends somewhat on its size. With a large left-to-right shunt, the F_A/F_1 ratio rises more rapidly and, if this is greater than perhaps 80% of the ventricular output, induction may be more rapid. Generally, with left-to-right shunts less than 50%, the rate of induction is minimally affected. Most large shunts to some degree have directional mixing, and the exact impact of intracardiac shunting (especially in patients with complex congenital heart disease) on the rapidity of inhalational induction cannot be predicted for the individual patient. Cautious vigilance by the anesthesiologist regarding anesthetic effect and depth of anesthesia, with an awareness that the usual duration of induction may be altered, is necessary during inhalational anesthesia in these children. **The use of elevated levels of inhalational anesthesia to speed induction in patients with right-to-left shunts must be avoided. If high blood concentrations of anesthetics are achieved, the myocardial depression that occurs, with a consequent fall in cardiac output, may make it quite difficult to decrease the depth of anesthesia and therefore the myocardial depression. Catastrophic myocardial depression, bradycardia, and hypotension may cause serious problems in patients with congenital heart disease.**

Anesthetic Requirements

After the neonatal period, minimum alveolar concentration (MAC) is generally greater in infants and younger children than in adults.[74,95,97] The relationship between MAC and age is, however, biphasic. In premature infants and neonates the MAC, of isoflurane and halothane appear to be decreased (Figs. 79-6 and 79-7). For example, the MAC of isoflurane in premature infants of less than 32 weeks' gestation is approximately 1.3%, whereas in 1-month postnatal and full-term infants the MAC may approach 1.9%, compared with 1.2% MAC generally reported in adults.[95] This trend is also apparently true for IV anesthetics, as typified by thiopental.[175] Several factors account for these developmental changes in anesthetic requirements.

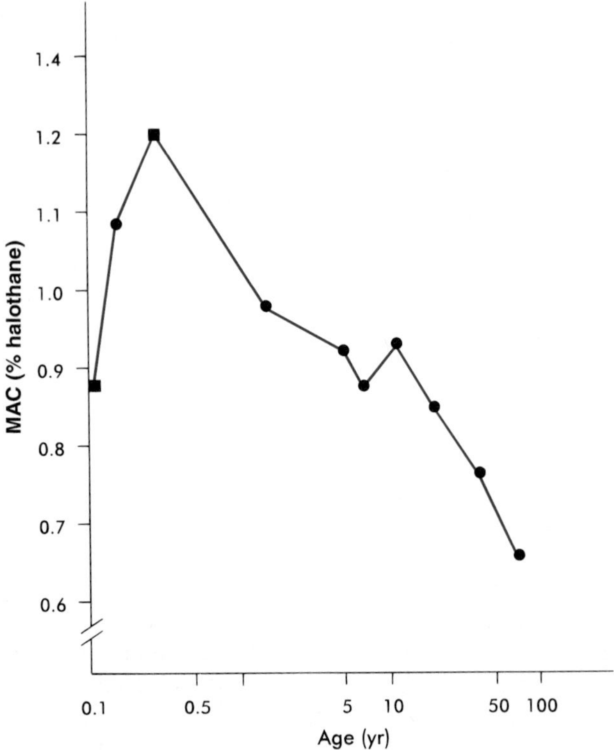

Fig. 79-6. MAC of halothane versus age on logarithmic scale. This demonstrates that MAC of anesthetic vapor is highest in early childhood, with a secondary peak in adolescence. Biphasic nature is characteristic of inhalational anesthetic agents.

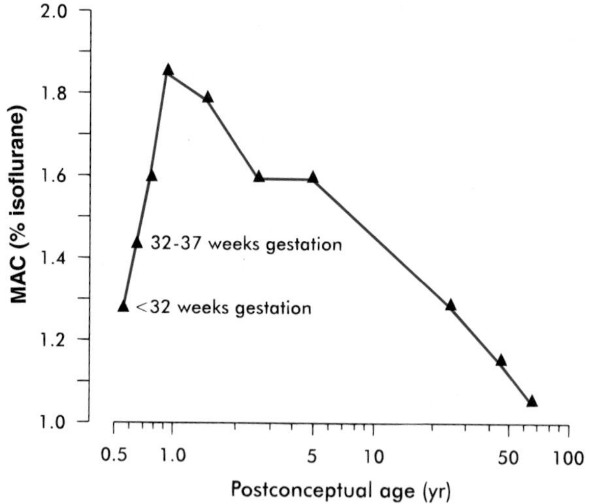

Fig. 79-7. MAC of isoflurane versus age. Again, as in Figure 74-6, characteristic biphasic relationship of MAC versus age is demonstrated. (From LeDez KM, Lerman J: The minimum alveolar concentration [MAC] of isoflurane in preterm infants, *Anesthesiology* 67:301, 1987.)

The development of the neonatal nervous system and nociception is discussed in Chapter 24. Even first trimester fetuses appear to be responsive to painful stimuli in that they withdraw from pain, grimace, and become tachycardic. Although in the past, it was believed that neonates and premature infants were insensitive to pain, this myth has recently largely been disproved.[2] Although maturation and myelination of the nervous system are absent, significant somatic and autonomic responses to painful stimuli still occur, even in the most premature neonate. Perhaps a major explanation for the apparent change in MAC with age is philosophical. One must consider the nature of MAC. Clearly the concentration of anesthetic in the central nervous system (CNS) and other nociceptive sites is the important issue. Alveolar concentration reflects this tissue concentration, but only in part. For example, at equivalent alveolar and arterial concentrations of anesthetic, neonates have higher tissue concentrations. This may partly explain the apparent decrease in MAC seen in premature infants and neonates. The concentration of inhaled anesthetics in the CNS may be relatively constant for a given level of anesthesia in all age groups; however, this remains to be demonstrated.

The general theories of the mechanism of anesthetic action indicate that a definite molar concentration of anesthetic vapors is required at the site of action to produce a given therapeutic effect.[112] Some evidence suggests that this is true in neonates, as shown by Cook et al.[24] The differences in MAC may be attributed to physical factors (e.g., blood), tissue and gas partition coefficients, water content, solubility, and protein binding, rather than to actual differences in sensitivity and receptor modulation by inhaled anesthetics.[96,111] This still does not explain the apparent biphasic MAC versus age curve of inhaled anesthetics (see Figs. 79-6 and 79-7). A potential explanation of the biphasic relationship could be an ever-increasing uptake caused by increasing solubility coefficients until infancy, followed by maturational changes in the CNS caused by changes in water content and percentage of cardiac output distribution, leading to a decreased equipotent alveolar concentration. It is not surprising, considering what is known of developmental differences in the characteristics affecting anesthetic uptake and distribution, that MAC varies with age; however, this does not necessarily imply that anesthetic concentration at the site of action is any different for a given effect.

Another potential cause of the difference in anesthetic requirements could be the presence of endogenous analgetic agents. The endorphin system has been shown to be quite active in premature infants and newborns, and intrinsic analgesia may decrease the need for inhaled anesthetics, as seen in the neonatal period.[3] Another potential cause could be the analgetic effects of maternal progesterone in the newborn circulation, which may decrease MAC in the first few days of life.[75] In critically ill neonates requiring anesthesia, the decreased metabolism of endogenous endorphins, increased concentration of progesterone, and other thus far unidentified endogenous analgetic systems could account for their decreased inhalational anesthetic needs.

The arguments that apply to depth of anesthesia also apply to the incidence of side effects. Just as a given alveolar concentration of anesthetic does not produce the same depth of anesthesia in patients of different ages, no reason exists to expect that anesthetics should have similar effects on the cardiovascular and respiratory systems at different ages. Comparison of side effects should be made at equianalgesic or equipotent concentrations of anesthetics rather than at arbitrarily chosen levels of inhalational anesthesia. Confusion regarding this point in the past has led to the teaching that neonates and infants are more susceptible to anesthetic depressant effects; however, they were not given equipotent doses. **The rapid rise in alveolar concentration and the uptake and distribution of anesthetics in neonates and infants puts them at greater risk for potential overdose.** Because the rise is more rapid, the child might quickly move from adequate anesthesia to deep anesthesia and multiple complications. This would give the apparent impression of increased sensitivity to the side effects of inhalational anesthetics. Thus overdosage may appear to occur more readily.

The anesthetic circuit also has an impact on the rapidity of induction. The use of a adult circle system with a soda-lime absorber and a large dead space leads to a slower rate of induction than the use of Mapelson D type of circuit with fresh gas flowing directly into the ET tube. Not surprisingly, attempts to determine the rapidity of induction (increase in F_A/F_I ratio) and MAC would have different results, depending solely on the anesthetic circuitry.

Respiratory Effects

As in adults, all inhalational anesthetics depress respiratory drive in a dose-dependent manner. Respiratory depression occurs at concentrations as low as 0.1% of inhaled anesthetic agent, with depression in hypoxic response and a shift to the right of the CO_2 response curve.[92] The effects of inhalational anesthesia are to decrease tidal volume, decrease minute ventilation, and decrease FRC, all of which may be greater in children.[118,155] Clearly, $Paco_2$ tends to increase. The clinical significance of these changes in infants and young children who already have decreased FRC (per kilogram), higher O_2 consumption, and difficult-to-manage airways is obvious. **During the use of inhalational anesthetics, controlled mechanical ventilation is preferable to spontaneous ventilation to avoid hypoventilation, respiratory acidosis, and hypoxemia.**

All inhaled anesthetics are bronchodilators. Although halothane has received the greatest attention, bronchodilatation is even an effect of ether.[154] Some debate has occurred over the years as to whether enflurane and isoflurane are as potent bronchodilators as halothane, but currently it appears that all, in equipotent doses, are equivalent. The decreased incidence of airway irritation on inhalational induction with halothane seems to make it the preferable anesthetic agent to use in asthmatic patients.[82,134] Sevoflurane is also characterized by minimal airway irritation and has the advantage over halothane of a reduced blood-gas partition coefficient which leads to a very rapid induction. Sevoflurane might easily replace halothane as the inhalation agent of choice for induction in asthmatics (and children in general) were it not for the significant cost differential.

Cardiovascular Effects

The cardiovascular depressant effects of inhalational anesthetics appear to be greater in infants and children than in adults. Numerous reports have demonstrated that cardiac arrest, bradycardia, and hypotension occur more often during the inhalational induction of anesthesia in younger patients.[57] All modern inhalational anesthetic agents depress myocardial contraction and lower heart rates.[59] Infants and small children are particularly dependent on heart rate. A decreased heart rate leads to a proportional decrease in cardiac output because of the inability of the pediatric heart to increase contractility. This is aggravated during inhalational anesthesia.[7,57,59] Further, baroreceptor reflex responses are quite sensitive to inhalational anesthetics.[37,38,119] Gregory[73] was perhaps the first to suggest that inhaled anesthetics inhibit baroreceptor activity in premature infants.[174] A caveat should be mentioned: One reason why the cardiovascular effects of the potent inhaled anesthetics appear greater in neonates than in adults may be that the alveolar and therefore arterial concentration of inhaled anesthetics rises more rapidly in children than in adults.

INDIVIDUAL INHALATIONAL ANESTHETICS

Halothane

Halothane remains the cornerstone of pediatric inhalational anesthesia. As with all anesthetics, halothane is an airway irritant and a mild sialagogue. Its use is associated with laryngospasm. Although this does not differ qualitatively from the other inhalational anesthetics (ethrane, isoflurane), as well as the newer anesthetics sevoflurane and desflurane, halothane is by far the least irritating. Halothane has a blood-gas partition coefficient of 2.4, which suggests a somewhat slower rate of increase in alveolar concentration than that of isoflurane (1.4) or even ethrane (1.8).[40] The lower-solubility coefficients suggest that these latter agents would have a more rapid rise in alveolar concentration, which could result in a more rapid induction of inhalational anesthesia in children. This has not proved clinically true.[53] Newer inhalational anesthetics have a monumentally successful inhalational anesthetic agent against which they must be compared.

Some of us may have forgotten what an advance halothane was for pediatric anesthesia. Although cyclopropane provided a rapid and smooth induction, its propensity for explosion eliminated its use in the United States. When compared to ether and chloroform for rapidity, smoothness of induction, airway irritability, and sialagogic effect, halothane was a revolutionary, infinitely preferable agent. Its potency, rapidity of induction, and cardiorespiratory depression earned it a reputation as a potentially difficult anesthetic; however, as anesthesiologists became familiar with it, the advantages of this drug far outweighed any of these concerns. The spluttering, choking, coughing, frothing, vomiting (i.e., stormy inductions) that occurred with the earlier agents (chloroform and ether) and which remain in the memories of our patients' parents are part of the past because of halothane. Any claims made for the newer inhalational induction agents must be compared with halothane, and it is unlikely that there will ever be another advance in inhalational agents for children as significant as halothane.

Several concerns surround the use of halothane. Halothane, like all inhalational anesthetics, is a direct myocardial depressant.[7,37,59,94] This myocardial depression occurs in all age groups and has significant implications in neonates and in children with congenital heart disease. Children with impaired myocardial contractility can become significantly hypotensive before they are adequately anesthetized, and an alternative induction technique must occasionally be chosen. The anesthesiologist should also remember that in children with low cardiac output, alveolar concentrations rise more rapidly and are difficult to reverse. Cardiac depression may readily occur. Baroreceptor reflexes are depressed by inhalational anesthetics, particularly in younger animals.[73,174] This significantly influences heart rate, contractility, and vascular resistance. Halothane is also a direct peripheral vasodilator, although to somewhat less of a degree than the other agents, and this also contributes to hypotension.

A further concern about inhalational anesthetics is that they sensitize the myocardium to endogenous and exogenous circulating catecholamines. This effect is aggravated by acidosis, especially respiratory acidosis,[86] and may be the underlying mechanism for the occurrence of ventricular extrasystole and bigeminy in children breathing spontaneously during halothane anesthesia. **The most likely cause of dysrhythmias during inhalational anesthesia is inadequate depth of anesthesia, thus leading to increased circulating catecholamines, or inadequate ventilation with CO_2 retention. Thus initial therapy for ventricular ectopy in anesthetized children is hyperventilation.** This clears CO_2, decreases respiratory acidosis, and increases the depth of anesthesia. The administration of exogenous catecholamines for ENT, neurosurgical, and orthopedic procedures to decrease blood loss during halothane anesthesia is permissible.[170] Most evidence seems to indicate that up to 10 μg/kg can be administered safely subcutaneously or injected extravascularly in children with very minimal risk of cardiac dysrhythmias.[85]

A major concern of every anesthesiologist is the risk of halothane hepatitis.[61] The literature contains recommendations that range from avoiding repeated exposure of halothane in children[88] to statements that deny the existence of halothane hepatitis in children.[172] The exact incidence of halothane hepatitis is not clear, although it must be very low in the pediatric population. However, there are a few reported deaths of children that clearly seem to be related to halothane hepatitis.[156] Halothane or its metabolites cause impairment of hepatic function, especially in patients with hypoxia or ischemia. Finally, a few episodes of hepatitis may be attributed to repeated use of halothane anesthetics.[61,88] If halothane hepatitis were a significant clinical risk, one would have expected dozens of deaths and hundreds of cases of hepatitis for an agent that is so widely used. The safety record of halothane after thousands, and perhaps millions, of uses worldwide is better than most drugs in use today. **The results of National Halothane Study, published in 1966, remain pertinent.[167] The study reported a virtual absence of halothane hepatitis in infants and prepubertal children.** Although the anesthesiologist needs to be aware of this issue, the impact on the selection of anesthetic agent is minimal. One might consider choosing another inhalational anesthetic agent in children with liver impairment or limiting the repeated use of halothane to four or five times per 6-month period in the same child.

Enflurane

Enflurane, introduced in 1972, has little application in pediatric anesthesia because it is a strongly pungent, irritating anesthetic and is not suitable for inhalational induction. In addition to this, enflurane has been demonstrated to lower the seizure threshold, especially in hypocapnic patients, and this has tended to make this drug less popular in pediatric anesthesia.[139] Enflurane appears to have no advantages over halothane.

Isoflurane

The introduction of isoflurane in 1981 was heralded by the theoretic advantage of a more rapid induction because of its relatively lower blood-gas partition coefficient.[40] Unfortunately, this did not occur in clinical practice. Isoflurane proved to be too irritating, causing respiratory pauses, coughing, choking, and occasionally laryngospasm and resulted in slower, not more rapid, inductions in children.[131] Thus isoflurane has not become an agent of choice for inhalational induction in children. Its value following IV induction and airway intubation is essentially the same as that for halothane and may be associated with slightly more rapid awakening.[134]

Isoflurane is somewhat less of a myocardial depressant than halothane but may be a more potent peripheral vasodilator than the other frequently used inhalational anesthetic agents.[161,181] In general, cardiac function appears to be better maintained with isoflurane than with halothane. Even though blood pressure may be decreased with isoflurane, its better maintenance of heart rate and myocardial contractility tends to maintain cardiac output. This suggests a slight advantage for isoflurane in children with congenital heart disease or in cases where a controlled hypotensive technique may be desirable. Isoflurane also may have an advantage in anesthetizing patients with elevated intracranial pressure or CNS lesions. It has been demonstrated that the cerebral metabolic rate of O_2 ($CMRO_2$) is decreased more with isoflurane than with halothane.[109] This appears to be accompanied by less effect on cerebral blood flow, because isoflurane does not appear to be as potent a cerebral vasodilator as halothane.[122]

Desflurane

Desflurane has even lower blood-gas (0.42) and tissue-blood partition coefficients than isoflurane. This led to hopes of its use to speed inhalational induction, but it is even more of an airway irritant than isoflurane with a 73% incidence of laryngospasm and a 58% incidence of coughing. This resulted in its rejection for inhalational induction.[184] The use of desflurane does, however, speed emergence when compared to other inhalational agents, including isoflurane. Emergence can be characterized by bucking and coughing, which can be ameliorated by the judicious use of small amounts of narcotic before the end of surgery. In children, emergence from desflurane can be associated with a high incidence of delirium with prolonged agitation. The use of narcotics or sedatives to modify these emergence phenomena may negate the rapid emergence from desflurane. Desflurane is associated with a decreased incidence of postoperative vomiting when compared with other inhalation agents.[184]

Similar to the other inhalational agents, MAC and cardiovascular effects of desflurane vary with patient age, but these age-related differences are of much lower magnitude than those seen with halothane and isoflurane.[168] Because of its extraordinarily low solubility, MAC of desflurane is the highest of all potent inhalational agents, being 9.2% in neonates, 9.4% and 9.2% in infants 1 to 6 and 6 to 12 months, respectively, and 8.0% in children 1 to 12 years of age.

Desflurane has cardiovascular effects which are similar to isoflurane: mild myocardial depression and a marked decrease in systemic vascular resistance (SVR), balanced by an increase in heart rate, leading to little net change in cardiac index.[20] Desflurane has been associated with an increase in blood pressure and heart rate when inhaled concentrations are rapidly increased.[184] This property is less problematic in children than it is in adult patients, where there are concerns about coronary artery disease (CAD). In any case, this response can be easily avoided by slowly increasing the inhaled concentration of desflurane. Desflurane does not sensitize the myocardium to catecholamines.

Sevoflurane

Sevoflurane is the most recently introduced volatile anesthetics. It, like desflurane, is characterized by a low blood-gas partition coefficient of 0.6 to 0.69.[166] **In contrast to desflurane, it is comparable to halothane in its extremely low incidence of airway irritation, leading to the recommendations of its use for mask inhalational induction in children. Because of its low solubility characteristics, its use is associated with an extremely rapid induction, even in the absence of N_2O.**

Sevoflurane's hemodynamic effects and MAC have been studied in children of all ages. The MAC is less variable with age than some of the other agents, being 3.3% and 3.2% in neonates and infants, respectively, and 2.5% in children 1 to 12 years of age.[98] The hemodynamic effects are similar to other inhalational agents, with a significant decrease in blood pressure at 1 MAC prior to incision. This effect was found through the use of transesophageal echocardiography (TEE) to be due to a small decrease in myocardial contractility leading to a decrease in ejection fraction and a decrease in SVR. These effects are balanced by an increase in heart rate, resulting in little change in cardiac index. Sevoflurane results in less cardiovascular depression than either isoflurane or halothane. Sevoflurane does not sensitize the myocardium to epinephrine.[121]

There are two concerns with sevoflurane. The first is related to its degradation in soda lime.[117] This can be avoided by using a Mapleson circuit or using moderate-to-high flows in a semiclosed breathing circuit. The second is the generation of inorganic fluoride ion during the course of its metabolism. The amount of fluoride generated under conditions of normal use has not been associated with evidence of renal toxicity[60] and use of sevoflurane for 15 MAC hours has been deemed safe in adults.[149]

Hepatitis has been reported in Japan in patients who have received sevoflurane, but the role of sevoflurane in these cases is unclear. It has been suggested that sevoflurane-related hepatic microsomal induction and possible related hepatotoxicity is no greater than that seen with isoflurane.[164] Sevoflurane has been associated with cases of malignant hyperthermia, when used alone or in combination with succinylcholine.[126] The relative importance of these issues will require further use and clarification in the next few years.

Extensive studies have shown that 7% sevoflurane with nitrous oxide results in smooth and rapid induction of anesthesia ($\leq$ 4 breaths) with excellent intubating conditions and less cardiovascular depression than halothane.[132] Some practitioners induce with sevoflurane then switch to a lower cost agent for the remainder of the anesthetic, but the continued use of sevoflurane results in faster emergence and shorter time to discharge from PACU.[120] Like desflurane, however, the rapid emergence may be associated with agitation or delirium in children. The resulting requirement for sedation may negate the rapid emergence advantages of sevoflurane and result in prolonged recovery time.[72]

PREMEDICATION AND INDUCTION

The primary goal of anesthetic induction in children is to transport the child from the awake to the anesthetized state in a way that is calm and stress free for the child, parent, and anesthesiologist. The range of techniques for the induction of anesthesia routinely used in children is much greater than those in adults. This difference stems from the special physiologic and psychologic needs of children and their families. The wide range of available techniques makes it possible for the anesthesiologist to modify the induction method to the needs of the individual child rather than attempting to force the child into a preconceived induction plan. The goals of anesthetic management are similar in adults and children (i.e., amnesia, analgesia, good operating conditions for the surgeon, and patient safety). In addition, the child's emotional needs must be addressed (which should be considered more often in adults as well) because hospitalization, anesthesia, and surgery have been shown to have an enduring emotional impact on children (see Chapter 25).[33] Therefore, an additional goal in the anesthetic management of children is to minimize the psychologic trauma of surgery and anesthesia within the parameters of an anesthetic plan that is safe for the patient.

Premedication

Formulation of a plan for anesthetic management should include the consideration of preoperative drug administration. The traditional goals of administration of preoperative medication include: (1) decreasing airway secretions; (2) blockade of detrimental autonomic (vagal) reflexes; (3) provision of sedation/anxiolysis; (4) facilitation of the smooth induction of general anesthesia; (5) supplementation of general anesthetic technique; (6) provision of preoperative analgesia to patients with pain; and (7) diminution of volume and acidity of gastric contents.

In children, the negative aspects of traditional premedication (e.g., IM injection, respiratory depression, possible airway obstruction), less-pungent volatile anesthetic agents eliminating the routine need for an antisialagogue, and the effectiveness of psychologic preparation and parental support have led to a decline in the use of classic premedication. In addition, the increase in outpatient surgery demands the elimination of premedications that outlast the duration of surgery, prolong somnolence, and therefore, delay discharge. In the era of IM premedication, the injection was frequently the most painful and terrifying experience of the child's stay in the hospital. The pain of an IM injection may persist even after the discomfort from the surgery wanes. Increasingly, education of the parent and child during the preoperative anesthetic visit has been substituted for the premedication needle. Despite the decreasing use of premedication, premedication is beneficial for some children, although seldom via the IM route.

In the days of ether anesthesia, preoperative treatment with an antisialagogue was essential. The modern potent inhalational agents are much less irritating to the airway, and therefore drying of secretions is necessary only in patients who have excessive airway secretions or who required antisialagogues for other reasons (airway endoscopy or laser surgery).[44] Atropine is also useful to prevent vagal reflexes, which include the oculocardiac reflex in children undergoing eye muscle surgery, bradycardia in response to halothane or succinylcholine, and the vagal responses to laryngoscopy in infants and children less than 6 years of age. This latter effect is especially important in infants less than 1 year of age, in whom cardiac output depends on heart rate because stroke volume is relatively fixed.[138] In most patients, atropine may be administered IV following induction of anesthesia (0.02 mg/kg; minimum dose, 0.15 mg) to prevent bradycardia. If a drying effect is desired preoperatively, oral atropine (0.05 mg/kg) 1 hour before surgery is effective. Atropine in the same dosage is also effective when added to rectally administered drugs.

If psychologic preparation of parent and child fails to render the child cooperative and relatively calm, sedative premedication may be desirable. This occurs most often in adolescents, children who have had extensive hospitalizations with multiple prior procedures, and children in preoperative pain. Many oral premedication "cocktails" have been found to be safe and as effective as IM premedications, and when properly administered, will not delay discharge after outpatient surgery.[17,123]

Sedative premedication is unnecessary in healthy infants less than 8 months of age because they have little anxiety, being unable to perceive what is to occur. Infants less than 6 months of age are more prone to airway obstruction and respiratory depression after sedation. Sedative premedication should be avoided in children with CNS disease (abnormal central ventilatory control mechanisms, hypoventilation, increased intracranial pressure [ICP]) or airway abnormalities.

Narcotic premedication still has a role in children older than 1 year of age who are in pain and in children with congenital heart disease who are at risk from undesirable hemodynamic responses to pain and anxiety. In contrast to the preceding caution about CNS disease, children with intracranial aneurysms or vascular malformations without increased ICP benefit from preoperative narcotic premedication to smooth anesthetic induction and avoid hypertension.

Older children (especially adolescents) are the group for whom premedication is still most often administered. Adolescents, in addition to being anxious about the outcome of surgery, may have age-related fears regarding body image and loss of autonomy. In adolescents, the effects of a usual adult oral dose of diazepam (0.15 mg/kg) are quite variable, with some patients being calm and others totally unaffected. More consistent sedation has been seen when quite large doses (0.3 to 0.5 mg/kg) are administered, but postoperative sedation may be prolonged, especially when the surgery is relatively brief. Droperidol has been studied and found to be an effective oral premedication in children in a dose of 0.2 mg/kg. It has the advantages of being an antisialagogue and antiemetic with effects that persist into the postoperative period. The incidence of CNS side effects (dysphoria, restlessness, extrapyramidal reactions) has resulted in decreased use of droperidol in adult patients, but these side effects rarely occur in children. In older children, discussing premedication options is often helpful. Many adolescents are more distraught by "feeling weird" and out of control than by anticipation of their surgery and prefer no premedication.

Recently, newer techniques of sedation have been studied in which relatively fast-acting drugs have been administered via innovative routes just before anesthetic induction with the patient in close proximity to the operating room (preinduction sedation). They include intranasal and oral (lollipop) administration of narcotics (fentanyl, sufentanil).[45,81] Although the use of these has been found to reduce perioperative analgetic requirements, they also have been associated with complications of chest rigidity and delayed emergence with higher doses. Oral, rectal, and nasally administered midazolam has been found to be safe, rapidly renders children calm and happy, and is not associated with airway obstruction or hypoventilation.[144,159,178] Subsequent mask induction is smooth and pleasant to both child and parent.

Induction Techniques

No single anesthetic induction technique is best for all children. No matter which technique is used, the goals of the ideal anesthetic induction are to minimize unpleasant experiences and morbidity while ensuring the patient's safety and expediting the achievement of good operating conditions for the surgeon. The risks of anesthetic induction are much more serious than simply prolonged emotional upset. They include airway obstruction, vomiting and aspiration, hypotension, dysrhythmias, and death. Psychologic preparation, premedication, and parental presence can contribute to a safe induction of anesthesia because calm, cooperative children have less stormy inductions. Nevertheless, the serious risks should be preeminent in the anesthesiologist's mind. Regardless of the technique chosen for induction, all monitoring, airway, and IV equipment and the anesthesia machine, circuit, and gas supplies should be thoroughly checked and ready for any eventuality before induction is begun.

Many institutions perform the induction of anesthesia in an area that may be contiguous with or separate from the operating room. This allows induction to occur in an environment that may be less threatening without the full array of operating room equipment. It also allows parents to be present for induction while not actually having them in the operating room. Adequate personnel and equipment must be available in these locations outside the operating room. Monitoring for transport from the induction area to the operating room usually consists only of a precordial stethoscope.

The major categories of anesthetic induction are IV, inhalational, and rectal. The agents and doses used for various modes of induction are listed in Table 79-2. Although IM induction is possible, it is rarely used because it is less safe without venous access and frightening and painful to the patient. IV induction of anesthesia is fast, reliable, and safe in the healthy, normovolemic child. IV induction is used less often than other methods because most children (and some adults) are terrified of the "big needle." IV placement of a very small (27-gauge) butterfly needle can be accomplished almost painlessly by an experienced anesthesiologist, and some practitioners prefer this technique to all others. Use of such a small-gauge needle for induction is safe only when the patient is normovolemic and no problems with induction are anticipated, because its small gauge does not allow the rapid administration of drugs or fluids. However, even with the use of a topically applied eutectic mixture of local anesthetics (EMLA), which reliably and painlessly renders the

Table 79-2 Agents for various modes of anesthesia induction

Drug	Dose (mg/kg)	Onset (min)	Comments
Intravenous			
Thiopental (2.5%)	4–6	1–2	Pain on injection
Methohexital (1%)	1–2	1–2	Avoid in patients with epilepsy
Ketamine (10%)	1–3	1	Catecholamine release; administer atropine (increased secretions); prolonged awakening after short procedure; dysphoria (administer benzodiazepine); increased intraocular and intracranial pressures
Propofol (1%)	2–3	1	Pain on injection; mix with lidocaine (final concentration 2 mg/ml); use large veins
Etomidate	0.3–0.4	1	Myoclonic jerks; inhibits steroid synthesis
Inhalational			
See text			
Intramuscular			
Ketamine	2–3 (sedation) 8–10 (general anesthesia)	5	Increased intraocular pressure, intracranial pressure; administer atropine; may be used intramuscular for rapid-sequence method
Methohexital (5%)	10	3	Pain on injection; avoid in patients with epilepsy; large volume required
Rectal			
Thiopental (10%)	40	5–15	Hiccough
Methohexital (10%)	25–30	5–15	Hiccough; avoid in patients with epilepsy; may sting on injection
Ketamine (5%)	6–10	7–15	Same under intravenous and intramuscular; may administer atropine rectally

planned venipuncture site numb, many children still view the experience as "painful" and remain uncooperative.[158]

In children over 5 years of age, it is important psychologically to give the child some choice in the manner in which he or she will go to sleep, and many will not choose a "shot" even if it is guaranteed to be painless. Risks of IV induction include extravascular infiltration of anesthetic agents; with thiopental, this may lead to tissue loss. The other major risk of IV induction occurs in patients with unrecognized abnormalities in airway anatomy (e.g., laryngeal cysts) who may be difficult to ventilate once asleep.

In cooperative older children, preoxygenation consisting of five large breaths should precede IV induction. In younger, uncooperative, but healthy children, preoxygenation may be omitted. **After sleep is induced, care should be taken to avoid assisted ventilation of the patient until he or she is clearly deep enough (e.g., absent lash reflex, conjugate gaze). Premature ventilation may lead to coughing, hiccoughing, or possibly laryngospasm.** The introduction of volatile anesthetic agents should be gradual. IV, rapid-sequence induction may be indicated in patients with "full stomachs" (intestinal obstruction, insufficient fasting time, gastroesophageal reflux). In these patients, preoxygenation for 2 minutes is mandatory before the rapid-bolus administration of the induction agent and muscle relaxant.

IV induction agents are listed in Table 79-2. For children with increased ICP (blocked shunt, tumor), IV induction using thiopental and lidocaine is the method of choice. Thiopental and methohexital are similar in onset, but methohexital has a shorter duration of action. Methohexital should be avoided in children with a history of seizures because it may be epileptogenic. Although it causes histamine release, thiopental has been shown not to precipitate bronchospasm. Because it lacks analgetic properties, however, intubation after a relatively small dose of thiopental (4 mg/kg) may cause bronchospasm because of light anesthesia. Therefore, asthmatic patients should receive a sufficient induction dose of thiopental (5 to 6 mg/kg) to attain an adequate depth of anesthesia before intubation. IV lidocaine (1 to 1.5 mg/kg) should also be administered to blunt airway reflexes. Alternatively, increased depth of anesthesia can be achieved with increasing concentrations of inhalation agent, either via spontaneous, assisted, or controlled ventilation.

Because of its catecholamine-stimulating properties, ketamine may be chosen for IV induction in children who are hypovolemic or hemodynamically unstable.[173] In addition, it is frequently used in children with cyanotic congenital heart disease in whom decreased SVR, as caused by thiopental, is undesirable. Ketamine is also used in children with asthma for its bronchodilating properties.[169] Asthmatic children in whom a rapid-sequence induction is indicated may be most safely induced with ketamine because it provides rapid attainment of profound analgesia and bronchodilatation. When ketamine is administered by any route, it should be preceded or accompanied by the administration of atropine or glycopyrrolate to attenuate the increase in airway secretions. The addition of a benzodiazepine is recommended to lessen the dysphoric emergence from anesthesia that may occur with ketamine.

Etomidate may be used for IV induction in children at risk for hemodynamic instability (hypovolemia) when the hypertension and tachycardia caused by ketamine are unacceptable (increased intraocular or ICP). As with thiopental and methohexital, etomidate may cause pain on injection, which can be very disturbing to the child. This pain may be attenuated by the prior injection of lidocaine.

Midazolam has been used as an IV induction agent in children. It has been found to be safe and effective but has not been found to reliably or rapidly render patients unconscious.[83]

The newest IV induction agent is propofol.[13,77] Its use is associated with pain on injection. This may be attenuated by adding 2% lidocaine to the drug immediately before administration (1:10 dilution; final concentration of lidocaine, 2 mg/ml). Slow injection and the use of larger (e.g., antecubital) veins are also associated with decreased pain. In children, propofol causes the smooth onset of loss of consciousness, which may be accompanied by large muscle movements. Mild hypotension may occur after rapid-bolus injection. The use of propofol is associated with amnesia but little analgesia. Propofol is rapidly distributed after bolus administration. The elimination half-life is very short. These pharmacokinetic characteristics lead to a very rapid decline in serum concentration after administration by bolus or infusion and are associated with rapid emergence from anesthesia.

Inhalational induction

Everyone who anesthetizes children should be an expert at mask inhalational inductions. Children's fear of needles and the anesthesiologist's desire to avoid patient discomfort make inhalational inductions a mandatory skill. Instilling confidence and a calm expectation in the child and parent is the first important step. The calm support of a familiar and loved person during induction can be very comforting for the child. We allow parents into the operating room until the child is obtunded and unable to be comforted by parental presence. Inhalational induction of anesthesia is well tolerated and accepted by healthy infants 1 to 6 months of age and by well-prepared children older than 4 years. An inhalational technique has the advantage of being painless, and the child can be assured of "no needles."

The key to mask inhalational induction is to maintain a calm child. Psychologic preparation of the child and parent is essential to enable them to feel comfortable with the mask. Humor, confidence, playfulness, the telling of stories can be helpful. The anesthesiologist should be a friend to the child. Friendly interaction during placement of the monitors is essential. One should try to keep the child smiling. Likening the mask to a jet pilot's mask may catch the interest of 5- to 10-year-old children. The challenge of blowing up the balloon may intrigue some older children. Some anesthesiologists use a mouthpiece adapter for the circuit to avoid the initial use of the mask.[12] Alternatively, if the mask is anxiety provoking, the cupped hand or even a bare anesthetic circuit elbow may be used in place of the mask. When the mask is used, allowing the patient to choose which smell of "sleepy air" he or she prefers gives the child some sense of control of the process. A single drop of food flavoring (Lorann Oils, Inc., Lansing, MI) may be applied in the elbow of the anesthetic circuit to obscure the odor of the inhalation agent. The flavoring should not be placed on the inner surface of the mask itself, because staining of the face (especially when grape is used) or dermatitis may result. Flavored lip gloss is an alternative source of smell for the mask.

The child's and parent's level of anxiety increases exponentially with every waking minute in the operating room. A child can be brave for only so long. When the child is brought into the room, the anesthesiologist and others present must be prepared to proceed immediately with induction. The child should not be allowed to stare at the equipment while the anesthesiologist is occupied with other tasks. The physician should focus attention on the child. A quiet, calm, pleasant, loving atmosphere in the induction area or operating room is mandatory. All staff must know that loud noises, talking, or rapid movement can sabotage the smoothest induction. Although the ambience should appear unhurried, speed is important; no child should be asked to be a hero any longer than necessary. Anything that distracts attention from the rapid induction of anesthesia once the child is present must be assiduously avoided.

The induction should be begun using 70% N_2O by holding the mask close to, but not on, the patient's face. Storytelling or singing may calm the child. The parents may be asked to participate in this aspect of the induction, and they should be encouraged to be in physical contact with the child. Older children may be encouraged to hold their own masks. The child may be allowed to sit on the operating table initially, then lowered to a supine position as he or she loses consciousness. Although it may seem less threatening to begin the induction with the child held in the parent's lap, the potential for airway obstruction when the child is not in a position for optimal airway management is worrisome. Monitoring of the healthy child 6 months of age or older during mask induction may be limited to a precordial stethoscope until the child is stunned, after which the pulse oximeter probe, ECG leads, and blood pressure cuff may be applied. The process of applying these monitors should not distract the anesthesiologist's attention from the child, and primary focus should be on breath sounds and respiratory pattern, heart sounds, and color.

The liberal, prolonged use of N_2O should be encouraged. The most common error in an inhalational induction is a too-rapid introduction of anesthetic vapors. They all stink, they are all pungent, and they all irritate. Three to five minutes of 70% N_2O inhibits smell and taste and allows a smooth introduction of the potent agent. In addition, N_2O induces a calm, playful, often laughing child, to the relief of the child, parents, operating room staff, and anesthesiologist. It also anesthetizes a child so that stage II can be rapidly traversed once the potent agent is introduced. The time spent (3 to 5 minutes) with N_2O is worthwhile by avoiding the agitation, fear, coughing, and patient resistance that may occur if the potent agent is introduced too early. Although mask inductions may be satisfactory and rewarding for most children requiring elective surgery, there are exceptions. Children undergoing urgent surgery, those with full stomachs, or those unable to tolerate inhalational induction may require IV or IM induction.

The major complication that occurs during inhalational induction is airway obstruction. As the patient becomes progressively anesthetized, airway tone is lost. The tongue and pharyngeal muscles, large tonsils, and floppy epiglottis may all obstruct the airway. A simple jaw thrust with extension often removes this obstruction in small children. In infants, care must be taken not to overextend the neck, which may actually cause airway obstruction. An oral or nasal airway should remove any residual upper airway obstruction.

The other major cause of airway obstruction is laryngospasm. Airway irritability is enhanced during stage II of an inhalation induction. Sudden, absolute glottic closure can occur. Corrective measures should be rapidly undertaken. Positive airway pressure from 10 to 20 cm H_2O pressure may help and should be maintained. If the laryngospasm has not improved within seconds or if saturation is falling, succinylcholine should be administered, mask ventilation used to restore oxygenation, and the airway intubated. Attempts to intubate without paralysis are dangerous and likely to be futile. Patients with upper respiratory infections and increased secretions are at greater risk for laryngospasm. Elective procedures should be postponed in these patients.

Halothane has been the preferred agent for inhalational induction because of its less pungent odor and lower degree of airway irritation compared with enflurane and especially isoflurane. The halothane is started at 0.5% and increased in 0.5% increments every 3 to 4 breaths up to 4% if the patient remains hemodynamically stable. When the patient is sufficiently under anesthesia, an IV catheter is placed if one is required for the surgical procedure. Although enflurane, isoflurane, and desflurane have lower solubility than halothane and theoretically are less blood soluble than halothane and offer the advantage of faster induction and emergence, their greater irritation of the airways causes a higher incidence of coughing and laryngospasm compared with halothane for inhalational induction.[53,131,184]

Sevoflurane has replaced halothane for inhalational induction in Japan. If cost were not a consideration, it would likely do so in the Western hemisphere. Extensive studies have shown that 7% sevoflurane with N_2O results in smooth and rapid induction of anesthesia ($\leq$ 4 breaths) with excellent intubating conditions and less cardiovascular depression than halothane.[132] Some practitioners induce with sevoflurane then switch to a lower-cost agent for the remainder of the anesthetic, but the continued use of sevoflurane results in faster emergence and shorter time to discharge from postanesthesia care unit.[120] Like desflurane, however, the rapid emergence may be associated with agitation or delirium in children. The resulting requirement for sedation may negate the rapid emergence advantages of sevoflurane and result in prolonged recovery time.[72]

Some children, especially those 4 to 6 years of age, may display great bravado with regard to the mask when they are in the induction area. These children are frequently concealing great fear, or they may sense parental anxiety. They may lose control when faced with the actual induction process in the operating room. These children may be quickly anesthetized with a "single-breath" halothane induction by flooding the circuit with 4% halothane in 70% N_2O and 30% O_2 and applying the mask to the face.[140] Induction time is decreased to 2 minutes, and the excitement stage is considerably shortened. The halothane concentration may then be reduced to 2% to 3% and regulated according to blood pressure, pulse, respiratory pattern, and the patient's response to stimulation. In this situation, some practitioners would prefer to proceed with an IM induction. This may be necessary especially in children too strong to hold down for the time required for them to go to sleep with this rapid-inhalational technique.

Infants less than 6 months of age may easily accept a nurse in place of the parent for comfort in the operating room. The incidence of airway complications is higher in this age group; therefore, parents of children in this age group may be asked to separate from them outside the operating room. The infant may be allowed to suck on the lower edge of the mask or a pacifier while breathing the anesthetic gas mixture through the nose. Because most infants this age are nose breathers, this presents no problem as long as the nose is not congested or otherwise obstructed. The pacifier may be removed and the mask placed more firmly on the infant's face after the child is calmed by 2 to 3 minutes of the 70% N_2O mixture.

Intramuscular induction

IM induction may be chosen for those children who: (1) are uncooperative or unresponsive to psychologic preparation (mental retardation); (2) lose control during attempted inhalational induction; (3) become agitated

rather than sedated after premedication; or (4) require rapid-sequence induction but have no venous access.

The most frequently used drug for IM induction is ketamine (8 to 10 mg/kg, 10% solution). It should be combined with atropine (0.02 mg/kg) to reduce secretions and may be administered in the same syringe with succinylcholine (4 mg/kg) for rapid-sequence induction. A smaller dose of ketamine (2 to 3 mg/kg) may be used to calm children who are uncooperative for subsequent mask induction or IV catheter placement. When the larger dose of ketamine is used for the induction of anesthesia, prolonged emergence with the necessity of maintaining postoperative intubation may occur after short surgical procedures. On the other hand, because of its superior analgetic properties only N_2O needs to be administered concomitantly for short procedures. In addition to atropine, a small dose of midazolam (0.05 mg/kg) should be administered IV to ameliorate any emergence delirium caused by the ketamine. This emergence delirium occurs more often in older children.

Methohexital (5%) may also be used for IM induction.[42,111] A dose of 10 mg/kg has been used both for induction of anesthesia and for sedation during nonpainful procedures (e.g., radiotherapy, CT scans, arteriograms). The large volume required may lead to a high incidence of postoperative pain at the injection site, and it is recommended that methohexital be given as a deep IM injection. IM methohexital is associated with a much quicker recovery than IM ketamine.

Complications of IM induction include pain at the injection site, sterile abscess formation, and unpredictable uptake of drug from tissue, especially in patients with decreased peripheral perfusion.

Rectal induction

Children between the age when they first develop separation fears (about 8 months of age) and the "age of reason" (5 to 6 years of age) are frequently poor candidates for smooth mask induction. These children are at greatest risk for long-lasting psychologic effects from their experience in the operating room. In addition, the child's inability to comprehend or cooperate may increase the anxiety of the parent who views a "brutal" inhalational induction. Children in this age group, if healthy, are ideal candidates for rectal induction of anesthesia. The use of the rectal route is usually well accepted because it is similar to "taking a temperature," it avoids both mask and needle, and the child may fall asleep peacefully in the parent's arms in the induction area, with no memory of struggle in the operating room. After the drug is administered, the anesthesiologist must continuously observe the child for signs of airway obstruction, coughing, and apnea until the child is asleep and ready to be taken into the operating room. On transfer to the operating table, primary attention should be devoted to the maintenance of a patent airway and deepening the level of anesthesia by mask while an assistant or nurse attends to monitor placement.

Thiopental, methohexital, and ketamine have all been used for rectal induction (see Table 79-2). Rectal administration of anesthetic agents is associated with a 10% to 15% incidence of defecation, which usually does not interfere with the onset of sleep. The parent's lap should be protected by a waterproof pad placed beneath the child. Drugs are administered via syringe through a 14-French suction catheter that has been lubricated and cut to 10 cm in length. A volume of air is instilled from the syringe to flush all the agent from the catheter into the rectum, and the parent holds the child's buttocks together for 2 minutes to encourage retention of the medication.

Methohexital is the most frequently used rectal induction agent. It has been traditionally administered as a 10% solution, but Forbes and Vandewalker[54] have demonstrated that using the same milligram per kilogram dose of a 2% solution is associated with higher blood levels and slightly faster induction times. The likely reason for the higher blood levels is that a larger area of mucosa is available for drug absorption. Recently, administration of 25 mg/kg of a 1% methohexital solution has been shown to have a faster induction time (6 minutes).[90] Using a more dilute solution may also be advantageous because rectally administered 10% methohexital has been shown to cause mucosal inflammation and ulceration in mice, and some children who receive the drug complain that their bottom burns. Thiopental (40 mg/kg, 2.5% solution) may be administered in a manner similar to that described for methohexital, and the time course for induction is similar. In children taking phenobarbital for seizure control, the dose of rectally administered barbiturate to induce sleep may need to be increased because of hepatic enzyme induction and increased first-pass metabolism.

Ketamine (10 mg/kg, 5% solution) may be used as described for methohexital, but may be associated with prolonged emergence from anesthesia. It also has been used in combination with rectal diazepam (0.5 mg/kg).[84]

MUSCLE RELAXANTS

Much has been learned about the developmental aspects of the neuromuscular junction and neuromuscular function.[70] Differences occur in the density and sensitivity of the postsynaptic acetylcholine receptor, in the rapidity of neuromuscular transmission, and in muscle fiber type.[63,102] Also, because differing distribution of cardiac output and inherent differences in muscle tone exist between adults and infants, numerous studies have failed to yield consistent answers to the question of whether infants are more sensitive to neuromuscular blockade than adults.[30] Another underlying factor that may also confound these data is that at equal end-tidal inhalational anesthetic concentrations, muscle concentrations of anesthetics may differ. Because all inhalational anesthetics partly potentiate the effect of neuromuscular blockade, at equal end-tidal alveolar anesthetic concentrations, the effect of neuromuscular blockade may demonstrate developmental differences. Clearly, studies that compare the effect of neuromuscular blockade in neonates, infants, and adults must control many variables.

Physiologically, the neonatal response to tetanic stimulation appears to fade more rapidly than that in adults.[30] This may have some impact on the assessment of neuromuscular function. Synaptic transmission also appears to be slower in neonates than in adults.[62] The underlying physiologic differences and varying methodologic approaches have made it difficult to determine the exact mechanism of these underlying differences. **Most recent studies, especially those by Fisher et al.[52] which closely control these methodologic differences, appear to indicate that neonates do have increased sensitivity to nondepolarizing neuromuscular-blocking agents but require the same dose when indexed to body surface area because of their larger volume of distribution.** This complex situation basically has led to an empiric approach to assessing the need for neuromuscular blockade in pediatric anesthesia. Somewhat surprisingly, the newer nondepolarizing muscle relaxants (e.g., vecuronium) seem to demonstrate the greatest developmental difference.[51]

Neuromuscular-Blocking Agents

Long-acting, nondepolarizing neuromuscular agents have been the cornerstone of neonatal anesthesia. The ability to provide immobility, ideal intubating conditions, and controlled ventilation, thus ensuring adequate oxygenation and CO_2 removal as well as optimal surgical conditions, while at the same time not requiring potentially hazardous concentrations of inhalational anesthetics, has improved the safety and efficacy of neonatal anesthesia. The difficulty in controlling potent inhalational anesthetics and the low margin of safety between cardiorespiratory depression and MAC has been largely overcome by the use of neuromuscular blockade.

Until recently, N_2O, O_2, and muscle relaxation were the standard approach for neonatal anesthesia. This allowed maximal cardiorespiratory stability and optimal surgical conditions. Unfortunately, it did not always provide sufficient analgesia, and whether consciousness was obtunded and amnesia secured was problematic.[4] Currently, this technique is often supplemented with small amounts of potent inhalational agents (below 0.5%) to provide adequate analgesia, hemodynamic stability, and amnesia. Alternatively, supplementation of the paralysis using an N_2O/O_2 technique with narcotics such as fentanyl has increasingly replaced the use of inhalation agents and provides remarkable hemodynamic stability.[137]

Pancuronium. The most widely used long-acting neuromuscular-blocking agent in pediatric anesthesia practice today is pancuronium bromide, mainly because of its vagolytic effect and its recognized release of catecholamines.[19,141] This generally leads to an increased heart rate in small infants and children. This is beneficial for two reasons: (1) cardiac output in children is, as mentioned, sensitive to changes in heart rate, and the best way to increase output and maintain blood pressure is to increase heart rate. Therefore, pancuronium provides a protective effect; (2) inhalational agents tend to decrease heart rate, and therefore the combination of a vagolytic agent with an inhalational anesthetic is complementary in providing hemodynamic stability.[8,124] This tachycardic effect may be unpredictable and occasionally difficult to manage, and marked tachycardias may be seen in children after the administration of pancuronium.[19,141]

The recommended dose for pancuronium bromide during halothane/N_2O is 0.1 mg/kg, although 0.06 mg/kg provides a 95% reduction in twitch height.[69] For intubation, 0.15 mg/kg provides a rapid, smooth onset of muscle relaxation. Doses in this range have a duration of effect from 50 to 70 minutes. This duration is quite variable. Neonates who have been receiving pancuronium over time appear to have some degree of tachyphylaxis and may require doses as frequently as every 30 minutes.[66] This variability necessitates neuromuscular blockade monitoring when using this potent neuromuscular relaxing agent. The onset of action of pancuronium has been reported as ranging from 1.5 to 3 minutes.[69] Doses of 0.15 to 0.2 mg/kg in neonates have a much more rapid onset, and optimal intubating conditions may be reached within 30 to 45 seconds, rivaling the onset of succinylcholine in these large doses.[32] Pancuronium is an ideal neuromuscular-blocking agent for prolonged paralysis in neonates and older children. Difficulty with reversibility after prolonged paralysis can be overcome.[8] After many weeks, an effect on neuromuscular function, similar to disease atrophy, may occur, and then slow weaning from mechanical ventilation may be required.[142]

***d*-Tubocurarine.** Much experience has been accumulated with the use of *d*-tubocurarine (curare) in infants and young children.[157] As previously mentioned, the neonate is more sensitive to curare but has a greater volume of distribution, and therefore, the dosage requirements appear to be the same.[51] Curare releases histamine and is associated with hypotension in infants and children just as in adults. The absence of a vagolytic effect and thus support of heart rate makes curare a rarely used drug in neonatal and infant anesthesia today. In this age group, its use has been virtually supplanted by pancuronium. Use of curare in older children during inhalational anesthesia is not accompanied with the same tachycardia seen with pancuronium. In general, because of vasodilatory and nontachydysrhythmic effects, heart rate and blood pressure are generally lower at equipotent concentrations of anesthetic agents than with pancuronium.[125] This fact may be used to advantage if hypotension is desired, and thus curare is a useful adjunct to hypotensive anesthesia for major orthopedic and neurosurgical procedures. These hypotensive effects of curare have become less troublesome as intraoperative monitoring has improved. The ability to closely monitor blood pressure and heart rate intraoperatively lessens the risk of undetected hypotension with curare.

Vecuronium. Vecuronium is a steroidal neuromuscular relaxing agent similar to pancuronium and has relatively few cardiac effects.[127] No change in heart rate or blood pressure seems to occur with vecuronium administration in all age groups. This may tend to decrease its usefulness in neonatal anesthesia; however, in older children, vecuronium is becoming established as a useful neuromuscular-blocking agent. The usefulness of vecuronium arises from its somewhat shorter action than pancuronium and curare in children.[106] These advantages disappear in infants, in whom the duration of blockade and recovery time are quite prolonged compared with those of older children and adults.[51,68] The duration of effect of vecuronium from time of injection to 90% recovery was 73 minutes in infants, 35 minutes in older children, and 53 minutes in adults.[51,105,108] The use of vecuronium for short surgical procedures in children over 2 years of age has become increasingly popular.

Rocuronium. Rocuronium is a steroidal, nondepolarizing muscle relaxant similar to vecuronium. It differs from vecuronium by being less potent and inducing a quicker onset of paralysis. Bolus administration of 0.6 mg/kg results in complete neuromuscular blockade and good intubating conditions in 50 and 80 seconds in infants and children, respectively. A dose of 0.8 mg/kg reduced the time to paralysis to an average of 30 seconds.[128] This rapid onset of action associated with minimal hemodynamic effects makes rocuronium an excellent alternative to succinylcholine for rapid-sequence intubation in children. The duration of action (time to reversibility of neuromuscular blockade [T25]) is prolonged in infants when compared with children 1 to 5 years of age (45 vs. 27 minutes after a dose of 0.6 mg/kg) and is similar to what is seen with vecuronium. The duration of action of the 0.8 mg/kg dose is prolonged further, being greater than 60 minutes in infants and 45 minutes in children. **Caution should be exercised when using rocuronium for rapid-sequence induction when thiopental is the induction agent. Rocuronium, like pancuronium and vecuronium, will precipitate and form a concretion in the IV line if the line is not flushed with fluid between the administration of pentothal and the relaxant. This can result in loss of the IV in the middle of the induction—a potential disaster.**

Atracurium. Atracurium is a shorter-acting anesthetic agent with a slower onset of paralysis than the other nondepolarizing anesthetics and a shorter duration of action.[48] Neonates are particularly sensitive to atracurium.[64] The median effective dose (ED_{50}) for atracurium is the least in neonates, followed by children and adolescents.[16] An ED_{95} dose of atracurium appears to last 25 to 35 minutes, making it useful for shorter surgical procedures in older children. The ED_{95} of atracurium appears to vary from 0.3 mg/kg in neonates to 0.5 mg/kg in older children.[14,116] Histamine release also occurs, although this has not been reported to be a problem in infants and neonates.[71] Atracurium is eliminated by Hoffman degradation, which releases laudanosine. This has been reported to lower the seizure threshold in older patients,[48] but has not been a problem in pediatric anesthesia. Because of the novel method of elimination of atracurium, its use in patients with renal or hepatic impairment is recommended. It does not rely on hepatic metabolism or renal excretion for its termination of its action. The decreased renal clearance (in neonates compared with adults) of other nondepolarizing muscle relaxants (e.g., vecuronium, pancuronium, or curare) may account for their longer duration of action. On the other hand, recovery from atracurium blockade does not appear to change with age.[14,43,116]

Mivacurium. Mivacurium is distinguished from other nondepolarizing muscle relaxants by its unique metabolism, which results in its short duration of action. The drug is metabolized by plasma cholinesterase. Because of this, the action of mivacurium is terminated by metabolism and reversal of its neuromuscular blockade by cholinesterase inhibitors is unnecessary (and may indeed prolong its action).[148]

The ED_{95} of mivacurium in infants and children is 85 and 95 μg/kg respectively.[179,180] The usual dose recommended for intubation is 0.2 mg/kg (approximately twice the ED_{95}). Use of this dose will not usually result in a rapid attainment of intubating conditions satisfactory for rapid-sequence intubation. Increasing the dose to 0.4 mg/kg will result in adequate intubating conditions almost as rapidly as succinylcholine, but at this dose there is a high incidence of mild-to-moderate hypotension caused by histamine release, similar to that seen with *d*-tubocurarine and atracurium. Its use for rapid sequence should be limited to patients who are hemodynamically stable and volume replete. Recovery (T25) from the 0.2-mg/kg dose of mivacurium is extremely rapid, and as with other relaxants, is faster in infants than in children (6.3 vs. 10 minutes, respectively). The use of the 0.4-mg/kg dose approximately doubles the duration.

Mivacurium may be given by continuous infusion, at a dose of approximately 8 to 18 μg/kg/min. Infants and children require a higher infusion rate than adults because their larger volume of distribution is associated with a faster effective clearance of the drug. No matter the duration of the infusion, spontaneous recovery will normally occur approximately 10 to 15 minutes after cessation of the infusion if a neuromuscular blockade monitor is used to maintain one twitch in the train-of-four during infusion.[15,107] If plasma cholinesterase activity is decreased (genetic, liver disease), the duration of action of mivacurium will be prolonged, as has been shown in adults.[22,67]

Other new neuromuscular-blocking agents, such as doxacurium and pipecuronium, are currently under investigation in pediatric patients. They confirm that dose, duration, and potency show significant developmental difference in children.[133,147]

Succinylcholine. Succinylcholine is the only clinically used depolarizing muscle relaxant.[39] In children less than 1 year of age, 2 mg/kg is the recommended dose. Other experts have suggested even higher doses in neonates.[104] This is almost certainly caused by an increased volume of distribution, despite decreased pseudocholinesterase activity in infants. Complete, reliable muscle relaxation occurs within 90 seconds. Recovery starts to occur within 5 to 7 minutes and is complete within 10 to 15 minutes.[39] In general, children appear to have a shorter duration of action with succinylcholine than do adults.[104] Succinylcholine may also be administered IM in doses of 4 to 5 mg/kg; reliable muscle relaxation occurs within 4 to 7 minutes. One should remember that when the dose has been administered IM, the effect is quite prolonged and 20 to 30 minutes should be allowed before complete recovery is expected. In an emergency situation when IV access is not available, succinylcholine can be administered intraosseously quite effectively or into a muscle with high blood flow, such as intralingually.[99] In a patient with a full stomach, rapid-sequence intubation, cricoid pressure, and gentle manual ventilation may be required to avoid serious hypoxemia following IM administration of succinylcholine due to its relatively slow onset.

Many side effects from succinylcholine occur in children. The increased sensitivity to the vagal effects of succinylcholine, with profound bradycardia and asystole occasionally occurring in children, is a major concern.[103] The administration of atropine is generally recommended even before the first administration of succinylcholine because of its propensity for causing vagally induced dysrhythmias.[100] This occurs infrequently after the first dose, but it does happen.[26] **A repeat dose of succinylcholine is virtually always associated with a decreased heart rate and is likely to cause a profound bradycardia and subsequent hypotension. Succinylcholine should never be used without atropine being immediately available, and a second dose should never be administered without atropine given beforehand.** IV atropine is required to abrogate these effects; IM premedication with atropine is less efficacious. Atropine is not apparently as critical when succinylcholine is administered IM.[78]

The occurrence of fasciculations with succinylcholine has been reported to be less of a problem in children than in adults.[18] Clinical observations, however, show that fasciculations occur occasionally even in young infants and that children over 2 years of age virtually always demonstrate fasciculations when careful observation is practiced. These fasciculations are also associated with increases in intraocular and intragastric pressures.

Infants have approximately half of the plasma pseudocholinesterase activity of older children and adults.[115] Pseudocholinesterase deficiency occurs as a genetic defect or in liver disease and may significantly prolong the activity of succinylcholine. Also, atypical enzymes occur that may result in the normal dibucaine number but inadequate hydrolysis of succinylcholine, therefore prolonging its activity, and may lead to prolonged paralysis following succinylcholine use.[130,171]

Rhabdomyolysis, myoglobinuria, myoglobinemia, renal injury, hyperkalemia, masseter spasm, and pulmonary edema are all concerns with the use of succinylcholine in children.[23,113,143] Malignant hyperthermia (see Chapter 94) is a significant concern in pediatric anesthesia and may be seen more frequently in children because of the routine use of inhalational anesthetics and succinylcholine.[55] The incidence of life-threatening hyperkalemia in children with neuromuscular disease precludes the use of succinylcholine in burned[150] or traumatized[56] children and in those with muscle diseases,[6,89] although apparently not in those with cerebral palsy.[36] All these complications have called into question the routine use of succinylcholine in children.[34]

The previously unrestricted use of succinylcholine for virtually every intubation in pediatric anesthesia has largely been abandoned.[34] ET intubation can be equally safely facilitated after an inhalational or IV induction in children by the use of nondepolarizing muscle relaxants, with sufficient care to provide ventilation when awaiting full onset of paralysis before intubation. This method may take a few minutes longer for routine anesthesia, but surgical muscle relaxation is achieved concomitantly. It should be a general practice, when muscle relaxation is planned as part of the anesthesia, to use a nondepolarizing agent for intubation rather than succinylcholine. This is somewhat more problematic when a rapid-sequence intubation may be required. In infants, the options include an awake intubation or the use of a 0.2-mg/kg IV bolus of pancuronium, which has an onset of action only slightly longer than that of succinylcholine.[32] In older children, awake intubation can be extremely difficult, and application of the priming principles or administration of a large dose of nondepolarizing agent may be effectively used. Nevertheless, succinylcholine, despite its risks, still remains the most rapid way to ensure muscle relaxation and ideal intubating circumstances when speed is essential. Weighing the potential risks and benefits for the use of succinylcholine is increasingly limiting its use to the emergency and rapid-sequence situation.

Reversal of Neuromuscular Blockade

Widespread use of prolonged nondepolarizing neuromuscular blockade in pediatric anesthesia necessitates familiarity with the principles of antagonism of neuromuscular blockade.[66,146] **Virtually every child who is to be extubated and is expected to maintain spontaneous ventilation independently and who has received nondepolarizing neuromuscular blockade should have the blockade antagonized or reversed at the end of the procedure.** This is especially true in infants and small children, in whom it has been demonstrated that the duration of neuromuscular blockade can be quite variable and prolonged. Reversal of blockade in children who are hypothermic (less than 35.5° C) also can be quite difficult.[125] There are essentially only two neuromuscular blockade–reversing agents from which to choose: neostigmine and edrophonium. Both agents have their proponents. Neostigmine has the advantage of being a familiar agent with time-honored use, whereas many experts report that edrophonium has a much more rapid onset, thus allowing quicker reversal of neuromuscular blockade.

The time for 50% reversal of neuromuscular blockade from a continuous curare infusion differs between adults and children.[49] In infants and children, 15 μg/kg of neostigmine were effective to produce a 50% antagonism, whereas in adults 23 μg/kg were required. The time to 70% antagonism of the blockade was 5 to 8 minutes. The duration of antagonism appeared to be equally long in all age groups. Similarly, the ED_{50} of edrophonium was found to be 145 μg/kg in infants, 233 μg/kg in children, and 128 μg/kg in adults.[50] The volume of distribution appeared to be similar in all age groups; however, the elimination half-life was shorter in infants than in the other groups. In infants, the duration of block reversal with edrophonium was shorter and the onset slower than that in adults. This tends to limit the use of edrophonium, making the use of this drug less attractive in infants than in older children and adults. In older children, the onset of action of edrophonium occurred within 1 minute. It has also been reported that when complete antagonism occurred, no differences were seen in the level of antagonism 10 minutes after the agents were administered. These data suggest that either neuromuscular reversal agent is equally effective and that use may be guided by other factors, such as personal preference and cost.[93] The recommended dose ranges are 35 to 70 μg/kg for neostigmine and 0.5 to 1.0 mg/kg for edrophonium.

Not surprisingly, both edrophonium and neostigmine have a significant vagomimetic effect, and this always should be antagonized by the administration of atropine. It is recommended that the atropine precede the reversal agent. For neostigmine, a somewhat larger dose of atropine is required—15 to 30 μg/kg. For edrophonium, 10 to 20 μg/kg is the appropriate dose.[28] No dose less than 0.15 mg should ever be administered to any child, because paradoxic bradycardia can occur at a lower dosage.

TEMPERATURE MAINTENANCE

As discussed in Chapter 25, thermal protection for the child undergoing surgery cannot be stressed too strongly. The usual cold, dry atmosphere of operating rooms is ideal for increasing both heat and evaporative losses. Further, the naked, exposed, immobile child undergoing surgery loses heat rapidly, even in an environment that may be too warm for their adult caregivers. Every means of decreasing heat and water loss intraoperatively must be used, as outlined in Table 79-3. Each of these approaches to maintain the child's thermal integrity should be considered and effectively employed. Although this is critical in premature and newborn infants, it is also important in older children and adults.

The use of warmed, humidified gases, apart from addressing a major source of heat loss intraoperatively, also minimizes difficulty with secretions, plugged ET tubes, atelectasis, dried airways, and mucosal damage.[10] A variety of flow-over, warm water humidifiers are available for operating room use and should be considered for every pediatric patient. Warming a child with a hot water pad to decrease conductive losses is essential for all children under 5 years of age. Maintaining this circulating water at 37° C and ensuring that it is in contact with the child's bare skin contribute significantly to temperature protection. Constant attention to keeping the child covered whenever possible and, if necessary, especially in infants and smaller children, using plastic wrap or bags for the limbs and head are worthwhile.[152] Maintaining the ambient humidity greater than 80% decreases evaporative losses dramatically. In addition, maintaining the room temperature at 22° to 25° C will decrease convective, conductive, and radiant heat loss.

Table 79-3 Heat loss in children

Problem	Solution
Respiratory heat loss	Heated, humidified inspiratory gases
Conductive heat loss	Thermally padded operating room table with circulating water water
Convective heat loss	Patient covered (plastic or bubble wrap); reflective coverings; warmed, ambient environment
Radiant heat loss	Operating room drapes, warmed environment
Wound losses	Intestines wrapped in warm, wet sponges; warmed irrigation solutions used

MONITORING

Standards for intraoperative monitoring of adults is discussed in Chapter 40. The challenges of their smaller size and developing physiology suggest several aspects in which monitoring may differ in children. These differences do not justify decreased vigilance. Children should be as intensively monitored intraoperatively as adults.

The provision of routine monitoring (Box 79-1) is possible in all ages and all sizes of children. Automatic blood pressure monitoring systems permit accurate, continuous, automatic monitoring of blood pressure, even in the smallest baby. Core temperature can be monitored rectally, orally, esophageally, or nasally and should be monitored in every child undergoing anesthesia. Pulse oximetry is a standard means of care for all anesthetized children.[25]

For long procedures, surgery during which blood loss may be excessive, and when cardiorespiratory disease is present, invasive hemodynamic monitoring may be indicated

BOX 79-1
ROUTINE MONITORING OF CHILDREN

Precordial stethoscope	Inspired O_2 tension (FIO_2)
Breath sounds	Temperature
Heart sounds	Cardiogram
Color	Blood pressure
Perfusion status	Oxygen saturation

BOX 79-2
ANCILLARY MONITORING OF CHILDREN

Capnography
Anesthetic vapor concentration
Urine output
Invasive monitoring

(Box 79-2). Arterial lines should be considered for all surgery in premature infants. Twenty-four-gauge catheters can be inserted in even the smallest premature infant's arteries. Central venous pressure (CVP) monitoring can also be readily achieved; catheters are available for even the smallest child. The compliance of the child's heart and the responsiveness of the circulatory system, however, generally make CVP monitoring a poor indicator of volume status. Nevertheless, access to the central circulation is useful if severe cardiorespiratory compromise is present or large blood loss is anticipated. Urine output measurement, to continually assess renal perfusion, is essential for lengthy procedures.

The advent of improved capnometry allows CO_2 sampling even in small children. In-line capnometry is of value in circle systems but is less useful when using Mapleson D systems. Aspiration techniques are available and can be used in children, but their interpretation must compensate for the withdrawal flow. ET tubes are designed with catheter adapters, which can be inserted through the lumen of the ET tube, or the sampling catheter may be integral to the ET tube lumen. This allows distal sampling for accurate end-tidal CO_2 monitoring. The addition of inhalational agent monitoring via several techniques, including Raman spectroscopy, has permitted closer monitoring of end-tidal CO_2 inspired and expired O_2 tension and anesthetic vapor concentration.

No justification exists for undermonitoring children.[177] These patients deserve the same level of monitoring as adults and frequently require that monitoring be more meticulous. **The hemodynamic status in children may be well compensated until severe hypovolemia occurs, and blood pressure may then rapidly and catastrophically fall, accompanied with decreasing heart rate. The infant's and child's heart is quite sensitive to hypoxia and hypotension, and bradycardia may frequently herald a cardiorespiratory catastrophe and should never be ignored.**

FLUID MANAGEMENT

Children undergoing routine elective surgery and anesthesia who have fasted preoperatively will have a mild fluid deficit. Children who have greater fluid deficits and require emergency surgery should be resuscitated as much as possible preoperatively to achieve a normal heart rate, blood pressure, peripheral perfusion, and skin turgor. This can be assessed by inspection of the mucous membranes, ocular tension, and anterior fontanelle tension in younger infants. Every effort should be made to ensure adequate volume status and hemodynamic stability before the induction of anesthesia. A few minutes spent preoperatively resuscitating critically ill children may avoid cardiovascular collapse on induction of anesthesia. When this cannot be done, replacement of deficit should be an ongoing priority in the child's surgical management.

The average child requires per day 1500 ml/m^2 H_2O, 2 to 4 mEq/kg of sodium, 1 to 3 mEq/kg of potassium, and 3 to 5 mEq/kg of chloride. This routine maintenance fluid is approximated by an estimate of maintenance fluid requirements on a weight basis (Table 79-4). For healthy children, this maintenance fluid could be in the form of a 5% glucose-containing solution and 0.25 to 0.5 normal saline. If surgery is prolonged (longer than 4 to 6 hours), determination of the child's glucose concentration and electrolytes is indicated.[110]

Routine replacement maintenance fluids for the fasting period in general consists of half this fluid being replaced in the first 1 to 2 hours of surgery while continuing to give maintenance fluid and replace ongoing losses. Calculating the deficits, the maintenance needs, and the losses frequently gives a greater volume of fluid than is necessary to maintain adequate heart rate and blood pressure in a child. However, any sign of hemodynamic instability, decreased urine output, tachycardia, borderline hypotension, or decreased perfusion should be initially treated with volume to be certain of restoration of all calculated needs before introducing other therapies or attributing tachycardia and hemodynamic instability to other causes. Thus the sum of deficit plus maintenance plus losses provides the bottom limit of replacement before aggressive fluid therapy or pressors are indicated intraoperatively. Replacement of losses is discussed in Chapter 25. Blood can be replaced by crystalloid solution (generally Ringer's lactate or normal saline) on a 3:1 basis. When the hematocrit is unacceptably low, blood transfusion is indicated on a milliliter-for-milliliter basis. Every attempt should be made to quantitate blood loss by the use of pediatric suction bottles, weighing sponges, and accurate estimation of blood losses in the operative field. In small children, blood removed for diagnostic purposes may

Table 79-4 Estimate of child's maintenance fluid requirements

Weight	Water per hour	Water per day
First 10 kg	4 ml/kg	100 ml/kg
10–20 kg	40 ml + 2 ml/kg > 10 kg	1000 ml + 50 ml/kg > 10 kg
> 20 kg	60 ml + 1 ml/kg > 20 kg	1500 ml + 25 ml/kg > 20 kg

make a significant contribution to blood loss; this should be limited and replaced as necessary. In infants and small children who have a blood volume that may only be several hundred milliliters, blood loss must be closely monitored and strict attention paid to fluid management.

Third-space losses must also be estimated and are generally related to the type and duration of surgery. Immobility and trauma alter the endothelium's and subendothelial tissue's ability to maintain vascular integrity. Water and salt leak into the interstitium. Even during the most trivial surgery, this third-space loss can be 1 to 3 ml/kg/hour. When more extensive surgery is undertaken, greater loss can be expected. Thoracotomy can be associated with losses of 3 to 5 ml/kg/hour; third-space losses during laparotomy can be associated with 5 to 7 ml/kg/hour. Large tissue exposure, large areas of tissue trauma, and handling of the bowel may increase third-space losses to 7 to 10 ml/kg/hour. These third-space losses can exceed those for maintenance fluid requirements. Although third-space fluid losses will result in postoperative edema, especially in dependent tissues, this is not the result of aggressive fluid therapy but rather is an indication for aggressive fluid therapy.

Detailed notation of fluids given and calculation of deficits and losses should be part of every anesthetic record. Postoperative fluid management may be influenced by the intraoperative fluid management, and knowledge of this should be available to the postoperative caregivers. Postoperatively, urine output, hemoglobin, and electrolyte status should be reviewed within 24 hours to assess the adequacy of intraoperative fluid management.

ANESTHETIC MANAGEMENT OF COMMON PEDIATRIC CONDITIONS

Acute Airway Obstruction

Causes of acute airway obstruction include laryngotracheobronchitis ([LTB], croup), the now rarely seen epiglottitis and foreign-object aspiration.[9] Pediatric anesthesiologists may be involved in emergent airway management and providing general anesthesia for endoscopy of these children.[35] Preoperative evaluation should include analysis of airway patency and the degree of respiratory distress; and observation for chest retractions, nasal flaring, and audible respiratory sounds consistent with obstruction. Stridor signifies airway obstruction. **Inspiratory stridor is the hallmark of upper airway, supraglottic, and glottic obstruction; whereas wheezing generally indicates intrathoracic airway obstruction.** It should be noted that this differentiation becomes blurred in younger age groups. Infants with upper airway obstruction (croup) can have prolonged expiration and audible wheezes, whereas infants with intratracheal foreign objects may have inspiratory stridor. Examination of the child's level of consciousness, respiratory rate and pattern, perfusion and color, as well as oxygen saturation by pulse oximetry, give an indication of the severity of respiratory distress. It should be remembered that acute upper-airway obstruction leads to profoundly negative intrathoracic pressures. This, through increased myocardial (left ventricular) afterload, can lead to hypoperfusion and, when extreme, pulmonary edema. Indeed, most children who require ET intubation for croup have some degree of interstitial pulmonary edema.

Generally, the three causes of acute airway obstruction may be differentiated by history and physical examination (see Table 79-5).[9,27,35] The astute clinician should always be aware that one condition may masquerade as the other. With the increasing incidence of hemophilus influenza type B immunization in the community, the incidence of acute epiglottitis in children has decreased markedly.[27] Acute epiglottitis is a life-threatening airway disease which, in our opinion (especially with its increasing rareness) requires laryngoscopic confirmation. Apart from the characteristic history and physical examination, a radiograph may reveal a characteristic flattened or thickened epiglottis which is wider at its base than it is tall, or not visualized at all, with thickened aryepiglottic folds and often, hypopharyngeal air trapping. In the absence of clearcut visualization of a normal epiglottis, epiglottitis should be suspected. An x-ray is not necessary to confirm the need for laryngoscopy. Suspicion is adequate. Delay for obtaining a radiograph may prove fatal. Although cautious observation of children with epiglottitis in the pediatric intensive care unit, with the capability of rapid airway manipulation, has been recently advocated by some, we feel that this is not a safe approach for small children with epiglottitis.[9,31,183] The decreasing incidence of epiglottitis gives rise to the serious risk of missing other potentially life-threatening diagnoses. For these reasons, in suspected epiglottitis, children are taken to the operating room where they are anesthetized, their airway is secured, and they can be further evaluated.

The anesthetic management of children with epiglottitis requires the immediate availability of a physician skilled in airway management and the equipment necessary to secure an airway. Even in the most skilled hands, it is occasionally not possible to visualize the glottic opening or pass an ET tube into the trachea if the supraglottic region is severely inflamed. For this reason, anesthetic management and induction mandates the presence of an otolaryngologic surgeon

Table 79-5 Upper airway obstruction in children

	Foreign object	Croup	Epiglottitis
Etiology	Aspiration	Viral	Bacterial
Age	6 mos–5 yrs	6 mos–4 yrs	1 yr–adult
Onset	Usually acute	Days (gradual)	Hours
Dysphagia	Possible	Rare	Usual
Drooling	Possible	None	Usual
Posture	Sitting or prone	Lying or sitting	Sitting
Obstruction	Supra or subglottic	Subglottic	Supraglottic
Cough	Usually none	Barking or brassy	Muffled
Voice	Clear	Hoarse	Muffled
Respiratory rate	Normal	Rapid	Normal
Sound	Wheezing	High pitch, inspiratory stridor	Low pitched, vibratory stridor
Season	None	Winter	None

who is immediately prepared to operatively secure the airway, by performing a tracheotomy should airway patency be lost. Coordinated management during this and other airway emergencies requires prospective planning among otolaryngologists, pediatricians, and pediatric anesthesiologists.[9,35]

Anesthetic induction is classically performed by an inhalational technique.[35] Children with epiglottitis have generally been on a no oral intake status for some period of time because of the sore throat. Nevertheless, as in all febrile ill children, a full stomach may be present. Regardless, the fear of losing the airway with paralysis and being unable to ventilate or intubate overrides the concern for a full stomach. **A slow, gentle, inhalational induction followed by intubation to secure the airway, only then followed by paralysis, is the preferred approach.** Either halothane or more recently sevoflurane in oxygen can be used. Pulse oximetry, ECG, a calm environment, and careful observation of the respiratory status of the child is essential. As the child becomes increasingly obtunded, some continuous positive airway pressure, and even skillful, gently assisted ventilation will help deepen the anesthetic. An IV can be started at this time. The classic teaching is to maintain spontaneous ventilation when performing a gentle laryngoscopy with the child deeply anesthetized with halothane. In a febrile child who has suffered for some period of time with dysphagia, intravascular volume expansion will be necessary to minimize the hypotension that will result from a deep inhalational induction. Alternatively, anesthesia may be deepened with ketamine after the IV has been initiated. This will maintain spontaneous ventilation and support the blood pressure. The supraglottic structures are extremely friable, and any irritation may lead to complete airway obstruction, from laryngospasm or soft tissue swelling. For this reason, the first visualization should be performed by a skilled practitioner to optimize the likelihood of ET intubation. It is not the role of the otolaryngologist to perform either a direct or indirect laryngoscopy at this point, but rather to be on stand-by to operatively secure the airway rapidly should the need arise. If the airway is lost during induction, the situation is desperate. The surgeon should immediately prepare for a tracheostomy. The administration of succinylcholine to facilitate ventilation and intubation may be worthwhile. The anesthesiologist should attempt to visualize the aryepiglottic folds and vocal cords and intubate the trachea as quickly and atraumatically as possible.[9,35] Once the airway is secured, further examination can be performed. Some experts have advocated that these children should be nasally intubated.[27,151] It may be preferable after securing the airway to change the orotracheal tube to a nasotracheal tube to provide for comfort and tube security in the intensive care unit for the next 24 to 48 hours.[151] Antibiotics should be administered as soon as the IV is initiated. Either ampicillin and chloramphenicol or a third-generation cephalosporin, such as ceftriaxone, is recommended.[27]

With regard to acute laryngotracheobronchitis (croup) in young children, airway intubation and examination only becomes necessary in the advanced states or if intubation is prolonged. Children with croup do not often require endoscopy unless intubation is prolonged or symptoms fail to resolve. The indication for intubation of these children is airway obstruction severe or prolonged enough to lead to respiratory muscle exhaustion and failure. Because of the propensity of children to become apneic in the advanced stages of respiratory failure, hypoxia is the major concern. When the diagnosis of LTB is certain, airway intubation with a rapid-sequence technique is feasible in the intensive care unit. The supraglottic structures will appear normal, and there will be narrowing in the subglottic region. If there is some question of the diagnosis, and the otolaryngologist wishes to examine the airway, an inhalational induction is possible; however, one must remember that in small, frail infants, a "full stomach" may be present. For this reason, we would still rapidly secure the airway, empty the stomach, provide adequate paralysis, and then allow thorough endoscopic examination of the airway, if this diagnosis is in question. Children who require intubation for croup generally have a very high incidence of bacterial LTB, especially staphylococcal, which requires appropriate antibiotics.

Foreign objects in the airway frequently provide a challenge for the anesthesiologist.[9] The acute onset of airway obstruction with stridor may indicate supraglottic or glottic obstruction or lower airway obstruction with wheezing and absent breath sounds on one side. There may be a clear history of an aspiration event. Occasionally, this may have occurred days to weeks prior to presentation. If the foreign object is subglottic, examination may reveal unequal breath sounds, and unilateral hyperresonance. A chest radiograph is useful. With the child adequately oxygenated, if it is certain that the foreign object is subglottic or distal to the carina, rapid-sequence induction or ET intubation followed by bronchoscopy is indicated. If there is concern that the foreign object is supraglottic, then a rapid-sequence induction could theoretically result in complete loss of the airway with inability to intubate. Although it is controversial, many experts would perform an inhalational induction to induce a state of deep anesthesia, provide IV access, and perform gentle, upper-airway endoscopy, removing the foreign object if possible, or securing the airway and bypassing it if not. If, when securing the airway for a foreign object, airway obstruction is worsened, it may be necessary to insert an ET tube, thus, dislodging the foreign object into one or the other mainstem bronchi to provide critical oxygenation. For small infants with distal foreign objects who will require rigid bronchoscopy, a rapid-sequence induction, and intubation with muscle relaxants, are performed prior to bronchoscopy. Alternatively, the child may undergo rigid bronchoscopy with an apneic technique or using a ventilating bronchoscope. The use of steroids is controversial.

Few challenges in pediatric anesthesia are more harrowing than dealing with airway obstruction. Cautious, individually tailored patient management, and an anesthesiologist skilled at airway intubation and sensitive to the needs of children, is critical. Rarely is it as possible to convert an acutely life-threatening situation to complete resolution as when managing acute airway obstruction. Rarely are the stakes so high.

Pyloric Stenosis

Pyloric stenosis is a common (1 in 500 white patients, 1 in 2000 African American patients) newborn disease which is caused by thickening of the circular musculature of the newborn pylorus. This generally leads to gastric outflow obstruction and episodes of nonbilious, projectile vomiting. Characteristically, pyloric stenosis presents in the first-born male child, between 2 and 4 weeks of age. The diagnosis, however, may be delayed. The child then may be malnourished with several weeks' history of vomiting, presenting a further anesthesic challenge. In addition, aspiration occasionally complicates the picture. Typically, when the vomiting has been severe, hypochloremic alkalosis caused by gastric acid loss occurs. Dehydration, decreased urine output, and hypokalemia also occur. In severe cases, renal sodium conservation and paradoxic aciduria complicate the alkalosis. In general, these metabolic abnormalities can be rapidly corrected in 12 to 24 hours by IV therapy. **The emergent therapy for pyloric stenosis is to give the child no oral intake status, metabolically reconstitute the child with IV therapy (glucose, NaCl, K^+), confirm the diagnosis either by ultrasound or radiology, and perform a pyloromyotomy.**

The anesthetic considerations include correction of the metabolic abnormalities with sodium chloride and potassium and adequate rehydration to achieve hemodynamic stability. Respiratory status should be documented with chest radiograph look for pneumonia. These children have full stomachs caused by gastric outlet obstruction and often have had radiologic studies with the instillation of barium. Both inhalational induction and rapid-sequence induction have been advocated. The stomach should be aspirated prior to induction. In general, children will have a functioning IV and there are generally no anatomic airway concerns. For these reasons, we advocate rapid-sequence induction to address the concerns of a full stomach. This, of course, necessitates a practitioner familiar with the neonatal airway who can reliably secure the infant's airway. Volume restitution should have returned the child to euvolemia, and the use of sodium pentothal should not be a concern. This surgery is generally short (from 15 to 30 minutes), and the addition of a short-acting muscle relaxant, such as mivacurium or rocuronium, provides optimal surgical conditions. Anesthesia can be maintained with either inhalational anesthesia or propofol. The use of N_2O during this intra-abdominal surgery is generally not an issue, because it is a brief operation through a small incision.

Following surgery it should be possible to extubate the infant. CNS alkalosis which has been aggravated by hyperventilation intraoperatively, may result in postoperative lethargy and respiratory depression. This is less of a problem in children who have been metabolically corrected preoperatively. Postoperative pain is generally mild, and analgesia can be provided either with the instillation of local anesthesia or the use of parenteral nonsteroidal anti-inflammatory agents.

Ventricular Shunts

The anesthesia for children requiring emergent ventricular-peritoneal shunts is performed in the setting of neurologic impairment and concerns about elevated ICP. Children requiring ventricular shunts have either internal or external hydrocephalus. This may result from neonatal illness, such as intraventricular hemorrhages or meningitis leading to blockage of the aqueductus Sylvius and the lateral foramina of Luschka and Magendie, or by congenital abnormalities of the base of the skull such as an Arnold-Chiari malformation, which is so common in children with myelodysplastic syndromes as to be virtually ubiquitous. Although these ventricular shunts have radically altered the life expectancy and neurologic outcome of children with hydrocephalus, they frequently give rise to complications (e.g., obstruction, infection) leading to the need for their externalization or replacement. Acute obstruction can lead to obtundation and elevated ICP. If not readily treated, permanent neurologic injury is certain.

All children requiring shunt replacement should be thoroughly assessed for the presence of intracranial hypertension. In infants, alteration in the level of consciousness can manifest as virtually any neurologic change, from the overt dramatic onset of seizures to profound obtundation and dilated pupils. Crying, irritability, sudden personality change, sudden behavior change, sleepiness, and lethargy may all indicate elevated intracranial hypertension and a potentially life-threatening situation. These symptoms virtually always precede the dramatic onset of Cushing's triad; bradycardia, hypertension, and respiratory abnormalities (apnea). In addition, any history of vomiting in children with a ventricular shunt should be taken as an indication of elevated ICP. The triad of vomiting, obtundation, or behavioral change and sun-setting eyes (the sclera visible between the upper level of the iris and the eyelid) indicates elevated ICP. In those infants who have an open fontanelle, ICP can be directly evaluated. This should always be part of an assessment.

Even in the absence of signs of elevated ICP, it is necessary to consider that general anesthesia and alterations in the child's respiratory pattern many increase ICP in children with obstructed shunts. One should remember the continuous need for neuroresuscitation in managing children with obstructed shunts. As discussed elsewhere, the neonate and infant's cerebral blood flow (and thus ICP) directly respond to changes in P_{CO_2}. Elevations in P_{CO_2} will lead to elevations in ICP and must be avoided in managing children with elevated ICP or who are suspected of having it. **Hyperventilation is effective therapy for *acute* rises in ICP. It does this at the cost of lowering cerebral perfusion. Not all children requiring ventricular shunts should be hyperventilated, rather only those patients suspected of having elevated ICP.** Then mild hyperventilation is indicated. Hyperventilation is best reserved for those acute elevations in ICP, which are manifest by acute neurologic changes.

Adequate analgesia is also an important cornerstone in the management of elevated ICP. Adequate depth of anesthesia with either inhalational (isoflurane) or IV (fentanyl, thiopental anesthesia) agents, is necessary to prevent the elevation in ICP seen with painful stimuli and tracheal intubation.[58] Nondepolarizing neuromuscular blockade prevents coughing and bucking which can lead to transient elevations in ICP, which then may be potentially life threatening in children with obstructed shunts with preexisting elevated ICP. The use of succinylcholine in patients with elevated ICP has been controversial.[58,114] If a child is suspected of having a full stomach, a rapid-sequence induction can generally be performed safely with a sufficient dose of thiopental and IV lidocaine. When succinylcholine can be avoided, an alternative nondepolarizing agent is recommended. The duration of most shunt operations permits rapid-sequence intubation with vecuronium or rocuronium in children with normal airways and normal oxygenation.

An additional concern in children with potentially elevated ICP is maintenance of adequate mean arterial pressure. Careful attention to adequate perfusion pressure maintenance is essential in managing children with elevated ICP. Cerebral perfusion pressure is the difference between mean arterial pressure and ICP. Thus induction agents which lead to hypotension should be cautiously used. Ketamine elevates ICP, and is not recommended in this setting.[29] Children with elevated ICP may have been treated with mannitol and diuretics to lower ICP and may have decreased intravascular volume.

If there is a question of significantly elevated ICP, discussion with the neurosurgeon concerning ways to lower ICP prior to anesthesia should be undertaken. Tapping the shunt or placing a spinal needle through what is believed to be a proximally obstructed shunt may be indicated to acutely decompress the intraventricular space. If a child has become acutely obtunded and is demonstrating Cushing's triad, urgent steps should be taken to decrease ICP, including drainage of cerebrospinal fluid (CSF) prior to the induction of anesthesia.

Herniorrhaphy Repair

Herniorrhaphy is the most common surgery performed in children (after circumcision) in the United States. In children under 1 year of age, this is frequently performed as a herniorrhaphy and exploration of the contralateral side. For an elective herniorrhaphy, routine general anesthesia with inhalational or IV induction is indicated. In small infants (< 6 months of age), ET intubation and mechanical ventilation is generally indicated, even for these brief operations. This is because of their decreased FRC compared with closing volumes, fatiguability, relative difficulty to maintain the airway, and the potential for acute airway obstruction. **Although herniorrhaphy seems a minor procedure, it should be remembered that it is an intraperitoneal procedure, and that there may be traction on the spermatic cord. This can be a profound stimulus which, in the unintubated airway, can lead to laryngospasm and loss of the airway.** In older children, mask anesthesia or laryngeal mask airway (LMA) are suitable alternatives. The use of nondepolarizing muscle relaxants to intubate the trachea, provide optimal surgical conditions, and minimize the use of inhalational anesthesia is routine practice. Postoperative analgesia can be provided either by a 'single-shot' caudal, a caudal-epidural catheter, ilioinguinal nerve blocks, nonsteroidal anti-inflammatory agents, or local infiltration of the wound.

Management of an acutely obstructed hernia is the same as that for any acute abdominal emergency. The patient should be treated as a full-stomach patient: a rapid-sequence IV induction and intubation is indicated. The child's stomach should be evacuated. The child should be extubated when fully awake.

Adenotonsillectomy

Adenotonsillectomy remains a common surgical procedure in children, which has been recently complicated by the trend to evaluate airway obstruction and obstructive sleep apnea.[80] Preoperative evaluation of these children should include a general physical examination. Loose or missing teeth should be noted and mentioned to the parents. Loose teeth may be extracted intraoperatively, but they should not become "missing" teeth. Evidence of airway obstruction, and a detailed history concerning snoring and apnea episodes, is essential. Episodes less than 20 seconds in duration, not accompanied by bradycardias or cyanotic spells, do not raise any special concerns.[80] Chronic airway obstruction may, with time, lead to right ventricular strain, cor pulmonale, pulmonary hypertension, and present a serious complication to anesthesiologists and the intraoperative management of these children. In extreme cases, chest radiograph, an ECG, and even an echocardiogram, may be indicated if airway obstruction is profound or prolonged. **If a sleep study demonstrates significant apneas greater than 20 seconds with desaturations to less than 90%, accompanied by changes in heart rate, then postoperative monitoring for at least 24 hours following tonsillectomy is indicated.[80] This monitoring should consist of apnea monitoring and pulse oximetry.** With the increasing trend toward outpatient adenotonsillectomies, caution needs to be exercised in screening for sleep apneas. Children with significant apnea who require monitoring, are not ideal candidates for outpatient anesthesia. Definition and agreement varies from institution to institution, but it is important for a consensus to be reached between the pulmonologist, otolaryngologist, and anesthesiologist in the management of these patients. The large majority of children requiring adenotonsillectomy can be managed on an outpatient basis and can be discharged safely.

Anesthetic induction for the majority of children requiring adenotonsillectomy can be either inhalational or IV, and may follow preinduction sedation. Inhalational inductions are generally smooth; an IV can be started after induction and muscle relaxation used to facilitate ET intubation. A short- or intermediate-acting nondepolarizing agent is usually selected. With resumption of spontaneous breathing succinylcholine can also be used.[9] Inhalational induction in children with severe tonsillar hypertrophy and symptoms of airway obstruction may require an alternative approach. During inhalational induction in some of these children, airway reflexes will be lost, and the airway may become obstructed. As the child fails to become deeper anesthetized with the inhalational agent, airway management can become difficult, and laryngospasm may supervene. This may be resolved with gentle CPAP to maintain pharyngeal and airway patency; however, these inductions can still be quite stormy. For this reason, starting an IV and performing an IV modified rapid-sequence induction may be preferred. The airway may be much more rapidly secured with an IV induction and succinylcholine than during an inhalational induction. The obstruction is caused by a known soft tissue enlargement (the adenoid and tonsils) and the tonsillar hypertrophy should not complicate intubation performed in a routine fashion.

Maintenance anesthesia can be provided by nearly any means. There are advocates, especially in Europe, of inhalational induction, spontaneous breathing with halothane, deep extubation with the child in the tonsil position, resulting in a patient who awakens with no irritation or coughing to impair hemostasis in the immediate postoperative period.[176] In this country, most clinicians use muscle relaxation, light fentanyl narcotic analgesia (1 to 2 μg) and N_2O maintenance, followed by awake extubation.[182] Regardless of which technique is chosen, strict attention to airway patency, hemostasis, and observation until the child is thoroughly awake and in control of his or her own secretions and airway, is necessary. The "tonsil sucker" should never be used carelessly. Postoperative analgesia can be provided with a local injection of the tonsillar fossa with lidocaine or bupivacaine, postoperative narcotics, and nonsteroidal anti-inflammatories. Acetominophen and codeine combinations are useful at home.

In rare instances, secondary hemorrhage 2 to 7 days following adenotonsillectomy may occur. In general, there has been slow bleeding, thus the child may be severely anemic and volume depleted. Further, the patient may have active bleeding into an airway, while at the same time have blood in the stomach. Thus, the child presents hemodynamic compromise with a full stomach and is at risk for aspiration of blood and gastric contents.[9] Frequently, no IV is present. Bleeding may also be quite brisk and shock may supervene. Obviously, intraoperative management necessitates intravascular access. An IV must be started with volume restitution and blood transfusion, as indicated by the child's general condition, hematocrit, and hemodynamic status. After the child is adequately volume resuscitated, a rapid-sequence induction is necessary to avoid aspiration. All preparations are critical. Good free-flowing IV access should be ensured. There should be two large-bore suction catheters available, extra laryngoscope blades, and multiple sizes of ET tubes that are styletted and lubricated. The airway may be difficult to manage. Swelling, clots, crusts, scarring, and retained secretions may obstruct the view of the larynx. Everyone in the operating theater should be aware of the gravity of the situation. Laryngeal distortion is unlikely, and the obstructions to visualizing the vocal cords can be readily removed with adequate suction, which must always be on hand. The child may bleed briskly at this stage, and the airway should be rapidly secured, probably with a cuffed ET tube. Adequate intravascular resuscitation must be ensured. It may even be necessary to use type-specific or uncrossed matched or O Rh negative blood, in cases of profound hemodynamic instability. Few emergencies are more harrowing than a hypotensive patient with a bleeding tonsil. If vascular access is difficult, either central access with an internal jugular or subclavian line is indicated, or in extreme circumstances, resuscitation by a intraosseous needle approach. When possible the child should be preoxygenated and atropine administered prior to induction. Consideration of the use of ketamine in hemodynamically compromised patients is wise. Following airway intubation the child's gastric contents should be suctioned through a large-bore tube. After hemostasis is ensured, the child may be extubated when fully awake.

CONCLUSION

Pediatric anesthesia is guided by the child's development. Confidence, flexibility, and concern for the child and family are essential. The principles discussed apply to all anesthetics used for children and should be reviewed for every child. Application of appropriate techniques, drugs, and approaches to each child will minimize the trauma for the child and maximize the rewards for the anesthesiologist.

KEY POINTS

- The unique physiologic characteristics of children require familiarity with equipment specifically designed for anesthetizing them, including masks, airways, and breathing circuits.
- Expertise with maintenance of the airway and mask ventilation is critical in the anesthetic management of children.
- Uncuffed, appropriately sized ET tubes, with an air leak of 10 to 30 cm of water pressure when inserted, are required for ET intubation in children less than 8 years of age.
- Many specialized laryngoscope blades have been designed for pediatric use; however, in general, a Miller 0 or 1 blade is sufficient for neonates and infants and a MacIntosh 2 or 3 blade for older children.
- Management of the difficult pediatric airway requires differentiation between an airway that is difficult to ventilate and one that is difficult to intubate. The ability to recognize a difficult-to-intubate airway is essential and relies on recognition of common patterns of malformation.
- Significant developmental differences in anesthetic uptake and distribution determined by alveolar ventilation, cardiac output, distribution of cardiac output, and partition coefficients underlie basic understanding of inhalational anesthesia in pediatrics. MAC varies with age, reaching a peak within the first few months of life and declining until senescence except for a small peripubertal rise.
- Halothane has the largest margin of safety, is the most familiar to use, causes the least amount of airway irritation, and is therefore the cornerstone of pediatric inhalational anesthesia.
- Preanesthetic sedation and anesthetic induction form a continuum in pediatric anesthesia. The selection of oral, rectal, IV, or inhalational induction must be tailored to each child and depends on the anesthesiologist's familiarity with the options available.
- The use of succinylcholine as part of routine anesthesia in children is losing favor. The risks of malignant hyperthermia, myoglobinemia and myoglobinuria, diffuse muscle fasciculation, and hyperkalemia seriously limit its usefulness.
- Nondepolarizing muscle relaxants have a different spectrum of action in children than in adults, which results from the immature neuromuscular system, volume of distribution, and developmental aspects of pharmacology. The increasing use of narcotics with balanced anesthesia and neuromuscular-blocking agents necessitates being familiar with the agents available. Neuromuscular blockade monitoring is essential when using neuromuscular blocking agents in children.
- Pancuronium has traditionally been used in infants and small children because it increases heart rate, supports blood pressure, and provides excellent, deep neuromuscular blockade.
- Perioperative maintenance of temperature is critical and a basic skill in the provision of medical care to all children. Thermal protection cannot be too strongly stressed.
- The ideal maintenance fluid for children is D5 half-normal saline provided at a rate of 150 mg/m^2/24 hours. This is approximately equivalent to 4 mg/kg/hr for the first 10 kg, 2 mg/kg/hr for 10 to 20 kg, and 1 mg/kg/hr over 20 kg.
- When anesthetizing children, rapport must be achieved not only with the child but with the parent who is the immediate support for the child. Maximizing parental involvement is useful in overall management of children undergoing anesthesia.

KEY REFERENCES

Anand KJS, Hickey PR: Pain and its effects in the human neonate and fetus, *N Engl J Med* 317:1321, 1987.

Berry FA, Yemen TA: Pediatric airway in health and disease, *Pediatric Clin North Am* 41:153–180, 1994.

Bickler P, Sessler DI: Airway humidification, *Anesth Analg* 71:415, 1990.

Delphin E, Jackson D, Rothstein P: Use of succinylcholine during elective pediatric anesthesia should be reevaluated, *Anesth Anal* 66:1190, 1987.

Garvin JP, Warner EJ: Halothane and children: the first quarter century, *Anesth Analg* 63:838, 1984.

Goudsouzian NG, Standaert FG: The infant and the myoneural junction, *Anesth Analg* 65:1208, 1986.

Gregory GA: The baroresponses of preterm infants during halothane anaesthesia, *Can Anaesth Soc J* 29:105, 1982.

Gregory GA, Eger EI II, Munson ES: The relationship between age and halothane requirement in man, *Anesthesiology* 30:488, 1969.

Helfaer MA, Wilson MD: Obstructive sleep apnea, control of ventilation and anesthesia in children, *Pediatric Clin North Am* 41:131–151, 1994.

Knill RL, Gelb AW: Ventilatory responses to hypoxia and hypercarbia during halothane sedational anesthesia in man, *Anesthesiology* 49:244, 1978.

Lerman J, Sikich N, Kleinman S, et al: The pharmacology of sevoflurane in infants and children, *Anesthesiology* 80: 814–824, 1994.

Murat I, Lapeyre G, Saint Maurice C: Isoflurane attenuates baroreflex control of heart rate in human neonates, *Anesthesiology* 70:395, 1989.

Nicholson SC, Betts EK, Jobes DR, et al: Comparison of oral and intramuscular preanesthetic medication for pediatric inpatient surgery, *Anesthesiology* 71:8, 1989.

Sarner JB, Levine M, Davis PJ, et al: Clinical characteristics of sevoflurane in children. A comparison with halothane, *Anesthesiology* 82:38–46, 1995.

Taylor RH, Lerman J: Minimum alveolar concentration of desflurane and hemodynamic responses in neonates, infants, and children, *Anesthesiology* 75:975–979, 1991.

Wetzel R, editors: *Pediatric anesthesia. Pediatric Clinics of North America*, vol 41, 1994.

Wolf WJ, Neal MB, Peterson MD: The hemodynamic and cardiovascular effects of isoflurane and halothane anesthesia in children, *Anesthesiology* 64:328, 1986.

Zwass MS, Fisher DM, Welborn LG, et al: Induction and maintenance characteristics of anesthesia with desflurane and nitrous oxide in infants and children, *Anesthesiology* 76:373–378, 1992.

REFERENCES

1. Alexander JP: Clinical comparison of the Bain and Magill anaesthetic systems during spontaneous respiration, *Br J Anaesth* 54:1031, 1982.
2. Anand KJS, Hansen DD, Hickey PR: Hormonal-metabolic stress responses in neonates undergoing cardiac surgery, *Anesthesiology* 73:661, 1990.
3. Anand KJS, Hickey PR: Pain and its effects in the human neonate and fetus, *N Engl J Med* 317:1321, 1987.
4. Anand KJS, Sippell WG, Aynsley-Green A: Randomised trial of fentanyl anaesthesia in preterm neonates undergoing surgery: effects on the stress response, *Lancet* 1:243, 1987.
5. Ayre P: Anaesthesia for hare lip and cleft palate operations in babies, *Br J Surg* 25: 131, 1937.
6. Azar I: The response of patients with neuromuscular disorders to muscle relaxants: a review, *Anesthesiology* 61:173, 1984.
7. Barash PG, Glanz S, Katz JD, et al: Ventricular function in children during halothane anesthesia: an echocardiographic evaluation, *Anesthesiology* 49:79, 1978.
8. Bennett EJ, Daugherty MJ, Bowyer DE, et al: Pancuronium bromide: experience in 100 pediatric patients, *Anesth Analg* 50: 798, 1971.
9. Berry FA, Yemen TA: Pediatric airway in health and disease, *Pediatr Clin North Am* 41:153–180, 1994.
10. Bickler P, Sessler DI: Airway humidification, *Anesth Analg* 71:415, 1990.
11. Black AE, Hatch DJ, Nauth-Misir N: Complications of nasotracheal intubation in neonates, infants and children: a review of 4 years' experience in a children's hospital, *Br J Anaesth* 65:461, 1990.
12. Boezaart AP, Van Hassett CH: Induction of anaesthesia in children, *S Afr Med J* 71: 643, 1987.
13. Borgeat A, Popovic V, Meier D, et al: Comparison of propofol and thiopental/halothane for short-duration ENT surgical procedures in children, *Anesth Analg* 71: 511, 1990.
14. Brandom BW, Cook DR, Woelfel SK, et al: Atracurium infusion requirements in children during halothane, isoflurane, and narcotic anesthesia, *Anesth Analg* 64:471, 1985.
15. Brandom BW, Sarner JB, Woelfel SK, et al: Mivacurium infusion requirements in pediatric surgical patients during nitrous oxide-halothane and during nitrous oxide-narcotic anesthesia, *Anesth Analg* 71:16–22, 1990.
16. Brandom BW, Woelfel SK, Cook DR, et al: Clinical pharmacology of atracurium in infants, *Anesth Analg* 63:309, 1984.
17. Brzustowicz RM, Nelson DA, Betts EK, et al: Efficacy of oral premedication for pediatric outpatient surgery, *Anesthesiology* 60:475, 1984.
18. Bush GH, Roth F: Muscle pains after suxamethonium chloride in children, *Br J Anaesth* 33:151, 1961.
19. Cabal LA, Siassi B, Artal R, et al: Cardiovascular and catecholamine changes after administration of pancuronium in distressed neonates, *Pediatrics* 75:284, 1985.
20. Cahalan MK, Weiskopf RB, Eger EI, II, et al: Hemodynamic effects of desflurane/nitrous oxide anesthesia in volunteers, *Anesth Analg* 73:157–163, 1991.
21. Chodoff P, Helrich M: Factors affecting pediatric endotracheal tube size: a statistical analysis, *Anesthesiology* 28:779, 1967.
22. Cook DR, Freeman JA, Lai AA, et al: Pharmacokinetics of mivacurium in normal patients and in those with hepatic or renal failure, *Br J Anaesth* 69:580–585, 1992.
23. Cook DR, Westman HR, Rosenfeld L, et al: Pulmonary edema in infants: possible association with intramuscular succinylcholine, *Anesth Analg* 60:220, 1981.
24. Cook NR, Brandom BW, Shiu G, et al: The inspired median effective dose, brain concentration at anesthesia and cardiovascular index for halothane in young rats, *Anesth Analg* 60:182, 1981.

25. Cote CJ, Rolf N, Liu LMP, et al: A single-blind study of combined pulse oximetry and capnography in children, *Anesthesiology* 74:980, 1991.
26. Craythorne NWB, Turndorf H, Dripps RD: Changes in pulse rate and rhythm associated with the use of succinylcholine in anesthetized children, *Anesthesiology* 21: 465, 1960.
27. Cressman WR, Myer CM, III: Diagnosis and management of croup and epiglottitis, *Pediatr Clin North Am* 41:265–276, 1994.
28. Cronnelly R, Morris RB: Antagonism of neuromuscular blockade, *Br J Anaesth* 54: 183, 1982.
29. Crumrine RS, Nulsen FE, Weiss MH: Alterations in ventricular fluid pressure during ketamine anesthesia in hydrocephalic children, *Anesthesiology* 42:758–761, 1975.
30. Crumrine RS, Yodlowski E, II: Assessment of neuromuscular function in infants, *Anesthesiology* 54:29, 1984.
31. Crysdale WS, Sendi K: Evolution in the management of acute epiglottitis: a 10-year experience with 242 children, *Int Anesthesiol Clin* 26:32, 1988.
32. Cunliffe M, Lucero VM, McLeod ME, et al: Neuromuscular blockade for rapid tracheal intubation in children: comparison of succinylcholine and pancuronium, *Can Anaesth Soc J* 33:760, 1986.
33. Davenport HT, Werry JS: The effect of general anesthesia, surgery, and hospitalization on the behavior of children, *Am J Orthopsychiatry* 40:806, 1970.
34. Delphin E, Jackson D, Rothstein P: Use of succinylcholine during elective pediatric anesthesia should be reevaluated, *Anesth Analg* 66:1190, 1987.
35. Diaz JH: Croup and epiglottitis in children: the anesthesiologist as diagnostician, *Anesth Analg* 64:621–633, 1985.
36. Dierdorf SF, McNiece WL, Rao CC, et al: Effect of succinylcholine on plasma potassium in children with cerebral palsy, *Anesthesiology* 62:88, 1985.
37. Duke PC, Fownes D, Wade JG: Halothane depresses baroreflex control of heart rate in man, *Anesthesiology* 46:184, 1977.
38. Duncan PG, Gregory GA, Wade JG: The effect of nitrous oxide on baroreceptor function in newborn and adult rabbits, *Can Anaesth Soc J* 28:339, 1981.
39. Durant NN, Katz RL: Suxamethonium, *Br J Anaesth* 54:195, 1982.
40. Eger EI: Uptake and distribution. In Miller RD, editor: *Anesthesia,* ed 3, New York, 1990, Churchill-Livingstone.
41. Ellis DG, Jakymec A, Kapplan RM, et al: Guided orotracheal intubation in the operating room using a lighted stylet: a comparison with direct laryngoscopic technique, *Anesthesiology* 64:823, 1986.
42. Elman DS, Denson JS: Preanesthetic sedation of children with intramuscular methohexital sodium, *Anesth Analg* 44:494, 1965.
43. Fahey MR, Rupp SM, Fisher DM, et al: The pharmacokinetics and pharmacodynamics of atracurium in patients with and without renal failure, *Anesthesiology* 61: 699, 1984.
44. Falick YS, Smiler BG: Is anticholinergic premedication necessary? *Anesthesiology* 43:472, 1975.
45. Feld LH, Champeau MW, van Steennis CA, et al: Preanesthetic medication in children: a comparison of oral transmucosal fentanyl citrate versus placebo, *Anesthesiology* 71:374, 1989.
46. Finholt DA, Audenaert SM, Stirt JA, et al: Endotracheal tube leak pressure and tracheal lumen size in swine, *Anesth Analg* 65:667, 1986.
47. Finucane BT, Santora AH: *Principles of airway management,* Philadelphia, 1988, FA Davis.
48. Fisher DM, Canfell PC, Fahey MR, et al: Elimination of atracurium in humans: contribution of Hofmann elimination and ester hydrolysis versus organ-based elimination, *Anesthesiology* 65:6, 1986.
49. Fisher DM, Cronnelly R, Miller RD, et al: The neuromuscular pharmacology of neostigmine in infants and children, *Anesthesiology* 59:220, 1983.
50. Fisher DM, Cronnelly R, Sharma M, et al: Clinical pharmacology of edrophonium in infants and children, *Anesthesiology* 61: 428, 1984.
51. Fisher DM, Miller RD: Neuromuscular effects of vecuronium (ORG NC45) in infants and children during N_2O, halothane anesthesia, *Anesthesiology* 58:519, 1983.
52. Fisher DM, O'Keefe C, Stanski DR, et al: Pharmacokinetics and pharmacodynamics of *d*-tubocurarine in infants, children and adults, *Anesthesiology* 55:203, 1982.
53. Fisher DM, Robinson S, Brett CM, et al: Comparison of enflurane, halothane, and isoflurane for diagnostic and therapeutic procedures in children with malignancies, *Anesthesiology* 63:647, 1985.
54. Forbes RB, Vandewalker GE: Comparison of two and ten per cent rectal methohexitone for induction of anaesthesia in children, *Can J Anaesth* 35:345, 1988.
55. Foster CA: Muscle pain that follows administration of suxamethonium, *Br Med J* 2:24, 1960.
56. Frankville DD, Drummond JC: Hyperkalemia after succinylcholine administration in a patient with closed head injury without paresis, *Anesthesiology* 67:264, 1987.
57. Friesen RH, Henry DB: Cardiovascular changes in preterm neonates receiving isoflurane, halothane, fentanyl, and ketamine, *Anesthesiology* 64:238, 1986.
58. Friesen RH, Honda AT, Thieme RE: Changes in anterior fontanel pressure in preterm neonates during tracheal intubation, *Anesth Analg* 66:874–878, 1987.
59. Friesen RH, Lichtor JL: Cardiovascular depression during halothane anesthesia in infants: a study of three induction techniques, *Anesth Analg* 61:42, 1982.
60. Frink EJ, Jr, Ghantous H, Malan TP, et al: Plasma inorganic fluoride with sevoflurane anesthesia: correlation with indices of hepatic and renal function, *Anesth Analg* 74:231–235, 1992.
61. Garvin JP, Warner EJ: Halothane and children: the first quarter century, *Anesth Analg* 63:838, 1984.
62. Goudsouzian NG: Maturation of neuromuscular transmission in the infant, *Br J Anaesth* 52:205, 1980.
63. Goudsouzian NG: The physiology and pharmacology of neuromuscular transmission in infants and children. In Steward DJ, editor: *Some aspects of paediatric anaesthesia,* Amsterdam, 1982, Elsevier/North-Holland Biomedical Press.
64. Goudsouzian NG: Atracurium infusion in infants, *Anesthesiology* 68:267, 1988.
65. Goudsouzian N, Cote CJ, Liu LMP, et al: The dose-response effects of oral cimetidine on gastric pH and volume in children, *Anesthesiology* 55:533, 1981.
66. Goudsouzian NG, Crone RD, Todres ID: Recovery from pancuronium blockade in the neonatal intensive care unit, *Br J Anaesth* 53:1303, 1981.
67. Goudsouzian NG, d'Hollander AA, Viby-Mogensen J: Prolonged neuromuscular block from mivacurium in two patients with cholinesterase deficiency, *Anesth Analg* 77:183–185, 1993.
68. Goudsouzian NG, Martyn JJA, Liu LM, et al: Safety and efficacy of vecuronium in adolescents and children, *Anesth Analg* 62:1083, 1983.
69. Goudsouzian NG, Ryan JF, Savarese JJ; The neuromuscular effects of pancuronium in infants and children, *Anesthesiology* 41:95, 1974.
70. Goudsouzian NG, Standaert FG: The infant and the myoneural junction, *Anesth Analg* 65:1208, 1986.
71. Goudsouzian NG, Young ET, Moss J, et al: Histamine release during the administration of atracurium or vecuronium in children, *Br J Anaesth* 58:1229, 1986.
72. Greenspun JC, Hannallah RS, Welborn LG, Norden JM: Comparison of sevoflurane and halothane anesthesia in children undergoing outpatient ear, nose, and throat surgery, *J Clin Anesth* 7:398–402, 1995.
73. Gregory GA: The baroresponses of preterm infants during halothane anaesthesia, *Can Anaesth Soc J* 29:105, 1982.
74. Gregory GA, Eger EI, II, Munson ES: The relationship between age and halothane requirement in man, *Anesthesiology* 30:488, 1969.
75. Gregory GA, Wade JG, Beihl DR, et al: Fetal anesthetic requirement (MAC) for halothane, *Anesth Analg* 62:9, 1983.
76. Grundfast KM, Camilon FS Jr, Barber CS, et al: Prospective study of subglottic stenosis in intubated neonates, *Ann Otol Rhinol Laryngol* 99:390, 1990.
77. Hannallah RS, Baker SB, Casey W, et al: Propofol: effective dose and induction characteristics in unpremedicated children, *Anesthesiology* 74:217, 1991.
78. Hannallah RS, Oh TH, McGill WA, et al: Changes in heart rate and rhythm after intramuscular succinylcholine with or without atropine in anesthetized children, *Anesth Analg* 65:1329, 1986.
79. Hawkins DB: Pathogenesis of subglottic stenosis from endotracheal intubation, *Ann Otol Rhinol Laryngol* 96:116, 1987.
80. Helfaer MA, Wilson MD: Obstructive sleep apnea, control of ventilation and anesthesia in children, *Pediatr Clin North Am* 41:131–151, 1994.
81. Henderson JM, Brodsky DA, Fisher DM, et al: Pre-induction of anesthesia in pediatric patients with nasally administered sufentanil, *Anesthesiology* 68:671, 1988.
82. Hirshman CA, Edelsteinn G, Peets S, et al:

Mechanism of action of inhalation anesthesia on airways, *Anesthesiology* 56:107, 1982.

83. Holloway AM, Jordaan DG, Brock-Utne JG: Midazolam for the intravenous induction of anaesthesia in children, *Anaesth Inten Care* 10:340, 1982.
84. Idvall J, Holsek J, Stenberg P: Rectal ketamine for induction of anaesthesia in children, *Anaesthesia* 38:60, 1983.
85. Karl HW, Swedlow DB, Lee KW, et al: Epinephrine-halothane interactions in children, *Anesthesiology* 58:142, 1983.
86. Katz RL, Matteo RS, Papper EM: The injection of epinephrine during general anesthesia. 2. Halothane, *Anesthesiology* 23: 597, 1962.
87. Keep PJ, Manford MLM: Endotracheal tube sizes for children, *Anaesthesia* 29: 181, 1974.
88. Kenna JG, Neuberger J, Mieli-Vergani G, et al: Halothane hepatitis in children, *Br Med J* 294:1209, 1987.
89. Kepes ER, Martinez LR, Andrews IC, et al: Anesthetic problems in hereditary muscular abnormalities, *NY State J Med* 72:1051, 1972.
90. Khalil SM, Florence FB, Van den Nieuwenhuyzen MCO, et al: Rectal methohexital: concentration and length of rectal catheters, *Anesth Analg* 70:645, 1990.
91. Kleeman PP, Jantzen JPAH, Bonfils P: The ultrathin bronchoscope in the management of the difficult paediatric airway, *Can J Anaesth* 34:606, 1987.
92. Knill RL, Gelb AW: Ventilatory responses to hypoxia and hypercarbia during halothane sedational anesthesia in man, *Anesthesiology* 49:244, 1978.
93. Kopman AF: The current status of edrophonium: have we come "full circle?" *Can J Anaesth* 38:145, 1991.
94. Krane EJ, Su JY: Comparison of the effects of halothane on newborn and adult rabbit myocardium, *Anesth Analg* 66:1240, 1987.
95. LeDez KM, Lerman J: The minimum alveolar concentration (MAC) of isoflurane in preterm neonates, *Anesthesiology* 67:301, 1987.
96. Lerman J, Gregory GA, Willis MM, et al: Age and solubility of volatile anaesthetics in blood, *Anesthesiology* 61:139, 1984.
97. Lerman J, Robinson S, Willis MM, et al: Anesthetic requirements for halothane in young children 0–1 month and 1–6 months of age, *Anesthesiology* 59:421, 1983.
98. Lerman J, Sikich N, Kleinman S, Yentis S: The pharmacology of sevoflurane in infants and children, *Anesthesiology* 80:814–824, 1994.
99. Liu LMP, DeCook TH, Goudsouzian NG, et al: Dose-response to intramuscular succinylcholine in children, *Anesthesiology* 55:599, 1981.
100. Lupprian KG, Churchill-Davidson HC: Effect of suxamethonium on cardiac rhythm, *Br Med J* 4:1774, 1960.
101. Mapleson WW: The elimination of rebreathing in various semi-closed anesthetic systems, *Br J Anaesth* 26:323, 1954.
102. Matthews-Bellinger LA, Salpeter MM: Fine structural distribution of acetylcholine receptors at developing mouse neuromuscular functions, *J Neurosci* 3:644, 1983.
103. McLeskey CH, McLeod DS, Hough TL, et al: Prolonged asystole after succinylcholine administration, *Anesthesiology* 49: 208, 1978.
104. Meakin G, McKiernan EP, Morris P, et al: Dose-response curves for suxamethonium in neonates, infants and children, *Br J Anaesth* 62:655, 1989.
105. Meistelman C, Agoston S, Kersten UW, et al: Pharmacokinetics and pharmacodynamics of vecuronium and pancuronium in anesthetized children, *Anesth Analg* 65: 1319, 1986.
106. Meistelman C, Loose JP, Saint-Maurice C, et al: Clinical pharmacology of vecuronium in children, *Br J Anaesth* 58:996, 1986.
107. Meretoja OA, Olkkola KT: Pharmacodynamics of mivacurium in children, using a computer-controlled infusion, *Br J Anaesth* 71:232–237, 1993.
108. Meretoja OA, Wirtavuori K, Neuvonen PJ: Age-dependence of the dose-response curve of vecuronium in pediatric patients during balanced anesthesia, *Anesth Analg* 67:21, 1988.
109. Michenfelder JD, Sundt TM, Fode N, et al: Isoflurane when compared to enflurane and halothane decreases the frequency of cerebral ischemia during carotid endarterectomy, *Anesthesiology* 67:336, 1987.
110. Mikawa K, Maekawa N, Goto R, et al: Effects of exogenous intravenous glucose on plasma glucose and lipid homeostasis in anesthetized children, *Anesthesiology* 74: 1017, 1991.
111. Miller JR, Stoelting VK, Darin MV: A preliminary report of the use of methohexital sodium (Brevital) for pediatric anesthesia, *Anesth Analg* 59:64, 1973.
112. Miller KM, Palon WDM, Smith EB, et al: Physiochemical approaches to the mode of action of anesthetics, *Anesthesiology* 36:339, 1972.
113. Miller RD, Way WL, Hamilton WK, et al: Succinylcholine-induced hyperkalemia in patients with renal failure? *Anesthesiology* 36:138, 1972.
114. Minton MD, Grosslight K, Stirt JA, Bedford RF: Increases in intracranial pressure from succinylcholine: prevention by prior nondepolarizing blockade, *Anesthesiology* 65:165–169, 1986.
115. Mirakhur RK, Elliott P, Lavery TD: Plasma cholinesterase activity and the duration of suxamethonium apnaea in children, *Ann R Coll Surg* 66:43, 1984.
116. Montgomery CJ, Steward DJ: A comparative evaluation of intubating doses of atracurium, *d*-tubocurarine, pancuronium and vecuronium in children, *Can J Anaesth* 35:36, 1988.
117. Morio M, Fujii K, Satoh N, et al: Reaction of sevoflurane and its degradation products with soda lime. Toxicity of the byproducts, *Anesthesiology* 77:1155–1164, 1992.
118. Motayama EK, Hen J, Tamas L, et al: Spirometry with positive airway pressure: a simple method to evaluate obstructive lung disease in children, *Am Rev Respir Dis* 126:766, 1982.
119. Murat I, Lapeyre G, Saint Maurice C: Isoflurane attenuates baroreflex control of heart rate in human neonates, *Anesthesiology* 70:395, 1989.
120. Naito Y, Tamai S, Shingu K, Fujimori R, Mori K: Comparison between sevoflurane and halothane for paediatric ambulatory anaesthesia, *Br J Anaesth* 67:387–389, 1991.
121. Navarro R, Weiskopf RB, Moore MA, et al: Humans anesthetized with sevoflurane or isoflurane have similar arrhythmic response to epinephrine, *Anesthesiology* 80:545–549, 1994.
122. Newburg LA, Milde JH, Michenfelder JD: The cerebral metabolic effects of isoflurane at and above concentrations that suppress cortical electrical activity, *Anesthesiology* 59:23, 1983.
123. Nicolson SC, Betts EK, Jobes DR, et al: Comparison of oral and intramuscular preanesthetic medication for pediatric inpatient surgery, *Anesthesiology* 71:8, 1989.
124. Nightingale DA, Bush GH: A clinical comparison between tubocurarine and pancuronium in children, *Br J Anaesth* 45:63, 1973.
125. Nugent SK, Laravuso R, Rogers MC: Pharmacology and use of muscle relaxants in infants and children, *J Pediatr* 94:481, 1979.
126. Ochiai R, Toyoda Y, Nishio I, et al: Possible association of malignant hyperthermia with sevoflurane anesthesia, *Anesth Analg* 74:616–618, 1992.
127. O'Connor JP, Ramsay JG, Wynands JE, et al: The incidence of myocardial ischemia during anesthesia for coronary artery bypass surgery in patients receiving pancuronium or vecuronium, *Anesthesiology* 70:230, 1989.
128. O'Kelly B, Fiset P, Meistelman C, Ecoffey C: Pharmacokinetics of rocuronium bromide in paediatric patients, *Eur J Anaesthesiol Suppl* 9:57–58, 1994.
129. Orlowski JP, Ellis NG, Amin NP, et al: Complications of airway intrusion in 100 consecutive cases in a pediatric ICU, *Crit Care Med* 8:324, 1980.
130. Pantuck EJ, Pantuck CB: Cholinesterases and anticholinesterases. In Katz RL, editor: *Muscle relaxants,* Amsterdam, 1975, Excerpta Medica.
131. Phillips AJ, Brimacombe JR, Simpson DL: Anaesthetic induction with isoflurane or halothane: oxygen saturation during induction with isoflurane or halothane in unpremedicated children, *Anaesthesia* 43: 927, 1988.
132. Piat V, Dubois MC, Johanet S, Murat I: Induction and recovery characteristics and hemodynamic responses to sevoflurane and halothane in children, *Anesth Analg* 79:840–844, 1994.
133. Pittet J-F, Tassonyl E, Morel DR, et al: Neuromuscular effect of pipecuronium bromide in infants and children during nitrous oxide-alfentanil anesthesia, *Anesthesiology* 72:432, 1990.
134. Pounder DR, Blackstock D, Steward DJ: Tracheal extubation in children: halothane versus isoflurane, anesthetized versus awake, *Anesthesiology* 74:653, 1991.
135. Rees GJ: Anaesthesia in the newborn, *Br Med J* 2:1419, 1950.
136. Roa TLK, Madhavareddy S, Chinthagada M, et al: Metoclopramide and cimetidine to reduce gastric fluid pH and volume, *Anesthesiology* 63:1014, 1984.
137. Robinson S, Gregory GA: Fentanyl-air-oxygen anesthesia for ligation of patent

ductus arteriosus in preterm infants, *Anesth Analg* 60:331, 1981.
138. Rogers MC, Richmond JB: The autonomic nervous system. In State U, Weech AA, editors: *Perinatal physiology,* New York, 1978, Plenum Press.
139. Rosen I, Soderbug M: Electroencephalographic activity in children under enflurane anesthesia, *Acta Anaesthesiol Scand* 19:361, 1975.
140. Ruffle JM, Snider MT, Rosenberger JL, et al: Rapid induction of halothane anaesthesia in man, *Br J Anaesth* 57:607, 1985.
141. Runkle B, Bancalari E: Acute cardiopulmonary effects of pancuronium bromide in mechanically ventilated newborn infants, *J Pediatr* 104:614, 1984.
142. Rutledge ML, Hawkins EP, Langston C: Skeletal muscle growth failure induced in premature newborn infants by prolonged pancuronium treatment, *J Pediatr* 109:883, 1986.
143. Ryan JF, Kagen LJ, Hyman AI: Myoglobinuria after a single dose of succinylcholine, *N Engl J Med* 285:824, 1971.
144. Saarnivaara L, Lindgren L, Klemola UM: Comparison of chloral hydrate and midazolam by mouth as premedicants in children undergoing otolaryngological surgery, *Br J Anaesth* 61:390, 1988.
145. Salanitre E: The kinetics of inhalation gas exchange in children. In Steward DJ, editor: *Some aspects of paediatric anaesthesia,* Amsterdam, 1982, Elsevier/North-Holland Biomedical Press.
146. Salanitre E, Rackow H: Respiratory complications associated with the use of muscle relaxants in young infants, *Anesthesiology* 22:194, 1961.
147. Sarner JB, Brandom BW, Cook DR, et al: Clinical pharmacology of doxacurium chloride (BW A938U) in children, *Anesth Analg* 67:303, 1988.
148. Sarner JB, Brandom BW, Woelfel SK, et al: Clinical pharmacology of mivacurium chloride (BW B1090U) in children during nitrous oxide-halothane and nitrous oxide-narcotic anesthesia, *Anesth Analg* 68:116, 1989.
149. Sarner JB, Levine M, Davis PJ, et al: Clinical characteristics of sevoflurane in children. A comparison with halothane, *Anesthesiology* 82:38–46, 1995.
150. Schaner PJ, Brown RL, Kirsey RD, et al: Succinylcholine induced hyperkalemia in burned patients, *Anesth Analg* 48:764, 1969.
151. Schuller DE, Birckh G: The safety of intubation in croup and epiglottitis: an eight-year follow-up, *Laryngoscope* 85:33–46, 1975.
152. Sessler DI, McGuire J, Sessler AM: Perioperative thermal insulation, *Anesthesiology* 74:875, 1991.
153. Sherman JM, Lowitt S, Stephenson C, et al: Factors influencing acquired subglottic stenosis in infants, *J Pediatr* 109:322, 1986.
154. Shnider WM, Papper EM: Anesthesia for asthmatic patients, *Anesthesiology* 22:886, 1961.
155. Shulman D, Bar-Yishay E, Beardsmore C, et al: Determinants of end expiratory volume in young children during ketamine or halothane anesthesia, *Anesthesiology* 66: 636, 1987.
156. Smith RM: Pediatric anesthesia in perspective, *Anesth Analg* 59:186, 1978.
157. Smith SM: The use of curare in infants and children, *Anesthesiology* 8:176, 1947.
158. Soliman IE, Broadman LM, Hannallah RS, et al: Comparison of the analgesic effects of EMLA (Eutectic Mixture of Local Anesthetics) to intradermal lidocaine infiltration prior to venous cannulation in unpremedicated children, *Anesthesiology* 68: 804, 1988.
159. Spear RM, Yaster M, Berkowitz ID, et al: Preinduction of anesthesia in children with rectally administered midazolam, *Anesthesiology* 74:670, 1991.
160. Squire R, Brodsky L, Rossman J: The role of infection in the pathogenesis of acquired tracheal stenosis, *Laryngoscope* 100:765, 1990.
161. Stevens WC, Cromwell TH, Halsey MJ, et al: The cardiovascular effects of a new inhalation anesthetic, forane, in human volunteers at constant arterial carbon dioxide tension, *Anesthesiology* 35:8, 1971.
162. Stiles CM: A flexible fiberoptic bronchoscope for endotracheal intubation in infants, *Anesth Analg* 53:1017, 1974.
163. Stocks JG: The management of respiratory failure in infancy, *Anaesth Intens Care* 1:486, 1973.
164. Stoelting RK, Blitt CD, Cohen PJ, Merin RG: Hepatic dysfunction after isoflurane anesthesia, *Anesth Analg* 66:147–153, 1987.
165. Strong RM, Passy V: Endotracheal intubation: complications in neonates, *Arch Otolaryngol* 103:329, 1977.
166. Strum DP, Eger EI, II: Partition coefficients for sevoflurane in human blood, saline, and olive oil, *Anesth Analg* 66:654–656, 1987.
167. Summary of the National Halothane Study, *JAMA* 197:775, 1966.
168. Taylor RH, Lerman J: Minimum alveolar concentration of desflurane and hemodynamic responses in neonates, infants and children, *Anesthesiology* 75:975–979, 1991.
169. Tobias JD, Martin LD, Wetzel RC: Ketamine by continuous infusion for sedation in the pediatric intensive care unit, *Crit Care Med* 18:819, 1990.
170. Ueda W, Hirakawa M, Mao O: Appraisal of epinephrine administration to patients under halothane anesthesia for closure of cleft palate, *Anesthesiology* 58:574, 1983.
171. Viby-Mogensen J: Correlation of succinylcholine duration of action with plasma cholinesterase activity in subjects with a genotypically normal enzyme, *Anesthesiology* 53:517, 1980.
172. Wark HJ: Postoperative jaundice in children: the influence of halothane, *Anaesthesia* 38:237, 1983.
173. Waxman K, Shoemaker WC, Lipmann M: Cardiovascular effects of anesthetic induction with ketamine, *Anesth Analg* 59:355, 1980.
174. Wear R, Robinson S, Gregory GA: The effect of halothane on the baroresponse of adult and baby rabbits, *Anesthesiology* 56: 188, 1982.
175. Westrin P, Jonmarker C, Werner O: Thiopental requirements for induction of anesthesia in neonates and in infants one to six months of age, *Anesthesiology* 71:344, 1989.
176. Wetzel RC: Optimal anesthesia for tonsil surgery: inhalational anesthesia. *Anesth Rep* 1:78–79, 1988.
177. Wetzel RC, Rogers MC, Pediatric hemodynamic monitoring. In Shoemaker WC, Thompson WL, editors: *Critical care—state of the art,* vol 2, Fullerton, 1981, The Society of Critical Care Medicine.
178. Wilton NC, Leigh J, Rosen DR, et al: Preanesthetic sedation of preschool children, using intranasal midazolam, *Anesthesiology* 69:972, 1988.
179. Woelfel SK, Brandom BW, McGowan FX, Jr, Cook DR: Clinical pharmacology of mivacurium in pediatric patients less than one years old during nitrous oxide-halothane anesthesia, *Anesth Analg* 77:713–720, 1993.
180. Woelfel SK, Brandom BW, Sarner JB, et al: Potency of mivacurium chloride (BW B1090U) during halothane nitrous oxide anesthesia in children, *Anesth Analg* 67:S261, 1988.
181. Wolf WJ, Neal MB, Peterson MD: The hemodynamic and cardiovascular effects of isoflurane and halothane anesthesia in children, *Anesthesiology* 64:328, 1986.
182. Yaster M: Optimal anesthesia for tonsil surgery: narcotic anesthesia, *Anesth Rep* 1:79–82, 1988.
183. Zulliger JJ, Schuller DE, Beach TP, et al: Assessment of intubation in croup and epiglottitis, *Ann Otol Rhinol Laryngol* 91:403–406, 1982.
184. Zwass MS, Fisher DM, Welborn LG, et al: Induction and maintenance characteristics of anesthesia with desflurane and nitrous oxide in infants and children, *Anesthesiology* 76:373–378, 1992.

CHAPTER 80

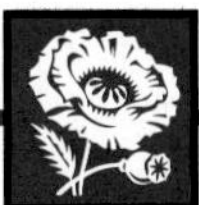

Anesthesia for Orthopedic Surgery

MERCEDES CONCEPCION

Dramatic changes in the practice of orthopedic surgery have occurred in the past 20 years. Advances in medicine, which have changed the treatment and prognosis of many medical conditions, have markedly changed the role of the orthopedic surgeon. Some diseases, such as poliomyelitis, which in the past required orthopedic intervention, have been almost totally eradicated. Others, such as rickets and scurvy, are usually detected early and treated successfully.

Probably the greatest advances in orthopedic surgery have occurred in the field of joint replacement for arthritic conditions. Aside from an increased understanding of the pathology of the musculoskeletal system and subsequent management, the greatest factors have been the introduction of new materials, such as metals and plastics, and knowledge of the human body's response to such foreign materials.

The outcome of a surgical procedure is intimately related to the anesthetic technique. The rapid evolution of orthopedic surgery has been paralleled by concomitant advances in anesthesia. The following should assure a good outcome for the orthopedic surgical patient: (1) understanding the surgical procedure and its potential physiologic effect; (2) application of appropriate anesthetic technique; (3) knowledge of the well-documented benefits of certain anesthetic techniques for orthopedic surgery; and (4) the use of sophisticated monitoring.

An important consideration in orthopedic anesthesia is the increasing age of the population. Approximately 10% of patients admitted for surgery are over the age of 75. Physiologic organ function decreases with age. The geriatric population is often affected by significant medical illness with multiple organ systems involved. Because orthopedic surgery is frequently performed in the elderly, careful consideration of these patients is essential.

Finally, an increased number of automobile and industrial accidents has resulted in an increase in trauma surgery. Changes have occurred in the way fractures are treated, increasing the number of open reduction and internal fixation procedures. Thus, the anesthesiologist must understand the sophistication and implications of the new surgical techniques and carefully assess and understand the variety of medical problems that may coexist in the orthopedic surgical patient. This chapter will discuss specific problems associated with certain orthopedic procedures, as well as the choice of the best anesthetic techniques for common procedures.

PREOPERATIVE ASSESSMENT

It is important to emphasize the value of a good preoperative evaluation because it can elicit relevant information such as the patient's present state of health, past medical history, prior anesthetic history, and other pertinent information. The information obtained allows the anesthesiologist to formulate a plan that offers the patient the appropriate anesthetic technique.

A large number of orthopedic procedures are performed in the elderly. Morbidity and mortality in this population appear to be related to concomitant medical problems, thus a careful medical assessment is mandatory in this patient group.

Patients with rheumatoid arthritis (RA) and ankylosing spondylitis (AS) frequently undergo multiple orthopedic reconstructive and corrective procedures and often present a challenge to the anesthesiologist.

Patients with RA may present with significant extra-articular manifestations involving multiple systems such as the cardiovascular and pulmonary systems, which may influence the choice of anesthesia or type of monitoring. Other systems may be indirectly involved as a result of the multiple medications used to treat these patients. Patients with AS may also experience significant systemic involvement. Assessment of patients with RA and AS requires a thorough history and physical examination. Table 80-1 summarizes common systemic manifestations of RA. For a detailed preoperative evaluation of these patients, the reader is referred to Chapter 16.

POSITIONING

Orthopedic procedures require a wide variety of positions; some of which may be unacceptable to an awake, unanesthetized patient. Because the majority of these positions must be adopted after the patient is anesthetized, a team approach is necessary. Anesthesiologists, surgeons, and other operating room staff must understand the position required and agree on the positioning procedure. An awake patient can participate during positioning. On the other hand, the anesthetized patient is unable to feel the extreme discomfort of certain positions that alter the normal mechanics of the body. Vulnerable parts, such as the ulnar nerve at the elbow and other peripheral nerves, must be especially protected to avoid injury by pressure or stretching. In the prone position, the eyes are protected by taping them closed and using padding to avoid corneal abrasion. The prone position may produce increased abdominal pressure, which will result not only in impairment of ventilation but also in increased bleeding from epidural veins and, potentially, in the formation of an epidural hematoma postoperatively. Hence, in-

Table 80-1 Pathophysiologic evaluation of the patient with rheumatoid arthritis

Considerations	Pathophysiology	Complications	Anesthesia concerns
Airway	Cervical spine fusion/subluxation	Fused or unstable cervical spine	Difficult intubation
	Temporomandibular joint involvement	Overbite, small mouth opening	
	Cricoarytenoid joint arthritis	Inflammation, immobilization of vocal cords	
Pulmonary involvement	Pleural effusions, nodules, interstitial fibrosis, pneumonitis, arteritis	Impaired alveolar capillary gas exchange, ↓ diffusion capacity, pulmonary hypertension	Small endotracheal tube
Cardiac manifestations	Pericarditis, myocarditis, endocardial disease (valves), conduction defects, coronary arteritis, granulomatous aortitis	Coronary arteritis, may lead to myocardial infarction	
Vasculitis	Distal arteritis, cutaneous ulceration, venulitis	Peripheral neuropathy Mild: distal sensory deficit Severe: sensory deficit and motor weakness	Patient positioning
Hematologic manifestations	Normocytic-hypochromic anemia, eosinophilia	Hgb, seldom < 10 g/dl	
	Thrombocytosis	May be associated with active intravascular coagulation, ↑	
Drug therapy	Nonsteroidal antiinflammatories, steroids, gold salts, methotrexate	bleeding, renal insufficiency, fragile blood vessels, skin discoloration, mimicking of hypoxemia, lung involvement	Difficult IV placement Drug interaction

creased abdominal pressure must be avoided to facilitate venous drainage from the operative site.

It is essential to appreciate the effect of positioning on physiologic functions and to protect the patient against potential injury and complications. For a complete discussion of positioning in surgery, the reader is referred to Chapter 35.

CHOICE OF ANESTHETIC TECHNIQUE

Several factors should be considered in choosing an anesthetic technique. These factors include the patient's physical and mental status, the surgical procedure, and the anesthesiologist's proficiency with various techniques.

Although general anesthesia continues to be frequently used for orthopedic surgery, the use of regional anesthesia has increased considerably. Scientific information concerning the choice of one anesthetic technique over another for specific surgical procedures has been unavailable in the past. Nonetheless, the influence of anesthetic technique on the intraoperative and postoperative periods has, in the past few years, been the subject of numerous studies.

For example, Sculco and Ranawat[137] and Thornburn[153] have shown that intraoperative blood loss during total hip replacement is significantly lower with spinal anesthesia than with general anesthesia. The same significant decrease in blood loss has been shown to occur with epidural anesthesia compared to general anesthesia.[72,98] In addition, several investigators[27,86,98,100,153] have reported a significant decrease in the incidence of thromboembolism in patients undergoing total hip replacement receiving regional anesthesia. Thus it appears that, at least in orthopedic surgery and particularly in hip surgery, regional anesthesia offers greater advantages over general anesthesia.

Data also exist on the influence of regional anesthesia on the metabolic and endocrine changes that occur during surgery.[70] Surgical stress gives rise to nociceptive stimuli that are transmitted to the hypothalamus and cerebral cortex, resulting in a series of efferent impulses that in turn stimulate various endocrine organs. The endocrine and metabolic alterations observed during surgery are known as "surgical stress." The majority of the surgically induced endocrine and metabolic changes can be inhibited by adequate afferent blockade. Plasma levels of epinephrine and norepinephrine have been shown to decrease following epidural anesthesia. These changes in catecholamine levels seem to be related to the level of the block. The neural blockade must extend to the midthoracic or upper thoracic dermatomes to produce a fall in catecholamine levels.

The release of metabolic products, such as glucose, lactate, free fatty acids, glycerol, and ketones is also inhibited by epidural anesthesia extending to midthoracic or upper thoracic levels. Inhibition of the metabolic and endocrine response to surgery by epidural anesthesia probably occurs as a result of blockade of afferent or efferent pathways or both. For example, inhibition of pituitary hormones release probably results from afferent pathway blockade, whereas inhibition of adrenal cortical hormones may result from the blockade of efferent pathways or inhibition of corticotropin (ACTH) release from the pituitary. Decrease of catecholamine release from the adrenal medulla and insulin by the pancreas is probably secondary to blockade of efferent autonomic fibers by epidural anesthesia. The relevance of this altered metabolic and endocrine response to surgery has not been clearly elucidated.

Other potential benefits of regional anesthesia include a shorter convalescence time and a shorter hospital stay. In addition, regional anesthesia employed for surgery as a continuous technique (e.g., epidural, continuous brachial plexus, or continuous femoral nerve blockade) can be extended into the postoperative period to provide prolonged analgesia.

SPINAL SURGERY

Laminectomy and discectomy are probably the most common spinal surgical procedures. Correction of spinal deformities, fusion, and stabilization, however, are also relatively common procedures involving more complicated anesthetic management.

The majority of spinal surgery requires the prone position. The prone position provides a stable posture that does not allow for movement when force is applied and facilitates exposure by straightening the lumbar lordosis.[91] Several problems are associated with the prone position:

- Chest pressure leads to decreased chest wall compliance and expansion and impaired respiration. Diaphragmatic excursion can also be impaired by abdominal pressure.
- Abdominal pressure leads to inferior vena cava (IVC) compression, which impedes venous return. This, in turn, forces retrograde venous flow into the vertebral venous plexus, resulting in epidural venous engorgement. Increased bleeding, difficulty in achieving hemostasis, and potential development of epidural hematoma may occur secondary to increased intra-abdominal pressure.
- Hence the abdomen must be allowed to hang free to facilitate respiratory movement and a decrease in bleeding.
- Peripheral nerve damage can occur as a result of excessive pressure or traction.
- Eyes, ears, and nose must be protected from excessive pressure.
- Pressure necrosis could occur in the nipples of the women patient. Genitalia in men also must be protected from pressure.

Several devices have been developed to optimize the prone position. Devices such as the Wilson and Relton frames are frequently used. Occasionally, simple blanket rolls will lift the body to free the chest and abdomen. In the knee-chest position introduced by Smith et al.[145] the patient is placed in the kneeling position on the surface of the operating table. Although this position provides good abdominal decompression, the considerable hip flexion required may compromise arterial and venous circulation.[30]

Modifications of the knee-chest position placing the patient on a frame have been introduced. An example is the Andrews frame which is now widely used.[124] On the Andrews frame, the patient's chest rests on pillows or pads placed on the operating table and the hips are supported by a plate. Lateral thigh supports or straps are used for stabilization. The foot section of the operating table is lowered to a vertical position, and a horizontal plate is attached to the lower end. The feet are then strapped to the padded plate (Fig 80-1).

The Andrews frame provides excellent abdominal decompression, which leads to ease of ventilation and decreased intraoperative bleeding. In addition, it allows easy protection of pressure points. Allowing the patient to sit back against a gluteal support partially neutralizes the lumbar lordosis. Lordosis can be easily restored if required for surgical fusion of the lumbar spine. Hyperlordosis relaxes the paraspinal musculature, and it is particularly important when posterolateral or lumbosacral fusion is being performed.

One potential disadvantage of the Andrews frame is the difficulty of obtaining posteroanterior x-ray films. The flexed thighs prevent proper positioning of the film cassette.

Cervical Spine

Posterior fusion

Posterior fusion of the cervical spine is frequently used to correct an unstable neck. Cervical subluxation of C1 over C2 and at other levels is commonly associated with rheumatoid arthritis. Whether the cervical instability is secondary to rheumatoid arthritis, trauma, malignancy, or any other cause, a major concern in the anesthesia planning will be airway management.

These patients are often managed preoperatively by neck traction, on a Stryker frame, with traction maintained by skull tongs. Endotracheal intubation is often difficult. In the past, endotracheal intubation was accomplished by a blind nasal approach; presently, fiberoptic-aided intubation is recommended. As more skill is gained in the use of the fiberoptic bronchoscope, its use has become more generalized.

A retrospective study of 128 consecutive posterior cervical spine fusions was conducted to assess the incidence of postoperative ventilatory complications and the frequency of postoperative reintubation. Risk factors leading to ventilatory complications were also determined. All patients had RA and presented with various degrees of cervical spine instability. The only significant risk factor was the mode of intubation. The frequency of postoperative respiratory complications and postoperative reintubation was significantly lower in patients intubated with the aid of a fiberoptic scope.[167]

An awake, sedated intubation is recommended, as maintenance of the airway in an unconscious nonintubated patient may prove very difficult. In addition, an awake intubation allows for intubation of the trachea to be achieved without manipulation of the unstable cervical spine. Nasotracheal intubation is usually easier than oral intubation because the nasopharynx, oropharynx, and glottis are commonly in the same axis. A nasotracheal tube is also easier to tolerate if postoperative intubation is required. Awake, fiberoptic nasotracheal intubation is described in Chapter 49.

Once endotracheal intubation has been accomplished and general anesthesia induced, the patient is turned to the prone position. Because the head rest has a horseshoe shape and

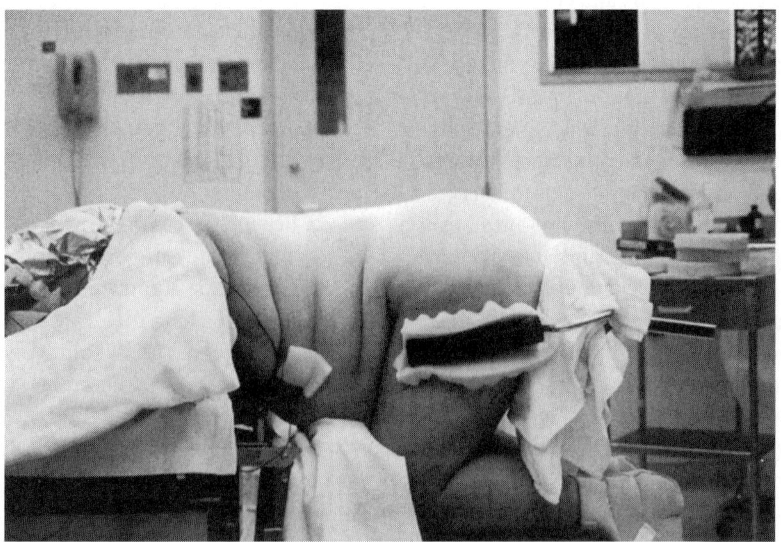

Fig. 80-1. Patient in prone position on the Andrews Frame. Chest and iliac crests are supported by blankets. Knees rest on a shelf attached to the lowered foot piece of the operating table.

the endotracheal tube hangs down, it is important to secure the tube tightly. An indwelling arterial catheter for invasive blood pressure monitoring is used routinely during orthopedic surgery for cervical fusion.

During a posterior approach to the cervical spine, the arms are restrained against the patient's side, hindering access to peripheral venous lines or pulses. The anesthesiologist should be aware that interference with intravenous (IV) lines and pressure monitoring devices could occur intraoperatively.

Anterior cervical discectomy and fusion

Cervical spine surgery is also performed by the anterior or the transoral approach.

When the anterior approach is chosen for cervical discectomy, the supine position is most frequently employed. Quite often, however, the sitting position is used. This position prevents venous engorgement resulting in a relatively bloodless field and an improved surgical exposure. Nonetheless, the risk of venous air embolism (VAE) associated with the sitting position is certainly present. Aside from routine intraoperative monitors, indwelling arterial and central venous catheters are recommended. Often the surgical approach involves the right side of the neck, necessitating central venous pressure (CVP) placement on the left side. Recommended monitors are shown in Box 80-1.

Anterior cervical fusion is potentially associated with significant risks. Major arteries and veins are in the vicinity of the surgical site and the potential for significant bleeding exists. The recurrent laryngeal nerve may be injured. This is less likely with a left-sided approach. Injuries to the sympathetic nervous system may also occur.

Cervical osteotomy

Ankylosing spondylitis, and quite often rheumatoid arthritis are associated with severe flexion deformities of the cervical spine. Although the spinal cord adapts to the anatomic distortion of the spine, neurologic function remains intact. The flexion deformity is a result of fibrosis and ossification, which usually begins at the ligament insertion sites.

Surgical correction, or osteotomy, is often necessary (lumbar and thoracic osteotomy are performed in patients with ankylosing spondylitis). In the past, cervical osteotomy was performed under local anesthesia with supplemental intravenous sedation.[53,155] The technique of local anesthesia and IV sedation has also been reported for lumbar osteotomy.[135,155]

In this technique, after sterile preparation of the area, the neck is anesthetized with local anesthetic infiltration and IV sedation with supplemental oxygen is administered. Once the surgeon has exposed the cervical spine, brief inhalation of N_2O can be used for correction of the deformity, which involves forcible disruption of the anterior spinal ligaments. With this technique, an awake patient serves as his/her own monitor of spinal cord function. In addition, the airway is maintained without the need for an often difficult endotracheal intubation. Lumbar osteotomy under local anesthesia has also been reported.[143,164]

Two developments have changed the anesthetic management of these patients. First, the use of flexible fiberoptic bronchoscopy for endotracheal intubation has become widespread, and the majority of anesthesiologists are skillful in the technique. The airway of these patients can be safely secured with fiberoptic endoscopy while they are still awake and capable of maintaining their airway. Adequate topical anesthesia of the nostril and nasopharynx, in association with the judicious use of IV sedation, is recommended. The second development is the use of spinal-cord monitoring by somatosensory-evoked potentials (SEPs). The use of spinal cord monitoring lessens the risk of postoperative neurologic damage.

A technique of general anesthesia for cervical osteotomy has been reported by Ovassapian et al.[109] Fig. 80-2 shows a patient with ankylosing spondylitis who underwent cervical osteotomy under general anesthesia.

BOX 80-1
RECOMMENDED MONITORS FOR ANTERIOR CERVICAL DISCECTOMY AND FUSION IN THE SITTING POSITION

Arterial line
Central venous pressure
Chest Doppler
End-tidal CO_2 and N_2
Esophageal stethoscope

Scoliosis: Surgical Correction

Scoliosis is a spinal deformity characterized by both lateral curvature of the spine and vertebral rotation. The vertebrae and spinous processes rotate in the area of the curvature toward the concave side of the curve (Fig. 80-3).[75]

The ribs on the convex side are pushed and badly deformed by the rotating spine, whereas on the concave side, the ribs are crowded together. In addition, scoliosis causes structural changes in the vertebrae and related structure. The vertebral bodies become wedge shaped and are thicker on the convex side. The discs are also wider on the convex side. On the other hand, the concave side exhibits shorter and thinner pedicles and laminae, and the vertebral canal becomes narrower. Scoliosis is occasionally associated with kyphosis.

The severity of the scoliosis is usually related to the angle of the curvature; the more severe the scoliosis, the larger the angle. The angle of the curvature is usually measured by the Cobb method. The upper- and lower-end vertebrae of the curvature are determined (the end vertebrae are those that tilt most severely toward the concavity). A horizontal line is traced across the superior border of the upper-end vertebra

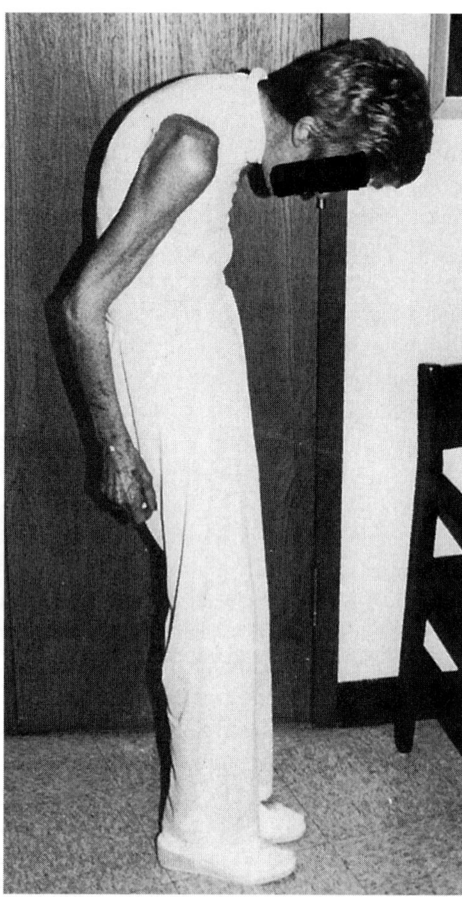

Fig. 80-2. Patient with ankylosing spondylitis who underwent a cervical osteotomy under general endotracheal anesthesia. (From Concepcion MA: Anesthesia for orthopedic procedures. In Goldberg V, editor: *Orthopaedic knowledge update 3, Home study syllabus,* Park Ridge, 1990, American Academy of Orthopaedic Surgeons.)

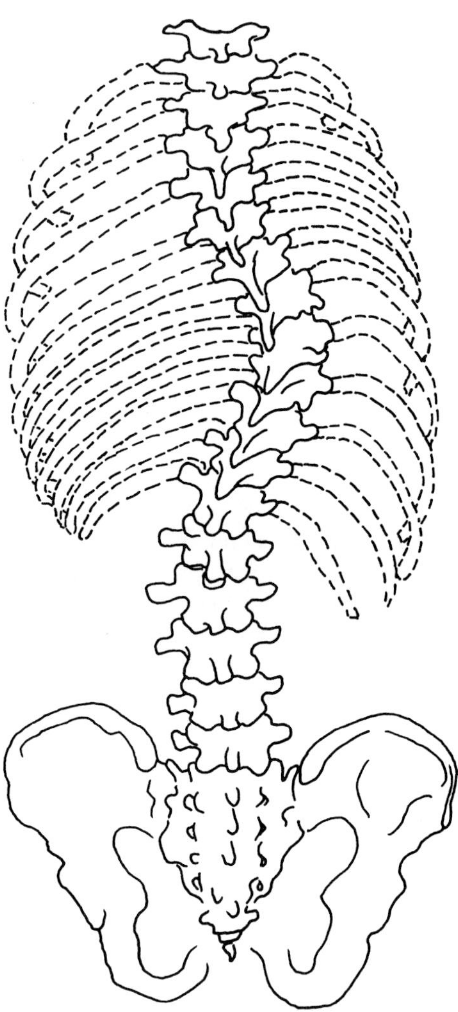

Fig. 80-3. Illustration demonstrating lateral curvature and vertebral rotation in scoliosis. Vertebral and spinous processes rotate in the direction of the concavity. Ribs are crowded together on the concave side and are flattened and further apart on the convex side of the curvature. (Courtesy of Diane Raeke.)

and another horizontal line across the inferior border of the lower-end vertebra. Perpendicular lines are then drawn from each of the horizontal lines, and the intersecting angles are measured (Fig. 80-4). Scoliosis is seldom associated with cardiopulmonary complications when the angle of the curvature is 60° or less.

Scoliosis can be broadly classified into structural and nonstructural types. Corrective surgery is required in structural scoliosis (Box 80-2). Idiopathic scoliosis is by far the most common form of structural scoliosis, occurring in approximately 70% of all cases. Adolescent scoliosis affects men and women, but 70% of persisting cases occur in women. In adolescent scoliosis, the major spinal curvature is most frequently to the right.

Cardiopulmonary involvement

Scoliotic deformity significantly affects respiratory mechanics, gas exchange, pulmonary vasculature, and chemical regulation of ventilation. As the degree of the curvature progresses, the severity of pulmonary and cardiovascular involvement increases, often resulting in respiratory failure, pulmonary hypertension, and cor pulmonale.

The earliest manifestation of abnormal pulmonary function is a restrictive pattern of lung volumes with a significant reduction in vital capacity (VC). Several factors are believed to play a role in the changes of lung volumes and decreased respiratory compliance. These include the abnormal development of the thoracic cage with a direct effect on the elastic properties of the respiratory system. In addition, the deformity will also affect the development of inspiratory and expiratory muscle forces.[64]

The major abnormality in gas exchange is a ventilation-perfusion maldistribution. Generalized alveolar hypoventilation results in hypoxia. There is also an increase in the dead space/tidal volume ratio (VD/VT) and in the alveolar-arterial oxygen difference (A-aDo_2). As the age of the scoliotic patient increases, the age-associated deterio-

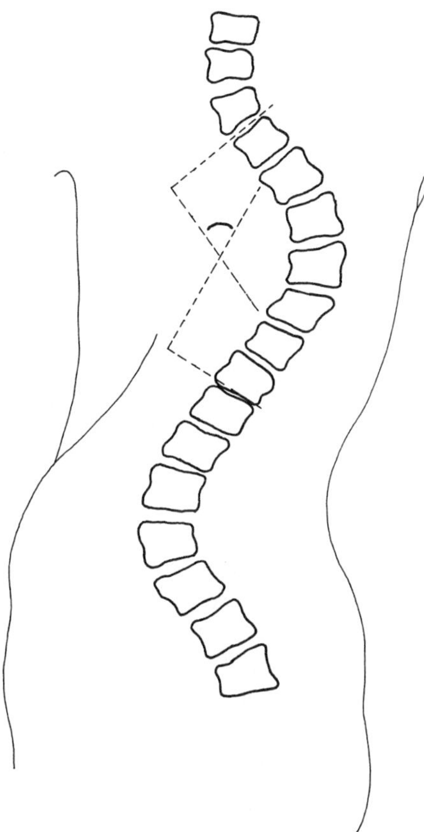

Fig. 80-4. Measurement of the angle of scoliotic curvature by the Cobb method. (Courtesy of Diane Raeke.)

BOX 80-2
CLASSIFICATION OF STRUCTURAL SCOLIOSIS

I. Idiopathic (genetic)
  A. Infantile (< 3 years of age)
  B. Juvenile (3–10 years of age)
  C. Adolescent (10 years to maturity)
II. Congenital scoliosis (probably not genetic)
  A. Vertebral
    1. Open with posterior spinal defect
    2. Closed with no posterior spinal defect
III. Scoliosis associated with neuromuscular disease
  A. Neuropathic forms
    1. Poliomyelitis
    2. Cerebral palsy
    3. Syringomyelia
  B. Myopathic forms
    1. Progressive (muscular dystrophy)
    2. Static (amyotonia congenita)
  C. Other (Friedreich's ataxia)
IV. Neurofibromatosis (von Recklinghausen's disease)
V. Other etiologic factors
  A. Mesenchymal disorders (congenital and acquired)
  B. Trauma (fractures, irradiation, burns, surgery)

Modified from Klein HA: Scoliosis. In Trench AH, editor: *Clinical symposia,* Summit, NJ, 1978, CIBA.

ration in blood gases, believed to be the result of diminished mechanical lung properties, will be superimposed on the existing $\dot{V}/\dot{Q}$ abnormalities. With the worsening of $\dot{V}/\dot{Q}$ abnormalities, ventilatory demands will increase. Failure to meet these requirements will be manifest by hypercapnia and eventually respiratory failure. In addition to these mechanical changes, it has been postulated that there is an impaired development of pulmonary vasculature as a result of rib cage deformity,[64] and that the number of vascular units/unit volume of lung is reduced.[26] Increased pulmonary vascular resistance will then lead to pulmonary hypertension (Fig. 80-5).[1]

Other problems

Scoliosis associated with neuromuscular disease may present other anesthetic concerns in addition to those associated with respiratory and cardiovascular problems. For example, patients with scoliosis associated with some types of muscular dystrophy or with poliomyelitis may exhibit muscle weakness (i.e., respiratory muscles), which will lead to inadequate cough and inadequate defense of the upper airway. These abnormalities will further impair pulmonary function.

Anesthesia in these patients has also been associated with malignant hyperthermia, hyperkalemia, and cardiac dysrhythmias. Although cases of malignant hyperthermia have been reported with idiopatic scoliosis,[14,125] the complications mentioned previously are rare and are more directly associated with specific types of muscular dystrophy or myopathies, such as Duchenne's muscular dystrophy.[77,138]

Management

Conservative management of moderate curves has been attempted. The Milwaukee brace has been the most successful nonsurgical management of idiopathic scoliosis.[10,71] When conservative management fails to prevent progression of the curvature or when it is determined that severe impairment of respiratory and cardiovascular functions are imminent, surgical correction is necessary. Harrington's surgical technique uses the posterior approach,[52] whereas other techniques, such as Dwayer's, use the anterior approach.[32]

The anterior approach is used in a variety of conditions, some of which require correction of deformities, stabilization, or decompression. Still others require a combined anterior and posterior stabilization usually carried out in two stages.

Correction of severe deformities by the anterior approach involves several major risks. These potential risks include excessive bleeding and damage to the spinal cord by extreme and rapid correction of deformities. **Excessive distension of the cord could interfere with its circulation and lead to anterior spinal artery syndrome. Therefore significant morbidity may be associated with the anterior**

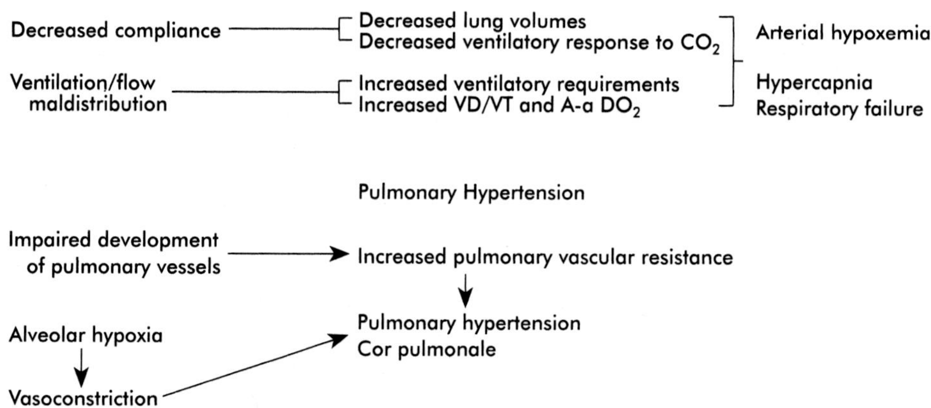

Fig. 80-5. Respiratory abnormalities associated with scoliosis.

approach to spinal surgery. If the transthoracic approach is selected for anterior spinal decompression and fusion, a double lumen tube is indicated, and one-lung anesthesia should be conducted until surgical decompression or correction has been achieved. A left thoracotomy is often preferred as the aorta is easier to handle than the relatively thin-walled vena cava. Although spinal cord blood supply is generally found to enter from the left, a direct relationship between the site of entry and subsequent spinal cord function has not been found.[150]

Preoperative preparation

In the patient with scoliosis, coexistent respiratory or cardiac disease must be determined in the preoperative assessment, as well as any type of associated neuromuscular disease. The angle of the curvature will give an approximate quantitative measure of the severity of scoliosis.

Electrocardiographic (ECG) abnormalities consistent with pulmonary disease are late in appearance and include right atrial dilatation and/or right ventricular hypertrophy. A prolonged interval between pulmonary valve closure and tricuspid valve opening was identified by phonocardiography and reported by Schnelerson et al.[135] Echocardiography (ECHO) to determine ventricular wall thickness and cavity dimensions may provide a useful noninvasive method for assessing right ventricular function. In addition, the following lung volumes and functions must be measured: VC (seated and supine), FEV_1, FEV_1/VC, response to bronchodilators, and room/air arterial blood gases. Aside from the ECG and lung volumes studies, chest radiographs and other indicated laboratory studies should be performed preoperatively (Box 80-3).

Premedication should be chosen by the anesthesiologist but should be guided by the patient's physical status. Consideration of any superimposed medical problems is important. Generally these patients should be well sedated. The use of a narcotic and a benzodiazepine for amnesia is recommended. These patients may have significant respiratory and cardiovascular embarassment and smaller than usual doses of a sedative or narcotic may significantly depress their ventilation.

Intraoperative management

It is important to plan an anesthetic technique that takes into consideration all the potential problems associated with spinal fusion. Aside from consideration of respiratory and cardiovascular functions, two major areas of concern are notable: blood loss and spinal cord function.

Deliberate hypotension Scoliosis surgery is usually associated with significant blood loss. Deliberate hypotension to decrease blood loss has been successfully used in a variety of surgical procedures and is frequently used in scoliosis surgery. Numerous techniques of deliberate hypotension have been employed.[73,116,170]

Hypotension is usually induced using direct-acting venous or arterial vasodilators, such as ganglionic-blocking drugs, alpha-adrenergic antagonists, combination of alpha- and beta-adrenergic blockers, and calcium channel blockers. The most commonly used drugs are sodium nitroprusside and nitroglycerin. The hypotensive effect of these drugs in children and adolescents was studied by Yaster et al.[170] Both drugs produced a decrease in heart rate. Cardiac output increased with nitroprusside; PaO_2 increased and the alveolar-arterial oxygen diffusion gradient decreased with both drugs. However, nitroglycerin failed to reduce mean arterial pressure to the desired level in a significant number of patients. Results suggest that nitroprusside is the agent of choice for reliable induction of hypotension. Nitroprusside consistently decreased blood pressure even in subjects who did not respond to nitroglycerin. Inhalation agents have also been used to induce hypotension. Patel et al.[116] reported the use of moderate hypotension for scoliosis surgery using enflurane supplemented by fentanyl.

Although deliberate hypotension has been advocated to reduce blood loss and to improve operative conditions, a major concern is the effect of hypotension on spinal cord blood supply. Animal studies have suggested an additive effect of hypotension and surgical pressure on the spinal cord in producing neurologic complications.[15] In

BOX 80-3
PREOPERATIVE TESTS FOR SCOLIOSIS SURGERY

Pulmonary function tests
 VC, FEV_1, FEV_1/VC
Arterial blood gases
Chest radiograph
Electrocardiogram
Echocardiogram*

*If evidence of pulmonary hypertension and cor pulmonale exist.

dogs, Griffith et al.[46] have shown that cord compression can alter dorsal column conduction at perfusion pressures that did not affect blood flow.

Grundy et al.[48] studied the effect of moderate hypotension for spinal fusion, monitoring spinal cord function with SEPs. Hypotension significantly reduced blood loss and improved the operative conditions. The authors suggest that continuous spinal cord monitoring should be used because it may decrease the risks of hypotension-related neurologic damage.[48]

Regardless of the technique used to induce hypotension, fine adjustments of the anesthetic technique will aid in achieving the desired effect of the hypotensive agent. Adequate and vigilant monitoring is essential to avoid complications associated with deliberate hypotension. An arterial line for blood pressure monitoring and blood gas determinations, urine output, routine intraoperative monitoring, and frequent assessment of blood loss are mandatory. Pulmonary artery (PA) pressures should be monitored when evidence of pulmonary hypertension and cor pulmonale exist.

Autologous blood transfusion Increasing concern regarding the risks associated with homologous blood transfusion has resulted in the development and use of alternative techniques. In addition to the increased use of anesthetic techniques known to reduce blood loss (e.g., deliberate hypotension and epidural anesthesia), different forms of autologous blood transfusion are widely used. Perioperative salvage of blood with isovolemic hemodilution and retransfusion of blood have been successfully used for a number of years. Deposition of autologous blood immediately before surgery is a safe and simple technique that is increasingly accepted by surgeons and patients.

The first report of banked autologous transfusion was by Grant in 1921.[45] Later investigations have suggested that patients with adequate iron stores will have a fourfold or greater increase in hematopoiesis following a series of phlebotomies.[38,51] The use of previously deposited autologous blood has been extensively reported in orthopedic surgery in children[23] and in adults.[5,152,169] In association with intraoperative salvage of blood, previously deposited autologous blood is now the most common method of autologous blood transfusion for major orthopedic procedures.

Monitoring spinal cord function. Neurologic deficit is the most feared complication associated with spinal fusion surgery. It has been postulated that traction of the cord during instrumentation occludes arterial blood supply and produces ischemia.

In a study by the Scoliosis Research Society reported by McEwen et al.[83] the incidence of acute neurologic complications was 0.72% (57 of 7885 patients). Monitoring of spinal cord activity by the "wake-up test" was first reported by Vauzelle et al.[159] This test consists of awakening the patient enough to permit motion of hands and feet on command. If movement does not occur in the lower extremities but is clear in the hands, the instrumentation is removed and the command repeated. Potential hazards of this test include accidental extubation if the patient raises his/her head, a sudden deep inspiration may lead to air embolism, and finally, violent motion of the patient may potentially dislodge the instrumentation. In addition, the "wake-up test" only provides information regarding the anterior spinal cord (motor function) but does not test function of the dorsal column (sensory). Further, the test is not easily applicable to patients with severe psychologic problems or to mentally retarded patients.

Electrophysiologic monitoring of spinal cord function is now used to monitor cord function.[34,47,48,103,139,147] Evoked cortical responses to somatosensory peripheral nerve stimulation (SSEP) allows for continuous assessment of spinal cord activity. **Monitoring SSEP, however, only reflects the function of sensory pathways.** Evoked potential signals can be affected by a variety of factors. Blood pressure, temperature, and anesthetic agents may affect the response. To prevent some of the effects of anesthetic agents on SSEP monitoring, a continuous narcotic infusion has been recommended.[117]

Ideally, both sensory and motor activity should be monitored. Techniques to monitor motor tracts, such as electrical and magnetic stimulation of the motor cortex, have been developed. These techniques, although still considered experimental, will probably become effective clinical tools.

Postoperative management

Patients with significant pulmonary impairment before surgery will probably require postoperative ventilation. Although corrective surgical procedures prevent the progression of the most deleterious effects associated with spinal deformities, the long-term effect of surgery on respiratory and cardiovascular functions is controversial. In fact, deterioration of respiratory function immediately following surgery is not uncommon.

A common and uncomfortable complication of scoliosis surgery is the development of paralytic ileus. A nasogastric tube is usually inserted following induction of anesthesia.

Lumbar Discectomy, Laminectomy, and Fusion

The most common surgical procedures of the spine are discectomy, laminectomy, and fusion. Approximately 5% to

10% of patients suffering from a herniated disc and sciatica will require surgery. Limited disc excision seems to be the procedure of choice, rather than discectomy and fusion.[65]

In addition to an open surgical approach, other methods of surgical treatment are occasionally used. Microdiscectomy is a limited procedure associated with less surgical trauma and limited scarring, resulting in shorter hospitalization. Percutaneous discectomy is performed under fluoroscopy, using a suction device to remove disc material. This procedure is usually performed with local anesthesia with IV sedation. Chemonucleolysis, which consists of the injection of chymopapain (a drug that lyses mucopolysaccharides) has been used to decrease the size of the herniated mass. Although chemonucleolysis was approved by the Food and Drug Administration (FDA) in 1982, it still remains a controversial mode of therapy, and its use is clearly waning. General or local anesthesia can be used, although local anesthesia is preferred by many experts. The injection of chymopapain may result in an anaphylactic reaction, which occurs more frequently in women. Injection of chymopapain in conjunction with discographic contrast media is not advised. Laboratory and clinical evidence suggest that an unintentional intrathecal injection of these two drugs may result in serious neurologic complications such as transverse myelitis.[65] Spinal stenosis and spondylolisthesis are other indications for spinal laminectomy and fusion.

These procedures are most often performed under general anesthesia. This allows the surgeon to obtain better exposure by putting the patient in a prone position. Any technique of general anesthesia can be used. A fully paralyzing dose of muscle relaxant is not recommended because muscle response to nerve root stimulation is required in many cases. Although the use of muscle relaxants may facilitate surgical exposure, complete abolition of neuromuscular transmission is unnecessary.

A major concern associated with this type of surgery is the potential embarrassment of circulation and respiration by the prone position, as discussed earlier.

Although general anesthesia is most commonly used for surgical procedures on the spine, spinal and epidural anesthesia have also been successfully employed.[94,131] Nonetheless, anesthesiologists may be reluctant to use regional anesthesia because it may limit surgical exposure.

UPPER EXTREMITY SURGERY

Regional anesthesia is probably the most frequently used method of providing anesthesia for surgery of the upper extremity. It can be achieved via IV regional anesthesia (IVRA), brachial plexus blockade, or blockade of more peripheral nerves (e.g., elbow and wrist blocks).

Intravenous regional anesthesia

IVRA is a simple and easy technique indicated for relatively short surgical procedures. It is easily applicable to children and adults. Although most local anesthetics available have been used, lidocaine is currently the only FDA-approved drug. Lidocaine (without epinephrine) at a concentration of 0.5% produces rapid and adequate anesthesia. In a comparison study of lidocaine and prilocaine for IVRA, Bader et al.[4] reported blood levels of prilocaine significantly lower than those of lidocaine following tourniquet deflation. Tissue redistribution and rapid metabolism are believed to be responsible for the lower blood levels. In addition, it appears that prilocaine is quickly taken up by peripheral tissues following the IV injection. Following tourniquet deflation, the drug is then slowly released into the systemic circulation.[36]

Despite this potential margin of safety, prilocaine is rarely used in the United States because of manufacturing limitations. Bupivacaine (0.25% and 0.5%) has also been used. The use of bupivacaine for IVRA is not recommended because of the potential for cardiotoxicity if accidental tourniquet deflation occurs. **The advantages of IVRA over brachial plexus block include simplicity and reliability of technique, rapid onset of anesthesia, controllable duration of action, and rapid return of function. The disadvantages are continuous use of a tourniquet, the potential for toxic reactions, and the lack of postoperative analgesia.**

Brachial plexus block

Surgery of the upper extremity from the shoulder to the hand can be performed under brachial plexus blockade. A thorough understanding of the anatomy and anatomic relationships of the brachial plexus is essential. Different approaches to the brachial plexus have been employed to produce anesthesia. The choice of a specific approach is related to the surgical site. For example, an interscalene approach is preferable for shoulder surgery. On the other hand, this particular approach may be less desirable for surgery at or below the elbow where blockade of C8 and T1 is essential. Although many techniques for brachial plexus blockade have been described,[16,35,123,166] they all provide adequate anesthesia, depending on the skills of the anesthesiologist.

By choosing the appropriate approach, the volume of local anesthetic can be limited, minimizing the potential for toxicity. Table 80-2 serves as a guideline for the choice of technique.

Factors other than site of surgery must be considered. For example, the axillary approach should be considered if one is concerned about the possibility of an accidental pneumothorax. Local anesthetic drug choice depends on the length of the procedure and the need for postoperative analgesia. Long-acting drugs are not recommended for ambulatory surgical patients.

Shoulder Surgery

Different regional anesthetic techniques have been used for shoulder surgery. Peterson described the use of an interscalene approach in combination with paravertebral blocks at the C8 through T4 levels.[115] The use of cervical epidural

Table 80-2 Choice of various techniques for brachial plexus blockade

Surgical site	Approach	Local anesthetic volume
Shoulder	Interscalene	25–30
	Subclavian perivascular (supraclavicular)	40
Upper arm	Interscalene, subclavian perivascular	25–30
Elbow	Subclavian perivascular	25–30
	Intraclavicular	
	Interscalene	40
	Axillary	40
Forearm	Subclavian perivascular	
Wrist	Infraclavicular	25–30
Hand	Axillary	40
	Interscalene	40

Table 80-3 Regional anesthetic techniques for surgery of the lower extremity

Surgical site	Regional anesthesia technique
Hip	Spinal, epidural, lumbar plexus block
Knee	Epidural, spinal, "3-in-1 block," femoral, sciatic blocks
Lower leg	Spinal, epidural, sciatic block (Labat or Winnie's technique and popliteal fossa), femoral-sciatic blocks (if use of tourniquet is expected), sciatic and saphenous nerve block at knee
Ankle	Spinal, sciatic (as above)
Foot	Spinal, sciatic, ankle block, transmetatarsal block, IV regional

anesthesia for shoulder surgery has been reported by Zablocki et al.[171]

Interscalene blockade provides excellent anesthesia and muscle relaxation for shoulder surgery. Shoulder arthroscopy, for example is often performed under brachial plexus block (interscalene approach) with the patient awake in the sitting position. This position allows the surgeon to manipulate the patient's arm freely. Interscalene blockade plus IV sedation can also be employed for other shoulder procedures such as the Bankhart procedure. Interscalene blockade in combination with light general anesthesia is used for major shoulder surgery such as, total shoulder arthroplasty. The regional anesthesia must extend to the C3 to C4 dermatomes to produce cervical plexus blockade. Occasional neurologic complications associated with shoulder surgery include suprascapular nerve injury, which may occur in arthroscopic surgery. Musculocutaneous nerve injury has been reported during an anterior approach to shoulder replacement surgery.[9] Assessment of neurologic function in the early postoperative course is requested by many surgeons.

Elbow Surgery

Elbow surgery can be easily performed under regional anesthesia. Elbow reconstructive surgery may be associated with ulnar nerve palsy. A 3% incidence of ulnar neuropathy has been reported by Bell et al.[7] although a higher incidence has been reported with some surgical techniques. In an attempt to identify the cause of ulnar nerve palsy, Alvine et al.[1] studied 6500 patients. They concluded that a subclinical ulnar neuropathy could be present in many patients preoperatively and that this becomes symptomatic following surgical maneuvers and tourniquet application.[1] Hence, an early assessment of neurologic function is desirable.

Reimplantation Surgery

Regional anesthesia alone or in combination with general anesthesia is the technique of choice for reimplantation surgery. **The main indication for a regional technique is to produce sympathetic blockade in an attempt to improve blood flow to the injured limb.** It is also believed that the deafferentation produced by the blockade decreases vasoconstrictor tone in the injured vessels.[140] Either a long-acting local anesthetic drug, such as bupivacaine, or a continuous technique is recommended. The advantage of a continuous technique is not only to provide postoperative analgesia but also to prolong the sympathetic blockade beyond surgery and thus increase flow to the reimplanted digit or limb.

Although Shanahan et al.[141] recommended regional anesthesia alone, these procedures are predictably long, and a light general anesthesia in association with the block will make the procedure more tolerable to the patient. In addition to routine monitoring a Foley catheter should be inserted. Large-bore peripheral IV lines are necessary; blood loss may be significant with early replacement required.

LOWER EXTREMITY SURGERY

Surgery of the lower extremity can be completely performed under regional anesthesia. Table 80-3 shows the regional anesthetic techniques applicable to surgery of the lower extremity. The choice of the anesthetic technique should always be guided by the patient's physical and mental status, the surgical procedure, and the surgical needs. For example, a total hip revision may easily be performed under regional anesthesia. However, the procedure may be a lengthy one and blood loss may be significant. Under these circumstances the use of light general anesthesia in addition to a regional anesthetic technique (epidural, spinal) would be advisable.

Why is regional anesthesia so highly recommended? For years investigators have attempted to determine if regional anesthesia is associated with less morbidity and mortality than general anesthesia. So far, the available data suggest little difference between general and regional anesthesia in terms of postoperative mortality. **Sufficient data do exist to suggest that, at least in orthopedic surgery, regional anesthesia does afford certain benefits in terms of perioperative morbidity, such as decreased blood loss and decreased incidence of thromboembolic phenomena following hip surgery.** More extensive and well-controlled studies are necessary to determine whether one type of anesthesia is better than another, especially in patients with significant medical problems undergoing major orthopedic surgery.

Epidural and spinal anesthesia can be used for any surgical procedure of the lower limb. Continuous epidural techniques can be extended into the postoperative period to provide postoperative analgesia. This is particularly important in knee surgery, which can be associated with a significant degree of pain. Another type of patient that may benefit from a continuous epidural technique is the patient undergoing extensive vascular graft procedures. The continuous sympathetic blockade may improve blood flow to the area.

On the other hand, for ankle surgery spinal anesthesia may be a more suitable choice. The nerve supply to the ankle originates almost entirely from the sacral plexus. (Skin of upper medial aspect is supplied by the saphenous nerve.) The sacral roots and lower lumbar roots, specifically S1, L5, and S2, are the thickest roots in the body and are not easily penetrated by local anesthetics injected epidurally.[39] Local anesthetic drugs of high lipid solubility (e.g., etidocaine) will exhibit a shorter latency in producing anesthesia in these roots. Subarachnoid injection, however, will produce a complete block in a relatively short time.

When regional anesthesia has been chosen, the judicious use of IV sedation will maintain the patient comfortable and drowsy. This can be achieved by incremental doses of benzodiazepines (midazolam, diazepam) and opioids (fentanyl).

Arthroscopy

The use of arthroscopy for joint examination has become increasingly popular during the last 15 years. The diagnostic value of arthroscopy is well established. In the late 1970s, arthroscopic surgery was restricted primarily to the knee joint, but recently it has been extended to other joints as well (Fig. 80-6).

Arthroscopy and arthroscopic surgery, which are usually performed in healthy young individuals, are not completely free of complications. The Arthroscopic Association of North America (AANA) sponsored a survey of complications in arthroscopy in 1983. In this retrospective survey, the overall complication rate was 0.6% and included thromboembolic phenomena, infection, and hemarthrosis. Of particular interest was the finding of occasional injury to the popliteal artery and vein and to the posterior tibial and peroneal nerves.[144] When surgical procedures involving the knee were analyzed, the complication rate was greater than 1%. Procedures in other joints also carried a greater than 1% complication rate. With anterior staple capsulorrhaphy of the shoulder, a complication rate of 5.3% has been reported. A second prospective study was designed, and in 1987 preliminary findings showed an overall complication rate of 1.8% in more than 8500 procedures. These findings clearly show that, although arthroscopic surgery is a less-invasive procedure, it can be associated with significant complications.

All types of anesthesia have been used for arthroscopy

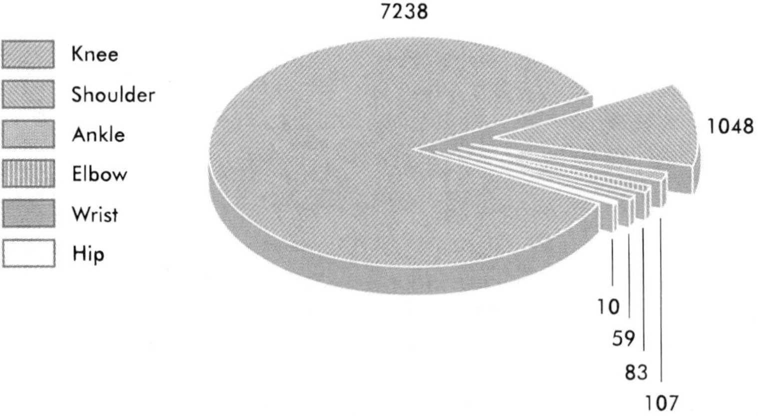

Fig. 80-6. Distribution of 8545 arthroscopic procedures in registry. (From Small N: Overview of arthroscopic complications. In Sprague NE III, editor: *Complications in arthroscopy,* New York, 1989, Raven Press.)

and arthroscopic surgery. Local, general, and regional anesthesia have all been used successfully.

Arthroscopic procedures of the knee joint are often carried out under local anesthesia. In addition to local infiltration of the area to facilitate insertion of the arthroscope, local anesthetic is injected intra-articularly. This may consist of a single injection or a continuous irrigation of a local anesthetic solution. Local anesthesia has been reported as safe, reliable, inexpensive, and acceptable to patients and surgeons.[8,24,74] Potential complications associated with general or regional anesthesia can be avoided. Further, it has been found that the accuracy of diagnosis is not diminished. Nonetheless, patients under local anesthesia may have inadequate muscle relaxation. Crane has reported a 10% higher rate of failure for arthroscopic procedures when local anesthesia is employed.[24]

Several local anesthetics or combinations of local anesthetics have been used. Intra-articular injection of bupivacaine is now widely used not only to produce surface anesthesia but also in an attempt to provide postoperative analgesia. Following intra-articular injection, systemic absorption of bupivacaine produces detectable plasma levels. Bupivacaine has been used in 0.25%, 0.5%, and 0.75% concentrations and in volumes varying from 20 to 40 ml. Two groups of investigators have reported bupivacaine pharmacokinetics following intra-articular injection.[42,70] The maximal plasma concentration (C_{max}) occurred between 30 and 40 minutes with all concentrations used, and the levels started to decline at approximately 60 minutes. The intra-articular injections of 20 ml of the 0.75% concentration produced a C_{max} of 1.06 μg/ml. Lower C_{max} values were found with 0.25% and 0.5% bupivacaine. No significant differences in patient comfort with the different concentrations were reported. Thus, it is recommended that 0.25% and 0.5% bupivacaine be used for intra-articular injection. More recently, the use of intra-articular morphine has been reported to provide some degree of postoperative analgesia.[61]

As already discussed, the majority of arthroscopic procedures are performed in young healthy patients. Hence the choice of general or regional anesthesia is often dictated by the patient's condition or the anesthesiologist's preferences. Proponents of regional anesthesia will argue that minor complications associated with general anesthesia (i.e., sore throat, injury to teeth, nausea and vomiting, etc.), could be prevented by the use of regional anesthesia.[122]

In terms of regional anesthesia, spinal or epidural anesthesia is often the choice in many centers. For spinal anesthesia, a small-gauge (26 to 25) spinal needle and short-acting local anesthetics are recommended, because these procedures are usually performed in ambulatory patients. Glucose-free 2% lidocaine is recommended for outpatients having spinal anesthesia. This will produce excellent anesthesia, the duration of which increases with the amount of local anesthetic administered. A duration of 60 to 90 minutes is usually obtained with 60 mg of 2% lidocaine. Duration will extend to 120 to 180 minutes by increasing the dose to 70 to 80 mg.[78] Additions of epinephrine will prolong duration of anesthesia in the lumbosacral roots.

In a recent study comparing hyperbaric 5% and isobaric 2% lidocaine for spinal anesthesia in knee arthroscopy, we found that patients receiving 2% lidocaine were discharged earlier than those receiving 5% lidocaine. Headache following spinal anesthesia is a potential complication in this young population of ambulatory patients. Although the incidence of such a headache is not significantly increased in ambulatory patients, it is recommended that subarachnoid block not be performed in patients who live a long distance from a major hospital, in case a headache develops following spinal anesthesia.

Epidural anesthesia provides adequate anesthesia with excellent muscle relaxation. This is the anesthesia of choice in some institutions for patients of all ages. By using local anesthetic drugs of short or intermediate duration (e.g., chloroprocaine, lidocaine), recovery time can be shortened and the potential of postdural puncture headache prevented.

Peripheral neural blockade may also be employed for arthroscopic procedures on the knee. The nerve supply of the lower extremity originates from the lumbosacral plexus. The knee joint is primarily supplied by the lumbar plexus although the sciatic nerve (sacral plexus) provides articular branches to the posterior aspect of the knee. **The three major nerves originating from the lumbar plexus and contributing to leg and knee innervation are the lateral femoral cutaneous (LFC), the obturator, and the femoral nerves.** These three nerves can be easily blocked by the "3-in-1 block" described by Winnie.[167] This technique of regional anesthesia has been successfully used for diagnostic and surgical arthroscopic procedures of the knee. The "3-in-1 block" requires the use of 20 to 30 ml of local anesthetic to produce adequate blockade of the three nerves. The LFC is occasionally missed. The LFC can be easily blocked separately by 5 to 10 ml of local anesthetic solution injected two fingerbreadths medial and two fingerbreaths caudal to the anterior superior iliac spine (Fig. 80-7). The "3-in-1 block" provides an excellent mode of anesthesia for knee arthroscopy when extensive manipulation of the posterior aspect of the joint is not required. Supplementation with IV fentanyl and midazolam will minimize posterior knee discomfort. Two groups of investigators have now reported the use of this technique for knee arthroscopy.[115,161] An important finding reported by Patel et al. was the significant decrease in the discharge time from the ambulatory center for patients in whom this technique of regional anesthesia was employed. When extensive work on the posterior knee joint is expected, a combination of femoral-sciatic nerve blockade is recommended. Capellino et al.[18] recently reported the successful use of femoral-sciatic blockades for knee arthroscopy. For ankle joint arthroscopy, general, spinal, or sciatic nerve block can be used.

Regional anesthesia can also be employed for arthro-

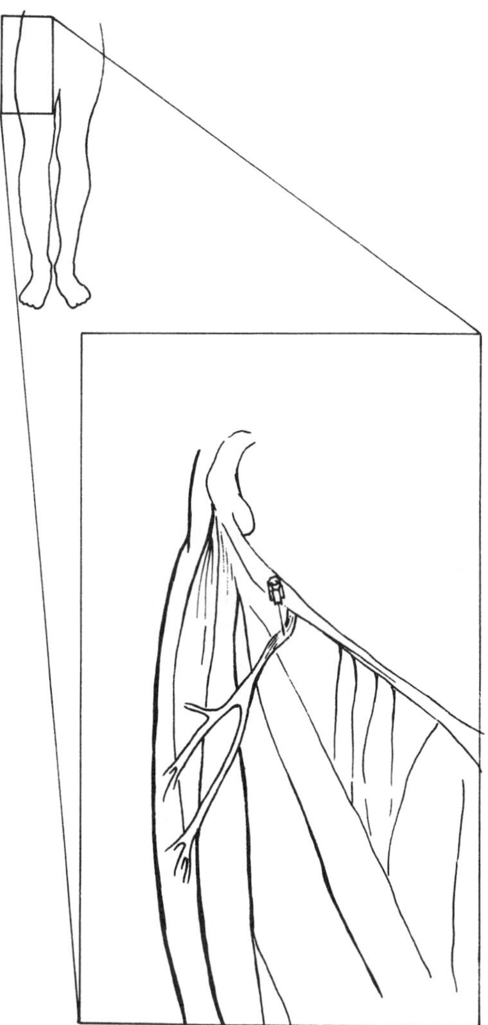

Fig. 80-7. Technique of lateral femoral cutaneous nerve block. Needle inserted perpendicular to the skin two fingerbreadths medial and two fingerbreadths caudal to the anterosuperior iliac spine. (Courtesy of Diane Raeke.)

scopic procedures of the upper extremity. In shoulder arthroscopic procedures, however, the posterior site of arthroscope incision is not reliably blocked by an interscalene blockade. In that event the block can be supplemented with local anesthesia infiltration of the incision site.

Amputations

Amputation of a limb or part of a limb is often performed in elderly patients who have significant medical problems. Occasionally amputations because of malignancy or trauma are necessary in young patients.

Spinal anesthesia is often preferred in the elderly with the expectation that various organ systems will be less affected. McLaren et al.[88] suggested that spinal anesthesia would be the anesthesia of choice for lower limb surgery. On the other hand, Mann et al.[90] found no significant differences between general and spinal anesthesia in the outcome of patients undergoing lower limb amputation. In the young patient, these procedures may be associated with significant psychologic trauma and the use of general anesthesia may be preferable.

A frequent sequela associated with limb amputation is that of phantom limb and/or phantom limb pain. A group of investigators in Denmark reported the effect of epidural anesthesia on phantom limb pain.[3] Epidural anesthesia with bupivacaine and morphine was established for 72 hours before surgery. This was compared with a group receiving general anesthesia. Six months following amputation, all patients in the epidural group were free of phantom limb pain. This was significantly different from the patients receiving general anesthesia. At the end of 1 year, patients in the epidural group were still free of pain, although the difference was not significant from those receiving general anesthesia. Although this study involved a small number of patients, it suggests that a preoperative sympathetic blockade may modulate phantom limb pain. At the very least, an intraoperative and postoperative neural blockade may be beneficial in these patients.

Tourniquets

A pneumatic tourniquet is often employed in surgery of the extremities to decrease bleeding and to provide a bloodless field. Tourniquet cuffs are usually inflated to a pressure of approximately 100 mm Hg above systemic arterial pressure. **Nerve injury and damage to blood vessels and skeletal muscle have been reported with tourniquets.**[50] **The potential injury resulting from the use of a tourniquet is a function of tourniquet pressure and the duration of inflation.**[50,59,76]

There is a variety of opinion regarding what is an appropriate inflation pressure for a tourniquet. In general, a greater pressure is used for a lower limb tourniquet than for an upper limb, because of the larger mass of the lower limb. In addition, femoral systolic pressure is higher than brachial pressure. It has been suggested that a cuff pressure of 100 mm Hg above systolic pressure is adequate for the lower extremity and 50 mm Hg above systolic pressure is adequate for the arm.[67] The duration of tourniquet inflation has also been a subject of controversy. Recommendations vary from 30 minutes to 4 hours. Following 1 hour of ischemia, depletion of glycogen granules in sarcoplasm has been shown by electron microscopy. After 2 hours of ischemia, mitochondrial swelling, myelin degeneration, and Z-line lysis occur.[118] It has been shown that these changes are reversible for tourniquet inflation times of between 1 and 2 hours.

It is essential that tourniquets be properly maintained with periodic checks on the accuracy of the pressure gauge. Tourniquets should be properly applied. The cuff should have a width 20% to 50% greater than the limb diameter. It should be applied over smooth padding and should overlap to ensure uniform pressure around the limb. The tourniquet should be protected from skin preparation solutions by an impermeable plastic drape. Complications from a tourniquet that is properly maintained, applied, and monitored should be minimal.[67]

The use of a tourniquet is also associated with hemodynamic and metabolic changes. In terms of hemodynamic changes, increases in systemic blood pressure and CVP have been reported. Minimal increases in blood pressure after inflation of the tourniquet have been reported using regional anesthesia. Nonetheless, marked increases in blood pressure of greater than 30% above control were reported in 53% of patients under general anesthesia.[157] The changes in blood pressure occurred without changing the depth of anesthesia, which included enflurane at or above 1 MAC, muscle relaxants, and fentanyl 1 to 2 μg/kg. Kaufman et al.[69] reported an overall 30% blood pressure increase in 11% of patients in whom tourniquets were used without distinguishing the type of anesthesia.

An increase in CVP following tourniquet inflation has been reported by Bradford.[12] Increases in blood volume following inflation of a tourniquet are difficult to estimate. It has been suggested that approximately 15% of the total blood volume is shifted to the general circulation following exsanguination of the lower limb.[157] Although changes in blood volume of 10% or less can occur without changes in CVP, changes greater than 10% will produce an increase in CVP. Bradford reported an increase in CVP of 14.5 cm H_2O when bilateral tourniquets were applied.[12] Following tourniquet deflation, a significant decrease in blood pressure may occur. These changes will require adaptation of the myocardium and alterations in cardiac output. These changes can be easily tolerated by young healthy patients; however, in older patients and patients with decreased myocardial reserve, these alterations could be significantly detrimental. Bilateral lower extremity surgery is being conducted with increased frequency; caution should be used with regard to inflating bilateral tourniquets simultaneously.

In addition to hemodynamic changes, metabolic changes have also been reported following tourniquet deflation; these include transient metabolic acidosis and increase in carbon dioxide.[82] These transient changes have no significant effects on the healthy patient or when one tourniquet is used. However, prolonged inflation and simultaneous release of two tourniquets may be detrimental in the poor-risk patient.

Tourniquet pain

Another potential problem associated with the use of a tourniquet—and a subject of considerable importance to the anesthesiologist—is that of tourniquet pain. Tourniquet-induced pain is an ill-defined pain occurring 45 to 60 minutes after tourniquet inflation. It is frequently described as a dull ache, the intensity of which increases until it becomes unbearable. Tourniquet pain has been reported in a significant number of patients under regional anesthesia despite an otherwise adequate blockade.[21,33,127] The cause of tourniquet pain remains obscure. **Tourniquet pain under spinal anesthesia has been related to the dose of local anesthetic used, the level of sensory anesthesia, the baricity of the local anesthetic solution, and the local anesthetic itself.**[13,20,28,33,128]

Several theories have been postulated in an attempt to explain the cause of tourniquet-induced pain. For example, Cole proposed that tourniquet pain was probably caused by compression and/or ischemia of the sciatic nerve. He suggested that the pain was of deep origin, because it occurred during an otherwise adequate spinal block. He proposed several mechanisms, such as "a progressive increase in the intensity of the stimulus, a fall in the concentration of local anesthetic until it could no longer block the stimulus, progression of ischemia to an intensity sufficient to produce pain, or the spinal block may be replaced by pressure anesthesia."[19]

Egbert and Deas[33] proposed that tourniquet pain involved activation of nociceptive fibers larger than those transmitting other types of pain. Following induction of a neural blockade, the concentration of local anesthetic in those larger fibers decreases rapidly until it is not sufficient to block the tourniquet stimulus. Egbert and Deas[33] were able to decrease the incidence of tourniquet pain by increasing the dose of tetracaine used for spinal anesthesia.

Whereas these theories relate to the concentration of local anesthetics in large fibers, DeJong and Cullen[28] proposed that tourniquet pain was transmitted by small unmyelinated fibers. These fibers would travel along sympathetic trunks before entering the cord at a level cephalad to the sensory block level. The incidence of tourniquet pain does not appear to be related to the sensory level of anesthesia. Tourniquet pain has been reported during both spinal and epidural anesthesia in the presence of high thoracic and cervical levels of sensory anesthesia.[21,127]

Although tissue ischemia has also been suggested as the cause of tourniquet pain, Hagenouw et al.[49] observed in a volunteer study that the pain subsides immediately following tourniquet deflation, which would be inconsistent with tissue ischemia.

It is generally accepted that pain is transmitted by small fibers. The smallest myelinated A fibers (A-delta) are responsible for the so-called fast pricking pain, consistent with incisional pain, whereas slow, persistent poorly localized pain is transmitted by unmyelinated C fibers. Tourniquet pain seems more consistent with pain sensation carried by C fibers. The work of Gissen et al. suggests that C fibers are more resistant to local anesthetic conduction blockade than the larger A fibers. At high concentrations of local anesthetics the action potentials of both types of fibers were equally suppressed. As the concentration of local anesthetic decreased, the amplitude of the C fiber action potential returns to baseline earlier than that of the A fibers.[42]

The tourniquet-induced pain occurring during spinal anesthesia could be a clinical manifestation of these *in vitro* results. Following intrathecal administration of an adequate dose of local anesthetic, conduction in both A and C fibers would be inhibited. As the concentration of local anesthetic in the cerebrospinal fluid (CSF) falls, conceivably C fibers would become active before the A fibers, resulting in tourniquet pain. In terms of the role of the local anesthetic drug on the occurrence of tourniquet pain, several clinical reports indicate that the incidence of tourniquet pain is significantly greater with tetracaine than with bupivacaine. Likewise, the differential effects on C and A fibers reported by Gissen were greater with tetracaine than with bupivacaine. This may explain the difference in the incidence of tourniquet pain observed between the two drugs.

Other possibilities have been postulated. Strichartz et al.[150] have shown that local anesthetic activity in an isolated nerve is enhanced by increasing the frequency of nerve stimulation, resulting in a frequency dependent block. Differences exist between the various local anesthetics with regard to frequency-dependent block. The potency of bupivacaine, for example, is markedly enhanced by an increase in the rate of nerve stimulation.[148] This could explain the reduced frequency of tourniquet pain with bupivacaine. The constant pressure of the tourniquet may result in an increased rate of firing by nociceptive fibers. Low concentrations of bupivacaine in those fibers may be sufficient to produce conduction blockade in some patients. On the other hand, because the anesthetic activity of tetracaine seems to be less influenced by the rate of stimulation, a low concentration of this agent would be insufficient to block nociceptive fibers activated by the tourniquet.

The study of Stewart et al.[148] on the frequency-dependent blocking characteristics of bupivacaine and tetracaine would support that theory. Their findings suggest that at 15 Hz the frequency-dependent conduction block is greater with bupivacaine than with tetracaine. These researchers suggest that if the perception of tourniquet pain is, at least, partially influenced by the frequency of action potentials conducted, then the greater frequency-dependent blockade produced by bupivacaine may contribute to the decreased incidence of tourniquet pain reported during spinal anesthesia with bupivacaine. Box 80-4 summarizes different theories proposed to explain tourniquet pain.

Once tourniquet pain develops, it is necessary to treat it early. The use of IV narcotics is somewhat disappointing. Increasing doses at frequent intervals are necessary to lessen the pain to a tolerable level. The induction of general anesthesia is often necessary, especially when tourniquet pain appears early in the procedure. The only efficacious treatment of tourniquet pain is releasing the pressure in the cuff.

It is now accepted that the addition of narcotics to local anesthetic-induced subarachnoid or epidural blockade improves the quality of anesthesia. Rucci et al. reported a 30% incidence of tourniquet pain in patients undergoing lower extremity surgery under epidural anesthesia with 0.5% bupivacaine with epinephrine. The authors reported a decrease of tourniquet pain to 8% when 200 μg of fentanyl were added to the epidural injection. Nonetheless, the efficacy of adding fentanyl to reduce tourniquet pain reached statistical significance only during the first 30 minutes of tourniquet inflation.[132] It is possible that the addition of other narcotics to epidurally injected local anesthetics may decrease the frequency of tourniquet pain for a longer period.

BOX 80-4
THEORIES OF TOURNIQUET PAIN

Transmitted by nerve fibers larger than those carrying other types of pain, running along the classical anatomic segmental distribution.
- Cole: Compression or ischemia of the sciatic nerve of sufficient intensity to "penetrate" the spinal block
- Egbert: Inadequate block (low concentration of local anesthetic in "large fibers" transmitting pressure pain)

Impulses arising in small fibers (A-delta and C).
Some of these impulses enter the cord at a level cephalad to that of the sensory block, along paraspinal pathways in the sympathetic trunks (De Jong, Collins)

Different nerve fibers (A-delta and C) sensitivity to the the effect of local anesthetic drug. With decreasing concentration of local anesthetic, the amplitude of C fiber action potential returns to normal, while the A fiber action potential is still suppressed

Frequency dependent block. The activity of local anesthetic in isolated nerves is enhanced as the frequency of nerve stimulation increases; the frequency-dependent block produced by bupivacaine is greater than that produced by tetracaine

Fracture of the Hip

With the exception of traumatic fractures in the young, hip fractures occur most often in the elderly. Concomitant medical problems, often affecting important organ systems, are frequent in this age population. Careful preoperative evaluation is of utmost importance. Some of these problems are correctable or partially correctable, and the patient's condition should be optimized prior to surgery. Although preoperative preparation is essential, excessive delay of surgical correction will increase the incidence of complications leading to increased mortality.

Of particular importance is the assessment of blood volume. **These patients are often debilitated and dehydrated. A large extravasation of blood at the fractured site may be undetected. A high or normal hematocrit may simply represent a constricted blood volume in a dehydrated patient.** Hence, careful evaluation is necessary. Urine output, specific gravity and osmolarity, and measurement of central venous pressure may be useful tools to determine volume status in these patients. If a decreased blood volume is suspected, careful hydration and restoration of intravascular volume is essential before induction of anesthesia.

The choice of anesthetic technique is controversial. It is widely believed that a regional anesthetic technique is preferable. This is not completely supported by the available literature.

Table 80-4 Summary of mortality studies following surgery for the fractured hip

Author	Incidence of death (%) Regional anesthesia	General anesthesia	Significance
Couderc (1977)	7/50–14	12/50–21	NS
McLaren (1978)	1/26–3.6	9/29–31	< 0/01
McKenzie (1980)	5/49–10	8/51–16	NS
White (1980)	0/20–0	0/20–0	NS
Davis (1982)	3/64–5	9/68–13	NS
McLaren (1982)	4/56–7	17/60–28	< 0.005
Wickstrom (1982)	2/32–6	6/97–6	NS
McKenzie (1984)*	3/73	12/25	< 0.05
	14/73	14/75	NS
Valentin (1987)	6%	8%	NS

The 3/73 incidence of death following regional anesthesia reported by McKenzie (1984) was over a period of 2 weeks; the 14/73 incidence was over a period of 2 months.

Mortality associated with surgery for hip fractures is high. Several studies have been carried out to determine the mortality following surgical correction of hip fractures under general and spinal anesthesia (Table 80-4). McLaren et al.[88] demonstrated a significantly lower mortality with spinal anesthesia at the end of 1 month. Other studies have also found mortality to be lower in the early postoperative period following spinal anesthesia. McKenzie et al. showed a statistically significant lower mortality rate with spinal than with general anesthesia. This difference was only significant 2 weeks following the procedure. At the end of 2 months, the mortality rate was the same with both anesthetic techniques.[87]

The high short-term mortality associated with fractured hip is related to age, gender (men greater than women), and site of fracture (trochanteric > femoral neck), whereas long-term mortality is related to male gender and ASA physical status.[148]

Hypoxemia may play an important role in the high mortality rate associated with hip fractures. Elderly patients with a fractured hip have been found to have significant hypoxemia.[93] Using the formula by Raine and Bishop to calculate the predicted Pao_2 levels, Sari et al.[134] found that in a group of 20 patients with femoral neck fracture, all exhibited Pao_2 levels well below that predicted for their age. Hole et al.[57] reported that postoperative hypoxemia was significantly greater and of longer duration in patients who have received general anesthesia than in those given regional anesthesia. Among other factors, fat embolism appears to play an important role in the development of hypoxemia.

Fat embolism syndrome

Fat embolism as a subclinical event occurs in all cases of long bone fractures. Monitoring of blood gases is the best tool to quantitate its clinical effects. Fat embolism syndrome (FES), on the other hand, is evident in 0.5% to 2% of long bone fractures. The incidence of FES increases sharply in multiple fractures and in association with pelvic injuries.[129] The most significant manifestations of FES occur at the level of the lungs. Fat globules impair perfusion in small vessels and cause endothelial damage in the pulmonary capillaries. This leads to vascular congestion, interstitial hemorrhage, alveolar wall damage, and airway collapse, resulting in ventilation/perfusion mismatch.

BOX 80-5
FAT EMBOLISM SYNDROME

Rapid fall in hematocrit
Erythrocyte aggregation
Platelet aggregation
Thrombocytopenia
Elevation of fibrinogen degradation products
Prolonged PT and PTT

A rise in serum lipid, particularly free fatty acids (FFA) and triglycerides, has been demonstrated in humans following trauma.[89,95] A rise in FFA and serum lipase activity was also demonstrated by Riseborough et al.[126] in patients with lower extremity fractures. These changes were associated with decreased Pao_2 and increased (A-aDo_2), increased platelet aggregation, thrombocytopenia and increased levels of fibrinogen degradation products. Therefore, significant coagulation abnormalities also occur in FES (Box 80-5). **Arterial hypoxemia may be the only clinical manifestations of subclinical fat embolism, whereas hypoxemia, tachycardia, and fever are early signs preceding the development of FES.**[44]

Petechiae in the anterior chest, axilla, neck, and conjunctivae are present in about 50% to 60% of cases and appear at 24 to 48 hours following the trauma. Lipuria is present in a similar number of cases. Although alterations of the clotting system are frequent, development of a clinical bleeding disorder is rare.[11] Chest radiographic findings are inconsistent. Electrocardiography demonstrates ST segment changes consistent with ischemia. Abnormalities consistent with right-sided heart strain may also be present.[120]

The frequency of fat embolism determined by autopsy was reported to be 2.4% to 3.3% in subcapital fractures and 0.7% to 0.8% in subjects with trochanteric fractures. In subjects treated conservatively, the incidence was 4.1% to 7% compared with 0.9% to 1% among subjects treated surgically.[139]

Although clinically FES is a relatively infrequent complication of trauma, once the syndrome has developed, it is associated with a relatively high mortality (10% to 15%). Thus, it is essential to have a high index of suspicion when caring for patients with lower extremity fractures.

Total Hip Replacement

Joint replacement has been the greatest advance in orthopedic surgery in the past two to three decades. Replacement of the hip, knee, shoulder, and finger have contributed to improved function and relief of pain in many patients, particularly those with rheumatoid arthritis.

Total hip replacement (THR) is by far the most successful reconstructive surgery for patients with rheumatoid arthritis and osteoarthritis. Changes in technique, type of prosthesis, mode of fixation, and other factors have occurred since Charnley performed the first hip arthroplasty in 1962.

THR is usually restricted to patients with marked functional limitations and/or substantial pain in whom other conservative therapies have not proved satisfactory. Patients over the age of 60 tend to obtain the best results. The majority of these procedures are carried out in patients with osteoarthritis and rheumatoid arthritis. THR may provide excellent benefits in other conditions, such as Paget's disease, ankylosing spondylitis, avascular necrosis, and congenital hip dislocation.

The surgical procedure is most commonly performed in the lateral decubitus position. It consists of enlarging the acetabulum and inserting an artificial cup usually made of high density polyethylene in a metal hemisphere. The femoral head is replaced by a metal sphere attached to a stem that is inserted in the femoral canal. Femoral components are generally made from superalloys of chromium-cobalt or titanium-aluminum-vanadium to provide maximum biocompatibility.[54]

At present, two different modes of fixing the components to the bone are employed—bone cement and bony ingrowth. Bone cement is an acrylic plastic, methylmethacrylate, which really consists of two components, a liquid (monomer) and a powder (polymer). The mixing of these components produces a chemical reaction that results in polymerization of the monomer. This exothermic reaction releases heat as the cement hardens. The only alternative to the use of bone cement requires that part or all of the artificial component has a porous surface that is placed against bone. Then bone or fibrous tissue grows into the pores of the component, providing a biologic fixation.

THR is a major surgical procedure that can be associated with severe complications. Severe hypotension, hypoxia, and cardiovascular collapse associated with insertion of the prothesis have been reported. Blood loss can be significant. The incidence of deep venous thrombosis and pulmonary embolism is uniquely high. In addition, major complications associated with the procedure include nerve damage[163] and femur fracture, both of which occur intraoperatively. Loosening of the components, hip dislocation,[168] infection, and heterotopic ossification may also occur following surgery.

Infection is a feared complication of joint replacement. The high incidence, 13%, which occurred in the early years of hip replacements[165] has been significantly decreased. The rate of deep-wound infection is now less than 1% for primary hip replacement and less than 3% for subsequent surgery.[133,136] Numerous approaches have been used to decrease the incidence of infection, such as the use of ultraviolet lights, laminar airflow enclosures, body exhaust systems,[80,133,136] and strict adherence to aseptic techniques. Whereas some of these methods may be unusual, the administration of prophylactic antibiotic agents is generally accepted as routine practice and has probably made a great contribution to the decreased incidence of infection. Second-generation cephalosporin drugs administered before or during the operation are the prophylactic antibiotics of choice.[54] Reoperation or hip revision is necessary in 10% to 30% of patients within 10 years of the original surgery. This is due almost completely to loosening of the components.

Hypotension, hypoxia, and cardiovascular collapse following prosthesis insertion have been reported.[43,99,111,119] These hemodynamic changes usually occur following insertion of the femoral components. Some authors have attributed these events to direct vasodilatory effects of the monomer,[111,119] whereas others consider that these hemodynamic changes are secondary to diffuse pulmonary fat emboli from bone marrow tissue.[25,139] In addition, air embolism has been implicated in the hemodynamic changes.[2,37,105] Although the cause is controversial, it is probably a multifactorial event.

In the early years of THR, it was believed that the hypotension resulted from a direct vasodilation produced by the monomer component of the cement. Experimental studies in dogs[99] showed that intravenous infusions of acrylic monomers caused no alterations of PaO_2 or $PaCO_2$. PA blood levels of the monomer significantly higher than those encountered in clinical situations were necessary to produce small and transient hypotension. Johansen et al. reported a significant cardiovascular effect of the methylmethacrylate. They reported significant decreases in cardiac output (CO), myocardial contractility (dp/dt), systemic vascular resistance (SVR), and arterial pressure, while pulse rate and left ventricular end-diastolic pressure (LVEDP) remained constant. The maximal cardiovascular effects occurred within 1 minute following insertion of the cement. Pulmonary vascular resistance and wedge pressure also increased significantly but at a later time period. The authors concluded that methylmethacrylate causes a direct pulmonary injury as opposed to particle embolization.[62]

In 1975, Modig et al.[99] conducted a study to determine the role of different mechanisms proposed to be responsible for the cardiovascular and respiratory events associated with THR.

PA blood showed fat particles in all patients following insertion of the femoral prosthesis. In over half the group, large amounts were found. However, they found a poor correlation between the presence of fat globules and the decrease in PaO_2 and hypotension. On the other hand, they found a significant release of tissue thromboplastic products following impaction of the femoral component, which could lead to platelet and fibrin aggregation in the pulmonary circulation. Platelet aggregation results in release of vasoactive substances, such as adenine nucleotides, which cause systemic vasodilation and hypotension. Platelet and fibrin aggregation also form microemboli in the pulmonary circulation resulting in hypoxemia.

Air embolism has been implicated as the probable cause of hemodynamic changes during THR. A number of reports have shown that air emboli are relatively common in THR.[2,37,60,96,105] Venous air emboli have been found to be common throughout the surgical procedure but become clinically significant during insertion of the femoral prosthesis. The source of this air is believed to be that remaining in the femoral canal after rimming the femoral shaft. This air would be entrapped and pressurized by the cement packed in the cavity.[67] It also has been proposed that during polymerization a significant amount of heat is released, which may increase the temperature of the blood resulting in the formation of gases.[2] Small air emboli are usually benign, but a potentially serious sequela could be parodoxic air embolism in the presence of an atrial septal defect.[17]

Several maneuvers have been recommended to reduce the amount of air entrapped in the femoral canal (e.g., femoral shaft venting[56,60] and carbon dioxide insufflation of the femoral canal before insertion of the cement).[55] In addition, Evans et al.[37] found that air embolism occurred less frequently when a long nozzled gun was used to insert the cement as compared with hand insertion of the cement.

Doppler ultrasonography, which is a sensitive method of detecting air emboli, has demonstrated that the presence of air in the right heart is common during THR.[2,97] Other very sensitive methods of diagnosing air emboli include esophageal echocardiography, esophageal Doppler ultrasonography and end-tidal nitrogen determination.[31,56,92] Changes in blood pressure, heart rate, increased central venous pressure, dysrhythmias, and decreased $PETCO_2$, are less sensitive methods and are usually late findings.

Anesthetic management

Close observation and monitoring of the cardiovascular status of patients with THR is of utmost importance. Frequent blood pressure determinations, especially at the time of cement insertion, are required. Blood pressure changes usually occur within the first minute of prothesis insertion and are generally transient. Although a noninvasive blood pressure device usually suffices, an indwelling arterial catheter is recommended for hip revision surgery, particularly if concomitant medical problems exist. Continuous ECG monitoring of lead II and V lead should be employed to detect myocardial ischemia.

Mass spectrometry would be helpful in detecting end-tidal nitrogen or a decrease in end-tidal CO_2, which is usually a late finding. An esophageal stethoscope should be used as a routine monitor, although the sensitivity of this device to detect air embolism is low. In addition, other routine monitoring such as pulse oximetry and body temperature should be used.

Close observation of volume status is necessary with prompt replacement of losses. Hypotension associated with cement insertion is more severe in hypovolemic patients.

The choice of anesthetic technique must be guided by the patient's physical and mental status. Data suggest that regional anesthesia offers significant advantages as compared with a general anesthetic technique for hip surgery, particularly with respect to blood loss and thromboembolism.

Blood loss

Blood loss can be significant during THR. Induced hypotensive anesthesia has been used extensively to reduce blood loss and the frequency of blood transfusion.[6,29,130,151,160] Nonetheless, deliberate hypotensive anesthesia may be contraindicated in some patients. Regional anesthesia is particularly useful in the elderly with significant medical problems. Sculco and Ranawat[137] and Thornburn et al.[153] have reported that **patients undergoing THR under spinal anesthesia have significantly lower blood loss and blood transfusion requirements than patients receiving general anesthesia.** Similar results have also been reported with epidural anesthesia.[72,98,100] Table 80-5 lists a number of studies on blood loss during THR.

A combination of factors is probably responsible for the decreased blood loss that accompanies regional anesthesia. A redistribution of blood flow to the major vessels of the lower limb and away from the operative field has been proposed by Modig.[102] Modig[101] also reported significant differences in some hemodynamic parameters between epidural anesthesia and general anesthesia. Mean arterial pressure (MAP), mean pulmonary artery pressure (MPAP), and peripheral venous pressure (PVP) were all significantly lower in patients under epidural anesthesia as compared with patients under general anesthesia and controlled ventilation undergoing THR.

Epidural anesthesia causes vasodilation of arteries, arterioles, and veins in the blocked area, resulting in a decreased MAP. This leads to decreased arterial oozing. The lower MPAP and particularly lower PVP will reduce venous oozing from the surgical area. Spontaneous respiration, which is not associated with an increase in intrathoracic pressure, will also contribute to decreased oozing.

Thromboembolism

The incidence of venous thromboembolism is significant following total hip replacement. Deep venous thrombosis

Table 80-5 Blood loss during regional (RA) and general (GA) anesthesia: summary of studies

Author	Number of patients		Decrease in blood loss in RA group (%)	Significance
	RA	GA		
Keith (1977)	10	17	50	S
Hole (1980)	29	31	20	NS
Modig (1981)	15	15	37	S
Chin (1982)	21	21	39	S
Hole (1982)	9	9	22	NS
Modig (1983)	30	30	28	S

(DVT) occurs in approximately 40% to 60% of patients. Proximal DVT, the precursor of pulmonary embolism (PE), occurs in 20% to 30% of subjects, whereas PE occurs in 2% to 3% of cases.[63,146] Preventive measures have been disappointing in the past. More recently, preoperative anticoagulant prophylaxis has been reported to decrease the frequency of DVT. For example, low-dose warfarin, low-dose subcutaneous heparin, and low-molecular weight heparin have been used to decrease the frequency of DVT following THR.[79,110,154] Hull et al.[58] demonstrated that intermittent leg compression significantly reduced the frequency of proximal vein and calf thrombosis.

The incidence of DVT and PE has also been shown to be significantly reduced when regional anesthesia is used. Thornburn found a significantly lower incidence of DVT following spinal anesthesia for THR.[153] Other authors have reported similar findings with epidural anesthesia (Table 80-6). Modig et al. compared the effects of continuous epidural anesthesia and general anesthesia on the incidence of thromboembolism following THR. They found a significantly lower frequency of DVT when epidural anesthesia was employed. The incidence of proximal vein thrombosis was 13% with epidural anesthesia and 67% with general anesthesia. PE occurred in 10% of patients in whom epidural anesthesia was employed, compared with 33% in the general anesthesia group.[100] Several factors contribute to thrombus formation. These include increased platelet aggregation and adhesiveness, blood hypercoagulability secondary to activation of clotting factors, vessel wall damage, and stagnation of blood. All of these factors are present during hip surgery.

Several studies have suggested the mechanisms by which continuous epidural anesthesia may decrease the incidence of thromboembolism. Local anesthetics, particularly lidocaine and other amides, may exert an antithrombolic effect by reducing adhesion of leukocytes to vessel walls.[22,41,81,149]

A hypercoagulable state is associated with surgery. Modig[98,100] found that the coagulative and fibrinolytic response to surgery was altered by afferent and efferent neural blockade. Patients with epidural anesthesia demonstrated higher resting levels of plasminogen and an increased capacity of releasing plasminogen activators as compared with patients in the general anesthesia group. In addition, fibronolysis inhibition activity associated with surgery was significantly lower in patients given epidural anesthesia.

Finally, hyperkinetic blood flow occurred in the lower extremities of patients under epidural anesthesia. Venous plethysmography showed that arterial inflow, venous capacity, and venous emptying rate were all significantly greater in the epidural anesthesia group.[102]

Thus, it would appear that continuous epidural anesthesia offers considerable advantages over general anesthesia in patients undergoing THR.

Table 80-6 Effect of regional (RA) and general (GA) anesthesia on the frequency of thromboembolism

Author	Regional anesthesia technique	Incidence of thromboembolism (% of patients)		
		RA	GA	Significance
Thornburn (1980)	Spinal	29	53	S
Davis (1981)	Epidural	46	77	S
Modig (1981)	Epidural	20	73	S
Modig (1981)	Epidural	40	77	S

Total Knee Arthroplasty

Total knee arthroplasty (TKA) is one of the most commonly performed joint replacement surgeries. It has been estimated that more than 140,000 patients underwent TKA in 1990.[104] TKA may be associated with severe, occasionally fatal complications. The incidence of DVT in TKA is 80%, which is higher than that associated with THR. PE occurs in 1% to 5% of patients. Both DVT and PE have been thought of as occurring postoperatively, with rare reported cases of PE during limb exsanguination before tourniquet inflation. These latter cases probably occur as a result of dislodgement of preexisting thrombus. Several cases of intraoperative fatal and near fatal PE following tourniquet deflation have been recently reported.[84,107]

These cases have lead several investigators to examine the incidence of intraoperative embolic phenomena during TKA, employing transesophageal echocardiography (TEE). Although McGrath et al.[85] demonstrated emboli in only 8 of 30 patients undergoing lower extremity procedures with the use of a tourniquet, Parmet et al.[112] reported echogenic emboli associated with tourniquet deflation in 100% of patients undergoing TKA.

Parmet et al. described two distinctive patterns of emboli released into the right atrium and right ventricle after tourniquet deflation: (1) showers of small venous emboli resembling a miliary pattern (which appeared in 100% of patients); and (2) larger discrete particles superimposed on a miliary pattern. The latter pattern has been found in 77% of patients. TEE does not allow determination of the nature or etiology of the embolic material, but several factors may contribute to its formation. Possibilities include fat originating from bone marrow manipulation, methylmethacrylate, air, or fresh thrombus.

In an attempt to determine the nature of the emboli, Parmet et al. placed a femoral venous catheter on the surgical side from which blood was aspirated following tourniquet deflation. Solid material was found in 5 of the 10 patients, which was identified as fresh thrombus. No air, fat, or bone marrow content was demonstrated in the aspirated blood. The authors speculate that these emboli represent thrombi formed during tourniquet inflation.[113] Ischemia, stasis, and cooling produced by the inflated tourniquet may contribute to thrombus formation. In addition, bone cement or methylmethacrylate has been shown to activate the coagulation cascade and to induce platelet aggregation. These effects may play a significant role in thrombus formation.

Parmet et al. also evaluated various hemodynamic parameters, and documented an increase in MPAP and increased pulmonary vascular resistance index (PVRI), but only in patients with larger-particle emboli. Cardiac output was unchanged. In addition, there was a transient decrease in mixed venous blood and oxygen saturation (SVO_2) and an increased end-tidal CO_2. These latter changes are present in all patients and are the result of deoxygenated blood and metabolites release from the ischemic limb. PVRI remained elevated long after SVO_2 returned to baseline. Thus, it is unlikely that decreased SVO_2 is a contributing factor in the increase in PVRI. **Increased PVRI may be the result of pulmonary vascular occlusion produced by embolic material.**[113]

In a subsequent study, Parmet et al. investigated the incidence of embolic phenomena during extramedullary guided knee arthroplasty, which avoids manipulation of the tibia marrow cavity. The incidence of small and large emboli released into the venous circulation was similar to that reported with intramedullary guided TKA.[114] **These findings suggest that the tourniquet may have a thrombogenic effect, and support the authors' previous conclusions that the embolic material observed after tourniquet release represented fresh thrombus.**

Patients with patent foramen ovale (PFO) undergoing TKA could potentially experience paradoxic emboli. Three subjects in Parmet's investigation demonstrated small emboli in the left atrium and left ventricle. Further, paradoxic air emboli resulting in near fatal cardiovascular collapse has been reported during THR.[17]

Anesthetic management

The influence of anesthetic technique during TKA has not been extensively investigated. Nonetheless, regional anesthesia seems to offer some advantages over general anesthesia.

For example, several authors have demonstrated the inability of general anesthesia to prevent tourniquet-induced hypertension.[69,157] A regional anesthesia technique (e.g., subarachnoid block or epidural anesthesia) significantly reduces or completely abolishes tourniquet-induced hypertension. In addition a continuous epidural technique can provide postoperative analgesia.

The influence of regional anesthesia on the incidence of postoperative DVT or PE following TKA has not been as well documented as with THR. Two studies have shown that postoperative DVT following TKA is significantly reduced by epidural anesthesia. In 1990, Nielsen et al. conducted a small prospective study of patients undergoing TKA, which demonstrated that the risk of postoperative DVT was significantly reduced by epidural anesthesia, as compared with general anesthesia.[106] Similar findings were reported by Sharrock et al.[142] in a more extensive retrospective study, involving more than 600 patients.

Nonetheless, the influence of anesthetic technique on the incidence of intraoperative embolic phenomena has not been investigated. All the investigations demonstrating echogenic emboli associated with tourniquet release employing TEE, have been conducted in patients undergoing TKA under general anesthesia. Further studies will be necessary to determine anesthetic effect and the role of antithrombotic therapy during tourniquet inflation.

KEY POINTS

- Several problems are associated with the prone position for patients undergoing surgery on the spine: (1) impairment of respiration; (2) abdominal pressure leading to inferior vena cava compression and impeded venous return; (3) excessive pressure or traction on the extremities leading to peripheral nerve damage; (4) excessive pressure on the eyes, ears, and nose; and (5) pressure necrosis of the nipples of women or the genitalia of men.
- The correction of severe spinal deformities by the anterior approach involves several major risks, including excessive bleeding and damage to the spinal cord. Distension of the cord can interfere with its circulation and lead to anterior spinal artery syndrome. If the transthoracic approach is selected for anterior spinal decompression and fusion, a double lumen endotracheal tube is indicated, and one-lung anesthesia should be conducted until surgical decompression or correction has been achieved.
- For cervical spinal fusion, awake intubation of the trachea is recommended, as maintenance of the airway in an unconscious, nonintubated patient may prove very difficult. In addition, intubation of the trachea in an awake patient usually avoids manipulation of the unstable cervical spine.
- In patients with scoliosis, the major abnormality in gas exchange is a ventilation/perfusion ($\dot{V}/\dot{Q}$) maldistribution. Generalized alveolar hypoventilation results in hypoxia. There is also an increase in the dead space:tidal volume ratio and in alveolar-arterial oxygen difference.
- Regional anesthesia is probably the most frequently used method of anesthesia for surgery of the upper extremity. This can be achieved with IV regional anesthesia (IVRA), brachial plexus blockade, or blockade of peripheral nerves at elbow and wrist.
- The advantages of IVRA over brachial plexus block include simplicity of technique, rapid onset of anesthesia, controllable duration of action, and rapid return of func-

tion. Disadvantages include the requirement that a tourniquet be used continuously, the potential for toxic reactions, and the absence of postoperative analgesia.

- Regional anesthesia alone or in combination with general anesthesia is the technique of choice for reimplantation surgery. The main advantage of a regional technique is sympathetic blockade, which may improve blood flow to the injured limb. The advantages of a continuous technique are not only postoperative analgesia, but also prolonged sympathetic blockade beyond surgery if desired.
- Elderly patients with a fractured hip have been found to have significant hypoxemia. Hypoxemia may play an important role in the high mortality rate that is associated with hip fractures. Among other factors, fat embolism appears to play an important role in the development of hypoxemia. Postoperative hypoxemia was reported to be more severe and of longer duration in patients who received general anesthesia that in those who were given regional anesthesia.
- A number of reports have shown that air emboli are relatively common in THR. Air embolism has been implicated as a probable cause of hemodynamic changes during THR. Clinically significant air embolism occurs most commonly during insertion of the femoral prosthesis.
- Release of embolic material into the central venous circulation occurs frequently following tourniquet release during lower limb surgery. Two TEE patterns have been described: (1) a miliary pattern; and (2) larger-particle emboli superimposed on a miliary pattern. The nature of these emboli has not been clearly determined, but it appears that the embolic material represent fresh thrombus.
- The most significant hemodynamic changes associated with tourniquet release and larger emboli are increased MPAP an increased PVRI. It is likely that embolic material produces pulmonary vascular occlusion, which leads to increased PVRI.

KEY REFERENCES

Concepcion MA, Lambert DH, Welch KA, et al: Tourniquet pain during spinal anesthesia: a comparison of plain solutions of tetracaine and bupivacaine, *Anesth Analg* 67:828, 1988.

Grundy BL, Nash CL, Brown RH: Deliberate hypotension for spinal fusion: prospective randomized study with evoked potential monitoring, *Can Anaesth Soc J* 29:452, 1982.

Harris WH, Sledge CB: Total hip and total knee replacement, *N Engl J Med* 323:12, 1990.

Kafer ER: Respiratory and cardiovascular functions in scoliosis and the principles of anesthetic management, *Anesthesiology* 52:339, 1980.

Ovassapian A, Land P, Schaefer MF, et al: Anesthetic management for surgical correction of severe flexion deformity of the cervical spine, *Anesthesiology* 58:370, 1983.

Parmet JL, Berman AT, Horrow JC, et al: Thromboembolism coincident with tourniquet deflation during total knee arthroplasty, *Lancet* 341(8852):1057–1058, 1993.

Patel NJ, Flashburg MH, Paskin S, et al: A regional anesthetic technique compared to general anesthesia for outpatient knee arthroscopy, *Anesth Analg* 64:185, 1986.

Valli H, Rosenberg PH: Effects of three anaesthesia methods on haemodynamic responses connected with the use of thigh tourniquet in orthopedic patients, *Acta Anaesth Scand* 29:142, 1985.

REFERENCES

1. Alvine RG, Schurrer ME: Postoperative ulnar nerve palsy: are there predisposing factors, *J Bone Joint Surg* 69A:255, 1987.
2. Anderson KH: Air aspirated from the venous system during total hip replacement, *Anaesthesia* 8:1175, 1983.
3. Bach S, Noreng MF, Tjellden NU: Phantom limb pain in amputees during the first 12 months following limb amputation, after preoperative lumbar epidural blockade, *Pain* 33:297, 1988.
4. Bader AM, et al: Comparison of lidocaine and prilocaine for intravenous regional anesthesia, *Anesthesiology* 69:409, 1988.
5. Bailey TE, Mahoney OM: The use of banked autologous blood in patients undergoing surgery for spinal deformity, *J Bone Joint Surg* 69A:329, 1987.
6. Barbier-Bohm G, et al: Comparative effects of induced hypotension and normovolaemic haemodilution on blood loss in total hip arthroplasty, *Br J Anaesth* 52:1039, 1980.
7. Bell S, Gschwand N, Steiger U: Arthroplasty of the elbow: experience with the Mark III BSB prosthesis, *Aust NE J Surg* 56:823, 1986.
8. Besser MI, Stahl S: Arthroscopic surgery performed under local anesthesia as an outpatient procedure, *Arch Orthop Trauma Surg* 105:296, 1986.
9. Bigliani LV, Flatow EL, Craig EV: Shoulder reconstruction. In Herndon J, editor: *Orthopaedic knowledge update 3, Home study syllabus,* Park Ridge, 1990, Academy of Orthopaedic Surgeons.
10. Blount WP, Moe JH: *The Milwaukee brace,* Baltimore, 1973, Williams & Wilkins.
11. Bradford DS, Foster RR, Nossel HL: Coagulation alterations, hypoxemia, and fat embolism in fracture patients, *J Trauma* 10:307, 1970.
12. Bradford EMW: Haemodynamic changes associated with the application of lower limb tourniquet, *Anaesthesia* 24:190, 1969.
13. Bridenbaugh PO, et al: Addition of glucose to bupivacaine in spinal anesthesia increases the incidence of tourniquet pain, *Anesth Analg* 65:1181, 1986.

14. Britt BA, Kalow W: Malignant hyperthermia: a statistical review, *Can Anaesth Soc J* 17:293, 1970.
15. Brodkey JS, et al: Reversible spinal cord trauma in cats. Additive effects of direct pressure and ischemia, *J Neurosurg* 37: 591, 1972.
16. Burnham PJ: Regional block of the great nerves of the upper arm, *Anesthesiology* 19:281, 1958.
17. Camann WR, et al: Nearly fatal cardiovascular collapse during total hip replacement: probable coronary arterial embolism, *Anesth Analg* 72:245, 1991.
18. Cappellino A, Jokl P, Ruwe PA: Regional anesthesia in knee arthroscopy: a new technique involving femoral and sciatic nerve blocks in knee arthroscopy, *J Arthro Related Surg* 12(1)120–123, 1996.
19. Cole F: Tourniquet pain, *Anesth Analg* 31:63, 1952.
20. Concepcion MA, Lambert DH, Welch KA, et al: Tourniquet pain during spinal anesthesia: a comparison of plain solutions of tetracaine and bupivacaine, *Anesth Analg* 67:828, 1988.
21. Concepcion MA, Maddi R, Francis D, et al: Vasoconstrictors in subarachnoid block. A comparison of epinephrine and phenylephrine, *Anesth Analg* 63:134, 1984.
22. Cooke ED, et al: Intravenous lignocaine in prevention of deep venous thrombosis after elective hip surgery, *Lancet* 2:797, 1977.
23. Cowell HR, Swickard JW: Autotransfusion in children's orthopaedics, *J Bone Joint Surg* 56A:908, 1973.
24. Crane L: Arthroscopic surgery under local anesthesia, *Orthopedics* 7:748, 1984.
25. Dandy DJ: Fat embolism following prosthetic replacement of the femoral head, *Injury* 3:85, 1971.
26. Davies G, Reid L: Effects of scoliosis in growth of alveoli and pulmonary arteries and on the right ventricle, *Arch Dis Child* 46:623, 1971.
27. Davis FM, Quince M, Laurenson VG: Deep vein thrombosis and anaesthetic technique in emergency hip surgery, *Br Med J* 2:1528, 1980.
28. Davis NJ, Jennings JJ, Harris WH: Induced hypotensive anesthesia for total hip replacement, *Clin Orthop* 101:93, 1974.
29. Dejong R, Cullen SC: Theoretical aspects of pain. Bizarre pain phenomena during low spinal anesthesia, *Anesthesiology* 24: 628, 1963.
30. Delong WB: Operative positioning for low back surgery. In White A, Rothman RH, Raj CD, editors: *Lumbar spine surgery, techniques and complications,* St. Louis, 1987, CV Mosby.
31. Drummond JC, Prutow RJ, Scheller MS: A comparison of the sensitivity of pulmonary artery pressure, end-tidal carbon dioxide, and end-tidal nitrogen in the detection of venous air embolism in the dog, *Anesth Analg* 64:688, 1985.
32. Dwayer AF, Shafer MF: Anterior approach to scoliosis. Results of treatment in fifty-one cases, *J Bone Joint Surg* 56A:218, 1974.
33. Egbert BD, Deas TC: Causes of pain from a pneumatic tourniquet during spinal anesthesia, *Anesthesiology* 23:87, 1962.
34. Engler GL, et al: Somatosensory evoked potentials during Harrington instrumentation for scoliosis, *J Bone Joint Surg* 60A: 528, 1978.
35. Eriksson E: Brachial plexus block: axillary approach. In Eriksson E, editor: *Illustrated handbook of local anaesthesia,* Philadelphia, 1980, WB Saunders.
36. Evans CJ, et al: Residual nerve block following intravenous regional anesthesia, *Br J Anaesth* 46:668, 1974.
37. Evans RD, Palazzo GA, Ackers JWL: Air embolism during total hip replacement: comparison of two surgical techniques, *Br J Anaesth* 62:243, 1989.
38. Finch S, Haskins D, Finch CA: Iron metabolism, hematopoiesis following phlebotomy. Iron as a limiting factor, *J Clin Invest* 29:1078, 1950.
39. Galindo A, Hermandez J, Benavides O: Quality of spinal extradural anesthesia: the influence of spinal nerve root diameter, *Br J Anaesth* 47:41, 1975.
40. Gerber H, et al: Intraarticular absorption of bupivacaine during arthroscopy. Comparison of 0.25%, 0.5% and 0.75% solution, *Anesthesiology* 63:A217, 1985.
41. Gidden DB, Lindhe J: In vivo quantitation of local anesthetic suppression of leukocyte adherence, *Am J Pathol* 68:327, 1972.
42. Gissen AJ, Covino BG, Gregus J: Differential sensitivities of mammalian nerve fibers to local anesthetic agents, *Anesthesiology* 53:467, 1980.
43. Gooding JM, Smith RA, Weng JT: Is methylmethacrylate safer than previously thought? *Anesth Analg* 59:542, 1980.
44. Gossling HR, Pellegrim VD: Fat embolism syndrome. A review of the pathophysiology and physiological basis of treatment, *Clin Orthop* 165:68, 1982.
45. Grant FC: Autotransfusion, *Ann Surg* 74:253, 1921.
46. Griffiths IR, Trench JE, Crawford RA: Spinal cord blood flow and conduction during experimental cord compression in normotensive and hypotensive dogs, *J Neurosurg* 50:353, 1979.
47. Grundy BL, Nash CL, Brown RH: Arterial pressure manipulation alters spinal cord function during correction of scoliosis, *Anesthesiology* 54:249, 1981.
48. Grundy BL, Nash CL, Brown RH: Deliberate hypotension for spinal fusion: prospective randomized study with evoked potential monitoring, *Can Anaesth Soc J* 29:452, 1982.
49. Hagenow R, et al: Tourniquet pain: a volunteer study, *Anesth Analg* 65:175, 1986.
50. Hamilton WK, Sokoll MD: Tourniquet paralysis, *JAMA* 199:37, 1967.
51. Hamstra RD, Block MH: Erythropoiesis in response to blood loss in man, *Blood* 34: 357, 1969.
52. Harrington PR: Treatment of scoliosis. Correction and internal fixation by spine instrumentation, *J Bone Joint Surg* 44A: 591, 1962.
53. Harris AG, Heron JS, Renwick WA: Anaesthesia for posterior cervical osteotomy, *Can Anaesth Soc J* 22:84, 1975.
54. Harris WH, Sledge CB: Total hip and total knee replacement, *N Engl J Med* 323:12, 1990.
55. Harvey PB, Smith JA: Prevention of air emboli in hip surgery. Femoral shaft insufflation with carbon dioxide, *Anaesthesia* 37:714, 1982.
56. Heinrich H, et al: Transesophageal two-dimensional echocardiography during total hip replacement, *Anaesthesia* 34:118, 1985.
57. Hole A, Terjesen T, Breivik H: Epidural versus general anaesthesia for total hip arthroplasty in elderly patients, *Acta Anaesth Scand* 24:279, 1980.
58. Hull RD, et al: Effectiveness of intermittent pneumatic leg compression for preventing deep vein thrombosis after total hip replacement, *JAMA* 263:2313, 1990.
59. Hurst LN, et al: The pneumatic tourniquet, *Plast Reconst Surg* 67:648, 1981.
60. Hyland J, Robins RHC: Cardiac arrest and bone cement, *Br Med J* 3:326, 1970.
61. Jaurequito JW, Wilcox JF, Cohn SJ, et al: A comparison of intra-articular morphine with bupivacaine for pain control after outpatient knee arthroscopy. A prospective randominized double-blind study, *Am J Sports Med* 23(3):350–353, 1995.
62. Johansen I, Benumof JL: Methylmethacrylate: a myocardial depressant and peripheral dilator (abstract), *Anesthesiology* 51:577, 1979.
63. Johnson R, et al: Deep venous thrombosis following Charnley arthroplasty, *Clin Orthop* 132:24, 1978.
64. Kafer ER: Respiratory and cardiovascular functions in scoliosis and the principles of anesthetic management, *Anesthesiology* 52:339, 1980.
65. Kahanovitz N: Lumbar spine. In Herndon J, editor: *Orthopedic knowledge update 3, Home study syllabus,* Park Ridge, 1990, American Academy of Orthopedic Surgeons.
66. Kallos T, et al: Intramedullary pressure and pulmonary embolism of femoral medullary contents in dogs during insertion of bone cement and a prothesis, *J Bone Joint Surg* 56A:1363, 1974.
67. Kallos T, Smith T: Anesthesia and orthopedic surgery. In Barash PG, editor: *Clinical anesthesia,* Philadelphia, 1988, JB Lippincott.
68. Katz J, et al: The pharmacokinetics of bupivacaine when injected intraarticularly following knee arthroscopy, *Reg Anesth Supp* 13:15, 1988.
69. Kaufman RD, Walts LF: Tourniquet induced hypertension, *Br J Anaesth* 54:333, 1982.
70. Kehlet H: The stress response to anesthesia and surgery—release mechanism and modifying factors, *Clin Anaesth* 2:315, 1984.
71. Keiser RP, Shufflebarger HL: The Milwaukee brace in idiopathic scoliosis, *Clin Orthop* 118:19, 1974.
72. Keith I: Anaesthesia and blood loss in total hip replacement, *Anaesthesia* 32:444, 1977.
73. Khambatta HJ, et al: Hypotensive anesthesia for spinal fusion with sodium nitroprusside, *Spine* 3:171, 1978.
74. Kikerby OJ, Aase S: Knee arthroscopy and arthrotomy under local anesthesia, *Acta Orthop Scand* 58:133, 1987.
75. Klein HA: Scoliosis. In Trench Att, editor: *Clinical symposia,* vol 30, Summit, 1978, CIBA.

76. Klenerman L: Tourniquet time—how long? *Hand* 12:231, 1980.
77. Larsen U, et al: Complications during anaesthesia in patients with Duchenne's muscular dystrophy (a retrospective study), *Can Anaesth J* 36:428, 1989.
78. Lawrence VS, et al: Spinal anesthesia with isobaric lidocaine 2% and the effect of phenylephrine, *Reg Anaesth* 9:17, 1984.
79. Leyvraz PF, et al: Adjusted versus fixed-dose subcutaneous heparin in the prevention of deep-vein thrombosis after total hip replacement, *N Engl J Med* 315:925, 1983.
80. Lidwell OM, et al: Effect of ultraclean air in operating rooms on deep sepsis in the joint after total hip or knee replacement: a randomized study, *Brit Med J* 285:10, 1982.
81. Luostarinen V, et al: Antithrombotic effects of lidocaine and related compounds on laser-induced micro-vascular injury, *Acta Anaesthesiol Scand* 25:9, 1981.
82. Lynn AM, et al: Systemic responses to tourniquet release in children, *Anesth Analg* 65:865, 1986.
83. MacEwen ED, Bunnell WP, Sriram K: Acute neurological complications in the treatment of scoliosis: a report of the Scoliosis Research Society, *J Bone Joint Surg* 57A:404, 1975.
84. McGrath BJ, Hsai J, Epstein B: Massive pulmonary embolism following tourniquet deflation, *Anesthesiology* 74:618–620, 1991.
85. McGrath BJ, Hsai J, Boyd A, et al: Venous embolization after deflation of lower extremity tourniquets, *Anesth Analg* 78(2) 349–393, 1994.
86. McKenzie PJ, Wishart HY, Gray I, et al: Effects of anaesthetic technique on deep vein thrombosis. A comparison of subarachnoid and general anaesthesia, *Br J Anaesth* 57:853, 1985.
87. McKenzie PJ, Wishart HY, Smith G: Long-term outcome after repair of fractured neck femur. Comparison of subarachnoid and general anaesthesia, *Br J Anaesth* 56:581, 1984.
88. McLaren AD, Stockwell MC, Reid VT: Anaesthetic technique for surgical correction of fracture neck of femur. A comparative study of spinal and general anaesthesia in the elderly, *Anaesthesia* 33:10, 1978.
89. McNamara J, et al: Lipid metabolism after trauma. Role in the pathogenesis of fat embolism, *J Thorac Cardiovasc Surg* 63:968, 1972.
90. Mann RAM, Bisset WIK: Anaesthesia for lower limb amputation. A comparison of spinal analgesia and general anaesthesia in the elderly, *Anaesthesia* 38:1185, 1983.
91. Martin JT: *Positioning in anesthesia and surgery,* Philadelphia, 1978, WB Saunders.
92. Martin RW, Colley PS: Evaluation of transesophageal Doppler detection of air embolism in dogs, *Anesthesiology* 58:117, 1983.
93. Martin VC: Hypoxemia in elderly patients suffering from fractured neck of femur, *Anaesthesia* 32:852, 1977.
94. Matheson D: Epidural anaesthesia for lumbar laminectomy and spinal fusion, *Can Anaesth Soc J* 7:149, 1960.
95. Meek RN, Woodruff MB, Allardyce DB: Source of fat macroglobules in fractures of the lower extremity, *J Trauma* 12:432, 1972.
96. Michael R: Air embolism in hip surgery, *Anaesthesia* 35:858, 1980.
97. Michenfelder JD, Miller RH, Gronert GA: Evaluation of an ultrasonic device (Doppler) for the diagnosis of venous air embolism, *Anesthesiology* 36:164, 1972.
98. Modig J, Borg T, Karlström G, et al: Thromboembolism after total hip replacement: role of epidural and general anesthesia, *Anesth Analg* 62:174, 1983.
99. Modig J, Busch C, Olerud S, et al: Arterial hypotension and hypoxaemia during a total hip replacement: the importance of thromboplastic products, fat embolism and acrylic monomers, *Acta Anaesthesiol Scand* 19:28, 1975.
100. Modig G, Hjelmstedt A, Sahlstedt B, et al: Comparative influences of epidural and general anaesthesia on deep venous thrombosis and pulmonary embolism after total hip replacement, *Acta Chir Scand* 247:125, 1981.
101. Modig J, Karlstrom G: Intra- and post-operative blood loss and haemodynamics in total hip replacement when performed under lumbar epidural versus general anaesthesia, *Eur J Anaesth* 4:345, 1987.
102. Modig J, Malmberg P, Karlstrom G: Effect of epidural versus general anaesthesia on calf blood flow, *Acta Anaesth Scand* 24:305, 1980.
103. Nash CL, et al: Spinal cord monitoring during operative treatment of the spine, *Clin Orthop* 126:100, 1977.
104. National Center for Health Statistics: The detailed diagnosis and procedures. National hospital discharge series 13, number 113, vital and vital and health statistics series, Hyattsville, 1990, United States Department of Health and Human Services.
105. Ngai SH, Stinchfield FE, Triner LK: Air embolism during total hip arthroplasties, *Anesthesiology* 40:405, 1974.
106. Nielsen PT, Jorgensen LN, Albretch-Beste E, et al: Lower thrombosis risk with epidural blockade in knee arthroplasty, *Acta Orthop Scand* 61:29, 1990.
107. Orsini EC, Richards RR, Mullen JMB: Fatal fat embolism during cemented total knee arthroplasty. A case report, *Can J Surg* 29:385–386, 1986.
108. Ovassapian A, Dykes M: The role of fiberoptic endoscopy in airway management, *Semin Anesth* 2:93, 1987.
109. Ovassapian A, Land P, Schaefer MF, et al: Anesthetic management for surgical correction of severe flexion deformity of the cervical spine, *Anesthesiology* 58:370, 1983.
110. Paiement G, et al: Low dose warfarin versus external pneumatic compression for prophylaxis against thromboembolism following total hip replacement, *J Arthroplasty* 2:23, 1987.
111. Park WY, et al: Changes in arterial oxygen tension during total hip replacement, *Anesthesiology* 39:642, 1973.
112. Parmet JL, Berman AT, Horrow JC, et al: Thromboembolism coincident with tourniquet deflation during total knee arthroplasty, *Lancet* 341(8852):1057–1058, 1993.
113. Parmet JL, Horrow JC, Singer R, et al: Echogenic emboli upon tourniquet release during total knee arthroplasty: pulmonary hemodynamic changes and embolic composition, *Anesth Analg* 79(5):940–945, 1994.
114. Parmet JL, Horrow JC, Pharo G, et al: The incidence of venous emboli during extramedullary guided total knee arthroplasty, *Anesth Analg* 81(4):757–762, 1995.
115. Patel NJ, Flashburg MH, Paskin S, et al: A regional anesthetic technique compared to general anesthesia for outpatient knee arthroscopy, *Anesth Analg* 65:185, 1986.
116. Patel NJ, Patel BS, Paskin S, et al: Induced moderate hypotensive anesthesia for spinal fusion and Harrington-rod instrumentation, *J Bone J Surg* 67A:2384, 1985.
117. Pathak KS, et al: Continuous opioid infusion for scoliosis fusion surgery, *Anesth Analg* 62:841, 1983.
118. Patterson D, Klenerman L: The effect of pneumatic tourniquets on ultra-structure of skeletal muscle, *J Bone Joint Surg* 61B: 178, 1979.
119. Peebles DJ, et al: Cardiovascular effects of methylmethacrylate cement, *Br Med J* 1:349, 1972.
120. Peltier LF: The diagnosis and treatment of fat embolism, *J Trauma* 11:661, 1971.
121. Peterson DO: Shoulder block anesthesia for shoulder reconstruction surgery, *Anesth Analg* 64:373, 1985.
122. Pitkanen M, Rosenberg PH: Minor complications following anaesthesia in young adults for orthopaedic surgery of the lower extremity, *Ann Chir Gynaecol* 76:99, 1988.
123. Raj PP, et al: Infraclavicular brachial plexus block. A new approach, *Anesth Analg* 52:897, 1973.
124. Ray CD: Positioning the patient for lumbar decompressions or fusions. In White A, Rothman RH, Raj CD, editors: *Lumbar spine surgery, techniques and complications*, St. Louis, 1987. CV Mosby.
125. Relton JES, et al: Hyperpyrexia in association with general anaesthesia in children, *Can Anaesth Soc J* 13:419, 1966.
126. Riseborough EJ, Herndon JH: Alterations in pulmonary function coagulation and fat metabolism in patients with fractures of the lower limbs, *Clin Orthop* 115:248, 1976.
127. Rocco AG, et al: A double blind evaluation of intrathecal bupivacaine without glucose and a standard solution of hyperbaric tetracaine, *Reg Anesth* 9:137, 1984.
128. Rocco AG, et al: Double blind evaluation of intrathecal bupivacaine and tetracaine, *Reg Anesth* 9:183, 1984.
129. Rokkanen P, et al: The syndrome of fat embolism: analysis of 30 consecutive cases compared with trauma patients with similar injuries, *J Trauma* 10:299, 1970.
130. Rosberg B, Fredin H, Gustafson C: Anesthetic techniques and surgical blood loss in total hip arthroplasty, *Acta Anaesth Scand* 26:189, 1982.
131. Rosenberg MK, Berner G: Spinal anesthesia in lumbar disc surgery: review of 200 cases, with a case history, *Anesth Analg* 44: 419, 1965.
132. Rucci FS, Trafficante FG, Pippa P: Fentanyl and bupivacaine mixture for extradural blockade in orthopaedic surgery: effects on haemodynamic responses and pain related to the use of thigh tourniquet, *Eur J Anaesthesiol* 4:167, 1987.
133. Salvati EA, et al: Infection rates after 3175 total hip and total knee replacements performed with and without a horizontal unidirectional filtered air-flow system, *J Bone Joint Surg* 64A:525, 1982.

134. Sari A, et al: The magnitude of hypoxemia in elderly patients with fractures of the femoral neck, *Anesth Analg* 65:892, 1986.
135. Schneerson JM, Venco A, Prime FJ: A study of pulmonary artery pressure, electrocardiography and mechanocardiography in thoracic scoliosis, *Thorax* 32:700, 1977.
136. Schutzer SF, Harris WH: Deep wound infection after total hip replacement under contemporary aseptic conditions, *J Bone Joint Surg* 70A:724, 1988.
137. Sculco TP, Ranawat C: The use of spinal anaesthesia for total hip replacement arthroplasty, *J Bone Joint Surg* 57A:173, 1975.
138. Seay AR, Ziter FA, Thompson JA: Cardiac arrest during induction of anesthesia in Duchenne muscular dystrophy, *J Pediatr* 93:88, 1978.
139. Sevitt S: Fat embolism in patients with fractured hips, *Br Med J* 2:257, 1972.
140. Sewell IA: *Circulation in the tissues.* In Scurr C, Feldman S, editors: *Scientific foundations of anaesthesia*, Chicago, 1974, Year Book Medical Publishers.
141. Shanahan PT, Kleinert HE: Anesthesia management of upper extremity reimplantation surgery, *Anesthesiol Rev* 5:10, 1983.
142. Sharrock NE, Haos SB, Hargett MJ, et al: Effects of epidural anesthesia on the incidence of deep-vein thrombosis after total knee arthrosplasty, *J Bone Joint Surg (AM)* 73:502, 1991.
143. Simmons EH: Surgery of the spine in rheumatoid arthritis and ankylosing spondylitis. In Evarts CM, editor: *Surgery of the musculoskeletal system,* vol 2, New York, 1983, Churchill-Livingstone.
144. Small N: Overview of arthroscopic surgery complications. In Sprague N III, editor: *Complications in arthroscopy,* New York, 1989, Raven Press.
145. Smith RH: The prone position. In Martin JT, editor: *Positioning in anesthesia,* Philadelphia, 1978, WB Saunders.
146. Stamatakis JD, et al: Femoral vein thrombosis and total hip replacements, *Br Med J* 2:223, 1977.
147. Starr A: Sensory evoked potentials in clinical disorders of the nervous system, *Ann Rev Neurosci* 1:103, 1978.
148. Stewart A, et al: Decreased incidence of tourniquet pain during spinal anesthesia with bupivacaine. A possible explanation, *Anesth Analg* 67:833, 1988.
149. Stewart GJ, et al: Inhibition of leukocyte locomotion by tacainide, a primary amide analog of lidocaine. A study of indium-labeled leukocytes and scanning electron microscopy, *Lab Invest* 42:302, 1980.
150. Strichartz G, Zimmerman M: An explanation for pain originating from tourniquets during regional anesthesia, *Reg Anesth* 94:44, 1984.
151. Thompson GE, et al: Hypotensive anesthesia for total hip arthroplasty: a study of blood loss and organ functions (brain, heart, liver and kidney), *Anesthesiology* 18: 91, 1978.
152. Thomson JD, et al: Prior deposition of autologous blood in elective orthopaedic surgery, *J Bone Joint Surg* 69A:320,1987.
153. Thornburn R, Louden JR, Vallance R: Spinal and general anaesthesia in total hip replacement: frequency of deep vein thrombosis, *Br J Anaesth* 52:1117, 1980.
154. Turpie AGG, et al: A randomized controlled trial of low molecular weight heparin (enoxaparin) to prevent deep-vein thrombosis in patients undergoing elective hip surgery, *N Engl J Med* 315:925, 1986.
155. Urist MR: Osteotomy of the cervical spine, *J Bone Joint Surg* 40A:833, 1958.
156. Valentin N, et al: Spinal or general anaesthesia for surgery of the fractured hip? A prospective study of mortality in 578 patients, *Br J Anaesth* 58:248, 1986.
157. Valli H, Rosenberg PH: Effects of three anaesthesia methods on haemodynamic responses connected with the use of thigh tourniquet in orthopaedic patients, *Acta Anaesth Scand* 29:142, 1985.
158. VandenBrink KD, Edmonson AS: The spine. In Edmonson AS, Crenshaw AH, editors: *Campbell's operative orthopaedics,* St Louis, 1980, CV Mosby.
159. Vauzelle C, Stagnara P, Jouvinrouk P: Functional monitoring of spinal cord activity during spinal surgery, *Clin Orthop* 93: 173, 1973.
160. Vazeery AK, Skeil S, Anda O: Changes in cardiac output and systemic arterial pressure after insertion of acrylic cement during trimethaphan sodium nitroprusside and glycerol trinitrate-induced hypotension. A comparison with changes during normotension, *Br J Anaesth* 55:783, 1983.
161. Warren SB, Brand L, Kiernan HA: Knee arthroscopy under regional anesthesia. The inguinal paravascular technique, *Am J Knee Surg* 3:74, 1990.
162. Wattenmaker I, Concepcion M, Hibberd P, et al: Upper airway obstruction and perioperative management of the airway in patients managed with posterior operations on the cervical spine for rheumatoid arthritis, *J Bone Joint Surg* 76A:3:360–365, 1994.
163. Weber ER, Daube JR, Coventry MB: Peripheral neuropathies associated with total hip arthroplasty, *J Bone Joint Surg* 58A:66, 1976.
164. Wills DG: Anaesthetic management of posterior lumbar osteotomy, *Can Anaesth Soc J* 32:248, 1985.
165. Wilson PD, et al: Total hip replacement with fixation by acrylic cement: a preliminary study of 100 consecutive McKee-Farrar prosthetic replacement, *J Bone Joint Surg* 54A:207, 1972.
166. Winnie AP: Plexus anesthesia. In Hakansson L, editor: *Perivascular techniques of brachial plexus block,* Philadelphia, 1983, WB Saunders.
167. Winnie A, Ramamurthy S, Durrani A: The inguinal paravascular technique of lumbar plexus anesthesia: the "3 in 1 block," *Anesth Analg* 52:989, 1973.
168. Woo RY, Morrey BF: Dislocations after total hip arthroplasty, *J Bone Joint Surg* 64A:1295, 1982.
169. Woolson ST, Marsh JS, Tanner JB: Transfusion of previously deposited autologous blood for patients undergoing hip replacement surgery, *J Bone Joint Surg* 69A: 325, 1987.
170. Yaster M, et al: A comparison of nitroglycerine and nitroprusside for inducing hypotension in children: a double blind study, *Anesthesiology* 65:175, 1986.
171. Zablocki AD, et al: Cervical epidural anesthesia for surgery of the shoulder, *Orthop Rev* 2:65, 1987.

CHAPTER 81

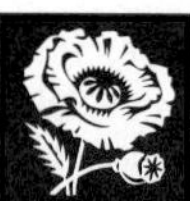

Trauma Anesthesia

CHRISTOPHER M. GRANDE
CHARLES E. SMITH
JOHN K. STENE

Trauma has become a national health concern over the past decade in many countries, and is the leading cause of death and disability in young, productive populations worldwide. **In the United States it is now the third leading cause of death at any age, behind only atherosclerosis and cancer. Every year approximately 145,000 die from trauma in the United States, and disability from traumatic injury is staggering. Of the 60 million injuries that occur annually in the United States, nearly 9 million are disabling, and 300,000 result in permanent disabilities.**[2] More lost work years occur as a result of trauma than from cancer and heart disease combined, because of the predominance of young victims. Direct cost of trauma care represents 7% of all health care expenditures.[115] **One third of all hospital admissions (19 million hospital days) result from trauma.** This represents more hospital days than required by all heart disease patients and four times the number needed by patients hospitalized for cancer care.[162]

Mortality from trauma is age related. Although the number of trauma victims is greater among the younger generation, elderly persons are likely to suffer most. **The elderly generation consumes nearly 33% of health care trauma**

resources and these patients are five times more likely to die of an equivalent injury than are younger people.[93] If elderly trauma victims survive, they often face a major decrement in the quality of life.[121]

Trauma deaths occur in a trimodal pattern.[162] It is believed that, in general, 50% of deaths happen within 1 hour of injury. These "immediate" fatalities are usually due to lacerations of the heart, great vessels, aorta, or brain stem. Few of these injuries are amenable to medical therapy. "Early" deaths, believed to be largely preventable, occur within a few hours of injury (the "golden hour"), due to airway emergencies, splenic or liver lacerations, subdural hematoma, hemothorax, or other injuries associated with major blood loss. "Late" deaths occur days to weeks after injury and constitute approximately 20% of all trauma deaths (Fig. 81-1). As trauma resuscitation has improved, devastating systemic complications, such as sepsis and multiorgan system failure, have assumed increased importance and are the subject of many diverse fields of investigations, such as immunomodulation.[150]

It is postulated that in cases where trauma patients survive the "golden hour" only to succumb to a late death, initial resuscitation, stabilization, and perioperative critical care was good, but not good enough to alter patient outcome. More sophisticated and sensitive indicators of tissue or cellular hypoxia and the ability to favorably alter the critical balance between oxygen supply and demand to prevent or treat "oxygen debt" in the trauma patient are required. The focus of the next decade must be on issues such as these in an effort to reduce late-phase trauma deaths. Anesthesia care providers have opportunities to play essential roles in early (emergency room and operating room) institution of sophisticated monitoring, and to perform inpatient interventions. This is one facet of the currently expanding "perioperative physician" role of anesthesia providers.[71]

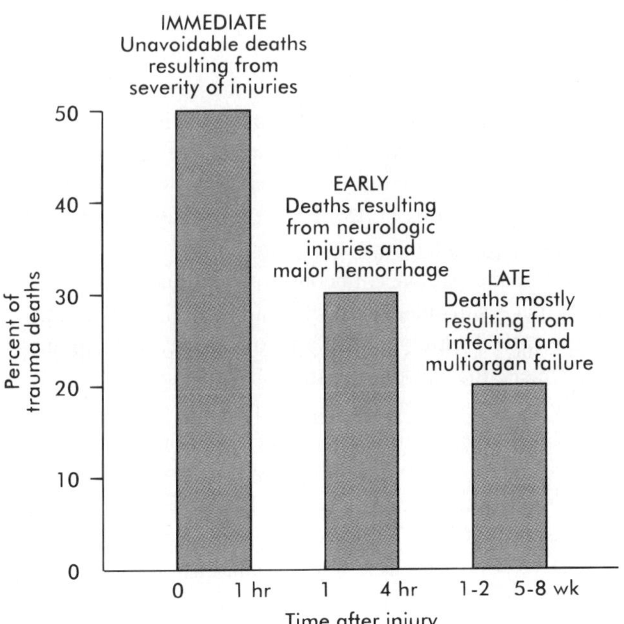

Fig 81-1. Trimodal distribution of trauma deaths.

Significant reduction in morbidity and mortality can be attained by integrated community approaches to trauma care, with attention to prehospital care, field triage and transport, acute care at an appropriate hospital, and subsequent rehabilitation.

Traumatized patients often require surgery with varying degrees of urgency—immediately, urgently, and even electively—but frequently outside normal working hours. To minimize mortality and morbidity from trauma, it is essential to have a proper understanding of special problems that trauma patients present. Indeed, many trauma centers require specific and continuous structured training in trauma as part of the credentialling process for clinicians and other providers.

One way of acquiring training in trauma management is to attend and be certified in the Advanced Trauma Life Support (ATLS) course, developed by the Committee on Trauma of the American College of Surgeons.[2] This course is open to anesthesia providers and gives a well-organized and practical approach in the management of trauma patients, although some of the principles taught may be controversial. The International Trauma Anesthesia and Critical Care Society (ITACCS), which was founded in 1988 to focus on and nurture the development of anesthesia providers as perioperative traumatologists, continues to recommend certification in ATLS. Recognizing that many anesthesia providers already possess expertise in many areas of primary focus in ATLS, such as airway control, fluid resuscitation, and critical care transport, ITACCS has thus taken a "beyond ATLS" approach to its course offerings, which are now also available in a programmed format, featuring didactic portions and specific advanced skills development workshops.

PREOPERATIVE ASSESSMENT AND PREPARATION FOR ANESTHESIA

Urgency of surgery will dictate time available for preoperative assessment of trauma patients, but often surgery should be delayed until adequate fluid resuscitation has occurred. The patient's physical status can be evaluated as completely as in the elective surgical patient if the patient's condition is stable. Full evaluation includes overall assessment of extent of the patient's injuries, which will indicate the approximate length and complexity of surgery, degree of blood loss, efficacy of initial resuscitative measures, and adequacy of ventilation. In emergency situations, it is not always possible to obtain much of this information. If the anesthesia provider is involved in the resuscitation phase, he or she will have an improved opportunity to gather important data during that period. If not, a brief summary from the previous caregiver will be very helpful.

Most investigations should be completed by the time the trauma patient enters the operating room. Some of these investigations are particularly important to the anesthesia provider. For example, the computed tomographic (CT) scan of the patient's head might reveal evidence of increased intracranial pressure or basilar skull fracture. The lateral neck radiograph might show cervical spine fractures or subcutaneous air. The chest x-ray might reveal fractured ribs, pneumothorax, hemothorax, widened mediastinum, improperly positioned endotracheal or gastric tube, and mediastinal or subcutaneous air. A focus on the "mechanism(s) of injury" will reveal details about how the trauma occurred and its magnitude and will assist in anticipating pitfalls during anesthetic management. Other useful information is the patient's age, height, and weight—data used to estimate fluid and drug requirements. A more detailed discussion of preoperative assessment of the trauma patient can be found in Chapter 31.

PREEXISTING ILLNESS

Anesthetic and surgical risk is altered by underlying disease in trauma patients. Operative mortality in those patients with preexisting medical illnesses was found to be 7.2%, compared with an overall trauma mortality of 5.3%.[36,134] Mortality was even higher—approaching 10%—in those patients with cardiovascular, neurologic, or hematologic disease.[36,134] Although many clinicians believe that invasive hemodynamic monitoring using a pulmonary artery (PA) catheter can reduce the incidence of perioperative complications and improve outcome in critically ill patients with severe hemodynamic disorders, these benefits have been difficult to demonstrate.[4,142] Nonetheless, PA catheter is often considered useful to guide the administration of fluids, blood products and vasoactive agents, especially in severely injured geriatric patients, patients with pre-existing cardiovascular disease, and in patients with multiple injuries and persistent shock, all of whom are likely to manifest an increasingly complicated and deteriorating clinical picture.

Preoperative and intraoperative management of trauma patients with underlying respiratory disease varies little from that of other trauma patients. Often, the only clue to underlying lung disease is body habitus, nicotine stains on fingertips and nails, nail clubbing, or presence of cigarettes or pulmonary medication in a pocket or purse. A major concern in these patients is weaning from the ventilator. Any additional lung injury such as adult respiratory distress syndrome (ARDS), contusion, or infection will likely make the process even more difficult. Maintenance of intake of bronchodilator agents, such as beta-adrenergic agents or aminophylline, and corticosteroids in patients with reversible obstructive lung diseases is useful to facilitate weaning from the ventilator.

Diabetes mellitus, thyroid disease, and other endocrine disorders are encountered occasionally in trauma victims. The stress of the trauma and operation may lead to uncontrolled hyperglycemia and may precipitate diabetic ketoacidosis, especially in Type I diabetics. Close monitoring of blood glucose, electrolytes, and acid-base status is crucial.

PREINDUCTION PERIOD

Before induction of anesthesia, the anesthesia provider should have obtained as much information as possible about the patient, as explained previously. He or she should also be certain of the availability of adequate venous access for resuscitation, because cardiac output may be further depressed by anesthetic agents, and significant bleeding may occur from expected and unexpected sites during surgery. If the patient's trachea is not already intubated, the unstable nature of the trauma patient warrants continuous reassessment of the airway in the perioperative period. The airway may be under control in the emergency room, but during transport to the operating room, the patient may develop airway obstruction due to loss of consciousness from head injury, hemodynamic instability, injury to the airways, or maxillofacial injuries with subsequent edema or hematoma.

AIRWAY MANAGEMENT

Airway management can be complex in trauma patients, and several factors contribute to the difficulty. Unlike the patient undergoing elective surgery, the trauma patient may have revealed and/or concealed injuries to the cervical spine, face and mouth, neck, and upper and lower respiratory tract, and frequently has a full stomach. Full extent of injuries is usually unknown, and there may be insufficient time to investigate their range and severity before committing to one of several options to achieve airway control. In addition, trauma patients may also present those characteristics which typically predispose to difficult airway management (e.g., receding jaw, large tongue, small space between tongue base and epiglottis, etc.) in any elective patient—characteristics which should be factored into the airway management plan.

On meeting the trauma patient, the anesthesia provider should encourage the patient to speak if his or her trachea has not been intubated. Ability to speak virtually guarantees a patent airway and confirms the patient's ability to breathe, at least for the moment. If the patient is unable to speak, the anesthesia provider must ascertain the presence of a patent airway. If the patient is unconscious but shows respiratory effort that results in air moving in and out of the lungs, there is time to formulate a plan for airway management. Conversely, the anesthesia care team must act emergently to secure an airway if the patient is unconscious and apneic.[1]

All maneuvers must be performed with protection of neurologic function in mind until cervical spine instability has been ruled out by radiographs, clinical criteria, dynamic fluoroscopy, CT scan, or magnetic resonance imaging (MRI).[40,75] Cervical spine fracture and instability may result from relatively "minor" events such as bicycling accidents or sports injuries. It is therefore important that the cervical spine be protected whenever possible until injury is officially ruled out. Although it is important to stress the issue of cervical spine protection, this consideration should occur within the context of the particular mechanism(s) of injury. A trauma patient with a penetrating injury to the abdomen does not need cervical spine precautions, whereas a patient who has been in a high-speed motor vehicle accident and was unrestrained does. These issues are elaborated upon in Chapter 31.

Airway Control Options

Airway obstruction normally results from the tongue falling back against the posterior pharynx (soft tissue obstruction) or a foreign body stuck in the pharynx or respiratory tract. Maneuvers such as chin lift or jaw thrust may be employed to relieve the soft tissue obstruction. These useful maneuvers should not hyperextend the neck. They may dramatically improve oxygenation and ventilation prior to obtaining a definitive airway. Flexion of the neck and extension of the head, which aligns the oral, pharyngeal, and laryngeal axis in the optimal "sniff" position are inappropriate for a trauma patient who has a suspected cervical spine injury. Establishment of an airway may be aided by using an artificial nasopharyngeal or oropharyngeal airway, but the caregiver must consider the accompanying risks, including agitation, retching, coughing, vomiting, and bleeding, that may contribute to complications such as elevated intracranial pressure (ICP) or pulmonary aspiration of gastric contents.

Inability to obtain and/or maintain a patent airway by these maneuvers may indicate foreign-body obstruction. Exploration with a finger or a Yankauer suction device may clear the airway. If these procedures are not immediately successful, attempts should be made to visualize the pharynx and larynx to identify and remove the foreign body. Laryngoscopy should be performed with the precautions described in the following paragraphs whenever cervical spine injury is suspected.

If the cervical spine has not yet been properly "cleared" or if the cervical spine radiograph shows bony injury, yet the airway is not under control and needs more definitive measures, the following options must be considered.

Nasal intubation

Awake fiberoptic nasal intubation in a properly prepared cooperative patient[131] is considered by many to be the method of choice for management of the difficult airway or of patients with cervical spine injuries. Adequate equipment and technical skills, in addition to topical anesthesia, conscious sedation, and an antisialagogue drug are elements of awake fiberoptic intubation.[122] Awake intubation allows evaluation of the patient's neurologic status after intubation, before inducing general anesthesia. This method may be difficult and even dangerous in a confused patient, because further damage to the cervical spine may occur with sudden inappropriate movements. For this reason, cervical spine stabilization must be maintained. Inadequate surface anesthesia or nerve block may cause retching and vomiting when the endotracheal tube is manipulated into the pharynx and larynx. This may result in a significant increase in ICP and/or cause laryngospasm and bronchospasm.

Some consider blind nasal intubation the method of choice in a patient with restricted neck movement, but this technique is not without important complications such as epistaxis, hypertension, vomiting, aspiration, and unsuccessful intubation.[44,72,96] Patients with cervical spine injuries may also have head injury accompanied by basilar skull fracture with disruption of the cribriform plate of the ethmoid bone deep inside the nose, in which case nasal intubation (or insertion of a nasopharyngeal airway) is contraindicated because the endotracheal tube or airway may traverse the fractured cribriform plate and disrupt the brain substance, or at least pose a major infection liability in the presence of a cerebral spinal fluid leak. Blind nasal intubation is contraindicated in the apneic patient, and whenever severe midface fractures exist. Although there is no doubt that blind nasal intubation has a place in airway management of patients with cervical spine injuries, the risk of causing upper-airway bleeding and compromised subsequent fiberoptic efforts with an initial blind attempt should be considered.

Oral intubation

Direct laryngoscopy is the most rapid method of securing the airway in a trauma patient. The major concern with direct laryngoscopy and oral intubation in a patient with suspected cervical spine injury is that movement of the head and neck, especially with an anesthetized paralyzed patient, may cause further cervical cord injury. Concerns about intubation in the patient with suspected cervical spine injury have been reviewed.[74] There are no controlled studies that suggest that any one method of intubation is better than another in terms of preventing compromise to the spinal cord as long as there is no neck movement.

Protection of the neck in patients with suspected cervical spine injury during direct laryngoscopy and intubation can be obtained with "manual in-line axial stabilization" (MIAS) (Fig. 81-2), a technique accepted by the American College of Surgeons as part of the ATLS protocol for emergency intubation.[2,155] Most trauma patients are now routinely transported from the field on a long spineboard. The head is immobilized between two sandbags (or other device) using head straps or tape, and the neck is stabilized with a rigid cervical collar. Before oral intubation is attempted, the anterior portion of the cervical collar is removed, and MIAS is applied by a person experienced in the management of cervical spine injury. Removal of the anterior cervical collar allows for full mouth opening, optimal external laryngeal manipulation to improve the laryngoscopic view of the glottis, and also provides access to the anterior neck should a surgical airway be needed.

Because all trauma patients are considered to have full stomachs, most anesthesia providers recommend cricoid pressure[143] until the trachea is intubated. Properly applied cricoid pressure requires a force of 44 Newtons to prevent

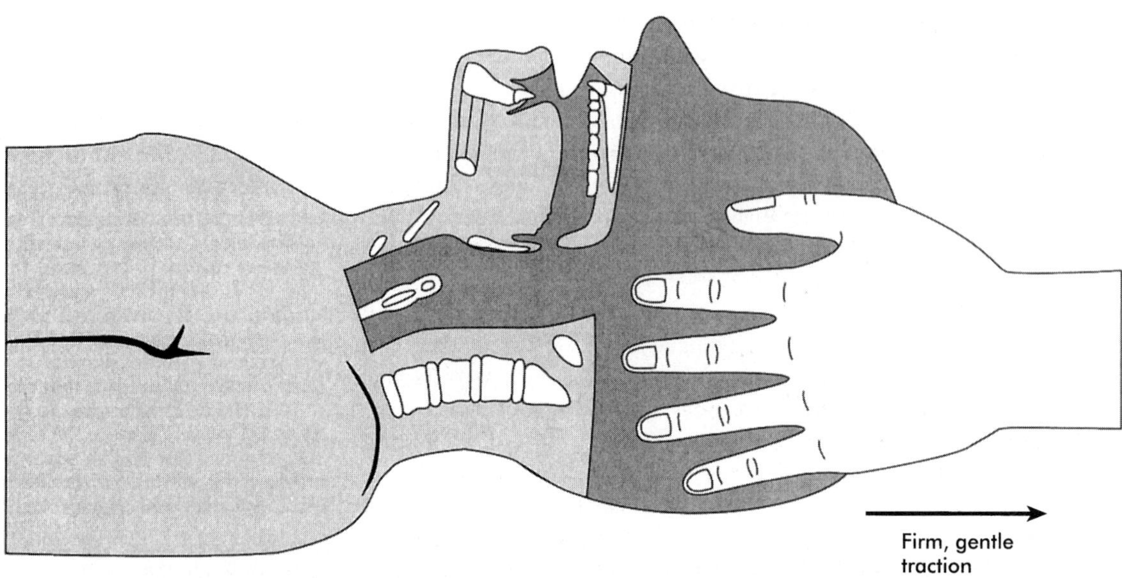

Fig 81-2. Manual in-line axial stabilization (MIAS) applied for immobilization of the cervical spine during endotracheal intubation.

regurgitation of gastric contents.[172] This force is approximately equivalent to the amount of pressure to cause pain when pressing on the bridge of one's nose. There is concern that too great a force on an unstable cervical spine fracture may cause further cervical cord injury. The "correct amount" of cricoid pressure should be used only after careful thought has been given to the risks of further cervical spine injury versus aspiration pneumonia. If the patient has an indwelling nasogastric (NG) tube, it may be prudent to connect it to continuous suction, while having a second large-bore suction available during the intubation sequence.

Manual ventilation of the patients' lungs should be performed with 100% oxygen using inflation pressures < 20 cm H_2O in order to prevent (or treat) hypoxemia and hypercapnia prior to and between intubation attempts. This "modified rapid induction" technique, shown in Box 81-1, is extremely unlikely to introduce any air into the stomach, and is especially important in the trauma setting because many patients are difficult to preoxygenate, and exhibit oxygen desaturation and CO_2 accumulation due to varying degrees of hypoventilation, airway obstruction, chest trauma, and ventilation-perfusion mismatch. Failure of oral intubation with manual in-line axial stabilization for the trauma patient with cervical spine injury after induction of anesthesia and paralysis usually requires establishment of an emergency surgical airway.

Surgical options

If nasal or oral intubation is technically difficult and is not successful despite a reasonable number of attempts by an experienced clinician, some type of surgical airway must be obtained. The number of attempts considered reasonable will depend on the specific conditions of each trauma patient and the skill and experience of the anesthesia provider.

Oxygen jet insufflation can be provided with a 14-gauge catheter inserted through the cricothyroid membrane or through the tracheal wall and attached directly to the gas outlet of the anesthetic machine. (This apparatus must be set up in advance and the trauma team must be familiar with its operation.) This setup can then be used similarly to a jet injector by intermittently pressing on the oxygen valve to provide an oxygen flow at 50 psi pressure.[13] The Venturi effect created entrains air that, together with the oxygen flow, produces inflation of the lungs. Complications of this technique usually result from pulmonary barotrauma and/or obstruction to gas outflow through the larynx.[13] Such oxygen insufflation is only a temporary alternative until a more permanent cricothyroidotomy or tracheostomy is performed.

Cricothyroidotomy is preferred to the more formal tracheostomy for the true emergency situation, because it is less time consuming, easier to perform, associated with fewer complications, and more likely to result in a dependable airway. It may later be converted to a tracheostomy under more controlled conditions. The prepackaged cricothyroidotomy "kits" available today contain the necessary equipment and may save time and confusion during resuscitation, but the user must become familiar with a particular kit before the emergency to avoid misuse and loss of precious time. If no prepackaged kit is available, an emergency cricothyroidotomy may be accomplished using a #11 surgical blade in a stabbing motion, hemostats (or scissors, tracheal expanders, etc.) to enlarge the wound, followed by the insertion of a #7 tracheostomy tube or a 5- to 6-mm ET tube through the surgical opening.

When considering the "surgical option," the anesthesia provider should realize that few surgeons have ever performed a true rescue surgical airway under emergency conditions, even if they may have performed many elective tra-

BOX 81-1
MODIFIED RAPID SEQUENCE INDUCTION AND INTUBATION FOR TRAUMA PATIENTS

1. Be familiar with evaluation of the difficult airway and the American Society of Anesthesiologists practice guidelines for management of the difficult airway.[3,102]
2. Be familiar with noninvasive and invasive techniques of airway management.
3. Evaluate the airway and be prepared to execute multiple contigency plans.
4. Preoxygenate the patient with 100% O_2 by facemask.
5. Remove anterior portion of the cervical spine collar and apply MIAS of the head and neck if suspected cervical spine injury.
6. Give appropriate medications IV, as indicated by the clinical setting and hemodynamic status:
   –Lidocaine, 1.5 mg/kg, if suspected head injury
   –Sedative-hypnotics (see Table 81-6)
   –Muscle relaxants (see Table 81-8)
7. Apply cricoid pressure until intubation completed.
8. Manually ventilate the patients' lungs with 100% O_2 using inflation pressures < 20 cm H_2O to prevent (or treat) hypoxemia and hypercarbia prior to (or in between) intubation attempt(s). Continue cricoid pressure during bag-mask ventilation.
9. Confirm correct position of endotracheal tube by visualizing tube passing through cords, sustained presence of end-tidal CO_2, auscultation of breath sounds, self-inflating bulb, etc.
10. After successful intubation, administer additional increments of sedative-hypnotics and analgesics, or begin a potent volatile agent, as dictated by clinical need. Consider using a longer acting relaxant once the effects of succinylcholine have worn off, if this agent was used.

ET—endotracheal; MIAS—manual in-line axial stabilization.

cheostomies. Moreover, a surgeon may not be immediately available to perform the technique. It thus behooves anesthesia providers working in the trauma setting to be prepared to undertake surgical airway techniques. These skills can be learned during mannikin and cadaver laboratory/workshop training.

Other options

Fiberoptic oral intubation, with the aid of a specialized oral airway guide and facemask may be useful in selected patients. This technique allows for the introduction of a fiberscope through a port in the mask, while at the same time maintaining bag-mask ventilation. The same concerns as addressed previously for fiberoptic nasal intubation apply here.

The Bullard intubating *fiberoptic laryngoscope* is an anatomically-shaped rigid fiberoptic instrument designed for *oral indirect visualization* of the larynx. The major advantage of the Bullard laryngoscope (Circon Acmi, Stamford, CT) is that virtually no head and neck movement is required to obtain a clear view of the vocal cords,[76] and the time to glottic visualization and endotracheal intubation is faster compared with standard oral fiberoptic techniques.[33] Three other fiberoptic laryngoscope devices, the Upsherscope (Upsher Scope Corp., Foster City, CA), the Wuscope (Pentax Precision Instruments, Orangeburg, NY), and the Rapiscope have recently become available. However, peer-reviewed publications have not yet appeared in the literature with respect to their utility in airway management of the acute trauma patient.

Transillumination of the soft tissues of the neck using a flexible lightwand device may also be useful in selected patients.[79] The lightwand is placed inside an ET tube during intubation. If the tube is advanced through the glottic opening (as opposed to the esophagus), there is a well-defined circumscribed glow that is readily appreciated in the anterior neck just below the thyroid prominence. This "light-guided" technique minimizes upper cervical spine movement and has been used successfuly to perform blind orotracheal intubation in patients with difficult airways.[80] The Augustine Guide (AG) (Augustine Medical Inc., Eden Praire, MN) is a recently introduced *anatomically-designed blind guide device* that consists of a molded plastic handle with a channel for an endotracheal tube containing a preinseted stylet.[28] The AG is inserted blindly until it "locks" into place in the glossoepiglottic fold. The stylet is then advanced into the larynx, and a 35-ml syringe attached to it is aspirated to confirm air return, characteristic of intratracheal placement. The endotracheal tube is then threaded over the sylet. This technique does not require any head and neck movement, and is not adversely affected by blood or secretions in the airway. As with all "blind" techniques, creation of a false passage from improper use of the stylet or an improperly directed tracheal tube can occur.

Retrograde intubation is another method for securing the airway in certain situations. This technique requires retrograde placement of a guidewire or catheter via the cricothyroid membrane into the trachea and between the cords into the oropharynx. An orally or nasally placed endotracheal tube (or fiber optic bronchoscope via the suction port, or a tube changer followed by an endotracheal tube) is then threaded over the guidewire and into the trachea.[77]

Both the *laryngeal mask airway* (LMA) and the *tracheo-esophageal Combitube* (Sheridan Catheter Corp., Argyle, NY) can be used to facilitate oxygenation and ventilation in the "cannot ventilate, cannot intubate scenario."[14,50] Advantages of the LMA in the trauma setting include increased speed and ease of placement,[27] minimal hemodynamic effects, no increase in intraocular pressure, and a satisfactory airway in terms of oxygen saturation.[23,97] The LMA has also been shown to be an excellent conduit to the larynx for fiber optic intubation. The Combitube can be inserted blindly, quickly, and requires a relatively low level of skill. The Combitube enters the esophagus 99% of the time, and after proper inflation of the smaller esophageal and larger oropharyngeal cuffs, ventilation is directed to the lungs by the multiple small pharyngeal openings. Unlike the LMA, a properly placed Combitube may help protect against pulmonary aspiration.[10,116] However, both the LMA and the Combitube are supraglottic ventilatory devices that cannot relieve laryngospasm or other glottic and subglottic problems.[14] Because the LMA covers both the esophageal and laryngeal orifices, this device does not protect against pulmonary aspiration. Major disadvantages of a properly positioned Combitube are that it does not permit suctioning of the trachea, and it is not well tolerated in the semiconscious patient.

RESUSCITATION

Assessment

Determining adequacy of intravascular volume begins with palpation of a peripheral pulse and measurement of arterial blood pressure (Table 81-1). Simultaneously, the patient's general skin condition and mental status should be assessed. The acutely volume-depleted trauma patient will have cool, moist, pallid, or cyanotic skin, especially at the extremities. A major goal in resuscitating these patients is to replete intravascular volume to maximize tissue oxygen delivery. **Cardiac output and oxygenated blood flow to the vital organs are the important determinants of outcome, and not blood pressure. Vasopressor agents must therefore be used sparingly, if at all, and only with the intention of temporarily gaining a little time until hypovolemia can be corrected.** Use of the pneumatic antishock trousers (also known as military antishock trousers, MAST) during resuscitation is no longer recommended by the American College of Surgeons or the American College of Emergency Physicians, except for field stabilization of pelvic fractures.[2]

Vascular Access Options

As volume status is being assessed, other members of the team are evaluating venous access. If necessary, open surgical cannulation of a peripheral vein should be performed without hesitation. There is controversy as to whether the saphenous vein or the antecubital vasculature is the preferred location.[112,146] The disadvantages of using the lower-limb venous system are that the veins may be smaller or occluded from chronic venous disease and there may be intrapelvic or abdominal bleeding, which may render such fluid replacement ineffective or even deleterious.

The problems with cutdown at the antecubital fossa are that it is technically more difficult and that resuscitation of intravascular volume may not be effective with unsuspected bleeding from the superior vena cava. When a cutdown is necessary, it is preferable to establish venous access rapidly with the saphenous vein first and then proceed to the veins of the upper limbs, if indicated.

Severely injured patients with inadequate vascular cannulation often require insertion of large-bore central venous catheters (8.5-French introducer or equivalent), using the Seldinger technique. The subclavian vein is generally a reliable approach, but it may present some difficulties in terms of interfering with other ongoing resuscitation efforts. The femoral vein is also a reliable route for a large-bore introducer catheter. The internal jugular vein, which may be the most familiar for many anesthesia providers, can also be used, but the rigid cervical collar limits access to the veins of the neck, and the risk of cervical spine injury limits contralateral neck rotation. Neutral head position during cannulation is therefore required. This position has been shown by two-dimensional ultrasound to produce less overlap between the internal jugular vein and carotid artery,[157] which theoretically should reduce

Table 81-1 American College of Surgeons classes of acute hemorrhage

Factors	Class I	Class II	Class III	Class IV
Blood loss (ml)*	Up to 750	750–1500	1500–2000	2000 or more
Blood loss (% BV)*	Up to 15%	15%–30%	30%–40%	40% or more
Pulse rate	> 100	> 100	> 120	140 or higher
Blood pressure	Normal	Normal	Decreased	Decreased
Pulse pressure (mm Hg)	Normal or increased	Decreased	Decreased	Decreased
Capillary refill test	Normal	Positive	Positive	Positive
Respiratory rate	14–20	20–30	30–40	> 35
Urine output (ml/hr)	30 or more	20–30	5–15	Negligible
CNS (mental status)	Slightly anxious	Mildly anxious	Anxious confused	Confused lethargic
Fluid replacement (3:1 rule)	Crystalloid	Crystalloid	Crystalloid + blood	Crystalloid + blood

*For a 70-kg man.
Courtesy the American College of Surgeons, 55 East Erie Street, Chicago, Illinois 60611.

the risk of accidental carotid artery puncture. In children less than 6 years of age, intraosseus needle access can be performed instead of central line insertion.

It should be noted that the ATLS protocol recommends against attempting central venous cannulation in hypovolemic trauma patients because of the risk of pneumothorax, venous air embolism, arterial puncture, lower success rate, multiple needle sticks, and other complications. Experience with central line insertion can help minimize, but not totally eliminate, these risks. Literature review indicates approximately a 5% rate of catheter-related sepsis.[99] In the majority of cases, the catheter initially becomes colonized by the patient's own cutaneous flora invading the insertion site. Careful aseptic placement is therefore of great importance during the period of resuscitation and induction of general anesthesia, in an effort to reduce late mortality from sepsis and multiorgan system failure.

Fluid Warming Devices

Rapid resuscitation of the trauma victim is best accomplished with large-gauge IV catheters, and effective fluid warmers with high thermal clearances.[111,123,164] Other considerations include length and size of the infusion set, set point of the warmer, and flow resistance of fluid warmers when rapid infusion is needed. Because alterations in red cell integrity are not apparent until 46° C,[163] the American Association of Blood Banks has recently changed its guidelines so that fluid warmers with set points of 42° C may be used. Thus, countercurrent water and other fluid warmers using 42° C set points will not damage red cells, will result in consistently warmer fluid delivery, and will allow the clinician to maintain thermal neutrality with respect to fluid management over a wide range of flow rates (Table 81-2).

Fluid options

There continues to be controversy about which solutions, colloid or crystalloid, should be used for resuscitation. The data available at present are confusing and conflicting.[53,61,129,138] Different study designs, difficulties in measuring small changes in pulmonary function, and different patient populations may account for the fact that opposite conclusions have been reached in these studies. During hemorrhage the interstitial space, in addition to the intravascular compartment, is diminished with the compensatory increase in reabsorption of fluid into the capillaries (Starling equilibrium of capillary exchange). To replete the intravascular and interstitial compartment rapidly and efficiently, both colloid and crystalloid should be given (Table 81-3).[147] Although there are no data on the "correct" combination of colloid and crystalloid, one reasonable approach is to start with a 1:1 ratio until the patient's condition is more stable or until specific laboratory data becomes available to guide more informed choices.

There is also considerable interest in administration of hypertonic fluids for resuscitating trauma patients, especially for prehospital use and in patients with burns and head injury. These fluids may provide rapid volume expansion, improved hemodynamics, decreased tissue edema, decreased intracranial pressure (ICP), decreased brain water and improved cerebral blood flow (see Table 31-5 in Chapter 31).[84] Lesser amounts of hypertonic and hyperoncotic fluids than 0.9% saline in hypotensive injured patients can improve blood pressure and cardiac output, at least transiently, because of osmotic translocation of extracellular and intracellular water. Because the intravascular half-life of hypertonic saline is similar to that of isotonic saline,[161] these fluids can be combined with colloid solutions such as hetastarch or dextran to prolong their plasma volume expansion effects. Hemoglobin solutions are also currently being investigated for resuscitation of hemorrhagic shock,[128] but none are yet approved in the U.S.

Table 81-2 Flow rate (ml/min) through level one fluid warmer*

Cannula size†	Crystalloid	Packed erythroctyes
Flow rates (ml/min with constant 300 mm Hg pressure)		
18 g	250	150
16 g	480	220
14 g	600	300
8.5 Fr	950	475
Flow rates (ml/min) with gravity (39-in drop)		
18 g	110	40
16 g	150	50
14 g	260	70
8.5 Fr	345	90

*Figures given by Level One Technology.
†18 g × 1.25 inch long; 16 g × 1.25 inch long; all by Jelco. 8.5 Fr × 4 inch long, by Argon.

Endpoints of Fluid Resuscitation

Fluid resuscitation of the patient is continued until improved perfusion and restoration of organ function occur or until vital organ monitoring indicates that cardiac failure is incipient. In the awake patient, mental status usually improves as hypovolemic shock resolves. Other manifestations of improved cardiac output include increased pulse pressure, decreased heart rate, increased urine output, resolution of lactic acidosis, and brisk capillary refill. Direct arterial pressure monitoring may allow early detection of intravascular volume deficits. Degree of systolic pressure variation with each mechanical breath correlates positively with the amount of hemorrhage. Trends in cardiac filling pressures (CVP or pulmonary capillary wedge pressure [PWP]), rather than absolute numbers, will also be helpful in fluid management.

More recently, the use of large (traditional) quantities of fluids for immediate resuscitation of victims of penetrating trauma before hemorrhage is controlled by surgical means has been questioned.[16] The concern is that vigorous infusion of fluids may disrupt or decrease resistance to flow around a partially formed thrombus and cause secondary hemor-

Table 81-3 Comparisons between crystalloid and colloid

Factors	Crystalloid	Colloid
Volume required for resuscitation	Two to four times the volume of colloid necessary; large volume shift into ISF	Faster administration and resuscitation; relatively small volume shift into interstitial fluid
COP	COP-IOP gradient maintained by dilution of IOP	COP and COP-PCWP gradient maintained with colloid; albumin stays inside pulmonary capillary and draws water out of the interstitium
Edema	Significant edema decreases wound healing and nutrient transport	Not significant

ISF—interstitial fluid; COP—colloid oncotic pressure; IOP—interstitial oncotic pressure; PCWP—pulmonary capillary wedge pressure.

rhage. This has led to a randomized, prospective trial of "delayed fluid resuscitation" in patients with isolated, penetrating torso injuries.[16] In the study, there were no differences in outcome with either delayed (fluids infused only during operative intervention) or conventional (fluids infused during transport, emergency room, and operating room) resuscitation, implying that delayed resuscitation was just as "safe" as conventional fluid protocols. Although these results are interesting and provocative, it is important to note that the study was conducted within the environs of the Houston, Texas, Emergency Medical System, one that is characterized by a very rapid response time and short scene and transport time. Moreover, the study was limited to isolated penetrating torso trauma, and the receiving trauma center had an operating room on stand-by and a trauma surgeon ready to operate. Therefore, results of this study[16] cannot be extrapolated to other types of injuries such as blunt trauma, head injury, or multiple sites of penetrating trauma. The results of this study also can not be extrapolated to trauma systems that lack rapid response capabilities, or that have long scene and transport times (remote access), or without immediate stand-by operating room teams. Further studies are required before one can safely advocate delaying fluid resuscitation to injured patients in shock.[118]

BLOOD TRANSFUSIONS

If the patient has lost large amounts of blood and is in shock (Classes III and IV of acute hemorrhage [Table 81-1]), blood administration is required. Available options are type O-negative, low titer; type-specific; typed and screened; or typed and crossmatched blood. The initial choice will depend on the degree of hemodynamic instability. Type O-negative erythrocytes have no major antigens and can be given reasonably safely to patients of any blood type; the accompanying serum may contain antibodies to A and B antigens. Even packed erythrocytes may have a significant amount of serum present, but the risk of a major hemolytic transfusion reaction remains low. Unfortunately, only 8% of the population has O-negative blood, and blood bank reserves on O-negative, low antibody titer blood are usually very low. For this reason, O-positive erythrocytes are frequently used. This is a reasonable approach in men, but may be a problem in childbearing-aged women who are Rh negative.

If 50% to 75% of the patient's blood volume has been replaced with type O blood, one probably should continue to administer type O blood. Otherwise, risk of a major crossmatch reaction increases, because the patient may have received enough anti-A or anti-B antibodies to precipitate intravascular hemolysis if A, B, or AB units are subsequently given. Fortunately, uncrossmatched type O blood is rarely given or needed today. Temporizing measures can almost always gain the 5 minutes necessary to obtain type-specific blood. The use of type-specific blood in this setting has been reported to be a reasonably safe and valid use of blood bank resources.[69] If one can wait 15 minutes, typed and screened blood should be available. When blood is typed and screened, the patient's blood group is identified and the serum is screened for major blood group antibodies. A full crossmatch generally requires about 45 minutes and involves mixing donor cells with recipient serum to rule out any antigen-antibody reactions.

COMPLICATIONS OF MASSIVE TRANSFUSIONS

Hypothermia

Hypothermia is a major problem during massive blood transfusions and is discussed under the heading of Intraoperative Problems. Hypothermia is a common cause of coagulopathy in trauma patients. Prevention and treatment of hypothermia is outlined in Table 81-4.

Impaired Oxygen Release from Hemoglobin

The ability of the erythrocyte to store and release oxygen is impaired after storage. The erythrocytic levels of 2,3-diphosphoglyceric acid (2,3 DPG) decrease both with CPD and CPDA-1 stored blood (Table 81-5). Low levels of 2,3 DPG will shift the blood's oxygen dissociation curve to the left (i.e., the erythrocyte will have a higher affinity for oxy-

Table 81-4 Methods to prevent and treat hypothermia in trauma patients[151]

Passive	
Higher ambient room temperatures, warm blankets, insulating blankets, dry off wet skin	Reduces heat loss by several mechanisms-radiation, convection, conduction, evaporation Relies on patients' internal heart production (0.5–1 kcal/kg/hr) for rewarming
Active external	
Convective warming	Intraoperative (vasodilated): provides 30 kcal/hr in adult patients Postoperative (vasoconstricted): rewarmed adults at rate of 0.86° C/hr Efficacy depends on amount of surface area covered
Circulating heated water mattress	Provides 2.7–5.2 kcal/hr in surgical patients and up to 35 kcal/hr in volunteers;[52] efficacy depends on amount of surface area covered and degree of vasoconstriction
Radiant warmers	Provides 17.7 kcal/hr
Active internal	
Heated humidified gases	Limited to tracheally intubated patients: provides 7–13 kcals/hr
Warmed intravenous fluids	10 l of 38° C fluid into 32° C patient provides 60 kcal 1 l crystalloid at 20° C corresponds to 17 kcal loss in 37° C patient 1 4° C blood corresponds to 30 kcal loss in 37° C patient
Continuous arteriovenous rewarming	Provides 90–150 kcal/hr Requires large-bore arterial and venous catheters and BP > 80 mm Hg Does not require heparinization
Cardiopulmonary bypass	Most effective heat exchange device, providing 700 kcal/hr Requires cannulation, heparinization, and perfusionist
Body cavity lavage with warmed fluids	Provides 30–40 kcal/hr provided that high enough flow rates are maintained (> 5 1/hr); pleural lavage may be more effective than peritoneal lavage

*Approximately 50–70 kcal are required to raise the temperature of a 70-kg patient by 1° C.

Table 81-5 Biochemical changes of blood stored in CPD and CPDA-1

	CPD		CPDA-1			
Biochemical changes	**Whole blood**		**Whole blood**	**Erythrocytes**	**Whole blood**	**Erythrocytes**
Variable (days of storage)	**0**	**21**	**0**	**0**	**35**	**35**
Viable cells (% at 24-hr posttransfusion)	100.0	80.0	100.0	100.0	79.0	71.0
pH (measured at 37° C)	7.20	6.84	7.6	7.55	6.98	6.71
ATP (% of initial value)	100.0	86.0	100.0	100.0	56.0 (± 16)	45.0 (± 12)
2.3-DPG (% of initial value)	100.0	44.0	100.0	100.0	< 10.0	< 10.0
Plasma K^- mmol/l	3.9	21.0	4.2	5.1	27.3	78.5*
Plasma Na^- mmol/l	168.0	156.0	169.0	169.0	155.0	111.0
Plasma hemoglobin mg/l	17	191	82	78	461	6580*

*Values for plasma hemoglobin and potassium concentrations may appear somewhat high in 35-day stored erythrocyte units; the total plasma in these units is only about 70 ml.

Data from the American Association of Blood Banks, 1117 North 19th Street, Arlington, Virginia 22209.

gen at physiologic PO_2 and will release less oxygen at a given tissue PO_2). A higher blood flow may then be needed to compensate for the lower oxygen extraction rate. Although, on a theoretic basis, tissue hypoxia may occur when trauma patients with marginal cardiac reserves are given stored blood for resuscitation, there is no evidence that clinically relevant impairment in oxygen consumption or changes in cardiac index occur in these patients.[21,165]

Coagulopathy

Dilutional thrombocytopenia may occur in trauma victims, but it rarely becomes a problem until at least 150% to 200% of the patient's blood volume has been replaced. Platelet activity in stored blood is only 5% to 10% of normal after 48 or 24 hours of storage, respectively. Thus infusion of CPD blood stored beyond 24 hours dilutes the endogenous platelet pool. The platelet count should be monitored and probably maintained at or greater than 50,000/ul to achieve adequate surgical hemostasis.[120]

Most coagulation factors are stable in stored blood except factors V and VIII.[110] These factors gradually decrease to 15% and 50% of normal, respectively, after 21 days of storage. Because only 5% to 20% of factor V and 30% of factor VIII is needed for adequate hemostasis during surgery, massive blood transfusion rarely lowers coagulation factors below critical levels by simple dilution. It is nonetheless advisable that prothrombin time, activated partial thromboplastin time, fibrinogen, and fibrin degradation products be monitored because deficiencies may be present due to other causes, including preexisting defects or disseminated intravascular coagulopathy resulting from tissue injury.[154]

Electrolytes and Acid-Base Abnormalities

Either hyperkalemia or hypokalemia can occur with massive blood transfusion in trauma victims. Potassium level in stored blood rises with length of storage and can be as high as 78 mmol/l after 35 days (see Table 81-5). Hyperkalemia does not usually present a problem, because potassium rapidly reenters the erythrocytes when they warm to body temperature, but the potential for clinically important hyperkalemia still exists in patients with renal failure or severe acidosis.[83] Hypokalemia occurs when metabolic or respiratory alkalosis (often iatrogenically induced during resuscitation) favors a potassium shift into the cell in exchange for hydrogen ions and/or when endogenous cathecholamines released in response to shock activate the Na^+-K^+ pump and transport K^+ into cells.

The acidosis seen in stored blood is partly respiratory and partly metabolic. The respiratory component is of little consequence with adequate patient ventilation. The metabolic component is also not considered to be clinically harmful.[83] It would seem unwise to administer sodium bicarbonate on an empiric basis, because there is already a pool of bicarbonate generated from the metabolism of citrate, which is of necessity present in large quantities in stored blood. The acid-base status should preferably be investigated before bicarbonate therapy is initiated.

Citrate Toxicity

Citrate toxicity is due to acutely decreased serum ionized calcium, which occurs because citrate chelates calcium. Despite rapid infusion rates of stored blood, it has been reported that serum ionized calcium decreases for only a few minutes and returns to normal shortly after the end of transfusion in patients whose circulatory volumes are well maintained.[36,86] Although there is controversy about whether calcium should be given routinely in patients receiving massive transfusions,[11,43,86] most clinicians believe that empiric administration of calcium is not warranted unless ionized serum calcium is low, especially when hypothermia or liver disease is present. Administration of calcium is also probably not indicated in patients with low outflow state who also have low-serum ionized calcium, because ionized calcium levels will return to normal when hemodynamic status is improved with an inotropic agent and fluids.[45] Despite the above judicious boluses of 100 to 200 mg $CaCl_2$ can dramatically improve deteriorating hemodynamics during massive transfusion situations, at least to gain time to "catch-up," if possible.

Microaggregates

Microaggregates begin forming after approximately 2 days of blood storage. During the first 7 days, microaggregates are mostly platelets or platelet debris. After the first week, the larger fibrin-leukocyte-platelet aggregates begin to accumulate.[6] Whether these microaggregates contribute to lung dysfunction during blood transfusion and whether they need to be removed by micropore filters have long been matters of controversy.[9,48,135,136] Although there is some suggestion, there is yet no conclusive evidence that micropore filters must be used with every blood transfusion. One important disadvantage of the micropore filters is that they decrease the maximal rate of blood transfusion. Pending further clinically relevant studies, it is probably advisable to use micropore filters unless the delay in the administration of blood is harmful to a rapidly bleeding patient.

Infection

The risks of transmisson of viral disease, particularly hepatitis C, is a major current concern. Type B hepatitis—once the major cause of posttransfusion hepatitis (PTH)—now occurs in less than 1% of transfused patients, because screening for hepatitis B surface antigen has proven so effective. Hepatitis C accounts for more than 90% of PTH. Every year, at least 2600 patients develop cirrhosis as a result of hepatitis after blood transfusions.[174] Each unit of fresh frozen plasma or platelets has the same risk of infection as a unit of packed erythrocytes. Recent estimates of infectious rates per unit transfused include hepatitis C—$<$ 1/3000, hepatitis B—1/200,000, HIV—1/225,000 and HTLV I or II—1/50,000.[31,46]

Other types of infectious diseases, such as toxoplasmosis, cytomegalovirus, Epstein-Barr virus, malaria, and bacterial infections, have been described in recipients of blood transfusions.[25,62,158]

Blood transfusion therapy is also associated with allosensitization, immunosuppression, and an increased incidence of postoperative infections.[90] These effects may be mediated by reduced lymphocyte function, down-regulation of macrophage function, and altered cytokin production and activity.[90]

PERIOPERATIVE MONITORING

During resuscitation of patients with major injuries, monitoring should be as simple as possible and as complex as necessary.

Noninvasive Monitoring

Monitoring the level of consciousness, ECG, pulse volume and rate, pulse oximetry, blood pressure by automated oscillometer, and urine output is often adequate initially.

Electrocardiograph monitoring is used to track heart rate and electrical rhythm, whereas cardiac pumping action and the intravascular volume are monitored via arterial blood pressure. The pulse oximeter measures the arterial oxygen saturation, an indicator of pulmonary gas exchange as well as peripheral tissue O_2 delivery. It also provides a continuous capillary pulse wave form, which is a reasonable reflection of adequate microcirculatory flow. Important parameters to monitor in the respiratory system are breath sounds through an esophageal stethoscope (provided the esophagus is thought to be intact), capnography, and inspiratory and expiratory tidal volumes.

"Gold standards" for identifying correct endotracheal tube placement are visualization of the tube passing through the cords followed by the sustained presence of CO_2 in expired gas.[17,102] This is because CO_2 is not produced by or contained within the esophagus or stomach, whereas CO_2 produced by cellular respirations is excreted by the lungs with each breath.[81] It should be noted that similar CO_2 wave forms can be *initially* obtained with "esophageal ventilations."[156] However, the CO_2 , if present initially, will be washed away rapidly, and will not be sustained on infrared capnography nor colorimetric capnometry after five or six breaths.[81] A low level of CO_2 recorded from the trachea during cardiac arrest or during low cardiac output states may falsely convince the caregiver that the tube is not intratracheal. This is because the concentration of end-tidal CO_2 depends not only depends on CO_2 production and alveolar ventilation, but also on circulation. **Thus, in conditions of low flow or cardiac arrest, absence of end-tidal CO_2 neither confirms or excludes proper tracheal tube insertion.** In these situations, use of a self-inflating bulb fitted with a standard 15-mm adaptor may differentiate between tracheal and esophageal intubation.[141] The bulb connected to a properly placed tracheal tube will instantaneously reinflate because the trachea is held open by rigid cartilaginous rings. The bulb connected to a tracheal tube in the esophagus will usually stay collapsed since the esophagus readily collapses when a negative pressure is applied to its lumen.[141] Comparing the expired and inspired tidal volumes has also been found to be a reliable way of assessing correct endotracheal tube placement with an intact lung.[156] Continuous monitoring of end-tidal CO_2 is a useful indicator of the effectiveness of cardiopulmonary resuscitation because during conditions of constant minute ventilation and metabolism, end-tidal CO_2 is closely related to pulmonary blood flow, which in turn is related to cardiac output.[81] **In the absence of sufficient CO_2 production, the only "gold standard" for assurance of proper endotracheal tube placement is direct visualization of tracheal rings via a bronchoscope (and proper tube location relative to the cariva).**

Invasive Monitors

Invasive monitors should be considered when the patient's condition permits or demands their insertion.

An *indwelling urinary catheter* allows urine output and specific gravity to be monitored. Low urine output with high specific gravity may indicate prerenal oliguria secondary to inadequate shock resuscitation.

Other invasive monitors that may be indicated are arterial, central venous, and PA catheters. *Directly measured arterial pressure* allows beat-to-beat arterial pressure monitoring, especially in a severely hypovolemic patient when blood pressure may not be obtainable with an automated oscillometer. Monitoring the trends in CVP gives an indication of the intravascular volume status. A PA catheter may be indicated if the patient has known or suspected left ventricular dysfunction, or has sustained multiple trauma with shock.

The *PA catheter* may allow for early normalization of cardiac output and ventricular filling pressures, measurement of mixed venous oxygen saturation, and calculation of oxygen delivery and consumption variables. Maintenance of supranormal values of oxygen delivery may be of benefit to certain subsets of patients following traumatic injuries.[55] Reaching supranormal circulation values (cardiac index > 4.5 l/min/m^2, DO_2 > 600 ml/min/m^2, and oxygen consumption > 160 ml/min/m^2), especially within 24 hours of injury, may improve survival and decrease the frequency of organ failure in severely injured trauma patients.[18] The early increase in cardiac index, oxygen delivery, and oxygen consumption appears necessary to compensate for the increased metabolic requirements related to severe trauma, and to repay the accumulated oxygen debt from prolonged tissue hypoxia.[18,55] There are patients who do not achieve supranormal values, yet survive, and there are those patients who reach these values, only to die. A prospective, randomized trial of hemodynamic therapy aimed at achieving supranormal values of cardiac index or normal values for mixed venous oxygen saturation did not reduce morbidity or mortality of critically ill patients compared with a control group in which the target was a normal cardiac index.[63] It may also be correct to say that the ability to generate supranormal values is simply a marker for organ reserve, which in turn, predicts survival.

Transesophageal echocardiography (*TEE*) can provide a direct and rapid assessment of hemodynamics and aortic injury in trauma victims.[26] TEE may be especially useful for guiding fluid and inotropic therapy. It is anticipated that the role of TEE in the perioperative setting will continue to evolve, especially in patients with chest trauma.

INDUCTION AND MAINTENANCE OF ANESTHESIA

Inducing anesthesia for trauma patients in stable condition may be no different than for patients having elective surgery, but the hypovolemic patient with multisystem injuries can present a challenge. In general, the most seriously injured patients in profound shock require minimal amounts of anesthetic or amnestic agents, muscle relaxants, and ventilation with 100% oxygen.

Although there has been much discussion about which induction agents are best—sodium thiopental, ketamine, etomidate, midazolam, or propofol[35]—none are ideal (Table 81-6).

Because of its cardiac depressant effect, sodium thiopental should be given in small increments for induction of anesthesia in trauma patients until the patient becomes unresponsive. Ketamine has the advantage of providing excellent analgesia with sympathetic stimulation, but the accompanying increase in ICP makes it undesirable in patients with suspected closed head injury. Ketamine elevates systemic blood pressure and heart rate through the release of norepinephrine from sympathetic nerve terminals; on occasion it actually decreases myocardial contractility and causes hypotension in patients whose vital signs are already being monitored with high sympathetic nervous activity.

Small doses of midazolam (1 to 2 mg IV) are very useful for amnestic, sedative, and anxiolytic effects, and have minimal, if any, hemodynamic effects. Incremental doses of midazolam are frequently indicated for conscious sedation during a wide variety of procedures including awake intubation. Induction doses of midazolam (0.2 to 0.3 mg/kg) may be associated with hypotension and do not appear to offer any advantage over standard doses of thiopental.

Although the cardiovascular depressant properties of propofol are similar to or greater than those of sodium thiopental,[168] this agent has been used in carefully titrated dosage during the acute phase of trauma. Considerable care must be taken to address cardiovascular and volume status when using this agent to induce anesthesia in the hypovoemic patient. Volume loading can, to a large extent, offset some of the cardiovascular effects associated with propofol. Because of its rapid clearance and short duration of action, propofol has many applications in trauma anesthesia, and has been successfully used in military battle casualties[170] and for the many follow-up surgical interventions and procedures that trauma patients often require (dressing changes, radiologic investigations, orthopedic adjustments). In head-injured patients, propofol tends to cause cerebral vasoconstriction and a reduction in ICP, cerebral blood flow (CBF) and cerebral metabolic rate for O_2 ($CMRO_2$). Continuous infusion of propofol, 10 to 50 μg/kg/min, is very useful for IV sedation during transport and in the intensive care unit because it provides a titratable level of sedation and a rapid recovery, which allows for frequent evaluation of neurologic status and cognitive function.[117,159]

Etomidate has minimal or absent cardiac depressant effects, compared with thiopental and propofol.[64] The lack of cardiovascular effects are most likely due to etomidate's lack of effect on the sympathetic nervous system and autonomic reflexes.[87] Administration of etomidate generally results in a stable or minimally decreased heart rate blood pressure, and systemic vascular resistance. There is a reduction in $CMRO_2$, CBF, and ICP, leading to an overall increase in cerebral pertusion pressure (CPP).[58,109] Etomidate's greatest benefit would thus appear to be for induction of anesthesia in trauma cases with shock or unstable cardiopulmonary status and in multiple trauma patients with head injury. Problems with etomidate include irritation and phlebitis in the injected vein, extrapyramidal movements on induction (which can confound the ongoing neurologic examination), and a higher incidence of nausea and vomiting in the postoperative period. Myoclonic movements and pain on injection with etomidate can be minimized with lidocaine, small doses of midazolam, and rapid-acting neuromuscular blocking agents. Although adrenal suppression following single doses of etomidate is reported, the suppression is apparently short-lived, incomplete, and of doubtful clinical significance.[37,59,87,167]

Unresponsive, hemodynamically unstable trauma patients often receive ventilation with 100% oxygen, neuromuscular blockade, and minimal amounts or no anesthetic agent. As soon as the patient's condition becomes more stable, an inhalation anesthetic agent and/or IV opioid in combination with an amnestic or hypnotic agent must be administered to alleviate pain and prevent awareness. No particular anesthetic technique (e.g., total inhalational or IV) has been shown to produce better outcome in these patients. The opioid agents most commonly used in the United States are fentanyl or sufentanil, because they have minimal direct depressant effects on the cardiovascular system (see Table 81-6).[35,56]

Inhalation Agents

Inhalational agents are generally used for maintenance of anesthesia, although both halothane and sevoflurane are suitable for inhalational induction, especially in pediatrics (Table 81-7). Although sevoflurane has only recently become available in the U.S., anectodal reports indicate that it may have a useful place in trauma. This is because sevoflurane has the attractive characteristics of being nonirritating

Table 81-6 Induction and adjuvant agents for trauma anesthesia

Agent	Standard dose (mg/kg)	Trauma dose* (mg/kg)	BP	CPP
Thiopental	3–5	0.5–2.0	Decreased	Decreased or stable
Comments: Rapid onset barbiturate hypnotic with short duration. Most popular induction agent for head trauma. May produce hypotension due to myocardial depression and vasodilation and therefore should be used in reduced or divided doses. Decreases C_{MRO2}, CBF, and ICP.				
Etomidate	0.2–0.3	0.1–0.2	Stable	Increased
Comments: Rapid onset imidazole hypnotic with short duration. Enhanced cardiovascular stability with well-maintained blood pressure. Decreases C_{MRO2}, CBF, and ICP. Associated with myoclonus (may mimic seizure).				
Ketamine	1–2	0.5–1.0	Stable	Stable or decreased
Comments: Rapid onset hypnotic with potent analgesia. Enhanced cardiovascular stability with well-maintained BP. Increases C_{MRO2}, CBF, and ICP. Can also be given IM, 5–10 mg/kg with onset of 5 minutes.				
Propofol	1.5–2.5	0.5–1.0	Decreased	Decreased or stable
Comments: Rapid onset nonbarbiturate hypnotic with short duration and extremely high clearance. May produce hypotension due to myocardial depression and vasodilation and therefore should be used in reduced doses. Decreases C_{MRO2}, CBF, and ICP. Drug of choice for total intravenous anesthesia (50–150 μg/kg/min).				
Midazolam	0.1–0.2	0.05–0.1	Stable	Stable or increased
Comments: Potent water soluble benzodiazepine. Small incremental doses are very useful in hemodynamically unstable patients for amnesia and sedation.				
Lidocaine	1.5–2.0	1.0–1.5	Stable	Stable or increased
Comments: Useful adjuvant agent for blunting airway reflexes. Also blunts BP, ICP and IOP response to intubation, and myoclonic response to etomidate. Decreases injection pain from propofol and etomidate.				
Fentanyl	3–10 μg/kg	1–3 μg/kg	Stable	Stable
Comments: Potent opioid analgesic with minimal hemodynamic or cerebrovascular effects. Useful adjuvant agent for procedures associated with pain, such as direct laryngoscopy and tracheal intubation. Combination of fentanyl with a hypnotic induction agent results in a synergistic interaction, such that the dose of hypnotic for loss of consciousness is reduced. May cause bradycardia (central vagal stimulation) and occasionally hypotension in patients with high sympathetic tone. Infusion rates of 0.02–0.10 μg/kg/min achieve stable analgesic plasma concentrations following a loading dose, with approximately a 50% reduction in minimum alveolar concentration (MAC) of volatile agents.[70]				
Sufentanil	0.5–1.0 μg/kg	0.1–0.5 μg/kg	Stable	Stable
Comments: Similar to fentanyl, but faster onset and offset. Infusion rates of 0.003–0.01 μg/kg/min achieve stable analgesic plasma concentrations following a loading dose, with approximately a 50% reduction in MAC of volatile agents.[70]				

*Hypnotic drugs are useful to induce general anesthesia in trauma patients who require rapid sequence intubation and/or emergency surgery. Actual response of any patient to these drugs depends on a number of factors such as degree of hemorrhage, presence of shock, and underlying sympathetic tone. Unresponsive patients with systolic BP $<$ 60 mm Hg do not usually require induction agents.

CBF—cerebral blood flow; C_{MRO2}—cerebral metabolic requirement for oxygen; IOP—intraocular pressure; ICP—intracranial pressure; BP—blood pressure; CPP—cerebral perfusion pressure = mean BP − ICP.

to the airway, as well as "quick on–quick off" pharmacokinetics. Nitrous oxide should probably not be used in the patient with multiple acute trauma because it may aggravate a pneumothorax or pneumocephalus. Nitrous oxide may also decrease cardiac output and exacerbate hypotension when used in conjunction with potent opioids.[51]

All the volatile anesthetic agents produce dose-related decreases in blood pressure due to alterations in vascular tone and/or cardiac output. The volatile agents also produce dose-related increases in CBF and uncoupling of the normal close relation between CBF and $CMRO_2$. The increase in CBF and cerebral blood volume may result in an increase in ICP. If there is concern about elevated ICP, hypocapnia may attenuate or block the increase in ICP. Although isoflurane is the least potent cerebral vasodilator of the volatiles, even this agent should be avoided in patients with critically elevated ICP.[7,8]

The relatively low solubility of desflurane and sevoflurane may allow rapid alterations in alveolar concentrations, thereby improving control of the depth of anesthesia during maintenance. Sevoflurane has the added advantage of minimal airway irritation, which makes this agent suitable for inhalational induction.[94] Desflurane has the advantage of having almost no metabolism (0.02%), which makes this agent particularly appealing for long cases.

Neuromuscular Blocking Agents

Succinylcholine **has the obvious advantage of rapid onset and offset and is commonly the muscle relaxant of choice for a "rapid sequence induction."** After an intubating dose

Table 81-7 Inhalational agents for trauma

Agent	Blood solubility	MAC (%)	Metabolism (%)	CV
Depression				
Desflurane	0.42	6	0.02%	Dose-related
Comments: Rapid uptake and elimination-rapid emergence; may cause sympathetic stimulation.[49] Associated with airway irritation. Requires special vaporizer because vapor pressure close to atmospheric at room temperature.				
Enflurane	1.8	1.68	2%, fluoride	Dose-related
Comments: May be associated with seizure activity. Nephrotoxicity a concern with prolonged surgery or renal dysfunction				
Halothane	2.5	0.75	10%–20%	Dose-related
Comments: Potent agent without airway irritation—useful for inhalational induction in pediatrics. Associated with decreased cardiac output, ventricular ectopy, and hepatic biotransformation.				
Isoflurane	1.4	1.15	Minimal, 0.2%	Dose-related
Comments: Potent peripheral vasodilator; Cardiac output, heart rate, and rhythm usually well maintained.				
Nitrous oxide	0.47	105	None	Minimal
Comments: Rapid uptake and elimination with little cardiac or respiratory depression. Useful for prehospital analgesia; potential for expansion of closed air spaces limits use in trauma				
Sevoflurane	0.69	2	2%–5%, fluoride, compound A	Dose-related
Comments: Rapid induction and emergence; agent of choice for inhalational induction. Theoretical concern for nephrotoxicity.[24]				

of succinylcholine (1.0 to 1.5 mg/kg), the actual time that a patient will resume adequate spontaneous respirations is approximately 5 to 10 minutes. Thus, succinylcholine is not rapidly reversible in the instance of the "can't intubate, can't ventilate" scenario. An alternative method of oxygenation/ventilation may have to be selected (e.g., LMA, Combitube, surgical airway, *see* above). Alternatively, a lower dose of succinylcholine may be used (e.g., 0.5 mg/kg) with repeated single twitch monitoring to document onset and offset of neuromuscular blockade. Care must be exercised before using succinylcholine in a trauma patient because of complications such as hyperkalemia, arrhythmias, and increased intracranial and intraocular pressures.[15,73] In rare instances, succinylcholine may cause masseter muscle rigidity and trigger malignant hyperthermia.[15]

Succinylcholine has long been considered contraindicated in patients with open-eye injuries, because it is associated with increased intraocular pressure (IOP) and possible extrusion of ocular contents. There is, however, some evidence to suggest that succinylcholine may be safely used in patients with eye injuries.[95] There is also experimental evidence that administration of succinylcholine does not result in loss of intraocular contents in a cat model of ocular trauma, despite IOP increases of 10 mm Hg.[113]

The literature strongly suggets that succinylcholine be avoided after 24 hrs of injury in patients with burns, massive trauma, crush injuries, spinal cord injuries, stroke, severe abdominal infections, tetanus, and neuromuscular disease because of the risk of hyperkalemic cardiac arrest. The clinician should also be aware that hyperkalemia after succinylcholine can occur on the first day in cases involving crush and degloving injuries, burns, trauma, and abdominal sepsis, and that the so-called "safe period" for succinylcholine may not be as long as previously believed. It may sometimes be difficult to accurately pinpoint the actual time of injury and to correctly calculate the "safe period," especially if the trauma patient is being received at a secondary or tertiary referral center. The administration of small defasciculating doses of nondepolarizing muscle relaxants prior to succinylcholine does not reliably prevent the development of life-threatening hyperkalemia.

Succinylcholine-induced bradyarrhythmias, including asystole, may occur following repeat doses of this agent in any patient, even with the initial dose in children, and in conditions of hypoxia or hypercapnia. Use of succinylcholine is controversial in patients with elevated ICP.[88] It is likely that ventilation, oxygenation, and absence of coughing and bucking are more important determinants of ICP than the onset of a depolarizing block.

Rocuronium is the first nondepolarizer alternative for succinylcholine in terms of onset, but has a clinical duration similar to vecuronium. In simulated rapid sequence inductions, it has been found that rocuronium in doses of 0.9 and 1.2 mg/kg produced similar onset times and intubating conditions to that of succinylcholine.[100] In contrast to succinylcholine, rocuronium does not cause hyperkalemia, elevated ICP, or IOP.[103] There is a potential for mild vagolysis with rocuronium, especially in lightly anesthetized patients. Ablation of the facial nerve–orbicularis oculis response to train-of-four stimulation appears to be an excellent predictor of good intubating conditions with nondepolarizing muscle relaxants (Table 81-8).[41,105,125]

Vecuronium's onset of action is delayed compared with rocuronium and succinylcholine. Vecuronium has the advantage of being a "clean drug" in terms of cardiovascular

Table 81-8 Muscle relaxants for trauma anesthesia[153]

Relaxant	ED_{95} (mg/kg)	Intubating dose (mg/kg)	Onset time (min)	Clinical duration of intubating dose* (min)
Atracurium	0.25	0.5–0.6	2–4	35–60
Comments: Histamine release and hypotension when given quickly; metabolized by Hoffman elimination and ester hydrolysis with short half-life (20 min) and predictable elimination.				
Cisatracurium	0.05	0.10	5	45
Comments: Stereoisomer of atracurium with predictable elimination. Metabolized by Hoffman elimination and ester hydrolysis; no histamine release or cardiovascular effects.				
Doxacurium	0.03	0.08	6–11	60–120
Comments: Not recommended for rapid sequence because of slow onset. Benzylisoquinolinium structure without histamine release or cardiovascular effects; eliminated in urine.				
Mivacurium	0.08	0.25–0.30	2–4	20–30
Comments: Histamine release and hypotension when given quickly; metabolized by plasma cholinesterase with ultra short half-life (3–4 min) and predictable elimination				
Org 9487	1.2	1.5	1	8
Comments: Low potency steroidal nondepolarizer currently undergoing clinical trials. May be candidate to replace succinylcholine.[169]				
Pancuronium	0.05	0.10–0.15	2–4	60–120
Comments: No histamine release; vagolytic effect and sympathetic stimulation (tachycardia). Metabolized by liver, eliminated in bile and urine.				
Rocuronium	0.3	0.9–1.2	0.75–1.5	45–90
Comments: Nondepolarizer of choice for rapid sequence intubation; no histamine release. Possible mild vagolysis; metabolized by liver, eliminated in bile and urine.				
Succinylcholine	0.30	1.0–1.5	0.5–1.0	5
Comments: Drug of choice for rapid sequence intubation, but depolarizing bloc and potential for bradycardia, hyperkalemia, increased intraocular and intracranial pressure, masseter muscle spasm, and malignant hyperthermia. Metabolized by plasma cholinesterase.				
Vecuronium	0.05	0.15–0.3	1.5–4	45–120
Comments: No histamine release; no cardiovascular effects. Metabolized by liver, eliminated in bile and urine.				

*Time to 25% first twitch recovery.

effects even when large doses are rapidly administered. Use of "high dose" vecuronium, 0.3 mg/kg or 6x effective dose for 95% twitch depression (ED_{95}) has been advocated. Doxacurium and pipecuronium are two long-acting nondepolarizers without cardiovascular effects. Pancuronium is also available for long-acting nondepolarizing muscle relaxation with well-documented cardiovascular effects such as tachycardia.

Both atracurium and mivacurium have the advantage of organ-independent elimination, although these agents may be associated with histamine release and hypotension. Cisatracurium, a more potent stereoisomer of atracurium, may be a useful drug in trauma because of predictable elimination without histamine release.

ROLE OF REGIONAL ANESTHESIA IN TRAUMA

Regional anesthesia in appropriately selected trauma patients with isolated injuries may provide beneficial effects such as decreased sympathetic tone, decreased stress response, decreased incidence of deep vein thrombosis, decreased blood loss, increased blood supply to the extremities, and increased blood flow following reimplantation procedures. Regional anesthesia allows the patient to be awake during the procedure (if desired), which facilitates sequential evaluation of neurologic and mental status, and allows the patient to maintain and protect their own airway. The regional technique can easily be extended into the postoperative period for prolonged analgesia.

When considering regional, one must take into consideration the requirements of the surgery (duration and number of operative sites), desires of the patient, contraindications of the technique, and the presence of neurologic and vascular injuries. For example, the use of regional anesthesia is inappropriate for the head-injured patient with low Glasgow Coma scale who has sustained extremity, chest, and/or abdominal trauma requiring urgent or emergency surgery. Patients such as these need intubation and airway protection, oxygenation, and ventilation. Use of regional anesthesia is also not advisable in hemodynamically unstable patients or in patients with altered mental status, respiratory distress, sepsis, or coagulopathy.

Nonetheless, regional anesthesia can provide excellent operative conditions for many parts of the body. The administration of a regional anesthetic requires thorough knowledge of applied anatomy, the clinical pharmacology of the anesthetic, and possible complications of the technique. Regional anesthetics may be administered via topical application, local infiltration, field block, block of individual nerves, plexus block, or central axis block (spinal-epidural).[145,160,171]

Upper-extremity blocks are ideally suited for trauma patients requiring repair of fractures, digital reimplants, debridement, tendon ruptures, and other procedures. Axillary blocks are used most often for procedures at the hand up to the elbow, whereas interscalene blocks are more useful for proximal procedures. An indwelling catheter can provide long-lasting pain relief. Use of insulated needles and a nerve stimulator capable of delivering low amperages (down to 0.1 to 0.2 mA) can greatly facilitate success of these blocks. IV regional anesthesia can also be used in selected cases.

Lower-extremity and abdominal surgery can be performed with various techniques such as spinals or epidurals. Nerve blocks may be helpful for lower-extremity surgery (e.g., femoral, lateral femoral cutaneous, obturator, sciatic, three-in-one block).

The main drawback to instilling local anesthetics into the epidural and subarachnoid spaces is the risk of hypotension with sympathetic outflow block, unwanted motor block, and urinary retention. Neuraxial anesthesia is also contraindicated in a trauma patient with coagulopathy. Because the risk of hypotension is so great in trauma patients with hypovolemia, epidural-spinal blocks with a local anesthetic are contraindicated until the fluid status and hemodynamics are under control. The unwanted motor and sensory block may also interfere with the initial and ongoing neuroassessment of the acute trauma patient. Some of these disadvantages may be avoided by using narcotics in the epidural or subarachnoid space.[98] The main side effects of epidural-spinal narcotics are late respiratory depression, nausea and vomiting, urinary retention, and itching. Neuraxial anesthesia has many appropriate applications in the stable, resuscitated trauma patient undergoing follow-up/repeat elective surgery.

INTRAOPERATIVE PROBLEMS

Awareness During Trauma Anesthesia

Priorities exist when administering anesthesia to trauma patients. Although hemodynamic resuscitation is clearly more immediately important than the concern of awareness, the latter issue should not be neglected. In one study, 43% of trauma patients who required discontinuance of the anesthetic agents for more than 20 consecutive minutes had awareness.[20] One of our goals is to resuscitate patients adequately so that their cardiovascular systems can tolerate sufficient anesthetic agents to blunt awareness and recall. Often in unstable patients, satisfactory hemodynamic resuscitation cannot be performed without a surgical procedure. The occurrence of awareness and recall does not necessarily mean that the anesthetic was inadequate. **Trainees are often concerned about this and may continue to give anesthetic agents in the face of severely deteriorating hemodynamics; the latter of course is exacerbated by the anesthetics. This vicious cycle must be avoided. The anesthesia provider's primary duty is to keep the patient alive.** Nonetheless, small doses of midazolam and/or scopolamine (both with minimal hemodynamic effects), and low doses of a volatile agent (e.g., isoflurane, 0.3%), can help prevent awareness in unstable patients without unduly jeopardizing hemodynamic stability.

Intraoperative Hypotension

Hemorrhage and hypovolemia are the most common causes of shock and hypotension in the trauma patient, although other causes, such as anaphylaxis, should be carefully considered.

Cardiogenic shock may occur due to contusion, tamponade, air embolism, valvular rupture, coronary ischemia, and infarction. Elevations in CK-MB enzymes or cardiac troponin T levels may signify myocardial injury or contusion.[5] Cardiac tamponade most often occurs in association with penetrating trauma, but has occassionally occurred after blunt trauma, and is diagnosed by signs of low cardiac output together with increased venous pressure, diminished heart sounds, and pulsus paradoxus. Cardiac contusion may result in subendocardial or subepicardial hemorrhage, intramyocardial hemorrhage or injury to a branch of coronary artery. Cardiac contusion very often entails conduction disturbances or arrhythmias.

Tension pneumothorax can result from pulmonary laceration, rupture of the trachea or major bronchus, esophageal rupture, or from inadequate sealing of an open pneumothorax. The clinical signs are hypoxia and hyperresonance of the chest wall with diminished breath sounds. If untreated, mediastinal shock follows with progressively reduced venous return, contralateral displacement of the mediastinum, and eventual compression of the intact lung combined with torsion and compression of the vena cava. Immediate decompression is life saving. A very high index of suspicion is often pivotal in making this diagnosis.

High spinal cord lesions may also produce hypotension due to anatomic sympathectomy. Other evidence pointing to a diagnosis of spinal shock includes bradycardia, warm skin, bounding pulses, priapism, and associated neurologic deficit. Treatment is supportive, and consists of fluids and vasopressors. High-dose methylprednisolone is recommended to improve neurologic deficit following acute spinal cord injuries.[22]

Renal Failure

Renal failure in the trauma patient is associated with high mortality and is often the principal determinant of survival in patients with multiorgan system failure. Recognition of patients at high risk and meticulous attention to optimization of hemodynamics is paramount in attempting to prevent acute renal failure. Renal function can be clinically monitored by urine output, and laboratory analysis of serum and urine from which creatinine clearance (Ccr) can be derived. Ccr is a measure of glomerular filtration rate (GFR) and is a very sensitive indicator of posttraumatic renal failure. Renal failure can be defined according to rate of urine formation: anuric ($\leq$ 50 ml/day), oliguric ($\leq$ 500 ml/day), and nonoliguric ($\leq$ 6000 ml/day). In the trauma patient, as in any surgical patient, decreased renal perfusion is the most common cause of acute renal dysfunction.[106] The kidney will vasoconstrict and reduce both total renal blood flow and GFR in response to reduced blood volume. Intrarenal failure is caused by direct kidney injury during trauma, by nephrotoxic drug administration, or by acute tubular necrosis after prolonged shock or precipitation of hemoglobin or myoglobin crystals (Box 81-2). In the patient who has had a difficult abdominal closure due to massive distension of the midgut, oliguria may signify compression of the renal veins. In this case, return to the operating room to remove packs, evacuate clot, or change to alternative closure techniques such as towel clips, may dramatically reduce intra-abdominal pressure, restore renal blood flow, as well as improve cardiorespiratory function.[54]

The differentiation of prerenal from renal parenchymal dysfunction (Table 81-9) is important in the trauma patient because the therapy differs. Prerenal failure will respond to appropriate increases in intravascular volume. Intrarenal failure is treated by careful monitoring of the intravascular volume and use of diuretics to try to convert oliguric to nonoliguric renal failure.

BOX 81-2
CAUSES OF POSTTRAUMATIC RENAL FAILURE

Prerenal

Inadequate fluid resuscitation
Cardiac failure
Liver failure
High airway pressure
Abdominal compartment syndrome
Intra-abdominal hematoma
Hepatorenal syndrome
Sepsis

Renal

Pre-existing renal disease
Myoglobinuria/hemoglobinuria
Renal trauma
Renal vascular occlusion
Nephrotoxic drugs such as aminoglycosides, amphotericin, cephalosporins, catecholamines, vancomycin
Sepsis and toxic cellular metabolites

Postrenal

Ureteral obstruction (rare)

Once renal failure has become obvious, treatment consists of controlling the concentrations of metabolic products in the patient's blood and controlling fluid balance through dialysis and careful limitation of nutritional protein load. Hemodialysis is more efficient in removing electrolytes and nitrogenous waste than is peritoneal dialysis. It can either be instituted on an everyday or an every-other-day schedule, depending on the patient's production of urea and performed for 1 to 2 hours with adequate removal of nitrogenous waste, potassium, and water.

Multiple Surgical Teams

Trauma patients often undergo multiple operations by different surgical teams simultaneously or in series. For example, the neurosurgeon may be trying to place a monitoring bolt or even evacuate a cerebral hematoma, whereas general and orthopedic surgeons are trying to stop bleeding from a lacerated liver and a pelvic fracture. The anesthesia team may have limited physical access. Utmost care and vigilance must be observed to avoid airway disconnection and other mechanical problems during anesthesia. Monitors may stop working intraoperatively if not established properly at the start. In hectic times, the primary anesthesia provider may need assistance from additional anesthesia care providers, and should not hesitate to make these requirements known. In the operating room, the anesthesia provider should take the leading role in the patient's resuscitation, and solid medical judgment must determine individual priorities. For example, formal resection and reconstructions in patients with abdominal trauma and exsanguinating hemorrhage may lead to irreversible physiologic insult due to hypothermia, coagulopathy, and acidosis. It may be prudent to have the surgeon obtain control of the bleeding and hollow visceral spillage, apply a temporary abdominal closure, and delay definitive repair until after the patient has been stabilized.[78]

Hypothermia

Hypothermia decreases oxygen consumption and has allowed for long ischemic times in cardiac and neurologic surgery. Application of moderate cooling after isolated closed head injury is currently being studied with encouraging results.[30,101] Although hypothermia decreases metabolic function of the body and is cerebroprotective, hy-

Table 81-9 Differentiation of renal failure

	Normal	Prerenal	Intrarenal
Urine (mEq/l)	20–40	< 20	> 40
BUN (mg/dl)	4–25	↑	↑
Creatinine (mg/dl)	0.5–1.4	↑	↑
BUN/Cr ratio	5–15	> 15	< 10
Urine/serum osmolality	1.5–4	> 1.8	< 1.1

pothermia most often results in deleterious effects in multiple trauma patients.[127]

Hypothermia (core temperature < 35° C) occurs in traumatized individuals because of impaired thermoregulation, decreased heat production and increased heat loss. In the field, the trauma patient may have extended exposure to adverse ambient environments. During rapid evacuation and transport, significant wind chill factors can be generated, especially with helicopter transport and decreased ambient temperatures associated with increasing altitude. In the emergency department, the injured patient is completely undressed as part of the evaluation process. In the operating room, prolonged surgery with an open abdomen, massive blood and fluid transfusions, and exposure of large body surface areas are common occurrences. All of these factors contribute significantly to the development of hypothermia.[152]

The adverse effects of hypothermia in the trauma patient include major coagulation derangements, peripheral vasoconstriction, metabolic acidosis, compensatory increased oxygen requirements during rewarming, and impaired immune response.[57,89,144,151] Standard coagulation tests are temperature corrected to 37° C and may not reflect hypothermia-induced coagulopathy.[132,133,166] Hypothermia impairs coagulation because of slowing of enzymatic rates and reduced platelet function. Hypothermia can cause cardiac dysrhythmias and even cardiac arrest due to electromechanical dissociation, standstill, or fibrillation, especially with temperatures below 30° C. Hypothermia also impairs citrate, lactate, and drug metabolism; increases blood viscosity, impairs erythrocyte deformability; increases intracellular potassium release, and causes a leftward shift of the oxyhemoglobin dissociation curve. Collectively, these adverse effects have been associated with an increased morbidity and mortality in hypothermic trauma patients.[127] A mortality of 100% has been reported in trauma patients whose body temperature fell to below 32° C, regardless of severity of injury, degree of hypotension, or fluid replacement.[85] Hence, every effort should be made to avoid hypothermia by increasing ambient temperature (> 22° C), using convective and/or radiant heat, and warming all fluids and blood transfusions to 37° C (see Table 81-4). Evaporation from the respiratory tract can be prevented by use of active airway humidifiers or passive heat and moisture exchangers.

The importance of fluid warming in the multiple trauma patient cannot be underestimated. It requires 16 kcal of energy to raise the temperature of 1 l of crystalloid infused at 21° C to body temperature (37° C), and 30 kcal to raise the temperature of cold (4° C) blood to 37° C. Infusion of 4.3 l of crystalloid at room temperature to an anesthetized adult trauma patient who cannot increase heat production can result in a decrease of 1.5° C in core temperature. Similarly, infusion of 2.3 l of erythrocytes could result in a core temperature decrease of between 1° and 1.5° C.[47,67,108] Because the thermal stress of infusing fluids at normothermia is essentially zero, it follows that use of effective fluid warming devices (outlet temperature > 37° C) would permit more efficient rewarming of hypothermic trauma patients using other methods such as the patient's own metabolically generated heat, or externally provided heat (e.g, convective warming, radiant heat).[144]

Active core rewarming refers to the use of various techniques such as peritoneal and hemodialysis, body cavity lavage, and cardiopulmonary bypass. Active or internal rewarming restores normothermia at a faster rate than surface methods and has been associated with more rapid normalization of coagulation, cardiac output and ECG, and a decreased risk of rewarming shock.[65,66,92] These methods of core rewarming are generally appropriate for severely injured hypothermic patients (< 28° C), but may also be extremely useful for moderately hypothermic patients (28° to 32.1° C) with cardiovascular instability and hypothermia-induced coagulopathy.

Although cardiopulmonary bypass is the most effective means of rewarming severely hypothermic patients,[137] in multiply injured trauma patients, use of cardiopulmonary bypass and systemic heparinization is unlikely to be possible due to the risk of bleeding. Nonclotting circuits with heparin coating or heparin bonding would be of great advantage in this setting. Peritoneal or mediastinal lavage with heated crystalloid at an exchange rate of 6 l/min may increase core temperature at a rate of 2° to 3° C/hr, and has been shown to be beneficial in patients sustaining environmental or exposure hypothermia.[39] Peritoneal and mediastinal lavage may be inappropriate in patients with abdominal or thoracic injuries. Another described technique involves connection of a percutaneously placed femoral arterial line to a countercurrent fluid warmer.[65,66,67] The patient's blood volume flows through the warmer and returns to the patient via large-bore venous tubing, such that a fistula is created through the heating warmer. This technique, known as continuous arteriovenous rewarming (CAVR), has been shown to rapidly rewarm hypothermic patients by providing 94 to 157 kcal/hr of heat, sufficient to raise core temperature in adults by 1.3° to 2.2° C/hr.[67] Advantages of CAVR include nonrequirement for heparinization and rapid reversal of hypothermia.

Multiple Repeat Surgery

Trauma patients often require multiple repeat surgery due to the nature of their injuries. Such multiple repeat surgery introduces undesirable potential consequences, which include coagulopathy, anemia, stress, and malnutrition leading to disturbance in plasma protein patterns, multiorgan system failure and sepsis, ARDS, and the need for multiple medications via many IV lines and infusion controllers (pumps).

With frequent repeat surgery the bone marrow and the liver will not have time to replenish the blood with the various necessary blood components. Nevertheless, use of blood products should be minimized to diminish the risk of transfusion-associated diseases and immunosuppression. Asanguineous fluids such as colloids and crystalloids should replace blood component therapy whenever possible. It has been shown that acute intraoperative normovolemic hemodilution to a hematocrit level of 22% was well tolerated even in patients with multisystem disease but without cardiac disease.[140] The lowest acceptable level of hemoglobin during the postoperative period varies with each patient, and anesthesia providers should therefore not be aiming for a specific level of hemoglobin. The ability of the patient's cardiovascular system to compensate is probably the most important determinant of how low the level of hemoglobin can be allowed to drop,[139] although there is evidence that marked hemodilution (hemoglobin 6 g/dl) may exacerbate neurologic injury.[130] Patients with coronary artery disease (CAD) and/or aortic stenosis or those receiving beta blockers may not be capable of increasing their cardiac output adequately and will experience diminished oxygen delivery with isovolemic anemia. Organs with a high oxygen extraction ratio such as the heart are likely to be most vulnerable, and the lack of oxygen supply may lead to organ failure or infarction.

During the rehabilitative phase, patients return for plastic surgery and/or orthopedic reconstructive procedures, such as delayed removal of internal or external hardware used for fracture fixation (usually 6 to 18 months after injury). Repeat elective operations on stable patients usually present no additional anesthetic problems, because the patients' cardiopulmonary and nutritional states are improved and there is time for a thorough history and examination.

POSTOPERATIVE CARE

Postoperative problems in trauma patients can be divided into general and specific. General problems—as in the routine elective surgical patient—include nausea and vomiting, pain management, central nervous system (CNS) depression, agitation, and complications of unsuspected drug abuse. Specific posttraumatic complications include ARDS, multiorgan system failure, and sepsis, the last two being the major late causes of death in trauma. Pain management is also an important component of postoperative trauma care.

Ventilatory Management

Trauma patients with multiple injuries who survive the "golden hour" usually require prolonged postoperative ventilation and critical care treatment to prevent and manage multiorgan system failure as they recover from their injuries. Extubation of trauma patients in the immediate postsurgical period should not be considered until the following conditions are ruled out:

- Actual and potential gas-exchange disturbances (e.g., in severe direct lung injury)
- Upper-airway obstruction: fracture of the larynx, cricoid or thyroid cartilage; edema of tongue, pharynx, or larynx
- Severe brain injury (e.g., patient may need to be ventilated to prevent secondary brain injury, protect the airway, and control ICP)

Pain Management in Trauma Patients

The effect of pain and the related stress response is almost always detrimental to the trauma patient. Immediate effects of pain are mediated by metabolic and neurohumoral mechanisms, and can result in increased plasma catecholamine and antidiuretic hormone levels, accelerated protein catabolism and lipolysis, hyperglycemia, delayed wound healing, and hypercoagulability.[32] Clinical effects of these metabolic and neurohumoral mechanisms manifest as salt and water retention, tachycardia, hypertension, deep venous thrombosis, pulmonary embolism, reduced gastroinstestinal motility, infections, immobility, ventilation-perfusion mismatch, and hypoxia.

Optimal pain management in trauma patients requires consideration of the entire clinical picture so that an effective perioperative approach can be undertaken. For example, in patients experiencing thoracic trauma, the goal is to allow the patient to take a deep breath and cough effectively in order to mobilize and clear secretions, and to improve ventilatory mechanics. In patients with major vascular disruption, techniques to reduce sympathetic overactivity and provide pain relief will be of benefit. Other goals of pain management are to restore function and mobility (e.g., extremity injuries, pelvic reconstruction), and prevent the development of chronic pain syndromes such as myofascial pain, sympathetically mediated pain (reflex sympathetic dystrophy or causalgia), phantom limb pain, and posttraumatic headaches.

It is important to recognize that trauma patients frequently present with injuries to multiple areas of the body. This necessitates flexibility when designing pain management plans. The need to continuously monitor mental status and neurologic function, and the presence of abnormalities such as coagulopathy, bacteremia, spinal cord injury, and hemodynamic instability will all influence the perioperative pain-management plan.

It is also important to note that the ideal method of pain relief may change depending on the evolving nature of the trauma patients' active problems. The use of sedatives as well as nonsteroidal anti-inflammatory agents, such as ketorolac, and other drugs, such as carbamazepine, may greatly help control pain in the trauma setting (Table 81-10).

Adult Respiratory Distress Syndrome

Adult respiratory distress syndrome is considered as the pulmonary component of a generalizaed panendothelial inflammation that affects multiple organs.[149] Trauma frequently leads to ARDS. Risk factors for developing ARDS include multisystem trauma, high injury severity score, hypotension, transfusion requirement greater than 1500 ml within 1 hour of hospital admission, and initial $Pa{O_2}$ less than 70 mm Hg. The clinical diagnosis of ARDS is made in the setting of tachypnea, dyspnea, hypoxemia, diffuse alveolar infiltrates,

Table 81-10 Methods of pain management in acute trauma patients[126]

Method (agent)	Advantages and disadvantages
IV opioids (morphine, fentanyl)	Suitable for all types of patients, although may not provide optimal analgesia because of inherent temporal variability in dose requirements. Most often used during acute phase of trauma, head injuries, neurologic injuries, etc.
IV PCA (morphine, fentanyl)	Reduces the pain and oversedation cycles that are associated with continuous or intermittent IV opioid infusions. Not suitable for patients with altered mental status.
Brachial plexus catheter (local anesthetic)	Ideal for upper-extremity injuries and revascularizations. Reduces sympathetic activity, improves blood flow and provides excellent pain relief. Cannot be used if frequent nerve checks are required.
Intercostal block (local anesthetic)	Ideal for rib fractures. Chief limitations are temporary pain relief (6–12 hrs), positioning, and risk of pneumothorax.
Interpleural catheter (local anesthetic)	Useful for thoracic pain. Problems include inadequate analgesia, relatively high plasma levels of local anesthetic agent, loss of agent via thoracostomy suction, and migration or movement of catheter tip.
Thoracic epidural catheter (local anesthetic and/or opioid)	Method of choice for thoracic pain but many contraindications, such as spinal cord injury, sepsis, coagulopathy, hemodynamic instability. Risk of spinal cord or epidural hematoma. Continuous infusions of bupivacaine with morphine are very useful. Motor and sensory block from local anesthetics may interfere with neurologic monitoring and early detection of compartment syndromes.
Lumbar epidural catheter (local anesthetic and/or opioid)	Very useful for abdominal and lower extremity pain. Epidural morphine is excellent for thoracic analgesia (rostral spread). Fentanyl has limited thoracic analgesia because of high systemic absorption. Similar contraindications/problems as with thoracic epidural.
Patient-controlled epidural analgesia	Can be used with either thoracic or lumbar route in selected, cooperative patients.
Peripheral nerve block (local anesthetic)	Indicated in many diverse situations. The triple nerve block (femoral, obturator, lateral femoral cutaneous) can provide excellent relief after repair of fractured femurs (lidocaine, bupivicaine)

IV—intravenous; PCA—patient controlled analgesia.

decreased lung compliance, and absence of cardiac failure. In the setting of trauma, ARDS may be caused by sudden changes in microvascular permeability from direct or indirect lung insults, such as contusion, aspiration, disseminated intravascular coagulation, sepsis, pneumonia, long-bone fractures, blast injury, neurogenic factors, and upper-airway obstruction.

Treatment goals include optimization of oxygen delivery (DO_2 = cardiac output $\times$ oxygen content of arterial blood), prevention of barotrauma, prevention of oxygen toxicity, treatment of the underlying cause, if possible, and prevention of nosocomial pneumonias. Pressure support ventilation with varying levels of oxygen and PEEP (or CPAP) are the cornerstones of therapy for severe ARDS. High mean airway pressures may promote damage of nonaffected lung tissues and prevent affected lung areas from healing. Permissive hypercapnia may be useful in select groups of patients without head injury.[68] The administration of large amounts of colloid fluid may accumulate in lung interstitium and worsen pulmonary edema. High levels of PEEP often mandate the use of a PA catheter to optimize filling pressures, cardiac output, and oxygen delivery-demand relationships. Although a variety of drugs have been used in the treatment of ARDS, such as free radical scavengers, antiproteases, prostaglandin inhibitors, and corticosteroids, none have sufficient therapeutic value as to be in widespread clinical use. Inhaled N_2O may soon prove to be a useful technique in the treatment of acute pulmonary hypertension that often accompanies severe ARDS.[19]

Sepsis/Multisystem Organ Failure

Sepsis is the leading cause of multisystem organ failure (MSOF), and accounts for the majority of "late deaths" in trauma. In one study,[60] sequential pulmonary, hepatic, gastrointestinal, and renal failure followed the diagnosis of infection within 10 days. Failure of two organ systems resulted in a mortality rate of 60%, whereas failure of three or four systems resulted in mortality rates of 85% and 100%, respectively.

There are many sources for infection in trauma patients. Contamination can occur from the initial injury (e.g., penetrating and blunt trauma, lacerations, open fractures, aspiration) and from any indwelling line (e.g., peripheral IVs, arterial lines, central lines, pulmonary artery catheters, chest tubes, Foley catheter, gastric tube, tracheal tube, ICP monitor, S_jO_2 catheter). Infection can also occur during surgical procedures and as a result of medications and other products that can harbor pathogens (e.g., contaminated blood, propo-

Table 81-11 Approach to sepsis in the trauma patient[150]

Alterations	Considerations
Disrupted skin and mucosal barriers	Clean and debride wounds; promptly resuscitate from shock and hypothermia. Restore tissue perfusion; meticulous line and tube care. Appropriate antibiotics.
Disrupted gastrointestinal barriers	Preserve normal gastric acidity; cytoprotection with sucralfate preferable to H_2 blockers.
Immune dysfunction after trauma	Preserve tissue blood flow and O_2 delivery; establish early enteral nutrition and nutritional supplements.
Exaggerated inflammatory response (macrophages, polymorphonuclear leukocytes)	All of the above, and eradication of occult infections; antiendotoxin strategies, mediator inhibition, and/or immunologic blockade.*

*Considered investigational.

fol).[12] Gastric colonization may also be a source of infection, particularly in patients receiving agents that alter gastric pH.

Prevention and treatment of sepsis and MSOF are of major concern in the care of the trauma patient. Strategies to prevent sepsis and the systemic inflammatory response are currently undergoing intense investigation in the laboratory and the clinical setting. At the present time, the most useful approaches are summarized in Table 81-11.

Septic shock represents a complex array of circulatory and metabolic derangements that ultimately leads to inadequate cellular energy use. Changes in levels of N_2O may mediate pathologic vasodilation, which is the primary hemodynamic abnormality seen in patients with septic shock.[119] Therapy for septic shock includes ventiltory support, correction of electrolyte abnormalities, maintenance of arterial pH above 7.30, nutritional support, infection control, and hemodynamic management directed at maximizing DO_2.[104] Invasive monitoring using a PA catheter is necessary to guide fluid and inotropic or vasopressor therapy. Maintenance of supranormal values of DO_2 may enhance survival.[18,55,148]

Severe Head Injury

Severe head injury is defined as a Glasgow Coma Scale (GCS) score of less than or equal to 8 after resuscitation. Severe head injury renders the brain more susceptible to secondary insults, particularly to hypotension and hypoxia (see also Chapter 31).[29] The mechanisms underlying this enhanced vulnerability include factors such as reduced CBF, impaired CBF autoregulation, abnormal CBF–cerebral metabolism coupling, and increased neuronal sensitivity to mediators of ischemia.[42]

Prevention and treatment of secondary brain insults requires vigilant monitoring and aggressive treatment to insure adequate CPP, DO_2, and normovolemia.[173] Monitoring ICP and mean blood pressure often serves as a bedside index of cerebral perfusion because CPP = MAP − ICP. A CPP level of at least 70 mm Hg is believed to be necessary to maintain adequate CBF in severely head-injured patients.[91] Aggressive hyperventilation can cause or exacerbate secondary brain injury due to hypocapnic cerebral vasoconstriction, and has been associated with worse outcomes.[114] Therefore, $PaCO_2$ should be maintained at normal levels, unless ICP, CPP, CBF, or cerebral metabolism measurements dictate otherwise. Cerebral oxygenation can be continuously monitored by inserting a fiber optic catheter into the jugular bulb, similar to mixed venous O_2 saturation monitoring using a PA catheter. The underlying concept behind continuous jugular bulb venous hemoglobin saturations (S_jO_2) monitoring is that the brain compensates for decreased or inadequate CBF by increasing O_2 extraction, which is reflected by a decrease in S_jO_2. Continuous S_jO_2 monitoring may therefore help guide therapy aimed at improving cerebral perfusion.[38]

Other Problems

Acute acalculous cholecystitis (hydrops of the gallbladder, increased mural thickening, and "sludge") is a well-known complication in severely traumatized inviduals that requires cholecystectomy.[82]

Trauma patients with prolonged immobilization are at increased risk for deep venous thrombosis. Prophylaxis against this devastating complication should be routine (sequential compression devices, low-dose anticoagulation). Slow depletion of fibrinogen with ancrod may also be useful in preventing or treating thromboembolic complications.[34]

Hypercalcemia of immobilization may occur in patients with spinal cord injury or multiple fractures and may cause urinary lithiasis and renal failure.[107]

CONCLUSIONS

Management of trauma patients is often complex, because multiorgan systems may be simultaneously involved. The importance of a clear understanding of the pathophysiology of the different systems in trauma patients cannot be overemphasized to improve final outcome for these often tragically injured patients. The early and continuous involvement of the anesthesia care team is likely to have a positive impact on improved patient outcome.

KEY POINTS

- Early involvement of the anesthesia provider in the perioperative care of the trauma patient will benefit the patient. A full understanding of the mechanisms of injury, preexisting medical conditions, requirements for airway management, fluid and blood resuscitation, and medications will thus be gained. Also, likely pitfalls in management will be avoided.
- The anesthesia caregiver should carefully consider whatever background medical conditions the trauma patient has and factor these issues into the perioperative care plan.
- Evaluation of the airway in trauma patients includes asking patients to speak and trying to assess whether the larynx and/or trachea have been injured.
- The anesthesia care team must understand the necessity of evaluating the patient's cervical spine, how it is performed in the specific hospital, and the exact meaning of clinical and radiologic "clearing" of the cervical spine. The anesthesia care team also must understand how to obtain and maintain a patent airway in a patient whose cervical spine has not yet been "cleared."
- Direct laryngoscopy can be performed in the presence of cervical spine injury, provided proper "manual in-line axial stabilization" is maintained. It is not by any means mandatory to move immediately to fiberoptic intubation, blind nasal intubation, or surgical airway. However, it is mandatory to have a series of contingency plans ready to be executed in the given patient, should the initial airway management strategy fail or not be fully satisfactory.
- Caregivers who often deal with emergency trauma patients must be facile with the full range of airway management techniques, including "surgical options" and should be familiar with the concepts and techniques of both "classic" and "modified" rapid sequence induction and the implications of each in the setting of acute trauma management.
- Every trauma patient should be considered to have a full stomach, no matter what time that he or she had the last meal.
- Caregivers should be thoroughly familiar with the complications of massive transfusion, which include hypothermia, impaired O_2 release, coagulopathies, electrolyte and acid-base abnormalities, and citrate intoxication.
- Anesthesia providers should have a solid plan for preoperatively assessing the volume status of any traumatized patient. Simply glibly thinking that a "tilt test" can be performed on a patient in whom one is unsure of the volume status is a prescription for disaster. (Incidentally, this is often a poorly answered question on the board examinations.)
- Use of succinylcholine for burns and other nonthermal injuries and its contraindications should be thoroughly understood in situations of massive trauma, spinal cord injury, burns, open eyes, and so forth. Hyperkalemia after succinylcholine can occur on the first day in cases involving crush and degloving injuries, burns, trauma, and abdominal sepsis. The so-called "safe period" for succinylcholine may not be as safe as previously believed.
- Awareness is a definite possibility in severely hemodynamically unstable trauma patients during anesthesia and surgery. Although the clinician may well be concerned about awareness, the primary duty is to keep the patient alive. Use of "cardiostable agents" may facilitate a compromise. On the other hand, rational use of amnestic agents should not be neglected.
- Intravenous fluid administration should not be restricted in patients with head injury and elevated ICP if there is evidence of hypovolemia. The goal is to insure normovolemia and adequate MAP and CPP (i.e., CPP = MAP − ICP).
- Prevention of renal failure is both difficult and important. Simply administering diuretics will not suffice. Adequately assessing volume status, in addition to replacing and maintaining circulating blood volume, is key.
- Standard coagulation tests are temperature corrected to 37° C and may not reflect hypothermia-induced coagulopathy. Hypothermia impairs coagulation because of slowing of enzymatic rates and reduced platelet function. The treatment of hypothermia-induced coagulopathy is rewarming, not fresh frozen plasma or platelets.
- Preventing hypothermia is extremely important during trauma resuscitation and surgery. The anesthesia provider should be thoroughly aware of the complications induced when hypothermia supervenes, as well as advantages and disadvantages of the various modalities used to prevent and treat hypothermia.
- The effect of pain and the related stress response is almost always detrimental to the trauma patient. Methods of pain relief range from simple continuous or on-demand IV opioids, to more sophisticated techniques such as regional and neuraxial blocks. Use of adjuvant drugs may decrease opioid dose and improve analgesia. Instituting effective postoperative analgesia should emphasize pain control during movement as well as at rest.
- Hyperventilating head-injured patients may cause regional or global cerebral ischemia due to hypocapnia-induced cerebral vasoconstriction and has been shown to worsen outcome after head trauma. Measurements of ICP, in conjunction with S_jO_2 monitoring, may help guide therapy aimed at improving cerebral perfusion.
- The anesthesia provider should consider early placement of invasive monitors in severely injured trauma patients to measure and optimize cardiac and metabolic parameters.

Patients who attain supranormal values of cardiac index, oxygen delivery, and oxygen consumption may have enhanced survival and decreased organ failure because of the ability to meet the increased metabolic requirements of trauma and the ability to repay a previous "oxygen debt."

KEY REFERENCES

Abrams KJ, Grande CM, editors: *Perioperative trauma anesthetic and critical care management of neurologic injury,* Armonk, Futura Publishing, 1997.

Adams AP, Grande CM, Hewitt PB: *Emergency anaesthesia,* ed 2, London, Arnold Publishers, 1997.

American College of Surgeons Committee on Trauma: *Advanced trauma life support course for physicians,* Student and Instructor Manual, Chicago, 1993, American College of Surgeons.

Berman JM, Hall J, editors: *Pediatric trauma anesthesia and critical care,* Armonk, Futura Publishing, 1996.

Capan LM, Miller S, Turndorf H, editors: *Trauma: anesthesia and intensive care,* Philadelphia, 1990, JB Lippincott.

Hastings RH, Marks JD: Airway management for trauma patients with potential cervial spine injuries, *Anesth Analg* 73:471, 1991.

Falk JL, Rackow ER, Weil MH: Colloid and crystalloid fluid resuscitation. In Shoemaker WC, Ayres S, Grenvik A, et al, editors: *Textbook of critical care*, Philadelphia, 1989, WB Saunders.

Fragen RJ, Avram MJ: Comparative pharmacology of drugs used for the induction of anesthesia. In Stoelting RK, Barash PG, Gallagher TJ, editors: *Advances in anesthesia,* Chicago, 1986, Year Book Medical Publishers.

Giesecke AH, editor: *Anesthesia for the surgery of trauma,* Philadelphia, 1976, FA Davis Company.

Grande CM, editor: Resuscitation and trauma anesthesia, *Curr Opin Anaesthesiol* 7(2), London, Current Science, 1994.

Grande CM, Stene JK, Berhard WN, editors: Overview of trauma anesthesia and critical care, *Crit Care Clin* 6(1), 1990.

Grande CM, Barton CR, Stene JK: Appropriate techniques for airway management of emergency patients with suspected spinal cord injury, *Anesth Analg* 67:714, 1989.

Grande CM, editor: *Textbook of trauma anesthesia and critical care,* St. Louis, 1993, Mosby–Year Book.

Greene NM, editor: *Anesthesia for emergency surgery,* Philadelphia, 1963, FA Davis Co.

Hanowell LH, Grande CM, editors: Trauma anesthesia for thoracic injury, *Semin Anesth* 13(2), 1994.

Hanowell LH, Grande CM, editors: Critical care management of the ill and injured, *Semin Anesth* 13(4), 1994.

Katz RL, editor: Emergency and trauma I, *Semin Anesth* 8(3), 1989.

Katz RL, editor: Emergency and trauma II, *Semin Anesth* 8(4), 1989.

Kirby RR, Brown DL, editors: Anesthesia for trauma, *Intl Anesth Clin* 25(1), 1987.

Matjasko MJ, Shin B: Anesthesia and trauma, *Probl Anesth* 4(3), 1990.

Meyer AA, editor: Critical care management of the trauma patient, *Crit Care Clin* 2(4), 1986.

Rosenberg AM, Bernstein R, Grande CM, editors: Trauma anesthesia and critical care for orthopedic injuries, *Probl Anesth* 8(3), 1994.

Rosenberg AM, Bernstein R, Grande CM, editors: *Perioperative pain management and regional anesthesia for the trauma patient,* 1997, London, WB Saunders.

Schou J: *Prehospital emergency medicine,* Lorrach, 1992, Alix Publishers.

Stene JK, Grande CM, editors: *Trauma anesthesia,* Baltimore, 1991, Williams & Wilkins.

REFERENCES

1. Abrams KJ: Airway management and mechanical ventilation, *New Horiz* 3:479, 1995.
2. American College of Surgeons Committee on Trauma: *Advanced trauma life support program for physicians, Student and Instructor Manual,* Chicago, 1993, American College of Surgeons.
3. American Society of Anesthesiologists Task Force on Management of the Difficult Airway: Practice guidelines for management of the difficult airway, *Anesthesiology* 78:597, 1993.
4. American Society of Anesthesiologists Task Force on Pulmonary Artery Catheterization: Practice guidelines for pulmonary artery catheterization, *Anesthesiology* 78:380, 1993.
5. Antman EM, Grudzien C, Sacks DB: Evaluation of a rapid bedside assay for detection of serum cardiac troponin T, *JAMA* 273:1279, 1995.
6. Arrington P, McNamara JJ: Mechanism of microaggregate formation in stored blood, *Ann Surg* 179:146, 1974.
7. Artru A: Relationship between cerebral blood volume and CSF pressure during anesthesia with halothane or enflurance in dogs, *Anesthesiology* 58:533, 1983.
8. Artru A: Relationship between cerebral blood volume and CSF pressure during anesthesia with isoflurane or fentanyl in dogs, *Anesthesiology* 60:575, 1984.
9. Barrett J, Tahir AH, Litwin MS: Increased pulmonary arteriovenous shunting in humans following blood transfusion, *Arch Surg* 113:947, 1978.
10. Bartlett RL, Martin SD, Perina D, et al: The pharyngeotracheal lumen airway: an

assessment airway control in the setting of upper airway hemorrhage, *Ann Emerg Med* 16:145, 1987.

11. Bashour TT, Ryan C, Kabbani SS, et al: Hypocalcemic acute myocardial failure secondary to rapid transfusion of citrated blood, *Am Heart J* 108:1040, 1984.
12. Bennett SN, McNeil MM, Blank LA, et al: Postoperative infections traced to contamination of an intravenous anesthetic, propofol, *N Engl J Med* 333:147, 1995.
13. Benumof JL, Scheller MS: The importance of transtracheal jet ventilation in the management of the difficult airway, *Anesthesiology* 71:769, 1989.
14. Benumof JL: The ASA difficult airway algorithm: new thoughts/considerations, *ASA Refresher Course Lectures* 253:1, 1995.
15. Bevan DR: Complications of muscle relaxants, *Semin Anesth* 14:63, 1995.
16. Bickell WH, Wall MJ, Pepe PE, et al: Immediate versus delayed fluid resuscitation for hypotensive patients with penetrating torso injuries, *N Engl J Med* 331: 1105, 1994.
17. Birmingham PK, Cheney FW, Ward RJ: Esophageal intubation: a review of detection techniques, *Anesth Analg* 65:886, 1986.
18. Bishop MH, Shoemaker WC, Appel PL, et al: Relationship between supranormal circulatory values, time delays, and outcome in severely traumatized patients, *Crit Care Med* 21:56, 1993.
19. Body SC, Hartigan PM, Shernan SK, et al: Nitric oxide: delivery, measurement, and clinical application, *J Cardiothorac Vasc Anesth* 9:748, 1995.
20. Bogetz MS, Katz JA: Recall of surgery for major trauma, *Anesthesiology* 61:6, 1986.
21. Bowen JC, Fleming WH: Increased oxyhemoglobin affinity after transfusion of stored blood: evidence for circulatory compensation, *Ann Surg* 180:760, 1974.
22. Bracken MB, Shepard MJ, Collins WF, et al: A randomized controlled trial of methylprednisolone or naloxone in the treatment of acute spinal cord injury, *N Engl J Med* 322:1405, 1990.
23. Brimacombe J: The advantages of the LMA over the tracheal tube or facemask: a meta-analysis, *Can J Anaesth* 42:1017, 1995.
24. Brown B: Sevoflurane: introduction and overview, *Anesth Analg* 81:S1, 1995.
25. Buchholz DH, Young VM, Friedman NR, et al: Bacterial proliferation in platelets products stored at room temperature, *N Engl J Med* 285:429, 1971.
26. Buckmaster MJ, Kearney PA, Johnson SB, et al: Further experience with transesophageal echocardiography in the evaluation of thoracic aortic injury, *J Trauma* 37:989, 1994.
27. Calder I, Ordman AJ, Jackowski A, et al: The brain laryngeal mask airway. An alternative to emergency tracheal intubation, *Anaesthesia* 45:137, 1990.
28. Carr R, Reyford H, Belani K, et al: Evaluation of the Augustine Guide for difficult tracheal intubation, *Can J Anaesth* 42:1171, 1995.
29. Chestnut RM: Secondary brain insults after head injury: clinical perspectives, *New Horiz* 3:366,1995.
30. Clifton GL: Hypothermia and hyperbaric oxygen as treatment modalities for severe head injury, *New Horiz* 3:474, 1995.
31. Cohen ND, Munoz A, Reitz BA, et al: Transmission of retroviruses by transfusion of screened blood in patients undergoing cardiac surgery, *N Engl J Med* 320(18):1172, 1989.
32. Cohen S, Alagesan R, Alagesan R, et al: Acute and chronic posttraumatic pain, *Probl Anesth* 8(3):489, 1994.
33. Cohn AI, Zornow MH: Awake endotracheal intubation in patients with cervical spine disease: a comparison of the Bullard laryngoscope and the fiberoptic bronchoscope, *Anesth Analg* 81:1283, 1995.
34. Cole CW, Shea B, Bormanis J: Ancrod as prophylaxis or treatment for thromboembolism in patients with multiple trauma, *Can J Surg* 38:249, 1995.
35. Corssen G, Reeves JG, Stanley TH: *Intravenous anesthesia and analgesia,* Philadelphia, 1988, Lea & Febiger.
36. Crighton HC, Giesecke AH: One year's experience in the anesthetic management of trauma, *Anesth Analg* 45:835, 1966.
37. Crozier TA, Schlaeger M, Wuttke W, et al: TIVA with etomidate-fentanyl versus midazolam-fentanyl. The perioperative stress of coronary artery surgery overcomes the inhibition of cortisol synthesis caused by etomidate-fentanyl anaesthesia, *Anaesthetist* 43:605, 1994.
38. Cruz J, Miner ME, Allen SJ, et al: Continuous monitoring of cerebral oxygenation in acute brain injury: injection of mannitol during hyperventilation, *J Neurosurg* 73:725, 1990.
39. Danzl DF, Pozos RS: Accidental hypothermia, *N Engl J Med* 331:1756–1760, 1994.
40. Davis JM, Parks SN, Detlefs CL, et al: Clearing the cervical spine in obtunded patients: the use of dynamic fluoroscopy, *J Trauma* 39:435, 1995.
41. Debaene B, Beaussier M, Meistelman C, et al: Monitoring the onset of neuromuscular block at the orbicularis oculi can predict good intubating conditions during atracurium-induced neuromuscular block, *Anesth Analg* 80:360, 1995.
42. Dewitt DS, Jenkins LW, Prough DS: Enhanced vulnerability to secondary ischemic insults after experiemental traumatic brain injury, *New Horiz* 3:376, 1995.
43. Dehlinger JK, Narhwold ML, Gibbs PS, et al: Hypocalcemia during rapid blood transfusion in anaesthetized man, *Br J Anaesth* 48:995, 1976.
44. Dronen SC, Mergian KS, Hedges JR, et al: A comparison of blind nasotracheal and succinylcholine-assisted intubation in the poisoned patient, *Ann Emerg Med* 16:650, 1987.
45. Drop LJ, Laver MB: Low plasma ionized calcium and response to calcium therapy in critically ill man, *Anesthesiology* 43:300, 1975.
46. Donahue JG, Munoz A, Ness PM: The declining risk of post-transfusion hepatitis C virus infection, *N Engl J Med* 327:369, 1992.
47. Dubois EF: *Basal metabolism in health and disease,* Philadelphia 1924, Lee & Febiger.
48. Durtschi MB, Haisch CE, Reynolds L, et al: Effect of micropore filtration in pulmonary function after massive transfusion, *Am J Surg* 138:8, 1979.
49. Ebert TJ, Muzi M: Sympathetic hyperactivity during desflurane anesthesia in healthy volunteers, *Anesthesiology* 79;419, 1993.
50. Eichenger S, Schreiber W, Heinz T, et al: Airway management in a case of neck impalement: Use of the oesophageal tracheal combitube airway, *Br J Anaesth* 68:534, 1992.
51. Eisele JH: Cardiovascular effects of nitrous oxide. In Eger EI II, editor: *Nitrous oxide* *(N_2O)*, New York, 1985, Elsevier.
52. English MJM, Farmer C, Scott WAC: Heat loss in exposed volunteers, *J Trauma* 30:422–425, 1990.
53. Falk JL, Rackow ER, Weil MH: Colloid and crystalloid fluid resuscitation. In Shoemaker WC, Ayres S, Grenvik A, et al, editors: *Textbook of critical care,* Philadelphia, 1989, WB Saunders.
54. Feliciano DV, Rozycki GS: The management of penetrating abdominal trauma, *Adv Surg* 28:1, 1995.
55. Fleming A, Bishop M, Shoemaker W, et al: Prospective trial of supranormal values as goals of resuscitation in severe trauma, *Arch Surg* 127:1175, 1992.
56. Fragen RJ, Avram MJ: Comparative pharmacology of drugs used for the induction of anesthesia. In Stoelting RK, Barash PG, Gallagher TJ, editors: *Advances in anesthesia,* Chicago, 1986, Year Book Medical Publishers.
57. Frank SM, Myers TP, Olson KF: Hemostatic, metabolic, and cardiovascular implications of perioperative hypothermia. In Smith CE, Grande CM, editors: *Etiology, prevention and treatment of hypothermia in the trauma patient,* ITACCS Monograph, New York, 1995, McMahon Group.
58. Frizzell RT, Fichtel FM, Jordan MB, Weprin BE: Effects of etomidate and hypothermia on cerebral metabolism and blood flow in a canine model of hypoperfusion, *J Neurosurg Anesth* 5:104, 1993.
59. Frost EA: Etomidate in trauma anesthesia. In Smith CE, Grande CM, editors: *The use of etomidate in the trauma patient,* ITACCS Monograph, New York, 1997, McMahon Group, in press.
60. Fry DE, Pearlstein L, Fulton RL, Polk HC: Multiple system organ failure: the role of uncontrolled infection, *Arch Surg* 115:136, 1980.
61. Gallagher JD, Moore RA, Kerns D, et al: Effects of colloid or crystalloid administration on pulmonary extravascular water in the postoperative period after coronary artery bypass grafting, *Anesth Analg* 64: 753, 1985.
62. Garfield MD, Ershler WB, Malu DG: Malaria transmission by platelets concentrate transfusion, *JAMA* 240:2285, 1978.
63. Gattinoni L, Brazzi L, Pelosi P, et al: A trial of goal-oriented therapy in critically ill patients, *N Engl J Med* 333;1025, 1995.
64. Gauss A, Heinrich H, Wilder-Smith OHG: Echocardiographic assessment of the haemodynamic effects of propofol: a comparison with etomidate and thiopentone, *Anaesthesia* 46:99, 1991.

65. Gentilello LM, Cortes V, Moujaes S, et al: Continuous arteriovenous rewarming: experimental results and thermodynamic model simulation of treatment for hypothermia, *J Trauma* 30:1436, 1990.
66. Gentilello LM: Practical approaches to hypothermia, *Adv Trauma Crit Care* 9:39, 1994.
67. Gentilello LM, Moujaes S: Treatment of hypothermia in trauma victims: thermodynamic considerations, *J Intens Care Med* 10:5, 1995.
68. Gentilello LM, Anardi D, Mock C, et al: Permissive hypercapnia in trauma patients, *J Trauma* 39:846, 1995.
69. Gervin AS, Fischer RP: Resuscitation of trauma patient with type-specific uncrossmatched blood, *J Trauma* 24:327, 1984.
70. Glass PSA: Intravenous anesthesia: new drugs and techniques, *ASA Refresher Course Lectures* 163:1, 1994.
71. Grande CM, editor: Resuscitation and Trauma Anesthesia, *Curr Opin Anaesth* 7 (2), 1994.
72. Grande CM, Barton CR, Stene JK: Appropriate techniques for airway management of emergency patients with suspected spinal cord injury, *Anesth Analg* 67: 714, 1989.
73. Gronert GA, Theye RA: Pathophysiology of hyperkalemia induced by succinylcholine, *Anesthesiology* 43:89, 1975.
74. Hastings RH, Marks JD: Airway management for trauma patients with potential cervial spine injuries, *Anesth Analg* 73: 471, 1991.
75. Hastings RH, Kelley SD: Neurologic deterioration associated with airway management in a cervical spine-injured patient, *Anesthesiology* 78:580, 1993.
76. Hastings RH, Vigil AC, Hanna R, et al: Cervical spine movement during laryngoscopy with the Bullard, Macintosh, and Miller laryngoscopes, *Anesthesiology* 82: 859, 1995.
77. Hines MH, Meredith JW: Modified retrograde intubation technique for rapid airway access, *Am J Surg* 159:597, 1990.
78. Hirshberg A, Mattox KL: Planned reoperation for severe trauma, *Ann Surg* 222:3, 1995.
79. Hung OR, Stewart RD: Lightwand intubation: I—a new lightwand device, *Can J Anaesth* 42:820, 1995.
80. Hung OR, Pytka S, Morris I, et al: Lightwand intubation: II—Clinical trial of a new lightwand for tracheal intubation in patients with difficult airways, *Can J Anaesth* 42:826, 1995.
81. Idris AH: End-tidal carbon dioxide physiology and monitoring during resuscitation, *Anesth Clin North Am* 13(4):785, 1995.
82. Imhof M, Raunest J, Rauen U, Ohmann C: Acute acalculous cholecystitis is severely traumatized patients: a prospective sonographic study, *Surg Endosc* 6:68, 1992.
83. Insalaco SJ: Massive transfusion, *Lab Med* 15:325, 1984.
84. Jacobs LM, Panic S: Prehospital care: what works, what does not, *Adv Trauma Crit Care* 9:1, 1994.
85. Jurkovich GH, Greiser WR, Luterman A, et al: Hypothermia in trauma victims: An ominous predictor of survival, *J Trauma* 27:1019, 1987.
86. Kahn RC, Jasco HD, Carlon GC, et al: Massive blood replacement: correlation of ionized calcium, citrate, and hydrogen ion concentration, *Anesth Analg* 58:274, 1979.
87. Kingsley CP: Perioperative use of etomidate for trauma patients. In Smith CE, Grande CM, editors: *The use of etomidate in the trauma patient,* ITACCS Monograph, New York, 1997, McMahon Group.
88. Kovarik WD, Mayberg TS, Lam Am, et al: Succinylcholine does not change intracranial pressure, cerebral blood flow velocity, or the electroencephalogram in patients with neurologic injury, *Anesth Analg* 78: 469, 1994.
89. Kurz A, Sessler DI, Lenhardt R, et al: Perioperative normothermia to reduce the incidence of surgical-wound infection and shorten hospitalization, *N Engl J Med* 334: 1209, 1996.
90. Landers DF, Hill GE, Wong KC, Fox IJ: Blood transfusion-induced immunomodulation, *Anesth Analg* 82:187, 1996.
91. Lang EW, Chestnut RM: Intracranial pressure and cerebral perfusion pressure in severe head injury, *New Horiz* 3:400, 1995.
92. Larach MG: Accidental hypothermia, *Lancet* 345:493–498, 1995.
93. Lauer AR: Age and sex in relation to accidents, *Traf Safety Res Rev* 3(4):21, 1959.
94. Lerman J: Sevoflurane in pediatric anesthesia, *Anesth Analg* 81:S4, 1995.
95. Libonati MM, Leahy JJ, Ellison N: The use of succinylcholine in open eye surgery, *Anesthesiology* 62:637, 1985.
96. Ligier B, Buchman TG, Breslow MJ, Deutschman CS: The role of anesthetic induction agents and neuromuscular blockade in the endotracheal intubation of trauma victims, *Surg Gynecol Obstet* I73: 477, 1991.
97. Logan ASC: Use of the laryngeal mask in a patient with an unstable fracture of the cervical spine, *Anaesthesia* 46:987, 1991.
98. Mackersie RC, Shackford SR, Hoyt DB, et al: Continuous epidural fentanyl analgesia: ventilatory function improvement with routine use in treatment of blunt chest injury, *J Trauma* 27:1207, 1987.
99. Maki DG, Cobb L, Garman JK, et al: An attachable silver impregnated cuff for prevention of infection with central venous catheters: a prospective randomized multicenter trial, *Am J Med* 85:307, 1988.
100. Magorian T, Flannery KB, Miller RD: Comparison of rocuronium, succinylcholine, and vecuronium for rapid-sequence induction of anesthesia in adult patients, *Anesthesiology* 79:913, 1993.
101. Marion DW, Obrist WD, Carlier PM, Penrod LE, Darby JM: The use of moderate therapeutic hypothermia for patients with severe head injuries: a preliminary report, *J Neurosurg* 79:354–362, 1993.
102. McIntyre JWR: The difficult tracheal intubation, *Can J Anaesth* 34:204, 1987.
103. McGeachie V, Norko P, Alisoglu R, et al: The effect of rocuronium on intraocular pressure, 8th Annual Trauma Anesthesia and Critical Care Symposium, 1995.
104. McGuire GP, Pearl RG: Trauma and sepsis. In Grande CM, editor: *Textbook of trauma anesthesia and critical care,* St. Louis, 1993, Mosby–Year Book.
105. Meistelman C, Debaene B, Billard V, Giraud O: Monitoring of the orbicularis oculi can predict onset of paralysis at the vocal cords during mivacurium-induced neuromuscular block, *Anesthesiology* 83: A888, 1995.
106. Meyer A: Acute renal failure. In Wilmore DW, Brennan MF, Harken AH, et al, editors: American College of Surgeons case of the surgical patient, vol 1, New York, 1988, Scientific American.
107. Meythaler JM, Tuel SM, Cross LL: Successful treatment of immobilization hypercalcemia using calcitonin and etidronate, *Arch Phys Med Rehab* 74:316, 1993.
108. Mendlowitz M: The specific heat of human blood, *Science* 107:97, 1948.
109. Milde LN, Milde JH, Michenfelder JD: Cerebral functional, metabolic and hemodynamic effects of etomidate in dogs, *Anesthesiology* 63:371, 1985.
110. Miller RD: Complications of massive blood transfusions, *Anesthesiology* 39:82, 1973.
111. Millihan JS, Cain TL, Hansbrough J: Rapid volume replacement for hypovolemic shock: a comparison of techniques and equipment, *J Trauma* 26:428, 1984.
112. Moore EE: Resuscitation and evaluation of the injured patient. In Zidema GD, Rutherford RB Ballinger WF, editors: *The management of trauma,* ed 4, Philadelphia, 1985, WB Saunders.
113. Moreno RJ, Kloess P, Carlson DW: Effect of succinylcholine on the intraocular contents of open globes, *Ophthalmology* 98: 636, 1991.
114. Muizelaar JP, Marmarou A, Ward JD, et al: Adverse effects of prolonged hyperventilation in patients with severe head injury: a randomized clinical trial, *J Neurosurg* 77: 15, 1992.
115. Munoz E: Economic cost of trauma, United States, 1982, *J Trauma* 24:237, 1986.
116. Niemann JJ, Rosborough JP, Myers R, et al: The pharyngeotracheal lumen airway: preliminary investigation of a new adjunct, *Ann Emerg Med* 13:591, 1984.
117. Nolan J: Pharmacology of propofol in the trauma patient. In Grande CM, Smith CE, editors: *Propofol in trauma anesthesia: An evolving perspective,* ITACCS Monograph, New York, 1996, Intamed Educational Group.
118. Nolan JP: Resuscitation of the trauma patient, *Care Crit Ill* II(6):222, 1995.
119. Ochoa JB, Udekwu AO, Billior TR, et al: Nitrogen oxide levels in patients after trauma and during sepsis, *Ann Surg* 214: 621, 1991.
120. Office of Medical Applications of Research, National Institutes of Health: Perioperative red cell transfusion, *JAMA* 260(18):2700, 1988.
121. Oreskovich MR, Howard JD, Copass MK, et al: Geriatric trauma: injury patterns and outcome, *J Trauma* 24:565, 1984.
122. Ovassapian A, Mesnik PS: The art of fiberoptic intubation, *Anesth Clin North Am* 13(2):391, 1995.
123. Patel N, Smith CE, Pinchak AC: Clinical comparison of blood warmer performance during simulated clinical conditions, *Can J Anaesth* 42:636, 1995.

124. Patel N, Knapke D, Smith CE, et al: Simulated clinical evaluation of conventional and newer fluid warming devices, *Anesth Analg* 82:517, 1996.
125. Patel N, Smith CE, Pinchak AC: Emergency surgery and rapid sequence intubation: Rocuronium vs succinylcholine, *Anesthesiology* 83;A914, 1995.
126. Patel N, Smith CE, Grande CM: Pain management in trauma. In Grande CM, editor: *Perioperative trauma anesthesia,* World Federation of Societies of Anesthesiologists Monograph, 1997, in press.
127. Pavlin EG: Hypothermia and trauma: incidence and outcome. In Smith CE, Grande CM, editors: *Etiology, prevention and treatment of hypothermia in the trauma patient,* ITACCS Monograph, New York, 1995, McMahon Group.
128. Poli de Figuerido LF, Tao W, Watson WC, et al: Small volume resuscitation of hemorrhagic shock with diaspirin crosslinked hemoglobin, 8th Annual Trauma Anesthesia and Critical Care Symposium, 1995.
129. Rackow EC, Falk JL, Fein IA, et al: Fluid resuscitation in circulatory shock: a comparison of the cardiorespiratory effects of albumin, hetastarch, and saline solutions in patients with hypovolemic and septic shock, *Crit Care Med* 11:839, 1983.
130. Reasoner DK, Ryu KH, Hindman BJ, et al: Marked hemodilution increases neurologic injury after focal cerebral ischemia in rabbits, *Anesth Analg* 82:61, 1996.
131. Reed AP: Preparation of the patient for awake flexible fiberoptic bronchoscopy, *Chest* 101:244, 1992.
132. Reed RL, Johnston TD, Hudson JD, Fischer RP: The disparity between hypothermic coagulopathy and clotting studies, *J Trauma* 33:465–470, 1992.
133. Reed RL, Bracey AW, Hudson JD, et al: Hypothermia and blood coagulation: dissociation between enzyme activity and clotting factor levels, *Circ Shock* 32:141, 1990.
134. Rembert FC: State of health at time of injury. In Giesecke AH, editor: *Anesthesia for surgery and trauma,* Philadelphia, 1976, FA Davis.
135. Reul GJ Jr, Beall AC Jr, Greenberg SD: Profile screen blood filtration, *Chest* 66:4, 1974.
136. Reul GJ Jr, Greenberg Sd, Lefrak EA, et al: Prevention of post-traumatic pulmonary insufficiency, *Arch Surg* 106:386, 1973.
137. Reynolds HN, Habashi N, Borg U: New directions and applications for extracorporeal cardiopulmonary support, *Adv Trauma Crit Care* 9:99, 1994.
138. Rodman GH, Kirby RR: Post traumatic respiratory failure: role of fluid therapy. In Brown BR, editor: *Contemporary anesthetic practice: fluid and blood therapy,* Philadelphia, 1983, FA Davis.
139. Robertie PG, Gravlee GP: Safe limits of isovolemic hemodilution and recommendations for erythrocyte transfusion, *Intl Anesthesiol Clin* 28:197, 1990.
140. Rose D, Coutsoftides T: Intraoperative normovolemic hemodilution, *J Surg Res* 31: 375, 1981.
141. Salem MR, Wafai Y, Joseph NJ, et al: Efficacy of the self-inflating bulb in detecting esophageal intubation, *Anesthesiology* 80:42, 1994.
142. Scalea TM, Simon HM, Duncan AO, et al: Geriatric blunt multiple trauma: improved survival with early invasive monitoring, *J Trauma* 30;129, 1990.
143. Sellick BA: Cricoid pressure to control regurgitation of stomach contents during induction of anaesthesia, *Lancet* 2:404, 1961.
144. Sessler DI: Perianesthetic thermoregulation and heat balance in humans, *FASEB J* 7:638–644, 1993.
145. Shackford SR, Virgilo RW, Peters RM: Selective use of ventilator therapy in flail chest injury, *J Thorac Cardiovasc Surg* 81:194, 1981.
146. Shires T: Initial care of the injured patient, *J Trauma* 10:940, 1970.
147. Shoemaker WC: Comparison of the relative effectiveness of whole blood transfusions and various types of fluid therapy in resuscitation, *Crit Care Med* 4:71, 1976.
148. Shoemaker WC, Appel PL, Kram HB, et al: Prospective trial of supranormal values of survivon as therapeutic goals in high-risk surgical patients, *Chest* 94:1176, 1988.
149. Silverman HJ: Pharmacologic approach in patients with pulmonary failure. In Chernow B, editor: *The pharmacologic approach to the critically ill patient,* ed 3, Baltimore, 1994, Williams & Wilkins.
150. Simons RK, Hoyt DB: Immunomodulation, *Adv Trauma Crit Care* 9:135, 1994.
151. Smith CE, Patel N: Hypothermia in adult trauma patients: anesthetic considerations, *Am J Anesthesiol* 23:283, 1996.
152. Smith CE, Patel N: Risk factors for hypothermia in the trauma patient. In Smith CE, Grande CM, editors: *Etiology, prevention and treatment of hypothermia in the trauma patient,* ITACCS Monograph, New York, 1995, McMahon Group.
153. Smith CE, Peerless JR: Rational use of neuromuscular blocking agents for emergency airway management in the trauma patient. In Smith CE, Grande CM, editors: *Muscle relaxants in the trauma patient,* ITACCS Monograph, New York, 1995, McMahon Group.
154. Sohmer PR, Scott RL: Massive transfusion, *Clin Lab Med* 2(1):21, 1982.
155. Stene JK: Anesthesia for the critically ill trauma patient. In Siegel J, editor: *Trauma, emergency surgery and critical care,* New York, 1987, Churchill-Livingstone.
156. Sum-Ping ST, Mehta MP, Anderton JM: A comparative study of methods of detection of esophageal intubation, *Anesth Analg* 69:627, 1989.
157. Sulek CA, Gravenstein N, Blackshear RH, et al: Head rotation during internal jugular vein cannulation and the risk of carotid artery puncture, *Anesth Analg* 82:125, 1996.
158. Tegtmeier GE: Transfusion-transmitted cytomegalovirus infections: significance and control, *Vox Sang* 51(1):22, 1986.
159. Thierbach A, Lipp MD, Daublander M: Propofol in trauma: an overview. In Grande CM, Smith CE, editors: *Propofol in trauma anesthesia: an evolving perspective,* ITACCS Monograph, New York, 1996, Intamed, in press.
160. Tinkle JK, Richardson JD, Franz JL, et al: Management of flail chest without mechanical ventilation, *Ann Thorac Surg* 19:355, 1975.
161. Tonnesen AS: Crystalloids and colloids. In Miller RD, editor: *Anesthesia,* ed 4, New York, 1994, Churchill Livingstone.
162. Trunkey DD: Trauma, *Sci Am* 249:28, 1983.
163. Uhl L, Pacini DG, Kruskall MS: The effect of heat on in vitro parameters of red cell integrity, *Transfusion* 33:60S, 1993.
164. Uhl L, Pacini D, Kruskall MS: A comparative study of blood warmer performance, *Anesthesiology* 77:1022–1028, 1992.
165. Valeri CR, Collins FB: Physiologic effects of 2,3-DPG-depleted red cells with high allecity for oxygen, *J Appl Physiol* 31:823, 1971.
166. Valeri CR, MacGregor H, Cassidy G, et al: Effects of temperature on bleeding time and clotting time in normal male and female volunteers, *Crit Care Med* 23:698–704, 1995.
167. Wagner RL, White PF, Kan PB, et al: Inhibition of adrenal steroidogenesisby the anesthetic etomidate, *N Engl J Med* 310: 1415, 1984.
168. White PF: Propofol: pharmacokinetics and pharmacodynamics, *Semin Anesth* VII 1(1):4, 1988.
169. Wierda JM, Van Den Broek L, Proost JH, et al: Time course of action and endotracheal intubating conditions of Org 9487, a new short-acting steroidal muscle relaxant: a comparison with succinylcholine, *Anesth Analg* 77:579, 1993.
170. Wilson RJ, Ridley SA: The use of propofol and alfentanil by infusion in military anaesthesia, *Anaesthesia* 47:231, 1992.
171. Worthley LI: Thoracic epidural in the management of chest trauma. A study of 181 cases, *Intens Care Med* 11:312, 1985.
172. Wraight WJ, Chamney AR, Howells TH: The determination of an effective cricoid pressure, *Anaesthesia* 38:461, 1983.
173. Zornow MH, Prough DS: Fluid management in patients with traumatic brain injury, *New Horiz* 3:488, 1995.
174. Zuck TF, Sherwood WC, Bove JR: A review of recent events related to surrogate testing of blood to prevent non-A, non-B posttransfusion hepatitis, *Transfusion* 27:203, 1987.

CHAPTER 82

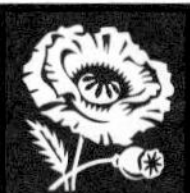

Anesthesia for Patients with Major Burns

KENT S. PEARSON
WILLIAM R. FURMAN

Burns are terrifying. They are also alarmingly common. Of the more than 1.25 million people who suffer burn injury annually, approximately 51,000 will require hospitalization and 5500 will die.[12] Burn injury is the second leading cause of accidental death in the United States, following only automobile accidents. Because of the high incidence of burn injury, it is very likely that most anesthesia providers will be involved at some point in the care of burn-injury patients.

Burn injury is a specific form of trauma in which the largest organ in the body, the skin, is damaged. **Major burns cause subtotal destruction of the skin and mucous membranes and are associated with severe metabolic, cardiovascular, and respiratory disorders. Burn patients require many life-saving, function-preserving, and appearance-saving surgical procedures. Many such operations cannot be delayed until the underlying systemic disorders are corrected.** Much of the metabolic, cardiovascular, and respiratory dysfunction associated with burn injury is perpetuated by the burn wound and thus cannot be fully corrected until the burn wound has been excised and grafted.

These factors make it necessary to anesthetize critically ill burn patients many times during course of treatment and also make it impossible to completely reverse their underlying ailments before surgery. One useful way to handle the discomfort inherent in this need to provide anesthesia to metabolically imbalanced patients is to view their transfer to the operating room as another aspect of their intensive care. In this respect, the anesthesia provider's responsibility is to continue (and modify as needed) metabolic, cardiovascular, and respiratory support during transport to the operating room, during surgery, and return transport to the burn unit. To effectively perform that role, it is necessary to understand the biology of burn injury, the direct and indirect metabolic, hemodynamic, and pulmonary consequences of burns and the logistic problems these consequences impose. These factors are considered in the preoperative visit.

BIOLOGY AND CONSEQUENCES OF BURN INJURY

Burns may be directly caused by heat or by the energy generated by chemicals, electricity, or ionizing radiation. This energy directly injures the skin and may also affect mucous membranes. Chemical mediators and vasoactive substances are released after burn injury, and many of the metabolic, cardiovascular, and pulmonary abnormalities that subsequently develop may be attributable to the effects of these mediators.

Characterization of Burns

Burns are classified according to their severity, by energy source, and by the presence of associated inhalational injury. The severity of a burn is related to its depth and extent. **The depth of skin destruction is characterized as first-, second- or third-degree, based on whether there is superficial, partial-thickness, or full-thickness destruction of the skin and its appendages.** The term *fourth-degree* is sometimes used to identify burns that injure structures beneath the skin, such as muscle and fascia. The extent of the burn is the percentage of the total body surface area (TBSA) that is affected, usually estimated by use of the Lund and Browder chart (Fig. 82-1).[65,79,88]

In terms of prognosis, it is helpful to make a single distinction between first- or second-degree burns and deep second- or third-degree burns because the latter do not heal spontaneously or do so with poor cosmetic and functional result. Superficial partial-thickness burns involve only the epidermis and outer dermis, resulting in only minor physiologic changes. The burned areas appear blistered, with pink or red epidermis below the blister (Table 82-1). The burned skin is very painful because of exposed still-functional nerve endings. Deep partial-thickness burns extend further into the dermis, but spare portions of the epidermal skin appendages (e.g., hair follicles, nerve endings, sweat glands, and sebaceous glands). These burns appear white but are soft and elastic to touch. Full-thickness burns spare no epithelial remnants in the wound and appear hard, dry, and white- or tan-colored. Pain is usually absent in areas of full-thickness burns because the nerve endings have been destroyed.

Deep second- and third-degree burns require surgical debridement and coverage, whereas more superficial burns generally do not. Mortality from thermal injury is related to the area involved by deep second- or third-degree burns. **Other factors associated with mortality are age, the presence of inhalational injury,[51,52,90] and the presence of a burn caused by high-voltage (> 1000 V) electrical shock.**[64] The decision to refer a patient to a regional burn center after resuscitation and initial stabilization is usually based on the determination that the burn is major. In adults, major burns are usually considered to be those involving 20% or more of the TBSA in deep partial-thickness or full-thickness burns (5% to 10% TBSA in infants and children) as well as those complicated by smoke inhalation or large facial, hand, or perineal burns. High-tension electrical burns are also considered major.

Direct Effects of Burn Injury

Injury to the skin

Mediator release. Thermal injury to skin and its microvasculature incites an inflammatory response consisting of activation of leukocytes and release of biologic response mediators (BRMs).[86] In general terms, this response consists of the cellular processes that localize injury, combat infection, and promote healing of the wound. Local blood flow increases and leukocytes migrate into the affected area. Complement is activated, and prostaglandins (PG), interleukins, platelet-aggregating factor, interferons, colony-stimulating factors, and other leukocyte-derived polypeptides (cytokines) are released into the wound and the bloodstream.[10,38,39,49]

Patients with burn wounds typically present with three concentric zones of injury. The central zone of coagulation contains necrotic tissue and thrombosed blood vessels and is nonviable. The outer zone of hyperemia is viable, but develops a significant increase in capillary permeability and tissue edema. The clinical course of the intermediate zone of stasis evolves over the first 48 hours after the burn injury; this zone may survive or suffer tissue death, depending on the type of burning medium and the duration of exposure.[11] The occlusion of blood vessels, increases in capillary permeability, and vasodilation that occur in these three zones are believed to be mediated by locally released biologic response modifiers (BRMs). These BRMs also have profound systemic effects, which contribute to alterations in metabolism, hemodynamics, and pulmonary function.

Local edema. Edema formation and resultant loss of plasma volume are primary reasons why burn victims require copious fluid resuscitation. An immediate increase in microvascular permeability to large molecular weight proteins occurs in the burn wound.[28,47] Although this is partly related to the thermal insult, histamine, prostaglandins (PGE_2 and prostacyclin), serotonin, and oxygen-free radicals are known to be released into the wound[86] and are probably also involved.

Direct injury to the respiratory system

Inhalational injury comprises carbon monoxide (CO) poisoning, upper airway swelling and obstruction, and damage to the lower respiratory tract (Box 82-1). Each of these can lead to respiratory failure and the requirement for early endotracheal intubation. **Inhalational injury is a serious complication of burn exposure because when present, on the average, it increases mortality rates by 40%.**[52,93]

Carbon monoxide poisoning. Carbon monoxide poisoning occurs at the scene of the injury and exerts its adverse effects in the first few hours. Carbon monoxide causes tissue hypoxia, despite a high Po_2, because it binds to hemoglobin 200 times more readily than oxygen, thus reducing the oxygen-carrying capacity of the blood. The reduction in oxygen-carrying capacity leads to a decrease in oxygen delivery, which is compounded by the fact that carbon monoxide also increases the stability of the oxyhemoglobin molecule and thus impedes release of oxygen to the tissues.[33,61]

Carbon monoxide poisoning should be suspected in victims of closed-space fires (buildings and automobiles). Clinical signs and symptoms of hypoxia may be present, such as headache, shortness of breath, nausea, angina

ADMISSION BURN EVALUATION SHEET

Date of Admission: ______________________ Weight: ______________________

AREA	PERCENT OF BURN					SEVERITY OF BURN		TOTAL PERCENT
	0-1 Year	1-4 Years	5-9 Years	10-15 Years	ADULT	2°	3°	
Head	19	17	13	10	7			
Neck	2	2	2	2	2			
Ant. Trunk	13	17	13	13	13			
Post. Trunk	13	13	13	13	13			
R. Buttock	2½	2½	2½	2½	2½			
L. Buttock	2½	2½	2½	2½	2½			
Genitalia	1	1	1	1	1			
R.U. Arm	4	4	4	4	4			
L.U. Arm	4	4	4	4	4			
R.L. Arm	3	3	3	3	3			
L.L. Arm	3	3	3	3	3			
R. Hand	2½	2½	2½	2½	2½			
L. Hand	2½	2½	2½	2½	2½			
R. Thigh	5½	6½	8½	8½	9½			
L. Thigh	5½	6½	8½	8½	9½			
R. Leg	5	5	5½	6	7			
L. Leg	5	5	5½	6	7			
R. Foot	3½	3½	3½	3½	3½			
L. Foot	3½	3½	3½	3½	3½			
				Total				

Code: Blue areas indicate 2°
Red areas indicate 3°

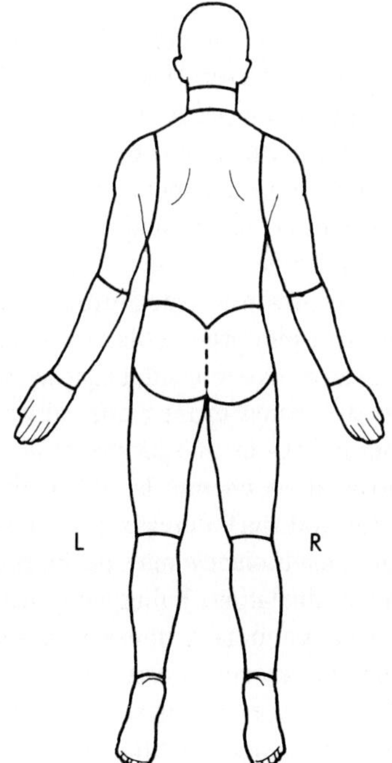

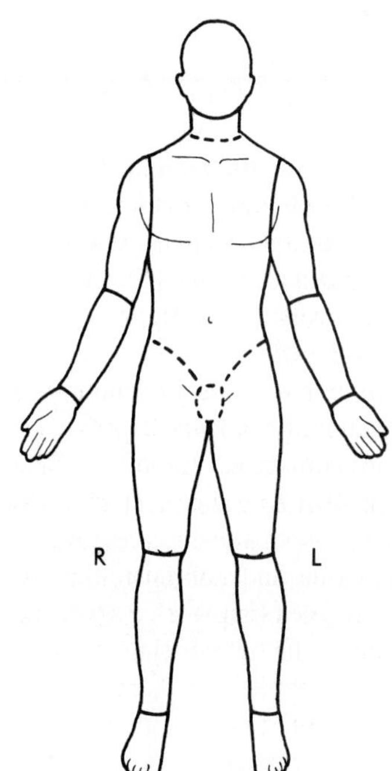

Fig. 82-1. Lund and Browder Chart for calculating the extent of burn injury, as adapted for use at the Baltimore Regional Burn Center. Only second- and third-degree burns are considered when making this determination.

Table 82-1 Classification of burn depth

Burn type	Characteristics
First degree	Only epidermis damaged Painful erythema Minimal local edema Spontaneous healing in 48–72 hours
Superficial second degree (superficial partial-thickness)	Outer layers of dermis destroyed Vesicles formed Erythema, blanching with pressure
Deep second degree deep partial-thickness)	Only deepest dermal appendages not damaged Skin pale, blistered, edematous
Third degree (full-thickness)	All of epidermis and dermis destroyed Burned area is anesthetic, dry, anc charred or white

BOX 82-1
TYPES OF DIRECT RESPIRATORY INJURY IN BURN PATIENTS

Carbon monoxide poisoning
Upper-airway obstruction
Subglottic thermal and chemical injury

pectoris, tachypnea, and mental status changes; however, the patient will not have cyanosis. Standard (two-wavelength) pulse oximetry does not distinguish between the oxyhemoglobin and the carboxyhemoglobin molecules. Newer three-wavelength devices capable of such distinction are being developed.[5]

The diagnosis of carbon monoxide poisoning is made by measuring the carboxyhemoglobin level, expressed as a percent saturation of hemoglobin in arterial blood. Saturations in excess of 15% are usually toxic, and those exceeding 50% are almost always lethal. The treatment is removal from the source of carbon monoxide and administration of 100% oxygen. Use of 100% oxygen displaces carbon monoxide from the hemoglobin molecule by reducing the half-life for dissociation of carbon monoxide from hemoglobin from 5 hours (breathing room air) to 45 to 60 minutes. Hyperbaric oxygen therapy has been recommended as a treatment for carbon monoxide poisoning because it can further reduce this half-life to 23 minutes. Hyperbaric oxygen therapy is not available in all burn centers and is controversial because outcome studies have not consistently shown it to be beneficial.[43,80,89] Even with appropriate treatment and despite apparent initial recovery from the acute effects of carbon monoxide poisoning, delayed neurologic symptoms may develop after several weeks. This is more common in elderly patients and in those with especially high initial carbon monoxide levels.[18]

Upper airway injury. Inhaled flames, toxic chemicals, and hot air can injure the upper airway and lower respiratory tract.[75] Inhalational injury is common in victims of structural fires (buildings and vehicles). Life-threatening swelling of the tissues of the upper airway, defined as those structures above the true vocal cords, occurs in 20% to 30% of patients with inhalational injury.[21,45] In these patients, the direct injury is initially manifested as erythema, blistering, and necrosis of the epithelium. After a latent period of 4 to 48 hours, however, significant edema of the epiglottis and laryngeal structures develops.[8,84]

The diagnosis of evolving airway obstruction is best made by examination of the upper airway. The clinical signs of facial burns, sooty oral or nasal secretions, hoarseness, and a swollen, erythematous tongue are suggestive but not diagnostic.[46,89] When clinical suspicion is high, a fiberoptic nasopharyngoscopy or direct laryngoscopy is required.[56,77] If upper-airway damage is confirmed, the safest course is to secure the airway for at least 72 hours with an endotracheal tube.[61] Although it is easier to diagnose this problem than to exclude it, pulmonary flow-volume loops that are consistently normal or mildly abnormal and do not worsen when repeated at frequent intervals (every 2 to 3 hours) correlate well with the absence of physiologically significant obstruction.[44]

If only minimal damage is observed, reexamination at frequent intervals is an alternative to immediate intubation of the airway; however, this approach incurs an increased risk of failure or complications. The implication of the delay inherent in reexamination is that the intubation may be performed under more difficult conditions after the swelling has become more severe and the anatomic structures less easily recognizable.

Lower respiratory tract injury. Direct thermal injury to the lower respiratory tract is rare, except when live steam or burning gases are inhaled, because the thermal energy of hot air is dissipated in the upper airway.[21,75] However, the tracheobronchial tree and lungs are not protected from exposure to noxious chemicals and particulates contained in smoke. Respiratory failure related to chemically mediated pulmonary insufficiency may develop as early as 3 hours after smoke inhalation. Pulmonary edema, associated with an increase in pulmonary transvascular fluid flux, and bronchopneumonic infections may follow.

Smoke exposure unassociated with burns can cause noncardiogenic pulmonary edema, usually within the first 2 to 5 days after the burn injury. Initially, mucociliary clearance and pulmonary surfactant activity are impaired, and histamine, kinins, and other BRMs are released within the lungs. Abnormalities of gas exchange develop because of bronchospasm, local atelectasis, and pulmonary edema. After several hours, depending on the chemicals contained in the smoke, pseudomembranous tracheobronchitis may develop and hyaline membrane formation, fibrin deposition, intra-alveolar hemorrhage, and pulmonary edema follow. Surface burns, especially if greater than 25% TBSA, can be synergistic with smoke in producing pulmonary injury.[95]

Special aspects of electrical injury

The passage of electrical current through the body generates heat in proportion to the square of the current flow (amperage). High-voltage exposures are particularly dangerous because although the amperage is proportional to the voltage, the heat produced is proportional to the voltage squared. The majority of heat production occurs in tissues with the highest electrical resistance. Almost all internal tissues (except bone) offer very low resistance, but skin resistance is relatively high.[40,85] As a result, considerable heat is produced in the body at points of entrance and exit of electric current, causing extensive damage to the skin and underlying blood vessels, muscles, and nerves.[14,40,85] Ignition of clothing and subsequent flame burns also often occur during electrical injury.

Significant deep tissue destruction, disproportionate to the amount of surface burn, is common after high-tension injury. For this reason, extremely aggressive fluid resuscitation is recommended (7 ml/kg/percent of TBSA burned) during the first day of therapy.[85,86] Compartment syndromes frequently develop in these patients, and they require fasciotomies or amputations because of the tissue destruction that occurs in the limbs.[55,64]

Two important visceral sequelae of electrical injury are myocardial damage and renal failure. Myocardial damage appears more likely to occur in larger burns caused by high-tension exposure when the electricity actually passes through the heart. A major risk factor is a vertical pathway of current flow (e.g., entrance and exit wounds on opposite sides of the pubic symphysis).[16] Skeletal muscle damage is associated with hypermyoglobinemia, myoglobinuria, and renal failure. Although it is not proved that heme pigments are causative of renal dysfunction, measures to alkalinize and increase the volume of the urine continue to be recommended as the treatment of choice for pigmenturia after electrical injury.

Systemic Effects of Burn Injury

Metabolic effects

Hypermetabolism, usually beginning toward the end of the first week after burn injury, is a prominent feature of burn injury with the degree of increase in metabolic rate directly related to burn size. Oxygen consumption is elevated to as much as 2.5 times predicted baseline levels, and heat production, body temperature, and protein catabolism also increase.[4] Increased levels of catecholamines, cortisol, glucagon, and growth hormone are all seen after burn injury. Collectively, they stimulate gluconeogenesis, and despite elevated insulin levels, glucose transport into tissues is impaired, often leading to hyperglycemia.[9,103]

Hypermetabolism and hyperthermia are common after burn injury. Circulating catecholamines appear to play a role in mediating the inherent temperature elevation seen in burn patients and their preference for a warmer environment.[104] Skin disruption in burned areas constitutes a breakdown of normal barriers to evaporative heat and fluid loss. Excessive heat loss can lead to shivering, which further increases oxygen consumption. **As a consequence of hypermetabolism, there is a dramatic increase in caloric requirements; more than 4000 kcal may be required daily to prevent protein catabolism.** At the time of the preoperative visit, the anesthesia provider should consider continuing the patient's enteric feedings as long as possible to minimize the length of the starvation interval.

Edema forms in both burned and nonburned tissue after burn injury[26] and is probably multifactorial in origin. Hypoproteinemia typically develops during the first week, when large volumes of intravenous (IV) fluid are being administered. In addition, the BRMs that promote local edema at the burn site are also released into the bloodstream. There is speculation that they may also act systemically to increase vascular permeability and fluid flux in nonburned areas.[86] Plasma protein levels are typically depressed after burn injury and remain depressed for a prolonged period.

Cardiovascular effects

Death from burn shock is now quite rare as a result of the widespread appreciation among health care providers that burn victims require between 2 and 4 ml/kg of fluid in the first 24 hours for each 1% of TBSA burned. Several effective formulas for preventing burn shock have been developed; all involve administration of large quantities of crystalloid fluids.

Edema formation after burn injury proceeds for approximately 24 to 36 hours, with most edema developing during the first 6 hours.[26] Large quantities of exogenously administered fluids and solutes are required during the first 2 days to maintain the plasma volume and cardiac preload. Spontaneous resorption of fluid begins thereafter, and fluid requirements decrease.

Cardiac output declines in the first 24 hours, often before the decrease in filling pressures. Circulating myocardial depressant factors have been implicated as the reason for this decrease in myocardial contractility, which may be mediated by oxygen-derived free radicals. These factors have yet to be identified, however.[32,83] Animal studies have suggested that decreased affinity of beta-adrenergic receptors for catecholamines may also lead to myocardial dysfunction.[99] Cardiac output usually increases toward normal after the first 24 hours, and later exceeds normal during the hypermetabolic phase if coronary artery disease (CAD) does not limit myocardial oxygen supply.

Pulmonary effects

Pulmonary complications of burns may be temporally divided into early, delayed, and late events. Early complications occur in the first 24 to 48 hours and include carbon monoxide exposure, upper-airway swelling, and noncardiogenic pulmonary edema. The adult respiratory distress syndrome (ARDS) usually develops at an intermediate time, within 2 to 5 days, and is a principal cause of death in hospitalized burn patients.[1,19] Important late complications are pneumonia, with and without atelectasis, and pulmonary emboli.

Adult respiratory distress syndrome can develop after surface burns unassociated with inhalational injury. A primary defect in pulmonary vascular permeability may be causative; however, the exact mechanism remains unknown.[6,48] The complement cascade, cytokines, oxygen-derived free radicals, and eicosanoids (products of leukocytes) have all been implicated and may interact in a multifactorial manner. In addition, endotoxemia may also be involved in activating leukocytes and causing them to aggregate in the lung.[95]

Burn patients who survive into the second week are especially susceptible to pneumonia and atelectasis, even in the absence of inhalational injury. These patients' immune systems are suppressed in direct proportion to the magnitude of the burn injury.[78] Patients are often immobilized during treatment and commonly have bacteremia. Development of pulmonary emboli is another potential pulmonary complication that occurs after burn injury in up to 30% of patients.[20] Risk factors for this complication may include immobilization and hypercoagulability. The latter is evidenced by thrombocytosis and elevated levels of factors V and VII.[95]

PREOPERATIVE CONCERNS FOR BURN PATIENTS

Surgery may be needed for burn patients at any time during their hospital stay. The most frequently performed surgical procedures involve wound debridement and coverage. In some centers, excision and grafting are begun as early as the first 24 hours after injury. Other procedures required in the course of recovery from burn injury include escharotomies, fasciotomies, tracheostomies, fracture repairs, and exploratory procedures related to blunt trauma associated with the burn.

During the acute phase, patients generally are metabolically compromised with hemodynamic and pulmonary dysfunction, yet the surgical procedure is necessary and may not be delayed in expectation of recovery. In cases of wound debridement and grafting, the surgery is viewed as the treatment. The anesthesia provider in such cases should understand the degree of physiologic compromise that exists and can be expected to complicate anesthetic care and be prepared to meet the challenges imposed by it. Burn patients' unique care includes altered responses to muscle relaxants, potentially massive transfusion requirements, difficulties encountered in patient positioning, airway management, ventilatory management, difficulties encountered in monitoring and intravascular access, and the details of safe transport to and from the operating room (Box 82-2).

BOX 82-2
MAJOR PREOPERATIVE CONSIDERATIONS IN BURN WOUND DEBRIDEMENT AND GRAFTING PROCEDURES

Altered muscle relaxant pharmacology
Potential for massive blood loss
Anticipated position of the patient during surgery
Airway management
Ventilatory management
Monitoring
Intravascular access
Safe transport to and from the operating room

Monitoring and Intravascular Access

During the preoperative visit, the specific plans as to how blood pressure, electrocardiogram (ECG), and oxygen saturation are to be monitored should be planned, especially if there are burns of the extremities and chest. Blood pressure cuffs can be applied on any nonburned arm or leg, but, when all four limbs are involved, use of a percutaneous arterial cathether is usually required. Arterial lines are often inserted for monitoring the initial fluid resuscitation and maintained for use during surgical procedures. A nonburned site of insertion is preferred; radial and femoral arteries are most commonly used. Use of an axillary artery is an alternative choice.

Standard ECG electrode placements are difficult when the chest and arms have been burned. The electrodes will not adhere to moist surfaces. To minimize the risks of contamination, an effort is usually made to avoid applying electrodes to burned or debrided dermis. Resulting nonstandard lead arrangements may make diagnosis of dysrhythmias more difficult. **In near-total burns, it is impossible to monitor the ECG, yet avoid placing electrodes in burned areas. Sterile skin staples may be applied over the chest or arms, with sterile "alligator" clips used to achieve electrical contact.** If the arms are not part of the operative field, a gauze wrap may be used to hold electrodes in place on the arms. Topical antibacterial ointments are reasonable electrical conductors.

Pulse oximeters have become an important part of intraoperative monitoring during anesthesia, and burn patients who frequently suffer respiratory disease are not exceptions. Unfortunately, burns of the extremities and face make it impossible to obtain a signal from an oximeter probe and preclude the use of this valuable technology in situations when it could be most useful. More frequent measurements of arterial blood gases are sometimes necessary because of this.

Other standard monitoring modalities are generally unaffected by burn injury, and difficulties with their application are not usually anticipated. Capnometry, auscultation of heart tones and breath sounds, and urine output and body temperature measurements can and should be used for other surgical procedures.

Ventilator management if the patient's airway is already intubated

Planning for intraoperative management of the patient who is already being treated for respiratory failure begins with a survey of the current ventilator settings (e.g., rate, tidal volume, inspired oxygen percentage, and level of positive end-expiratory pressure, if any). Oxygen consumption and carbon dioxide production are increased after thermal injury in proportion to the burn size, and inhalational injury impairs oxygenation and increases the dead space/tidal volume ratio.[87] For these reasons, burn patients usually require an elevated minute volume. An adult patient with a large burn may need more than 20 l/min. In larger patients, minute volumes greater than 30 l/min, which exceeds the capability of some standard anesthesia machine ventilators, may be required.

At the time of the preoperative visit, an estimate is usually made regarding the patient's postoperative ventilatory support needs. The decision to wean from mechanical support and extubate a burn patient is based on the same principles as in any intensive care setting. Weaning is not attempted in the presence of cardiovascular instability, hypothermia, significant metabolic derangement, sepsis, or signs of worsening pulmonary function. Extubation is delayed until the patient is alert enough to protect the upper airway from obstruction or aspiration of secretions.

Extensive debridement and grafting procedures in a patient with a major burn may represent such physiologic trespass as to warrant postoperative ventilatory support. This ensures adequacy of oxygenation and ventilation during a period of potential risk for hypoxia or hypoventilation. Another situation when a patient with airway mechanics suitable for extubation might require continued postoperative intubation is when grafts have been applied to the patient's back and the postoperative plan calls for the patient to remain prone after surgery. Reintubation in the event of decompensation would require turning the patient supine and would compromise the grafts.

Safe Transport to and from the Operating Room

Transportation to and from the operating room can be extremely hazardous for patients who have hemodynamic instability and/or respiratory failure. Measures should be taken to ensure the safety of these critically ill patients in hallways, corridors, and other areas where help may be unavailable. Often, transfer necessitates use of an elevator, which completely isolates the transport team. The transport team therefore should be able to provide emergency medical care in isolation and be prepared to perform reintubation and advanced cardiac life support.

At least two anesthesia transport personnel are usually required to manage the airway, observe the monitors, and administer medications. In preparation for transport, consideration should be given to how pulse, blood pressure, and oxygen-saturation monitoring will be established and how ventilatory support is to be continued during this difficult interval (Box 82-3). If the patient is combative, the use of sedatives and muscle relaxants should also be contemplated.

BOX 82-3
CONSIDERATIONS WITH RESPECT TO TRANSPORT OF CRITICALLY ILL BURN PATIENTS TO THE OPERATING ROOM

Monitoring

Vital signs
Oxygen saturation

Oxygen delivery to lungs

High-flow system
Ability to provide high inspiratory pressures
Ability to provide positive end-expiratory pressure
Sufficient volume of oxygen to withstand high flows and unexpected delays
Successfull trial of oxygen delivery system before departure from burn unit

Monitoring and ventilatory support

Consideration should be given to using continuous displays of ECG, arterial pressure, and arterial oxygen saturation (SaO_2) via portable battery-powered instruments during transport. Special attention should be given to the means by which oxygenation and ventilation will be accomplished during transport because of the severe nature of pulmonary dysfunction that occurs in patients with surface burns complicated by inhalational injury. It is often necessary to use a system capable of delivering high flows of 100% oxygen, positive end-expiratory pressure (PEEP), and very high inspiratory pressures for an extended period.

An anesthesia gas delivery apparatus, such as a Mapleson "D" system, is a good choice because it avoids many of the problems encountered in the standard manual resuscitators. Most standard bag-valve systems cannot provide 100% oxygen unless high-flow rates are used and a reservoir component is added to the system, and most cannot provide PEEP. One oxygen tank may be inadequate for transfer of a burn patient to the operating room because it is not uncommon for a burn patient to require as much as 30 l/min of fresh gas flow to support ventilation. To provide such a high flow, two tanks may be yoked together because the standard regulators are limited at 15 to 20 l/min. In addition, a standard E cylinder of oxygen contains only 620 l when filled (20 minutes at 30 l/min).

For patients with severe pulmonary disease, it is advisable to perform a 5-minute trial of oxygenation and ventilation in the intensive care unit with the breathing system that will be used during transport. If there is any doubt about the adequacy of the portable breathing system at that point, arterial blood gases can be obtained for confirmation. Occasionally, the degree of pulmonary dysfunction is so great that respiratory function simply cannot be supported during transfer to the operating room and surgery remains impossible until clinical improvement occurs.

Patients can also be sufficiently combative that effective ventilation and oxygenation are impeded, and safe transfer to the operating room can only be accomplished if sedatives and muscle relaxants are administered. Use of benzodiazepines is safe in these patients if amnesia is desired. If muscle paralysis is indicated, only nondepolarizing muscle relaxants should be used.

RECONSTRUCTIVE PROCEDURES

For months to years after the burn wounds have been successfully grafted, there follows a reconstructive phase during which repeated surgical procedures are performed to remove or reduce scar tissue and so improve both functional and cosmetic outcomes. In general, these patients can be treated as most other plastic surgery patients, although the safety of using succinylcholine during the first 1 to 2 years after the burn injury remains controversial.[71]

For this patient group, the most important ongoing anesthetic problems relate to the physical effects of scar contractures and the psychologic effects of repeated hospitalizations (especially in burn-injured children). Intubation of the trachea continues to be difficult in patients with scar contractures of the face and neck until these scars have been released.

ACUTE MANAGEMENT OF THE BURNED PATIENT

Metabolic Support

Burns cause major shifts in metabolic demands. Immediately after injury, the body enters an "ebb" phase characterized by decreased oxygen delivery and nutrient flow to cells.[23] Within 24 to 48 hours, the patient then enters a dramatic hypermetabolic state, which can cause a doubling of metabolic rate if a patient has sustained large TBSA burns.[102] The exact cause of this hypermetabolic state remains unclear, but it is certainly related to heat loss from burn tissue and increased intrinsic sympathetic nervous system activity.[105] Wilmore et al.[104] demonstrated that the metabolic rate of burned patients could be decreased by raising ambient temperature. Even if a patient remains in a temperature-neutral environment, some hypermetabolism persists. This has been shown in animals and humans to be due to increased endogenous catecholamine activity.[103,106] This hypermetabolism results in extreme catabolic activity, with elevated free fatty acids, glycogen depletion, insulin resistance, and gluconeogenesis.[24] Anesthetic planning should be tailored to this hypermetabolic state. It is our goal to minimize the period of preoperative fasting before any surgical procedure. This specifically means some changes in the usual "rules" on this subject (see following paragraphs).

Evaluation

All burn-injured patients need complete medical evaluations at the time of initial resuscitation. It is easy to focus attention on the burn and overlook other important injuries. A burned patient requires the same detailed initial assessment as any other trauma patient. Initial evaluation should include assessment of airway patency and adequacy of circulation, including evaluation of resuscitation and adequacy of respiration. This should then be followed by a detailed assessment of the entire patient to determine the extent, if any, of associated injuries.[59] After this assessment, a plan can be developed and priorities established for optimal patient care and resuscitation.

Airway management

Early patient evaluation must rule out acute hypoventilation or partial airway obstruction. As mentioned earlier, risk of mortality is significantly increased if inhalation injury is present in association with a burn injury.[108] Airway edema can increase dramatically after injury; therefore careful upper-airway evaluation and possibly early intubation may be required before referral of a severely burned patient to an appropriate burn treatment center.

Fluid resuscitation

Early, aggressive fluid resuscitation is required after major burns, with IV fluid resuscitation necessary for patients with burns affecting more than 15% to 20% of TBSA.[98] Rapid advances in recognition of the importance of fluid resuscitation during the 1960s and early 1970s led to significant decreases in burn-associated mortality and morbidity.[7] Controversy remains as to appropriate resuscitation fluid(s) with publication of multiple formulas to estimate fluid requirements of the burned patient. Table 82-2 lists currently used fluid resuscitation protocols. Initial crystalloid resuscitation with a balanced salt solution will provide adequate replacement of lost fluid and sodium.[7] Currently, the Baxter formula for crystalloid resuscitation is widely employed.[29] With this formula, lactated Ringer's solution is given at a rate of 4 ml/kg per total body surface area (TBSA) burned during the initial 24 hours after the injury. Half of this volume is given in the initial 8 hours postinjury, with the remaining volume given over the next 16 hours. Fluid infusion is adjusted to maintain urine output of 0.5 to 1.0 ml/kg/hr.

Demling et al.[26] and Pruitt[83] have suggested that resuscitation can be improved by altering the composition of this resuscitation fluid (i.e., adding colloid). Large volumes of crystalloid may lead to significant tissue edema in both burned and normal tissue.[54] Proponents of this colloid resuscitation believe that the addition of a protein solution to the

Table 82-2 Three fluid resuscitation formulas for burn patients

Formula	First 24 hours	Second 24 hours
Brooke		
Crystalloid	2 ml lactate Ringer's/percent/burn/kg Half in first 8 hr Half in next 16 hr	D_5W maintenance
Colloid	None	0.5 ml/% burn/kg
Parkland		
Crystalloid	4 ml lactate Ringer's/percent/burn/kg Half in first 8 hr Half in next 16 hr	D_5W maintenance
Colloid	None	0.5 ml/% burn/kg
MGH		
Crystalloid	1.5 ml lactate Ringer's/percent/burn/kg Half in first 8 hr Half in next 16 hr	Not specified
Colloid	0.5 ml/percent/burn/kg None in first 4 hr Half in second 4 hr Half in next 16 hr	Not specified

resuscitation fluid after the first day of resuscitation will decrease fluid requirements considerably.[26,83] Administration of colloid is begun after reduction of cellular leak present in the first day after the injury. The use of a colloid decreases the amount of tissue edema, but as Tranbaugh et al.[97] demonstrated, there was no difference in the incidence of pulmonary edema whether either crystalloid or colloid solutions were used for resuscitation. Hypertonic saline solutions have also been used for fluid resuscitation. Monafo et al.[72] demonstrated that adequate fluid resuscitation could be carried out with hypertonic sodium (250 mEq/l of sodium). They found reductions of estimated fluid requirements for burn resuscitation of 20% to 25% per patient compared with standard crystalloid resuscitation.[72] Use of hypertonic saline is problematic because of potentially serious electrolyte disturbances. Considerable caution and careful monitoring must be employed during resuscitation with hypertonic saline solution.

Regardless of the fluid chosen for resuscitation, careful patient monitoring is required. Although it is necessary to individualize the types of monitors required during resuscitation, it is necessary to continually assess response to therapy. The easiest monitor to follow is the patient's sensorium. In the absence of carbon monoxide poisoning or head injury, the patient should remain lucid and responsive throughout resuscitation. The patient's sensorium can become acutely clouded with early hypovolemia. Routine monitoring of blood pressure and pulse can also be useful, although elevated levels of endogenous catecholamines can raise the blood pressure during the acute postinjury period.[83] **The most accurate index of the adequacy of resuscitation is urine output. Experimental and clinical evidence have demonstrated that tissue perfusion is adequate if urine output is maintained at 0.5 to 1.0 ml/kg/hr.**[3,31] Critically ill burn patients with associated cardiac or pulmonary disease may benefit from invasive monitoring of cardiac filling pressures during resuscitation.[2] Pulmonary artery (PA) monitoring is rarely required, and avoidance of this catheter will prevent potential complications.[30] If such catheters are necessary, they should be placed using strict aseptic technique to avoid potential infectious complications.[35]

OPERATIVE MANAGEMENT OF THE BURNED PATIENT

The goal of current burn therapy is to rapidly restore skin integrity after the burn injury. This is done through early excision of burn eschar and grafting of the burn wounds. This approach has been shown to decrease mortality, improve functional and cosmetic outcome, and shorten hospitalization time, as compared with earlier nonoperative treatment of burn wounds.[13,27,30,37] Although affording better results, early operative treatment of burn wounds can present major problems for the anesthesia provider. Excisions of burn eschar usually start within 3 days of injury. This means that the burned patient has just been resuscitated from the original burn shock, and then is exposed to dramatic physiologic changes during repeated burn debridements. A knowledge of applied physiology makes the anesthetic management of these patients possible.

Burn debridements are extraordinarily bloody operations. The blood loss can be deceptively large. The goal of current methods of wound management is to remove layers of burn eschar until briskly bleeding dermis is reached.[50] **It is possible for the surgical team to remove the eschar so rapidly that it is difficult to keep up with the massive blood loss, resulting in a suddenly hypovolemic patient.** To avoid such a catastrophe, two approaches are very useful: (1) good communication between surgeons and anesthesia providers is mandatory because burn excision should be a team effort; (2) it is wise to limit the area of burn excised at each burn debridement. Heimbach and Engrav[50] recommend limiting excision to 20% TBSA burned or limiting excision to 2 hours and, if possible, limiting excision to a four-unit blood loss. This strategy limits the amount of stress, hypothermia, and shock that the patient endures during each operation.

Attention to blood component therapy is always required during burn wound excision and grafting. Chang and associates[17] demonstrated significant decreases in burn patients' platelets, fibrinogen, and factors V, VIII, and IX immediately following surgery. Thus, close monitoring of the coagulation system will be necessary during debridement of large burns.

Careful planning is necessary to manage hemorrhage. Two large peripheral IV catheters are often necessary for transfusion. These may be introduced through burned tissue, but any catheter placed through burned tissue should be removed as soon as possible after surgery. Use of central venous or pulmonary artery monitoring catheters depends on underlying patient disease. Pulmonary artery catheter introducers can be useful for both infusion and central venous pressure (CVP) monitoring in patients with large burns. It is mandatory to have blood ready for transfusion before burn excision is begun. As Moran et al.[74] point out, almost 200 ml of blood is lost for each 1% of TBSA excised and grafted. This implies that three to four units of blood might be lost by a 70-kg man (blood volume approximately 5250 ml) undergoing a debridement of an 8% TBSA burn. It is impossible to catch up with such great blood loss without preparation before blood loss begins. This blood loss is often hidden in the drapes, sponges, and on the floor, making exact quantitation of blood loss very difficult.

It is also possible to be lulled into a false sense of security immediately after eschar incision. Often, gauzes soaked in a vasoconstrictor (e.g., epinephrine or phenylephrine) are placed on the newly excised wound.[59] This can result in systemic absorption of vasoconstrictor, causing elevation of the patient's blood pressure, even in the face of hypovolemia. Surgeons may apply epinephrine-soaked gauze pads after debridement (before grafting) to achieve local control of bleeding. Greater systemic absorption of this agent has been demonstrated.[68] This is predictable, because each pad may contain 1 to 2 mg of the drug, based on a content of 100 to 200 ml of 10 μg/ml solution of epinephrine in saline (10 ml of 1:1000 epinephrine in 1000 ml NaCl.) Although epinephrine supports the blood pressure during periods of rapid blood loss, excessive levels of epinephrine can cause ventricular dysrhythmias, especially if the myocardium has been sensitized by the administration of halothane. Infants and children may be most susceptible to this complication, because their high surface area-to-volume ratio may facilitate the absorption of great amounts of epinephrine. A nondysrhythmogenic alternative drug is phenylephrine. Systemic absorption of part of the 1 to 2 mg per gauze pad of a 10 μg/ml solution (1 ml of 1% phenylephrine in 1000 ml NaCl) would not be expected to cause dysrhythmias. As in the initial resuscitation, an indwelling urinary catheter demonstrating good urinary output is a valuable monitor of ongoing fluid resuscitation intraoperatively. If very extensive debridement is necessary, a second anesthesia provider is useful in helping to manage fluid administration during excision.

Positioning the Patient

When burns involve the patient's back or all available ventral skin-graft donor sites have been exhausted, part or all of the procedure may be performed with the patient in the prone position. Femoral and subclavian vascular catheter insertion sites and tracheostomies are hard to access in any prone patient, and if they malfunction during surgery, troubleshooting them can be difficult.

Fractured limbs may require special attention during positioning for surgery. Long-bone fractures are associated with burns when deceleration injury occurs. The two most common scenarios that involve this mixture of burns and blunt trauma are motor vehicle accidents in which the victim is trapped in a burning automobile and situations wherein the victim jumps from a window to escape a burning building.[107]

Securing the Airway if Not Already Intubated

The inducton of anesthesia and intubation of the airway of a burn-injured patient who has not sustained an inhalational injury is straightforward, apart from altered muscle relaxant pharmacology. A potential exception to this is the patient with facial and neck burns. Topical antibiotic creams applied to the face can make airtight application of an anesthesia mask difficult, and contractures of skin of the neck and around the lips may limit exposure of even a normal larynx.

When the face and neck have been burned, the plan for securing the airway may require gas induction by mask to ensure the ability to control the airway or an awake intubation, either orally or nasally, depending on the severity of the burns or contractures. A fiberoptic bronchoscope is a very useful adjunct for an awake intubation in this setting. A surgical release of burn scar contracture may also facilitate intubation. Such a release may be performed under local anesthesia or under inhalation anesthesia delivered through a mask.[60,61]

Pulmonary and Metabolic Management

Intraoperative care of a burn-injured patient requires attention to significant physiologic alterations present during the patient's rehabilitation. Careful attention should be paid to the continuing metabolic needs of these critically ill patients. Significant pulmonary dysfunction also may be present after injury. If wound debridements become necessary, ventilation of the patient intraoperatively could be extremely difficult using only the conventional anesthesia ventilator. Marks et al.[67] studied the efficacy of anesthesia ventilators and concluded that such ventilators could not meet the needs of critically ill patients. They suggested use of a critical-care ventilator with pressure-independent inspiratory flow for patients requiring minute ventilation of greater than 15 l/min or peak airway pressure over 50 cm of water.[67] **High levels of minute ventilation are required in critically ill burn patients due to their high metabolic rates and resultant high rates of carbon dioxide production.[50]** Pulmonary injury from smoke inhalation will result in acutely noncompliant lungs that require high peak inspiratory pressures to achieve adequate gas exchange. Both of these problems can be overcome through the use of critical-care ventilators during operative procedures. During these procedures, patients may be successfully maintained on the same ventilator settings that have been proven adequate in the burn unit perioperatively. Unless specially modified ventilators with anesthetic vaporizers are available, a total IV anesthetic is administered. This provides for adequate analgesia and amnesia during surgery. Continuation of muscle relaxation and narcotics until the end of surgery can facilitate postoperative transfer back to the burn unit.

Burn patients have tremendous metabolic demands that should be met at all times, including the perioperative period. These caloric needs approach twice the patient's basal metabolic rate.[23,98,106] The nutritional needs of burned patients can be calculated by formulas that adjust feedings to reflect size of burn injury.[22] **Using such a formula, we can calculate that severely burned patients may require over 4000 kcal daily to ensure adequate nutrition.** This nutritional requirement is usually met through continuous enteral feedings if a patient does not have an adequate oral intake.

The necessity for continued adequate caloric intake cannot be ignored during the preanesthetic evaluation. Due to the importance of nutrition, it is unwise to arbitrarily stop enteral feedings the night before surgery. This can result in an excessive loss of calories, especially if the patient must undergo multiple burn debridements in a short period. We have found that it is safe to stop tube feedings 1 hour before transport to the operating room.[82] To ensure the safety of anesthetic induction, it is necessary to carefully monitor enteral feedings in the perioperative period. We routinely check for high residual gastric volumes and discontinue feedings at the first appearance of elevated residual gastric volumes. On admission to the operating room, the patient's nasogastric tube is suctioned, then anesthetic induction is tailored to ensure rapid protection of the airway. If the patient possesses normal upper-airway anatomy, a rapid-sequence intubation is usually performed; if abnormal anatomy is present, awake intubation is our usual choice. This approach guarantees the delivery of large caloric loads accompanied by minimal risk of aspiration during anesthetic induction. After the patient is returned to the ward, enteral feeding is resumed when the patient is fully awake.

INTRAOPERATIVE ANESTHETIC MANAGEMENT

Choice of intraoperative monitors should be governed by the severity of burn and the time elapsed from the burn injury. Minimal monitoring should include ECG, blood pressure, end-tidal carbon dioxide, temperature, volume of ventilation, and oxygen saturation. These follow suggested standards for intraoperative monitoring.[36] We have found end-tidal carbon dioxide to be very useful in adjusting ventilatory parameters to compensate for the large carbon dioxide production present in patients during the hypermetabolic phase of burn injury. Creativity in application of monitors is often necessary in patients with massive burns. Nonstandard configurations of ECG leads may be used to avoid burn tissues, or needle electrodes may be used to secure ECG leads in burned tissue.

Extensive debridement or critical injury demands more extensive monitoring. In these patients, continuous monitoring of arterial blood pressure via interarterial catheters is very useful. This allows for continuous observation of arterial blood pressure during debridements, as well as easy access for obtaining blood samples for the analysis of arterial blood gas concentrations or other laboratory studies that may be necessary. Addition of a CVP monitoring catheter may provide valuable additional information in the perioperative period. Observation of changes in central pressure can serve to fine-tune resuscitation fluid administration during debridements. The central catheter can also be used for additional access for transfusions. Other patients with significant cardiovascular disease may benefit from pulmonary artery catheterization for resuscitation and intraoperative management. Aikawa et al.[2] believe that use of the Swan-Ganz catheter improved outcome in an uncontrolled series of 39 patients with severe burns. Use of a pulmonary artery catheter in burn patients is associated with many potential complications.[35] **Because of the increased risks of catheter-associated sepsis in burn patients, Demling**[30] **recommends that these catheters be inserted only in patients with significant associated diseases or injury.** Choice of insertion site is dictated by the extent of burn wounds. If at all possible, the catheter should be inserted through unburned tissue. These catheters should be removed as soon as possible after hemodynamic stabilization in the postoperative period. This will limit possible septic complications.

CHOICE OF ANESTHETIC AGENTS AND TECHNIQUES

There is no single "best" anesthetic technique for burned patients. As in all other types of cases, the anesthesic should be tailored to individual patient diseases and needs. Choice of appropriate anesthetic technique will depend on multiple factors. Only after complete preoperative assessment is performed can an anesthetic plan be implemented.

A key point is the evaluation is the airway. As discussed earlier, severe edema may be present in the early postinjury period, and significantly decreased range of motion of the neck and jaw may be present later in the postinjury period. If any potential airway compromise is possible, utmost care must be taken to guarantee airway patency during anesthesic induction. If doubt exists regarding the ability to ventilate a patient with bag and mask, an awake intubation using either a blind approach or fiberoptic bronchoscope should be performed after appropriate sedation and administration of a topical anesthesic.

Choice of agents for anesthetic induction and maintenance will also depend on preferences of the anesthesia provider. Virtually every agent has been successfully applied to burn patients, if appropriate allowances are made for physiologic alterations. **Ketamine is a phencyclidine derivative that has been widely used as an anesthetic in a variety of burn procedures.** Ketamine is a potent drug that produces a dissociative anesthetic state of relative short duration.[101] This drug can be used in low doses (1 to 2 mg/kg intramuscularly) during debridements of superficial burns,[91] or in larger doses (4 to 6 mg/kg intramuscularly) for more extensive procedures.[25] Repeated use of ketamine is associated with rapid development of tolerance, necessitating large doses of drug during repeated administration of the anesthetic. This tolerance, plus the occasional emergence delirium, limits the use of this drug to relatively brief cases.[101]

Potent inhalation anesthetics have often been chosen as the principle anesthetic agents for burn debridements. Gronert et al.[41] reported on the use of halothane for 1770 anesthetics in 408 burned patients. They found that it was a safe and effective agent, and in addition, burn patients do not appear to be at risk for halothane-associated hepatitis.[41] Martyn[68] reported similar results in over 10,000 patients anesthetized with halothane. Presently, our personal bias is to choose isoflurane for the majority of our burn debridements, because it only minimally depresses cardiac output.[53] Isoflurane does not sensitize the myocardium to ventricular dysrythmias induced by systemic absorption of exogenous catecholamines.[57] This potential advantage is useful if topical catecholamines are applied to achieve hemostasis during burn debridements.

Muscle relaxant pharmacology is dramatically altered in burned patients. Use of the depolarizing muscle relaxant succinylcholine has been associated with sudden cardiac arrest and even death shortly after induction of anesthesia.[63] As Tolmie et al.[96] first pointed out, cardiac arrest usually occurs when anesthesia is attempted several weeks after injury, and is due to massive increases in plasma potassium concentration that lead to ventricular dysrhythmias. This hyperkalemia probably results from a spread of acetylcholine receptors over the entire muscle membrane in the weeks after a burn.[42] Succinylcholine will then cause depolarization and potassium release from the entire muscle membrane, rather than causing depolarization of only the endplate.[42] **Exactly when the patient is at risk of hyperkalemia after burn injury is uncertain.** As Busch et al.[15] point out, all published cases of cardiac arrest occurred more than 21 days after injury. This does not imply that succinylcholine can be safely administered until that time. Prudent practice would suggest that succinylcholine should be avoided in patients with burns more than 8 to 12 hours after injury. Endotracheal intubations performed for the treatment of carbon monoxide poisoning invariably take place within the first few hours postinjury, making succinylcholine still useful, if a relaxant is required. Similarly, the need to intubate for upper-airway obstruction is usually recognized early. If the swelling is not severe and a muscle relaxant is appropriate (as opposed to the use of an awake technique), succinylcholine may be used safely in this setting as well. It is also unclear when succinylcholine may be administered safely after the healing of the burn wounds. Martyn et al.[69] used indirect evidence of prolonged resistance to nondepolarizing relaxants to suggest that succinylcholine not be used until at least 1 year after the injury. **Therefore, it is also prudent to avoid succinylcholine until complete recovery from a burn is evident.** The safest generalization is to avoid succinylcholine at almost all times in the burn-injured patient. The drug is absolutely contraindicated from approximately 10 days postinjury until complete closure of wounds takes place.

Dramatic changes in dose of nondepolarizing muscle relaxants are also necessary in burn patients. Several authorities have reported resistance to nondepolarizing relaxants in these patients.[66,69,70] To ensure adequate muscle relaxation, very large doses in high serum concentrations of nondepolarizing relaxants are necessary.[34] This effect is due mainly to pharmacodynamics of the relaxant rather than to changes in plasma protein binding or alteration in pharmacokinetics.[62,66] The mechanism, like that of succinylcholine-induced hyperkalemia, is probably related to spread of acetylcholine receptors away from the nerve terminal.[58] Recent evidence suggests that plasma of burn victims may have an anticurare effect.[94] In contrast to the other nondepolarizing agents, mivacurium has minimal alterations in pharmacodynamics in burn patients. Complete neuromuscular blockade was found with normal intubating doses of 0.15 mg/kg BW.[100] Additionally, duration of action was slightly prolonged compared to nonburned control patients. Werba and colleagues[101] postulated that these findings may be due to reduced $alpha_1$ glycoprotein binding, coupled with decreased levels of serum cholinesterases in severely burned patients. The net result from these pharmacodynamic alterations is that a large dose of nondepolarizing relaxant should be administered to facilitate intubation and ensure adequate operative muscle relaxation. Monitoring of neuromuscular transmission is necessary to facilitate dosage adjustments to meet individual requirements.

Careful attention should be paid to perioperative heat loss. The burned patient is at great risk for hypothermia due to the loss of the protective skin layer.[13] Heat loss occurs through four mechanisms: radiation, evaporation, conduction, and convection.[92] Radiant heat loss is a loss of heat due to the transmission of infrared energy from the body to the environment, especially to colder objects even if distant. Conductive heat loss occurs from direct contact between the patient's body and the environment.[81] These two causes of heat loss can be minimized by completely warming the operating room well before beginning an operation involving a burn-injured patient. Evaporative and convective heat losses are from the loss of liquid molecules to the air and from circulation of air over fluids.[81] These losses can be minimized by using warm skin preparation solutions and decreasing the amount of air exchanges in the operating room during surgery. In addition, fluid warmers and airway heater humidifiers should be employed to minimize heat loss.[76] Wilmore et al.[104] demonstrated decreased hypermetabolism in burn-injured patients cared for in areas with higher environmental temperature. These patients had decreased metabolic rates, as compared with those patients nursed in an area with normal ambient temperature. Careful attention to intraoperative temperature control may decrease some of the postoperative complications in burn patients.

CONCLUSIONS

Patients with major burns present the anesthesia provider with many challenges. From the time of injury until completion of rehabilitation, these patients undergo multiple physiologic changes that should be recognized and addressed when planning and carrying out anesthetic support for multiple operations. The patient who will undergo early wound debridement 1 day after burn injury will have entirely different physiologic changes 1 month later, and these changes should be treated when he or she undergoes reconstructive surgery. Of primary importance is that more than any other type of patient, burn-injured patients deserve the physician's empathy. These patients undergo multiple painful procedures during their hospital stays. Anything that we as anesthesia providers can do to lessen their suffering will be remembered and appreciated by these critically ill patients.

KEY POINTS

- Assessment of the size of the patient's burn, most often using the "rule of nines," is an important help in understanding the magnitude of injury.
- Upper-airway injury should be anticipated in anyone with facial burns, but it should not be surprising that airway or lung injury can occur in any burned patient.
- A currently popular formula for crystalloid resuscitation uses 4 ml/kg total body surface area (TBSA) burned during the first 24 hours, with half of this given in the initial 8 hours and the other half over the following 16 hours. This formula is used in an attempt to maintain urinary output between 0.5 and 1.0 ml/kg/hr. There are also proponents of colloid-based resuscitation. Various formulas are given.
- The potential for blood loss during burn debridement is often unappreciated by beginning anesthesia providers. The surgical team can easily get ahead of the anesthesic team with respect to adequacy of volume replacement.
- Soaking burn eschar debridement sites with vasoconstrictor-soaked gauzes can lead to a false sense of security on the part of the anesthesia provider.
- Positioning, airway management, and IV access, not to mention invasive monitoring, are all difficult during the administration of anesthetics in the burn-injured patient.
- In recent years, it has been understood that burn patients' caloric intake requirements are enormous. This intake should not be stopped arbitrarily before surgery. We believe that it is safe to stop tube feedings 1 hour before transport to the operating room.
- It is well known that succinylcholine can cause massive potassium release and death shortly after induction of anesthesia. This should never be forgotten. Nondepolarizing muscle relaxants are not without their own problems in burn-injured patients. For example, there tends to be major physiologic resistance to these medications. The anesthesia provider should carefully understand this problem.

KEY REFERENCES

Demling RH: Management of the burn patient. In Shoemaker WC, editor: *Textbook of critical care,* ed 2, Philadelphia, 1989, WB Saunders.

Demling RH, Kramer G, Harmes B: Role of thermal injury-induced hypoproteinemia on fluid flux and protein permeability in burned and nonburned tissue, *Surgery* 95:136, 1984.

Fein A, Leff A, Hopewell PC: Pathophysiology and management of the complications resulting from fire and the inhaled products of combustion: review of the literature, *Crit Care Med* 8:94, 1980.

Fong Y, Moldawer LL, Shires GT, et al: The biologic characteristics of cytokines and their implication in surgical injury, *Surg Gynecol Obstet* 170:363, 1990.

Haponik EF, Meyers DA, Munster AM, et al: Acute upper airway injury in burn patients: serial changes on flow-volume curves and nasopharyngoscopy, *Am Rev Respir Dis* 135:360, 1987.

Lowenstein E: Succinylcholine administration in the burned patient, *Anesthesiology* 27:494, 1966.

Martyn JAJ, Matteo RS, Szfelbein SK, et al: Unprecedented resistance to neuromuscular blocking effects of metocurine with persistence after complete recovery in a burned patient, *Anesth Analg* 61:614, 1982.

Wilmore DW, Long JM, Mason AD Jr, et al: Catecholamines: mediator of the hypermetabolic response to thermal injury, *Ann Surg* 180:653, 1974.

Wilmore D, Mason AD, Johnson DW, et al: Effect of ambient temperature on heat production and heat loss in burn patients, *J Appl Physiol* 38:593, 1975.

Young CJ, Moss J: Smoke inhalation: diagnosis and treatment, *J Clin Anesth* 1:377, 1989.

REFERENCES

1. Achauer BM, Allyn PA, Furnas DW, et al: Pulmonary complications of burns: the major threat to the burn patient, *Ann Surg* 177:311, 1973.
2. Aikawa N, Martyn JA, Burke JF: Pulmonary artery catheterization and thermodilution cardiac output determination in the management of critically burned patients, *Burn Manage* 135:811, 1978.
3. Asch RS, et al: Regional blood flow in the burned unanesthetized dog, *Surg Forum* 22:55, 1971.
4. Aulick LH, Hander EH, Wilmore DW, et al: The relative significance of thermal and metabolic demands on burn hypermetabolism, *J Trauma* 19:559, 1979.
5. Barker SJ, Tremper KK, Hufstedler S, et al: The effects of carbon monoxide inhalation on noninvasive oxygen monitoring, *Anesth Analg* 65:S12, 1986.
6. Bartlett RH: Types of respiratory injury, *J Trauma* 19:918, 1979.
7. Baxter CR: Fluid volume and electrolyte changes in the early postburn period, *Clin Plast Surg* 1:693, 1974.
8. Beal DD, Conner GH: Respiratory tract injury: a guide to management following thermal and smoke injury, *Laryngoscope* 80:25, 1970.
9. Bessey PQ, Watters JM, Aoki TT, et al: Combined hormonal infusion simulates the metabolic response to injury, *Ann Surg* 200:264, 1984.
10. Border J: Hypothesis: sepsis, multiple systems organ failure, and the macrophage, *Arch Surg* 123:285, 1988.
11. Boykin JV, Eriksson E, Pittman RN: *In vivo* microcirculation of scald burn and the progression of postburn dermal ischemia, *Plast Reconstr Surg* 66:191, 1980.
12. Brighan PA, McLoughlin E: Burn incidence and medical care use in the United States: estimates, trials and data sources, *J Burn Care Rehab* 17:95, 1996.
13. Burke J, Quinby W, Bondoc CC: Early excision and prompt wound closure supplemented with immunosuppression, *Surg Clin North Am* 58:1141, 1978.
14. Burke JF, Quinby WC Jr, Bondoc C, et al: Patterns of high tension electrical injury in children and adolescents and their management, *Am J Surg* 133:492, 1977.
15. Bush GH, Graham HAP, Littlewood AHM: Danger of suxamethonium and endotracheal intubation in anesthesia for burns, *Brit Med J* 1081, 1962.
16. Chandra NC, Siu CO, Munster AM: Clinical predictors of myocardial damage after high voltage electrical injury, *Crit Care Med* 18:293, 1990.
17. Chang P, Murray D. Olson J, et al: Analysis of changes in coagulation factors after post-operative blood loss in burn and nonburn patients, *Burns* 21:432, 1995.
18. Choi IS: Delayed neurologic sequelae in carbon monoxide intoxication, *Arch Neurol* 40:433, 1983.
19. Clark WR, Monaventura M, Myers W: Smoke inhalation and airway management at a regional burn unit: 1974-1983, *J Burn Care Rehab* 10:52, 1989.
20. Coleman JB, Chang FC: Pulmonary embolism: an unrecognized event in severely burned patients, *Am J Surg* 130:697, 1975.
21. Crapo RO: Smoke-inhalation injuries, *JAMA* 246:1694, 1981.
22. Curreri PW, Luterman A, et al: Nutritional support of the burned patient, *Surg Clin North Am* 58:1151, 1978.
23. Cuthbertson DP: Post-shock metabolic response, *Lancet* 1:433, 1942.
24. deCampo T, Aldrete JA: The anesthetic management of the severely burned patient, *Inten Care Med* 7:55, 1981.
25. Demling RH, Ellerbee S, Janett F: Ketamine anesthesia for tangential excision of burn eschar: a burn unit procedure, *J Trauma* 18:269, 1978.
26. Demling RH, Harms B, Kramer GC: Role of thermal injury induced hypoproteinemia on fluid flux and protein permeability, *Surgery* 95:136, 1984.
27. Demling RH, La Londe C: Management of the burn wound. In Demling RH, editor: *Burn trauma,* New York, 1989, Thiene Medical Publishers.
28. Demling RH, Will JA, Belzer FO, et al: Effect of major thermal injury on the pulmonary microcirculation, *Surgery* 83:746, 1978.
29. Demling RH: Fluid resuscitation after major burns, *JAMA* 250:1438, 1983.
30. Demling RH: Improved survival after massive burns, *J Trauma* 23:179, 1983.
31. Demling RH: Management of the burn patient. In Shoemaker WC, editor: *Textbook of critical care,* ed 2, Philadelphia, 1989, WB Saunders.
32. Demling RH: Pathophysiological changes after cutaneous burns and approach to initial resuscitation. In Martyn JAJ, editor: *Acute management of the burned patient,* Philadelphia, 1990, WB Saunders.
33. Dreisbach RH: *Handbook of poisoning: diagnosis and treatment,* Los Altos, 1974, Lange Medical.
34. Dwersteg JF, Pavlin EC, Heimbach DM: Patients with burns are resistant to atracurium, *Anesthesiology* 65:517, 1986.
35. Ehrie M, Morgan AP, Moore FD, et al: Endocarditis with the indwelling balloon-tipped pulmonary artery catheter in burn patients, *J Trauma* 18:664, 1978.
36. Eichhorn JH, Cooper JB, Cullen DJ, et al: Standards for patient monitoring during anesthesia at Harvard Medical School, *JAMA* 256:1017, 1989.
37. Engrav L, Steinbach D, Reus J: Early excision and grafting vs. nonoperative treatment of burns of indeterminate depth: a randomized prospective study, *J Trauma* 23:1001, 1983.
38. Faist E, Mewes A, Strasser T, et al: Alteration of monocyte function following major injury, *Arch Surg* 123:287, 1988.
39. Fong Y, Moldawer LL, Shires GT, et al: The biologic characteristics of cytokines and their implication in surgical injury, *Surg Gynecol Obstet* 170:363, 1990.
40. Gilmore JP, Fozzand HA: Mechanism of acute erythrocyte loss following burns, *Am J Physiol* 198:487, 1960.
41. Gronert GA, Schaner PI, Gunther RC: Multiple halothane anesthetics in burn patients, *JAMA* 205:878, 1968.
42. Gronert GA, Theye NA: Pathophysiology of hyperkalemia induced by succinylcholine, *Anesthesiology* 43:89, 1975.
43. Grube BJ, Marvin JA, Heimbach DM: Therapeutic hyperbaric oxygen: help or

hindrance in burn patients with carbon monoxide poisoning? *J Burn Care Rehab* 9:249, 1988.
44. Haponik EF, Meyers DA, Munster AM, et al: Acute upper airway injury in burn patients: serial changes of flow-volume curves and nasopharyngoscopy, *Am Rev Respir Dis* 135:360, 1987.
45. Haponik EF, Munster AM, Wise RA, et al: Upper airway function in burn patients: correlation of flow-volume curves and nasopharyngoscopy, *Am Rev Respir Dis* 129: 251, 1984.
46. Haponik EF: Clinical and functional assessment. In Haponik EF, Munster AM, editors: *Respiratory injury: smoke inhalation and burns,* New York, 1990, McGraw-Hill.
47. Harms BA, Bodai BI, Kramer GC, et al: Microvascular fluid and protein flux in pulmonary and systemic circulations after thermal injury, *Microvasc Res* 23:77, 1982.
48. Head JM: Inhalation injury in burns, *Am J Surg* 139:508, 1980.
49. Heggers JP, Loy GL, Robson ML: Histological demonstration of prostaglandin and thromboplastin in burned tissues, *J Surg Rev* 28:110, 1980.
50. Heimbach DM, Engrav L: Excision and donor site techniques. In Heimbach D, editor: *Surgical management of the burn wound,* New York, 1985, Avon.
51. Heimbach DM: Smoke inhalation: current concept. In Wachtel TL, Kahn V, Frank HA, editors: *Current topics in burn care,* Rockville, 1983, Aspen Systems.
52. Herndon DN, Thompson PB, Linares HA, et al: Postgraduate course: respiratory injury, part I, *J Burn Care Rehab* 7:184, 1986.
53. Heughan C, Niinikoski J, Hunt TK: Effect of excessive infusion of saline solution in tissue oxygen transport, *Surg Gynecol Obstet* 135:257, 1972.
54. Hickey RF, Eger EI: Circulatory pharmacology of inhaled anesthetics. In Miller RD, editor: *Anesthesia,* ed 2, New York, 1986, Churchill Livingstone.
55. Holliman CJ, Saffle JR, Kravitz M, et al: Early surgical decompression in the management of electric injuries, *Am J Surg* 144:733, 1982.
56. Hunt JL, Agee RN, Pruitt BA: Fiberoptic bronchoscopy in acute inhalational injury, *J Trauma* 15:641, 1975.
57. Johntson RR, Eger EI, Wilson C: A comparative interaction of epinephrine with enflurane, isoflurane and halothane in man, *Anesth Analg* 55:709, 1976.
58. Jones WG, Madden M, Finkelstein J, et al: Tracheostomies in burn patients, *Ann Surg* 209:471, 1989.
59. Kealy GP, Cram AE: Thermal injuries. In Liechtz RD, Soper RT, editors: *Fundamentals of surgery,* ed 6, St Louis, 1989, Mosby–Year Book.
60. Kreulen M, Mackie DP, Kreis RW, et al: Surgical release for intubation purposes in post-burn contractures of the neck, *Burns* 22: 310, 1996.
61. Lamb JD: Anaesthetic considerations for major thermal injury, *Can Anaesth Soc J* 32:84, 1985.
62. Leibel WS, Martyn JA, Szfelbein SK, et al: Elevated plasma binding cannot account for burn-related d-tubocurarine hyposensitivity, *Anesthesiology* 54:378, 1981.
63. Lowenstein E: Succinylcholine administration in the burned patient, *Anesthesiology* 27:494, 1966.
64. Luce EA, Gottlieb SE: "True" high-tension electric injuries, *Ann Plast Surg* 12:321, 1984.
65. Lund CC, Browder NC: Estimates of area of burns, *Surg Gynecol Obstet* 79:352, 1944.
66. Marathe PH, Dwersteg JF, Paulin EG, et al: Effect of thermal injury on the pharmacokinetics and pharmacodynamics of atracurium in humans, *Anesthesiology* 70:752, 1989.
67. Marks JD, Shapera A, Kraemer RW, et al: Pressure and flow limitation of anesthesia ventilators, *Anesthesiology* 71:403, 1989.
68. Martyn J: Clinical pharmacology and drug therapy in the burned patients, *Anesthesiology* 65:67, 1986.
69. Martyn JAJ, Matteo RS, Szfelbein SK, et al: Unprecedented resistance to neuromuscular blocking effects of metocurine with persistence after complete recovery in a burned patient, *Anesth Analg* 61:614, 1982.
70. Martyn JAJ, Szfelbein SK, Ali HH, et al: Increased d-tubocurarine requirement following major thermal injury, *Anesthesiology* 52:352, 1980.
71. Marytn JA, Goldhill DR, Goudsouzian NG: Clinical pharamcology of muscle relaxants in burned patients, *J Clin Pharmacol* 26:680, 1986.
72. Monafo WW, Chuntrasakul C, Ayvazian V: Hypertonic sodium solutions in the treatment of burn shock, *Am J Surg* 126:778, 1973.
73. Monti F, Sepulchre C, Miskulin M, et al: Pharmacologic properties of a cardiotonic factor isolated from the blood serum of burned patients, *J Pathol* 127:147, 1979.
74. Moran KT, O'Reilly TJ, Furman W, et al: A new algorithm for calculation of blood loss in excisional burn surgery, *Am Surg* 54: 207, 1988.
75. Moritz AR, Henriques FC, McLean R: The effects of inhaled heat on the air passages and lungs, *Am J Pathol* 21:311, 1945.
76. Morrison RC: Hypothermia in the elderly, *Int Anesthiol Clin* 25(2):124, 1988.
77. Moylan JA, Adib K, Birnbaum M: Fiberoptic bronchoscopy following thermal injury, *Surg Gynecol Obstet* 140:541, 1975.
78. Munster AM, Eurenius K, Katz RM, et al: Cell-mediated immunity after thermal injury, *Ann Surg* 177:139, 1973.
79. Munster AM: Burn wound. In Cameron JL, editor: *Current surgical therapy,* St Louis, 1986, CV Mosby.
80. Norkol DM, Kirkpatrick JN: Treatment of acute carbon monoxide poisoning with hyperbaric oxygen: a review of 115 cases, *Ann Emerg Med* 14:1168, 1985.
81. Owens WD: Temperature regulation during anesthesia. International Anesthesia Research Society 1990 review course lectures, New York, 1990, Elsevier.
82. Pearson KS, From RP, Symreng T, et al: Continuous enteral feeding and short fasting periods enhance perioperative nutrition in patients with burns, *J Burn Care Rehab* 13:477–481, 1992.
83. Pruitt BA: Fluid and electrolyte replacement in the burned patient, *Surg Clin North Am* 58:1291, 1978.
84. Reed GF, Camp HL: Upper airway problems in severely burned patients, *Ann Otolaryngol Rhinol Laryngol* 78:741, 1969.
85. Remensnyder JP: Acute electrical injuries. In Martyn JAJ, editor: *Acute management of the burned patient,* Philadelphia, 1990, WB Saunders.
86. Riley-Paull KL, Munster AM: The role of cytokines in thermal injury, *Crit Care Rep* 2:4, 1990.
87. Robinson NB, Hudson LD, Robertson HT, et al: Ventilation and perfusion alterations after smoke inhalation injury, *Surgery* 90:352, 1981.
88. Robson MC, Kucan JO: The burn wound. In Wachtel TL, Kahn V, Frank HA, editors: *Current topics in burn care,* Rockville, 1983, Aspen Systems.
89. Sendak MJ, Furman WR: Anesthetic aspects. In Haponik EF, Munster AM, editors: *Respiratory injury: smoke inhalation and burns,* New York, 1990, McGraw-Hill.
90. Shirani KL, Pruitt BA, Mason AD: The influence of inhalational injury and pneumonia on burn mortality, *Ann Surg* 205:82, 1987.
91. Slogoff S, Allen CW, Wessels JV, et al: Clinical experience with subanesthetic ketamine, *Anesth Analg* 53:354, 1974.
92. Starr MS, West GB: Bradykinin and oedema formation in heated paws of rats, *Br J Pharmacol Chemother* 31:178, 1967.
93. Stephenson SF, Essis B, Polk H: The pathophysiology of smoke injury, *Ann Surg* 182:652, 1975.
94. Storella RJ, Martyn JAJ, Birnkamprn GC: Anti-curare effect of plasma from patients with thermal injury, *Life Sci* 43:35, 1988.
95. Strongin J, Hales CA: Pulmonary disorders in the burn patient. In Martyn JAJ, editor: *Acute management of the burned patient,* Philadelphia, 1990, WB Saunders.
96. Tolmie JD, Joyce TH, Mitchell GD: Succinylcholine danger in the burned patient, *Anesthesiology* 28:467, 1967.
97. Tranbaugh RF, Lewis FR, Christensen JM, et al: Lung water changes after thermal injury, *Ann Surg* 192:479, 1980.
98. Turner WW, Ireton CS, Hunt JL, et al: Predicting energy expenditure in burned patients, *J Trauma* 25:11, 1985.
99. Wang C, Martyn JAJ: Burn injury alters β adrenergic receptor and second messenger function in rat ventricular muscle, *Crit Care Med* 24:118, 1996.
100. Werba AE, Neiger FX, Bayer GS, et al: Pharmacodynamics of mivacurium in severely burned patients, *Burns* 22:62, 1996.
101. White P, Way WL, Trevor AJ: Ketamine—its pharmacology and therapeutic uses, *Anesthesiology* 56:119, 1982.
102. Wilmore DW, Aulich LH: Metabolic changes in burned patients, *Surg Clin North Am* 58:1173, 1978.
103. Wilmore DW, Long JM, Masur AD: Catecholamines: mediator of the hypermetabolic response to thermal injury, *Ann Surg* 180:653, 1974.
104. Wilmore DW, Mason AD, Johnson DW, et al: Effect of ambient temperature on heat

production and heat loss in burn patients, *J Appl Physiol* 38:593, 1975.

105. Wolfe RR, Durkot MJ: Evaluation of the role of the sympathetic nervous system in the response of substrate kinetics and oxidation to burn injury, *Circ Shock* 9:395, 1982.
106. Wolfe RR: Caloric requirements of the burned patient, *J Trauma* 21:712, 1981.
107. Wong L, Grande CM, Munster AM: Burns and associated nonthermal trauma: an analysis of management, outcome, and relation to the Injury Severity Score, *J Burn Care Rehab* 10:512, 1989.
108. Zawacki BE, Azen SP, Imbus SH, et al: Multifactorial probit analysis of mortality in burned patients, *Ann Surg* 189:1, 1979.

CHAPTER 83

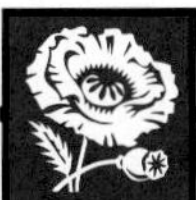

Anesthesia for Ophthalmic Surgery

STANLEY W. STEAD
CHRISTOPHER D. BEATIE
MARY A. KEYES

Ophthalmic surgery presents challenges to the anesthesiologist not seen in other surgical areas. Some of these challenges are presented in Box 83-1. Blind or potentially blind patients are especially apprehensive prior to surgery, and discussion of anesthetic procedures and expectations is extremely valuable. Ophthalmic surgery patients are especially likely to benefit from preoperative screening, because they tend to be at the extremes of age, have a high incidence of systemic disease, and are frequently managed in an outpatient setting. In this chapter, we will review the anatomy and physiology of the eye, preoperative medical preparation, regional and general anesthetic techniques, and anesthetic management of specific pediatric and adult surgical procedures.

OCULAR ANATOMY

A working knowledge of ocular anatomy is necessary for the anesthesiologist to understand ophthalmic procedures, perform and evaluate ophthalmic regional nerve blocks, evaluate and manage complications from these blocks, and appreciate the importantce of intraocular pressure (IOP).

The eyes lie within two bony cavities of the skull (termed *orbits*). The orbit is pear shaped with the orbital entrance approximately 35 mm in height and 45 mm in width, giving a volume of approximately 30 ml. The depth of the orbit varies with race and gender but averages slightly more than 40 mm. The optic foramen is located in the apex of the orbit. The optic nerve, ophthalmic artery, and sympathetic fibers from the carotid plexus pass through the optic foramen. Just lateral to the optic foramen is the superior orbital fissure. It is 22 mm long and conducts the lacrimal, frontal, and nasociliary branches of cranial nerve (CN) V, CN IV, CN III, CN VI; the superior ophthalmic vein; and sympathetic nerve plexus. The maxillary and pterygoid branches of CN V, a nerve from the pterygopalatine ganglion and the inferior ophthalmic vein, pass through the inferior orbital fissure, which is located just below the superior fissure and extends laterally.

The adult globe averages 24 mm in diameter.[13,40] The nor-

BOX 83-1
SPECIAL CONCERNS IN OPHTHALMIC ANESTHESIOLOGY

Elderly patients with multiple systemic diseases
Pediatric patients, often premature with congenital syndromes
Patients anxious from their loss of vision
Limited access to the airway
Oculocardiac reflex
Intraocular pressure and anesthetic interactions
Systemic effects of ophthalmic medications

mal anteroposterior diameter varies between 21 and 26 mm. At birth, the anteroposterior diameter is approximately 16 mm but reaches approximately 23 mm by 3 years of age. The globe reaches maximum size at puberty.

The transparent cornea occupies the center of the anterior pole of the globe and is approximately 11 to 12 mm in diameter. The cornea, lens, and aqueous humor form the main refractive elements of the eye. The curvature of the cornea contributes approximately one third of the refractive power of the eye, whereas the lens and aqueous humor contribute the remaining two thirds of the refractive power. The limbus borders the cornea and is gray and translucent in appearance. The sclera is opaque and white and covers the remaining 80% of the globe. Tendons of the rectus muscles insert into the superficial scleral collagen.

The wall of the globe is composed of three layers: (1) the sclera; (2) the uveal tract; and (3) the retina (Fig. 83-1). The middle layer is the uveal tract. It is composed of three specialized structures: (1) the iris; (2) the ciliary body located in the anterior uvea; and (3) the choroid located in the posterior uvea. The iris contains dilator and sphincter muscle fibers that control the central aperture, the pupil. Parasympathetic stimulation originating from the CN III nucleus contracts iris sphincter fibers, causing pupillary constriction or miosis. Conversely, sympathetic fibers traveling with the ophthalmic division of CN V stimulate iris dilator fibers, dilating the pupil. Directly adjacent and behind the iris is the ciliary body. The ciliary body has two primary functions: production of aqueous humor and accommodation. Ciliary muscles within the ciliary body are responsible for fine-tuning visual focus by releasing tension on the suspensory fibers or zonules of the lens, increasing the refractive power of the lens. The contraction of ciliary muscles also opens space for increased aqueous drainage. The posterior part of the uveal tract is a layer of blood vessels and capillaries called the choroid. These vessels nourish the outer portion of the retina, providing oxygen and nutrients. **Bleeding from the choroid layer can cause catastrophic intraoperative expulsive hemorrhage.**

The retina is a thin, transparent structure that differentiates from the optic cup and constitutes the inner layer of the

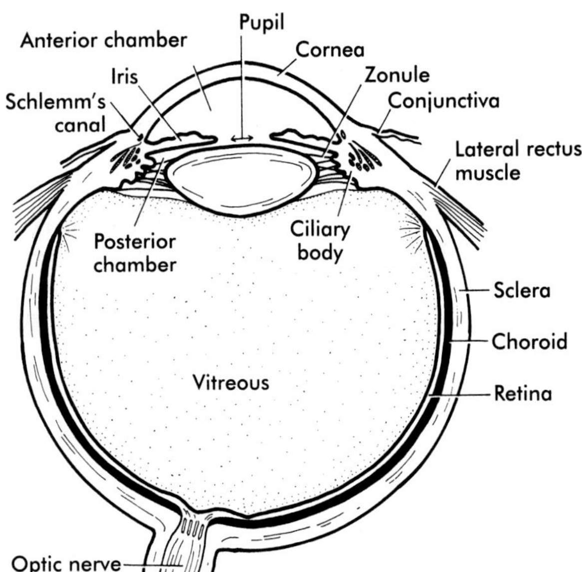

Fig. 83-1. Anatomy of the eye. (From Bruce RA Jr, McGoldrick KE, Oppenheimer P: *Anesthesia for ophthalmology,* Birmingham, 1982, Aesculapius.)

medioposterior wall of the globe. Photoreceptors of the retinal layer convert light into neural signals, which are processed and carried to the brain via the optic nerve.

The vitreous cavity occupies more than 80% of the volume of the globe. The transparent vitreous humor is important in the metabolism of the intraocular tissues; it provides a passageway for metabolites used by the lens, the ciliary body, and the retina. Although it has a gel-like structure, the vitreous is composed of 99% water. Vitreous is twice as viscous as water, principally due to mucopolysaccharides and hyaluronic acid. Vitreous adheres to the retina peripherally at the vitreous base, the disc margin, and onto the posterior margin. Separation of the vitreous from the inner retina proceeds with age and is the most common event associated with retinal detachment. Scarring, bleeding, or opacification of the vitreous is treated by its removal, or vitrectomy.

Extraocular muscles arise from a fibrous ring at the orbital apex and insert on the sclera approximately 6 mm posterior to the limbus. These muscles produce eye movements within the orbit. Together, they form what has been termed a "cone" within the orbit, which contains the optic nerve, ophthalmic artery and vein, oculomotor and abducens nerves, and ciliary ganglion. The extraocular muscles are comprised of two differing types of cells: Fibrillenstruktur and Felderstruktur. Fibrillenstruktur muscle fibrils are believed to produce fast or twitch movements. The Felderstruktur muscle fibers are responsible for slow or tonic movements. Felderstrukturs appear to control the resting position of the extraocular muscles and may keep the eyes conjugate. These muscles are sensitive to the effects of acetylcholine and have been implicated in the exaggerated IOP response to succinylcholine and other depolarizing muscle relaxants. Extraocular movements are used to assess the success of ophthalmic nerve blocks. A summary of the function and innervation of the extraocular muscles is seen in Table 83-1.

The conjunctiva is a mucous membrane that lines the inner surface of the eyelids and covers the anterior surface of the globe between the cornea and limbus. The bulbar extension of the conjunctiva fuses with Tenon's capsule and inserts into the limbus.

Tenon's capsule is an incomplete fascial layer composed of collagen fibers and fibroblasts. Anteriorly, it fuses with the conjunctiva and extends posteriorly where it is perforated by the optic nerve sheath and the posterior ciliary vessels and nerves. Tenon's capsule and the intermuscular fibrous membranes surrounding the four rectus muscles fuse to form a type of fibrous sling or support. This structure may also be called the "cone," but it is important to understand that the cone is not continuous.

The eyelids are composed of an outer layer of skin, a muscle layer, a cartilaginous tarsal plate, and an inner layer of conjunctiva. The upper lid can be raised 15 mm by the action of the levator palbebrae superiorus muscle which is innervated by CN III. The orbicularis oculi muscle, innervated by CN VII, allows tight closure of the eyelids.

The lacrimal gland is located in a shallow depression within the orbital portion of the frontal bone. Tears are formed here by the serous secretion of acinar and myoepithelial cells. Under both reflex and psychogenic stimulation, tears pass from the surface of the eye via the puncta, through either the upper or lower canaliculi to the lacrimal sac and duct, and drain into the nasopharynx below the inferior turbinate.

The blood supply to the ocular structures is primarily the ophthalmic artery. The ophthalmic artery is a branch of the internal carotid artery just before the circle of Willis. Venous drainage flows through the superior and inferior ophthalmic veins directly to the cavernous sinus.

The cranial nerves innervate ocular structures. The optic nerve (II) carries the sensory information from the retina. Cranial nerves III, IV, and VI supply the extraocular muscles.

The optic nerve is a special sensory nerve, but it is not a true nerve. Developmentally speaking, both the retina and optic nerve are part of the brain. The optic nerve extends from the retina and enters the cranial cavity through the optic canal (optic foramen). The intraorbital part of the optic nerve is approximately 25 mm long. The optic nerve is enclosed by three sheaths which are continuous with the meninges of the brain. These sheaths extend as far as the back of the globe. The thick outer sheath is continuous with the dura mater of the brain and the sclera of the eye. The thin intermediate sheath is continuous with the arachnoid of the brain and is separated from the outer sheath by the subdural space and from the inner sheath by the subarachnoid space. The vascular inner sheath is continuous with the pia mater of the brain and closely invests the optic nerve. The inner sheath sends connective tissue partitions and blood vessels into the nerve. The central artery and vein of the retina pierce the dural and arachnoid coverings of the optic nerve approximately 1 cm behind the globe and after a short course in the subarachnoid space, penetrate the optic nerve and run within it to the inner aspect of the retina.

Table 83-1 Innervation and function of extraocular muscles

Muscle	Innervation	Function
Superior rectus	III (oculomotor)	Elevation
Inferior rectus	III (oculomotor)	Depression
Medial rectus	III (oculomotor)	Adduction
Inferior oblique	III (oculomotor)	Elevation/ abduction
Superior oblique	IV (trochlear)	Depression/ adduction
Lateral rectus	VI (abducens)	Abduction

The oculomotor nerve (CN III) is the somatic motor nerve to four of the six muscles that move the eye and to the levator palpebrae superioris, the muscle that raises the eyelid. The oculomotor nerve was so named because it supplies most of the muscles that move the eye. It also contains parasympathetic fibers to the involuntary muscles that constrict the pupil and change the curvature of the lens (accommodation).

The trochlear (CN IV) nerve has the fewest nerve fibers of any cranial nerve, but it has the longest intracranial course. The trochlear nerve enters the orbit through the superior orbital fissure. It then extends superiorly to innervate the superior oblique muscle. This location of the nerve, outside of the muscle cone, delays the abolition of depression and adduction of the globe following retrobulbar block.

The trigeminal nerve (CN V) provides sensory innervation to the skin and conjunctiva of the lower lid via the maxillary nerve and the upper lid and conjunctiva via the frontal branch of the ophthalmic nerve. The nasociliary branch of the ophthalmic nerve provides sensory innervation to the medial canthus, lacrimal sac, and canaliculi and sends sensory fibers to the ciliary ganglion.

The ciliary ganglion provides sensory innervation of the cornea, iris, and ciliary body. Parasympathetic motor fibers originating from the oculomotor nerve synapse in the ciliary ganglion before innervating the sphincter muscle of the iris and the ciliary muscle. Sympathetic motor fibers originating from the carotid plexus travel through the ciliary ganglion to innervate the dilator muscle of the iris.

The abducens nerve (CN VI) passes through the superior orbital fissure to innervate the lateral rectus muscle on its ocular surface. There appear to be no sympathetic or parasympathetic fibers that accompany the motor fibers.

The facial nerve (CN VII) is a mixed nerve, but is predominantly motor in function. It was given its name because of large motor branches that spread across the face. The facial nerve exits the skull through the stylomastoid foramen (along with the internal carotid artery) and passes into the substance of the parotid gland where it divides into five branches which supply the muscles of facial expression. The orbicularis oculi muscle, innervated by the zygomatic branch of the facial nerve, allows the patient to close the eyelid tightly. Local anesthetic blockade of the facial nerve can be important in intraocular surgery by eliminating squeezing caused by contraction of the orbicularis oculi.

OCULOCARDIAC REFLEX

The oculocardiac reflex is caused by traction on the extraocular muscles, manipulation of the globe or an increase in IOP. It is most commonly described as occurring during eye muscle surgery, but it is also prevalent during retinal detachment repair and enucleation. The oculocardiac reflex has even been observed following retrobulbar block and retrobulbar hemorrhage. The oculocardiac reflex is most commonly manifested as bradycardia, but may also appear as bigeminy, ectopic beats, nodal rhythms, atrioventricular (AV) block or asystole. These dysrhythmias may persist as long as the stimuli is present. Repeated stimuli cause fatigue with diminished vagal effects.

The oculocardiac reflex's afferent pathway is via the ciliary ganglion to the ophthalmic division of the trigeminal nerve, through the gasserian ganglion to the trigeminal nucleus in the fourth ventricle. The efferent pathway is exclusively through the vagus nerve. It is the vagus innervation to the abdominal viscera that causes nausea and vomiting which can accompany the cardiac manifestations. Alexander reported that 90% of patients experienced the oculocardiac reflex (OCR) during traction of the extraocular muscles.[2] The reported incidence of other cardiac dysrhythmias varies between 32% and 82%.

Diagnosis of the OCR relies upon continuous monitoring of the electrocardiogram (ECG). Treatment varies based upon the severity of the reflex. If the reflex manifests itself as bradycardia or infrequent ectopic beats, and the blood pressure remains stable, no treatment may be sufficient. If the dysrhythmias become significant, cessation of the surgical stimuli is indicated. Often the procedure may resume after a brief pause. The OCR fatigues easily and usually there is little or no OCR after a brief pause in surgical stimuli. When the OCR is severe, treatment with anticholinergics (glycopyrrolate or atropine) is indicated. Caution must be exercised with large doses of atropine, because more severe, prolonged tachydysrhythmias may result.[44]

ANESTHESIA AND INTRAOCULAR PRESSURE

IOP is the pressure exerted by the contents of the eye upon the cornea and sclera of the globe. The sclera is inelastic, making the compliance of the globe low; small changes in volume result in large changes in pressure. The volume of the globe is principally determined by the aqueous humor and the blood vessels of the eye, particularly of the choroid. Aqueous humor volume is determined by the production and drainage of aqueous. Excessive increases in IOP interfere with choroidal and retinal blood supply as well as corneal metabolism, potentially causing retinal ischemia and corneal opacification. Decreased IOP or hypotony increases the risk for retinal detachment and vitreous hemorrhage.

The blood vessels of the choroid constitute a large and variable volume in the eye. Because choroidal vessels of the eye act much like intracranial vessels, it is useful to think of anesthetic effects upon IOP as being similar to anesthetic effects upon intracranial pressure (ICP). Choroidal vessels constrict with hyperventilation (hypocapnia) and cause a decrease in IOP. Hypoventilation (hypercapnia) causes vasodilatation and an increase in IOP. Similarly, hypoxia may contribute to increased IOP through vasodilatation of intraocular vessels.

The normal IOP is 16 ± 5 torr in the sitting position and is generally maintained within this narrow range. IOP undergoes normal minor fluctuations because of: (1) changes in body position (+1 torr supine); (2) diurnal rhythm (2 to 3 torr); (3) blood pressure oscillations (1 to 2 torr); and (4) respiration (deep inspiration decreases IOP by 5 torr). Changes in blood pressure are reflected in IOP—hypotension decreases IOP, whereas hypertension increases IOP.

The most severe increases in IOP are usually caused by blockage of aqueous outflow by acute venous congestion. Any straining, bucking, breath holding, or obstructed airway during the induction or emergence of general anesthesia will increase venous congestion in the ophthalmic veins and therefore raise IOP. Coughing, valsalva maneuvers, or straining can increase IOP to 30 to 40 torr. Endotracheal intubation is also a potent stimuli for increasing IOP. External pressure from face mask, fingers, orbital tumors, contraction of the orbicularis oculi muscle, or retrobulbar hemorrhage will also increase IOP.

Aqueous humor is formed by the ciliary body, which is the vascular component of the uveal tract located in front of the pars plana and behind the fibers of the suspensory ligament of the lens (Figure 83-2). The ciliary body is folded over into a series of 80 folds, each 2 to 3 mm, termed processes which extend to the posterior aspect of the iris. This structure is supplied by a vascular plexus and covered with epithelium that is impervious to proteins and high molecular weight substances.

Aqueous humor is the major transport system in the eye for oxygen, glucose, proteins, medications, and inflammatory cells. It provides the nourishment for the lens and the corneal endothelium. Approximately half of the cornea's oxygen supply comes from aqueous, with the remainder from diffusion with the air. Drugs may enter the eye with aqueous humor via the cellular pumping action of the ciliary body, but as noted above there is a distinct blood-aqueous barrier preventing high molecular weight drugs from entering aqueous from the blood.

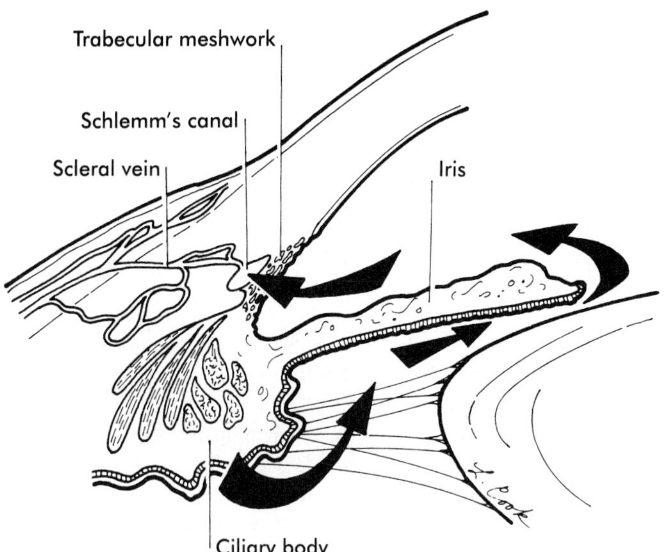

Fig. 83-2. Anatomy of aqueous flow. (From Bruce RA Jr, McGoldrick KE, Oppenheimer P: *Anesthesia for ophthalmology,* Birmingham, 1982, Aesculapius.)

The aqueous flows forward from the suspensory ligament of the lens and passes between the anterior capsule of the lens and posterior surface of the iris through the pupil to the anterior chamber. Flow then proceeds laterally to the meshwork of the trabeculum and into the circular canal of Schlemm. This lateral drainage area is termed the "angle." Episcleral veins drain aqueous to the venous system. Approximately one third of the aqueous produced is reabsorbed through the veins in the iris and choroid.

Altered circulation of aqueous can produce an increase in IOP, termed glaucoma, or a decrease in IOP, termed *phthisis.* Glaucoma is usually caused by obstruction to outflow of aqueous humor. Glaucoma is rarely caused by an abnormal increase in aqueous production. In these cases vascular abnormalities or diseases lead to increased vascularity of the eye.

Acute glaucoma is the sudden occlusion of the drainage angle. This occlusion is often associated with a narrow anatomical angle, a pupil dilated by atropinergic compounds, or an iris propelled anteriorly. There is often a history of an episode of coughing or straining.

The onset of *chronic glaucoma* is insidious. Although peripheral vision is gradually lost in the early stages of the disease, the angle is found open and the trabeculum appears to operate normally. Chronic glaucoma may be congenital, associated with a familial diathesis, or increasing age.

IOP is clinically measured indirectly. Invasive measurements are not common because of the risk of eye damage, the danger of infection, and the likelihood that the measurement itself may alter IOP. IOP is measured via an indentation technique (Schiotz) or applanation (Goldmann).

The Schiotz technique uses a plunger activated by a small weight to indent the cornea. The plunger is connected to a lever which points to a number on an arbitrary scale. This number, along with the weight used in the measurement, allows the determination of IOP from a normogram. A small amount of aqueous is forced out of the eye with each indentation. Because of this and because of the mechanical friction of the tonometer, Schiotz readings decrease as the measurements are repeated. The applanation method exerts graduated pressures to a cornea and results in a more reproducible IOP measurement.

Many drugs alter the production or drainage of aqueous and consequently IOP (Table 83-2). The method and speed of administration of drugs is important. Inhalational and intravenous drugs have the most rapid and pronounced effect upon IOP. Medications taken intramuscularly, orally or rectally have less influence upon IOP. Most medications exhibit a "dose-response" relationship with IOP; initial dosing has minimal effects, then a rapid linear response occurs leading to a plateau effect, where increasing dosages have little or no effect upon IOP.

Deep inhalational or thiopental anesthesia reduces IOP 30% to 40% in a dose-related manner.[25,26] Narcotics generally cause a small decrease in IOP. Atropine in usual doses is not a problem, even in patients with open-angle glaucoma. Ketamine may cause a modest-to-significant increase in IOP. Most of this increase can be explained by increased blood pressure.[3]

Succinylcholine causes a 6 to 12 mm increase in IOP, which can be sustained for 5 to 10 minutes.[16,52,66,82] This increase has been ascribed to the contraction of the extraocular muscles leading to compression of the globe. This contraction could potentially extrude globe contents in a patient with an open globe injury. Kelley and colleagues[45] studied patients undergoing elective enucleation and compared IOP following the administration of succinylcholine between the normal eye and the diseased eye which had all extraocular muscles detached.[45] No difference between the two eyes was found in baseline or peak IOP. Nonetheless, both eyes exhibited a precipitous rise in IOP, leading the authors to conclude that extraocular muscle contraction does not contribute to the increase in IOP after succinylcholine. "Self-taming" doses,[57,79] precurarization,[56] diazepam,[28] and lidocaine[53] do not completely abolish the response. **The use of succinylcholine for induction in cases of open-globe injury is controversial although vitreous loss in precurarized patients due to succinylcholine has not been reported.**

SYSTEMIC EFFECTS OF OPHTHALMIC DRUGS

Some ophthalmic medications given in the perioperative period are sufficiently potent to have systemic effects. Ocular drugs applied topically can act as readily as if given intravenously. Although the medication is absorbed slowly from the conjunctival sac, much more rapid absorption can occur via the mucosal surfaces of the nasolacrimal duct. Systemic absorption may be altered in a diseased or postsurgical eye.

Table 83-2 Anesthetic drugs and intraocular pressure

	Dose	Route	Comments
Drugs that increase intraocular pressure			
Ketamine	1–2 mg/kg	IV	Increase
Ketamine	5 mg	IM	Slight increase
Succinylcholine	1–2 mg/kg	IV	18% increase
No effect or unknown			
Alfentanil	5 μg/kg	IV	No effect
Atracurium	0.4–0.5 mg/kg	IV	No effect
Atropine	0.4–1.0 mg	IM	No effect
Desflurane	6%–12%	Inhalation	Unknown, probable decrease
Flumazenil	0.0025 mg/kg	IV	No effect
Glycopyrrolate	0.2–0.4 mg	IV	No effect
Meperidine	50–100 mg	IM	May increase, normally no effect
Nitrous oxide	70%	Inhalation	No effect
Remifentanil	0.5 μg/kg	IV	No effect
Scopolamine	0.4 mg	IM	No effect
Vecuronium	0.08–0.1 mg/kg	IV	No effect
Drugs that decrease intraocular pressure			
Chlorpromazine	10–25 mg	IM	20%–30% decrease
Curare	0.5–0.6 mg/kg	IV	Slight decrease
Dexmedetomidine	1 μg/kg	IV	40% decrease
Diazepam	10 mg	IV	Decrease
Dilaudid	1–2 mg	IV	Decrease
Droperidol	5–10 mg	IV	12% decrease
Enflurane	1% with N_2O	Inhalation	35%–40% decrease
Etomidate	0.3 mg/kg	IV	30% decrease
Fentanyl	50–100 μg	IM	20% decrease
Haloperidol	0.5 mg	IV	15% decrease
Halothane	1 MAC	Inhalation	14%–33% decrease
Isoflurane	1%–3%	Inhalation	40% decrease
Lidocaine	1.5 mg/kg	IV	Decrease
Methohexital	6 mg/kg	IV	Decrease
Metocurine	0.3–0.4 mg/kg	IV	Slight decrease
Midazolam	0.15 mg/kg	IV	25% decrease
Morphine	8–15 mg	IM	Decrease
Pancuronium	0.05 mg/kg	IV	Slight decrease
Pentothal	3–5 mg/kg	IV	30% decrease
Propofol	1–2 mg/kg	IV	Decrease
Sevoflurane	1%–3% with N_2O	Inhalation	40% decrease
Sufentanil	1–2 μg/kg	IV	Decrease
Thiamylal	4–5 mg/kg	IV	Decrease
Thiopentone	2.5 mg/kg	IV	30% decrease

Phenylephrine is commonly used as a mydriatic. There is little increase in mydriasis when solutions with concentrations greater than 5% are used.[35] This is important, because significant complications have been reported with 10% phenylephrine. A single drop of this high concentration solution may contain 5 mg of phenylephrine (100 mg/ml ÷ 20 drops/ml). Complications seen include myocardial infarction (MI), hypertension, reflex bradycardia, and cardiac dysrhythmias.[30]

Topical application of 2% *epinephrine* solution to the eye causes a decrease in aqueous secretion and improves outflow, both which act to reduce IOP in open angle glaucoma. Complications include hypertension, tachycardia, dysrhythmias, and fainting. Since a single drop of 2% solution contains 0.5 to 1.0 mg of epinephrine, it is reasonable to expect systemic complications to occur. *Intraocular* epinephrine administered during halothane anesthesia is poorly absorbed and has no significant cardiac effects.[72]

Beta adrenergic antagonists (e.g., timolol) are used in the treatment of glaucoma. This class of medication acts to reduce aqueous humor secretion, with minimal effects on aqueous outflow. Pupillary size is not affected. Patients may complain of lightheadedness, fatigue, disorientation, and may exhibit a general depression of central nervous system function. Excessive dosage of beta-adrenergic antagonists may lead to cardiovascular dysfunction including bradycardia, palpitations, syncope, increase in heart block, and congestive heart failure (CHF).[46] Rare exacerbations of asthma have also been reported.[41] Particular caution should be exercised with neonates receiving timolol eye drops, because cases of apnea have been reported.[8]

Apraclonidine is a relatively new alpha$_2$-adrenergic agonist which has found a role as a topical antiglaucoma medication. Like epinephrine, it causes a decrease in aqueous formation and improves aqueous outflow. Systemic absorption may cause significant sedation and drowsiness. Hypotension is a possible complication, but has not been reported. Acute withdrawal from long-term therapy may result in rebound hypertension.

Echothiophate iodide is a long-acting anticholinesterase drug still used to treat glaucoma. The pupil is constricted and aqueous drainage is increased. Its duration of action is 4 to 6 weeks. Three weeks after the cessation of treatment with echothiophate, plasma cholinesterase activity remains at 50% of normal.[20] If a patient receives succinylcholine, a relative overdose of succinylcholine leads to two to three times the usual duration of action. Careful titration of succinylcholine with the use of a peripheral nerve stimulator will avoid prolonged paralysis. The effects of ester local anesthetics (procaine and chloroprocaine) may also be significantly prolonged. Amide-type local anesthetics may be a better choice for regional anesthesia.

Muscarinic agonists are given to cause prolonged mydriasis. A drop of *atropine* 1% solution contains 0.2 to 0.5 mg of the drug. One drop of 0.5% *scopolamine* contains 0.2 mg of the drug. Systemic reactions have been seen in both young and elderly patients following the administration of topical ocular atropine or scopolamine. These reactions are manifest by tachycardia, flushing, thirst, and dry skin. Elderly patients may show agitation. CNS excitement and agitation can be treated with incremental doses of physostigmine 0.15 mg/kg, IV.

The carbonic anhydrase inhibition of *acetazolamide* interferes with the formation of the aqueous humor and lowers IOP. Aside from a metabolic acidosis with depletion of sodium and potassium, long-term therapy may result in dyspepsia. Given rapidly IV, the patient may exhibit an acute decrease in blood pressure. Caution should be exercised in patients with renal disease, dehydration, and sodium or potassium depletion.

PREOPERATIVE EVALUATION

The importance of a thorough preoperative evaluation cannot be overemphasized. Only through effective communication between the patient, anesthesiologist, surgeon, and medical consultants can plans be made to manage chronic medical problems perioperatively and conduct a safe anesthetic. In a study of malpractice litigation in cataract surgery, failure of the anesthesiologist, ophthalmologist, and internist to coordinate perioperative patient care resulted in litigation that accounted for 16% of the indemnity.[49]

Ophthalmic surgery patients tend to be at the extremes of age and therefore represent a high-risk population. Adult patients tend to be elderly. Many will have multiple coexisting diseases, such as hypertension, diabetes, chronic obstructive pulmonary disease (COPD), atherosclerosis, coronary artery disease (CAD), arthritis, anemia, osteoporosis, cerebrovascular disease, Parkinsonism, dementia, malignancy, renal insufficiency and hepatic disease. Children presenting for ophthalmic surgery may have problems associated with prematurity, such as bronchopulmonary dysplasia and apneic episodes. Children who present with congenital anomalies of the eye may have associated anomalies in other organ systems. Patients with congenital strabismus have an increased incidence of myopathies and are at increased risk for malignant hyperthermia.

Most ophthalmic surgery procedures, however, are relatively low risk. They are generally not associated with significant physiologic derangements or fluid shifts caused by blood loss or third-spacing. Therefore, mortality for ophthalmic surgery is significantly lower than for general surgery despite the high-risk population.[38,66,67,77] Where does this leave the anesthesiologist with the high-risk patient having low-risk surgery? The following principles may provide helpful guidance:

1. Every patient undergoing a surgical procedure must have an appropriate and thorough medical history and physical examination, preferably performed by the patient's personal physician. Ideally, every patient seeing a physician for treatment of chronic medical problems should visit *that* physician preoperatively. The purpose of the visit is to ensure that all reversible medical conditions (e.g., bronchospasm, hypertension, CHF, etc.) are optimized and that the patient is not acutely ill. Written documentation of the visit should include a concise history and physical examination, a complete problem list with a comment on the status of each problem, a list of current medications and any recent pertinent laboratory data. A statement that the patient is simply "cleared for surgery" or "cleared for general anesthesia" is not acceptable.
2. In addition to preoperative consultation with the patient's personal physician, a preanesthetic interview with the individual who will anesthetize the patient is also desirable. The purposes of this interview are: (1) To review the patient's medical history and laboratory data; (2) To determine whether further testing or consultations are required; (3) To formulate a perioperative anesthetic plan; and (4) To discuss this plan with the patient. Blind, or potentially blind patients and

their families are often particularly apprehensive prior to surgery and will derive great psychologic benefit from a preanesthetic interview with their anesthesiologist. This interview should preferably take place prior to the day of surgery to avoid unnecessary delays, cancellations and other disruptions.

3. Ordering routine batteries of laboratory studies is not an efficient method of preoperative screening. Unnecessary testing is economically wasteful and may lead to unnecessary work-up and/or therapy initiated on the basis of false positive results. Medical history and physical examination should guide all preoperative testing. More extensive laboratory testing and consultations may be indicated by the results of the initial work-up.
4. The special sense of vision is a profoundly important one, and is tied to strong emotions in most patients. Some individuals would rather die than be blind. The anesthesiologist therefore may sometimes have to cope with a patient in poor medical condition who requires an urgent sight-saving procedure. Top priority should be given to optimizing the patient's overall medical condition prior to even the most emergent ophthalmic procedures. Occasionally, however, a patient with severe, chronic, life-threatening disease will demand ophthalmic surgery even if there is an increased risk of a major complication or death. Our practice is to carefully explain the risks of anesthesia in these situations, and to be as certain as possible that a detailed informed consent is obtained. If the patient understands the risks and wishes to proceed, then his or her wishes are honored. The procedure is performed under local anesthesia and monitored anesthesia care if possible, so as to minimize hemodynamic changes and stress responses.

MONITORED ANESTHESIA CARE

Ophthalmic procedures traditionally performed under general anesthesia are now routinely performed under monitored anesthesia care (MAC). Topical or nerve block anesthesia coupled with MAC is highly effective for ophthalmic procedures. Today, quality and efficiency have become primary focuses. Anesthesiologists have sought agents that provide a rapid and smooth onset of action, good surgical conditions, and rapid recovery with an absence of side effects.

The desire to provide sedation during the injection of local anesthetics is not based solely upon aesthetics. The performance of some local anesthetic blocks can be a brief, but very painful experience. Failure to block the clinical response to this stimulus can initiate catecholamine-mediated sequelae including anxiety, tachycardia, and hypertension,[69] which may produce significant morbidity and mortality in the patient.[68]

Patients can also respond to a local anesthetic injection by moving away from the stimulus, making the block more difficult and dangerous. Thus, the primary goals of monitored anesthesia care are hemodynamic stability and immobility. These can be achieved by providing analgesia and central nervous system depression.

Table 83-3 Suggested ophthalmic block sedation regimen

	Alfentanil dose	Propofol dose
Alfentanil/propofol bolus		
Age:		
< 50 yrs	5 μg/kg	0.40 mg/kg
50–70 yrs	4 μg/kg	0.32 mg/kg
> 70 yrs	3 μg/kg	0.24 mg/kg
Alfentanil/propofol infusion rate		
Type of local injection:		
Discrete nerve block(s)	0.75 μg/kg/min	60 μg/kg/min
Large field blocks	1.00 μg/kg/min	80 μg/kg/min

Emotional stress and anxiety can trigger the same sympathetic responses elicited by physical pain, therefore sedation and anxiolysis are worthwhile goals. Providing amnesia for the patient often will improve the perioperative experience. Many patients want to have no recall of the operating room and are dissatisfied if they do. The final goal of monitored anesthesia care is rapid recovery. This has become much more important recently as more and more surgical procedures are performed on an outpatient basis.

At Jules Stein Eye Institute, we combine propofol and alfentanil to accomplish most of the goals of monitored anesthesia care.[12] Alfentanil provides a brief period of intense analgesia that maintains stable hemodynamics during stress and painful stimuli. Because it is combined with propofol, very small doses can be used and side effects are avoided. Propofol provides additional sedation, decreased awareness, antiemesis (counteracting the emetic effects of alfentanil) and amnesia. Using this technique patients remain responsive and cooperative while they are sedated. They show cardiopulmonary stability and return to baseline mental status within 10 minutes. Patients generally do not need any further sedation and are ready for discharge when they leave the operating room. Patient acceptance and ophthalmologist satisfaction have reinforced the use of this technique in nearly all MAC cases. A summary of our dosing guidelines is given in Table 83-3.

REGIONAL ANESTHETIC TECHNIQUES

Topical Anesthesia

There is a great deal of confusion over the terminology of types of anesthesia used in ophthalmic surgery. Originally, topical anesthesia referred to the technique of placing cocaine crystal either on the globe or in the cul-de-sac. Instillation anesthesia referred to instilling a solution of local anesthetic into the conjunctival sac or upon the cornea. Today, crystals are not routinely used for anesthesia and topical anesthesia refers to instilling drops of local anesthetic solution onto the globe.

Topical anesthesia is becoming increasingly popular for less invasive and short duration ophthalmic surgery. However, only the conjunctiva and cornea are anesthetized. The patient still has sensations of pressure and eyelids may transmit sensations of splashing irrigation. The patient must be carefully instructed regarding these sensations, and continuous verbal contact with the patient maintained during the procedure.

Topical anesthesia is initiated with proparacaine 0.03% to 0.5%, tetracaine 0.5%, or bupivacaine 0.75% eye drops. Anesthesia may be enhanced by additional drops of tetracaine 0.5% or lidocaine 4.0% every 5 or 10 minutes. This anesthesia may be supplemented by subconjunctival injection lidocaine 1.0% 1 to 2 ml or by orbital injection anesthesia if necessary.[29]

Injection Anesthesia

The safety and efficacy of injection anesthesia for cataract surgery have been enhanced by studies of orbital anatomy, computerized tomography (CT) imaging of orbital injection needles in situ, and CT imaging of orbital anesthetic solution spread. Anatomical factors include orbital size and shape, eye size, optic nerve and ophthalmic artery position, and orbital fascial compartments. CT images of orbital injection needles *in situ* have demonstrated the advantages of fixation in the primary position of gaze during inferior temporal orbital injections.[76] Anesthetic solutions in the retrobulbar and peribulbar space have been shown to spread into all parts of the retrobulbar space and anteriorly into the preseptal area of the eyelids.[70]

There are a multitude of terms used to describe injection anesthesia for ophthalmic anesthesia. Normally infiltration anesthesia describes subcutaneous or intraplanar deposits of local anesthesia, whereas nerve blocks refer to placement of local anesthesia immediately adjacent to a specific nerves. The term "*retrobulbar anesthesia*" has been adopted to indicate deposition of a local anesthetic solution in the "cone" immediately behind the globe, providing anesthesia to CN III, IV, and VI.

Unfortunately, there is no space behind the globe in which a membrane links each of extraocular muscles and encapsulates a neurovascular bundle. Rather, there is a retrobulbar space limited anteriorly by the equator of the globe and extending posteriorly to include the optic nerve, the rectus muscles and all of the tissue between them. Posteriorly, the rectus muscle converges sufficiently to define a retrobulbar conal space. Atkinson described a retrobulbar block in which the ciliary ganglion and ciliary nerves within this muscular cone were blocked. Spread of local anesthetic extended the block to include the extraocular muscles.

Alternatively, if an injection of local anesthetic is placed outside of the "cone," but the spread of the local anesthetic extends sufficiently to produce akinesia and anesthesia, then the block may be termed "peribulbar," but the block really anesthetizes the same structures as a retrobulbar block.

The dura splits into two layers at the entrance of the optic nerve. The parietal dura becomes the periorbita. The visceral layer of dura covers the optic nerve and becomes the optic sheath continuing forward as Tenon's capsule. Thus, any block between the orbital apex and the orbital septum functions as an orbital epidural block.

Knapp is first credited with publishing the method of retrobulbar anesthesia, in association with local anesthesia for enucleation.[47] Atkinson described a method in which the sensory nerves of the conjunctiva and orbit were blocked in addition to a retrobulbar injection into the muscular cone.[5]

A retrobulbar injection is any injection in which the needle passes behind the equator of the globe. The anesthetic then passes directly into the "retrobulbar space." All such injections, regardless of initial approach can be considered retrobulbar injections. All sensory nerves to the globe and the orbit, as well as all of the extraocular muscles transverse the retrobulbar space. Even if the local anesthetic does not block the abducens, the oculomotor or trochlear nerves, it may still produce adequate operative anesthesia.

A number of needles have been optimized for use in ophthalmic nerve blocks. These needles have a difference of bevel, length and gauge compared with those used by other physicians. The angle of the point of the needle, or bevel, is an important differentiation point. The longer the bevel (shallower angle), the "sharper" the needle and the less force is needed for penetration of the tissue. A shorter bevel is duller and may in fact core tissue. A needle may have multiple faces cut so that it penetrates skin without coring. The Atkinson needle was expressly developed for ophthalmic blocks. It has a short bevel, with multiple faces so that it makes a nearly flat incision through the skin without coring.

In our institution we use a 25-gauge, 36-mm disposable Atkinson retrobulbar needle for retrobulbar anesthesia. This needle has the characteristic of easy entrance through the skin and smooth placement in the orbit. We use an equal mixture of lidocaine 2.0% with epinephrine and bupivacaine 0.75% with hyaluronidase (5.0 turbidity units per ml) as our anesthetic solution.

Injection, performed with the eye in the primary position, commences at the inferior orbital margin approximately 5 mm nasal to the lateral orbital margin. The needle is aimed at the inferior edge of the superior orbital fissure and inserted 31 mm. The needle remains in the inferior temporal orbit and always stays inferior and lateral to the optic nerve, ophthalmic artery, and optic axis (Fig. 83-3).

Aspiration of the needle is followed by slow injection (1 ml per 10 sec) of 3.0 to 3.5 ml of anesthetic solution. Needle movement during the injection is minimized and an additional 1.0 ml of anesthetic solution is injected slowly (1 ml per 20 sec) anterior to the orbital septum upon with-

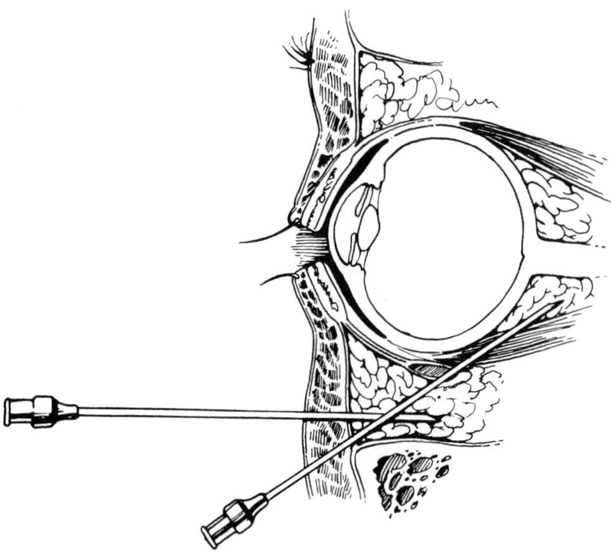

Fig. 83-3. Retrobulbar block. (From Spaeth GL: *Ophthalmic surgery: principles and practice,* Philadelphia, 1982, WB Saunders.)

drawal of the needle. Immediately after completion of the injection, moderate pressure is applied to the eye and orbit through closed lids for 3 to 5 minutes.

Outcome of the injection is evaluated 10 minutes after the injection and supplementation using the same technique may be necessary in about 10% of patients. The complication rate of orbital injection anesthesia has been reported in a number of large series. Among these reports are a report of 12,000 orbital anesthetic injections,[36] a description of 12,500 consecutive retrobulbar injections[27] and a report of over 50,000 orbital injections.[33] Complications of a significant nature are rare if attention is given to case selection, orbital anatomy and injection procedure. **Major complications include scleral perforation or globe penetration, optic nerve injury, extraocular muscle paresis, severe retrobulbar hemorrhage, intraocular vascular occlusion, and central spread of the local anesthesia to the brain stem (retrobulbar apnea syndrome).** The latter requires respiratory and cardiovascular support until the effects of anesthesia wear off. Special care must be taken in the presence of adverse anatomical factors, particularly in the presence of a large myopic globe with an axial length greater than 26 or 27 mm, and in patients with severe or inadequately controlled systemic vascular disease.[24]

Some physicians apply manual compression to assist the spread of local anesthesia following ophthalmic nerve blocks. Manual compression, or a mechanical compression device (such as a Honen's balloon) may also be used to produce a "soft eye" (decrease IOP) before eye surgery. Compression has been used with great safety over a number of years, however, case reports can be found implicating orbital compression as the cause of postoperative ptosis and more importantly, impairing retinal circulation.[6,42] Postoperative ptosis is a complication that can be seen both after ophthalmic and nonophthalmic surgery. After ophthalmic surgery, it can be caused by edema of the upper lid from local anesthesia, pressure applied to the globe or orbital rim either by a lid speculum or by a face mask.[42] When compression on the globe is used, the pressure exerted should be substantially below diastolic pressure to ensure that vascular impairment does not occur.

Facial Nerve Blocks

Despite an eyelid retractor, patients may squeeze their eyelids shut during ophthalmic surgery. The orbicularis occuli is the muscle that mediates the squeeze. It is innervated by branches of the facial nerve. Various facial nerve blocks have been developed to ensure akinesia of the eyelids (Fig. 83-4). These blocks include:

- **Modified van Lint.**[78] The needle is inserted 1 cm lateral to the lateral orbital rim, and 2 to 4 ml of anesthetic is injected deeply on the periosteum just lateral to the superolateral and inferolateral orbital rim.
- **O'Brien.**[64] The mandibular condyle is palpated inferior to the posterior zygomatic process and anterior to the tragus of the ear as the patient opens and closes the jaw. The needle is inserted perpendicular to the skin about 1 cm to the periosteum. As the needle is withdrawn, 3 ml of anesthetic is injected.
- **Nadbath-Rehman.**[62] A 12-mm, 25-gauge needle is inserted perpendicular to the skin between the mastoid process and the posterior border of the mandible. The needle is advanced its full length, and after careful aspiration, 5 ml of anesthetic is injected. This blocks the entire trunk of the facial nerve as it exits the skull at the stylomastoid foramen. As noted previously, the facial nerve exits the stylomastoid foramen accompanied by the internal carotid artery. Careful aspiration and stabilization of the needle during the injection is essential for patient safety. The patient should be told to expect a lower facial droop for several hours postoperatively.

The local anesthetic solution used most at our institution for facial nerve block is a combination of bupivacaine 0.75% and lidocaine 2% in a 1:1 ratio with epinephrine. Hyaluronidase is added to speed tissue penetration. Alternately, mepivicaine 2% with epinephrine may be used. In all cases injection should be slow (1 ml per 10 sec) to minimize discomfort to the patient.

GENERAL ANESTHESIA

General anesthesia is used in approximately 35% of the ophthalmic surgery cases at our institution, the most common of which are lengthy retinal surgery and pediatric strabismus surgery. Indications for general anesthesia include:

- Inability of the patient to coöperate with MAC (e.g., children, adults with mental or psychologic deficits, tremor, inability to lie supine, etc.).
- Complete ocular akinesia desired by surgeon.

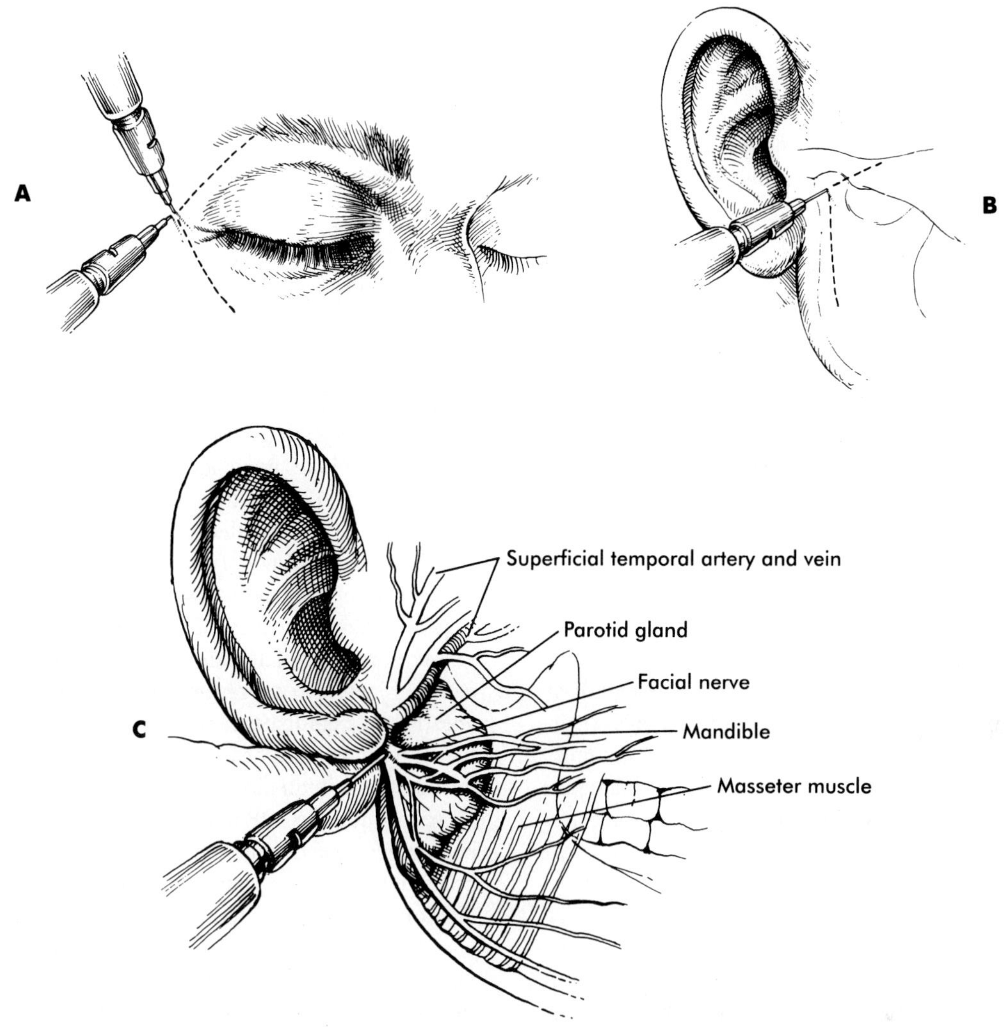

Fig. 83-4. Facial nerve blocks. **A,** van Lint; **B,** O'Brien; **C,** Nadbath. (From Spaeth GL: *Ophthalmic surgery: Principles and practice,* Philadelphia, 1982, WB Saunders.)

- Lengthy procedure (> 3 to 4 hours).
- Surgical field not amenable to regional, local, or topical anesthesia.
- Regional block technically difficult or contraindicated (e.g., large myopic globe, coagulopathy, etc.).
- Intrathecal or intravascular injection of local anesthetic.
- Surgeon or patient preference.

Controversy exists as the relative safety of general and regional anesthesia in ophthalmic surgery. The two techniques have shown no postoperative differences with regard to memory,[43] cognitive function,[15] or oxygen saturation.[54] The incidences of mortality and major complications are also similar.[52] Regional anesthesia has been reported to be associated with fewer episodes of intraoperative oxygen desaturation, hemodynamic fluctuation,[15] postoperative nausea and vomiting (PONV),[52] and less initial postoperative pain.[48] Regional anesthesia for ophthalmic surgery has also been shown to be free of the hormonal stress response associated with general anesthesia.[9,10] With these considerations in mind, it would seem prudent to avoid general anesthesia if possible, in patients with severe cardiovascular or pulmonary disease, as well as those who are particularly prone to PONV.

The goals of general anesthesia for ophthalmic surgery include a smooth induction with stable IOP, avoidance or treatment of severe oculocardiac reflexes, maintenance of a motionless field, a smooth emergence, and avoidance of PONV. These goals can be accomplished in a variety of ways, using inhalation anesthesia, IV agents, or a combined technique. Muscle relaxants are especially useful during intraocular microsurgery, when the slightest patient movement can be disastrous (see section on anesthesia-related eye injuries).

"Deep extubation" is a term we use to describe the extubation of a patient before complete awakening has occurred. Other centers may define "deep extubation" somewhat differently. It is indicated whenever there is a compromised globe, intravitreal gas, or whenever it is essential to avoid an increase in IOP from tracheal stimulation. Deep extubations are performed just after the patient has passed through stage 2, which is classically described as "delirium" to stage 1—"analgesia." This stage of anesthesia is characterized by slow regular breathing with diaphragm and intercostal muscles, and the presence of a lid reflex. A patient extubated at this time experiences amnesia, analgesia, and sedation. Extubations at this point have a minimum of tracheal stimulation, but there is a small possibility of aspiration, because airway reflexes have not completely returned. As such, patients with full stomachs (having recently ingested food or drink prior to surgery) or patients with a compromised airway are not good candidates for deep extubation.

OPEN GLOBE, FULL STOMACH

The ocular trauma patient presents a dilemma for the anesthesiologist who wishes both to protect the patient from aspirating stomach contents and to protect the eye from losing vitreous. A rapid-sequence intravenous induction is needed to protect the airway, but theoretic concerns have arisen about the use of succinylcholine. The classic rapid-sequence induction using succinylcholine will provide excellent intubating conditions in less than 1 minute. Paralysis will dissipate in 4 to 6 minutes. Succinylcholine does, however, increase IOP by 6 to 12 mm Hg for approximately 5 minutes[65] and has been implicated in the loss of vitreous during ocular surgery.[22,51] Following initial reports in 1955, most anesthesiologists avoided the use of succinylcholine in patients with open eye injuries. In 1968, Miller et al.[58] published a technique for avoiding succinylcholine-induced intraocular hypertension by pretreating with nondepolarizing muscle relaxants. Precurarization has since become a commonly accepted method of dealing with the open globe/full stomach situation. There have been no published reports of loss of intraocular contents linked to its use.[50,60]

Modifications of the classic rapid-sequence induction which use nondepolarizing muscle relaxants in place of succinylcholine have also been proposed. Typically these have involved using high doses of relaxant to achieve a rapid onset. A priming method, in which one third of non-depolarizing muscle relaxant is administered several minutes before induction, followed by the remaining dose immediately after the induction agent is given has also been described.[75] These techniques generally result in good intubating conditions within 60 to 90 seconds from loss of consciousness, but paralysis lasts far longer than with succinylcholine. Depending on the agent and technique employed and the length of the surgical procedure, temporary postoperative mechanical ventilation may be required. New nondepolarizing muscle relaxants are being continuously developed in an effort to duplicate succinylcholine's speed without the side effects. Currently, the agent that comes the closest in terms of onset is rocuronium. A 1.2-mg/kg dose will allow intubation in approximately 1 minute with minimal side effects. Unfortunately, paralysis will last for more than 1 hour at this dose.

If rapid-sequence induction is indeed indicated, succinylcholine with precurarization and rocuronium are both effective and safe for the eye. Succinylcholine has the advantage of rapid offset, whereas rocuronium has fewer side effects and provides better hemodynamic stability. Thus, the decision of which relaxant to use should be based on the anticipated length of surgery and the presence of risk factors for the use of succinylcholine.

ANESTHESIA FOR PEDIATRIC OPHTHALMOLOGY

Anesthesia for pediatric ophthalmology encompasses a diverse group of patients and procedures. It has been said that pediatric ophthalmic anesthesiology can be considered a separate subspecialty.[4] Patients range from newborns with medical problems associated with prematurity, to children with congenital syndromes, to the healthy adolescents. The procedures that the pediatric ophthalmic patient undergoes are also diverse. Many of the ophthalmic procedures that are performed in adults with Monitored Anesthesia Care (MAC) require general anesthesia in the pediatric population.

Measurement of IOP in the awake child is difficult because of lack of cooperation and frequently requires general anesthesia (examination under anesthesia [EUA]). IOP is affected by most anesthetic drugs and practices such as laryngoscopy and intubation. Therefore, most ophthalmologists prefer to measure IOP before a deep level of anesthesia has been reached and intubation has been performed. It is our practice to allow measurement of the IOP soon after the induction of anesthesia and before instrumentation of the airway has taken place. This is accomplished by positioning the mask and hand of the anesthesiologist so that the ophthalmologist has unobstructed access to the eye. Instillation of topical anesthetic drops into the eye may allow earlier IOP measurement than otherwise possible. If necessary, the mask can be removed to allow IOP measurement and then replaced. If further examination is required (e.g., ultrasound, gonioscopy), the patient is either intubated or a laryngeal mask airway is inserted.

Measurement of IOP in the pediatric patient is performed to diagnose glaucoma or to follow the efficacy of therapy. Congenital glaucoma can be associated with several systemic syndromes (e.g., rubella, oculocerebrorenal [Lowe] syndrome). In addition, Sturge-Weber disease or congenital capillary hemangioma may effect the skin of the face, neck, mucous membranes, meninges, and choroid plexus. If the affected areas include the distribution of the fifth cranial nerve, glaucoma is commonly found. These patients also have seizure disorders. Children with Sturge-Weber disease come to the operating room for frequent examinations under anesthesia to follow efficacy of surgical and medical interventions. Good rapport and appropriate use of premedicants allow a smooth induction of anesthesia and the most accurate measurement of IOP.

Strabismus surgery is the most common type of ophthalmic surgery performed in children. **The incidence of postoperative nausea and vomiting has been reported to**

be greater than 50% in numerous studies. Many different anesthetic techniques and antiemetic regimens have been used in an attempt to decrease this high incidence of nausea and vomiting. Abramowitz et al.[1] showed that 75 μg/kg of droperidol was effective in reducing nausea and vomiting following strabismus surgery. This dose may cause profound sedation and contribute to a delayed discharge.[37] Watcha et al.[80] found that patients receiving propofol alone after a mask induction with halothane had an incidence of emesis in the first 24 hours of 23% versus 50% in those receiving halothane, N_2O, or droperidol. All of the patients in the study received perioperative opioids, which may have contributed to the high incidence of emetic symptoms. In addition, emergence from anesthesia, time to oral intake, ambulation and fitness for discharge were more rapid in those receiving propofol for maintenance of anesthesia. Propofol has become widely used in outpatient surgical settings because of these characteristics. Whether propofol has intrinsic antiemetic properties is controversial. It has become common practice at this institution to discontinue halothane following induction and use a propofol infusion for maintenance of anesthesia.

The choice of patients who should received prophylactic antiemetics is controversial. Postoperative emesis is multifactorial in origin, including many nonanesthetic factors. The incidence of emesis is higher in the pediatric population. A history of motion sickness, previous postoperative nausea, obesity, and anxiety have been found to be correlated. In this institution, only those patients with risk factors for emesis are given prophylaxis. If risk factors are present, ondansetron, a selective $5HT_3$ receptor antagonist, is used in the dose of 0.1 mg/kg. This regimen has been shown to be more effective in reducing the incidence of emesis in pediatric ambulatory patients when compared with 75 μg/kg of droperidol.[19] Patients receiving ondansetron also had shorter hospital stays than those receiving droperidol. If sedation is desired, then droperidol is a good alternative.

The OCR is frequently elicited during strabismus surgery by traction on the extraocular muscles. The incidence of OCR appears to be higher in patients receiving propofol anesthesia when compared with halothane.[80]

Nasolacrimal duct (NLD) probing for obstruction is another common procedure performed in pediatric ophthalmic patients. Successful relief of obstruction diminishes after the first year of life, so many of these patients are infants. The use of the laryngeal mask airway (LMA) provides unobstructed access to the patient for the surgeon and protects the airway from the fluorescein dye that is injected into the nasolacrimal duct.

When an infant or young child presents with poor vision but normal ocular structures, electroretinography can help differentiate between retinal disorders. This procedure is generally performed in a completely dark laboratory and requires a period of approximately 20 minutes for the retina to dark adapt. General anesthesia or sedation are required as the child is usually not able to cooperate for the examination. Prior to the beginning of the procedure, the anesthesiologist must become familiar with where the various pieces of equipment and power outlets are located, and be completely satisfied with the setup.

Retinopathy of prematurity (ROP), previously called *retrolental fibroplasia* usually occurs in premature infants. Although a disease of complex etiologies, it is believed to be primarily related to hyperoxic periods during neonatal intensive care. Nonetheless, full-term infants can have this condition as well as premature infants who have never had oxygen therapy. Following initial examinations in the intensive care unit, the child may come to the operating room for multiple EUAs and vitreoretinal procedures such as scleral buckling or vitrectomy. The care of the ex-premature infant is complex and must start with a thorough history and physical examination. Important historical data include gestational age at birth, birth weight, duration of intubation, and ventilation, history of apneic episodes, and other congenital anomalies.[63] Hyaline membrane disease (HMD) occurs in 60% to 80% of infants born less than 28 weeks gestation. HMD may progress to the chronic pulmonary disease of prematurity called *bronchopulmonary dysplasia* (BPD). Although BPD improves with growth and development, these children should be considered at risk for having increased airway reactivity.

If an inhalation induction is chosen, intravenous or inhalation anesthesia may be used for maintenance. Intravenous access is rapidly secured so that the amount of inhalational agent can be decreased and muscle relaxants administered. For retinal cases, paralysis is maintained throughout the procedure, as a motionless field is critical. Conservative amounts of opioids, most commonly fentanyl, are administered. In the very premature infant, who had required intubation and controlled ventilation after birth and who has recently been extubated, it may be difficult to extubate at the end of retinal surgery. Although extubation should be the goal at the conclusion of surgery, the endotracheal tube should be left in place if the child does not have a regular respiratory pattern or is much less vigorous than preoperatively.

In 1982, anesthesiologists were first alerted to the occurrence of postoperative apnea in the ex-premature infant recovering from minor surgical procedures after general anesthesia.[73] Exactly when these infants are no longer at risk is not definitely known;[17] however, it is known that the incidence of apnea is strongly related to gestational age and postconceptual age. **Criterion for hospital admission for apnea monitoring after general anesthesia varies from institution to institution. A conservative range would be admission for those infants less than 50 to 54 weeks postconceptual age.**

In pediatric patients, it is especially important to calculate the amount of local anesthetic drug that is allowable to prevent toxicity. It is also important to know whether these solutions contain epinephrine and the amount contained within. The dosages are calculated on a per-kilogram basis and can be easily exceeded in the very small child. The recommended safe maximal dose of the commonly used local anesthetics in ophthalmology are:

lidocaine—7 mg/kg;

bupivacaine—3 mg/kg; and

cocaine—2 mg/kg. In a patient anesthetized with halothane, 1.5 μg/kg epinephrine should not be exceeded; when isoflurane is used, up to 3 μg/kg are acceptable. These dosages of epinephrine are conservative and may be repeated after 10 minutes if there have been no untoward effects.

As noted earlier, there are systemic effects of drugs used in ophthalmology. Most of these drugs come in varying concentrations, and the least concentrated effective form should be used in small children to avoid toxicity. One drug that is used often in the operating room to produce mydriasis is phenylephrine hydrochloride. Only the 2.5% solution should be used in pediatrics, because excessive absorption can cause hypertension.

OPHTHALMIC PROCEDURES

Strabismus

Strabismus means ocular misalignment or deviation of one eye relative to the visual axis of the other. The etiology may be related to abnormalities in binocular vision or neuromuscular problems of ocular motility. A detailed nomenclature has evolved to describe the various patterns of strabismus. The prefix "*eso-*" denotes deviation nasally, whereas "*exo-*" denotes temporal deviation. The suffix "*-phoria*" describes the tendency of one eye to turn outward and "*-tropia*" describes inward deviation.

The surgical correction of strabismus is a repositioning of the extraocular muscles. To strengthen a muscle, a resection is performed. To weaken a muscle, a recession is performed. In severe cases, a resection may be performed on one muscle, and a recession on the opposing muscle. Because visual maturation occurs by 5 years of age, strabismus correction is usually attempted early in childhood. If left uncorrected, amblyopia, or a defect in central vision occurs. Adjustable sutures are sometimes used to improve the chances of alignment with a single operation. The adjustment is performed in the immediate postoperative period, when the patient is fully awake and able to focus.

Pediatric patients undergoing strabismus surgery require general anesthesia. As noted before, some adult patients do well with a regional technique and intravenous sedation. Most patients prefer general anesthesia and have a particularly satisfactory result with propofol which seems to decrease PONV.

Cornea

Penetrating keratoplasty

Penetrating keratoplasty (PKP) refers to surgical replacement of a portion of the cornea with donor tissue. If donor tissue is from the patient, it is called an *autograft.* If the tissue is from another person, it is called an *allograft.* The indications for this procedure are many—corneal opacity, keratoconus, infection, and scarring are a few. Either regional or general anesthesia may be appropriate for this procedure.

Pterygium

A pterygium is a fold of conjunctiva and fibrovascular tissue that has invaded the superficial cornea. There is a strong association with ultraviolet exposure. Excision is indicated when vision becomes impaired or the lesion causes irritation. Topical anesthesia or injection anesthesia, with or without intravenous sedation, is satisfactory for removal.

Radial keratotomy

Radial keratotomy (RK) is the surgical procedure used to correct myopia. Recall that the cornea contributes approximately 30% of the refractive element of vision. Under topical anesthesia, a series of incisions is made in the cornea in a spokelike manner, causing a positive diopter change in vision. The indications and rationale for RK remain controversial. Typically, these procedures are performed with topical anesthesia only.

Cataracts

Cataracts are a common cause of visual impairment in older individuals. The pathogenesis of cataracts is multifactorial, but basically results in opacity of the lens. Extracapsular cataract extraction (ECCE) is the preferred method of routine cataract extraction. The procedure is performed through a smaller incision and is less traumatic to the corneal endothelium. Removal of the lens with an intact posterior capsule provides for better positioning of an intraocular lens implant. Phacoemulsification is an ECCE technique performed through a 3- to 4-mm incision. The nucleus of the cataract is fragmented by an ultrasonic needle and then aspirated. Intracapsular cataract extraction (ICCE) is a technique that completely removes the lens with the capsule through a much larger incision. ICCE is performed in selected cases and in locations where sophisticated equipment is not available. Cataract extraction is usually performed with a retrobulbar or peribulbar injection and a facial nerve block. Intravenous sedation and analgesia may be given for the placement of the block. In selected patients, a rapid and skilled surgeon can perform the procedure under topical anesthesia.

Glaucoma

Glaucoma is a general term for a group of eye diseases characterized by an increased IOP. Goniotomy is a procedure performed to treat infantile glaucoma. A superficial incision is made in the trabecular meshwork to improve outflow of aqueous humor from the anterior chamber. Infants and children require general anesthesia for this procedure. Trabeculectomy is the most commonly performed filtering procedure in adults. A block of limbal tissue is removed beneath a scleral flap that permits outflow of aqueous. Antimetabolites, such as mitomycin, can be injected intraoperatively to help prevent surgical failures secondary to scarring. Many different tubes or shunts have been used to divert aqueous (e.g., Molteno valve). These implants are generally reserved for cases that have not responded to other management. Those in current use have a plastic tube placed in the anterior chamber connected to a plate placed posterior to the limbus. Iridectomy is usually performed with a YAG laser, however, an incisional iridectomy may occasionally be required. Iridectomy is the definitive treatment in angle-closure glaucoma.

Anesthesia for glaucoma surgery in adults is usually performed with retrobulbar or peribulbar injection and a facial nerve block. Intravenous sedation and analgesia is typically given for placement of the blocks.

Vitreoretinal Surgery

Vitrectomy refers to surgical extraction of the contents of the vitreous chamber and their replacement with a physiologic solution. An anterior segment vitrectomy is performed for vitreous loss during cataract surgery and for late anterior segment vitreous complications. A posterior segment vitrectomy would be indicated for the removal of an intraocular foreign body, to manage complicated retinal detachments with intraocular membranes, to remove media opacities, and to alleviate vitreous traction on the retina. Because the surgery may be prolonged and many of the patients have medical problems (e.g., diabetes), vitrectomy can offer difficult challenges to the anesthesiologist.[62]

General anesthesia has been traditionally used for vitreoretinal surgery. However, using local anesthesia with MAC has become an attractive alternative. A retrobulbar block or perilimbal block under MAC offers several advantages to the ophthalmologist.[14] Following retrobulbar block, there is usually an absence of the OCR. The rapid recovery associated with MAC allows early prone positioning in the recovery room after posterior chamber gas injection. Patient comfort is also increased, because there is less nausea and vomiting along with a diminution of pain postoperatively.[59] Unfortunately, MAC is not suitable for long procedures. Procedures lasting longer than 3 to 4 hours exceed the tolerance of patients to lie supine and motionless. If necessary, a retrobulbar block can be supplemented during surgery by a sub-Tenon's injection with a blunt, 19-gauge needle.[55,71]

General anesthesia is appropriate for longer cases. It is also a useful technique when communication is difficult with the patient (e.g., young, hard of hearing, infirmed). General anesthesia has some disadvantages. There may be an increase in IOP, risking the retinal repair, at induction and during extubation. The OCR is much more common during general anesthesia, frequently requiring anticholinergic treatment. Following general anesthesia, patients require more systemic postoperative analgesics and antiemetics. Somnolence, pain, and nausea may delay the proper positioning of patients postoperatively.

When general anesthesia is used, there are significant advantages to the use of long-acting retrobulbar blockade. Retrobulbar "irrigation" with 0.75% bupivacaine greatly reduces the need for parenteral analgesics within the first 24 hours following surgery.[23] In a prospective double-masked study of patients receiving general anesthesia with or without retrobulbar block with 0.5% bupivacaine, the group receiving the bupivacaine had significantly less pain and nausea postoperatively.[34] Alternatively, under direct vision, a blunt 19-gauge cannula can be used to directly inject the anesthetic agent into the retrobulbar space via a sub-Tenon's approach.[59] This technique minimizes risk of scleral perforation.

Laryngoscopy and endotracheal intubation are the anesthesia practices most likely to significantly increase IOP (10 to 20 torr).[61] The mechanism probably relates to the sympathetic cardiovascular response to tracheal intubation. Pretreatment with lidocaine (1.5 mg/kg) or sufentanil (0.05 to 0.15 μg/kg) administered 3 to 5 minutes before induction can blunt the IOP response to tracheal stimulation.[7] Pretreatment with oral administered clonidine (5 μg/kg) given 1 hour prior to surgery will also blunt the IOP response.[31]

It is important to recognize the danger of using nitrous oxide when intravitreal gas is administered. To provide internal tamponade of the retina after reattachment, an intravitreal gas bubble (e.g., air, SF_6, or C_3F_8) replaces some of the vitreous. Nitrous oxide (N_2O) is a very insoluble gas in blood, but is 117 times more soluble than SF_6. N_2O enters the intraocular gas bubble more rapidly than SF_6 can exit. If N_2O continues to be administered after the injection of SF_6 gas into the vitreal cavity, the size of the injected gas can expand up to three times its original size.[74] Similar effects can be seen when C_3F_8 is used. Within 19 minutes in a closed eye, the IOP will increase by 14 to 30 torr. If nitrous is then discontinued, the bubble size will decrease by half within 18 minutes.[81] The resulting decrease in IOP can lead to redetachment of the retina. **Washout of N_2O from the lungs is 90% complete within 10 minutes, but to provide a margin of safety, N_2O should be discontinued at least 20 minutes *before* the intravitreal injection of gas.** It is important that patients returning for surgery within 3 to 4 weeks caution anesthesiologists that they have had an intravitreal gas injection. A similar hazard exists in air transport of patients. Because the aircraft cabin is pressurized to an altitude of approximately 2000 m above sea level, the gas bubble will expand, resulting in elevated IOP. Patients should therefore avoid air travel for 3 to 4 weeks following injection of intravitreal gas.[21]

Oculoplastic Surgery

All of the oculoplastic procedures listed below can be performed on adult patients with regional anesthesia.

Ectropion repair

An ectropion results from excess, loose eyelid tissue or scarring which causes the margin of the lid to turn outward, away from the globe (eversion). Repair is made by excising excess tissue and tightening the remaining lid, or by release of the related scar tissue.

Entropion repair

An entropion is usually caused by senile or involutional changes, primarily in the lower eyelids that result in weakening of the lid retractor muscles and horizontal laxity. The lid margin is turned inward toward the globe (inversion). The goal of surgical repair is to increase the tension of the

Table 83-4 Categories of ophthalmic emergencies

Category	Time frame	Examples
True emergencies	Therapy must be instituted within minutes	Chemical burns of cornea Central retinal artery occlusion
Urgent situations	Therapy should be instituted within hours	Penetrating injuries to globe Endophthalmitis Acute narrow-angle glaucoma Acute vitreal hemorrhage Pupillary block glaucoma Acute macular detachment Acute retinal tear w/hemorrhage Corneal foreign body Cavernous sinus thrombosis Hyphema Corneal ulcer Lid laceration
Semiurgent situations	Therapy should be instituted within days	Ocular tumors Acute exophthalmos Blow-out fracture Congenital cataract Old retinal detachment

retractor muscles (e.g., by reattaching them) and tighten any horizontal laxity.

Ptosis repair

Ptosis is a congenital or acquired drooping of the eyelid. It is most often repaired by shortening or reattaching the levator palpebrae aponeurosis. In cases in which levator function is inadequate, the upper lid can be suspended from the frontalis by means of a sling of fascia lata.

Blepharoplasty

Blepharoplasty is any plastic surgery of the eyelids, usually to remove redundant tissue. The procedure is performed to remove visual field obstruction and for cosmesis.

Dacrocystorhinostomy

Dacrocystorhinostomy (DCR) is the creation of a communication between the lacrimal sac and the nasal cavity to allow for tear drainage. A Jone's tube is sometimes used to bypass the canaliculi and form a conjunctivorhinostomy. Nasolacrimal duct probing is performed in children with congenital nasolacrimal duct obstruction. The duct is probed with a wire, then dye is injected into the duct and aspirated from the nasal cavity to test the patency of the duct. Silicon tubes may be inserted to act as stents.

Orbital Surgery

Most orbital surgery requires general anesthesia unless the procedure is limited to the anterior orbit and does not involve the bones of the orbit.

Orbitotomy

An orbitotomy is performed to gain surgical access to the orbit. Approaches include transconjunctival, transseptal, and transperiosteal. Indications for orbitotomy include tumor, abscess, foreign body, and orbital fractures.

Orbital decompression

Orbital decompression is indicated for correction of exophthalmos resulting from Grave's disease. Access to the orbit is obtained either by a transconjuntival or transperiosteal approach. Some surgeons use a coronal incision with reflection of the scalp anteriorly to the level of the orbit. Cases can be lengthy (4+ hours) and blood loss can be large enough to require transfusion.

Ophthalmic Emergencies

Most ophthalmic procedures are not emergencies. This is important to understand because the anesthetic plan depends on the patient's "nothing-by-mouth" (NPO) status and general condition. If the patient has a full stomach or a condition that can be reversed or improved by nonsurgical means, surgery should be delayed. This does not apply to true emergencies where therapy must be instituted within a matter of minutes (e.g., chemical burns of the cornea and central retinal artery occlusion). Many ophthalmic conditions are considered urgent, wherein therapy should be instituted within several hours. Ophthalmic conditions where therapy can be instituted within days or sometimes within weeks are considered semiurgent. Ophthalmic emergencies are categorized in Table 83-4.

ANESTHESIA-RELATED EYE INJURIES

There are many reported cases of iatrogenic ophthalmic injuries. At a reported incidence of 44% in the unprotected eye, corneal abrasion is the most common complication of both nonophthalmic and ophthalmic surgery.[11] Closed claims analysis has shown that permanent injury is relatively rare (16%).[32] In the case of nonophthalmic surgery, it is usually associated with failure to tape the eyelids shut (with or without ointment) until the patient has returned to consciousness. In the case of ophthalmic surgery, the patient who has undergone a local anesthetic block is at particular risk, because the cornea is insensitive in the postoperative period. Additionally, lacrimal gland function may be suppressed by either local or general anesthesia, making the cornea more susceptible to damage.[18] When lid function is impaired, the operated eye should be patched until sensation and motor function return.

Corneal abrasions can be prevented by placing a sterile lubricant over the cornea and/or taping the eyelids closed immediately after loss of consciousness. This prevents the dry gas mixture, which can leak from a poorly fitted mask, from coming into contact with the eyes and prevents contact between the exposed eye and an improperly held mask. If a patient emerges from general anesthesia complaining of a foreign body sensation, one should suspect a corneal abrasion and treat it promptly.[11] Left untreated, a corneal abrasion can develop into a corneal ulcer.

A second major category of eye injury results from patient movement during ophthalmic surgery. Closed claims analysis show these types of injuries to be associated with high severity of injury (blindness was the end result in all cases), relatively high levels of plaintiff compensation and a high incidence of deviations from the standard of care, especially in those injuries that occurred under general anesthesia.[32] These findings underscore the importance of vigilance on the part of the anesthesiologist during ophthalmic surgery. Movement-related eye injuries under general anesthesia should be preventable by a vigilant anesthesiologist.

Anesthesiologists must also be aware of the possible damage that can result from ocular compression. Patients at risk include those undergoing surgery in the supine position with a face mask, or those positioned lateral or prone. **If a patient emerges from general anesthesia complaining of visual impairment, it must be considered and treated as an emergency, because eye compression can cause central retinal artery (CRA) occlusion.** This can result in irreversible blindness because the CRA, a branch of the ophthalmic artery, supplies the optic nerve and the bipolar and ganglion cell layers of the retina. When using a face mask, one must be certain not to apply pressure to the eyes. When the patient is in the lateral or prone position, extreme care should be taken during positioning to make certain that the dependent eye or eyes are not compressed. The eyes should also be checked during the course of the anesthetic, because the position of an anesthetized patient can shift. **Systemic hypotension has also been associated with visual loss by decreasing retinal perfusion pressure.** Thus, avoiding ocular compression and systemic hypotension will help to prevent CRA occlusion and vision loss from occurring during general anesthesia.[39]

KEY POINTS

- An understanding of the anatomy and physiology of the eye along with the indications for ophthalmic procedures is essential in preparing an appropriate anesthetic plan. Likewise, a knowledge of the systemic effects of ophthalmic drugs is vital in determining and proceeding with this plan.
- Pressure on the globe or traction on the extraocular muscles can result in a trigeminovagal reflex (also known as OCR) that can manifest as bradycardia, AV block, ventricular ectopy, or asystole.
- The blood supply to the retina and optic nerve depends on the intraocular perfusion pressure. IOP is predominantly determined by the aqueous humor and choroidal blood volume. An increase in either constituent can lead to impedance of capillary blood supply to these vital structures.
- Deep inhalational or thiopental anesthesia decreases IOP, whereas ketamine or succinylcholine increases IOP and can result in extravasation of intraocular contents in an open globe injury.
- Although ophthalmic surgical procedures are considered "low-risk" in terms of blood loss, third-spacing of fluids, and postoperative pain, the patient population as a whole tends to be a "high-risk" group, which necessitates appropriate preoperative medical consultation.
- Most ophthalmic surgery requires akinesis of the eyelids and ocular muscles along with profound anesthesia of the surgical site.
- Facial nerve block produces akinesis of the eyelid and can result in temporary lower facial droop.
- Complications of retrobulbar block include retrobulbar hemorrhage, globe perforation, increased IOP, accidental ophthalmic artery injection causing convulsions, and subarachnoid injection via the optic nerve sheath with resultant obtundation and respiratory arrest.
- Neither regional nor general anesthesia has been demon-

strated to be safer in ophthalmic surgery; however, regional offers some advantages, such as less postoperative nausea and vomiting, greater cardiopulmonary stability, quicker return to ambulation, and prolonged postoperative analgesia.

- Nitrous oxide should not be used for 20 minutes before the use of intravitreal gas in vitreoretinal surgery and should be avoided for 3 to 4 weeks thereafter to prevent bubble expansion and a significant increase in IOP.
- Pediatric ophthalmic anesthesiology can be considered a separate subspecialty because of the multitude of potential anesthetic risks and complications that can occur in patients with underlying congenital syndromes.
- Whereas true emergencies such as chemical burns of the cornea and central retinal artery occlusions require immediate therapy, urgent situations such as penetrating injuries to the globe can often be delayed for several hours, to allow time for optimization of the general condition of the patient.
- Eye compression caused by a face mask or positioning can result in central retinal artery occlusion or corneal abrasion.

KEY REFERENCES

Barker JP, Vafdis GC, Robinson PN, Hall GM: Plasma catecholamine response to cataract surgery: a comparison between general and local anaesthesia, *Anaesthesia* 46:642, 1991.

Campbell DNC, Lim M, Kerr Muir M, O'Sullivan G, Falcon M, Fison P, Woods R: A prospective randomized study of local versus general anaesthesia for cataract surgery, *Anaesthesia* 48:422–428, 1993.

Donlon JV: Local anesthesia for ophthalmic surgery: patient preparation and management, *Ann Ophthalmol* 12:1183, 1980.

Duncalf D: Anesthesia and intraocular pressure, *Bull NY Acad Med* 51:374, 1975.

McGoldrick KE, editor: *Anesthesia for ophthalmic and otolaryngologic surgery,* Philadelphia, 1992, WB Saunders.

Stead SW: Complications in ophthalmic anesthesiology, *Semin Anesth,* 15:171–182, 1996.

REFERENCES

1. Abramowitz MD, Oh TH, Epstein BS, Ruttiman UE, Friendly DS: The antiemetic effect of droperidol following outpatient strabismus surgery in children, *Anesthesiology* 59:579–583, 1983.
2. Alexander JP: Reflex disturbance of cardiac rhythm during ophthalmic surgery, *Br J Opthalmol* 59:518–522, 1975.
3. Antal M: Ketamine aneaesthesia and intraocular pressure, *Ann Ophthalmol* 10 (9), 1281–1289, 1978.
4. Arthur DS, Dewar KMS: Anaesthesia for eye surgery in children, *Br J Anaesth* 52: 681, 1980.
5. Atkinson WS: Local anesthesia in ophthalmology, *Tr Am Ophth Soc* 32:399–451; 1934.
6. Atkinson WS: Akinesia of the orbicularis, *Am J Ophthalmol* 26:1255–1258, 1953.
7. Badrinath SK, Vacery A, McCarthy RJ, et al: Alfentantil and sufentanil prevent the increase in IOP from succinylcholine, *Anesth Analg* 67:S5, 1988.
8. Bailey PL: Timolol and postoperative apnea in neonates and young infants [letter]. *Anesthesiology* 61(5):622, 1984.
9. Barker JP, Robinson GC, et al: Local analgesia prevents the cortisol and glycaemic response to cataract surgery, *Br J Anaesth* 64: 442, 1990.
10. Barker JP, Vafdis GC, Robinson PN, Hall GM: Plasma catecholamine response to cataract surgery: a comparison between general and local anaesthesia, *Anaesthesia* 46: 642, 1991.
11. Barta KY, Bali MI: Corneal abrasions during general anesthesia, *Anesth Analg* 56:363, 1977.
12. Beatie CD, Stead SW: Cardiorespiratory stability and amnesia with propofol and alfentanil sedation, *Anesthesiology* 77(3A), 1992.
13. Bruce RA Jr: Ocular anatomy. In Bruce RA Jr, McGoldrick KE, Oppenheimer P, editors: *Anesthesia for ophthalmology,* Birmingham, 1982, Aesculapius Publishing.
14. Brucker AJ, Saran BR, Maguire AM: Perilimbal anesthesia for pars plana vitrectomy, *Am J Ophthalmol* 117(5):599–602, 1994.
15. Campbell DNC, Lim M, Kerr Muir M, O'Sullivan G, Falcon M, Fison P, Woods R: A prospective randomized study of local versus general anaesthesia for cataract surgery, *Anaesthesia* 48:422–428, 1993.
16. Cook JH: The effect of suxamethonium on intraocular pressure, *Anaesthesia* 36:359, 1981.
17. Cote' CJ, Zaslavsky A, Downes JJ, Kurth CD, Welborn LG, Warner LO, Malviya SV: Postoperative apnea in former preterm infants after inguinal herniorrhaphy, *Anesthesiology* 82, 809–822, 1995.
18. Cross DA, Krupin T: Implications of the effect of general anesthesia on basal tear production, *Anesth Analg* 56:35, 1977.
19. Davis PJ, McGowan FX Jr, Landsman I, Maloney K, Hoffmann P: Effect of antiemetic therapy on recovery and hospital discharge time, *Anesthesiology* 83:956–960, 1995.
20. De Roeth A, Dettbarn WD, Rosenberg P: Effect of phospholine iodide on blood cholinesterase levels, *Am J Ophthalmol* 59: 586, 1965.
21. Dieckert JP, O'Connor PS, Schaklett DE, et al: Air travel and intraocular gas, *Ophthalmology* 93:642, 1986.
22. Dillon JB, Sabawala P, Taylor DB, Gunter R: Action of succinylcholine on extraocular muscles and intraocular pressure, *Anesthesiology* 18:44, 1957.
23. Duker JS, Nielsen J, Vander JF, et al: Retrobulbar bupivacaine irrigation for postoperative pain after scleral buckling surgery, *Ophthalmology* 98:514, 1991.
24. Duker JS, Belmont JB, Benson WE, Brooks HL, Brown GC, Federman JL, et al: Inadvertent globe perforation during retrobulbar and peribulbar anesthesia: patient characteristics, surgical management, and visual outcome, *Ophthalmology* 98:519–526, 1991.
25. Duncalf D, Foldes FF: Effect of anesthetic drugs and muscle relaxants on intraocular pressure, *Int Ophthalmol Clin* 13:21, 1973.
26. Duncalf D, Weitzner SW: The influence of ventilation and hypercapnia on intraocular

pressure during anesthesia, *Anesth Analg* 42:232, 1963.
27. Edge KR, Nicoll JMV: Retrobulbar hemorrhage after 12,500 retrobulbar blocks, *Anesth Analg* 76:1019–1022, 1993.
28. Feneck RO, Cook JH: Failure of diazepam to prevent the suxamethonium-induced rise in intraocular pressure, *Anaesthesia* 38:120, 1983.
29. Fichman RA: Fichman technique for topical anesthesia. Ophthalmic Anesthesia. In Gills JP, Hustead RF, Sanders DR, editors: *Ophthalmic anesthesia,* Thorofare, NJ, 1993, Slack.
30. Fraunfelder FT, Scafidi AF: Possible adverse effects from topical ocular 10% phenylephrine, *Am J Ophthalmol* 85(4): 447–453, 1978.
31. Ghignone M, Noe C, Calvillo O, et al: *Anesthesia for ophthalmic surgery in the elderly, Anesthesiology* 68:707, 1988.
32. Gild WM, Posner KL, Caplan RA, Cheney FW: Eye injuries associated with anesthesia. A closed claims analysis, *Anesthesiology* 76:204, 1992.
33. Gills JP, Loyd T: Anesthesia for ophthalmic surgery. In Gills JP, Hustead RF, Sanders DR, editors: Thorofare, NJ, 1993, Slack.
34. Gottfreothsdottir MS, Gislason I, Stefansson E, et al: Effects of retrobulbar bupivacaine on post-operative pain and nausea in retinal detachment surgery, *Acta Ophthalmica* 71(4):544–547, 1993.
35. Haddad NJ, Moyer NJ, Riley FC Jr: Mydriatic effect of phenylephrine hydrochloride, *Am J Ophthalmol,* 70(5):729–733, 1970.
36. Hamilton RC, Gimbel HV, Strunin L: Regional anaesthesia for 12,000 cataract extraction and intraocular lens implantation procedures, *Can J Anaesth* 35:615–623, 1988.
37. Hardy JF, Charest J, Girouard G, Lepage Y: Nausea and vomiting after strabismus surgery in preschool children, *Can Anaesth Soc J* 33:57–62, 1986.
38. Hovi-Viander M: Death associated with anaesthesia in Finland, *Br J Anaesth* 52:483, 1980.
39. Jampol LM, Goldblum M, Rosenberg M: Ischemia of posterior ciliary artery circulation from ocular compression, *Arch Ophthalmol* 93:1311, 1975.
40. Jay JL: Functional organization of the human eye, *Br J Anaesth* 52:649, 1980.
41. Jones FL Jr, Ekberg NL: Exacerbation of asthma by timolol [letter], *New Engl J Med* 301(5):270, 1979.
42. Kaplan LJ, Jaffes NS, Clayman HM: Ptosis and cataract surgery, *Ophthalmology* 92: 237–242, 1985.
43. Karhunen U, Jonn G: A comparison of memory function following local and general anesthesia for extraction of senile cataract, *Acta Anaesthesiol Scand* 26:291, 1982.
44. Katz RL, Bigger JT: Cardiac Arrhythmias during anesthesia and operation, *Anesthesiology* 33(2):193–213, 1970.
45. Kelly RE, Dinner M, Turner LS, et al: Succinylcholine increases intraocular pressure in the human eye with the extraocular muscles detached, *Anesthesiology* 79(5): 948–952, 1993.
46. Kim JW, Smith PH: Timolol-induced bradycardia, *Anesth Analg* 59(4):301–303, 1980.
47. Knapp H: On cocaine and its use in ophthalmic and general surgery, *Arch Ophthalmol* 13:402, 1884.
48. Koay P, Laing A, Adams K, Branney S, Mathison J, Freeland F, Studley M, Black H: Ophthalmic pain following cataract surgery: a comparison between local and general anesthesia, *Br J Ophthalmol* 76(4):225–227, 1992.
49. Kraushar MF, Turner MF: Medical malpractice litigation in cataract surgery, *Arch Ophthalmol* 105:1339, 1987.
50. Libonati MM, Leahy JJ, Ellison N: The use of succinylcholine in open eye surgery, *Anesthesiology* 62:637, 1985.
51. Lincoff HA, Breinin GM, DeVoe AG: The effect of succinylcholine on extraocular muscles, *Am J Opthalmol* 43:440, 1957.
52. Lynch S, Wolf GL, Berlin I: General anesthesia for cataract surgery: a comparative review of 2217 consecutive cases, *Anesth Analg* 53:909, 1974.
53. Mahajan RP, Grover VK, Munjal VP, et al: Double-blind comparison of lidocaine, tubocurarine and diazepam pretreatment in modifying intraocular pressure increases, *Can J Anaesth* 34:41, 1987.
54. McCarthy, GJ, Mirakhur RK, Elliott P: Postoperative oxygenation in the elderly following general or local anaesthesia for ophthalmic surgery, *Anaesthesia* 47:1090–1092, 1992.
55. Mein CE, Woodcock MG: Ocular anesthesia for cataract surgery: A direct sub-tenon's approach, *Retina* 10:47, 1990.
56. Meyers EF, Krupin T, Johnson M, et al: Failure of nondepolarizing neuromuscular blockers to inhibit succinylcholine induced increased intraocular pressure, *Anesthesiology* 48:149, 1978.
57. Meyers EF, Singer P, Otto A: A controlled study of the effect of succinylcholine self-taming on intraocular pressure, *Anesthesiology* 53:72, 1980.
58. Miller RD, Way WL, Hickey RF: Inhibition of succinylcholine-induced intraocular hypertension by non-depolarizing muscle relaxants, *Anesthesiology* 29:123, 1968.
59. Murat J, Chauvaud D: Evaluation of a simplified protocol of local regional anesthesia for the surgery of the posterior segment, *J Franc D Ophtalmol* 16(4):254, 1993.
60. Murphy DF, Davis MJ: Succinylcholine use in emergency eye operations, *Can J Anaesth* 34:101, 1987.
61. Murphy DF: Anesthesia and intraocular pressure, *Anesth Analg* 64:250, 1985.
62. Nadbath RP, Rehman I: Facial nerve block, *Am J Ophthalmol* 55:143, 1963.
63. Nelson WE, Vaughan VC III, McKay RJ Jr, Behrman RE: *Textbook of pediatrics,* ed 14, Philadelphia, 1992, WB Saunders.
64. O'Brien CS: Local anesthesia in ophthalmic surgery, *Trans Sect Ophthalmol AMA* 237:253, 1927.
65. Pandey K, Badola RP, Kumar S: Time course of intraocular hypertension produced by suxamethonium, *Br J Anaesth* 44:191, 1972.
66. Petruscak I, Smith RB, Breslin P: Mortality related to ophthalmical surgery, *Arch Ophthalmol* 89:106, 1973.
67. Quigley HA: Mortality associated with ophthalmic surgery: a twenty year experience, *Am J Ophthalmol* 77:517, 1974.
68. Roizen, MF, Lampe GH, Benefiel DJ, et al: Is increased operative stress associated with worse outcome? *Anesthesiology* 67(3A):A1, 1987.
69. Roizen MF, Horrigan RW, Frazer BM: Anesthetic doses blocking adrenergic (stress) and cardiovascular response to incision–MAC BAR, *Anesthesiology* 54:390–398, 1981.
70. Ropo A, Nikki P, Ruusuvaara P, Kivisaari L: Comparison of retrobulbar and periocular injections of lignocaine by computerised tomography, *Br J Anaesth* 75:417–420, 1991.
71. Simcock PR: Combined peribulbar injection and blunt cannula infiltration for vitreoretinal surgery, *Ophthal Surg* 25(4):232, 1994.
72. Smith RB, Douglas H, Petruscak J, Breslin P: Safety of intraocular adrenaline with halothane anaesthesia, *Br J Anaesth* 44(12): 1314–1317, 1972.
73. Steward DJ: Preterm infants are more prone to complications following minor surgery than are term infants, *Anesthesiology* 56: 304–306, 1982.
74. Stinson TW III, Donlon JV Jr: Interaction of intraocular air and sulfur hexafluoride with nitrous oxide, a computer simulation, *Anesthesiology* 56:385, 1982.
75. Taboada JA, Rupp SM, Miller RD: Redefining the priming principle for vecuronium during rapid-sequence induction of anesthesia, *Anesthesiology* 64:243, 1986.
76. Unsold R, Stanley J, et al: The CT topography of retrobulbar anesthesia, *Albrecht von Graefes Arch Klin Ophthalmol* 217:125–126, 1981.
77. Vacanti CH, VanHouten RJ, Hill RC: A statistical analysis of the relationship of physical status to postoperative mortality in 68,388 cases, *Anesth Analg* 49:564, 1970.
78. Van Lint: Paralysis palperbrale temporaire provoquee dans l'operation de la cataracte, *Ann Occul* 151:420, 1914.
79. Verma RS: "Self-taming" of succinylcholine-induced fasciculations and intraocular pressure, *Anesthesiology* 50:245, 1979.
80. Watcha WF, Simeon RM, White PF, Stevens JL: Effect of propofol on the incidence of postoperative vomiting after strabismus surgery in pediatric outpatients, *Anesthesiology* 75:204–209, 1991.
81. Wolf GL, Capuano C, Hartung J, et al: Nitrous oxide increases intraocular pressure after intravitreal sulfur hexafluoride injection, *Anesthesiology* 59:547, 1983.
82. Wynands JE, Crowell DE: Intraocular tension in association with succinylcholine and endotracheal intubation, *Can Anaesth Soc J* 7:39, 1960.

CHAPTER 84

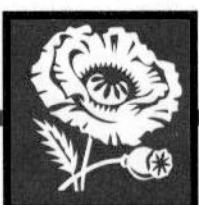

Anesthesia for Ear, Nose, and Throat Surgery

MARY M. JOSEPH

Anesthesia for ear, nose, and throat (ENT) surgery presents numerous challenges for the anesthesiologist. This field encompasses a wide variety of surgical procedures ranging from laser surgery of the vocal cords to major head and neck cancer resections. Frequently, the surgeon and anesthesiologist are competing for the same territory, namely the airway. Often the anesthesiologist cannot be positioned near the patient's head. The continually evolving use of laser technology demands up-to-date technical knowledge. In addition, most otolaryngologic surgeries today are performed on an outpatient or "same-day admit" basis, further taxing the anesthesiologist's skills of preoperative readiness. This chapter is designed to provide the knowledge needed for the anesthesiologist to meet these challenges.

ENDOSCOPIC PROCEDURES

Laryngoscopy and Microlaryngoscopy

Some of the greatest airway management challenges occur during anesthesia for direct laryngoscopy. The patient's airway is shared continuously by the surgeon and the anesthesiologist; thus communication in the operating room is of utmost importance. Laryngoscopy and bronchoscopy are performed for both diagnosis and therapy. With children, indications include evaluation of stridor (particularly in infants), foreign body retrieval, and treatment of laryngeal papillomatosis. With adults, laryngoscopy is employed for the evaluation of hoarseness, hemoptysis, neck masses, and also in treatment of vocal cord pathology. These pathologic processes may compromise the airway, so care must be taken with induction of anesthesia (see Head and Neck Cancer section). Sedative premedication should be avoided in any patient with a questionable airway. An antisialagogue may be used to help dry secretions in the surgical field.

Microlaryngoscopy differs from laryngoscopy in that the surgeon uses an operating microscope to visualize the glottis. The laryngoscope handle is attached to an extension that allows the laryngoscope to be suspended from either a Mayo stand or a bracket secured to the operating room table (Fig. 84-1). This frees the surgeon's hands for instrument or laser manipulation while visualizing the glottis through the operating microscope.[38]

Anesthetic techniques

It is possible to anesthetize the pharynx, larynx, and trachea with local and/or topical anesthesia for laryngoscopy and minor procedures such as vocal cord stripping. Adequate local anesthesia can be achieved with bilateral superior laryngeal nerve blocks near the greater cornu of the hyoid bone, glossopharyngeal block at the posterior tonsillar pillars, and a transtracheal injection. These blocks can be supplemented with intravenous (IV) sedation. Because the recurrent laryngeal nerve is not blocked, the surgeon can ask the patient to voluntarily phonate during Teflon® (polytetrafluoroethylene—E.I. DuPont de Nemours & Co., Inc.) injection of the vocal cords to check for paralytic dysphonia.[12]

The goals of general anesthesia for laryngoscopy are to provide an immobile patient, decreased laryngeal reflexes, relaxation of jaw musculature to allow airway instrumentation, adequate ventilation and oxygenation, attenuation of cardiovascular responses, and rapid awakening and return of airway reflexes following surgery.[33] **Laryngoscopy can produce considerable stimulation resulting in hypertension, tachycardia, and possible myocardial ischemia or infarction.[122] Also, a reflex pathway exists between the afferent fibers of the superior laryngeal nerve and the cardioinhibitory fibers of the vagus. Under light anesthesia, bradycardia and dysrhythmias can be produced by laryngeal stimulation.[122]**

It is possible to accomplish these goals with various techniques and anesthetic agents. Muscle relaxants are often necessary to provide adequate operating conditions. An intermediate-acting, nondepolarizing relaxant such as atracurium, vecuronium, rocuronium or mivacurium may be used. A continuous infusion of succinylcholine has the advantage of allowing quick reversal of profound neuromuscular blockade and rapid return of airway reflexes at the end of the case.[115]

Ventilation

The ventilation mode chosen is critical to anesthetic management during laryngoscopy. Although the airway is "shared" between surgeon and anesthesiologist, each has different concerns. One method to control the airway is to use a small, cuffed endotracheal tube (e.g., 5.0 to 6.0 mm for an adult). For the anesthesiologist, advantages of an endotracheal tube include a secure airway with easily controlled ventilation, the ability to use respiratory gas monitoring such as end-tidal CO_2 or mass spectrometry, and a cuff to protect the lower airway from debris. Major drawbacks include the potential for complications during laser surgery (see Laser Airway Surgery section), and interference with the operative field by the endotracheal tube. However, for many laryngoscopic procedures, ventilation with an endotracheal tube is possible and safe. Special microlaryngeal tracheal (MLT) tubes (manufactured by Mallinckrodt Critical Care, Glen Falls, NY) are available. These are 4.0- to 6.0-mm size tubes with cuffs comparable in size to a larger endotracheal tube to accommodate an adult.[128]

Another option is to have the surgeon repeatedly remove the endotracheal tube, operate during a brief period of apnea and then allow the anesthesiologist to reintubate and venti-

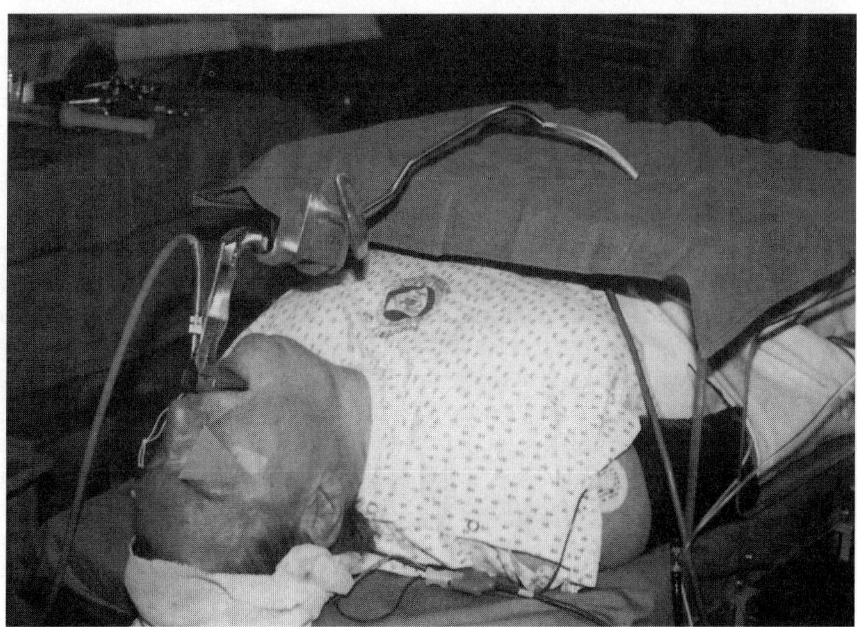

Fig. 84-1. Patient in suspension laryngoscopy.

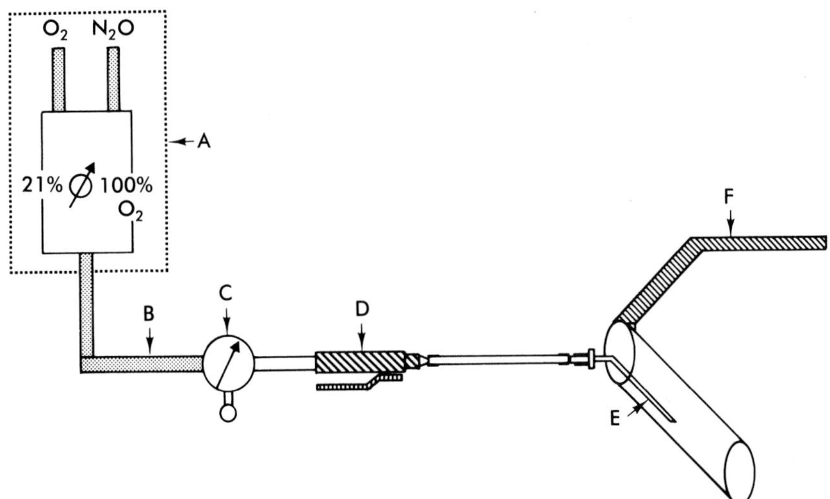

Fig. 84-2. Schematic drawing of Venturi jet ventilation apparatus. Concentration of oxygen and nitrous oxide are controlled by a blender **(A)**. High pressure tubing **(B)** delivers gas mixture to pressure regulator **(C)**. Hand-operated valve **(D)** allows intermittent delivery of gas to blunt needle **(E)**, which fits into a side channel of laryngoscope **(F)**. (Modified from Van Der Spek AFL, Spargo PM, Norton ML: The physics of lasers and implications for their use during airway surgery, *Br J Anaesth* 60:708, 1988.)

late the patient. When using an intermittent apnea technique such as this, it is important to closely monitor the oxygen saturation with a pulse oximeter. Disadvantages of this approach are that it is time consuming because the procedure must be interrupted frequently to ventilate the patient and that the airway is unprotected while the endotracheal tube is removed. One important advantage of either the intermittent apnea or standard endotracheal tube technique for laryngoscopy is that no special equipment is needed.

Jet ventilation has been used extensively for laryngeal surgery.[5,14,80,82,94,95,118] This technique was first described by Sanders in 1967,[101] and numerous modifications have been made since then. Basically, O_2 and N_2O are supplied from central sources to a mixer, such as a Bird® O_2-N_2O blender (Bird Corporation, Palm Springs, CA). A pressure regulator provides the correct pressure, and intermittent gas delivery is controlled by a hand-operated toggle valve (Fig. 84-2).[22] Jet ventilators that automate some of the manual functions of older devices are available.

Gas from the jet ventilator can be delivered to the patient via the subglottic or supraglottic routes. In subglottic jet ventilation, the gas may be delivered translaryngeally by either a long needle[100] or a long, flexible tube such as that described by Carden[14] or Hunsaker.[55] **If there is a large airway mass above the level of delivery of the gas jet, a "ball-valve" phenomenon can occur, wherein gas is forced down the trachea during inspiration but is trapped during expiration. This air trapping can lead to increased airway pressure, subcutaneous emphysema, and pneumothorax.**[22]

Supraglottic jet ventilation is performed by placing a blunt needle (approximately 14 gauge), down the side channel of one of several straight laryngoscope blades (e.g., a Dedo) used by ENT surgeons.[5,103] Gas under high pressure exits from the needle and entrains ambient air for ventilation (Venturi principle, Fig. 84-3).[129] Adequacy of ventilation is assessed by observing chest movement, because accurate respiratory gas monitoring is difficult with jet ventilation. Pulse oximetry is extremely helpful for following oxygenation. Using blood gas analysis, various studies have documented the efficacy of jet ventilation for laryngoscopic procedures.[14,95,102,118] Anesthesia is primarily maintained with IV agents[49] because volatile anesthetics cannot be reliably delivered with jet ventilator systems. Nitrous oxide may be used safely,[13] but inspired concentrations of both N_2O and O_2 are diluted because of room air entrainment.[102] Also, operating room pollution with N_2O is a concern with this open system.

The main advantages of Venturi jet ventilation for laryngoscopy are a clear operating field for the surgeon and safety during laser surgery. **Jet ventilation carries the risk of barotrauma, which can result in subcutaneous emphysema, pneumothorax, or pneumomediastinum.**[59,90] **The needle should never be allowed to lie on or near the mucosa.** The initial jet pressure should be limited to 20 psig for adults and 10 psig for children.[21] Peak pressures may then be slowly adjusted upward as required for adequate chest rise. Gastric distention may occur with supraglottic jet ventilation, especially if the jet is directed by the surgeon slightly toward the esophagus rather than directly at the vocal cords.[16] Blowing debris down the unprotected trachea can also occur. Each jet ventilation breath causes the vocal cords to flutter, which may be distracting to the surgeon. During lengthy procedures, the vocal cords may become

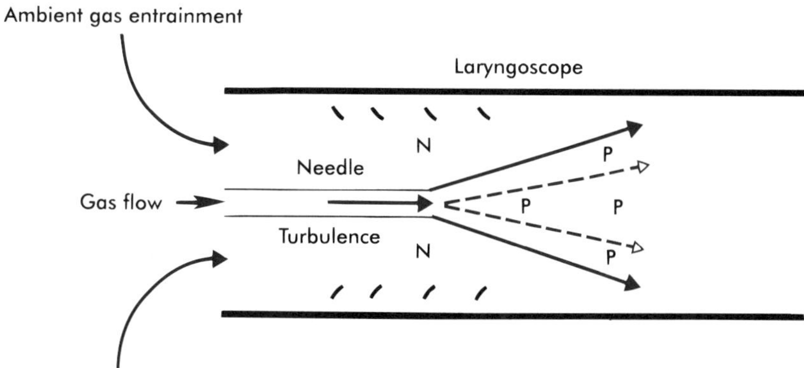

Fig. 84-3. Diagram of Venturi effect. Gas exits under high pressure from a needle placed in laryngoscope lumen. The pressure distal to tip of the needle is relatively higher than the pressure proximal to the jet exit site. Because of this pressure gradient, ambient gas is entrained. P, high pressure area; N, relatively negative pressure when compared with P. (Redrawn from Van Der Spek AFL, Spargo PM, Norton ML: The physics of lasers and implications for their use during airway surgery, *Br J Anaesth* 60:708, 1988.)

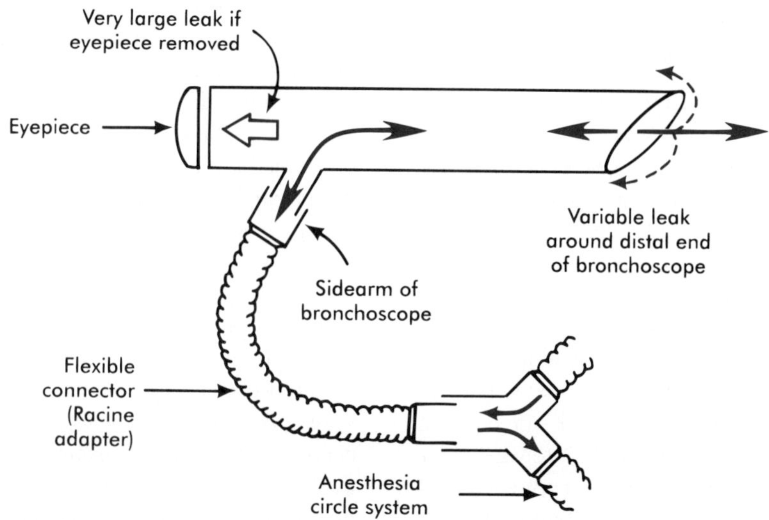

Fig. 84-4. Ventilation through a rigid bronchoscope using the circle system. The leak around the distal end of the bronchoscope depends on the fit of the bronchoscope in the trachea. If the surgeon removes the eyepiece to suction or pass an instrument, a large leak in the system will be created. (Redrawn from Benumof JL: *Anesthesia for thoracic surgery,* Philadelphia, 1987, WB Saunders.)

desiccated. Finally, jet ventilation may be difficult or impossible in extremely obese patients (heavy chest wall) or patients with poor pulmonary compliance.[22]

Bronchoscopy

Anesthesia for bronchoscopy shares many of the same principles and problems as that for laryngoscopy. Most flexible fiberoptic bronchoscopy is performed under topical anesthesia, but rigid bronchoscopy usually requires general anesthesia. The rigid ventilating bronchoscope (Fig. 84-4) has a side port that allows direct connection to an anesthesia circuit or to a flexible connector known as a Racine adaptor. There is a variable amount of leak around the distal end of the bronchoscope because the latter does not fit tightly against the trachea. To compensate for this leak, it may be necessary to use high gas flows or a pharyngeal pack. When the eyepiece is removed for suctioning or passing instruments, a large gas leak will occur out of the proximal end of the scope, making ventilation impossible. Ventilating pressures can be high through the smaller diameter pediatric bronchoscopes.[6] Rigid Venturi bronchoscopes operate on principles similar to those described for laryngoscopy.[101,117]

Complications of bronchoscopy include bronchospasm during light anesthesia, hypercapnia, and hypoxemia. Cardiac arrhythmias are frequent and can develop secondary to light anesthesia, low Po_2, or increased Pco_2.[6] Carinal stimulation may lead to patient "bucking," requiring careful attention to muscle relaxation and anesthetic depth.

Esophagoscopy

Esophagoscopy has both diagnostic and therapeutic indications and can be performed with either a flexible or rigid esophagoscope. General anesthesia is preferred for rigid esophagoscopy and is used for removal of foreign bodies and localization of massive esophageal bleeding or tumors. If aspiration is a risk at induction, intubation may be performed with succinylcholine and an infusion may be used for short procedures. **A serious complication is perforation of the esophagus, therefore, adequate muscle relaxation is of utmost importance. A common site of perforation is the hypopharynx and has a mortality rate of 34% to 84%.**[121] Other complications seen during the procedure are dysrhythmias, occlusion of ET tube, and aspiration. Flexible esophagoscopy can be performed under IV sedation and monitoring.

LASER AIRWAY SURGERY

LASER is an acronym for Light Amplification by Stimulated Emission of Radiation. It was first discovered by American physicists Townes and Schawlow in 1958 for which they were awarded the Nobel prize. The CO_2 laser was discovered by Patel in 1964 and then used by Jako in 1968 on a canine larynx and then in clinical practice in 1972. Various types of lasers are available for medical purposes, but microlaryngeal surgery is performed exclusively with the CO_2 laser. The neodymium-yttrium-aluminum-garnet (Nd:YAG) laser is used for airway tumor debulking. The potassium-titanyl phosphate laser (KTP) emits green light with a wavelength of 532 nm and it can be propagated by fiberoptic filaments. The KTP laser is used on otolaryngeal surgery for myringotomy, stapedectomy, and tympanoplasty.

Laser Technology

Some knowledge of laser physics is necessary for the anesthesiologist to understand the use and hazards of laser technology in the operating room. This topic has been reviewed in depth by Van Der Spek et al.[129] Lasers produce coherant radiation, a form of light which has three special characteristics:

1. Coherence—all waves travel in phase.
2. Collimation—all waves are parallel to each other and do not diverge.
3. Monochromaticity—all waves are of the same wavelength or color.

The potential uses and side effects of a laser vary with its wavelength, which is determined by the medium in which the laser beam is generated. For example, the carbon dioxide laser uses CO_2 gas molecules to produce its coherent radiation. Stimulation of a gas, liquid, or solid "medium" by an energy source, such as an electrical spark, produces laser light. The energy causes electrons in these molecules or atoms to reach a higher energy state ("excited state"). These electrons have the tendency to drop back to the lower or "ground" state. When this occurs, a packet of energy or a photon of a specific wavelength will be given off. This radiation will cause other molecules in the medium to produce photons of identical wavelengths. This process takes place in a cylindric chamber that has reflective mirrors at each end (Fig. 84-5), allowing amplification of the light beam. A laser produces light of the same wavelength in phase and traveling in parallel. This coherent beam can be focused into an extremely small spot, producing high-power density.[53]

$$\text{Power density} = \text{Watts/Spot size}(\text{Cm}^2)$$

Energy produced by the laser is absorbed by biologic tissues and converted to heat. The specific wavelengths produced by each type of laser medium have different effects on tissue. The longer the wavelength, the more absorption of energy will occur. For example, the CO_2 laser has a relatively long wavelength in the far infrared portion of the electromagnetic spectrum (10.6 nm). The CO_2 laser beam is almost entirely absorbed by the surface of the tissue and destroys tissue by vaporizing cellular water. This is important when precise cutting is needed, as in excision of vocal cord lesions. On the other hand, the Nd:YAG laser has a

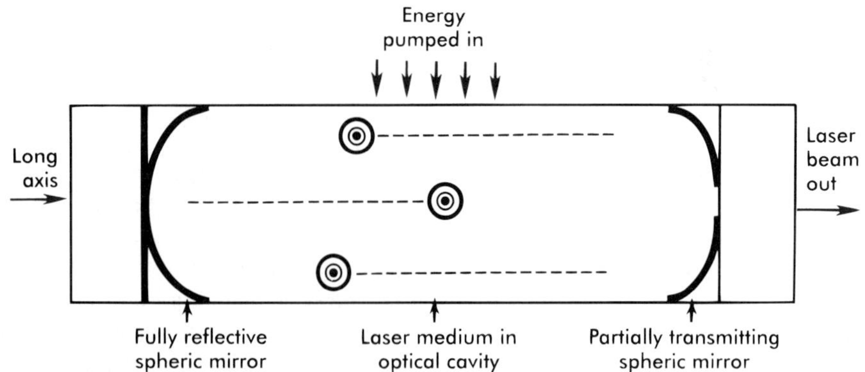

Fig. 84-5. Simplified diagram of laser operation. (Redrawn from Van Der Spek AFL, Spargo PM, Norton ML: The physics of lasers and implications for their use during airway surgery, *Br J Anaesth* 60:709, 1988.)

wavelength one tenth that of the CO_2 laser. The energy is absorbed deeper by pigment-containing tissue. For this reason, the Nd:YAG laser works well for deep thermal tumor debulking.[90] Also, the shorter wavelength of the Nd:YAG laser allows its beam to be conducted through channels in flexible fiberoptic instruments, whereas the CO_2 laser beam must be aimed directly.[60] Both the CO_2 and Nd:YAG wavelengths are outside the visible spectrum, so a separate, lower energy, visible laser beam is necessary for aiming. In contrast, the green beam of the KTP laser is transmitted through clear tissues but is absorbed by pigments such as hemoglobin and melanin. The commonly used wavelengths, their respective lasing media, and their general characteristics are listed in Table 84-1.

Risks Associated with Laser Procedures

Lasers offer many advantages to the surgeon: precise cutting, freedom from instruments in the field, and decreased edema and bleeding in the patient. However, there are serious disadvantages and hazards associated with use of lasers. The American National Standards Institute (ANSI)[2] has classified lasers based upon their optical emission into classes I through IV such that the potential hazards of the laser increase with classes; class 4 lasers are the most hazardous. Most lasers used in the operating room are class 4 lasers.[90]

The greatest fear during laser surgery is fire in the endotracheal tube. Other complications include corneal ulcerations and scars and inhalation of smoke (laser plume) produced by tissue vaporization. The laser plume may contain infectious particles such as viral DNA and may be mutagenic like cigarette smoke.[90] High intensity exposure of skin may results in burns. The risk of accidents caused by laser use can be reduced by implementing a hospital laser safety program overseen by a laser safety committee. The responsibilities of the laser safety committee include strategic planning, physician credentialing, safety policies, protocol formulation, and inservice education of health care personnel. Operating rooms in which lasers are in use should have warning signs posted at all entrances. The personnel in the operating rooms must protect their eyes by wearing goggles appropriate for the wavelength in use. For CO_2 lasers, any type of glass or plastic will be protective. Prescription eyeglasses generally lack side protectors, however, so plastic goggles should be worn over them. The color of protective goggles needed with other lasers are as follows: Orange for an Argon laser; green for a Nd:YAG laser; and orange-red for a KTP laser. The patient's eyes should be protected with wet gauze. The incidence of laser fires has been reported as high as 1.5% in patients undergoing laryngeal surgery with a CO_2 laser.

General precautions to reduce the risk of fire include:

- Use lowest possible fraction of inspired oxygen (FIO_2) because oxygen supports combustion (N_2O also supports combustion).
- Use water-soluble ointments because oil-based ointments are flammable.[55]
- Keep paper drapes away from operative field.
- Use laser on lowest effective power setting; always use laser in intermittent mode because continuous mode allows heat buildup.[91]

Fire in the airway is the most serious and life-threatening complication of laser surgery. There have been numerous reports of airway fire,[10,21,107] with the greatest risk being ignition of the endotracheal tube. Penetration of the endotracheal tube allows the beam to reach the interior of the tube. **Propagation of the flame along the oxygen-enriched at-**

Table 84-1 Lasers commonly used in the operating room

Laser	Wavelength (nm)	General characteristics
Argon	488/515 (blue/green)	Absorbed selectively by hemoglobin and melanin or other similar pigments Transmitted through clear substances Tissue penetration: 0.5–2 mm
KTP (frequency-doubled YAG)	532 (green)	Strongly absorbed by hemoglobin, melanin, and similar pigments Transmitted through clear substances Tissue penetration: 0.5–2 mm
Nd:YAG	1065 (near infrared)	More readily absorbed by dark tissue Transmitted through clear fluids Tissue penetration: 2–6 mm
CO_2	10,600 (far infrared)	Strongly absorbed by water and, thus, by all tissue (pigmented or not)
HeNe	632 (red)	Used as a low-power coaxial aiming beam for nonvisible lasers (CO_2 and Nd:YAG) Has no significant tissue interaction

From Pashayan AG: Anesthesia for laser surgery, *ASA Refresher Courses in Anesthesiology,* Philadelphia, 1995, JB Lippincott, p 276.

mosphere of the tube can cause a "blowtorch" type of flame because of the presence of all three of the elements needed for a fire—combustible material, ignition source, and an atmosphere that supports combustion.

Anesthetic techniques to reduce the risk of fire (CO_2 laser)

Endotracheal tube fire can be avoided by using a nonintubation technique such as jet ventilation or intermittent apnea. The jet or Venturi ventilation technique has been well described for CO_2 laser surgery of the larynx.[100,102] This technique allows removal of flammable materials from the path of the laser beam but there is an increased risk of blowing smoke and debris down the trachea into an unprotected lower airway. It is possible for the laser beam to perforate the trachea or a bronchus.[35] Jet ventilation can be especially helpful in small children, where an endotracheal tube can obscure a large portion of the surgical field.

If endotracheal intubation is chosen to manage ventilation during laser surgery, it is important to understand that all endotracheal tubes not made of metal are capable of combustion. There exists some controversy over which tubes are most flammable. Patel and Hicks found that standard polyvinyl chloride (PVC) tubes ignited more easily than red rubber tubes.[91] Wolf and Simpson performed in vitro flammability tests and found PVC tubes to be less flammable than silicone or red rubber tubes.[135] (Ignition refers to the amount of energy needed to ignite a tube, whereas flammability refers to the ability to sustain a flame.) Because PVC is a thermoplastic material, it will melt at a lower temperature than silicone or red rubber. This allows the beam to enter the tube and produce the previously described "blow-torch" effect.[90] In addition, PVC burns to produce molten debris and hydrogen chloride gas, which is toxic to the airway. In contrast, ignited red rubber tubes tend to char rather than melt.

All-metal endotracheal tubes are available, but there are several drawbacks to the use of these tubes. There is no cuff, and the tubes are bulky and relatively nonpliable. They are potentially traumatic to the vocal cords. Also, the laser beam can reflect off the tube, potentially damaging adjacent airway tissue.[90]

In the past, attempts were made to wrap tubes with saline-soaked gauze or muslin to protect against ignition. Unfortunately, the risk of fire recurred when the material dried out.[91] A better option is to wrap a tube (usually a red rubber tube) with metallic tape (Fig. 84-6, *top*) to decrease the risk of penetration and ignition. In an in vitro experiment, Sosis compared six types of metallic tape to assess their ability to protect endotracheal tubes. With 100% O_2 flowing through the tube, the CO_2 laser beam on highest power and continuous mode was aimed directly at the tube. The best protection was provided by 3M tape No. 425. Other tapes either allowed penetration of the beam or had a flammable adhesive backing.[116]

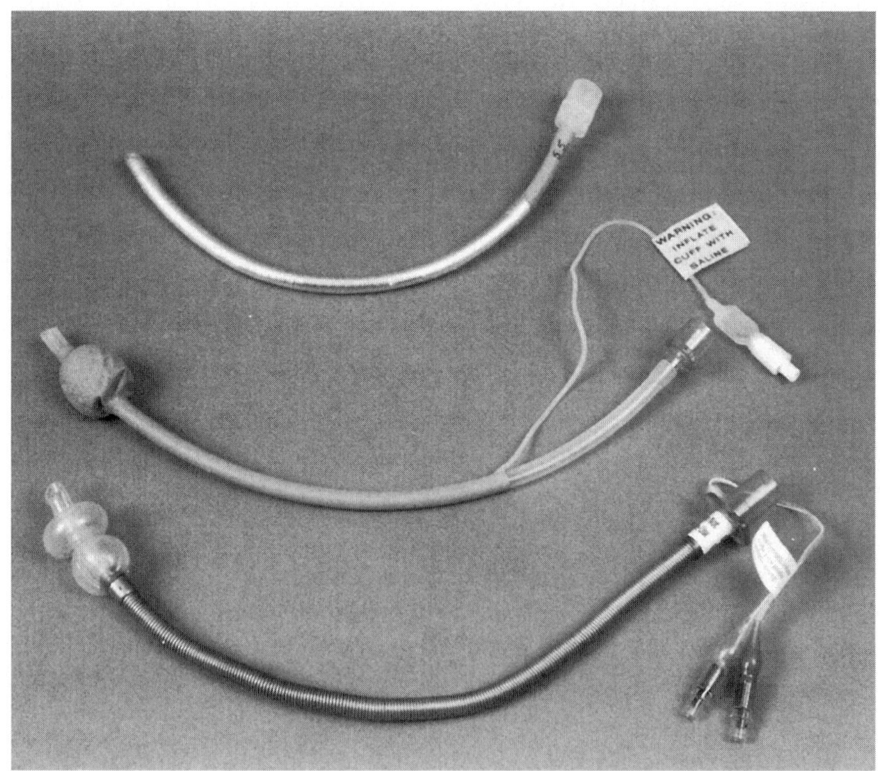

Fig. 84-6. Endotracheal tubes for CO_2 laser airway surgery: red rubber tube with metallic wrap (*top*), Xomed Laser Shield (*middle*), and Mallinckrodt Laser-Flex (*bottom*).

When using metallic tape to protect an endotracheal tube, the tape should be carefully applied. Wrapping too tightly can kink a soft red rubber tube. Rough tape edges can cause damage to mucosal surfaces, and pieces of tape may break off and be aspirated. Any gaps will leave portions of the tube unprotected.[53] One part of the endotracheal tube that cannot be protected by wrapping is the cuff. Unfortunately, the cuff is made of thinner material and may even be more vulnerable to laser beam penetration than the body of the tube. One option is to pack the cuff area with a saline-soaked gauze. A more popular practice is to fill the cuff with saline or water rather than air. The fluid will act as a heat sink,[64] and if the cuff is penetrated, streams of the liquid may help quench any fire.[80] Methylene blue can be added to the cuff, so if the cuff is penetrated by the laser beam, the surgeon will be warned by the presence of dye in the airway.[38]

Laser-Guard (Americal Corporation, Mystic, CT) is a new product that also protects conventional endotracheal tube shafts. It consists of two layers: a silver foil layer covered with a thin absorbent sponge layer that acts as a heat sink when moistened. The foil is corrugated to provide diffused laser beam reflection. This product is designed to be more easily applied than metallic tape; however, like tape, it cannot protect the cuff. In an in vitro study, Sosis et al. demonstrated that the Laser-Guard® covering protected PVC endotracheal tube shafts from combustion during continuous exposure to CO_2 laser radiation of 70 W for 60 seconds.[109]

There are also several endotracheal tubes manufactured specifically for CO_2 laser surgery of the airway. The Xomed-Treace Laser Shield II (Xomed, Jacksonville, FL) is a silicon tube covered with metallic particles (Fig. 84-6, *middle*). This tube actually has a cuff with a metallic covering that is not as dense as the tube body.[52] The Fome-Cuf® (Bivona, Inc., Gary, IN) consists of a flexible aluminum tube with a silicon sheath. It has a silicon cuff filled with a spongelike material, which acts as a heat sink when filled with liquid. The inner foam cuff will retain its shape even if the outer silicon cuff is struck by the laser. The Laser-Flex™ (Mallinckrodt Medical Inc., St. Louis, MO) (Fig. 84-6, *bottom*) has a body composed entirely of flexible stainless steel, but its two cuffs are made of PVC and thus are still vulnerable to the laser beam. If the proximal cuff deflates, the distal cuff remains inflated to protect the distal airway.

Sosis and Heller compared these three endotracheal tubes with red rubber tubes wrapped with metallic tape (3M No. 425). The CO_2 laser was aimed at the body of the tube (but not the cuff) in continuous mode, high power with 100% O_2 flowing through the tube. This experiment is designed to be more severe than usual clinical situations. The Laser-Flex and the 3M No. 425 tape–wrapped red rubber tubes were judged safe, whereas the Bivona and Xomed tubes burned.[114] This does not imply that this would occur if the laser was used in the intermittent mode with limited FIO_2. Also, only the bodies of the tubes were tested, not the cuffs. The Laser Flex® tube has PVC cuffs, and the Xomed tube cuff has been reported to have undergone combustion during CO_2 laser surgery.[115] **Therefore there is no ideal cuffed "laser-proof" tube available at this time for use with the CO_2 laser. The main difficulty exists in manufacturing a cuff that can be resistant to penetration and yet remain pliable and able to seal the airway.**

Use of helium mixed with oxygen has been suggested to reduce the risk of airway fire. Helium has a high "thermal diffusivity," which means that it inhibits increases in temperature around the site of laser exposure. Theoretically, this decreases the chance of ignition.[88] Pashayan et al. devised a protocol using special unmarked, unwrapped PVC ET tubes ($FIO_2 \leq 0.4$, helium ≥ 0.6), and CO_2 laser in the intermittent mode with limited power (≤ 10.0 W). One fire in 523 cases was reported when the oxygen flush valve was inadvertently pushed while laser resection continued.[86] Using a mixture of 70% helium and 30% oxygen has been suggested to prevent this type of mishap. Pashayan and Gravenstein also examined the endotracheal tubes after their use and found a high rate of occurrence of laser beam contact with the tubes, although no actual fire occurred.[89] At the present time, the safety of using unprotected PVC tubes for CO_2 laser surgery remains controversial. If a fire does occur, the products of combustion are toxic and the tube may burn with a blow torch type of flame.[113] Also, an in vitro study showed helium to be ineffective in reducing endotracheal tube flammability.[105]

The anesthesiologist needs to be aware of the limitations and benefits of different anesthetic techniques for CO_2 laser surgery. Decisions regarding appropriate anesthetic management for laser airway surgery need to be based on current technical information and clinical experience. As new products or techniques become available, it is absolutely necessary to critically review literature about their safety.

Because all anesthetic techniques for laser surgery have some fire risk, knowledge of how to manage an airway fire is important (Table 84-2). In the event of a fire, the following management is appropriate. It is important that the anesthetist understand that these airway fires can occur with extreme suddeness (i.e., suddenly it appears that the entire tube is aflame). Careful thought ahead of time on the part of the anesthesiologist can prevent severe complications.

Eye damage

The energy of the CO_2 laser is absorbed primarily by the water-containing tissue of the cornea, whereas the Nd:YAG beam mainly reaches the pigmented retina. The following precautions should be taken to prevent eye damage:

- The operating room should have a warning sign posted outside indicating a laser is in use.
- All operating room personnel must wear goggles specific for absorbing the wavelength light of the laser in use.
- The patient's eyes should be protected with moistened gauze.

Table 84-2 Response algorithm for airway fire during laser operations on the airway

	Steps	Measures
Immediate	First	Disconnect oxygen source at Y piece and remove burning objects from the airway
	Second	Irrigate site with water if fire is still smoldering
	Third	Ventilate the patient by mask or reintubate the patient and ventilate with as low a fraction of inspired oxygen as possible
Secondary	Fourth	Evaluate extent of injury by bronchoscopy and laryngoscopy
	Fifth	Reintubate the patient or perform a tracheostomy if needed
	Sixth	Monitor with oximetry and arterial blood gas analysis and serial chest radiograms
	Seventh	Use ventilatory support, steriods, and antibiotics as needed

From Pashayan AG: Anesthesia for laser surgery, *ASA Refresher Courses in Anesthesiology,* Philadelphia, 1995, JB Lippincott, p276.

- Nonreflective instruments (matte finish) should be used to help disperse the beam.
- The laser should be in stand-by mode when not in use.
- In addition to eye damage, skin may also be burned by the laser; all tissues adjacent to the field should be protected with moistened gauze or towels to dissipate heat.[53,90]

Noxious fumes

Tissue combustion by the laser produces a smoke composed of carbonized cell fragments, water vapor, and hydrocarbons called the laser plume. The use of lasers to treat malignant growths and human papilloma virus has raised concern regarding the transmission of pathogens through the smoke. Although the pathogenicity of particles in laser smoke has not been conclusively demonstrated, it may be prudent to assume such and use suction to scavenge the smoke,[90] and wear protective surgical face masks.

The risk of Nd:YAG laser surgery

The Nd:YAG laser is used for palliative debulking of unresectable endobronchial tumors that are causing airway obstruction, collapse, or infection. As mentioned previously, this laser can be passed through a fiberoptic bronchoscope channel to reach lesions in the tracheobronchial tree because of its relatively short wavelength. As described for the CO_2 laser, airway fire is a major hazard. All endotracheal tubes are believed vulnerable.[44] Clear, unmarked PVC tubes are relatively resistant to the Nd:YAG laser beam compared with the CO_2 laser, but soiling with blood or debris renders these tubes vulnerable.[44,108] **None of the specialized laser tubes described previously are marketed for use with the Nd:YAG laser and are not known to provide protection.**[112] It was previously believed that wrapping endotracheal tubes offered no protection,[44] but Sosis and Heller recently showed 3M No. 425 tape to be an adequate protectant.[111] The safest way to use the Nd:YAG laser may be to pass a flexible fiberoptic bronchoscope through a rigid bronchoscope rather than through an endotracheal tube. Ventilation can be accomplished by attaching the circuit to the side port of the bronchoscope.[6] The fiberoptic bronchoscope itself may be ignited by the Nd:YAG laser.[90]

Other complications of Nd:YAG airway surgery include perforation of the trachea or bronchi and bronchospasm. Perforation of the airway may lead to penetration of the great vessels and fatal, uncontrolled bleeding.[131,132]

ADENOTONSILLECTOMY

Tonsillectomy and adenoidectomy are common pediatric surgical procedures usually performed on an outpatient basis. Adenoidectomy is a treatment for adenoid hyperplasia which may cause nasopharyngeal obstruction and is often accompanied by tonsillectomy.

Preoperative Evaluation

The major indications for tonsillectomy are chronic or recurrent tonsillitis, obstructive tonsillar hyperplasia, and peritonsillar abscess.[25] Tonsillectomy is also combined with uvulopalatopharyngoplasty (UPP) to alleviate sleep apnea in patients with Pickwickian syndrome. During rapid eye movement (REM) sleep, the pharyngeal muscles of patients with obstructive sleep apnea relax, causing airway obstruction. Adults with this problem are usually obese and have abundant pharyngeal soft tissue which is treated by UPP involving uvulectomy with limited resection of redundant pharyngeal tissue. In extreme cases, tracheostomy may be required.[18,38] If left untreated, it may lead to recurrent episodes of hypoxemia resulting in pulmonary hypertension, cor pulmonale, and congestive heart failure (CHF). Electrocardiographic and echocardiographic evidence of left ventricular hypertrophy has been observed in 30% of children with sleep apnea and tonsillectomy is effective in relieving sleep apnea in 66% of cases.[38,96] Chest radiograph shows cardiomegaly. Sudden death during sleep in patients with sleep apnea is probably caused by fatal arrythmias that occur secondary to asphyxia. Preoperative preparation consists of stabilization of cardiovascular status and detection of cor pulmonale or CHF. Preoperative evaluation should include a careful history to screen for personal or family bleeding tendencies (e.g., hemophilia or Von Willebrand's disease) and use of over-the-counter medication (e.g., aspirin or compounds that contain aspirin which affect platelet function). Patients with a history of sleep apnea should not receive sedative premedication.

Intraoperative Management

In children, anesthesia is induced with halothane or sevoflurane, oxygen and nitrous oxide by mask. Endotracheal intubation is achieved by either deep inhalation anesthesia or combined with short-acting nondepolarizing muscle relaxants. The use of succinylcholine is avoided in children. Intubation is accomplished with an appropriately sized oral right angle endotracheal (RAE) tube which is placed in the groove in the midline of the tongue blade of the Crowe-Davis gag used to keep the mouth open (Fig. 84-7). The endotracheal tube can easily be compressed or kinked by the mouth gag, so it is important to check breath sounds and to note peak airway pressures after the gag is placed. Unintentional extubation can occur during placement of the mouth gag. Continuous monitoring of end-tidal CO_2 and airway compliance is mandatory. Maintenance of anesthesia can be accomplished by inhalation agents. All muscle relaxation should be completely reversed prior to extubation of the trachea.

At the end of these cases, most anesthesiologists prefer to have a patient who is awake with intact protective airway reflexes. Some practitioners extubate tonsillectomy patients while they are still deeply anesthetized, but the risk of laryngospasm may be greater with this technique.[4] Lidocaine 1.0 to 1.5 mg/kg IV has been advocated to help suppress cough and laryngospasm at the time of extubation.[44] Infiltration of the tonsillar capsule with local anesthetic has been suggested to reduce bleeding, aid in dissection, and contribute to postoperative pain relief. Bupivacaine has been shown to be superior to lidocaine by providing longer pain relief in tonsillectomy patients.[85]

Blood loss during tonsillectomy averages 4 ml/kg and must be carefully monitored, especially in pediatric patients. The pharynx must be suctioned thoroughly at the end of surgery. After extubation, the patient is placed in the "tonsil position," on one side with the head lower than the hips. This allows blood and secretions to drain out of the mouth rather than drip onto the vocal cords causing laryngospasm. Most morbidity from adenotonsillectomy is due to unrecognized bleeding and airway obstruction in the recovery period.

Post-tonsillectomy Bleed

Crysdale and Russel[23] reviewed 9409 operations and found that 202 patients had problems with bleeding postoperatively; six (0.6% of all patients) of those required reoperation for control of bleeding. Ninety percent of the patients who bled did so in the first 9 hours postoperatively.[23] Usually, blood loss after adenotonsillectomy consists of slow oozing rather than brisk bleeding. **These patients may swallow large volumes of blood before the bleeding is detected. At this point, the patient may be hypovolemic with tachycardia and orthostatic hypotension. Before reanesthetizing such a patient, intravascular volume should be restored.** Serial hematocrits should be checked and the patient transfused if necessary.[4] Deaths have occurred during ill-timed anesthetic inductions in patients who were rushed to the operating room while still hypovolemic. Intravenous induction with pentothal may result in hypotension and cardiac arrest.[26,125] These patients may be hypoxemic secondary to blood in the airway. Proper management of the patient with bleeding tonsils requires consideration that the stomach is full of blood. Alternatives include awake intubation or rapid sequence induction with either ketamine 1 to 2 mg/kg or etomidate 0.2 to 0.3 mg/kg IV. A wide-bore suction apparatus should be immediately available to clear the pharynx. After the patient is anesthetized, a nasogastric (NG) tube should be passed to empty the stomach of blood and clots, which may help decrease postoperative nausea and emesis.

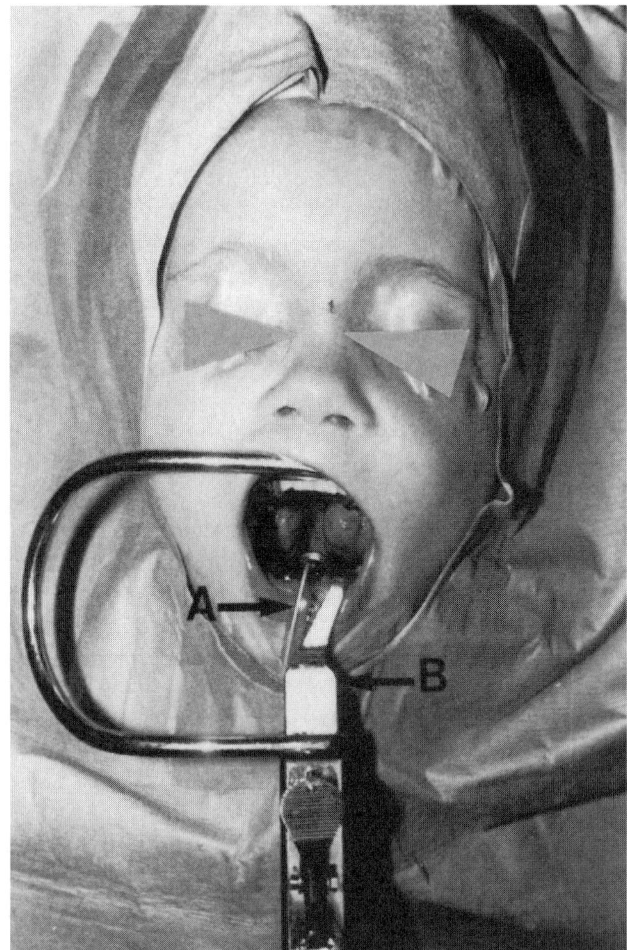

Fig. 84-7. Patient positioned for adenotonsillectomy. A right angle endotracheal tube (*A*) is held in place by Crow-Davis mouth gag (*B*).

Postoperative hemorrhage after adenotonsillectomy is the main reason many hospitals do not perform this procedure on an outpatient basis, although outpatient tonsillectomies are becoming more common. These patients must be observed carefully while recovering, with frequent pharyngeal checks for evidence of bleeding.[9]

NASAL AND SINUS SURGERY

Nasal and sinus procedures include: drainage procedures for chronic sinusitis, such as the Caldwell-Luc procedure (radical maxillary sinusotomy); polyp removal; and cosmetic or reconstructive surgery, such as repair of a deviated septum. Endoscopic techniques are now being used frequently for sinus surgery. The candidates for these procedures are generally young, healthy adults, but it is important to note that patients with sinusitis may also frequently have reactive airway disease.

The main consideration in sinus surgery is blood loss because the mucosa is highly vascular. Head elevation (15° to 20°) and use of potent inhalation agents to lower systolic blood pressure are helpful.[75] The application of cocaine to the mucosa is frequently used to help control bleeding.[75] Cocaine is an ester-type local anesthetic. In addition to its local anesthetic properties, it also produces local vasoconstriction by blocking reuptake of norepinephrine in adrenergic nerve terminals. In addition, cocaine prevents uptake of exogenous epinephrine, so cocaine and epinephrine are somewhat synergistic in their sympathetic effects. Cocaine is well absorbed from mucous membranes, especially those of the trachea and pharynx. Excessive systemic absorption is manifested by autonomic symptoms including hypertension and tachycardia. The awake patient may complain of restlessness or anxiety. Severe toxicity may manifest as seizures or coronary spasm leading to myocardial ischemia and/or severe arrhythmias.[36]

To avoid toxicity, the total cocaine dose should be limited to 3 mg/kg. Cocaine is often prepared as a 4% solution. Five ml of this solution will contain 200 mg or the equivalent of 3 mg/kg in a 70-kg patient. As an ester-linked local anesthetic, cocaine is hydrolyzed by plasma pseudocholinesterase. Therefore, pseudocholinesterase deficiency or drugs that inhibit pseudocholinesterase, such as echothiophate eye drops, will decrease the metabolism and increase the risk of systemic toxicity. The hypertension and tachycardia of cocaine toxicity can be treated by titrating propranolol or use of an esmolol infusion.[51,103]

Endoscopic sinus surgery can be performed either with general anesthesia or local anesthesia supplemented with IV sedation. General anesthesia is usually preferred by patients. Supplemental local anesthesia with vasoconstrictors (e.g., epinephrine and cocaine) lowers the requirement for postoperative narcotic in postanesthesia care unit and decreases bleeding.

Because the sinus cavities are closed spaces, nitrous oxide diffuses rapidly into them. However, there have been no reports of problems with increased pressure in sinus surgery in contrast with middle ear surgery (see Ear Surgery section).[77]

Surgical complications include venous air embolism, cerebrospinal fluid (CSF) leak, ecchymosis and hematoma of the eye lids, proptosis, pain in the eye, and loss of vision due to intraorbital and retrobulbar hematoma causing an increase in intraocular pressure, vascular obstruction, and ischemia. Perforation of the lamina papyracea may cause disturbances of eye movements due to trauma to the medial rectus muscle.[70] Anesthetic management may have a bearing on the incidence of bleeding and orbital hematoma. Control of blood pressure during surgery and at emergence may help lower this incidence.

Reinhart and Anderson[97] reported a fatal complication of endoscopic sinus surgery that presented as hemodynamic instability with electrocardiographic evidence of ischemia. It was associated with excessive bleeding, failure to emerge from anesthesia, and a focal neurologic deficit.

The complications of endoscopic surgery are infrequent, and the type of anesthesia (i.e., local or general) does not make a significant difference except a higher risk of aspiration and laryngeal spasm with general anesthesia. Blackwell and colleagues[7a] reported significant ($p < 0.01$) decreased bleeding with propofol infusion (110 ml blood) compared with isoflurane anesthesia (250 ml) studied retrospectively on 25 patients. Patients who have undergone previous surgery do not show an increase in complications. The complication rate increases significantly if the middle turbinate is removed. Another rare complication reported is toxic shock syndrome which can be avoided by not packing the nose postoperatively.[136]

At the end of sinus surgery, the posterior pharyngeal pack must be removed. After suctioning the pharynx well, the patient should be extubated awake when airway reflexes are intact. Some clinicians elect to extubate these patients while they are still deeply anesthetized in order to decrease the likelihood of coughing on the endotracheal tube and bleeding. The disadvantage of this deep extubation technique is a potentially increased risk of aspiration.

HEAD AND NECK CANCERS AND RECONSTRUCTIVE SURGERY

Most cancers of the upper respiratory tract are squamous cell carcinomas. Total laryngectomy is performed when there is invasion of the laryngeal musculature or cartilage. Neck dissection is often required when there is local tumor extension.

Preoperative Evaluation

Oropharyngeal and laryngeal carcinoma account for 3% to 5% of human cancers and approximately 75% of patients are over 60 years of age. Men are affected more than women by 2.5:1 and blacks greater than whites by 8:1. Chick et al.[17] reported the incidence of complications from head and neck surgery to be 65% in patients over 65 years of age (n = 31) and 49% in patients under 65 years of age (n = 90). He reviewed 1000 consecutive surgeries performed on patients over 70 years of age and noted a nonfatal anesthetic morbidity in 36% of the patients.

Goldman and associates[45] estimate the risk of perioperative cardiac mortality to be increased tenfold in patients over 70 years of age.

Site of tumor

Lip carcinoma accounts for 20% to 30% of all oral cavity tumors. Other frequent sites are the floor of the mouth, ventral or lateral tongue surface, and the soft palate. Risk factors include tobacco smoking and alcohol consumption.

Oropharyngeal carcinomas (soft palate, tongue base, uvula, retromolar, trigone, and tonsil) have a lower survival rate (i.e., 40% to 70%) because of advanced local disease at presentation and increased incidence of metastases.

Laryngeal carcinomas account for 2% to 3% of malignancies. The incidence is higher in men than women (5.5:1). Eighty percent occur in patients 50 to 80 years of age. Most frequent risk factors are smoking and alcohol consumption. Laryngeal tumors are classified as supraglottic, glottic, or subglottic. The tumors of the glottis account for 50% to 60% of laryngeal cancers. Subglottic lesions constitute 20% to 30% and true glottic tumors constitute 1%. Hoarseness is the hallmark of glottic carcinoma. Its onset is delayed with supra- and subglottic tumors. Common symptoms include weight loss, dysphagia, odynophagia, and cough.

Preexisting medical conditions that may contribute to complications are cardiac, vascular, pulmonary, or renal disease, history of smoking with chronic obstructive airway disease, alcohol abuse, and malnutrition. **Most of these patients are older and are frequently men with long histories of heavy smoking and alcohol abuse. Associated medical problems may include chronic obstructive pulmonary disease, hypertension, coronary artery disease, and alcohol withdrawal.** Because of decreased appetite and poor swallowing ability, these patients may be in poor nutritional condition or even cachectic. Preoperative evaluation centers on investigation of these problems.

Airway management

The technique used to secure the airway is based on the site of tumor and type of surgery. Possible techniques include direct laryngoscopy, awake fiberoptic bronchoscopy, or tracheostomy. Topical anesthesia and vasoconstriction of the nostril is achieved with either 1% lidocaine with 0.25% neosynephrine or 4% cocaine (3 mg/kg maximum). If transtracheal and superior laryngeal nerve blocks are not desirable due to the site of tumor, 4% lidocaine may be delivered with a hand-held nebulizer.

Types of microvascular flap[104]

Head and neck reconstruction is an integral part of surgery for removal of head and neck tumors. Sites of defects most commonly requiring reconstruction are oral cavity (i.e., tongue, floor of mouth, lip), mandible, laryngopharynx, craniofacial, and facial skin.

Traditional methods of reconstructing head and neck defects include regional pedicle flaps, such as pectoralis major myocutaneous flap or trapezius flap, or local rotational flaps, such as forehead flap and nasolabial flap. In recent years, microvascular free tissue transfer has significantly improved the functional outcome of reconstruction head and neck defects and has become an integral part of head and neck reconstruction in many centers. The advantages of free flaps are that major reconstruction can be achieved in a single stage and a defect can be "custom-fitted" with tissue of appropriate size and composition. Commonly used microvascular free flaps for head and neck reconstruction are radial forearm, rectus, lateral thigh and latissimus dorsi for soft tissue coverage, and fibula, iliac crest and scapula for osseous reconstruction. The radial forearm free flap has become a workhorse flap for intraoral soft tissue reconstruction, as it provides pliable, thin skin which facilitates restoration of floor of mouth sulci and tongue mobility. This flap is easy to use and extremely reliable due to its large-caliber vessels. The rectus flap is used to reconstruct large soft tissue defects, such as radical maxillectomy or total glossectomy. The fibula free flap is currently the most commonly used flap for mandible reconstruction, although iliac crest also is used commonly. The fibula flap is popular because it can easily provide up to 20 cm of bone, adapts well to restore mandibular contour, has large-caliber vessels for anastomosis, and is easy to harvest. The thin skin paddle also offers the same advantages as the radial forearm flap for oral cavity reconstruction.

Success rates of 90% to 95% are expected with head and neck free tissue transfer. In a large series, comprised of 206 patients (follow-up of 14.2 months), the vessel thrombosis rate was 6.8% with a salvage rate of 19%, resulting in an ultimate flap survival rate of 94.5%.[103] The overall complication rate for microvascular free tissue transfer was 36%. Delay in recognition of arterial insufficiency or venous congestion, failure to return to the operating room immediately to address the problem of vascular compromise, use of interposition vein graft, and persistent hypotension are predisposing factors to flap loss.

The anesthesia team plays a very important role in maximizing the overall success rate of the free flap.[3,58,99] It is imperative that the anesthesiologist and the surgeon work as a team perioperatively for these types of cases. **The anesthesiologist must communicate with the surgeon regarding the planned donor site, which will limit the available sites for the anesthesiologist to place the lines necessary for monitoring and venous access.** For example, a pectoralis myocutaneous flap would preclude the use of an ipsilateral subclavian line. Most surgeons prefer to use the left arm for the radial forearm free flap, and therefore, one should not perform any venopuncture or place a line in that arm. No lines should be placed in the neck, as the internal jugular vein must be spared for the surgeon for use as a recipient vein. The advisability of placing a femoral line should be discussed ahead of time if the surgeon is planning an iliac crest or rectus flap.

Intraoperative Management

Intraoperative monitoring for these procedures should include an arterial line for serial hematocrit and blood gas determinations. Central venous or pulmonary artery monitoring is performed if the patient's cardiovascular status merits it. The internal jugular approach should be avoided because of proximity to the surgical field. The subclavian route is possible, but an intraoperative chest radiograph is necessary to rule out pneumothorax. Placement of a long central venous catheter through the basilic vein in the antecubital fossa is preferable because it remains away from the surgical field, but a pulmonary artery catheter may be difficult to place with this approach.[38] The femoral vein may be used if other sites are not available.

Maintenance of anesthesia is often accomplished with an inhalation agent and supplemental narcotics. The inhalation agent may be beneficial in patients with reactive airway disease; it also helps to blunt airway reflexes. The use of nondepolarizing muscle relaxants should be discussed with the surgical team preoperatively because a nerve stimulator is frequently used during neck dissections.

Significant intraoperative blood loss can be a problem. Elevating the head slightly may help reduce bleeding. At least one, but preferably two, large-bore IV lines should be started. Because these procedures often require many hours, a fluid warmer and humidifier should be used to help maintain patient temperature. A Foley catheter is used for collecting urine output.

In these types of cases, the goal is to maintain adequate intravascular volume and blood pressure to facilitate good perfusion to the flap. Generally, this can be achieved with fluids, although every effort must be made not to fluid overload the patient. A large positive fluid balance in the early postoperative period can result in severe edema and congestion in the flap, which can predispose to vascular compromise. In general, use the minimal amount of fluid needed to maintain the patient's baseline blood pressure and a urine output of 0.5 to 1 ml/kg/hr. Use of vasoconstricting agents ($alpha_1$ agonists) must be avoided. Any blood transfusion should be discussed with the surgeons, as their preference in these cases is to keep the hematocrit in the range of 27% to 30% to minimize thrombosis. Dextran 40 is used by some surgeons for reducing platelet aggregability.

Before a tracheostomy or total laryngectomy is performed during the surgical procedure, the anesthesiologist should make sure the patient is receiving 100% oxygen. Next, the trachea is transected while the anesthesiologist backs out the oral endotracheal tube. A spiral reinforced or J-tube (Fig. 84-8) is placed in the distal airway by the surgeon and connected to the anesthesia machine by a fresh, sterile breathing circuit. **At this point, bilateral breath sounds should be checked and end-tidal CO_2 waveforms verified. Occasionally, the tube will be placed down a mainstem bronchus because of the short distance to the carina. Also, the cuff may herniate around the distal end of the tube. Bronchospasm may occur because of tracheal stimulation during light anesthesia.** After satisfactory tube placement, the cuff may be sutured to the chest wall for the duration of the surgery. After surgical closure, the reinforced tube may be switched to a metal or Shiley tracheostomy cannula.[75]

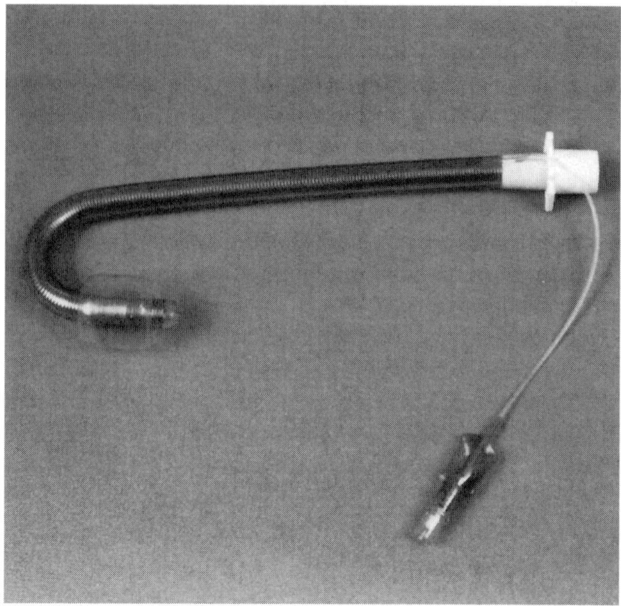

Fig. 84-8. Spiral reinforced J-tube for use with a tracheostomy. The tube may be sutured to the patient's chest, which allows the surgeon convenient access to the head and neck.

Complications

Complications of head and neck microvascular reconstructive surgery are systemic and local.[57] As mentioned earlier, systemic complications may be increased by preexisting medical conditions. Intraoperative complications may be related to the nature of surgery or anesthetic management of a prolonged surgery on an older age group with multiple medical problems.

Head and neck surgery such as laryngectomy and radical neck dissection combined with a microvascular free flap may last 8 to 12 hours or more and may involve substantial blood loss.[71,17,106]

During tracheostomy, possible complications include pneumothorax, subcutaneous emphysema, false passage, damage to recurrent laryngeal nerve, bleeding, aspiration, tracheoesophageal fistula, and tracheal fires due to a high FIO_2.

The operative sites are exposed for long periods so prophylactic antibiotics are administered. The patient's temperature is maintained by using a heated water mattress, a forced air flow blanket, and warming IV infusions and blood.

In the postoperative period, one problem is tracheal mucosal ulceration from prolonged intubation which may lead to stenosis. Other problems include myocardial infarction, stroke, pulmonary edema, difficulty in weaning from the ventilator, postoperative mental confusion, delirium tremons, and metabolic and electrolyte disorders. **Desaturation and hypoventilation after extubation in the intensive care unit is not uncommon and extubation should be done under controlled conditions with a fiberoptic bronchoscope available for reintubation.**

Other complications reported include:

1. *Increased intracranial pressure following bilateral neck dissection and radiotherapy.* Interruption of major venous drainage of the head and neck occurs in radical neck dissection. Bilateral neck dissection is usually staged to minimize complications which include facial and conjunctival edema, cyanosis, hemorrhage, wound infection and flap necrosis. Visual problems such as diplopia, papilledema, and decreased acuity are rare. Radiotherapy has been shown to promote thrombosis of small blood vessels. Kiers and King[61] reported a clinical syndrome of pseudotumor cerebri occurring in a man who had undergone staged radical neck dissection combined with radiotherapy. He was found to have left sigmoid sinus thrombosis at postmortem.
2. *Bilateral posterior optic neuropathy after bilateral radical neck dissection and hypotension.*[79] Ischemic optic neuropathy may occur in an anterior form that is associated with optic disc swelling or in posterior form that is associated initially with an optic disc of normal appearance. Both forms may occur in association with conditions that impair cerebral blood flow to the optic nerve which includes acute blood loss, hypovolemia, systemic hypotension, anemia, pre-existing arteriosclerosis and atherosclerosis and perhaps facial edema after bilateral radical neck dissection.
3. *Blindness following bilateral neck dissection.*[30] Bilateral neck dissection is an uncommon operation, as only 5% of these tumors metastasize to both sides of the neck. Major physiological changes occur during bilateral neck dissection. Ligation of both internal jugular veins cause dilation of the vertebral venous plexus, occipital veins, posterior jugular veins, deep cervical veins, pharyngoesophageal plexus and the pterygoid plexus. The collateral system may be poorly developed resulting in a rise of cerebral venous pressure. Unilateral ligation of the jugular vein may cause venous pressure to rise 300% and bilateral ligation may produce a rise of 500%.[123,127] Positioning of the patient with a slight head-up tilt may counteract venous engorgement. Positioning the patient with pads between the scapulae to aid neck dissection for improved access to the field may compress venous system and contribute to a rise in pressure.
4. *Thromboembolic risk factors in patients undergoing maxillofacial surgery for malignancies.*[133] Venous thromboembolism is a common complication in patients undergoing major surgery. Some of the risk factors associated with thromboembolism such as interoperative tissue damage, long duration of surgery, or damage to large vessel occur in these patients. Watzke and Watzke[133] found reduced antithrombin III level and increased level of fibrinogen in a series of 16 patients studied.
5. *Large visible gas bubbles in the internal jugular vein.*[98] Unexplained undesirable intraoperative events (e.g., hypotension, arrhythmia, and hyperemia) during radical neck dissection could be a result of venous air emboli or paradoxical air embolus which have a high frequency of occurrence. Rice and Gonzalez[98] found grossly visible gas bubbles in 42% of supine modified radical neck dissection. Positive pressure ventilation of the lungs decreases the likelihood of venous air embolism.
6. *Laryngeal edema induced by neck dissection and catheter thrombosis.* There are many possible causes of airway edema in a patient being treated for squamous cell carcinoma of the head and neck. These include radiation changes, anaphylaxis, venous and/or lymphatic obstruction secondary to mechanical compression resulting from infection, recurrent tumor, or anatomic distortions. Venous obstruction secondary to a thrombosed left-sided central venous catheter in a patient who had undergone prior right radical neck dissection, as described by Stropper and Calcaterra.[119] A functional neck dissection preserving the internal jugular vein when the size and location of a patient's tumor permits may circumvent complete obstruction of the venous drainage of larynx.
7. *Prolonged QT syndrome following right radical neck dissection.* Prolonged QT syndrome with subsequent cardiac arrest was reported by Otteni et al.[81] Any neck dissection, whether radical, modified, or selective, affects the deep cervical fascia and elevates carotid sheath structures and the sympathetic chain which could result in transient or partial disruption of sympathetic neural transmission. Strickland et al.[120] have described a patient who underwent partial glossectomy with supraomohyoid neck dissection which caused a transient decrease in right cervical sympathetic activity augmenting the prolongation of the QT interval resulting in ventricular fibrillation.
8. *Giant negative T waves after maxillofacial surgery.* Kim et al.[62] reported giant T waves in almost all leads and a prolonged QT following maxillofacial surgery 2 days postoperatively which returned to normal 4 months later. The possible causes for such abnormalities are ischemic heart disease, metabolic disturbances (K^+ or Ca^{++}), cerebral disturbances, drug effects, surgical damage to sympathetic innervation of the heart, hypertrophic cardiomyopathy, bradycardia, Stokes Adams syndrome associated with complete heart block, right ventricular hypertrophy, and right bundle branch block.
9. *Loss of hypoxic ventilatory responses following bilateral neck dissection.*[74] Two of five patients showed flattened responses compared with preoperative measurements

due to denervation of their carotid bodies. This may contribute to morbidity and mortality of patients following bilateral neck dissection especially in the presence of other factors such as primary disease, metastatic disease, extensive surgery, radiation, and chemotherapy.

10. *Adult respiratory distress syndrome (ARDS).* Ezri et al.[36] reported the development of ARDS a few hours following neck surgery in a patient without any apparent indication of sepsis.

Postoperatively, patients who have undergone major head and neck procedures should be monitored overnight in the intensive care unit. Controlled ventilation may be required in the immediate postoperative period. Problems in the recovery period include pneumothorax, airway impingement because of restrictive neck dressings or hematoma development, and communication difficulties after laryngectomy.[75] An endotracheal ventilation catheter may be used in the management of difficult extubations.[20] Reintuations should be performed with fiberoptic bronchoscopy to avoid damage to the microvascular flap.

PHONOSURGERY (VOCAL CORD FUNCTION RESTORATION)

The most common indication for phonosurgery remains vocal cord paralysis, either unilateral or bilateral, following thyroidectomy. Vocal cord paralysis may also occur following procedures of the neck or chest endoscopy, cardiac surgery, anterior approaches to the cervical spine, and injury of the base of the skull. Other causes may be neurogenic in origin due to central nervous system (CNS) lesions of the cerebral cortex or the brain stem.[121] Involvement of the tenth cranial nerve may occur anywhere along its course. The treatment depends on whether vocal cord paralysis is unilateral or bilateral.

Unilateral vocal cord paralysis usually requires no therapy and may compensate in 6 months to 1 year. If by then the larynx has not regained adequate function, injection of Teflon, fat emulsion, or silicone may be performed for medialization of the cord. This may be accomplished with IV sedation and local or general anesthesia with a small ET tube (5 to 6 mm). Surgical medialization consists of thyroplasty which can be performed using local anesthesia and IV sedation. Patient cooperation is needed for phonating an "E" sound to adjust the tension on the vocal cord. Fiberoptic bronchoscopy is performed to check the medialization. Bilateral abductor vocal cord paralysis usually requires surgical intervention (e.g., tracheostomy or surgical lateralization). The procedure can be performed either by external approach or endoscopically removing the arytenoid by microdissection or with the CO_2 laser.

TRACHEAL RESECTION AND RECONSTRUCTION

Tracheal resections and reconstructions are usually performed for tracheal stenosis caused by prolonged intubation. Giffen et al.[42] described 31 patients who underwent tracheal reconstructive surgery. The stenotic part of the trachea is resected and divided ends mobilized and anastomosed. General anesthesia is administered using two endotracheal tubes[42,50] or high frequency jet ventilation during the anastomosis. The intraoperative complications include barotrauma, aspiration, hypoxemia, and hypercapnia.

Postoperative complication are wound dehiscence, mucosal ulceration from pressure by the endotracheal tube which may cause recurrence of stenosis. Eckhardt et al.[32] reported a case where a laryngeal mask airway was used as a blocker during tracheoplasty.

MAXILLOFACIAL TRAUMA

LeFort[63a] determined the common fracture lines of the midface by experimentation on cadavers in 1901. The fractures are divided into LeFort I, II, and III[47] (Fig. 84-9). LeFort I is a dental alveolar fracture of the maxilla passing above the floor of the nose, involving the lower third of the nasal septum, and mobilizing the palate, maxillary alveolar process, the lower third of the pterygoid plates and part of the palatine bone. There is little airway compromise and patients may be intubated orally or nasally. The LeFort II fracture is pyramidal, involving the thick upper part of the nasal bone, then beneath the zygomaticomaxillary suture, crossing the lateral wall of the atrium and then posteriorly through the pterygoid plate. Nasotracheal intubation is relatively contraindicated because of the presence of a fractured nose. In a LeFort III fracture, a thin line of fracture runs parallel to the base of the skull separating the midface. The midface is often distracted posteriorly. **Fracture of the base of the skull is an absolute contraindication to nasotracheal intubation.**

Preoperative Evaluation

Preoperative evaluation of the patient with maxillofacial trauma center on three areas:

- airway assessment: fractures limit jaw mobility after upper airway trauma by producing pain, edema, and mechanical impairment of the zygomatic arch.
- assessment of associated injuries: intracranial (15% incidence), chest injuries (flail chest and pneumothorax), fracture dislocation of the cervical spine (1% to 6%); fractures of extremities; and ruptured spleen or liver.
- assessment of concurrent medical problems: acute or chronic alcoholism, drug intoxication, myocardial infarction, or stroke.

Repair of facial fractures is frequently not an emergency procedure and can be delayed hours to days, depending on the nature of the fracture and degree of swelling.[27,75]

Intraoperative Management

Tracheostomy may be indicated for unrelieved airway obstruction, inability to intubate, basal skull fracture and se-

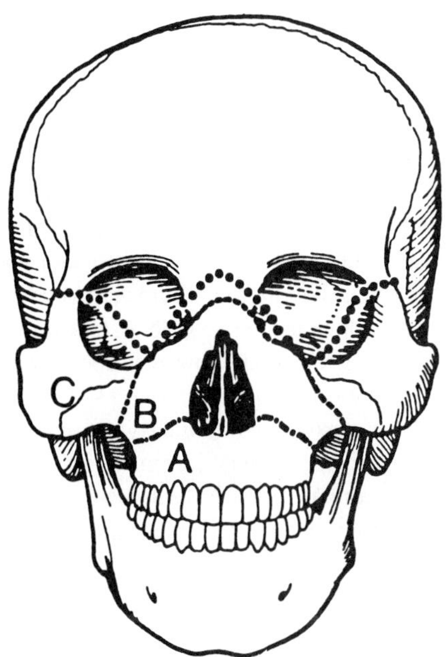

Fig. 84-9. La Forte I (**A**), II (**B**), and III (**C**) maxillary fractures (From Gotta A: Maxillofacial trauma: anesthetic considerations, *ASA Refresher Courses* 15:39–50, 1987.)

vere nasal fracture. Tracheostomy may be performed using local anesthesia or after securing the airway orally with a fiberoptic intubation. It is important to be knowledgable about these types of facial fractures because these can influence anesthetic management. Mandibular fractures usually occur at the condyles or rami and result in limited jaw movement because of trismus or pain. Midface or maxillary fractures are commonly classified according to the Le Fort scheme. Le Fort I fractures involve the lower aspect of the maxilla, causing separation of the hard palate, alveolar processes, and upper teeth from the maxilla. Le Fort II fractures extend close to the malar-maxillary suture lines, ending at the anterior part of the inferior orbital floor, leaving most of the maxilla free floating. Le Fort III fractures involve more or less complete bony separation of the midface from the skull and extend through the orbits and the nasoethmoidal region. With this type of fracture, a CSF leak is not unusual because of damage to the ethmoid plate.[39]

For many patients with facial fractures, nasal intubation is indicated because it allows better surgical access. Nasal intubation is contraindicated if there is a CSF leak or if the nasal passages are severely disrupted. If nasopharyngeal integrity is in doubt, the anesthesiologist can first intubate orally. Anesthesia is induced with an IV agent and maintained with inhalation agents taking precautions to avoid any increase in intracranial pressure associated with head injury. After anesthetic induction the nasopharynx can be examined; if appropriate, the oral tube can be replaced with a nasal tube. Blindly passing a nasotracheal tube into a disrupted nasopharynx can result in the tip of the tube being directed into the orbit, sinus, submucosally into the hypopharynx or even intracranially. Once the patient is intubated, intraoperative care includes careful attention to ventilation, preferably with continuous end-tidal CO_2 monitoring. A nasal tube is very useful (assuming it is possible) because the proximity of an oral endotracheal tube to the surgical site greatly increases the risk of accidental dislodgement or cutting into the tube.

Monitoring includes arterial line and central venous pressure for optimal fluid and electrolyte management. Blood loss, urine output, and maintainence must be continually assessed.

ORTHOGNATHIC SURGERY

Orthognathic surgery is performed electively by oral and maxillofacial surgeons primarily on healthy adolescents and young adults to treat dental malocclusion and balance facial proportions. The most common procedure is the sagittal split osteotomy of the mandible to either advance or setback the lower jaw. Le Fort I or II osteotomies are also used to move the maxilla en bloc. The maxilla may be moved in any direction (most commonly forward) or segmented to change transverse dimensions. Occasionally, combined maxillary and mandibular osteotomies are performed.[76] Many of these patients have anatomic features that make intubation difficult, such as retrognathia, maxillary protrusion (overbite), or limitation in mouth opening.[78] In addition, most such patients will have orthodontic appliances in place as part of their treatment.

Intraoperative Management

Orthognathic surgery requires the patient to be nasotracheally intubated because all incisions are made intraorally. Either a nasal RAE tube or a standard endotracheal tube modified with a curved connector and a malleable extension can be used. Care must be taken to avoid pressure on the nasal tip, because this can lead to pressure necrosis. Arranging the breathing circuit to come down behind the top of the patient's head allows easy surgical access to the mouth (Fig. 84-10).

Expected blood loss varies with the type of orthognathic surgery. With sagittal split osteotomy of the mandible, blood loss averages 300 ml. In maxillary surgery, more significant blood loss is possible. This usually occurs during the down fracture of the maxilla, at which time the greater palatine arteries can be torn. Preoperative autologous blood donation should be encouraged for maxillary surgery because blood loss can approach 2000 ml.[78]

Controlled hypotension has been advocated to attempt to decrease blood loss and to improve the operative field in orthognathic surgery.[41] Fromme et al.[40] studied sodium nitroprusside-induced hypotension and found no improvement in blood loss or operating conditions despite mean arterial pressures of 55 to 60 mm Hg.[40] In contrast, Lessard et al. lowered blood pressure to similar levels with isoflurane and found significant improvement in both blood loss and in the

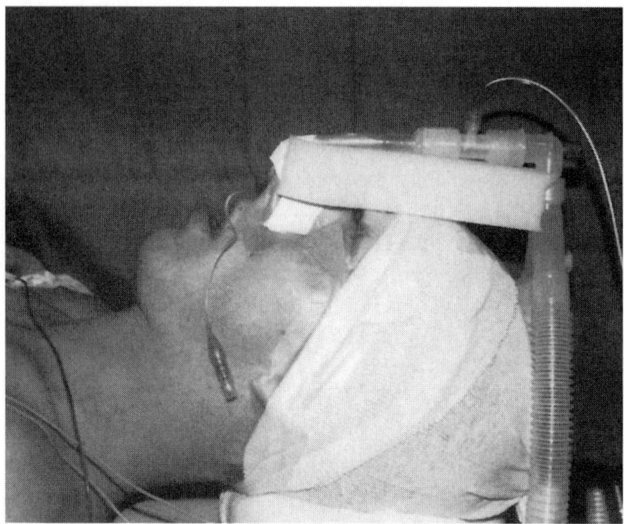

Fig. 84-10. Patient positioned for orthognathic surgery. A nasal right angle endotracheal tube is taped over the forehead with the breathing circuit coming down behind the top of the patient's head.

quality of the surgical field.[65] Blau et al.[8] compared esmolol with sodium nitroprusside in reducing blood loss in orthognothic surgery and found the former to be more effective. Labetalol has also been used for deliberate hypotension in orthognathic surgery but has not been subjected to a controlled trial.[72] Maxillary procedures justify the use of induced hypotension[43] but not mandibular surgery alone.

One unusual, but life-threatening complication during orthognathic surgery is direct damage to the nasotracheal tube by cutting instruments. This can occur when the medial wall of the maxillary sinus is cut during a maxillary osteotomy. The tube and pilot tube can be cut completely, requiring quick action to reestablish the airway.[37]

A pharyngeal pack is placed at the beginning of surgery to keep blood, secretions, and foreign bodies, such as wire or screws, from reaching the pharnyx. At the conclusion of surgery, this pack is removed and the pharynx well suctioned. A nasogastric tube is placed to drain the stomach of secretions and blood. Extubation should be performed only after the patient is fully awake with airway reflexes intact.[78]

In the past, most patients having orthognathic surgery were placed in intermaxillary fixation at the end of surgery. Intermaxillary fixation means that upper and lower teeth are held together by either wires or elastics to stabilize the jaws. This impedes access to the airway, hinders suctioning, and makes reintubation difficult. **If the patient is placed in intermaxillary fixation, the anesthesiologist needs to have appropriate cutting tools *at the bedside at all times* in case of an airway emergency.** The introduction of so-called rigid internal fixation methods has changed management. Titanium or stainless steel screws and plates are often now used to stabilize both maxillary and mandibular osteotomies; therefore, the patient does not have his or her upper and lower jaws "wired shut." Rigid internal fixation is obviously more comfortable for the patient in the weeks postoperatively.[76,78]

DENTAL ANESTHESIA

The majority of dental anesthesia is administered in dentists offices to outpatients in a dental chair (Fig. 84-11). Anesthesia may be achieved by local nerve blocks that may be combined with IV sedation (i.e., midazolam or an infusion of propofol or methohexital).[1,67] Dembo[29] and Meyers[73] compared the two infusions and showed propofol was superior for dental extraction and postoperative psychomotor recovery. The sedation may be combined with oxygen alone or with nitrous oxide which can be administered via nasal mask, nasopharyngeal airway or laryngeal mask airway (LMA). Airway management with LMA was shown to be superior compared with the other two techniques. Third molar surgery is frequently carried out under general anesthesia on an outpatient basis. IV sedation is an alternative modality.[48] The techniques of local anesthesia used are (Fig. 84-12):

- Topical-sensory—topical anesthesia is produced when a local anesthetic is placed on the free nerve endings.
- Injections—can be submucosal, paraperiosteal, or subperiosteal.

EAR SURGERY

Patients for ear surgery are often young healthy people undergoing procedures, such as tympanoplasty, mastoidectomy, myringotomy, or placement of pressure-equilization tubes. Daum and O'Reilly[24] have described the use of the LMA for myringotomies (62 patients) and major ear surgeries (52 patients). General anesthesia using a face mask for myringotomies and an endotracheal tube for longer surgeries is more commonly used.

Stapedectomy, a procedure performed more often for older patients, is frequently performed under local anesthesia. Communicating with patients having ear surgery may be difficult because of their decreased hearing ability. It may be helpful to have a set of cards with written instructions in the operating room for communication purposes. Also, some patients may have vertigo associated with their hearing loss (i.e., Meniere's disease).

Intraoperative Management

In ear surgery the anesthesiologist must be concerned primarily with the effect of nitrous oxide on the middle ear, facial nerve preservation, and control of bleeding. The KTP laser is used for middle ear surgery (see Laser Airway Surgery). Postoperative nausea and vomiting frequently occur with ear surgery and may be treated with droperidol 0.625 to 1.25 mg[75] or 4 mg IV odensetron.

Nitrous Oxide and Middle Ear Pressure

Nitrous oxide is 34 times more soluble in blood than nitrogen.[77] The gas diffuses into the middle ear across mucosal

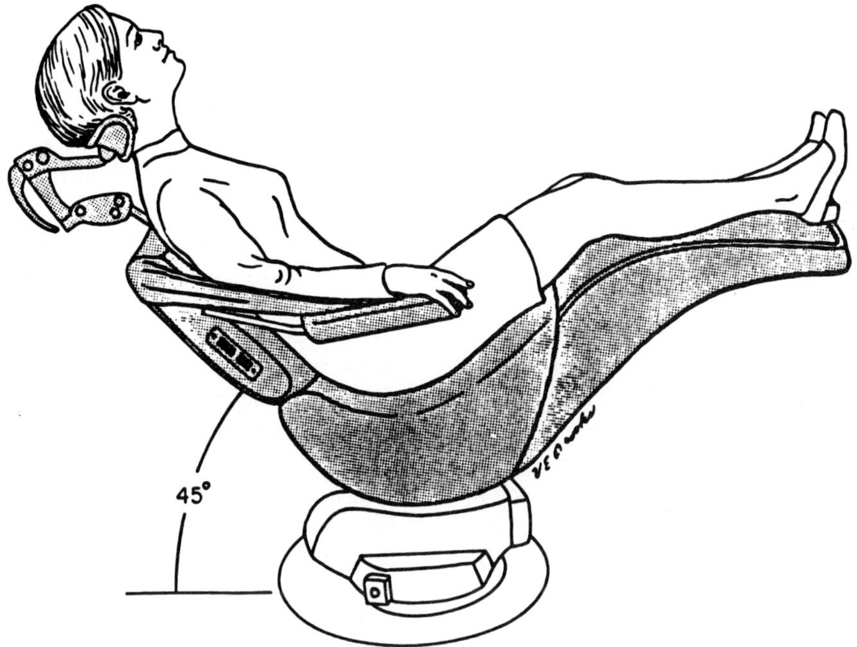

Fig. 84-11. In dental anesthesia and analgesia, the position of the patient in the contour dental chair is of importance in proper airway maintenance. The 45° position is the best compromise between cardiovascular and other considerations. (From Allen GD: *Dental Anesthesia and Analgesia,* ed 3, Baltimore/London, 1983, Williams & Wilkins.)

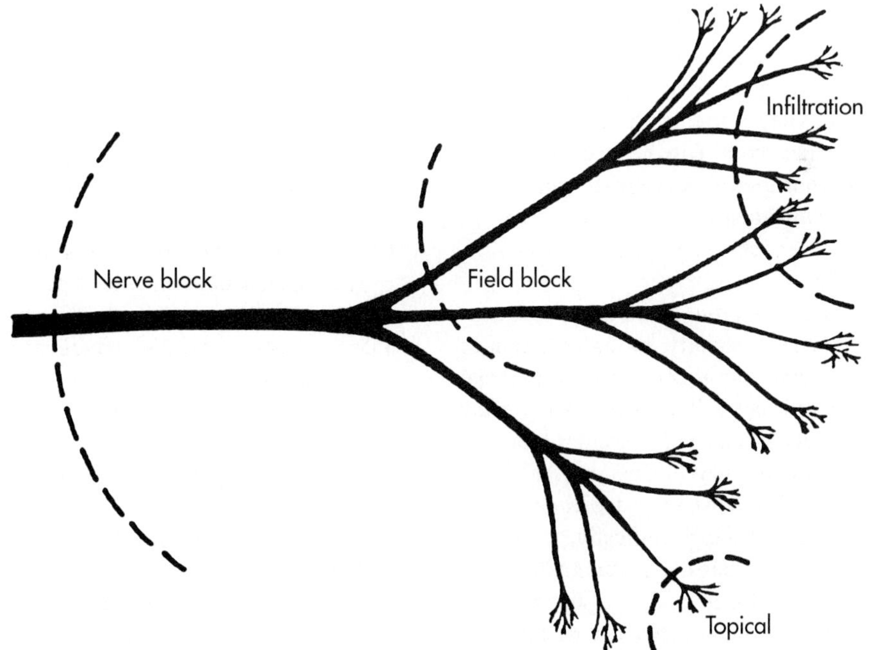

Fig. 84-12. Anatomical classification of techniques of local dental anesthesia. (From Allen GD: *Dental Anesthesia and Analgesia,* ed 3, Baltimore/London, 1983, Williams & Wilkins.)

blood vessels much more rapidly than nitrogen can leave. This causes the overall pressure in the middle ear to increase. In a normal ear, this pressure increase is vented by the eustachian tube into the nasopharynx. Yawning and swallowing actively open the eustachian tubes, but these cannot occur in anesthetized patients. During anesthesia, when the middle ear pressure increases to a certain point, the eustachian tube passively opens. In a diseased ear, however, scarring may disrupt even this passive venting.[83]

Many studies have documented increased middle ear

pressure during nitrous oxide administration.[28,69,93,126,134] With 70% nitrous oxide administration, there is a rapid rise of middle ear pressure of approximately 10 to 20 mm H_2O/min. Passive venting occurs at 200 to 300 mm H_2O via eustachian tubes. The increase in middle ear pressure depends on the following factors: duration of anesthesia, percentage of N_2O used, an intact tympanic membrane, and the functioning of the eustachian tube.

Complications resulting from this increased pressure include displacement of tympanoplasty grafts and tympanic membrane rupture. For example, tympanic membrane rupture in a patient anesthetized for a gynecologic procedure was discovered by noticing bright red blood in the ear canal. The patient had a history of middle ear disease and prior surgery.[83] Also, disruption of prior middle ear surgical repair has been reported when nitrous oxide was administered for subsequent surgery. The resulting hearing loss was noted on emergence from anesthesia.[68,93]

Middle ear pressure changes have been implicated in postoperative nausea and vomiting, although this has never been conclusively proven. When nitrous oxide is discontinued at the end of the case, negative pressure develops secondary to rapid diffusion of the nitrous oxide out of the middle ear.[135] The eustachian tube better equilibrates middle ear pressure when it is below ambient pressure than when it is greater.[7] Subatmospheric middle ear pressure has been implicated as a cause of transient hearing loss postoperatively and may contribute to serous otitis media.[7,135] **For a tympanoplasty procedure the middle ear remains open until the surgeon places the graft over the tympanic membrane. Nitrous oxide can be used until approximately 10 to 15 minutes before graft placement and then should be discontinued.**

Facial nerve preservation

Identification and preservation of the facial nerve is a concern during otologic surgery especially during resection of an acoustic neuroma. A nerve stimulator is used, and facial movement is monitored visually. For this reason, many anesthesiologists commonly avoid neuromuscular blocking drugs during ear surgery. Studies have shown, however, that there is a difference in sensitivity between facial and ulnar nerves to train-of-four stimulation. Specifically, there is a greater twitch decrement with ulnar nerve stimulation than with facial nerve stimulation for a given dose of relaxant.[11,92] Ho et al.[54] examined facial movement response to direct intracranial stimulation in patients undergoing acoustic neuroma surgery. They found that facial movement to intracranial stimulation preceded return of the ulnar train-of-four response. At the earliest hint of ulnar train-of-four recovery they also found that the facial twitch response to intracranial stimulation was already strong. **Thus, it can be concluded that reliable intraoperative facial nerve monitoring may be performed despite significant neuromuscular blockade as monitored by conventional ulnar train-of-four monitoring.** Although there may be little theoretic reason to avoid nondepolarizing relaxants during ear surgery, most anesthesiologists continue to avoid their use.

Control of bleeding

During microscopic ear surgery, even a small drop of blood can make the procedure difficult. Injecting the ear with an epinephrine-containing solution is the primary means used to control such bleeding. Elevating the patient's head can improve venous drainage.[75] More controversial is the use of deliberate hypotension. Many surgeons contend that lowering the arterial pressure is helpful. In contrast, Eltringham et al.[34] found no correlation between degree of hypotension and surgical estimate of bleeding during middle ear surgery. Profound hypotension with systolic blood pressure less than 50 mm Hg in healthy patients has been advocated for ear surgery. No morbidity and mortality was reported in a series of healthy patients using this technique.[60] Numerous complications of hypotensive anesthesia have been reported, especially in older patients.[19] Because younger patients without evidence of cardiopulmonary disease tolerate deliberate hypotension well, it may be reasonable to lower the *mean* arterial pressure to the 60- to 70-mm Hg range for middle ear surgery, but more drastic measures are not recommended.

Given these considerations, volatile anesthetics are often a good choice for middle ear surgery. Volatile agents in sufficient concentrations prevent movement without use of muscle relaxants. They can be used to produce deliberate hypotension, and they can provide adequate anesthesia without nitrous oxide.[38]

Glomus Tumors

Glomus tumors are paragangliomas[56] of the head and neck which present multiple anesthetic risks including:

1. Involvement of cranial nerves IX, X, XI, and XII causing dysphagia, aspiration, and upper airway obstruction.
2. Highly vascular and can lead to major blood loss.
3. May secrete catecholamines producing symptoms of pheochromocytoma.
4. May secrete serotonin producing symptoms of carcinoid syndrome.
5. Prophylactic embolization may trigger a cerebrovascular accident.
6. Surgical treatment may be associated with cerebrospinal fluid leak, venous air embolism, or gastroparesis after tumor resection due to elevated baseline cholecystokinin levels.

SUMMARY

The skills required for airway management during ear, nose, and throat surgery are considerable and are applicable to many other aspects of anesthesia practice. When faced with a difficult and/or shared airway, it is always important for the anesthesiologist to have "back-up" plans. Communication with the surgeon is vital during these cases. Remembering these principles will enhance patient safety and contribute to quality of care.

KEY POINTS

- Endoscopic procedures are usually brief but may trigger acute sympathetic responses during airway manipulation which could be detrimental to patients with coronary artery disease.
- The anesthesiologist should understand the rationale and technique of superior laryngeal nerve block and glossopharyngeal nerve block.
- Ventilation for surgical laryngoscopy can be achieved by using a small, cuffed endotracheal tube that is either left in or intermittently removed (intermittent apnea) or by using jet ventilation.
- Laser fires are real; they burn endotracheal tubes (and therefore tracheas), but they can also burn surgeon's gowns, gloves, drapes, and fill the entire operating room with flames and smoke.
- Metallic tape (3M No. 425) can be used to wrap flammable endotracheal tubes, but it is not a perfect solution. On the other hand, the metallic tubes that don't burn may reflect the laser beam and do damage elsewhere.
- Airway fires can occur with incredible suddenness. The procedure for prevention and dealing with such fires should be planned ahead.
- The patient who is returned to the operating room for bleeding from tonsillectomy must be considered to have a full stomach and may be severely hypovolemic.
- The toxicity of cocaine must be well understood. The maximum dose of 3 mg/kg is approximately 5 ml of the usual 4% solution. Although this drug is being applied topically, there is a real danger of toxicity, especially in patients with coronary artery disease.
- Major head and neck cancer surgery is usually combined with a microvascular flap for reconstruction. The viability of the flap is dependent upon surgical and anesthetic management.
- The anesthesiologist should plan a safe establishment of the airway in maxillofacial trauma. That depends on the type of facial trauma present.
- During oral orthognathic surgery, it is possible for the surgeon to cut the pilot tube to the cuff on the nasal RAE tube. There should be a back-up plan for this possibility.
- The risk of use of nitrous oxide in middle ear surgery should be understood and discussed with the surgeon.
- During various kinds of otologic surgery, it may be necessary to have a nonparalyzed patient because of the proximity of the facial nerve.

KEY REFERENCES

Crockett DM, Scamman FL, McCabe BF, et al: Venturi jet ventilation for microlaryngoscopy: technique, complications, pitfalls, *Laryngoscope* 97:1326, 1987.

Gotta AW: Management of the traumatized airway, *ASA Refresher Courses,* vol 23, 1995.

Hunsaker DH: Anesthesia for microlaryngeal surgery: the case for subglotic jet ventilation, *Laryngoscope* 104:Aug p1, 1994.

McGolderick KE: Complications associated with otohinologic anesthesia surgery. In McGoldrick KE, editor: *Anesthesia for Ophthalogic and Otolaryngologic Surgery,* Philadelphia, 1992, WB Saunders.

Malamed SF, Quinn CL: Techniques of intravenous Sedation. In *Sedation—A Guide to Patient Management,* ed 34, Philadelphia, 1995, Mosby–Year Book.

Pashayan AG: Anesthesia for laser surgery, *ASA Refresher Courses,* 276, 1995.

Schusterman MA, Miller MJ, Reece GP, et al: A single center's experience with 308 free flaps for repair of head and neck cancer defects, *Plas Reconstr Surg* 93:472, 1994.

Sosis MB: Evaluation of five metallic tapes for protection of endotracheal tubes during CO_2 laser surgery, *Anesth Analg* 69:392, 1989.

Van Der Spek AFL, Spargo PM, Norton ML: The physics of lasers and implications for their use during airway surgery, *Br J Anaesth* 60:709,1988.

REFERENCES

1. Allen GD: *Dental Anesthesia and Analgesia (Local and General),* ed 3, Baltimore/London, 1983, Williams & Wilkins.
2. American National Standarda Institute: American National Standard for the safe use of lasers. *ANSI* 136:1, 1986.
3. Aps O, Cox RG, Mayou R, et al: The role of anaesthetic management in enhancing peripheral blood flow in patients undergoing free flap transfer. *Ann R Coll Surg Engl* 67:177, 1985.
4. Badrinath SK, et al: Anesthesia for tonsillectomy and adenoidectomy. In Brown BR, editor: *Anesthesia and ENT surgery,* Philadelphia, 1987, FA Davis.
5. Barr NL, Istscoitz S, Chan C, et al: Oxygen injection in suspension laryngoscopy, *Arch Otolaryngol* 93:606, 1971.
6. Benumof JL: *Anesthesia for thoracic surgery,* Philadelphia, 1987, WB Sanders.
7. Blackstock D, Gettes MA: Negative pressure in the middle ear in children after nitrous oxide anaesthesia, *Can Anaesth Soc J* 33:32, 1986.

7a. Blackwell KE, Ross DA, Kapur P, et al: Propofol for maintenance of general anesthesia: a technique to limit blood loss during surgery, *Am J Otolaryngol* 14:262, 1993.

8. Blau WS, Kafer ER, Anderson JA: Esmolol is more effective than sodium nitroprusside in reducing blood loss during Orthognathic surgery, *Anath Analg* 75;172,1992.

9. Brown BR: The outpatient and ENT surgery. In Brown BR, editor: *Anesthesia and ENT Surgery,* Philadelphia, 1987, FA Davis.

10. Burgess GE, LeJeune FE: Endotracheal tube ignition during laser surgery of the larynx, *Arch Otolaryngol* 105:561, 1979.

11. Caffrey RR, Warren ML, Becker KE: Neuromuscular blockade monitoring comparing the orbicularis oculi and adductor pollicis muscles, *Anesthesiology* 65:95, 1986.

12. Calcaterra TC, House J: Local anesthesia for suspension microlaryngoscopy, *Ann Otolaryngol* 85:71, 1976.

13. Carden E, Schwesinger WB: The use of nitrous oxide during ventilation with the open bronchoscope, *Anesthesiology* 39: 551, 1973.

14. Carden E, Vest HR: Further advances in anesthetic techniques for microlaryngeal surgery, *Anesth Analg* 53:584, 1974.

15. Carnie J: Continuous suxamethonium infusion for microlaryngeal surgery, *Br J Anaesth* 54:11, 1982.

16. Chang JL, Meeuwis H, Bleyaert A: Severe abdominal distention following jet ventilation during general anesthesia, *Anesthesiology* 49:216, 1978.

17. Chick LR, Walton RL, William R, Colen L, Sasmor M: Free flaps in the elderly. *Plas Reconst Surg,* 90(1):87, 1992.

18. Chung F, Crago RR: Sleep apnoea syndrome and anaesthesia, *Can Anaesth Soc J* 29:439, 1982.

19. Condon HA: Deliberate hypotension in ENT surgery, *Clin Otolaryngol* 4:241, 1979.

20. Cooper RM: The use of an endotracheal ventilation catheter in the management of difficult extubations. *Can J Anaesth* 43(1): 90–93, 1996.

21. Cozine K, Rosenbaum LM, Askanazi J, et al: Laser-induced endotracheal tube fire, *Anesthesiology* 55:583, 1981.

22. Crockett DM, Scamman FL, McCabe BF, et al: Venturi jet ventilation for microlaryngoscopy: technique, complications, pitfalls, *Laryngoscope* 97:1326, 1987.

23. Crysdale WD, Russel D: Complications of tonsillectomy and adenoidectomy in 9409 children observed overnight, *Can Med Assoc J* 135:1139, 1986.

24. Daum REO, O'Reilly BJ: The laryngeal mask airway in ENT surgery, *J Laryngol Otolaryngol* 106:28–30, 1992.

25. Davidson TM, Calloway CA: Tonsillectomy and adenoidectomy, its indications and its problems, *West J Med* 133:451, 1980.

26. Davies DD: Re-anaesthetizing cases of tonsillectomy and adenoidectomy because of persistent postoperative haemorrhage, *Br J Anaesth* 36:244, 1964.

27. Davies RM, Scott JG: Anaesthesia for major oral and maxillofacial surgery, *Br J Anaesth* 40:202, 1968.

28. Davis I, More JRM, Lahiri SK: Nitrous oxide and the middle ear, *Anaesthesia* 34:147, 1979.

29. Dembo JB: Methohexital versus propofol for outpatients anesthesia, Part II: Propofol is superior. *J Oral Maxillofac Surg* 53:816, 1995.

30. Dodd FM: Blindness Following Bilateral Neck Dissection. *Eur J Anaesthesiol* 10: 37, 1993.

31. Donlon JV: Anesthesia for eye, ear, nose and throat surgery. In Miller RD: *Anesthesia,* ed 3, New York, 1990, Churchill-Livingstone.

32. Eckhardt WF, Forman S, Denman W, Grillo HC, Muehrcke D: Another use for the laryngeal mask airway-as a blocker during tracheoplasty, *Anesth Analg* 80: 622–624, 1995.

33. El-Naggar M, et al: Jet ventilation for microlaryngoscopic procedures: a further simplified technique, *Anesth Analg* 53:797, 1974.

34. Eltringham RJ, Young PN, Fairbairn ML, et al: Hypotensive anaesthesia for microsurgery of the middle ear. A comparison between enflurane and halothane, *Anaesthesia* 37:1028, 1982.

35. Emery RE: Laser perforation of a main stem bronchus, *Anesthesiology* 64:120, 1986.

36. Ezri T, Szmuk P, Shklar B, Poria I, Schattner A, Soroker D: Clinical Reports: adult respiratory distress syndrome after radical neck dissection. *Can J Anaesth* 40: 658, 1993.

37. Fagraeus L, Angelillo JC, and Dolan EA: A serious anesthetic hazard during orthognathic surgery, *Anesth Analg* 59:150, 1980.

38. Feinstein RF, Owens WD: Anesthesia for ENT. In Barash PG, Cullen BF, Stoelting RK, editors: *Clinical Anesthesia,* Philadelphia, 1992, JB Lippincott.

39. Fergusson NV: Anesthesia for head and neck surgery. In DeKornfeld TJ, editor: *Anesthesiology,* New York, 1986, Medical Examination Publishing.

40. Fromme GA, MacKenzie RA, Gould AB Jr, et al: Controlled hypotension for orthognathic surgery, *Anesth Analg* 65:683, 1986.

41. Gallagher DM, Milliken RA: Induced hypotension for orthognathic surgery, *J Oral Surg* 37:47, 1979.

42. Geffin B, Bland J, Grillo HC: Anesthetic management of tracheal resection and reconstruction, *Anesth Analg* 48:884, 1969.

43. Geffin B, Shapshay SM, Bellack GS, et al: Flammability of endotracheal tubes during Nd-YAG laser application in the airway, *Anesthesiology* 65:511, 1986.

44. Gefke K, Andersen LW, Friesel E: Lidocaine given intravenously as a suppressant of cough and laryngospasm after tonsillectomy, *Acta Anesthesiol Scand* 27:111, 1983.

45. Goldman L, Caldera DL, Nussbaum SB, et al: Multifactorial index of cardiac risk in noncardiac surgical procedures, *N Engl J Med* 297:843, 1977.

46. Goode RL: Sleep disorders. In Cummings CW, Fredrickson JM, Harker LA, et al, editors: *Otolaryngology—Head and Neck Surgery,* St Louis, 1986, CV Mosby.

47. Gotta AW: Management of the traumatized airway, *ASA* 23:103, 1995.

48. Grainger JK: Intravenous sedation for third molar surgery. *Anesth Pain Con Dentistry* 2:98, 1993.

49. Gussack GS, Evans RF, Tacchi EJ: Intravenous anesthesia and jet ventilation for laser microlaryngeal surgery, *Ann Otol Rhinol Laryngol* 96:29, 1987.

50. Hannallah MS: The optinal breathing tube for tracheal resection, *Anesthesiology,* 83:2, 1995.

51. Hashisaki GT, Johns ME: Cocaine applications in otorhinolaryngologic anesthesia. In Brown BR, editor: *Anesthesia and ENT Surgery,* Philadelphia, 1987, FA Davis.

52. Hayes DM, Gaba DM, Goode RL: Incendiary characterstics of a new laser-resistant endotracheal tube, *Otolaryngol Head Neck Surg* 95:37, 1986.

53. Hermens JM, Bennett MJ, Hirshman CA: Anesthesia for laser surgery, *Anesth Analg* 62:218, 1983.

54. Ho LC, Crosby G, Sundaram P, et al: Ulnar train-of-four stimulation in predicting face movement during intracranial facial nerve stimulation, *Anesth Analg* 69:242, 1989.

55. Hunsaker DH: Anesthesia for Microlaryngeal Surgery: The case for subglotic jet ventilation. *Laryngoscope* 104:1, 1994.

56. Jensen FN:Glomus tumors of the head and neck: anesthetic considerations. *Anesth Analg* 78:112, 1994.

57. Joseph MM, Kaufman WA, Shindo ML: Complications of anesthesia for head-neck and reconstructive surgery, *Semin Anesth* 15(3):203–211, 1996.

58. Joseph MM, Narahari SL: Review of Anesthetic Management of Patients Undergoing Free Flap Reconstructive Surgery Following the Resection of Head and Neck Tumors, 11th World Congress of Anaesthesiologists, Sydney, Australia, April 14–20, 1996 (abstract).

59. Keon TP: Anesthetic considerations for laser surgery, *Int Anesth Clin* 26:50, 1988.

60. Kerr AR: Anaesthesia with profound hypotension for middle ear surgery, *Br J Anaesth* 49:447, 1977.

61. Kiers L, King JO: Increased intracranial pressure following bilateral neck dissection and radiotherapy, *Aust NZ J Surg* 61:459, 1991.

62. Kim Y, Shibutani T, Hasuaki H, Tomonori H, Hideo M: Giant negative T waves after maxillofacial surgery, *Anesth Prog* 39:28, 1992.

63. Lau S, Pinosky ML, Cooke JE, Halstead LA: The laryngeal mask airway in a patient with an endotracheal stent, *Am J Anesthesiol* 22:318–320, 1995.

63a. LeFort R: Etude experimentale sur les fractures de la machoire supérieure, *Rev Chir* 23:208–227, 360–379, 479–507, 1901.

64. LeJeune FE, Guice C, Letard F, et al: Heat sink protection against lasering endotracheal cuffs, *Ann Otol Rhinol Laryngol* 91: 606, 1982.

65. Lessard MR, Trepanier CA, Gourdeau M, et al: Isoflurane-induced hypotension in orthognathic surgery, *Anesth Analg* 69:379, 1989.

66. Linder A, Lindholm CE: Vocal fold lateralization using carbon dioxide laser and fibrin glue. *J Laryngol Otol* 106:226–230, 1992.
67. Malamed SF, Quinn CL: Techniques of intravenous sedation. In Sedation: A Guide to Patient Management, ed 3, St Louis, Mosby–Year Book, 1995.
68. Man A, Segal S, Ezra S: Ear injury caused by elevated intratympanic pressure during general anesthesia, *Acta Anesthesiol Scand* 24:224, 1980.
69. Matz GJ, Rattenborg CG, Holaday DA: Effects of nitrous oxide on middle ear pressure, *Anesthesiology* 28:948, 1967.
70. McGolderick KE. Complications Associated with Otorhinologic Anesthesia and Surgery. In McGoldrick KE, editor: *Anesthesia for Ophthalmic and Otolaryngologic Surgery,* Philadelphia, 1992, WB Saunders.
71. McGowen FX: Anesthesia for Major Head and Neck Surgery. In McGoldrick KE, editor: *Anesthesia for Ophthalmic and Otolaryngologic Surgery,* Philadelphia, 1992, WB Saunders.
72. McNulty S, Sharifi-Azad S, Farole A: Induced hypotension with labetalol for orthognathic surgery, *J Oral Maxillofac Surg* 45:309, 1987.
73. Meyers CJ: Comparison of propofol and methohexital for deep sedation, *J Oral Maxillofac Surg* 52:444, 1994.
74. Moorthy SS, Sullivan TY, Fallon JH, Dierdorf SF, Radpour S, DeAtley RE: Loss of hypoxic ventilatory response following bilateral neck dissection, *Int Anesth Res Soc,* 76:791, 1993.
75. Morrison JD, Mirakhur RK, Craig HJL: *Anaesthesia for Eye, Ear, Nose and Throat Surgery,* ed 2, Edinburgh, 1985, Churchill-Livingstone.
76. Munro IR: Craniofacial surgery: airway problems and management, *Int Anesth Clin* 26:72, 1988.
77. Munson ES: Transfer of nitrous oxide into body air cavities, *Br J Anaesth* 46:202, 1974.
78. Murphy A, Donoff B: Anesthesia for orthognathic surgery, *Int Anesth Clin* 27:98, 1989.
79. Nawa Y, Jaques JD, Miller NR, Palermo RA, Green RW: Bilateral posterior optic neuropathy after bilateral radical neck dissection and hypotension, *Graefe's Arch Exp Ophthalmol* 230:301, 1992.
80. Norton ML, Strong MS, Vaughan CW, et al: Endotracheal intubation and Venturi (jet) ventilation for laser microsurgery of the larynx, *Ann Otol Rhinol Laryngol* 85: 656, 1976.
81. Otteni JC, Pottecher T, Bronner G, et al: Prolongation of the Q-T interval and sudden cardiac arrest following right radical neck dissection, *Anesthesiology* 59:358, 1983.
82. Oulton JL, Donald DM: A ventilating laryngoscope, *Anesthesiology* 35:540, 1971.
83. Owens WD, Gustave F, Sclaroff A: Tympanic membrane rupture with nitrous oxide anesthesia, *Anesth Analg* 57:283, 1978.
84. Paes ML: General anaesthesia for carbon dioxide laser surgery within the airway, *Br J Anaesth* 59:1610, 1987.
85. Pappas AL, Sukhani R, Bowie JR: Post tonsillectomy analgesia and recovery: narcotics versus local anesthetics, *Anesthesiology* 71:A694, 1989.
86. Pashayan AG, Gravenstein JS, Cassisi NS, et al: The helium protocol for laryngotracheal operations with CO_2 laser: a retrospective review of 523 cases, *Anesthesiology* 68:801, 1988.
87. Pashayan AG, Gravenstein JS: Airway fires during surgery with the carbon dioxide laser (letter), *Anesthesiology* 71:478, 1989.
88. Pashayan AG, Gravenstein JS: Helium retards endotracheal tube fires from carbon dioxide lasers, *Anesthesiology* 62:274, 1985.
89. Pashayan AG, Gravenstein N: High incidence of CO_2 laser beam contact with the tracheal tube during operations on the upper airway, *J Clin Anesth* 1:354, 1989.
90. Pashayan AG: Anesthesia for laser surgery. *ASA Refresher Courses* 276, 1995.
91. Patel KF, Hicks JN: Prevention of fire hazards associated with the use of carbon dioxide lasers, *Anesth Analg* 60:885, 1981.
92. Pathak D, et al: A comparison of the response of hand and facial muscles to non-depolarizing relaxants, *Anesthesiology* 65:A299, 1986.
93. Patterson ME, Bartlett PC: Hearing impairment caused by intratympanic pressure changes during general anesthesia, *Laryngoscope* 86:399, 1976.
94. Prybus DA, O'Connor AF, Henville JD: Anaesthesia for laryngoscopy: a technique using the Nuffield anaesthetic ventilator, *Br J Anaesth* 50:501, 1978.
95. Rajagopalan R, Smith F, Ramachandran PR: Anaesthesia for microlaryngoscopy and definitive surgery, *Can Anaesth Soc J* 19:83, 1972.
96. Reilly JS: Tonsillar and adenoid airway obstruction: modes of treatment in children, *Int Anesth Clin* 26:54, 1988.
97. Reinhart DJ, Anderson JS: Fatal outcome during endoscopic sinus surgery: anesthetic manifestation, *Anesth Analg* 77(1): 188 , 1993.
98. Rice JH, Gonzalez RM: Large visible gas bubbles in the internal jugular vein: A common occurrence during supine radical neck surgery? *J Clin Anesth,* 4:21, 1992.
99. Robins DW: The anaesthetic management of patients undergoing free flap transfer, *Br J Plas Surg* 36:231, 1983.
100. Ruder CB: Anesthesia for carbon dioxide laser microsurgery of the larynx, *Otolaryngol Head Neck Surg* 89:732, 1981.
101. Sanders DR: Two ventilating attachments for bronchoscopes, *Del Med J* 39:170, 1967.
102. Scamman FL, McCabe BF: Supraglottic jet ventilation for laser surgery of the larynx in children, *Ann Otol Rhinol Laryngol* 95: 142, 1986.
103. Schenck NL: Cocaine: Its use and misuse in otolaryngology, *Trans Am Acad Ophthalmol Otolaryngol* 80:343, 1975.
104. Schusterman MA, Miller MJ, Reece GP, Kroll SS, Marchi M, Goepfert H: A single center's experience with 308 free flaps for repair of head and neck cancer defects, *Plas Reconst Surg* 93:472, 1994.
105. Simpson JI, Wolf GL: Helium does not reduce endotracheal tube flammability, *Anesth Analg* 68:S266, 1989.
106. Singlis M, Edwards JM, Robbie DS, et al: The anaesthetic management of patients undergoing free flap reconstructive surgery following resection of head and neck neoplasms - a review of 64 patients. *Ann R Coll Surg Engl* 70:235, 1988.
107. Snow JC, Norton ML, Saluja TS, et al: Fire hazard during CO_2 laser microassurgery on larynx and trachea, *Anesth Analg* 55:146, 1976.
108. Sosis M, Dillon F, Heller S: Hazards of a new clear unmarked polyvinylchloride tube designed for use with the Nd-YAG laser, *Anesthesiology* 71:A420, 1989.
109. Sosis M, Dillon F, Heller S: Prevention of CO_2 laser induced endotracheal tube fires with the Laser-Guard protective coating, *Anesthesiology* 71:A419, 1989.
110. Sosis M, Dillon F, Heller S: Saline filled cuffs help prevent laser-induced polyvinylchloride endotracheal tube fires, *Anesthesiology* 71:A421, 1989.
111. Sosis M, Dillon F: What is the safest foil tape for endotracheal tube protection during Nd-YAG laser surgery? A comparative study, *Anesthesiology* 72:553, 1990.
112. Sosis M, Heller S: A comparison of special endotracheal tubes for use with the Nd-YAG laser, *Anesth Analg* 68:S271, 1989.
113. Sosis M: Polyvinylchloride endotracheal tubes are hazardous for CO_2 laser surgery (letter), *Anesthesiology* 69:801, 1988.
114. Sosis MB, Heller S: A comparison of special endotracheal tubes for use with the CO_2 laser, *Anesthesiology* 69:A251, 1988.
115. Sosis MB: Airway fire during CO_2 laser surgery using a Xomed laser endotracheal tube, *Anesthesiology* 72:747, 1990.
116. Sosis MB: Evaluation of five metallic tapes for protection of endotracheal tubes during CO_2 laser surgery, *Anesth Analg* 68:392, 1989.
117. Spoerel WE, Grant PA: Ventilation during bronchoscopy, *Can Anaesth Soc J* 18:178, 1971.
118. Spoerel WE, Greenway RE: Technique of ventilation during endolaryngeal surgery under general anesthesia, *Can Anaesth Soc J* 20:369, 1973.
119. Storper IA, Calcaterra TC: Laryngeal edema induced by neck dissection and catheter thrombosis, *Am J Otolaryngol* 13 (2):101, 1992.
120. Strickland RA, Stanton MS, Olsen KD: Case report - Prolonged QT syndrome: perioperative management, *Mayo Clin Proc* 68:1016–1020, 1993.
121. Strome M, Kelly JH, Fried MP: *Manual of Otolaryngology,* ed 1, Boston/Toronto, Little Brown and Company.
122. Strong MS, Vaughn CW, Mahler DL, et al: Cardiac complications of microsurgery of the larynx: Etiology, incidence and prevention, *Laryngoscope* 84:908, 1974.
123. Sugarbaker ED, Wiley HM: Intracranial pressure studies incident to resection of the internal jugular veins, *Cancer* 4:242, 1951.
124. Takata M, Benumof JL, Ozaki GT: Confirmation of endotracheal intubation over a jet stylet: In vitro studies, *Anesth Analg* 80:800–805, 1995.
125. Tate N: Deaths from tonsillectomy, *Lancet* 2:1090, 1963.
126. Thomsen KA, Terkildsen K, Arnfred I:

Middle ear pressure variations during anesthesia, *Arch Otolaryngol* 82:609, 1965.
127. Tobin HA: Increased cerebrospinal fluid pressure following unilateral radical neck dissection, *Laryngoscope* 82:817, 1972.
128. Torres LE, Reynolds RC: Experiences with a new endotracheal tube for microlaryngeal surgery, *Anesthesiology* 52:357, 1980.
129. Van Der Spek AFL, Spargo PM, Norton ML: The physics of lasers and implications for their use during airway surgery, *Br J Anaesth* 60:709, 1988.
130. Vleming M, Middelweard RJ, Vries ND: Complications of endoscopic sinus surgery, *Arch Otolaryngol Head Neck Surg* 118: 617, 1992.
131. Vourc'h G, Tannieres ML, Toty L, et al: Anaesthetic management of tracheal surgery using the neodymium-yttrium-aluminum-garnet laser, *Br J Anaesth* 52:993, 1980.
132. Warner ME, Warner MA, Leonard PF: Anesthesia for neodymium-YAG (Nd-YAG) laser resection of major airway obstructing tumors, *Anesthesiology* 60:230, 1984.
133. Watzke I, Watzke H: Thromboembolic risk factors in patients undergoing maxillofacial surgery for malignancies, *Oral Surg Oral Med Oral Pathol* 67:137, 1989.
134. Waun JE, Sweitzer RS, Hamilton WK: Effects of nitrous oxide on middle ear mechanics and hearing acuity, *Anesthesiology* 28:846, 1967.
135. Wolf GL, Simpson JI: Flammability of endotracheal tubes in oxygen and nitrous oxide enriched atmosphere, *Anesthesiology* 67:236, 1987.
136. Younis RT, Gross CW, Lazaer RH: Toxic Shock syndrome following endoscopic sinus surgery: a case report, *Head and Neck* 13:247, 1991.

CHAPTER 85

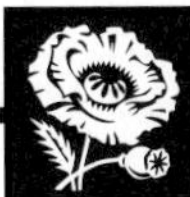

Outpatient Anesthesia

L. REUVEN PASTERNAK

The dramatic growth of ambulatory surgery programs during the past several years represents a unique phenomenon for both the extent and speed with which it has transformed the practice of surgery and anesthesiology. During the past decade, the volume of outpatient surgery has virtually quadrupled, to comprise over 60% of all adult surgery and as much as 80% of all pediatric surgery performed in the United States.

The extent to which one views this as a new phenomenon depends on the depth of historic perspective taken in examining this subject. In an excellent summary of the history of this field, Davis[22] traces the development of ambulatory surgery facilities from ancient civilization to the present. However, as with surgery in general, only in the nineteenth century were three critical forces combined to define this field as it is currently known. These innovations were the introduction of anesthesia, aseptic technique, and the use of common recovery facilities for postoperative patients. Before these developments, hospitals were regarded as crowded buildings of questionable cleanliness for treatment of indigent patients and a final place for desperate efforts before inevitable death. As a result of these revolutionary changes, the performance of surgery was placed on a new level, representing a science requiring the combination of specialized medical services and a setting dedicated to this task. The fundamental identity of the hospital had now changed to one of an environment offering painless, sterile surgical technique of increasing sophistication and success.

As the hospital gained a positive association with good health, an associated and unproven perception grew, linking longer preoperative and postoperative stays with better outcomes. Nicoll[77] is credited with taking an opposing viewpoint in his review of 8988 patients from the Glasgow Royal Hospital from 1899 to 1909. This survey included his experience with operations on patients with cleft palate, spina bifida, pyloric stenosis, depressed skull fracture at birth, mastoid empyema, ligation or resection of the internal jugular vein during radical mastoid procedures or excision of cervical glands, and varied hernia repairs. In his advocacy of outpatient surgery, Nicoll stated that "we keep similar cases in adults too long in bed" and that "sucklings and young children should remain with their parents after surgery." Regarding results of ambulatory surgery, he stated these were "at a tithe of the costs are equally good."[77] Included in this work was a discussion of the legal liability of discharging patients on the same day of operation, but the author noted that the testimony of experts as to its safety should remove any such concerns.

Herzfeld[43] echoed these sentiments in her report of 1000 outpatient hernia procedures on children under 12 years of age at the Royal Hospital for Sick Children in Edinburgh, Scotland. She found outpatient management to be safe and effective and added that ". . . it is important in operating on young infants not to keep them in hospitals."[43] In 1899, Ries[97] wrote of his extensive experience with early ambulation following abdominal surgery, noting that "very soon I found that the period for which it was advisable to confine such cases to bed could be counted by hours instead of days, so that of late I have allowed my patients to get up within 24 to 48 hours and to leave the hospital in four to six days. . . . I could not fail to notice that these same patients did not present the picture of listlessness and muscular weakness." In 1907, Boldt[9] confirmed these results with gynecologic surgery, as did Kelley[48] at Johns Hopkins Hospital. However, the strong reservations of Halstead, a Hopkins contemporary of Kelley and chief of surgery, about allowing ambulation during the initial weeks following operation delayed the use of this technique.

Although early criticism of ambulatory surgery related more to potential compromise of the patient's surgical repair than anesthesia risk, experience disproved this concept as ambulatory surgery continued to be performed in several locations. Among the first ambulatory surgery facilities in the United States was Waters' Down-Town Anesthesia Clinic[125] in Sioux City, South Dakota, during World War I. Reporting in 1918 at the fourth annual meeting of the Interstate Association of Anesthetists in Indianapolis, Waters noted the clinic's convenient location in the central part of town, where local and general anesthesia for circumcision, abscess incision and debridement, fracture setting, dental, and other less demanding procedures could be performed.

The first modern hospital-based program was established at Butterworth Hospital in Grand Rapids, Michigan, in 1961, with the first academic unit established soon thereafter at the University of California at Los Angeles. Dornette,[26] speaking in 1968 of the free-standing unit established in association with the Children's Hospital in Vancouver, British Columbia, the first such facility in North America, was prophetic in setting the tone of the dialogue in this issue. In his address before the American Society of Anesthesiologists (ASA), he commented that:

"One facility about which little has been written is outpatient service offering general anesthesia for minor surgical procedures. Such a facility, properly designed, staffed, and operated, has several advantages. A significant patient load is removed from the inpatient bed and operating facilities. There is a distinct savings in the cost to the patient or to the patient's hospitalization insurance carrier. But a safe and efficient facility for performance of general anesthesia and minor surgical procedures need not be affiliated either administratively or geographically with a hospital."

The classic model for free-standing facilities is credited to Ford and Reed[33] with the establishment of the Surgicenter in Phoenix. Opened in 1970 in response to a general need of patients, employers, insurers, and local government to find a way to perform procedures on a safe yet less expensive basis, this facility has served as the prototype of ambulatory surgical units throughout the U.S.

Although the early pioneers in ambulatory surgery based their efforts on clinical perspectives and patient convenience, the rapid growth of this specialty finds its true origins in what has previously been a nonmedical basic science—that of economics. **Unlike other advances in health care that arose in response to new technologies or breakthroughs in research and technique, ambulatory surgery has developed largely as a response to financial concerns** from private and government third-party payers, health provider organizations, and the private economic sector to control the rising costs of health care.

That ambulatory surgery has found its greatest use in the U.S. should not come as a surprise when one considers that health care is the largest industry in the U.S. today, comprising more than 15% of the domestic national product (DNP)—more than any other nation. As the largest industry and the single-largest budget item for federal and state governments and major corporations, health care was naturally the target of intense scrutiny. Despite an increasing commitment of resources, a belief arose that an entirely new approach to health care was needed that entailed a careful reexamination of the need for various aspects of traditional care. These considerations led to the single greatest impetus for ambulatory surgery, the Omnibus Reconciliation Act of 1980, in which the federal government recognized ambulatory surgery as an appropriate alternative to inpatient management.

In this spirit, procedures were mandated to be performed on an outpatient basis by government agencies, with private parties soon following suit. The medical establishment largely was caught unprepared for this change and was compelled to adjust rapidly to the changing environment as hospitals found themselves without facilities and knowledgeable staffs able to direct these efforts. However, ambulatory surgery has been found to be of great benefit to hospitals in need of reducing their dependence on inpatient staff and facilities. Pineault et al.[88] purported to demonstrate no patient or economic advantage for patients undergoing tubal ligation, hernia repair, and meniscectomy. However, the patient population and associated anesthetic techniques could not be called characteristic of current practice. In contrast, Kitz et al.[49] (Table 85-1) revealed significant savings with ambulatory procedures compared with inpatient procedures (e.g., surgical arthroscopy, diagnostic laparoscopy, tubal ligations) based on reduced laboratory testing and more efficient surgery and anesthesia. Laffaye[53] revealed a savings of $2000 per case for patients undergoing six common procedures, with a corresponding significant reduction in hospital days, a finding confirmed by Keithley et al.[47] for same-day admission procedures. Lakhani et al.[54] reported that the performance of procedures on an ambulatory basis allowed for closing of 15% of the surgical beds in Great Britain, whereas Roos[99] found a similar potential and associated savings for hospitals in Manitoba, Canada. As the ability to maintain hospital activities for inpatients becomes increasingly difficult, ambulatory surgery will free up these resources for use by patients who have the greatest need.

Despite its origins in economic imperatives, ambulatory surgery has been recognized to have significant advantages for patients as well as hospitals and third-party payers. After overcoming an initial perception of ambulatory surgery as "bargain basement" medicine, patients are increasingly expressing a preference for this method. A survey of patients[44] has revealed that more than 74% prefer their procedures to be done on an outpatient basis whenever possible. The reason for this and similar findings is patients' preference to recover in the familiar surroundings of their home, which, in addition to convenience, also minimizes the disruption of return visits to the hospital for other family members. Further, studies in children, such as that of Campbell et al.[13] have shown a beneficial psychologic effect. In their study of 70 children, these authors found that children having outpatient surgery required less attention during the first postoperative week and, at 3 months postoperatively, had significantly less psychologic trauma associated with their surgery.

Ambulatory surgery thus represents one of the most profound changes in the practice of medicine during the past decade. These decisions have usually been based on the presumed complexity of the surgical procedure without consideration of the patient's medical condition and the associated anesthetic risk. Although previously restricted to minor procedures, ambulatory anesthesia increasingly involves complex surgery, in some centers including laser surgery of the airway and, in the near future, such procedures as outpatient cholecystectomy. Practitioners of this specialty are thus facing challenges as formidable as their counterparts in other areas and are called on to address issues of preoperative evaluation and perioperative management innovatively.

PROGRAM AND FACILITY DESIGN

The success of ambulatory surgery depends on a well-designed and efficiently operating system that recognizes the inherent differences between ambulatory and inpatient surgery. These include appropriate facilities, preoperative preparation, perioperative management, and reasonable protocols for recovery, discharge, and follow-up of patients. Planning for an ambulatory surgical program thus requires all the careful preparation and commitment of staff and resources given to any other anesthesia or critical care program. Surgical, anesthesia, and nursing staff should be included in planning and development at the project's earliest stages.

Coordination of anesthesia preoperative evaluations, surgical scheduling, nursing staff availability and policies, and appropriate operating facilities is mandatory. It is better to delay a program for several months to ensure proper planning than rush into a poorly organized system with the attitude of "working things out as we go along" with its inevitable confusion, conflicts, and ad hoc revisions.

Facilities

Ambulatory surgical systems are either free-standing, office-based, or hospital-based, and are characterized as single

Table 85-1 Mean operating and recovery room time (minutes) for day surgery (DSU) patients and inpatients per surgical procedure

	Surgical arthroscopy		Level I laparoscopy		Level II laparoscopy	
Time period	DSU patients	Inpatients	DSU patients	Inpatients	DSU patients	Inpatients
Operating room						
Time (min)	83*	128	58*	83	65*	85
Labor costs	$39.25*	$66.38	$28.28*	$41.24	$30.69*	$43.30
Recovery room						
Time (min)	101*	76	115*	63	125*	78
Labor costs	$11.85	$8.99	$13.48*	$7.47	$14.65	$9.31

*$p < 0.001$.

From Kitz DS, Slusarz-Ladden C, Lecky JH: Hospital resources used for inpatient and ambulatory surgery, *Anesthesiology* 69:383, 1988.

or multispecialty. Free-standing facilities, although at times associated with hospitals, are separate and fully autonomous buildings, whereas hospital-based units are located within the hospital itself, often with separate entrances and parking. Office-based surgery usually refers to procedures performed in a surgeon's office, often without benefit of anesthesia coverage. Single-specialty facilities refer to those that exclusively serve one surgical specialty, whereas multispecialty units are used by diverse surgical groups.

Foremost in the planning is the assignment of dedicated facilities, including a preoperative area, operating rooms, and recovery rooms. It is well recognized that aggregation of outpatients into one area enhances efficiency, since anesthesia, surgical staff, and nursing staff function in a more coordinated fashion with a view toward the efficient performance of procedures.[49] In addition, such an arrangement eliminates the likelihood that outpatient surgery will be delayed or canceled because of emergencies or inpatient procedures lasting longer than their scheduled times.

An orderly flow of patients is key to the efficient operation of the preoperative facility. As with the operating room suite, patient traffic should flow in a smooth pattern that minimizes back-and-forth movement, with the patient progressing through the facility in an orderly fashion. The preoperative visit should be relaxed and not expose the patient to individuals being prepared for or recovering from operation. A preoperative evaluation center located close to the operating suite is preferable, with separate entrances that do not impede the flow of patients to and from the operating rooms, preparatory areas, or recovery areas. A separate pediatric area with appropriate decor can make the visit less traumatic for children and parents while not disturbing adult patients who prefer a quieter environment.

The preparatory and recovery areas should be located immediately adjacent to the operating rooms. Such a system permits easy communication with operating room staff concerning potential problems, availability of appropriate medical personnel in the event of postoperative difficulties, and the administration of preoperative sedation, when needed, in a monitored setting. As with the preoperative area, a separate area for pediatric patients is appropriate for both the preparatory and the recovery room sites, allowing parents to remain with their children.

Patients and their families should be discouraged from bringing additional family members for the preoperative evaluation and on the day of surgery. Adults should be accompanied by one other responsible adult and children only by their parents or guardians. Arrangements should be made for the care of siblings because they tend to distract attention from the patient, who is more in need of parental support.

Staff

Designated staff familiar with the nuances of outpatient surgery should be assigned to work in the outpatient area. Although anesthesiologists' responsibilities may not be exclusively in this domain, anesthesia care is enhanced by those who perform these procedures regularly. Similarly, nursing staff in the outpatient operating room are also better prepared to handle the rapid turnover of patients and special needs of surgeons and anesthesiologists. As with intraoperative management, recovery room care for outpatients requires a distinctively different approach than that for inpatients, with nursing and ancillary staff dedicated to this area.

A medical director of ambulatory surgery must be designated as the person responsible for coordinating activities relating to the operating rooms and general policy issues. Because surgeons may be using many operating room sites among different hospitals, the director of anesthesia is usually called on to serve as medical director. The medical director must work closely with the surgeons, the director of nursing, and administrators in a formal structure to enhance the orderly functioning of the unit.

Scheduling

Whenever possible, patients should be scheduled several days before the operation to allow adequate preparation by the anesthesia staff, the facility, the patients and their families. Often, in a rush to fill open operating room time, hospital staff forget that patients and their families need to make arrangements for time away from work, transportation, and *day care* for other children. All paperwork, including consents and financial approval, should be taken care of before surgery so as not to distract the staff on the day of surgery and delay the procedure.

Although convenience for patients and surgeons is a major consideration, the tendency to place the marketing of ambulatory surgery on a par with routine consumer purchases demeans the nature of the medical practice and invites a relaxation of standards that may compromise appropriate patient care. Discretion should be employed in allowing last-minute additions to the schedule. When they occur, they should be completed in a way that is safe for the patient and consistent with standards of practice.

Preoperative evaluations and operation should be scheduled with reasonable assurance to patients that they will be seen at that time. The practice of scheduling large numbers of people for the same time invariably results in unnecessary waiting and patient dissatisfaction. Every effort should be made to adhere to scheduled appointments, with hours that are convenient to patients and that minimize disruption of daily activities. Often, this entails evening and weekend hours for the facility to see patients preoperatively.

Medical and Emergency Support

Even the most diligently administered anesthetic for a minor procedure carries with it the risk for serious patient complications. Before any procedure is performed in the outpatient surgical unit, arrangements should be made with the nearest hospital for management of patients requiring admission and major intervention. The ambulatory surgery facility should be prepared to support the patient with appropriate transport, usually an ambulance, immediately available.

Staffing arrangements should include sending medical and nursing staff with patients to their appropriate destinations.

Preoperative and Postoperative Lodging

Patients travelling a long distance for their surgery may prefer lodging before or after their procedure to avoid extensive trips before surgery or during their recovery. It is advantageous to both the surgical facility and the patient that arrangements be made with a nearby hotel or motel for these accommodations. Frequently, favorable rates and transportation to the surgical unit can be arranged, and the use of one lodging site facilitates communication with patients. Many larger facilities have found it convenient and profitable to manage such a facility on their own, with special arrangements with third-party payers to assist patients in defraying the costs.

PREOPERATIVE EVALUATION

The practice of ambulatory surgery employs a great diversity of techniques and approaches that represent an evolution of its practitioners' experience. Although the relative merits of alternative anesthetic techniques provide for lively debate, the issue of appropriate preoperative evaluation of outpatients for surgery remains ambiguous and largely unexplored. Regulatory bodies that have thrived on providing explicit, detailed guidelines in other areas have yet to venture into this area with anything more than vaguely worded advisories. At present, these groups merely require that an appropriate work-up by the anesthesiologist—including physical examination and laboratory tests—be on the chart before commencing with the procedure. As a result, physicians and other health care providers looking for definitive guidance in this area find themselves frustrated and relying on the ad hoc experience and impressions of other ambulatory surgery units.

It is unlikely that any single system will emerge as the standard or ideal for preoperative evaluation. The diversity of health and reimbursement systems, surgical procedures, geographic locations, and patient populations will dictate the organization of the appropriate system. A more reasonable standard should require that whatever system emerges adequately address a uniform set of issues in a manner that is safe, convenient, and efficient for providers and consumers. Anesthesiologists, in setting up their systems, are well advised to allow for a measure of flexibility. While adhering to a strong standard of appropriate care, reasonable judgment in complying with that care is preferable to unyielding policies.

The preoperative examination process is designed to ensure that patients are appropriately prepared for their procedure. Although the surgeon retains the opportunity to examine and assess the patient before the scheduling of surgery, the anesthesiologist operates under a deadline to resolve many issues before the procedure. These include identifying risk factors that may affect the patient's clinical management; obtaining appropriate, timely laboratory results; and educating patients about issues relevant to their anesthesia. In their final analysis, **the selection of procedures by third-party payers to be performed on an outpatient basis is generally determined by complexity of the procedure, not on the patient's other underlying medical problems or potential issues associated with anesthesia.** Because the administration of anesthesia often carries greater risk for the patient than the operation itself, the preoperative process is a crucial first step that may affect the clinical safety and viability of the ambulatory surgery unit.

Philosophy of Preoperative Visit

The preoperative evaluation should address those issues relevant for the safe administration of anesthesia. Therefore the rule is to do what is reasonable rather than engage in preparation for every remote circumstance. Histories, physical examinations, and laboratory tests should be obtained on the basis of their usefulness to anesthesia and surgical staff and not as a general medical screening. The temptation to use this setting as a screening clinic for the investigation of unrelated primary care problems should be avoided and referred back to the patient's surgeon and primary care provider, who can institute appropriate, consistent care.

Agreement among the anesthesia staff about the content and conduct of appropriate preoperative assessments is very important, especially when performed by ancillary staff under their supervision. No issue will cause greater ire among surgeons and patients than to have a patient cleared by one anesthesiologist, only to be canceled by another. These occurrences portray the anesthesia staff and preoperative system as being in disarray and serve as a major incentive to circumvent the system and shop for the group's most compliant member. Therefore, although sufficient art exists in the practice of anesthesiology to allow for individual variation in practice, **it is imperative that the anesthesia group reach a consensus on major issues. These concern such matters as required laboratory tests, accepted values for these tests, and causes for cancellation, such as nothing by mouth (NPO) violations, upper respiratory infections, and significant abnormalities on physical examination.** These policies should be labelled as guidelines rather than rules to allow some discretion by the anesthesiologist on a case-by-case basis.

Time of Examination

The appropriate timing and location of preoperative assessments vary considerably between centers; no definitive indications exist in this area. Preoperative visits provide an opportunity for teaching and evaluation by anesthesia staff, but many patients prefer not having to take the time to make an additional visit before the day of surgery. In this circumstance, convenience must be balanced against appropriate medical care.

A common system employed in some centers is to have

patients evaluated by their primary care physician, with recommended laboratory tests performed at that time. This method is especially popular with managed health plans, such as health maintenance organizations (HMOs), which may have special arrangements with laboratories and other facilities to perform tests at rates less than those of the hospital or ambulatory surgery facility. Such an arrangement requires close communication among primary care providers, surgeons, and anesthesiologists. A sound first step is to provide a standard form (Fig. 85-1) to the primary care provider or surgeon to be completed and returned to the ambulatory surgery unit. The use of such a form provides standardized information that is readily reviewed to identify problems.

The availability of this form before the day of surgery may be difficult but is considerably facilitated with the use of facsimile transmission (FAX) devices. The proliferation of these machines in offices, clinics, and laboratories is making this an increasingly viable alternative to the vagaries of relying on the mail or patients to deliver these documents and allows for review before the day of the procedure. Lacking such a system, it must be emphasized to the surgeon and primary care provider that clearance for operation

PREOPERATIVE EVALUATION/HISTORY AND PHYSICAL

DATE: ______ TIME ______ AGE ______ SEX ______ RACE ______

PROCEDURE ______

DIAGNOSIS ______

MEDICATIONS ______

ALLERGIES ______

USE BALLPOINT PEN

PAST MEDICAL HISTORY AND REVIEW OF SYSTEMS

YES NO **CARDIOVASCULAR**
□ □ MI
□ □ HYPERTENSION
□ □ ARRHYTHMIA
□ □ ANGINA
□ □ CHF
□ □ VALVULAR DISEASE
□ □ PERIPHERAL VASC. DISEASE
□ □ PAST CARDIAC SURGERY
□ □ OTHER

PULMONARY
□ □ SMOKING Hx
□ □ ASTHMA
□ □ COPD/EMPHYSEMA/BPD
□ □ OTHER

RENAL
□ □ RENAL FAILURE
□ □ OTHER

YES NO **HEPATIC**
□ □ HEPATITIS
□ □ OTHER

ENDOCRINE
□ □ DIABETES
□ □ OTHER

INFECTIOUS
□ □ SEPSIS
□ □ OTHER

NEUROLOGIC
□ □ SEIZURE
□ □ ELEVATED ICP
□ □ CEREBROVASC. DISEASE
□ □ NEUROMUSCULAR DISORDER
□ □ OTHER

GASTROINTESTINAL
□ □ G.E. REFLUX/HIATAL HERNIA
□ □ BOWEL OBSTRUCTION
□ □ OTHER

YES NO **HEMATOLOGIC**
□ □ SICKLE CELL
□ □ COAGULOPATHY
□ □ PREGNANCY/TRANSFUSION WITHIN LAST 3 MONTHS Y/N
□ □ OTHER

PEDIATRICS
□ □ PREMATURITY
□ □ CONGENITAL ABN.
□ □ APNEA
□ □ OTHER

OBSTETRICS
□ □ PREECLAMPSIA/ECLAMPSIA
□ □ PREMATURITY
□ □ PLACENTA PREVIA/ABRUPTIO
□ □ LMP ______
□ □ OTHER

ANESTHETIC DIFFICULTIES
□ □ DIFFICULT INTUBATION
□ □ FAMILY HISTORY
□ □ OTHER

DRUG USE
□ □ ETOH
□ □ OTHER

□ HISTORY UNKNOWN EXCEPT AS NOTED ABOVE

EXPLANATION OF POSITIVE DATA ______

PHYSICAL EXAMINATION BP (RANGE): ______ P ______ R ______ T ______ WT ______ (lbs.) (Kg.)

LABS:

H&P PERFORMED BY ______

ECG FINDINGS: ______

RISK FACTORS:
HEMODYNAMIC COMPROMISE ______ OTHER ______
CRITICAL AIRWAY ______
FULL STOMACH ______ LAST PO ______

IMPRESSION: ASA STATUS 1 | 2 | 3 | 4 | 5 | E ______

REVIEWED BY: ______ M.D. | DATE ______ TIME ______

CHART COPY

Fig. 85-1. Preoperative evaluation form.

depends on the anesthesiologist's consideration of information provided by these physicians, and that an increased risk of cancellation or delay is part of the convenience of not requiring a preoperative visit to the ambulatory surgery unit.

Although this system may be convenient for the patient, a visit to the ambulatory surgery unit before the day does offer definite advantages. Studies demonstrating no alleviation of anxiety with a preoperative visit are limited in their scope and cannot yet be viewed as applicable to the general patient population. Among the current studies, one did not specify the nature of the procedure or health status of the patient,[100] and three only evaluated healthy women undergoing termination of pregnancy and therapeutic abortion[2,122,123] or laser procedures to the cervix and vagina[122] on presumably otherwise healthy, young patients. Of these, only one involved general anesthesia,[122] and none of these studies addressed issues relating to pediatric patients, those patients with more extensive medical problems, or those patients undergoing more invasive procedures. The studies also did not address cancellations or delays associated with previously unknown or inappropriately evaluated conditions or missing laboratory data. The use of telephone surveys to identify at-risk patients had some success for pediatric[87] and some adult[126] patients, but no guarantee exists that patients will be available by phone, and this method does not allow for full preoperative testing or familiarization with the facility.

The preoperative visit can be used by patients and their families to familiarize themselves with the facilities and not be compelled to add navigation through a new system to their list of anxieties on the day of operation. The availability of all relevant information can also be ensured and appropriate instructions given for preoperative preparation, including those relating to guidelines for use of prescription medications. Preoperative teaching can be performed in this setting, and especially anxious patients can be identified for further instruction and preoperative medication, if needed. In scheduling the visit, it is preferable that patients be seen at a time that allows for retrieval of laboratory tests before the day of operation and to address any unresolved issues to avoid last-minute delays or cancellation. This practice also provides the surgeon the opportunity to fill cancelled time with another patient rather than leaving gaps in the operating room schedule.

In balancing the virtues of this extra visit, one must remember that operating rooms represent the most resource-intensive area of a hospital or ambulatory care facility. Delays caused by addressing issues on the day of operation can limit the number of procedures performed and divert staff from their regular tasks, leaving the operating room idle. The performance of many laboratory tests on the day of operation may also place an undue burden on the laboratory system, add to the communication difficulties at a time when staff should be efficiently preparing patients for the operating room, and enhance the risk of cancellation because of an abnormal laboratory value. Patient apprehension is only intensified in these circumstances. Because some patients may have had to arrange for care of their children or coverage at work, avoidable delays or cancellations may result in needless patient expense and inconvenience.

When requiring a preoperative evaluation, the facility and staff must provide this in a way convenient for the patient. The availability of this service during evening hours and weekends can minimize disruption of the patient's home and work schedules. Patients should have a reasonable assurance that they will be seen at a scheduled time. Scheduling visits every 15 minutes is sufficient and allows for last-minute "walk-ins" and more complicated preoperative evaluations. Appropriate laboratory facilities should also be available to handle tests obtained at these times. Ambulatory surgery facilities located close to surgeons' offices may find it to their advantage to have the patient sent directly for their preoperative assessment. Such a practice prevents an additional trip and allows for timely discussion of preoperative concerns. To allow for these unscheduled visits, block time can be set aside for a particular surgeon or surgical service.

At times, patients may travel considerable distances to a specialized facility for outpatient procedures, making communication with their primary care provider somewhat difficult. These individuals should have a note from their primary care provider to assist in the evaluation. A telephone interview in this instance is advised to avoid potential problems in patients undertaking this at considerable expense and time.

Although it is always safest and best for preoperative evaluations to be completed before the day of operation by anesthesia staff, common sense would also dictate that the likelihood of problems in healthy patients would be minimal and easily addressed on the day of operation. This group includes healthy patients (American Society of Anesthesiologists class I [ASA I] rating) undergoing minor procedures. Some with minimal dysfunction medical problems (ASA II) may also be evaluated on the day of operation if all appropriate information is available at that time. Some centers have found that ensuring the availability of these data is sufficiently difficult as to make the preoperative visit a more efficient way of managing these patients.

In balancing patient convenience with appropriate care, it must be emphasized that the anesthesiologist assumes the ultimate responsibility for the patient, regardless of how many other physicians of health care have seen the patient beforehand. Although surgeons, internists, pediatricians, and family practitioners are in a position to provide valuable information, the anesthesiologist retains the unique perspective of how anesthetic techniques and agents are selected and interact with the patient's medical conditions. As the acute condition of patients undergoing ambulatory surgery increases, it also should be emphasized that low-risk surgery does not necessarily imply low-risk anesthesia. Consequently, certain medical conditions are of sufficient concern to warrant preoperative evaluation by anesthesia staff or their extended group before surgery (Box 85-1). At times,

BOX 85-1
CONDITIONS FOR WHICH PREOPERATIVE EVALUATION IS RECOMMENDED BEFORE DAY OF SURGERY

Cardiocirculatory

- History of angina
- History of coronary artery disease
- History of myocardial infarction
- Past cardiac surgery
- Symptomatic dysrhythmias (atrial and/or ventricular)
- Hypertension (diastolic > 110, systolic > 160)
- History of congestive heart failure

Hematopoietic

- Sickle cell disease or other hemoglobinopathy, coagulopathy
- Coagulation disorder

Respiratory

- Asthma: chronic bronchodilator or steroid dependent and/or acute episode within 1 month
- Significant chronic obstructive pulmonary disease
- Past major airway surgery
- Other significant respiratory disease or history
- Upper- and/or lower-airway tumor or obstruction

Endocrine

- Non-diet-controlled diabetes (insulin or oral hypoglycemic agents)
- Adrenal disorders
- Active thyroid disease

Neuromuscular

- History of seizure disorder
- History of significant central nervous system disease
- History of myopathy or other muscle disorders

Hepatic

- Ascites
- Other active hepatobiliary disease or compromise

Musculoskeletal

- Kyphosis and/or scoliosis causing functional compromise
- Temporomandibular joint disorder
- History of cervical or thoracic spine injury or surgery

Oncology

- Patients receiving chemotherapy
- Other oncology process with significant physiologic residual

Gastrointestinal

- Massive obesity (> 140% ideal body weight)
- Hiatal hernia
- Symptomatic gastroesophageal reflux

surgeons and primary care providers may question the need for this step. In this circumstance, a diplomatic reminder that the anesthesiologist assumes the responsibility and liability for guiding the patient through the procedure is appropriate.

Preoperative Assessment Staff

Preoperative assessments can be performed by various providers, provided that they are well trained and supervised with appropriate support by anesthesiologists. Some groups have anesthesiologists leave the operating room for preoperative examinations, but this system places a stress on the interview, because the anesthesiologist faces the pressure of expediting the process to return to the anesthetized patient.

At our institution we have used a staff of *nurse practitioners* and *physician assistants* to perform the initial history and physical examination, consulting with the anesthesia staff as necessary for patients with more complicated conditions. This issue in this system, as with allowing primary care physicians to provide evaluations, is the extent to which anesthesiologists can delegate their traditional responsibility of evaluating patients. A review of more than 3000 patients at our institution whose preoperative assessments were performed by ancillary staff found a 15% discrepancy in ASA classification, in all instances by one classification category, evenly divided between underestimating and overestimating the ASA status. More importantly, cancellations because of problems improperly assessed by these individuals were less than 1% and allowed the anesthesiologists to devote their attention to patients in the operating room. One drawback of this system is the anesthesiologist's inability to speak personally with the patient before the procedure. However, consultations for patients with more complicated conditions and good preoperative education can alleviate this situation.

When using such a system, extended staff must have immediate access to an anesthesiologist to evaluate specific problems, such as potentially difficult airway management. Failure to have this backup available will compromise the integrity and purpose of the preoperative evaluation. In addition, it should be emphasized to staff performing this function that the anesthesiologist will make the final determination of anesthetic technique. Although they should be able to explain some of the alternatives to the patient, they should advise the patient that the anesthesiologist will discuss the anesthetic technique on the day of operation. Under no circumstances should extended staff members compromise the anesthesiologist's position by promising that a certain technique or agents will be used. They may reassure the patient that their concerns will be brought to the attention of the anesthesiologist for discussion on the day of operation.

An additional note of caution: the previous proposals to enhance patient convenience and the efficiency of the anesthesia staff all entail, to some extent, anesthesiologists surrendering part of their traditional roles. Once surrendered, such activities could prove very difficult to regain should the staff think they should do so. Therefore, the anesthesia staff should consider carefully these issues and the general philosophy of practice before developing the preoperative system.

Physical Examination

A patient questionnaire (Figs. 85-2 and 85-3) **to determine the presence of medical problems or past history of anesthetic complications is often useful.** Although such documents may add to the overall paperwork of the system at our institution, we have found them beneficial in directing the interview, especially when ancillary staff perform this task. The interview and physical examination should then be performed in a private setting. The patient should be reas-

The Johns Hopkins Hospital
SAME DAY CARE CENTER
Adult Preanesthesia Evaluation, p. 1

INSTRUCTIONS: This form helps the anesthesiologist to evaluate your health. Please answer all questions by indicating with a check or writing your answer in the space provided.

1. Name ______ Sex ____ Age ____
   Weight ____ Height ____ Occupation ______
2. Besides the reason for your current hospitalization, are you under a doctor's care for any other conditions? yes ____ no ____ Doctor's name ______
3. Approximate date of last physical examination? ______
4. Approximate date of last chest x-ray? ______
5. Approximate date of last electrocardiogram (ECG)? ______
6. Your physical activity level now: little ____ moderate ____ very active ____
   Can you climb stairs? yes ____ no ____ Number of flights: 1 ____ 2 ____ 3 ____
   Has there been a change in your activity level within the last 6 months? yes ____ no ____
7. Have you had a cold or flu within the last month? yes ____ no ____
8. Family History

	Yes	No	Don't Know
a. Do any family members have a tendency to bleed excessively?	____	____	____
b. Have any family members had unusual reactions to anesthesia?	____	____	____
c. Have any family members had unexplained fevers during or following surgery?	____	____	____

Your Medical History

9. Please list all hospitalizations or operations:

Reason	Year
______	____
______	____
______	____
______	____
______	____

10. Have you ever had a blood transfusion? yes ____ no ____ Year ______

Fig. 85-2. Adult patient questionnaire.

The Johns Hopkins Hospital
SAME DAY CARE CENTER
Pediatric Preanesthesia Evaluation, p. 1

INSTRUCTIONS: This questionnaire is to help the anesthesiologist evaluate your child's health and aid in the selection of anesthetic techniques and medicines for his/her procedure. Please indicate by a check your answer to each question.

CHILD'S NAME ______ NICKNAME ______
YOUR NAME ______ RELATIONSHIP ______
YOUR HOME PHONE ______ WORK OR OTHER NUMBER ______

CHILD'S MEDICAL HISTORY

1. Have you noticed any changes in your child's medical condition since surgery was decided upon? yes ____ no ____ If so, what? ______
2. Has your child ever had an operation? yes ____ no ____
   If yes, why? (or what?) ______ When ______ Where ______
3. Has your child ever had problems after having anesthesia? yes ____ no ____
   If yes, what happened? ______
4. Does your child have any allergies to medicine, food, or other substances? yes ____ no ____
   If yes, to what ______
5. Has your child ever had a blood transfusion? yes ____ no ____
6. BIRTH HISTORY
   Was your child: (Answer Yes or No)
   Full Term yes ____ no ____
   Premature yes ____ no ____ If yes, how early? ______
   Born by cesarean section (C-section) yes ____ no ____
   Was your child:
   On oxygen yes ____ no ____ If yes, how long? ______
   A respirator/ventilator (breathing machine) yes ____ no ____
   If yes, how long? ______
   In a Neonatal Intensive Care Unit (NICU) yes ____ no ____
   If yes, how long? ______
7. What was his/her birth weight ______ birthplace ______
8. Has your child ever been on an apnea monitor at home? yes ____ no ____
   When? ______
9. Who is your child's pediatrician and/or what clinic does your child usually attend? ______
   ______ Phone number ______
10. Are your child's immunizations up to date? yes ____ no ____

Fig. 85-3. Pediatric patient questionnaire.

sured that ambulatory surgery is not "bargain basement" medicine. A pleasant, private setting establishes an appropriate start for the process and allows for more candid and accurate histories, and more complete physical examinations.

If it is determined from the history or physical examination that the patient is not appropriate for ambulatory management, the patient can be referred back to the surgeon or primary care physician without going through the remainder of the evaluation process. **The patient questionnaire and history will generally direct the examination, with attention to appropriate organ systems. Auscultation of the heart and lungs and examination of the airways are routine, as is any observation of gross abnormalities or issues relevant to specialized anesthetic techniques, such as regional anesthesia.** As with any preoperative assessment, careful documentation of findings is important. The history and physical examination results should be included on the same form provided by primary care providers, allowing for easy scrutiny and identification of relevant problems.

Laboratory Testing

Some centers advocate obtaining laboratory tests before the history and physical examination. In practice, the results are rarely available in time for interpretation when the patient is being evaluated. In addition, the history and examination may reveal a need for additional testing, necessitating the patient's return to the laboratory and additional venipuncture. Even worse, one may find in the course of the examination that some of the tests are unnecessary, resulting in needless patient expense and discomfort.

Laboratory tests beyond those ordered by the surgeon should be performed on the basis of their potential usefulness to the anesthesiologist. The focus of such tests should be on the patient's medical condition and the likely form of anesthesia for the procedure. Appropriate data should be available, but numbers should not be generated solely on the basis of obscure possibilities or curiosity. In this, more than any other area, anesthesia staff must arrive at a consensus to provide direction for surgeons, their own assistants, and primary care providers. Although the physical examination is somewhat standard, the nature of appropriate laboratory testing remains flexible. The issue is the extent to which laboratory tests should be established as protocol or performed only on the basis of individual need. Because preoperative assessments have generally been performed by individuals other than the staff member providing anesthesia, protocol testing has evolved to relieve the examiner of the decision-making responsibility and to ensure the availability of all required tests on the day of operation.

However, such a practice has a strong tendency to result in excessive testing, subjecting the patient to potential invasive procedures and added costs. Kaplan et al.[46] reviewed the records of 2000 patients undergoing elective operations who received a routine battery of complete blood cell count (CBC), differential cell count, prothrombin time (PT), partial thromboplastin time (PTT), platelet count, glucose level, and six-channel chemistry studies. They found that 60% of these tests would not have been performed if they had been done only on the basis of the patient's clinical indication and, of these, only 0.22% revealed abnormalities that might have affected perioperative management (Tables 85-2 through 85-4 and Fig. 85-4). Interestingly, none of these were acted on or affected surgical or anesthetic management.

In a more recent study, Wyatt et al.[130] studied two groups of ambulatory patients over 1 year. Group 1 received selective tests based on demonstrated need, and group 2 received routine biochemical profile, CBC, and urinalysis. Both groups had electrocardiograms (ECGs) if patients were over age 40, chest radiographs if patients were over age 50, and PT and PTT if patients were receiving anticoagulant therapy. Cancellation rates for the two groups were virtually unchanged (6.9% versus 6.4%). In the group receiving routine laboratory tests, 99% of the 4058 tests were normal, with only 1% resulting in abnormality requiring cancellation. Of the ECGs, 99.93% were normal, as were 99.97% of chest radiographs (Tables 85-5 through 85-8). Unfortunately, this study included no breakdown of this patient population by age, clinical condition, or ASA status. The results are probably as much a demonstration of the selection of young, healthy patients as they are of the limited benefit of routine laboratory tests. Obtaining ECGs on all patients over 40 years of age and chest radiographs for those over 50 years of age represents a more conservative approach than followed in most centers, enhancing the potential savings noted in this study if adapted to current standards.

A more relevant examination of preoperative testing was performed by Kitz et al.[49] who examined preoperative chemistries, ECGs, and chest radiographs obtained for patients undergoing elective diagnostic arthroscopy or laparoscopy as outpatients or inpatients (Table 85-9). The outpatients received testing based on need, as determined by anesthesiology staff, whereas inpatients were tested by the surgical service on the basis of need and protocol. The authors found that laboratory tests performed on the basis of need rather than protocol reduced the frequency of ordering by 58% to 100%. In addition to demonstrating the appropri-

Table 85-2 Action limits for preoperative tests

Test	Adult reference range	Action limits*
Prothrombin time (seconds)	10.5–12.5	10.0–13.0
Partial thromboplastin time (seconds)	24.0–38.0	22.0–40.0
Platelet count (1000/mm³)	140–450	115–800
Complete blood cell count		
Hematocrit (%)	M: 41–53 F: 36–46	30–55
Hemoglobin (g/dl)	M:13.5–17.5 F: 12.0–16.0	10.0–18.0†
White blood cell count (1000/mm³)	3.1–11.0	3.0–15.0
Differential cell count		
Polymorphonuclear leukocyte count (1000/mm³)	2.6–9.18	< 1.5
Abnormal white blood cells‡ (%)	0	≤ 1
Nucleated red blood cells (per 100 white blood cells)	≤ 1	≤ 1
Six-factor automated multiple analysis		
Sodium (mEq/L)	136–144	130–150
Potassium (mEq/L)	3.5–5.3	3.2–5.8
Creatinine (mg/dl)	0.5–1.2	≤ 1.5
Glucose (mg/dl)	65–110	50–180

*Test results are considered normal if they are within the action limits. For example, a prothrombin time of 12.5 seconds would be normal; one of 13.0 seconds would not.

†For patients not expected to require a transfusion.

‡Abnormal white blood cell indicates any white blood cell except band forms and metamyelocytes not usually found in peripheral blood.

From Kaplan EB et al: The usefulness of preoperative laboratory screening, *JAMA* 253:3576, 1985.

Table 85-3 Indication for preoperative tests

Test	Indications
Prothrombin time/partial thromboplastin time	Known coagulation disorder, anticoagulant therapy, hemorrhage, anemia; liver disease, malabsorption, malnutrition, or other potentially relevant diseases (e.g., systemic lupus erythematosus)
Platelet count	Known platelet abnormality, hemorrhage, purpura, hypersplenism, hematologic malignancy (e.g, leukemia), radiation/chemotherapy, thrombosis, some anemias (e.g., aplastic), other potentially relevant diseases (e.g., systemic lupus erythematosus, paroxysmal nocturnal hemoglobinuria, renal transplant rejection)
Hemoglobin	Potentially bloody procedure (determined by need for preoperative cross-match), chronic renal failure, known anemia, bleeding disorder, hemorrhage, hematologic malignancy, rediation/chemotherapy, or other potentially relevant diseases (e.g., some infections, liver disease, malnutrition)
Erythrocyte count and differential cell count	Infection, diseases of erythrocytes (including leukemia), radiation/chemotherapy, immunosuppressive therapy, hypersplenism, aplastic anemia, or other potentially relevant abnormalities (e.g., rheumatoid arthritis)
Six-factor automated multiple analysis	Age 60 years or over, diuretic use, renal disease, other fluid/electrolyte abnormalities (e.g., diarrhea, syndrome of inappropriate secretion of antidiuretic hormone, diabetes insipidus, severe liver disease), or other potentially relevant abnormalities (e.g., convulsions)
Glucose	Diabetes mellitus, hypoglycemia, steriod treatment, pancreatic disease (e.g., pancreatitis, carcinoma, glucagonoma), pituitary disease (e.g., acromegaly), hypothalamic disease, or adrenal disease

From Kaplan EB, et al: The usefulness of preoperative laboratory screening, *JAMA* 253:3576, 1985.

Table 85-4 Indication for preoperative tests

Tests	No. of tests per year	No. of tests in sample	No. (%) of tests without indication	No (%) of abnormal results in sample	No. (%) of unindicated abnormal results	No. (%) of unindicated SSA results	Confidence limits† (95%) (%)
Prothrombin time	650	201	154 (77)	2 (1.0)	0 (0)	0 (0)	0–1.8
Partial thromboplastin time	650	199	154 (77)	1 (0.5)	0 (0)	0 (0)	0–1.8
Platelet count	1320	407	366 (90)	3 (0.7)	2 (0.5)	1 (0.2)	0–1.4
Complete blood cell count	4660	610	293 (48)	22 (3.6)	2 (0.3)	0 (0)	0–0.6
Differential cell count	1480	390	324 (83)	2 (0.5)	1 (0.3)	0 (0)	0–0.9
Six-factor automated multiple analysis	3200	514	174 (34)	41 (8.0)	1 (0.2)	1. (0.2)	0–1.1
Glucose	3100	464	361 (78)	25 (5.4)	4 (0.9)	2 (0.4)	0–1.6
Sample totals	—	2785	1828	96	10	4	—
Yearly totals‡	15,060	—	9164 (61)	618 (4.1)	59 (0.4)	23 (0.15)	0–0.4

*Unindicated SSA results mean unindicated (potentially) surgically significant abnormal results.
†Confidence limits: 95% upper and lower confidence limits for the true fraction of unindicated SSA results.
‡Yearly totals are the projections based on expected tests per year.
From Kaplan EB, et al: The usefulness of preoperative laboratory screening, *JAMA* 253:3576, 1985.

ateness of ordering on the basis of need, this study revealed the potential benefit of testing on the basis of an anesthesiologist's assessment before the day of operation.

Routine urinalyses[132] and hematocrits[39,79] are of questionable value, except when indicated by a urologic surgical procedure or by the patient's medical condition, such as a urologic or metabolic disorder. Routine chest radiographs[18] and pulmonary function testing[131] have not been found to add any information beyond that of the history and physical examination in patients without significant respiratory distress.

A consensus is developing concerning a dramatically more conservative approach to preoperative testing. This consensus includes raising the age at which routine ECGs are obtained for healthy patients from 40 to 50 years of age and eliminating serum chemistry and hematology studies for patients without a medical history in-

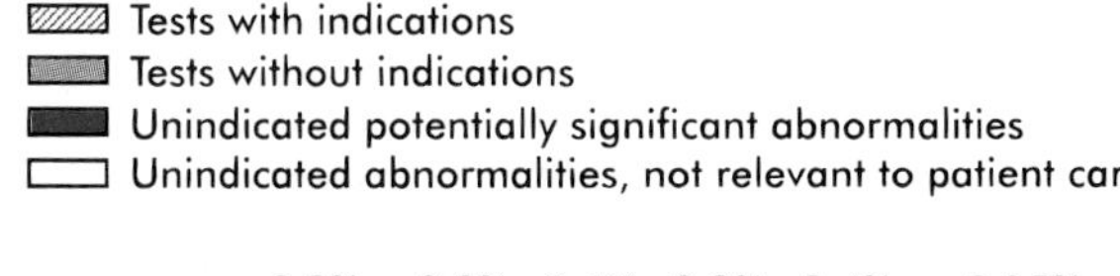

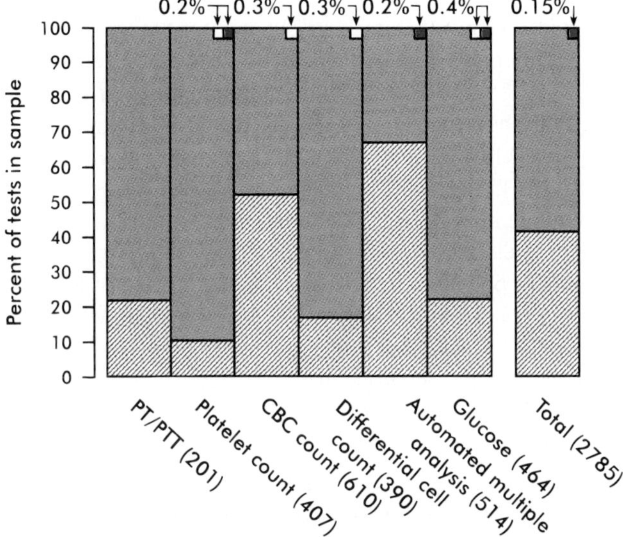

Fig. 85-4. Usefulness of preoperative screening. (From Kaplan EB, et al: The usefulness of preoperative laboratory screening, *JAMA* 253:3576, 1985.)

Table 85-5 Causes of ambulatory surgery cancellations

	Group 1 (n = 127): no. of patients (%)	Group 2: (n = 261): no. of patients (%)
Laboratory abnormalities	41 (32)	38 (15)
Electrocardiographic changes	5 (4)	4 (1.5)
Chest radiographic changes	3 (2)	1 (0.5)
Miscellaneous	54 (34)	173 (66)
Unknown	24 (19)	45 (17)
Total	127	261

From Wyatt WJ, Reed DN, Apelgren KN: Pitfalls in the role of standardized preadmission laboratory screening for ambulatory surgery, *Am Surg* 55:343, 1989.

dicating their need (Table 85-10). **Chest radiographs are not required for any patient without a history of respiratory disease,** regardless of age, and are only obtained in patients whose respiratory conditions: (1) are either resolving from a recent acute event; (2) are progressing in severity over the past year; or (3) were recently diagnosed. In the latter two cases, a radiologist's report within the last 3 months is acceptable. Pulmonary function testing, previously obtained in all patients with moderate or severe chronic respiratory problems, is now only obtained in patients whose condition is progressive or whose disability creates two-pillow orthopnea or makes them unable to walk a flight of

Table 85-6 Laboratory abnormalities causing ambulatory surgery cancellation

Biochemical profile	Patients (%)
Potassium	43 (54.4)
Glucose	11 (13.9)
Liver function tests	1 (1.2%)
Calcium	1 (1.2)
Phosphorus	—
Sodium	—
Blood urea nitrogen	—
Creatinine	—
Carbon dioxide	—
Chloride	—
Uric acid	—
Cholesterol	—
Other tests	
Prothrombin time/partial thromboplastin time	11 (13.9)
Complete blood count	10 (12.6)
Ethanol (ethyl alcohol)	1 (1.2)
Cardiac enzymes	1 (1.2)
Total	79 (100)

From Wyatt WJ, Reed DN, Apelgren KN: Pitfalls in the role of standardized preadmission laboratory screening for ambulatory surgery, *Am Surg* 55:343, 1989.

Table 85-7 Comparison of costs for standardized screening versus selective ordering

Standardized preadmission screening program		Selective ordering	
Chemical profile	$ 59.00	Serum potassium	$ 13.00
Complete blood count	17.00	Serum glucose	10.00
Urinalysis	8.00	Blood count	17.00
	$ 84.00		$ 40.00
PT/PTT	$ 13.00		
ECG*	67.00		
Chest radiograph†	69.00		
Maximum cost	$233.00		$189.00

*≥ 40 years.
†≥ 50 years
From Wyatt WJ, Reed DN, Apelgren KN: Pitfalls in the role of standardized preadmission laboratory screening for ambulatory surgery, *Am Surg* 55:343, 1980.

stairs or a city block without distress. In these circumstances, patients should also have arterial blood gases (ABG) measured and be evaluated by an anesthesiologist to determine their fitness for outpatient management.

An additional area of interest concerns serum levels of medications, specifically anticonvulsants, bronchodilators, and digitalis preparations. Previously, patients were required to demonstrate therapeutic levels of these medications, regardless of their clinical status, before undergoing outpatient procedures. Medical specialists, however, note that because of the wide range of patient response to these agents, management is titrated to clinical presentation rather than to laboratory values to prevent patient toxicity. Anesthesiologists also agree that the value is of interest, but it rarely contributes to the anesthetic plan in a manner not already determined by the patient's history and clinical condition. Subsequently, these tests are likely to be eliminated in the near future as well.

Therefore, the only required test for patients without a positive history or physical examination aside from the specific surgical concern is an ECG for individuals over 50 years of age. Further testing is performed on the basis of the patient's medical condition or as indicated by the procedure. Blood type and screen tests are obtained for patients whose procedure may result in a blood loss greater than 500 ml, with blood available in the blood bank for losses anticipated to exceed 1000 to 1500 ml. Clearly, procedures causing the latter blood loss would probably not be scheduled on an outpatient basis.

The use of these criteria for testing is believed to be consistent with good medical care and indicates the need for continual review of these practices. The value of physician knowledge of costs, and the ability to decrease testing without compromising patient care, have been demonstrated in the medical area[188] and will likely apply to ambulatory surgery as well.

Table 85-8 Cost-effectiveness of tests

Test	Normal percent and cost	Abnormal percent and cost
Laboratory	99.1% $337,680.00	0.9% $3192.00
Chest radiograph	99.97% $248,124.00	0.03% $275.00
Electrocardiogram	99.93% $149,745.00	0.07% $603.00

From Wyatt WJ, Reed DN, Apelgren KN: Pitfalls in the role of standardized preadmission laboratory screening for ambulatory surgery, *Am Surg* 55:343, 1980.

Medical Consultation and Support

In the event that medical consultation is necessary, a well-defined system is required to obtain consultations from either primary care physicians or appropriate specialty services. When obtaining consultation before operation is not feasible, the procedure should be delayed so as to ensure proper evaluation and any additional required evaluation. Although these procedures are elective, some may be performed under a time constraint that requires resolution within a short period. Examples include the diagnosis and staging of potential malignancies in anticipation of more invasive therapy or procedures and patients who have travelled considerable distances and arranged overnight lodging in anticipation of operation. In these circumstances, arrangements with the various services to accommodate these needs are important so that these procedures can be performed.

As the proportion of managed-care patients increases, the ability to obtain needed consultations and evaluations for unresolved medical issues becomes more difficult. Frequently, these programs require that their staffs do further assessments. Surgeons also frequently deal with a preferred group of primary care and specialty physicians. Thus, when further evaluation is indicated, surgeons should be approached about any preferences for referral. If they have none, or if the managed health care system is not accessible from the ambulatory surgery unit's location, the alternative of the existing arrangements should be offered. A unit with an appropriately used preoperative screening system should find that these circumstances seldom arise.

Preoperative Instructions

Following the history and physical examination, written and verbal instructions are given to patients and their families, including NPO instructions, arrival times, and what to expect on the day of operation. All patients are advised of the need to be escorted home by a responsible adult and of the advisability of having an adult immediately available for assistance at their postdischarge location. The possibility of unscheduled admission is also discussed, regardless of how minor the operation or healthy the patient. Plans should be

Table 85-9 Percent of day surgery (DSU) patients and inpatients with each preoperative test per surgical procedure

	Surgical arthroscopy		Level I laparoscopy		Level II laparoscopy	
Preoperative test	DSU patients (n = 62)	Inpatients (n = 61)	DSU patients (n = 49)	Inpatients (n = 24)	DSU patients (n = 46)	Inpatients (n = 42)
Chest radiograph	12%*	30%	24%*	58%	0%*	79%
Electrocardiogram	11%*	30%	12%*	50%	2%*	83%
Panel 6	3%*	92%	0%*	75%	2%*	86%

*$p < 0.05$.
From Kitz DS, Slusarz-Ladden C, Lecky JH: Hospital resources used for inpatient and ambulatory surgery, *Anesthesiology* 69:383, 1988.

Table 85-10 Recommended laboratory tests

Test	Indications
Hematocrit	All patients
Erythrocyte count, platelets, prothrombin time, partial thromboplastin time	Oncology therapy Anticoagulant therapy
Type and screen	As per surgery
Sickle cell test	At-risk patients without prior documented results
Sodium (Na), potassium (K)	Diuretic therapy without renal compromise
Na, K, chlorides (Cl), blood urea nitrogen (BUN), creatinine, glucose	Renal compromise Diabetes mellitus Hepatic dysfunction
Urinalysis	Renal compromise Genitourinary infection Urologic procedure
Electrocardiogram	Age > 50 years History of cardiac disease or dysrhythmia
Chest radiograph	Thoracic procedure History of aspiration Seizure disorders with history of aspiration Progressive, severe cardiorespiratory disease
Theophylline levels	Symptomatic History of difficult management
Anticonvulsant levels	Symptomatic History of difficult management

made for the possible care of children or dependent adults in the event that admission is required.

Nothing-by-mouth status

Preoperative fasting is aimed at reducing the risk of aspiration on induction of anesthesia and the risk of postoperative emesis, with the duration of fasting balanced against the risk of hypoglycemia and dehydration. Although specific recommendations vary among centers, most recommendations are relatively similar, requiring NPO by adult patients after midnight, regardless of scheduled procedure time.

This standard assumption, however, is being reevaluated. Recent studies in adults demonstrate reduced gastric contents when patients are given 150 ml of clear fluid 2 hours before operation.[94] In their study of 211 patients, Scarr et al.[105] found that patients who were permitted to have 150 ml of tea, coffee, apple juice, or water up to 3 hours before anesthesia had no difference in gastric volume or pH than those who were NPO for the traditional 8-hour period. Schreiner et al.[106] evaluated this same issue in pediatric patients, comparing those with routine NPO status with those allowed to take clear liquids up to 2 hours before operation, with the only limitation in volume being the last intake (8 ounces). The study group taking oral fluids was found to be less anxious and less irritable at the time of induction while not having any statistically significant difference in gastric volume or pH. Similarly, Sandhar et al.[104] evaluated oral intake of liquids (5 ml/kg) with and without ranitidine (2 mg/kg) and ranitidine alone up to 2 to 3 hours before operation in patients 1 to 14 years of age. The use of fluids alone did not appear to place patients at risk, and their combination with ranitidine was found to be beneficial.

These findings increasingly suggest that **the 8-hour NPO rule for outpatients may be subjecting many low-risk individuals, especially children, to unwarranted discomfort and that allowing clear liquids up to 2 to 3 hours before operation may be preferable.** Until further studies confirm these findings, however, it is still advised that patients remain NPO for the traditional 8 hours before surgery. Although new information may lead to changes in the practice of preoperative fasting, current guidelines at our center are consistent with the general practice of requiring NPO past midnight. An issue often overlooked is the practice of some patients to have a late dinner or snack in anticipation of morning hunger, with large volumes of solid foods only 8 to 10 hours before general anesthesia. Such a practice may increase the risk of aspiration and postoperative nausea. It is preferable that patients be advised not to have any solids after 9 PM to better ensure that these foods have been adequately digested before induction of anesthesia.

The NPO guidelines for children involve more careful consideration of their age. Special consideration should be given to the scheduling of infants and young children in consideration of their NPO status. The hunger associated with prolonged denial of food enhances their anxiety and can cause a more difficult induction. In addition, the common practice of not administering intravenous (IV) fluids until after induction of anesthesia also places them at special risk for dehydration, as well as extreme hypotension on induction of volatile agents. The best method of avoiding these situations is to make every effort to place infants and children first on the operating room schedule and, if delayed because of unforeseen problems in their scheduled room, to give them preference for any other operating room opening. Breast milk is treated as a clear liquid for purposes of NPO before operation.

Medications

Specific medications are addressed in the following section on patient selection. As a rule, patients should be advised to bring their prescription medications on the day of operation. In addition to the issues raised under the specific conditions, unscheduled admission or delay is always a possibility, and discontinuation of needed medications should be avoided.

Time of arrival

Patients should be instructed to arrive at a time that ensures their availability in the event the operating room is available earlier than planned, but without having them wait a long time before operation. Arrival 2 hours before the scheduled start of the procedure usually allows adequate time for preparation, with the patient ready if the operating room timetable is ahead of schedule. Facilities with a well-established system often find that arrival 1 hour before surgery is sufficient; each center should decide its best time. Discharge criteria are reviewed at the preoperative visit so that patients know what to expect postoperatively regarding discharge. Patients should also be instructed to call the ambulatory surgery unit if an acute illness develops before the scheduled procedure. This practice decreases delays, cancellations, and frustrations on the day of operation.

PATIENT AND PROCEDURE SELECTION

Indications for outpatient surgery include that patients be medically stable, that the procedure be brief in duration (preferably less than 3 hours), and that the possibility of significant postoperative complications be unlikely from either the operation or the anesthetic. Proscriptions concerning the procedure are that blood loss be minimal (less than 500 ml), that patient discomfort be adequately controlled with oral medications, and that postoperative care not require any resources beyond those usually available within the home.

Contrary to early perceptions that ambulatory surgery could be performed only on the healthiest patients, the assignment of a patient to ASA class III or IV should not itself preclude outpatient surgery. However, these patients must be under the care of a primary care physician or appropriate specialist and must comply with prescribed therapy. As with laboratory testing, definitive guidelines concerning requirements for preoperative and postoperative admission are based on common sense and assumptions rather than definitive data.

Admission to the hospital before or after ambulatory surgery should be viewed as an unusual event, required by the need either for preoperative evaluation or preparation that can be performed only on an inpatient basis, or for postoperative management not appropriate in the home setting. Indications for preoperative admission include the need to perform further preoperative diagnostic tests, therapeutic preparation (e.g., hydration, pulmonary toilet), or preparation for special anesthetic techniques that cannot be performed on an outpatient basis. Admission merely for the convenience of the surgeon, anesthesiologist, or patient must be strongly discouraged. Such a practice results in inappropriate use of increasingly scarce inpatient facilities and staff, decreases the care for patients more in need of these services, and places reimbursement for the procedure in jeopardy, because third-party payers may disallow the entire stay. When faced with extensive paperwork to justify admission, some medical staff have resorted to planning "emergency" admissions to circumvent the system. A request for admission is rarely denied if accompanied by an appropriate note from the surgeon or anesthesiologist clearly stating the reason for that action.

The anesthesia for outpatient surgery should be regarded with the same concern as the inpatient procedures. Not only is the perioperative risk for the patient still present, but the additional concern of postoperative recovery in a nonmedical environment mandates careful attention to the patient's medical status. The following clinical conditions, although not exhaustive, represent those most often encountered in the outpatient setting. When faced with less frequent medical conditions, the anesthesiologist and surgeon should address these issues on a case-by-case basis. A generally good rule is that any reasonable concern about the patient's ability to recover should be addressed with the reservation of a hospital bed postoperatively.

Age

Geriatric patients

There is no inherent upper age limit for ambulatory surgery. The limiting factor in these individuals is determined by their medical condition and the extent to which they are debilitated. When choosing anesthetic technique, the anesthesiologist should consider issues specific to geriatric patients: decreased respiratory and cardiac reserve, decreased renal clearance, altered volume of distribution, and susceptibility to narcotics and sedatives. Patients who are disorientated preoperatively are not appropriate candidates for outpatient management and should be observed overnight after the procedure. Even those who are normally self-sufficient may find themselves unable to appropriately handle postoperative drowsiness or other distress. If living alone, these patients should be strongly advised to make arrangements to recover in a location with appropriate support, such as with family or friends, if this is not available in their usual residence.

Infants

Controversy exists over the advisability of ambulatory surgery in young infants. Recommendations and common practice for minimal age for outpatient surgery range from 1 to 60 weeks. **The more conservative approach is based on the predisposition of infants to develop apnea and bradycardia following general anesthesia.** These findings are believed to result from the relative immaturity of the infant's respiratory and cardiac physiologic responses to hypoxia, hypercapnia, hypotension, and bradycardia. Although older children and adults increase ventilatory drive and cardiac output in response to these conditions, infants are at risk of developing further cardiorespiratory compromise. Preterm infants undoubtedly are at greater risk for apnea before 60 weeks,[38,52,58,112] but debate has generally centered on whether this danger is averted at 48 or 60 weeks of age. Mestad et al.[69] added some interesting controversy to this issue when they established that infants 40 weeks of age without a history of apnea or lung disease are appropriate candidates for ambulatory surgery (Table 85-11). However, the authors agreed with other studies that prematurity is a contraindication to outpatient management.

Table 85-11 Significant clinical differences between infants with and without apnea and relationship among postconceptual age, history of lung disease or apnea, and development of postoperative apnea

Parameter	Apnea	No apnea
Postconceptual age (weeks)*	38.4 ± 2.0	40.8 ± 2.6
Gestational age (weeks)*	28.2 ± 1.8	32.1 ± 3.2
Weight (kg)*	2.3 ± 0.3	3.3 ± 1.2
History of apnea†	89%	35%
History of lung disease	72%	38%

$p < 0.05$ by Student's t-test.
†$p < 0.05$ by chi-square analysis.

	History of apnea or lung disease	No history of apnea or lung disease
Postsurgical apnea (n = 18)	●●●●●●●●●●●● ■■■■■	●
No Postsurgical apnea (n = 82)	●●●●●●●●●●●●●●● ■■■■■■■■■■ ■■■■■■■■■■ ■■■■■■	●●●●●●●●●●● ■■■■■■■■■■ ■■■■■■■■■■ ■■■■■■■■■■

● Postconceptual age less than 40 weeks (n = 39)
■ Postconceptual age greater than or equal to 40 weeks (n = 61)
From Mestad PH, Glenski JA, Binda RE: When is outpatient surgery safe in preterm infants? *Anesthesiology* 69:A744, 1988.

Lacking more definitive studies, and because these procedures are usually elective, outpatient surgery should be deferred until the infant is at least 48 weeks and, if possible, 60 weeks of age. If operation must be performed earlier than this, postoperative admission with apnea monitoring is indicated.

Other criteria for outpatient surgery in children involve family-related factors. The parent or primary care provider must be able to understand and follow the instructions for preoperative and postoperative care of the pediatric patient. Home health care workers can assist the family and ensure adequate resources for providing optimal care. As noted earlier, every effort should be made to place these children on the operating room schedule first to avoid dehydration resulting from prolonged NPO before induction of anesthesia and placement of an IV line.

Respiratory Status

Reactive airway disease ("asthma")

After conditions resulting from cigarette use, reactive airway disease, alternatively referred to as "asthma," is the most common chronic respiratory condition found in the ambulatory setting. It can vary from mild, easily controlled episodes of bronchospasm to fatal episodes of respiratory failure. Reactive airway disease refers to a predisposition for bronchospasm associated with allergies, infection, or other medical conditions, such as chronic obstructive pulmonary disease (COPD). Whatever the etiology, intraoperative events such as endotracheal (ET) intubation or surgical stimulation may provoke bronchospasm;[80] therefore, the patient with asthma should be optimally treated preoperatively. Patients with wheezing at the preoperative assessment should be referred to their primary care provider unless all reasonable measures have been taken to stop the wheezing.

A serum theophylline level is necessary only in those patients who have had a recent acute event or have a history of susceptibility to episodes of severe bronchospasm that place them at risk for complication perioperatively. When obtained, the time of sampling should be noted, as well as its association with the time of drug administration, to provide an appropriate interpretation of the patient's status. Similarly, a chest radiograph and pulmonary function studies, including ABG, are indicated only in patients in significant distress or who have marked progression of disease during the past 6 months. The pulmonary function tests should include administration of bronchodilator therapy, with a 15% or greater improvement indicating reversible disease for which further medical therapy should be instituted before surgery. Patients with symptomatic compromise should be seen before surgery by their primary care provider and an anesthesiologist. Patients who, through poor compliance or other causes, are not receiving optimal medical management or who remain symptomatic should be referred to appropriate medical staff for management before undertaking the stress of anesthesia and operation.

All chronic medications, including bronchodilators, steroids, and inhalants, are continued through the day of surgery. Patients receiving nebulized bronchodilator therapy should receive treatment immediately before going to the operating room. Individuals who are steroid dependent should also receive their medication as scheduled on the day of operation, with additional "stress" doses of 100 mg hydrocortisone administered immediately preoperatively and 4 hours later, even in patients whose steroid therapy has been discontinued within the past 12 months. Some clinicians have advised administration of prophylactic steroids to patients in anticipation of bronchospasm associated with manipulation of the airway. Evidence to support this practice is lacking, and judicious anesthesia induction and maintenance perioperatively are usually sufficient.

Chronic obstructive pulmonary disease

Patients with COPD are managed similar to those with reactive airway disease. Patients with severe COPD must be under a physician's continuing care, with appropriate medical management to address the problems of reactive airways, pulmonary infection, hypoventilation, hypoxemia and hypercapnia. Although preoperative admission for pulmonary toilet is rarely indicated, patients experiencing dyspnea at rest or with minimal activity should be advised of possible postoperative admission and should have their procedure performed in an operating room associated with an inpatient facility.

Sleep apnea

Many children with a history of sleep apnea may be scheduled for tonsillectomy and adenoidectomy for presumed upper-airway obstruction. A careful history should be taken for any indication of apnea as a possible manifestation of seizure activity. **Children whose sleep apnea is sufficiently severe to require awakening or stimulation to breathe should undergo sleep studies to verify sleeping respiratory patterns, including documentation of oxygen (O_2) saturation. Because these children are prone to develop pulmonary hypertension, an ECG and echocardiogram are advised to assess right-sided heart function.**

Children with a history of sleep apnea or who are on monitors should be free of apnea and off monitors for 6 months before consideration for outpatient surgery. Children with current apnea, who are on apnea monitors, or who have indications of pulmonary hypertension, compromised right-sided heart function, or marked desaturation ($< 80\%$) should be admitted postoperatively for observation. Intraoperative management for these patients is a challenge, because they may be prone to develop postoperative airway obstruction and subsequent pulmonary edema. Observation should at least include a monitored bed with intensive care observation for those with significant preoperative respiratory or cardiac dysfunction.

Upper respiratory infections

The viral upper respiratory tract infection (URI) is usually a mild, self-limiting disease that does not preclude routine activities. However, the URI that may be deemed trivial by the surgeon or patient represents a more significant issue for the anesthesiologist. Considerable controversy persists about the advisability of anesthesia for patients with current or resolving URIs. **Complications associated with anesthesia in patients with URIs are bronchospasm,[77] intraoperative hypoxemia with an increased alveolar-arterial O_2 gradient,[24,25,67,116,117] and postoperative hypoxemia.[25] Children with acute URIs have a complication rate more than three times that of healthy children (5.3% versus 1.6%).[115]**

After the acute phase, increased risk also exists during the recovery phase. Increased bronchial reactivity and compromised lung bactericidal activity have been shown to continue for as long as 6 weeks after a URI.[28,59] This is the presumed basis for the finding of a small but statistically significant increase in respiratory complications in the asymptomatic child who has recently recovered from a URI. These patients, although in no distress before operation, may manifest all the complications of the acute phase with manipulation of the airway and stimulation under anesthesia.

Recently, some have speculated that a URI does not constitute a contraindication to general anesthesia and that anesthesia may even have a salutary effect. Animal studies have purported to show a beneficial effect of anesthetics on morbidity and mortality during viral challenge.[50] A recent report concluded that halothane may beneficially alter the course of URIs in children by reducing both the prevalence and the duration of symptoms.[115] However, two of these studies[85a,115] evaluated children undergoing mask anesthesia for myringotomy tube placement, and a third[112] did not mention the nature of the procedures. More definitive studies are needed to evaluate the response to ET intubation and more prolonged anesthesia before adopting these guidelines.

It is generally agreed that productive or "croupy" cough, fever, purulent nasal discharge, malaise, or abnormal chest radiographs are indications for postponing elective outpatient procedures. At our institution, we generally proceed with anesthesia in otherwise healthy individuals with clear rhinorrhea who are afebrile and have no other evidence of distress.

The anesthesiologist may make exceptions based on the individual patient's medical history. Many anesthesiologists anesthetize children who have recently recovered from a URI because some children develop URIs with such frequency that it is nearly impossible to find intervals when the patient is asymptomatic. This situation is frequently encountered in children undergoing myringotomy for placement of tubes because of chronic otitis media. Although the decision to proceed may be further complicated in patients who have travelled significant distances for their operation or for whom a delay would pose a significant hardship, subjecting these individuals to avoidable risks is not in their best interests. Some may consider this an overly cautious recommendation; this conservative approach is warranted in elective procedures, at least until appropriate studies prove otherwise.

Cystic fibrosis

Cystic fibrosis (CF) is the most common fatal genetic disorder, occurring in approximately 1 in 2000 live births in whites. This systemic disease **involves mucus-secreting glands, resulting in chronic pulmonary disease or exocrine pancreatic dysfunction. Less common but significant manifestations include cirrhosis of the liver and coagulopathy secondary to vitamin K deficiency.** The increasing longevity of these patients has increased the likelihood that they will be candidates for outpatient procedures.

The clinical spectrum of CF ranges from the asymptomatic individual to the patient dying of pulmonary insufficiency. Many of the anesthetic considerations pertaining to children with asthma apply to children with CF. Performing outpatient surgery on these individuals thus depends on their clinical condition. Patients with debilitating respiratory and other diseases are not appropriate outpatient candidates and should be admitted for preoperative respiratory therapy and hydration. Because of the respiratory conditions and vitamin deficiency–induced coagulopathy that may occur, **patients with CF should have preoperative chest radiographs, CBCs, coagulation studies, and serum electrolyte determinations**. When procedures are performed on an outpatient basis, a low threshold for admission should be maintained for any of these children who experience perioperative or postoperative distress.

Cardiocirculatory Status

The availability of outpatient procedures for patients with cardiocirculatory disease depends on the extent of the lesion and physiologic compromise. Patients whose cardiac disease, whether corrected or not, that leaves them in a debilitated state should not be considered for outpatient surgery; they are best observed overnight with discharge the following day. Patients with significant sequelae secondary to their cardiocirculatory disease, such as renal or central nervous system (CNS) dysfunction, should be evaluated by their primary care provider before the preoperative assessment.

Hypertension

Hypertension is the most frequently encountered cardiocirculatory condition. In general, systolic blood pressure should be below 180 mm Hg and diastolic below 110 mm Hg. Patient compliance with medical therapy is imperative, with referral for appropriate medical management for patients who have poor control or compliance. Sometimes, even with maximal medical management, control is not achieved. These patients may arrive the day of operation, with admission indicated postoperatively for those who have significant perioperative changes that persist through the recovery period.

Because hypertension is associated with cardiac, renal, and cerebrovascular compromise, thorough evaluation and laboratory tests, including an ECG, are indicated. Serum sodium and potassium values must be determined for patients receiving diuretic therapy and, as with the ECG, should be obtained within the week before operation. Hypokalemia (less than 3.0 mEq/l potassium) is a relative contraindication to anesthesia because of the enhanced risk of dysrhythmias, although further assessment may change this level to 2.5 mEq/l. Correction of the serum potassium by IV boluses of potassium on the day of operation is inappropriate because it does not address the need to reestablish intracellular stores.

Patients should take their regular medication on the morning of operation to ensure appropriate control through the perioperative period. Because of their NPO status, diuretic therapy may be withheld to avoid intravascular depletion. It is better for patients bring their medication and take it in the ambulatory surgery center, where fluid intake can be controlled. Otherwise, patients should be instructed to take their medications with sips of water at the usual time.

Coronary artery disease and angina

Coronary artery disease (CAD) is the second most frequently cardiocirculatory condition encountered in adults. Patients who have had a coronary artery bypass graft with subsequent relief from all symptoms and no evidence of change on the ECG are managed routinely. Unstable angina, defined as angina at rest or episodes of changing frequency or severity, should be treated as a relative contraindication to outpatient management. Patients with stable angina are best advised to visit their cardiologist or primary care provider before their anesthesia evaluation and to have an ECG within 1 week of the procedure. A change in symptoms or on the ECG within the past 6 months indicates the need for consultation with an internist or cardiologist before consideration for outpatient management. In these patients, clearance for ambulatory management depends on the determination that the change does not represent evidence of recent infarct or ischemia. Postoperative admission of these patients is indicated only when significant perioperative or postoperative distress occurs. These patients should be admitted to a location that allows for continual monitoring.

As with patients taking antihypertensive medication, established drug regimens for patients with stable angina should be continued through the day of operation, including beta blockers, calcium channel blockers, and nitroglycerin patches. Continuation of diuretic therapy for these patients through the day of surgery is generally discouraged because, with their NPO status and potential postoperative emesis, diuresis may predispose them to intravascular depletion. Anesthetic management for these patients requires scrupulous attention to avoid hypertension, tachycardia, and hypoxia.

Patients with stable angina who successfully complete their procedure and recovery without difficulty may be discharged to care at home.

Dysrhythmias

As with patients who have other cardiocirculatory problems, patients with dysrhythmias undergoing ambulatory surgery should be optimally managed before their procedure. New-onset dysrhythmias must be evaluated before proceeding with anesthesia. **The presence of symptomatic or potentially malignant dysrhythmias, such as new-onset atrial fibrillation or multifocal ventricular ectopy, are contraindications to ambulatory surgery; patients should be observed postoperatively in a monitored setting.**

A 12-lead ECG with rhythm strip should be obtained at the preoperative evaluation. The anesthesiologist may consult with the cardiologist or internist to decide on the management plan.

Patients with asymptomatic atrial fibrillation of at least 3 months' duration are reasonable candidates for ambulatory surgery, as are patients with asymptomatic premature ventricular ectopic beats that are unifocal and less than 7 to 10 beats per minute. Individuals with first-degree atrioventricular block usually tolerate outpatient procedures well; however, this finding should alert the anesthesiologist to seek the etiology of the condition.

Patients with pacemakers may undergo outpatient procedures, but one must verify proper functioning of the pacemaker, preoperatively. Patients with dysrhythmias who have no evidence of distress or dysfunction perioperatively or postoperatively should be allowed to go home, per routine discharge criteria.

Valvular heart disease

Patients with asymptomatic valvular heart lesions are usually reasonable candidates for outpatient surgery. Symptomatic lesions should be evaluated by a cardiologist before operation.

Congestive heart failure

Congestive heart failure (CHF) is a contraindication to outpatient surgery for all but the most minor procedures. Such procedures include those performed with local anesthesia and mild sedation. More invasive outpatient procedures, or the requiring general or major regional anesthesia, should be performed in a facility within a hospital setting.

Neurologic Status

Seizure disorders

Seizure disorders should be well controlled before consideration of outpatient or elective surgery. Patients with intractable seizures, those with seizures based on metabolic derangements, or those who require extensive continual nursing care are not appropriate candidates for outpatient surgery and should be admitted postoperatively. As with other conditions, clinicians increasingly tend to rely more on clinical presentation more than on pharmacologic data. Patients whose seizures are well controlled generally do not need determination of serum anticonvulsant levels. The exceptions to this rule are patients with a history of seizures despite careful medical management and children, who because of their rapid rate of growth require frequent adjustment of their dose. These two groups of patients are advised to see the physician managing their disorders immediately before operation.

Patients with cerebral palsy and seizure disorders are at risk for aspiration. Episodes of choking, cyanosis, or other related distress increase the risk for aspiration of stomach contents under anesthesia. A chest radiograph should be obtained to determine the extent to which chronic aspiration or pneumonia may have resulted in residual damage.

Mental retardation

Patients with mental retardation are appropriate for outpatient management only if they attain baseline status before discharge and have full support in their discharge location. The preoperative evaluation is otherwise done as for patients with associated medical conditions, with scrupulous attention to the nature of the postdischarge destination. The possible inability of these individuals to identify their distress or to seek appropriate medical attention should indicate a low threshold for postoperative admission.

Hematologic Disorders

Sickle cell disease

Patients with sickle cell disease are at particular risk for crises when they have dehydration, acidosis, or hypoxia. Therefore, prolonged NPO status can predispose these patients to unnecessary risks. Although initially requiring that all patients with sickle cell disease be admitted preoperatively, studies have found that the broad spectrum of this condition allows outpatient procedures to be performed on selected patients. Appropriate candidates include patients who have no history of crisis within the previous 12 months, who are otherwise in good health, and who are without significant associated end-organ disease.

The preoperative evaluation and preparation of patients with sickle cell disease offer interesting challenges for the anesthesiologist. Because 9% of all black children are carriers of the sickle gene, screening for this condition in all children at risk is indicated, regardless of family history or absence of anemia.

Screening for the presence of sickle cell disease should be complete before proceeding with operation.

A major consideration and point of debate involves recommendations about preoperative transfusion in patients with sickle cell disease. The general consensus is that avoidance of predisposing risk factors should result in an uncomplicated procedure. However, even the most carefully performed anesthesia carries the still-undetermined risk of hypotension, laryngospasm, hypoxemia, and other distress. Previous guidelines provided for preoperative transfusion for elective outpatient procedures were based on a presumption that the risks and costs of transfusion were more than offset by the avoidance of sickling crises should complications arise. Increasing experience has shown the scrupulous attention to hydration and ventilation can preclude the need for this intervention for those patients undergoing outpatient and many inpatient procedures.

Preoperative dehydration from extended NPO status has usually been cited as the reason for preoperative admission. These patients generally do well at home sleeping through the night without IV fluids, repleting themselves with normal oral intake during the following morning and throughout the day. Unless they have significant respiratory compromise, hypoxia is also not present when breathing room air. Finally, as long as dehydration, hypotension, and hypoxia are absent, acidosis is also an extremely unlikely event. With hydration the only remaining preoperative concern, patients should arrive at the ambulatory surgery preparation site early on the morning of operation, where IV access is immediately established to ensure adequate hydration. The procedure should then be scheduled to start no less than 2 hours later to ensure adequate time for administration of fluids before surgery and for preoperative observation. Although many pediatric patients may receive IV access after sedation or anesthesia induction in the operating room, those with sickle cell should receive IV fluids on arrival in the preoperative preparation area.

Anticoagulant therapy

Patients receiving anticoagulant therapy should have demonstrated reversal of anticoagulation by measurement with PT, PTT, and bleeding time before initiation of surgery.

Metabolic Disorders

Patients with disorders of the thyroid and adrenal gland are managed similar to inpatients. Specifically, careful management and control must be established before proceeding with elective surgery.

Diabetes mellitus

Diabetes mellitus is the most common endocrine problem managed in the ambulatory surgical setting. **Because of the high incidence of end-organ disease, especially in adults with longstanding insulin-dependent diabetes mellitus (IDDM), one must determine the extent of associated conditions such as renal or cardiocirculatory compromise.**

A principal concern in managing diabetic patients is the avoidance of hyperglycemia and hypoglycemia. Patients with IDDM should have their operation scheduled in the morning, at a time that allows adequate preoperative preparation and postoperative recovery. Administration of insulin to an NPO patient before arrival at the surgical facility places them at significant risk for hypoglycemia. Consequently, they should arrive at the preoperative preparation site no later than 8 AM. Their insulin is then administered after obtaining an estimate of blood glucose (which can be obtained with a "dip stick" method) and starting an IV solution containing glucose, usually dextrose 5% in lactated Ringer's solution. One half the normal dose of insulin is administered if the glucose is greater than 150 mg/dl, and one third the amount for glucose values of 90 to 150 mg/dl.

Patients taking oral hypoglycemic agents are instructed not to take their medication on the day of operation, because the extended half-life of these medications is longer than 24 hours. Balancing appropriate management is difficult in diabetic patients. The stress of the procedure increases serum glucose by several mechanisms, and careful attention to this issue should include a glucose determination during the perioperative and recovery periods. Sliding-scale insulin is used as necessary for these and insulin-dependent diabetic patients, based on glucose estimates obtained perioperatively and postoperatively. At our institution, we generally do not need to administer insulin to these patients.

Hepatorenal Disorders

Patients with renal or hepatic failure should be accepted for ambulatory surgery only after consultation with an anesthesiologist. The advisability of proceeding with outpatient operation is made on a case-by-case basis depending on the extent of physiologic compromise and the type of operation and anesthesia to be administered. Patients undergoing renal dialysis should receive a dialysis treatment within 24 hours of the scheduled procedure, with a CBC and electrolyte panel provided after dialysis. In our institution, dialysis patients who are alert, oriented, and normotensive with normal electrolyte values do quite well with ambulatory surgical procedures. Patients not fulfilling these criteria should receive further medical evaluation before operation; if these conditions are not correctable, inpatient postoperative observation is indicated.

Individuals with significant hepatic compromise often pose more of a challenge. **Fulminant hepatic failure (FHF) is generally a contraindication to ambulatory surgery except for the most minor procedures.** Symptomatic compromise, such as malaise or neurologic disturbances, is an absolute contraindication. Serum electrolyte measurements and liver function studies should be obtained within 1 day of the procedure and compared with earlier values to determine the extent of disease progression.

Substance Abuse

Unfortunately, substance abuse, whether alcohol or narcotics, is often encountered in the ambulatory surgical setting. The anesthetic management of these patients is particularly challenging in both the chronic and the acute phases of their substance abuse.

Individuals engaging in substance abuse are especially prone to violations of preoperative instructions, whether concerning drugs or NPO status. Nonetheless, the use of inpatient facilities and resources to guarantee their compliance with preoperative protocols or to adjust their narcotic abuse is rarely appropriate. If considered coherent enough to understand and give consent to a surgical procedure, these individuals should be able to understand the risks associated with violations of preoperative protocols. **A low threshold for cancellation should be maintained for those who arrive on the day of operation with any indication of substance use or abuse. This should especially should apply to individuals using cocaine and its various derivatives. The susceptibility of these patients to serious ventricular dysrhythmias—especially with stimulation or administration of epinephrine with local anesthetics—places them at major risk during even minor procedures.**

This final word of caution is somewhat controversial. Because of the physiologic alterations involved with acute cessation of substance abuse, anesthesiologists may advise their patients to continue their routine use of narcotics through the day of operation. Although the perioperative concerns are understandable, these physicians should be aware that in so doing, they are encouraging continuation of a practice that is not only illegal but potentially fatal and that is frequently supported by theft or violence against others. These physicians may not be liable, but such a recommendation to continue these activities does involve some moral responsibility. The preoperative assessment is better used to educate patients about the potential risk of their habit rather than to lend tacit support to this practice.

PREOPERATIVE PREPARATION: DAY OF OPERATION

Arrival Time

Patients should be instructed to arrive at the surgical facility at a time that allows adequate preparation and ensures their availability at the operating room if operations are ahead of schedule. This must be balanced against the patient waiting for prolonged periods before going to surgery. When preoperative evaluations have been completed before the day of operation, arrival 60 to 90 minutes before scheduled procedure is usually sufficient, with another 30 minutes added for patients being evaluated on the day of operation.

Some patients should be scheduled at the start of the day and brought to the unit early in the morning because of special circumstances relating to medications (diabetes) and hydration (sickle cell disease). In older children and adults, IV fluids are begun. Hydration for patients in whom hypovolemia is not a major concern should be gradual, without attempting to replace the entire fluid deficit in 1 hour. Lactated Ringer's solution or normal (0.9%) saline is generally accepted as appropriate for adults, but the selection of fluids for pediatric patients is the subject of debate, especially concerning dextrose concentrations.

Prophylaxis for Aspiration, Nausea, and Emesis

The need for adherence to NPO guidelines is one of the most important and, at times, most difficult aspects of ambulatory practice. Unlike the restrictions placed on the inpatient, the ambulatory patient is presented with many temptations and opportunities to violate the NPO standard. Patients, surgeons, and other medical staff must understand the importance of this issue, especially with regard to patient morbidity.

The most significant condition causing perioperative morbidity is aspiration pneumonitis, a potentially fatal complication in even the healthiest patients undergoing anesthesia. Following Mendelson's classic description of aspiration pneumonitis in 1946,[65] further studies have demonstrated the severity of this phenomenon. Bynum and Pierce,[12] in their series of 50 surgical inpatients with aspiration, noted an initial mortality rate of 12%; 26% demonstrated initial improvement, which was followed by bacterial pneumonia and mortality within this group of 60%, for an overall mortality rate exceeding 25%. Although this mortality rate may be somewhat greater than that reported by others, it highlights the need for careful attention to this complication. Contrary to the belief that intraoperative emesis and aspiration are rare and are clearly manifested during the procedure, Blitt et al.[9] used an orally administered dye in the pharynx as an indicator to document silent regurgitation in 68 (9.0%) of 734 patients undergoing general anesthesia. Of these, six had been presumed to have aspirated based on the presence of dye in the trachea. Interestingly, regurgitation and aspiration were greatest in patients undergoing upper-abdominal, neurosurgical, or otolaryngologic procedures and in those whose airways were "protected" with an ET tube (Tables 85-12 through 85-14). Based on these findings, anesthesiologists must not underestimate the importance of regurgitation and aspiration in the ambulatory care setting.

The conditions that predispose to aspiration are more common than one might suspect. Studies have shown that patients with a gastric pH less than 2.5 and, for adults, gastric volumes greater than 25 ml place patients at special risk.[6,114] Ong et al.[81] demonstrated a greater incidence of larger volumes and lesser gastric pH in outpatients than in their inpatient counterparts (Figs. 85-5 and 85-6). Manchikanti et al.[62] studied 125 outpatients undergoing general anesthesia and receiving various forms of premedication, including none, placebo, and combinations of diazepam, hydroxyzine, and meperidine. They found that 88% to 96% had a gastric pH less than 2.5 and that 36% to 56% had gastric volumes greater than 25 ml, with no significant differ-

Table 85-12 Influence of surgical procedures on regurgitation and aspiration

Surgical procedure	No. of patients	Regurgitations (%)	Aspirations
Upper abdominal	90	16 (17.8)	2
Neurosurgical	30	5 (16.7)	0
Ear, nose, throat	57	6 (11.4)	2
Lower abdominal	124	9 (7.4)	0
Superficial and examination under anesthesia	443	31 (7.0)	2
Chest	18	1 (5.6)	0
Eye	138	2 (1.4)	0

From Blitt CD, et al: Silent regurgitation and aspiration during general anesthesia, *Anesth Analg* 49:707, 1970.

Table 85-13 Influence of airway management on regurgitation and aspiration

Method of securing airway	No. of patients	Regurgitations (%)	Aspirations (%)
Endotracheal tube	472	58 (12.3)	4 (7)
Mask alone	74	3 (4.5)	1 } (17)
Mask and oral airway	209	9 (4.4)	1 }
None (local standby or blocks)	144	0	0

From Blitt CD, et al: Silent regurgitation and aspiration during general anesthesia, *Anesth Analg* 49:707, 1970.

Table 85-14 Influence of patient's position on regurgitation and aspiration

Position	No. of patients	Regurgitations (%)	Aspirations
Sitting	6	2 (33.4)	0
Prone	16	4 (25.0)	0
Jackknife	8	1 (12.5)	0
Lateral	38	3 (7.9)	1
Supine	619	45 (7.3)	8
Lithotomy	213	15 (7.0)	2

From Blitt CD, et al: Silent regurgitation and aspiration during general anesthesia, *Anesth Analg* 49:707, 1970.

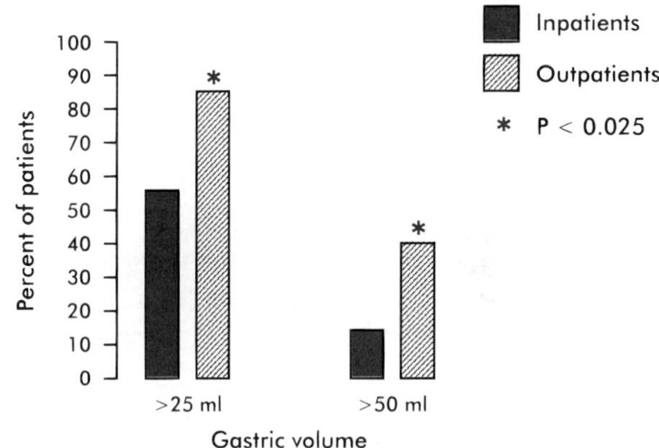

Fig. 85-6. Frequency of occurrence of large gastric volumes among hospital inpatients and outpatients. (From Ong BY, Palahniuk RJ, Cumming M: Gastric volume and pH in out-patients, *Can Anaesth Soc J* 25:36, 1978.)

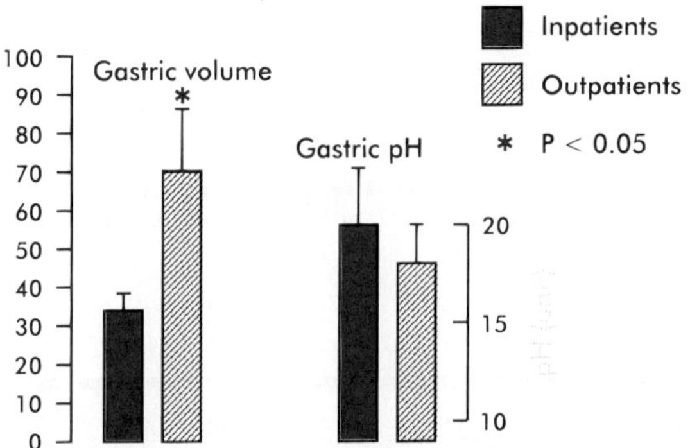

Fig. 85-5. Mean gastric volume and pH of hospital inpatients and outpatients. (From Ong BY, Palahniuk RJ, Cumming M: Gastric volume and pH in out-patients, *Can Anaesth Soc J* 25:36, 1978.)

ence between the various groups (Tables 85-15 through 85-17). These studies not only confirm the extent to which patients are at risk, but also cast doubt on assertions that premedication with benzodiazepines or narcotics reduces these risk factors.

Considering the prevalence of patients with increased gastric volumes and decreased pH, one could argue that aspiration prophylaxis should be performed for all patients, and certainly for those with obesity, hiatal hernia, duodenal or gastric ulcers, gastroesophageal reflux, pregnancy, or swallowing disorders secondary to neurologic or anatomic abnormalities. Cricoid pressure with rapid-sequence induction may be used to prevent aspiration. However, this technique poses considerable hazards to patients with compromised airways and to those at risk for the tachycardia and increased blood pressure associated with this technique. Therefore, preparation before induction is the best approach.

Management of aspiration prophylaxis begins with an appropriate NPO status. Further reduction in risk for aspiration should ideally involve increasing the gastric pH and a reduction, or at least no increase, in gastric fluid volume. Those who believe that acidity is more critical than volume have often administered Bicitra® (sodium citrate and citric acid) because of its simplicity and ease of administration. However, many studies have shown that this practice denies the high-risk patient the added value of other medical regimens. Manchikanti et al.[60] compared patients taking various combinations of Bicitra (15 and 30 ml orally) and metoclopramide (10 mg IV) with a control group to assess volume and acidity of gastric secretions. Although Bicitra alone increased gastric pH, gastric volume remained the same or was increased (Tables 85-18 through 85-20), whereas metoclopramide alone reduced gastric volume and increased gastric pH. The best result occurred with Bicitra (15 ml orally) and metoclopramide (15 mg IV), with larger Bicitra doses providing no additional benefit. However, the authors com-

Table 85-15 Patient characteristics and fasting periods for patients receiving premedication

Patient group	No. of patients	Sex distribution (male/female)	Age (years)*	Height (cm)*	Weight (kg)*	Fasting period (hrs)*
Group 1: no premedication	25	11/14	33.3 ± 2.7	172.1 ± 1.6	70.8 ± 2.8	11.51 ± 0.62
Group 2: meperidine and hydroxyzine, IM	25	15/10	27.6 ± 2.2	173.3 ± 1.6	72.0 ± 3.2	11.16 ± 0.53
Group 3: meperidine and prochlorperazine, IV	25	14/11	31.7 ± 2.7	173.1 ± 2.1	72.6 ± 3.5	10.63 ± 0.43
Group 4: diazapam and prochlorperazine, IV	25	11/14	30.7 ± 2.7	171.8 ± 2.2	68.9 ± 3.7	10.60 ± 0.42
Group 5: diazepam and hydroxyzine, orally	25	12/13	33.5 ± 2.8	170.3 ± 1.4	67.9 ± 2.6	13.50 ± 0.85

*Values are mean ± SEM.
IM—Intramuscularly; IV—intravenously.
From Manchikanti L, et al: Assessment of effect of various modes of premedication on acid aspiration risk factors in outpatient surgery, *Anesth Analg* 66:81, 1987.

Table 85-16 Gastric pH data for patients receiving premedication

Patient group	pH		Patients with pH ≤ 1.5	Patients with pH ≤ 1.8	Patients with pH ≤ 2.5
	Mean ± SEM	Range			
Group 1: no premedication	1.86 ± 0.11	1.28 – 3.64	5 (20%)	19 (76%)	22 (88%)
Group 2: meperidine and hydroxyzine, IM	2.10 ± 0.23	1.12 – 6.47	4 (16%)	16 (64%)	20 (80%)
Group 3: meperidine and prochlorperazine, IV	1.94 ± 0.12	1.27 – 4.30	5 (20%)	14 (56%)	23 (92%)
Group 4: diazepam and prochlorperazine, IV	1.90 ± 0.12	1.26 – 4.31	4 (16%)	16 (64%)	23 (92%)
Group 5: diazepam and hydroxyzine, orally	1.82 ± 0.10	1.28 – 2.73	4 (16%)	14 (56%)	24 (96%)

IM—Intramuscularly; IV—intravenously.
From Manchikanti L, et al: Assessment of effect of various modes of premedication on acid aspiration risk factors in outpatient surgery, *Anesth Analg* 66:81, 1987.

Table 85-17 Gastric volume data for patients receiving premedication

Patient group	Volume (ml)		Patients with volume ≥ 25 ml	Patient with volume ≥ 25 ml and pH ≤ 1.5	Patients with volume ≥ 25 ml and pH ≤ 1.8	Patients with volume ≥ 25 ml and pH ≤ 2.5
	Mean ± SEM	Range				
Group 1: no premedication	30.0 ± 4.1	5 – 80	15 (60%)	5 (20%)	12 (48%)	14 (56%)
Group 2: meperidine and hydroxyzine, IM	26.2 ± 4.0	2 – 90	12 (48%)	3 (12%)	9 (36%)	12 (48%)
Group 3: meperidine and prochlorperazine, IV	25.7 ± 4.6	5 – 100	9 (36%)	3 (12%)	8 (32%)	9 (36%)
Group 4: diazepam and prochlorperazine, IV	30.0 ± 4.9	5 – 100	11 (44%)	4 (16%)	10 (40%)	11 (44%)
Group 5: diazepam and hydroxyzine, orally	26.0 ± 4.7	8 – 100	9 (36%)	2 (8%)	7 (28%)	9 (36%)

IM—Intramuscularly; IV—intravenously.
From Manchikanti L, et al: Assessment of effect of various modes of premedication on acid aspiration risk factors in outpatient surgery, *Anesth Analg* 66:81, 1987.

Table 85-18 Gastric pH characteristics of patients administered Bicitra and metoclopramide

Patient group	pH		H^+ concentration (gEq/L) (mean ± SEM)	Patients with pH ≤ 2.5
	Mean ± SEM	Range		
1. Control	2.12 ± 0.23	1.27–6.85	0.018 ± 0.002	22 (88%)
2. Bicitra, 15 ml orally	3.20 ± 0.21	1.56–4.74	0.005 ± 0.002	8 (32%)
3. Bicitra, 30 ml orally	3.72 ± 0.17	1.75–4.64	0.002 ± 0.001	4 (16%)
4. Metoclopramide, 10 mg IV	2.41 ± 0.25	1.42–6.16	0.013 ± 0.002	18 (72%)
5. Bicitra, 15 ml orally, and metoclopramide, 10 mg IV	3.40 ± 0.29	1.56–7.89	0.006 ± 0.002	9 (36%)
6. Bicitra, 30 ml orally, and metoclopramide, 10 mg IV	3.71 ± 0.30	1.48–7.68	0.004 ± 0.002	7 (28%)
Direction and significance of values (groups)	1 = 4 < 2 = 3 = 5 = 6		1 = 4 > 2= 3 = 5 = 6	1 = 4 > 2 = 3 = 5 = 6

IV—Intravenously.
From Manchikanti L, et al: Bicitra and metoclopramide in outpatient anesthesia for prophylaxis against aspiration pneumonitis, *Anesthesiology* 63:378, 1987.

Table 85-19 Characteristics of gastric volume in patients administered Bicitra and metoclopramide

Patient group	Volume (ml)		Patients with volume ≥ 25 ml	Patients with volume ≥ 50 ml	Patients with pH ≤ 2.5 and volume ≥ 25 ml
	Mean ± SEM	Range			
1. Control	32.7 ± 7.6	5–180	9 (36%)	5 (20%)	9 (36%)
2. Bicitra, 15 ml orally	32.4 ± 5.5	5–100	14 (56%)	4 (16%)	3 (12%)
3. Bicitra, 30 ml orally	58.4 ± 8.9	2–210	21 (84%)	14 (56%)	3 (12%)
4. Metoclopramide, 10 mg IV	15.6 ± 2.6	1–50	5 (20%)	2 (8%)	5 (20%)
5. Bicitra 15 ml orally, and metoclopramide, 10 mg IV	21.8 ± 4.1	3–100	7 (28%)	4 (16%)	1 (4%)
6. Bicitra, 30 ml orally, and metoclopramide, 10 mg IV	26.0 ± 5.5	3–100	9 (36%)	5 (20%)	2 (8%)
Direction and significance of values (groups)	3 > 1 – 6		1 = 2 2 > 4 3 > 1 = 4 – 6 3 = 2	3 > 1– 6	1 = 2 – 6 1 > 5 = 6 2 = 3 – 6

IV—Intravenously.
From Manchikanti L, et al: Bicitra and metoclopramide in outpatient anesthesia for prophylaxis against aspiration pneumonitis, *Anesthesiology* 63:378, 1987.

pared these results with those of two previous studies[63,64] that examined the use of ranitidine (150 mg orally) and cimetidine (300 mg orally). Both these drugs were superior to either of the other combinations, and ranitidine was the most effective of all.

Others have demonstrated the effectiveness of the H_2-receptor antagonists, cimetidine and ranitidine, in significantly increasing pH and reducing volume. Summarizing 12 articles in this area, Joyce[45] reviewed the IV and oral administration of these agents. In general, IV administration of 50 mg of ranitidine or 150 mg of cimetidine resulted in peak effects at 45 to 60 minutes, with no increase in effect with larger doses. The IV formulation was carefully administered over 20 minutes to avoid the hypotensive effect caused by rapid infusion. Oral administration of 150 mg of ranitidine and 300 mg of cimetidine required 90 minutes to 3 hours for peak effects.

Manchikanti et al.[61] assessed the combination of glycopyrrolate with cimetidine. Because glycopyrrolate provided no added benefit compared with cimetidine alone and required intramuscular (IM) administration, glycopyrrolate was not recommended.

Table 85-20 Comparison of effects in patients administered Bicitra, cimetidine, ranitidine, or Bicitra and metoclopramide

	Gastric pH					
Patient group	Mean ± SEM	Time-interval from drug administration to sampling (min)	Patients with gastric pH ≤ 2.5	Gastric volume (ml) (mean ± SEM)	Patient with gastric volume ≥ 25 ml	Patient with pH ≤ 2.5 and volume ≥ 25 ml
1. Bicitra, 15 ml orally (n = 25)	3.20 ± 0.21	45.4 ± 3.5	8 (32%)	32.4 ± 5.5	14 (56%)	3 (12%)
2. Bicitra, 30 ml orally (n = 25)	3.72 ± 0.17	45.6 ± 3.5	4 (16%)	58.4 ± 8.9	21 (84%)	3 (12%)
3. Cimetidine, 300 mg orally (n = 25)	5.04 ± 0.44	146.2 ± 9.9	4 (16%)	13.0 ± 2.4	3 (12%)	1 (4%)
4. Ranitidine, 150 mg orally (n = 20)	6.40 ± 0.44	153.9 ± 13.4	2 (10%)	9.6 ± 2.0	2 (10%)	1 (5%)
5. Bicitra, 15 ml orally, and metoclopramide, 10 mg IV (n = 25)	3.40 ± 0.29	50.0 ± 3.5	9 (36%)	21.8 ± 4.1	7 (28%)	1 (4%)
6. Bicitra, 30 ml orally, and metoclopramide, 10 mg IV (n = 25)	3.71 ± 0.30	50.4 ± 3.6	7 (28%)	26.0 ± 5.5	9 (36%)	2 (8%)
Direction and significance of values (groups)	1 > 3 4 > 1 = 2 = 5 = 6 3 > 1 = 2 = 5 = 6	3 = 4 > 1 = 2 = 5 = 6	No significant difference	2 > 1 = 5 = 6 2 > 3 = 4 = 5 = 6 1 > 3 = 4	1 > 3 = 4 2 > 3 = 4 = 5 = 6 1= 2 1 = 5 = 6	No significant difference

IV—Intravenously; n—number of patients.
From Manchikanti L, et al: Bicitra and metoclopramide in outpatient anesthesia for prophylaxis against aspiration pneumonitis, *Anesthesiology* 63:378, 1987.

In deciding which of the H_2-receptor antagonists to use, one should consider the side effects of cimetidine, including decreased hepatic clearance of certain drugs. In comparing cimetidine and ranitidine, Gonzalez et al.[36] randomly assigned ASA class I patients undergoing arthroscopy to receive either 150 mg of ranitidine or 400 mg of cimetidine on awakening in the morning. Both the ranitidine and the cimetidine groups had a significantly greater pH and decreased gastric volume than a placebo group at induction of anesthesia, but the raniditine group maintained this advantage through 1.2 hours of anesthesia better than did the cimetidine group. Although 46% of those receiving cimetidine were considered at risk (pH less than 2.5 or gastric volume greater than 20 ml), only 15% of those receiving ranitidine were included in this category at the end of the procedure, mainly because of maintaining a higher pH.

Because patients are usually requested to arrive 1 to 2 hours before their scheduled induction time, the use of ranitidine (150 mg orally) appears to provide the best protection against aspiration. In the Lerman et al.[57] study, the authors used no premedication, ranitidine alone (2 mg/kg), metoclopramide alone (0.1 mg/kg), or both agents together. Ranitidine alone provided advantages over other single or combination modalities (Figs. 85-7 and 85-8). Although these medications were given 4 hours before operation, Guay et al. found similar results with medication given 2 hours preoperatively (Fig. 85-9).

Nausea and emesis represent the two most common factors for delay of discharge from the outpatient surgical unit and for admission of pediatric patients. Thus successful management of these two issues can potentially enhance patient safety, comfort, and efficiency. Pandit et al.[84] in studying 140 adult women undergoing outpatient laparoscopy, found that metoclopramide (5 and 10 mg) given orally 30 minutes before operation did not reduce nausea and emesis. However, IV droperidol (5, 10, and 20 μg/kg) had some beneficial effect in decreasing nausea and vomiting (Tables 85-21 and 85-22). This effect was statistically

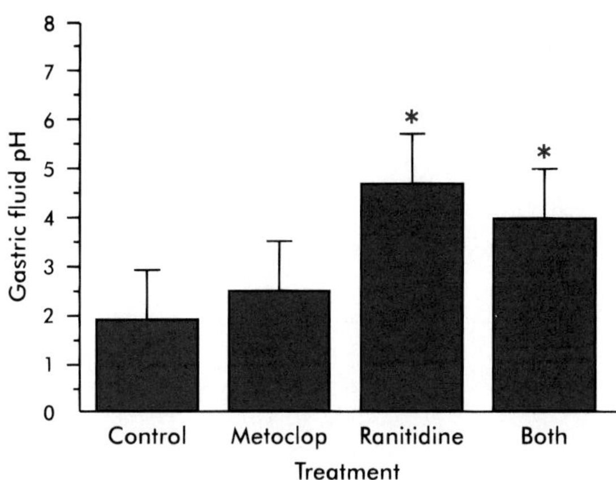

Fig. 85-7. Effect of ranitidine on gastric fluid pH. (From Lerman J, Christensen SK, Farrow-Gillespie AC: Effects of metoclopramide and ranitidine on gastric fluid pH and volume in children, *Anesthesiology* 69(3A):A748, 1988.)

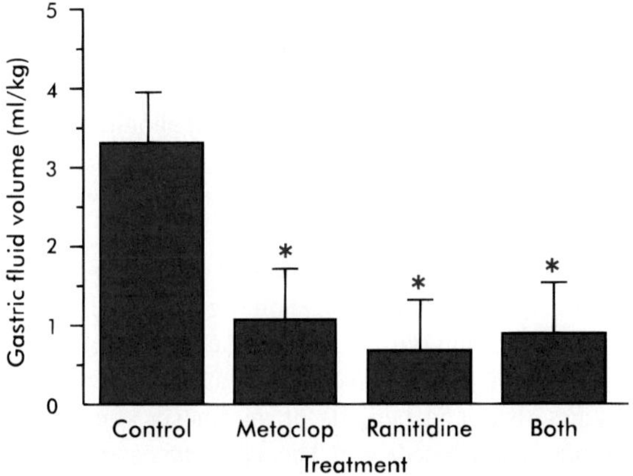

Fig. 85-8. Effect of ranitidine on gastric fluid volume. (From Lerman J, Christensen SK, Farrow-Gillespie AC: Effects of metoclopramide and ranitidine on gastric fluid pH and volume in children, *Anesthesiology* 69:(3A)A748, 1988.)

significant for droperidol in doses of 10 and 20 μg/kg, and 20 μg was especially useful in eliminating any postoperative need to treat nausea and emesis.

Christenson et al.[19] in comparing droperidol with lidocaine for pediatric patients undergoing ophthalmologic surgery, reported similar findings. Patients received either droperidol (75 μg/kg), lidocaine (1.5 mg/kg), or both (droperidol, 25 μg/kg; lidocaine, 1.5 mg/kg) at anesthesia induction. Of the group receiving only high-dose droperidol, 22% had nausea, compared with 50% of the lidocaine group. The combination of the two drugs provided no significant advantage. These studies contrast with the findings of Broadman et al.[11] who found that administration of metoclopramide (0.15 mg/kg) in the recovery period reduced the incidence of nausea and emesis from 60% to 41% in patients undergoing strabismus surgery.

A recent report found that transdermal scopolamine applied the evening before operation and worn for 3 days post-

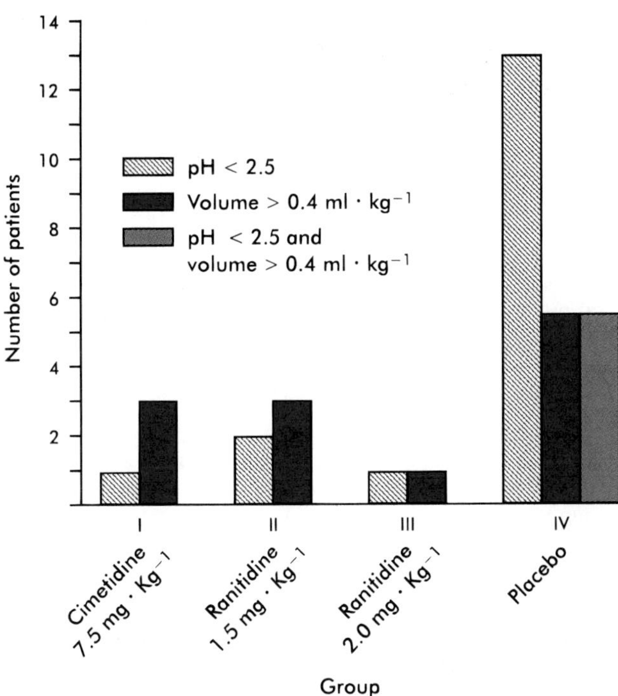

Fig. 85-9. Number of patients having either pH less than 2.5, gastric volume greater than 0.4 ml/kg, or both. Group IV was statistically different from groups I, II, and III for gastric pH and for combination of both factors ($p < 0.001$). (From Guay J, Santerre L, Gaudreau HP, et al: Effects of oral cimetidine and ranitidine on gastric pH and residual volume in children, *Anesthesiology* 71:547, 1989.)

operatively was more effective than a placebo in ameliorating postoperative nausea and emesis and reducing the need for antiemetic medication.[3] Unfortunately, scopolamine was not compared with agents other than the placebo. In addition, the side effects of dry mouth and, on rare occasion, dysphoric reactions, have diminished the attraction of this method. Finally, the logistics of requiring patients to take new medications at home before operation are best avoided in those circumstances where anesthesiologists or their staff do not have the opportunity to interview the patient prior to the day of operation.

Interpreting these studies is difficult because of the widely varying doses, routes of administration, time intervals and procedures. Current recommendations include the use of ranitidine for adults (150 mg orally) and children (2 mg/kg) for aspiration prophylaxis, with droperidol (20 μg/kg) at anesthesia induction for postoperative nausea and emesis. Further studies focusing on metoclopramide and other medications postoperatively may provide additional data in this area.

Sedation

Preoperative sedation is administered to allay the patient's fears and anxieties, permit a smooth induction of and emergence from anesthesia, and lead to a more pleasant and shorter recovery time. A wide selection of

Table 85-21 Frequency of nausea and vomiting (as percentage of 20 patients in each group) in recovery room*

Patient group	No nausea or vomiting (%)	Nausea only (%)	Nausea and vomiting (%)	Any nausea/vomiting (%)
1. Metoclopramide, 5 mg, and placebo	45	30	25	55
2. Metoclopramide, 10 mg, and placebo	55	25	20	45
3. Placebo and droperidol, 5 μg/kg	60	20	20	40
4. Placebo and droperidol, 10 μg/kg	75	20	5	25†
5. Placebo and droperidol, 20 μg/kg	80	10	10	20†
6. Placebo and placebo	35	25	40	65
7. Metoclopramide, 10 mg, and droperidol 10 μg/kg	75	20	5	25†

*Chi-square tests were performed with raw data. Group 6 was significantly different from groups 4, 5 and 7.
†$p < 0.05$.
From Pandit SK, Kothary SP, Pandit UA, et al: Dose-response study of droperidol and metoclopramide as antiemetics for outpatient anesthesia, *Anesth Analg* 68:798, 1989.

Table 85-22 Percentage of patients requiring additional antiemetic therapy in recovery room*

Patient group	No additional treatment (%)	One additional treatment (%)	Two or more additional treatments (%)
1. Metoclopramide, 5 mg	70	25	5
2. Metoclopramide, 10 mg	75	10	15
3. Droperidol, 5 μg/kg	90	10	0
4. Droperidol, 10 μg/kg	85	15	0
5. Droperidol, 20 μg/kg	100†	0	0
6. Placebo	60	35	5
7. Metoclopramide, 10 mg, and droperidol, 10 μg/kg	90	10	0

*Chi-square tests were performed with raw data. Only group 5 was significantly different from placebo (group 6).
†$p < 0.05$.
From Pandit SK, Kothary SP, Pandit UA, et al: Dose-response study of droperidol and metoclopramide as antiemetics for outpatient anesthesia, *Anesth Analg* 68:798, 1989.

medications and alternative approaches exist regarding dosage and time and route of administration. However, regardless of which medication is chosen, the anesthesiologist must consider several issues when using these agents.

Providing appropriate assistance and management for patients receiving preoperative sedation is the foremost issue. Even the mildest sedative can cause drowsiness, which requires that the patient be observed. The preoperative waiting area at least should include reclining chairs in which patients may relax close to the operating room with a family member or nursing staff in attendance. The patient should be afforded some privacy, even if by a simple partition or curtain. Transport to the operating room, even for those who appear completely awake, should be by wheelchair to protect the patient from potential injury caused by unsteady ambulation.

A second consideration is the timing of the sedation in relation to discussion with the anesthesia staff about the procedure. Some may not consider the patient to be competent to discuss risks and benefits of anesthesia after receiving heavy preoperative sedation. The anesthesia staff should arrange to see the patient *before* sedation to ensure that these discussions are held with an alert, understanding individual. This will also help the anesthesia staff to determine whether the patient needs premedication and, if so, to choose the appropriate agent.

Finally, although preoperative sedation is beneficial to certain patients, little scientific or empiric support exists for its universal administration to all patients, except possibly for younger children, who are usually fearful of their unusual surroundings and activities. Egbert and Baird[27] and later Leigh et al.[56] showed that a preoperative visit by an anesthesiologist is more useful in allaying anxiety than medication alone or information in a booklet.

Candidates for preoperative sedation include children under 5 years of age, adults who demonstrate anxiety despite discussions with the anesthesia staff, and patients whose conditions necessitate avoidance of anxiety and associated physiologic changes, such as tachycardia and increased blood pressure. These include patients with CAD, hypertension, or severe anxiety disorders and those with impaired mental capacities who may have difficulty cooperating. **Contraindications to preoperative sedation include impaired airways, significant respiratory distress, and altered mental status, as evidenced by somnolence.**

Patients who may have compromised drug elimination, such as those with major renal or hepatic conditions, also should not be sedated.

When selecting agents and routes of administration, one should remember that, unlike with inpatients, a limited time is available to administer medication to ambulatory surgical patients. Assuming the patient arrives 2 hours before the scheduled operation and then expeditious management is provided, the anesthesiologist may only have a window of 60 to 90 minutes in which to administer a medication and achieve the desired effect. Further, the route of administration, especially in children, should serve to alleviate rather than promote anxiety and fear. Specifically, one might consider alternatives to IM injections to spare the patient the sight and discomfort of another needle.

When selecting appropriate agents, the clinician generally can choose among benzodiazepines, barbiturates, or a combination of these, with or without other agents (e.g., antisialogogues). In the past, narcotics and barbiturates were used because they were routinely administered to inpatients and showed promise in preanesthetic sedation.

Pandit and Kothary,[82] in comparing sufentanil, fentanyl, morphine, and a placebo, found that sufentanil was somewhat better than the other narcotics for sedation and analgesia. Although more than half the patients were lightheaded after IV injection, sedation (as measured by anxiety scores) had begun to disappear in all except the sufentanil group at the start of anesthesia induction, the time sedation is perhaps needed the most (Table 85-23). In an earlier assessment of these same agents, the authors,[83] although advocating the use of sufentanil because of its sedative properties, found that narcotics did not prolong the anesthetic or recovery periods when compared with a placebo. They also found a greater incidence of nausea and vomiting with all the narcotics except sufentanil. Although some advocate the use of narcotics to assist in postoperative pain management, these authors reported that the incidence of postoperative pain was virtually identical in all the groups (Tables 85-23 through 85-25).

The use of narcotics is being supplanted by benzodiazepines, especially midazolam, because they achieve better sedation than barbiturates while avoiding the side effects associated with narcotics (including dysphoria, nausea, vomiting, and respiratory depression). Benzodiazepines also have less potential for overdosage, especially when given orally, than the narcotic agents. In two comparisons of benzodiazepines with narcotics, the former demonstrated a consistent advantage over both narcotics and placebos. Raeder and Breivik[91] compared IM midazolam, morphine, and scopolamine, and a placebo for sedation and associated side effects, and found that midazolam was superior in regard to all parameters. Investigating the use of IM midazolam combined later with a narcotic, Shafer et al.[108] found that midazolam provided better anxiolysis compared with a placebo. When anesthesia was supplemented with narcotics intraoperatively, patients had a smoother intraoperative course, as measured by absence of respiratory compromise (hiccups, laryngospasm) and no increase in recovery time. However, the midazolam-narcotic group had more nausea and emesis postoperatively than the midazolam-placebo group (42% and 18%, respectively).

Although effective, IM administration of these agents is at least uncomfortable and an additional concern for patients who are already anxious. Oral premedication has been found to be very effective, such as diazepam in doses of 0.25 mg/kg to a maximum of 15 mg[6] administered 1 hour or more before operation. However, conflicting data surround the de-

Table 85-23 Anxiety scores

Premedicant	Baseline	15 minutes*	Before induction
Morphine	50.7 ± 26.91	28.3 ± 24.62	39.6 ± 29.51
Meperidine	44.7 ± 24.57	21.3 ± 19.46†	30.9 ± 29.29†
Fentanyl	65.1 ± 26.32	32.7 ± 19.23†	45.5 ± 27.88†
Sufentanil	52.0 ± 26.03	27.1 ± 23.91	29.6 ± 28.68†
Placebo	51.9 ± 27.02	43.5 ± 29.20	48.7 ± 26.89

*Analysis of variance: group differences significant, $p < 0.05$.
†Compared with baseline, $p < 0.05$, t-test with Bonferoni correction.
From Pandit SK, Kothary SP: Intravenous narcotics for premedication in outpatient anesthesia, *Acta Anesthesiol Scand* 33:353, 1989.

Table 85-24 Recovery time in minutes (mean ± SD)* (see also Table 85-23)

Premedicant	Orientation	Ambulation	Discharge
Morphine	21.4 ± 6.63	148.4 ± 49.33	210.3 ± 65.84
Meperidine	19.2 ± 6.54	135.2 ± 30.02	187.0 ± 50.87
Fentanyl	19.9 ± 7.41	145.8 ± 51.73	187.9 ± 67.73
Sufentanil	19.7 ± 8.19	134.2 ± 44.05	181.5 ± 62.01
Placebo	20.2 ± 7.69	156.0 ± 54.05	200.0 ± 69.12

*Analysis of variance: no significant differences among groups.
From Pandit SK, Kothary SP: Intravenous narcotics for premedication in outpatient anesthesia, *Acta Anesthesiol Scand* 33:353, 1989.

Table 85-25 Side effects in recovery room (see also Tables 85-23 and 85-24)

Premedicant	Nausea/vomiting	Drowsiness	Pain
Morphine	25	15	45
Meperidine	20	20	45
Fentanyl	15	15	45
Sufentanil	10	15	40
Placebo	10	15	45

*Chi-square test: no significant differences among groups.
From Pandit SK, Kothary SP: Intravenous narcotics for premedication in outpatient anesthesia, *Acta Anesthesiol Scand* 33:353, 1989.

bate on whether midazolam is superior to diazepam. Barclay et al.[5] compared 0.23 mg/kg of diazepam with 0.115 mg/kg of midazolam and found them to have equally good sedative properties; however, the midazolam group had deeper amnesia and less postoperative drowsiness than the diazepam group. O'Boyle et al.[78] obtained different results when comparing oral midazolam (15 mg) with oral diazepam (10 mg), with midazolam having a more rapid onset of action but patients having slower recovery. Raybould and Bradshaw[94] found 7.5 mg of oral midazolam to be ineffective but 15 mg to be very effective in providing sedation; however, they also found significant postoperative sedation 2 hours after operation. Similar conflicting results are found in comparing midazolam with other benzodiazepines, such as temazepam[37,42] and triazolam.[6]

A good summation of the debate concerning adult premedication would be to note that, when needed, oral benzodiazepines have been shown to be effective when administered at least 1 hour before operation. Diazepam, in an oral dose of 10 to 15 mg, appears to be a good sedative when administered 60 to 90 minutes before operation, although it may delay recovery somewhat.

Sedation in pediatric patients

Preoperative sedation in pediatric patients presents a different set of issues. Usually, pediatric patients are unable to comprehend the unusual and potentially threatening activity about them, and cannot have their anxiety allayed by comprehensive discussion. Those under 5 years of age often do not have IV access and require a mask induction with its attendant distress. Although the need for adequate sedation is greater, the margin of error in these smaller patients is decreased. Thus, sedation must be approached cautiously.

The best anxiolysis may come from keeping the child with at least one parent when awake, including during anesthesia induction and immediate postoperative care. Having the parent in the induction facility has been shown to provide minimal disruption, with smoother induction and less psychologic trauma to the child.[34] Similarly, a parent in the recovery room can comfort and communicate with the child on emergence.

When preoperative sedation is to be used, the first consideration is that sedation not cause further distress. Sedation refers to the achievement of anxiolysis before transport to the induction area. Rectal midazolam or methohexital and other agents administered by this route are usually induction agents, not preoperative sedation. The use of IM injections also defeats the purpose and, with the bioavailability of oral benzodiazepines, is not indicated. Feld et al.[31] demonstrated that oral midazolam in a dose of 0.5 mg/kg was virtually as effective as IM injections of 0.1 to 0.2 mg/kg, and, if necessary, midazolam could be given in doses up to 1 mg/kg. Recovery times were not significantly prolonged, and the anesthesia staff reported induction as being smoother. Although intranasal midazolam[128] has been shown to be effective, its irritating effect to children, potential difficulty in administration, and lack of clear advantage over oral premedication make it a poor alternative.

Diazepam and droperidol have been found to be effective,[35,55] but neither offers the convenience of midazolam. A controversial innovation has been the use of a lollipop containing fentanyl citrate. Studies using the lollipops[2,30,111,114] have consistently found that doses of 15 to 20 μg/kg provided excellent sedation and smooth induction of anesthesia in children 2 years of age and older. Common side effects are those expected for narcotics, including decreased respirations, nausea and emesis, and pruritis. The controversy stems from the belief of some that children will develop a pleasant association with the narcotic effect. Because no evidence suggests that narcotic administration, either acutely or chronically in any form, leads to narcotic dependence, this concern should not decide this issue. However, as with adults, the evidence indicates that a benzodiazepine is more efficacious and less prone to cause postoperative difficulties than a narcotic.

PERIOPERATIVE MANAGEMENT

The perioperative care of the ambulatory surgery patient requires scrupulous attention to issues of safety, comfort, convenience, and efficiency. Selection of anesthetic technique must ensure a cooperative patient. The anesthesiologist must use a method that provides rapid induction and emergence from anesthesia, with the patient feeling little discomfort in the recovery period and thus allowing for a reasonably quick discharge. The margin for error is considerably smaller in outpatient procedures, because little time is available to stabilize a patient during the perioperative period if one discovers excessive or insufficient depth of anesthesia.

Therefore, the anesthesia staff should be thoroughly familiar with the actions and interactions of anesthetic agents. It is often stated that it is better to know much about a few agents than little about many agents; this adage applies in outpatient anesthesia practice, where familiarity will lead to improved results.

As with any procedure, the anesthetic technique should be discussed with the patient and the discussion documented in the medical record. Potential complications should be discussed, and patients should be advised of alternative plans that may ensue. These plans are usually in the form of general anesthesia in the event that other techniques are insufficient for completion of the procedure. Because of the variations in surgical technique, it is best to discuss the planned technique with the surgeon, both to ensure agreement and to prevent conflicting messages to the patient.

Monitoring and Anesthesia Equipment

A fully operational anesthesia system must be available for outpatient general anesthesia, including all the monitoring that is standard for the inpatient setting. This monitoring includes pulse oximetry, capnography, ECG, blood pressure measurement, and precordial stethoscope. Although some devices are initially expensive, the ability to monitor inspiratory and expiratory inhalation agents is proving to be of significant value in modifying anesthetic technique to allow for smooth induction and rapid emergence. Attempts to decrease costs through the assignment of antiquated equipment from other areas to the ambulatory surgery suite convey a misplaced perception of the care needs for outpatients.

Monitored Sedation

Although at times derided as a boring or unchallenging, monitored sedation (monitored anesthesia care [MAC]) often provides the safest, most comfortable, and most efficient anesthetic management for outpatients. It is especially desirable in patients whose medical condition (e.g., major cardiorespiratory disease) makes them unsuitable candidates for general anesthesia. Whereas regional and general anesthesia may provide deep anesthesia over a large body area and allow leeway to both anesthesiologist and surgeon, monitored sedation requires scrupulous technique by both.

Procedures that can often be performed by experienced surgeons include breast biopsies, inguinal hernia repairs, limited superficial procedures on the skin and subcutaneous tissue, ophthalmic procedures such as cataract extraction, and procedures on the digits amenable to a local block by the surgeon. A full listing of the procedures is not possible, partly because these depend on the skills and experience of the surgeon. Operation performed with local anesthesia require a site that is limited and amenable to local infiltration, a procedure that can be performed rapidly, and one that does not require excessive doses of either local anesthesia or sedation. Surgical skill is critical; attempts to perform invasive procedures such as tonsillectomy or laparoscopy with sedation and local anesthesia is fraught with potential disaster if the operator is not experienced and skilled in such procedures.

Patient cooperation is best secured through constant communication, as well as advance notice of medication administration so as not to surprise the patient. All staff in the operating room should be aware that sedation is being administered to an awake patient and alerted to the need to maintain appropriate decorum; placement of a sign to this effect on the operating room door is advised to prevent staff from entering the room and making comments inappropriate to the situation.

In general, sedation allows a patient to achieve a more relaxed state and permits a more pleasant and rapid completion of the procedure. A wide array of drugs is employed. The technique that has generally worked well involves the use of a benzodiazepine with a short-acting narcotic, replacing the past practice of relying on barbiturates (Fig. 85-10). Midazolam causes less postoperative drowsiness than diazepam; combined with its faster onset of action and less venous irritation, it is the mainstay of current technique. Midazolam is routinely administered in increments of 0.5 to 1.0 mg, or 0.01 mg/kg, to provide a relaxed but easily arousable patient. Contrary to conventional wisdom, the retrograde amnesia associated with midazolam is minimal and is marked by impaired ability to integrate events into long-term memory.[20,35,90]

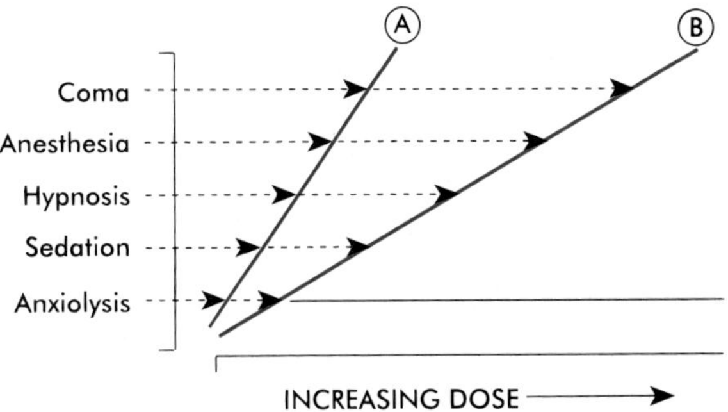

Fig. 85-10. Spectrum of central nervous system (CNS) activity. Sedative-hypnotics produce dose-dependent spectrum of CNS depression. In this schematic, drug A might represent a barbiturate (e.g., pentobarbital), whereas drug B might represent a benzodiazepine (e.g., diazepam). (From White PF: Pharmacologic and clinical aspects of preoperative medication, *Anesth Analg* 65:963, 1986.)

Administration of short-acting narcotics, such as fentanyl (1 to 2 μg/kg), can supplement the sedative effects of the midazolam, with the anesthesiologist checking closely for any impaired or compromised ventilation. Alfentanil (10 to 20 μg/kg) is also effective and provides more rapid onset and shorter duration of action than fentanyl. As with all procedures, varying levels of stimulation occur, usually associated with initial and subsequent injections of local anesthetic into the surgical site. Administration of 25 to 50 mg of a short-acting barbiturate or 10 to 20 mg of propofol immediately before local infiltration may preclude the need for larger doses of longer-acting agents. Frequent need for such medication indicates the need for deeper sedation.

An alternative approach to sedation involves the use of propofol, a rapid-onset, short-acting hypnotic. After an initial dose of 1 mg/kg, increments of 0.25 mg/kg up to a total dose of 2.5 mg are used to achieve sedation. A continuous infusion of 20 μg/kg is then used to maintain sedation, adjusting to the patient's level of sedation and vital signs. Propofol is a hypnotic and not an analgesic. Therefore, its success depends on appropriate local anesthesia.

The anesthesiologist should be familiar with the operative procedure and the specific points of intense but transient stimulation, so that sedation needs can be met prospectively. Points of stimulation may include the preparation of the skin with cold solutions, examination before commencing with the procedure, and initial injection of local anesthetic. In these circumstances, incremental doses of thiopental (25 to 75 mg) or propofol (10 to 20 mg) are useful to provide transient deeper sedation.

Patient discomfort that persists despite sedation in the unstimulated state may indicate the need for more local anesthetic infiltration or alteration of technique. If major sedation and local infiltration do not provide a satisfactory surgical patient, then general anesthesia may be necessary to complete the procedure. When this occurs, the patient should be informed calmly that general anesthesia is required, and the induction is performed immediately.

Regional Anesthesia

In addition to epidural and spinal techniques, the practitioner of outpatient anesthesia should be well acquainted with regional anesthesia, especially anesthesia of the extremities, ranging from digital, ankle, and wrist blocks to axillary, supraclavicular, interscalene, and femoral blocks.

Regional anesthesia offers potential major benefits. Although this is especially true for those patients in whom general anesthesia may pose a significant risk, regional anesthesia also provides advantages for the general patient population. The most frequently cited criticisms of regional anesthesia, other than spinal, is the time required to establish analgesia—usually 20 to 30 minutes—and the perceived risk of failure requiring general anesthesia.

In assessing the usefulness of regional anesthesia, one must consider recovery time and the patient's postoperative comfort. In a review of 543 brachial plexus blocks, Davis[23] found a success rate of 93% for anesthesiologists performing such blocks regularly, with the greatest success among those using the transarterial technique. Bowe et al.[9] and Baysinger et al.[6,7] demonstrated that brachial plexus anesthesia for carpal tunnel release and upper extremity procedures did not significantly differ from general anesthesia in total operating room and recovery room time. However, the incidence of postoperative nausea, emesis, and pain requiring medication was less than half that found in patients who had general anesthesia.

Similar findings have been found for arthroscopy of the knee performed under epidural or spinal anesthesia, with administration of neuraxial narcotic for prolonged analgesia.[10,57,86,93] As with brachial plexus blockade, the incidence of nausea, emesis, and postoperative pain were significantly less than with general anesthesia. Parnas et al.[86] although finding a frequency of postoperative pain of 20.3% versus 27.0% in patients under regional or general anesthesia, respectively, found significantly less nausea and emesis (4.1% versus 16.5%, respectively). Bowe et al.[10] found an even greater difference in postoperative pain (27% versus 65% for regional versus general) and nausea with emesis (1.5% versus 25% for regional versus general). In all studies, neither operating room nor recovery times were significantly different between these two groups. Of interest is the additional finding of Randel et al.[93] that epidural anesthesia results in a decreased recovery time to 123 minutes, as compared with 164 minutes for general anesthesia.

These studies were performed using inhalational anesthetic techniques. Comparisons using newer general anesthetic techniques, including total IV anesthesia, may alter these findings. Nonetheless, practitioners of outpatient anesthesia are finding regional anesthesia to be an increasingly useful tool. The use of an anesthesia induction room while the previous surgery is underway is one method to provide regional anesthesia without interfering with the orderly progression of the schedule.

Epidural anesthesia

Epidural anesthesia has been found to provide significant benefit and safety for peripheral vascular, urologic, gynecologic, and arthroscopic surgery.[73,93,96] Randel et al.[93] showed that the additional time required for placement of the block could be compensated for by reduced time to oral intake, ambulation, voiding, and discharge (Tables 85-26 and 85-27). Although the incidence of moderate-to-severe headache was less than with either general or spinal anesthesia, patients undergoing epidural anesthesia did have a greater incidence of moderate-to-severe backache. This side effect should be considered when evaluating this technique in those with preexisting lower-back pain. Whether using the "single-shot" or continuous catheter technique, it is best to avoid using long-acting local anesthetics (e.g., bupiva-

Table 85-26 Recovery times after general, spinal, and epidural anesthesia (minutes mean ± SD)

	General	Spinal	Epidural
Intake	98 ± 46	81 ± 33	68 ± 32*
Ambulation	133 ± 47	135 ± 50	97 ± 26*†
Void	137 ± 49	145 ± 54	106 ± 35*†
Discharge	164 ± 58	168 ± 51	123 ± 36*†

*Analysis of variance with Bonferoni correction: $p = 0.0003$ (epidural vs. general).
†$p = 0.0003$ (epidural vs. spinal).
From Randel et al: Epidural anesthesia is superior to spinal or general for outpatient knee arthroscopy, *Anesthesiology* 71:A769, 1989.

Table 85-27 Incidence of headache and backache in patients after general, spinal, and epidural anesthesia*

	General	Spinal	Epidural
Headache			
Mild	21.3%	14.8%	25.8%
Moderate	8.2%	9.8%	5.2%
Severe	0.0%	5.2%	0.0%
Backache			
Mild	21.3%	37.7%	22.4%
Moderate	6.6%	19.7%	36.2%
Severe	0.0%	3.3%	6.9%

*Combined data from days 1 to 5 after surgery.
From Randel et al: Epidural anesthesia is superior to spinal or general for outpatient knee arthroscopy, *Anesthesiology* 71:A769, 1989.

caine), to prevent prolonged recovery while the block recedes. Most catheter procedures can be performed using 1.5% lidocaine, with or without epinephrine, with redosing as needed during operation.

Spinal Anesthesia

Although offering the benefit of rapid and intense block, the risk of spinal headache and subsequent distress is a major concern for outpatient anesthesia. Three aspects of spinal headache are particular concerns in the ambulatory setting: (1) it often occurs 2 to 3 days postoperatively, after routine follow-up has already been accomplished; (2) it incapacitates the patient for several days thereafter; and (3) it increases the potential for readmission or further intervention with a blood patch. Because these events can transform an outpatient procedure into a protracted, expensive period of discomfort and inconvenience for the patient, the anesthesiologist should carefully weigh the advantages before proceeding with spinal anesthesia. Advocates of spinal anesthesia point out the low incidence of postoperative spinal headache as a justification for its use. This incidence ranges from 4% to 37% in published data when a 25-gauge needle is used, which is much greater than[32,73,88] the generally accepted unscheduled admission rate of 2% or less.

Some advocates, such as Mulroy,[73] have maintained that alteration in technique and appropriate patient selection can reduce these figures to a more acceptable 2% or less, and that maintenance of a recumbent position does not help avoid headache[15,120] and may simply delay its onset. The use of 27-gauge needles and use of Greene "pencil-point" needles or Whitacre side-port needles has reduced the incidence of postdural puncture headache to less than 1%. The clinical advantages of the 27-gauge Whitacre is making it the standard for ambulatory surgery. The ability to select patients appropriately is also a consideration in light of the study of Perz et al.[89] (Tables 85-28 through 85-30), which showed a fourfold difference in headache rate between women (16.6%) and men (4%), both greater than the 2% goal that Mulroy has set. In addition, the incidence of backache associated with spinal procedures is greater than that with general anesthesia.

In summary, the issue of spinal anesthesia is still controversial, and resolution awaits further study and refinement in technique. In the meantime, practitioners are still advised to approach this method with caution and to avoid using spinal anesthesia in young women and patients with preexisting back pain or injury unless it presents a clear advantage in the patient at risk for general anesthesia. Even in these latter patients, epidural anesthesia may remain the most viable and appropriate option.

Table 85-28 Procedures and position of men and women patients (number) undergoing spinal anesthesia

	Arthroscopy	Laparoscopy	Other lithotomy	Other supine	Other phone
Men	57	0	32	34	2
Women	25	42	78	16	2

From Perz RR, Johnson DL, Shinozaki T: Spinal anesthesia for outpatient surgery, *Anesth Analg* 67:S168, 1988.

Table 85-29 Headache data from patients who underwent spinal anesthesia

	No headache	Grade 1	Grade 2	Grade 3	Grade 4	Grade 2 or greater (%)
Men	113	7	3	2	0	4
Women	127	9	12	6	9	16.6

From Perz RR, Johnson DL, Shinozaki T: Spinal anesthesia for outpatient surgery, *Anesth Analg* 67:S168, 1988.

Table 85-30 Backache data from patients who underwent spinal anesthesia

	No backache	Grade 1	Grade 2	Grade 3	Grade 4	Grade 2 or greater (%)
Men	87	9	21	8	0	23
Women	86	12	48	12	5	40

From Perz RR, Johnson DL, Shinozaki T: Spinal anesthesia for outpatient surgery, *Anesth Analg* 67:S168, 1988.

Regional supplementation of general anesthesia

There is increasing use of regional anesthesia to supplement general anesthesia for postoperative analgesia. The most significant of these has been the use of caudal anesthesia in pediatric patients undergoing genitourinary or lower-extremity procedures. Caudal anesthesia has found widespread favor in alleviating the postoperative discomfort associated with inguinal hernia repairs, orchiopexies, and other procedures.[95,104] Although the delayed discharge associated with caudal anesthesia has been a principal objection, the use of 0.125% bupivacaine has diminished the incidence of postoperative urinary retention while maintaining adequate analgesia.[96]

Local infiltration with anesthetics is also useful in diminishing postoperative pain. Placing local anesthetics into the wound is an increasingly popular technique. Casey et al.[17] found that simple instillation of 0.25% bupivacaine was as effective as a more elaborate ilioinguinal or iliohypogastric block with bupivacaine for children having inguinal hernia repair. Studies have reported a significant reduction in postoperative pain in patients having bilateral tubal ligation, with injection of 5 ml of 1% etidocaine into the banded portion of the tube.[4] Narchi et al.[75] obtained similar results in patients undergoing laparoscopy, with 80 ml of 0.5% lidocaine or 0.5% bupivacaine applied to the right subdiaphragmatic area. Local anesthetics or narcotics can be instilled in the knee joint during arthroscopy also.

General Anesthesia

General anesthesia, should be administered in a way that allows for rapid induction and emergence from anesthesia. **Principal problems associated with the otherwise successful general anesthesia are somnolence, nausea and emesis, postoperative pain, and associated delays in discharge and possible hospital admission.** As the number of procedures performed with sedation and regional anesthesia increases, general anesthesia may be required less frequently. Nonetheless, it remains the mainstay of outpatient anesthetic practice, and considerable progress has been made to reduce the associated problems.

Monitoring for patients under general anesthesia follows the routine format. Humidification and airway heating at one time was believed to be beneficial for even short procedures, but Goldberg et al.[36] have shown that these techniques neither reduce postoperative distress nor decrease recovery time. When brought into the room, patients frequently experience increasing distress because of the imminence of the procedure, the number of staff in the room, and the unfortunate lack of modesty often associated with patient positioning. Allowing patients to wear scrub pants into the operating room, although a minor inconvenience after induction, helps preserve their self-respect and their warmth in the cold operating room environment. Application of monitors and induction of anesthesia should proceed quickly in the stable patient.

Attempts to administer sedatives immediately before induction are usually self-defeating. Not only is the patient awake longer and allowed to experience more anxiety in this foreign environment, but the anesthesiologist runs the risk of giving an agent whose duration of action may exceed the duration of the procedure and contribute to delayed awakening and postoperative somnolence. Anxious patients should be given preoperative sedation before they come to the operating room, and anesthesia should be induced promptly on arrival in the operating suite.

Induction

Most patients are healthy and able to tolerate anesthesia induction without undue distress. However, the hemodynamic changes and bronchial irritation associated with general anesthesia, whether with intubation or mask, are special concerns for some patients, such as those with CAD, hypertension, and reactive airways. In these individuals, induction must achieve an appropriate depth of anesthesia before manipulating the airway or starting the procedure.

After administering the induction agent and establishing the airway, the depth of anesthesia should be established with either IV or inhalation agents before proceeding further. In patients at risk for complications of tachycardia (e.g., those with CAD), administration of esmolol (100 mg) has been shown to blunt undesirable hemodynamic responses[87] without untoward perioperative side effects; increasing the dose offers no additional benefit (Fig. 85-11). This technique may also allow the anesthesiologist to use less anesthetic to prevent the hemodynamic response and thus prevent postoperative distress from excessive medication.

Induction in pediatric patients who are too young for prior IV placement should begin with an inhalation technique. Rectal midazolam[130] produces a cooperative patient when given in a dose of 1 mg/kg, but it still subjects the child to the unpleasant experience of rectal administration and prolongs induction time. Similarly, the routine use of IM ketamine[41] involves a needle stick in a child who may be otherwise cooperative. As with adults, preoperative anxiety is best treated with preoperative sedation and rapid induction.

Before the introduction of propofol, sodium was the mainstay for induction. Considerable evidence now shows that propofol offers distinct advantages. Sampson et al.[102] in an analysis of the two agents, compared 4 mg/kg of thiopental with 2.5 mg/kg of propofol followed by 100% O_2 for termination of pregnancy. The recovery time until patients were comfortable postoperatively was considerably shorter for the patients receiving propofol than for those receiving thiopental (Fig. 85-12). These findings of reduced recovery time, less nausea, and greater postoperative alertness have also been reported consistently in other studies.[21,71,92,103,107,114] Anecdotal information from practitioners also notes smoother emergence, almost bordering on a transient pleasant euphoria. Marais et al.[65] and Sung et al.,[113] in separate studies indicative of future cost-benefit analyses, also found that propofol was effective in reducing costs by decreasing patient stay and postoperative symptoms.

Two major drawbacks to propofol, however, are its tendency to cause bradycardia and hypotension and venous irritation. When compared with thiamylal, propofol had a uniformly more pronounced effect on the cardiocirculatory system (Fig. 85-13), as measured by bradycardia, hypotension, and decreased systemic vascular resistance (SVR).

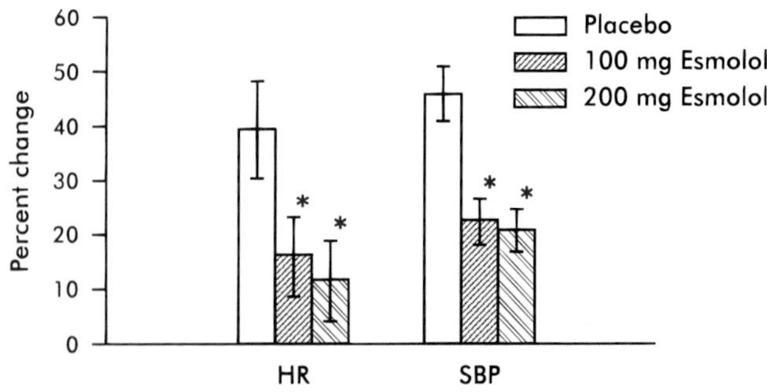

Fig. 85-11. Maximum percent changes from baseline in heart rate (HR) and systolic blood pressure (SBP) following intubation (mean ± SEM). Asterisk indicates significant difference between placebo and group treated with esmolol. (From Parnas S, et al: Single dose esmolol for prevention of hemodynamic changes of intubation in an ambulatory surgery unit, *Anesthesiology* 71:A12, 1989.)

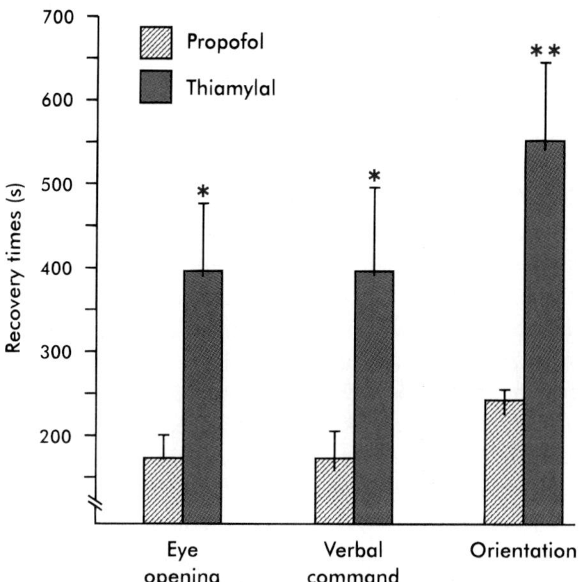

Fig. 85-12. Recovery times (mean, SEM bars) from discontinuation of anaesthesia (N_2O turned off) until eye opening, response to verbal command, and orientation. $*p < 0.05$; $**p < 0.01$. (From Sampson IH, et al: Comparison of propofol and thiamylal for induction and maintenance of anesthesia for outpatient surgery, *Br J Anaesth* 61:707, 1988.)

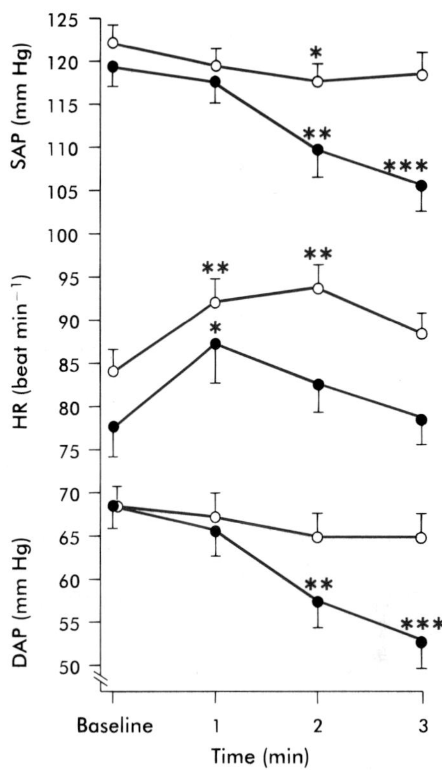

Fig. 85-13. Changes in systolic arterial pressure (SAP), diastolic arterial pressure (DAP), and heart rate (HR) (mean, SEM bars) after administration of propofol (*solid circles*) or thiamylal (*open circles*). Within group differences (measured from baseline): $*p < 0.05$; $**p < 0.01$; $***p < 0.001$. (From Sampson IH: Comparison of propofol and thiamylal for induction and maintenance of anaesthesia for outpatient surgery, *Br J Anaesth* 61:707, 1988.)

However, the magnitude of these changes was not deemed clinically significant in the otherwise stable patient. Venous irritation, found in smaller vessels, is caused mainly by the carrier agent and can be ameliorated by adding 10 to 20 mg of lidocaine to the propofol solution.

Maintenance of anesthesia

The availability of newer agents has altered perspectives on maintenance of anesthesia. Specifically, the short-acting neuromuscular agents atracurium, cis-atracurium, and mivacurium; the short-acting narcotics fentanyl, alfentanil, and sufentanil; and the newer inhalation agents desflurane and sevoflurane are allowing new approaches to general anesthesia for outpatients.

Before the availability of these agents, the major issue was whether an inhalational technique or a balanced technique with narcotics and nitrous oxide (N_2O) was preferred. In assessing volatile agents, little has been found to differentiate among them as to postoperative drowsiness, headache, myalgia, nausea and vomiting,[16,34,84] or perioperative stability.

In assessing the preference for narcotics versus volatile agents, increasing evidence suggests that balanced technique with narcotics results in better postoperative comfort and less nausea and other distress. Roetman et al.[98] found that fentanyl (2 and 10 μg/kg) with N_2O was safe and provided better analgesia in infants. Although Enright and Pace-Florida[29] found that patients receiving volatile agents had better recovery, as measured by the Bender Gestalt test, the narcotic dosage was not specific and did not include the use of alfentanil or sufentanil. Haley et al.[40] compared alfentanil (15 μg/kg), fentanyl (1.5 μg/kg), and thiopental with enflurane for short gynecologic procedures. In contrast to Enright and Pace-Florida, Haley et al. found that the narcotics resulted in faster recovery, with alfentanil the fastest, but also found an increased incidence of adverse perioperative events, most significantly chest wall rigidity, which was easily managed with succinylcholine.

At present, the choice of fentanyl, alfentanil, or sufentanil as the principal narcotic for ambulatory surgery is under investigation. The immediate onset and short duration of alfentanil makes this agent very useful in the ambulatory setting and provides benefits over morphine and fentanyl. However, its potency also carries some potential problems and its short duration of action also means less coverage for postoperative pain for patients undergoing procedures in which pain is a major concern; in tubal ligation, for example, ischemia of the tubes can cause considerable distress. When using alfentanil, the anesthesiologist should be prepared to manage pain in the recovery room.

Total intravenous anesthesia

The introduction of short-acting hypnotics and narcotics—specifically, propofol and alfentanil—has assisted in the development of total IV anesthesia (TIVA) as a means of providing general anesthesia. In two studies, propofol in a continuous infusion of 12 mg/kg/hour was compared with enflurane[85] and isoflurane. In both instances, patients receiving propofol had significantly less nausea and emesis, less recovery time, and less need for intervention for these problems in the recovery room. Although one study has found that narcotics did not enhance TIVA,[72] many strongly advocate the continuous infusion of propofol and alfentanil both separately and in combination.

When using continuous infusion techniques, it is best to use infusion pumps that allow for delivery of controlled volumes. Newer infusion pumps use microprocessor technology to permit delivery by specific doses in micrograms per kilogram. When using propofol, an induction dose of 2.5 mg/kg is followed by a continuous infusion of 150 to 200 μg/kg/minute for 10 minutes and then gradually reduced to 50 to 100 μg/kg/minute. Maintenance of the pulse and blood pressure within 20% of preinduction values is used as the principal guide in dosing, with the infusion turned off 5 to 10 minutes before the end of the procedure. This infusion is usually performed in association with 70% N_2O and midazolam (2 mg).

Although an excellent hypnotic, propofol is not an analgesic. Consequently, propofol infusion is often supplemented with a short-acting narcotic, such as fentanyl (100 μg) or alfentanil. Administration of alfentanil should be performed judiciously. Its rapid onset is also associated with bradycardia, hypotension, and chest wall rigidity when administered too rapidly. The bradycardia is easily treated with atropine and the rigidity with succinylcholine. When used with propofol, an initial dose of 50 μg/kg of alfentanil provides analgesia for 30 to 40 minutes, with an abrupt cessation of action that results in light anesthesia if the anesthesiologist is not vigilant. An alternative technique for procedures longer than 30 minutes is continuous infusion of alfentanil. After a 50- to 100-μg/kg loading dose, an infusion of 0.5 to 3 μg/kg/minute with N_2O generally provides excellent anesthesia. With this technique, careful communication with the surgeon is important, because the infusion of alfentanil should be discontinued 15 to 20 minutes before the end of the procedure to prevent respiratory depression.

Total intravenous anesthesia is especially useful when administration of inhalational agents is compromised by interruption of the patient's airway, as in diagnostic and laser procedures of the airway, or when use of volatile agents is limited by lack of scavenging systems, such as anesthesia in locations outside the operating room. Many anesthesiologists also use continuous-infusion muscle relaxants with hypnotics or narcotics. Although intriguing, maintaining more than two continuous infusions may tax the anesthesiologist's ability to monitor the patient appropriately. Nevertheless, whichever combination is used, the newer systems are becoming increasingly simple, and their use will likely increase in the future.

Comparisons of TIVA with the newer inhalation agents, desflurane and sevofluane, have not yet established definitive evidence as to preferred choice. Although desflurane and sevoflurane may have shorter emergence times than TIVA or other inhalation techniques, they have not yet been found to significantly alter the overall perioperative and postoperative course of outpatients.[55]

Muscle relaxants

The use of muscle relaxants in ambulatory surgery patients has been made safer and easier with the advent of atracurium, cis-atracurium, and vecuronium, which are distinguished by relatively short durations of action and, with vecuronium and cis-atracurium, by absence of hemodynamic and other side effects. Because most procedures are short, muscle relaxants are best used only as required to allow surgical exposure or to prevent catastrophic consequences of abrupt patient movement. Pancuronium is likely to lead to prolonged neuromuscular blockade in outpatients. Although some advocate continuous infusion of succinylcholine, it requires an additional set of functions to monitor the patient continually in a fast-paced situation, and there is the continued risk of phase II block.

Reversal of neuromuscular blockade should be performed on completion of the procedure, regardless of the time from the last dose or the neuromuscular blocking drug used.

The principal source of controversy in the area of neuromuscular blockade is the extent to which succinylcholine is responsible for postoperative myalgia and whether preadministration of a nondepolarizing agent prevents this phenomenon. It is difficult to assess the true extent of this phenomenon given the current literature, and advocates for succinylcholine appropriately note that this drug should not be contraindicated, for it can be efficient and occasionally life-saving.

RECOVERY

After the selection of anesthetic techniques that provide an alert patient with little postoperative distress, the recovery period should be relatively brief. This is often easier said than done, and the management of the patient in the recovery unit often requires intervention to provide relief from distress while simultaneously not unduly prolonging the postoperative stay.

Postoperative care of the outpatient is best completed in a two-stage process, with the first in a standard recovery room. This care includes routine ECG monitoring and pulse oximetry for those who have had general anesthesia or sedation. Use of O_2 for transport and initial recovery is appropriate for patients who have received general anesthesia or significant sedation, because hypoxia is no less a problem for outpatients than for inpatients.[14,74,124] In a study of 164 patients, Murray et al.[74] found a 7% incidence of hypoxia, with an O_2 saturation less than 92%; they found no association with type of anesthesia used or preoperative history. Because these patients demonstrated no overt evidence of hypoxia, the authors appropriately advised that one should monitor O_2 saturation if supplemental O_2 is not administered. Because the cost and difficulty in doing this may be prohibitive and the risk of hyperoxia is virtually nil, simple O_2 administration should be sufficient.

In the second stage of postoperative care, patients who are reasonably alert and able to take sips of fluids should be placed in a step-down recovery unit in reclining chairs, where ambulation, voiding, and further oral intake are encouraged. This area should be in immediate proximity to the primary recovery room and also staffed with nurses who can attend to patient needs. Clear fruit juices or soda are the best fluids; crackers or cookies may be given after the patient demonstrates adequate oral intake. Patients who have received no sedation or who are very alert and oriented with no distress following a minor procedure may be placed directly in this location.

On admission to the recovery facility, every effort should be made to reunite children with their parents to allay their anxieties and enhance recovery. If at all possible, children should recover in an area apart from adults to ensure mutual privacy.

Pain

The two principal problems encountered in the recovery setting are postoperative pain and nausea with or without emesis. Pain management is often best addressed through attention to the surgical site in the operating room and use of local blocks. Studies[66,95,101,129] have demonstrated that caudal block with 0.125% bupivacaine and 1:200,000 epinephrine in a dose of 0.75 to 1.0 ml/kg provides excellent analgesia with minimal motor block in pediatric patients undergoing circumcision or orchiopexy repair. Similar findings have been documented for inguinal hernia repair in children[109] and adults.[110] In children, iliohypogastric nerve blocks with 0.5% bupivacaine and 1:200,000 epinephrine provided adequate comfort without need for further medication in 3 of 81 children; 74 of 75 control subjects without block needed pain medication. In the study of adults,[110] lidocaine aerosol in the surgical site resulted in improved ambulation and less pain, compared with those who received a placebo spray. Similar findings have been reported with laparoscopic tubal ligation[119] using 0.5% bupivacaine. Studies are currently underway to determine the efficacy of instillation of local anesthetics and narcotics into joints during arthroscopic procedures, and these approaches are used by numerous outpatient practitioners.

When the pain persists, the choice of medication should include agents that provide prompt relief but also allow for prompt discharge. Patients receiving IV analgesics should be observed for at least 30 minutes following administration to ensure that no side effects occur; this period is extended to 60 minutes for patients receiving IM agents. Although oral acetaminophen may be helpful, immediate treatment with narcotics usually provides the most rapid relief. Codeine, 1 mg/kg for children up to 12 years of age or increments of 30 mg IV for adults repeating every 15 to 20 minutes until relief is achieved, usually suffices, as does morphine (0.1 mg/kg) or fentanyl (1 μg/kg). In general, it is better to avoid IM injections, because these often must be repeated, to the discomfort of a patient already in some distress. When pain medication is administered to children, they should be held by the parent to minimize the distress caused by separation.

Patients who have onset of pain in the step-down recovery facility should receive whatever oral medication the surgeon has prescribed for use at home. This practice allows one to determine the adequacy of the prescription and to adjust doses or choose another agent if necessary.

Nausea and Emesis

Nausea and emesis prolong recovery time and costs. Metter et al.[70] found increases of almost 50% in both time and cost for patients who experienced these problems. Natof[76] reported an incidence of only 4% in his 1980 study of complications associated with ambulatory surgery. However, other reports place this number much higher, at 12% to 54% in adults and as high as 85% in children,[1] with nausea and emesis noted as one of the most frequent causes of unscheduled admissions.

Regional anesthesia and the newer general anesthetic agents significantly reduce the incidence of nausea and emesis. However, nausea and emesis persist as a problem in the recovery period. Despite the importance of this problem, determinations of etiology and appropriate perioperative and postoperative management remain somewhat confused and vague.

Although possible in all surgical situations, nausea and emesis are most significantly associated with ocular, intraabdominal, and ear procedures, as well as with hypotension, gastric air or fluid, and general anesthesia. As with pain management, the best treatment is prevention. Agents used to reduce gastric volume and acidity are beneficial in this regard. Droperidol (25 to 75 μg/kg) has been useful, but the potentially sedating effect and reports of dysphoria found with this drug have caused it to be used with greater caution. Kraynack and Bates[51] and others have found that preoperative ranitidine, 300 mg orally administered 2 to 3 hours before operation, reduces nausea and emesis after laparoscopy from 63% of control subjects to 4%. Suctioning the stomach of intubated patients is also a standard part of this regimen, to eliminate remaining air and fluid. The arrival of an alert, comfortable patient into the recovery room may prompt the nursing staff to engage in immediate preparation for discharge. However, these patients may become dizzy or hypotensive, with subsequent nausea and emesis. Patients should be kept in a resting, recumbent position in a bed or reclining chair for at least 20 minutes after arrival in the recovery facility.

When nausea and emesis occur, use of prochlorperazine (Compazine) suppositories may provide adequate relief. Until recently, droperidol (10 to 20 μg/kg) was the mainstay for treatment of portoperative neausea. However, the required dose often caused drowsiness, delay of discharge, and concerns about concomitant administration of narcotic. The antiserotonic drug, ondansetron, has rapidly replaced droperidol and other agents. Initially used for patients receiving chemotherapy, **the routine administration of ondansetron (4 mg IV) in the recovery room for patients undergoing laparoscopy reduced the incidence of nausea and emesis from in excess of 75% for selected procedures to less than 20%.**[8] The combination of ondanstetron and anesthetic techniques that decrease nausea should result in an even greater reduction in this problem. With proper management, hospital admission for control of nausea and vomiting should be rare. Patients who have nausea but are able to take sips of liquids and are well hydrated, as evidenced by stable blood pressure and voiding, may be discharged. These patients, including children, usually do better at home in a more comfortable environment. When discharged, patients should be advised to return if they remain unable to take increasing volumes of liquids.

DISCHARGE

The criteria for discharge of patients from the facility should include their ability to be transported home and maintained in reasonable comfort with good oral intake. Because of the consequences of operation and anesthesia, it is inappropriate to hold patients until they are "street ready," because this represents a status that will not be achieved until at least the following day. Rather, **patients should be ready for discharge when they have achieved a reasonable return to functional status, including no cardiorespiratory distress, unlabored respirations, orientation to time and place, demonstrated ability to tolerate oral fluids and solids, ability to ambulate except as limited by the operation, stable wound site, and reasonable control of nausea and pain.** This last consideration is difficult to gauge and, although many scoring systems are available to assist in this effort, they are generally cumbersome and not applicable to many ambulatory surgery patients. A commonsense approach would indicate that a patient who is able to rest and tolerate oral fluids without visible distress is in reasonably good condition for discharge (Box 85-2).

Discharge should be on a physician's order in accordance with Joint Commission on Accreditation of Hospitals (JCAH) protocols. **No patient should be discharged unless in the company of a responsible adult who will assist the patient to their destination, where an individual must be available to provide further aid, if needed. Written instructions should be provided and reviewed with the patient and the accompanying individual, including precautions specific to the procedure and the individual(s) to be called in the event of distress.** Arrangements for postoperative pain relief, if needed, should be made, with a prescription for appropriate pain medications and a means for this order to be filled. Once discharged, patients should be taken by wheelchair to their vehicle and assisted into the vehicle by ambulatory surgery staff.

BOX 85-2
DISCHARGE CRITERIA FOR AMBULATORY SURGERY PATIENTS

Stable vital signs
No airway difficulties
No respiratory distress
Return to usual state of alertness
Return to usual ambulatory status (except as limited by surgery)
Stable wound site
Ability to retain fluids
Responsible adult caretaker to accompany patient

Discharge should be based on achievement of these criteria and not on a routine protocol for recovery times. Williams and Epstein[127] reported that recovery times often depend on the time of day the operation is performed; patients undergoing afternoon procedures recovered more quickly than those having earlier surgery, controlling for type of anesthesia used and patient condition. These findings point to the ability of surgical units to shorten recovery stays without adverse effects.

Follow-Up

In addition to satisfying a concern for rendering complete patient care, regulatory mandates increasingly require that patients be telephoned the day after operation to determine if any problems have arisen. If they have, the anesthesia staff should be available to speak with the patient and, if necessary, to see the patient on a return visit to the facility.

Postoperative follow-up should be formal and noted on the medical record, with specific symptoms listed, including their severity and extent of resolution (Fig. 85-14). Failure to attend to this important function can negate all the careful preparation and scrupulous perioperative attention. This written follow-up should be an integral part of the outpatient's complete management.

CONCLUSION

The practice of outpatient surgery and anesthesia remains a rapidly expanding field, limited only by the imagination of its practitioners. As new procedures, such as laparoscopic cholecystectomies, become part of ambulatory surgery, anesthesiologists will increasingly be called on to provide highly sophisticated support and leadership in this area.

The Johns Hopkins Hospital
SAME DAY CARE CENTER
Outpatient Followup

Telephone: ( ) ____________

Date of procedure: ____________

Procedure: ____________

Date: ______ Time: ______ ___ No Answer ___ Message Left
Time: ______ ___ No Answer ___ Message Left
Date: ______ Time: ______ ___ No Answer ___ Message Left
Time: ______ ___ No Answer ___ Message Left
Person Contacted: ____________

Problem	Rating 0 = no problem 1 = mild 2 = moderate 3 = severe	Treatment	Decreased 1 Day POP	Resolved 1 Day POP
1. Appetite/nausea	______	______	Yes No	Yes No
2. Vomiting	______	______	Yes No	Yes No
3. Sore throat	______	______	Yes No	Yes No
4. Headache	______	______	Yes No	Yes No
5. Backache	______	______	Yes No	Yes No
6. Muscle ache	______	______	Yes No	Yes No
7. Pain at operative site	______	______	Yes No	Yes No
8. a. Temperature-touch	______	______	Yes No	Yes No
b. Temperature-reading	______	______	Yes No	Yes No
9. Bleeding	______	______	Yes No	Yes No
10. Drowsiness	______	______	Yes No	Yes No

11. Pediatric patients: alterations in comfort/pain ____________

12. Other problems ____________

Other things to look at: ____________

Physician followup required regarding problems found? Yes No

Signed ____________

Physician review by: ____________

Fig. 85-14. Follow-up form for the ambulatory surgery patient.

KEY POINTS

- Ambulatory surgery developed largely in response to financial concerns, with the greatest impetus noted as the Omnibus Reconciliation Act of 1980. Ambulatory operation has significant advantages for patients as well as hospitals and third-party payers.
- Ambulatory surgical systems are free-standing, office based, or hospital based and are characterized as single or multispecialty. Dedicated facilities, including a preoperative area, operating rooms, and recovery rooms, which should be located immediately adjacent to each other, characterize these units.
- The medical director of ambulatory surgery is responsible for coordinating activities related to operating rooms and general policy issues; the director of anesthesia usually serves in this role.
- Whenever possible, operations are scheduled several days

ahead of time to allow adequate preparation by the staff, patient, and family. Before any procedure is performed in the outpatient surgical unit, arrangements are made with the nearest hospital for admission and intervention as needed.

- Third-party payers select procedures to be performed on an outpatient basis based on the procedure's presumed complexity and not on the patient's underlying medical problems or issues associated with anesthesia.
- Laboratory testing is based on what is necessary rather than on preparation for every remote circumstance.
- Commonly, patients are evaluated by the primary care physician and recommended laboratory tests are preformed at that time. Although this is convenient for the patient, a visit to the ambulatory surgery unit before the procedure provides definite advantages.
- In balancing patient convenience with appropriate care, the anesthesiologist assumes responsibility for the patient, retaining a unique perspective of how anesthetic techniques and agents are selected and how they interact with the patient's medical conditions.
- Low-risk operation does not necessarily imply low-risk anesthesia, thus even minor procedures may be inappropriate for the outpatient unit in some patients, because of extremes of age or associated disease(s).
- Nonphysician staff must have immediate access to an anesthesiologist to evaluate specific problems.
- Laboratory tests beyond those needed by the surgical procedure should be performed based on their usefulness to the anesthesiologist.
- The only test required for patients with no medical problems is an ECG for individuals over 50 years of age. Blood type and screen is obtained when blood loss may exceed 500 ml, with blood products available for losses anticipated to exceed 1000 to 1500 ml.
- Special consideration should be given to infants and young children, placing them first on the operating room schedule.
- Patients for outpatient surgery must be medically stable, the procedure should be brief (less than 3 hours), and significant postoperative complications should be highly unlikely.
- The assignment of a patient to ASA class III or IV should not itself preclude outpatient surgery.
- Admission to the hospital before or after outpatient operation should be viewed as unusual.
- The limiting factor for ambulatory surgery in older individuals is determined by their medical condition and the extent to which they are debilitated.
- Young infants should be treated conservatively, based on their greater predisposition to develop apnea and bradycardia after general anesthesia. Preterm infants are at greater risk for apnea until 60 weeks of age.
- If outpatient surgery is done on children, the parent or primary care provider must be able to understand and follow the instructions for preoperative and postoperative care.
- Preoperative sedation is administered to allay the patient's fears and anxieties, to permit a smooth induction of and emergence from anesthesia, and to lead to a more pleasant and shorter recovery. Candidates of preoperative sedation include children under 5 years of age, adults who demonstrate anxiety despite discussions with the anesthesia staff, and patients whose conditions necessitate avoidance of anxiety and associated physiologic changes, such as tachycardia and increased blood pressure. Contraindications to preoperative sedation include impaired airways, significant respiratory distress and altered mental status, as evidenced by somnolence. Patients who may have compromised drug elimination, such as those with major renal or hepatic conditions, should not be sedated.
- Postoperative care of the outpatient is best completed in a two-stage system, with the first in a standard recovery room. In the second stage, patients who are reasonably alert and able to tolerate sips of fluids should be placed in a step-down recovery unit in reclining chairs, where ambulation, voiding, and further oral intake are encouraged.
- Patients are ready for discharge when they have achieved a reasonable return to functional status, including no cardiorespiratory distress, unlabored respiration, orientation to time and place, and ability to ambulate except as limited by the operation, stable wound site, and reasonable control of nausea and pain. No patient should be discharged unless in the company of a responsible adult who will assist the patient to their destination, where an individual should be available to provide continued aid, if needed.
- Follow-up should be formal and noted on the medical record, with specific symptoms listed, including their severity and extent of resolution.

KEY REFERENCES

Bowe EA, et al: Subarachnoid blockade versus general anesthesia for knee arthroscopy in outpatients, *Anesthesiology* 73:A45, 1990.

Kaplan EB, et al: The usefulness of preoperative laboratory screening, *JAMA* 253:3576, 1985.

Manchikanti L, Roush JR, Colliver JA: Effect of preanesthetic ranitidine and metoclopramide on gastric contents in morbidly obese patients, *Anesth Analg* 65:195, 1986.

Pandit SK, Kothary SP: Intravenous narcotics for premedication in outpatient anesthesia, *Acta Anaesthesiol Scand* 33:353, 1989.

Pandit SK, Kothary, Pandit UA, et al: Dose-response study of droperidol and metoclopramide as antiemetics for outpatient anesthesia, *Anesth Analg* 68:798, 1989.

Randel GI, et al: Epidural anesthesia is superior to spinal or general for outpatient knee athroscopy, *Anesthesiology* 71:A769, 1989.

Wyatt WJ, Reed DN, Apelgren KN: Pitfalls in the role of standardized preadmission laboratory screening for ambulatory surgery, *Am Surg* 55:343, 1989.

REFERENCES

1. Abramowitz MD, et al: The effect of droperidol in reducing vomiting in pediatric strabismus outpatient surgery, *Anesthesiology* 65:322, 1981.
2. Ashburn MA, et al: Clinical evaluation of oral transmucosal fentanyl citrate, OTFC, for use as a premedication in pediatric outpatient surgery, *Anesthesiology* 71:A1172, 1989.
3. Bailey PL, Streisand JB, East KA, et al: Differences in magnitude and duration of opioid-induced respiratory depression and analgesia with fentanyl and sufentanil, *Anesth Analg* 70:8, 1990.
4. Baram D, Smith C, Stinson S: Intraoperative topical etidocaine for reducing postoperative pain after laparoscopic tubal ligation, *J Reprod Med* 35:407, 1990.
5. Barclay JK, Hunter KM, McMillan W: Midazolam and diazepam compared as sedatives for outpatient surgery under local analgesia, *Oral Surg* 59:349, 1985.
6. Baughman VL, Becker GL, Ryan CM, et al: Effectiveness of triazolam, diazepam, and placebo as preanesthetic medications, *Anesthesiology* 71:196, 1989.
7. Baysinger CL, et al: Brachial plexus blockade and general anesthesia for carpal tunnel release in ambulatory patients (abstract), *Proc Fifth Annu SAMBA Conf,* Baltimore, 1990.
8. Bodner M, White P: Anitemetic effect of ondansetron after outpatient laparoscopy, *Anesth Analg* 73:250,1993.
9. Boldt HJ: The management of laparotomy patients and their modified after treatment, *NY Med* J 85:145, 1907.
10. Bowe EA, et al: Subarachnoid blockade versus general anesthesia for knee arthroscopy in outpatients, *Anesthesiology* 73:A45, 1990.
11. Broadman LM, Ceruzzi W, Patane PS, et al: Metoclopramide reduces the incidence of vomiting following strabismus surgery in children, *Anesthesiology* 69:A747, 1988.
12. Bynum LJ, Pierce AK: Pulmonary aspiration of gastric contents, *Am Rev Respir Dis* 114:1129, 1976.
13. Campbell IR, Scaife JM, Johnstone JMS: Psychological effects of day case surgery compared with inpatient surgery, *Arch Dis Child* 63:415, 1988.
14. Canet J, Ricos M, Vidal F: Early postoperative arterial oxygen desaturation, *Anesth Analg* 69:207, 1989.
15. Carbat PAT, van Crvel H: Lumbar puncture headache: controlled study on the preventive effect of 24 hours bed rest, *Lancet* 1:1133, 1981.
16. Carter JA, Dye AM, Cooper GM: Recovery after day-case anesthesia: The effect of different inhalational anaesthetic agents, *Anaesthesia* 40:545, 1985.
17. Casey WF, Rice LJ, Hannallah RS, et al: A comparison between bupivacaine instillation versus ilioinguinal/iliohypogastric nerve block for postoperative analgesia following inguinal heriorraphy in children, *Anesthesiology* 72:637, 1990.
18. Charpak Y, Blerg C, Chastang C, et al: Prospective assessment of a protocol for selective ordering of preoperative chest x-ray, *Can J Anaesth* 35:259, 1988.
19. Christensen S, Farrow-Gillespie A, Lerman J: Incidence of emesis and postanesthetic recovery after strabismus surgery in children: a comparison of droperidol and lidocaine, *Anesthesiology* 70:251, 1989.
20. Cope DK, et al: Impaired learning and recall after IV sedation: implications for outpatients, *Anesth Analg* 70:S69, 1990.
21. Cork RC, et al: Propofol infusion vs. thiopental/isoflurane for outpatient anesthesia, *Anesthesiology* 69:A563, 1988.
22. Cote CJ, Goldstein EA, Cote MA, et al: A single blind study of pulse oximetry in children, *Anesthesiology* 68:184, 1988.
23. Davis WJ: Outpatient brachial plexus anesthesia, *Anesthesiology* 73:A25, 1990.
24. DeSoto H, et al: Changes in oxygen saturation following general anesthesia in children with "URI" symptoms, *Anesthesiology* 66:A443, 1986.
25. DeSoto H, Patel RI, Soliman IE, et al: Changes in oxygen saturation following general anesthesia in children with upper respiratory infection signs and symptoms undergoing otolaryngologic procedures, *Anesthesiology* 68:276, 1988.
26. Dornette WNL: *Planning tomorrow's hospital today,* paper presented at ASA meeting, Washington, DC, October 1968.
27. Egbert W, Baird WLM: Preoperative anxiety—a study of the incidence and aetiology, *Br J Anaesth* 39:5003, 1967.
28. Empey DW, et al: Mechanisms of bronchial hyperactivity in normal subjects after upper respiratory tract infection, *Am Rev Respir Dis* 113:131, 1976.
29. Enright AC, Pace-Florida A: Recovery from anesthesia in outpatients: a comparison of narcotic and inhalation techniques, *Can Anaesth Soc J* 24:618, 1977.
30. Feld LH, Champeau MW, van Steennis CA, et al: Preanesthetic medication in children: a comparison of oral transmucosal fentanyl citrate versus placebo, *Anesthesiology* 71:374, 1989.
31. Feld LH, et al: Premedication in children: oral versus intramuscular midazolam, *Anesthesiology* 69:A745, 1988.
32. Flaaten H, Raeder J: Spinal anaesthesia for outpatient surgery, *Anaesthesia* 40:1101, 1985.
33. Ford F, Reed W: The surgicenter—an innovation in the delivery and cost of medical care, *Ariz Med* 26:801, 1969.
34. Forrest JB, Rehder K, Goldsmith CH, et al: Multicenter study of general anesthesia, *Anesthesiology* 72:252, 1990.
35. Ghoneim MM, Mewaldt SP: Benzodiazepines and human memory: a review, *Anesthesiology* 72:926, 1990.
36. Goldberg ME, Jan R, Gregg CE, et al: The heat and moisture exchanger does not preserve body temperature or reduce recovery time in outpatients undergoing surgery and anesthesia, *Anesthesiology* 68:122, 1988.
37. Greenwood BK, Bradshaw EG: Preoperative medication for day-case surgery: a comparison between oxazepam and temazepam, *Br J Anaesth* 55:933, 1983.
38. Gregory GA, Steward DJ: Life-threatening perioperative apnea in the ex-"premie," *Anesthesiology* 59:495, 1983.
39. Hackman T, Steward DJ: What is the value of preoperative hemoglobin determinations

in pediatric outpatients? *Anesthesiology* 71:A1168, 1989.
40. Haley S, Edelist G, Urbach G: Comparison of alfentanil, fantanyl, and enflurane as supplements to general anaesthesia for outpatient gynecologic surgery, *Can J Anaesth* 35:6, 1988.
41. Hannallah RS, Patel RI: Low-dose intramuscular ketamine for anesthesia preinduction in young children undergoing brief outpatient procedures, *Anesthesiology* 70:598, 1989.
42. Hargreaves J: Benzodiazepine premedication in minor day-case surgery: comparison of oral midazolam and temazepam with placebo, *Br J Anaesth* 61:611, 1988.
43. Herzfeld G: Hernia in infancy, *Am J Surg* 39:422, 1938.
44. Jensen J, Jackson B: Consumers prefer same-day surgery to inpatient care for minor procedures, *Mod Healthcare* 10:76, 1985.
45. Joyce TH: Prophylaxis for pulmonary acid aspiration, *Am J Med* 83:46, 1987.
46. Kaplan EB, et al: The usefulness of preoperative laboratory screening, *JAMA* 253: 3576, 1985.
47. Keithley J, Glandon GL, Llewellyn J, et al: The cost-effectiveness of same day surgery, *Nurs Econ* 7:90, 1989.
48. Kelley HD: Getting up early after grave surgical operations, *Surg Gynecol Obstet* 13:78, 1911.
49. Kitz DS, Slusarz-Ladden C, Lecky JH: Hospital resources used for inpatient and ambulatory surgery, *Anesthesiology* 69: 383, 1988.
50. Knight PR, et al: Alterations in influenza virus pulmonary pathology induced by diethyl ether, halothane, enflurane and pentobarbital anesthesia in mice, *Anesthesiology* 58:209, 1983.
51. Kraynack BJ, Bates MF: Antiemetic action of ranitidine in outpatient laparoscopy under propofol-isoflurane anesthesia, *Anesthesiology* 73:A13, 1990.
52. Kurth CD, Spitzer AR, Broennle AM, et al: Postoperative apnea in preterm infants, *Anesthesiology* 66:483, 1987.
53. Laffaye HA: The impact of an ambulatory surgical service in a community hospital, *Arch Surg* 124:601, 1989.
54. Lakhani S, Leach RD, Jarrett PEM: Effect of a surgical day unit on waiting lists, *J R Soc Med* 80:628, 1987.
55. Lebenbom-Mansour MH, Pandit SJ, Kothary SP, et al: Desflurane versus propofol anesthesia: a comparative analysis in outpatients, *Anesth Analg* 76:936, 1993
56. Leigh JM, Walker J, Janaganathan P: Effect of preoperative anaesthetic visit on anxiety, *Br Med J* 2:987, 1977.
57. Lerman J, Christensen SK, Farrow-Gillespie AC: Effects of metoclopramide and ranitidine on gastric fluid pH and volume in children, *Anesthesiology* 69(3A): A748,
58. Liu LMP, et al: Life-threatening apnea in infants recovering from anesthesia, *Anesthesiology* 59:506, 1983.
59. Manawadu BR, Mostow SR, LaForce FM: Pulmonary antibacterial defense mechanisms are depressed by halothane, *Anesth Analg* 58:505, 1979.
60. Manchikanti L, Roush JR: Effect of glycopyrrolate and cimetidine on gastric fluid pH and volume in outpatients, *Anesth Analg* 63:40, 1984.
61. Manchikanti L, Roush JR, Colliver JA: Effect of preanesthetic ranitidine and metoclopramide on gastric contents in morbidly obese patients, *Anesth Analg* 65:195, 1986.
62. Manchikanti L, et al: Assessment of effect of various modes of premedication on acid aspiration risk factors in outpatient surgery, *Anesth Analg* 66:81, 1987.
63. Manchikanti L, et al: Bicitra and metoclopramide in outpatient anesthesia for prophylaxis against aspiration pneumonitis, *Anesthesiology* 63:378, 1987.
64. Manchikanti L, et al: Evaluation of ranitidine as an oral antacid in outpatient anesthesia, *South Med J* 78:818, 1985.
65. Marais ML, et al: Reduced demands on recovery room resources with propofol (Diprivan) compared with thiopental-isoflurane, *Anesthesiol Rev* 16:29, 1989.
66. Mazoit JX, Denson DD, Samii K: Pharmacokinetics of bupivacaine following caudal anesthesia in infants, *Anesthesiology* 68:387, 1988.
67. McGill WA, Coveler LA, Epstein BS: Subacute upper respiratory infection in small children, *Anesth Analg* 58:331, 1979.
68. Mendelson CL: The aspiration of stomach contents into the lungs during obstetic anesthesia, *Am J Obstet Gynecol* 191, 1946.
69. Mestad PH, Glenski JA, Binda RE: When is outpatient surgery safe in preterm infants? *Anesthesiology* 69:A744, 1988.
70. Metter SE, et al: Nausea and vomiting after outpatient laparoscopy: incidence, impact on recovery room stay and cost, *Anesth Analg* 66:S116, 1987.
71. Millar JM, Jewkes CF: Recovery and morbidity after daycase anaesthesia, *Anaesthesia* 43:738, 1988.
72. Mingus ML, et al: Droperidol dose-response in out-patients following alfentanil-nitrous oxide anaesthesia (abstract), *Proc Fifth Annu SAMBA Conf,* Baltimore, 1990.
73. Mulroy MF: Is spinal anesthesia appropriate for outpatient? *SAMBA Newslett* 4:1, 1989.
74. Murray RS, Raemer DB, Morris RW: Supplemental oxygen after ambulatory surgical procedures, *Anesth Analg* 67:697, 1988.
75. Narchi P, et al: Intraperitoneal local anesthetics and scapular pain following daycase laparoscopy, *Anesthesiology* 73:A5, 1990.
76. Natof HE: Complications associated with ambulatory surgery, *JAMA* 244:1116, 1980.
77. Nicoll JH: The surgery of infancy, *Br Med J* 2:753, 1909.
78. O'Boyle CA, Harris D, Barry H, et al: Comparison of midazolam by mouth and diazepam IV in outpatient oral surgery, *Br J Anaesth* 59:746, 1987.
79. O'Connor ME, Drasner K: Preoperative laboratory testing of children undergoing elective surgery, *Anesth Analg* 70:176, 1990.
80. Olsson GL: Bronchospasm during anaesthesia: a computer-aided incidence study of 136,929 patients, *Acta Anaesthesiol Scand* 31:244, 1987.
81. Ong BY, Palahniuk RJ, Cumming M: Gastric volume and pH in out-patients, *Can Anaesth Soc J* 25:36, 1978.
82. Pandit SK, Kothary SP: Intravenous narcotics for premedication in outpatient anaesthesia, *Acta Anaesthesiol Scand* 33:353, 1989.
83. Pandit SK, Kothary SP: Should we premedicate ambulatory surgical patients? *Anesthesiology* 65:A352, 1986.
84. Pandit SK, Kothary SP, Pandit UA, et al: Dose-response study of droperidol and metoclopramide as antiemetics for outpatient anesthesia, *Anesth Analg* 68:798, 1989.
85. Pandit SK, et al: Recovery after outpatient anesthesia: propofol versus enflurane, *Anesthesiology* 69:A565, 1988.
85a. Pandit UA, et al: Perioperative respiratory complications in children with upper respiratory infections, *Anesthesiology* 71: A1011, 1989.
86. Parnas SM, et al: A prospective evaluation of epidural versus general anesthesia for outpatient arthroscopy (abstract), *Proc Fifth Annu SAMBA Conf,* Baltimore, 1990.
87. Parnas SM, et al: Single dose esmolol for prevention of hemodynamic changes of intubation in an ambulatory surgery unit, *Anesthesiology* 71:A12, 1989.
88. Patel RI, Kasprzak S, Hannallah RS: Preoperative telephone screening in pediatric ambulatory surgery, *Am Acad Pediatr Sci Sess* 6, 1986.
89. Perz RR, Johnson DL, Shinozaki T: Spinal anesthesia for outpatient surgery, *Anesth Analg* 67:S168, 1988.
90. Philip BK: Supplemental medication for ambulatory procedures under regional anesthesia, *Anesth Analg* 64:1117, 1985.
91. Raeder JC, Breivik H: Premedication with midazolam in out-patient general anaesthesia: a comparison of morphine, scopolamine and placebo, *Acta Anaesthesiol Scand* 31:509, 1987.
92. Raeder JC, Misvaer G: Comparison of propofol induction with thiopentone or methohexitone in short outpatient general anaesthesia, *Acta Anaesthesiol Scand* 23: 607, 1988.
93. Randel GI, et al: Epidural anesthesia is superior to spinal or general for outpatient knee arthroscopy, *Anesthesiology* 71:A769, 1989.
94. Raybould D, Bradshaw EG: Premedication for day case surgery, *Anaesthesia* 42:591, 1987.
95. Rice LJ, Pudimat MA, Hannallah RS: Timing of caudal block placement does not affect duration of postoperative analgesia in pediatric ambulatory surgical patients, *Anesthesiology* 69:A771, 1988.
96. Rice LJ, et al: Intraoperative and postoperative analgesia in children undergoing inguinal herniorrhaphy: a comparison of caudal bupivacaine 0.125% and 0.25%, *Anesthesiology* 73:A3, 1990.
97. Ries E: Some radical changes in the after-treatment of celiotomy cases, *JAMA* 33:454, 1899.
98. Roetman KJ, et al: Evaluation of awakening and recovery characteristics of fentanyl versus halothane anesthesia for short outpatient procedures in term infants, *Anesthesiology* 71:A1012, 1989.

99. Roos NO: What is the potential for moving adult surgery to the ambulatory setting? *CMAJ* 138:809, 1988.
100. Rosenblatt MA, Bradford C, Miller R, Zahl K: A preoperative interview by an anesthesiologist does not lower preoperative anxiety in outpatients, *Anesthesiology* 71: A926, 1989.
101. Saint-Raymond S, O'Donovan F, Ecoffey C: Criteria for safe ambulation following caudal block in children, *Anesthesiology* 69:A769, 1988.
102. Sampson IH, et al: Comparison of propofol and thiamylal for induction and maintenance of anaesthesia for outpatient surgery, *Br J Anaesth* 61:707, 1988.
103. Sanderson JH, Blades JF: Multicentre study of propofol in day case surgery, *Anaesthesia* 43:70, 1988.
104. Sandhar BK, et al: The effect of oral liquids and ranitidine on gastric fluid volume and pH in children undergoing outpatient surgery, *Anesthesiology* 71:327, 1989.
105. Scarr MS, et al: Volume and acidity of residual gastric fluid after oral fluid ingestion before elective ambulatory surgery, *CMAJ* 141:1151, 1989.
106. Schreiner MS, Triebwasser A, Keon TP: Ingestion of liquids compared with preoperative fasting in pediatric outpatients, *Anesthesiology* 72:593, 1990.
107. Sebel PS, Lowdon JD: Propofol: a new intravenous induction agent, *Anesthesiology* 71:260, 1989.
108. Shafer A, et al: Outpatient premedication: use of midazolam and opioid analgesics, *Anesthesiology* 71:495, 1989.
109. Shandling R, et al: Regional analgesia for postoperative pain in pediatric outpatient surgery, *Pediatr Surg* 15:477, 1980.
110. Sinclair R, et al: Topical anesthesia with lidocaine aerosol in the control of postoperative pain, *Anesthesiology* 68:895, 1980.
111. Stanley TH, et al: Oral transmucosal fentanyl citrate (lollipop) premedication in human volunteers, *Anesth Analg* 69:21, 1989.
112. Steward DJ: Preterm infants are more prone to complications following minor surgery than are term infants, *Anesthesiology* 56:304, 1982.
113. Sung YF, Reiss N, Tillette T: The differential cost of anesthesia and recovery with propofol-nitrous oxide anesthesia versus thiopental-nitrous oxide (abstract), *Proc Fifth Annu SAMBA Conf,* Baltimore, 1990.
114. Sung YF, et al: Comparison of propofol and thiopental anesthesia in outpatient surgery: Speed of recovery, *Anesthesiology* 69: A562, 1988.
115. Tait AR, Knight PR: The effects of general anesthesia on upper respiratory tract infection in children, *Anesthesiology* 67:930, 1987.
116. Tait AR, McLear MA, Knight PR: Anesthesia and the common cold: why not sleep on it? *Anesthesiology* 65:A492, 1984.
117. Tait AR, et al: Anesthesia and upper viral infections, *Anesthesiology* 67:A450, 1987.
118. Teabeault JR: Aspiration of gastric contents, *Am J Pathol* 28:51, 1952.
119. Thompson RE, Wechtler BV, Alexander CD: Infiltration of the mesosalpinx for pain relief after laparoscopic tubal sterilization with Yoon rings, *J Reprod Med* 32:537, 1987.
120. Thornberry EA, Thomas TA: Posture and post-spinal headache, *Br J Anaesth* 60:195, 1988.
121. Tverskoy M, et al: Postoperative pain after inguinal herniorrhaphy with different types of anesthesia, *Anesth Analg* 70:29, 1990.
122. Twersky RS, Frank D, Lebovits AH: Preop anesthesia evaluation of the ambulatory surgery patient: is it really worth it (abstract)? Part two, *Proc Fifth Annu SAMBA Conf,* Baltimore, 1990.
123. Twersky RS, Lewis M, Lebovits AH: Early evaluation of patients in an ambulatory surgical setting: does it really help? *Anesthesiology* 71:A1186, 1989.
124. Vijayakumar HR, Metriyakool K, Jewell MR: Effects of 100% oxygen and a mixture of oxygen and air on oxygen saturation in the immediate postoperative period in children, *Anesth Analg* 66:181, 1987.
125. Waters RM: The down-town anesthesia clinic, *Am J Surg* 33:7, 1919.
126. Wechtler BV: Ambulatory surgery: patient selection criteria for 1987, *AORN* 45:30, 1987.
127. Williams JJ, Epstein RH: Dependence of recovery time on operating room start time in outpatient surgery, *Anesthesiology* 71: A931, 1989.
128. Wilton NC, et al: Preanesthetic sedation of preschool children using intranasal midazolam, *Anesthesiology* 69:972, 1988.
129. Wolf AR, et al: Bupivacaine for caudal analgesia in infants and children, *Anesthesiology* 69:102, 1988.
130. Wyatt WJ, Reed DN, Apelgren KN: Pitfalls in the role of standardized preadmission laboratory screening for ambulatory surgery, *Am Surg* 55:343, 1989.
131. Zibrak JD, O'Donnell CR, Marton K: Indications for pulmonary function testing, *Ann Intern Med* 112:763, 1990.
132. Zilva JF: Is unselective biochemical urine testing cost effective? *Br Med J* 291:323, 1985.

CHAPTER 86

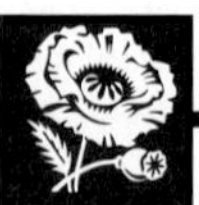

Monitored Anesthesia Care

THEODORE E. M. HANLEY
REBECCA S. TWERSKY

DEFINITION OF MONITORED ANESTHESIA CARE

In 1986, the House of Delegates of the American Society of Anesthesiologists (ASA) defined "Monitored Anesthesia Care" (MAC) as those "instances in which an anesthesiologist has been called upon to provide specific anesthesia services to a particular patient undergoing a planned procedure, in connection with which a patient receives local anesthesia or, in some instances, no anesthesia at all. In such a case, the anesthesiologist is providing specific services to the patient and is in control of his or her nonsurgical or nonobstetrical medical care, including the responsibility of monitoring his or her vital signs, and is available to administer anesthetics or provide other medical care as appropriate."[4] The term MAC was intended to replace the inaccurate term of "local standby." The statement by the ASA also notes that the provision of MAC shall be requested by the surgeon, the request shall be made known to the patient, and the request will be preceded by an appropriate preoperative evaluation and prescription of medical care.[4] The policy further mandates that the patient be personally attended by the anesthesiologist or another qualified anesthesia provider under the medical direction of an anesthesiologist and that ". . . all institutional regulations pertaining to anesthesia shall be observed, and all the usual services performed by the anesthesiologist shall be furnished . . ."[4] including, as a minimum, noninvasive monitoring, O_2 therapy, and pharmacologic interventions.

This description of MAC is perhaps cumbersome for everyday use, but it contains all the essential elements of MAC. **The primary components of MAC are generally**

those contained in provision of any other type of anesthetic care. This includes preoperative evaluation, selection of monitors, continuous presence of an anesthesia provider, and pharmacologic interventions to achieve suitable operating conditions for the surgeon or diagnostician while maintaining safety and comfort for the patient.

GUIDELINES FOR SEDATION AND ANALGESIA (CONSCIOUS SEDATION)

The term "conscious sedation" has been used to describe the provision of MAC outside the operating room by anesthesiologists or frequently by nonanesthesiologists to patients undergoing diagnostic or therapeutic procedures. To this end, an ASA Task Force developed guidelines for Sedation and Analgesia by Non-Anesthesiologists that were approved at the ASA House of Delegates in October 1995.[5] Sedation and analgesia, as opposed to the imprecise term "conscious sedation," describes a state which allows patients to tolerate unpleasant procedures while maintaining adequate cardiorespiratory function with minimally reduced level of consciousness. **Patients should maintain ability to respond purposefully to verbal command and or tactile stimulation.** Patients whose only response is reflex withdrawal from painful stimulus are sedated to a greater degree than encompassed by sedation and analgesia. **For purposes of consistency, the term "conscious sedation" will be substituted with "sedation and analgesia."**

ASA practice guidelines for sedation and analgesia contain all the essential components of MAC. These includes preprocedure evaluation and patient preparation, selection of monitors, continuous presence of an anesthesiologist or appropriately credentialled nonphysician anesthesia provider and pharmacologic interventions to achieve suitable therapeutic, diagnostic or operating conditions while also maintaining patient safety and comfort.

The role of the anesthesia department is pivotal in developing policies and promoting education related to sedation and analgesia. These policies contain the primary components of MAC with sedation and analgesia and guide other credentialed providers in performing procedures with sedation/analgesia in nonoperating room settings. These policies should also address selection of appropriate drugs, identify components of intra- and postprocedure monitoring and recovery of patients, and delineate physician and nonphysician responsibilities. Provisions for emergency equipment and training of personnel should also be included in the institution's policies.

ASA guidelines for sedation and analgesia are applicable to procedures performed in a variety of settings (e.g., hospitals, free-standing clinics, physicians' offices) by practitioners who are not specialists in anesthesiology. The guidelines specifically exclude the following: (1) Patients not undergoing a diagnostic or therapeutic procedure (e.g., postoperative analgesia, sedation for treatment of insomnia); (2) otherwise healthy patients receiving peripheral nerve blocks, local or topical anesthesia, and/or no more than 50% N_2O with O_2, with no other sedative or analgesia agents administered by other routes; (3) situations where it is anticipated that the required sedation will eradicate the purposeful response to verbal commands or tactile stimulation (distinct from reflex withdrawal from a painful stimulus); (4) perioperative management of patients undergoing general anesthesia or major conduction anesthesia (spinal or epidural blockade).

As the numbers and complexity of procedures outside of the operating room continue to expand, anesthesiologists will not only be called upon to design policy, but they themselves will have to leave the comfort and perceived safety of the operating room and adapt to delivering MAC outside the operating room. It is predicted that 40% to 50% of all ambulatory surgery procedures will be shifted to nonoperating room practice in the twenty-first century.[35] Therefore, the guidelines for sedation and analgesia for nonanesthesiologists are just as applicable for practicing anesthesiologists as more operating room procedures move to areas outside the operating room. Because many of those cases would be performed under MAC, familiarity with current standards of care will facilitate expansion into new environments.

Scope of Institutional Policies

The scope of the policy should delineate (four) key elements:

(1) Types of procedures—In the changing economic environment with unpredictable reimbursement patterns, the policy should allow for flexible expansion of procedures. These may include procedures such as: orthopedic (reduction of fractures); urologic or gynecologic procedure; upper and lower gastrointestinal (GI) endoscopy; arteriography; diagnostic and electroconvulsive therapy; interventional radiologic procedures; pulmonary artery (PA) catheterization; cardiac catheterization; bronchoscopy; and oral surgical procedures. (Table 86-1).

(2) Location—Appropriate locations for sedation and analgesia should be determined and clearly defined in the scope of the policy. Each location should be outfitted with appropriate monitoring and resuscitative equipment which should be specified in the policy. Procedures requiring sedation and analgesia can be performed in such locations as the radiology suite, emergency room, critical care areas, GI suites, and various other units.

(3) Patient Characteristics—Because not every patient is an acceptable candidate for sedation and analgesia, a preprocedure interview is essential. "At-risk" patients for sedation/analgesia are listed in Box 86-1. If a decision is made to proceed, these patients require strict adherence to sedation and analgesia guidelines as outlined in the hospital policy.

(4) Sedating Conditions—The policy should clearly state under which conditions adherence is required. It may be

Table 86-1 Clinical areas administering sedation or analgesia

Location	Procedure
Critical care units	Endoscopy, intubation, cardioversion pacemaker insertion, PEG, bronchoscopy, Swan-Ganz insertion
Pediatric unit	Bronchoscopy, line insertion, lumbar puncture, intubation, bone marrow biopsies, aspiration
Cardiac lab	Cardiac catheterization, pacemaker insertion, cardioversion
Pulmonary lab	Bronchoscopy
Neurology lab	EEG, EMG
Gastroenteroloy suite	EGD, PEG, ERCP, colonoscopy, esophageal dilation
Radiology suite	Interventional procedures, embolization, angiography, MRI, CT
Psychiatric unit	ECT

EEG — electroencephalogram; EMG — electromyograph; EGD — esophagogastroduodenoscopy; PEG — purcutaneous endoscopic gastrostomy; ERCP — endoscopic retrograde cholangiopancreatography; MRI — magnetic resonance imaging; CT — computed tomography; ECT — electroconvulsive therapy.

BOX 86-1
"AT RISK" PATIENTS FOR SEDATION OR ANALGESIA

- The American Society of Anesthesiologists physical status risk classification of 3 or greater
- Critical car patients
- Extremes of age (< 1 or > 70 years of age)
- Patients with chronic respiratory diseases, chronic obstructive pulmonary disease, emphysema
- History of sleep apnea
- Mentally and neurologically handicapped patients
- Patients at risk for aspiration (i.e., hiatal hernia with regurgitation, diabetes with gastroparesis)
- Altered mental status

erroneously assumed that these guidelines may be applicable only for parenterally administered medication. Sedation/analgesia when given to "at-risk" patients, regardless of route, should follow the guidelines and be specified in policy. Application of these guidelines should also be considered when there is altered level of consciousness secondary to already administered oral or intramuscular (IM) medications.

Patient Evaluation and Preparation

Once the appropriate candidates have been selected, a thorough preanesthesia evaluation should be completed. Pre-

BOX 86-2
AIRWAY ASSESSMENT FOR SEDATION AND ANALGESIA—HISTORY

- Previous problems with anesthesia or sedation
- Stridor, snoring, or sleep apnea
- Dysmorphic facial features (e.g., Pierre-Robin syndrome, trisomy 21)
- Advanced rheumatoid arthritis

BOX 86-3
AIRWAY ASSESSMENT—PHYSICAL EXAMINATION

- Habitus — significant obesity (especially involving the neck and facial structures)
- Head and neck — short neck, limited neck extension, decreased hyoid-mental distance (< 3 cm in an adult), neck mass, cervical spine disease or trauma, tracheal deviation
- Mouth — small opening (< 3 cm in an adult); edentulous; protruding incisors; loose or capped teeth, high, arched palate; macroglossia; tonsillar hypertrophy; nonvisible uvula
- Jaw — micrognathia, retrognathia, trismus, significant malocclusion

procedure counseling about MAC appears to improve patient satisfaction and reduces risk, although data are lacking that link outcome with patient preparation. Patients should also be informed about the risks, benefit, and alternatives of the sedation technique as well as its limitations. Patients should be willing to accept the limitations of sedation/analgesia, and not be mislead into expecting a general anesthetic.

All patients should have documentation of pertinent medical history and physical examination prior to the procedure, equivalent to that performed for a general anesthetic. Clinicians administering MAC/sedation and analgesia should be familiar with the relevant aspects of the patient's medical history including: (1) Abnormalities of major organ systems; (2) Previous adverse experience with MAC as well as regional and general anesthesia; (3) Current medications and drug allergies; (4) Time and nature of last oral intake; (5) History of tobacco, alcohol, and antidepressant medications or substance use or abuse.

Each patient should also undergo a focused physical examination including auscultation of the heart and lungs and evaluation of the airway (see Box 86-2 and Box 86-3). Any preprocedure laboratory examination should be guided by the patient's underlying condition and the resulting effect on the conduct of MAC. The ASA supports the concept that no routine laboratory or diagnostic screening test is necessary for preanesthetic screening of patients, unless guided by patient history and physical examination.

Preprocedure laboratory testing

An extensive body of literature has accumulated regarding efficacy of current preoperative evaluation practices in the healthy ambulatory surgery population.[45,58,66] Many authors have found that much routine preoperative laboratory testing in asymptomatic patients did not fulfill its avowed purpose of providing "screening" for undiagnosed disease that might be of consequence to the patient in the perioperative period.[66,77] Just a review of the patient's medical record can predict most preoperative laboratory findings. In the Kaplan et al.[37] study of preoperative laboratory tests, roughly 60% of such tests obtained were not indicated by review of available patient data. Indeed, only four abnormal laboratory tests of potential surgical importance were found, and none of them were associated with any additional perioperative morbidity. Blery et al.[12] found in a prospective trial that ordering only indicated tests was clinically acceptable and effective. They concluded that only 0.2% of tests not ordered would have been useful, and that no additional morbidity or mortality could be ascribed to not ordering additional tests. Other schema that are useful involve analysis of standardized questionnaire responses to determine which tests to order preoperatively. Routine preoperative chest radiographs, electrocardiograms (ECGs), and internal medicine consultations are also suspect.[16,30,55,74] Macpherson et al.[47] found that reference to previous laboratory tests could also safely decrease need for preoperative laboratory testing. In their analysis of 7549 tests ordered before elective surgery, 47% duplicated tests performed in the preceding year. Only 0.4% of the tests that were previously normal were abnormal on preoperative testing, and almost all these abnormalities were predicted from patient history and physical examination. Only 17% of the previously abnormal values were still out of the normal range at time of scheduled surgery. They concluded that previously normal tests should not be repeated unless clinically indicated. Ordering more tests as medicolegal protection should not be condoned and indeed is not protective. The history and physical examination performed by the anesthesiologist and/or surgeon are the most sensitive tools for preoperative evaluation of healthy patients. Findings of the history and physical examination can then be used to direct ordering of appropriate tests (Fig. 86-1).

Preprocedure fasting

Instructions regarding no oral intake (NPO) status and preprocedure medications should be provided, preferably as written instructions during the preprocedure visit. If a telephone method is used, equivalent level of preparation should be met. Knowledge of current medications including possible drug interactions with sedatives should be sought. Because sedatives and analgesics tend to impair airway reflexes in a dose-dependent manner, the patient should un-

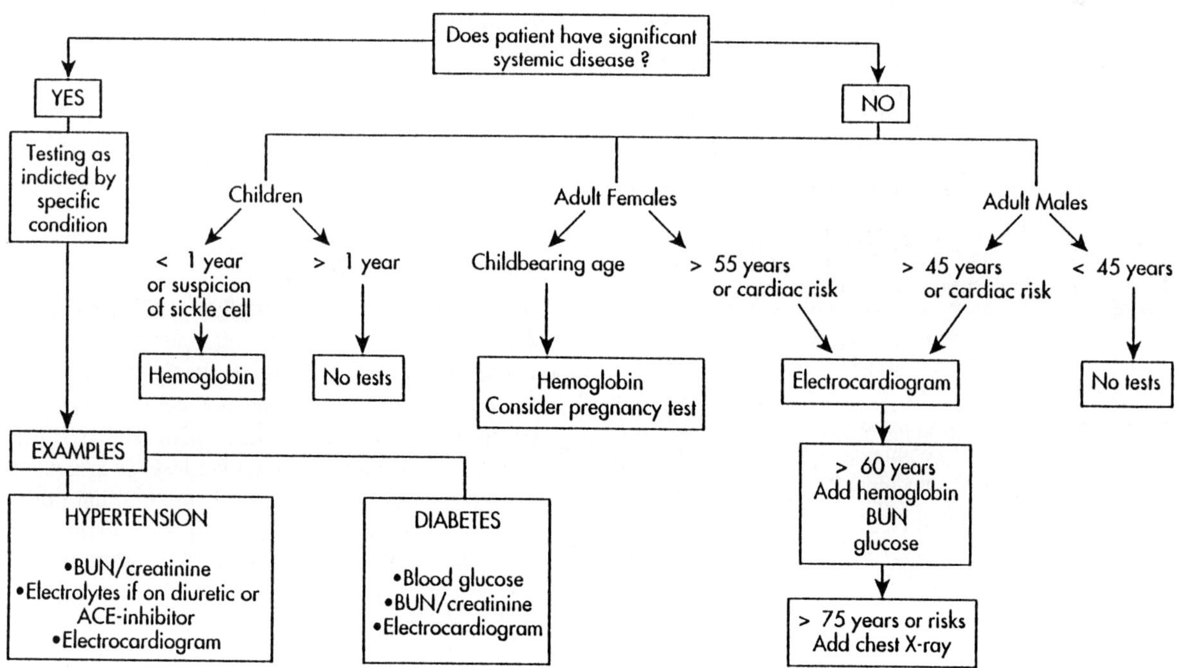

Fig. 86-1. Preoperative Testing Algorithm. From Everett LL, Kallar SK: Presurgical Evaluation and Laboratory Testing. In Twersky RS, editor: *The ambulatory anesthesia handbook,* St. Louis, 1995, Mosby–Year Book.

derstand the importance of adherance to fasting protocols that are prescribed (Table 86-2).

PATIENT SELECTION

A primary concern with MAC, as with any other type of anesthesia care, is fitness of the cardiovascular and pulmonary systems. The category of patients that may require more in-depth preoperative evaluation and periprocedure monitoring are those patients who are ASA 3 and greater. Some of these patients may have a combination of cardiovascular, respiratory and other systemic diseases that can alter responses to commonly used sedative analgesic medications. In patients present greater complexity with respect to preoperative evaluation. Although some of their known medical problems are presumably addressed, the hospitalized patient's health is generally less robust than the outpatient's. Indeed, patients receiving MAC are frequently the oldest and sickest patients. Perhaps this explains the data, reported in a review of 100,000 anesthetics, that MAC was associated with the highest mortality rate of 209 per 100,000 deaths.[17]

Considerations

Age

Although cardiovascular disease is a major cause of death in the elderly, it is difficult to state categorically that age alone, and not dysfunction in other organ systems, is the primary process. Age appears less of a predictor than presence of coexisting disease.[34,52]

ASA physical status

The ability of ASA physical status rating to predict cardiovascular- or anesthetic-specific mortality is fairly weak, but its predictive value in terms of overall outcome is remarkably good given its subjective nature.[18] Whereas use of the ASA physical status is not particularly productive to predict specific complications or forecast short-term outcomes, a good correlation of greater morbidity and mortality with higher ASA scores is a consistent finding in general. Higher ASA scores may encourage greater intensity of monitoring and other anesthesia-related care aspects.

Table 86-2 Fasting protocol for sedation and analgesia for elective procedures (in patients not at risk for aspiration)

	Solids and nonclear liquids*	Clear liquids
Adults	6–8 hours or nothing after midnight**	2–3 hours
Children > 36 months old	6–8 hours	2–3 hours
Children 6–36 months old	6 hours	2–3 hours
Children < 6 months old	4–6 hours	2 hours

*This includes milk, formula, and breast milk (high fat content may delay gastric emptying).
** There are no data to establish whether a 6- to 8-hour fast is equivalent to an overnight fast prior to sedation/analgesia.

Cardiovascular risk

Mangano et al.[49,50] reviewed preoperative assessment of cardiovascular risk in detail. Although the problem of perioperative myocardial ischemia and myocardial infarction (MI) is pervasive, answers to questions of whom and how to evaluate and treat remain elusive. The problem is amplified by the fact that roughly 50% of detected ischemic events or infarctions were not associated with chest pain.[40] It is not clear whether perioperative ischemic patterns are affected adversely, favorably, or not at all by anesthesia and surgery, but common sense dictates that any such disturbance of the status quo might be problematic. It is also unclear which diagnostic studies should be performed and which specific interventions should be undertaken to reduce the risk of cardiac events in the perioperative period. The history and physical examination can identify some patients at risk.

Previous myocardial infarction

A history of previous MI is one of the stronger and more consistently observed indicators of increased perioperative risk, especially if the MI is recent.[64] Many studies support the principle that myocardial reinfarction risk increases with temporal proximity to the original cardiac event. A previous MI does represent a marker for serious cardiac disease and dictates need for extra care during the perianesthetic period. Elective surgery should still be postponed, preferably for 6 months if possible, after an MI. Because of this widespread practice, data are lacking to determine whether patients that receive MAC within 6 months of an MI are also at risk of reinfarction. Only under nonelective circumstances should MAC be considered.

Congestive heart failure

Evidence of congestive heart failure (CHF), especially in association with a previous MI is an ominous outcome predictor; patients with CHF have markedly increased mortality rates compared with patients not demonstrating CHF.[10,57] CHF likewise appears associated with increased perioperative risk in patients undergoing surgery using general or regional anesthesia. Goldman et al.[32] found that preoperative CHF was a consistent predictor of postoperative CHF. New development of CHF was seen in almost 60% of the postoperative CHF group, in concert with a 40% mortality rate from cardiac causes.

Other cardiac risk factors

Numerous investigations have addressed other physiologic conditions believed to be associated with increased cardiac risk with controversial results. Angina, presence of peripheral vascular disease, hypertension, preexisting dysrhythmia, diabetes, type of surgery, and type of anesthetic have all been evaluated in this context. Although all of these elements have been found to be predictors of perioperative morbidity and mortality in at least one study, none have been as consistent as the presence of previous MI and CHF.

Pulmonary risk

Although cardiac risks of surgery are present even during procedures employing MAC that involve minimal hemodynamic disturbance and physiologic trespass, pulmonary risks vary depending on site and severity of the surgical procedure. Thoracic and upper-abdominal procedures are associated with as much as a 20% incidence of postoperative pulmonary complications, but peripheral procedures usually have much lower pulmonary complication rates.[3] Patients with suspected or known pulmonary impairment can be evaluated effectively with bedside spirometry and arterial blood gases.[76] Spirometric parameters associated with increased risk of pulmonary complications have been studied for abdominal procedures; studies using CO_2 retention as a predictor for postoperative pulmonary complications are less conclusive. No definite guidelines exist for procedures performed using MAC, but general principles of preoperative preparation of any patient who has pulmonary disease are appropriate here as well.

Preoperative treatment of pulmonary infections should be vigorously pursued to reduce hypoxemia and coughing, which could be especially dangerous in the patient undergoing an ophthalmologic or awake intracranial procedure using MAC.

Bronchodilator therapy should be optimized in patients with reactive airways undergoing any surgical procedure. Patients with chronic obstructive pulmonary disease (COPD) may also benefit from bronchodilator therapy, particularly from $beta_2$-agonists or ipratropium, which are just as effective and much less toxic than theophylline.[24]

Pulmonary manifestations of CHF should be addressed with appropriate diuretic/vasodilator therapy. The serious perioperative implications of CHF in the patient undergoing any type of procedure were discussed previously. For patients undergoing MAC, reduction in dyspnea and work of breathing associated with achievement of adequate cardiac function may permit an otherwise marginal patient to have a procedure performed without the use of general anesthesia and invasive monitors.

The positive effect of preoperative smoking cessation may be limited by the time interval. Cessation the night before surgery may result in an excess postoperative bronchorrhea; however, it may also increase O_2-carrying capacity. Six weeks or more of cessation in the heavy smoker may be necessary to minimize perioperative problems.

Special Considerations

The pregnant patient

In addition to the possible airway management difficulties and a greater risk for aspiration because of the normal physiological changes of pregnancy, the pregnant patient's pulmonary reserve is also diminished, increasing the potential for rapid desaturation following administration of sedatives, narcotics, and potent respiratory depressants. Drugs should be administered during MAC with due consideration regarding transmission to the fetus, their effects on maternal protective reflexes, and the effects on utero-placental perfusion; these drugs should be titrated to produce little or no maternal respiratory depression.

The pediatric patient

Drugs should have minimal effects on the cardiovascular system, especially in infants, whose cardiac output is dependent on heart rate to a greater extent than in adults and older children. Neonates have altered metabolism and/or excretion, with a larger volume of distribution, both resulting in different pharmacokinetic profiles than in adults. The respiratory depressant effects may be more profound in younger children, whose higher metabolic rate may result in more rapid destauration.

The patient with renal failure

Drug degradation should result in both inactive and nontoxic metabolites which are not required to be excreted by the kidney. Drugs should be dialyzable and should have a short elimination half-life. Renal patients often need a higher initial dose of sedative in order to reach effect because they have a higher volume of distribution; however, it should also be noted that the clearance of drug is decreased so that the effect of any dose is likely to be prolonged.

The patient with hepatic disease

As with renal patients, drug degradation should result in both inactive and nontoxic metabolites that are not required to be metabolized by the liver or excreted by the biliary tract. Drugs should have a short elimination half-life. They should have minimal or no effect on blood pressure to reduce the possibility of further liver compromise secondary to hypotension and reduced blood flow.

The substance abuser

There may be a cross tolerance with abused drugs. Enzyme induction may alter drug metabolism and decrease duration of action. Acute use (i.e., within past 24 hours) may enhance the effects of drugs used for conscious sedation, including the effects on cardiovascular and respiratory systems.

The psychiatric patient on psychotropic drugs

Almost all psychotropic drugs have additive effects when combined with drugs used for conscious sedation. Hypotension may occur with the combination of major tranquilizers and drugs for conscious sedation.

The obese patient

The volume of distribution may be altered so that drugs which bind to lipids may require increased dosages. There is a greater risk for aspiration and pulmonary reserves are decreased resulting in a greater potential for rapid desaturation. There is also a greater potential for airway problems in the obese patient.

Other considerations

As with regional anesthesia techniques, MAC involves provision of anesthesia care to awake patients during surgical or diagnostic procedures. The anesthesiologist should assess the patient's psychologic ability to deal with the operating or treatment room environment. Very little data are available regarding preoperative psychologic assessment. A study by Domar et al.[21] found that adults accompanied by a support person were more anxious than those without; women were more anxious than men; age, type of surgery, possibility of cancer, and previous surgical experience were not predictive of preoperative anxiety. Preoperative and postoperative contact with a specific anesthesia care provider was found to be useful in another study.[25]

SAFETY

How safe are MAC, sedation, and analgesia? Mortality and morbidity may occur with sedation techniques. This may be caused by unanticipated drug reactions, aspiration, airway obstruction, bronchospasm, or cardiovascular events related to hypertension and arrhythmias. In 1984, a Federated Ambulatory Surgery Association (FASA) Study of 87,000 patients undergoing elective ambulatory procedures in freestanding facilities, the complication rate was 1 of 106 cases with MAC procedures, compared with a higher rate for other techniques: 1 of 120 for general anesthesia, 1 of 268 for local only, 1 of 277 for regional anesthesia.[59] Another study by Campbell[14] reported a mortality rate of 1 of 314,000 for MAC versus 1 of 324,000 following general anesthesia in dentistry procedures. A landmark article by Caplan et al.[15] analyzed occurrences of unexpected cardiac arrest with death or severe residual neurologic damage in 14 healthy patients undergoing surgery with spinal anesthesia and intravenous (IV) sedation.[15] The patients were attended continuously by qualified anesthesia providers and were sedated to the point where spontaneous verbalization was suppressed. Monitoring included a blood pressure cuff in all cases, an ECG in all but one case, and precordial stethoscopes in approximately 50% of the cases; advanced monitors (pulse oximetry, capnography) were not used. Bradycardia, hypotension, and finally cyanosis presaged full-blown cardiac arrest in these cases. Tinker et al.[75] reviewed the large, closed-claims database maintained by the ASA to determine whether additional monitoring, if available or not at the time of the occurrence, could have prevented adverse outcomes during anesthesia. They found that 31.5% of the adverse outcomes (ranging from emotional distress without physical injury to death) could have been prevented by pulse oximetry and/or capnometry. More important, the worst outcomes (brain damage and death) were those judged most preventable by additional monitoring. The determination that pulse oximetry and capnometry used together could have prevented 93% of the negative outcomes that were considered preventable at all underscores the value of these noninvasive monitors.

MONITORING FOR MAC

The most versatile and valuable monitor for MAC or sedation/analgesia procedures is a dedicated caregiver, but appropriate selection and use of additional monitors can markedly enhance monitoring effectiveness. Monitoring selection for MAC should take into consideration the patient's underlying diseases and type of procedure being performed. In addition, it is critical that the individual performing the procedure be separate and distinct from the qualified individual who is responsible for monitoring the procedure and recording cardiorespiratory and sedation variables. Selection of basic and invasive monitoring for MAC should be governed by the same considerations used to select monitors for any other type of procedure. ASA has developed standards for basic intraoperative monitoring with the goal of improved patient safety. For sedation and analgesia procedures in nonoperating room locations, intraprocedure monitoring should include at least the following (Box 86-4): Ventilation, Oxygenation, Circulation, and Level of Consciousness.

Ventilation

ASA standards mandate that clinical signs of adequacy of ventilation (chest movement, reservoir bag movement, aus-

BOX 86-4
MAC/MONITORING FOR SEDATION AND ANALGESIA

Ventilation

Respiratory rate electronically or manually

Oxygenation

Pulse oximetry or equivalent to ensure adequate oxygenation of the patient
Supplemental O_2 as needed

Circulation

Continuous display of heart rate, using an EKG monitor for rhythm when necessary
Arterial blood pressure, either automated or manual

Level of consciousness

Alert and responding
Asleep but arousable
Uncooperative/restless/delirious
Voluntary movements

cultation) be continually assessed during the course of anesthesia. During the conduct of general anesthesia, rigorous measurement of ventilation is undertaken. During MAC, accurate measurement of expiratory CO_2 is difficult, because the airway generally is not isolated from the atmosphere by an endotracheal tube or airtight mask. The capnometer can be employed as a qualitative monitor of respiratory rate during MAC by sampling done through a soft cannula near the external nares.[31] Expiratory CO_2 determinations made in this fashion cannot be relied on to ensure adequacy but supply evidence of some ventilation.[23,80] This is not mandated by ASA standards. Transcutaneous CO_2 monitors are limited by slow response times and by calibration drift with use. **There is currently no satisfactory expired CO_2 monitor for the patient undergoing MAC; assessing the adequacy of respiratory exchange thus depends on vigilance of anesthesia providers and use of traditional methods such as precordial stethoscopes and observation of chest motion.**

Oxygenation

The ASA has reported data that strongly suggest detection of hypoxemia using oximetry during sedation and analgesia decreases the likelihood of adverse outcomes such as cardiac arrest and death.[5] A device to measure inspired O_2 should be used during every anesthetic. Illumination and exposure of the patient should be sufficient to assess skin color. **Use of a pulse oximeter is not specifically required by ASA standards but is strongly preferred over a transcutaneous monitor (TCM), the only other readily available device for continuous tissue oxygenation monitoring.** Although TCM devices are available to measure both O_2 and CO_2 tension, the values measured may not accurately reflect adequacy of arterial oxygenation because of variances in patient temperature and circulating blood volume. Most pulse oximeters are somewhat less prone to signal failure from vasoconstriction than TCM devices, but are themselves subject to error from other sources such as patient motion, ambient light, organic dyes, or interference by hemoglobin species other than oxyhemoglobin or deoxyhemoglobin. At present, only pulse oximetry combines constant rapid assessment of arterial hemoglobin O_2 saturation with a qualitative measure of perfusion.

Circulation

ASA standards specify that blood pressure and heart rate should be measured and recorded at least every 5 minutes and that an ECG should be continuously displayed while anesthesia is in progress. Choice of methods used to measure these parameters should be based on the anesthesiologist's assessment of the method's risk versus benefit of detection of circulatory changes and myocardial ischemia or arrythmias. ECG detection of myocardial ischemia continues to evolve. An early study found that a majority (89%) of myocardial ischemic events were detected by monitoring lead V5 alone and that monitoring lead II with lead V5 increased the sensitivity to 96%.[11] Another comparison of two-lead monitoring with a 12-lead system (using echocardiographic measurement of regional wall motion as a control) found that the 12-lead system detected about 20% more ischemic events than a two-lead monitor during coronary angioplasty procedures.[85] Findings in the coronary angiography laboratory or on the treadmill may not be directly applicable to MAC because the surgical field may encompass part or all the area where electrodes would be placed for 12-lead ECG monitoring. The sheer volume of information from continuous monitoring of all 12 leads simultaneously is not currently manageable in the operating room. An alternative to this approach is use of recently developed computerized analysis of ST segment changes for detection of changes in myocardial O_2 supply-demand balance. At least one such system in use has been reported considerably more sensitive than reliance on visual observation alone.[41] Incidence of myocardial ischemia during MAC is unknown, but the stress associated with surgery and anesthesia of any kind can be expected to precipitate cardiac ischemia in individuals at risk. Use of these computerized systems appears to represent improvement in noninvasive detection of myocardial ischemia. It is recognized that sophisticated monitoring for ischemia may not be available in all anesthetizing locations and at the minimum measurement of blood pressure and when appropriate heart rate and rhythm should be conducted.

Procedures selected for MAC usually do not involve major blood loss, fluid shifts, or hemodynamic changes. Generally, noninvasive monitoring of blood pressure with an automated oscillometric blood pressure cuff is sufficient. Invasive monitoring of arterial pressure can be used in settings where adverse intraoperative changes in blood pressure can be anticipated or where infusions of vasoactive agents (vasopressors/inotropes or vasodilators) may be required. Use of central venous pressure (CVP) or pulmonary artery catheters can be considered in the same fashion as use of an arterial catheter, although they are unlikely to be used in a MAC case. If the procedure involves use of diuretics or large amounts of fluids and if urine output is not likely to be a reliable indicator of systemic perfusion (as is sometimes the case in vascular surgery or neurosurgery), placement of a catheter to measure central pressure is reasonable.

Level of Consciousness (See Box 86-4)

Verbal responses to commands during procedures performed under MAC with sedation and analgesia serve as guide to level of consciousness. Several scoring systems can be used to determine the extent of central nervous system (CNS) depression. Spoken responses confirm that phonation is occurring and provides an indication that the patient is breathing. Patients whose only response is reflex withdrawal from painful stimuli are most likely deeply sedated and are approaching the continuum of CNS depression consistent with general anesthesia, which should be treated appropriately. **A critically important monitoring modality for patients under MAC is the response of the awake patient to**

verbal or physical stimulation. This monitoring may be valuable during episodes of symptomatic myocardial ischemia, where the patient's pain or dyspnea can alert the anesthesia provider to the need to institute appropriate therapeutic interventions. Another example where monitoring may be useful is during carotid endarterectomy (CEA) under local anesthesia, where changes in mental performance may be noted before electroencephalographic (EEG) changes are present. The disadvantage of a fully awake patient is that the possibility exists of untoward psychologic response to pain or surgical preparations such as placement of drapes over the face. **The anesthesia provider should maintain a high index of suspicion whenever the patient complains of discomfort or becomes unruly during the course of a procedure. Agitation during MAC should be considered to be reflective of hypoxia, hypercapnia, or inadequate perfusion of the brain or myocardium until proved otherwise.**

Temperature

ASA standards state that a device to measure temperature should be available whenever changes in temperature are expected. Most of the time, the patient undergoing MAC can report whether the temperature under the drapes is satisfactory or not, which is often sufficient. Cold procedure rooms or cold fluids may cause hypothermia, even in patients whose thermoregulatory mechanisms are not impaired by general anesthesia, resulting in shivering that may be severe enough to interfere with the procedure and which will be quite distressing to the patient. The elderly patient is particularly susceptible to cold stress because basal heat production is reduced compared with younger patients and ability to compensate for heat loss is thereby reduced.[56] **Prevention of hypothermia involves maintaining operating room or diagnostic area temperatures sufficiently warm for the patient's comfort.** During surgery, much heat lost is radiant heat loss. Intravenous (IV) fluid warmers should be used whenever large skin or mucosal surfaces will be exposed. Keeping the patient dry can also eliminate large evaporative heat losses. If hypothermia is severe enough to generate uncontrollable shivering, myocardial ischemia, respiratory insufficiency, or metabolic acidosis, general anesthesia with controlled ventilation and muscle relaxation will likely need to be instituted and maintained at least until the patient is sufficiently rewarmed to alleviate these adverse responses.

Hypothermia is an important problem in anesthetized patients or in patients undergoing MAC, but the problem of hyperthermia also deserves consideration. The patient who complains of being unusually warm during MAC should be evaluated carefully before assuming that there are too many layers of drapes in place. The feeling of heat may reflect sympathetic activation that may accompany hypoxia, hypercapnia, myocardial ischemia, sepsis, or pulmonary edema. The possibility of malignant hyperthermia is remote under MAC, because triggering agents (e.g., volatile anesthetics and succinylcholine) are seldom used, but it should also be considered along with other rare entities such as thyroid storm, malignant neuroleptic syndrome, or an adverse drug interaction in the patient taking monoamine oxidase (MAO) inhibitors. In most cases, however, the basis for hyperthermia is simply overzealous insulation of the patient from the operating room atmosphere. This problem is easily corrected by removing blankets and/or cooling the room a few degrees.

Recording of Monitored Parameters

The patient's level of consciousness, respiratory function and hemodynamics should be monitored and recorded before, during, and after the procedure and anesthesia. The use of a standardized Flow Sheet facilitates the monitoring and recording of the variables. Fig. 86-2 illustrates a "conscious sedation" flow sheet that was instituted at the Long Island College Hospital in an effort to standardize hospital-wide monitoring of patients receiving sedation and analgesia. The record also serves as a database for continuous quality improvement and as an educational tool to nursing and physician staff not regularly accustomed to anesthesia monitoring. With each entry, dedicated monitoring personnel can identify any deviation from the patient's baseline status and intervene when appropriate. Intrasedation vital signs, O_2 saturation, sedation scale and ECG rhythm should be monitored 5 minutes after each medication administration and at least every 15 minutes through recovery. The documentation tool also facilitates patient recovery and discharge, as discussed further.

RECOVERY AND DISCHARGE

Each patient-care facility in which sedation/analgesia is administered should develop recovery and discharge criteria which are suitable for its specific patients and procedures. Some of the basic principles which might be incorporated into the recovery period are enumerated below.

1. **Duration of recovery—all patients receiving sedation/analgesia should be monitored until appropriate discharge criteria are satisfied.** Duration of monitoring should be individualized depending upon the level of sedation achieved, the overall condition of the patient, and the nature of the intervention for which sedation/analgesia was administered.
2. Monitoring—Level of consciousness and vital signs (including frequency and depth of respiration in the absence of stimulation) should be recorded at regular intervals during recovery. The responsible practitioner should be notified if vital signs fall outside limits previously established for each patient.
3. Equipment—the recovery area should be equipped with appropriate monitoring and resuscitation equipment.
4. Personnel—A nurse or other trained individual should be in attendance until discharge criteria are fulfilled. An individual capable of establishing a patent airway

NAME:

MR #:

CONSCIOUS SEDATION FLOW RECORD

DATE	TIME	☐ OUTPATIENT ☐ INPATIENT UNIT ______ ☐ ED	AGE

PHYSICIAN ASSESSMENT

CURRENT PROBLEM	PROCEDURE:
PAST MEDICAL HISTORY:	
PREVIOUS SURGICAL/ANESTHESIA HISTORY:	
HEENT/NECK:	CHEST:
HEART:	GYN: ☐ N/A PREGNANT: ☐ YES ☐ NO ☐ N/A
NPO SINCE:	
CONSENT OBTAINED: ☐ YES ☐ NO - EXPLAIN	☐ ON CHART

TIME	MEDICATION/DOSE	ROUTE	SIGNATURE/TITLE

PROCEDURE STARTED: ______
PATHOLOGY: ☐ BIOPSY______
☐ POLYP______
☐ NA ☐ OTHER ______
SPECIMEN SENT TO LAB: ☐ YES ☐ NO
PROCEDURE FINISHED: ______
PUNCTURE SITE:______
LOCAL ANESTHETIC:______

TIME	B/P	PULSE	EKG RHYTHM	RESP.	O_2 SAT.	O_2 SUPPLEMENT	*SEDATION SCALE LOC			COMMENTS

*** SEDATION SCALE - LOC CODE**

0 = WIDE AWAKE	1 = DROWSY	2 = SLEEPING, AROUSABLE	3 = DIFFICULT TO AROUSE	4 = NOT ABLE TO AWAKEN

1786 PHM768 (1/95)

Page 1 of 2

WHITE - MEDICAL RECORD CANARY - DEPARTMENT COPY

Fig. 86-2. Conscious Sedation Flow Record.

Continued

Conscious Sedation Flow Record

Name: ______________________

M.R. No.: ______________________

IV FLUIDS

I.V. SITE: ______________________

☐ N/A ☐ FROM UNIT

☐ INSERTED _______ ANGIO _______ HEPLOCK _______ CENTRAL LINE

TIME	SOLUTION	RATE	ADDITIVES	AMT INFUSED
			TOTAL	

ALDRETE SCORE - MODIFIED	0 - 2	PRE	IMMEDIATE POST PROCEDURE	UPON DISCHARGE	DISCHARGE CRITERIA
ACTIVITY: Able to move on command Impaired movement Not moving	 2 1 0				* All patients must achieve a score of "2" in the Respiration and Circulation Category prior to discharge. ** All patients must achieve a TOTAL score of "9" prior to discharge.
RESPIRATION: * Able to breathe freely * Dyspnea or limited breathing Apneic	 2 1 0			SaO2: _____ % Resp.: _____	
CONSCIOUSNESS: Fully awake Arousable on calling Not responding	 2 1 0				
CIRCULATION: * B/P, Pulse within normal range for pt. Impaired Circulation Unstable	 2 1 0			Pulse: _____ B/P: _____	
PAIN NAUSEA AND/OR VOMITING: Minimal Moderate, having required treatment Severe, requiring treatment	 2 1 0				
TOTAL SCORE **					

1. Written instructions given: ☐ Yes
2. Verbal instructions given: ☐ Yes
3. Responsible adult escort for ambulatory patients ☐ Yes
4. Patient discharged: ☐ Home _______ AM PM ☐ Unit _______ AM PM

Verbal report given to: ______________________ (For inpatients only)
NAME

COMMENTS:

____

____

____

MD Signature: ______________________ M.D. Nurse Signature: ______________________ R.N.

Print Name: ______________________ M.D. Print Name: ______________________ R.N.

F1786 PHM768 (1/95)

Page 2 of 2

Fig. 86-2, *continued.* Conscious Sedation Flow Record.

and providing positive pressure ventilation should be immediately available.

Guidelines for Discharge

Criteria for discharge following MAC in both operating room and nonoperating room settings are similar to those undergoing ambulatory surgical procedures and should be applied accordingly. These include return to baseline level of orientation, return of vital signs within 20% of baseline values, ambulating without dizziness (when appropriate), minimal pain, nausea and vomiting, and availability of an adult escort. Some special considerations are discussed in the following paragraphs.

Patients whose mental status was initially abnormal should have returned to their baselines. Practitioners should be aware that pediatric patients are at risk for airway obstruction should the child's head fall forward while the child is secured in a car seat. Sufficient time (up to 2 hours) should have elapsed following the last administration of reversal agents (naloxone, flumazenil) to ensure that patients do not become resedated after reversal effects have worn off. Outpatients must be discharged in the presence of a responsible adult who will accompany them home and be able to report any postprocedure complications. Inpatients returning to the floor should have a complete report provided to the staff who will continue the recovery of the patient. Outpatients should be provided with written instructions regarding postprocedure diet, medications, activities, and a phone number to call in case of emergency.

To evaluate the patient and determine that he or she has fully recovered from the effects of sedation, either physician evaluation on rigorous application of approved medical staff discharge criteria can be used and documented in the medical record.

AVAILABILITY OF EMERGENCY EQUIPMENT AND REVERSAL AGENTS

Appropriately sized emergency airway and resuscitative equipment should be immediately available during administration of sedation and analgesia (see Boxes 86-5 through 86-7). Pharmacologic support, drug antagonists, as well as a cardiac defibrillator should be included in the emergency set-up in any anesthetizing location. The ASA also strongly supports placement of an IV access, regardless of the route of sedation, and maintaining that access until the patient is no longer at risk from the risks of sedative/analgesic drugs.

Naloxone and flumazenil are specific antagonists for narcotics and benzodiazepines respectively. Naloxone reverses opioid-induced sedation and ventilatory depression, but acute reversal of opioid-induced analgesia may result in pain, hypertension, tachycardia, or pulmonary edema.[27] It may be possible to titrate naloxone such that depression of ventilation is sufficiently antagonized with maintenance of analgesia. Administration of 1 to 4 μg/kg IV naloxone promptly reverses opioid-induced analgesia and ventilatory depression. Its short duration of action of 30 to 45 minutes is presumed to be caused by the prompt removal of the drug from the brain, and repeat administration may be needed so as to prevent return of respiratory depression.

Flumazenil has been shown to reverse sedation and ventilatory depression caused by benzodiazepines.[72] When there has been concomitant administration of opioids, the effectiveness of flumazenil in reversing ventilatory depression is

BOX 86-5
EMERGENCY EQUIPMENT FOR SEDATION AND ANALGESIA

Basic airway management equipment
Source of compressed O_2 (tank with regulator or pipeline supply with flowmeter)
Source of suction
Suction catheters (pediatric suction catheters)
Yankauer-type suction
Face masks (infant/child face masks)
Self-inflating breathing bag-valve set (pediatric bag-valve set)
Oral and nasal airways (infant/child sized airways)
Lubricant

BOX 86-6
ADVANCED AIRWAY MANAGEMENT EMERGENCY EQUIPMENT

Laryngoscope handles (tested)
Laryngoscopy blades (pediatric laryngoscope blades)
Endotracheal tubes—cuffed 6.0, 7.0, 8.0 mm i.d. (uncuffed 2.5, 3.0, 3.5, 4.0, 4.5, 5.0, 5.5, 6.0 mm i.d.)
Stylet (appropriately sized for endotracheal tubes)

BOX 86-7
INTRAVENOUS EMERGENCY EQUIPMENT

Gloves
Tourniquets
Alcohol wipes
Sterile gauze pads
Intravenous catheters (24, 22 gauze)
Intravenous tubing (pediatric 'microdip'—60 drops/ml)
Intravenous fluid
Three-way stopcocks
Assorted needles for drug aspiration, IM injection (intraosseous bone marrow needle)
Appropriately sized syringes
Tape

problematic. The duration of action of flumazenil is brief. Return of the benzodiazepine effect may require repeated doses. Administration of 8 to 15 μg/kg IV flumazenil reverses the CNS effects of benzodiazepine agonist within 2 minutes. This antagonism is not followed by acute anxiety, hypertension, tachycardia, or neuroendocrine evidence of a stress response.[38,83]

AGENTS FREQUENTLY ADMINISTERED DURING MAC

The variety of agents administered during MAC sedation and analgesia usually include local anesthetics, narcotic analgesics, anxiolytics, sedative-hypnotics, and occasionally other agents. Generally, agents from one or more of these categories will be used in combination to achieve a specific effect. The pharmacologic properties of commonly used agents are discussed.

Local Anesthetics

MAC may involve administration of local anesthesia during the procedure. Lidocaine is frequently selected for several of the following reasons: (1) predictability of action; (2) low allergic reaction potential; (3) relative safety even in large doses or with inadvertent IV injection; (4) ready availability; (5) duration of action appropriate to most MAC procedures; and (6) low cost. Infiltration anesthesia with lidocaine can be expected to provide anesthesia for 1 to 2 hours; peripheral nerve blocks may last slightly longer. In some cases, a longer-acting local anesthetic is preferred for long-lasting perioperative analgesia or for those procedures expected to last for extended periods. Bupivacaine is usually selected because it allows 2 to 4 hours of local anesthesia with infiltration and up to 12 hours' duration with peripheral nerve block. Its value is limited by its cardiotoxicity, which is related to its kinetics in cardiac sodium channels. This has been a major problem only with inadvertent IV injection of large doses of bupivacaine, but nevertheless, a less toxic, long-acting local anesthetic is still desirable. One such agent currently under development is ropivacaine. This agent differs from bupivacaine only in the presence of a propyl rather than butyl group on its amine nitrogen. Studies have shown it to be slightly less potent than bupivacaine but with a similar duration of action. Its cardiotoxic potential seems to be approximately 50% of its parent compound, bupivacaine, and there also appears to be a wider difference between the dose that induces convulsions and the cardiotoxic dose. Whether ropivacaine will replace bupivacaine in anesthetic practice remains to be seen.

Opioid Analgesics—Morphine, Meperidine, Fentanyl, Sufentanil, and Alfentanil

Opioid analgesics are often administered at some point during anesthesia, irrespective of whether the anesthesia is general, regional, or MAC. Which agent is selected depends on qualities such as speed of onset and duration of action as well as propensity for production of side effects such as histamine release.

Morphine and meperidine

Morphine, the prototype for this class of drugs, has been in clinical use for centuries. It has several properties that render it less than ideal for use in brief procedures or in other situations where the plan includes a short duration of sedation and analgesia followed by a rapid return to normal mentation. Highly water-soluble drugs like morphine are very slow to penetrate lipid membranes, including the blood–brain barrier and hence tend to have slow onset of action. Because morphine has a relatively long elimination half-life but does not redistribute widely and rapidly to other tissues, its duration of action is prolonged as well. Meperidine is more lipid soluble than morphine and thus has a somewhat faster onset but has liabilities of its own, including anticholinergic properties that can cause tachycardia and delirium, especially in elderly patients. The dosage required for sedation and analgesia varies among different patients and a minimum plasma concentration of 0.7 μg/ml of meperidine would be expected to provide analgesia in approximately 95% of patients.[6] Doses of 0.5 to 1.0 mg/kg usually provides adequate sedation and analgesia with varying levels of respiratory depression. Caution should therefore be exercised when the drug is being titrated during the course of sedation.

Fentanyl

Fentanyl and its analogs, alfentanil and sufentanil, have many excellent properties for brief procedures. Because these drugs are highly lipid soluble, their onset of action is rapid. Duration of effect is relatively short, because redistribution from the CNS to other tissues is the primary mechanism for termination of effect in low doses used in outpatient anesthesia or MAC. Fentanyl, a phenylpiperidine derivative, is the most widely used narcotic for MAC with sedation and analgesia. It produces analgesia, drowsiness, sedation, and euphoria but not amnesia. The drug is injected in 25- to 50-μg increments at 1- to 2-minute intervals to usual loading dose of 1 to 3 μg/kg. Its onset is within 5 minutes, its peak is at 10 minutes and its effect lasts 45 to 60 minutes. Over time, progressive saturations of inactive sites leads to increased duration of analgesics and respiratory depression. Although peak respiratory effect with small dose is at 30 minutes, respiratory depression comparable with that produced by morphine may last as long as 4 hours. This can become a problem later in the recovery period, when the drug redistributes from inactive tissue sites. Shift in the ventilatory response curve to CO_2, increase in end-tidal CO_2, decrease in PO_2 and depression of hypoxic ventilatory drive, occur with narcotic doses too small to alter consciousness. Those effects are heightened during sleep or when external stimuli are reduced.

Alfentanil

Alfentanil is the shortest-acting narcotic currently available. It is one fifth as potent and has one third the duration of fentanyl. Sedatives and euphoria may be more profound than fentanyl, but respiratory depression is briefer.

At physiologic pH, alfentanil is unionized and has a rapid onset and redistribution. Its low lipid solubility, high protein binding and small volume of distribution make it available for rapid elimination within 1 to 2 hours. It is cumulative only after prolonged administration or large doses; clearance is decreased in the obese, in the elderly, in patients with liver disease and in the presence of erythromycin.[78] A bolus or infusion loading dose of 5 to 10 μg/kg, has an onset within 1 to 2 minutes, with a duration of about 20 minutes.

Sufentanil

Sufentanil is a thiamyl analog of fentanyl, and is the most potent opioid currently in use. It is approximately 5 to 10 times more potent than fentanyl, and has a more rapid onset and a slightly shorter elimination half-life. Compared with fentanyl, it is more fat soluble, more highly protein bound, and has a small volume of distribution. Initial dose for sedation is 0.1 to 0.5 μg/kg. Its respiratory depressant effect is considered less than that of fentanyl and it has increased analgesic and amnestic properties. Other than bradycardia, cardiovascular side effects are minimal. Although its pharmacokinetic and pharmacodynamic properties seem ideal for MAC/sedation, sufentanil has not achieved popularity for sedation and analgesia because of the frequent occurrence of chest wall rigidity, when compared with fentanyl or alfentanil.

Mixed Agonist-Antagonists

In hopes of avoiding some of the side effects associated with the administration of pure narcotic agonists, such as morphine and fentanyl, drugs that act as partial narcotic agonists or mixed agonist-antagonists have been developed. These agents have varying effects on the subtypes of opioid receptors and lead to differing clinical responses. Several of the mixed agonists-antagonists may have a role in MAC.

The pharmacology of the opioid receptors is complex, and knowledge of the various subtypes of receptors is rapidly evolving. Analgesia is believed to involve activation of the supraspinal mu receptor and spinal cord kappa receptors; there may also be activation of the delta receptors. Activation of these delta receptors produces mild analgesia and respiratory depression.[65] Activation of the mu receptor also results in euphoria, miosis, and respiratory depression. Simulation of the kappa receptor results in analgesia but less respiratory depression and miosis compared with that of the mu receptor.[65] In contrast to these receptors, activation of the sigma receptor results in dysphoria and hallucinations.[8] Agonist-antagonist agents possess agonist activity at the kappa and sigma receptors, while exhibiting antagonist behavior at the mu receptors. Their hemodynamic effects are noted in Table 86-3.

The first widely used agonist-antagonist was pentazocine. This drug has one fourth to one half the potency of morphine and also has similar respiratory depression effect comparable with equivalent doses of morphine. It also possesses agonist properties at the sigma receptor that may lead to dysphoria with high doses. Because of these properties, there is little to recommend use of pentazocine as an adjunctive agent for MAC.

Table 86-3 Hemodynamic effects of agonist-antagonist compounds compared with morphine

Drug	Cardiac workload	Blood pressure	Heart rate	Pulmonary artery pressure
Morphine	↓	↓	= ↓	= ↓
Buprenorphine	↓	↓	↓	?
Nalbuphine	↑	= ↑	=	↑
Butorphanol	↓	=	= ↓	=
Pentazocine	↑	↑	↑	↑

Nalbuphine is a kappa agonist and a mu antagonist with potential utility for MAC. Its activation at the kappa receptor results in moderate analgesia combined with a ceiling effect in respiratory depression.[19] Klein[39] reported that satisfactory sedation was achieved using a combination of 30 mg of nalbuphine with 2.5 mg of droperidol administered before surgery. Sury and Cole[73] reported that nalbuphine doses of up to 0.2 mg/kg combined with 0.05 mg/kg of midazolam provided reliable deep sedation while causing minimally increased end-tidal CO_2 coupled with a mild decrease in response to CO_2 rebreathing. These investigators did, however, note that several of the patients developed short periods of apnea immediately after infusion of the drugs. Because of its mixed agonist-antagonist action, nalbuphine may interfere with analgesia produced by mu agonists such as morphine.[42] It should be administered with caution to patients who have recently received morphine or other mu agonists.

Dezocine has partial agonist activities at mu and delta receptors.[67] Because of these actions, dezocine potentiates the analgetic effects of the mu agonist agents. Gal et al.[29] also found moderate increases in partial pressure of alveolar carbon dioxide ($PACO_2$) similar to that seen after morphine administration. The use of this drug as an adjunctive agent for MAC has yet to be determined.

Propofol

The substituted alkyl-phenol agent, propofol, has achieved wide acceptance for use as a sedative-hypnotic during MAC procedures. It possesses no analgesic properties. Its cardiovascular and respiratory depressant effects should limit its use to practitioners knowledgeable in its pharmacologic properties and who are able to manage an obstructed airway and/or provide a general anesthetic, if necessary. The drug's short duration and brief distribution half-life provide the practitioner with an agent that can be rapidly titrated to provide a desired level of sedation, which is followed by rapid recovery once infusion is stopped.[46] Monk et al.[53] reported that adequate levels of patient comfort and sedation for lithotripsy were achieved with two bolus doses of 1.5 μg/kg of fentanyl in conjunction with a loading dose of 0.5 mg/kg of propofol followed by a continuous propofol infusion starting at 50 μg/kg/min, then titrated according to patient response. This regimen produced excellent analgesia, minimal hemodynamic alterations, and excellent patient satisfaction. It is necessary to continually adjust these recommended anesthetic doses in response to surgical stimulus and patient responses. **Typical doses for sedation and analgesia range from 3.5 mg/kg/hr to 5 mg/kg/hr.** These continuous subanesthetic doses produced sedation similar to N_2O, without hemodynamic or respiratory changes.[60] Level of sedation should not exceed easy arousability or response to command. To date, propofol has been extensively studied for use under MAC, and consistently result in rapid return to baseline after short procedures following subanesthetic doses.[84,86] In addition, its effects on mood and psychomotor cognitive performance give it an advantage compared with other available sedative-hypnotics and anxiolytics.[38a,84]

Sedative-Hypnotics

Most potent opioids have some inherent sedative properties, but when used alone as sedatives or as preoperative medication in the absence of pain, they frequently produce disturbing dysphoric reactions. When sedation alone is desired, use of a sedative-hypnotic is more logical. Barbiturates, such as pentobarbital, were once used in this fashion, but their long duration of action are unsatisfactory for the short procedures usually performed during MAC. Lorazepam (a benzodiazepine) also is slow in onset and long acting and hence not particularly useful for MAC. Diazepam and especially midazolam are commonly used as sedative-hypnotic agents in healthy patients undergoing MAC procedures. **For intraoperative sedation, midazolam has almost completely replaced diazepam.** In nonoperating room locations, or when anxiolysis and sedation is administered by nonanesthesiologists, diazepam may still be used.

Diazepam has long been employed as a component of sedation regimens in patients undergoing medical or surgical procedures. It has a rapid onset of action (2 to 3 minutes) after IV administration. Duration of effect is dose dependent. The parent drug is eliminated slowly (half-life in hours roughly equals the patient's age in years after age 20).[48] Unfortunately, the metabolites of diazepam are active and are eliminated even more slowly. In low doses, redistribution of diazepam rapidly terminates its effect while generating minimal levels of active metabolites, so that its clinical duration of effect is relatively short. Increased drowsiness and secondary peaks in serum concentration have been found 6 to 8 hours after initial administration.[9] Patients given diazepam should be cautioned about possible recurrent sedation after their discharge from the hospital. A 10-mg dose in adult patients has been associated with a 90% incidence of amnesia from time of injection lasting at least 30 minutes.[22] The formulation which uses propylene glycol as the solvent causes pain on injection and phlebitis in roughly 40% of patients.

Midazolam is the only benzodiazepine that is water soluble at acid pH and becomes highly lipophilic above pH 6.0. It possesses the rapid onset of sedation and amnesia of diazepam but causes little phlebitis or pain on injection. It does not produce any active metabolites and has an elimination half-life of 2 to 3 hours.[63,78] It is two to three times as potent as diazepam with respect to sedation and amnesia and has largely displaced diazepam as the sedative-hypnotic of choice in most procedures performed during regional anesthesia or MAC. Although recovery from sedation with midazolam is usually faster than that with diazepam, there are two reasons why this is not always the case. First, termination of effects of small doses of midazolam depend on redistribution as with diazepam. Second, the receptor kinetics of diazepam and midazolam are virtually identical despite different plasma pharmacokinetic profiles.[20] Perhaps because of greater lipid solubility of midazolam and easier penetration of the blood–brain barrier, a better correlation exists between plasma levels and clinical effect than exists with diazepam.[62] Midazolam is effective and relatively easy to administer if the difference in potency relative to diazepam is kept in mind and if the anesthesia provider understands the well-known propensity of combinations of opiates and benzodiazepines to produce hypotension. As Bailey et al.[7] emphasize, the combination of midazolam with a narcotic agent can be dangerous. They found that 11 of 12 volunteers who received a combination of fentanyl and midazolam experienced serious hypoxia, whereas hypoxia was present in only 6 of 12 volunteers receiving fentanyl alone and in none of the volunteers receiving only midazolam.[7] They also noticed short episodes of apnea in 6 of the 12 patients who received both drugs. As these data clearly indicate, it is necessary to carefully monitor patients receiving a combination of opiates and narcotics in the perioperative period. In most healthy, pain-free patients, a benzodiazepine alone will provide adequate sedation for most procedures. In elderly or debilitated individuals, even small doses of benzodiazepine may cause unacceptable hemodynamic side effects. Elderly patients also seem more likely to become disoriented when benzodiazepines are administered. In this setting, use of an antihistamine, such as diphenhydramine, is an excellent alternative that provides mild sedation without major hemodynamic change.

SEDATION TECHNIQUES

Administration of small increments of sedative and analgesic drugs until the desired level of sedation is achieved is preferable to a single-bolus dose based on the patient's size, weight, or age. Sedation and analgesia is an art that develops over time and experience. It was first developed by oral surgeons for office procedures and now has become a very popular technique for operative and nonoperative procedures. The goal of sedation is to provide a fine balance between patient comfort without compromising patient safety while preventing cardiovascular or respiratory compromise or delay in recovery.

Component drugs are primarily delivered intraoperatively by the IV route; however, one or more drugs may be administered as premedication via oral, IM, transmucosal, or rectal routes.

Administration of Drugs

The administration of drugs ideal for sedation/analgesia would possess the characteristics outlined in Box 86-8. These drugs should possess a small volume of distribution, short elimination half-life, and rapid clearance. Table 86-4 highlights drugs and dosages commonly used for sedation and analgesia.

Techniques

Bolus sedation techniques

Benzodiazepines, opioids, sedative-hypnotics, and inhalational agents may be used in various combination to enhance sedation amnesia and analgesia (Table 86-5). Drug combinations are administered to achieve the desired effects. The anxiolytic is usually administered first, followed by the narcotic, and finally by the sedative-hypnotic. Drugs may be administered by bolus or by infusion. The initial dose is determined by clinical judgement depending on length of the procedure and the patient's weight, physical conditions, anxiety level, and drug history. Kallar[36] has described a useful technique for MAC during operative procedures which consist of the following: First 2 to 3 mg of midazolam is administered, followed by 250 to 500 μg of alfentanil, or 50 to 100 μg of fentanyl, with 20 to 30 mg of methohexital or 10 to 20 mg propofol given at the time of the local anesthesia or block. The endpoint is titration to divergent pupils or nystagmus, accompanied by spontaneous respiration, maintenance of SpO_2 greater than 95%. Another technique may include using almost the same method, al-

BOX 86-8
THE IDEAL DRUG FOR INTRAVENOUS SEDATION

- Water soluble, nonirritating, stable
- Rapid onset
- Specific, identifiable, and readily titratable effect
- Short, reliable duration of action
- Ease of administration
- Absence of cardiovascular or respiratory depressant effects
- No hypersensitivity reactions
- Non–organ dependent elimination
- Absence of toxicity
- Pharmacokinetic independence of altered physiology
- Rapid recovery
- Favorable cost-benefit ratio

Reproduced from Greenberg CP, DeSoto H: Sedation Techniques. In Twersky RS, editor: *The ambulatory anesthesia handbook,* St. Louis, 1995, Mosby–Year Book

Table 86-4 Dosages of drugs for conscious sedation

Drug	Loading dose (μg/kg)	Maintenance infusion rate (μg/kg/min)	Plasma drug level
Thiopental	1000–3000	100–300	4–8 μg/ml
Methohexital	250–1000	10–50	2–5 mg/ml
Diazepam	50–150		
Midazolam	25–100	0.25–1	40–100 ng/ml
Droperidol	5–17		
Propofol	250–1000	10–50	1–2 μg/ml
Ketamine	500–1000	10–20	0.1–1 μg/ml
Etomidate	100–200	7–14	100–300 ng/ml
Fentanyl	1–3	0.01–0.03	1–2 ng/ml
Alfentanil	10–25	0.25–1	25–75 ng/ml
Sufentanil	0.1–0.5	0.005–0.01	0.02–0.2 ng/ml
Butorphanol	0.01–0.03		
Nalbuphine	0.07–0.2		

Reproduced from Greenberg CP, DeSoto H: Sedation Techniques. In Twersky RS, editor: *The ambulatory anesthesia handbook,* St. Louis, 1995, Mosby–Year Book.

Table 86-5 Intravenous bolus sedation techniques

Procedure	Drug
Dental[69]	Alphaprodine 30 mg, Atropine 0.6 mg, Hydroxyzine 50 mg, Methohexital 30–60 mg
Dental/ENT[68]	Diazepam 10–20 mg, Fentanyl 50-μg increments, Scopolamine 0.25 mg
Oral surgery[61]	Midazolam 0.12 mg/kg, Fentanyl 100 μg
Neuroradiology[1]	Midazolam 2.5–20 mg, Fentanyl 50–300 μg *or* Propofol 100–150 mg, Fentanyl 50–125 μg
Endoscopy[13]	Diazepam 10 mg, Meperidine 50–75 mg
Endoscopy[51]	Midazolam 0.05 mg/kg, Alfentanil 5 μg/kg
Multiple ambulatory surgery procedures[36]	Midazolam 2–3 mg Alfentanil 250–500 μg *or* Fentanyl 50–100 μg, Methohexital 20–30 mg *or* Propofol 10–20 mg

Reproduced from Greenberg CP, DeSoto H: Sedation Techniques. In Twersky RS, editor: *The ambulatory anesthesia handbook,* St. Louis, 1995, Mosby–Year Book.

though modified, using 25 to 50 mg of diphenhydramine, followed by 4 to 10 mg of morphine or 50 μg of fentanyl, and a bolus of propofol, usually 0.5 mg/kg. Table 86-5 lists several IV bolus sedation techniques, which may be adjusted for different procedures.

Combinations of drugs exert synergistic effects, which allows for lower doses of each drug, and thus a better quality of sedation and more rapid recovery. Although bolus doses achieve the desired result for short procedures, the need for rebolusing during prolonged procedures can lead to accumulation of the drugs with concomitant untoward side effects.

Continuous infusion techniques

Continuous infusion techniques offer an advantage over bolus techniques because a steady state is better achieved, peaks and valley of anesthetic levels are minimized, and the total amount of drug required to produce anesthesia or sedation is reduced. Infusions can sometimes be administered simply and inexpensively via Buretrol, but more efficiently and accurately via volumetric or syringe pumps (see Table 86-6). Computerized volumetric pumps can deliver precise dosages of infusions, based on patient's weight and concentration of drug. They can be calibrated for optimal delivery rate for a particular medication, and the rate can be set in ml/hr, μg/kg/min, mg/kg/min or mg/kg/hr.

Table 86-7 displays examples of procedures and infusion dosages of drugs commonly used for outpatient procedures. Infusion techniques can be tailored to deliver multiple sedation and analgesic drugs, while achieving the level of sedation consistent with the desired procedure. Infusion techniques have been shown to be superior to bolus techniques, and as more "smart" pumps become available greater control and safety of sedation and analgesia will be achieved.

Pediatric Sedation

Pediatric sedation is probably the most challenging undertaking for anesthesiologists and nonanesthesiologists alike. Because successful sedation and analgesia usually requires a cooperative and consenting patient, the sedation of a child requires patience, understanding, and creativity. Often, sedation and analgesia is administered to pediatric patients for procedures that may require them to lay still for either frightening or painful procedures. Radiologic procedures, such as magnetic resonance imaging (MRI) or computed tomography (CT) scans, require the patient to be absolutely still, while gastroenterologic or pulmonary procedures require a cooperative and comfortable patient. It is important that the physicians administering sedation and analgesia to this patient group understands the differences in the pharmacokinetic profiles of the drugs, and are also credentialed in pediatric airway management. As discussed earlier, **the individual responsible for observing and monitoring the child should be distinct from the person performing the procedure (operator).** Although parents may assist during the procedure, they should in no way be depended upon for monitoring and ongoing evaluation. Pediatric airway and resuscitative equipment with proper drug doses, laryngoscope blades, pediatric airway and endotracheal tubes should be available. It should be understood by the personnel involved that the same degree of vigilance and

Table 86-6 Comparison of techniques available for administration of intravenous anesthetic agents

	Syringe	Buretrol	Volumetric pump	Syringe pump	Computer-assisted continuous infusion
Bolus	+			+	
Infusion		+	+	+	+
Inexpensive	+	+			
Flexible dosing	+	+	+	+	+
Established dosing methods	+	+	+	+	?
Conceptual appeal					+
Convenient instrumentation	+	+	+	+	?
User friendly	+	+	+	+	+
Data provided by device					
Cumulative dose (ml)				+	+
Cumulative dose (mg)				+	+
Cumulative volume (ml)	+	+	+	+	+
Infusion rate			+	+	+
Theoretical plasma level					+
Predictive capability					+
Availability	+	+	+	+	+
Accuracy	+	+	+	+	?

Reproduced from Greenberg CP, DeSoto H: Sedation Techniques. In Twersky RS, editor: *The ambulatory anesthesia handbook,* St. Louis, 1995, Mosby–Year Book.

Table 86-7 Intravenous infusion sedation techniques

Procedure	Drug	Bolus	Infusion
Multiple procedures with local/regional anesthesia[84]	Midazolam	3–6 mg	3–14 mg/hr
	Propofol	45–95 mg	80–450 mg/hr
Multiple procedures with local/regional anesthesia[81]	Methohexital	30–90 mg	115–245 mg/hr
	Etomidate	4.5–21 mg	20–44 mg/hr
	Midazolam	2–5 mg	3–12 mg/hr
Ovum retrieval[70]	Mixture of 50 ml propofol (10 mg/ml) plus 4 ml alfentanil (500 μg/ml)	—	2 ml/kg/hr, then 1 ml/kg/hr
Knee arthroscopy[43]	Alfentanil	8 μg/kg	0.75 μg/kg/min
	Propofol	1 mg/kg	*or* 50 μg/kg/min
Extracorporeal shock wave lithotripsy[53]	Midazolam	0.05 mg/kg	
	Alfentanil	10 μg/kg	1 μg/kg/min
	or		
	Fentanyl	1.5 μg/kg	
	Propofol	0.5 mg/kg	50 μg/kg/min
Extracorporeal shock wave lithotripsy[54]	Midazolam	4–9 mg	
	Alfentanil	10 μg/kg	0.5–2 μg/kg/min
	or		
	Midazolam	4–14 mg	25–50 μg/kg/min
	Ketamine	0.4 mg/kg	

Reproduced from Greenberg CP, DeSoto H: Sedation Techniques. In Twersky RS, editor: *The ambulatory anesthesia handbook,* St. Louis, 1995, Mosby–Year Book.

monitoring for MAC in adults most certainly applies to the pediatric population.[2]

Children can be sedated by the oral, rectal, IM or IV route. Because children generally fear needles, the oral or rectal route is the most accepted.

Nonparenteral routes

Administration of 25 to 50 mg/kg of chloral hydrate[44] has been used successfully for sedation in children less than 12 months old, so long as high doses are avoided. Because desired effects are frequently not achieved, interest is high among nonanesthesiologists as to the ways anesthesiologists have developed for premedication and sedation. Table 86-8 lists several oral sedation techniques in children. Ketamine and midazolam are good and safe choices in children older than 1 year of age.[26,79] Transmucosal (oral) fentanyl has been found to produce adequate sedation at doses of 5 to 15 μg/kg. Higher doses were associated with respiratory depression, serious pruritis, and emetic symptoms.[28] Depending on the extent of the procedure, this oral sedation may be sufficient to allow the child to separate from the parents, after which further IV, IM, or even inhalational sedation may required. Midazolam is probably the most commonly used drug for oral premedication and sedation in children. With doses of 0.5 to 1.0 mg/kg, a well-relaxed and cooperative child is often apparent in 15 to 30 minutes. Midazolam administered orally is not very pleasant and the taste should be masked by other palatable fluids. It can be mixed with cherry flavored fluids or apple juice. The volume of oral administration should be as low as possible to reduce risk of aspiration.

Table 86-8 Oral sedation techniques in children

Drug	Usual dose
Chloral hydrate	25–50 mg/kg (for small infants up to 12 months)
	25–75 mg/kg (for children older than 12 months)
Ketamine	5–10 mg/kg (above 1 year)
Midazolam	0.5–1.0 mg/kg orally
	0.2–0.3 mg/kg intranasally (above 1 year)
Fentanyl (Oralet)	5–15 μg/kg transmucosally (for children weighing more than 15 kg)

Reproduced from Greenberg CP, DeSoto H: Sedation Techniques. In Twersky RS, editor: *The ambulatory anesthesia handbook,* St. Louis, 1995, Mosby–Year Book.

IM and IV sedation

Because children are universally afraid of needle sticks, the intramuscular and intravenous routes requires a little more creativity on the part of the anesthesiologist if they must be used at all. **The availability of EMLA (eutectic mixture of local anesthetic: lidocaine and prilocaine) has allowed successful performance of painless venipuncture in children.**[71] Its use in sedation has to be carefully planned be-

Table 86-9 Intramuscular sedation techniques in children

Drug	Usual dose
Ketamine	2–5 mg/kg
Midazolam	0.08 mg/kg
Pentobarbital	4–5 mg/kg (Injection can be painful)
DPT cocktail	
Meperidine	2 mg/kg
Promethazine	1 mg/kg
Chlorpromazine	1 mg/kg

Reproduced from Greenberg CP, DeSoto H: Sedation Techniques. In Twersky RS, editor: *The ambulatory anesthesia handbook,* St. Louis, 1995, Mosby–Year Book.

cause it requires at least 1 hour of contact time with the skin under occlusive dressing to have full effect. It has been recommended that EMLA be applied to two sites so that an alternative site is available if the first venipuncture is not successful.

Table 86-9 and 86-10 demonstrate IM and IV sedation techniques in children. The most popular IM drug is ketamine which is administered in doses of 2 to 5 mg/kg.[33] It usually lasts between 15 and 30 minutes and is ideal for uncooperative or mentally challenged children.

Because of its water solubility, midazolam is ideal for IM use and it is administered in 0.8 mg/kg dose. This dose produces good predictable sedation and lasts approximately 30 minutes.

IV sedation is performed with the usual drugs approved for adult usage. Barbiturates, bezodiazepines, propofol, ketamine, and narcotics are the most commonly used drugs.

Propofol has become popular for use in pediatric sedation.[82] It is used in doses of 1 to 2 mg/kg, followed by an infusion of 4 to 8 mg/kg/hr. Ketamine, at doses 0.5 to 1.0 mg/kg followed by repeated boluses as needed has been shown to provide excellent sedation and analgesia in children.[33]

Table 86-10 Intravenous sedation techniques in children

Drug	Usual dose
Pentobarbital	2.5 mg/kg; may repeat up to 7.5 mg/kg; watch for apnea
Methohexital	0.5 to 1.0 mg/kg; may repeat as needed; watch for apnea
Midazolam	0.08 mg/kg; may follow with infusion at 0.04 to 0.12 mg/kg/hr
Propofol	1 to 2 mg/kg; may follow with infusion at 4 to 8 mg/kg/hr
Ketamine	0.5 to 1.0 mg/kg; may repeat as needed
Fentanyl	0.5 to 2.0 μg/kg

Reproduced from Greenberg CP, DeSoto H: Sedation Techniques. In Twersky RS, editor: *The ambulatory anesthesia handbook,* St. Louis, 1995, Mosby–Year Book.

SUMMARY

Performing sedation and analgesia during MAC requires vigilance and expertise equal to that of any other anesthesia technique. A complete preanesthetic evaluation is necessary which permits sufficient evaluation of the patient's medical and psychologic issues, before the procedure is undertaken. Drugs should be chosen with care and administered to provide the desired effect while attention should be paid to possible drug-induced side effects. Most important, MAC with sedation and analgesia should never become an uncontrolled general anesthetic. Understanding of all basic anesthetic principles are necessary for MAC with sedation and analgesia. If these principles are followed, a satisfactory result will be obtained for both the practitioner and the patient.

KEY POINTS

- The anesthesiologist should clearly understand that some MAC situations can involve the oldest, youngest, and/or most ill patients.
- Monitored anesthesia care is an opportunity to review the toxicity of local anesthetics, the total doses that should not be exceeded, and preparation for treatment of local anesthetic toxicity, including seizures and cardiovascular collapse.
- The challenge for the MAC provider is to ensure that "sedation" does not become "general anesthesia." If a deeper plane of anesthesia is required, practitioners should understand that sedation is a continuum, gain control of the airway and convert MAC into general anesthesia rather than risking hypoxia, hypoventilation, hypotension airway obstruction, or aspiration.
- It is important to review the pharmacology of the various sedatives as discussed in this and other chapters before participating in MAC.
- The vigilance requirement for MAC is at least as great if not greater than for other kinds of anesthesia.
- The opportunity exists for anesthesiologists to take the lead role in developing policies and providing services for "conscious sedation" outside the operating room and in nontraditional settings.

KEY REFERENCES

American Society of Anesthesiologists: Position on monitored anesthesia care, Park Ridge, 1986.

The American Society of Anesthesiologists: Guidelines for sedation and analgesia by non Anesthesiologists, Park Ridge, 1995.

Bailey PL, Pace NL, Ashburn MA, et al: Frequent hypoxemia and apnea after sedation with midazolam and fentanyl, *Anesthesiology* 73:826, 1990.

Cohen MM, Duncan PG, Tate RB: Does anesthesia contribute to operative mortality? *JAMA* 260:2859, 1988.

Kestin IG, Harvey PB, Nixon, et al: Psychomotor recovery after three methods of sedation during spinal anaesthesia, *Br J Anesth* 64:675, 1990.

Stoelting RK: *Pharmacology and physiology in anesthetic practice,* ed 2, Philadelphia, 1991, JB Lippincott.

Twersky RS: The Pharmacology of Anesthetics Used for Ambulatory Surgery, The American Society of Anesthesiologists, Vol 21, Philadelphia, 1993, JB Lippincott.

Urguhart ML, White PF: Comparison of sedative infusions during regional anesthesia-methohexital, etomidate, and midazolam, *Anesth Analg* 68:249, 1989.

White PF, Negus JB: Sedative infusions during local and regional anesthesia: a comparison of midazolam and propofol, *J Clin Anesth* 3:32, 1991.

REFERENCES

1. Allan MWB, Laurence AS, Gunawardena WJ: A comparison of two sedation techniques for neuroradiology, *Eur J Anesthesiol* 6:379, 1989.
2. American Academy of Pediatrics Committee on Drugs and Committee on Environmental Health: Use of chloral hydrate for sedation in children, *Pediatrics* 92:471, 1993.
3. Ali J, Weisel RD, Layug AB, et al: Consequences of postoperative alterations in respiratory mechanics, *Am J Surg* 128:376, 1974.
4. American Society of Anesthesiologists: Position on monitored anesthesia care, Park Ridge, 1986.
5. American Society of Anesthesiologists: Guidelines for sedation and analgesia by non-Anesthesiologists, Park Ridge, 1995.
6. Austin KL, Stapleton JV, Mather LE: Relationship between blood meperidine concentrations and analgesic response, *Anesthesiology* 53:460, 1980.
7. Bailey PL, Pace NL, Ashburn MA, et al: Frequent hypoxemia and apnea after sedation with midazolam and fentanyl, *Anesthesiology* 73:826, 1990.
8. Bailey PL, Stanley TH: Narcotic intravenous anesthetic. In Miller RD et al, editors: *Anesthesia,* ed 4, New York, 1994, Churchill-Livingstone.
9. Baird ES, Hailey DM: Delayed recovery from a sedative: correlation of the plasma levels of diazepam with clinical effects after oral and intravenous administration, *Br J Anaesth* 44:803, 1972.
10. Bigger JT, Fleiss JL, Kleiger R, et al: The relationships among ventricular arrhythmias, left ventricular dysfunction, and mortality in the two years after myocardial infarction, *Circulation* 69:250, 1984.
11. Blackburn H, Katigbak R: What ECG leads to monitor after exercise, *Am Heart J* 67:184, 1964.
12. Blery C, Charpak Y, Szatan M, et al: Evaluation of a protocol for selective ordering of preoperative tests, *Lancet* 1:139, 1986.
13. Boldy DAR, English JSC, Lang, et al: Sedation for endoscopy. A comparison between diazepam plus pethidine with naloxone reversal, *Br J Anesth* 56:1109; 1994.
14. Campbell RL: Prevention of complications associated with intravenous sedation and general anesthesia, *J Oral Maxillofac Surg* 44:289, 1986.
15. Caplan RA, Ward RJ, Posner K, et al: Unexpected cardiac arrest during spinal anesthesia: a closed claims analysis of predisposing factors, *Anesthesiology* 68:5, 1988.
16. Charpak Y, Blery C, Chastang C, et al: Prospective assessment of a protocol for selective ordering of preoperative chest x-rays, *Can J Anaesth* 35:259, 1988.
17. Cohen MM, Duncan PG, Tate RB: Does anesthesia contribute to operative mortality? *JAMA* 260:2859, 1988.
18. Cohen MM, Duncan PG: Physical status score and trends in anesthetic complications, *J Clin Epidemiol* 41:83, 1988.
19. De Souza DB, Schmidt WK, Kukor MJ: Nalbuphine: an autoradiographic opioid receptor binding profile in the central nervous system of an agonist/antagonist analgesic, *J Pharmacol Exp Ther* 244:391, 1988.
20. Dixon J, Power SJ, Grundy EM, et al: Sedation for local anaesthesia. Comparison of intravenous midazolam and diazepam, *Anaesthesia* 39:372, 1984.
21. Domar AD, Everett LL, Keller MG: Preoperative anxiety: is it a predictable entity? *Anesth Analg* 69:763, 1989.
22. Dundee JW, Pandit SK: Anterograde amnesic effects of pethidine, hyoscine, and diazepam in adults, *Br J Pharmacol* 44:593, 1972.
23. Dunphy JA: Accuracy of expired carbon dioxide partial pressure sampled from a nasal cannula, II, *Anesthesiology* 68:960, 1988.
24. Easton PA, Jadue C, Dhingra S, et al: A comparison of the bronchodilating effects of a beta-2 adrenergic agent (albuterol) and an anticholinergic agent (ipratropium bromide) given by aerosol alone or in sequence, *N Engl J Med* 315:735, 1986.
25. Elsass P, Duedahl H, Friis B, et al: The psychological effects of having a contact-person from the anesthesia staff, *Acta Anesthesiol Scand* 31:584, 1987.
26. Feld LH, Negus JB: Oral midazolam for pre anesthetic medication in pediatric patients, *Anesthesiology* 73:831, 1990.
27. Flacke JW, Flacke WE, Williams GD: Acute pulmonary edema following naloxone reversal of high dose morphine anesthesia, *Anesthesiology* 47:376, 1977.
28. Frieseu RH, Lochart CH: Oral transmucosal fentanyl citrate for preanesthetic medication of pediatric day surgery patients with and without droperidol as prophylactic antiemetic, *Anesthesiology* 76:46, 1992.
29. Gal TJ, Di Fazio CA: Ventilatory and analgesic effect of dezocine in humans, *Anesthesiology* 61:716, 1984.
30. Gold BS, Young ML, Kinman JL, et al: The utility of preoperative electrocardiogram in the ambulatory surgery patient, *Arch Intern Med* 152:301, 1992.
31. Goldman JM: A simple, easy, and inexpensive method for monitoring $EtCO_2$ through nasal cannulae, *Anesthesiology* 67:606, 1987.
32. Goldman L, Caldera DL, Southwick FS, et al: Cardiac risk factors and complications in noncardiac surgery, *Medicine* 57:357, 1978.
33. Green SM, Johnson NE: Ketamine sedation for pediatric procedures: review and implications, *Ann Emerg Med* 19:1033, 1990.
34. Greenberg AG, Saik RP, Pridham D: Influence of age on mortality of colon surgery, *Am J Surg* 150:65, 1985.

35 Health Care Advisory Board: Ambulatory

Care: The movement of ambulatory surgery procedures to less-intensive settings, Issue Tracking Service Project #3, Chicago, July 1995.
36. Kallar SM: Conscious Sedation in Ambulatory Surgery, *Anesth Rev* 17(supp 2):45, 1990.
37. Kaplan EB, Sheiner LB, Boeckmann AJ, et al: The usefulness of preoperative laboratory screening, *JAMA* 253:3576, 1985.
38. Kaukinen S, Kataja J, Kaukinen L: Antagonism of benzodiazepine-fentanyl anesthesia with flumazenil, *Can J Anaesth* 37:40, 1990.
38a. Kestin IG, Harvey PB, Nixon, et al: Psychomotor recovery after three methods of sedation during spinal anaesthesia, *Br J Anesth* 64:675, 1990.
39. Klein DS: Nalbuphine and droperidol combination for local standby sedation, *Anesthesiology* 43:397, 1982.
40. Knight AA, Hollenberg M, London MJ, et al: Perioperative myocardial ischemia: importance of the preoperative ischemic pattern, *Anesthesiology* 68:681, 1988.
41. Kotter GS, Kotrly KJ, Kalbfleisch JH, et al: Myocardial ischemia during cardiovascular surgery as detected by an ST-segment trend monitoring system, *J Cardiothorac Anesth* 1:190, 1987.
42. Krishnan A, Tolhurst-Cleaver CL, King B: Controlled comparison of nalbuphine and morphine for post-tonsillectomy pain, *Anaesthesia* 40:1178, 1985.
43. Lee W, Worthington J, Zahl K: An evaluation of alfentanil vs propofol for sedation in monitored anesthesia care during arthroscopy (abstract), Eighth SAMBA Annual Meeting, 1993.
44. Lichenstein R, King JC, Bice D: Evaluation of chloral hydrate for pediatric sedation, *Clin Pediatr* 32:632, 1993.
45. Macario A, Roizen MF, Thisted RA, et al: Reassessment of preoperative laboratory testing has changed the test-ordering patterns of physicians, *Surg Gynecol Obstet* 175:539, 1992.
46. Mackenzie N, Grant IS: Propofol for intravenous sedation, *Anaesthesia* 42:3, 1987.
47. Macpherson DS, Snow R, Lolfgren RP: Preoperative screening: value of previous tests, *Ann Intern Med* 113:969, 1990.
48. Mandelli M, Tognoni G, Garattini S: Clinical pharmacokinetics of diazepam, *Clin Pharmaco* 3:72, 1978.
49. Mangano DT, Goldman L: Current concepts: preoperative assessment of patients with known or suspected coronary disease, *N Engl J Med* 333:1750, 1995.
50. Mangano DT: Perioperative cardiac morbidity, *Anesthesiology* 72:153, 1990.
51. Milligan KR, Howe JP, McLoughlin J, et al: Midazolam sedation for outpatient fiberoptic endoscopy: evaluation of alfentanil supplementation, *Ann R Coll Surg Engl* 70:303, 1988.
52. Mohr DN: Estimation of surgical risk in the elderly: a correlative review, *J Am Geriatr Soc* 31:99, 1983.
53. Monk TG, Boure B, White PF, et al: Comparison of intravenous sedation—analgesic techniques for outpatient immersion lithotripsy, *Anesth Analg* 62:616, 1991.
54. Monk TG, Rater JM, White PF: Comparison of alfentanil and ketamine infusions in combination with midazolam for outpatient lithotripsy, *Anesth Analg* 74:1023, 1991.
55. Mooman JR, Hlatky MA, Eddy DM, et al: The yield of the routine admission electrocardiogram: a study in a general medical service, *Ann Intern Med* 103:590, 1985.
56. Morrison RC: Hypothermia in the elderly, *Intern Anesthesiol Clin* 26:124, 1988.
57. Multicenter Postinfarction Research Group: Risk stratification and survival after myocardial infarction, *N Engl J Med* 309:331, 1983.
58. Narr BJ, Hansen TR, Warner M: Preoperative laboratory screening in health Mayo patients: cost-effective elimination of tests and unchanged outcomes, *Mayo Clin Proc* 66:155, 1991.
59. Natof HE: Federated Ambulatory Surgery Association: Special Study 1, Alexandria, 1986.
60. Oei-Lim VL, Kalkman CJ, Bouvy-Berends EC, et al : A comparison of effects of propofol and nitrous oxide on the electroencephalogram in epileptic patients during conscious sedation for dental procedures, *Anesth Analg* 75:708, 1992.
61. Ochs MW, Tucker MR, White RP: A comparison of amnesia in outpatients sedated with midazolam or diazepam alone or in combination with fentanyl during oral surgery, *J Am Dent Assoc* 113:894, 1986.
62. Persson MP, Nilsson A, Hartvig P: Relationship of sedation and amnesia to plasma concentrations of midazolam in surgical patients, *Clin Pharmacol Ther* 43:324, 1988.
63. Persson P, Nilsson A, Hartvig P, et al: Pharmacokinetics of midazolam in total IV anesthesia, *Br J Anaesth* 59:548, 1987.
64. Rao TK, Jacobs KH, El-Etr AA: Reinfarction following anesthesia in patients with myocardiac infarction, *Anesthesiology* 59:499, 1983.
65. Reisine T, Pasternak G: Opioid analgesics and antagonists. In Hardman JG, Lee E, Limbrid, editors: *Goodman & Gilman's, The pharmacological basis of therapeutics,* ed 9, New York, 1995, McGraw-Hill.
66. Roizen MF, et al: The relative roles of the history and physical examination, and laboratory testing in preoperative evaluation for outpatient surgery: the "Starling" curve of preoperative laboratory testing, *Anesth Clin North Am* 5:15, 1987.
67. Rowlingson JC, Moscicki JC, Di Fazio C: Anesthetic potency of dezocine and its interaction with morphine in rats, *Anesth Analg* 62:899, 1983.
68. Scamman FL, Klein SL, Chio WW: Conscious sedation for procedures under local or topical anesthesia, *Ann Otol Rhinol Laryngol* 94:21, 1985.
69. Shane SM: *Conscious sedation for ambulatory surgery,* Baltimore, 1983, University Park Press, pp. 1–11.
70. Sherry E: Admixture of propofol and alfentanil. Use for intravenous sedation and analgesia during transvaginal oocyte retrieval, *Anaesthesia* 47:477, 1992.
71. Soliman IE, Broadman LM, Hannallah RS, McGill WA: Comparison of analgesic effects of EMLA (eutectic mixture of local anesthetics) to intradermal lidocaine infiltration prior to venous cannulation in unpremedicated children, *Anesthesiology* 68: 804, 1988.
72. Stoelting RK: *Pharmacology and physiology in anesthetic practice,* ed 2, Philadelphia, 1991, JB Lippincott, p. 131.
73. Sury MRJ, Cole PV: Nalbuphine combined with midazolam for outpatient sedation, *Anaesthesia* 43:281, 1988.
74. Tape TG, Mushlin AI: The utility of routine chest radiographs, *Ann Intern Med* 104:63, 1986.
75. Tinker JH, Dull DL, Caplan RA, et al: Role of monitoring devices in prevention of anesthetic mishaps: a closed claims analysis, *Anesthesiology* 71:541, 1989.
76. Tisi GM: Preoperative evaluation of pulmonary function: validity, indications, and benefits, *Am Rev Resp Dis* 119:293, 1979.
77. Turnbull JM, Buck C: The value of preoperative screening investigations in otherwise healthy individuals, *Arch Intern Med* 147:1101, 1987.
78. Twersky RS: *The pharmacology of anesthetics used for ambulatory surgery,* The American Society of Anesthesiologists, Vol 21, Philadelphia, 1993, JB Lippincott.
79. Twersky RS, Berger BJ, McClain J, Beaton C: Midazolam enhances anterograde but not retrograde amnesia in pediatric patients, *Anesthesiology* 78:51, 1993.
80. Urmey WF: Accuracy of expired carbon dioxide partial pressure samples from a nasal cannula, I, *Anesthesiology* 68:959, 1988.
81. Urguhart ML, White PF: Comparison of sedative infusions during regional anesthesia-methohexital, etomidate, and midazolam, *Anesth Analg* 68:249, 1989.
82. Vangerven M, Van Hemelrijck J, Wouters B, et al: Light anaesthesia with propofol for paediatric MRI, *Anaesthesia* 47:706, 1992.
83. White PF, Shafer A, Boyle WA, et al: Benzodiazepine antagonism does not evoke a stress response, *Anesthesiology* 70:636, 1989.
84. White PF, Negus JB: Sedative infusions during local and regional anesthesia: a comparison of midazolam and propofol, *J Clin Anesth* 3:32, 1991.
85. Wohlgelernter D, Cleman M, Highman HA: Regional myocardial dysfunction during coronary angioplasty: evaluation by two dimensional echocardiography and 12-lead electrocardiography, *J Am Coll Cardiol* 7:1245, 1986.
86. Zacny JP, Lichtor JL, Coalson DW, et al: Subjective and psychomotor effects of subanesthetic doses of propofol in healthy volunteers, *Anesthesiology* 76:696, 1992.

CHAPTER 87

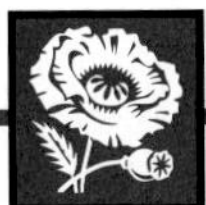

Anesthesia for Nonsurgical Procedures

ROBERT B. FORBES

Advances in medical technology have provided physicians and their patients with a rapidly growing variety of new sophisticated diagnostic and therapeutic techniques. These procedures, such as computed tomography (CT), magnetic resonance imaging (MRI), interventional angiography, and external-beam radiation therapy allow detailed anatomic imaging of pathologic states and precise treatment of a variety of medical problems. Although they are extremely useful, these procedures are not without risk and present physicians with a variety of clinical problems that should be overcome. Increasingly, anesthesia providers are called upon to care for patients undergoing these types of procedures, usually in locations far from the main operating room suite (and therefore distant from rapidly available colleague assistance in the event of difficulty). The demands placed on the anesthesia care team range from monitored anesthesia care (MAC) in a conscious patient to intravenous (IV) sedation or general anesthesia. Providing anesthesia in these remote, often unfamiliar, areas can be a difficult and intimidating task. **The challenge for the anesthesia team is to overcome the obstacles encountered and ensure that safe, effective anesthesia care is provided. Because there are solid medical reasons for the procedures and examinations and because the equipment needed to perform them can seldom be moved to our familiar anesthetizing locations, we should be prepared to provide quality services under challenging conditions.**

GENERAL CONSIDERATIONS FOR ANESTHESIA CARE OUTSIDE THE OPERATING ROOM

Indications for Anesthesia Involvement

There are a number of reasons why anesthesia teams become involved in care for patients undergoing procedures outside the operating room. Although most of these procedures are not painful, sufficient discomfort may occur, even in adults and older children, that patients require appropriate doses of sedatives or analgesics. In younger children, effective sedation is often difficult to achieve, is unpredictable in duration, and may be associated with troublesome side effects. Indeed, general anesthesia may be required to ensure not only that the patient will tolerate the procedure, but also remain sufficiently still for the time required to allow successful completion of the study. General anesthesia may also be required for children or adults who become claustrophobic when placed in scanning equipment (which can occur without warning), and for patients who are either mentally impaired or for whom communication and cooperation is difficult. Patients with movement disorders that interfere with a scanning procedure or painful conditions that prevent them from lying still for prolonged periods also may require general anesthesia. The same is true for some patients with serious medical problems or traumatic injuries requiring intense monitoring during the procedure. Patients who are at risk for serious allergic reactions to the contrast material used to augment many diagnostic scans may also require anesthesia care team attention.

Facilities

Several factors combine to make anesthesia providers uncomfortable when caring for patients in locations outside the operating room. In most instances, the room to be used was not designed with the needs of the anesthesia team in mind. In addition to being distant from the main operating suite, "satellite" anesthetizing locations may lack pipeline O_2, N_2O, suction and gas evacuation systems. Before providing care in such conditions, each potential problem should be identified and resolved. This may entail modification of the existing structure and equipment. In addition, the anesthesia provider may be required to transport necessary anesthesia equipment from the central operating room. Sometimes, there is a tendency for the anesthesia provider to simply try to "fit in" (i.e., "not make waves"). This situation could prove tragic (and costly).

The size and design of the procedure room, and the presence of the radiation source, cameras, angiographic equipment, fluoroscopy C-arms, scanners, and laser devices can make access to the patient difficult. It is imperative, therefore, to have a clear understanding of the procedure, including: (1) the patient's position; (2) need for contrast material; (3) placement of anesthesia gas machine; (4) whether or not the anesthesia provider can remain in the room during the procedure; and (5) the effect the diagnostic or therapeutic equipment may have on essential anesthesia monitoring. Patient monitoring will be further complicated if the room should be kept dark. Suitable lighting to observe the patient, the anesthesia machine, and the monitors should be provided. This condition is something that should be insisted upon by the anesthesia provider. An answer of, "Just a minute, we'll turn the lights on" will not suffice. Finally, nonanesthesia personnel employed in these areas are usually less familiar with the needs of the anesthetized patient than are operating room personnel and so may be less able to provide adequate support in the event of a medical emergency or when anesthesia equipment fails.

Anesthesia Equipment

Anesthesia equipment and supplies required to care for patients in remote locations should be of the same standard as the equipment and supplies used in the main operating room and should receive identical preventive maintenance. The common tendency of some administrators to place older outmoded equipment in these areas because of relatively infrequent usage is a violation of JCAH standards. It also violates common sense, because an emergency or equipment failure in a remote location with less help than can usually be called upon in the main operating room suite, is a potential disaster. Many administrators now understand that state-of-the-art equipment needs to be used in these remote areas. Also, the cost of a modern anesthesia machine should be compared with even rather ordinary radiologic equipment.

Absence of pipeline gases may require working with cylinder-supplied machines and provision for rapid replacement of depleted cylinders should be made. Suction and evacuation for waste gases also should be available. A mobile anesthetic cart that contains necessary drugs and equipment for airway management, IV placement, monitoring, induction and maintenance of anesthesia, recovery, and patient resuscitation and transport is extremely useful. Limitations imposed on the function of existing monitoring systems when working near an MRI should be considered when choosing anesthesia equipment. The equipment may be permanently located at the remote location or may be portable and transported to the area when needed. The frequency with which anesthesia is provided in a remote location determines which arrangement is most appropriate. **The practice of using "hand-me-down," obsolete equipment in these areas should be condemned. The anesthesia provider working so far from colleagues who can help in true emergencies needs the best possible equipment.**

Monitoring

The American Society of Anesthesiologists (ASA) standards for basic monitoring during general anesthesia or MAC are the same for all patients regardless of where the procedure is performed.[7,87,103,107] The American Academy of Pediatrics (AAP) and the American Academy of Pediatric Dentistry (AAPD) have developed similar guidelines.[61,63] In certain circumstances, for example during MRI and external-beam radiation, some of the basic monitoring techniques may be ineffective or impractical. Every effort should be made to ensure that the patient is appropriately monitored during the procedure. This includes assessments of oxygenation, ventilation, circulation, and body temperature.

Appropriate monitoring of oxygenation requires adequate illumination and access so that the patient's color can be assessed. A dark room makes recognition of cyanosis difficult. The anesthesia machine should include an O_2 analyzer. Pulse oximetry is highly desirable if not mandatory. Adequacy of ventilation may be evaluated using clinical signs which include chest movement, observation of reservoir bag, and auscultation of breath sounds. Quantitative techniques, such as measurement of the volume of expired gas or end-tidal CO_2, are also recommended. If capnometry is in use for general anesthesia in the operating room then it is reasonable and proper that the same standard should be applied in remote anesthetizing locations. If an endotracheal tube is used, correct placement should be verified and when ventilation is controlled, a modern disconnect alarm should be incorporated into the breathing circuit. Circulatory function should be monitored with continuous electrocardiography (ECG), auscultation of heart sounds, and frequent determinations of blood pressure and pulse. Because these "satellite" areas are air-conditioned to protect the computerized components of the CT or MRI scanner, changes in body temperature should be anticipated and patient temperature monitored.

During external-beam radiation, all personnel should leave the room during the period of radiation exposure. Monitoring should continue from outside the room, either through a window or with remote-controlled cameras that provide views of both the patient and monitoring equipment. A microphone or electronic stethoscope allows breath sounds to be monitored in sedated or anesthetized patients,[70] when the anesthesia provider is outside the room. Simply "hoping" that the patient's condition will not change during the "short time" of the procedure, with the anesthesia provider waiting blindly outside the procedure room, is unacceptable.

Preanesthesia Evaluation

Patients who require monitored anesthesia care, sedation, or general anesthesia for diagnostic or therapeutic procedures outside the main operating room require the same preanesthetic evaluation as patients undergoing surgical procedures. Ideally, the evaluation and preparation of these patients should be discussed with the physicians in charge of the patient's ongoing care so that an organized approach to scheduling, preanesthetic evaluation, informed consent, and postanesthetic recovery can be established. This prevents unnecessary delays and avoids compromises in patient care that can occur when organization has been neglected and left to the last minute. It is not valid to hope that a "standard" sedation method will work, and expect anesthesia personnel to respond immediately, without prior notice, if this method is unsuccessful.

Postanesthesia Care

After anesthesia or sedation, patients cared for outside the operating room require the same recovery care as other surgical patients.[7,87,103] Recovery may take place in a postanesthesia care unit at the remote site or patients may be transported to the main operating room's postanesthesia care unit. Simply "observing" patients out in the hallway is unacceptable. The postanesthesia care unit may be a long distance and involve transportation of the patient in an ambulance, elevator, or other areas away from support services and personnel. During transport, appropriate monitoring should be continued. Gurneys or other transport equipment that facilitate use of monitors, supplemental O_2 and airway equipment, IV infusions, plus resuscitative drugs and equipment will likely be required. Adequately trained personnel should be available to ensure that transport is safely and efficiently completed. The same criteria for discharge from the recovery area that apply to surgical patients should be used for patients recovering outside the main operating room.[7,61,63,87,107]

These problems should be resolved before initiating anesthetic services in any remote area. Modification of existing facilities, provision of necessary support services and equipment, education of involved personnel, and establishment of agreed-upon scheduling of procedures should be accomplished before these "satellite" services are undertaken. When the problems of unfamiliar surroundings, procedures, and personnel have been solved, attention can be focused on the requirements of individual patients.

SPECIFIC PROCEDURES

Radiology: Diagnostic and Interventional

Computed tomography

Principles. Computed tomography has been available for more than 25 years and has improved the diagnosis of many disorders by providing rapid, noninvasive evaluations.[1,145] CT produces an image using ionizing radiation that detects variations in densities of different body tissues.[146] The x-ray sources and the detectors are mounted opposite each other on a gantry with the patient situated between them. During a single scan, multiple readings of radiation transmission through a single body plane are taken; then the system rotates in small increments and the process is repeated until a rotation of 180° has occurred. Individual readings of transmission are collected and stored. When all "cuts" have been completed, the data are processed by computer to produce images. CT scanning is extremely sensitive to changes in tissue density, recognized as small differences in absorption. It is this capacity to differentiate variations in tissue density that is the major advantage of CT scanning over conventional radiography and permits precise visualization of anatomic structures.

Clinical uses. Computed tomography was first used for scanning the head and was useful in diagnosis of neoplasms, vascular abnormalities, intracranial bleeding or infarction, cerebral edema, contusion, and hydrocephalus.[96] Over the years, CT scanning has been extended to all body parts and can be used, for example, to diagnose thoracic and mediastinal masses,[134] lung abscesses,[144] aortic injuries,[56] and determine the patency of coronary artery bypass grafts.[55] CT scanning is also useful in evaluation of intra-abdominal pathologic conditions, including traumatic injuries,[42] abscesses,[44] staging of gastrointestinal tract malignancies,[136] and imaging of pancreas,[83] liver, and biliary tract.[77] The kidney and retroperitoneum[74] can also be evaluated with CT scans, as can spinal or pelvic fractures and prolapsed intervertebral discs.[147] Because CT scanning is used in such a diverse group of conditions, patients who require anesthesia care during CT scanning will present wide varieties of medical problems.

Although CT scanning is not painful, the patient should remain still to prevent image degradation by motion artifact. Early scanners required more than 4 minutes to complete a single "cut." Newer units can complete each "cut" in less than 2 seconds. With rapid imaging of this type, excellent CT scans can usually be completed in less than 30 minutes, but this can be a very long time for some patients.

Anesthetic considerations. Because CT is a short, painless procedure that usually requires less than 30 minutes to complete, few adults require anesthesia when undergoing routine CT scanning. Young children, patients unable to cooperate, and patients with movement disorders, severe pain, or traumatic or medical conditions that require intensive monitoring during the procedure, may benefit from anesthetic intervention. Although many techniques can provide good conditions for CT scanning, some agents have been associated with problems. Ferrer-Brechner and Winter found that use of ketamine was associated with profuse salivation and unpredictable, involuntary movements that sometimes resulted in technically unsatisfactory scans.[43] Similar problems have occurred when etomidate was used.[99]

In an attempt to avoid use of general anesthesia, radiologists and cardiologists frequently try to develop a sedation "recipe" that can be used for most pediatric patients. There are a variety of such "recipes" for sedating or anesthetizing children for CT scanning and each has its advocates. The youngest children (i.e., less than 6 months of age) can often be satisfactorily immobilized by bundling them snugly in a blanket and allowing them to suck on a pacifier without using any pharmacologic sedation. In older children (up to approximately 5 years of age), some type of sedation or general anesthesia is frequently required.[62,106] Although many different sedation regimens have been reported with enthusiasm, all have unsatisfying failure rates and all are also associated with potentially serious complications.[92,137,141,150] Chloral hydrate has been used for many years, but supplemental medication or restraints may often be required to adequately immobilize children who receive only chloral hydrate.[43,92,137] Large doses of chloral hydrate almost always result in sedation greatly prolonged after the procedure, with discharge delayed. Recent concerns regarding the use of chloral hydrate for sedation of children have resulted in the publication of new cautions and recommendations.[133,138]

Numerous combinations of medications have been used for sedation before scans, including narcotics, barbiturates, anticholinergics, major tranquilizers, and benzodiazepines.[4,16,82,137] These "lytic cocktails" have varying degrees of success, numerous adverse reactions, and often produce deepest sedation after the procedure has been completed. Thompson et al.[137] reported that the average time required to achieve adequate sedation with the combination of intramuscular (IM) atropine, meperidine, promethazine, and secobarbital was 53 minutes; more than 10% of the children required supplemental sedation, and in 12% of patients, the CT scan was unsatisfactory. Burckart et al.[16] found that 14% of CT scans were unsatisfactory in children who received a combination of chlorpromazine, promethazine, and meperidine. In these children, the duration of sedation exceeded 7 hours. Mitchell et al.[92] reported serious adverse reactions following various types of premedication for CT scanning in 13 of 106 pediatric patients 5 hours to 16 years of age. Life-threatening cardiorespiratory depression occurred in four of the children, and other adverse reactions included CNS depression, behavioral changes, and vomiting. Severe adverse reactions were most likely to occur in children less than 3 months of age and in children who received large doses of medication or combinations of several drugs. The usefulness of lytic cocktails that combine opioids, antihistamines, and phenothiazines has repeatedly and recently been questioned, and new recommendations have been published.[25,110,131]

Use of IM for children undergoing CT scanning has been reported safe and effective. Varner et al.[139] reported a sleep time of 3.3 minutes after administration of 10 mg/kg IM methohexital. Although four of 50 children required supplemental medication for movement during the scan, no complications, except pain on injection, were noted. The children were awake and alert after an average of 86 minutes.

Rectal methohexital is also safe and effective for anesthetizing children.[48,49,50,57,85] It is simple, with relatively rapid onset, appropriate duration of action, and minimal effect on respiratory[81] and cardiovascular function[49] in healthy children. With either rectal or IM methohexital (once the child is asleep), care should be taken so that airway obstruction does not occur. Occasionally, patients who receive rectal methohexital become apneic, and its use has been associated with seizures in susceptible patients.[115] Rectal methohexital does not provide analgesia; patients may respond to painful stimuli, such as placement of an IV catheter. Response to venipuncture can be minimized by the application of EMLA cream—a eutectic mixture of lidocaine and prilocaine—to the skin 30 to 60 minutes prior to placing the IV catheter.[65,113,126] To improve the local anesthetic effect and increase penetration into the dermis, an occlusive dressing should be placed over the cream. Prolonged exposure and application of large amounts of EMLA should be avoided because the prilocaine can cause methemoglobinemia.[51] Also, EMLA should not be applied to mucous membranes.[98]

Rectal methohexital should be considered a general anesthetic, not simply sedation, and appropriate monitoring should be used throughout the scanning procedure. Equipment to control the airway and maintain ventilation and oxygenation should be available.

In addition to IM or IV sedation[2,118,135] and rectal methohexital, general anesthesia with N_2O and/or a potent inhalation agent[43] is also effective to ensure that patients remain immobile during the diagnostic procedure. General anesthesia avoids long induction times and important failure rates associated with rectal or IM medication, has a low incidence of side effects, and provides prompt recovery and discharge from the hospital when the procedure is completed.[94] Anesthesia may be maintained using a continuous IV infusion of propofol or a volatile agent administered by face mask, laryngeal mask airway (LMA), or endotracheal tube, depending on the clinical circumstances. The incidence of complications associated with general anesthesia for CT scanning is no greater than that seen with most sedation regimens and the incidence of technical artifacts or nondiagnostic scans is less.

Contrast media. The images produced by CT and a variety of other radiologic techniques can often be enhanced by administration of contrast media. Because of their physiologic effects and the high incidence of untoward and/or allergic reactions, it is important that anesthesia providers be familiar with effects of contrast media and possible side effects. Approximately 5% to 8% of radiographic studies using contrast media are complicated by adverse systemic reactions.[54,122] The incidence of reactions depends on the specific radiographic study, the type and dose of dye, the method of injection, and the patient's history of allergic and/or cardiovascular disease. Until 1984, adverse reactions to contrast media during general anesthesia were rarely reported. Since then, reactions to both ionic and nonionic contrast media have also been noted in patients during general anesthesia. Although most adverse reactions are mild and require no treatment, severe and fatal reactions can occur.[123]

Contrast media are salts formed by combining iodine-containing anions with a variety of different cations.[46] The contrast effect is related to the density of the compound. Iodine is a basic constituent (24% to 99%) of most contrast media because of its high density and low toxicity. Ninety-nine percent of the iodine is rapidly bound to organic cations that are filtered at the glomerulus and do not undergo renal tubular reabsorption. Many dyes are hypertonic with an osmolarity that may exceed 2000 mOsm/l.

Among the most important effects of hypertonic contrast media are changes in intravascular volume and osmolality that result in hemodynamic changes unrelated to other systemic reactions. Following infusion of a hypertonic radiographic contrast solution, there is an initial, transient hypertensive response. This is accompanied by an increase in intravascular volume, central venous pressure (CVP), pulmonary artery (PA) pressure, and cardiac output as well as by decreased systemic vascular resistance.[24,72] Serum osmolality may be increased, and the hemoglobin and hematocrit may decrease.[19,93] The increased osmolarity causes an osmotic diuresis, which may later lead to relative hypovolemia and/or acute bladder distention. Equilibration of intravascular and extracellular fluid compartments occurs over 10 minutes after contrast injection, as the medium is excreted by the kidney, and osmolality and intravascular volume return to normal. Excretion of contrast media may be delayed in patients with renal dysfunction. These hemodynamic changes are most important in patients with impaired cardiovascular function.

Radiographic contrast material can also affect the cardiovascular system through mechanisms unrelated to hypertonicity. These effects include dysrhythmias and ischemia in healthy patients and decreased ionized calcium levels producing a negative inotropic effect and interfering with conduction.[72,105,149] The incidence of side effects is substantially greater in patients with preexisting heart disease.[5] Other important side effects of the contrast agents include shrinking and clumping of erythrocytes, competition for protein-binding sites with other medications, and interference with complement and coagulation systems by binding to and activating system proteins.[19,120,127] Contrast material is also known to penetrate the blood–brain barrier leading to seizures and can cause pulmonary edema and cardiac arrest. The effect of contrast on the hypothalamus contributes to chills, fever, nausea, vomiting, dysrhythmias, and bronchospasm, all of which are manifestations of contrast toxicity.[80]

Of great concern during use of contrast agents are the idiosyncratic reactions that occur. Nausea, vomiting, and urticaria seen frequently after intravascular injection of contrast media are usually benign and short-lived, but can be prodromal signs of a severe anaphylactic reaction. Chills, fever, and cutaneous flushing are also common reactions that may be accompanied by feelings of anxiety and restlessness in awake patients. Although these initial symptoms usually do not progress to more serious reactions, it is important that they are noticed by the anesthesia provider, particularly when monitoring a sedated patient covered with drapes in a dark room.

The most serious idiosyncratic reactions include hypotension, tachycardia, or dysrhythmias, which may be the first signs of acute toxic responses.[79] Anaphylactic shock and airway edema are serious manifestations that can occur immediately upon injection of contrast agent or may appear several hours after the procedure. These changes may progress rapidly to airway obstruction and bronchospasm, compromising oxygenation and ventilation, and rarely can result in death.[75,122,123]

Patients who have experienced previous reactions or who have histories of allergic or cardiovascular disease may be at greater risk of having severe systemic reactions to contrast material. Although it has been suggested that a small test dose or use of prophylactic medication may prevent life-threatening reactions, neither pretesting nor use of premedication has, in fact, been shown to decrease or prevent occurrence of adverse reactions. Therefore, all studies that require contrast media carry the risk of adverse, potentially life-threatening reactions. Prior history of successful contrast media exposure is certainly no guarantee of similar nonreaction next time. A well-equipped emergency cart and appropriate resuscitation equipment should be immediately available to personnel proficient in the diagnosis and treatment of reactions to contrast material.

Mild reactions to contrast media are effectively treated with fluid replacement, observation, and patient reassurance. More severe reactions, including hypotension, bronchospasm, or anaphylaxis, require more aggressive monitoring and treatment. Blood pressure, pulse, and ECG should be monitored and IV access ensured. Oxygen should be administered to all such patients. Depending on the patient's condition, medications frequently recommended for the management of anaphylactoid reactions to contrast media include adrenergic agonists, methylxanthines, anticholinergics, antihistamines, and corticosteroids.[54]

In recent years, several new low-osmolality agents have become available, and although expensive, may be safer and better tolerated by patients.[30,34,128,142,148] Some radiologists believe there is a significant reduction in the incidence of nausea and vomiting, flushing and urticaria, cardiovascular reactions, and central nervous system (CNS) symptoms, particularly in high-risk patients, when low-osmolality contrast medium is used. Other radiologists contend that improved patient safety with low-osmolality contrast media remains unproved. Numerous studies have found no significant differences between high-osmolality agents and the newer low-osmolality media when incidences of serious reactions, such as renal failure, bronchospasm, or anaphylaxis, were compared. Low-osmolality agents may be indicated in patients with hemoglobinopathies, ischemic heart disease with shock or heart failure, pulmonary hypertension, or a history of previous reaction to high-osmolality agents.

Magnetic resonance imaging

Principles. MRI is a diagnostic technique that has become increasingly important during the past 10 years because it does not use ionizing radiation, it produces high-resolution, multiplane cross-sectional images of the body, it requires little preparation, and it is well accepted by most patients.[23,26] MRI uses the magnetic properties of atomic nuclei to generate images and to provide information about the characteristics of the tissues imaged.

All nuclei possess an intrinsic angular momentum or "spin" caused by the rotation of protons or neutrons. In nuclei with equally paired neutrons or protons, a balance occurs producing a net spin of zero. In contrast, nuclei with an odd number of protons (e.g., ^{1}H, ^{31}P, ^{23}Na, ^{13}C) have an associated electrical charge; the net rotation of these elements produces a magnetic field. Unless influenced by an outside force, the individual magnetic fields surrounding these nuclei are randomly oriented, but when placed in a strong magnetic field, the nuclei align themselves (and therefore their electric charges) parallel to the static magnetic field.

MRI makes use of this phenomenon by placing the patient into a powerful cylindrical magnet. Within this magnetic tube are coils surrounding the patient that transmit radio waves and also act as a radio receiver. To produce nuclear resonance, specific radio frequency (RF) pulses are directed toward the patient from the transmitter coil. The RF pulse exerts torque on the aligned nuclei, displacing them from their orientation parallel to the static magnetic field. When the pulse is terminated, the nuclei return to their magnetic alignment positions. It takes a known, specific period of time for this return to occur, during which an electromagnetic (radio frequency) signal is emitted by the nucleus and detected by the receiver coil. This RF signal is used to produce the MRI. These "return to alignment" or "recovery" times are sensitive to inherent tissue properties and can be used to distinguish normal from pathologic tissue. Specific atomic nuclei respond (i.e., resonate), to certain radio frequencies and the response is proportional to the strength of the static magnetic field. By placing the patient in a gradient magnetic field, the response to a specific frequency can be used to define a distance along the body. This allows the body to be scanned in successive cuts, similar to CT scans. An image is constructed by computer from received signals. Resolution of the image depends on strength of the magnetic field (most are 0.5 to 1.5 Tesla). It is the great strength of this static magnetic field that introduces numerous problems and hazards for the anesthesia personnel who must care for patients during MRI.[100,141]

Clinical uses. MRI is a revolutionary technique for evaluation of the CNS because fine-resolution and multiplane images can be obtained.[28,84] It is of particular value for evaluating posterior fossa tumors because of the absence of bony artifacts and for detecting and localizing cerebral infarction. MRI is also useful in the assessment of head trauma, dementia, and intracranial infections[29] and has been used to study the effects of anesthesia on the brain.[97,143]

MRI of the spinal canal has advantages over myelography because it provides a direct, noninvasive image.[28] MRI can also be used for imaging the heart and great vessels because a unique signal is generated by movement of blood. This allows visualization of cardiac chambers and vessel lumina without use of contrast medium. It does require ECG–gated or cine MRI and does not replace coronary angiography in evaluation of ischemic heart disease.[27,47] MRI can also be used to evaluate a variety of intrathoracic[13] or intra-abdominal[132] disorders and because of excellent soft tissue resolution, it is useful in evaluation of traumatic injuries, especially to muscles and ligaments.[23]

Anesthetic considerations during MRI. Problems that complicate the anesthetic management of any patient outside the operating room also exist for patients requiring anesthesia or sedation for MRI.[100] Usually the MRI suite is located far from the operating room and may have been designed with little consideration of anesthetic needs. The MRI suite may lack pipeline gases, suction, and waste anesthetic exhaust capabilities. In addition, the size and design of the room and the MRI equipment are not conducive to anesthesia care. As with other satellite anesthetizing locations, MRI personnel may be unfamiliar with the needs of anesthetized patients, making assistance during emergencies problematic.

In addition to these problems, which again are common to all remote anesthetizing locations, providing anesthesia for patients undergoing MRI is further complicated by major problems unique to the MRI suite. These problems include the severe constraints created by the powerful magnetic field generated by the imager and by the physical structure of the unit itself. Access to the patient is difficult, as is airway control. Much standard anesthesia equipment and monitoring devices commonly used in other anesthetizing locations may not function effectively (or at all) in the MRI environment.

Three major problems encountered during administration of anesthesia in the MRI suite are related to the powerful magnetic fields and the RF pulses produced by the scanner. The power of these forces (both RF and magnetic) is inversely related to the square of the distance away from the generating source. Anything near the scanner that contains ferromagnetic material will be attracted toward the scanner and can even become a truly dangerous flying projectile that can injure the patient or others in the room. These materials include laryngoscopes, stethoscopes, scissors, IV poles, gas cylinders, and anesthesia machines themselves. Also, most electronic anesthesia equipment and monitoring devices do not function properly in close proximity to the magnet. Specially designed monitoring techniques and/or equipment should be substituted or the monitors should be shielded. Finally, metal objects and electronic monitors reflect and/or produce RF waves that interfere with the image generated by the MRI scanner resulting in a degraded, nondiagnostic image. **Insistence on use of a monitoring device that renders the examination less than optimal defeats the purpose of performing the scan in the first place.**

Although MRI is a very effective diagnostic tool, to obtain images free of movement artifacts, patients should remain motionless throughout the time required to make each cut. In most current MRI individual cuts take several minutes and the total scanning period may last up to 2 hours. Although most adults can tolerate remaining still, many younger children cannot. Adults who are claustrophobic or mentally handicapped may also be unable to cooperate and with increasing frequency, patients requiring intensive monitoring are being scheduled for MRI. All these patients may benefit from the expertise of an anesthesia care team to ensure that a useful image is obtained in a safe and efficient manner. Patients may require monitored anesthesia care, sedation, or general anesthesia. The technique chosen depends on the age and medical condition of the patient, design and size of the scanner, and the specific type of scan to be completed.

Both sedation and general anesthesia are used in MRI units. If sedation is chosen, any of the techniques described for CT scanning can also be used effectively for MRI scanning. Because of the longer duration of MRI compared with CT scanning, it is usually necessary to have an IV infusion in place to allow administration of additional sedation, either as intermittent boluses or a continuous infusion. **Because patients are almost out of sight and out of reach when they are in the scanner and therefore access to the airway is difficult, many prefer to employ general anesthesia with endotracheal intubation or placement of an LMA.** This minimizes the problem of limited patient access and difficulty with airway control that can result in airway obstruction and hypoventilation in heavily sedated patients.

Whether sedation or general anesthesia is used, it is often best to induce anesthesia outside the MRI unit, away from the effects of the magnet, because most metallic anesthesia equipment contains some ferromagnetic material that will be attracted by the MRI magnet. The larger the magnet in the MRI unit and the closer the item is to the magnet, the greater the attraction will be. IV poles, stylets, scissors, metal connectors, O_2 and N_2O tanks, pens, stethoscopes, and anesthesia machines all may contain sufficient ferromagnetic material to be attracted by the magnet and can be suddenly pulled across the room into the magnet. Vaporizers and mechanical ventilators contain little ferromagnetic material and generally function as designed when taken into the MRI suite. Ferromagnetic items should not be taken into the scanning room. Nonmagnetic alternatives should be substituted.[102] MRI–compatible anesthesia machines and monitors are now available.[52,108,109,129] There is a great variation among MRI scanners; any equipment to be used in an MRI unit should be tested to ensure that it functions safely and effectively before patient use.

A variety of anesthetic techniques have been used for patients during MRI scans, including IM ketamine,[140] IV techniques with thiopental, midazolam or propofol,[17] and inhalation anesthesia with a volatile agent.[97,100,118] After IV access has been established, anesthesia induced and the airway secured, the patient can be transported into the scanning unit. All basic monitors used in the operating room should be used when anesthetizing a patient for an MRI.[7,87] Unfortunately, the magnetic field interferes with many electronic monitors, so considerable care may be required to ensure that adequate monitoring can be achieved.

The ECG is grossly distorted by the scanner because the lead wires pass through the time-varying magnetic field and capacitance-coupled currents are generated. Blood flowing through the magnetic field acts as a conductor and is also capacitance-coupled; again, this can alter the ECG vector.[15] Therefore, the ECG may be of little value in the diagnosis of ischemia, for example, during MRI procedures. Although it is possible to reduce interference using RF filters or telemetry, these methods are not completely successful.[117,118] Therefore, cardiac monitoring should be achieved with an esophageal or nonmetallic precordial stethoscope. Even then, heart sounds may be difficult to hear over the noise generated by the scanner. Doppler systems have also been used to successfully amplify the pulse if it cannot be heard or palpated manually.[17]

Monitoring blood pressure may also be difficult during MRI scanning. A mercury manometer can be effective, as can a sphygmomanometer, if it is kept away from the scanner. Both these methods are hampered by difficulty hearing Korotkoff's sounds in the scanner. Automated blood pressure machines do work if carefully placed in the room to avoid interference from the magnetic field. Although the tubing on these units can be lengthened, this may adversely affect the accuracy of the readings obtained.

Temperature control of patients in the MRI may be difficult, particularly in infants and small children. To protect the computer, MRI suites are heavily air-conditioned. Small children and infants may cool rapidly in this environment. Conversely, inside the MRI unit during the scanning process, the changing magnetic and RF fields produce sufficient heating to actually increase a patient's temperature.[15,33] Therefore, temperature should be monitored on all patients undergoing MRI scans. Localized heating can also occur and has resulted in patient burns because of heating of pulse oximetry and temperature probes.[10,64]

Once the patient is in the scanner, monitoring respiration is also difficult. Breath sounds may be difficult to hear, so an end-tidal CO_2 monitor with an extended sampling tube is the most effective method to assess the adequacy of ventilation in both anesthetized and sedated patients.

MRI–compatible pulse oximeters can be used in most scanners, although the internal microprocessor may be damaged by the magnetic field if it is not adequately shielded. In addition, RF waves emitted by the oximeter probe and cable can cause deterioration in the quality of the image obtained.[97,100] None of the available monitors is completely reliable when used too close to the imaging magnet. Each should be carefully evaluated to confirm effectiveness in the MRI suite before use with patients. Devices that work well with one scanner may not be effective when used in another unit. This places an extra burden on the anesthesia provider to maintain vigilant patient observation.

After monitoring has been adequately established, the MRI scanning procedure can begin. If sedation only is required, it can be maintained with any of the short-acting IV agents, including ketamine, methohexital, midazolam, or propofol. During general anesthesia, an elongated anesthetic circuit can be used with spontaneous or controlled ventilation to maintain oxygenation and ventilation. Although volatile and IV agents both provide excellent conditions for obtaining a diagnostic image, use of propofol and the LMA during MRI may provide several specific advantages. The onset and recovery from anesthesia with propofol is rapid, and clinically significant cardiorespiratory depression is unusual.[11,88,130] There is also evidence that propofol is associated with less postoperative emesis when compared with other volatile or IV agents.[89] The incidence of nausea and vomiting in children following MRI is low no matter which anesthetic techniques is used.[94] Scavenging of volatile agents and N_2O may also be problematic in these locations.

Use of the LMA during MRI provides a stable airway and avoids the need for endotracheal intubation,[8,104] but coughing or laryngospasm can occur if depth of anesthesia is not adequate. This is commonly seen in response to repositioning the patient's head during the scanning procedure, unless the depth of anesthesia is not briefly increased. Propofol appears to suppress the pharyngeal and laryngeal reflexes better than thiopental, facilitating placement of an LMA.[90] One drawback to use of an LMA during MRI is the presence of a small metallic spring in the pilot valve that can cause artifacts to appear in the images obtained.

In addition to the problems encountered in providing anesthesia and monitoring patients during MRI scanning, there are other hazards associated with MRI that affect not only the patient but also anyone working near the scanner. These hazards are related to the static magnetic field, the time-varying magnetic field, and the RF waves generated by the scanner. There have been no documented adverse effects from static magnetic fields below 2.0 Tesla[15] (most MRI scanners use 0.5 to 2.0 Tesla), except in patients with implanted metallic devices, such as cerebrovascular clips,[95] cochlear implants, or cardiac pacemakers.[101] Many vascular clips are ferromagnetic and the force exerted on them by the static magnetic field is sufficient to create a risk of clip dislodgment and hemorrhage or cerebral injury by displacement of the clip without dislodgment.[124] Clips with greater nickel contents (10% to 14%) do not appear to be a hazard. Imaging artifacts may also be a problem in patients with implanted medical or dental devices, including dentures and orthodontic braces.[125] Both the static and time-varying magnetic fields can affect cardiac pacemakers. Demand pacemakers may be converted to the asynchronous mode. The time-varying magnetic field and the RF waves generated by the scanner may be interpreted as cardiac activity by the pacemaker, which could inhibit demand pacemakers. Stainless steel pacemakers may even be displaced or the leads fractured. Patients with pacemakers should avoid MRI scans.[101,117,118] Of no medical concern, but rather of considerable practical importance, is the damage done to pocket calculators, watches, pagers, and credit cards with magnetic strips when they are exposed to the magnetic field.

Following an MRI, patients require standard postanesthesia recovery care. Ideally, this should be provided in an area close to the MRI suite. Facilities with skilled recovery personnel may not be available, in which case patients should be transferred to the main recovery room. This may involve traveling a considerable distance. Adequate equipment and personnel should be available during the transfer to ensure it is quickly and safely performed and that emergencies that arise during transport can be adequately handled. Depending on the clinical situation, the patient may be awakened and extubated in the MRI suite, then transported to the recovery room or the patient can be transported anesthetized and intubated so that recovery and extubation can take place in a more familiar environment. **In today's high-pressure hospital environment, radiology personnel should understand that anesthesia care cannot be discontinued until safe transfer to competent recovery room personnel is accomplished. Pressure to decrease the oft-decried "turnaround time" may result in tragedy.**

Angiography

Angiography involves injection of contrast material into an artery to visualize anatomic abnormalities.[91] After arterial cannulation and injection of contrast material, a series of images are taken as the dye passes through the vascular network. Although any artery may be evaluated, anesthesia is commonly required for cerebral angiography in patients who have subarachnoid hemorrhage, cerebral aneurysm, arteriovenous malformation, or tumor. Cerebral angiography can also be used to assess intracerebral and extracerebral arteries in patients with transient ischemic attacks or other evidence of carotid atherosclerosis. Local anesthesia plus light IV sedation are all that is usually needed for adults in such situations. Placement of the arterial catheter can be painful, the patient should remain motionless while the radiographs are taken, and the contrast material may cause an unpleasant, burning sensation. Therefore, most children and some adults require general anesthesia to ensure a successful study. Although many different anesthetic techniques have been effective in patients undergoing cerebral angiography, there are a number of specific factors that should be considered when caring for these patients. These include airway control and ventilation, circulatory changes associated with angiography, and complications of the procedures.

During cerebral angiography, access to the patient's airway is difficult. Also, personnel should move away from the patient during exposure of the radiographs. This makes endotracheal intubation or an LMA essential in patients undergoing cerebral angiography under general anesthesia. When choosing an anesthetic technique for angiography, CT scanning, or MRI, the patient's pathologic condition should be considered. With increased intracranial pressure (ICP), subarachnoid hemorrhage, cerebral aneurysm, or arteriovenous malformation, the technique chosen should minimize changes in both ICP and blood pressure during intubation and throughout the procedure. In particular, hypertension, which may increase the risk of intracranial bleeding, should be avoided during endotracheal intubation.

In addition to providing a secure airway, endotracheal intubation and mechanical ventilation also provide better control of $Pa{CO_2}$.[18] This is important for two reasons. Many patients with intracranial pathology undergoing cerebral angiography have increased ICP. Hyperventilation, by reducing $Pa{CO_2}$, causes cerebral vasconstriction and reduces cerebral blood flow and ICP. Even in patients without increased ICP, hyperventilation and cerebral vasoconstriction slow transit time of the contrast medium as it passes through the brain. This increases the contrast concentration in cerebral vessels, allowing abnormal vessels to be better visualized.[39] Dallas and Moxon[32] reported that high-quality images were achieved when $Pa{CO_2}$ was maintained between 30 and 35 mm Hg. Hypocapnia below 20 mm Hg may cause severe vasoconstriction and cerebral ischemia and should be avoided. This implies strongly that capnography is needed. Again, the message to administrators is the same: do not underestimate the quality and quantity of anesethesia and monitoring equipment needed in these locations. General anesthesia with potent volatile anesthetics may cause cerebral vasodilation. This can increase cerebral blood flow and ICP; therefore the addition of N_2O, a narcotic, and a muscle relaxant combined with hyperventilation may offer advantages over a pure inhalation anesthesia. Propofol also may be used during neuroradiologic procedures because it causes significant reductions in CMR_{02}, CBF, and ICP. Nevertheless, hemodynamic changes that occur following induction of anesthesia with propofol can reduce the cerebral perfusion pressure.[130] Because leakage around the cuff of an LMA is common during positive pressure ventilation, it is not a useful technique in patients who require hyperventilation to reduce ICP.[35]

Circulatory changes in response to cerebral angiography are common. Tachycardia or bradycardia exceeding 20% of control levels occurred in 22% of patients undergoing cerebral angiography in one study.[69] Intracranial hemorrhage can cause marked changes in the ECG. T-wave inversions occur or T waves may appear widened and continuous with large U waves. These changes may be accompanied by bradycardia. Injection of contrast material can induce undesirable circulatory effects related to its hyperosmolarity. Infants with large cerebral arteriovenous malformations associated with cardiac failure and ischemic myocardial damage may not tolerate the circulatory effects[31,73,78] associated with contrast material. In all patients, it is important that the maximum dose of contrast material that can be safely administered during a procedure be determined in advance to minimize risk of circulatory or toxic complications.

Neurologic complications are relatively common after cerebral angiography and may be transient or permanent. Earnest et al.[37] reported complications in 8.5% of patients. In 2.6% of patients, the complications were neurologic, and in 0.33%, the deficit was permanent. Neurologic complications occur more frequently in the elderly and in patients with a previous stroke, transient ischemic attacks (TIAs), hypertension, diabetes, and renal insufficiency. Prolonged procedures that require larger volumes of contrast material and considerable catheter manipulation are also associated with greater incidences of neurologic complications.[36] The anesthetic technique chosen for a patient undergoing cerebral angiography should allow prompt awakening so that neurologic changes can be quickly identified.

Interventional radiology

Development of sophisticated intravascular catheters, new embolic materials, and improved imaging techniques have resulted in their increased use for treatment of serious conditions such as arteriovenous fistulas, cerebral aneurysms, or arteriovenous malformations.[20] These are often long, complex procedures that require general anesthesia, particularly in children. The goal of embolization therapy is to occlude the arterial origins of a vascular malformation or tumor but preserve vascular supply to normal tissue. This is achieved by injecting embolic material as close as possible to the abnormal vessels. New microcatheters allow precise localization into very distal vessels. A variety of embolic agents, including detachable balloon systems, tissue adhesives (such as isobutyl-2-cyanoacrylate polyvinyl alcohol, and silicon spheres) are available for primary occlusion of vascular malformations, preoperative tumor devascularization, and treatment of intractable bleeding.[20]

Because of the technical complexity of these cases and the serious risk of severe bleeding if a large arteriovenous malformation is perforated, close communication with the radiologist and vigilant patient monitoring is essential. Some patients may require somatosensory (SEP) or motor-evoked potential (MEP) monitoring during the procedure. Choice of anesthetic technique should take into account its effect on the quality of evoked potentials obtained.[21] It is likely that the anesthesia provider's role will become increasingly important as these techniques are applied to a wider variety of pathologic conditions.

Radiotherapy

Pediatric radiotherapy

Anesthetic considerations. Radiotherapy is used in the treatment of many different kinds of pediatric malignancy, including acute lymphoblastic leukemia, brain tumors, sarcomas, lymphomas, and neuroblastomas. The beam of ionizing radiation used to destroy tumor cells should be precisely delivered to the affected area so that only malignant cells are destroyed and damage to surrounding tissue is minimized. Patients should remain motionless throughout the treatment period, which may last as little as 30 to 60 seconds. During a single-treatment session, up to four different fields may be irradiated, some requiring that the patient be turned to the prone position. The patient may require one or two treatments per day, repeated daily for several weeks. Although adults and older children are able to cooperate and remain still during exposure to the ionizing radiation, younger children are rarely able to remain motionless even for the time required to complete these brief treatments. Children under 6 years of age usually require general anesthesia throughout the course of their radiotherapy. Their anesthetic requirements can be demanding. When planning the anesthetic care of such patients, several important factors should be considered. First, treatments are generally very brief. Agents chosen should provide rapid onset and adequate depth of anesthesia to ensure that the patient remains immobile while being exposed to radiation. Second, it is desirable that recovery be prompt, with few unpleasant side effects, because most such patients are outpatients. Some may receive treatments twice daily. It is important to maintain adequate nutrition over the weeks required to complete the radiotherapy. Anesthetic techniques that produce prolonged sedation or serious postanesthetic nausea and vomiting impair proper feeding. Because numerous treatments are usually required, it is desirable to avoid repeated painful or invasive procedures and to be sensitive to the emotional needs of the family who is dealing with a child afflicted with cancer. Therefore, it is helpful to limit the number of different anesthesia personnel to whom the family is exposed so that continuity of care is maintained, rapport is established with the family, and a level of confidence and trust develops. Because daily treatments are often required for several weeks at a time, it may be preferable to avoid intubating the patient for every procedure. This can make airway control difficult when the patient is in the prone position. Use of an LMA can be advantageous in these children.[58] To protect health care personnel from ionizing radiation, during the time the patient is exposed to the electron beam, everyone should leave the treatment room, which further complicates airway control and monitoring. The patient should be continually observed from outside the treatment room via an observation window and/or a remote camera that allows views of both patient and monitors.

Although it would be preferable to perform radiotherapy without general anesthesia, in young children this is usually not possible. Many different sedation regimens have been tried. It is difficult to consistently achieve adequate results with any of the more common sedatives, either alone or in combination. Effects are often unpredictable, so that immobility cannot be ensured or, if sedation is adequate, recovery is prolonged. **General anesthesia is, in fact, required for most young children.**

Many anesthetic techniques have been tried for radiation therapy in young children. Ketamine has been favored in the past because of rapid onset, short duration of action, cardiovascular stability, and ease with which it can be administered either IM or IV.[3,38,45] There are a number of drawbacks to the use of ketamine that impair its usefulness for radiotherapy. Purposeless movements are common during ketamine anesthesia. Salivation, which may be profuse, complicates airway management. Apnea has been reported during use of ketamine in children with posterior fossa or brain stem tumors. Nausea, vomiting, and emergence delirium can be important postanesthetic problems. Although delirium and hallucinations associated with ketamine are attenuated by use of benzodiazepines, many parents are disturbed by the behavior and/or affect on their child after the use of ketamine. Also, the benzodiazepines may prolong sedation, interfering with nutrition.

Rectal administration of thiopental or methohexital has been recommended in the past for radiotherapy, but large doses are required, resulting in prolonged sedation. Up to 15% of children may fail to fall asleep with a single dose.[68] Proctitis has been reported after repeated use in some children,[68] and rectal administration of medication in a child who is immunocompromised could increase the risk of systemic infections.

Harrison and Bennet[68] described advantages of halothane anesthesia for the radiotherapy of children in 1963. Onset and recovery from anesthesia were relatively rapid, nausea and vomiting were infrequent, and adequate immobility was ensured. The researchers administered the drug by insufflation, avoiding use of a face mask or endotracheal intubation. Pollution of the treatment area with volatile anesthetics administered by insufflation complicates this technique, but no patient complications were reported.

In recent years, widespread use of long-term indwelling central venous catheters in children with malignancies has simplified their anesthetic care.[14,66,71] By permitting a smooth, painless induction, patients' fears and resistance are greatly reduced and radiotherapy is better accepted by the family. Although complications, including thrombosis, air embolism, catheter disruption, and infection can occur, these complications are unlikely with diligent attention to appropriate aseptic technique. Parents are usually well versed in the procedures used in gaining access to the central line and can be extremely helpful in assisting the anesthesia provider. They can also be quite critical of anesthesia personnel when accepted aseptic technique is not followed and often exhibit protective attitudes toward the catheter.

Glauber and Audenaert[53] described use of a central venous line in children for IV induction using thiopental followed by inhalation of halothane or isoflurane through a face mask taped to the face. This technique provided predictable immobility during irradiation, rapid recovery, few complications or side effects, and good acceptance by parents who remained with their child during the induction and recovery. They reported that accumulation of thiopental over time did not occur, despite daily use for several weeks. Anesthesia can also be maintained with repeated boluses or continuous infusion of a short-acting barbiturate or benzodiazepine. Propofol is an excellent agent for children undergoing radiotherapy, especially because of its antinausea properties.

Monitoring during radiotherapy should include ECG, blood pressure, pulse oximetry, capnography, and assessment of heart and breath sounds. Because the anesthesia provider should leave the treatment room during radiation exposure, a window or remote video camera should be available to allow constant observation of the patient and the monitors. Resuscitation equipment should be available, and, if a serious, problem arises during the treatment, the radiation should be stopped immediately and the problem resolved.

Total body irradiation

Anesthetic considerations. Total body irradiation of children before bone marrow transplantation presents many of the same problems encountered during craniospinal radiotherapy. These children may be extremely ill. Precautions required during use of linear acceleration make monitoring difficult, and facilities are often not well suited to administration of general anesthesia. In addition, unlike craniospinal radiotherapy, which involves short bursts of radiation, total body irradiation requires 30 to 60 minutes of exposure time. This is usually given in 15-minute blocks with the patient positioned first supine and then prone. Because the patient cannot be directly monitored, care should be taken to ensure a secure airway and reliable monitoring of vital signs from outside the treatment room, including remote TV camera observation. General anesthesia and monitoring for total body irradiation can be provided using any of the techniques described for craniospinal radiotherapy.[58,66,67,70,86]

Complications of ionizing radiation. Radiation injuries may develop acutely in patients undergoing radiotherapy, or complications may be delayed. Both the acute and late effects of radiotherapy can have important implications for anesthesia care. The acute effects of total body irradiation include nausea, vomiting, fever, and hypotension. This syndrome usually resolves within hours and requires only symptomatic treatment. Other acute effects of total body irradiation and localized radiotherapy that complicate anesthesia include laryngeal and subglottic edema, leading to airway obstruction, and suppression of bone marrow, affecting erythrocytes, leukocytes, and platelets.

Late complications of radiotherapy may appear months or years after treatment and can involve any major organ system. Radiation to the thorax for treatment of lymphomas and breast or lung tumors may cause pericarditis, pericardial effusions, and myocardial fibrosis.[6,41] In addition, changes in the lung are common following thoracic radiation, including radiation pneumonitis, pulmonary fibrosis, and pleural effusions. Diffusion capacity may be impaired and arterial saturation reduced, although many patients remain asymptomatic despite radiographic changes.[59] Liver and kidneys may also be affected by radiation injury to the microvasculature, resulting in hepatitis[111] or nephritis.[60] Other complications of radiation include endocrine dysfunction, leukoencephalopathy, and secondary malignancies. Careful airway evaluation is critical in patients who have received radiation for head and neck tumors. Fibrosis of the tissues of neck, oropharynx, and tongue may make direct laryngoscope and endotracheal intubation extremely difficult. This should be recognized before induction of anesthesia, so that alternate methods of intubation can be planned and available.

Complications of chemotherapy. Current treatment of many malignancies includes surgery, radiotherapy, and chemotherapy in varying combinations, and patients who require general anesthesia for radiation treatment may also have received chemotherapy. These medications affect not only malignant cells but also have toxic effects on normal tissues, which produce physiologic problems of concern to the anesthesia provider. Awareness of problems associated with the use of chemotherapeutic agents is important in planning the anesthetic management of a patient undergoing radiotherapy.[22,76,114,121]

A common side effect is bone marrow depression that occurs with almost all chemotherapeutic agents and affects erythrocytes, leukocytes, and platelet precursors. It is usually reversible within weeks of discontinuing chemotherapy. Bone marrow function should be evaluated before anesthesia with complete blood and platelet counts. In addition to thrombocytopenia, other coagulation defects may be encountered in patients receiving nitrogen mustard, l-asparaginase, and mithramycin. Immunosuppression also occurs with the majority of chemotherapeutic agents and requires that diligent attention to asepsis be observed in all aspects of the anesthetic management of these patients, particularly when indwelling central venous catheters are used. GI side effects, particularly nausea and vomiting, are also common.[9] Propofol in subanesthetic doses has been used to treat nausea and vomiting associated with chemotherapy.[119]

Cardiotoxicity may be seen in patients receiving doxorubicin[112] and several other antineoplastic drugs. Congestive heart failure (CHF) with cardiomegaly, pleural effusion, and dysrhythmias are common manifestations and mortality is high. Patients who have also received radiation therapy are particularly sensitive to cardiotoxicity with these drugs, which is often manifested by diminution in QRS complex size. This suggests that widespread myocardial damage exists. Other nonspecific ECG changes occur in approximately 10% of patients receiving doxorubicin and include ST-T wave abnormalities and a variety of conduction defects. These changes, unlike the decreased QRS voltage, usually resolve when the drug is stopped.

The alkylating agents—methotrexate, bleomycin, and cytarabine—have all been shown to induce pneumonitis that may progress to pulmonary fibrosis.[12] A chest radiograph and arterial blood gas analysis may be useful in such patients, especially those with a history of dyspnea.

Hepatotoxicity or nephrotoxicity may occur with a variety of chemotherapeutic agents. Evidence of impaired liver and kidney function should be sought in cancer patients. CNS and autonomic nervous system toxicity and peripheral neuropathies may be seen during chemotherapy with nitrogen mustard, vincristine, and cisplatin, and evidence of neurologic dysfunction should be documented.[116] The anticholinesterase effects of the alkylating agents represent another important interaction the anesthesia provider should consider.[151]

There are many toxic chemotherapeutic agents currently in use. Patients often receive combinations of four to eight different drugs. The risks of major side effects are high. Complications may appear in several different organ systems. Familiarity with the side effects and potential interactions of these drugs plus careful preoperative patient evaluation is critical in selecting an appropriate anesthetic technique in the care of patients undergoing radiation therapy.

Other Procedures

Occasionally, deep sedation or general anesthesia is requested for other diagnostic or therapeutic procedures in offices or clinics throughout the hospital. These include GI endoscopy, positron emission tomography, cryotherapy for retinopathy of prematurity, and laser treatment of port-wine stain hemangiomas.[40] Typically, the request occurs because the patient is a child and/or has a medical or behavioral disorder that prevents the study from being completed in the standard way. As with radiographic procedures, these studies are performed far from the familiar operating room environment with equipment and personnel that also may be unfamiliar. When providing anesthesia care in different areas throughout the hospital, the same principles apply. The anesthesia provider should ensure that facilities, anesthesia equipment, monitors, and personnel are adequate to provide the care required. **These patients should receive the same quality of preoperative evaluations, anesthetic care, transportation, and postanesthesia recovery provided to patients in the main operating room. Advance interdepartmental planning, with regular problem-solving conferences, is best. Last-minute requests to calm a struggling or panicked patient are not considered components of quality patient care. Services that only occasionally use anesthesia services cannot be expected to understand the problems and requirements without advance education and planning.**

KEY POINTS

- Satellite anesthesia is an increasing requirement in remote sites throughout the hospital. MRI and other kinds of complex CT are among the techniques that cannot be performed in a traditional operating room setting.
- A major problem with delivery of anesthesia in remote locations is that immediate help from experienced anesthesia personnel in the event of a disaster is not necessarily available.
- Quality portable equipment (not old, outdated equipment) should be available.
- Scheduling remote procedures means involving nonsurgeons in the surgical scheduling process. This is never easy and should be done in advance.
- The anesthesia provider should be knowledgeable about the use of sedation versus general anesthesia, especially for children.
- Contrast media are hypertonic and can cause osmotic diuresis. Allergic reactions can also occur.
- Understanding the magnetic properties of anesthesia equipment is critical in performing competent anesthesia in the MRI environment.
- Provisions should be made for postanesthetic care.
- The role of anesthesia in the various new interventional radiographic procedures is still evolving. These procedures often require patients to lie on hard tables in darkened rooms for long periods of time and may involve pain or great anxiety. The anesthesia provider can help to alleviate these problems.
- Developing an anesthetic plan that allows multiple treatments for children who need numerous radiographic procedures for cancer requires teamwork among the radiologists, radiotherapists, and the anesthesia team providing care for these children. Continuity of health care personnel reduces parental anxiety and promotes patient cooperation.

KEY REFERENCES

American Academy of Pediatrics Committee on Drugs: Guidelines for monitoring and management of pediatric patients during and after sedation for diagnostic and therapeutic procedures, *Pediatrics* 89:1110, 1992.

American Academy of Pediatric Dentistry: Guidelines for the elective use pharmacologic conscious sedation and deep sedation in pediatric dental patients, *Pediatr Dent* 15:297, 1993.

American Society of Anesthesiologists: *American Society of Anesthesiologists Standards, Guidelines and Statements,* Park Ridge, 1995.

American Society of Anesthesiologists: *Manual for Anesthesia Department Organization and Management,* Park Ridge, 1994.

American Society of Anesthesiologists: *Practice guidelines for sedation and analgesia by non-anesthesiologists.* A report by the American Society of Anesthesiologists task force on sedation and analgesia by non-anesthesiologists, *Anesthesiology* 84:459, 1996.

Chung F: Cancer, chemotherapy and anaesthesia, *Can Anaesth Soc J* 29:364, 1982.

Coté CJ: Sedation for the pediatric patient: a review, *Pediatr Clin North Am* 41:31, 1994.

Council on Scientific Affairs: Fundamentals of magnetic resonance imaging, *JAMA* 258:3417, 1987.

Goldberg M: Systemic reactions to intravascular contrast media, *Anesthesiology* 60:45, 1984.

Mitchell AA, Loui KC, Lacouture P, et al: Risks to children from computed tomographic scan premedication, *JAMA* 247:2385, 1982.

Patterson SK, Chesney JT: Anesthetic management for magnetic resonance imaging, *Anesth Analg* 74:121, 1992.

Selvin BL: Cancer chemotherapy: implications for the anesthesiologist, *Anesth Analg* 60:425, 1981.

Shellock FG, Morisoli S, Kanal E: MR procedures and biomedical implants, materials and devices. 1993 update, *Radiology* 189:587, 1993.

REFERENCES

1. Abrams HL, McNeil BJ: Medical implications of computed tomography ("CAT scanning"), *N Engl J Med* 298:310, 1978.
2. Aidinis SJ, Zimmerman RA, Shapiro HM, et al: Anesthesia for brain computer tomography, *Anesthesiology* 44:420, 1976.
3. Amberg HL, Gordon G: Low-dose intramuscular ketamine for pediatric radiotherapy: a case report, *Anesth Analg* 55:92, 1976.
4. Anderson RE, Osborn AG: Efficacy of simple sedation for pediatric computed tomography, *Radiology* 124:739, 1977.
5. Ansell G, Tweedie MC, West CR, et al: The current status of reactions to intravenous contrast media, *Invest Radiol* 15:532, 1980.
6. Applefeld MM, Slawson RG, Hall-Craigs M, et al: Delayed pericardial disease after radiotherapy, *Am J Cardiol* 47:210, 1981.
7. American Society of Anesthesiologists: *American Society of Anesthesiologists Standards, Guidelines and Statements American Society of Anesthiologists,* Park Ridge, 1995.
8. Asai T, Morris S: The laryngeal mask airway: its features, effects and role, *Can J Anaesth* 41:930, 1994.
9. Bakowski MT: Advances in anti-emetic therapy, *Cancer Treat Rev* 11:237, 1984.
10. Bashein G, Syrory G: Burns associated with pulse oximetry during magnetic resonance imaging, *Anesthesiology* 76:152, 1992.
11. Bloomfield EL: Propofol for sedation of pediatric patients, *Radiology* 186:580, 1993.
12. Blum RH, Carter SK, Agre K; A clinical review of bleomycin—a new antineoplastic agent, *CA* 31:903, 1973.
13. Brasch RC, Gooding CA, Lallemand DP, et al: Magnetic resonance imaging of the thorax in childhood, *Radiology* 150:463, 1984.
14. Broviac JW, Cole JJ, Scribner BH: A silicone rubber atrial catheter for prolonged parenteral nutrition, *Surg Gynecol Obstet* 136:602, 1973.
15. Budinger TF: Nuclear magnetic resonance (NMR) *in vivo* studies: known thresholds for health effects, *J Comput Assist Tomogr* 5(6):800, 1981.
16. Burckart GJ, White TJ III, Siegle RL, et al: Rectal thiopental versus an intramuscular cocktail for sedating children before computerized tomography, *Am J Hosp Pharmacol* 37:222, 1980.
17. Burk NS: Anesthesia for magnetic resonance imaging, *Anesth Clin North Am* 7:(3)707, 1989.
18. Campkin TV: General anaesthesia for neuroradiology, *Br J Anaesth* 48:783, 1976.
19. Chaplin H, Carlson E: Changes in human red blood cells during in vitro exposure to several roentgenologic contrast media, *Am J Roentgenol* 86:1127, 1961.
20. Choi IS, Berenstein A: Surgical neuroangiography of intracranial lesions, *Radiol Clin North Am* 26:1143, 1988.
21. Choi IS, Berenstein A: Surgical neuroangiography of the spine and spinal cord, *Radiol Clin North Am* 26:1131, 1988.
22. Chung F: Cancer, chemotherapy and anaesthesia, *Can Anaesth Soc J* 29:364, 1982.
23. Consensus Conference: Magnetic resonance imaging, *JAMA* 14:2132, 1988.
24. Coté CJ, Greenhow DE, Marsall BE: The hypotensive response to rapid administration of hypertonic solutions in man and in the rabbit, *Anesthesiology* 50:30, 1979.
25. Coté CJ: Sedation for the pediatric patient: a review, *Pediatr Clin North Am* 41:31, 1994.
26. Council on Scientific Affairs: Fundamentals of magnetic resonance imaging, *JAMA* 258:3417, 1987
27. Council on Scientific Affairs: Magnetic resonance imaging of the cardiovascular system. Present state of the art and future potential, *JAMA* 259:253, 1988.
28. Council on Scientific Affairs: Magnetic resonance imaging of the central nervous system, *JAMA* 259:1211, 1988.
29. Council on Scientific Affairs: Magnetic resonance imaging of the head and neck region, *JAMA* 260:3313, 1988.
30. Cumberland DC: Low osmolality contrast media in cardiac radiology, *Invest Radiol* 19:S301, 1984.
31. Cumming GR: Circulation in neonates with intracranial arteriovenous fistula and cardiac failure, *Am J Cardiol* 45:1019, 1980.
32. Dallas SH, Moxon CP: Controlled ventilation for cerebral angiography, *Br J Anaesth* 41:597, 1969.
33. Davis PL, Crooks L, Arakawa M, et al: Potential hazards in NMR imaging: heating effects of changing magnetic fields and RF fields on small metallic implants, *AJR* 13: 857, 1981
34. Dawson P: New contrast agents. Chemistry and pharmacology, *Invest Radiol* 19:S293, 1984.
35. Dewitt JH, Wenstone R, Noel AG, et al: The laryngeal mask airway and positive-pressure ventilation, *Anesthesiology* 80: 550, 1994.
36. Dion JE, Gates PC, Fox AJ, et al: Clinical events following neuroangiography: a prospective study, *Stroke* 18:997, 1987.
37. Earnest F IV, Forbes G, Sandok BA, et al: Complications of cerebral angiography: prospective assessment of risk, *AJR* 142: 247, 1984.

38. Edge WG, Morgan M: Ketamine and paediatric radiotherapy, *Anaesth Inten Care* 5:153, 1977.
39. Edmonds-Seal J, duBoulay G, Bostick T: The effect of intermittent positive pressure ventilation upon cerebral angiography with special reference to the quality of the films—a preliminary communication, *Br J Radiol* 40:957, 1967.
40. Epstein RM, Brummett RR, Lask GP: Incendiary potential of the flash-lamp pumped 585-nm tunable dye laser, *Anesth Analg* 71:171, 1990.
41. Fajardo LF, Stewart JR, Cohn KE: Morphology of radiation-induced heart disease, *Arch Pathol* 86:512, 1968.
42. Federle MP: Abdominal trauma: the role and impact of computed tomography, *Invest Radiol* 16:260, 1981.
43. Ferrer-Brechner T, Winter J: Anesthetic considerations for cerebral computer tomography, *Anesth Analg* 56:344, 1977.
44. Ferrucci JT, van Sonnenberg E: Intra-abdominal abscesses: radiologic diagnosis and treatment, *JAMA* 246:2728, 1981.
45. Filshie J, Harrison CA: Paediatric radiotherapy. In Filshie J, Robbie DS, editors: *Anesthesia and malignant disease,* Dobbs Ferry, 1989, Sheridan House.
46. Fischer HW: Catalog of intravascular contrast media, *Radiology* 159:561, 1986.
47. Fletcher BD, Scoles PV, Nelson AD: Gated magnetic resonance imaging of congenital cardiac malformations, *Radiology* 150:137, 1984.
48. Forbes RB, Murray DJ, Dillman JB, et al: Pharmacokinetics of two percent rectal methohexitone in children, *Can J Anaesth* 36:160, 1989.
49. Forbes RB, Murray DJ, Dull DL, et al: Haemodynamic effects of rectal methohexitone for induction of anaesthesia in children, *Can J Anaesth* 36:526, 1989.
50. Forbes RB, Vandewalker GE: Comparison of two and ten percent rectal methohexitone for induction of anaesthesia in children, *Can J Anaesth* 35:345, 1989.
51. Fragling IM, Addison GM, Chattergee K, et al: Methemoglobinemia in children treated with prilocaine-lignocaine cream, *BMJ* 301:153, 1990.
52. Geiger RS, Cascorbi HF: Anesthesia in an NMR scanner, *Anesth Analg* 63:619, 1984.
53. Glauber DT, Audenaert SM: Anesthesia for children undergoing craniospinal radiotherapy, *Anesthesiology* 67:801, 1987.
54. Goldberg M: Systemic reactions to intravascular contrast media, *Anesthesiology* 60:45, 1984.
55. Goodwin JD, Califf RM, Korobkin M, et al: Clinical value of coronary bypass graft evaluation with CT, *AJR* 140:649, 1983.
56. Goodwin JD, Korobkin M: Acute disease of aorta, diagnosis by computed tomography and ultrasonography, *Radiol Clin North Am* 21:551, 1983.
57. Goresky GV, Steward DJ: Rectal methohexitone for induction of anaesthesia in children, *Can Anaesth Soc J* 26:213, 1979.
58. Grebeuk CR, Ferguson C, White A: The laryngeal mask airway in pediatric radiotherapy, *Anesthesiology* 47:446, 1990.
59. Gross NJ: Pulmonary effects of radiation therapy, *Ann Intern Med* 86:81, 1978.
60. Grossman BJ: Radiation nephritis, *J Pediatr* 47:424, 1955.
61. American Academy of Pediatrics Committee on Drugs: Guidelines for monitoring and management of pediatric patients during and after sedation for diagnostic and therapeutic procedures, *Pediatrics* 89: 1110, 1992.
62. American Academy of Pediatrics Committee on Drugs Section on Anesthesiology: Guidelines for the elective use of conscious sedation, deep sedation, and general anesthesia in pediatric patients, *Pediatrics* 76:312, 1985.
63. American Academy of Pediatric Dentistry: Guidelines for the elective use pharmacologic conscious sedation and deep sedation in pediatric dental patients, *Pediat Dent* 15:297, 1993.
64. Hall SC, Stevenson GW, Saresh S: Burns associated with temperature monitoring during magnetic resonance imaging, *Anesthesiology* 76:152, 1992.
65. Halperin DL, Koren G, Attias D, et al: Topical skin anesthesia for venous subcutaneous drug reservoir and lumbar punctures in children, *Pediatrics* 84:281, 1989.
66. Harrison CA, Filshie J: The use of Hickman Broviac catheters for paediatric radiotherapy, *Ann R Coll Surg Engl* 68:312, 1986.
67. Harrison CA: Total body irradiation and intraoperative radiotherapy. In Filshie J, Robbie DS, editors: *Anesthesia and malignant disease,* Dobbs Ferry, 1989, Sheridan House.
68. Harrison GG, Bennet MB: Radiotherapy without tears, *Br J Anaesth* 35:720, 1963.
69. Hayakawa K, Nishimura Y, Yosida M, et al: ECG changes during cerebral angiography: an analysis of 334 patients—942 cerebral angiographies, *Neuroradiology* 26:369, 1984.
70. Henneberg S, Nilsson A, Hok B, et al: Anesthesia and monitoring during whole body radiation in children, *J Clin Anesth* 2:76, 1990.
71. Hickman RO, Buckenr CD, Clift RA, et al: A modified right atrial catheter for access to the venous system in marrow transplanted recipients, *Surg Gynecol Obstet* 148:871, 1979.
72. Higgins CB: Overview of cardiovascular effects of contrast media. Comparison of ionic and non-ionic media, *Invest Radiol* 19:S187, 1984.
73. Jedeikin R, Rowe RD, Freedom RM, et al: Cerebral arteriovenous malformation in neonates, *Pediatr Cardiol* 4:29, 1983.
74. Jeffrey RB, Fedele MP: CT and ultrasonography of acute renal abnormalities, *Radiol Clin North Am* 21:515, 1983.
75. Kim SJ, Salem MR, Joseph NJ, et al: Contrast media adversely affect oxyhemoglobin dissociation, *Anesth Analg* 71: 33, 1990.
76. Klein DS, Wilds PR: Pulmonary toxicity of antineoplastic agents: anaesthetic and postoperative implications, *Can Anaesth Soc J* 30:399, 1983.
77. Knopf DR, Torres WE, Fajman WJ, et al: Liver lesions: comparative accuracy of scintigraphy and computed tomography, *AJR* 138:623, 1983.
78. Knudson RP, Alden ER: Symptomatic arteriovenous malformation in infants less than 6 months of age, *Pediatrics* 64:238, 1979.
79. Lalli AF: Contrast media reactions: data, analysis and hypothesis, *Radiology* 134:1, 1980.
80. Lampke KF, James G, Erbesfeld M: Cerebrovascular permeability of a water-soluble contrast material, Hypaque (sodium diatrizoate): experimental study in dogs, *Invest Radiol* 5:79, 1970.
81. Larsson LE, Nilsson K, Andreasson S, et al: Effects of rectal thiopentone and methohexitone on carbon dioxide tension in infant anaesthesia with spontaneous ventilation, *Acta Anesthesiol Scand* 31:227, 1987.
82. Laub M, Sjogren P, Holm-Knudson R, et al: Lytic cocktail in children: rectal versus intramuscular administration, *Anaesthesia* 45:110, 1990.
83. Lawson TL: Acute pancreatitis and its complications: computed tomography and sonography, *Radiol Clin North Am* 21:495, 1983.
84. Levene MI, Whitelaw A, Dubowitz V, et al: Nuclear magnetic resonance imaging of the brain in children, *Br Med J* 285:774, 1982.
85. Liu LMP, Gaudreault P, Friedman PA, et al: Methohexital plasma concentrations in children following rectal administration, *Anesthesiology* 62:567, 1985.
86. Lo JN, Buckley JJ, Kim TH, et al: Anesthesia for high-dose total body irradiation in children, *Anesthesiology* 61:101, 1984.
87. American Society of Anesthesiologists: *Manual for Anesthesia Department Organization and Management,* Park Ridge, 1994.
88. Martin ML, Pasternak LR, Pudimat MA: Total intravenous anesthesia with propofol in pediatric patients outside the operating room, *Anesth Analg* 74:609, 1992.
89. Martin TM, Nicolson SC, Bargas MS: Propofol anesthesia reduces emesis and airway obstruction in pediatric outpatients, *Anesth Analg* 76:144, 1993.
90. McKeating K, Bali IM, Dundee JW: The effects of thiopentone and propofol on upper airway integrity, *Anaesthesia* 43:638, 1988.
91. McMillan JH, Batnitzky S: Neurodiagnostic imaging, In Porter S, editor: *Problems in anesthesia,* vol 4, Philadelphia, 1984, JB Lippincott.
92. Mitchell AA, Loui KC, Lacouture P, et al: Risks to children from computed tomographic scan premedication, *JAMA* 247: 2385, 1982.
93. Morissette M, Gagnon RM, Lamaureux J, et al: Effects of angiographic contrast media on colloid oncotic pressure, *Am Heart J* 100:319, 1980.
94. Murray DJ, Schmid CM, Forbes RB: Anesthesia for magnetic resonance imaging in children: A low incidence of protracted post procedure vomiting, *J Clin Anesth* 7:232, 1995.
95. New PF, Rose BR, Brady TJ, et al: Potential hazards and artifacts of ferromagnetic surgical and dental materials and devices in nuclear magnetic resonance imaging, *Radiology* 217:139, 1983.
96. New PFJ, Scott WR, Schnur JA, et al: Computerized axial tomography with the EMI scanner, *Radiology* 110:109, 1974.
97. Nixon C, Hirsch NP, Ormerod IEC, et al: Nuclear magnetic resonance: its implications for the anaesthetist, *Anaesthesia* 41:131, 1986.
98. Norman J, Jones PL: Complications of the

use of EMLA, *Br J Anaesth* 64:403, 1990.
99. Patel A, Dallas SH: A trial of etomidate infusion anaesthesia for computerized axial tomography, *Anaesthesia* 34:509, 1979.
100. Patterson SK, Chesney JT: Anesthetic management for magnetic resonance imaging, *Anesth Analg* 74:121, 1992.
101. Pavlicek W, Geisinger M, Castle L, et al: The effects of nuclear magnetic resonance on patients with cardiac pacemakers, *Radiology* 147:149, 1983.
102. Pavlicek W: Safeguards help minimize potential MRI hazards, *Diagn Imag* 7:166, 1985.
103. American Society of Anesthesiologists: *Peer Review in Anesthesiology,* Park Ridge, 1989.
104. Pennant JH, White PF: The laryngeal mask airway. Its uses in anesthesiology, *Anesthesiology* 79:144, 1993.
105. Pfister RC, Hutter AM: Cardiac alterations during intravenous urography, *Invest Radiol* 15:5239, 1980.
106. Piedalue RJG, Milnes A: An overview of non-pharmacological pedodontic behavior management techniques for the general practitioner, *Can Dent Assoc J* 56:137, 1990.
107. American Society of Anesthesiologists: Practice guidelines for sedation and analgesia by non-anesthesiologists. A report by the American Society of Anesthesiologists task force on sedation and analgesia by non-anesthesiologists, *Anesthesiology* 84: 459, 1996.
108. Ramsay JG, Gale L, Sykes MK: A ventilator for use in nuclear magnetic resonance studies, *Br J Anaesth* 58:1181, 1986.
109. Rao CC, McNiece WL, Emhardt J: Modification of an anesthesia machine for use during magnetic resonance imaging, *Anesthesiology* 68:640, 1988.
110. American Academy of Pediatrics Committee on Drugs: Reappraisal of lytic cocktail/demorol, phenergan, and thorazine (DDT) for sedation of children, *Pediatrics* 95:598, 1995.
111. Reed GB, Cox AJ: The human liver after radiation injury, *Am J Pathol* 48:597, 1966.
112. Rinehart JL, Lewis RP, Balcerzak SP: Adriamycin cardiotoxicity in man, *Ann Intern Med* 81:475, 1974.
113. Robieux I, Gliopoulous C, Hwang P, et al: Pain perception and effectiveness of the eutectic mixture of local anesthetics in children undergoing venipuncture, *Pediatr Res* 32:520, 1992.
114. Robinson PN: Chemotherapy and anaesthesia. In Filshie J, Robbie DS, editors: *Anesthesia and malignant disease,* Dobbs Ferry, 1989, Sheridan House.
115. Rockoff MA, Goudsouzian NG: Seizures induced by methohexital, *Anesthesiology* 54:333, 1981.
116. Rosenthal S, Kaufman S: Vincristine neurotoxicity, *Ann Intern Med* 80:733, 1974.
117. Roth JL, Nugent M, Gray JE, et al: Patient monitoring during magnetic resonance imaging, *Anesthesiology* 62:80, 1985.
118. Samra SK: Anesthesia for diagnostic procedures and nonsurgical treatment in children with brain tumors, *J Neurosurg Anesth* 1:145, 1989.
119. Scher CS, Amar D, McDowall RH, et al: Use of propofol for prevention of chemotherapy-induced nausea and emesis in oncology patients, *Can J Anaesth* 39:170, 1992.
120. Schulze G: Swine proteases as mediators of radiographic contrast media toxicity, *Invest Radiol* 15:518, 1980.
121. Selvin BL: Cancer chemotherapy: implications for the anesthesiologist, *Anesth Analg* 60:425, 1981.
122. Shehadi WH: Contrast media adverse reactions: occurrence, recurrence, and distribution patterns, *Radiology* 143:11, 1982.
123. Shehadi WH: Death following intravascular administration of contrast media, *Acta Radiol Diagn* 26:457, 1985.
124. Shellock FG, Crues JV: High-field-strength MR imaging and metallic biomedical implants: an *ex vivo* evaluation deflection farces, *AJR* 151:389, 1988.
125. Shellock FG, Morisoli S, Kanal E: MR procedures and biomedical implants, materials and devices. 1993 update, *Radiology* 189:587, 1993.
126 Sims C: Thickly and thinly applied lignocaine-prilocaine cream prior to venipuncture in children, *Anaesth Intensive Care* 19:343, 1991.
127. Skalpe IO: Complications in cerebral angiography with iohexol (Omnipaque) and meglumine metrizoate (Isopaque cerebral), *Neuroradiology* 30:69, 1988.
128. Smith DC, Yahiku PY, Maloney MD, et al: Three new low-osmolality contrast agents: a comparative study of patient discomfort, *AJNR* 9:137, 1988.
129. Smith DS, Askey P, Young ML, et al: Anesthetic management of acutely ill patients during magnetic resonance imaging, *Anesthesiology* 65:710, 1986.
130. Smith I, White PF, Nathanson M, Gouldson R: Propofol: an update on its clinical use, *Anesthesiology* 81:1005, 1994.
131. Snodgrass WR, Dodge WF: Lytic/"DPT" cocktail: time for national and safe alternatives, *Pediatr Clin North Am* 36:1285, 1989.
132. Stark DD, Moss AA, Goldberg HI, et al: Magnetic resonance and CT of the normal and diseased pancreas: a comparative study, *Radiology* 150:153, 1984.
133. Steinberg AD: Should choral hydrate be banned? *Pediatrics* 92:442, 1993.
134. Stones PJ, Torres Jr WE, Colvin RS, et al: Effectiveness of CT in evaluating intrathoracic masses, *AJR* 139:469, 1982.
135. Strain JD, Harvey LA, Foley LC, et al: Intravenously administered pentobarbital sodium for sedation in pediatric CT, *Radiology* 161:105, 1986.
136. Thoeni RF, Moss AA, Schnyder P, et al: Detection and staging of primary rectal and rectosigmoid cancer by computed tomography, *Radiology* 141:135-138, 1981.
137. Thompson JR, Schneider S, Ashwal S, et al: The choice of sedation for computed tomography in children: a prospective evaluation, *Radiology* 143:475, 1982.
138. Academy of Pediatrics Committee on Drugs and Committee on Environmental Health: Use of chloral hydrate for sedation in children, *Pediatrics* 92:471, 1993.
139. Varner PD, Ebert JP, McKay RD, et al: Methohexital sedation of children undergoing CT scan, *Anesth Analg* 64:643, 1985.
140. Welborn SG: Anesthesia for EMI scanning in infants and small children, *South Med J* 69:1294, 1976.
141. Weston G, Strunin L, Amundson GM: Imaging for anaesthetists: a review of methods and anaesthetic implications of diagnostic imaging techniques, *Can Anaesth Soc J* 32:552, 1985.
142. White RI, Halden WJ: Liquid gold: low-osmolality contrast media, *Radiology* 159:559, 1986.
143. Whitfield A, Douglas RH: Effect of general anaesthesia on the magnetic resonance imaging signal from the brain, *Br J Anaesth* 62:694, 1989.
144. Williford ME, Goodwin JD: Computed tomography of lung abscesses and empyema, *Radiol Clin North Am* 21:575, 1983.
145. Wittenberg J, Fineberg HV, Ferrucci Jr, JT, et al: Clinical efficacy of computed body tomography, II, *AJR* 134:1111, 1980.
146. Wittenberg J: Computed tomography of the body, I, *N Engl J Med* 309:1160, 1983.
147. Wittenberg J; Computed tomography of the body, II, *N Engl J Med* 309:1224, 1983.
148. Wolf GL: Safer, more expensive iodinated contrast agents: how do we decide? *Radiology* 159:557, 1986.
149. Wolpers HG, Hunneman DH, Stellwaag M, et al: Calcium binding by arteriographic contrast media, *J Pharm Sci* 70:231, 1981.
150. Yaster M, Nichols DG, Deshpande JK, et al: Midazolam-fentanyl intravenous sedation in children: case report of respiratory arrest, *Pediatrics* 86:463, 1990.
151. Zsigmond EG, Robins G: The effect of a series of anticancer drugs on plasma cholinesterase activity, *Can Anaesth Soc J* 19:75, 1972.

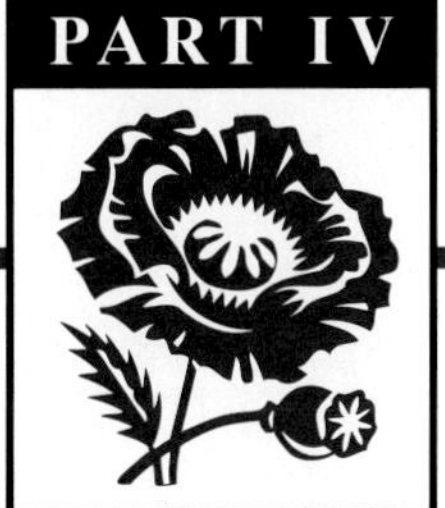

Postoperative Recovery and Complications

CHAPTER 88

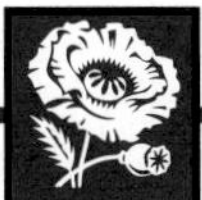

Postanesthesia Care Unit

BRIAN A. ROSENFELD
TANYA L. OYOS*

Successful completion of a procedure in the operating room does not ensure a smooth and uneventful recovery from anesthesia and surgery. Individualized monitoring and assessment are necessary to ensure adequate recovery. Postoperative complications severe enough to require treatment occur in 7% to 10% of general postanesthesia care unit (PACU) admissions.[25] The magnitude of this treatment frequently depends on the patient's underlying medical problems and the rapidity with which the problem is identified. Although surgical bleeding or preexisting medical conditions complicate early postoperative recovery, many PACU problems are the result of adverse physiologic and pharmacologic effects of anesthetic drugs and techniques. Careful communication of information from anesthesia provider to PACU nurse, and monitoring of anesthetized patients needs to continue until the effects of anesthesia have been satisfactorily reversed and protective reflexes reestablished. In this chapter, we examine: (1) admission and discharge criteria; (2) specific problems commonly encountered in the PACU; and (3) organ system problems often seen in PACU patients.

ADMISSION CRITERIA

The decision to admit a patient to the PACU is determined by the magnitude of the surgical procedure, the anesthetic technique, and the patient's underlying medical condition. Healthy patients undergoing superficial procedures with local anesthetic infiltration frequently do not require observation in the PACU. Most other patients, including patients receiving minimal intravenous (IV) sedation, should be observed for a period of time postoperatively.

The role of the PACU has expanded in recent years. New procedures in interventional radiology, for example, have increased demand to monitor postanesthesia/sedated patients who have not had surgery. The PACU, with its trained staff, is the ideal location to monitor these patients. Whatever the reason for admission to the PACU, the transition of patient care should be accomplished in the safest possible manner. Responsibility should not be turned over to the PACU staff until hemodynamic, ventilatory, and airway status are appropriately stable and secure. Caregivers transferring care to the PACU staff should be readily accessible or should clearly designate another qualified practitioner who will handle any emergency problem. Safe transfer to the PACU requires that important information concerning patients be communicated to the receiving staff. This information, which constitutes the

*Revised for the second edition by Dr. Oyos.

BOX 88-1
COMPONENTS OF A PACU ADMISSION REPORT

Preoperative history

Medication allergies or reactions
Underlying medical illness
Chronic medications (when last dose received)
Acute problems (ischemia, acid-base, dehydration)
Premedications
Vital signs

Intraoperative factors

Surgical procedure
Surgeon
Type of anesthetic
Relaxant/reversal status
Unexpected surgical or anesthetic events
Intraoperative vital signs ranges
Intraoperative laboratory findings
Estimated blood loss
Urine output
Type/amount intravenous fluids
Drugs given
Time/amount opioid administration

Assessment and report of current status

Heart rate and rhythm
Systemic blood pressure
Temperature
Ventilatory adequacy
Level of consciousness
Endotracheal tube position
Function of invasive monitors
Anesthetic equipment (e.g., epidural catheters)
Overall impression

Postoperative instructions

Acceptable vital signs ranges
Anticipated cardiovascular problems
Expected airway and ventilatory status
Location of responsible physician
Diagnostic tests to be secured
Acceptable urine output and blood loss
Orders for therapeutic interventions
Surgical instructions (positioning, wound care)
Therapeutic goals and endpoints before discharge

PACU admission report (Box 88-1), includes relevant history and physical findings, as well as details about the intraoperative course, especially medications received, operation, surgeon, anesthetic technique, blood loss, fluid administration, and neuromuscular status. In this report, the anesthesia provider should outline immediate postoperative plans and potential adverse clinical events.

Patients admitted to the PACU are monitored, including respiratory rate and character, heart rate and rhythm, blood pressure, temperature and mental status. Qualitative observations including skin color, level of consciousness, and airway patency are also made. These observations are repeated at intervals dictated by the patient's condition, but seldom less frequently than every 15 minutes. Patients should be continuously monitored by electrocardiogram (ECG) for dysrhythmias and by pulse oximetry for oxygen saturation. Myocardial ischemia can be monitored using a precordial or modified V5 in those at risk for coronary artery disease (CAD).[57]

DISCHARGE CRITERIA

When patients satisfy preestablished criteria (Box 88-2), they are considered for PACU discharge. Many patients will not satisfy all discharge criteria, requiring individual assessment before discharge. Knowledge of the patient's preoperative status can be important in decisions regarding discharge. For example, patients with preoperative mental obtundation would not be expected to be oriented postoperatively before discharge. Diabetic patients should have blood sugar levels checked. When indicated, pulmonary status should be evaluated with arterial blood gas levels, chest radiographs, and spirometry. Patients who fail to satisfy discharge criteria and/or whose condition differs significantly from their preoperative status warrant further observation in the PACU or transfer to an intensive care setting.

Before discharging patients, PACU caregivers should determine whether a "margin of safety" exists (e.g., Can the patient increase his or her minute ventilation in response to increased oxygen consumption? Is intravascular volume sufficient to tolerate ongoing blood loss?) If there is doubt about whether this margin of safety exists, further clinical evaluation or prolonged observation may be necessary. Similarly, if a patient's O_2 saturation level is borderline (low 90s on room air), the patient should be transferred with supplemental O_2 to provide a margin of safety.

Patients recovering from regional anesthesia should demonstrate evidence of resolving neurologic blockade. Another important criterion prior to PACU discharge in these patients is hemodynamic stability. Using orthostatic blood pressures, Alexander et al.[2] demonstrated that hemodynamic stability does not correlate with the level of block. They suggested that patients may be discharged sooner than previously recommended.

Interest in cost containment and reduction has prompted investigation of the way anesthetic agents influence duration of the patient's stay in the PACU. A meta-analysis of literature studies by Dexter and Tinker[29] indicated outpatients who received propofol were discharged from recovery sooner than patients who received desflurane. Patients who received desflurane followed commands in the PACU sooner than patients who received isoflurane.

PROBLEMS COMMONLY ENCOUNTERED IN THE POSTANESTHESIA CARE UNIT

Ischemic Heart Disease

Surgery is today performed on sicker, older patients, making CAD more common in PACU patients. Because intra-

BOX 88-2
GUIDELINES FOR PACU DISCHARGE

Overall condition

- Oriented to person, place, and time
- Follows simple instructions
- "Acceptable" color without cyanosis, splotchiness, paleness
- Adequate muscular strength and mobility for minimal self-care
- Suitable control of nausea and emesis
- Destination unit appropriate for patient's status

Cardiovascular condition

- Within ± 20% resting preoperative values for heart rate and blood pressure
- Cardiovascular status relatively constant for at least 30 minutes
- Resolution of any new sustained dysrhythmia
- Acceptable intravascular volume status
- Any suspicion of myocardial ischemia rectified

Airway maintenance

- Protective reflexes (swallow, gag) intact
- Absence of stridor, retraction, or partial obstruction
- No further need for artificial airway support

Ventilation and oxygenation

- Ventilatory rate greater than 10, less than 30
- Adequate ability to cough and clear secretions
- Acceptable work of breathing (clinical assessment)

Pain control

- Adequate analgesia
- Observation since last narcotic administered
  - 30 minutes if IV
  - 60 minutes if IM/SQ
  - 30 minutes if peripheral PCA
  - 60 minutes if epidural fentanyl PCA

Renal function

- Urine output approximately 30 m/hr^{-1} (catheterized patients)
- Appropriate color and appearance of urine, evaluation of hematuria
- Follow-up orders regarding output if spontaneous voiding has not occurred

Regional anesthesia

- Resolving sensory block with level no higher than T12
- Evidence of lower extremity motor function (toe movement)
- Able to void spontaneously if not catheterized

Ambulatory patients

- Regional block totally resolved
- Ability to ambulate without dizziness, hypotension, or support
- Suitable control of nausea and vomiting after ambulation
- Tolerating oral intake
- Voiding spontaneously

operative ischemia and infarction can remain undetected,[44] recognition of these events in the immediate postoperative period is important. High-risk patients may develop myocardial ischemia on emergence from anesthesia and in the immediate postoperative period. This can be particularly dangerous because myocardial infarction (MI) occurring in the perioperative period has a greater mortality than in nonsurgical settings.[86,108]

Between 0.5 and 4.0% of PACU patients may experience a cardiovascular complication in the recovery room.[51] Hines et al.[51] reported that MI occurred in 0.3% of PACU patients. The presence of factors detrimental to myocardial O_2 (MVO_2) supply and demand occur frequently in the immediate postoperative period and contribute to the development of PACU cardiovascular complications. (Fig. 88-1). Increased catecholamine levels resulting from surgical stress, pain, shivering, and emergence delirium can all lead to myocardial ischemia. Anemia, hypoxemia, fever, and hypovolemia can cause tachycardia, the most frequent perioperative hemodynamic event precipitating myocardial ischemia.[69] Other hemodynamic causes of myocardial ischemia include hypotension, increased preload, and increased afterload. Moderate increases in preload and afterload are well tolerated by patients with CAD and normal myocardial function; these changes in patients with

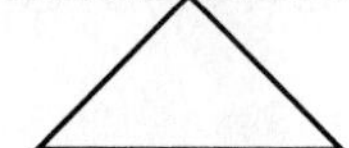

Fig. 88-1. Detrimental changes in myocardial oxygen balance. Note that tachycardia and increased preload affect both sides of the balance. (From Thys D: Cardiovascular physiology. In Miller RD, editor: *Anaesthesia,* ed 3, New York, 1990, Churchill-Livingstone.)

poor left ventricular function frequently lead to ischemia.[31] The combination of hypotension and tachycardia can be especially deleterious in all patients with CAD.[18]

Diagnosing postoperative myocardial ischemia is often complicated by absence of symptoms and the presence of nonspecific ECG changes. Studies on postoperative MI demonstrate that only 15% to 20% of patients complain of anginal pain.[7,10] This is probably due to the overriding pain of surgery, narcotic administration, and residual anesthesia/sedation. Other patients undergo silent myocardial ischemia during the early postoperative period.[85] Loss of anginal pain as a diagnostic tool means that certain cardiovascular events should raise suspicion for ischemia. Unexplained dysrhythmias, hypotension, oliguria, or increased filling pressures (central venous pressure [CVP] or pulmonary capillary wedge pressure [PCWP]) should be assessed with a 12-lead ECG to try to rule out myocardial ischemia. To obtain maximum benefit from ECG monitoring, lead V5 or modified V5 should be observed continuously (Fig. 88-2).[62] ECG changes should not be "overread." Breslow et al.[16] have shown that postoperative T-wave changes are nonspecific (Fig. 88-3).[16]

Pharmacologic therapy of myocardial ischemia depends on the specific cause (Table 88-1 and Box 88-3). Tachycardia may indicate volume, blood, antipyretics, analgesics, or ventilation, possibly combined with beta blockers. Nitrates should be used after intravascular volume is considered adequate. IV or sublingual nitroglycerin is preferred because transdermal nitrates may not be absorbed in hypothermic or vasocontricted postoperative patients. Sublingual nifedipine can also be used, but precipitous drops in blood pressure leading to MI have occurred.[82] Newer IV calcium channel blockers (e.g., nicardipine) may enable easier control of blood pressure.[54] Most narcotics have been used in postoperative patients, providing both analgetic and bradycardic effects.

Failure to Extubate

Several conditions may necessitate continued intubation after surgery, including: (1) epiglottitis: (2) localized edema of the upper airway secondary to surgery or trauma; (3) surgery causing damage to recurrent laryngeal nerves; (4) upper airway edema from massive intraoperative volume infusion in patients maintained in Trendelenburg position for prolonged periods; and (5) unstable hemodynamics or bleeding after major surgery.

Criteria for extubation include consciousness, return of protective airway reflexes, and adequate ventilatory function. Although subjective, level of consciousness is easily discerned. Patients who do not regain consciousness as expected should remain intubated and be evaluated further (see discussion of failure to awaken). **Recently published criteria establish physical tests that correlate with adequate airway protection.**[88] **Criteria for adequate ventilatory function have previously been established and include: (1) resting minute ventilation of < 10 l; (2) the ability to voluntarily double the resting minute ventilation; (3) peak negative pressure on maximal inspiration of > 30 cm of water; and (4) forced vital capacity > 10 to 15 ml/kg.**[101]

Difficulty extubating postoperative patients is primarily caused by surgical and anesthetic effects on underlying pulmonary abnormalities. Such preoperative abnormalities include obstructive or restrictive lung disease, myasthenia gravis, Eaton-Lambert syndrome, and obesity. Procedures involving the thorax and upper abdomen have greater effect on postoperative ventilation than lower abdominal or extremity procedures. Certain specific surgical procedures can also affect the ability to ventilate postoperatively. Placement of spinal rods changes the anatomic configuration of the chest wall, altering ventilation/perfusion matching, and ventral hernia closures increase intra-abdominal pressure, decreasing diaphragmatic excursion. Anesthetic factors affecting postoperative ventilation and ability to extubate include residual neuromuscular paralysis, central nervous system (CNS) depression from narcotics and inhalational agents, hypothermia, and inadequate pain control.

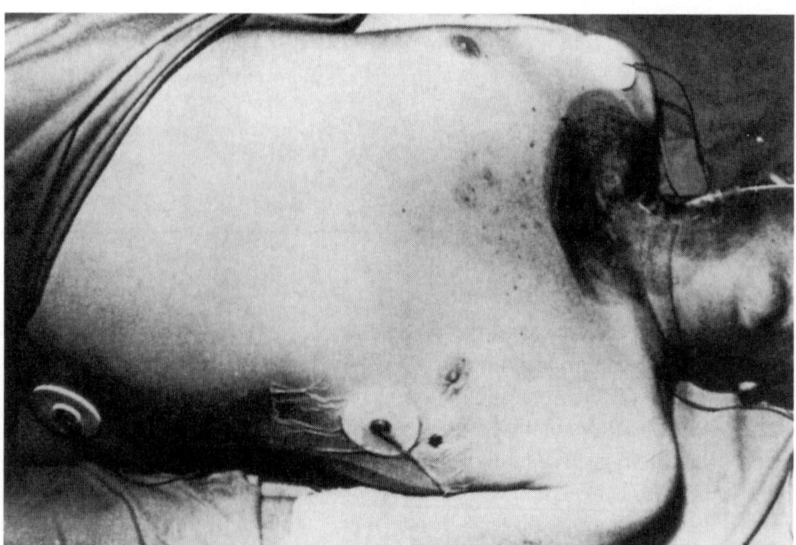

Fig. 88-2. CS5 lead arrangement. Standard lead I should be selected to monitor a modified V5 lead. (From Kaplan J, editor: *Cardiac anesthesia,* ed 2, New York, 1987, WB Saunders.)

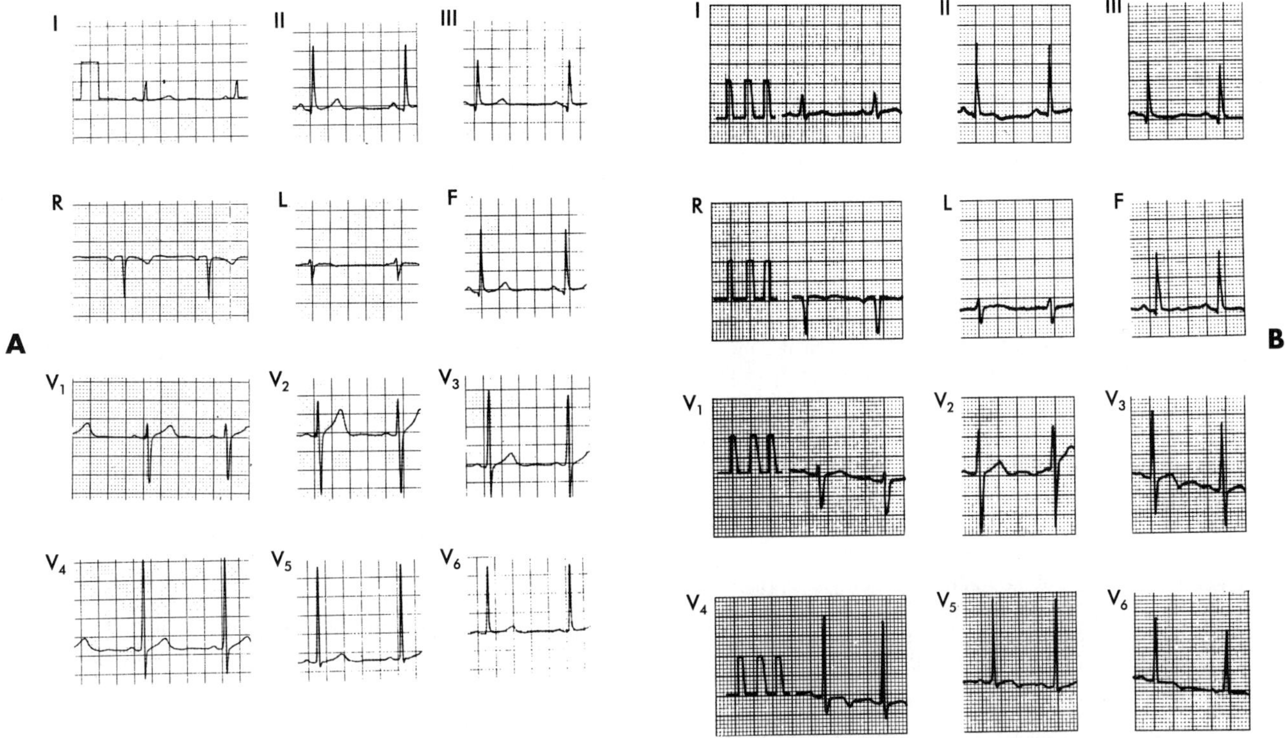

Fig. 88-3. A, Preoperative electrocardiogram. **B,** Immediate postoperative electrocardiogram. Note the T-wave changes in the inferior and lateral leads. This occurred in 14% to 20% of all (n = 394) postoperative patients. (From Breslow MJ, Miller CF, Parker SD, et al.: Changes in T-wave morphology following anesthesia and surgery: a common recovery room phenomenon, *Anesthesiology* 64:398, 1986.)

Table 88-1 Pharmacologic guidelines for treating hemodynamic changes in patients with ischemic heart disease

	Tachycardia*	Normal Heart Rate	Bradycardia
Hypertensive*	Labetalol Esmolol Propranolol	Labetalol Nifedipine SL Nipride Hydralazine Nicardipine	Nifedipine SL Nipride Hydralazine Nicardipine
Normotensive	Fluid bolus Esmolol Propranolol	Smile!	Smile! Atropine (HR < 40)
Hypotensive†	Fluid bolus Phenylephrine	Fluid bolus Phenylephrine	Fluid bolus Atropine

*Rule out pain and treat with analgetics.
†Rule out hypovolemia and treat wth fluid.

Complications that occur intraoperatively can also affect postoperative ventilation. For example, a primary CNS event, pneumothorax, hemothorax, collapse of single or multiple lung lobes from mainstem intubation or positioning, and rib fractures decrease ability to ventilate. An unusual cause of postoperative respiratory failure involves bilateral phrenic nerve damage.[99]

PACU patients unable to be extubated require close monitoring, physical examination and laboratory work-up, with special attention to neurologic and cardiopulmonary systems. Residual paralysis, CNS depression, chest wall abnormalities, and pulmonary parenchymal abnormalities should be sought. Laboratory examination may include arterial blood gas, chest radiograph, and bedside pulmonary mechanics.

Excessive Bleeding

The PACU patient who develops bleeding should be evaluated and treated expeditiously. Specific treatment is dictated by the rapidity, location, and cause of the bleeding. All rapid

BOX 88-3
DOSAGE OF MEDICATIONS USED TO TREAT MYOCARDIAL ISCHEMIA

Labetalol	20 mg in 20 ml over 20 min (repeat as needed up to 400 mg)
Esmolol	0.5 mg/kg load plus 50–200 mcg/kg/min (2500 mg in 100 ml start at 10 ml/hr), titrating to desired HR
Inderal	0.5–1.0 mg up to 0.1 mg/kg total
Phenylephrine	Titrate drip to BP (10 mg in 100 ml start at 10 ml/hr)
Hydralazine	5 mg boluses up to 20 mg (wait 15 min for effect of dose)
Nicardipine	2.5 mg bolus then 5–15 mg/hr
Atropine	0.5 mg as needed up to 2 mg
Analgetics	Titrate to pain relief avoiding respiratory depression.
Fluid boluses	500 ml of NS or RL, or blood as needed, keeping Hct > 30
Nifedipine	10-mg capsule given sublingually (can give up to 30 mg)
Nitroglycerine	Sublingual × 3 or IV titrated to effect

blood loss requires immediate treatment with crystalloid, colloid, and blood replacement. Bleeding from poor surgical hemostasis requires immediate reoperation, whereas other causes of bleeding require further diagnostic evaluation. Visible bleeding from wounds or surgical drainage is readily apparent, but internal bleeding into the gastrointestinal (GI) tract, thorax, retroperitoneum, pelvis, and thigh is more difficult to detect. Occult bleeding can be diagnosed by signs of hypovolemia (hypotension, poor peripheral perfusion, oliguria, and tachycardia), a falling hematocrit and a high index of suspicion. Hypotension in supine patients is a relatively late sign of hypovolemia and may already represent a major decrease in cardiac output (Table 88-2). Orthostatic signs (blood pressure and heart rate) can provide an earlier indication of intravascular volume status. Changing hematocrit values can be difficult to interpret and should be evaluated in conjunction with the rate of IV fluid infusion. Rapid crystalloid or colloid infusion in volume-depleted patients who are not bleeding lowers the hematocrit more rapidly than slow infusion in slowly bleeding patients. Further diagnostic studies in patients suspected of occult blood loss include CVP monitoring, chest radiograph, computed tomography (CT) scan, endoscopy, and arteriography. Location of bleeding occasionally requires urgent attention. Bleeding from a wound or venous cannulation site in the neck can obstruct the airway; bleeding into an extremity can lead to a compartment syndrome; and bleeding into the CNS can present with altered consciousness or focal deficits.

Postoperative bleeding can also indicate coagulation disorders. These may have been apparent preoperatively or may develop from complications of surgery. Coagulation disorders can represent problems of the intrinsic or extrinsic clotting system, platelet function, or fibrinolysis. Problems of the intrinsic or extrinsic system (Fig. 88-4) are caused by congenital or acquired factor deficiencies. Acquired deficiencies are usually caused by liver disease, but in hospitalized patients, these deficits may be due to vitamin K malabsorption or starvation in conjunction with antibiotic therapy.[91]

Table 88-2 Decreases in cardiac output and arterial pressure during graded hemorrhage in dogs

Blood volume removed (%)	Cardiac output (%)	Arterial pressure (%)
10	−21	−7
20	−45	−15

Modified from Hinshaw et al: Regional blood flow in hemorrhagic shock, *Am J Surg* 102:224, 1961.

The two drugs most commonly affecting coagulation are coumadin and heparin. Coumadin decreases the levels of vitamin K–dependent factors,[2,7,9,10] causing prolongation of prothrombin time (PT), which can be corrected with fresh frozen plasma (FFP). Heparin blocks conversion of factors 9 and 10 to their active forms and also by increasing the activity of antithrombin III. Anticoagulation with heparin causes prolongation of the activated partial thromboplastin time (aPTT). Another measure of heparin activity, the activated coagulation time (ACT), is affected by the amount of circulating heparin and can also be used to roughly estimate the dose of protamine necessary to reverse heparin-induced anticoagulation.[19]

Abnormalities of platelet number and function can lead to postoperative bleeding. Platelet counts less than 75,000/mm^3 have been associated with bleeding, particularly in massively transfused patients.[26] This thrombocytopenia has previously been attributed to a dilutional effect, but recent data have questioned this conclusion.[30] Platelet transfusions are indicated for patients with platelet counts less than 75,000/mm^3 who are actively bleeding. Bleeding patients with normal platelet counts may have a qualitative platelet dysfunction caused by uremia or drugs (Box 88-4). This may be demonstrated by an abnormal bleeding time, thromboelastogram, or platelet aggregometry.[57] Platelet dysfunction associated with uremia is treated with dialysis,[80] cryoprecipitate,[56] or vasopressin,[67] whereas drug-related dysfunction is treated with platelet transfusion.

Disorders producing increased fibrinolysis can cause bleeding in postoperative patients. Disseminated intravascular coagulation (DIC) is the classic pathologic fibrinolytic state. It can be seen in acute or chronic forms and is diagnosed by thrombocytopenia, hypofibrinogenemia, prolonged PT and aPTT, and elevated levels of both fibrin degradation products and D-dimer. Hemolytic transfusion reactions from blood given intraoperatively may be partially

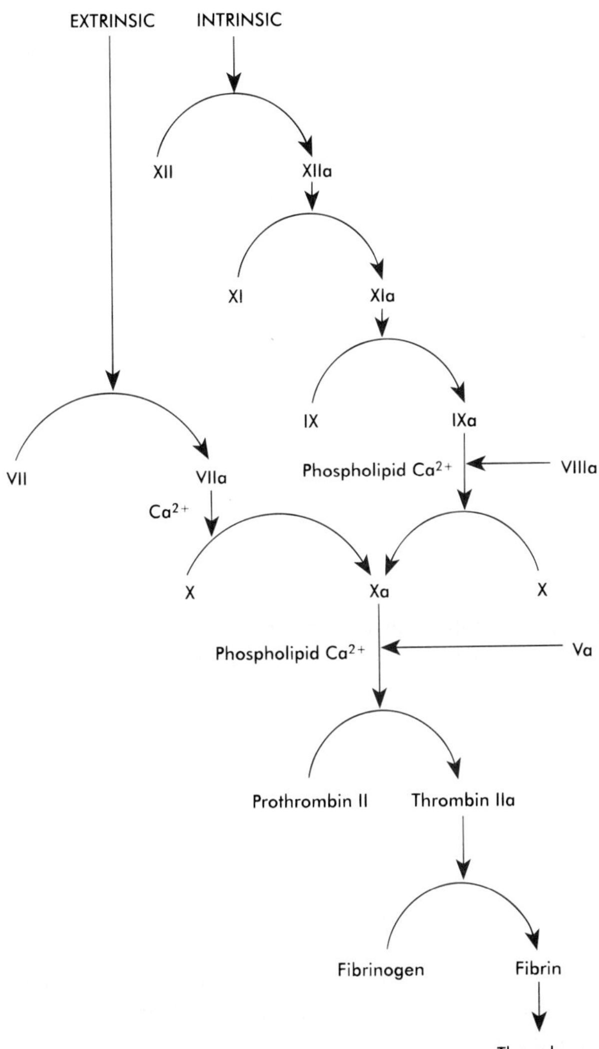

Fig. 88-4. Coagulation cascade. Extrinsic and intrinsic systems merge at factor X into the common pathway, ultimately leading to thrombus formation.

BOX 88-4
DRUGS THAT INHIBIT PLATELET FUNCTION

- Agents that affect prostanoid synthesis
  - Aspirin
  - Corticosteroids
  - Others (e.g., ketorolac, indomethacin, phyenylbutazone, ibuprofen, fenprofen, naproxen, sulfinpyrazone)
- Adenylate cyclase activators
  - Prostanoids (e.g., prostacyclin, PGE_1)
  - Others (e.g., isoprenaline, adenosine)
- Phosphodiesterase inhibitors
  - Pyrimidopyrimidines (e.g., dipyridamole)
  - Methyl xanthines (e.g., caffeine, theophylline, aminophylline, papaverine)
- Antimicrobial agents
  - Penicillins and cephalothins (e.g., carbenicillin, penicillin G, ticarcillin, ampicillin, cephalothin)
  - Others (e.g., nitrofurantoin, ristocetin, hydroxychloroquin)
- Membrane stabilizing agents
  - Local anesthetics (e.g., procaine, lidocaine)
  - Antihistamines (e.g., diphenhydramine, promethazine)
  - Tricyclic antidepressants (e.g., imipramine, nortriptyline)
- Beta blockers (e.g., propanolol)
- Anticoagulant agents
  - Heparin
  - Dextrans
  - Fibrinolytics
- Miscellaneous drugs
  - Ethanol
  - Nitroglycerin, nitroprusside
  - Quinidine, calcium channel blockers
  - Ticlopidine
- Other (e.g., phenothiazines, clofibrate, reserpine, tegretol, methysergide)

masked by anesthesia and can present with DIC in the PACU. Placement of shunts for intractable ascites and some genitourinary procedures are other causes of DIC that can occur postoperatively. In most instances of DIC, therapy is directed at stabilizing the bleeding diathesis with appropriate blood products and treating the underlying causes.

Failure to Awaken

The three major causes of failure to awaken after anesthesia are: (1) prolonged action of anesthetic agents; (2) metabolic abnormalities; (3) neurologic injury (Box 88-5). Delayed awakening after general anesthesia is most commonly caused by the effects of anesthetic drugs. Inhalational agents, narcotics, barbiturates, anticholinergics, and neuromuscular blockers can all result in delayed emergence. This may be the result of an absolute overdose of these agents or altered pharmacokinetic and pharmacodynamic effects. In the general population there is a wide variation in patient sensitivity to anesthetic agents. Factors that can further reduce anesthetic requirements and prolong emergence are advanced age, hypothermia, hypothyroidism,[34] liver and renal disease, and unsuspected illicit drug use. Anticholinergic agents (e.g., scopolamine) have CNS depressant effects, and high doses of atropine can also cause prolonged sedation.

Metabolic disturbances associated with postoperative CNS depression are listed in Box 88-5. **Hypoxia may present with delirium before obtundation and requires immediate diagnosis and treatment.** Hypercapnia causes CNS depression by its central acidotic effect, whereas the systemic effects prolong the action of neuromuscular blockers, creating a vicious cycle. Liver failure, renal failure, hypothyroidism, and adrenal failure (Addison's disease) can all cause coma. In postoperative patients, the primary effects of these diseases may be difficult to distinguish from their secondary effects on decreased drug metabolism and clearance. These disorders are usually diagnosed preoperatively,

BOX 88-5
DIFFERENTIAL DIAGNOSIS OF FAILURE TO REGAIN CONSCIOUSNESS AFTER ANESTHESIA

- Prolonged drug action
  - Overdose
  - Increased sensitivity
  - Decreased protein binding
  - Redistribution
  - Drug interaction
- Metabolic
  - Hypoxia or hypercapnia
  - Hepatic, renal, or endocrine end organ dysfunction
  - Hypoglycemia, hyperosmolar-hyperglycemia, diabetic ketoacidosis
  - Electrolyte imbalance (Na^+, CA^{++}, Mg^{++})
- Neurologic injury
  - Intracranial hemorrhage
  - Cerebral ischemia
  - Cerebral embolus
  - Cerebral contusion
  - Subclinical seizures
  - Enlarging pneumocephalus

and the anesthetic plan is altered accordingly, although hypothyroidism and Addison's disease can go unrecognized and result in postoperative coma.[76,77] Hypothyroidism is particularly difficult to diagnose in the PACU because hypothermia and/or bradycardia are common in PACU. Careful review of preoperative clinical findings may reveal evidence of hypothyroidism that was not appreciated.

Disorders of glucose homeostasis that prolong emergence include hypoglycemia; hyperosmolar, hyperglycemic, nonketotic coma (HHNK); and diabetic ketoacidosis (DKA). Although surgical stress generally increases blood glucose levels, dangerous hypoglycemia can occur intraoperatively. Patients with insulin-producing tumors, severe liver failure, and diabetics who are given insulin inadequately covered by glucose are at risk. HHNK leads to severe dehydration, hyperosmolarity, and CNS depression. Frequently found in patients with a history of mild noninsulin-dependent diabetes, HHNK can carry a mortality of up to 50%.[95] DKA usually occurs in insulin-dependent diabetic patients who have inadequate insulin coverage. Although the metabolic acidemia rarely causes CNS effects, treatment with bicarbonate can lead to a paradoxic increase in CNS acidosis and obtundation.[83] Minor electrolyte imbalances, which are common in postoperative patients, do not usually cause problems with arousal. Severe changes in electrolytes, however, can lead to depressed CNS function. The most common causes are acute hyponatremia and hypernatremia, which are usually caused by disorders of water balance (water intoxication in the transurethral prostatectomy syndrome or dehydration); hypercalcemia from malignancy; hypocalcemia from parathyroid surgery; and hypermagnesemia from magnesium sulfate therapy. Disorders of temperature can also cause delayed emergence (see discussion of abnormal temperature).

Primary central neurologic events (hemorrhage, ischemia, and embolus) that occur during surgery can cause postoperative coma. Undiagnosed CNS injuries in trauma patients, the effects of N_2O on pneumocephalus,[109] and subclinical status epilepticus can all cause failure to awaken.

Evaluation of PACU patients who fail to awaken from anesthesia in timely fashion involves close review of the history for preexisting diseases and drug intake, reviewing the intraoperative course for cardiopulmonary changes, and performing a meticulous neurologic examination. Further work-up can include electrolyte and blood chemistries, toxicology screening, arterial blood gases, and emergency CT scan of the head.

Supraventricular Tachycardia

Supraventricular tachycardia (SVT) is defined as any heart rate greater than 100 beats/min that originates at or above the atrioventricular node (AVN). These dysrhythmias are very common in PACU patients because of elevated postoperative catecholamine levels. In this situation, it is essential to determine whether the rhythm is sinus in origin. Regular heart rates of less than 130 beats/min are usually sinus, and identification of sinus node P-waves on the ECG should be relatively easy. Regular heart rates from 130 to 160 beats/min may be sinus, but they may also be atrial flutter with 2:1 block, accelerated ectopic, or reentrant supraventricular rhythms (Figs. 88-5 through 88-7). Appropriate management depends on making this differentiation. Changes in blood pressure and cardiac output may point to a nonsinus origin of the rhythm. With nonsinus supraventricular dysrhythmias, loss of the atrial contraction contribution to cardiac output can be important. Atrial contraction normally adds perhaps 15% to resting cardiac output. In patients with obstruction to left ventricular filling from valvular disease or noncompliant ventricles (diastolic dysfunction), loss of atrial contraction can result in a 20% to 40% decrease in cardiac output. If patients are stable, a 12-lead ECG should be obtained to rule out myocardial ischemia and identify the rhythm disturbance. When examining the 12-lead ECG, leads II and V1 should be evaluated for the presence and position of P waves. P waves are always upright in lead II with sinus rhythms but are inverted with low atrial or junctional rhythms (Fig. 88-8). Increasing the voltage and doubling the speed of the ECG can help to delineate the presence and morphology of P waves. Carotid sinus massage can be used as a diagnostic test to differentiate SVTs (Table 88-3) but is probably contraindicated in patients more than 60 years of age or in those with carotid vascular disease. Adenosine is now the agent of choice for diagnosis and treatment of patients with SVTs. Conversion of supraventricular dysrhythmias to sinus rhythm is occasionally associated with widespread T-wave inversions on the ECG. The mechanism

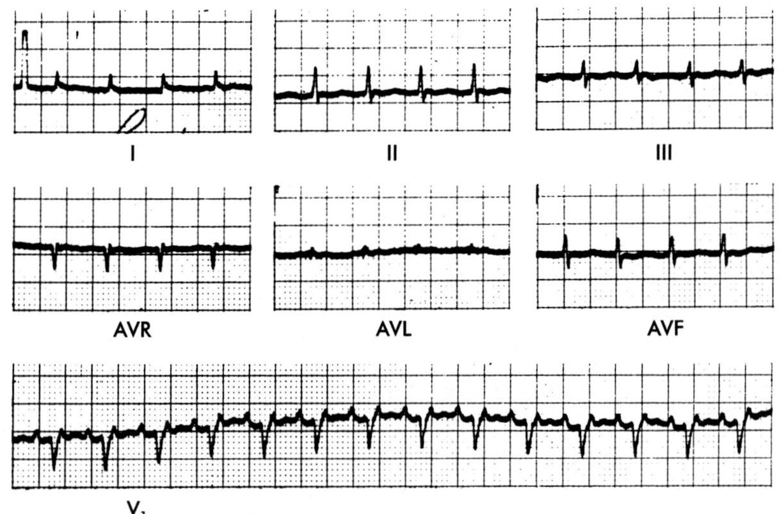

Fig. 88-5. Atrial flutter with 2:1 block. Ventricular rate is 150; atrial flutter waves are visible in V1.

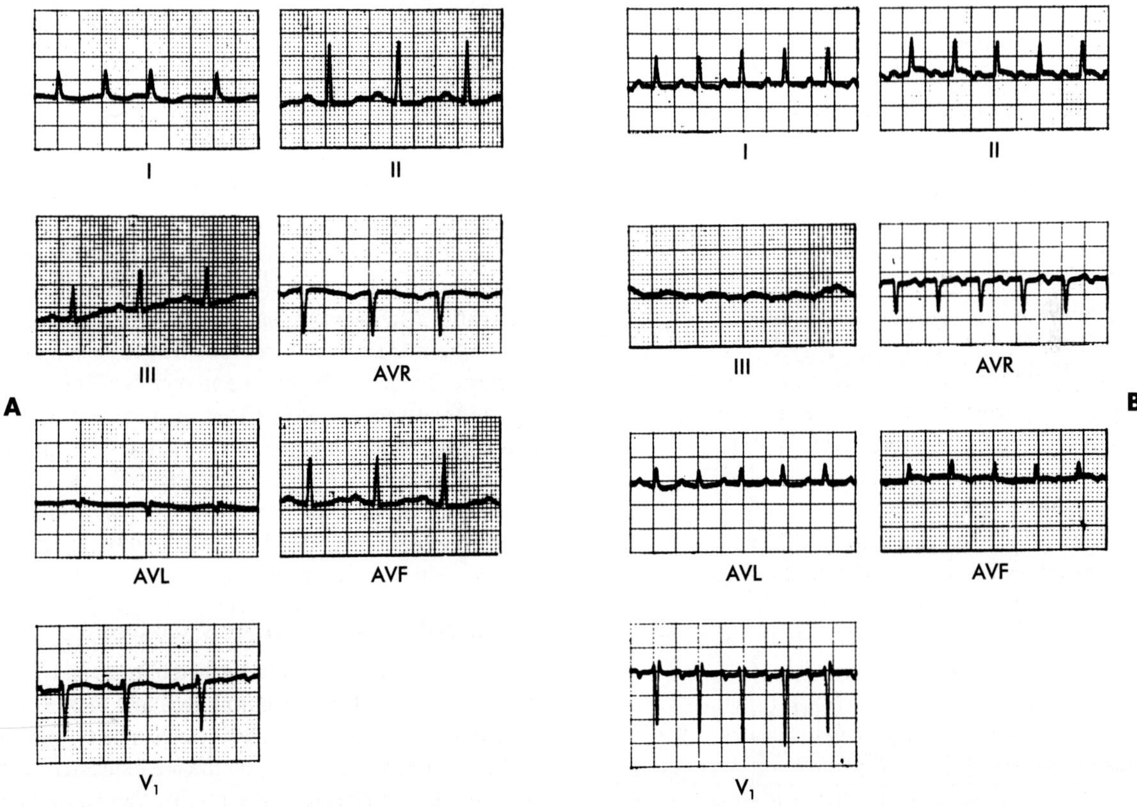

Fig. 88-6. **A,** Sinus rhythm before paroxysm. P wave morphology clearly seen in lead II. Atrial premature beats are seen in leads I and V1. **B,** Ectopic supraventricular tachycardia (rate 155). P wave morphology is different from sinus P waves.

of this phenomenon is unknown, but it occurs even in healthy hearts. There are no apparent sequelae, and these T-wave changes gradually recede over 2 to 7 days.

The most common SVT in PACU patients is sinus tachycardia, which has many etiologies (Box 88-6). It is important to identify and treat the cardiopulmonary causes. Rapid assessment of O_2 saturation, intravascular volume, hematocrit, and ventilation should be performed. Additional diagnostic tests, including CVP monitoring and arterial blood gas determination, may need to follow. Simple questioning and physical examination should also be conducted in a search for evidence of pain and visceral distension (bladder,

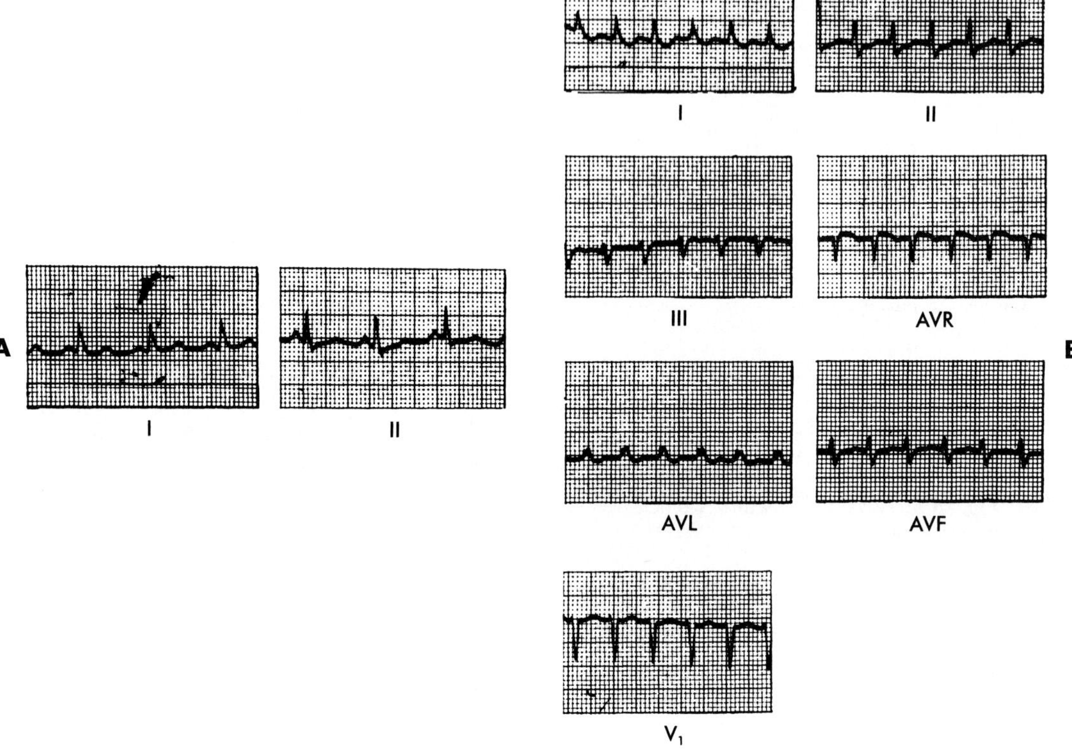

Fig. 88-7. A, Sinus rhythm with visible P waves. B, Reentrant SVT at rate of 160. P waves are not visible.

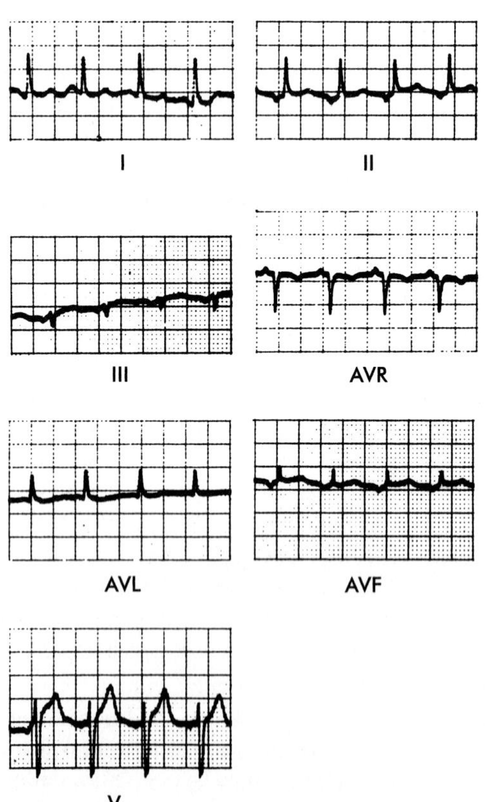

Fig. 88-8. Supraventricular dysrhythmia with a rate of 130. Note the inverted P waves in lead II and V1, denoting nonsinus origin.

gastric). Scrutiny of the preoperative and intraoperative medications frequently uncovers the most common causes and suggests treatment. Occasionally, patients will be tachycardiac without any apparent etiology. In this case, the decision to treat should be based on the patient's physical condition and underlying medical problems. Young patients, who are more prone to develop postoperative tachycardia, generally do not need treatment. Patients with ischemic heart disease, on the other hand, will likely require heart rate slowing with beta blockers.

Prolonged Neuromuscular Weakness

Patients who fail to meet established clinical and twitch monitor criteria of adequate neuromuscular function should remain intubated and ventilated. Occasionally, patients with borderline neuromuscular function are extubated in the operating room. On arrival in the PACU, these patients breathe shallowly and require airway support (e.g., jaw thrust). At this point, they are at risk for hypercapnic acidosis and aspiration. Assisted ventilation or reintubation and mechanical ventilation are indicated until the neuromuscular blockade resolves. Most patients with prolonged neuromuscular weakness arrive in the PACU intubated and ventilated. The most common cause of prolonged neuromuscular weakness is excessive use of neuromuscular blockers. Weakness occurs from an absolute overdose in patients with normal neuromuscular function or a relative overdose in patients with systemic disorders causing abnormal neuromuscular function.

Table 88-3 Response of regular supraventricular tachydysrhythmia to carotid sinus massage and adenosine

Rhythm	Sinus tachycardia	Accelerated ectopic atrial	Nodal reentrant	Atrial flutter 2:1
Rate	100–160	120–200	120–200	140–160
Response to carotid sinus massage	Minimal slowing	Minimal slowing	No response or Return to sinus	No response or Increased block, usually to 4:1
Response to intravenous adenosine	Marked slowing	Minimal slowing	Return to sinus	Increased block

BOX 88-6
CAUSES OF POSTOPERATIVE SINUS TACHYCARDIA

Hypovolemia, hypervolemia
Anemia
Fever
Hypercapnia
Hypoxemia (early sign)
Hyperthyroid, pheochromocytoma
Drug withdrawal (beta blockers, clonidine)
Drugs
- Theophylline
- Atropine
- Robinol
- Beta$_2$ agonists
- Epinephrine
- Cocaine
- Ketamine

Pain
Anxiety
Shivering
Bladder distension

Table 88-4 Dependence of various muscle relaxants on the kidney for their elimination

Drug	Precentage of injected dose
Gallamine	100
Decamethonium	100
Metocurine	80–100
Pancuronium	60–80
Alcuronium	70–90
Fazadinium	70–90
d-Tubocurarine	40–60
Vecuronium	10–20
Atracurium	< 5
Succinylcholine	0

Evaluating patients with prolonged neuromuscular weakness begins with a neurologic examination, review of the anesthetic record and the patient's medical history. The neurologic examination should assess the location and extent of paralysis (twitch monitor) and rule out a CNS or spinal cord etiology. Review of the anesthetic record may reveal a recent dose of neuromuscular blocker. This problem has decreased in recent years with the increased use of short-acting agents. Residual neuromuscular paralysis will frequently cause generalized jerking movements, which may be accompanied by considerable tachycardia and hypertension in conscious patients. Verbal reassurance at this point can be very beneficial, and mild sedation may be indicated before reversal. A level of paralysis inconsistent with the drugs listed on the anesthetic record should cause suspicion of another etiology.

Causes of prolonged neuromuscular blockade include metabolic and electrolyte abnormalities, acid-base disturbances, and drugs.[5,74] Liver disease decreases metabolic clearance; renal failure decreases drug excretion[66] (Table 88-4); and hypothermia decreases metabolism and excretion. Hypokalemia, hypocalcemia, hypermagnesemia, and metabolic alkalosis all prolong the effect of neuromuscular blockers. Respiratory acidosis ($Paco_2$ > 50 mm Hg) inhibits the action of neuromuscular blocker antagonists. This leads to a vicious cycle in which respiratory acidosis causes increased hypoventilation, augmenting the respiratory acidosis. Commonly used drugs such as aminoglycosides, furosemide, and antidysrhythmics (i.e., lidocaine, procainamide, and quinidine) all have been reported to potentiate the effect of neuromuscular blockers. Large doses of neuromuscular-blocker antagonists can cause a paradoxic response, increasing the neuromuscular block.[89] This effect is seen with dosages of neostigmine (> mg/70 kg) and pyridostigmine (> 20 mg/70 kg). **Succinylcholine phase II block markedly increases its duration of action.** Pseudocholinesterase deficiency causes prolongation of succinylcholine action. This can be seen in severe liver disease, malnutrition, pregnancy, and in patients undergoing plasmapheresis.

Neurologic problems predisposing to prolonged neuromuscular blockade include disorders of upper and lower motor neurons and the motor endplate. Upper–motor neuron lesions from strokes cause resistance to nondepolarizing agents and are easily managed if the nonaffected side is monitored intraoperatively. Amyotrophic lateral sclerosis

(ALS) involves upper and lower motor neurons and causes a prolonged response to nondepolarizing neuromuscular blockers. Patients with either myasthenia gravis or the myasthenic (Eaton-Lambert) syndrome are exquisitely sensitive to both nondepolarizing and depolarizing muscle relaxants. Familial periodic paralysis and hereditary hepatic porphyrias are other disorders in which patients demonstrate prolonged response to neuromuscular blockers.

Treatment of prolonged neuromuscular blockade is largely supportive, providing reassurance, sedation, and mechanical ventilation until the paralysis has been reversed. Correcting electrolyte abnormalities, acid-base disturbances, and hypothermia are beneficial. After partial return of function, a reversal dose of a neuromuscular-blocker antagonist is indicated to expedite extubation.

Abnormal Urine Output

Oliguria, polyuria, and hematuria are urinary abnormalities most frequently encountered in PACU patients. Oliguria (< 0.5 ml/kg/hr) is caused by anatomic obstruction of urine flow (postrenal), primary renal disease (intrarenal), decreased cardiac output, hypotension, or low intravascular volume (prerenal). Oliguria is exacerbated by elevated evels of antidiuretic hormone (ADH) seen in postoperative patients.

When presented with an oliguric patient, the PACU caregiver should first determine whether there is adequate drainage of urine. Bladder catheterization can be considered in patients who have not voided. Catheters already in place may need flushing or unkinking. Preoperative medical problems of the cardiovascular or renal system (congestive heart failure [CHF], cirrhosis, renal insufficiency) can predispose to postoperative oliguria, and routine use of diuretics preoperatively may signify "diuretic-dependent" urine output. The anesthetic record should be examined for intraoperative urine output and fluid administration that may demonstrate inadequate volume replacement.

The most common cause of postoperative oliguria is hypovolemia, which often presents with tachycardia and hemoconcentration in nonbleeding patients. Specific urine chemistries (Table 88-5) provide further evidence of prerenal azotemia. If hypovolemia is suspected in the otherwise healthy patient, a rapid fluid challenge with 500 ml of balanced salt solution is indicated. This should elicit a urinary response within 30 to 60 minutes. If the patient responds with an increased urine output and decreased heart rate, then hypovolemia is probably the cause and maintenance IV fluids should be increased. If the response is negligible or equivocal, a second 500-ml fluid challenge should be infused. If there is still no response, further evaluation should be conducted, looking for continued volume loss (e.g., bleeding, third spacing) or low cardiac output (e.g., dyspnea, elevated neck veins, S3 gallop). Patients suspected of being hypovolemic should not be given diuretics to induce urination. Subsequent fluid challenges may be given as needed, or a CVP catheter may be placed to assess intravascular volume. Further fluid resuscitation should then be based on the measured CVP. Patients with a high CVP and oliguria should have a Swan-Ganz catheter placed to measure left heart filling pressure, cardiac output, and systemic vascular resistance (SVR). Patients with low CVP should continue to receive fluid, and a search for the etiology should begin. Patients with low cardiac output (heart failure) or high cardiac output and low SVR (sepsis) require additional treatment. In these situations, therapy directed at increasing renal perfusion pressure with inotropes and pressors usually improves urine output. Chronic hypertensive patients with "relative hypotension" may require higher blood pressure to improve urine flow. In this situation, renal vascular autoregulation has been shifted, requiring a higher pressure to maintain urine output.

Intraoperative problems, including ureteral obstruction from surgical trauma, acute tubular necrosis from hypotension, and suprarenal aortic cross clamping, can cause postoperative oliguria. Infrarenal aortic cross-clamp procedures also cause redistribution of intrarenal blood flow, possibly leading to postoperative oliguria.[39] Patients with preoperative renal dysfunction (creatinine clearance < 40 ml/min) who are diuretic dependent will likely require postoperative diuretics to maintain urine flow.

Polyuria can be a problem when it is misinterpreted as evidence of adequate intravascular volume. In healthy patients, excessive volume infusion intraoperatively can cause polyuria in the PACU. Polyuria can also be caused by renal, metabolic, or drug-induced abnormalities that can lead to hypovolemia and free-water imbalance. Renal causes of

Table 88-5 Laboratory findings in oliguria

Findings	Prerenal	Renal
Concentration		
Specific gravity	> 1.015	1.010
Urine osmolality (mOsm/l)	> 400	250–350
Sodium reabsorption		
Urine Na (mEq/l)	< 20	> 40
Fractional excretion of Na	< 1%	> 2%
Creatinine		
U/P creatinine ratio	> 40	< 20
BUN creatinine ratio	> 10	10
Sediment	Negligible protein casts	Erythrocytes/Leukocytes
	Rare hyaline casts	Tubular cell and broad brown casts

polyuria are diabetes insipidus, hyposthenuria or isosthenuria, and postobstructive diuresis. Diabetes insipidus can develop in head trauma or other neurosurgery patients. Hyposthenuria is possible in patients with sickle-cell disease and other renal concentrating defects. Polyuria from postobstructive diuresis occurs in patients with elevated blood urea nitrogen (BUN) levels when the obstruction is relieved. The BUN acts as an osmotic diuretic in conjunction with tubular dysfunction (from the obstruction), leading to excessive urine output. Hyperglycemia and mannitol are both osmotic diuretics and cause a disproportionately large urine output relative to intravascular volume.

Hematuria can be the result of erythrocytes, heme pigments from intravascular hemolysis (hemoglobinuria), or pigments from rhabdomyolysis (myoglobinuria). Hematuria also is commonly caused by genitourinary trauma from surgery or Foley catheters and will be exaggerated by any coagulopathy. Intraoperative transfusion reactions can present in the PACU as hemoglobinuria. Myoglobinuria usually seen in trauma patients with rhabdomyolysis also presents as dark red urine. Differentiating hemoglobinuria from myoglobinuria is clinically important and requires specific diagnostic tests. Treatment of transfusion reactions and myoglobinuria involves maintaining adequate urine output with mannitol and diuretics and treating the underlying cause.

Abnormal Temperature

In the immediate postoperative period, patients are often hypothermic. Uncommonly, hyperthermia is present. Knowing the causes and physiologic consequences of both hypothermia and hyperthermia can direct management in PACU patients with abnormal temperatures.

Hypothermia occurs in postoperative patients more often than in any other patient population. It occurs in patients given both general and regional anesthesia, although patients under general anesthesia appear more susceptible.[37] The effects of anesthesia on the thermoregulatory system cause loss of temperature-sensing, regulating abilities and heat production. Heat loss also increases as a result of evaporation, convection, and radiation.

Hypothermia ($< 35°$ C) leads to physiologic changes that retard the patient's recovery from anesthesia. As body temperature drops, metabolic rate and drug excretion decrease, delaying removal of anesthetic and paralytic agents. CO_2 production and O_2 consumption decrease, causing a reduction in minute ventilation.[100] In mechanically ventilated patients, as temperature drops, ventilation should be corrected to prevent respiratory alkalemia. The O_2-hemoglobin dissociation is shifted left with hypothermia, exaggerating any decreased tissue O_2 delivery. Hypothermia also results in a mild nonprogressive hyperchloremic metabolic acidosis that is caused by a decrease in renal tubular reabsorption of bicarbonate. This nonanion gap acidosis is further increased in postoperative patients with large blood loss and fluid replacement. In this situation, the renal response is to maintain electroneutrality (reabsorb chloride preferentially), which normally does not require bicarbonate treatment. Bicarbonate therapy may be indicated in patients unable to provide respiratory compensation to maintain a pH ≥ 7.30.

The cardiovascular effects of mild hypothermia include increased SVR caused by cutaneous vasoconstriction and a slight decrease in heart rate.[100] The lower heart rate is due to intrinsic slowing of the sinoatrial (SA) node and reflex slowing from increased SVR. Stroke volume and contractility remain normal in mild hypothermia. With rewarming, increased cutaneous blood flow can lead to hypotension if additional fluids are not administered. (Shivering and its cardiopulmonary effects are discussed under Central Nervous System Abnormalities.)

Hypothermia may be responsible for increased bleeding and reduced leukocyte function leading to increased wound infections. Hypothermic patients should be rewarmed gradually to prevent sudden changes in vascular resistance, O_2 consumption, and CO_2 production. Patients who receive regional anesthesia rewarm more quickly than those given general anesthesia from similar levels of hypothermia.[37] Rewarming can be as simple as providing warmed blankets and IV fluids. More severe levels of hypothermia are treated with warmed forced air mattresses that surround the patient. Rewarming should be stopped before normothermia to avoid overshooting.[11]

Hyperthermia in PACU patients can be caused by infection, transfusion reaction, drug reaction, primary CNS disorder, or malignant hyperthermia. Patients usually arrive in the PACU normothermic (except for malignant hyperthermia) and then develop a fever.

Fever increases O_2 consumption, CO_2 production, heart rate, and fluid requirements, and causes peripheral vasodilation. Patients at risk when these symptoms occur include those with ischemic heart disease and poor cardiopulmonary reserve. Infection is the most common cause of immediate postoperative fever, and a search for its source should begin in the PACU. Usually the source of infection has been identified preoperatively or is discovered intraoperatively. If the infectious source is not apparent, specimens of urine, blood, sputum, and all intraoperative fluids should be cultured. Broad-spectrum antibiotics may be started, and antipyretics should be administered. Patients with transfusion reactions can present with fever, hemoglobinuria, wheezing, hypotension, and oliguria. Those with drug reactions may also present with fever in addition to rash, hypotension, and wheezing. These symptom complexes are very similar to one another and mimic other postoperative conditions. In any PACU patient, supportive therapy should always be instituted until the cause of the fever can be determined.

SYSTEMIC PROBLEMS

Central Nervous System Abnormalities

Emergence from general anesthesia is often accompanied by neurologic signs and symptoms that would be considered pathologic in nonsurgical settings. These include transient disorders of orientation and mentation, pathologic spinal reflexes, and movement disorders.

Emergence phenomena

Emergence excitement occurs in 5% to 30% of recovery room admissions.[32,40] It is characterized by tachycardia, restlessness, disorientation, altered pain responsiveness, crying, moaning, and irrational talking during recovery from general anesthesia. In some cases, patients are delirious, shout, scream, and thrash about, posing a danger to themselves and recovery room staff. In a series of more than 12,000 surgical patients, Eckenhoff et al.[32] observed emergence excitement in 5.3% of recovery room admissions. The incidence of excitement was higher after surgical procedures with emotional overtones (such as breast surgery with fear of mutilation or cancer) than after routine dental procedures. It was also more common in young patients. Anesthesia with either halogenated agents or ketamine is associated with a higher incidence of emergence excitement than spinal or narcotic-based general anesthetic techniques.[32,40] Paradoxical reactions to benzodiazepines can cause emergence excitement in susceptible patients. Scopolamine also causes delirium, hallucinations, memory disturbances, and agitation in postoperative patients.[53] Emergence excitement is transient and self-limited in most patients, and treatment is largely supportive. Analgetic therapy often aborts or decreases the severity of excitement.[32] Physostigmine, which penetrates the blood–brain barrier, reverses the central anticholinergic effects of scopolamine within 5 to 10 minutes of administration and markedly improves the mental status of affected patients.[53] Physostigmine and other stimulants (e.g., theophylline, caffeine) have been reported to have general CNS arousal properties,[12,13,115] but their use postoperatively is rarely indicated.

Marcantonio et al.[68] studied 1341 patients who underwent noncardiac procedures. Nine percent of patients had postoperative delirium. Factors independently associated included age over 70 years, a history of alcohol abuse, electrolyte abnormalities, glucose levels, thoracic and abdominal aneurysm surgery.

Disorders of mentation commonly occur in elderly patients recovering from anesthesia. These disorders include disorientation, short-term memory lapse, and problems with language ability. Immediate postoperative confusion in elderly patients is so common that studies of postoperative mental function demonstrate that after 6 hours, confusion is less in patients who received regional anesthesia (without sedation) than in those who received general anesthesia.[23] When regional anesthesia patients were given sedation (e.g., diazepam, fentanyl, droperidol) the incidence of confusion at 6 hours was no different between the two groups.[22] With the newer short-acting agents such as midazolam, the results at 6 hours might have been similar to patients receiving no sedation, but this needs to be confirmed.

Common neurologic findings

Emergence from anesthesia in healthy patients is often accompanied by transient symmetric neurologic changes (sustained and nonsustained ankle clonus, bilateral hyperreflexia, the Babinski reflex, and decerebrate posturing) that are otherwise believed to be pathologic reflexes.[98] These changes can often be detected within minutes of discontinuation of anesthesia when the patient is still poorly responsive to verbal commands. Nevertheless, these changes may persist for more than 40 minutes into the postoperative period. These abnormalities occur more frequently after enflurane/N_2O anesthesia than after halothane or narcotic-based anesthetics (Table 88-6). Their cause remains unexplained, but they are not associated with adverse clinical consequences. Discovery of *focal* neurologic deficits in a postoperative patient should point to possible acute CNS or peripheral nervous system injury.[84]

Postanesthetic shivering

Spontaneous shivering (postanesthetic tremor) is common during recovery from all types of general anesthesia. Uncontrolled motor activity can disrupt delicate surgical repairs and can result in dental damage. In addition, the subjective feeling of intense cold is often cited by patients as being the most uncomfortable PACU experience. Shivering increases metabolic rate and O_2 consumption, and may not be tolerated in patients with CAD and/or compromised cardiopulmonary function.[67,96]

Postanesthetic tremor is usually attributed to normal regulatory mechanisms that generate heat in response to intraoperative hypothermia. Hypothermia during anesthesia results from decreased metabolic heat production and loss of heat to the environment. Decreased hypothalamic thermal regulation produced by anesthetic agents inhibits compensatory responses to hypothermia such as vasoconstriction, shivering, and nonshivering thermogenesis. Postoperative shivering is usually caused by decreased body temperature, but shivering may also occur at normal body temperature after anesthesia, suggesting that mechanisms other than thermoregulation may contribute to postanesthesia tremor.[37,98,103] Recent evidence suggests that spontaneous tremor may be the result of increased spinal reflex activity during recovery from anesthesia. Electromyograms (EMGs)

Table 88-6 Neurologic changes after 20 minutes in the PACU

	Percentage of group		
Neurologic changes	Halothane (n= 8)	Ethrane (n= 12)	N_2O-narcotic (n= 9)
Hyperreflexia	25	58	0
Clonus	75	83	44
Sustained clonus	0	50	0
Babinski	0	50	0

Modified from Rosenberg H, Clofine R, Bialik O: Neurologic changes during awakening from anesthesia, *Anesthesiology* 54:125, 1981.

in shivering muscles after isoflurane anesthesia reveal tonic/clonic activity similar to that produced by pathologic clonus in patients with spinal cord transection. Because EMG clonus was not observed during cold-induced shivering in unanesthetized volunteers, Sessler et al.[103] suggested that a functional spinal cord transection (the brain remains "asleep" while the spinal cord is "awake") develops as the concentration of anesthetic decreases during recovery. EMG evidence of clonus occurs at end-tidal concentrations of isoflurane between 0.1% and 0.19%. Greater concentrations demonstrate little muscular activity, and at lesser concentrations normal thermogenic shivering predominates.[103] Although these conclusions have been questioned,[47] they do offer a reasonable explanation for postanesthesia tremor in normothermic patients and provide insight into potential mechanisms for other postoperative neurologic changes (e.g., clonus, Babinski reflex, hyperreflexia).

Postanesthesia tremor is prevented or treated by various techniques. Meperidine (10 to 25 mg IV) successfully suppresses visible shivering in most patients and is associated with subsequent reductions in O_2 consumption and CO_2 production.[64] Other less frequently used pharmacologic agents that may minimize shivering include methylphenidate (Ritalin), magnesium sulfate, calcium chloride, chlorpromazine, droperidol, and opiates. Stimulation of thermal receptors in blush areas appears to alter signals reaching the CNS because application of radiant heat to the face, neck, chest, and abdomen is reported to suppress shivering within minutes in postoperative patients, despite continuing low core temperatures.[79,104]

Postanesthetic seizures

Tonic/clonic seizure activity has been reported after propofol anesthesia. Causes are unknown, although the phenomenon appears to be temporary and may be associated with prior seizure disorder.[66]

Pulmonary Complications

Pulmonary complications after anesthesia are well-recognized problems. In one study, major adverse pulmonary events (excluding airway obstruction), occurred in 44 of 2293 (1.9%) patients.[8] The most frequently encountered pulmonary complications are airway obstruction, hypoventilation, and hypoxemia.

Airway obstruction

Airway obstruction may be caused by vomitus or secretions in the pharynx, the tongue, laryngospasm, or laryngeal edema. Airway obstruction by the tongue, a result of anesthetic-induced hypotonicity of the genioglossus muscle, is particularly common and can usually be alleviated by hyperextension of the neck and anterior displacement of the mandible. Placement of a nasal airway is occasionally required and may be preferable to an oral airway because it is less likely to induce gagging, laryngospasm, or vomiting if it can be placed without bleeding. Maintaining a protected patent airway is of major concern in the PACU. It was previously believed that the ability to ventilate was synonymous with airway protection in patients whose paralysis had been reversed. We now know this is not true. Pavlin et al.[84] demonstrated that despite vital capacity and maximum inspiratory pressure (MIP) sufficient to allow spontaneous ventilation, previously anesthetized volunteers could not swallow, perform a valsalva maneuver, protect their airway, or approximate their teeth. In these normal volunteers, swallowing returned at an MIP of -43 cm H_2O, approximation of teeth at -42 cm H_2O, patent airway at -39 cm H_2O, and the ability to perform a valsalva maneuver above -33 cm H_2O. The clinical responses that correlated best with adequate airway protection were the leg-lift and head-lift performed for 5 seconds. Thus, the ability to ventilate, which involves the diaphragm (and is relatively resistant to neuromuscular blockers), should not be accepted as evidence of acceptable airway skeletal muscle function.

Laryngospasm (spastic glottic closure) during anesthesia emergence is a protective reflex mediated by the superior laryngeal nerve resulting in constriction of the extrinsic muscles of the larynx. Airflow obstruction occurs as a result of opposition of the true and false vocal cords in the midline. The diagnosis of laryngospasm is usually made when airway obstruction persists despite usual measures to relieve upper-airway obstruction (proper head position, placement of an airway, and anterior displacement of the mandible). Treatment includes clearing secretions from the pharynx and frequent, steady small tidal volume positive pressure breaths using an Ambu-bag with properly fitting face mask. Succinylcholine should seldom be required. The combination of glottic obstruction and strong inspiratory attempts during laryngospasm can cause marked negative intrathoracic pressures that occasionally result in hydrostatic pulmonary edema.[116] The mechanism responsible for the pulmonary edema is similar to a Müller maneuver (inspiration against a closed glottis) where venous return is increased and left ventricular function is decreased (Fig. 88-9).[90] This form of pulmonary edema may occur various times after relief of laryngospasm, but commonly presents after arrival in the PACU.

Upper-airway obstruction caused by edema from surgical or anesthetic trauma is most common in patients with preexisting airway problems (e.g., oropharyngeal and laryngeal tumors). Incomplete obstruction can often be treated with head-up positioning, humidified O_2, He/O_2 mixtures, and nebulized epinephrine. IV steroids have also been shown to hasten the resolution of traumatic laryngeal edema.[14] Near complete or complete obstruction requires either intubation with a small endotracheal (ET) tube or tracheostomy. Prolonged surgery in a head-down position can result in marked pharyngeal swelling. Patients with such swelling are potentially at risk for airway obstruction, and continued intubation until the swelling decreases is advisable. Vocal cord paralysis from damage to recurrent laryngeal nerve(s), particularly after anterior neck

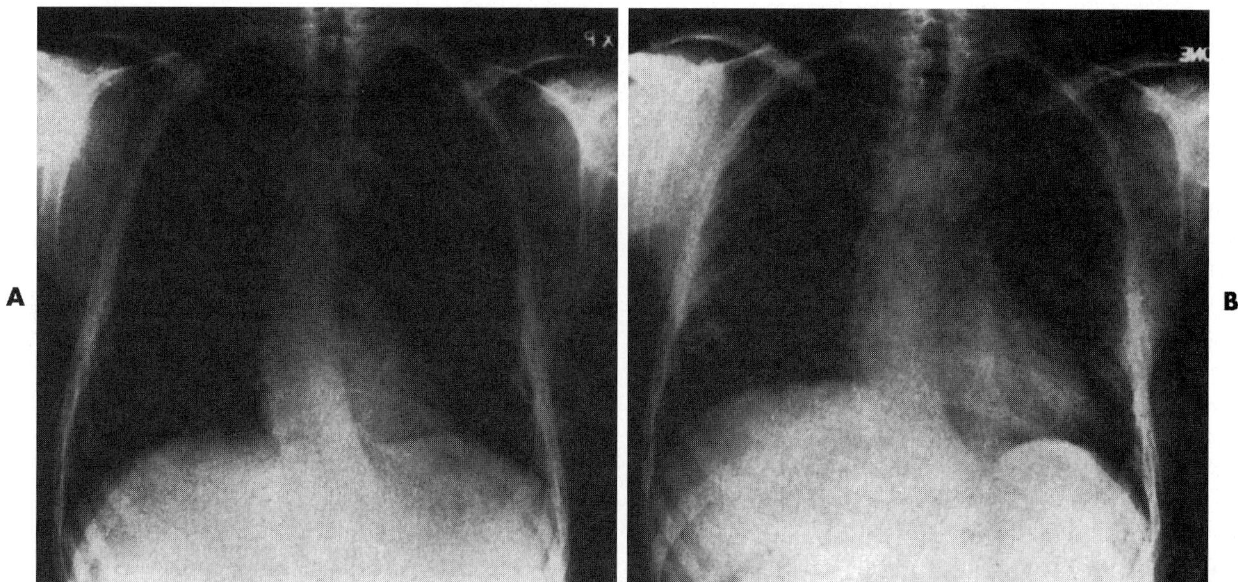

Fig. 88-9. Chest radiographs taken in the same subject sequentially. **A,** Standard PA radiograph at functional residual capacity. **B,** Radiograph taken just before concluding a 10-second vigorous Müller maneuver. There is a dramatic increase in pulmonary vascular markings, cardiomegaly, and dilation of the ascending aorta. (From Montenegro HD, editor: *Chronic obstructive pulmonary disease,* New York, 1984, Churchill-Livingstone.)

surgery, can cause airway obstruction. This situation may require a tracheostomy. Paradoxic vocal cord motion is a rare cause of airway obstruction that occurs in patients with a history of functional disorders and paroxysms of upper-airway obstruction.[44] Avoidance of intubation, if possible, or extubation in a deep plane of anesthesia may prevent paradoxical vocal cord motion. If the patient is alert, continuous positive airway pressure (CPAP) by mask may be of benefit.

Hypoventilation

In one large study, hypoventilation was reported to be the most common respiratory problem that occurred in PACU patients.[8] The cause of postoperative hypoventilation is the depressant effect of narcotics, benzodiazepines, and inhalational agents on CO_2 responsiveness.[81] This effect is usually apparent on the patient's arrival in the PACU, but may be delayed with some narcotics that produce biphasic respiratory depression.[9] Epidural and intrathecal morphine can also produce late respiratory depression, usually 2 to 6 hours after administration.[27] In intubated patients, end-tidal CO_2 can be used to noninvasively monitor ventilation. In nonintubated patients, respiratory rate and depth are unreliable, and the only way to monitor ventilation is to directly measure the pco_2 in arterial blood. Pulse oximetry cannot be used to assess ventilation, particularly when supplemental O_2 is being administered. Supplemental O_2 can result in high Pao_2 values, despite $Paco_2$ levels that are quite elevated.

Although, nasal cannulae have been used for monitoring end-tidal CO_2, sampling error is so great as to make this method unreliable.[3]

Narcotic-induced respiratory depression can be reversed by small incremental doses (e.g., 0.04 to 0.08 mg) of naloxone without precipitating pain.[93] The duration of action of naloxone (1 to 4 hours) is shorter than some narcotics (methadone, CNS morphine), and repeat doses or a continuous infusion of naloxone may be required.

Benzodiazepines can also lead to respiratory depression. The short-acting agent midazolam has attenuated this problem, and the recent development of a benzodiazepine antagonist (Flumazenil) was expected to alleviate the problem entirely. Unfortunately, Flumazenil appears to have less reversal effect on ventilation than on sedation.[75] Prolonged paralysis is another important cause of hypoventilation (see discussion of prolonged neuromuscular weakness).

Hypoxemia

Hypoxemia after anesthesia and surgery is common in patients who are not receiving supplemental O_2.[110] Using continuous pulse oximetry during transfer of ASA Class I and II patients from the operating room to the PACU, Tyler et al.[110] found that 30% of patients breathing room air had O_2 saturations below 90% and 12% had O_2 saturations less than 85%. There was a significant correlation between presence of hypoxemia and preoperative obesity or asthma. Accordingly, it is advisable for all patients to receive supplemental O_2 during transport from the operating room to the PACU and initially during their PACU stay.

Causes of hypoxemia in the early postoperative pe-

riod include drug-induced hypoventilation, V/Q mismatch, intrapulmonary shunting, pulmonary embolism, and aspiration. Inhalational agents alter respiratory muscle function by reducing functional residual capacity (FRC). The decrease in FRC is associated with diffuse microatelectasis in dependent lung regions, which can be seen on intraoperative CT scans.[17] These changes may be more severe in patients with preoperative pulmonary dysfunction (i.e., patients who are elderly, obese, or have COPD, pulmonary edema or pneumonia). Decreased FRC and hypoxemia usually reverse within 1 to 3 hours as inhalational anesthetic agents are eliminated from the body.[81] In spontaneously breathing patients, pulmonary dysfunction present after elimination of anesthetic agents is usually caused by pain-induced splinting and mechanical dysfunction. Mechanical dysfunction is caused by effects on the diaphragm from abdominal and thoracic incisions.[28]

Inhalational anesthetics and narcotics blunt normal responses to hypoxemia in postoperative patients (Figs. 88-10 and 88-11).[108] Continuous monitoring of arterial O_2 saturation with pulse oximetry is valuable for the early detection of hypoxemia. Treatment consists of increasing the inspired concentration of O_2, placing the patient in a head-up position and performing lung expansion maneuvers such as incentive spirometry.[35] Other causes of postoperative hypoxemia include cardiogenic and noncardiogenic pulmonary edema, pulmonary embolism, and bronchospasm.

Aspiration

Pulmonary aspiration of GI contents is an infrequent but potentially devastating cause of postoperative hypoxemia. Aspiration of gastric contents can lead to pneumonitis or pneumonia. Lack of widely accepted definitions, management strategies, and data collection has prevented assessment of the true incidence of aspiration. A 3-year review of 105,364 consecutive cases with general anesthesia at Mayo revealed 42 cases of aspiration (1:2509).[113] In this study, pulmonary aspiration was rigidly defined as presence of bilious secretions or particulate matter in the tracheobronchial tree. Major risk factors for aspiration included emergency procedures, patient age less than 2 years, and high ASA classification. Of the 41 patients who suffered aspiration, 1 died intraoperatively, 26 (63%) had no respiratory sequelae, and 15 (37%) needed intensive care unit observation, with 10 of these requiring mechanical ventilation. The clinical factors associated with the development of respiratory complications were a symptomatic cough, wheezing, hypoxemia on room air, or radiographic abnormalities within 2 hours of aspiration. The study demonstrates that, even with a strict definition of pulmonary aspiration, many patients do well. Clinical criteria in the PACU can be used to determine triage and prognosis.

Cardiovascular Complications

Cardiovascular complications developing in PACU patients can lead to serious morbidity and mortality. Changes in blood pressure, myocardial ischemia, and dysrhythmias constitute the major problems.

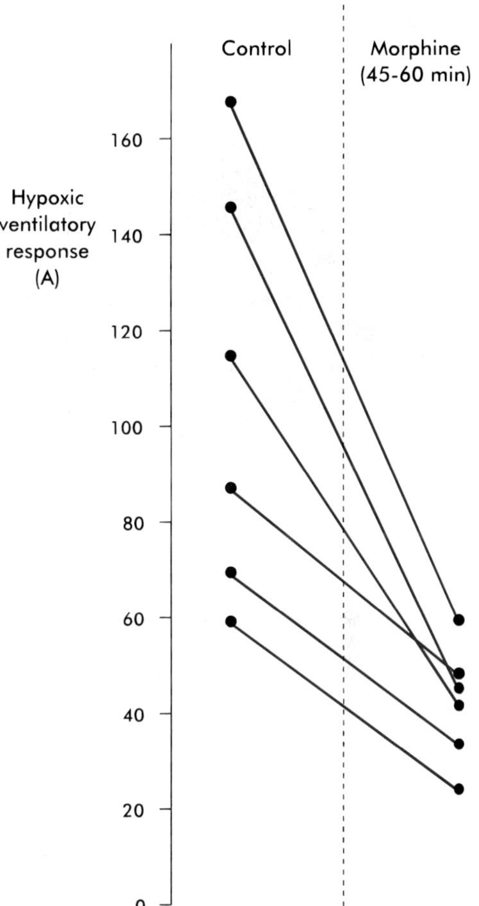

Fig. 88-10. Ventilatory response to hypoxia as measured by the shape parameter A (high values of A denote a vigorous ventilatory response) before and after the administration of morphine. Values after administration of 7.5 mg subcutaneous morphine were obtained by averaging the data at 45 and 60 minutes. The depression of hypoxic ventilatory drive was of considerable magnitude and highly consistent, in that it occurred in every subject. (From Weil JV, McCullough RE, Kline JS, et al: Diminished ventilatory response to hypoxia and hypercapnia after morphine in normal man, *N Engl J Med* 292:1103, 1975.)

Hypotension

Hypotension in the PACU is usually caused by residual effects of anesthesia. It is more common after regional than general anesthesia because of the more profound and prolonged vasodilator effect of regional techniques. Local anesthetics delivered into the epidural or subarachnoid space produce a "chemical sympathectomy" that results in arteriolar and venodilation. High sympathetic block involving the cardioaccelerator fibers (thoracic levels T1 to T4) blocks reflex increases in heart rate. Elderly patients are particularly susceptible to regional anesthetic-induced hypotension, which may be poorly tolerated because of underlying myocardial, renal, or cerebrovascular disease. Initial treatment of hypotension after spinal or epidural anesthesia

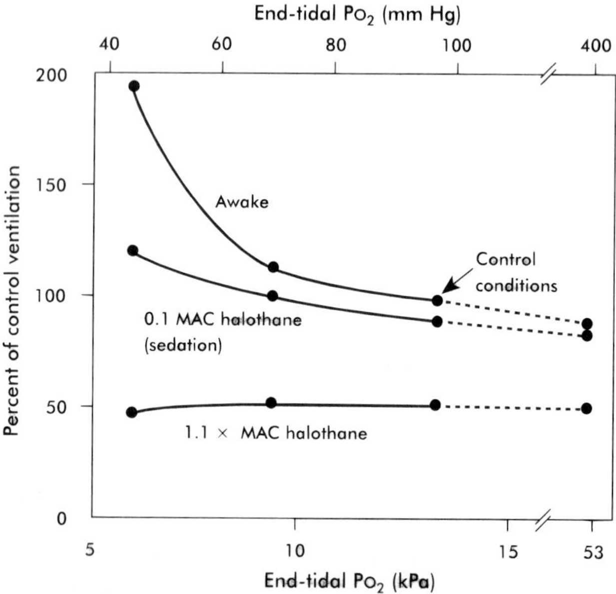

Fig. 88-11. Effect of halothane anesthesia on ventilatory response to hypoxia. Hypoxic drive is markedly attenuated at 0.1 MAC of halothane, a level of anesthesia frequently present in postanesthesia care unit patients. (From Nunn J: *Applied respiratory physiology,* Boston, 1987, Butterworths.)

is Trendelenburg positioning to augment venous return. Judicious volume replacement with adrenergic agonists are needed if hypotension persists.[20] Fluid administration should be individualized, because as the sympathetic block recedes and venous capacitance system regains tone, patients with marginal myocardial or renal function may be compromised by increased filling pressures.

Hypovolemia causes hypotension in normal unanesthetized patients. The residual effects of anesthetic agents (vasodilation, decreased myocardial contractility, and blunting of baroreceptor reflex activity) can further exacerbate the effect of hypovolemia on PACU patients. Patients may be hypovolemic as a result of inadequate intraoperative blood and fluid replacement, or they may become hypovolemic in the PACU from ongoing hemorrhage or third-space losses. The diagnosis of hypovolemia can be made by measuring urine output, urine osmolality, urine electrolytes, hematocrit, and heart rate. Uncertainty about the intravascular volume or fluid replacement may indicate measurement of central venous or pulmonary artery (PA) pressures. In rare instances, sepsis-induced hypotension develops intraoperatively or in the immediate postoperative period in patients undergoing surgery for perforated abdominal viscera or abscess drainage. Management of these patients includes administering antibiotics, fluids, and alpha agonists to increase SVR.

Hypertension

Transient arterial hypertension is common in the immediate postoperative period and has many etiologies (Box 88-7). Gal and Cooperman[38] observed postoperative hypertension (blood pressure > 190/100 mm Hg) in 60 (3.25%) of 1844 patients. In this group, hypertension developed 10 to 30 minutes after completion of surgery and resolved without specific antihypertensive therapy within 3 hours in 47 (78%) patients (Figs. 88-12 and 88-13). In the remaining 13 patients (22%), hypertension lasted beyond 3 hours, and six patients suffered complications secondary to hypertension. Preoperative hypertension was present in more than 50% of the patients who developed postoperative hypertension.

BOX 88-7
CAUSES OF POSTOPERATIVE HYPERTENSION

Preexisting hypertension
Withdrawal of antihypertensive medications
Hypercapnia
Volume overload
Bladder distension
Increased intracranial pressure
Pain
Drugs
- Pressors, epinephrine, cocaine, ketamine
- MSO_4 reversal with naloxone
- Indirect-acting vasopressor with chronic MAO use

Autonomic hyperreflexia
Pheochromocytoma
Carotid surgery

Hypertension can increase postoperative hemorrhage and third-space losses and increase myocardial wall tension, precipitating ischemia and dysrhythmias. It can also decrease cardiac output in patients with aortic and mitral regurgitation. Disruption of major vascular suture lines is an often-cited but never proven sequela of postoperative hypertension.

Accurate measurement of arterial pressure is important in making the diagnosis and avoiding overtreatment. An inappropriately small blood pressure cuff yields erroneously high readings. The width of the blood pressure cuff should be approximately 20% less than the diameter of the arm (Table 88-7). Blood pressures should be assessed in both arms and the leg if necessary. Improperly zeroed or calibrated transducers and excessive resonance in an arterial line system can also lead to inaccurate readings.

Withdrawal of antihypertensive medications can contribute to postoperative hypertension in patients with preexisting hypertension. Rebound hypertension is most often caused by withdrawal of beta blockers or clonidine.[72] Beta blockers can be administered IV in the PACU, but IV clonidine is not presently available. Although clonidine can be administered transdermally, it requires 48 hours to reach therapeutic levels,[105] and altered blood flow to the skin during the postoperative period may complicate absorption. If clonidine therapy has been discontinued, combined alpha- and beta-adrenergic blockade can be used to prevent increased adrenergic responsiveness. Excessive use of naloxone to reverse narcotic-induced respiratory depression can

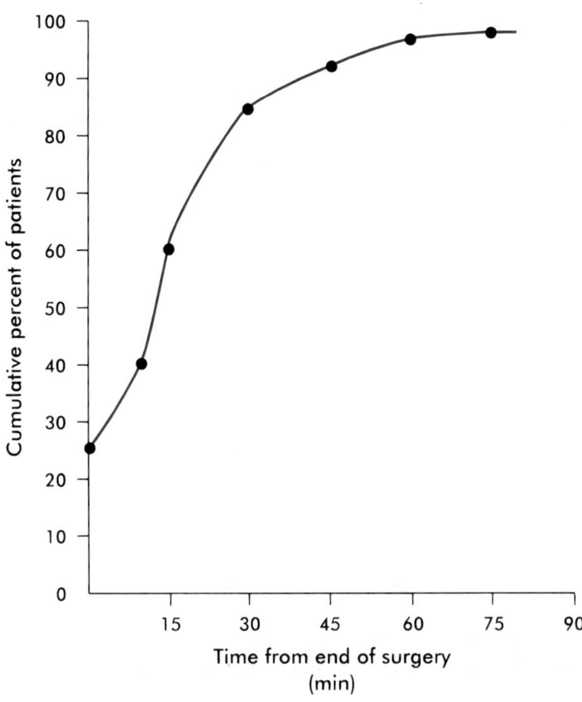

Fig. 88-12. Onset of hypertension after the end of surgery. (From Gal TJ, Cooperman LH: Hypertension in the immediate postoperative period, *Br J Anaesth* 47:70, 1975.)

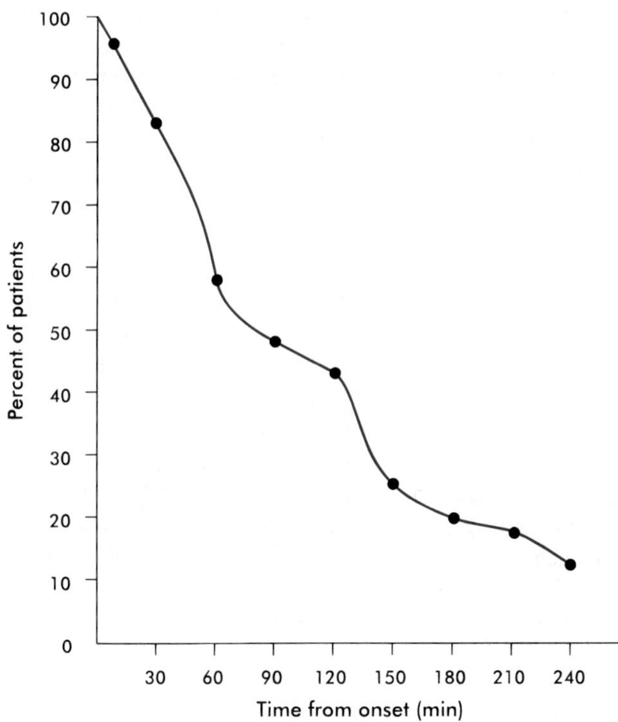

Fig. 88-13. Duration of postoperative hypertension in untreated patients. (From Gal TJ, Cooperman LH: Hypertension in the immediate postoperative period, *Br J Anaesth* 47:70, 1975.)

Table 88-7 Width of sphygmomanometer cuff bladder

	Bladder width (cm)	Length (cm)
Thigh	18.5	38.5
Obese	15	38
Adult	12.5	25
Child	8.5	18
Infant	6	12
Neonate	4	7.5

cause excessive sympathetic stimulation leading to severe hypertension and cardiac compromise. This can occur in patients without preexisting cardiac disease.[107] Hypertension can reflect problems such as hypoxemia, hypercapnia, and intracranial hypertension, which should be ruled out (or treated) immediately. Pain, intravascular volume overload, hypothermia, and bladder distension are other causes of hypertension requiring attention. If hypertension persists, specific antihypertensive medication should be administered according to the severity of the situation and the patient's medical history. Systemic vasodilators frequently elicit reflex tachycardia, which may be detrimental in patients with ischemic heart disease. In these patients a combined alpha-beta blocker (e.g., labetalol) or a vasodilator in conjunction with a beta blocker is preferred.

Less common causes of postoperative hypertension are autonomic hyperreflexia, pheochromocytoma, and carotid artery surgery. Autonomic hyperreflexia occurs in patients with spinal cord injury at or above the level of T7. Hyperreflexia is precipitated by bowel or bladder distention and presents with hypertension, diaphoresis, headache, and bradycardia above the level of the lesion. Denervation of carotid baroreceptors can cause hypertension after carotid endarterectomy (CEA).

Dysrhythmias

Dysrhythmias, particularly sinus tachycardia, are extremely common in PACU patients (see discussion of SVT). Other commonly encountered rhythm disturbances are sinus bradycardia, premature ectopic beats, and accelerated ectopic rhythms.

Causes of sinus bradycardia include: (1) beta blocker therapy; (2) neuromuscular blockade reversal agents; (3) local anesthetic effects on the cardioaccelerator fibers in patients receiving regional anesthesia; (4) underlying heart disease (sick sinus syndrome); and (5) hypothermia. Bradycardia can also be an ominous sign of severe hypoxemia that should always be ruled out. The neuromuscular blocker reversal agents (neostigmine, pyridostigmine, and edrophonium) cause bradycardia by increasing the available acetylcholine at all postganglionic receptors. To prevent bradycardia, muscarinic blockers (atropine or glycopyrolate) are given concomitantly. The net result is to increase acetylcholine only at the neuromuscular nicotinic receptors. Duration of action of acetylcholine esterase inhibitors tends to be longer than the muscarinic receptor antagonists. Theoretically, this could result in unopposed muscarinic receptor stimulation, possibly leading to sinus bradycardia and even escape rhythms. These dysrhythmias should be treated if they are hemodynamically significant; they spontaneously revert in time.

Other causes of bradycardia in the PACU include high spinal and epidural blocks that affect the cardioaccelerator sympathetic fibers (T1 to T4), leading to unopposed vagal stimulation. Extreme sinus bradycardia and asystole are more common in the operating room after spinal anesthesia[64] but may also occur in the PACU. Unopposed vagal stimulation and the Bezold-Jarisch reflex are believed responsible for this complication. Hypothermia to 33° C decreases sinus node activity and also increases peripheral vasoconstriction, which in turn reflexly slows heart rate.[100] Rewarming reverses these changes. More severe hypothermia can result in atrial and ventricular dysrhythmias.[100] Bradycardia which compromises the patient's hemodynamic status and remains unresponsive to pharmacologic therapy requires placement of a transvenous pacing wire.

Ectopic rhythms (e.g., ventricular tachycardia, junctional tachycardia, atrial fibrillation, and atrial flutter) occur infrequently in PACU patients. Electrolyte and acid-base disturbances, residual inhalational anesthetic agents, central venous catheters, and particularly elevated catecholamines all play important roles in generating and sustaining these dysrhythmias. Elevated postoperative catecholamines are probably the most important cause of PACU tachydysrhythmias. Catecholamines accelerate impulse conduction velocity, shorten the refractory period, augment calcium influx into myocardial cells, and increase amplitude of delayed afterpotentials, enhancing propensity for more dysrhythmias (Fig. 88-14).[92] Catecholamines increase the slope of phase-4 spontaneous depolarization of the action potential, which increases automaticity and the potential for ectopic beats and accelerated ectopic rhythms. Another cause of accelerated dysrhythmias involves residual inhalational anesthetics, particularly halothane, which increases the myocardial susceptibility to catecholamine stimulation.[50] Acute administration of theophylline compounds can also produce dysrhythmias by this mechanism, and these agents should be used cautiously in the immediate postoperative period.[62,97] Premature ventricular contractions and premature atrial contractions are the most common ectopic rhythm disturbances seen in postoperative patients. They are rarely of clinical significance unless associated with myocardial ischemia. The decision to treat these disturbances with antidysrhythmics should be based on the cause and clinical situation. Beta blockers have been used successfully in terminating ventricular ectopy and some accelerated rhythms caused by catecholamines.[49] In other situations, no therapy may be indicated. Accelerated dysrhythmias that are associated with major hemodynamic changes require treatment to slow and convert the rhythm disturbance. Dysrhythmias that cause hypotension, myocardial ischemia, or CHF should be treated immediately. In these cases, cardioversion may be required before the situation deteriorates.

Gastrointestinal Complications

Surgery and anesthesia can have profound effects on GI function. By far, the most common GI problem in PACU patients is nausea and vomiting.

Vomiting is caused by stimulation of the vomiting center, located in the dorsal part of the lateral reticular formation of the medulla. Autonomic afferents from the GI tract and mediastinum, vestibular component of the eighth cranial nerve, visual and cortical stimuli, and the chemoreceptor trigger zone all feed into the vomiting center (Fig. 88-15). Stimulation of the vomiting center causes reflex efferent activity, resulting in emesis. Causes of postoperative vomiting include drug effects, GI distention, intra-abdominal surgery, swallowed blood, pharyngeal stimulation, movement, and hypotension. Adriani et al.,[1] in 1961 reported an incidence of 23%, with persistent vomiting in 3.5% of patients. The incidence of postoperative emesis may be highest after ophthalmic and otologic surgery and is more common in women

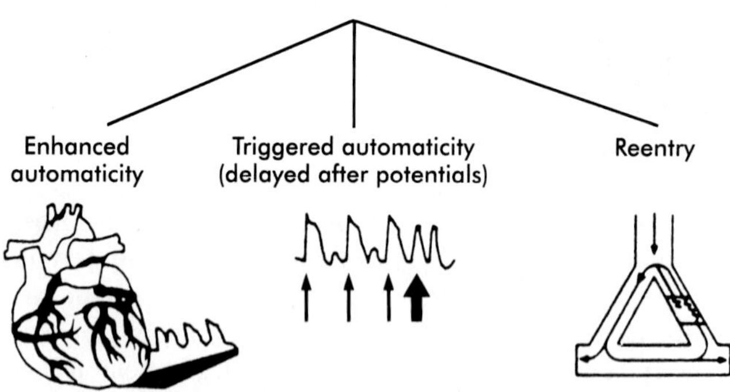

Fig. 88-14. Mechanisms of dysrhythmogenesis. The three proposed mechanisms are enhanced automaticity, triggered automaticity, and reentry. All three mechanisms are increased by elevated catecholamines. (From Podrid PJ, Vendetti FJ, Levine PA, et al: The role of exercise testing in evaluation of arrhythmias, *Am J Cardiol* 62:24H, 1988.)

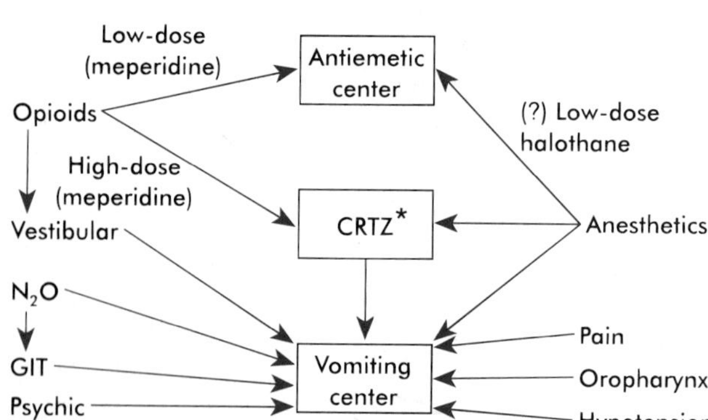

Fig. 88-15. Sites of action of stimuli related to surgery and anesthesia that are known to cause nausea and vomiting. (From Palazzo MG, Strunin L: Anaesthesia and emesis. I. Etiology, *Can Anaesth Soc J* 31:178, 1984.) *Chemoreceptor trigger zone.

and young healthy patients.[111] An increased incidence of postoperative nausea and vomiting occurs in patients with a history of motion sickness as well as in patients with previous episodes of postoperative emesis, suggesting that some patients may be predisposed to this problem.[77]

The association between morphine premedication and postoperative nausea and vomiting is well known.[94] Riding[94] observed a 22.4% incidence of nausea, retching, or vomiting in a study of unpremedicated women undergoing uterine curettage. When morphine was added as a premedication, the incidence increased to 67%. When atropine was combined with morphine for premedication, emetic symptoms occurred in only 37% of patients. The antiemetic effect of atropine was subsequently confirmed when preoperative administration of atropine alone reduced the incidence to 11.5%.[94] Narcotics do not always precipitate emesis. In fact, they may be antiemetic in certain postoperative situations. Andersen and Krogh[4] noted during the first 12 to 24 postoperative hours that only 10% of patients had pain without nausea compared with 58.6% of patients who experienced pain with nausea. These authors concluded that pain relief decreases the severity of nausea, and when pain relief is inadequate, nausea persists.

Avoiding postoperative emesis involves both preventive maneuvers and pharmacologic interventions. Minimizing gastric inflation during mask ventilation and gastric suctioning before extubation may decrease postoperative emesis.[52] Oropharyngeal packing can prevent blood from reaching the stomach during nasopharyngeal procedures. Because pharyngeal suctioning can provoke retching and vomiting, suctioning should be performed before reversal of muscle paralysis in the operating room. Excessive movement of patients who have received regional anesthesia or opioids can also provoke nausea and should be avoided. Adequate pain relief and hydration as well as preventing hypotension likely helps to decrease postoperative emesis. Anticholinergics, antihistamines, phenothiazines, sedatives, dopamine, and serotonin antagonists all have antiemetic properties (Table 88-8). Because these antiemetics are not innocuous, widespread prophylaxis is not recommended. Prophylaxis is indicated for patients in whom vomiting poses an excessive risk of aspiration or damage (e.g., oral surgery patients with jaw wiring, or patients undergoing eye or ear surgery). Phenothiazines are effective antiemetic agents because of antidopaminergic, antihistaminic, and anticholinergic properties; their routine use is limited by a high incidence of side effects. The butyrophenones (haloperidol and droperidol) have antidopaminergic properties that make this class of drugs especially effective against narcotic-induced vomiting. Droperidol is a useful antiemetic with proven prophylactic efficacy at low doses (0.005 to 0.07 mg/kg). Its duration of action (up to 24 hours) is longer than other agents that are commonly used, making it an attractive choice for the postoperative period. The use of small doses of droperidol (up to 1.25 mg) is associated with acute neurologic side effects,[60] particularly anxiety reactions.[70] Metoclopramide and domperidone are specific dopamine antagonists that cause very little sedation in normal doses (domperidone does not cross the blood–brain barrier).[60] For postoperative nausea and vomiting, prophylaxis with low-dose metoclopramide (10 to 20 mg) is effective when administered at the end of surgery. High-dose metoclopramide (1 to 2 mg/kg), similar to that used with chemotherapy, has not been evaluated in postoperative patients. This larger dose may be more effective and does not appear to increase the incidence of side effects.[42] Domperidone has no proved efficacy as a prophylactic agent but can be used to effectively treat active vomiting when given IV.[36,117]

A new class of drugs that are serotonin antagonists has recently become available. Ondansetron, a 5HT3 receptor antagonist, has shown considerable efficacy as an antiemetic in cancer chemotherapy patients. In postoperative patients it is safe, well tolerated, and better than a placebo.[15] Side effects secondary to ondansetron use appear to be mild and the time to discharge following its administration does not appear to be prolonged.[46,61] **Routine use of ondansetron for prophylaxis of postoperative nausea and vomiting may be precluded by its high cost, but it is clearly indicated today if a patient appears to be developing pathologic persistent postoperative vomiting.**

The causes of postoperative emesis in any one patient are likely multifactorial. Antiemetic prophylactic maneuvers, such as avoidance of oral airways and excessive movement, and the treatment of pain, should be used in PACU patients. Specific pharmacologic antiemetics should be used in patients with persistent nausea and vomiting. If the first drug used is ineffective, a second agent, preferably one with a different site of action, should be tried.

Green and Jonsson[43] in 1993 reported on 95 ambulatory patients given propofol versus isoflurane. Isoflurane was associated with more nausea or vomiting, and this complication was responsible for all three patients who were hospitalized overnight.

Genitourinary Complications

Postoperative oliguria, urinary retention, and the post-transurethral prostatic resection syndrome are the most common genitourinary problems of PACU patients. For a discussion of postoperative oliguria see the section on abnormal urine output.

Urinary retention

Acute urinary retention is a common postoperative complication. Surgical trauma to the detrusor muscle and damage to pelvic nerves can inhibit bladder emptying, and operations on genitourinary and other pelvic structures are associated with the highest incidence of urinary retention.[33] Delayed recovery of autonomic and somatic nerve function after spinal or epidural anesthesia does not appear to be a common cause of postoperative oliguria; the incidence of urinary retention is similar after either general anesthesia or regional techniques.[102] Obtunded postoperative patients may be unaware of acute bladder distension and may benefit from urethral catheterization but the risk of infection should

Table 88-8 Activity of antiemetic drugs at neurotransmitter receptor sites

Drug	Dopamine (D_2)	Muscarinic cholinergic	Histamine (H_1)	Serotonin (5-HT_3)
Anticholinergics				
Hyoscine	–	5+	–	–
Atropine	–	5+	–	–
Glycopyrrolate	–	5+	–	–
Antihistamines				
Promethazine	4+	5+	5+	–
Diphenhydramine	–	4+	5+	–
Cyclizine	1+	3+	5+	–
Phenothiazines				
Fluphenazine	5+	4+	5+	–
Prochlorperazine	5+	5+	4+	–
Chlorpromazine	5+	4+	5+	–
Butyrophenones				
Droperidol	5+	–	1+	–
Haloperidol	5+	–	1+	–
Miscellaneous				
Metoclopramide	4+	–	1+	2+
Domperidone	4+	–	–	–
Ondansetron	–	–	–	5+

1+, Least activity; 5+, strongest activity; –, no activity.

limit enthusiasm for the procedure. Perioperative use of parasympatholytic agents, such as atropine, scopolamine, and glycopyrrolate, may partially inhibit bladder contraction and contribute to postoperative urinary retention. Administration of parasympathomimetic agents (pilocarpine or bethanechol) can increase detrusor muscle tone and promote micturition, but these agents should be avoided in patients with obstructive urinary retention, in which case, bladder catheterization may be a better choice.

Transurethral prostatectomy syndrome

Exposure of large venous sinuses adjacent to the prostatic capsule during transurethral resection of the prostate (TURP) provides a conduit for absorption (infusion under pressure) of large quantities of irrigation solution into the intravascular space. Absorption of commonly used irrigants such as glycine results in TURP syndrome, which is characterized by neurologic changes (dizziness, restlessness, confusion, visual disturbances, seizures, coma), bradycardia, hypertension and intravascular volume overload. This isotonic solute-free solution is not associated with hemolysis, but may cause acute water intoxication with severe hyponatremia when absorbed in large volume. Hahn added small amounts of ethanol to the glycine irrigant and found the concentration of ethanol in the exhaled breath of patients undergoing TURP to correlate with the volume of glycine absorbed and the decrease in serum sodium levels.[45] Wang et al.[112] suggested that glycine acts as an inhibitory transmitter in the retina and may contribute to visual disturbances in the TURP syndrome. It remains a matter for speculation whether other neurologic aberrations are the result of hyperglycinemia, hyperammonemia, hyponatremia, or other unidentified factors. The incidence of clinically significant TURP syndrome was reported in 1989 to be 2%. Operative factors associated with the development of TURP syndrome are resection time greater than 90 minutes and gland size greater than 45 g.[70] In recent years, enthusiasm for the procedure itself has been dampened by criticisms of its high complication rate.

Immediate treatment of TURP syndrome is required as the fatality rate may exceed 1%.[106] Surgery should be terminated and O_2 administered. Patients should be observed closely in the PACU, with serum sodium levels repeatedly measured. Furosemide aids in excretion of excess free water and hastens the return of serum sodium levels to normal. Hypertonic saline can be cautiously administered if clinical signs of water intoxication are present (usually at serum sodium levels less than 120 mEq/l) but rapid correction of serum sodium levels should be avoided. Anticonvulsant therapy with benzodiazepines, barbiturates, or dilantin is indicated if seizure activity develops. Effective treatment of pulmonary congestion or shock may require invasive pulmonary catheter monitoring and transfer to an intensive care unit.

KEY POINTS

- Elevated levels of catecholamines, resulting from the stress response to surgery, can adversely affect the myocardial O_2 supply-demand ratio, leading to ischemia. Initial assessment of the physiologic causes of tachycardia include evaluation of intravascular volume status, adequacy of ventilation, hematocrit, fever, and evidence of pain from the surgical incision or from visceral distension.
- Several conditions make continued intubation necessary after surgery: (1) epiglottitis; (2) surgery or trauma to the upper airway associated with severe edema; (3) surgery on the neck that causes damage to the recurrent laryngeal nerves; and (4) massive intraoperative volume infusion in patients maintained in the Trendelenburg position for prolonged periods.
- Excessive blood loss can result from inadequate surgical hemostasis or coagulation disorders. Internal bleeding is usually first diagnosed by signs of hypovolemia and a falling hematocrit. Hypotension in supine patients is a late sign of hypovolemia and may already represent a 40% decrease in cardiac output.
- The three major causes of failure to awaken after general anesthesia are: (1) prolonged action of anesthetic agents (the most common cause); (2) metabolic abnormalities (e.g., hypoglycemia, hyponatremia, hypocalcemia, hypermagnesemia); and (3) neurologic injury.
- Evaluation of patients with prolonged neuromuscular weakness begins with a neurologic examination and close scrutiny of the anesthetic record. The most common cause of prolonged neuromuscular weakness is the excessive use of neuromuscular blockers. A level of paralysis that is inconsistent with the drug listed on the anesthetic record should cause the physician to suspect an anatomic or physiologic neuromuscular abnormality.
- Oliguria, polyuria, and hematuria are the most frequently encountered urinary abnormalities in the PACU. Oliguria can result from primary renal disease, prerenal pathology (decreased cardiac output or low intravascular volume), or postrenal (obstruction) causes. The most common cause of postoperative oliguria in healthy patients is hypovolemia. Hematuria can be caused by erythrocytes, intravascular hemolysis (hemoglobinuria), or presence of pigments from rhabdomyolysis (myoglobinuria).
- The incidence of hypothermia is greater in postoperative patients than in any other patient population. Hyperthermia in recovery room patients can be caused by infection (the most common cause), transfusion reaction, drug reaction, primary CNS disorders, and malignant hyperthermia.
- Transient disorders of mentation, pathologic spinal reflexes, and movement disorders such as shivering are common nervous system abnormalities observed in the PACU. Emergence excitement occurs in 5% to 30% of PACU admissions and is more common in very young and very old patients. Postoperative symmetric neurologic abnormalities do not appear to be associated with adverse clinical consequences. However, the discovery of focal neurologic deficits should point to possible acute CNS injury and warrant further investigation.
- Airway obstruction, which is common in postoperative patients, can result in hypoxemia and hypercapnia. It may be caused by vomitus or secretions in the pharynx, the tongue falling back onto the posterior pharynx, laryngospasm, or laryngeal edema. Clinical examinations that correlate best with adequate airway patency are sustained leg-lift and sustained head-lift for 5 seconds. Hypoxemia and hypercapnia can also result from the depressant effects of narcotics and inhalational agents on O_2 and CO_2 responsiveness, residual neuromuscular blockade, or ventilation-perfusion mismatch. All patients should receive supplemental O_2 during transport from the operating room to the PACU and during their initial PACU stay.
- Hypotension in the PACU is usually caused by the residual effects of anesthesia or by hypovolemia and is more common after regional than general anesthesia. Treatment includes Trendelenburg position, judicious volume replacement, and, if necessary, the administration of alpha- and beta-adrenergic agonists.
- Dysrhythmias, particularly sinus tachycardia, are extremely common in PACU patients. Other commonly encountered rhythm disturbances are sinus bradycardia, premature ectopic beats, and accelerated ectopic rhythms. Elevated postoperative catecholamines is probably the most important cause of recovery room tachydysrhythmias. Premature ventricular or atrial contractions are rarely of clinical significance unless associated with myocardial ischemia.
- Nausea and vomiting are by far the most common GI problems in the PACU. The causes of postoperative vomiting include drug effects, GI distension, intra-abdominal surgery, swallowed blood, pharyngeal stimulation, movement, and hypotension. Anticholinergics, antihistamines, phenothiazines, sedatives, and antidopaminergics all have antiemetic properties. Antiemetic prophylaxis is indicated only for patients in whom vomiting poses an excessive risk of aspiration or damage (e.g., oral surgery patients with jaw wiring or patients undergoing ocular and otologic procedures).

KEY REFERENCES

Breslow MJ, Miller CF, Parker SD, et al: Changes in T-wave morphology following anesthesia and surgery: a common recovery room phenomenon, *Anesthesiology* 64:398, 1986.

Camm AJ, Garratt CJ: Adenosine and supraventricular tachycardia, *N Engl J Med* 325:1621, 1991.

Knill RL, Gelb AW: Ventilatory responses to hypoxia and hypercapnia during halothane sedation and anesthesia in man, *Anesthesiology* 49:244, 1978.

Melnick B, Sawyer R, Karambelkar D, et al: Delayed side effects of droperidol after ambulatory general anesthesia, *Anesth Analg* 69:748, 1989.

Pavlin EG, Holle RH, Schoene RB: Recovery in airway protection compared with ventilation in humans after paralysis with curare, *Anesthesiology* 70:381, 1989.

Sessler DI, Israel D, Pozos RS, et al: Spontaneous postanesthetic tremor does not resemble thermoregulatory shivering, *Anesthesiology* 68:843, 1988.

Weil JV, McCullough RE, Kline JS, et al: Diminished ventilatory response to hypoxia and hypercapnia after morphine in normal man, *N Engl J Med* 292:1103, 1975.

REFERENCES

1. Adriani J, Summers FW, Antony SO: Is the prophylactic use of antiemetics in surgical patients justified? *JAMA* 175:666, 1961.
2. Alexander CM, Teller LE, Gross JB, et al: New discharge criteria decrease recovery room time after subarachnoid block, *Anesthesiology* 70:640, 1989.
3. Anderson JA, Clark PJ, Kafer ER: Use of capnography and transcutaneous oxygen monitoring during outpatient general anesthesia for oral surgery, *J Oral Maxillofac Surg* 45:3, 1987.
4. Anderson R, Krohg K: Pain as a major cause of postoperative nausea, *Can Anaesth Soc J* 23:366, 1976.
5. Argov Z, Mastaglia FL: Disorders of neuromuscular transmission caused by drugs, *N Engl J Med* 301:409, 1979.
6. Azzam FJ: A simple and effective method for stopping post-anesthesia clonus, *Anesthesiology* 66:98, 1987.
7. Baer S, NakhJavah F, Kajani M: Postoperative myocardial infarction, *Surg Gynecol Obstet* 1:315, 1965.
8. Beard K, Jick H, Walker AM: Adverse respiratory events occurring in the recovery room after general anesthesia, *Anesthesiology* 64:296, 1986.
9. Becker LD, Paulson BA, Miller RD, et al: Biphasic respiratory depression after fentanyl-droperidol or fentanyl alone used to supplement nitrous oxide anesthesia, *Anesthesiology* 44:291, 1976.
10. Becker RC, Underwood DA: Myocardial infarction in patients undergoing non-cardiac surgery, *Clev Clin J Med* 54:25, 1987.
11. Behnke AR, Yaglov CP: Physiological responses of man to chilling in ice water to slow and fast warming, *J Appl Physiol* 3:591, 1951.
12. Bidwai AV, Cornelius LR, Stanley TH: Reversal of Innovar-induced postanesthetic somnolence and disorientation with physostigmine, *Anesthesiology* 44:249, 1976.
13. Bidwai AV, Stanley TH, Rogers C, et al: Reversal of diazepam-induced postanesthetic somnolence with physostigmine, *Anesthesiology* 51:256, 1979.
14. Biller HF, Bone RC, Harvey JE, et al: Laryngeal edema: an experimental study, *Ann Otol Rhinol Laryngol* 79:1084, 1976.
15. Bodner M, Poler SM, White PF: Initial evaluation of ondansetron—a novel antiemetic, *Anesthesiology* 73:A328, 1990.
16. Breslow MJ, Miller CF, Parker SD, et al: Changes in T-wave morphology following anesthesia and surgery: a common recovery room phenomenon, *Anesthesiology* 64:398, 1986.
17. Brismar B, Hedenstierna G, Lundquist H, et al: Pulmonary densities during anesthesia with muscular relaxation—a proposal of atelectasis, *Anesthesiology* 62:422, 1985.
18. Buffington CW: Hemodynamic determinants of ischemic myocardial dysfunction in the presence of coronary stenosis in dogs, *Anesthesiology* 63:651, 1985.
19. Bull BS, Huse WM, Brauer FS, et al: Heparin therapy during extracorporeal circulation. II. The use of a dose-response curve to individualize heparin and protamine dosage, *J Thorac Cardiovasc Surg* 69:686, 1975.
20. Butterworth JF, Piccione W Jr, Berrizbeitia LD, et al: Augmentation of venous return by adrenergic agonists during spinal anesthesia, *Anesth Analg* 65:612, 1986.
21. Camm AJ, Garratt CJ: Adenosine and supraventricular tachycardia, *N Engl J Med* 325:1621, 1991.
22. Chung FF, Chung A, Meier RH, et al: Comparison of perioperative mental function after general anaesthesia and spinal anaesthesia with IV sedation, *Can J Anaesth* 36:382, 1989.
23. Chung F, Meier R, Lautenschlager E, et al: General or spinal anesthesia: Which is better in the elderly? *Anesthesiology* 67:422, 1987.
24. Clarke MM, Storrs JA: The prevention of postoperative vomiting after abortion; metoclopramide, *Br J Anaesth* 41:890, 1969.
25. Cooper JB, Cullen DJ, Nemeskal R, et al: Effects of information feedback and pulse oximetry on the incidence of anesthesia complications, *Anesthesiology* 67:686, 1987.
26. Counts RD, Haisch C, Simon TL, et al: Hemostasis in massively transfused trauma patients, *Ann Surg* 190:91, 1979.
27. Cousins MJ, Mather LE: Intrathecal and epidural administration of opioids, *Anesthesiology* 61:276, 1984.
28. Cuschieri RJ, Morran CG, Howie JC, et al: Postoperative pain and pulmonary complications: comparison of three analgesic regimens, *Br J Surg* 72:495, 1985.
29. Dexter F, Tinker J: Comparisons between desflurane and isoflurane or propofol on time to following commands and time to discharge, *Anesthesiology* 83:77–32, 1995.
30. Domen RE, Kennedy MS, Jones LL, et al: Hemostatic imbalances produced by plasma exchange, *Transfusion* 24:336, 1984.
31. Dunn RB, Griggs DM Jr: Ventricular filling pressure as a determinant of coronary blood flow during ischemia, *Am J Physiol* 244:H429, 1983.
32. Eckenhoff JE, Kneale DH, Dripps RD: The incidence and etiology of postanesthetic excitement. A clinical survey, *Anesthesiology* 22:667, 1961.
33. Egbert LD: Spinal anesthesia for anorectal surgery, *Int Anesthesiol Clin* 1:811, 1963.
34. Eger EI II, editor: *Anesthetic uptake and action,* Baltimore, 1974, Williams & Wilkins.
35. Fairley HB: Oxygen therapy for surgical patients, *Am Rev Resp Dis* 122:37, 1980.
36. Fragen RJ, Caldwell N: A new benzimidazole antiemetic, domperidone, for the treatment of postoperative nausea and vomiting, *Anesthesiology* 49:289, 1978.
37. Frank SM, Crowley H, Rock P, et al: Perioperative body temperature regulation in regional vs. general anesthesia (ASA abstract), *Anesthesiology,* 1990.
38. Gal TJ, Cooperman LH: Hypertension in the immediate postoperative period, *Br J Anaesth* 47:70, 1975.
39. Gamulin Z, Forster A, Morel D, et al:

Effects of infra-renal aortic cross-clamping on renal hemodynamics in humans, *Anesthesiology* 61:394, 1984.

40. Garfield JM, Garield FB, Stone JG, et al: A comparison of psychologic responses to ketamine and thiopental-nitrous oxide-halothane anesthesia, *Anesthesiology* 36:329, 1972.
41. Goold JE: Postoperative spasticity and shivering: a review with personal observations of 500 patients, *Anaesthesia* 39:35, 1984.
42. Gralla RJ, Itri LM, Pisko SE, et al: Antiemetic efficacy of high-dose metoclopramide: randomized trials with placebo and prochlorperazine in patients with chemotherapy-induced nausea and vomiting, *N Engl J Med* 305:905, 1981.
43. Green G, Jonsson L: Nausea: the most important factor determining length of stay after ambulatory anemia: comparison is Isoflurane vs Propopol *Acth Anes Scand* 37:742–746, 1993.
44. Griffin RM, Kaplan JA: Myocardial ischemia during non-cardiac surgery, *Anaesthesia* 41:155, 1987.
45. Hahn RG: Ethanol monitoring of irrigating fluid absorption in transurethral prostatic surgery, *Anesthesiology* 68:867, 1988.
46. Hall S, Ceuppens P: A study to evaluate the effect of ondansetron on psychomotor performance after repeated oral dosing in healthy subjects, *Psychopharmacology* 104:86, 1991.
47. Hamel HT: Anesthetics and body temperature regulation, *Anesthesiology* 68:833, 1988.
48. Hammer G, Schwinn D, Wollman H: Postoperative complications due to paradoxical vocal cord motion, *Anesthesiology* 66:685, 1987.
49. Hanna MH, Heap DG, Kimberly APS: Cardiac dysrhythmia associated with general anaesthesia for oral surgery, *Anaesthesia* 38:1192, 1983.
50. Hashimoto K, Hashimoto K: The mechanism of sensitization of the ventricle to epinephrine by halothane, *Am Heart J* 83: 652, 1972.
51. Hines R, Barash P, Watrous G, et al: Complications occurring in the postanesthesia care unit: a survey, *Anesth Analg* 74:503, 1992.
52. Holmes C: Postoperative vomiting after ether/air anaesthesia, *Anaesthesia* 20:199, 1965.
53. Holzgrafe RE, Vondrell JJ, Mintz SM: Reversal of postoperative reactions of scopolamine with physostigmine, *Anesth Analg* 52:921, 1973.
54. Intravenous Nicardipine Study Group: Efficacy and safety of IV nicardipine in the control of postoperative hypertension, *Chest* 99:393, 1991.
55. Iwamoto K, Schwartz H: Antiemetic effect of droperidol after ophthalmic surgery, *Arch Ophthalmol* 96:1378, 1978.
56. Janson PA, Jubelier SJ, Weinstein MJ, et al: Treatment of the bleeding tendency in uremia with cryoprecipitate, *N Engl J Med* 303:1318, 1980.
57. Kang YG, Martin DJ, Marquez J, et al: Intraoperative changes in blood coagulation and thromboelastographic monitoring in liver transplantation, *Anesth Analg* 64:888, 1985.
58. Kaplan J, editor: *Cardiac anesthesia,* ed 2, New York, 1986, Grune & Stratton.
59. Knill RL, Gelb AW: Ventilatory responses to hypoxia and hypercapnia during halothane sedation and anesthesia in man, *Anesthesiology* 49:244, 1978.
60. Korttila K, Kauste A, Auvinen J: Comparison of domperidone and metoclopramide in the prevention and treatment of nausea and vomiting after balanced general anaesthesia, *Anesth Analg* 58:396, 1979.
61. Kovac A, Steer P, Hutchinson M, et al: Effect of ondansetron on recovery time, sedation level, and discharge from ambulatory surgery, *Anesthesiology* 75:A7, 1991.
62. Levine JH, Michael JR, Guarnieri TK: Multifocal atrial tachycardia: a toxic effect of theophylline, *Lancet* 1:12, 1985.
63. London M, Hollenberg M, Wong MG, et al: Intraoperative myocardial ischemia: localization by continuous 12-lead electrography, *Anesthesiology* 69:232, 1988.
64. Macintyre PE, Pavlin EG, Dwersteg JF: Effect of meperidine on oxygen consumption, carbon dioxide production, and respiratory gas exchange in post-anesthesia shivering, *Anesth Analg* 66:751, 1987.
65. Mackey DC, Carpenter RL, Thompson GE, et al: Bradycardia and asystole during spinal anesthesia: a report of three cases without morbidity, *Anesthesiology* 70:866, 1989.
66. Makela JP, Livainen M, Pieninkeroinenl P, et al: Seizure associated with Propopol anesthesia. *Epilepsia:* 34:832–835, 1993.
67. Mannucci PM, Remuzzi G, Pusineri F, et al: Deamno-8-D-arginine vasopressin shortens the bleeding time in uremia, *N Engl J Med* 308:8, 1983.
68. Marcantonio ER, Goldman L, Mangrove CM, et al: A chemical prediction rule for delirium after elective noncardiac surgery, *JAMA* 271:134–139, 1994.
69. McCann RL, Clements FM: Silent myocardial ischemia in patients undergoing peripheral vascular surgery. Incidence and association with perioperative cardiac morbidity and mortality, *J Vasc Surg* 9:583, 1989.
70. Mebust WK, Holtgrewe HL, Cockett TK, et al: Transurethral prostatectomy: immediate and postoperative complications. A cooperative study of 13 participating institutions evaluating 3,885 patients, *J Urol* 141:243, 1989.
71. Melnick B, Sawyer R, Karambelkar D, et al: Delayed side effects of droperidol after ambulatory general anesthesia, *Anesth Analg* 69:748, 1989.
72. Metz S, Klein C, Morton N: Rebound hypertension after discontinuation of transdermal clonidine therapy, *Am J Med* 82:17, 1987.
73. Miller RD, Cullen DJ: Renal failure and postoperative respiratory failure: recurarization? *Br J Anaesth* 48:253, 1976.
74. Miller RD, Savarese JJ: Pharmacology of muscle relaxants and their antagonists. In Miller RD, editor: *Anesthesia,* ed 2, New York, 1987, Churchill-Livingstone.
75. Mora CT, Torjman M, White PF: Effects of diazepam and flumazenil on sedation and hypoxic ventilatory response, *Anesth Analg* 68:473, 1989.
76. Morss HL, Baillie TW: A case of postoperative respiratory insufficiency and prolonged unconsciousness, *Br J Anaesth* 30:19, 1958.
77. Muir JJ, Warner MA, Offord KP, et al: Role of nitrous oxide and other factors in postoperative nausea and vomiting: a randomized and blinded prospective study, *Anesthesiology* 66:513, 1987.
78. Murkin JM: Anesthesia and hypothyroidism: a review of thyroxine physiology, pharmacology, and anesthetic implications, *Anesth Analg* 61:371, 1982.
79. Murphy MT, Lipton JM, Loughren P, et al: Post-anesthetic shivering in primates: inhibition by peripheral heating and by taurine, *Anesthesiology* 63:161, 1985.
80. Nenci GG, Berrettini M, Agnelli G, et al: Effect of peritoneal dialysis, hemodialysis, and kidney transplantation on blood platelet function, *Nephron* 23:287, 1979.
81. Nunn JF, editor: Respiratory aspects of anesthesia. In Nunn JF: *Applied respiratory physiology,* ed 3, London, 1987, Butterworths.
82. O'Mailia JJ, Saunder GE, Giles TD: Nifedipine associated myocardial ischemia or infarction in the treatment of hypertensive urgencies, *Ann Intern Med* 107:185, 1987.
83. Ohman JL Jr, Marliss EB, Aoki TT, et al: The cerebrospinal fluid in diabetic ketoacidosis, *N Engl J Med* 284:283, 1971.
84. Oliver SB, Cucchiara RF, Warner MA, et al: Unexpected focal neurologic deficit on emergence from anesthesia: a report of three cases, *Anesthesiology* 67:823, 1987.
85. Ouyang P, Gerstenblith G, Furman WF, et al: Frequency and significance of early postoperative silent myocardial ischemia in patients having peripheral vascular surgery, *Am J Cardiol* 64:L1113, 1989.
86. Pasternak RC, Braunwald JA: Acute myocardial infarction. In Braunwald E, Isselbacher KJ, Petersdorf RG, et al, editors: *Harrison's principles of internal medicine,* ed 11, New York, 1987, McGraw-Hill.
87. Patton CM, Moon MR, Dannemiller FJ: The prophylactic antiemetic effect of droperidol, *Anesth Analg* 53:361, 1974.
88. Pavlin EG, Holle RH, Schoene RB: Recovery in airway protection compared with ventilation in humans after paralysis with curare, *Anesthesiology* 70:381, 1989.
89. Payne JP, Hughes R, Azawi SA: Neuromuscular blockade by neostigmine in anaesthetized man, *Br J Anaesth* 52:69, 1980.
90. Peters J, Kindred MK, Robotham JL: Transient analysis of cardiopulmonary interactions. II. Systolic events, *J Appl Physiol* 64:1518, 1988.
91. Pineo GF, Gallus AS, Hirsh J: Unexpected vitamin K deficiency in hospitalized patients, *CMA J* 109:880, 1973.
92. Podrid PJ, Venditti FJ, Levine PA, et al: The role of exercise testing in evaluation of arrhythmias, *Am J Cardiol* 62:24H, 1988.
93. Rawal N, Schott U, Dahlstrom B, et al: Influence of naloxone infusion on analgesia and respiratory depression following epidural morphine, *Anesthesiology* 64:194, 1986.
94. Riding JE: Postoperative vomiting, *Proc Royal Soc Med* 53:671, 1960.
95. Rossini AA, Mordes JP: The diabetic

comas. In Rippe JM, Irwin RS, Alpert JS, et al: editors: *Intensive care medicine,* Boston, 1985, Little Brown.

96. Rodriguez JL, Weissman C, Damask MC, et al: Physiologic requirements during rewarming: suppression of the shivering response, *Crit Care Med* 11:490, 1983.
97. Roizen MF, Stevens WC: Multiform ventricular tachycardia due to the interaction of aminophylline and halothane, *Anesth Analg* 57:738, 1978.
98. Rosenberg H, Clofine R, Bialik O: Neurologic changes during awakening from anesthesia, *Anesthesiology* 54:125, 1981.
99. Rossett RL: An unusual cause of postoperative respiratory failure, *Anesthesiology* 66:695, 1987.
100. Rueler JB: Hypothermia: pathophysiology, clinical settings, and management, *Ann Intern Med* 89:519, 1978.
101. Sahn SA, Lakshminarayan S: Bedside criteria for discontinuation of mechanical ventilation, *Chest* 63:1002, 1973.
102. Scarborough RA: Spinal anesthesia from the surgeon's standpoint, *JAMA* 168:1324, 1958.
103. Sessler DI, Israel D, Pozos RS, et al: Spontaneous post-anesthetic tremor does not resemble thermoregulatory shivering, *Anesthesiology* 68:843, 1988.
104. Sharkey A, Lipton JM, Murphy MT, et al: Inhibition of post-anesthetic shivering with radiant heat, *Anesthesiology* 66:249, 1987.
105. Shaw JE: Pharmacokinetics of nitroglycerin and clonidine delivered by the transdermal route, *Am Heart J* 108:217, 1984.
106. Sunderrajan S, Bauer JH, Vopat RL, et al: Post-transurethral prostatic resection hyponatremic syndrome: case report and review of the literature, *Am J Kid Dis* 4:80, 1984.
107. Taff RH: Pulmonary edema following naloxone administration in a patient without heart disease, *Anesthesiology* 59:576, 1983.
108. Tarhan S, Moffitt EA, Taylor WF, et al: Myocardial infarction after general anesthesia, *JAMA* 220:1451, 1972.
109. Toung T, Donham RT, Lehner A, et al: Tension pneumocephalus after posterior fossa craniotomy: report of four additional cases and review of postoperative pneumocephalus, *Neurosurgery* 12:164, 1983.
110. Tyler IL, Tantisira B, Winter PM, et al: Continuous monitoring of arterial oxygen saturation with pulse oximetry during transfer to the recovery room, *Anesth Analg* 64:1108, 1985.
111. Vance JP, Neill RS, Norris W: The incidence and aetiology of postoperative nausea and vomiting in a plastic surgical unit, *Br J Plast Surg* 26:336, 1973.
112. Wang JM, Creel DJ, Wong KC: Transurethral resection of the prostate, serum glycine levels, and ocular evoked potentials, *Anesthesiology* 70:36, 1989.
113. Weber JG, Warner MA, Warner ME: Perioperative pulmonary aspiration: incidence and risk factors, *Anesthesiology* 73:A1071, 1990.
114. Weil JV, McCullough RE, Kline JS, et al: Diminished ventilatory response to hypoxia and hypercapnia after morphine in normal man, *N Engl J Med* 292:1103, 1975.
115. Weinstock M, Davidson JT, Rosin AJ, et al: Effect of physostigmine on morphine-induced postoperative pain and somnolence, *Br J Anaesth* 54:429, 1982.
116. Wilms D, Shure D: Pulmonary edema due to upper airway obstruction in adults, *Chest* 94:1090, 1988.
117. Wilson DB, Dundee JW: Evaluation of the antiemetic action of domperidone, *Anaesthesia* 34:765, 1979.

CHAPTER 89

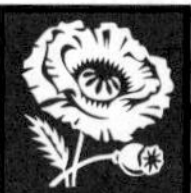

Acute Postoperative Pain Management

F. MICHAEL FERRANTE

A CONCEPTUAL BASIS FOR POSTOPERATIVE PAIN MANAGEMENT

The intramuscular administration of opioids has largely been abandoned as the mainstay of postoperative analgesic therapy. Despite the widespread acceptance and implementation of newer and more effective analgesic modalities, many practitioners still consider postoperative pain management in terms reminiscent of Erlich's "magic bullet": "use of a single technique will result in complete analgesia." Such a conceptualization of postoperative pain management is fraught with the potential for poor clinical outcomes, as it is predicated upon a basic misunderstanding of the physiologic processes surrounding nociception. Epidemiologic studies repeatedly demonstrated the failure of single modality therapy to produce complete analgesia.[33] Thus, we must use our enhanced understanding of nociception to formulate a new concept of analgesic therapy.[38,58]

Nociception

Pain is defined as "an unpleasant sensory and emotional experience associated with actual or potential tissue damage or described in terms of such damage."[80] Pain requires perception of a noxious event by a sentient being; it is operationally separate from the processes that bring about the "sensory and emotional experience." Between the site of tissue damage and the perception of pain lies a complex series of physiologic processes. Collectively, these processes are termed *nociception.* Four physiologic processes are involved in nociception (Fig. 89-1):[58]

Transduction is the process whereby noxious stimuli release a number of algesic neurotransmitters and translate these noxious stimuli into electrochemical events at sensory nerve endings (through a series of incompletely understood steps).

Transmission refers to the propagation of these electrical impulses through higher centers in both the peripheral nervous system (PNS) and central nervous system (CNS).

Modulation is the process whereby endogenous analgesic substances (e.g., opioids, serotonin, norepinephrine) exert an inhibitory influence upon transmission through the dorsal horn of the spinal cord.

Perception is the final process wherein all contributing influences interact to produce the final subjective and emotional experiences.

After transduction of noxious stimuli occurs at undifferentiated bare sensory nerve endings in the periphery, nociceptive transmission to the CNS occurs primarily through small myelinated Aδ and unmyelinated C fibers. Upon entering the spinal cord primarily through the dorsal roots, primary afferent nociceptors synapse in three of the six anatomically distinct layers of the dorsal horn. From the initial synapse, there are multiple interneuronal synaptic connections among all the layers of the dorsal horn (Fig. 89-2).

After decussation, nociceptive fibers ascend in the an-

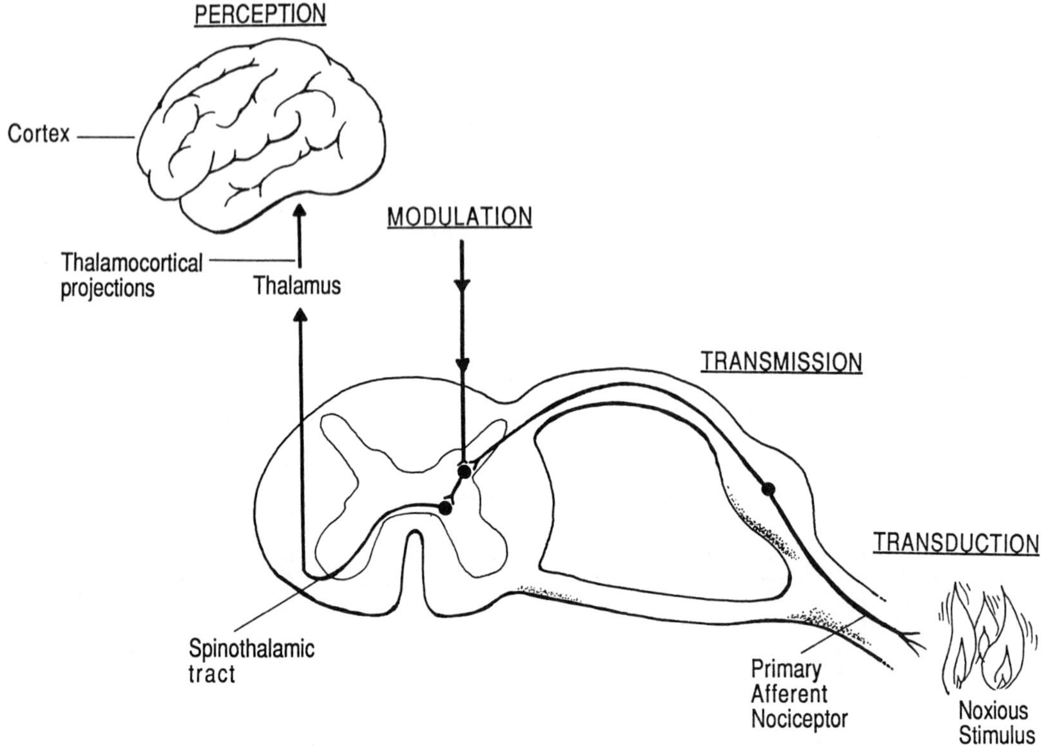

Fig. 89-1. The physiologic process of nociception. (From Katz N, Ferrante FM: Nociception. In Ferrante FM, VadeBoncouer TR, editors: *Postoperative pain management,* New York, 1993, Churchill-Livingstone.)

terolateral quadrant of the spinal cord forming the spinothalamic and spinoreticulothalamic tracts. Both tracts synapse in the thalamus. Nociceptive transmission then reaches the cortex via thalamocortical projections (Figs. 89-1 and 89-2).

Within the midbrain, pons, and medulla are discrete nuclear groups that contain endogenous analgesic substances including opioids, serotonin, and norepinephrine. Axons from these diverse nuclei and locations coalesce to form a descending modulating system and a tract, the *dorsolateral funiculus.* These axons synapse in the same six layers of the dorsal horn that receive primary afferent nociceptive transmission (Fig. 89-2).

The Gate Theory of Pain

The dorsal horn of the spinal cord is the focal point for the integration and modulation of nociception; it functions as a "gate" (Fig. 89-2). All the physiologic processes of nociception converge to affect the depolarization of dorsal horn neurons. **Factors that enhance excitability of dorsal horn neurons** (e.g., intense noxious stimuli) **"open the gate" and allow nociceptive transmission to higher centers. Factors that inhibit dorsal horn neuron excitability** (e.g., analgesics), **"close the gate" and interdict nociceptive transmission.** The descending modulating system, composed of nuclei and axons containing endogenous opioids, serotonin and norepinephrine, "closes the gate." **The concept of the dorsal horn as a "gate" that can be closed by pharmacologic manipulation of transduction, transmission, and modulation forms one of the underlying tenets for effective postoperative pain management.**[58]

Central hypersensitization

Surgical trauma results in an afferent barrage of nociceptive transmission that may alter the threshold for excitation as well as the magnitude of impulse generation in nociceptors.[18,127] Such sensitization may occur in both peripheral and central nociceptors after peripheral trauma. **This enhanced afferent transmission to the dorsal horn of the spinal cord may expand the receptive fields of dorsal horn neurons**[18] **as well as induce a progressive facilitation of dorsal horn neuronal discharge**[123] **(a process referred to as central hypersensitization or "wind-up,"** Fig. 89-3). Besides these electrophysiologic changes within the cord, postsynaptic morphology also is altered as a result of the afferent barrage.[112] These findings indicate that the nervous system is not merely an unchanging conduction system. Rather, **the nervous system is able to alter both structure and function in response to noxious stimuli, a process known as *neuroplasticity.***

Research to identify the chemical mediators of central hypersensitization demonstrated the pivotal role of the excitatory amino acids glutamate and aspartate in excitation of N-methyl-D-apartic acid (NMDA) receptors (Fig. 89-4).[93,129] The afferent barrage associated with noxious stimuli will result in bursts of glutamate release from presynaptic terminals. Glutamate receptors are of three types: (1) the NMDA

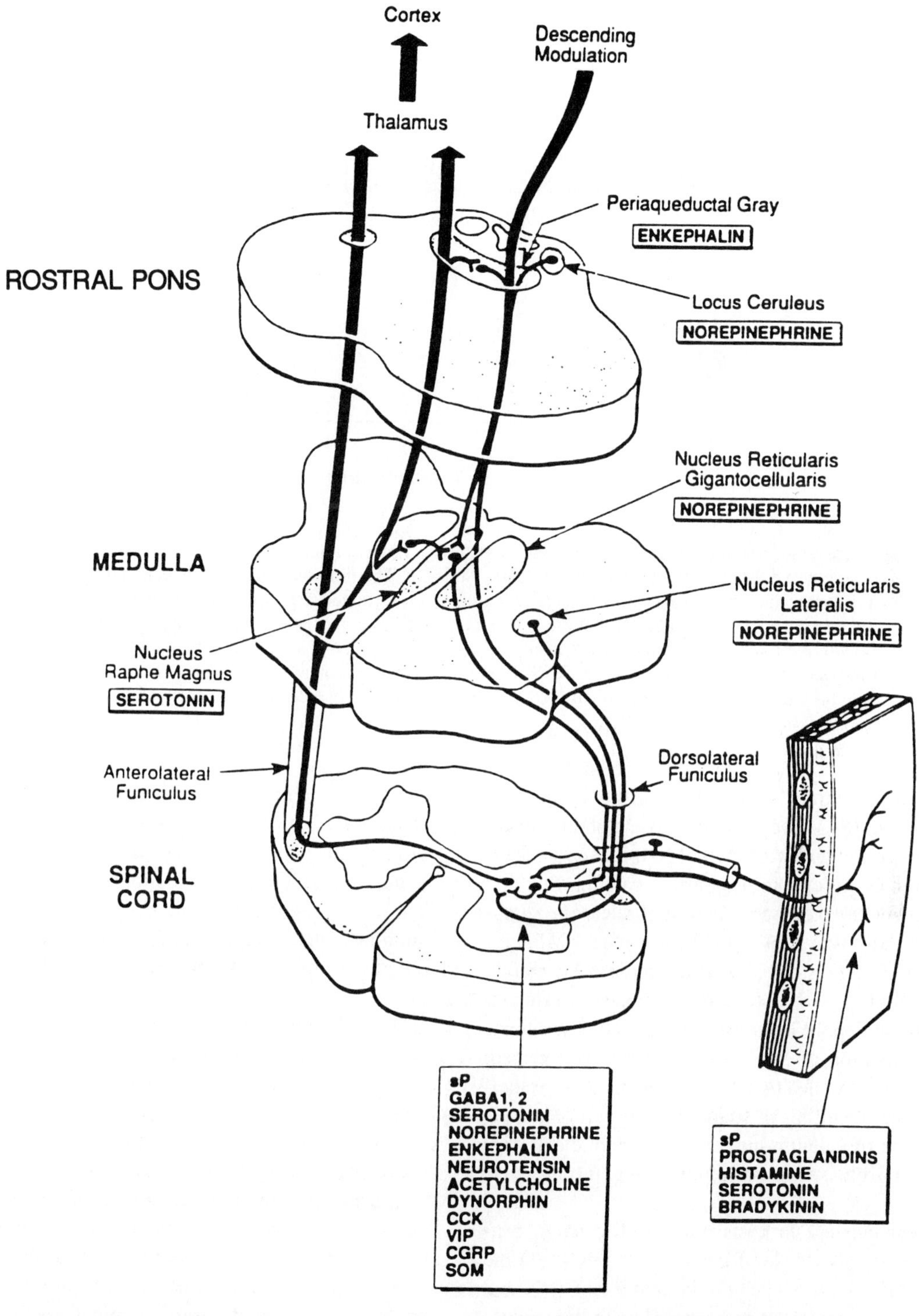

Fig. 89-2. Simplified schema of the process of nociception and the Gate Theory of Pain. Afferent nociceptive transmission from the periphery enters the dorsal horn of the spinal cord. Within the dorsal horn are multiple interneuronal synapses and multiple neurotransmitters of both excitatory and inhibitory types. Second order nociceptors send axons to cross to the opposite anterolateral quadrant and ascend to higher neural centers as the spinothalamic and spinoreticulothalamic tracts. Endogenous analgesic substances (enkephalin, serotonin, norepinephrine) are localized in discrete areas of the higher rostral centers and send axons to form a descending tract, the dorsolateral funiculus. These neurotransmitters form the descending modulating system that, when activated, "closes the gate," interdicting afferent nociceptive transmission. (From Cousins MJ, Bridenbaugh PO, editors: *Neural blockade in clinical anesthesia and management of pain,* ed 2, Philadelphia, 1988, Lippincott-Raven).

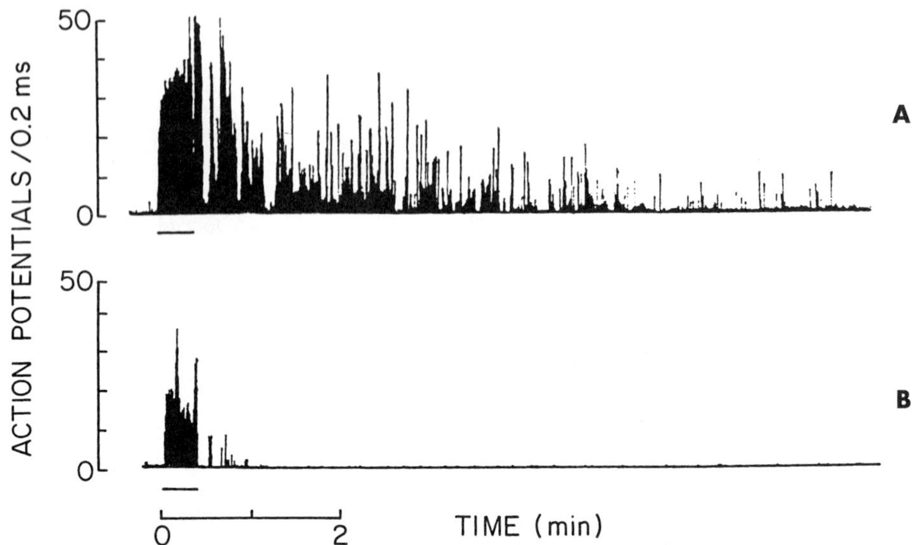

Fig. 89-3. Central hypersensitization or "wind-up." Frequency of discharge produced in posterior bicepsfemoris/semitendinous α-motor neurons of the rat by stimulation of a chronically sectioned sciatic nerve for 20 seconds at 10 Hz at C-fiber strength. The time of stimulation is denoted by horizontal lines under each recording. **A,** Stimulation of sectioned nerve produces an increase in the number of action potentials that are generated as well as a very long after-discharge (wind-up). **B,** Stimulation of intact sciatic nerve results in a smaller number of action potentials for a shorter time period. (From Wall PD, Woolf CJ: The brief and prolonged facilitatory effects of unmyelinated afferent input on the rat spinal cord are independently influenced by peripheral nerve section, *Neuroscience* 17:1199, 1986.)

receptor; (2) the α-amino-3-hydroxy-5-methyl-4-isoxazole propionic acid (AMPA) receptor; and (3) metabotropic receptors. Metabotropic receptors are not coupled to ion channels but activate G proteins in response to calcium flux and second messengers (see below). The initial release of glutamate activates the postsynaptic AMPA receptor. AMPA receptors open their cation channels resulting in postsynaptic cell depolarization caused by sodium and potassium flux. If the magnitude of depolarization is sufficient, magnesium-dependent inactivation of the NMDA receptor is reversed. Glutamate binding to NMDA receptors opens their associated ion channels resulting in sodium, potassium, and calcium flux. Influx of calcium into the postsynaptic cell triggers a further release of calcium from intracellular stores.[93,126,129]

The transient increase in postsynaptic cell calcium concentrations sets off a cascade of events (Fig. 89-4): (1) the postsynaptic cell releases arachidonic acid,[74] N_2O,[9,133] and CO,[133] which act as retrograde messengers upon the presynaptic cell; (2) the retrograde messengers cause more neurotransmitter release in response to succeeding presynaptic action potentials; (3) calcium-dependent enzymes (e.g., protein kinase C, calcium/calmodulin kinase, and cyclic-AMP-dependent protein kinase A are activated;[9] (4) activation of calcium-dependent enzymes results in phosphorylation of membrane proteins on receptors and ion channels; (5) the phosphorylation of membrane protein results in enhanced excitability of the postsynaptic cell; and (6) more AMPA receptors become available on the postsynaptic cell.[93,126,129]

Finally, central hypersensitization, with its cascade of electrochemical events, results in gene transcription with production of numerous cellular products (e.g., c-Fos, dynorphin, substance P, calcitonin gene-related peptide).[25] The consequences of this altered gene expression are largely unknown, but are believed to prolong (weeks to months) the duration of hypersensitization.[73]

Balanced analgesia

The clinical implications of the above-mentioned electrophysiologic changes associated with nociception are numerous: (1) the multiplicity of mechanisms associated with nociception, hypersensitization and hyperalgesia make it extremely unlikely that any single analgesic agent will provide complete pain relief in all patients; (2) because of the complex interrelationships among the chemical mediators of central hypersensitization, coadministration of analgesics affecting different physiologic processes of nociception or different chemical mediators of central hypersensitization may produce additive (if not synergistic) analgesic effects;[39] and (3) the process of central hypersensitization with resultant altered gene expression may be in some way related to "morbidity" on the molecular biologic level.[119] At least some of the manifestations of gene induction can be inhibited by analgesic therapy.[94] Thus, alteration of the aberrant and harmful effects of central hypersensitization via analgesic therapies may provide the link between analgesia and changes in morbidity and mortality.

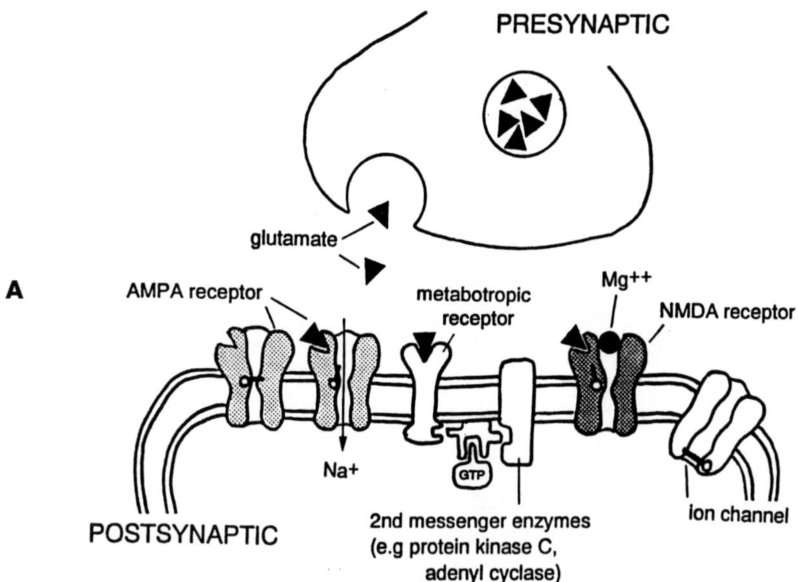

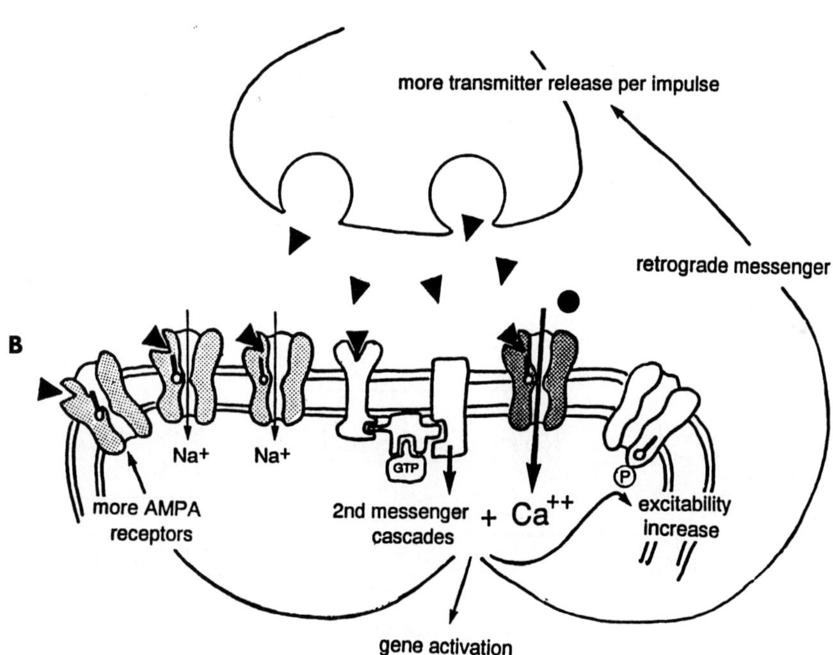

Fig. 89-4. Chemical mediation of central hypersensitization. **A,** Normal synaptic transmission. Depolarization of the presynaptic nerve terminal causes release of glutamate by exocytosis. Glutamate binds to three types of postsynaptic receptors: (1) AMPA receptors; (2) NMDA receptors; and (3) metabotropic receptors. Glutamate binding to AMPA receptors results in opening of Na^+ and K^+ channels and transient depolarization of the postsynaptic nerve terminal. Glutamate binding to metabotropic receptors causes binding of guanosine triphosphate (GTP) to G-proteins in cell membranes. This results in activation of second messenger enzymes such as protein kinase C and adenyl cyclase. Binding of glutamate to NMDA receptors opens Na^+, K^+, and Ca^{++} channels. There is no ion flux, however, as the channels are blocked by Mg^{++} ions in the extracellular fluid. **B,** Induction of central hypersensitization. Afferent barrage of nociceptive transmission causes release of glutamate of greater magnitude than in (**A**). More AMPA receptors are activated, and a larger postsynaptic depolarization is generated which ejects Mg^{++} from the NMDA receptor. Ca^{++} flux now occurs. The Ca^{++} interacts with second messenger enzymes, and a cascade of events occurs. Retrograde messengers (e.g., arachidonic acid, N_2O, CO) are released and act at presynaptic terminals to release more glutamate per depolarization. Activation of calcium-dependent enzymes results in phosphorylation of membrane proteins in ion channels. This phosphorylation of membrane proteins and the generation of more AMPA receptors makes the postsynaptic nerve terminal more excitable (see Fig. 89-3). The postsynaptic calcium surge also induces gene expression in the nucleus of the postsynaptic cell. (From Pockett S: Spinal cord synaptic plasticity and chronic pain, *Anesth Analg* 80:173, 1995.)

The above process requires a new concept of postoperative pain management. **Balanced analgesia[22] signifies the coadministration of analgesics that selectively affect the physiologic processes involved in nociception, transduction, transmission, modulation (i.e., the Gate Theory of Pain), or the chemical processes involved in central hypersensitization** (Fig. 89-5). There is much tangible evidence to suggest that use of such an approach may achieve more "complete" analgesia, and perhaps affect morbidity and clinical outcomes.[37,132]

Preemptive analgesia

If central hypersensitization results in aberrant electrophysiologic changes in the dorsal horn that may be harmful, would it be better to administer analgesics prior to the genesis of pain? Analgesia initiated prior to painful stimuli could be expected to reduce or eliminate the peripheral and central sensitization of nociceptors. Thus, the perception of pain may be significantly ameliorated for protracted periods even after the initial analgesic therapy.

The concept of *preemptive analgesia* (i.e., the treatment of postoperative pain by prevention of central hypersensitization) is tantalizing, and there are a number of animal studies that are consistent with the basic pharmacologic mechanisms underlying such a hypothesis.[24,39,44] For example, subarachnoid administration of μ-receptor opioid agonists can completely prevent the development of central hypersensitization.[24] Interestingly, **it takes one tenth the dose of morphine to prevent development of central hypersensitization as is required to abolish it** once it occurs.[130,131] Both subarachnoid[39] and intravenous (IV)[2] administration of local anesthetics have been shown to prevent central hypersensitization.

In animals, analgesic techniques have differential efficacy for preventing central hypersensitization. Whereas opioids[24,130,131] and local anesthetics[2,39] prevent the development of central hypersensitization, volatile anesthetics do not.[1] Moreover, inhalational anesthetics may directly antagonize the preemptive effects of other analgesics.[44] As would be predicted from the pivotal role of the NMDA receptor in establishment of central hypersensitization, the preemptive analgesic effects seen in animals result from direct or indirect blockade of NMDA receptor activation.[19,128]

Despite data in animals supporting the concept of preemptive analgesia, results of human studies are mixed.[128] This is largely the result of methodologic inconsistencies among the studies. However, the majority of studies involving the preoperative administration of single analgesics or combinations of analgesics have documented either decreased pain or decreased analgesic demand for a protracted time period after operation. Although inconclusive, the results of these studies and the protracted duration of the ef-

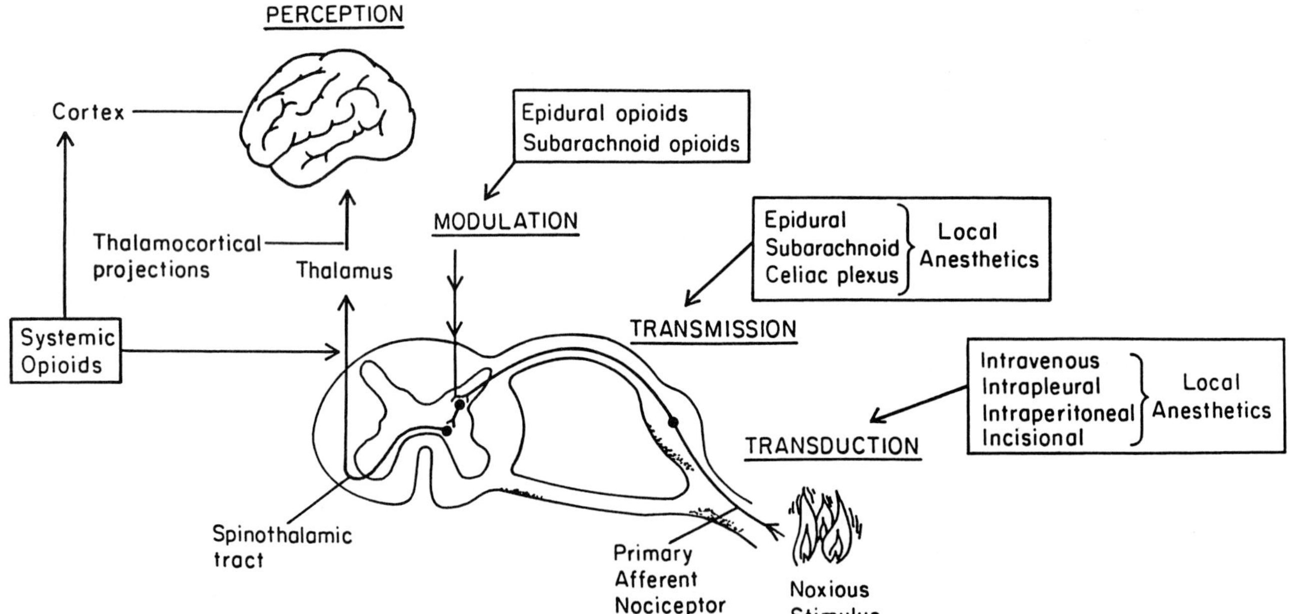

Fig. 89-5. The concept of balanced analgesia. The physiologic processes of transduction, transmission, and modulation converge and impact upon the discharge of nociceptors in the dorsal horn of the spinal cord. Summation of the processes will either facilitate or interdict nociceptive transmission or the development of central hypersensitization. Thus, the concept of *"balanced analgesia"* (polypharmacologic interdiction of nociception at discrete points in the nociceptive physiologic processes or the chemical mediation of central hypersensitization) forms the basis for effective postoperative pain management. (From Katz N, Ferrante FM: Nociception. In Ferrante FM, VadeBoncouer TR, editors: *Postoperative pain management,* New York, 1993, Churchill-Livingstone.)

fect are suggestive enough to warrant continued investigation into the clinical use of preemptive analgesia.

The neuroendocrine stress response

Discrete neural connections between nociceptive pathways and various endocrine organs are of great importance for autonomic, hormonal, and affective reactions to pain. The spinoreticulothalamic tract has synaptic connections with the hypothalamic paraventricular nucleus via the medial forebrain bundle.[114] The paraventricular nucleus of the hypothalamus is a major integrating center for global hormonal and autonomic responses.[114] In addition, a direct projection of nociceptors from the spinal cord to the hypothalamus has been identified as the spinohypothalamic tract.[15] Thus, **there are direct anatomic and physiologic links between afferent nociceptive transmission and autonomic and hormonal responses, collectively termed the *neuroendocrine stress response.***

Surgical stress consistently evokes a global, linked, endocrinologic, immunologic, and inflammatory response by activation of the sympathetic and somatic nervous systems and by local trauma.[16,59,60] **The neuroendocrine stress response results in reduced body mass and tissue reserve,[3] immunosuppression,[99] increased myocardial O_2 demand with vulnerability to arrthymogenesis,[65] impaired respiratory function,[59] enhanced risk or thromboembolism,[118] and an increased risk for postoperative morbidity and mortality.**[59,60,65] Blocking this neuroendocrine response by profound analgesia is desirable.

Analgesia *per se* is not necessarily synonymous with abolition of the neuroendocrine response to operation and improved outcome.[59,60,65] Inhibition of the stress response is best demonstrated with neuraxial administration of local anesthetics (and in particular, epidural analgesia).[59,60,65] The clearest inhibitory effects are seen for operations below the umbilicus.[60,65] For procedures of the upper abdomen and thorax, epidural analgesia has failed to inhibit the stress response despite excellent analgesia.[104,106] This finding is explained by the persistence of evoked potential responses to somatic stimulation during thoracic epidural anesthesia.[69]

ACUTE ANALGESIC MODALITIES

The previous discussion has outlined a rationale for postoperative pain management based upon an understanding of nociception, the Gate Theory of Pain, and the idea of balanced analgesia. We will now explore several of the individual modalities that allow the perioperative physician to achieve balanced analgesia.

Nonsteroidal Anti-inflammatory Drugs

Aside from their role in central hypersensitization as previously discussed, prostaglandins are generated by peripheral tissue trauma and sensitize first-order nociceptors in conjunction with other algesic chemical mediators. Prostaglandins play an important role in the genesis of inflammatory, pyretic, and algesic responses to local tissue injury.[21]

Oral nonsteroidal anti-inflammatory drugs (NSAIDs) have long been used in medicine for the treatment of inflammatory conditions, such as the arthritides, and for their antipyretic properties. Only recently have NSAIDs been used for postoperative analgesia.

NSAIDs are a structurally diverse group of agents (Table 89-1) that inhibit the enzyme cyclooxygenase (Fig. 89-6). Cyclooxygenase catalyzes the conversion of arachidonic acid to unstable cyclic endoperoxide intermediates from which the prostanoids are formed.[30] Although the anti-inflammatory, antipyretic, and analgesic properties of NSAIDs can be explained by inhibition of cyclooxygenase, the resulting analgesia cannot be explained solely by the traditional role in the periphery.[76,77] Indeed, numerous studies suggest both central and peripheral sites of analgesic action for NSAIDs.[76,77,82]

Side effects of NSAID use are both prostaglandin- and nonprostaglandin-mediated. Prostaglandin-mediated side effects include gastropathy, hemostatic defects, and nephrotoxicity.[21] The prostaglandin-mediated side effects are of major concern for the use of NSAIDs with respect to postoperative pain management. A variety of prostaglandins (e.g., PGE_1, PGE_2, and prostacyclin [PGI_2]) have been shown to be integral to gastric mucosal cytoprotection. Suppression of prostaglandin synthesis by NSAIDs would potentially lead to decreased mucosal cytoprotection, increased acid secretion, and perhaps, gastric ulceration. Symptoms of NSAID gastropathy include dyspepsia, epigastric pain, anorexia, and reflux esophagitis.[30,103]

NSAIDs inhibit platelet function by affecting the balance between inhibition of thromboxane (TxA_2) synthesis within platelets and inhibition of PGI_2 synthesis within endothelial cells. Acetylsalicylic acid (aspirin) will irreversibly inhibit platelet cyclooxygenase; all other NSAIDs reversibly inhibit the enzyme. Thus, for all NSAIDs except for aspirin, normal hemostasis will be restored after the drug is cleared from the body (approximately five half-lives). Refer to Table 89-1 for representative half-lives of the NSAIDs. The bleeding time will be prolonged for 6 to 10 days after ingestion of aspirin (i.e., the lifetime of the platelet).[30]

In the normal individual, renal blood flow and glomerular filtration are not prostaglandin-dependent. This relationship is changed for patients who are volume depleted or who have hepatic cirrhosis or congestive heart failure (CHF). Inhibition of prostaglandin synthesis in these disease states could produce nephrotoxicity.[30]

NSAIDs are most useful for postoperative pain management in their per rectal[124] or parenteral[71,72,98] formulations, although oral use prior to and after surgery should be encouraged for certain clinical scenarios. Ketorolac is the first parenteral NSAID preparation available for use within the United States.[71,72,98] It may be administered either by the intramuscular (IM)[71] or IV[98] routes of administration. Ketorolac has analgesic potency similar to opioids, but un-

Table 89-1 Representative nonsteroidal anti-inflammatory drugs

Drug	Dosage range (orally, mg/day)	Half-life (hr)	Doses per day
Carboxylic acids			
Salacylic acids			
Acetylsalicylic acid (aspirin)	1000–6000	4–15	2–4
Nonacetylated salicylates			
Choline magnesium trisalicylate (Trilisate)	1500–4000	4–15	2–4
Salicylsalicylate (Disalcid)	1500–5000	4–15	2–4
Diflunisal (Dolobid)	500–1500	7–15	2
Acetic acids			
Indoles			
Indomethacin (Indocin)	50–200	3–11	2–4
Sulindac (Clinoril)	300–400	16	2
Pyrrole acetic acids			
Tolmetin (Tolectin)	600–2000	1–2	3–6
Ketorolac (Toradol)	15–60 (intravenous)	3–8	4
Phenyl acetic acids			
Diclofenac (Voltaren)	100–200	2	2–4
Propionic acids			
Phenylpropionic acids			
Ibuprofen (Motrin)	1200–3200	2	3–6
Fenoprofen (Nalfon)	1200–3200	2	3–4
Flurbiprofen (Ansaid)	200–300	3–4	2–3
Ketoprofen (Orudis)	100–400	2	3–4
Naphthylpropionic acids			
Naproxen (Naprosyn, Anaprox)	250–1500	13	2
Anthranilic acids			
Fenamates			
Meclofenamate (Meclomen)	200–400	2–3	4
Pyrazoles			
Phenylbutazone (Butazolidin)	200–800	40–80	1–4
Oxicams			
Piroxicam (Feldene)	20	30–86	1

like opioids, ketorolac does not produce respiratory depression, reduction of gastrointestinal (GI) motility, psychomotor effects, or addiction.[30] Ketorolac should only be used for short-term therapy after operation because of the potential for the aforementioned prostaglandin-mediated side effects.

Patient-Controlled Analgesia

In common usage, patient-controlled analgesia (PCA) signifies the intermittent IV administration of opioids under direct patient control. In a broader sense, PCA is really a conceptual framework for administration of analgesics and is not strictly related to a single class of analgesics, route of administration, or the need for infusion apparatus. Opioids, local anesthetics,[40,41,72] and benzodiazepines[67] have all been used under patient control. Similarly, the sublingual,[109] transbuccal,[7] subcutaneous,[120] and epidural[31,34,36,40,41] routes of administration have been used for PCA.

In its broadest sense, PCA is a concept implying self-administration of analgesics. Therefore, the parameters affecting the "decision" to demand analgesia must be defined. There is a complex interplay of pharmacokinetic, pharmacodynamic, and psychologic factors that determine use of PCA. Patient characteristics influencing the effective use of PCA are best understood when considering intermittent demand dosing of opioids; discussion will be restricted to this model. However, before considering the factors that determine patients' effective use of PCA, it is best to discuss the practical application of PCA as an analgesic modality.

PCA as an operational system

To most practitioners, the use of PCA implies the presence of sophisticated "pump" technology. In his pioneering work on PCA, Sechzer[107] evaluated the analgesic response to small IV doses of opioid given on demand by nursing personnel and subsequently by a programmable mechanical device.[108]

However, the on-demand administration of analgesics to large numbers of patients by nursing personnel presents an insurmountable logistic problem. Therefore, prototype demand-analgesia devices were developed in the late 1960s.

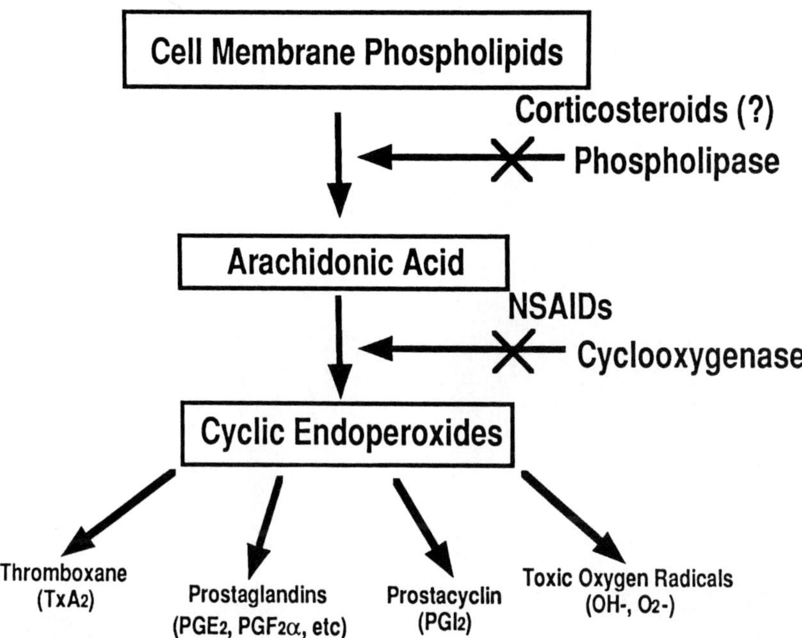

Fig. 89-6. Metabolism of arachidonic acid via the cyclooxygenase pathway. The prostanoids (e.g., thromboxanes, prostaglandins, and prostacyclins) are the active metabolites of the cyclooxygenase pathway. Arachidonic acid may also be metabolized by lipoxygenase (pathway not shown) to form the eicosanoids (the leukotrienes). (From Ferrante FM: Nonsteroidal anti-inflammatory drugs. In Ferrante FM, VadeBoncouer TR, editors: *Postoperative pain management,* New York, 1993, Churchill-Livingstone.)

The first widely used PCA infuser (the Cardiff Palliator,[29] Graseby Dynamics, Ltd. Herts, England) was introduced into clinical practice in the United Kingdom in 1976. Subsequently, newer infusers have included sophisticated computer programming and fail-safe systems (Fig. 89-7). From a bioengineering viewpoint, all PCA infusers use negative feedback control technology;[125] as patients use increasing amounts of analgesic, pain is reduced, and the demand for analgesia is decreased.

Definition of PCA modes and dosing parameters

The most common mode of PCA administration is demand dosing, in which a dose of fixed amount is self-administered. Constant-rate infusion plus demand dosing implies administration of a minimum background infusion determined by a physician; it can be supplemented by demand doses. The background infusion should be set at a minimum that does not ablate the necessity of patient demand. Otherwise, the risk of respiratory depression is enhanced.[78]

Less commonly available modes of administration include infusion demand (where demands are granted as an infusion) and variable-rate infusion plus demand dosing (where a microprocessor monitors demands and controls the infusion rate accordingly). These modes remain to be studied in detail.[51]

For each mode of PCA, there are basic variables: (1) loading dose; (2) demand dose; (3) lockout interval; (4) background infusion rate; (5) and 1- and 4-hour limits (Fig. 89-7 and Table 89-2). For the postoperative patient, PCA is preferably implemented in the postanesthesia care unit. At this time, analgesia is accomplished by administration of small loading doses of opioid. When patients recover sufficiently from general anesthesia, they may initiate patient demands.

Many opioids have been used via the PCA system. Guidelines for the administration of several common opioids are listed in Table 89-2. The demand dose (incremental or PCA dose) is the quantity of analgesic administered to the patient on activation of the PCA infuser demand button. To prevent overdosage by continual demand, all PCA systems use a lockout interval. The lockout interval is the length of time between patient demands in which the infuser will not administer analgesics. Some PCA devices allow determination of 1- and 4-hour limits. The use of these limits is controversial. Guidelines for use of PCA have been largely empiric. Research is needed to define the administration variables for each mode of PCA.

The PCA paradigm

PCA is increasingly used in lieu of IM opioids. The rationale for its increasing use lies in the relationship between opioid concentration and analgesia over time. This relationship was defined in two classic articles by Austin, Stapleton, and Mather.[4,5]

Analgesia is obtained when the plasma opioid concentration reaches a particular value, depending on the individual

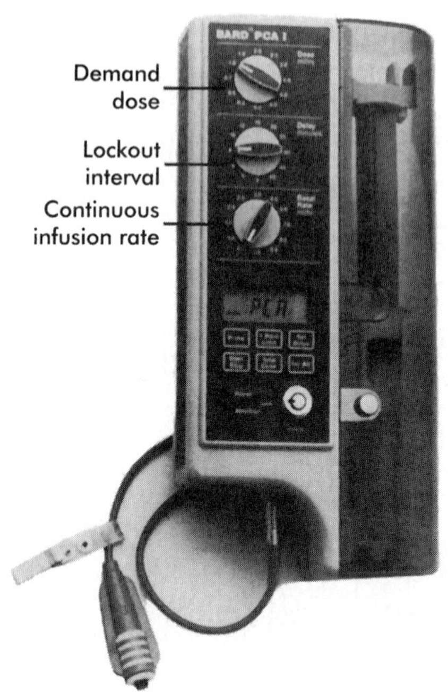

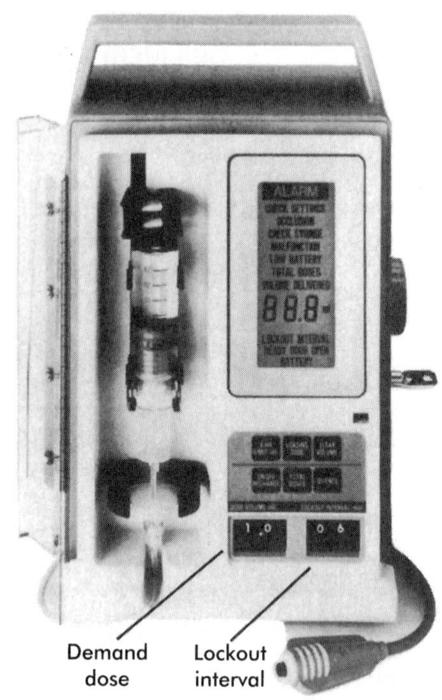

Fig. 89-7. Examples of commercially available PCA devices. Demand dose and lockout interval settings are common to nearly all systems; some units permit programming for continuous infusions and allow limitation of hourly opioid use.

Table 89-2 Guidelines for opioid administration with PCA

Drug (concentration)	Demand dose (mg)	Lockout interval (min)
Morphine (1 mg/ml)	0.5–3.0	5–12
Meperidine (10 mg/ml)	5.0–30	5–12
Fentanyl (0.01 mg/ml)	0.01–0.02	3–10
Hydromorphone (0.2 mg/ml)	0.05–0.25	5–10
Oxymorphone (0.25 mg/ml)	0.2–0.4	8–10
Methadone (1 mg/ml)	0.5–2.5	8–20
Nalbuphine (1 mg/ml)	1–5	5–10

Analgesic requirements vary widely among patients. Adjustment of dosage upward or downward because of age, severe disease, or individual patient needs is always necessary.

patient and opioid (Fig. 89-8). For a small increase in plasma opioid concentration, there is a rapid decrease in pain. The nadir of the perceived pain defines the minimum effective analgesic concentration (MEAC). For increasing concentrations above MEAC, there is no further increase in the intensity of analgesia. For small decreases in concentration below MEAC, there is rapid appreciation of pain. There is considerable interpatient variability of MEAC. This may explain the large interpatient variability in analgesic requirements.

The relationships among opioid concentration, analgesia, and dosing intervals define the therapeutic effectiveness of a particular method of opioid administration (Fig. 89-9). IM injections characteristically yield unpredictable plasma concentrations. In any particular individual, peak concentrations (C_{max}) with multiple IM injections can vary twofold, and time to peak concentration (T_{max}) can vary threefold.[4] Among patients in a given population, C_{max} can vary fivefold whereas T_{max} can vary sevenfold.[4] At the same time, plasma concentrations fluctuate in phase with the dosing interval (Fig. 89-9). It has been calculated that opioid concentrations are in excess of MEAC only 35% of the time during any 4-hour dosing interval.[4]

Use of PCA avoids these variable absorption phenomena by permitting on-demand, repetitive dosing of small doses of opioid. When the patient's plasma concentration falls below the MEAC, the patient rapidly appreciates pain (steep concentration-analgesic response relation). Thus, patients use PCA to "titrate" their plasma concentration of opioid around the MEAC. PCA provides more constant plasma concentrations of opioid[23,115,116] and more consistent analgesia.[35]

Individual analgesic requirements

PCA is a dynamic, flexible modality; it allows patients to give as little, or as much, opioid as they desire. PCA can therefore accommodate patients' widely divergent analgesic

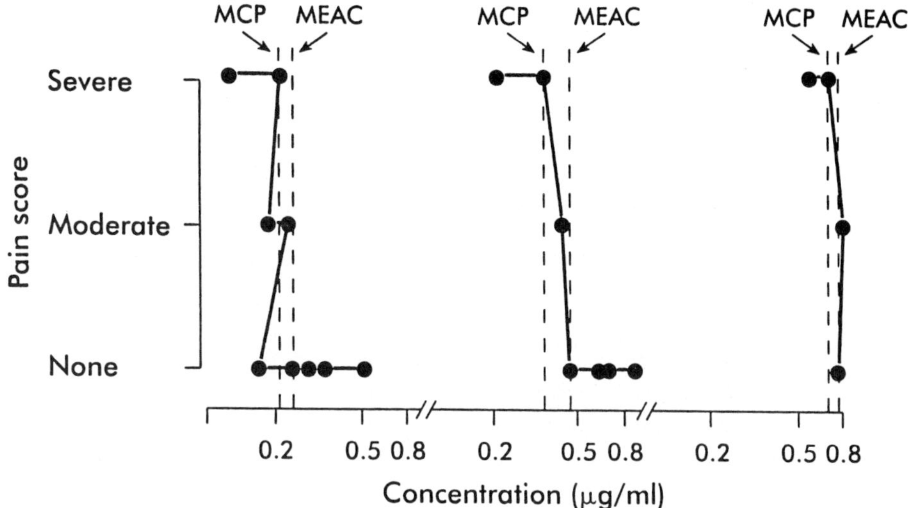

Fig. 89-8. The relationship between plasma concentration of opioid and analgesia. For a minimal increase in opioid concentration above the maximum concentration associated with severe pain (MCP), there is a rapid decrease in pain. The nadir of the perceived pain is called the minimum effective analgesic concentration (MEAC). (From Austin KH, Stapleton JV, Mather LE: Relationship between blood meperidine concentrations and analgesic response: a preliminary report, *Anesthesiology* 53:460, 1980.)

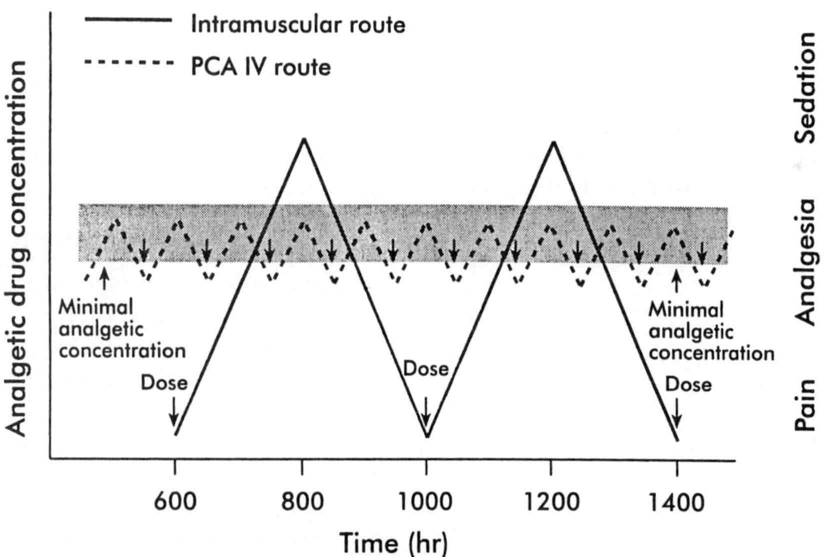

Fig. 89-9. The patient-controlled analgesia (PCA) paradigm versus standard intramuscular opioid analgesic therapy. (From Ferrante FM, Orav EJ, Rocco AG, et al: A statistical model for pain in patient-controlled analgesia and conventional intramuscular opioid regimens, *Anesth Analg* 67[5]:457, 1988.)

requirements. With PCA, individual differences in analgesic requirements are expressed in individual patterns of analgesic administration. Both pharmacokinetic and pharmacodynamic factors affect the proper use of PCA.

Pharmacokinetic factors. In a classic series of studies, Tamsen et al.[115,116] examined the influence of pharmacokinetic factors on analgesic requirements in patients using PCA. The volume of distribution, distribution rate constant, and elimination rate constant for meperidine,[116] ketobemidone,[115] and morphine[23] were determined in patients undergoing laparotomy. **For all opioids, pharmacokinetic parameters were found to have no relation to an individual's hourly analgesic requirement. The authors concluded that pharmacokinetic variations among patients had no influence on patients' hourly demand for opioid using PCA.** However, mean plasma opioid concentration and the MEAC were found to significantly correlate with individual hourly opioid use.

Pharmacodynamic factors. All opioids produce analgesia by mimicking the actions of endogenous opioids.[38] Thus, changes in levels of endogenous opioids or changes in opioid receptor numbers or affinities could influence analgesic requirements. Do preoperative endogenous opioid concentrations in the brain, spinal cord, or cerebrospinal fluid (CSF) affect the MEAC?

Tamsen et al.[117] addressed some of these questions in patients receiving meperidine by PCA after laparotomy. Before operation, lumbar puncture was performed, and a sample of CSF was obtained. Endogenous opioid content was determined using a radioreceptor assay. Patients received a standard anesthetic and PCA for postoperative pain relief. Another sample of CSF and a sample of central venous blood was obtained 24 hours after operation when patients used PCA. The concentration of meperidine was determined in these specimens.

A significant inverse relationship was discovered between preoperative endogenous opioid concentrations in the CSF and individual postoperative concentrations of meperidine in plasma and in CSF (Fig. 89-10). Patients with lesser concentrations of endogenous opioid in CSF administered more exogenous opioids postoperatively by PCA to maintain greater concentrations in the plasma. Similarly, the converse was true.[117]

Therefore, endogenous opioids interact with exogenously administered opioids to influence analgesic demand and the MEAC. According to the results of this study, individual analgesic demand during PCA is dictated by individual CSF endogenous opioid content. Therefore, only the patient should determine when and how much analgesia is required. This is the basic tenet of PCA.

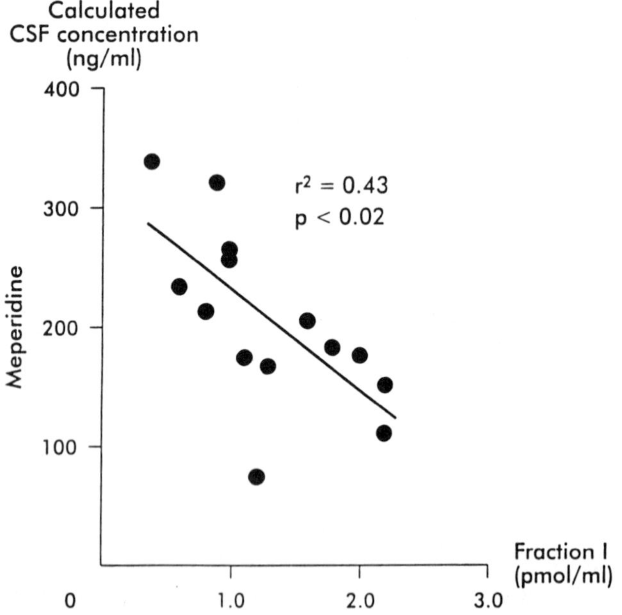

Fig. 89-10. Inverse linear relationship between preoperative cerebrospinal fluid concentration of endogenous opioids (Fraction I) and postoperative analgesic demand (CSF concentration of meperidine) while using patient-controlled analgesia (PCA). (From Ferrante FM, Ostheimer GW, Covino BG: *Patient-controlled analgesia,* Boston, 1990, Blackwell Scientific.)

Psychologic factors. If CSF endogenous opioid concentrations were the only determinant of how patients use PCA, then PCA would be flawlessly efficacious in all patients. However, experience with PCA indicates that other factors influence the demand for opioids also. Multiple components of an individual's psyche are involved in the way a particular patient uses PCA.

Although illness and pain behaviors have previously been hypothesized to be important in patient use of PCA, four studies provide the real definition of their effects.[42,55,56,91] Psychometric testing can be used to determine factors that affect patients' ability to derive maximum benefit from PCA. Further study of this concept is necessary for full application of these concepts to clinical practice, however.

Patient-controlled epidural analgesia

Patient-controlled epidural analgesia (PCEA) has included the use of opioids[75,110,122] or local anesthetics alone,[41,72] or in combination[31,34,36] by demand dosing[34,40,75,110] or continuous infusion plus demand dosing.[36,41,72] PCEA appears to be dose-sparing in both postoperative patients[27,110] and in obstetric patients.[31,34,36,40,41]

The optimal local anesthetic, opioid or combination for use with PCEA, as well as the volume-concentration relationships of the demand dose, have not been fully determined in various populations. Suggested dosing guidelines for general use of PCEA for postoperative analgesia are given in Table 89-3.

Epidural and Spinal Analgesia

The discovery of the spinal action of opioids in the late 1970s has led to the widespread use of epidural and subarachnoid opioids for the treatment of postoperative pain. The use of opioids alone or in combination with local anesthetics provides profound analgesia after most surgical procedures. By using continuous drug infusions or intermittent bolus injections through an indwelling epidural catheter, pain can be reliably attenuated or eliminated. The quality of analgesia is more intense than that achieved with parenteral opioids.

Epidural local anesthetics

Postsurgical analgesia can be maintained indefinitely by intermittent boluses of local anesthetics via an indwelling

Table 89-3 Dosing parameters for PCEA

Drug	Concentration	Demand dose	Lockout interval	Background infusion
Morphine	0.05–0.1 mg/ml	2–3 ml	20–30 min	3–5 ml
Fentanyl	5–10 μg/ml	2–3 ml	10–15 min	3–5 ml

epidural catheter. This technique produces profound analgesia but may be associated with unwanted side effects such as hypotension, blockade of motor function, and tachyphylaxis.[83–87] Bupivacaine is most often used because of its prolonged duration of action and its relative resistance to the development of tachyphylaxis.[85,87] However, even with low concentrations of bupivacaine (i.e., 0.125% or 0.25%), the requirement for large volumes of local anesthetic to maintain analgesia is associated with both hypotension and extensive sensory blockade.

In an attempt to maintain stable levels of analgesia without the need for intermittent boluses and their attendant side effects, several authors reported the use of continuous epidural infusions of bupivacaine.[83–86] In these early studies, 0.125% to 0.5% bupivacaine was infused continuously to provide pain relief after major abdominal operations. Low lumbar epidural catheters were used in all cases. With the exception of 0.125% bupivacaine,[83] all of the solutions resulted in an unpredictable regression of the initial sensory level of analgesia during the infusion.[84,86] Tachyphylaxis (a reduction in apparent effectiveness with continued administration) to bupivacaine occurred regardless of whether the infusion was large volume–low concentration or low volume–high concentration.[86] The regression of the cephalad level of sensory analgesia was always associated with an increase in the subjective pain score reported by the patient.

The phenomenon of tachyphylaxis during epidural analgesia has been shown to occur whether local anesthetic is given by intermittent injection or continuous infusion. Several theories have been proposed to explain tachyphylaxis: increased uptake of drug from the epidural space secondary to a drug-induced increase in epidural blood flow,[85] localized nerve edema,[88] down-regulation of local anesthetic receptors in nerve tissue,[85] and changes in afferent activity or spinal modulation of afferent impulses.[8]

Tachyphylaxis makes postsurgical pain management with epidural local anesthetics difficult, and the need for intermittent "top-up" doses of drug must be anticipated.

Epidural opioids

The application of opioid drugs to the dorsal horn of the spinal cord results in profound analgesia in humans.[20] **Epidural opioid analgesia produces segmental analgesia without the concomitant motor, sensory, or autonomic changes associated with the use of local anesthetics.**[20] The analgesia produced is usually intense and far exceeds that obtained when similar opioid doses are given systemically. A detailed review of the anatomic, physiologic, and pharmacologic basis of spinal opioid analgesia can be found in Chapter 64. The present review will emphasize the clinical application of these concepts in the management of postoperative pain. Table 89-4 lists the commonly used epidural opioids and their clinical profile after a single-bolus dose.

The physicochemical feature of opioids that best predicts their clinical behavior as epidural or subarachnoid analgesics is lipid solubility. The lipid-soluble drugs (e.g., fentanyl) penetrate the dura quickly and are also more easily absorbed into the epidural vasculature. Hence, they reach the spinal cord rapidly, and onset time is short. Morphine, a lipid-insoluble drug, penetrates the dura slowly, and therefore has a slower onset of analgesia.[45] The duration of analgesic action of an epidural opioid is inversely related to its lipid solubility.[92] Clearance of drug from CSF is related to uptake by spinal cord tissue and removal via spinal cord blood flow. The lipid-insoluble drugs are cleared from CSF slowly because they are not avidly absorbed by the lipid-rich spinal cord. Thus, analgesic concentrations of opioid remain in the CSF for long periods of time. Conversely, the lipid-soluble drugs are rapidly absorbed by spinal cord tissue and removed via the blood. Analgesia is therefore of short or intermediate duration.

Table 89-4 Guidelines for bolus dosing of epidural opioids

Drug	Dose	Analgesia onset (min)	Analgesia duration (hr)	Relative lipid solubility
Morphine	5 mg	30–45	12–24	1
Meperidine	50–100 mg	5–10	5–8	30
Fentanyl	100 μg	5–10	5–8	700
Hydro-morphone	1 mg	15	10–15	1
Methadone	5 mg	10–15	5–10	80

Lipid solubility also explains the peculiar ability of some opioids to produce analgesia in dermatomes far removed from the epidural site of application. Because of the slow clearance from CSF of the more polar drugs such as morphine, cephalad migration through the CSF can occur. As the rostral level of CSF opioid increases, progressively more cephalad levels of segmental analgesia are produced. This mechanism accounts for the clinical phenomenon of lumbar administration of epidural morphine producing analgesia in the thorax[111] and in the head and neck.[113]

The situation with the lipid-soluble opioids is more complex. Because these drugs migrate less in CSF, the epidural drug delivery should be as close as possible to the nerve roots mediating nociceptive transmission. Because of their enhanced lipid-solubility, opioids such as fentanyl and sufentanil gain easy access to the vasculature. Systemic blood levels of the lipid-soluble opioids approach concentrations approximating their minimal effective analgesic concentrations. A significant systemic contribution to analgesia has been demonstrated for fentanyl[28,47,48,68,105] and sutentanil.[81]

When lipid-soluble opioids are used for epidural analgesia, the injection site (whether via needle or epidural catheter) **should be as near as possible to the nerve roots mediating nociceptive transmission.** A high thoracic epidural catheter (between T4 and T8) should be placed for treating postthoracotomy pain with lipid-soluble opioids, because nociceptive transmission enters the spinal cord through these thoracic spinal roots. When the delivery site of lipid-soluble opioids is close to the nerve roots mediating nociceptive transmission, the contribution from segmental analgesia is increased relative to the contribution from systemic analgesia. If the epidural injection site is distant from the surgical incision, unusually large doses of lipid-soluble drug may be required. This may result in appreciable blood concentrations of opioid such that the systemic versus spinal contribution to pain relief is uncertain.

Side effects. The side effects of epidural opioid therapy are respiratory depression, nausea, pruritus, sedation, and urinary retention. The mechanisms responsible for these side effects have been extensively outlined in Chapter 64.

Respiratory depression after administration of epidural opioid is biphasic, with early and late phases of ventilatory compromise.[20] Early respiratory depression is believed to be secondary to increased blood concentrations of opioid following absorption via the epidural veins. It usually occurs within the first hour after epidural administration regardless of the drug used, and it is indistinguishable from the respiratory effects produced by an identical IV dose of the same opioid. **The delayed respiratory effects of epidural opioids are classically seen with lipid-insoluble drugs, such as morphine and hydromorphone. The time course of decreased respiratory responsiveness parallels that of increasing rostral levels of analgesia and the onset of nausea and vomiting.**[13] All of these changes are the result of increasing cephalad migration of morphine in the CSF. Decreased respiratory response to CO_2 may persist for up to 24 hours after a single bolus of epidural morphine.[13,61] Vigilant assessment of respiratory status is therefore necessary during this time period after epidural delivery of a lipid-insoluble opioid. Delayed respiratory depression is not seen after a single epidural bolus of lipid-soluble fentanyl (100 μg), underscoring the importance of lipid insolubility in the rostral spread of drug in CSF.[62] It has not been clearly shown whether continuous infusions of epidural fentanyl result in late respiratory depression because blood fentanyl levels may become appreciable in such situations.

The usual manifestations of respiratory depression (decreased rate of breathing and increased arterial CO_2 tension) are well tolerated in most patients. The onset of ventilatory depression is gradual. Often, it is accompanied by other clinical evidence of excessive opioid concentrations in the CSF: nausea, pruritus, or somnolence. These findings, combined with the results of a large-scale survey of epidural and subarachnoid opioid use in Sweden, suggest that routine observation on a general surgical ward is adequate for most patients after epidural opioid administration.[95] In the Swedish study, the incidence of delayed respiratory depression after epidural morphine was 0.09% (i.e., 11/14,000).

Nausea and vomiting occur in 12%[63] to 50%[12] of patients after administration of epidural morphine. This usually coincides with other evidence of cephalad migration of lipid-insoluble opioid in CSF and may reflect interaction of drug with the vomiting center and chemotactic trigger zone.[20] The lipid-soluble opioids may be expected to produce nausea when systemic concentrations are significant, but rostral CSF spread would be unusual in this case. Nausea and vomiting are not uncommon whenever parenteral opioids are used, and, because pain itself may produce nausea; the actual incidence of nausea associated with epidural administration of opioids is unclear. It appears that the incidence of nausea decreases after repeated epidural doses, probably reflecting some tolerance to this effect.[43]

Pruritus occurs commonly after epidural administration of opioids. The incidence may be greater than 50%, although severe pruritus probably occurs in only 1% of patients.[11]

Histamine release is not the mechanism of opioid-induced itching after epidural administration, because fentanyl (which does not result in histamine release) produces pruritus when administered epidurally.[102] Like nausea, tolerance to pruritus usually occurs with subsequent doses of opioid.

Urinary retention may also occur with epidural opioid use.[14] The mechanisms of this phenomenon were recently elucidated by Durant and Yaksh.[26] Administration of epidural morphine blocks volume-induced bladder contractions and inhibits the vesicle somatic reflex required for external sphincter relaxation.[26] The incidence of urinary retention is unknown.

Management of side effects. The side effects of epidural opioid therapy are easily reversed with the opioid antagonist naloxone. The key to successful treatment is careful titration of the naloxone dose so as to preserve as much analgesia as possible. Both incremental dosing and continuous infusion (5 μg/kg/hr) of naloxone have been shown to reverse respiratory and nonrespiratory side effects of opioids without completely reversing analgesia.[6,46,96] Some loss of analgesia should always be anticipated when opioid antagonists are administered in conjunction with lipid-soluble opioids.[46] Loss of analgesia does not occur with epidural administration of morphine, although duration of analgesia may be decreased after bolus dosing.[96]

Nalbuphine, an agonist-antagonist opioid, has also been used for treatment of epidural opioid-related side effects.[50] Because this drug is a κ-receptor agonist and a μ-receptor antagonist, analgesia is maintained to some extent when respiratory depression is reversed. As with naloxone, careful titration of nalbuphine (1- to 3-mg increments) is essential to preserve analgesia when lipid-soluble opioids have been administered.

When apnea or severe respiratory depression occur, IV naloxone should be administered immediately in doses adequate to promptly restore ventilation (0.2 to 0.4 mg). Patients should be monitored closely after naloxone therapy because respiratory depression may recur because of the short half-life of naloxone (approximately 55 minutes); repeat boluses, constant infusion or IM naloxone may be required.

The nonrespiratory side effects of epidural opioids are

often amenable to treatment without requiring opioid antagonists. Nausea may be ameliorated with the phenothiazine antiemetics or droperidol. Mild pruritus may respond to periodic injections of antihistaminics (e.g., diphenhydramine); severe itching usually requires administration of opioid antagonists. Although there have been no clinical trials, recent work on the cause of epidural opioid-induced bladder dysfunction suggests that beta-adrenergic and dopaminergic agonists, as well as alpha-adrenergic antagonists may be clinically useful in treating urinary retention.[26]

Subarachnoid opioids

The subarachnoid administration of opioids results in analgesia via the same mechanisms as described previously for the epidural route of administration. **The major differences between spinal and epidural administration of opioids are the size of the bolus doses and the incidence of side effects.** Because the drug is delivered directly into the CSF, tissue barriers for diffusion to the dorsal horn (e.g., dura mater, epidural fat) are greatly reduced or eliminated. As a result, **analgesic doses of subarachnoid opioids are a fraction of the usual epidural dose, depending on the drug.**

Because the highly lipid-soluble opioids may be absorbed by lipid-rich tissues other than the dura mater or dorsal horn, the fraction of the analgesic epidural dose required to produce subarachnoid analgesia is not always clear. Morphine, which is lipid-insoluble, has a fairly reliable dural transfer fraction (i.e., fraction of epidural dose delivered to CSF) of approximately 20%.[79] This is consistent with the clinical observation that 0.5 to 1.0 mg of subarachnoid morphine produces reliable and effective analgesia.[54] However, doses as low as 0.1 to 0.25 mg have proved efficacious[20] and subarachnoid doses $\leq$ 0.5 mg are recommended. In doses ranging from 6.25 to 50 μg, subarachnoid fentanyl produced effective analgesia for 3 to 4 hours, regardless of the dose used.[53] This may reflect extensive nonspecific binding of the lipid-soluble agents to tissues other than opioid receptors.[79]

As with the epidural route of administration, cephalad migration of drug combined with a low clearance from CSF permits lipid-soluble opioids to produce a long duration of analgesia over multiple spinal segments. Despite placement of drug directly into the CSF, the duration of action of liphophilic opioids after epidural and subarachnoid administration is similar.

Subarachnoid opioids may be administered alone for postoperative pain. Alternatively, they may be given at the same time as local anesthetic when spinal anesthesia is initiated. The choice of drug depends on the length of desired analgesia and the extent of the surgical incision. In this regard, guidelines are identical to those described previously for epidural opioids.

Side effects. The type and treatment of subarachnoid opioid-induced side effects are the same as described previously for the epidural route of administration. The incidence of pruritus, sedation, nausea, urinary retention, and respiratory depression has been reported to be greater for subarachnoid than for epidural administration.[20]

Epidural opioid-local anesthetic combinations

The most recent development in epidural analgesia is the use of dilute solutions of local anesthetic and opioid administered as a continuous epidural infusion. Early reports on the clinical use of this technique emphasized a need for limiting side effects as the motivation for combining subanalgesic doses of the two drugs.[66] Decreasing the local anesthetic concentration would hopefully limit hypotension, sensory block, and motor block, whereas lesser opioid doses might reduce the risk of respiratory depression, nausea, and pruritus.

The proposition that subanalgesic concentrations of opioid and local anesthetic might together produce pain relief was suggested by an investigation of the effects of combined epidural morphine and epidural bupivacaine.[52] All patients underwent abdominal operations. In this study, analgesia and dermatomal level of sensory analgesia to pinprick were maintained when morphine was added to patients' continuous epidural infusion of 0.5% bupivacaine. Patients who received only 0.5% bupivacaine invariably were removed from the study because of pain or a substantial decrement in their level of pinprick analgesia. The cephalad level of sensory analgesia to pinprick in the group receiving combined epidural opioid–local anesthetic therapy remained unchanged for the full 16-hour observation period after surgery. Prevention of the regression of sensory analgesia during continuous epidural local anesthetic infusion has also been demonstrated when IV morphine was administered to patients receiving epidural infusion of 0.5% bupivacaine.[70]

Hjortsø et al.[52] attributed this synergistic effect of epidural opioid and local anesthetic to an inhibition of the development of central hypersensitivity. According to their thesis, the afferent barrage of nociceptive transmission antagonizes the neural blockade of epidural bupivacaine. Clinically, this is perceived as a regression in the dermatomal level of pinprick analgesia (tachyphylaxis). The addition of either IV or epidural opioid (morphine) results in activation of descending modulating pathways or interdiction of the afferent nociceptive barrage locally at the level of the dorsal horn. This, in turn, restores analgesia and prevents the development of tachyphylaxis. Although the interaction of opioids and local anesthetics at the level of the spinal cord has not been clearly defined, a recent study by Penning, Nagasakath, and Yaksh[90] in laboratory animals suggests that such analgesic synergism occurs without producing significant effects on motor or sympathetic function.

Table 89-5 lists guidelines for the clinical use of opioid–local anesthetic combinations administered by epidural infusion.

Wound Infiltration and Peripheral Nerve Blocks

The placement of local anesthetic into surgical wound margins or in proximity to the nerve(s) innervating the surgi-

Table 89-5 Suggested use of epidural bupivacaine/opioid solutions for postoperative pain management

Drug	Concentration	Infusion rate	Special considerations
Bupivacaine with	0.1–0.25%	4–15 ml/hr with 0.1–0.125%	Less motor, sensory, sympathetic block
Fentanyl	5 μg/ml 10 μg/ml	4–15 ml/hr 3–10 ml/hr	> 100 μg/hr may result in high blood levels; may not be satisfactory for large surgical incisions
Meperidine	1–1.5 mg/ml 2.5 mg/ml	5–15 ml/hr 5–10 ml/hr	Better cerebrospinal fluid spread than fentanyl > 25 mg/hr may result in high blood levels
Morphine	0.05–0.1 mg/ml	5–10 ml/hr	> 1 mg/hr may produce excessive cephalad cerebrospinal fluid spread, side effects, etc.; probably best opioid for large surgical incisions

cal incision provides effective pain relief. The use of epinephrine-containing solutions of bupivacaine can provide analgesia of long duration. The intense sensory and motor blockade often produced by these techniques may make neurovascular evaluation and active motion of the affected part impossible. Therefore, prior to the use of neural blockade, it is imperative to determine whether the presence of neurovascular compromise (e.g., compartment syndrome) will need to be assessed and whether active motion of the operated part will be required for early postoperative rehabilitation.

Infiltration anesthesia/analgesia

Direct instillation of local anesthetic into surgical wound margins provides postoperative pain relief.[49,64] Reports of the use of this technique for analgesia after major operations are rare; most of the clinical experience associated with wound infiltration has been with minor surgical procedures, such as herniorrhaphy.[49] Administration of 0.25% bupivacaine with epinephrine is usually used for this technique.

Peripheral nerve block

Brachial plexus block. When epinephrine-containing solutions of bupivacaine are used for brachial plexus block, protracted profound analgesia of the upper extremity can usually be achieved. This can be performed at the time of operation or in the immediate postoperative period. Paramount to the decision of brachial plexus approach is the site of the surgical procedure. Shoulder and upper-arm operations usually require an interscalene approach. A supraclavicular (subclavian-perivascular) approach may be used for elbow and forearm procedures. The axillary approach to the brachial plexus is used for wrist or hand procedures.

Indwelling continuous brachial plexus catheters can be used for extended upper-extremity analgesia (see Chapter 61).[17] Single injections via a block needle or continuous infusions through a catheter should be administered as close as possible to the nerve root, nerve trunk, or peripheral nerve transmitting nociception. When an indwelling brachial plexus catheter is used, 0.25% bupivacaine can be administered in intermittent boluses of 10 to 20 ml, or administered as a continuous infusion of 6 to 15 ml/hr. The major obstacle to widespread use of indwelling catheters is the seeming inability to reliably secure the catheter within the brachial plexus sheath. Whether short plastic cannulas or thin epidural-type catheters are introduced, motion of the neck and arm tend to displace the catheter from its desired location. This has lead some authorities to advocate use of the infraclavicular approach, as the incidence of catheter dislodgement from the brachial plexus sheath is reduced.[17]

Femoral nerve block. Surgical procedures of the femur and knee are amenable to femoral nerve block for postoperative analgesia. Six to 12 hours of pain relief can be achieved through the use of 0.25% to 0.5% bupivacaine with epinephrine in a volume of 10 to 20 ml. Indwelling catheter techniques can be effective because the nerve is contained in a discrete sheath, and patient movement is unlikely to dislodge the catheter. Ambulation during femoral nerve block is contraindicated because of the resultant quadriceps muscle weakness. Analgesia for knee procedures is not complete because the knee joint also receives sensory innervation from the sciatic nerve.[37]

Sciatic nerve block. An underappreciated and rarely performed nerve block is the popliteal fossa approach to the sciatic nerve. Blockade of the two divisions of the sciatic nerve at this level (tibial and common peroneal) renders the entire leg analgesic below the knee, save for the skin of the medial calf and ankle. Because of extensive adipose tissue within the popliteal fossa, large volumes of local anesthetic (30 to 40 ml) are required. Ambulation is not permissible with this block because foot dorsiflexion and plantar flexion may be compromised.[37]

Intercostal nerve block. All surgical procedures involving the thoracic dermatomes are amenable to prolonged pain relief with intercostal nerve blocks. Analgesia of 8 to 12 hours in duration can be achieved when epinephrine-containing bupivacaine solutions are used. Limitations of this method are the requirement for repeated injections to sustain analgesia, confinement of analgesia to somatic structures (only the chest or abdominal wall are affected by the block), and the risk of pneumothorax or local anesthetic toxicity. Although repeated injections can be performed, it may be difficult to manage several patients simultaneously with this method. Pneumothorax is rare if the practitioner is skilled. Local anesthetic toxicity is usually a concern only when multiple bilateral nerve blocks are necessary for analgesia.[37]

Intercostal nerve block produces effective analgesia after major abdominal and thoracic surgery. Bilateral blocks are necessary for midline incisions. Improvements in pulmonary function (i.e., increased forced vital capacity, forced expiratory volume, and expiratory flow rate) have been demonstrated with intercostal nerve blocks following open cholecystectomy[97] or thoracotomy.[57] Significant reductions in postoperative opioid requirement have also been documented when intercostal nerve blocks are used after cholecystectomy.[89]

Interpleural analgesia. In 1986 Reiestad and Strømskag described the successful treatment of postoperative pain originating in the thoracic dermatomes with administration of local anesthetic into the ipsilateral chest cavity.[100] This interpleural (between the visceral and parietal pleura) technique was shown to be highly effective for pain relief after open cholecystectomy, nephrectomy, or mastectomy.[100] Although initial reports suggested extremely long analgesic duration following an interpleural bolus, subsequent work has shown that effective pain relief only lasts approximately 4 to 6 hours after a single injection of 0.5% bupivacaine.[10,121] Although effective for flank incisions, the technique has become less popular because of documented lack of efficacy for postoperative pain relief after thoracotomy[32,101] and the growing enthusiasm for thoracic epidural analgesia.

SUMMARY

The demonstrated safety and efficacy of epidural analgesia and PCA have made effective pain relief an achievable goal following nearly all surgical procedures. Although numerous issues remain to be resolved, widespread clinical application of these techniques is ongoing. Providing these services for large numbers of surgical patients can be a formidable task. Staffing and in-service education requirements are great and are mandatory if a safe and efficient service is to be maintained.

The apparent value of effective analgesia is recognized by patients, nurses, and other medical personnel, but it may create a moral dilemma for the acute pain management team. Can state-of-the-art analgesia be offered to all patients? If so, can this be accomplished without unreasonable requirements for nursing and anesthesia personnel, especially in an era of cost containment and clinical efficiency?

There are no clear answers to these questions. However, the perioperative practice of anesthesiology includes the prevention and treatment of pain. Therefore, it is logical that anesthesiologists provide the services to surgical and nonsurgical patients who require enhanced analgesia, especially after operation or trauma.

KEY POINTS

- Nociception consists of four physiologic processes: (1) transduction; (2) transmission; (3) modulation; and (4) perception. The dorsal horn of the spinal cord is the focal point for the integration and modulation of nociception; it functions as a "gate" for control of pain processes.
- Surgical trauma results in an afferent barrage of nociceptive transmission that may alter the threshold for excitation and the magnitude of action potential generation in both central and peripheral neurons. This enhanced afferent nociceptive transmission may expand the receptive fields of dorsal horn neurons, induce postsynaptic morphologic changes, and induce progressive facilitation of dorsal horn neuronal discharge (central hypersensitization or "wind-up").
- Central hypersensitization is mediated by the binding of excitatory amino acids (glutamate and aspartate) to the NMDA receptor.
- The multiplicity of mechanisms associated with nociception and central hypersensitization make it extremely unlikely that any single analgesic modality will provide complete pain relief in all patients.
- The concept of balanced analgesia implies the coadministration of analgesics that selectively affect the physiologic processes involved in nociception or the chemical mediators of central hypersensitization. Combined analgesic techniques facilitate achievement of more "complete" analgesia, and may decrease morbidity.
- Surgical stress evokes a global, linked, endocrinologic, immunologic, and inflammatory response that is harmful to homeostasis. Analgesia *per se* does not ablate the stress response, and inhibition of the stress response depends on the individual analgesic techniques (e.g., epidural or subarachnoid analgesia is more effective than systemic analgesia).
- Patient-controlled anesthesia signifies the intermittent IV administration of opioids under direct patient control.
- The most common mode of PCA administration is demand dosing wherein a fixed dose is self-administered. Constant-rate infusion plus demand dosing implies administration of a minimum background infusion that can be supplemented by patient demand. When using this mode, the background infusion must not ablate the need

for patient demand. Otherwise, the risk of respiratory depression is enhanced.

- Systemic analgesia is obtained when the plasma opioid concentration reaches a specific level in each patient. For a small increase in plasma opioid concentration, there is a rapid decrease in pain. The nadir of the perceived pain defines the MEAC.
- For opioids administered by PCA, pharmacokinetic parameters have no relation to an individual's hourly analgesic requirement. However, mean plasma opioid concentration and the MEAC correlate significantly with hourly opioid use.
- Opioids alone or in combination with local anesthetics produce profound postoperative analgesia when administered by continuous infusion or intermittent bolus injections through an indwelling epidural catheter. The advantage of this technique is segmental analgesia without concomitant motor, sensory, or autonomic changes. The analgesia produced is usually intense and far exceeds that obtained when similar doses are administered systemically.
- The onset time and duration of analgesic action of epidural opioids are inversely related to their lipid solubility.
- Respiratory depression after epidural opioid administration is biphasic, with early and late phases. Early respiratory depression is related to increased blood levels of opioid; it usually occurs within the first hour and is indistinguishable from the respiratory effects produced by an IV dose of the same opioid. Delayed respiratory depression is seen with lipid-insoluble drugs such as morphine; it results from cephalad migration of the opioid in the CSF.
- Respiratory depression may persist for up to 24 hours after a single epidural bolus of morphine. Vigilant assessment of respiratory status is therefore needed during this interval, although this can usually be accomplished in a regular postoperative nursing environment in healthy patients.
- Nausea and vomiting occur in 12% to 50% of patients after administration of epidural morphine. This usually coincides with other evidence of cephalad migration of the opioid and may reflect interaction of drug with the vomiting center and chemotactic trigger zone.
- The incidence of pruritus may be greater than 50% after epidural opioid, although severe pruritus probably occurs in only 1% of patients.
- Urinary retention occurs because spinal or epidural morphine blocks volume-induced bladder contractions and inhibits the vesicle somatic reflex required for external sphincter relaxation.
- The side effects of epidural opioid therapy are easily reversed by intravenous naloxone, but continued monitoring and repeat injections may be required, because of the short duration of opioid antagonism.
- The combination of dilute solutions of local anesthetic and opioid administered by continuous epidural infusion limits side effects by combining subanalgesic doses of the two drugs, yet provides effective analgesia.
- Surgical procedures involving the thoracic dermatomes are amenable to prolonged pain relief with intercostal nerve blocks. Analgesia of 8 to 12 hours in duration can be achieved with epinephrine-containing bupivacaine solutions. Limitations include the requirement for repeated injections to sustain analgesia, confinement of analgesia to somatic structures (only the chest or abdominal wall are affected by the block), and the risk of pneumothorax or local anesthetic toxicity.

KEY REFERENCES

Cousins, MJ, Mather LE: Intrathecal and epidural administration of opioids, *Anesthesiology* 61:276, 1984.

Ferrante FM, Ostheimer GW, Covino BG: *Patient-controlled analgesia,* Boston, 1990, Blackwell Scientific.

Ferrante FM, VadeBoncouer TR: *Postoperative pain management*, New York, 1993, Churchill-Livingstone.

Fields HL: *Pain*, New York, 1987, McGraw Hill.

Kehlet H: Surgical stress: the role of pain and analgesia, *Br J Anesth* 63: 189, 1989.

Liu S, Carpenter RL, Neal JM: Epidural anesthesia and analgesia: their role in postoperative outcome, *Anesthesiology* 82:1474, 1995.

Pockett S: Spinal cord synaptic plasticity and chronic pain, *Anesth Analg* 80:173, 1995.

Tverskoy M, Cozacov C, Ayache F, et al: Postoperative pain after inguinal herniorrhaphy with different types of anesthesia, *Anesth Analg* 70:29, 1990.

Woolf CJ: Evidence of a central component of post-injury hypersensitivity, *Nature* 306:686, 1983.

Woolf CJ, Thompson SWN: The induction and maintenance of central hypersensitization is dependent upon N-methyl-D-aspartic acid receptor activation; implications for the treatment of post-injury pain hypersensitivity states, *Pain* 44:293, 1991.

Woolf CJ, Chong MS: Pre-emptive analgesia—treating postoperative pain by preventing the establishment of central sensitization, *Anesth Analg* 77:362, 1993.

REFERENCES

1. Abram SE, Yaksh TL: Morphine, but not inhalation anesthesia, blocks post-injury facilitation. The role of preemptive suppression of afferent transmission, *Anesthesiology* 78:713, 1993.
2. Abram SE, Yaksh TL: Systemic lidocaine blocks nerve injury-induced hyperalgesia and nociceptor-driven spinal sensitization in the rat, *Anesthesiology* 80:383, 1994.
3. Asoh T, Shirasaka C, Uchida I, et al: Effects of indomethacin on endocrine responses and nitrogen loss after surgery, *Ann Surg* 206:770, 1987.
4. Austin KL, Stapleton JV, Mather LE: Relationship between blood meperidine concentrations and analgesic response: a preliminary report, *Anesthesiology* 53:460, 1980.
5. Austin KL, Stapleton JV, Mather LE: Multiple intramuscular injections: a major source of variability in analgesic response to meperidine, *Pain* 8:47, 1980.
6. Bailey PL, Clark NJ, Pace NL, et al: Antagonism of postoperative opioid-induced respiratory depression: nalbuphine versus naloxone, *Anesth Analg* 66:1109, 1987.
7. Bell MD, Murray GR, Mishin P, et al: Buccal morphine—a new route for analgesia? *Lancet* 1:71, 1985.
8. Bigler D, Lund C, Mogensen T, et al: Tachyphylaxis during postoperative epidural analgesia—new insights, *Acta Anaesthesiol Scand* 31:664, 1987.
9. Bliss TVP, Collingridge GL: A synaptic model of memory: long-term potentiation in the hippocampus, *Nature* 361:31, 1993.
10. Brismar B, Pettersson N, Tokics I, et al: Postoperative analgesia with intrapleural administration of bupivacaine adrenaline, *Acta Anaesthesiol Scand* 31:515, 1987.
11. Bromage PR, Camporesi EM, Durant PAC, et al: Non-respiratory side effects of epidural morphine, *Anesth Analg* 61:490, 1982.
12. Bromage PR, Camporesi EM, Durant PAC, et al: Rostral spread of epidural morphine, *Anesthesiology* 56:431, 1982.
13. Bromage PR, Camporesi EM, Leslie J: Epidural narcotics in volunteers: sensitivity to pain and carbon dioxide, *Pain* 9:145, 1980.
14. Brownridge PR: Epidural and intrathecal opiates for postoperative pain relief, *Anaesthesia* 38:74, 1983.
15. Burstein R, Cliffer, KD, Geisler Jr, GJ: Direct somatosensory projections from the spinal cord to the hypothalamus and telencephalon, *J Neurosci* 7:4159, 1987.
16. Cepeda MS, Carr DB: The neuroendocrine response to postoperative pain. In Ferrante FM, VadeBoncouer TR, editors: *Postoperative pain management,* New York, 1993, Churchill-Livingstone.
17. Concepcion MC: Continuous brachial plexus catheter techniques. In Ferrante FM, VadeBoncouer TR, editors: *Postoperative pain management,* New York, 1993, Churchill-Livingstone.
18. Cook AJ, Woolf CJ, Wall PD, et al: Dynamic receptive field plasticity in rat spinal cord dorsal horn following C-primary afferent input, *Nature* 325:151, 1987.
19. Cousins MJ: The injury response and prevention of postoperative pain, *Anesth Analg* 72 [Suppl]:47, 1991.
20. Cousins MJ, Mather LE: Intrathecal and epidural administration of opioids, *Anesthesiology* 61:276, 1984.
21. Dahl JB, Kehlet H: Non-steroidal anti-inflammatory drugs: rationale for use in severe postoperative pain, *Br J Anaesth* 66: 703, 1991.
22. Dahl JB, Rosenberg J, Dirkes WE, et al: Prevention of postoperative pain by balanced analgesia, *Br J Anaesth* 64:518, 1990.
23. Dahlström B, Tamsen A, Paalzow L, et al: Patient-controlled analgesic therapy, Part IV: pharmacokinetics and analgesic plasma concentration of morphine, *Clin Pharmacokinet* 7:266, 1982.
24. Dickenson AH, Sullivan AF: Subcutaneous formalin-induced activity of dorsal horn neurones in the rat: differential response to an intrathecal opiate administered pre- or post-formalin, *Pain* 30:349, 1987.
25. Dubner R, Ruda MA: Activity-dependent neuronal plasticity following tissue injury and inflammation, *TINS* 15:96, 1992.
26. Durant PAC, Yaksh TL: Drug effects on urinary bladder tone during spinal morphine-induced inhibition of the micturition reflex in unanesthetized rats, *Anesthesiology* 68:325, 1988.
27. Eisenach JC, Grice SC, Dewan DM: Patient-controlled analgesia following cesarean section: a comparison with epidural and intramuscular narcotics, *Anesthesiology* 68:444, 1988.
28. Ellis DJ, Millar WL, Reisner LS: A randomized double-blind comparison of epidural versus intravenous fentanyl infusion for analgesia after Cesarean section, *Anesthesiology* 72:981, 1990.
29. Evans JM, Rosen M, MacCarthy J, et al: Apparatus for patient-controlled administration of intravenous narcotics during labour, *Lancet* 1:17, 1976.
30. Ferrante FM: Nonsteroidal anti-inflammatory drugs. In Ferrante FM, VadeBoncouer TR, editors, *Postoperative pain management,* New York, 1993, Churchill-Livingstone.
31. Ferrante FM, Barber MJ, Segal M, et al: 0.0625% bupivacaine with 0.0002% fentanyl via patient-controlled epidural analgesia for pain of labor and delivery, *Clin J Pain* 11:121, 1995.
32. Ferrante FM, Chan VWS, Arthur BR, et al: Interpleural analgesia after thoracotomy, *Anesth Analg* 72:605, 1991.
33. Ferrante FM, Covino BG: Patient-controlled analgesia: a historical perspective. In Ferrante FM, Ostheimer GW, Covino BG, editors: *Patient-controlled analgesia,* Boston, 1990, Blackwell Scientific.
34. Ferrante FM, Lu L, Jamison SB, et al: Patient-controlled epidural analgesia: demand dosing, *Anesth Analg* 73:547, 1991.
35. Ferrante FM, Orav EJ, Rocco AG, et al: A statistical model for pain in patient-controlled analgesia and conventional intramuscular opioid regimens, *Anesth Analg* 67:457, 1988.
36. Ferrante FM, Rosinia FA, Gordon C, et al: The rate of continuous background infusions in patient-controlled epidural analgesia for labor and delivery, *Anesth Analg* 79:80, 1994.
37. Ferrante FM, VadeBoncouer TR: *Postoperative pain management,* New York, 1993, Churchill-Livingstone.
38. Fields HL: *Pain,* New York, 1987, McGraw-Hill.
39. Fraser HM, Chapman V, Dickenson AH: Spinal cord local anesthetic actions on afferent evoked responses and wind-up of nociceptive neurones in the rat spinal cord: combination with morphine produces marked potentiation of antinociception, *Pain* 49:33, 1992.
40. Gambling DR, McMorland GH, Yu P, et al: Comparison of patient-controlled epidural analgesia and conventional intermittent "top-up" injections during labor, *Anesth Analg* 70:256, 1990.
41. Gambling DR, Yu P, McMorland GH, et al: A comparative study of patient controlled epidural analgesia (PCEA) and continuous infusion epidural analgesia (CIEA) during labour, *Can J Anaesth* 35:249, 1988.
42. Gil KM, Ginsberg B, Muir M, et al: Patient-controlled analgesia in postoperative pain: the relation of psychological factors to pain and analgesic use, *Clin J Pain* 6:137, 1990.
43. Glynn CJ, Mather LE, Cousins MJ, et al: Peridural meperidine in humans: analgesic response, pharmacokinetics and transmission into CSF, *Anesthesiology* 55:520, 1981.
44. Goto T, Marota JJ, Crosby G: Nitrous oxide induces pre-emptive analgesia in the rat that is antagonized by halothane, *Anesthesiology* 80:809, 1994.
45. Gourlay GK, Cherry DA, Plummer JL, et al: The influence of drug polarity on the absorption of opioid drugs into CSF and subsequent cephalad migration following lumbar epidural administration: application to morphine and pethidine, *Pain* 31:297, 1987.
46. Gueneron JP, Coffey C, Carli P, et al: Effect of naloxone infusion or analgesia and respiratory depression after epidural fentanyl, *Anesth Analg* 67:35, 1988.
47. Guinard JP, Carpenter RL, Chassot PG: Epidural and intravenous fentanyl produce equivalent effects during major surgery, *Anesthesiology* 82:377, 1995.
48. Guinard JP, Mavrocordatos P, Chiolero R, et al: A randomized comparison of intravenous versus lumbar and thoracic epidural fentanyl for analgesia after thoracotomy, *Anesthesiology* 77:1108, 1992.
49. Hashemi K, Middleton MD: Subcutaneous bupivacaine for postoperative analgesia after herniorrhaphy, *Ann R Coll Surg Engl* 65:38, 1983.
50. Henderson SK, Cohen H: Nalbuphine aug-

mentation of analgesia and reversal of side effects following epidural hydromorphone, *Anesthesiology* 65:216, 1986.
51. Hill HF, Mackie AM, Jacobson RC: Infusion based patient-controlled analgesia systems. In Ferrante FM, Ostheimer GW, Covino BG, editors: *Patient-controlled analgesia,* Boston, 1990, Blackwell Scientific.
52. Hjortsø N-C, Lund C, Mogensen T, et al: Epidural morphine improves pain relief and maintains sensory analgesia during continuous epidural bupivacaine after abdominal surgery, *Anesth Analg* 65:1033, 1986.
53. Hunt CO, Naulty JS, Bader AM, et al: Perioperative analgesia with subarachnoid fentanyl-bupivacaine for cesarean delivery, *Anesthesiology* 71:535, 1989.
54. Jacobson L, Cirabal C, Brody MC: A dose-response study of intrathecal morphine: efficacy, duration, optimal dose, and side effects, *Anesth Analg* 67:1082, 1988.
55. Jamison RN, Taft K, O'Hara JP, et al: Psychosocial and pharmacologic predictions of satisfaction with intravenous patient-controlled analgesia, *Anesth Analg* 77:121, 1993.
56. Johnson LR, Magnani BJ, Chan V, et al: Modifiers of patient-controlled analgesia efficacy. I: locus of control, *Pain* 39:17, 1989.
57. Kaplan JA, Miller ED, Gallagher EG: Postoperative analgesia for thoracotomy patients, *Anesth Analg* 54:773, 1975.
58. Katz N, Ferrante FM: Nociception. In Ferrante FM, VadeBoncouer TR, editors: *Postoperative pain management,* New York, 1993, Churchill-Livingstone.
59. Kehlet H: Modification of responses to surgery by neural blockade: clinical implications. In Cousins MJ, Bridenbaugh PO, editors: *Neural blockade in clinical anesthesia and management of pain,* ed 2, Philadelphia, 1988, JB Lippincott.
60. Kehlet H: Surgical stress: the role of pain and analgesia, *Br J Anaesth* 63:189, 1989.
61. Knill RL, Clement JL, Thompson WR: Epidural morphine causes delayed and prolonged respiratory depression, *Can Anaesth Soc J* 28:537, 1981.
62. Lam AM, Knill RL, Thompson WR, et al: Epidural fentanyl does not cause delayed respiratory depression, *Can Anaesth Soc J* 30:578, 1983.
63. Lanz E, Theiss D, Reiss W, et al: Epidural morphine for postoperative analgesia: a double-blind study, *Anesth Analg* 61:236, 1982.
64. Levack ID, Holmes JD, Robertson GS: Abdominal wound perfusion for the relief of postoperative pain, *Br J Anaesth* 58:615, 1986.
65. Liu S, Carpenter RL, Neal JM: Epidural anesthesia and analgesia: their role in postoperative outcome, *Anesthesiology* 82:1474, 1995.
66. Logas WG, El-Baz N, El-Ganzouri A, et al: Continuous thoracic epidural analgesia for postoperative pain relief following thoracotomy: a randomized prospective study, *Anesthesiology* 67:787, 1987.
67. Loper KA, Ready LB, Brady M: Patient-controlled anxiolysis with midazolam, *Anesth Analg* 67:1118, 1988.
68. Loper KA, Ready LB, Downey M, et al: Epidural and intravenous fentanyl infusions are clinically equivalent after knee surgery, *Anesth Analg* 70:72, 1990.
69. Lund C, Hansen OB, Mogensen T, et al: Effect of thoracic epidural bupivacaine on somatosensory evoked potentials after dermatomal stimulation, *Anesth Analg* 66:731, 1987.
70. Lund C, Mogensen T, Hjortsø N-C, et al: Systemic morphine enhances spread of sensory analgesia during postoperative epidural bupivacaine infusion, *Lancet* 2:1156, 1985.
71. Lysak SZ, Anderson PT, Carithers RA, et al: Postoperative effects of fentanyl, ketorolac, and piroxicam as analgesics for outpatient laparoscopic procedures, *Obs Gynecol* 83:270, 1994.
72. Lysak SZ, Eisenach JC, Dobson CE II: Patient-controlled epidural analgesia during labor: a comparison of three solutions with a continuous infusion control, *Anesthesiology* 72:44, 1990.
73. Madison DV, Malenka RC, Nicoll RA: Mechanisms underlying long-term potentiation for synaptic transmission, *Ann Rev Neurosci* 14:379, 1991.
74. Malmberg AB, Yaksh TL: Hyperalgesia mediated by spinal glutamate or substance P receptor blocked by spinal cyclooxygenase inhibition, *Science* 57:1276, 1992.
75. Marlowe S, Engstrom R, White PF: Epidural patient-controlled analgesia (PCA): an alternative to continuous epidural infusions, *Pain* 37:97, 1989.
76. McCormack K: Non-steroidal anti-inflammatory drugs and spinal nociceptive processing, *Pain* 59:9, 1994.
77. McCormack K, Brune K: Dissociation between the antinociceptive and anti-inflammatory effects of the nonsteroidal anti-inflammatory drugs. A survey of their analgesic efficacy, *Drugs* 41:533, 1991.
78. McKenzie R: Patient-controlled analgesia (PCA) (letter), *Anesthesiology* 69:1027, 1988.
79. McQuay HJ, Sullivan AF, Smallman K, et al: Intrathecal opioids, potency and lipophilicity, *Pain* 36:111, 1989.
80. Merskey H: Classification of chronic pain: description of chronic pain syndromes and definition of pain terms, *Pain* 3[Suppl]:S1, 1986.
81. Miguel R, Barlow I, Morrell M, et al: A prospective, randomized, double-blind comparison of epidural and intravenous sufentanil infusions, *Anesthesiology* 81:346, 1994.
82. Minami T, Uda R, Horiguchi S, et al: Allodynia evoked by intrathecal administration of prostaglandin to conscious mice, *Pain* 57:217, 1994.
83. Mogensen T, Dirkes W, Bigler D, et al: No tachyphylaxis during postoperative continuous epidural 0.125% bupivacaine infusion, *Reg Anaesth* 13:117, 1988.
84. Mogensen T, Hjortsø N-C, Bigler D, et al: Unpredictability of regression of analgesia during the continuous postoperative extradural infusion of bupivacaine, *Br J Anaesth* 60:515, 1988.
85. Mogensen T, Hojgaard L, Scott NB, et al: Epidural blood flow and regression of sensory analgesia during continuous postoperative epidural infusion of bupivacaine, *Anesth Analg* 67:809, 1988.
86. Mogensen T, Scott NB, Hjortsø N-C, et al: The influence of volume and concentration of bupivacaine on regression of analgesia during continuous postoperative epidural infusion, *Reg Anaesth* 13:122, 1988.
87. Mogensen T, Simonsen L, Scott NB, et al: Tachyphylaxis associated with repeat epidural injections of lidocaine is not related to changes in distribution or the rate of elimination from the epidural space, *Anesth Analg* 69:180, 1989.
88. Myers RR, Kalichman MW, Reisner LS, et al: Neurotoxicity of local anesthetics: altered perineural permeability, edema and nerve fiber injury, *Anesthesiology* 70:721, 1989.
89. Nunn JF, Slavin G: Posterior intercostal nerve block for pain relief after cholecystectomy, *Br J Anaesth* 52:253, 1980.
90. Penning JP, Nagasakatt H, Yaksh TL: Intrathecal morphine and bupivacaine in the rat: analgesic synergy without augmentation of motor dysfunction or hypotension, *Can Soc J* 37:S49, 1990.
91. Perry F, Parker RK, White PF, et al: Role of psychological factors in a postoperative pain control and recovery with patient-controlled analgesia, *Clin J Pain* 10:57, 1994.
92. Plummer JL, Cmielewski PL, Reynolds GD, et al: Influence of polarity on dose-response relationships of intrathecal opioids in rats, *Pain* 40:339, 1990.
93. Pockett S: Spinal cord synaptic plasticity and chronic pain, *Anesth Analg* 80:173, 1995.
94. Presley RW, Menetrey D, Levine JD, et al: Systemic morphine suppresses noxious stimulus-evoked Fos protein-like immunoreactivity in the rat spinal cord, *J Neurosci* 10:323, 1990.
95. Rawal N, Arner S, Gustafsson LL, et al: Present state of extradural and intrathecal opioid analgesia in Sweden, *Br J Anaesth* 59:791, 1987.
96. Rawal N, Schött U, Dahlström B, et al: Influence of naloxone infusion on analgesia and respiratory depression following epidural morphine, *Anesthesiology* 64:194, 1986.
97. Rawal N, Sjöstrand UH, Dahlström B, et al: Epidural morphine for postoperative pain relief: a comparative study with intramuscular narcotic and intercostal nerve, *Anesth Analg* 61:93, 1982.
98. Ready LB, Brown CR, Stahlgren LH, et al: Evaluation of intravenous ketorolac administered by bolos or infusion for treatment of postoperative pain: a double-blind, placebo-controlled, multicenter study, *Anesthesiology* 80:1277, 1994.
99. Reichlin S: Neuroendocrine-immune reactions, *N Engl J Med* 329:1246, 1993.
100. Reiestad F, Strømskag KE: Interpleural catheter in the management of postoperative pain. A preliminary report, *Reg Anaesth* 11:89, 1986.
101. Rosenberg PH, Scheinin BM-A, Lepantalo MJA, et al: Continuous intrapleural infusion of bupivacaine for analgesia after thoracotomy, *Anesthesiology* 67:811, 1987.
102. Roscow CE, Moss J, Philbin DM, et al: Histamine release during morphine and

fentanyl anaesthesia, *Anesthesiology* 56: 93, 1982.
103. Roth SH, Bennett RE: Non-steroidal anti-inflammatory drug gastropathy: recognition and response, *Arch Intern Med* 147:2093, 1987.
104. Rutberg H, Hakanson E, Anderberg B, et al: Effects of extradural administration of morphine or bupivacaine on the endocrine response to upper abdominal surgery, *Br J Anesth* 56:233, 1984.
105. Sandler AN, Stringer D, Panos L, et al: A randomized, double-blind comparison of lumbar epidural and intravenous fentanyl infusions for post-thoracotomy pain relief, *Anesthesiology* 77:626, 1992.
106. Scott NB, Mogensen T, Bigler D, et al: Continuous thoracic extradural 0.5% bupivacaine with or without morphine: effect on quality of blockade, lung function and the surgical stress response, *Br J Anesth* 62:253, 1988.
107. Sechzer PH: Objective measurement of pain, *Anesthesiology* 29:209, 1968.
108. Sechzer PH: Studies in pain with the analgesic-demand system, *Anesth Analg* 50:1, 1971.
109. Shah MV, Jones DI, Rosen M: "Patient demand" postoperative analgesia with buprenorphine. Comparison between sublingual and IM administration, *Br J Anaesth* 58:508, 1986.
110. Sjöström S, Hartvig D, Tamsen A: Patient-controlled analgesia with extradural morphine or pethidine, *Br J Anaesth* 60:358, 1988.
111. Steidl LJ, Fromme GA, Danielson DR: Lumbar vs. thoracic epidural morphine for post-thoracotomy pain, *Anesth Analg* 63: 277, 1984.
112. Sugimoto T, Takemura M, Sakai A, et al: Rapid transneuronal destruction following peripheral nerve transection in the medullary dorsal horn is enhanced by strychnine, picrotoxin and biculline, *Pain* 30:385, 1987.
113. Sullivan SP, Cherry DA: Pain from an invasive facial tumor relieved by lumbar epidural morphine, *Anesth Analg* 66:777, 1987.
114. Swanson LW, Sawchenko PE: Hypothalamic integration: organization of the paraventricular and supraoptic nuclei, *Ann Rev Neurosci* 6:269, 1983.
115. Tamsen A, Bondesson V, Dahlström B, et al: Patient-controlled analgesic therapy, part III: pharmacokinetics and analgesic plasma concentrations of ketobemidone, *Clin Pharmacokinet* 7:252, 1982.
116. Tamsen A, Hartvig P, Fagerlund C, et al: Patient-controlled analgesic therapy, part II: individual analgesic demand and analgesic plasma concentrations of pethidine in postoperative pain, *Clin Pharmacokinet* 7:164, 1982.
117. Tamsen A, Sakurada T, Wahlstrom A, et al: Postoperative demand for analgesics in relation to individual levels of endorphins and substance P in cerebrospinal fluid, *Pain* 13:171, 1982.
118. Tuman KJ, McCarthy RJ, March RJ, et al: Effects of epidural anesthesia and analgesia on coagulation and outcome after major vascular surgery, *Anesth Analg* 73:696, 1991.
119. Tverskoy M, Cozacov C, Ayache M, et al: Postoperative pain after inguinal herniorrhaphy with different types of anesthesia, *Anesth Analg* 70:29, 1990.
120. Urquhart ML, Klapp K, White PF: Patient-controlled analgesia: a comparison of intravenous versus subcutaneous hydromorphone, *Anesthesiology* 69:428, 1988.
121. VadeBoncouer TR, Riegler FX, Gautt RS, et al: A randomized double-blind comparison of the effects of interpleural bupivacaine and saline on morphine requirements and pulmonary function after cholecystectomy, *Anesthesiology* 71:339, 1989.
122. Vercautern MP, Coppejans HC, ten Broecke PW, et al: Epidural sufentanil for postoperative patient-controlled analgesia (PCA) with or without background infusion: a double-blind comparison, *Anesth Analg* 80:76, 1995.
123. Wall PD, Woolf CJ: The brief and prolonged facilitatory effects of unmyelinated afferent input on the rat spinal cord are independently influenced by peripheral nerve section, *Neuroscience* 17:1199, 1986.
124. Watanabe S, Kondo T, Asakura N, et al: Intraoperative combined administration of indomethacin and buprenorphine suppositories as prophylactic therapy for post-open-cholecystectomy pain, *Anesth Analg* 79:85, 1994.
125. White PF: Patient-controlled analgesia: delivery systems. In Ferrante FM, Ostheimer GW, Covino BG, editors: *Patient-controlled analgesia,* Boston, 1990, Blackwell Scientific.
126. Wilcox GL: Spinal mediators of nociceptive neurotransmission and hyperalgesia: relationships among spinal plasticity, analgesic tolerance and blood flow, *APS Journal* 2:265, 1993.
127. Woolf CJ: Evidence for a central component or post-injury hypersensitivity, *Nature* 306:686, 1983.
128. Woolf CJ, Chong MS: Pre-emptive analgesia-treating postoperative pain by preventing the establishment of central sensitization, *Anesth Analg* 77:362, 1993.
129. Woolf CJ, Thompson SWN: The induction and maintenance of central hypersensitization is dependent upon N-methyl-D-aspartic acid receptor activation; implications for the treatment of post-injury pain hypersensitivity states, *Pain* 44:293, 1991.
130. Woolf CJ: A dissociation between the analgesic and antinociceptive effects of morphine, *Neurosci Lett* 64:238, 1986.
131. Woolf CJ, Wall PD: Morphine-sensitive and morphine-insensitive actions of C-fiber input on the rat spinal cord, *Neurosci Lett* 64:221, 1986.
132. Yeager MP, Glass DD, Neff RK, et al: Epidural anesthesia and analgesia in high-risk surgical patients, *Anesthesiology* 66:729, 1987.
133. Zhuo M, Small SA, Kandall ET, et al: Nitric oxide and carbon monoxide produce activity-dependent long-term synaptic enhancement in hippocampus, *Science* 260:1946, 1993.

CHAPTER 90

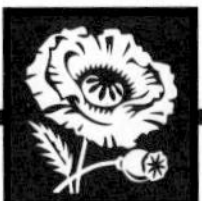

Pulmonary Complications of Anesthesia

RALPH T. GEER

Alterations in pulmonary function induced by anesthesia and surgery have historically been recognized as significant causes of perioperative morbidity and acute respiratory failure. In 1910, Pasteur described pulmonary changes after abdominal surgery.[71] In 1932, Beecher recognized that decreases in lung volumes were important in producing postoperative hypoxemia and that the functional residual capacity was a useful measure of pulmonary reserve.[7] In modern anesthetic practice, decreases in functional residual capacity associated with atelectasis and hypoxemia remain among the most common perioperative clinical abnormalities.[23,55,73,92,102]

Knowledge of the pathophysiologic changes associated with anesthesia and surgery provides the foundation for prevention, diagnosis, and treatment of pulmonary complications. This chapter describes the risk factors associated with pulmonary complications, the pulmonary changes expected with anesthesia and surgery, and common postoperative pulmonary complications.

RISK EVALUATION

Three factors that influence the development of perioperative pulmonary complications are: (1) the specific surgery and surgical incision performed; (2) individual characteristics of the patient; and (3) the anesthetic drug or technique used. For example, the incidence of pulmonary complications for all patients after all types of surgery is approximately 6%.[78,105] However, in patients with chronic obstructive pulmonary disease (COPD) undergoing upper abdominal surgery, the complication rate can be as high as 92%. In contrast, for healthy patients after nonabdominal, nonthoracic surgery, the rate of complications is as low as 0.6%.[73,78,95,105] Further, some patients with severe ($FEV_1 < 0.5$ l) pulmonary compromise, may recover extremely well following major abdominal surgery.[70]

The site of surgery is strongly associated with the pulmonary complication rate. Upper abdominal surgery has a 30% to 40% pulmonary complication rate, whereas lower abdominal surgery has only a 10% to 16% rate.[5,94] Nonthoracic, nonabdominal surgery is associated with a pulmonary complication rate less than 10%.[73,78,95,105]

The specific type of surgical incision can also be a risk factor for pulmonary complications. Vertical laparotomies are associated with more postoperative hypoxemia than are horizontal laparotomies. A lateral thoracotomy commonly results in lung trauma and compression that will produce perioperative pulmonary abnormalities. A median sternotomy, when compared with a lateral thoracotomy, is not as strongly associated with postoperative pulmonary dysfunction, perhaps because lung compression and trauma are less severe.[32,44,97]

Certain patient characteristics are associated with increased postoperative pulmonary complications. Among these characteristics are increased age, smoking,[20] nutritional status, obesity, chronic obstructive lung disease, asthma, and cardiac disease.[43] **Although pulmonary function testing may distinguish between patients at either very low or high risk, it is of limited value in predicting risk for those with moderate degrees of dysfunction based on airway flow rate measurements or depression of resting lung volumes. In such cases, degree of dysfunction based on assessment of blood gases and exercise tolerance may have more predictive value.**[3,69]

Finally, anesthetic factors influence postoperative pulmonary complications. Anesthesia duration of greater than 3.5 hours has been associated with increased pulmonary complications.[62,98] For most surgeries, subarachnoid or epidural anesthesia holds no proven advantage compared with general anesthesia in reducing pulmonary complications. However, peripheral surgery performed using a regional block is associated with a lower pulmonary complication rate than major conduction or general anesthesia.[35,81,98,100]

The risk factors just outlined are potentially additive in producing pulmonary complications perioperatively.[73] It is especially important to try to correct all easily reversible clinical abnormalities in high-risk patients and to select the surgical procedure and anesthetic presenting the least risk. For most surgical procedures, the type of anesthetic administered is less likely to modify the patient's postoperative condition than optimization of the preoperative condition and quality of the surgical outcome.[4,18]

EFFECT OF ANESTHESIA ON PULMONARY FUNCTION

It has been well established that general anesthesia and mechanical ventilation produce marked alterations in pulmonary function, lung volumes, and compliance. This is in part caused by the effects of general anesthesia on the motion of the chest wall and diaphragm.[8,83,90,101,104] **The shift of the diaphragm cephalad with induction of anesthesia decreases lung volumes, especially functional residual capacity.**[102] Using computed tomography (CT) scanning techniques, atelectatic changes can be detected in most patients within 5 minutes of induction of general anesthesia and muscle relaxation.[11] The alteration in diaphragmatic function is believed to be caused by a loss of tonic activity secondary to anesthetic-induced depression of the central nervous system (CNS).[102] This cephalad movement is most marked for the dependent portions of the diaphragm[8,30,83,90,101,104] and produces more pronounced airway closure in dependent portions of the lung, so that nondependent regions of the lung have relatively increased ventilation.[39,90] Thus the well-perfused, dependent lung regions are poorly ventilated, producing a ventilation/perfusion abnormality that results in hypoxemia.

The lung volume at which small airway closure begins to occur is termed the *closing capacity*. As lung volumes decrease during anesthesia and surgery, small airways (0.1 mm diameter) tend to close because they are supported by a negative transpulmonary pressure as opposed to the connective tissue and cartilage that support the large airways.[16,36] The supine position and general anesthesia produce decreased functional residual capacity with associated decreased chest wall and lung compliance.[23,102] The resulting closing capacity may lie within or even above the tidal volume range, leading to the collapse of alveoli and small airways. Associated physiologic abnormalities include a reduction in ventilation to affected areas, ventilation/perfusion abnormalities, increased intrapulmonary shunting, and hypoxemia.[68] In contrast, the prone position has less effect and may even be associated with improvement in functional residual capacity and improvement in oxygenation.[72]

Effects of mechanical ventilation on pulmonary function may contribute to postoperative morbidity. Specifically, morbidity related to pulmonary barotrauma may create difficulties in intraoperative and postoperative ventilation and circulatory stability. The cause of barotrauma is overdistention with resultant disruption of pulmonary parenchyma. Clinically, barotrauma may cause subcutaneous emphysema, pneumomediastinum, and pneumopericardium.[51] **In adults, the most significant complication of barotrauma is gas escape into the pleural space with development of pneumothorax causing ventilatory insufficiency, hypoxia, and hemodynamic collapse. Mechanical ventilation exacerbates cardiovascular changes associated with pneumothoraces, producing significant hypotension and depression of cardiac output.** Underlying pulmonary pathology may produce conditions making development of pulmonary barotrauma more likely. Acute airway obstruction from bronchoconstriction and secretions, or mechanical obstruction from endotracheal tube malposition may produce heterogenous movement of gas resulting in marked maldistribution of ventilation. This causes overdistention of well-ventilated lung during inspiration and/or gas trapping and overdistention during exhalation. Further, use of excessively large tidal volumes in lungs with limited compliance or with compliance heterogeneity may lead to overdistention and lung rupture in the most compliant portions.

Pulmonary function abnormalities can be produced by the pharmacologic effects of anesthetic drugs. Inhalation anesthetics inhibit hypoxic pulmonary vasoconstriction.[36] This inhibition has little effect on patients with normal lungs but could produce marked hypoxia in patients with significant preexisting lung disease and preoperative ventilation/perfusion mismatch. Ventilation with 100% O_2 eventually causes increased intrapulmonary shunting and decreased functional residual capacity.[9,27,96] Finally, inhalation anesthetics may impair mucociliary clearance, causing secretions to pool in atelectatic lung segments, particularly after prolonged abdominal surgery.[33]

EXPECTED POSTOPERATIVE ABNORMALITIES IN PULMONARY FUNCTION

After thoracic or upper and lower abdominal surgery, patients develop restrictive pulmonary dysfunction with a severely reduced vital capacity and functional residual capacity.[1,2,59] Although the degree of restriction is similar, the duration is several times longer for thoracic surgical procedures.[2] Because of reduced inspiratory capacity, these patients are unable to cough effectively, breathing rapidly with small tidal volumes. These changes are less consequential after lower abdominal surgery, and far less common after superficial or extremity surgery.[1,2,59]

General anesthetic-induced pulmonary dysfunction usually produces mild decreases in arterial oxygenation. It is well known that any of the factors adversely altering the balance between total body O_2 delivery (such as anemia or cardiac output depression) and metabolic rate may also affect arterial oxygenation.[52] Transient postoperative decreases in oxygenation are partly caused by increased O_2 consumption during rewarming without adequate compensatory increases in O_2 delivery. Further, in the immediate postoperative period, residual anesthetic effects can produce alveolar hypoventilation, diffusion hypoxia, depression of cardiac output, right-to-left shunting of blood, and ventilation/perfusion mismatch.[52] However, the strong association between site of surgery and postoperative pulmonary dysfunction suggests that changes in the anesthetic technique would not be expected to produce profound changes in the rate of postoperative pulmonary dysfunction.[23] In fact, most of the postoperative pulmonary effects expected with a general anesthetic probably subside within the first 2 hours after surgery.[52]

Postoperative abnormalities in oxygenation without hypercapnia that persist beyond 2 hours are probably secondary to pain, abdominal distension, and immobilization in bed, all of which impair the patient's ability to breathe deeply and cough effectively.[52] This leads to decreased functional residual capacity, increased closing capacity, atelectasis, and hypoxemia. These abnormalities in lung volume commonly progress over the first 24 hours postoperatively and may not return to normal for 7 to 10 days or even longer following thoracic surgery.[2]

GENERAL POSTOPERATIVE PULMONARY CARE

Major therapeutic goals in the postoperative period are effective breathing and coughing, maintenance of functional residual capacity, and prevention of atelectasis. The judicious use of intravenous (IV), intraspinal, and epidural narcotics as well as regional blocks and intrapleural installation of local anesthetics can minimize hypoventilation and help the patient maintain a more normal ventilatory pattern.[12,49,58,82,84,86,91,94] Each technique has risks and benefits, and none has been shown to be clearly superior.[13,28,58,76,86,91,94,108] Preoperative respiratory training, early mobilization, voluntary deep breathing, incentive spirometry, chest physical therapy, aerosol therapy, continuous positive airway pressure, and inspiratory pressure support are among the techniques that may help to maintain lung volumes.[19,67] Studies attempting to compare and evaluate these techniques have been conflicting.[9,67] The best choice is made after consideration of cost, benefit, and the technique which seems to work for an individual patient.[26,45,70]

COMMON CAUSES OF POSTOPERATIVE PULMONARY DYSFUNCTION

Despite general measures at postoperative pulmonary care, the physiologic abnormalities discussed previously can progress to severe pulmonary dysfunction and respiratory failure. The remainder of this chapter emphasizes some common diseases that contribute to the development of postoperative respiratory failure (Box 90-1). These diseases are categorized by cause and clinical presentation as follows: (1) extrapulmonary disease; (2) diseases that produce pulmonary infiltrates; (3) exacerbations of chronic pulmonary disease; and (4) venous thromboembolic disease.

Extrapulmonary Respiratory Failure

Pure extrapulmonary respiratory failure is characterized by a low PaO_2, a high $PaCO_2$, and a normal alveolar-arterial O_2 gradient.[79] However, many patients will have a combination of extrapulmonary and pulmonary disease, so clinicians

BOX 90-1
COMMON CAUSES OF POSTOPERATIVE PULMONARY DYSFUNCTION

- Extrapulmonary causes
  - Decreased central respiratory drive
  - Decreased respiratory muscle function
- Diseases causing pulmonary infiltrates
  - Atelectasis
  - Pulmonary edema
    - Cardiogenic
    - Adult respiratory distress syndrome
  - Aspiration of gastric contents
  - Pulmonary infection
- Exacerbation of chronic pulmonary disease
  - Chronic obstructive pulmonary disease
  - Asthma
- Pulmonary thromboembolism

should consider extrapulmonary causes in all patients with postoperative respiratory failure.

Decreased central respiratory drive

Respiratory center dysfunction is an expected effect of most opioids, barbiturates, benzodiazepines, and inhalation anesthetics. Opioids have direct dose-dependent depressant effects on brain stem respiratory centers and increase $Paco_2$. Doses of opioids that are too small to alter consciousness can produce respiratory depression. Large doses can produce respiratory arrest.[89] However, as previously mentioned, administration of opioids may also produce several beneficial pulmonary effects, because these drugs provide patient comfort, and may promote deep breathing and an effective cough in the postoperative period.[93] Barbiturates, benzodiazepines, and inhalation anesthetics also produce respiratory depression by decreasing the patient's ventilatory response to hypoxia and hypercapnia.[75,80] In large doses, they too may produce apnea.[80]

In addition to these anesthetic-induced abnormalities in central respiratory drive, brain stem abnormalities (e.g., infarction, neoplasm, infection), hypothyroidism, metabolic alkalosis, and sleep apnea syndromes may produce depression of the normal respiratory response perioperatively.[14]

Decreased respiratory muscle function

Residual muscle relaxation is a common cause of postoperative respiratory muscle dysfunction. Standard anesthetic practice dictates the use of only as much muscle relaxant as is necessary and an assessment of muscle strength (adequate inspiratory force, sustained head lift) or other evidence of full reversal of muscle relaxation (sustained response to tetanic stimulation) before extubation. These practices should reduce the rate of persistent perioperative muscle weakness caused by muscle relaxants. Further, for patients not immediately extubated postoperatively, residual muscle relaxation can be detected with a peripheral nerve stimulator and respiratory mechanics assessed before weaning from mechanical ventilation.[18]

Other less common causes of respiratory muscle dysfunction in the perioperative period include metabolic abnormalities (e.g., hypothermia, hypophosphatemia, hypokalemia, hypo- and hypermagnesemia, and hypercalcemia), myasthenia gravis and Eaton-Lambert syndrome, hypothyroidism, spinal cord lesions, and exacerbations of porphyria.[18] In addition, certain medications, such as antibiotics (including aminoglycosides, clindamycin, and neomycin) and local anesthetics, may cause or potentiate neuromuscular blockade.[99]

Diseases Causing Pulmonary Infiltrates

Box 90-2 lists conditions that clinicians should consider depending on the clinical setting, for patients found to have pulmonary infiltrates on chest radiograph in the postoperative period. Patients frequently have several of these disorders simultaneously (cardiogenic pulmonary edema, atelectasis, and pulmonary infection). Importantly, comparison of the preoperative and postoperative chest radiograph can help establish the cause by giving an indication of the time when the chest radiograph abnormality occurred.

BOX 90-2
POTENTIAL CAUSES OF PULMONARY INFILTRATES ON CHEST RADIOGRAPH

Atelectasis
Pulmonary edema
Aspiration of gastric contents
Pulmonary infection
Pulmonary contusion
Pulmonary hemorrhage
Hypersensitivity pneumonitis
Noninfectious inflammatory lung disease
Malignancy

Atelectasis

Atelectasis—the collapse of a normally inflated lung—is the most common cause of postoperative respiratory dysfunction and fever. Using CT scanning, it can be detected in as many as 90% of patients following abdominal surgery (see discussion of the effects of anesthesia on pulmonary function).[48] In addition to causes related to surgery and anesthesia, atelectasis can be caused by pathologic intrinsic or extrinsic proximal airway obstruction. As trapped gas is absorbed but not replaced, the distal alveoli collapse. This abnormality can be produced by an endobronchial carcinoma, aspiration of a foreign body, endobronchial intubation, or excessive mucus production. Atelectasis can cause severe hypoxemia out of proportion to the extent of collapse, particularly when substantial perfusion is maintained to areas of nonventilated lung (i.e., pulmonary shunt).[38,61]

Pulmonary edema

Pulmonary edema is the abnormal accumulation of fluid in the interstitial and alveolar spaces of the lung. Mechanisms that produce pulmonary edema include: (1) increased hydrostatic pressures favoring fluid flow into the pulmonary interstitium (cardiogenic pulmonary edema); (2) increased permeability across microvascular endothelium (noncardiogenic pulmonary edema—the adult respiratory distress syndrome [ARDS]); and more rarely, (3) decreased intravascular colloid oncotic pressure. Patients with pulmonary edema commonly present with hypoxia and diffuse bilateral pulmonary infiltrates.[54]

Postoperative patients most frequently develop pulmonary edema as a result of: (1) relative overhydration (e.g., pulmonary edema associated with irrigant absorption during transurethral prostatic resection); (2) myocardial dysfunction (e.g., cardiogenic pulmonary edema associated with a perioperative myocardial infarction [MI]); or (3) increased permeability (e.g., ARDS associated with sepsis, massive transfusion, or allergic reaction).

Cardiogenic pulmonary edema and fluid overload are associated with elevated central venous pressures (CVP) and pulmonary capillary wedge pressures (PCWP). These elevated pressures may be caused by primary myocardial dysfunction or excessive fluid administration relative to excretory capacity. MI or ischemia, hypertension, valvular heart disease (specifically mitral stenosis, mitral regurgitation, and aortic stenosis), diastolic dysfunction caused by hypertrophic cardiomyopathy, and dysrhythmias are common sources of cardiogenic pulmonary edema caused by myocardial dysfunction. Overhydration of patients with renal insufficiency and oliguria can produce cardiogenic pulmonary edema in patients with normal myocardial function.[54] Cardiogenic pulmonary edema commonly occurs shortly after the end of surgery. It is likely that metabolic stress imposed by rewarming and increased sympathetic tone associated with emergence from anesthesia are important precipitating factors. Treatment includes preload reduction (e.g., nitroglycerine), mechanical ventilation with positive end-expired pressure (PEEP), and supplemental O_2.

Patients with increased alveolar capillary permeability (ARDS) have diffuse alveolar damage and present with severe dyspnea, hypoxemia, decreased lung compliance, and diffuse pulmonary infiltrates. **Unlike cardiogenic pulmonary edema, CVP and PCWP are usually low or normal. ARDS is associated with sepsis, multiple trauma, tissue inflammation, intravascular coagulation, and some drug effects.**[10,31] Exacerbations of bleomycin-induced lung toxicity have been reported in patients who have been exposed to hyperoxic anesthetic mixtures for prolonged periods (see Chapter 21).[53] Treatment of ARDS is directed at the underlying illnesses (antibiotics for sepsis, etc.) while providing supplemental O_2 and mechanical ventilatory support. Close monitoring for pulmonary infection is imperative, as sepsis is the most common cause of death in patients with ARDS.[10,31]

Pulmonary edema has also been reported to occur in association with upper airway obstruction, particularly in children and healthy young adults.[50,106] The mechanism by which the edema is produced has not been definitely established, but probably involves changes induced by generation of negative intrapleural pressures creating acute and marked increases in left ventricular preload and afterload.[15] The treatment for this condition includes relief of airway obstruction and airway supportive measures (e.g., O_2, mechanical ventilation, etc.).

Gastric acid aspiration pneumonia

Aspiration pneumonia is a term used to describe pulmonary inflammation caused by the aspiration of gastric or nasopharyngeal secretions. A severe acute pneumonitis is associated with aspiration of large quantities of acidic gastric secretions (pH $<$ 2.5). However, aspiration of heavily infected nasopharyngeal contents can also initiate necrotizing pulmonary infection or lung abscess formation. Although the onset of severe sequelae related to acid aspiration is usually acute, aspiration of infected or particulate matter is usually more insidious. Nevertheless, patients who do not develop coughing, wheezing, or hypoxemia when exposed to room air within 2 hours after suspected aspiration are unlikely to develop significant pulmonary sequelae.[103] **Common conditions that predispose patients to aspiration pneumonia include conditions that impair consciousness (e.g., anesthetic induction, alcohol ingestion, head trauma) and those assosiated with abnormal gastrointestinal (GI) function (e.g., small bowel obstruction, hiatal hernia, gastroparesis).**[25,47,57,87,103]

The diagnosis of gastric acid aspiration may be difficult to prove unless the aspiration was witnessed and gastric contents are seen in the airway or suctioned from the endotracheal tube. Significant gastric acid aspiration causes severe dyspnea, hypoxemia, wheezing, and subsequently, lobar pulmonary infiltrates on chest radiograph (Mendelson's syndrome). Pathologic examination early in gastric acid aspiration shows hemorrhagic pulmonary edema and microatelectasis but typically no bacteria. However, patients with acid aspiration may develop secondary bacterial infections caused by a variety of aerobic gram-positive and gram-negative organisms and may even initially present with signs of pulmonary infection.[47]

Therapy for aspiration of gastric contents includes protection of the airway (i.e., intubation), tracheal toilet, positive pressure ventilation, oxygenation, fluid resuscitation, and hemodynamic support.[107] Bronchoscopy with lavage may be performed to remove food or other large particles from the segmental bronchi and to culture the aspirate. Following gastric acid aspiration, bronchial lavage is not efficacious, as the effect of acid on lung parenchyma is immediate. Prophylactic antibiotics are not recommended; however, if evidence of infection occurs (fever, purulent sputum, progression of chest radiograph abnormality, septic shock), appropriate antibiotics should be administered.[47] Clinical practice favors administering antibiotics to patients who aspirate grossly infected material and to immunocompromised, neutropenic patients. The majority of investigators believe that corticosteroids are of no benefit and are potentially harmful for patients with gastric acid aspiration.[87]

Pulmonary infection

Infectious agents are commonly introduced into the lung by inhalation down the tracheal-bronchial tree and less commonly by hematogenous spread through the bronchial and pulmonary circulations.[17] After aspiration of infected nasopharyngeal secretions, nonhospitalized patients can develop anaerobic pulmonary infections (pneumonia and lung abscesses).[17,25,29] In contrast, gram-negative rods are found to colonize the upper airways of most hospitalized patients who have been intubated for more than a few days. In addition, after several days of antibiotic therapy, many nonintubated patients will develop colonization with antibiotic-resistant strains of gram-negative bacteria. These colonizing organisms may eventually produce infection in patients with an impaired immune defense. For example, upper airway defense mechanisms are bypassed by endotracheal intubation, impaired cough, and reduced mucociliary clearance.[24]

Pulmonary infection after upper abdominal surgery most often presents 24 to 48 hours postoperatively and ranges in incidence from 5% to 70%, depending on the diagnostic criteria used. Radiographic criteria tend to overestimate the incidence.[4,25] Most recent studies agree on an overall incidence of approximately 20%.[6,56] In healthy patients having surgery distant from the chest or upper abdomen, postoperative pulmonary infections are unusual.[34] Prophylactic antibiotic administrations to patients undergoing abdominal surgery have not proved beneficial in preventing postoperative pulmonary infection and may have harmful effects by increasing the antimicrobial resistance of bacterial flora.[34] Various techniques of postoperative pain control have been investigated for their beneficial effects on postoperative pulmonary infection, but results have been inconsistent.[4,5,28,37,56,60,82,84,86,88,91,94,108]

Exacerbation of Preoperative Pulmonary Disease

Chronic obstructive pulmonary disease

Chronic obstructive pulmonary disease (COPD) includes a spectrum of pulmonary diseases characterized by chronic cough and progressive reduction in expiratory airflow. Chronic bronchitis and emphysema are the two most common forms of COPD and are associated with distinctive pathophysiologic changes in the airways and the lung parenchyma. Although the damage associated with emphysema is permanent (destruction of alveolar septa and enlarged terminal airspaces), many of the pathophysiologic changes of bronchitis (mucus hypersecretion, mucosal edema, increases in airway resistance) can and should be improved before elective surgery. Most patients have components of both chronic bronchitis and emphysema with some element of acute airway obstruction responsive to bronchodilators. Preoperative pulmonary function studies before and after bronchodilators may be helpful in assessing the value for additional bronchodilator therapy. Evidence of active infection (purulent sputum, exacerbation of symptoms, new pulmonary infiltrates on chest radiograph) should be treated with appropriate antibiotics for at least several weeks before elective surgery. Preoperative teaching of coughing and breathing exercises will help facilitate postoperative pulmonary toilet. Clinicians should look for and treat any precipitating event in patients who develop a perioperative exacerbation of chronic bronchitis (Box 90-3).

BOX 90-3
COMMON CAUSES OF EXACERBATIONS OF COPD AND ASTHMA

Pulmonary infection
Congestive heart failure
Dehydration
Malabsorption of medications
Noncompliance with medications
Climate changes
Airway instrumentation
Noxious airway stimuli
Pulmonary emboli

Exacerbation of asthma

Exacerbation of asthma is a common occurrence in the perioperative period and can produce life-threatening physiologic abnormalities (e.g., ventilatory obstruction, hypoxemia, pneumothorax). Pathophysiologic abnormalities include bronchial smooth muscle contraction, bronchial mucosal edema with hypertrophy and hypersecretion, and an inflammatory infiltrate (neutrophils and eosinophils) in the peribronchial tissue. Both allergic (atopic disease) and nonallergic (exercise, cold air, environmental irritants, tracheal irritation, endotracheal intubation, and recent viral respiratory tract infections) mechanisms are known to produce exacerbations. Usually, nonallergic mechanisms are more prevalent in the perioperative period.

Asthma symptomatology depends on the severity of the airflow obstruction. Bronchospasm may be perceived as a cough or chest tightness if mild. When severe, it may produce dyspnea, wheezing, and labored respirations. In extreme cases, there may be no more than deadspace ventilation. Attempts at positive pressure ventilation may produce high airway pressures and little tidal volume. **Wheezing is a symptom of obstruction; however, all wheezing is not asthma. Conversely, in the patient with extremely severe airway obstruction, wheezing may be absent because airflow is so reduced.** In the postsurgical patient, there are several life-threatening conditions that may mimic asthma (Box 90-4).[85] Expiratory capnography may be useful in showing the characteristic ramp pattern with a delayed rise that never attains the true end-tidal CO_2 value. This is due to gas mixing heterogeneity caused by small airway obstruction.

Pulmonary Thromboembolism

Pulmonary embolism is usually caused by the migration of a lower extremity venous thrombosis (a clot formed in the venous system above the popliteal vein) which obstructs branches of the pulmonary artery. The most common clinical manifestation of pulmonary embolism in the spontaneously breathing patient is dyspnea, although many pulmonary emboli do not produce any symptoms. With larger emboli or pulmonary infarction, patients may develop severe hypoxemia, chest pain, bronchospasm, pulmonary infiltrates, or atelectasis. Catastrophic pulmonary emboli cause acute cor pulmonale and shock resulting from pulmonary vascular obstruction. Thus, the clinical diagnosis of embolism is difficult and requires a high index of suspicion.[64]

BOX 90-4
CAUSES OF PERIOPERATIVE WHEEZING

Large airway obstruction
- Foreign body aspiration
- Epiglottitis
- Pharyngeal abscess
- Anterior mediastinal mass
- Pneumothorax
- Endotracheal tube obstruction
- Anaphylaxis

Small airway obstruction
- Pulmonary edema
- Asthma
- Chronic obstructive pulmonary disease
- Pulmonary thromboembolism
- Anaphylaxis
- Histamine release

Pulmonary embolism is unusual without antecedent venous thrombosis. In addition, thrombi that are confined to the calf veins are associated with a much lower risk of pulmonary embolism than thrombi that extend above the popliteal veins. Thus, if proximal deep venous thrombosis (DVT) can be prevented, pulmonary embolism will also be prevented.

It has been estimated that each year five million patients in the United States develop venous thrombosis. Of these, 10% (500,000) have a pulmonary embolism, and 10% of these 500,000 (or 50,000) patients die from pulmonary embolism. In the absence of prophylaxis, the frequency of fatal postoperative pulmonary emboli ranges from 0.1% to 0.8% of patients undergoing elective general surgery, from 0.3% to 1.7% of patients undergoing elective hip surgery, and from 4% to 7% of patients undergoing emergency hip surgery.[46]

In 1986, the National Institutes of Health Consensus Development Conference supported the widespread use of prophylactic measures to guard against DVT in high-risk patients.[66] Heparin is the most commonly used drug for DVT prophylaxis. This drug activates plasma antithrombin III, which blocks the activity of several activated clotting factors. Intermittent pneumatic leg compression is another form of DVT prophylaxis that may decrease venostasis by increasing venous return through the deep veins of the lower limb to the central circulation.[21,42] A major advantage of intermittent pneumatic compression compared with heparin is that it has no deleterious effects on hemostasis. In addition, lumbar epidural and subarachnoid anesthesia have been shown to decrease the frequency of DVT when compared with general anesthesia in patients undergoing open surgery on the prostate and hip surgery.[22,63,77]

Clinicians cannot assume that negative studies of the leg veins rule out the diagnosis of embolism, because approximately 30% of patients with acute embolism will have negative venous studies (e.g., venography, impedance plethysmography, or radiolabeled fibrinogen scanning).[41] The only study, other than pulmonary angiography, that can reasonably exclude pulmonary embolism is ventilation/perfusion lung scanning.[40] Abnormal lung ventilation/perfusion scans are often nonspecific and may be caused by multiple conditions not necessarily related to pulmonary thromboembolism. However, if a scan is normal, significant pulmonary embolism is unlikely. However, if the perfusion scan is neither normal nor diagnostic of pulmonary embolism, pulmonary angiography may be required for a definitive diagnosis.[40,65]

SUMMARY

In summary, the risk of pulmonary complications associated with anesthesia is multifactorial. Factors which may affect risk include individual patient characteristics, type and site of surgery, and anesthetic technique. Factors which may modify risk include preoperative evaluation, patient optimization, intraoperative avoidance of precipitating factors, and preparation of a plan for postoperative care and monitoring.

KEY POINTS

- Perioperative pulmonary complications are associated with three factors: (1) the specific surgery and surgical incision site; (2) patient characteristics such as age, smoking, obesity, presence of COPD or cardiac disease; and (3) anesthetic technique.
- The supine position and general anesthesia produce a cephalad shift of the diaphragm, leading to decreased lung volumes, especially the functional residual capacity.
- Inhalation anesthetics inhibit hypoxic pulmonary vasoconstriction.
- Prolonged anesthesia may impair mucociliary clearance.
- After thoracic or abdominal surgery, patients develop restrictive pulmonary dysfunction.
- Most of the pulmonary effects caused by a general anesthetic are resolved within the first 2 hours postoperatively.
- Atelectasis is the most common cause of postoperative respiratory dysfunction.
- Respiratory center dysfunction is an expected effect of most opioid, barbiturate, and inhalational anesthetics.

- Postoperative pulmonary edema is generally caused by: (1) relative overhydration; (2) myocardial dysfunction; or (3) increased alveolar capillary permeability.
- Cardiogenic pulmonary edema is associated with increased CVP and increased PCWP.
- Patients with increased alveolar capillary permeability or ARDS have diffuse alveolar damage and present with severe dyspnea and hypoxemia, decreased lung compliance, and diffuse pulmonary infiltrates.
- Therapy for aspiration includes bronchoscopy to remove particulates but does not include prophylactic antibiotics and/or corticosteroids.
- All wheezing does not indicate asthma.
- The most common manifestation of pulmonary embolus is dyspnea, but catastrophic pulmonary emboli may present as acute cor pulmonale and shock.
- Each year, five million patients develop deep vein thrombosis; 10% progress to pulmonary emboli and of these, 10% die—50,000 deaths each year in the United States.

KEY REFERENCES

Ali J, Weisel RD, Layug AB, et al: Consequences of postoperative alterations in respiratory mechanics, *Am J Surg* 128:376, 1974.

American College of Physicians: Preoperative pulmonary function testing, *Ann Intern Med* 112:793,1990.

Brussel T, Matthay MA, Chernow B: Pulmonary manifestations of endocrine and metabolic disorders, *Clin Chest Med* 10:645, 1989.

Garibaldi RA, Britt MR, Coleman ML, et al: Risk factors for postoperative pneumonia, *Am J Med* 70:677, 1981.

Hedenstierna G: New aspects on atelectasis formation and gas exchange impairment during anesthesia, *Clin Physiol* 9:407, 1989.

Moser KM: Venous thromboembolism: state of the art, *Am Rev Respir Dis* 141:235, 1990.

National Institutes of Health Conference on the Scientific Basis of In-Hospital Respiratory Therapy, *Am Rev Resp Dis* 122:1, 1979.

National Institutes of Health Consensus Development Conference Statement: Prevention of venous thrombosis and pulmonary embolism, *Arch Intern Med* 146:463, 1986.

Schwieger I, Gamulin Z, Suter PM: Lung function during anesthesia and respiratory insufficiency in the postoperative period: physiological and clinical implications, *Acta Anaesthesiol Scand* 33:527, 1989.

Tarhan S, Moffitt EA, Sessler AD, et al: Risk of anesthesia and surgery in patients with chronic bronchitis and chronic obstructive pulmonary disease, *Surgery* 74:720, 1973.

Wahba RWM: Perioperative functional residual capacity, *Can J Anaesth* 38:384 1991.

Wynne JW, Modell JH: Respiratory aspiration of stomach contents, *Ann Intern Med* 87:466, 1977.

REFERENCES

1. Alexander JI, Spence AA, Parikh RK, et al: The role of airway closure in postoperative hypoxemia, *Br J Anaesth* 5:34, 1973.
2. Ali J, Weisel RD, Layug AB, et al: Consequences of postoperative alterations in respiratory mechanics, *Am J Surg* 128: 376, 1974.
3. American College of Physicians: Preoperative pulmonary function testing, *Ann Intern Med* 112:793,1990.
4. Anderson WH, Dossett Jr BE, Hamilton GL: Prevention of postoperative pulmonary complications, *JAMA* 186:763, 1963.
5. Aull L, Woodward ER, Rout RW, et al: Analgesia and postoperative hypoxemia after gastric partition with and without bupivacaine wound infiltration, *Can J Anaesth* 37:S53, 1990.
6. Baxter WD, Levine RS: An evaluation of intermittent positive pressure breathing in prevention of postoperative pulmonary complications, *Arch Surg* 98:795, 1969.
7. Beecher HK: Effect of laparotomy on lung volume: demonstration of a new type of pulmonary collapse, *J Clin Invest* 12:651, 1932.
8. Behrakis PK, Higgs BD, Bevan DR, et al: Partitioning of respiratory mechanics in halothane-anesthetized humans, *J Appl Physiol* 58:285, 1985.
9. Benumof JL, Wahrenbrock EA: Local effects of anesthetics on regional hypoxic pulmonary vasoconstriction, *Anesthesiology* 43:525, 1975.
10. Bersten A, Sibbald WJ: Acute lung injury in septic shock, *Crit Care Clin* 5:49, 1989.
11. Brismar B, Hedenstierna G, Lundquist H, et al: Pulmonary densities during anesthesia with muscular relaxation—a proposal for atelectasis, *Anesthesiology* 62:422, 1985.
12. Brismar B, Tokics PL, Strandbert A, et al: Postoperative analgesia with intrapleural-administration of bupivacaine-adrenaline, *Acta Anaesthesiol Scand* 31:515, 1987.
13. Bromage PR, Campores EM, Durant PAC, et al: Non-respiratory side effects of epidural morphine, *Anesth Analg* 61:490, 1982.
14. Brussel T, Matthay MA, Chernow B: Pulmonary manifestations of endocrine and metabolic disorders, *Clin Chest Med* 10:645, 1989.
15. Buda AJ, Pinsky MR, Ingels NB, et al: Effect of intrathoracic pressure on left ventricular performance, *N Engl J Med* 301:453, 1979.
16. Burger EJ Jr, Macklem P: Airway closure: demonstration by breathing 100% O_2 at low lung volumes and by N_2 washout, *J Appl Physiol* 25:139, 1968.
17. Cameron EW, Appelbaum PC, Pudifin D, et al: Characteristics and management of chronic destructive pneumonia, *Thorax* 35:340, 1980.
18. Celli BR: Respiratory muscle function, *Clin Chest Med* 7:567, 1986.
19. Celli BR, Rodriguez KS, Snider GL: A controlled trial of intermittent positive pressure breathing, incentive spirometry,

and deep breathing exercises in preventing pulmonary complications after abdominal surgery, *Am Rev Respir Dis* 130:12, 1984.
20. Chalon J, Tayyab MA, Ramanathan S: Cytology of respiratory epithelium as a predictor of respiratory complications after operation, *Chest* 67:32, 1975.
21. Clarke-Pearson DC, Synan IS, Hinshaw WM, et al: Prevention of postoperative venous thromboembolism by external pneumatic calf compression in patient with gynecologic malignancy, *Obstet Gynecol* 63:92, 1984.
22. Covert CR, Fox GS: Anesthesia for hip surgery in the elderly, *Can J Anaesth* 36:311, 1989.
23. Craig DB: Postoperative recovery of pulmonary function, *Anesth Analg* 60:46, 1981.
24. Craven DE, Steger KA: Nosocomial pneumonia in the intubated patient. New concepts on pathogenesis and prevention, *Infect Dis Clin North Am* 3:843, 1989.
25. Dal Santo G: Acid aspiration pathophysiologic aspects, prevention and therapy, *Int Anesthesiol Clin* 24:31, 1986.
26. Dohi S, Gold MI: Comparison of two methods of postoperative respiratory care, *Chest* 73:592, 1978.
27. Don HF, Wahba M, Guadradol L, et al: The effects of anesthesia and 100% oxygen on the functional residual capacity of the lungs, *Anesthesiology* 32:521, 1970.
28. Ellis DJ, Millar WL, Resiner LS: A randomized double blind comparison of epidural versus intravenous fentanyl infusion for analgesia after cesarean section, *Anesthesiology* 72:981, 1990.
29. Fein AM, Feinsilver SH, Niederman MS, et al: When the pneumonia doesn't get better, *Clin Chest Med* 8:529, 1987.
30. Froese AB, Sryan AC: Effects of anesthesia and paralysis on diaphragmatic mechanics in man, *Anesthesiology* 41:242, 1974.
31. Fulkerson WJ, MacIntyre N, Stamler J, et al: Pathogenesis and treatment of the adult respiratory distress syndrome, *Arch Intern Med* 156:29, 1996.
32. Gaensler EA, Cugell D, Lindgren I, et al: The role of pulmonary insufficiency in mortality and invalidism following surgery for pulmonary tuberculosis, *J Thorac Surg* 29:163, 1959.
33. Gamsu G, Singer MM, Vincent HH, et al: Postoperative impairment of mucous transport in the lung, *Am Rev Respir Dis* 114:673, 1976.
34. Garibaldi RA, Britt MR, Coleman ML, et al: Risk factors for postoperative pneumonia, *Am J Med* 70:677, 1981.
35. Gold MI, Helrich M: A study of the complications related to anesthesia in asthmatic patients, *Anesth Analg* 42:283, 1963.
36. Graig DG, Wahba WM, Don MF, et al: "Closing volume" and its relationship to gas exchange in the seated and supine position, *J Appl Physiol* 31:717, 1871.
37. Grant RP, Dolman JF, Harper JA, et al: Patient controlled lumbar epidural fentanyl for post thoracotomy pain, *Can J Anaesth* 37:S45, 1990.
38. Hedenstierna G: New aspects of atelectasis formation and gas exchange impairment during anesthesia, *Clin Physiol* 9:407, 1989.
39. Hedenstierna G, Bindslev L, Santesson J, et al: Airway closure in each lung of anesthetized human subjects, *J Appl Physiol* 50:55, 1981.
40. Hull R, Hirsh J, Carter CJ, et al: Pulmonary angiography, ventilation lung scanning and venography for clinically suspected pulmonary embolism with abnormal perfusion scans, *Ann Intern Med* 98:891, 1983.
41. Hull R, Taylor DW, Hirsh J, et al: Impedance plethysmography: the relationship between venous filling and sensitivity and specificity for proximal vein thrombosis, *Circulation* 58:896, 1978.
42. Inada K, Koike S, Shirai N, et al: Effects of intermittent pneumatic leg compression for prevention of postoperative deep venous thrombosis with special reference to fibrinolytic activity, *Am J Surg* 155:602, 1988.
43. Jackson CV: Preoperative pulmonary evaluation, *Arch Intern Med* 148:2120, 1988.
44. Julian OC, Lopez-Belio M, Dye WS: The median sternal incision in intracardiac surgery with extracorporeal circulatiol: a general evaluation of its use in heart surgery, *Surgery* 42:753, 1957.
45. Jung R, Wight J, Nusser R, et al: Comparison of 3 methods of respiratory care following upper abdominal surgery, *Chest* 78:31, 1980.
46. Kakkar VV, Stamatakis JD, Bentley PG, et al: Prophylaxis for postoperative deep-vein thrombisis, *JAMA* 241:39, 1979.
47. Kirsch CM, Sanders A: Aspiration pneumonia. Medical management, *Otolaryngol Clin North Am* 21:677, 1988.
48. Lindberg P, Gunnarsson L, Tokics E, et al: Atelectasis and lung function in the postoperative period, *Acta Anesthesiol Scand* 36:546, 1992.
49. Logas WG, El-Baz N, I-Ganzouri, et al: Continuous thoracic epidural analgesia for postoperative pain relief following thoracotomy: a randomized prospective study, *Anesthesiology* 67:787, 1987.
50. Lorch DG, Sahn SA: Post-extubation pulmonary edema following complete upper airway obstruction. Are certain patients at increased risk? *Chest* 90:802, 1986.
51. Manning HL: Peak airway pressure: why the fuss? *Chest* 105:242, 1994.
52. Marshall BE, Wyche MQ: Hypoxemia during and after anesthesia, *Anesthesiology* 37:178, 1972.
53. Mathes D: Bleomycin and hyperoxia exposure in the operating room, *Anesth Analg* 81:624, 1995.
54. Matthay MA, Chatterjee K: Bedside catheterization of the pulmonary artery: risks compared with benefits, *Ann Intern Med* 109:826, 1988.
55. Matthay MA, Weiner-Kronish JP: Respiratory management after cardiac surgery, *Chest* 93:693, 1989.
56. McCabe R, Reid WM, Knox WG: Evaluation of the use of a temporary percutaneous endotracheal catheter in the treatment and prevention of postoperative pulmonary complications, *Ann Surg* 156:5, 1962.
57. McCammon RL: Prophylaxis for aspiration pneumonitis, *Can Anaesth Soc J* 33:S47, 1986.
58. McCormack JP, Warriner CB, Levine M, et al: The use of regularly scheduled oral morphine in the treatment of post surgical pain secondary to total hip arthroplasty, *Can J Anaesth* 27:S57, 1990.
59. Meyers JR, Lembeck L, O'Kane H, et al: Changes in functional residual capacity of the lung after operation, *Arch Surg* 110:576, 1975.
60. Miguel RA, Barlow I, Morrell M, et al: A prospective, randomozed, double-blind comparison of epidural and intravenous sufentanil infusions, *Anesthesiology* 81: 346, 1994.
61. Mintzer RA, Sakowicz BA, Blonder JA: Lobar collapse. Usual and unusual forms, *Chest* 94:615, 1988.
62. Mitchell C, Garrahy P, Peake P: Postoperative respiratory morbidity: identification and risk factors, *Aust NZ J Surg* 52:203, 1982.
63. Modig J, Borg T, Karlstrom G, et al: Thromboembolism after total hip replacement: role of epidural and general anesthesia, *Anesth Analg* 62:174, 1983.
64. Moser KM: Venous thromboembolism: state of the art, *Am Rev Respir Dis* 141:235, 1990.
65. Moser KM, Fedullo PF: Venous thromboembolism: three simple decisions, *Chest* 83:117, 1983.
66. National Institutes of Health Consensus Development Conference Statement: Prevention of venous thrombosis and pulmonary embolism, *Arch Intern Med* 146:463, 1986.
67. National Institutes of Health Conference on the Scientific Basis of In-Hospital Respiratory Therapy, *Am Rev Resp Dis* 122:1, 1979.
68. Nunn JF, Bergman NA, Coleman AJ: Factors influencing the arterial oxygen tension during anesthesia with artificial ventilation, *Br J Anaesth* 37:898, 1965.
69. Nunn J, Milledge D, Chen D, et al: Respiratory criteria of fitness for surgery, *Anaesthesia* 43:543 1988.
70. O'Donohue Jr, WJ: National survey of the usage of lung expansion modalities for the prevention and treatment of postoperative atelectasis following abdominal and thoracic surgery, *Chest* 87:76, 1985.
71. Pasteur W: Active lobar collapse of the lung after abdominal operations: a contribution to the study of postoperative lung complications, *Lancet* 2:1080, 1910.
72. Pelosi P, Croci M, Calappi E, et al: The prone positioning during general anesthesia minimally affects respiratory mechanics while improving functional residual capacity and increasing oxygen tension, *Anesth Analg* 80:955, 1995.
73. Pedersen T, Eliasen K, Henriksen E: A prospective study of risk factors and cardiopulmonary complications associated with anaesthesia and surgery: risk indicators of cardiopulmonary morbidity, *Acta Anaesthesiol Scand* 34:144, 1990.
74. Pflug AE, Bonica JJ: Physiopathology and control of postoperative pain, *Arch Surg* 112:773, 1977.
75. Pietak S, Weenig CS, Hickey RF, et al: Anesthetic effects on ventilation in patients with chronic obstructive lung disease, *Anesthesiology* 42:160, 1975.
76. Pillow KJ, Moote CA, Komar WE, et al: Postoperative pain management in patients

with inflammatory bowel disease, *Can J Anaesth* 37:S57, 1990.

77. Poikolainen E, Hendolin H: Effects of lumbar epidural analgesia and general anesthesia on flow velocity in the femoral vein and postoperative deep vein thrombosis, *Acta Chir Scand* 149:361, 1983.
78. Pontoppidan H: Mechanical aids to lung expansion in nonintubated surgical patients, *Am Rev Respir Dis* 122(suppl):109, 1980.
79. Pratter MR, Irwin RS: Extrapulmonary causes of respiratory failure, *J Intens Care Med* 1:197, 1986.
80. Rall TW: Hypnotics and sedatives; ethanol. In Gilman AG, Rall TW, Nies AS, Taylor P, editors: *The pharmacological basis of therapeutics,* ed 8, New York, 1990, Pergamon Press.
81. Ravin MB: Comparison of spinal and general anesthesia for abdominal surgery in patients with chronic obstructive pulmonary disease, *Anesthesiology* 35:319, 1971.
82. Ready LB: Spinal opioids in the management of acute and postoperative pain, *J Pain Sympt Manage* 5:138, 1990.
83. Rehder K, Sessler AD, Marsh HM: General anesthesia and the lung, *Am Rev Respir Dis* 112:541, 1975.
84. Reimer EJ, Badner NH, Moote CA, et al: Bupivacaine added to epidural fentanyl does not improve postoperative analgesia, *Can J Anaesth* 37:S54, 1990.
85. Rodriguez Roisin R, Ballester E, Roca J, et al: Mechanisms of hypoxemia in patients with status asthmaticus requiring mechanical ventilation, *Am Rev Respir Dis* 139: 732, 1989.
86. Rosenberg PH, Scheinin BMA, Lepantalo MJA, et al: Continuous intrapleural infusion of bupivacaine for analgesia after thoracotomy, *Anesthesiology* 67:811, 1987.
87. Russin SJ, Adler AG: Pulmonary aspiration. The three syndromes, *Postgrad Med* 85:155, 1989.
88. Sandler AN: Epidural opiate analgesia for acute pain relief, *Can J Anaesth* 37:Sxxxiii, 1990.
89. Santiago TV, Edelman NH: Opioids and breathing, *J Appl Physiol* 59:1675, 1985.
90. Schmid ER, Rehder K: General anesthesia and the chest wall, *Anesthesiology* 55:668, 1981.
91. Schulman M, Sandler AN, Bradley JW, et al: Postthoracotomy pain and pulmonary function following epidural and systemic morphine, *Anesthesiology* 61:569, 1984.
92. Schwieger I, Gamulin Z, Suter PM: Lung function during anesthesia and respiratory insufficiency in the postoperative period: physiological and clinical implications, *Acta Anaesthesiol Scand* 33:527, 1989.
93. Simonneau G, Simonneau G, Vivien A, Sartene R: Diaphragm dysfunction induced by upper abdominal surgery: role of postoperative pain, *Am Rev Respir Dis* 128: 899, 1983.
94. Spenca AA, Smith G: Postoperative analgesia and lung function. A comparison of morphine with extradural block, *Br J Anaesth* 43:144, 1971.
95. Stein M, Koota GM, Simon M, et al: Pulmonary evaluation of surgical patients, *JAMA* 181:765, 1962.
96. Suter PM, Fairly HB, Schlobohm RM: Shunt, lung volume, and perfusion during short periods of ventilation with oxygen, *Anesthesiology* 43:617, 1975.
97. Tammeling G, Lanos C: An analysis of the pulmonary function of ninety patients following pulmonectomy for pulmonary tuberculosis, *J Thorac Surg* 37:148, 1959.
98. Tarhan S, Moffitt EA, Sessler AD, et al: Risk of anesthesia and surgery in patient with chronic bronchitis and chronic obstructive pulmonary disease, *Surgery* 74: 720, 1973.
99. Taylor P: Neuromuscular blocking agents. In Gilman AG, Rall TW, Nies AS, Taylor P, editors: *The pharmacological basis of therapeutics,* ed 8, New York, 1990, Pergamon Press.
100. Tisi GM: Preoperative evaluation of pulmonary function, *Am Rev Respir Dis* 119:293, 1979.
101. Tusiewicz K, Bryan AC, Froese AB: Contributions of changing rib cage-diaphragm interactions to the ventilatory depression of halothane anesthesia, *Anesthesiology* 47:327, 1977.
102. Wahba RWM: Perioperative functional residual capacity, *Can J Anaesth* 38:384 1991.
103. Warner MA, Warner ME, Weber JG: Clinical significance of pulmonary aspiration during the perioperative period, *Anesthesiology* 78:56 1993.
104. Westbrook PR, Stubbs SE, Sessler AD, et al: Effects of anesthesia and muscle paralysis on respiratory mechanics in normal man, *J Appl Physiol* 34:81, 1973.
105. Wightman JAK: A prospective survey of the incidence of postoperative pulmonary complications, *Br J Surg* 55:85, 1968.
106. Willms D, Shure D: Pulmonary edema due to upper airway obstruction in adults, *Chest* 94:1090, 1988.
107. Wynne JW, Modell JH: Respiratory aspiration of stomach contents, *Ann Intern Med* 87:466, 1977.
108. Yeager MP, Glass DD, Neff RK, et al: Epidural anesthesia and analgesia in high risk surgical patients, *Anesthesiology* 66:729, 1987.

CHAPTER 91

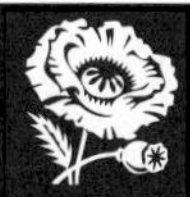

Protection of the Central Nervous System During Anesthesia and Surgery

DAVID S. WARNER
MICHAEL M. TODD

The human central nervous system (CNS) enjoys a structural and functional complexity of unparalleled proportions. To support its energetics, a substantial component of human physiology is dedicated to providing a continuous supply of substrate for neuronal metabolic requirements. Although the brain constitutes approximately 2% of adult body weight (i.e., 1500 g), 15% to 20% of cardiac output (expressed as cerebral blood flow [CBF]) is normally required to maintain viability. Despite this, the CNS exists in a precarious balance of metabolic supply versus demand because there are little or no tissue stores of critical metabolic substrates (i.e., O_2 and glucose). To compensate for this, the brain tightly couples blood flow (i.e., substrate delivery) to functional activity (i.e., metabolic requirements). Thus increases (or decreases) in metabolism result in increases (or decreases) in supply (Fig. 91-1).[158] Obviously, disease states that invoke surgical therapy, anesthetic effects that become necessarily coexistent, or preexisting neurologic disorders in surgical patients may perturb this delicate balance and can potentially threaten tissue viability. This chapter explores several factors relevant to minimizing neurologic complications of anesthesia and surgery. First, we will examine the epidemiology of CNS injury in surgical patients. This will be followed by a discussion of normal CNS physiology juxtaposed with pathophysiology associated with ischemia. Particular emphasis has been placed on factors that the anesthesia provider might manipulate and how these factors might relate to ischemic outcome.

EPIDEMIOLOGY OF PERIOPERATIVE CENTRAL NERVOUS SYSTEM ISCHEMIA

Depending on the surgical procedure and the patient population, patients undergoing anesthesia may be at either very low or very high risk for intraoperative ischemic insults to the brain or spinal cord. For example, in a multi-institutional prospective outcome analysis of 17,201 patients undergoing general anesthesia, Forrest et al.[51,52] reported only seven cases of cerebral infarction, yielding an overall stroke rate of 0.41/1000 patients (.04%). Although patients had been randomized to four discrete anesthetic agent regimens, the stroke rate was too low to allow outcome differences to be distinguished on the basis of anesthetic agent, if in fact, any existed at all.

The overall incidence of perioperative stroke appears to be exceedingly rare. The mean age of studied patients was

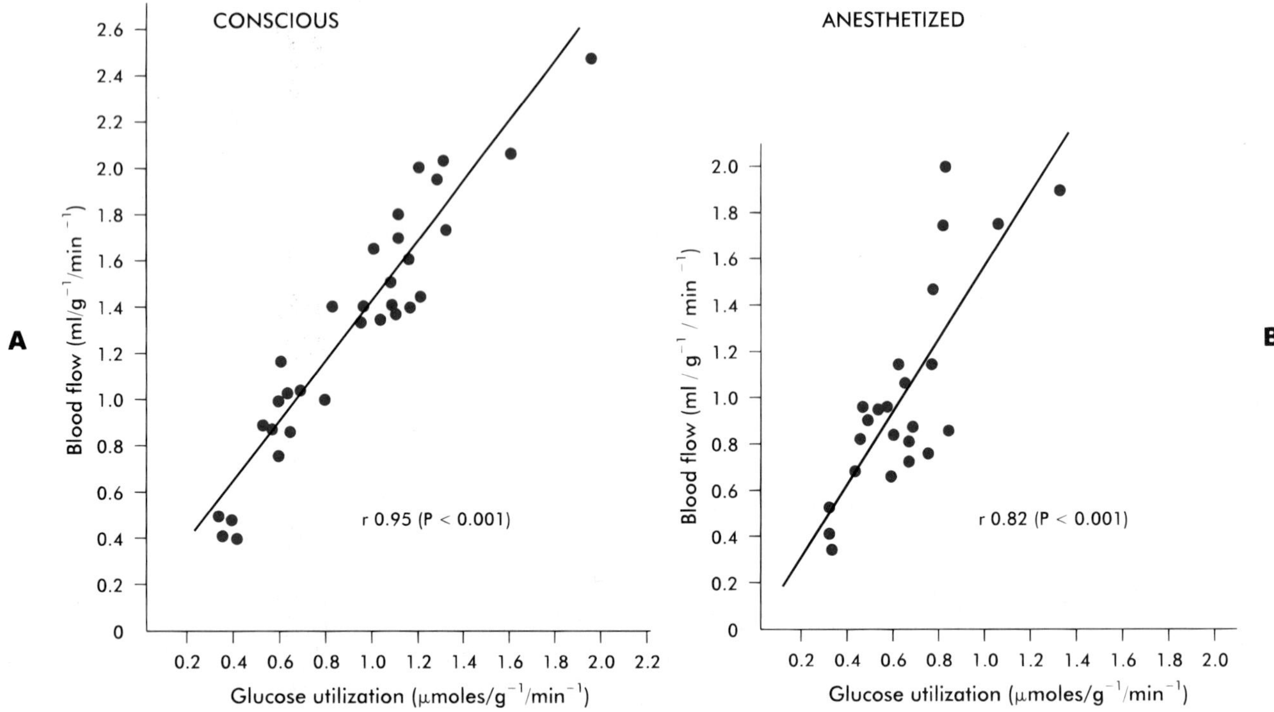

Fig. 91-1. Correlation between local cerebral blood flow, measured with the [^{14}C]iodoantipyrine technique (Sakaruda et al. 1978)[139] and local cerebral utilization of glucose measured with the [^{14}C]deoxyglucose technique (Sokoloff et al. 1977).[159] Each point represents a different structure in the brain. **A,** Normal conscious rat. Each point represents the mean local glucose use obtained from 10 rats and the mean local blood flow obtained from six rats. **B,** Animals under thiopental anesthesia. Each point represents the mean values of local glucose use and blood flow obtained from eight animals and six animals, respectively. (From Sokoloff L: Local cerebral energy metabolism: its relationships to local functional activity and blood flow. In Purves MJ, Elliot K, eds: *Cerebral vascular smooth muscle and its control,* CIBA Foundation Symposium, Amsterdam, 1978, Elsevier.)

43 years, allowing a distinct possibility that in an older patient population the stroke rate might be substantially different. In addition, only 5% of the procedures were neurologic in nature, again allowing the possibility that stroke rates may be different if specific procedures are evaluated. The follow-up interval was a maximum of 7 days. Although this seems adequate to identify sequelae directly attributable to intraoperative events, it would be inadequate to identify patients showing delayed signs of CNS injury that may be more subtle and therefore identifiable only when they attempt to resume normal activities.

There is evidence that the perioperative stroke rate for non-neurologic procedures is greater in a more elderly population. Larsen, Zaric, and Boysen[95] reported on 2463 general surgical patients, 40 years of age or older (mean age, 65 years), who were prospectively followed-up for occurrence of perioperative stroke after general surgery. Of those patients, nine showed new focal deficits. Four had major strokes, two had minor strokes, and three had transient ischemic attacks (TIAs). If those patients with TIAs were excluded, the risk of sustaining permanent neurologic sequelae was 0.2% (five times the 0.04% previously discussed). All nine patients had at least one preoperative manifestation of atherosclerosis. Symptoms tended to develop late in the postoperative course (range, 5 to 26 days after operation; mean, 10 days); no patient had evidence of stroke in the immediate postoperative period. Analysis of intraoperative events that may have presaged the strokes (e.g., hypotension) failed to identify risk factors of the anesthetic or surgery, with the exception of a bias for increased incidence of stroke in procedures that were emergent instead of elective. Postoperative factors associated with stroke included dehydration and atrial fibrillation. The authors also attempted to determine if this stroke rate was greater than would be observed in a demographically similar nonhospitalized group. Relying on a previous data base, it could be predicted that of 2463 nonhospitalized people with a mean age of 65, one person would have a stroke, whereas over the same interval of time six hospitalized patients had permanent injury. This confirms an increased rate of stroke attributable to surgical hospitalization.

As indicated, the incidence of perioperative neurologic complications also depends on the procedure. Whereas elderly general surgical patients have a stroke rate of 0.2%, the incidence of stroke associated with carotid endarterectomy (CEA) is approximately 3% to 5%.[69] For cardiopulmonary bypass, obvious neurologic deficits may occur in as many as 7.5% of the cases.[120] When more subtle psychometric analyses are applied, the incidence of neurologic sequelae has been reported to be as high as 60%.[15,76,145,157] Other procedures involving high risks of CNS injury include thoracic aortic aneurysm repair (up to 42%),[22,43,138,164] cerebral aneurysm clipping (18%),[168] craniotomy for excision of tumor (3% mortality, 20% neurologic morbidity),[49,171] and certain scoliosis procedures (1% to 17%).[100,189]

Although variations in reported incidence of neurologic sequelae seem to depend on the quality of medical care provided as much as any other factor, these statistics provide insight into the magnitude of the problem as well as the conditions under which ischemic CNS injury might occur. Perhaps the most convincing evidence that ischemic injury is to be meticulously avoided is the clinical experience gained by caring for patients who have sustained such a complication.

PHYSIOLOGY AND PHARMACOLOGY OF CEREBRAL ISCHEMIA

The brain tightly regulates the relationship between metabolic supply and demand. Superimposed on this is autoregulation (i.e., stable blood flow over a range of perfusion pressures), as well as reactivity to $Paco_2$ and hypoxia (Fig. 91-2).[144] The normal human brain uses approximately 75 mg glucose/min (25 μmol/100 g/min), which combined with a cerebral metabolic rate for O_2 use of 5 ml/100 g/min, provides sufficient energy to sustain both structure and function. When an agent, such as a barbiturate, is administered in a quantity sufficient to produce an isoelectric electroencephalogram (EEG), the metabolic requirements are reduced by approximately 50% (Fig. 91-3).[107] This, perhaps more than coincidentally, corresponds to the appearance of ischemic EEG changes that occur with a reduction of CBF by 50% to 60% from normal (Fig. 91-4).[7,106] Below this threshold for transmission of action potentials, the neuron also requires energy for maintenance of ionic electrochemical gradients between the intracellular and extracellular environments. Additional thresholds exist for energetic requirements associated with protein and lipid synthesis to maintain structural integrity. Although the brain may tolerate a transient reduction of flow below any of these thresholds, it seems clear that loss of ionic homeostasis (particularly for calcium) is most closely associated with eventual neuronal death.

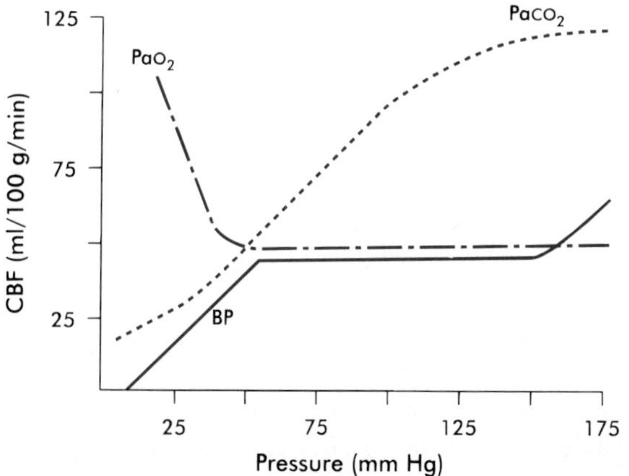

Fig. 91-2. Cerebral blood flow changes related to alterations in $Paco_2$, Pao_2, and blood pressure (*solid line*). The other two variables remain stable at normal values when the remaining variable is altered. (From Shapiro HM, Anesthesia effects upon cerebral blood flow, cerebral metabolism, and the electroencephalogram. In Miller RD, editor: *Anesthesia,* New York, 1981, Churchill-Livingstone.)

Calcium Homeostasis

The intracellular calcium ion concentration is used to regulate numerous intracellular functions. Because the extracellular/intracellular Ca^{++} concentration gradient is normally 10,000:1, considerable energy is required to maintain this gradient. The neuron has several mechanisms that allow transport of Ca^{++} into the cell. Intracellular concentrations may also be controlled by binding with calmodulin and sequestration of Ca^{++} into organelles. Finally, transport of Ca^{++} out of the cell occurs via energy-dependent processes (Fig. 91-5). It is clear that an overload of intracellular Ca^{++} leads to irreversible injury of the neuron,[175] and this has been suggested to be the final common pathway of ischemically mediated neuronal death.[151,152]

Not surprisingly, attention has focused on methods that might inhibit entry of Ca^{++} into the energy-deficient neuron. As can be observed in Fig. 91-5, Ca^{++} may enter via either voltage-sensitive Ca^{++} channels (VSCC), which are opened on neuronal depolarization (either physiologic or as a terminal event), or via agonist-operated channels (AOCC), which are activated by release of excitatory neurotransmitters from the presynaptic cell (i.e., glutamate or aspartate).[152] Pharmacologic agents have been identified that inhibit the influx of Ca^{++} through either portal of entry, and under some conditions, these agents improve outcome from ischemic events.

A prototypical VSCC antagonist is the dihydropyridine compound, nimodipine. This agent, which also exhibits preferential cerebrovascular dilation[8] (thus the simultaneous interest in this drug as treatment for cerebral vasospasm[15,131,143]), has been evaluated for efficacy in treating humans with brain ischemia under several different conditions. With respect to global ischemia, Forsman et al.[53] reported on the administration of nimodipine during out-of-hospital resuscitation from cardiac arrest. Although treated patients exhibited more rapid return to consciousness and greater CBF during subsequent evaluation, no improvement in final neuro-

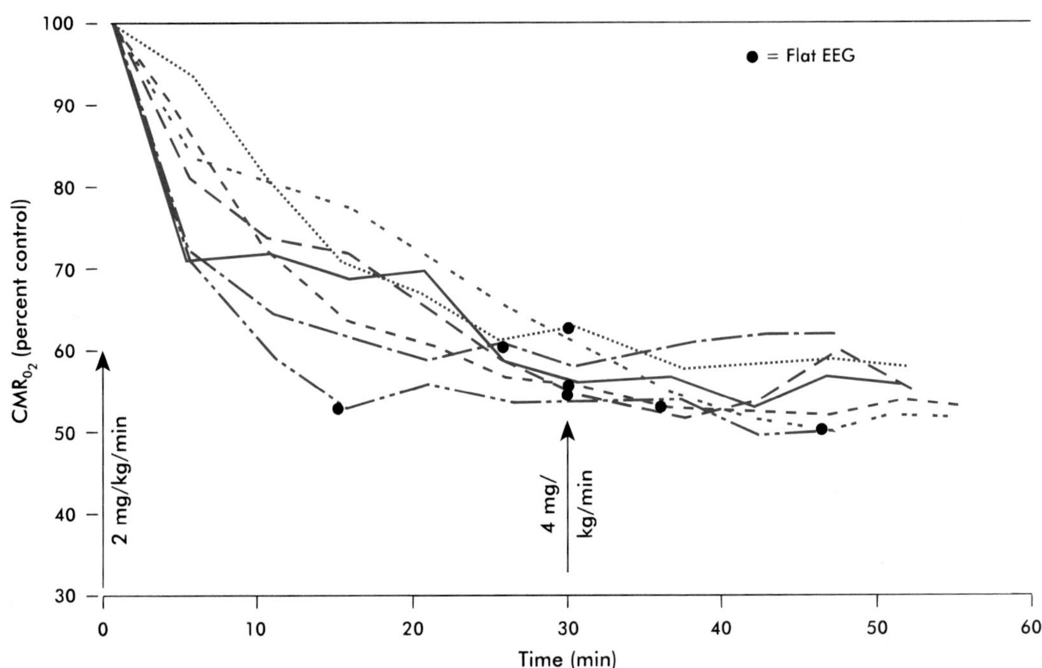

Fig. 91-3. Individual $CMRo_2$ values plotted as percentages of control (initial) values determined before initiating thiopental infusion but after establishing partial cardiopulmonary bypass. In each dog, $CMRo_2$ decreased progressively until EEG became isoelectric. At this point, $CMRo_2$ stabilized and despite continued infusion of thiopental, did not decrease further. (From Michenfelder JD: The interdependency of cerebral function and metabolic effects following massive doses of thiopental in the dog, *Anesthesiology* 41:231, 1974.)

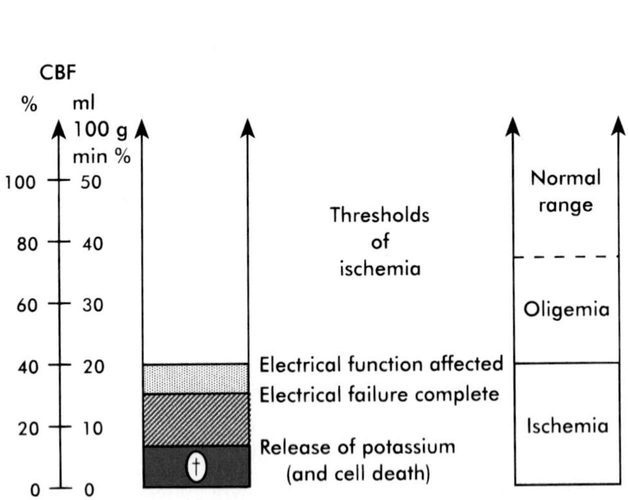

Fig. 91-4. Ischemic thresholds for electrical failure and for release of cellular K^+ (ion-pump failure). (From Astrup J, Symon L, Branston N, et al: Cortical evoked potential and extracellular K^+ and H^+ at critical levels of brain ischemia, *Stroke* 8:51, 1977.)

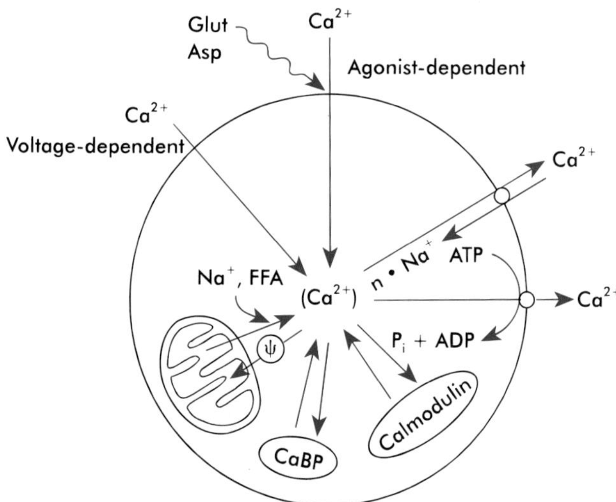

Fig. 91-5. Cellular influx of Ca^{++} via agonist- and voltage-dependent channels, Ca^{++} efflux by Na^+/Ca^{++} exchange and by Ca^{++}-ATPase activity, and sequestration of Ca^{++} by electrophoretic uptake into mitochondria and by binding to calmodulin and Ca^{++} binding protein (CaBP). Efflux of Ca^{++} from mitrochondria is shown to be enhanced by Na^+ and free fatty acids (FFA). (From Siesjö BK, Wieloch T: Molecular mechanisms of ischemic brain damage: Ca^{++}-related events. In Plum F, Pulsinelli W, editors: *Cerebrovascular diseases,* New York, 1985, Raven.)

logic status was observed when compared with those treated with placebo. The study was performed on a small group of patients. A larger similar study was completed in Finland, but again little benefit for nimodipine was observed.[137]

Nimodipine has also been evaluated in the context of focal ischemia (stroke) in humans.[23,60,103,125] Most of these studies can be criticized on methodologic grounds (e.g., small sample sizes, delayed institution of therapy), but the trend suggests modest improvement in outcome if nimodipine is administered (Fig. 91-6).[61] None of the studies found the administration of nimodipine to be detrimental (i.e., its systemic vasodilatory effects are well tolerated).[50] Nimodipine has also been found to be efficacious in the treatment of vasospasm caused by subarachnoid hemorrhage and has generally been accepted as a requisite therapy in the treatment of this disorder.[2,121] It remains unclear as to whether improved outcome is attributable to direct neuroprotection versus direct vascular effects of the drug. Nicardipine, an analog of nimodipine, has also been shown to reduce incidence of symptomatic vasospasm in patients with subarachnoid hemorrhage. Despite this, long-term neurologic outcome was not superior to treatment with hypertensive-hypervolemic therapy.[72,73] Clearly, the overall clinical effect of inhibition of Ca^{++} entry via VSCC is weak. This may be because antagonism of the VSCC does little to inhibit Ca^{++} entry via agonist-operated portals of Ca^{++} entry which provide high conductivity for Ca^{++} in the ischemic state.

Pharmacologic blockade of the AOCC has been achieved with numerous compounds. Such drugs may have activity at either the receptor for the excitatory neurotransmitters (competitive antagonists) or at the ion channels associated with these receptors (noncompetitive antagonists) (Fig. 91-7). Drugs exhibiting either property have been evaluated for protective efficacy. The prototype drug for noncompetitive antagonism of the N-methyl-D-aspartate (NMDA) receptor is dizocilpine (MK-801). This agent increases both blood flow and metabolism in a variety of cerebral structures, has been associated with ketaminelike psychotomimetic side effects and has anesthetic attributes.[91,128,141] In cats, dizocilpine is highly effective in reducing infarct

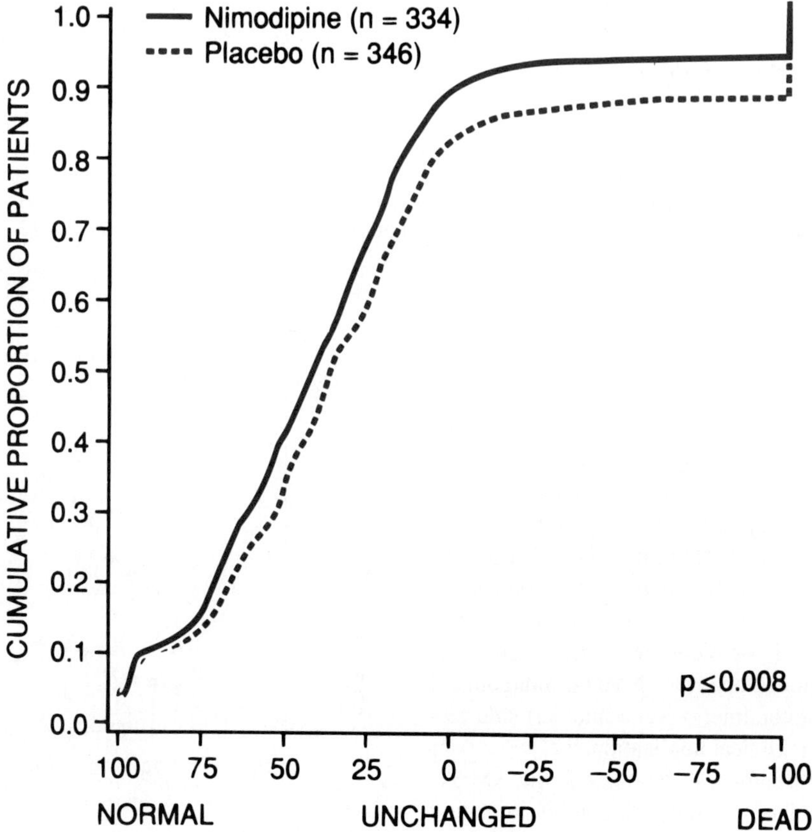

Fig. 91-6. A meta-analysis was performed on the results of five studies which examined the efficacy of nimodipine as a therapy for stroke in humans. This cumulative frequency histrogram depicts percentage change in neurologic impairment as a function of treatment group. Although a statistically significant benefit from the drug was found, the effect on the overall population was small. (From Gelmers HJ, Hennerici M: Effect of nimodipine on acute ischemic stroke: Pooled results from five randomized trials, *Stroke* 21 (suppl IV): IV-81, 1990.)

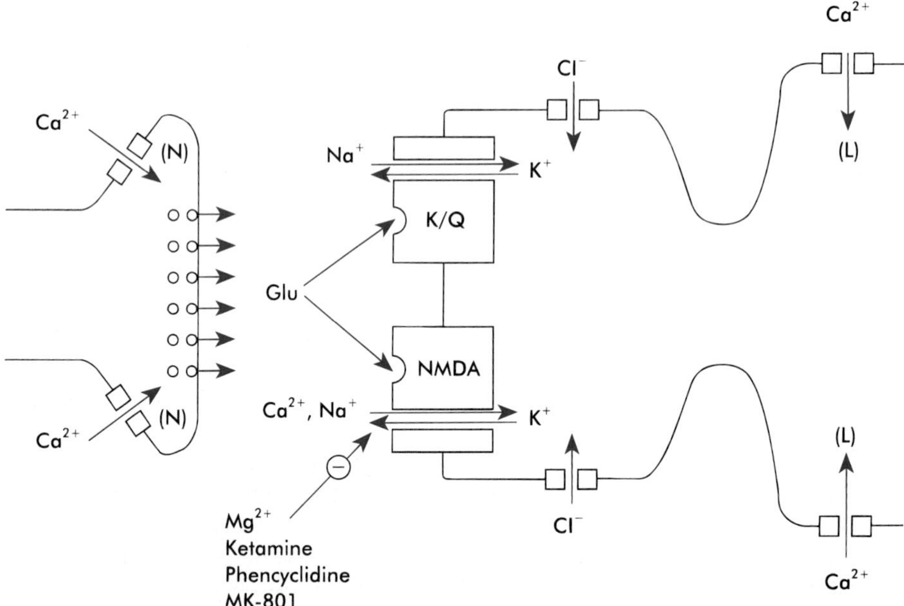

Fig. 91-7. Diagram illustrating presynaptic voltage-sensitive calcium channels (VSCCs) and postsynaptic agonist-operated calcium channels (AOCCs). Presynaptically, VSCCs involved in transmitter release are assumed to be the N type (*N*), which is not sensitive to calcium antagonists. At the postsynaptic site, kainate/quisqualate-operated channels (*K/Q*) are assumed to allow Na^+ influx and thereby to cause depolarization, whereas N-methyl-D-aspartate-operated channels (*NMDA*) are assumed to allow calcium influx. The ionic shifts at the K/Q and NMDA–gated channels occur when the K/Q and NMDA receptors are activated by glutamate (*Glu*), respectively. When Na^+ enters the cell postsynaptically, electrostatic forces are assumed to cause Cl^- influx along voltage-sensitive or agonist-operated channels. Na^+ and Cl^- entry is accompanied by osmotically obligated water that can result in swelling of apical dendrites. On the central dendrite or cell soma, VSCCs of the L type (*L*) are assumed to be located to allow Ca^{++} entry. (From Siesjö B, Bengttson F: Calcium fluxes, calcium antagonists, and calcium-related pathology in brain ischemia, hypoglycemia, and spreading depression: a unifying hypothesis, *J Cereb Blood Flow Metab* 9:127, 1989.)

volume resulting from permanent middle cerebral artery occlusion whether administered before or shortly after onset of the insult (Fig. 91-8).[124,126,127] In contrast, in well-controlled animal studies of global ischemia, dizocilpine has been found to offer no benefit.[93,108] Therefore, noncompetitive antagonism of the NMDA receptor presents a pattern of neuroprotection similar to that of barbiturates (i.e., efficacy in focal but not global ischemia). Competitive antagonism of glutamate at the NMDA receptor has also been shown to be effective in reducing focal ischemic injury.[130] Unfortunately, both competitive and noncompetitive NMDA antagonists have considerable psychotomimetic (ketaminelike) side effects that will likely limit clinical application.[70]

Another subtype of receptor for glutamate is the AMPA (formerly named quisqualate) receptor. Competitive antagonists for this receptor have been identified (e.g., NBQX). In contrast to antagonism of the NMDA receptor, competitive antagonism of glutamate neurotransmission at the AMPA receptor is efficacious in reducing damage resulting from both focal and global ischemia.[25, 26,117,146] The psychotomimetic properties of AMPA receptor blockade have not been determined, although it seems likely that effects will be minimal.

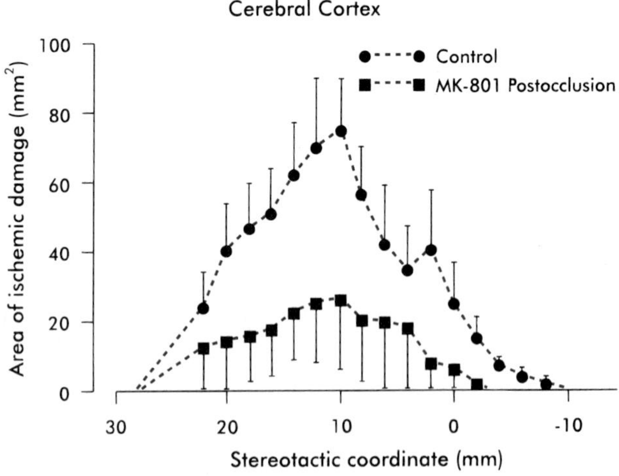

Fig. 91-8. The effect of dizocilpine (5 mg/kg, IV), administered 2 hours after middle cerebral artery occlusion, on the area of ischemic damage in the cerebral cortex at 16 defined coronal planes. Data (mean ± SEM) represent eight control and seven dizocilpine-treated cats. (From Park CK, Nehls D, Graham D, et al: Focal cerebral ischaemia in the cat: treatment with the glutemate agonist MK-801 after induction of ischaemia, *J Cereb Blood Flow Metab* 8:757, 1988.)

It is also possible to inhibit glutamatergic activation of the NMDA receptor by antagonizing glycine at its recognition site, and this has potential significance for the ischemic brain. Both glycine and glutamate are required to coactivate the NMDA receptor before the associated ionophore becomes permeable to calcium.[44,54,97] Glycine has been demonstrated to potentiate glutamate toxicity in cultured neurons.[84] Further, interstitial glycine concentrations become substantially increased during an ischemic insult and remain elevated for prolonged intervals after reperfusion.[12,68] In laboratory models of either ischemia or head trauma, a reduction in injury has been observed following use of glycine recognition site antagonists.[62,118,167,174,182] To date, adverse psychotomimetic effects of these compounds have not been observed, a potential distinct advantage over both competitive and noncompetitive NMDA receptor antagonists.[14,70] These same drugs have anesthetic potential allowing halothane minimum alveolar concentration (MAC) to be reduced to zero in rodent models.[104] Ongoing investigations may define the importance of this mechanistic approach to potential intraoperative neuroprotection.

Effects of Anesthetic Agents on the Ischemic Brain

The brain tightly couples metabolic requirements with substrate delivery. If delivery is insufficient, intracellular energy charge deteriorates and function fails. It has long been assumed that during ischemia, adverse sequelae of reduced supply can be at least temporarily offset by reduction in demand. Investigation of this therapeutic potential has essentially been the domain of anesthesia providers because of the efficacy of many anesthetic agents in decreasing cerebral metabolic rate (CMR), most commonly by virtue of a reduction in cerebral electrical activity. It became clear early on that such an approach would have specific limits. It has additionally become clear that simple pharmacologic reduction of CMR is insufficient to protect the brain. This section will review classical concepts of how anesthetic agents might provide protection (i.e., CMR reduction) and offer examples of emerging insights into other possible roles anesthetics may play.

A classic example of the limitations of pharmacologic reduction of brain electrical activity as a protective measure was provided by Michenfelder and Theye.[111] Dogs were either treated or untreated with large doses of barbiturate before onset of ischemia. Both groups received an ischemic insult (hemorrhagic hypotension), which was sufficiently severe to cause attenuation but not abolition of the EEG. Cerebral energy charge was better preserved in the barbiturate-treated group. In contrast, if the insult was produced by anoxia, wherein the EEG became isoelectric, barbiturates had no effect. Based on this observation, it was predicted that when outcome studies are performed, barbiturates (and perhaps other CMR depressants) will be beneficial only in circumstances when some electrical (i.e., synaptic) activity would prevail. This prediction makes sense: If a drug reduces metabolic demand by reducing electrical activity, there should be some electrical activity for the drug to suppress if any benefit is to occur.

This prediction has proven correct for barbiturates over two decades of research. For example, during focal ischemia when only part of the brain undergoes a reduction in flow (and that reduction is graded over a range of tissue), barbiturate therapy has repeatedly proved successful in improving outcome.[109,116,120,155,185] In contrast, during global ischemia, when the EEG is severely attenuated or isoelectric, barbiturates have failed to offer benefit.[24,65,160] This was well demonstrated in a human study wherein thiopental was administered immediately after successful cardiopulmonary resuscitation (CPR) following cardiac arrest.[24] There was no benefit from the therapy with respect to neurologic outcome or survival. There are few perioperative conditions when pharmacologic reduction in metabolic demand may be efficacious; such situations occur primarily in the domain of temporary intracranial vascular occlusion (e.g., aneurysm surgery) or perhaps during some conditions of normothermic cardiopulmonary bypass (e.g., open ventricular procedures) when emboli may elicit a pattern of focal ischemia.[120] It is of note that there is little or no experimental support for barbiturate therapy for the patient undergoing coronary artery bypass grafting during hypothermic cardiopulmonary bypass.[170,192]

Barbiturates produce simultaneous reductions in electrical activity and cerebral metabolic rate as well as an increased tolerance of the brain to focal ischemic challenges. It seems reasonable to conclude the mechanism of barbiturate protection rests on the CMR depressant effect. Extension of this logic suggests that other drugs that also substantially reduce CMR (e.g., isoflurane, etomidate, midazolam, propofol, lidocaine) will offer protection under similar circumstances. Unfortunately, this has not been the case, at least for isoflurane, which has been the most extensively evaluated nonbarbiturate CMR depressant. Early work indicated that, like barbiturates, isoflurane offers no benefit during near-complete global ischemia (even of brief duration).[178] It was an unexpected finding that isoflurane offers no greater benefit during focal ischemia than does halothane, a drug which produces only modest CMR reduction.[59,185] The neuroprotective potency of isoflurane was considerably less than that of thiopental in a baboon focal ischemia outcome study (Fig. 91-9).[116] Despite the fact that fewer episodes of EEG occur in humans anesthetized with isoflurane as opposed to enflurane or halothane while undergoing CEA, neurologic outcome is not improved.[110]

The failure of isoflurane to offer protection comparable with that of barbiturates is puzzling and raises several questions about anesthetic meditated neuroprotection. One possibility is that isoflurane produces an adverse effect which counteracts benefit from CMR reduction. Because the drug is a cerebrovasodilator, there is possibility of a blood flow steal from greater resistance vessels providing collateral flow to ischemic tissue. When the latter was examined in a

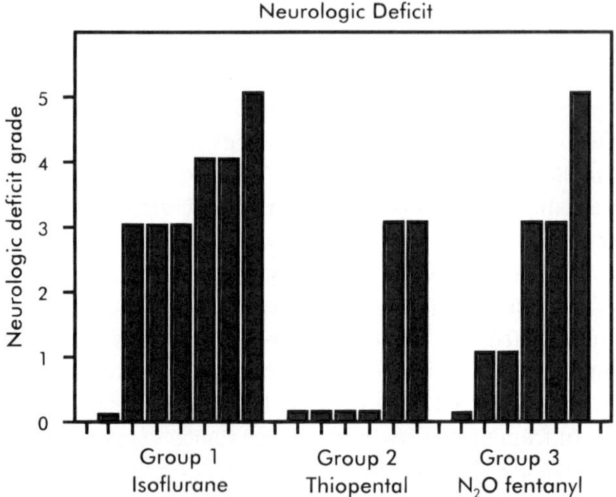

Fig. 91-9. Neurologic deficit scores assessed 7 days after recovery from 6 hours of middle cerebral artery occlusion in the baboon. Three anesthetic regimens administered during the ischemic insult were evaluated: deep isoflurane, deep thiopental, or N_2O/fentanyl. A score of "0" indicates a normal neurologic examination, whereas a score of "5" indicates death. (From Nehls D, Todd M, Spetzler, et al: A comparison of the cerebral protective effects of isoflurance and barbiturates during temporary focal ischemia in primates, *Anesthesiology* 66:453, 1987.)

rat model of middle cerebral artery occlusion, no evidence was found for a steal.[180]

Another possibility is that barbiturates have unique beneficial properties which contribute to their efficacy. Barbiturates do act as free-radical scavengers (a property not identified for isoflurane).[156] Barbiturates also produce antagonism of glutamate neurotoxicity.[122] Interestingly, however, both isoflurane and halothane have been shown to also be effective inhibitors of ion flux through glutamate-activated Ca^{++} channels although the relative potencies of volatile anesthetics and barbiturates is unknown.[6,191]

Regardless of mechanism, to date, the only clinically available pharmacologic CMR depressants that have been consistently demonstrated to improve the brain's tolerance to ischemia are in the barbiturate family. Other agents, such as propofol, midazolam, etomidate, or lidocaine, which offer CBF/CMR profiles similar to the barbiturates,[16,112,119] have only been partially evaluated during ischemia, and are not currently recommended as substitutes for barbiturates. Consequently, barbiturates remain the most reliable of the CMR depressants when brain ischemia is anticipated and even then only under very specific circumstances can a protective effect be anticipated.

The dose of barbiturate required to elicit maximal effect has often been believed to be that dose which provides complete suppression of the EEG. In fact, the experimental basis for this practice is weak. A few early studies examined the dose responsivity of barbiturate protection in focal ischemia models.[41,79] These studies were performed prior to recognition that critical physiologic factors (including brain temperature, blood pressure, and blood glucose) should be controlled for meaningful interpretation of neuroprotective efficacy. Given the fact that isoflurane offers protection inferior to that of barbiturates, despite similar reductions in CMR, it seems reasonable that maximal neuroprotection can be achieved with substantially lesser doses. In the rat focal ischemia model, this has been found to be the case (Fig. 91-10).[184] Most likely, the reason why EEG burst suppression has become an established endpoint for barbiturate administration is because it is discrete and easy to identify. A drug dose large enough to produce this EEG effect also means that a lengthy delay in emergence from anesthesia can be expected. Although it has been shown that most patients readily tolerate the hemodynamic effects of these large doses of barbiturate,[161,169] available theoretical and experimental evidence indicates that substantially lesser doses of barbiturates may be sufficient in providing maximal neuroprotective benefit.

There is an alternative hypothesis concerning how anesthetic agents might influence ischemic brain damage. This is derived from several experimental sources. Rats were exposed to transient spinal cord ischemia when either awake or anesthetized with a variety of agents. Regardless of drug, anesthetized animals had better neurologic recovery than those which were awake.[40] In another model of hemispheric ischemia (combined unilateral carotid artery occlusion and systemic hypotension) most every anesthetic examined provides superior neurologic/histologic outcome when compared with low doses of fentanyl and N_2O.[17,80,89] In a rat model of transient focal ischemia, halothane, sevoflurane, and pentobarbital all caused substantial improvement in neurologic/histologic outcome when compared with animals maintained awake during the ischemic insult (Fig. 91-11).[181,183,184]

What possible mechanistic basis explains this apparent ability of the state of anesthesia to provide neuroprotection given the disparity of pharmacologic effects of these various compounds? It has been proposed that this is attributable to obtundation of a stress response to ischemic injury. Evidence supporting this is derived again from the hemispheric incomplete ischemia model.[81,187] In one study, rats were administered the ganglionic blocker hexamethonium before ischemia.[187] This resulted in substantial reduction of circulating plasma catecholamines and a major improvement in histologic outcome. The beneficial neuroprotective effect of ganglionic blockade was reversed by intravenous (IV) infusion of epinephrine indicating an adverse effect of catecholamines on ischemic injury. Although others have found, to the contrary, that circulating catecholamines have beneficial effects on ischemic outcome,[71,90] interactions between anesthetic effects on the adrenergic nervous system and mechanisms of ischemic injury are of potential importance to understanding how anesthesia can modulate ischemic injury.

HYPOTHERMIA

Hypothermia as a strategy for intraoperative neuroprotection has been recognized for decades. It was largely abandoned

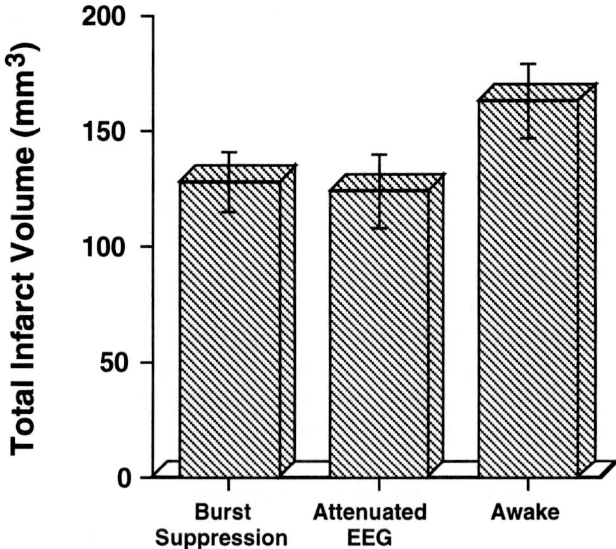

Fig. 91-10. Mean ± SEM infarct volumes in rats maintained either awake or anesthetized with pentobarbital so as to produce an attenuated EEG or EEG burst suppression during 90 minutes of temporary middle cerebral artery occlusion (MCAO). Low-dose pentobarbital resulted in a 25% reduction in total infarct volume compared with awake rats. A larger dose of pentobarbital provided no additional benefit (Warner DS, Takaoka S, Wu B, et al: Electroencephalographic burst suppression is not required to elicit maximal neuroprotection from pentobarbital in a rat model of focal cerebral ischemia, *Anesthesiology* 84:475–484, 1996).

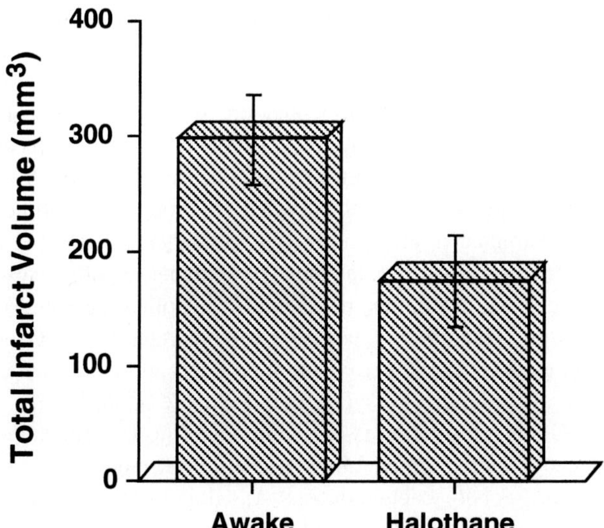

Fig. 91-11. Total infarct volumes (mean ± SEM) in rats undergoing 90 minutes of middle cerebral artery occlusion and 4-day recovery. In both awake and halothane-anesthetized rats, brain temperature was maintained at 38° C during the ischemic insult and early reperfusion period. Mean infarct volume was reduced by 46% in the anesthetized rats. (From Warner DS, Ludwig PS, Pearlstein R, et al: Halothane reduces focal ischemic injury in the rat when brain temperature is controlled, *Anesthesiology* 82:1237, 1995.)

because it was thought that the principle mechanism by which hypothermia protects is by reduction in CMR. This implied that deep levels of hypothermia are necessary to provide meaningful benefit. Cardiopulmonary bypass would likely be essential to avoid complications of dysrrhythmia and coagulopathy. Beside logistical issues, bypass requires administration of heparin which considerably increases the complexity of performing surgery on the brain.

Largely by accident, it became evident that mild levels of hypothermia can provide substantial and lasting protection in laboratory animals. Active investigation is now defining the relevance of these findings to the human condition. Further, advances in animal modeling have allowed clearer definition of mechanisms of hypothermic brain protection as well as limitations regarding efficacy. The discussion below reviews these developments. For the purpose of communication, clinical hypothermia is divided into: (1) mild hypothermia, 32° to 35° C; (2) moderate hypothermia, 26° to 31° C; (3) deep hypothermia 20° to 25° C; and (4) profound hypothermia, 14° to 19° C.[190]

Animal Studies Demonstrating Protection

The development of rodent models of cerebral ischemia was crucial to this issue. Those models provided opportunity for thorough examination of factors influencing ischemic outcome using disease-free, genetically consistent, and low-cost subjects. Dramatic reduction in neural injury was observed when brain temperature was reduced by only 3° to 5° C in models of focal ischemia,[32,123,135] global ischemia,[28,140] brain trauma,[36,46] or status epilepticus.[99]

Anesthesia providers promptly recognized the logical extension that mild hypothermia might also be beneficial in the care of patients at risk for perioperative ischemic insults. Mild hypothermia is easy to induce in the anesthetized patient and presumably the risk associated with this practice is small, particularly if the patient is rewarmed prior to emergence from anesthesia. Anesthesia providers were beginning to understand that hypothermia offers more potent neuroprotection than does anesthetic-mediated reduction in CMR. Thus, alternative therapies were actively sought. This was most clearly demonstrated by Sano et al. who observed that histologic outcome from global ischemia was similarly poor for halothane and isoflurane anesthetized rats (despite large differences in CMR). Virtually all damage was inhibited by reducing brain temperature by only 3° C (small effect on CMR).[140] This has caused those caring for patients with acute cerebral insults to seriously consider application of mild hypothermia as a tool for improving outcome.

There also is evidence that postischemic hypothermia is protective. Original work suggested that the therapeutic window may persist for only 30 minutes after reperfusion of the brain.[27] Later work indicates that the window for onset of hypothermia may extend up to 12 hours after reperfusion. This is true only if the duration of hypothermia lasts at least several hours.[37] There is strong evidence that the protective effect of postischemic hypothermia is long lasting.

Whether hypothermia truly offers protection or instead

causes only a delay in the cascade of pathophysiologic events which ultimately results in a similar outcome as observed for normothermic comparators has been controversial. Most laboratory studies of hypothermic protection have only evaluated animals as far out as several days after the ischemic event. Others who have examined animals at weeks to months after ischemia have observed that long-term hypothermic protective effects against histologic changes become small if the duration of hypothermia is 12 hours or less.[38,47] Perhaps a definitive study has recently been performed.[39] Gerbils with appropriate monitoring of brain temperature were exposed to mild hypothermia for 24 hours after global ischemia. Examination of histologic and neurologic changes at 6 months revealed persistent benefit from hypothermia. The clinical relevance of this is unknown, but should postischemic hypothermia be employed, prolonged intervals (up to 24 hours) may be required to obtain lasting benefit.

Human Studies Demonstrating Protection

Evidence that profound reduction of brain temperature can reduce injury resulting from prolonged intervals of ischemia is strong. Perhaps the most convincing example was provided by Silverberg et al.[154] who reported that adults undergoing cardiopulmonary bypass for cerebral aneurysm clipping were capable of sustaining up to one hour of circulatory arrest when core temperature was reduced to approximately 20° C.

While an extension from laboratory models to human efficacy for mild-or-moderate hypothermia may seem intuitive, it is not that simple. There is no uniform agreement that moderate hypothermia is of value in cardiac surgery despite enormous experience. The incidence of frank stroke was not different in a population of 1732 patients randomized to either "warm" (core temperature = 33° to 37° C) or "cold" (25° to 30° C) groups during coronary artery bypass grafting.[115] Even if hypothermia is efficacious, other factors involved with the surgical technique may have greater importance such as use of cardiac standstill versus low-flow bypass in pediatric heart surgery.[18] No data exists with respect to neurosurgical procedures, but it seems obvious that hypothermia will not protect against a variety of iatrogenic events such as surgical excision of an eloquent area of the brain. Of greatest relevance to the use of mild hypothermia in the neurosurgical patient were three reports made almost simultaneously in 1993. All three studies were only preliminary trials because of small sample size. Nevertheless, either a clear benefit or a trend toward benefit was observed in patients rendered mildly hypothermic in the acute phase after head injury.[35,101,149]

Until studies are performed that examine outcome in neurosurgical patients, the clinician should decide to use mild intraoperative hypothermia in the presence of sound animal evidence for efficacy but in the absence of direct human data to support that practice. Fortunately, risk associated with mild hypothermia is small. In a recent poll taken from members of the Society of Neurosurgical Anesthesia and Critical Care, 40% of clinicians practiced induced mild hypothermia in patients undergoing cerebral aneurysm surgery.[42]

Mechanisms of Hypothermia Protection

For several decades it was believed that the predominant mechanism by which hypothermia caused protection was by virtue of its effects on CMR. This theory has been called into question because mild hypothermia offers potent neuroprotection, although CMR is only minimally reduced. Other cellular and biochemical effects better explain how hypothermia protects. For example, during an ischemic insult, extracellular concentrations of glutamate become massively increased. Such increases in glutamate are believed to initiate an excitotoxic cascade ultimately resulting in cell death. Mild hypothermia effectively blocks this increase in glutamate (Fig. 91-12).[30,82,129] The mechanism is unknown, but postsynaptic events may be important. Energy failure is associated with a large influx of calcium into the neuron. *In vitro* studies have shown that mild hypothermia reduces calcium influx.[5,21] Presumably, such an effect causes decreased opportunity for intracellular calcium to accumulate to concentrations sufficient to exert toxic effects.

Undoubtedly, there are also numerous generalized effects of hypothermia on intracellular enzymatic activity. Mild reductions in brain temperature, despite having no effect during the early recirculation interval,[20] have been shown to hasten recovery of protein synthesis several hours after reperfusion.[188] Specific effects are also being defined. Protein kinase C (PKC), an enzyme involved in regulating neuronal excitability and neurotransmitter release, is activated in response to an increase in cytosolic calcium. Hypothermia has been demonstrated to diminish membrane-bound PKC activity in selectively vulnerable regions of the postischemic brain.[29]

Nitric oxide synthase activity in ischemic brain is also suppressed by hypothermia.[85] It is not clear whether this activity is beneficial or detrimental because of the variability in outcome results obtained when N_2O synthase inhibitors are examined in outcome models of ischemia.[45] If N_2O or other free-radical mechanisms are germane to pathogenesis of neuronal death, then the effects of hypothermia are again relevant. Hypothermia has been demonstrated to reduce accumulation of lipid peroxidation products and the consumption of free-radical scavengers in ischemic brain.[11,88]

Other information is available regarding free-radical effects of hypothermia. Using two different models of brain injury (global ischemia or trauma), Globus et al.[66,67] demonstrated that free-radical production persists for at least several hours after reperfusion or impact. The quantity of free-radical generated is reduced to near-normal values by moderate hypothermia.

Of interest are the electrophysiologic effects of hypothermia during focal ischemia. If monitored for direct current potential, tissue in the ischemic penumbra shows recurrent episodes of depolarization which have been associated with

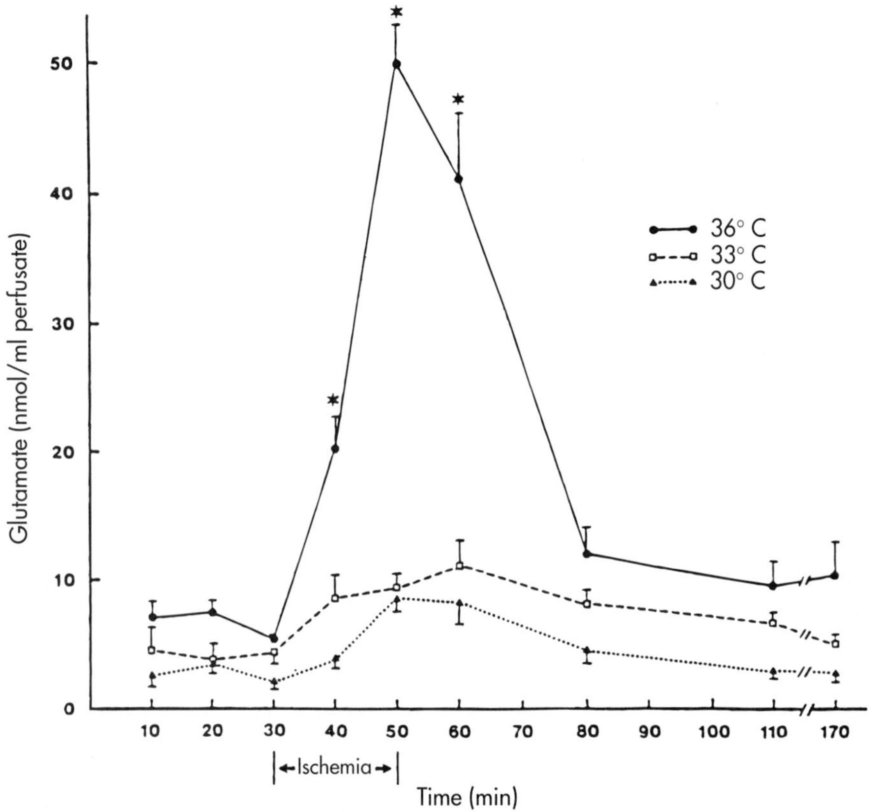

Fig. 91-12. Line plot of time-course changes in the perfusate levels of glutamate (nmol/ml) in rats whose intraischemic brain temperature was maintained at 36° C, 33° C, or 30° C. With animals in which intraischemic brain temperature was maintained at 36° C, a massive increase in extracellular glutamate was demonstrated. No major changes were found in animals in which intraischemic brain temperature was maintained at 33° C or 30° C. (From Busto R, Globus MY-T, Dietrich WD, et al: Effect of mild hypothermia on ischemia-induced release of neurotransmitters and free fatty acids in rat brain, *Stroke* 20:904, 1989.)

transient intervals of tissue hypoxia and depression of electrical activity.[10] If such events can be considered as insults secondary to the primary etiology of ischemia, then the observation that hypothermia greatly diminishes the frequency of such depolarizations provides an additional mechanistic basis for its protective effects.[33]

Clinical Implications

If one accepts that mild hypothermia is indicated in either the intraoperative period or intensive care environment, then questions regarding method(s) of cooling and monitoring of temperature arise. During craniotomy, the brain is differentially exposed to ambient temperature. Despite core normothermia, some regions of the brain may undergo substantial cooling, whereas other regions do not. Because it is difficult to define exactly which regions are at greatest risk (i.e., tissue under a retractor versus tissue distal to a cerebral artery potentially undergoing occlusion) it is virtually impossible to use core temperature to accurately define ideal conditions for specific tissue at risk. Some work has related brain temperature to core temperature, but most data is derived from the cardiopulmonary bypass literature. Stone et al.[162] directly measured cortical surface temperature during bypass cooling and rewarming in cerebral aneurysm surgery performed with circulatory arrest. Temperature from other measurement sites (e.g., nasopharynx, tympanic membrane, etc.) often varied by 2° to 3° C from brain temperature during various stages of cooling and rewarming. Although such differences might be negligible during profound hypothermia, if mild hypothermia is in use, such errors may encompass the entire therapeutic range. Various studies of cooling methods have been performed with respect to brain temperatures of patients in intensive care units. Intraventricular thermistors were used to compare brain temperature against rectal temperature.[105] During normothermia, rectal temperature was found to underestimate brain temperature by as much as 2° to 3° C although most often values were within 0.5° C. When attempts were made to specifically reduce brain temperature to 34° C, rectal temperature values (while tracking brain temperature) were often found to be at variance from the brain by 1° to 2° C.[105] The same study also showed that brain temperature in the comatose patient was surprisingly resistant to efforts of cooling and that only intensive total body surface cooling combined with pharmacologic therapy was effective in achieving that result. This data suggest a role for either intracranial pressure (ICP) monitors or ventriculostomy drains with incorporated thermistors to be made commercially available if induced hypothermia is to become routine practice and if maximal efficacy is desired.

With craniotomy, it is not clear what endpoint is ideal for induced hypothermia. An additional concern in the patient undergoing carniotomy is the practicality of cooling and rewarming in an interval of only several hours. One investigation of this practice reported that it is feasible to achieve core temperatures of approximately 34° C but that full rewarming to normothermia prior to emergence from anesthesia is unlikely.[13] Rewarming was most easily accomplished in adult patients who had low body surface areas. Overall, a rewarming rate of 0.7 ± 0.6° C/hr was obtained using standard surface rewarming techniques.

Mild hypothermia is not known to be associated with the life-threatening complications found with deep hypothermia (e.g., coagulopathy, arrhythmia). Nevertheless, there are several factors which have potential relevance to patient outcome and which may influence the decision whether to employ this technique. During emergence from anesthesia, myocardial ischemia may be a risk in patients who develop shivering in response to continued hypothermia. To date, this has not been associated with increased incidence of myocardial infarction (MI); but incidence of electrocardiographic (ECG) ischemic changes was nearly tripled when peripheral vascular patients were allowed to begin recovery from anesthesia with core temperatures less than 34.5° C.[55] Follow-up work in a similar patient population has shown that hypothermic patients exhibit greater peripheral vasoconstriction, increased norepinephrine concentrations, and greater blood pressures in the early postoperative period.[56]

The presence of mild hypothermia may also alter the dose of anesthetic required. Volatile anesthetic minimum alveolar concentration (MAC) is known to decrease with decreases in temperature.[176] The decrease in MAC with temperature has been shown to be rectilinear over the range of 39° to 20° C in the goat. At 20° C, hypothermia provides a sufficient state of anesthesia in and of itself.[3] It is unlikely that the effect on MAC is clinically relevant at temperatures of 33° to 35° C. In contrast, MAC for N_2O appears largely resistant to the effects of body temperature.[4]

Duration of action of muscle relaxants is increased by mild hypothermia. A twofold increase in duration of action of vecuronium was reported when body temperature was reduced from 36.8° C to 34.4° C.[77] This cause for this occurrence is unknown, although it is clearly not attributable to changes in a plasma concentration-effect relationship.[78] At the same time, neostigmine-induced reversal of neuromuscular blockade may be enhanced at lesser temperatures.[9]

There are three remaining concerns for complications from induced mild hypothermia. First, it is known that coagulopathies can occur at temperatures less than 30° C. Within the range of mild hypothermia, clinical evidence of coagulopathies in neurosurgical patients has been absent.[35,101,134,149] There is concern that mild hypothermia may suppress the patient's immune system allowing a greater chance of infection. Although there is evidence from animal studies that hypothermia during anesthesia may increase risk of dermal wound infection,[147] an increase in infections was not noted in any of the three trials of mild hypothermia in head-injury patients. [35,101,149] There is concern that rapid intraoperative rewarming may increase risk of thermal injury to the patient. Indeed, burns from warming devices used during anesthesia have constituted approximately 1% of anesthesia malpractice claims in the United States.[34] These cases were not those which employed induced hypothermia and active rewarming but instead were simply those where various methods were employed to maintain normothermia. Most of those injuries were attributable to placing heated saline bottles adjacent to the skin.

The short interval between completion of the high-risk phase of a neurosurgical procedure (e.g., temporary vascular occlusion during aneurysm clipping) and emergence from anesthesia requires that aggressive rewarming techniques be employed. It seems reasonable that simultaneous use of multiple heating devices including warmed IV fluid, forced air heating blankets, circulating warmed water blankets, and heated humidified inspiratory gases should be efficacious. The temperature of no single device should increase to a level where risk of thermal injury is present.

HYPERTHERMIA

Another series of laboratory-based observations have been made in recent years which have relevance to intraoperative neuroprotection. Hyperthermia has consistently been shown to cause adverse effects on both pathophysiologic processes as well as histologic/neurologic outcome from brain ischemia or trauma. Busto et al.[28] and others[113] have reported in the rat that increasing brain temperature during global ischemia from 36° C to 39° C caused approximately a 50% increase in neuronal injury.[28] Convincing data regarding global ischemia comes from a canine study conducted by Wass et al.[186] When dogs were subjected to transient global ischemia with brain temperature held at 37°, 38°, or 39° C, normothermic animals (37° C) were left essentially neurologically normal despite the ischemic insult. In contrast, hyperthermic animals (39° C) were either comatose or died.

With respect to focal ischemia, a similar pattern emerges. Infarct volumes in rats undergoing transient middle cerebral artery occlusion were almost tripled when brain temperature was increased from 37° C to 40° C.[33] We have demonstrated that an increase in brain temperature by as little as 1.2° C from normothermic values is sufficient to double size of a resultant infarct (Fig. 91-13).[183]

The mechanistic basis for this potent adverse effect of hyperthermia is not entirely known. Glutamate release in the penumbra of a rat focal ischemic lesion is increased by approximately tenfold when brain temperature is increased from 37° C to 39° C.[166] The frequency of spontaneous depo-

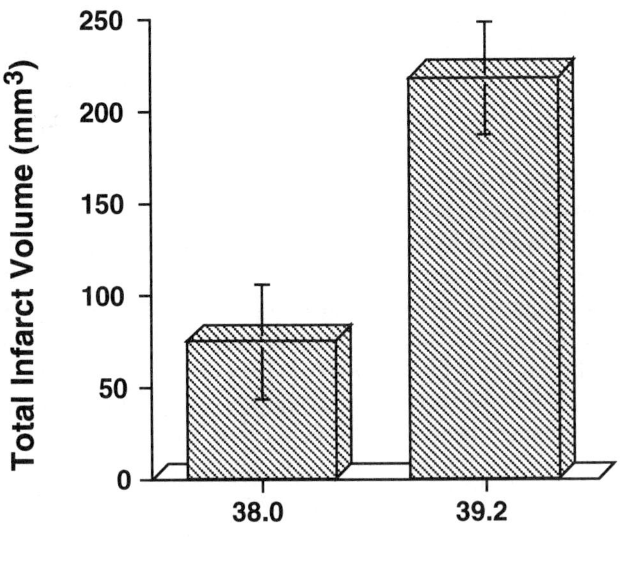

Fig. 91-13. Total infarct volumes (mean ± SEM) in normothermic (38° C) or hyperthermic (39.2° C) halothane-anesthetized rats after 90 minutes of middle cerebral artery occlusion and a 96-hour reperfusion interval. Infarct size was nearly doubled in the hyperthermic group. (From Warner DS, McFarlane C, Todd MM, et al: Sevoflurane and halothane reduce focal ischemic brain damage in the rat: Possible influence on thermoregulation, *Anesthesiology* 79:985, 1993).

larizations occurring in the ischemic penumbra is also markedly increased during mild hyperthermia. In both head injury and ischemia models, mild hyperthermia increases rate of free-radical formation.[66,67]

Although debate continues regarding the efficacy and role for mild hypothermia as a strategy for intraoperative neuroprotection, there is strong agreement that mild hyperthermia presents an adverse challenge to the injured brain. It is imperative that hyperthermia be guarded against in the anesthetized patient at risk for ischemic complications.

PLASMA GLUCOSE AND ISCHEMIC OUTCOME

Laboratory research has presented a dilemma to physicians dealing with cerebral ischemia. Although the normal brain is almost totally dependent on a continuous delivery of exogenous glucose for maintenance of cellular energy requirements, in the ischemic or hypoxic brain, continued glucose availability is detrimental. Pursuit of an explanation has yielded a large body of information, some of which has considerable clinical relevance. The initial observation that preischemic glucose infusion worsens ischemic outcome was serendipitous. Myers and Yamaguchi[114] designed an experiment to assess the effects of brief cardiac arrest on learned visual tasks in fasted primates. They recognized that successful cardiac resuscitation could be enhanced by prearrest IV volume loading, but although most animals recovered, two monkeys developed seizures and died early after reperfusion. Those two monkeys had received dextrose in their fluid boluses, whereas those that survived had not. This association between glucose infusion and worsened outcome from global ischemia was soon validated under more controlled conditions, and has subsequently been reported with remarkable consistency in numerous models, species, and research centers.

Before this discovery, other investigators had suggested an unfavorable relationship between cerebral acidosis and ischemic injury.[165] Such acidosis was soon linked to glucose administration.[133] With insufficient O_2 supply, cellular energy requirements may be partially supported by anaerobic glycolysis. Under conditions of hypoxemia or ischemia, relative hyperglycemia would be expected to force glycolytic ATP production at the cost of an enhanced accumulation of lactate. Lactate has a pKa of 3.83 (i.e., at physiologic pH virtually all of it is ionized), therefore causing an intracellular acidosis, which is considered the cause of the worsened outcome.[153]

Although laboratory experiments have provided a very consistent series of results, anesthesia providers may still be uncertain as to how this information should guide clinical practice. Laboratory protocols were designed to produce maximal effects (i.e., the animals were rendered hyperglycemic). Does this correlate with a modest glucose infusion, such as occurs with 1 l of dextrose-containing solution at the start of a surgical procedure? Lanier et al.[94] addressed this question by administering D_5W in clinically relevant amounts to monkeys before inducing a reversible global ischemic insult. Neurologic outcome in those monkeys was compared with a control group given normal saline. This dextrose infusion did not produce elevated blood glucose. Nevertheless, a significantly worsened neurologic outcome was observed in the animals given dextrose. Thus, hyperglycemia is not necessary to elicit the glucose effect, and as far as this primate model can predict, small doses of glucose may predispose patients to a worsened outcomes if a reversible global ischemic insult occurs.

Coincidence may have provided the surgical patient with a safeguard in that elective procedures are performed in patients with "no oral intake" status. This tends to minimize their ability to mount a hyperglycemic response to the stress of anesthesia and surgery. Conversely, does withholding dextrose predispose the fasted patient to the risk of hypoglycemia? This question has been addressed in patients undergoing craniotomy for supratentorial tumors.[150] Eight fasted patients received 5% dextrose in normal saline (D_5NS) whereas another eight patients received normal saline (NS) as intraoperative fluids. Throughout the procedure and for 24 hours postoperatively, the patients were monitored for plasma glucose and for evidence of starvation (e.g., ketones, base excess, urinary nitrogen). Intraoperatively, none of the patients in either group became hypoglycemic, although a difference in plasma glucose was identified between the groups (NS = 120 to 160 mg/dl; D_5NS = 200 to 242 mg/dl). No differences in base excess or arterial pH were observed.

Intraoperatively, free fatty acids, ketones, and urinary nitrogen levels were modestly elevated in those patients who did not receive dextrose. By 24 hours, however, all values had normalized without residual differences between groups.

These results support the conclusion that, although human metabolism recognizes the absence of intraoperative glucose, the price paid for withholding dextrose is small and justifiable in neurosurgical patients and others at risk for ischemia. Exceptions to this are patients with diabetes and neonates, in whom onset of hypoglycemia may be rapid and have severe consequences. In these patients, it is our practice to monitor blood glucose frequently and weigh the likelihood of cerebral ischemia against the risk of withholding dextrose. In cardiac surgical patients, it is routine practice in most centers to avoid priming the pump with dextrose-containing solutions.

Should insulin be administered to correct hyperglycemia when ischemia seems possible or likely? To date, there are no human studies to support this practice, but considerable laboratory evidence supports the concept that preischemic correction of hyperglycemia with insulin administration improves ischemic outcome (Fig. 91-14).[57,74,136,163,179] The concern with insulin administration is induction of profound hypoglycemia, which itself may augment ischemic brain damage. Before high-risk neurovascular procedures, if hyperglycemia is encountered, treatment of hyperglycemia with insulin should be considered. The level to which plasma glucose should be reduced has not been strictly defined. One carefully performed animal study and one human head-trauma trial showed major improvement in outcome if glucose concentrations were held to less than approximately 180 mg/dl.[92,98]

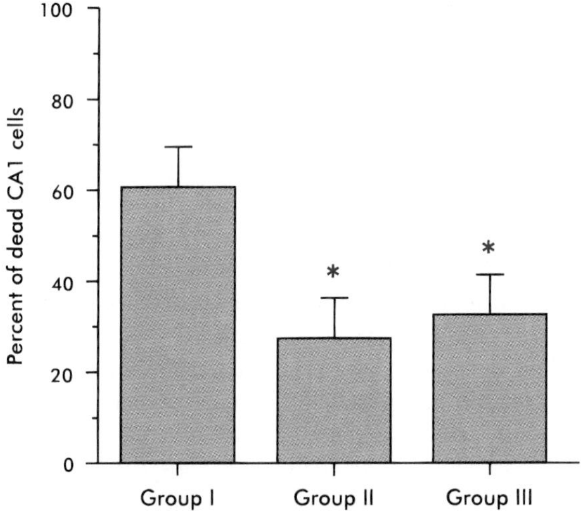

Fig. 91-14. Diabetic rats were exposed to 10 minutes of bilateral carotid artery occlusion combined with systemic hypotension, yielding a dense global ischemic insult. Rats in group I received no insulin and had a preischemic plasma glucose of 300 to 350 mg/dl. In group II, insulin was administered 90 minutes before ischemia to reduce PPG to 100 to 150 mg/dl. Group III were treated as group II, although in group III insulin administration was begun 30 minutes before ischemia. All rats were allowed 5 days of recovery. Depicted here are the percent of dead hippocampal CA1 neurons for each experimental group. In both of the insulin-treated groups, ischemic damage was significantly decreased ($p < 0.05$) as compared with the untreated control animals. (From Warner DS, Gionet TX, Todd MM, et al: Insulin-induced normoglycemia improves ischemic outcome in hyperglycemic rats, *Stroke* 1775, 1992.)

With focal ischemia (e.g., during occlusion of a major intracranial vessel), the effect of glucose administration on outcome is not as clear. There have been mixed experimental results. Satisfactory explanation compared with global ischemia has not been provided. These discrepancies may be attributable to variations in collateral flow to the ischemic penumbra.[63] Interest in focal ischemia has been largely in treatment of nonoperative stroke patients. Numerous studies have been reported comparing blood glucose values at time of hospital admission with outcome from stroke.[1,19,31,132,142] The majority of these studies did find a relationship (i.e., that patients who fared the worst neurologically also had the highest glucose values), but it cannot be determined whether the elevated glucose values represented reactive hyperglycemia, or rather truly caused worsened outcome. Also confusing is the occasional report that preischemic hyperglycemia may *actually improve* outcome from focal ischemia in some animal models.[64,193] The most convincing of these two studies used a rat model of cortical photochemical coagulation, reflecting a type of ischemia that is unlikely to occur intraoperatively.[64] Most evidence indicates aggressive management of the glycemic state during focal ischemic insults.

With to spinal cord ischemia, only one study has evaluated the effects of hyperglycemia on outcome.[48] Rabbits underwent a transient infrarenal balloon occlusion of the aorta. Before ischemia, either lactated Ringer's solution or D_5W was infused for 90 minutes. A much greater plasma glucose concentration was observed in those rabbits given the dextrose, which corresponded to worsened neurologic outcome.

INTRAVENOUS FLUIDS AND BRAIN EDEMA

Because the brain is housed in the rigid cranium, small increases in intracranial contents may result in increased ICP and decreased cerebral perfusion pressure. This is most relevant when normal compensatory mechanisms (i.e., reductions in CSF and venous volumes) are exhausted. Consequently, brain edema (i.e., increased brain water content) is often actively treated by either fluid restriction or administration of mannitol. In patients with intracranial tumors, the preoperative combination of restricted fluid intake and steroid therapy is believed to provide transient improvement in neurologic status by reducing brain water content.[58,148] This practice, along with the observation that large volumes of IV crystalloid solutions often cause edema in other organs (e.g., the bowel and thus presumably the brain), has led to the practice of keeping patients with intracranial pathologic conditions "dry." Unfortunately, this hypovolemia is not without consequence, which may be most evident on induction of anesthesia with vasodilating anesthetics, which can potentially result in hypotension with further decreases in cerebral perfusion pressure. This concern has led to careful analysis of the effects of IV fluid administration on brain water content. Information obtained has improved understanding of how various IV fluids might influence edema formation (in both the normal and injured brain) and has allowed rational modifications in practice.

With IV fluid therapy, three properties of blood can be manipulated: (1) hematocrit; (2) colloid oncotic pressure (owing to large molecules only); and (3) osmolality (owing to concentrations of large and small molecules). Laboratory studies have failed to demonstrate that decreases in hematocrit or oncotic pressure promote edema in either normal or injured brain. In contrast, osmolality plays a major role in determining brain water content; this is related to the blood–brain barrier (BBB), which is relatively impermeable even to ions (Fig. 91-15). When rabbits with uninjured brains underwent an isovolemic plasma exchange, resulting in a 70% reduction in plasma oncotic pressure, brain water content and ICP remained normal. In contrast, a 5% reduction in plasma osmolality under otherwise normal conditions resulted in brain edema and increased ICP.[194] These findings have been observed under conditions of severe anemia[173] and also have proved consistent when changes were either acute or chronic.[86,87] Similarly, with a cortical freeze injury (the pathophysiology of which resembles both tumors and trauma), neither hematocrit nor oncotic pressure affects brain water content, whereas plasma osmolality does (Fig. 91-16).[194] This work was extended to the case of implanted gliomas in the rat brain where, again, osmolality was found to be the driving force for water accumulation in peritumoral tissue.[75] Because severe elevations in ICP (as well as retractor pressure during craniotomy) may invoke ischemic pathophysiology, the corroborative findings that severe isotonic reduction in either hematocrit or plasma oncotic pressure has no effect on postischemic brain edema in the rat may also be relevant to patients with space-occupying lesions.[177]

Based on this information, it seems appropriate for the anesthesia provider to use crystalloid solutions if

PERIPHERAL CAPILLARY: oncotic gradient: no osmotic gradient

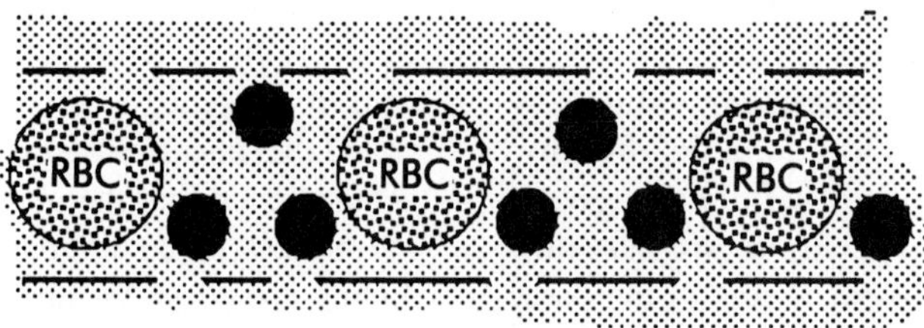

CEREBRAL CAPILLARY: small molecule (osmotic) and oncotic gradient

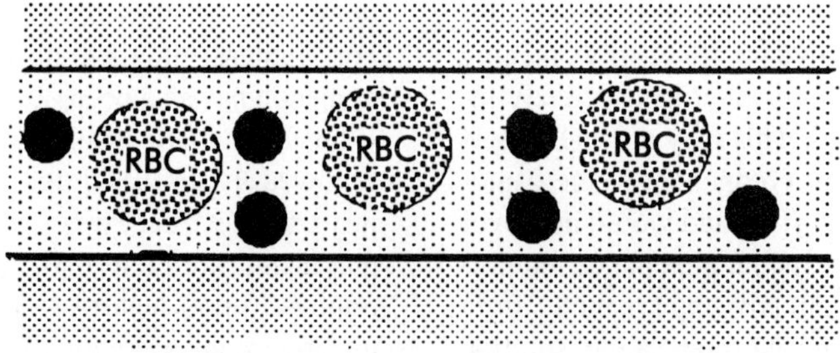

● = Colloid molecule ▒ = Small molecules (e.g., ions)

Fig. 91-15. The blood–brain barrier distinguishes cerebral from peripheral capillaries. The peripheral capillary is impermeable to macromolecules but permeable to most osmotically active constituents (e.g., ions) (note the relative numbers of large versus small molecules). The brain capillary is functionally permeable to neither. Because a concentration gradient is necessary for water to move between extravascular and intravascular compartments, ionic factors are neutral in the periphery but relevant in the brain. In contrast, oncotic pressure, although theoretically active in both systems, is only relevant in the periphery because 1 mOsm of osmotic pressure equals 19.3 mm Hg. Because colloid oncotic pressure is normally 18 to 20 mm Hg, fluid shifts of only a few mOsms dwarf any potential role for oncotic pressure to cause water movement. For these reasons, there is little concern for the colloidal properties of intravenous (IV) fluids when considering effects on brain water content. Instead, the patient's plasma osmolality is determined and fluids appropriate to stabilizing that value are administered.

DISPRUPTED BBB: no colloid gradient; no osmotic gradient

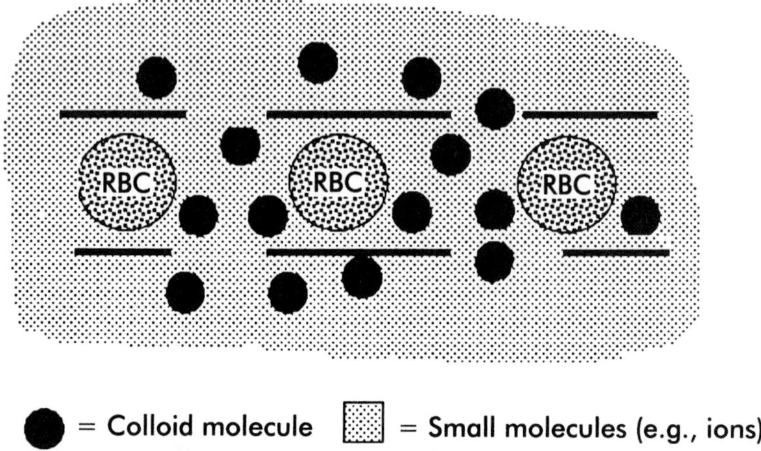

Fig. 91-16. In the case of the injured brain, when the blood–brain barrier becomes dysfunctional, the following conditions apply. Unlike either the peripheral or normal cerebral capillary, there is now permeability to both oncotic and ionic plasma constituents. Because of this permeability, no gradient between extravascular and intravascular compartments can be established. Consequently, manipulations in plasma oncotic and osmotic pressures have little to do with edema formation in injured tissue. It is important to recall, however, that normal tissue in other parts of the brain will continue to respond to changes in osmotic pressure.

deemed necessary to increase intravascular volume. A superb neuroanesthetic, with respect to fluid therapy, might be best assessed not by how little fluid was given, but rather by how stable cerebral perfusion pressure and plasma osmolality were maintained. If this is the case, what fluids seem most appropriate to treat hypovolemia and dehydration in neurosurgical patients? Certainly, severely hypotonic solutions (i.e., D_5W, D_5.45NS) should be avoided. In particular, it is prudent to avoid dextrose-containing solutions anyway because of their adverse effect in worsening ischemic outcome, and because free water is effectively introduced as dextrose is consumed. This may also be true of lactate, which contributes a major component to the osmolality in lactated Ringer's solution (LR) and would not favor large volumes of LR (i.e., greater than maintenance requirements), particularly in patients already hyperosmotic from dehydration or mannitol therapy. Normal saline solution (measured osmolality, 300 to 305 mOsm/kg) serves most appropriate when volumes of crystalloid above maintenance are needed. Determination of plasma osmolality may be helpful in making these decisions. Because oncotic pressure appears to play no role in the formation of brain edema, the question of whether to use isotonic crystalloid versus colloid solutions (e.g., hydroxyethyl starch) appears to rest on other considerations, such as general cardiopulmonary parameters, as well as the potential for a dilutional coagulopathy.

SECONDARY INSULTS

Secondary insults (i.e., insults [hemodynamic or hypoxic] superimposed on already injured brain), can substantially worsen outcome, even if those secondary insults ordinarily would be insufficient to cause damage. Tomida et al.[172] demonstrated that the gerbil brain is better able to tolerate 15 minutes of continuous ischemia than three isolated 5-minute episodes (15 minutes total), if the interval between each 5-minute insult is 1 hour. This 1-hour interval is associated with a residual postischemic hypoperfusion resulting from the previous insult, thus defining an interval when the brain may be particularly vulnerable to further challenge. For humans, this window is unknown. A similar phenomenon has also been observed in a rat brain injury model. When a traumatic insult (too mild to cause injury itself) was followed by an ischemic insult (also too mild to cause injury), the net effect was a seriously injured brain, indicating that insults are more than additive.[83] It is not difficult to extrapolate this scenario to the unstable trauma patient who undergoes an anesthetic induction. It appears prudent to rigorously treat hypotension or hypoxia in patients with preexisting brain injury.

CARE OF THE PATIENT WITH STROKE

Despite enormous advances in our understanding of the pathophysiology of CNS ischemia over the past several decades, there has been little change in care of patients with acute perioperative stroke or spinal cord ischemia. Practitioners begin with the fundamentals of maintaining adequate perfusion of nervous tissue with oxygenated blood; for the latter there is still no proven substitute. Initial approaches to the patient who awakens with neurologic deficit include maintenance and support of ventilation and blood pressure.

Surgical sources of injury that may be potentially correctable should be explored (e.g., misapplied aneurysm clip, carotid hematoma or thrombus, intravascular air, epidural hematomas). In the early stages of recovery, it is valuable for the anesthesia provider to contribute information with respect to potential effects of residual anesthetic agents on the neurologic examination. Glucose levels should be assessed to rule out hypoglycemia, and a CT scan should be obtained early. Although CT evidence of ischemia may not be present until many hours after onset of symptoms, intraparenchymal hematoma should be examined. Magnetic resonance imaging (MRI) may reveal ischemic tissue earlier than CT scan, but because MRI shows hematomas poorly, this is rarely a first-line approach.[96] Otherwise, as discussed throughout this chapter, pharmacologic approaches have either been disqualified or remain investigational. Possible exceptions include administration of nimodipine. Although outcome results have been mixed, experience with this agent in humans has indicated a wide margin of safety with respect to hemodynamic effects, especially if the patient is initially hemodynamically stable. A second possibility is use of tissue plasminogen activator (TPA). Recent work has demonstrated improvement in outcome from ischemic stroke (although there is risk of conversion to hemorrhagic stroke) when administered within the first several hours after onset of symptoms.[102] Use of this drug has not been extended to the postoperative environment by formal study and such therapy remains experimental.

KEY POINTS

- Appreciating the pathophysiology of cerebral ischemia involves understanding the brain's tight regulation of O_2 supply and demand, calcium homeostasis, and roles of excitatory neurotransmitters.
- The anesthesia provider should be familiar with the efforts undertaken over the past 20 years to limit cerebral damage by reducing cerebral O_2 demand, especially with barbiturates. Fundamentally, barbiturates can be expected to offer protection only under conditions where EEG activity persists which indicates metabolic activity amenable to suppression by the drug. Neuroprotection by barbiturates under these conditions is robust although the magnitude of benefit is small.
- It is not clearly understood why isoflurane, which does reduce cerebral O_2 demand, does not seem to provide the kind of protection against focal cerebral ischemia that is provided by thiopental. This calls into question the importance of causing metabolic suppression as a strategy for neuroprotection.
- The role of hypothermia in cerebral protection is complex, involving effects on excitatory amino acid neurotoxicity, free-radical formation, metabolic demand, and protein synthesis. Mild hypothermia is consistently protective in animal models of brain injury, but human evidence is scant.
- There is solid agreement that excessive levels of glucose, in the presence of cerebral ischemia, exacerbate that ischemia; therefore, close attention must be paid to keeping plasma glucose levels within reasonable values.
- Anesthesiologists should also be concerned about intravenous fluids and brain edema. There is considerable dogma that states that patients with intracranial pathologic conditions should be kept "dry." However, this practice does affect other organs. Use of crystalloid solutions to maintain reasonable intravascular volumes is a competent and appropriate practice if plasma osmolality is maintained stable. The practitioner should not sacrifice the other organs with the rationale that the brain is being protected.

KEY REFERENCES

Baker KZ, Young WL, Stone JG, et al: Deliberate mild intraoperative hypothermia for craniotomy, *Anesthesiology* 81:361, 1994.

Brain Resuscitation Clinical I Study Group: Randomized clinical study of thiopental loading in comatose survivors of cardiac arrest, *N Engl J Med* 314:397, 1986.

Clifton GL, Allen S, Barrodale P, et al: A phase II study of moderate hypothermia in severe brain injury, *J Neurotrauma* 10:263, 1993.

Haley EC, Kassell NF, Torner JC: A randomized controlled trial of high-dose intravenous nicardipine in aneurysmal subarachnoid hemorrhage, *J Neurosurg* 78:537, 1993.

Kaieda R, Todd MM, Warner DS: Prolonged reduction of colloid oncotic pressure does not increase brain edema following cryogenic injury in rabbits, *Anesthesiology* 71:554, 1989.

Lanier W, Stangland K, Scheithauer B, et al: The effects of dextrose infusion and head position on neurologic outcome after complete cerebral ischemia in primates: Examination of a model, *Anesthesiology* 66:39, 1987.

Mellergård P, Nordström CH: Intracerebral temperature in neurosurgical patients, *Neurosurgery* 28:709, 1991.

Michenfelder JD, Theye RA: Cerebral protection by thiopental during hypoxia, *Anesthesiology* 39:510, 1973.

Nehls DG, Todd MM, Spetzler RF, et al: A comparison of the cerebral protective effects of isoflurane and barbiturates during temporary focal ischemia in primates, *Anesthesiology* 66:453, 1987.

Nussmeier NA, Arlund C, Slogoff S: Neuropsychiatric complications after cardiopulmonary bypass: cerebral protection by a barbiturate, *Anesthesiology* 64:165, 1986.

Sano T, Drummond J, Patel P, et al: A comparison of the cerebral protective effects of isoflurane and mild hypothermia in a model of incomplete forebrain ischemia in the rat, *Anesthesiology* 76:221, 1992.

Sieber F, Smith DS, Kupferberg J, et al: Effects of intraoperative glucose on protein catabolism and plasma glucose levels in patients with supratentorial tumors, *Anesthesiology* 64:453, 1986.

Warner DS, Takaoka S, Wu B, et al: Electroencephalographic burst suppression is not required to elicit maximal neuroprotection from pentobarbital in a rat model of focal cerebral ischemia, *Anesthesiology* 84:475–484, 1996.

Wass CT, Lanier WL, Hofer RE, et al: Temperature changes of ≥ 1° C alter functional neurologic outcome and histopathology in a canine model of complete cerebral ischemia, *Anesthesiology* 83:325, 1995.

Werner C, Hoffman WE, Thomas C, et al: Ganglionic blockade improves neurologic outcome from incomplete ischemia in rats-partial reversal by exogenous catecholamines, *Anesthesiology* 73:923, 1990.

REFERENCES

1. Adams HP, Olinger C, Biller J, et al: Usefulness of admission blood glucose in predicting outcome after severe cerebral infarction, *Stroke* 18:297, 1987.
2. Allen GS, Ahn HS, Preziosi TJ, et al: Cerebral arterial spasm—a controlled trial of nimodipine in patients with subarachnoid hemorrhage, *N Engl J Med* 308:619, 1983.
3. Antognini JF: Hypothermia eliminates isoflurane requirements at 20° C, *Anesthesiology* 78:1152, 1993.
4. Antognini JF, Lewis BK, Reitan JA: Hypothermia minimally decreases nitrous oxide anesthetic requirements, *Anesth Analg* 79:980, 1994.
5. Arai H, Uto A, Ogawa Y, et al: Effect of low temperature on glutamate-induced intracellular calcium accumulation and cell death in cultured hippocampal neurons, *Neurosci Lett* 163:132, 1993.
6. Aronstam RS, Martin DC, Dennison RL: Volatile anesthetics inhibit NMDA-stimulated ^{45}Ca uptake by rat brain microvesicles, *Neurochem Res* 19:1515, 1994.
7. Astrup J, Symon L, Branston NM, et al: Cortical evoked potential and extracellular K^+ and H^+ at critical levels of brain ischemia, *Stroke* 8:51, 1977.
8. Auer LM: Pial arterial vasodilation by intravenous nimodipine in cats, *Arzneim Forsch/Drug Res* 31:1423, 1981.
9. Aziz L, Ono K, Ohta Y, et al: Effect of hypothermia on the *in vitro* potencies of neuromuscular blocking agents and on their antagonism by neostigmine, *Brit J Anaesth* 73:662, 1994.
10. Back T, Kohno K, Hossman K-A: Cortical negative DC deflections following middle cerebral artery occlusion and KCl-induced spreading depression: effect on blood flow, tissue oxygenation, and electroencephalogram, *J Cereb Blood Flow Metab* 14:12, 1994.
11. Baiping L, Xiujuan T, Hongwei C, et al: Effect of moderate hypothermia on lipid peroxidation in canine brain tissue after cardiac arrest and resuscitation, *Stroke* 25:147, 1994.
12. Baker AJ, Zornow MH, Scheller MS, et al: Changes in extracellular concentrations of glutamate, aspartate, glycine, dopamine, serotonin, and dopamine metabolites after transient global ischemia in the rabbit brain, *J Neurochem* 57:1370, 1991.
13. Baker KZ, Young WL, Stone JG, et al: Deliberate mild intraoperative hypothermia for craniotomy, *Anesthesiology* 81:361, 1994.
14. Balster RL, Mansbach RS, Shelton KL, et al: Behavioral pharmacology of two novel substituted quinoxalinedione glutamate antagonists, *Behav Pharmacol* 6:577, 1995.
15. Bashein G, Townes BD, Nessly ML, et al: A randomized study of carbon dioxide management during hypothermic cardiopulmonary bypass, *Anesthesiology* 72:7, 1990.
16. Baughman VL, Hoffman WE, Albrecht RF, et al: Cerebral vascular and metabolic effects of fentanyl and midazolam in young and aged rats, *Anesthesiology* 67:314, 1987.
17. Baughman VL, Hoffman WE, Thomas C, et al: Comparison of methohexital and isoflurane on neurologic outcome and histopathology following incomplete ischemia in rats, *Anesthesiology* 72:85, 1990.
18. Bellinger DC, Jonas RA, Rappaport LA, et al: Developmental and neurologic status of children after heart surgery with hypothermic circulatory arrest or low-flow cardiopulmonary bypass, *N Engl J Med* 332:549, 1995.
19. Berger L, Hakim A: The association of hyperglycemia with cerebral edema in stroke, *Stroke* 17:865, 1986.
20. Bergstedt K, Hu BR, Wieloch T: Postischaemic changes in protein synthesis in the rat brain: effects of hypothermia, *Exp Brain Res* 95:91, 1993.
21. Bickler PE, Buck LT, Hansen BM: Effects of isoflurane and hypothermia on glutamate receptor-mediated calcium influx in brain slices, *Anesthesiology* 81:1461, 1994.
22. Bloodwell RD, Hallman GL, Cooley DA: Partial cardiopulmonary bypass for pericardectomy and resection of descending thoracic aortic aneurysms, *Ann Thorac Surg* 6:46, 1968.
23. Bogousslavsky J, Regli F, Zumstein V, et al: Double-blind study of nimodipine in non-severe stroke, *Eur Neurol* 30:23, 1990.
24. Brain Resuscitation Clinical I Study Group: Randomized clinical study of thiopental loading in comatose survivors of cardiac arrest, *N Engl J Med* 314:397, 1986.
25. Buchan AM, Li Hui, Cho S, et al: Blockade of the AMPA receptor prevents CA1 hippocampal injury following severe but transient forebrain ischemia in adult rats, *Neurosci Lett* 132:255, 1991.
26. Buchan AM, Xue D, Huang ZG, et al: Delayed AMPA receptor blockade reduces cerebral infarction induced by focal ischemia, *Neuro Rep* 2:473, 1991.
27. Busto R, Dietrich WD, Globus MYT, et al: Postichemic moderate hypothermia inhibits CA1 hippocampal ischemic neuronal injury, *Neurosci Lett* 101:299, 1989.
28. Busto R, Dietrich WD, Globus MYT, et al: Small differences in intraischemic brain temperature critically determine the extent of neuronal injury, *J Cereb Blood Flow Metab* 7:729, 1987.
29. Busto R, Globus MYT, Neary JT, et al: Regional alterations of protein kinase C activity following transient cerebral ischemia: effects of intraischemic brain temperature modulation, *J Neurochem* 63: 1095, 1994.
30. Busto R, Globus MY-T, Dietrich WD, et al: Effect of mild hypothermia on ischemia-induced release of neurotransmitters and free fatty acids in rat brain, *Stroke* 20:904, 1989.
31. Candelise L, Landi G, Orazio E, et al: Prognostic significance of hyperglycemia in acute stroke, *Arch Neurol* 42:661, 1985.

32. Chen H, Chopp M, Zhang ZG, et al: The effect of hypothermia on transient middle cerebral artery occlusion in the rat, *J Cereb Blood Flow Metab* 12:621, 1992.
33. Chen Q, Chopp M, Bodzin G, et al: Temperature modulation of cerebral depolarization during focal cerebral ischemia in rats: correlation with ischemic injury, *J Cereb Blood Flow Metab* 13:389, 1993.
34. Cheney FW, Posner KL, Caplan RA, et al: Burns from warming devices in anesthesia: A closed claims analysis, *Anesthesiology* 80:806, 1994.
35. Clifton GL, Allen S, Barrodale P, et al: A phase II study of moderate hypothermia in severe brain injury, *J Neurotrauma* 10:263, 1993.
36. Clifton GL, Jiang JY, Lyeth BG, et al: Marked protection by moderate hypothermia after experimental traumatic brain injury, *J Cereb Blood Flow Metab* 11:114, 1991.
37. Coimbra C, Wieloch T: Moderate hypothermia mitigates neuronal damage in the rat brain when initiated several hours following transient cerebral ischemia, *Acta Neuropathol* 87:325, 1994.
38. Colbourne F, Corbett D: Delayed and prolonged post-ischemic hypothermia is neuroprotective in the gerbil, *Brain Res* 654:265, 1994.
39. Colbourne F, Corbett D: Delayed postischemic hypothermia: a six month survival study using behavioral and histologic assessments of neuroprotection, *J Neurosci* 15:7250, 1995.
40. Cole DJ, Shapiro HM, Drummond JC, et al: Halothane, fentanyl/nitrous oxide, and spinal lidocaine protect against spinal cord injury in the rat, *Anesthesiology* 70:967, 1989.
41. Corkill G, Sivalingam S, Reitan JA, et al: Dose dependency of the post-insult protective effect of pentobarbital in the canine experimental stroke model, *Stroke* 9:10, 1978.
42. Craen RA, Gelb AW, Eliazaw M, et al: Current anesthetic practices and use of brain protective therapies for cerebral aneurysm surgery at 41 North American centers (abstract), *J Neurosurg Anesth* 6:303, 1994.
43. Crawford ES et al: Progress in treatment of thoraco-abdominal and abdominal aortic aneurysms involving coeliac, superior mesenteric, and renal arteries, *Ann Surg* 188:404, 1978.
44. Dalkara T, Erdemli G, Barun S, et al: Glycine is required for NMDA receptor activation: electrophysiological evidence from intact rat hippocampus, *Brain Res* 576:197, 1992.
45. Dawson DA: Nitric oxide and focal cerebral ischemia: multiplicity of actions and diverse outcome, *Cerebrovasc Brain Metab Rev* 6:299, 1994.
46. Dietrich WD, Alonso O, Busto R, et al: Post-traumatic brain hypothermia reduces histopathological damage following concussive brain injury in the rat, *Acta Neuropathol* 87:250, 1994.
47. Dietrich WD, Busto R, Alonso O, et al: Intraischemic but not postischemic brain hypothermia protects chronically following global forebrain ischemia in rats, *J Cereb Blood Flow Metab* 13:541, 1993.
48. Drummond J, Moore S: The influence of dextrose administration on neurologic outcome after temporary spinal cord ischemia in the rabbit, *Anesthesiology* 70:64, 1989.
49. Fadul C, Wood J, Thaler H, et al: Morbidity and mortality of craniotomy for excision of supratentorial gliomas, *Neurology* 38:1374, 1988.
50. Fagan SC, Gengo FM, Bates V, et al: Effect of nimodipine on blood pressure in acute ischemic stroke in humans, *Stroke* 19:401, 1988.
51. Forrest JB, Cahalan MK, Rehder K, et al: Multicenter study of general anesthesia. II. Results, *Anesthesiology* 72:262, 1990.
52. Forrest JB, Rehder K, Goldsmith CH, et al: Multicenter study of general anesthesia: I. Design and patient demography, *Anesthesiology* 72:252, 1990.
53. Forsman M, Aarseth HP, Nordby HK, et al: Effects of nimodipine on cerebral blood flow and cerebrospinal fluid pressure after cardiac arrest: correlation with neurologic outcome, *Anesth Analg* 68:436, 1989.
54. Forsythe ID, Westbrook GL, Mayer ML: Modulation of excitatory synaptic transmission by glycine and zinc in cultures of mouse hippocampal neurons, *J Neurosci* 8:3733, 1988.
55. Frank SM, Beattie C, Christopherson R, et al: Unintentional hypothermia is associated with postoperative myocardial ischemia, *Anesthesiology* 78:468, 1993.
56. Frank SM, Higgins MS, Breslow MJ, et al: The catecholamine, cortisol, and hemodynamic responses to mild perioperative hypothermia: a randomized clinical trial, *Anesthesiology* 82:83, 1995.
57. Fukuoka S, Yeh H, Mandybur TI, et al: Effect of insulin on acute experimental cerebral ischemia in gerbils, *Stroke* 20:396, 1989.
58. Galicich JH, French LA, Melby JC: Use of dexamethasone in the treatment of cerebral edema resulting from brain tumors and brain surgery, *Am Pract* 12:169, 1961.
59. Gelb AW, Boisvert DP, Tang C, et al: Primate brain tolerance to temporary focal cerebral ischemia during isoflurane- or sodium nitroprusside-induced hypotension, *Anesthesiology* 70:678, 1989.
60. Gelmers HJ, Gorter K, De Weerdt CJ, et al: A controlled trial of nimodipine in acute ischemic stroke, *New Engl J Med* 318:203, 1988.
61. Gelmers HJ, Hennerici M: Effect of nimodipine on acute ischemic stroke pooled results from five randomized trials, *Stroke* 21:IV81, 1990.
62. Gill R, Hargreaves RJ, Kemp JA: The neuroprotective effect of the glycine site antagonist 3R-(+)-cis-4-methyl-HA966 (L-687,414) in a rat model of focal ischaemia, *J Cereb Blood Flow Metab* 15:197, 1995.
63. Ginsberg MD: Glycolytic metabolism in brain ischemia. In Weinstein PR, Faden AI, editors: *Protection of the brain from ischemia,* Baltimore, 1990, Williams & Wilkins.
64. Ginsberg M, Prado R, Dietrich W, et al: Hyperglycemia reduces the extent of cerebral infarction in rats, *Stroke* 18:570, 1987.
65. Gisvold SE, Safar P, Hendrickx HHL, et al: Thiopental treatment after global brain ischemia in pigtailed monkeys, *Anesthesiology* 60:88, 1984.
66. Globus MYT, Alonso O, Dietrich WD, et al: Glutamate release and free radical production following brain injury: effects of posttraumatic hypothermia, *J Neurochem* 65:1704, 1995.
67. Globus MYT, Busto R, Lin BW, et al: Detection of free radical activity during transient global ischemia and recirculation: effects of intraischemic brain temperature modulation, *J Neurochem* 65:1250, 1995.
68. Globus MYT, Ginsberg MD, Busto R: Excitotoxic index-a biochemical marker of selective vulnerability, *Neurosci Lett* 127: 39, 1991.
69. Goldstein LB, Hasselblad V, Matchar DB, et al: Comparison and meta-analysis of randomized trials of endarterectomy for symptomatic carotid artery stenosis, *Neurology* 45:1965, 1995.
70. Grotta J, Clark W, Coull B, et al: Safety and tolerability of the glutamate antagonist CGS 19755 (Selfotel) in patients with acute ischemic stroke, *Stroke* 26:602, 1995.
71. Gustafson I, Westerberg EJ, Wieloch T: Extracellular brain cortical levels of noradrenaline in ischemia: effects of desipramine and postischemic administration of idazoxan, *Exp Brain Res* 86:555, 1991.
72. Haley EC, Kassell NF, Torner JC: A randomized controlled trial of high-dose intravenous nicardipine in aneurysmal subarachnoid hemorrhage, *J Neurosurg* 78:537, 1993.
73. Haley E C, NF Kassell, JC Torner, et al: A randomized trial of two doses of nicardipine in aneurysmal subarachnoid hemorrhage, *J Neurosurg* 80:788, 1994.
74. Hamilton MG, Tranmer BI, Auer RN: Insulin reduction of cerebral infarction due to transient focal ischemia, *J Neurosurg* 82:262, 1995.
75. Hansen T, Warner DS, Traynelis V, et al: Plasma osmolality and brain water content in a rat glioma model, *Neurosurgery* 34:505, 1994.
76. Harrison MJ, Schneidau A, Ho R, et al: Cerebrovascular disease and functional outcome after coronary artery bypass surgery, *Stroke* 20:235, 1989.
77. Heier T, Caldwell JE, Sessler DI, et al: Mild intraoperative hypothermia increases duration of action and spontaneous recovery of vecuronium blockade during nitrous oxide-isoflurane anesthesia in humans, *Anesthesiology* 74:815, 1991.
78. Heier T, Caldwell JE, Sharma ML, et al: Mild intraoperative hypothermia does not change the pharmacodynamics (concentration-effect relationship) of vecuronium in humans, *Anesth Analg* 78:973, 1994.
79. Hoff JT, Smith AL, Hankinson HL, et al: Barbiturate protection from cerebral infarction in primates, *Stroke* 6:28, 1975.
80. Hoffman WE, Kochs E, Werner C, et al: Dexmedetomidine improves neurologic outcome from incomplete cerebral ischemia in the rat, *Anesthesiology* 75:328, 1991.
81. Hoffman WE, Pelligrino D, Werner C, et al: Ketamine decreases plasma catecholamines and improves outcome from incomplete cerebral ischemia in rats, *Anesthesiology* 76:755, 1992.
82. Illievich UM, Zornow MH, Choi KT, et al: Effects of hypothermia or anesthetics on

hippocampal glutamate and glycine concentrations after repeated transient global cerebral ischemia, *Anesthesiology* 80:177, 1994.

83. Jenkins LW, Moszynski K, Lyeth BG, et al: Increased vulnerability of the mildly traumatized rat brain to cerebral ischemia: the use of controlled secondary ischemia as a research tool to identify common or different mechanisms contributing to mechanical and ischemic injury, *Brain Res* 477:211, 1989.
84. Johnson JW, Ascher P: Glycine potentiates the NMDA response in cultured mouse brain neurons, *Nature* 325:529, 1987.
85. Kader A, Frazzini VI, Baker CJ, et al: Effect of mild hypothermia on nitric oxide synthesis during focal cerebral ischemia, *Neurosurgery* 35:272, 1994.
86. Kaieda R, Todd MM, Cook LN, et al: Acute effects of changing plasma osmolality and colloid oncotic pressure on the formation of brain edema after cryogenic injury, *Neurosurgery* 24:671, 1989.
87. Kaieda R, Todd MM, Warner DS: Prolonged reduction of colloid oncotic pressure does not increase brain edema following cryogenic injury in rabbits, *Anesthesiology* 71:554, 1989.
88. Karibe H, Chen SF, Zarow GJ, et al: Mild intraischemic hypothermia suppresses consumption of endogenous antioxidants after temporary focal ischemia in rats, *Brain Res* 649:12, 1994.
89. Kochs E, Hoffman WE, Werner C, et al: The effects of propofol on brain electrical activity, neurologic outcome, and neuronal damage following incomplete ischemia in rats, *Anesthesiology* 76:245, 1992.
90. Koide T, Wieloch T, Siesjö BK: Circulating catecholamines modulate ischemic brain damage, *J Cereb Blood Flow Metab* 6:559, 1986.
91. Kurumaji A, Nehls DG, Park CK, et al: Effects of NMDA antagonists, MK-801 and CPP, upon local cerebral glucose use, *Brain Res* 496:268, 1989.
92. Lam AM, Winn HR, Cullen BF, et al: Hyperglycemia and neurological outcome in patients with head injury, *J Neurosurg* 75:545, 1991.
93. Lanier WL, Perkins WJ, Karlsson BR, et al: The effects of dizocilpine maleate [MK-801], an antagonist of the N-methyl-D-aspartate receptor, on neurologic recovery and histopathology following complete cerebral ischemia in primates, *J Cereb Blood Flow Metab* 10:252, 1990.
94. Lanier W, Stangland K, Scheithauer B, et al: The effects of dextrose infusion and head position on neurologic outcome after complete cerebral ischemia in primates: examination of a model, *Anesthesiology* 66:39, 1987.
95. Larsen SF, Zaric D, Boysen G: Postoperative cerebrovascular accidents in general surgery, *Acta Anaesth Scand* 32:698, 1988.
96. Latchaw RE, Eelkema EA, Hecht ST: Imaging methods: CT, MR, xenon-enhanced CT, and SPECT. In Weinstein PR, Faden AI, editors: *Protection of the brain from ischemia,* Baltimore, 1990, Williams & Wilkins.
97. Lester RAJ, Tong G, Jahr CE: Interactions between the glycine and glutamate binding sites of the NMDA receptor, *J Neurosci* 13:1088, 1993.
98. Li P-A, Shamloo M, Smith M-L, et al: The influence of plasma glucose concentrations on ischemic brain damage is a threshold function, *Neurosci Lett* 177:63, 1994.
99. Lundgren J, Smith M-L, Blennow G, et al: Hyperthermia aggravates and hypothermia ameliorates epileptic brain damage, *Exp Brain Res* 99:43, 1994.
100. MacEwen GD, Bunnell WP, Spiram K: Acute neurological complications in the treatment of scoliosis, *J Bone Joint Surg* 57-A:404, 1975.
101. Marion DW, Obrist WD, Carlier PM, et al: The use of moderate therapeutic hypothermia for patients with severe head injuries: a preliminary report, *J Neurosurg* 79:354, 1993.
102. Marler JR, Brott T, Broderick J, et al: Tissue plasminogen activator for acute ischemic stroke, *N Engl J Med* 333:1581, 1995.
103. Martinezvila E, Guillen F, Villanueva JA, et al: Placebo-controlled trial of nimodipine in the treatment of acute ischemic cerebral infarction, *Stroke* 21:1023, 1990.
104. McFarlane C, Warner DS, Nader A, et al: Glycine receptor antagonism: effects of ACEA-1021 on the minimum alveolar concentration for halothane in the rat, *Anesthesiology* 82:963, 1995.
105. Mellergård P, Nordstöm CH: Intracerebral temperature in neurosurgical patients, *Neurosurgery* 28:709, 1991.
106. Messick JM Jr, Casement B, Sharbrough FW, et al: Correlation of regional cerebral blood flow (rCBF) with EEG changes during isoflurane anesthesia for carotid endarterectomy: critical rCBF, *Anesthesiology* 66:344, 1987.
107. Michenfelder JD: The interdependency of cerebral function and metabolic effects following massive doses of thiopental in the dog, *Anesthesiology* 41:231, 1974.
108. Michenfelder JD, Lanier WL, Scheithauer BW, et al: Evaluation of the glutamate antagonist dizocilipine maleate (MK-801) on neurologic outcome in a canine model of complete cerebral ischemia: correlation with hippocampal histopathology, *Brain Res* 481:228, 1989.
109. Michenfelder JD, Milde JH, Sundt TM: Cerebral protection by barbiturate anesthesia: use after middle cerebral artery occlusion in Java monkeys, *Arch Neurol* 33:345, 1976.
110. Michenfelder JD, Sundt TM, Fode N, et al: Isoflurane when compared to enflurane and halothane decreases the frequency of cerebral ischemia during carotid endarterectomy, *Anesthesiology* 67:336, 1987.
111. Michenfelder J D, Theye RA: Cerebral protection by thiopental during hypoxia, *Anesthesiology* 39:510, 1973.
112. Milde LN, Milde JH, Michenfelder JD: Cerebral functional, metabolic, and hemodynamic effects of etomidate in dogs, *Anesthesiology* 63:371, 1985.
113. Minamisawa H, Smith ML, Siesjö BK: The effect of mild hyperthermia and hypothermia on brain damage following 5, 10, and 15 minutes of forebrain ischemia, *Ann Neurol* 28:26, 1990.
114. Myers RE, Yamaguchi S: Nervous system effects of cardiac arrest in monkeys. Preservation of vision, *Arch Neurol* 34:65, 1977.
115. Naylor CD, Lichtenstein SV, Fremes SE, et al: Randomised trial of normothermic versus hypothermic coronary bypass surgery, *Lancet* 343:559, 1994.
116. Nehls DG, Todd MM, Spetzler RF, et al: A comparison of the cerebral protective effects of isoflurane and barbiturates during temporary focal ischemia in primates, *Anesthesiology* 66:453, 1987.
117. Nellgård B, Wieloch T: Postischemic blockade of AMPA but not NMDA receptors mitigates neuronal damage in the rat brain following transient severe cerebral ischemia, *J Cereb Blood Flow Metab* 12:2, 1992.
118. Newell DW, Barth A, Malouf AT: Glycine site NMDA receptor antagonists provide protection against ischemia-induced neuronal damage in hippocampal slice cultures, *Brain Res* 675:38, 1995.
119. Newman MF, Murkin JM, Roach G, et al: Cerebral physiologic effects of burst suppression doses of propofol during nonpulsatile cardiopulmonary bypass, *Anesth Analg* 81:452, 1995.
120. Nussmeier NA, Arlund C, Slogoff S: Neuropsychiatric complications after cardiopulmonary bypass: cerebral protection by a barbiturate, *Anesthesiology* 64:165, 1986.
121. Ohman J, Servo A, Heiskanen O: Long-term effects of nimodipine on cerebral infarcts and outcome after aneurysmal subarachnoid hemorrhage and surgery, *J Neurosurg* 74:8, 1991.
122. Olney JW, Price MT, Fuller TA, et al: The anti-excitotoxic effects of certain anesthetics, analgesics, and sedative-hypnotics, *Neurosci Lett* 68: 29, 1986.
123. Onesti ST, Baker CJ, Sun PP, et al: Transient hypothermia reduces focal ischemic brain damage in the rat, *Neurosurgery* 29:369, 1991.
124. Oyzuart E, Graham DI, Woodruff GN, et al: Protective effect of the glutamate antagonist, MK-801 in focal cerebral ischemia in the cat, *J Cereb Blood Flow Metab* 8:138, 1988.
125. Paci A, Ottaviano P, Trenta A, et al: Nimodipine in acute ischemic stroke: a double-blind controlled study, *Acta Neurol Scand* 80:282, 1989.
126. Park CK, Nehls DG, Graham DI, et al: Focal cerebral ischaemia in the cat: treatment with the glutamate antagonist MK-801 after induction of ischaemia, *J Cereb Blood Flow Metab* 8:757, 1988.
127. Park CK, Nehls DG, Graham DI, et al: The glutamate antagonist MK-801 reduces focal ischemic brain damage in the rat, *Ann Neurol* 24:543, 1988.
128. Park CK, Nehls DG, Teasdale GM, et al: Effect of the NMDA antagonist MK-801 on local cerebral blood flow in focal cerebral ischaemia in the rat, *J Cerebral Blood Flow Metab* 9:617, 1989.
129. Patel PM, Drummond JC, Cole DJ, et al: Differential temperature sensitivity of ischemia-induced glutamate release and eicosanoid production in rats, *Brain Res* 650:205, 1994.

130. PerezPinzon MA, Maier CM, Yoon EJ, et al: Correlation of CGS 19755 neuroprotection against *in vitro* excitotoxicity and focal cerebral ischemia, *J Cereb Blood Flow Metab* 15:865, 1995.
131. Pickard JD, Murray GD, Illingworth R, et al: Effect of oral nimodipine on cerebral infarction and outcome after subarachnoid haemorrhage: British aneurysm nimodipine trial, *Br Med J* 298:636, 1989.
132. Pulsinelli WA, Levy DE, Sigsbee B, et al: Increased damage after ischemic stroke in patients with hyperglycemia with or without established diabetes mellitus, *Am J Med* 74:540, 1983.
133. Rehncrona S, Rosen I, Siesjö B: Brain lactic acidosis and ischemic cell damage: 1. Biochemistry and neurophysiology, *J Cereb Blood Flow Metab* 1:297, 1981.
134. Resnick DK, Marion DW, Darby JM: The effect of hypothermia on the incidence of delayed traumatic intracerebral hemorrhage, *Neurosurgery* 34:252, 1994.
135. Ridenour TR, Warner DS, Todd MM, et al: Mild hypothermia reduces infarct size resulting from temporary but not permanent focal ischemia in the rat, *Stroke* 23:733, 1992.
136. Robertson CS, Grossman RG: Protection against spinal cord ischemia with insulin-induced hypoglycemia, *J Neurosurg* 67: 739, 1987.
137. Roine RO, Kaste M, Kinnunen A, et al: Nimodipine after resuscitation from out-of-hospital ventricular fibrillation, *JAMA* 264:3171, 1990.
138. Ross RT: Spinal cord infarction in disease and surgery of the aorta, *Can J Neurol Sci* 12:289, 1985.
139. Sakurada O, Kennedy C, Jehle J, et al: Measurement of local cerebral blood flow with iodo[14C]antipyrine, *Am J Physiol* 234:H59, 1978.
140. Sano T, Drummond J, Patel P, et al: A comparison of the cerebral protective effects of isoflurane and mild hypothermia in a model of incomplete forebrain ischemia in the rat, *Anesthesiology* 76:221, 1992.
141. Scheller MS, Zornow MH, Fleischer JE, et al: The noncompetitive N-methyl-D-aspartate receptor antagonist, MK-801 profoundly reduces volatile anesthetic requirements in rabbits, *Neuropharmacology* 28:677, 1989.
142. Schneider S, Tomasi L, Thompson J: Prognostic implications of hyperglycemia and reduced cerebral blood flow in childhood near-drowning, *Neurology* 40:820, 1990.
143. Seiler RW, Grolimund P, Zurbruegg HR: Evaluation of the calcium-antagonist nimodipine for the prevention of vasospasm after aneurysmal subarachnoid haemorrhage, *Acta Neurochir* 85:7, 1987.
144. Shapiro HM: Anesthesia effects upon cerebral blood flow, cerebral metabolism, and the electroencephalogram. In Miller RD, editor: *Anesthesia,* New York, 1981, Churchill Livingstone.
145. Shaw PJ, Bates D, Cartlidge NE, et al: Neurologic and neuropsychological morbidity following major surgery: comparison of coronary artery bypass and peripheral vascular surgery, *Stroke* 18:700, 1987.
146. Sheardown MJ, Nielsen EO, Hansen AJ, et al: 2,3-Dihydroxy-6-nitro-7-sulfamoyl-benzo(F) quinoxaline: a neuroprotectant for cerebral ischemia, *Science* 247:571, 1990.
147. Sheffield CW, Sessler DI, Hunt TK: Mild hypothermia during isoflurane anesthesia decreases resistance to *E. coli* dermal infection in guinea pigs, *Acta Anaesth Scand* 38:201, 1994.
148. Shenkin HA, Bezier HS, Bouzarth WF: Restricted fluid intake: rational management of the neurosurgical patient, *J Neurosurg* 45:432, 1976.
149. Shiozaki T, Sugimoto H, Taneda M, et al: Effect of mild hypothermia on uncontrollable intracranial hypertension after severe head injury, *J Neurosurg* 79:363, 1993.
150. Sieber F, Smith DS, Kupferberg J, et al: Effects of intraoperative glucose on protein catabolism and plasma glucose levels in patients with supratentorial tumors, *Anesthesiology* 64:453, 1986.
151. Siesjö BK: Cerebral circulation and metabolism, *J Neurosurg* 60:883, 1984.
152. Siesjö BK, Bengtsson F: Calcium fluxes, calcium antagonists, and calcium-related pathology in brain ischemia, hypoglycemia, and spreading depression: a unifying hypothesis, *J Cereb Blood Flow Metab* 9:127, 1989.
153. Siesjö BK, Smith ML, Warner DS: Acidosis and ischemic brain damage. In Raichle E, Powers WJ, editors: *Cerebrovascular diseases,* New York, 1987, Raven.
154. Silverberg GD, Reitz BA, Ream AK: Hypothermia and cardiac arrest in the treatment of giant aneurysms of the cerebral circulation and hemangioblastoma of the medulla, *J Neurosurg* 55:337, 1981.
155. Smith AL, Hoff JT, Nielsen SL, et al: Barbiturate protection in acute focal cerebral ischemia, *Stroke* 5:1, 1974.
156. Smith DS, Rehncrona S, Siesjö BK: Inhibitory effects of different barbiturates on lipid peroxidation in brain tissue *in vitro:* comparison with the effects of promethazine and chlorpromazine, *Anesthesiology* 53:186, 1980.
157. Smith PL, Treasure T, Newman SP, et al: Cerebral consequences of cardiopulmonary bypass, *Lancet* 1:823, 1986.
158. Sokoloff L: Local cerebral energy metabolism: Its relationships to local functional activity and blood flow. In Purves MJ, Elliot K, editors: *Cerebral vascular smooth muscle and its control,* Ciba Foundation Symposium, Amsterdam, 1978, Elsevier.
159. Sokoloff L, Reivich M, Kennedy C, et al: The [14C]deoxyglucose method for the measurement of local cerebral glucose utilization: theory, procedure, and normal values in the conscious and anesthetized albino rat, *J Neurochem* 28:897, 1977.
160. Steen PA, Milde JH, Michenfelder JD: No barbiturate protection in a dog model of complete cerebral ischemia, *Ann Neurol* 5:343, 1979.
161. Stone JG, Young WL, Marans ZS, et al: Cardiac performance preserved despite thiopental loading, *Anesthesiology* 79:36, 1993.
162. Stone JG, Young WL, Smith CR, et al: Do standard monitoring sites reflect true brain temperature when profound hypothermia is rapidly induced and reversed? *Anesthesiology* 82:344, 1995.
163. Strong AJ, Fairfield JE, Monteiro E, et al: Insulin protects cognitive function in experimental stroke, *J Neurol Neurosurg Psychiat* 53:847, 1990.
164. Svensson LG, Stewart RW, Cosgrove DM, et al: Intrathecal papaverine for the prevention of paraplegia after operation on the thoracic or thoracoabdominal aorta, *J Thorac Cardiovasc Surg* 96:823, 1988.
165. Swanson PD: Acidosis and some metabolic properties of isolated cerebral tissues, *Arch Neurol* 20:653, 1969.
166. Takagi K, Ginsberg MD, Globus M Y-T, et al: Effect of hyperthermia on glutamate release in ischemic penumbra after middle cerebral artery occlusion in rats, *Am J Physiol* 266:H1770, 1994.
167. Takano K, Formato JE, Tatlisumak T, et al: Effects of the glycine antagonist, ZD9379, on experimental focal ischemia in rats (abstract), *Stroke* 27:188, 1996.
168. Tempelhoff R, Modica PA, Rich KM, et al: Use of computerized electroencephalographic monitoring during aneurysm surgery, *J Neurosurg* 71:24, 1989.
169. Todd MM, Drummond JC, Sang U H: The hemodynamic consequences of high-dose thiopental anesthesia, *Anesth Analg* 64:681, 1985.
170. Todd MM, Hindman BJ, Warner DS: Barbiturate protection and cardiac surgery-A different result, *Anesthesiology* 74:402, 1991.
171. Todd MM, Warner DS, Sokoll MD, et al: A prospective comparative trial of three anesthetics for supratentorial craniotomy: fentanyl/propofol, isoflurane/N2O, and fentanyl/N2O, *Anesthesiology* 78:1005, 1993.
172. Tomida S, Nowak Jr TS, Vass K, et al: Experimental model for repetitive ischemic attacks in the gerbil: the cumulative effect of repeated ischemic insults, *J Cereb Blood Flow Metab* 7:773, 1987.
173. Tommasino C, Moore S, Todd MM: Cerebral effects of isovolemic hemodilution with crystalloid or colloid solutions, *Crit Care Med* 16:862, 1988.
174. Tsuchida E, Bullock R: The effect of the glycine site-specific N-methyl-D-aspartate antagonist ACEA1021 on ischemic brain damage caused by acute subdural hematoma in the rat, *J Neurotrauma* 12:279, 1995.
175. Uematsu D, Greenberg JH, Reivich M, et al: Direct evidence for calcium-induced ischemic and reperfusion injury, *Ann Neurol* 26:280, 1989.
176. Vitez TS, White PF, Eger EI: Effects of hypothermia on halothane MAC and isoflurane MAC in the rat, *Anesthesiology* 41:80, 1974.
177. Warner DS, Boehland LA: The effects of iso-osmolal hemodilution on post-ischemic brain water content in the rat, *Anesthesiology* 68:86, 1988.
178. Warner DS, Deshpande JK, Wieloch T: The effect of isoflurane on neuronal necrosis following near-complete forebrain ischemia in the rat, *Anesthesiology* 64:19, 1986.
179. Warner DS, Gionet TX, Todd MM, et al: Insulin-induced normoglycemia improves ischemic outcome in hyperglycemic rats, *Stroke* 1775, 1992.

180. Warner DS, Hansen TD, Vust L, et al: Distribution of cerebral blood flow during deep isoflurane vs. pentobarbital anesthesia in rats with middle cerebral artery occlusion, *J Neurosurg Anesth* 1:219, 1989.
181. Warner DS, Ludwig PS, Pearlstein R, et al: Halothane reduces focal ischemic injury in the rat when brain temperature is controlled, *Anesthesiology* 82:1237, 1995.
182. Warner DS, Martin HJ, Ludwig P, et al: *In vivo* models of cerebral ischemia: effects of parenterally administered NMDA receptor glycine site antagonists, *J Cereb Blood Flow Metab* 15:188, 1995.
183. Warner DS, McFarlane C, Todd MM, et al: Sevoflurane and halothane reduce focal ischemic brain damage in the rat: possible influence on thermoregulation, *Anesthesiology* 79:985, 1993.
184. Warner DS, Takaoka S, Wu B, et al: Electroencephalographic burst suppression is not required to elicit maximal neuroprotection from pentobarbital in a rat model of focal cerebral ischemia. *Anesthesiology* 84:475–484, 1996.
185. Warner DS, Zhou J, Ramani R, et al: Reversible focal ischemia in the rat: effects of halothane, isoflurane and methohexital anesthesia, *J Cereb Blood Flow Metab* 11:794, 1991.
186. Wass CT, Lanier WL, Hofer RE, et al: Temperature changes of ≥ 1° C alter functional neurologic outcome and histopathology in a canine model of complete cerebral ischemia, *Anesthesiology* 83:325, 1995.
187. Werner C, Hoffman WE, Thomas C, et al: Ganglionic blockade improves neurologic outcome from incomplete ischemia in rats-partial reversal by exogenous catecholamines, *Anesthesiology* 73:923, 1990.
188. Widmann R, Miyazawa T, Hossmann KA: Protective effect of hypothermia on hippocampal injury after 30 minutes of forebrain ischemia in rats is mediated by postischemic recovery of protein synthesis, *J Neurochem* 61:200, 1993.
189. Wilber RG, Thompson GH, Shaffer JW, et al: Postoperative neurological deficits in segmental spinal instrumentation, *J Bone Joint Surg* 66-A:1178, 1984.
190. Wong KC: Physiology and pharmacology of hypothermia, *West J Med* 138:227, 1983.
191. Yang J, Zorumski CF: Effects of isoflurane on N-methyl-D-aspartate gated ion channels in cultured rat hippocampal neurons, *Ann NY Acad Sci* 625:287, 1991.
192. Zaidan JR, Klochany A, Martin WM, et al: Effect of thiopental on neurologic outcome following coronary artery bypass grafting, *Anesthesiology* 74:406, 1991.
193. Zasslow MA, Pearl RG, Shuer LM, et al: Hyperglycemia decreases acute neuronal ischemic changes after middle cerebral artery occlusion in cats, *Stroke* 20:519, 1989.
194. Zornow MH, Scheller MS, Todd MM, et al: Acute cerebral effects of isotonic crystalloid and colloid solutions following cryogenic brain injury in the rabbit, *Anesthesiology* 69:180, 1988.

CHAPTER 92

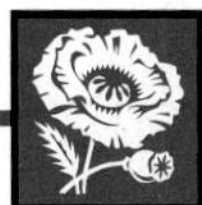

Anaphylactic Reactions and Anesthesia

ROBERT S. HOLZMAN
CAROL A. HIRSHMAN

Anaphylaxis is an acute, severe, and potentially life-threatening reaction. Because of its sudden onset and potential for catastrophic outcome, anaphylaxis may be the most important clinical allergic reaction. The first reported death from anaphylaxis was recorded in the year 2600 BC. Written in hieroglyphics, it tells the story of Menes,who died after a fatal Hymenoptera (bee) sting.[156] In 1902, Portier and Richet[156] reported that the second injection of sea anemone extract into dogs resulted in a fatal systemic reaction after a first injection had no direct observable effect. This result was totally unexpected at the time, and Richet coined the word *anaphylaxis* from the Greek *ana* ("contrary to") and *phylaxis* ("protection"). Thus, the term was initially used to describe a phenomenon in which repeated exposure to a foreign protein produced an adverse reaction rather than the intended immunization or prophylaxis. For his discovery of anaphylaxis, Richet won the Nobel Prize in 1913 (Fig. 92-1).

EPIDEMIOLOGY OF ANAPHYLAXIS DURING ANESTHESIA

Anaphylaxis during anesthesia may have a different epidemiology and etiology than nonanesthetic associated anaphylaxis. **The incidence of anaphylaxis during anesthesia is variable, but ranges between 0.5 and 16.3:10,000** (Table 92-1). Cardiovascular collapse has been described as the most common presenting problem. **Patients who react have a greater incidence of allergy, atopy, asthma, and previous reactions than nonreactors.** The higher incidence of allergy, atopy, and asthma has led to suggestions that these are significant predictive factors. Whereas a past history of drug allergy was found in 37% of cases, and atopy in 38%,[26] the majority of patients do not have such a history, and most patients with such a history do not react.[36] One

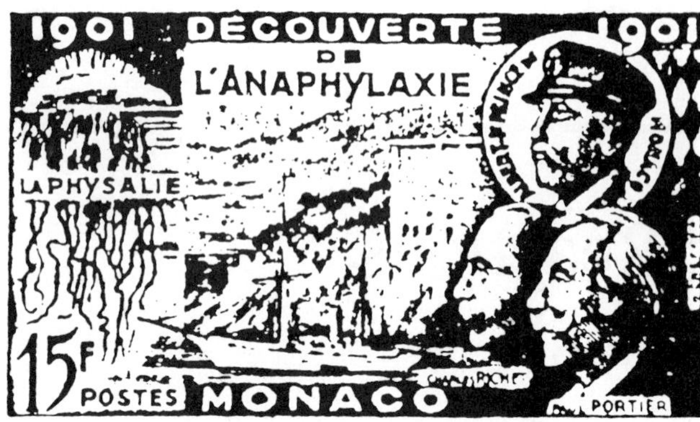

Fig. 92-1. Monaco stamp commemorating the discovery of anaphylaxis by Richet and Portier.

Table 92-1 Anaphylaxis during anesthesia: incidence

Location	Incidence	Mortality (%)	Reference
Australia	0.5–1:10,000	3.4	58
United States	3.3:10,000		215
France, single institution	16.3:10,000		213
France	1–2:10,000		55
Germany	0.5–3:10,000	3–6	200
Boston Collaborative Drug Program (United States, New Zealand, Scotland)	4.5:10,000	5	1

cannot then validate this hypothesis based on a higher incidence of allergic phenomena in reactors.[57] A multicenter survey carried out in France in 1990 and 1991 revealed that in a series of 1585 patients, reactions occurred mostly in adults (80%), but 9% were observed in children, and 86% of the reactions occurred in women.[213] Thus, **predisposing factors are more commonly associated with the women, preexisting allergy or atopy history, and previous anesthetic exposure** (Table 92-2).[22,55,61]

Causation of anaphylaxis during anesthesia in most reviews has been attributed to induction agents, and particularly, muscle relaxants. A review of 826 patients referred to an Anesthetic Allergy Clinic in Australia over a 17-year period revealed severe immediate anaphylactic reactions in 54%; in 59% a muscle relaxant was involved.[58] Four hundred fifty-two patients were evaluated in an allergy-anesthesia clinic in Nice, France; 62 patients experienced anaphylaxis, 57 due to muscle relaxants, 4 to latex and 1 to gelatine. By avoiding drug reexposure and offering alternate methods of anesthesia (e.g., regional block), subsequent allergic reactions were avoided.[152] A 20-year review of the French and English language literature (1964–

Table 92-2 Anaphylaxis during anesthesia: associated findings

	Previous history		
Reference	Allergy (%)	Atopy (%)	Female Gender (%)
26	37	38	
213	52		
21		48	86
117			62
58	45	39	80
108	72		76

1984) yielded 975 cases of immediate life-threatening anaphylactoid reactions due to parenterally administered anesthetic drugs. The greatest number of cases was caused by muscle relaxants (51%) and hypnotic drugs (42.3%).[26] In one series, the most frequently suspected drug was succinylcholine.[213] In a recent series, the substances involved were muscle relaxants (70%), latex (12.6%), hypnotics (3.6%), benzodiazepines (2.0%), opioids (1.7%), colloids (4.7%), and antibiotics (2.6%).[117] Although neuromuscular blocking drugs account for most of the cases of significant anaphylactoid reactions (59%–70%), particularly in Europe and Australia the incidence of latex-related reactions is increasing.[200]

Mosicki et al.[144] reported 27 patients who were referred for evaluation of anaphylaxis after induction of general anesthesia in which thiobarbiturates, muscle relaxants, or antibiotics were administered intravenously (IV). Skin tests were positive in 13 patients (thiobarbiturates in 5, muscle relaxants in 6, and antibiotics in 2 patients).[144] Twenty-eight adults with a history of a generalized allergic reaction during anesthesia were investigated by Binkley et al.[21]; 17 had positive thiopental skin tests, 14 had in IgE thiopental RAST value greater than two standard deviations above the mean for control sera from ragweed-allergic subjects. Allergy to thiopental as a possible basis for the reactions was confirmed in more than 50% of the patients who were investigated.[21] In a 20-year claims study, Kurtz et al.[108] reported 31 anaphylactic episodes during anesthetic induction out of 268 incidents partially or totally attributable to anesthesia. Thiopental-succinylcholine combined accounted for 60%, whereas alfadione-succinylcholine accounted for another 25%.[108] Clarke and Watkins[34] examined the pattern of drugs responsible for anaphylactoid reactions in Sheffield during 4 years and graded the reactions. They included only systemic, life-threatening, and potentially fatal reactions and determined that 120 to 150 reports per year occurred. Succinylcholine was involved in nearly 50% of the reactions, thiopental in more than 50%, and propofol in 23%.[34]

There were 57 reports of possible allergic reactions in the perioperative period reported to the Australian Incident Monitoring Study, representing approximately 3% of the first 2000 incidents. Nineteen were judged as "very likely allergic responses," which represented nearly 1% of the first 2000 incidents. Suspected causative agents included "induction drug" (38 of 58), antibiotic (19 of 57), nondepolarizing relaxant (14 of 57), opiate (12 of 57), blood/plasma/Haemaccel (11 of 57) or "other" (16 of 57). Forty (70%) were associated with two or more of the first three indicators (Table 92-3).[36]

Anaphylaxis has been estimated to occur in the United States at rates as high as once in every 3000 patients, and may account for more than 500 deaths annually.[215] These reactions resulted in a 3.4% mortality rate in Australia. Drug sensitization has likewise been implicated in 4.3% of deaths and 5.6% of cerebral damage in cases of anesthetic mishaps reported in the United Kingdom.[60] Undoubtedly, an increasing awareness of the existence of anaphylaxis during anesthesia has contributed to some changes in the recognition of its occurrence.[22] Although anaphylactic reactions are a rare event during anesthesia, the high incidence of morbidity and mortality make these reactions a major concern.

MAST CELL ACTIVATION

The activation of mast cells and basophils, with the generation and release of vasoactive and bronchoconstrictive mediators, is the central and penultimate step in the anaphylactic syndromes. Mediators released from mast cells and basophils cause severe and abrupt physiologic alterations, leading to urticaria, laryngeal edema, nausea, vomiting, abdominal pain, diarrhea, or bronchospasm with or without cardiovascular collapse. Classically, the term *anaphylaxis* has been employed to denote an IgE antibody-mediated reaction. The same clinical manifestations may occur consequent to non–IgE-mediated reactions, which have previously been termed anaphylactoid or "pseudoallergic" reactions. For simplicity, throughout the rest of this chapter, the term *anaphylaxis* will refer to the clinical syndrome, without implying a specific mechanism.

IgE-Mediated Anaphylaxis

Antigenic molecules (usually proteins) capable of stimulating IgE antibody production may cause IgE-mediated anaphylaxis after initial sensitization and subsequent reexposure. Haptens are molecules that are too small to stimulate immune responses themselves. However, haptens may bind to endogenous proteins, such as serum albumin, and become antigenic. Once produced, IgE antibodies become fixed to tissue mast cells and/or circulating basophils, both of which contain high-affinity IgE receptors.[135] Reexposure to antigens or haptens, with subsequent cross-linking of IgE antibody, causes the direct bridging of cell surface IgE-receptor molecules. This induces activation of membrane-associated enzymes, causing complex biochemical cascades that lead to an influx of extracellular calcium and a mobilization of intracellular calcium with subsequent release of

Table 92-3 Drugs associated with anaphylaxis during anesthesia*

Reference	Number of reactions	Succinylcholine (%)	Alcuronium (%)	Atracurium (%)	d-Tubocurarine (%)	Vecuronium (%)	Pancuronium (%)	Thiopental (%)	Propofol (%)	Etomidate (%)	Latex (%)
34	529	45	10	16	3	12	2	57	23	4	
213	21	38	5				5	10			
26	975	63	33	100	60			69			
152	62	65									6
21	23	0						74			4
117	1585	43	8	7		37	13	62	34		13
58	443	27	44	8	7	1	3	53	1		
108	35	91						60			

*The percent of total cases in which the drug was used. In most cases, multiple drugs were used.

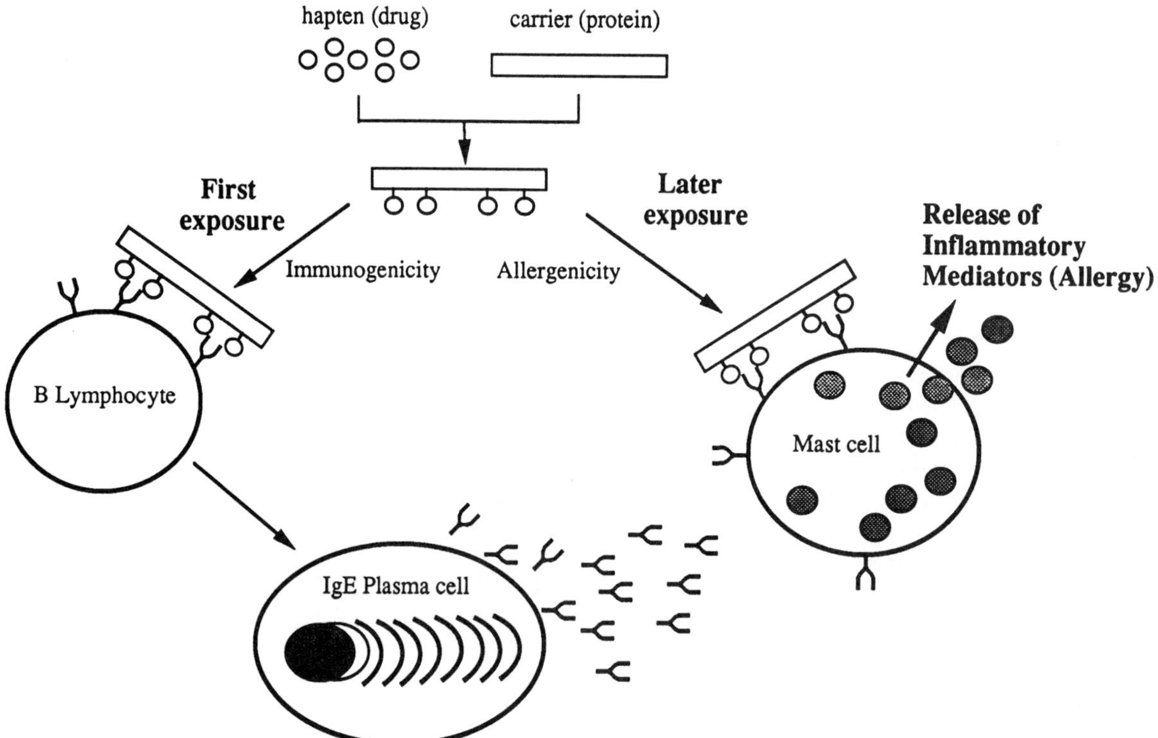

Fig. 92-2. The drug hapten combines with a carrier molecule to induce IgE antibody production against the drug. On subsequent exposure, hapten combines with IgE antibody on mast cell surface, leading to anaphylactic reaction.

preformed granule-associated mediators and the generation of new mediators from cell membrane phospholipids (Fig. 92-2).[93,181]

Complement-Mediated Reactions

Complement consists of a series of plasma and cell membrane proteins that lyse susceptible targets, promote phagocytosis and generate peptide mediators (anaphylotoxins) of the inflammatory response.[41,64] The anaphylatoxins are capable of causing mast cell and basophil mediator release, directly increasing vascular permeability, contracting smooth muscles, aggregating platelets, and stimulating macrophages to produce thromboxane (Fig. 92-3).[68,227] The complement cascade may be activated through either the classic pathway or the alternative pathway. Complement activation through the classic pathway can be initiated through IgG or IgM antibody-binding to antigens such as in hemolytic ABO-incompatible blood transfusion reactions. Heparin-protamine complexes have also been shown *in vitro*[167] and *in vivo*[19,104] to activate complement via the classic pathway. Injection of preformed immune complexes or IgG aggregates can activate complement and mimic clinical anaphylaxis.[215] Patients with selective IgA antibody deficiency may develop IgG anti-IgA antibodies after receiving multiple transfusions, which may result in complement activation and anaphylactic reactions.[214] Complement activation via the alternative pathway may be stimulated by lipopolysaccharides (endotoxins),[54] Althesin,[216] radiocontrast media,[73] and membranes used for cardiopulmonary bypass and dialysis.[35]

Pharmacologic (Nonimmunologic) Mast Cell Activators

Certain drugs can cause mast cell–mediator release by a nonimmunologic mechanism. The exact mechanism of nonimmunologic mediator release is poorly understood, but release is noncytotoxic. Drugs that induce nonimmunologic release include opiates (especially morphine and codeine)[48,87] and neuromuscular-blocking agents such as atracurium and d-tubocurarine.[150] Recent evidence suggests that neuromuscular-blocking agents such as atracurium, vecuronium, or succinylcholine may also induce mast cell–mediator release via IgE antibodies directed against quarternary or tertiary ammonium ion epitopes.[12,83,211]

Mediators of Anaphylactic Reactions

Any of the mechanisms described may lead to mast cell- and/or basophil-mediator release. Mediators released include those preformed and stored in granules and those newly generated on appropriate stimulation. Release of these mediators may cause various pathophysiologic responses that may result in life-threatening anaphylactic reactions. The variously preformed and newly generated mediators released by mast cells and/or basophils, along with

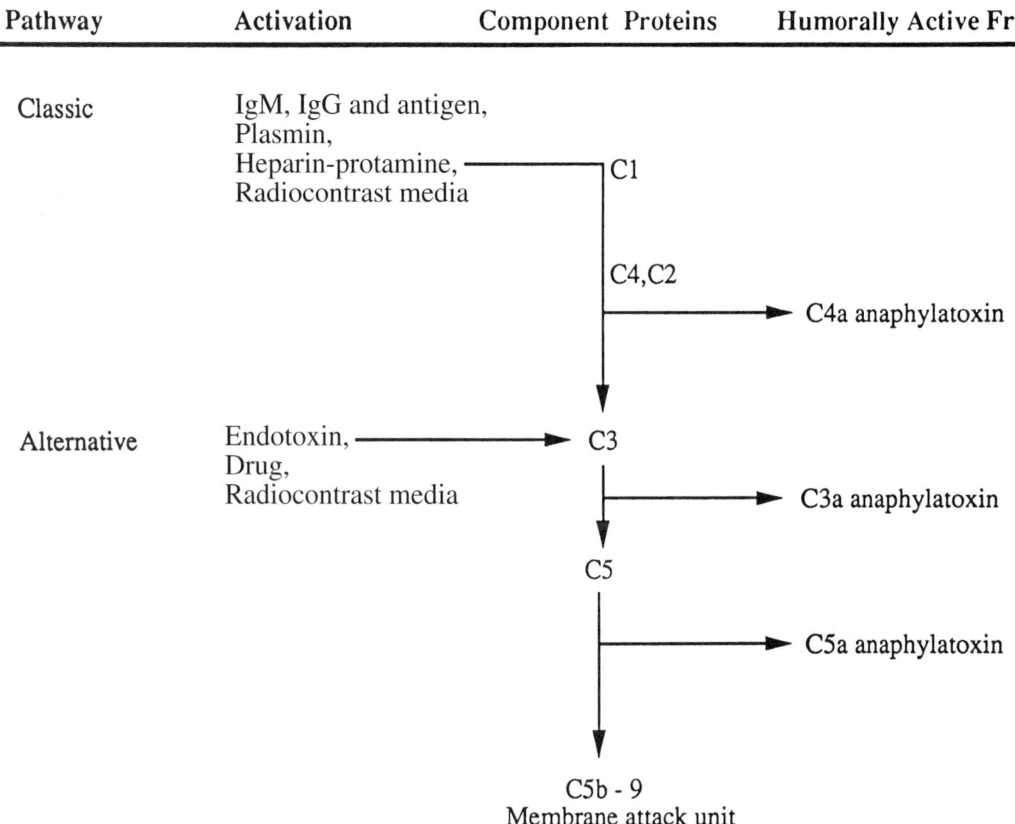

Fig. 92-3. Schematic diagram outlining pathways, stimuli, and humorally active fragments produced from complement activation. (Modified from Levy JH: *Anaphylactic reactions in anesthesia and intensive care,* Boston, 1986, Butterworths.)

their biologic actions and physiologic effects, are shown in Table 92-4.

CLINICAL MANIFESTATIONS OF ANAPHYLAXIS

Individuals vary in the onset and manifestations of anaphylaxis. In general, symptoms begin soon (within minutes) after introduction of the causative agent but can be delayed for 1 to 2 hours. Along with other symptoms, conscious patients frequently describe a sense of impending doom. **The primary anaphylactic target organs in humans are the cutaneous, gastrointestinal (GI), respiratory, and cardiovascular systems** (Table 92-5). Involvement of the respiratory and cardiovascular systems are of primary importance. In a large series of fatal anaphylactic reactions occurring outside of the operating room, 70% died from respiratory complications and 24% from cardiovascular complications.[14] **During general and regional anesthesia, or during deep sedation, cardiovascular signs predominate.**[59]

Cutaneous Manifestations

Initial signs and symptoms may include erythema, flushing, and pruritus (especially of the palms, soles, and groin), which often progress to urticaria and angioedema.

Gastrointestinal Manifestations

Gastrointestinal findings (in awake or easily arouseable patients) may include nausea, cramping abdominal pain, vomiting, and intense diarrhea that may be bloody.

Respiratory Manifestations

Upper respiratory tract involvement includes laryngeal edema, which may progress to asphyxia. This finding is of grave importance and must be carefully assessed. Early symptoms of laryngeal edema in the conscious patient include hoarseness, dysphonia, or a "lump in the throat." Lower respiratory tract involvement often manifests as chest tightness, shortness of breath, cough, wheezing, or difficulty in ventilating the patient because of an increase in airway pressures.

Cardiovascular Manifestations

Cardiovascular signs may include hypotension and tachycardia with symptoms of light-headedness, faintness, and syncope. Cardiovascular complications include myocardial infarction (MI), dysrhythmias, and cardiovascular collapse.

Intraoperative and Perioperative Anaphylaxis

Evaluation and treatment of patients who develop anaphylaxis in the operating room are challenging even for the ex-

Table 92-4 Biologic actions and physiologic manifestations of mast cell mediators

Mediators	Biologic action	Physiologic manifestations
Preformed		
Histamine	Smooth muscle contraction	Bronchospasm, abdominal pain, diarrhea, nausea, vomiting
	Vasodilation	Tachycardia, hypotension
	Increases vasopermeability	Edema, urticaria/angioedema, influx of inflammatory cells
	Stimulates mucus secretion	Excessive respiratory/gastrointestinal secretions, inspissation
ECF-A	Eosinophil chemotaxis	Inflammation
NCA	Neutrophil chemotaxis	Inflammation
Neutral proteases	Cleaves amino acids from proteins	
	? stimulate mucus secretion	
Proteoglycans (heparin and chondroitin sulfate)	Anticoagulant	?
Newly generated		
PGD_2	Smooth muscle contraction	Bronchospasm, abdominal pain, diarrhea, nausea, vomiting
	Vasodilation	Tachycardia, hypotension
	Stimulates mucus secretion	Excessive respiratory/gastrointestinal secretions, inspissation
	Inhibits platelet aggregation	?
	Enhances basophil mediator release	Potentiates reactions
$LTC_4/D_4/E_4$ (SRS-A)	Smooth muscle contraction	Bronchospasm, abdominal pain, diarrhea, nausea, vomiting
	Vasodilation	Tachycardia, hypotension
	Increases vasopermeability	Edema, urticaria/angioedema, influx of inflammatory cells
	Stimulates mucus secretion	Excessive respiratory/gastrointestinal secretions, inspissation
PAF	Smooth muscle contraction	Bronchospasm, abdominal pain, diarrhea, nausea, vomiting
	Vasodilation	Tachycardia, hypotension
	Increases vasopermeability	Edema, urticaria/angioedema, hypotension
	Decreases inotropy of heart	Hypotension
	Neutrophil stimulation	?
	Platelet aggregation	?

perienced physician. In the perioperative period, multiple medications are frequently given in close proximity, making temporal relationships more difficult to interpret. Patients are frequently unconscious and draped, potentially masking early signs and symptoms of anaphylaxis. Anesthetics themselves alter mediator release, possibly delaying early recognition of the syndrome.[101] **Often the only observed manifestation of anaphylaxis occurring during anesthesia is cardiovascular collapse,[122] a relatively late event in the syndrome.** In suspected anaphylactic reactions in patients undergoing hemodynamic monitoring, cardiovascular changes are characterized by decreases in systolic, diastolic, and mean arterial pressures. Systemic vascular resistance (SVR) also decreases, while cardiac output and stroke volume increase. Sudden decreases in pulmonary compliance may be manifested by an increase in airway pressures during positive-pressure ventilation. Cyanosis (associated with O_2 desaturation) also may be noted.[59]

DIFFERENTIAL DIAGNOSIS

In a conscious patient, anaphylaxis is most easily confused with a vasovagal reaction (Box 92-1). This usually occurs when a patient collapses after an injection or painful procedure. During a vasovagal reaction, the patient looks pale and complains of nausea before syncope but does not note pruritus or become cyanotic. Respiratory difficulty does not occur and symptoms are almost immediately relieved once the patient is supine. The syndrome is usually accompanied by profuse diaphoresis and bradycardia, without flushing, urticaria, angioedema, pruritus, or wheezing. The differential diagnosis of sudden collapse also includes dysrhythmias, MI, aspiration of food and foreign body, pulmonary embolism, seizure disorder, hypoglycemia, and stroke. In the presence of laryngeal edema, especially when accompanied by abdominal pain, the diagnosis of hereditary angioedema should be considered. *Globus hystericus* and fictitious asthma need to be considered when respiratory symptoms are present.

Serum sickness may present with urticaria similar to anaphylaxis, but it generally occurs from 6 to 21 days after the antigenic stimulation and is frequently associated with fever, lymphadenopathy, arthralgias, arthritis, nephritis, and neuritis. Other conditions that can mimic anaphylaxis include overdose of medication, cold urticaria (especially if generalized), idiopathic urticaria, carcinoid tumors, and systemic mastocytosis.

Table 92-5 Clinical manifestations of anaphylaxis

System	Signs and symptoms
Cutaneous	Pruritis
	Flushing*
	Erythema*
	Urticaria/angioedema*
Gastrointestinal	Nausea
	Abdominal pain
	Diarrhea
	Vomiting
Respiratory	Laryngeal edema
	Hoarseness
	Dysphonia
	"Lump" in throat
	Chest tightness
	Dyspnea
	Cough
	Wheezing*
	Cyanosis*
	Increase in peak airway pressure*
Cardiovascular	Light-headedness
	Faintness
	Syncope
	Tachycardia*
	Hypotension*
	Dysrhythmias*

*Most likely to occur in patients during anesthesia.

In an anesthetized patient, anaphylaxis may be confused with other catastrophes producing cardiovascular collapse and/or severe hypotension or bronchospasm. These include MI or dysrhythmias, drug overdose, pulmonary embolism, irritant-induced bronchospasm, pulmonary edema, and aspiration of gastric contents (see Box 92-1).

TREATMENT OF ANAPHYLAXIS

Anaphylactic reactions must be recognized early because death may occur within minutes.[96] The longer initial therapy is delayed, the greater the incidence of fatality.[13] Morbidity and mortality from anaphylactic reactions are primarily associated with compromised cardiovascular and respiratory function. Therefore close monitoring of vital signs—focusing on blood pressure, airway patency, and ventilation—is most important in assessing the severity of the reaction and response to therapy. Treatment of anaphylactic reactions can be divided into initial and secondary therapies (Box 92-2).

Initial Therapy

Initial therapy involves the following procedures:

- When possible, steps should be taken to interrupt further administration and absorption of the offending agent. Intravenous (IV) infusions of suspected allergens should be stopped immediately. The airway should be maintained and 100% O_2 should be administered; adequate arterial oxygenization should be monitored with arterial blood gas values and pulse oximetry. If the trachea is not already intubated and there is any suggestion of airway compromise secondary to laryngeal edema, the tracheal intubation should be accomplished immediately. If laryngeal edema is present, aerosolized epinephrine (three inhalations of 0.16 to 0.20 mg epinephrine/inhalation from a metered-dose inhaler) or by a nebulizer (8 to 15 drops of 2.25% epinephrine in 2 ml normal saline) may be useful. If laryngeal edema is refractory to these measures or is progressing too rapidly, a needle catheter cricothyrotomy or emergency surgical cricothyrotomy may be necessary.
- At the first signs of a severe reaction, intravenous access should be established (if not already in place), and blood pressure should be maintained with the administration of isotonic crystalloid (normal saline) solutions. Rapid administration of 25 to 50 ml/kg (2 to 4 l in an adult) of normal saline or lactated Ringer's solution is important in the initial therapy for these reactions. Military antishock trousers (MAST suit) can be useful in patients suffering hypotension secondary to anaphylaxis.[20,128] The MAST suit provides perfusion to vital organs and may also help obtain peripheral venous access in the upper extremities.[126]

BOX 92-1
DIFFERENTIAL DIAGNOSIS OF ANAPHYLAXIS

Vasovagal reaction
Dysrythmia
Myocardial infarction
Overdose of medication or illicit drugs
Pulmonary embolism
Seizure disorder
Cerebrovascular accident
Aspiration
Globus hystericus
Fictitious asthma
Hereditary angioedema
Physical or idiopathic urticaria
Serum sickness
Carcinoid tumors
Systemic mastosystosis

Epinephrine is the mainstay of initial pharmacologic treatment. In cases of severe hypotension or airway obstruction, 0.1-ml (100 μg) increments of 1:1000 (0.0001 to 0.001 mg/kg) epinephrine should be administered IV, usually not exceeding 0.5 mg total. Depending on the patient's condition, however, the dosage may need to be increased. Risks include cardiac dysrhythmias (especially during halothane

BOX 92-2
MANAGEMENT OF ANAPHYLAXIS

Inital therapy

Stop administration or reduce absorption of offending agent
- If antigen given subcutaneously:
  - Venous tourniquet proximal to site
  - Epinephrine (1:1000) into antigen site
- If latex is suspected:
  - Consider potential routes of administration, including mucosal contact and inhalation
  - Remove all latex from surgical field
  - Change to non-latex gloves

Maintain airway and administer 100% O_2
- Aerosolized epinephrine if not already intubated
- Intubation, cricothyrotomy, or tracheostomy

Rapid intravascular volume expansion
- 25 to 50 ml/kg (2 to 4 l) of crystalloid or colloid for hypotension

Administer epinephrine
- 0.01 ml/kg increments of 1:1000 IV—titrate as needed
- 10 ml of 1:10,000—endotracheal administration in adults

Discontinue all anesthetic agents

Consider use of MAST (lower body pressure suit)

Secondary therapy

Administer antihistamine
- Diphenhydramine 1 mg/kg IV or IM (maximal dose 50 mg)
- Ranitidine 1 mg/kg IV (maximal dose 50 mg)

Administer glucocorticoids
- Hydrocortisone—5 mg/kg initially and then 2.5 mg/kg q 4 to 6 hrs
- Methylprednisolone—1 mg/kg initially and 0.8 mg/kg q 4 to 6 hrs

Administer aminophylline
- Loading dose—5 to 6 mg/kg
- Continuous infusion—0.4 to 0.9 mg/kg/hr (check blood level)

Administer inhaled β_2-adrenergic agonists

Continuous catecholamine infusion
- Epinephrine—0.02 to 0.05 μg/kg/min (2 to 4 μg/min)
- Norepinephrine—0.05 μg/kg/min (2 to 4 μg/min)
- Dopamine—5 to 20 μg/kg/min

Administer sodium bicarbonate
- 0.5 to 1 mg/kg initially, titrate using ABGs

anesthesia), MI, or stroke. In the rare instance when an IV access is not present, 0.3 ml of 1:1000 epinephrine can be administered intramuscularly (IM) or 10 ml of 1:10,000 epinephrine can be administered through the endotracheal (ET) tube. However, when a patient is in shock, the absorption of IM or subcutaneous epinephrine is unreliable.

Inhalational anesthetics should be discontinued. Anesthetics have negative inotropic properties, may decrease SVR, and may interfere with the reflex compensatory response to hypotension. Halothane also sensitizes the heart to circulating catecholamines, required for the treatment of severe anaphylactic reactions.

Secondary Treatment

After the initial treatment of cardiovascular and respiratory abnormalities, the administration of other pharmacologic agents may be warranted.

An antihistamine, such as diphenhydramine, will be helpful for symptomatic relief of itching. Although there is no evidence demonstrating the effectiveness of histamine$_2$-receptor antagonists in the treatment of anaphylaxis, ranitidine (1 mg/kg IV) may be useful[129] when hypotension is persistent, because peripheral vasodilation may be exacerbated by the effects of histamine on endothelial histamine$_2$-receptors. The role of cimetidine is controversial.[121]

Glucocorticoids may be useful in preventing potential late-phase reactions and in treating persistent bronchospasm, but they will have no immediate effects. Hydrocortisone, 5 mg/kg (up to 200 mg initial dose) and then 2.5 mg/kg every 6 hours or methylprednisolone 1 mg/kg initially and every 6 hours as indicated, may be given.

For persistent bronchospasm, aminophylline—administered IV in a loading dose (5 to 6 mg/kg) followed by a continuous infusion (0.4 to 0.9 mg/kg/hour)—may be helpful. We have recently shown that aminophylline acutely releases catecholamines,[201] which may be responsible for the beneficial effects of aminophylline on airways. It may be more prudent to use beta$_2$-adrenergic agonists by aerosol.

For persistent hypotension, catecholamine infusions may be used. Epinephrine may be useful if both hypotension and bronchospasm persist. Suggested starting doses of epinephrine are indicated in Box 92-2. If greater than 8 to 10 μg/min are required, tachycardia may be a significant side effect and norepinephrine may be more effective. Suggested starting dose for norepinephrine is 0.05 μg/kg/min (2 to 4 μg/min) and should be titrated to maintain tissue perfusion. Dopamine may be used to maintain blood pressure. A dose of 5 to 20 μg/kg/min may help maintain cardiac output, thereby improving coronary, cerebral, renal, and mesenteric blood flow.

Treatment with bicarbonate is controversial and should probably be reserved for profound acidosis or accompanying severe cardiovascular instability.[16,76,147] If profound acidosis is suspected, sodium bicarbonate (0.5 to 1 mg/kg) should be administered initially. Acid-base status must be monitored using arterial blood gas levels to guide further therapeutic interventions.

Response to therapy is usually prompt, but despite all of the measures mentioned previously, some patients do not respond quickly. Treatment of anaphylaxis may be complicated by the increased use of beta-adrenergic-blocking agents (e.g., propranolol).[94] Treatment of anaphylaxis in patients who are taking beta-blocking drugs is not clear. A limited number of studies have suggested that in addition to the measures mentioned previously, use of the MAST suit and the administration of atropine or glucagon may also be of benefit.[215]

DETERMINING THE CAUSE OF ALLERGIC REACTIONS

Patients who have had anaphylactic reactions to drugs administered in the operating room require evaluation to identify the causal agents and to guide selection and use of future medications.

The evaluation starts with a detailed patient history, including concurrent illness and earlier allergic and anesthetic encounters (Box 92-3). It is helpful to prepare a flow diagram of the patient's reaction temporally depicting the clinical manifestations of the reaction and the medications received, including indications, when initiated, doses, and duration of therapy. Equally important information includes previous exposure to the same or structurally related medications, the effect of drug discontinuation, the response to treatment, and any previous diagnostic testing or rechallenge. Medications should be considered with regard to their known propensity for causing anaphylaxis. The proximity of drug administration to the onset of acute reactions should also be documented. In general, agents that have been used for long, continuous periods before the onset of an acute reaction are less likely to be implicated than agents recently introduced or reintroduced. However, in the perioperative period, patients commonly receive many medications in close temporal proximity, making a diagnosis by history alone difficult.

Immunodiagnostic Tests

Skin testing for immediate hypersensitivity reactions.

Although standardized and commonly used by allergists in the diagnosis of immediate hypersensitivity to aeroallergens and Hymenoptera allergy, the evaluation of drug allergy is hampered by the unavailability of relevant drug metabolites or appropriate multivalent testing reagents. However, **intradermal skin tests are still the most readily available and generally useful diagnostic test for drug allergy.** Skin testing clearly has an established role in the evaluation of IgE-mediated penicillin allergy[221] and is also useful in the evaluation of allergy to muscle relaxants,[56,211] barbiturates,[56,143] chymopapain,[71] streptokinase,[47] insulin,[82] latex,[141,182] and miscellaneous drugs. Specific protocols for skin testings are well documented[4,148] but will not be discussed in detail here.

For safety, a scratch or puncture (epicutaneous) test should be performed before the more definitive intradermal test.[4] Appropriate skin testing concentrations of medications commonly used in anesthesia practice have been published.[56,211] When skin testing with drugs or reagents that have not been well validated previously, all positive skin-test responses should be confirmed by skin testing five normal individuals as an appropriate control to rule out irritative, false-positive skin responses. It is prudent to discount negative skin-test results unless previous studies have established their reliability. Skin testing must be done in the absence of medications that will affect the skin test response (especially, H_1 antihistamines, tricyclic antidepressants, and sympathomimetic agents). Appropriate positive (histamine) and negative (diluent) controls should be used.

BOX 92-3
TECHNIQUES USED TO EVALUATE THE CAUSE OF ALLERGIC REACTIONS

Detailed history
In vivo tests
- Skin tests for immediate hypersensitivity reactions*
- Delayed type hypersensitivity skin tests
- Patch tests
- Incremental provocative challenge*

In vitro tests
- Total serum IgE
- Assays to measure complement activation
- Basophil histamine release
- Measurements of mediators — serum/urine
- Lymphocyte blast transformation
- Antigen-specific IgG, M antibody (ELISA, RIA)
- Antigen-specific IgE antibody (RAST)*

*Denotes the technique most often used to evaluate prior reactions.

Other in vivo *tests*

Delayed (tuberculinlike) skin tests have little if any place in the evaluation of drug allergy. Patch tests may be of value in cases of contact dermatitis, even if the eruption was provoked by systemic administration of a drug.

In vitro *tests*

Total serum IgE values. Although increases in total serum IgE have been reported after allergic reactions,[53] the total IgE concentration is rarely, if ever, helpful in establishing the diagnosis of an allergic drug reaction.

Assays to measure complement activation. Assays to measure complement activation include measuring decreases in complement components (e.g., C4, C3, or total hemolytic complement [C_H50]) and assays to measure the generation of products of complement activation (C3a, C4a, C5a, and so on). If positive, these assays may implicate complement activation in specific reactions.

Release of histamine and other mediators by basophils. Washed leukocytes containing basophils with IgE antibody on their cell surfaces will release histamine and other mediators when incubated with relevant antigens.[126,127] In general, results appear to correlate with those of direct immediate skin tests.[27,149] Although the *in vitro* basophil-histamine-release assay avoids exposing a patient to a drug, the assay is relatively laborious, requires whole blood drawn immediately before the test, and at present is limited in availability to research laboratories. This test has been used to demonstrate sensitivity to thiopental,[88] muscle relaxants,[210,211] and penicillins.[164] Because some agents induce nonimmunologic release of histamine, appropriate negative and positive controls are required.

Measurements of mediators. During or shortly after allergic reactions, blood may be obtained and analyzed for the release of various mediators such as histamine, PGD_2, or high molecular-weight neutrophil chemotactic factor.[10,184] Urine may also be analyzed for metabolites of histamine or PGD_2. Plasma histamine and PGD_2 levels remain elevated for only brief periods, limiting their clinical use. Bioassays to measure serum neutrophil chemotactic factor are cumbersome to perform and have large interassay variability. Recently assays to measure serum tryptase (a protease released specifically from mast cells) appeared promising in the clinical assessment of mast cell–mediated allergic reactions.[59,113,173,212] Serum tryptase may remain elevated for hours after release from mast cells.

Radioallergosorbent testing. A solid-phase radioimmunoassay, termed the radioallergosorbent test (RAST), was first introduced in 1967. The RAST measures circulating allergen-specific IgE antibody. The basic principle of the RAST is quite simple. The allergen is attached to a solid-phase (carbohydrate particle, paper disc, or the wall of polystyrene test tubes or plastic microtiter wells) and incubated with the serum under study, during which time a specific antibody of all immunoglobulin classes is bound. The particles are then washed, and a second incubation is undertaken with a radiolabelled, highly specific anti-IgE antibody. After washes, the bound radioactivity is directly related to the allergen-specific IgE antibody content in the original serum. When appropriately done, the RAST correlates well with skin test endpoint titration, basophil-histamine release, and provocation tests.[77,149,165] Results from the serum under study are compared with a positive reference serum and a negative control serum. RASTs have been developed to measure IgE antibody to insulin,[82] chymopapain,[71] muscle relaxants,[12,83] thiopental,[85] trimethoprim,[202] protamine,[223] and latex.[141,206,226] False-positive tests may occur because of high nonspecific binding, high total serum IgE levels, or poor technique.[81] False-negative tests may occur because of interference of high levels of IgG "blocking antibodies" or inability to maximize assay sensitivity.[231]

Requirement of Drug in the Future

If a patient has had an allergic reaction to a medication in the past but requires use of the medication again, the physician must weigh the risks and benefits of readministration. If equally effective and noncross-reacting alternative drugs are available, they should be used. If alternative drugs fail, induce unacceptable side effects, or are clearly less effective, then cautious administration of the drug using a premedication regimen or a desensitization protocol may be considered.

Premedication regimens have been tested, validated, and used most often in patients who have had previous reactions to radiocontrast media and again require the administration of radiocontrast.[73] These reactions are not IgE mediated. There is little evidence supporting the use of premedication with antihistamines or steroids to prevent IgE-mediated anaphylaxis, and therefore the use of these drugs is not recommended for reactions mediated by IgE antibodies.[133,174] Acute desensitization protocols have been developed and used in patients with allergic reactions to penicillin,[3,194,221] insulin,[159] sulfonamides,[185] heterologous antisera,[159] and aspirin.[190]

SPECIFIC ALLERGIC REACTIONS OFTEN SEEN BY THE ANESTHESIOLOGIST

Penicillin Antibiotics

Penicillin antibiotics constitute the most common medications causing allergic drug reactions.[25] Available data do not permit exact conclusions about the true frequency of allergic reactions to penicillin, but they are reported to occur from 0.7% to 8% of treatment cases in different studies.[23,179] Anaphylactic reactions occur in 0.004% to 0.015% of penicillin treatment cases.[92] Fatality from penicillin anaphylaxis occurs about once in every 50,000 to 100,000 treatment cases,[92] resulting in 400 to 800 deaths per year.[179] All four types of immunopathologic reactions described by Gell and Coombs[66] have been seen with penicillin (Table 92-6). Some reactions to penicillin have an obscure pathogenesis and have been labeled idiopathic. Among these are the common maculopapular rash, eosinophilia, Stevens-Johnson syndrome, exfoliative dermatitis, and toxic epidermal necrolysis (Table 92-6). For reasons presently unknown, ampicillin induces rashes with much greater frequency than does penicillin.[177,221] Pseudoanaphylactic reactions have been observed after IM or inadvertent IV injection of procaine penicillin. These reactions are most likely caused by a combination of a toxic and embolic phenomena from procaine.[65] IgE-mediated reactions may be the most important allergic reaction to penicillin clinically because of the risk of life-threatening anaphylaxis.

Penicillin (molecular weight = 356) is a low molecular-weight chemical and as such must first covalently combine with tissue macromolecules (presumably proteins) to produce multivalent hapten-protein complexes, which are required for both the induction of an immune response and the elicitation of an allergic reaction.[50] In the 1960s, Levine and Parker[118,158] showed that the beta-lactam ring in penicillins spontaneously opens under physiologic conditions, forming the penicilloyl group. Recent evidence suggests that this reaction may be facilitated by low molecular-weight molecules in serum.[42,193] The penicilloyl group has been designated the "major determinant" because approximately 95% of the penicillin molecules that irreversibly combine with proteins form penicilloyl moieties.[120] This reaction occurs with the prototype benzylpenicillin and virtually all semisynthetic penicillins.

Benzylpenicillin can also be degraded by other meta-

Table 92-6 Classification of immunopathologic reactions according to the scheme of Gell and Coombs

Type of reactions	Description	Antibody	Cells	Other	Clinical reactions
I	Anaphylactic (reagenic) Immediate hypersensitivity	IgE	Basophils, mast cells		Anaphylaxis, urticaria
II	Cytotoxic or cytolytic	IgG, IgM	Any cell with isoantigen	C′, RES	Coombs + hemolytic anemia; drug induced nephritis; transfusion reaction; Rh disease
III	Immune complex disease	Soluble immune complexes (Ag-Ab)	None directly	C′	Serum sickness; drug fever; glomerulonephritis
IV	"Delayed" or cell mediated hypersensitivity	None known	Sensitized T lymphocytes		Contact dermatitis
V	Ideopathic		?	?	Maculopapular eruptions
			?	?	Eosinophilia
			?	?	Stevens-Johnson syndrome
			?	?	Exfoliative dermatitis

C′ — complement; RES — reticuloendothelial system; Ag-Ab — antigen-antibody; (?) — indicates that the immunopathologic mechanism is in doubt.
From Weiss ME, Adkinson, NR, Jr., *Clin Allerg* 18:515 – 540, 1988.

bolic pathways to form additional antigenic determinants.[119] These derivatives are formed in small quantities and stimulate a variable immune response; hence, they have been termed the "minor determinants." Anaphylactic reactions to penicillin are usually mediated by IgE antibodies directed against minor determinants, although some anaphylactic reactions have occurred in patients with only penicilloyl-specific IgE antibodies.[119–121] Accelerated and late urticarial reactions are generally mediated by penicilloyl-specific IgE antibody (major determinant).[119]

Individuals with a history of previous penicillin reactions have a four- to sixfold increased risk for subsequent reactions to penicillin compared with those without previous histories.[186] However, most serious and fatal allergic reactions to penicillin and beta-lactam antibiotics occur in individuals who have never had a previous allergic reaction. Sensitization of these individuals may have occurred from their last therapeutic course of penicillin or (less likely) by occult environmental exposures.

Approximately 10% to 20% of hospitalized patients claim a history of penicillin allergy. However, studies have shown that many of these patients have been either incorrectly labeled as allergic to penicillin or have lost their sensitivity. The most useful single piece of information in assessing an individual's potential for an immediate IgE-mediated reaction is the skin-test response to major and minor penicillin determinants (Fig. 92-4).

Penicillin anaphylaxis has not been reported in patients with negative skin tests. Therefore, negative skin tests indicate that penicillin antibiotics may be safely given. A limited number of patients with positive skin tests have been treated with therapeutic doses of penicillin. The risk of an anaphylactic or accelerated allergic reaction ranges from 50% to 70% in such patients.[221] Therefore, if skin tests are positive, equally effective non–cross-reacting antibiotics should be substituted when available. If alternative drugs fail, induce unacceptable side effects, or clearly are less effective, then the administration of penicillin should be considered using a desensitization protocol to reduce the risk of anaphylaxis.

Cephalosporins

Like penicillins, cephalosporins possess a beta-lactam ring, but the five-membered thiazolidine ring is replaced by the six-membered dihydrothiazine ring. Shortly after cephalosporins came into clinical use, allergic reactions—including anaphylaxis—were reported and the question of cross-reactivity between cephalosporins and penicillins was raised.[75] Both animal and human studies have clearly demonstrated cross-reactivity between penicillins and cephalosporins using immuno- and bioassays to evaluate IgG, IgM, and IgE antibodies.[1,163,180] Primary cephalosporin allergy in nonpenicillin-allergic patients has also been reported, but the exact incidence is not clear.[2,153] Studies have been limited, because the haptenic determinants involved in cephalosporin allergy are unknown. **The exact incidence of clinically relevant cross-reactivity between penicillin and the cephalosporins is unknown and probably small but cannot be discounted on statistical grounds because life-threatening anaphylactic cross-reactivity has occurred. Therefore, patients with positive skin tests to any penicillin reagent should probably not receive cephalosporin antibiotics unless alternative drugs are clearly less desir-**

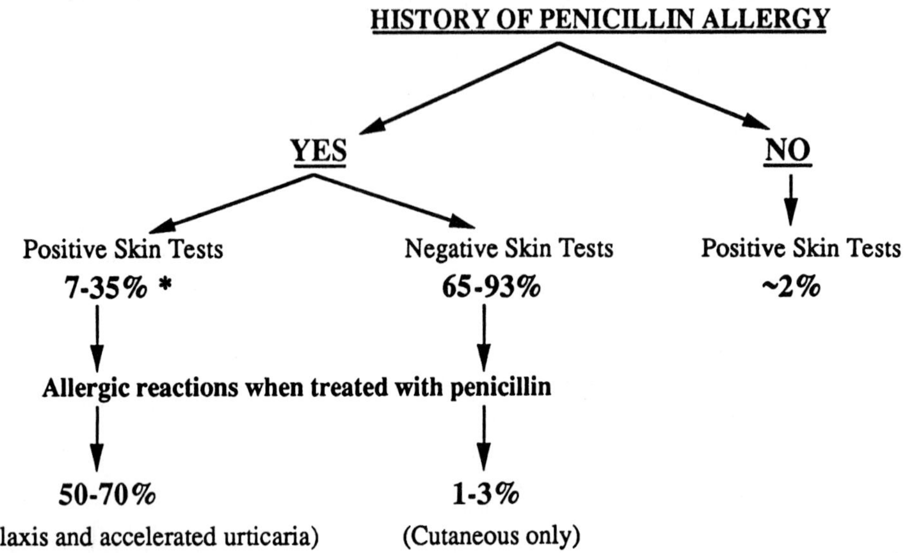

Fig. 92-4. Prevalence of positive and negative skin tests and subsequent allergic reactions in patients treated with penicillin (based on studies using both PPL and MDM as skin test reagents). (From Weiss ME, Adkinson NF Jr: Beta-lactam allergy. In Mandell GL, Douglas RG Jr, Bennett JE, editors: *Principles and practice of infectious disease,* ed 3, New York, 1989, Churchill-Livingstone.)

able. If cephalosporin drugs are used, they should be administered cautiously, possibly using a modified desensitization protocol.

New Beta-Lactam Antibiotics

Two new classes of beta-lactam antibiotics are the carbapenems (Imipenem) and monobactams (aztreonam). Initial studies suggest significant cross-reactivity between penicillin determinants and Imipenem, indicating the prudence of withholding carbopenems from patients with positive penicillin skin tests.[25,171,224] Initial investigations suggest weak cross-reactivity between aztreonam and other beta-lactam antibiotics and indicate that aztreonam may be administered safely to most, if not all, penicillin-allergic subjects.[5,11,105,218]

Vancomycin

Hypotension is the most serious immediate adverse effect associated with the use of vancomycin. Direct myocardial depression[188] and nonimmunologically mediated histamine release[123,209] have been reported as the mechanism of vancomycin-induced hypotension, not true anaphylaxis. In humans, hypotension occurs most commonly when the drug is rapidly infused or when it is administered in a concentrated solution.[188] Vancomycin-associated hypotension most commonly occurs intraoperatively and may be exacerbated by the concurrent use of other drugs that cause vasodilation or have a negative inotropic effects.[188] In addition to hypotension, vancomycin can produce a syndrome which consists of an intense erythematous discoloration of the upper trunk, arms, and neck and which may be associated with pruritus. Vancomycin has also been associated with the sudden development of throbbing pain or spasm in the chest or parasternal muscles without evidence of myocardial ischemia. To decrease the risk of reactions, vancomycin should be infused slowly (preferably over a period of at least 60 minutes) and in a dilute solution (500 mg/100 ml). Reactions should be treated by discontinuation of the vancomycin infusion, administration of an antihistamine, and the use of medications that counteract the hypotension.

Muscle Relaxants

Anaphylactic reactions, including cardiovascular collapse, tachycardia, urticaria, and bronchospasm, can occur after the administration of muscle relaxants.[159] Evidence supporting an IgE-mediated mechanism include positive Prausnitz-Kustner tests, basophil-histamine release studies, inhibition of basophil-histamine release after desensitization to anti-IgE, and the demonstration of drug-specific IgE antibodies in sera from patients who had adverse reactions to muscle relaxants.[12,84,210,211] It appears that IgE antibodies are directed against the quarternary or tertiary ammonium ions present in muscle relaxants.[12]

Extensive *in vitro* cross-reactivity has been reported between the muscle relaxants and other compounds that contain quarternary and tertiary ammonium ions.[12] In so far as these compounds occur widely in many drugs, foods, cosmetics, disinfectants, and industrial materials, patients may become sensitized through environmental contact with these various compounds. Sensitization to ammonium ion epitopes in cosmetics has been postulated to explain the predominance of reactions in women.[12] Molecules with ammonium ions less than 4 angstroms (Å) apart appear incapable of inducing histamine release, whereas the optimal length for cross-linking cell surface IgE appears to be less than 6Å.[40] Muscle relaxants with a rigid backbone between the two ammonium ions (such as pancuronium and vecuronium) appear to be less likely than flexible molecules to initiate anaphylaxis.[40] Atopy does not appear to be a significant risk factor for the occurrence of anaphylactic reactions to muscle relaxants.[31] Although the exact incidence of allergic reactions caused by muscle relaxants is unknown, reactions to muscle relaxants are less common in the United States as compared with France or Australia.

Barbiturates

Acute allergic reactions have been reported after the administration of thiobarbiturates, especially thiopental.[122] Proposed mechanisms for thiobarbiturate reactions include nonimmunologically induced mediator release and IgE-mediated reactions.[21,122] Positive immediate skin tests to thiopental have been reported in patients who had anaphylactic reactions after the induction of general anesthesia.[43,56,144] Recently, a thiopental RAST has been reported,[85] and mast cell histamine release to thiopental *in vitro* has been described.[88,89] The predictive value of the RAST to thiopental is presently uncertain and requires further study, but skin testing appears to be useful.[144]

Local Anesthetics

Despite patients commonly reporting adverse reactions to local anesthetics and being advised that they are "allergic" to these agents, **true allergic reactions to injected local anesthetics are exceedingly rare.** Reactions to local anesthetics are often the result of vasovagal reactions, toxic reactions (probably caused by inadvertent IV injection), side effects from epinephrine, or psychomotor responses such as hyperventilation. Toxic symptoms often involve the central nervous (CNS) and cardiovascular systems and may produce slurred speech, euphoria, dizziness, excitement, nausea, emesis, disorientation, or convulsions.[172] Vasovagal reactions are usually associated with bradycardia, sweating, pallor, and rapid improvement in symptoms when the patient is supine. Sympathetic stimulation, either from epinephrine or anxiety, may result in tremors, diaphoresis, tachycardia, and hypertension. Rarely, symptoms of reactions to local anesthetics are consistent with IgE-mediated reactions, such as urticaria, bronchospasm, and anaphylactic shock. However, acceptable documentation of IgE-mediated reactivity against local anesthetics in such patients is lacking, with few exceptions.[38] IgE-mediated sensitivity has, on rare occasions, also been reported to parabens, preservatives that are used in local anesthetics.[145]

Local anesthetics are divided into two chemical groups (Box 92-4). One group consists of chemicals containing benzoate esters that may cross-react with each other but not with the amide drugs. The second distinct group are mostly amides that do not substantially cross-react with each other.

Evaluation of a patient with a history of adverse reaction to local anesthetics should include a complete history of the episode, skin testing, and incremental drug challenge. The protocol used at Johns Hopkins University is listed in Table 92-7. An even more aggressive protocol is used at Northwestern University (Table 92-7). The local anesthetic tested should be appropriate for the proposed procedure and not expected to cross-react with the drug implicated in the pre-

BOX 92-4
CLASSIFICATION OF LOCAL ANESTHETICS

Group I: Benzoic acid esters	Group II: Amides (others)
Amydricaine (Alypin)	Antihistamines*
Butacaine (Butyn)	Bupivacaine (Marcaine)
Benzocaine	Dibucaine (Nupercaine)
Chlorprocaine (Nesacaine)	Dicycloine (Dyclone)
Cyclomethycaine (Surfacaine)	Lidocaine (Xylocaine)
Isobucaine (Kincaine)	Mepivicaine (Carbocaine)
Meprylcaine (Oracaine)	Oxethazine (Oxaine)
Metabulethamine (Oracaine)	Phenacaine (Holocaine)
Piperocaine (Metycaine)	Promoxine (Tronothane)
Procaine (Novocaine)	
Tetracaine (Pontocaine)	

*Antihistamines have minor anesthetic effect

Table 92-7 Examples of protocols for evaluation of local anesthetic allergy

Step*	Route	Volume (ml)	Dilution
Johns Hopkins University			
1	Intradermal	0.02	1:1000+
2	Intradermal	0.02	1:100
3	Intradermal	0.02	1:10
4	Intradermal	0.02	Undiluted
5	Subcutaneous	0.3	Undiluted

*Administer at 15-minute intervals; + If history is strongly suggestive of IgE mediation reaction, start with puncture at 1:1000 dilution.

Step*	Route	Volume (ml)	Dilution
Northwestern University			
1	Puncture		Undiluted
2	Subcutaneous	0.1	Undiluted
3	Subcutaneous	0.5	Undiluted
4	Subcutaneous	1.0	Undiluted
5	Subcutaneous	2.0	Undiluted

*Administer at 15-minute intervals.

vious reaction. If the previous drug is unknown, an amide anesthetic (frequently lidocaine) should be chosen. In a patient with history suggestive of an IgE-mediated reaction or possible paraben sensitivity, preparations without paraben should be used for testing, challenge, and treatment. Preparations without epinephrine should be used for skin testing, because they may mask a positive skin test[39] and may induce toxic effects.

Narcotics

Narcotics most commonly cause nonimmunologically mediated histamine release from skin mast cells, rather than anaphylaxis. Studies *in vitro* suggest that the skin mast cell is uniquely sensitive to narcotics, whereas the GI and lung mast cell and the circulating basophil do not release histamine when exposed to narcotics.[48,87,116] Most opioid-induced reactions are self-limiting and cutaneous, restricted to hives and pruritus or mild hypotension treated by fluid administration. Recent evidence suggests that IgE antibodies may be induced that bind epitopes contained in opiate narcotics.[17,83,232] However, the pharmacologic release of mediators induced by opiates is a far more common clinical occurrence than the rare reactions induced by morphine-specific IgE antibody.[219] Because codeine, morphine, and meperidine (Demerol) routinely cause positive skin responses secondary to nonimmunologic skin mast cell histamine release, skin tests must be interpreted cautiously and accompanied by the skin testing of normal control subjects.

Radiocontrast Media

The incidence of reactions induced by radiocontrast media (RCM) injections is between 5% to 8%.[73] Vasomotor reactions (e.g., nausea, vomiting, flushing, or warmth) occur in 5% to 8% of patients.[73] Anaphylactoid reactions (e.g., urticaria, angioedema, wheezing, dyspnea, hypotension, or death) occur in 2% to 3% of patients receiving IV or intra-arterial infusions.[160] Fatal reactions after RCM administration occur in approximately 1:50,000 IV procedures,[159] and it has been estimated that as many as 500 deaths/year are caused by RCM administration. Most reactions begin 1 to 3 minutes after intravascular administration. Patients with a previous reaction to RCM have approximately a 33% (range 17% to 60%) chance of reaction on reexposure.[159]

The causes of adverse reactions to RCM are unknown at present. Histamine release is a feature of most reactions, although elevations in plasma histamine have occurred without hemodynamic changes or anaphylactic reactions.[73] Activation of serum complement occurs after the intravascular injection of RCM,[74] either by the classic or the alternative pathway. Therefore, it has been suggested that production of anaphylatoxins with subsequent mast cell and basophil-mediator release is the cause of RCM reactions. Yet, RCM is capable of inducing nonimmunologic histamine release from mast cells and basophils in the absence of complement activation.[73] It has been suggested that the hypertonicity of RCM results in nonimmunologic mediator from mast cells and basophils.[73] There is no evidence that IgE-mediated mechanisms play a role in RCM reactions.

A patient who requires RCM administration and who has had a previous reaction to RCM has an increased (35% to 60%) risk for a reaction on reexposure (Table 92-8).[73] Pretreatment of these high-risk patients with prednisone (50 mg)[5,17] and diphenhydramine (50 mg) 1 hour before RCM administration reduces the risk of reactions to 9%.[99] Almost all reactions in pretreated patients are of no clinical importance (e.g., mild urticaria).[73] The addition of ephedrine (25 mg) 1 hour before RCM administration (in patients without angina, dysrhythmias, or other contraindications for ephedrine administration) resulted in a reaction rate of 3.1% in one study.[73]

A recent study showed that steroid pretreatment before the administration of hyperosmolar RCM is as effective in reducing the risk of RCM reactions (and much less expensive) as is the use of newer, nonhyperosmolar RCM.[114] A preliminary study, using historical controls, suggested that combining premedication with nonhyperosmolar RCM may be of added benefit in preventing reactions in high-risk individuals.[74]

Protamine

Protamine sulfate is a polycationic (strongly basic) small protein (molecular weight = 4300) extracted from salmon milt and used medicinally to reverse heparin anticoagulation and to retard the absorption of certain insulins (NPH and PZI). The use of IV protamine following cardiopulmonary bypass, cardiac catheterization, hemodialysis, and phoresis has resulted in increasing reports of life-threatening adverse reactions.

Diabetic patients receiving daily subcutaneous injections of insulins containing protamine have a 40- to 50-fold increased risk for life-threatening reactions when given IV protamine.[70,191] Another group at increased risk

Table 92-8 Premedication of patients with previous radiocontrast media reaction

Premedication with	Repeat reaction rate
A. No premedication	A—33% (range 17%–60%)
B. Prednisone (50 mg orally) 13, 7, and 1 hr before	
C. Diphenhydramine (50 mg intramuscular or orally) 1 hr before	B and C—9% (reactions mild)
D. Ephedrine (25 mg orally) 1 hr before	B, C, and D—3.1% (historical controls)
E. ? Ranitidine	

for protamine reactions are men who have undergone vasectomies. With disruption of the blood-testis barrier, studies have shown that 20% to 33% of such men develop hemaglutinating autoantibodies against protaminelike compounds.[169] Antiprotamine IgG antibodies are found in the sera of 34.5% of vasectomized men whereas none were found in age-matched controls.[6] No antiprotamine IgE antibodies were found in either vasectomized or control patient sera.

Another group at theoretic risk for protamine reactions are individuals with allergy to fish. Because protamine is produced from the matured testis of salmon or related species of fish belonging to the family Salmonidae or Clupeidae, it has been suggested that individuals allergic to fish may have serum antibodies directed against protamine. However, evidence supporting the increased risk for protamine reactions in fish-allergic patients is limited to rare case reports.[106]

Finally, previous exposure to IV protamine given for reversal of heparin anticoagulation may increase the risk for a reaction upon subsequent protamine administration.[178] No systematic study has been concluded evaluating the human immune response to protamine after IV administration.

The exact mechanisms by which acute protamine reactions occur are not completely understood. Animal studies initially suggested that protamine could cause direct, nonimmunologic release of histamine in hamster and rat peritoneal mast cells *in vitro*.[98] However, studies using human basophils and mast cells have been unable to demonstrate significant histamine release with protamine at concentrations up to 100 μg/ml.[63,170] Some protamine reactions may be associated with complement activation, either through protamine-heparin complexes[19,29,104,167] or through the interaction of protamine and complement fixing, antiprotamine IgG antibody,[112] leading to pulmonary artery (PA) pressure elevation through the generation of thromboxane.[37,142]

Lakin, et al.[112] provided evidence that protamine-specific IgG antibodies could cause protamine reactions by activating complement, whereas others have also reported the presence of protamine-specific IgG antibodies in small numbers of protamine reactors.[69,72] We conducted a case-control study and found that in both diabetic patients who had received protamine-insulin injections and those who had no previous exposure to them, the presence of serum antiprotamine IgG antibody was a significant risk factor for protamine reactions. The relative risk for the former group was 38, whereas that for the latter group was 25.[223] Using a double-antibody, radioimmunoprecipitation assay, Kurtz et al.[107] found that 38% to 91% of protamine-insulin-dependent diabetic patients had serum antiprotamine IgG antibodies. Using an enzyme-linked immunosorbent assay (ELISA), Nell and Thomas found that 38% of 319 neutral protamine. Hagedorn (NPH) insulin-treated diabetic patients and only 2.5% of 202 normal control subjects had antiprotamine IgG antibodies in their serum.[146] Recent data suggests that protamine could inhibit the ability of plasma carboxypeptidase N to convert the anaphylatoxins and bradykinins to the less-active des-arginine metabolites,[198] potentially allowing these vasoactive compounds previously generated to produce more significant hemodynamic manifestations.

We developed an agarose-based RAST to measure antiprotamine IgE antibodies and showed that in diabetic patients who had received protamine-insulin injections, the presence of serum antiprotamine IgE antibody was a significant risk factor for acute protamine reactions (relative risk = 95) (Table 92-9).[223] It appears that in protamine-insulin-

Table 92-9 Association of protamine reactions with the presence of serum IgE and IgG antibodies to protamine

Protamine-specific antibody	Cases (reaction)	Controls (no reaction)	Relative risk	Lower 95% confidence limit	p-value
With prior exposure to subcutaneous protamine-insulin preparations					
IgE present	9	0	95	6.6	1.0×10^{-5}
IgE absent	4	22			
IgG present	11	2	38	5	1.2×10^{-5}
IgG absent	2	20			
No prior exposure to subcutaneous protamine-insulin preparations					
IgE present	0	0	N/A	N/A	0.99
IgE absent	14	21			
IgG present	5	0	25	1.6	0.006
IgG absent	9	21			

N/A — not applicable. From Weiss, et al: *N Engl J Med* 320:886–892, 1989.[222]

dependent diabetic patients, antibody-mediated mechanisms are the likely cause for the increased risk of protamine reactions seen in this group. Prescreening high-risk patients (protamine-insulin-dependent diabetics) for the presence of antiprotamine antibodies before elective procedures that would involve the administration of IV protamine may be worthwhile. We have observed and others have suggested that if such antibodies are present, special precautions could be taken or alternative heparin antagonists—such as hexadimethrine (which, at present, is approved only for compassionate use by the Food and Drug Administration [FDA])—could be substituted.[44]

Skin testing with protamine does not appear to be useful in discriminating between subjects with significant serum antiprotamine IgE antibody and control subjects.[217,221,222] It is possible that protamine may be an incomplete or univalent antigen that first must combine with a tissue macromolecule or possibly heparin to become a complete, multivalent antigen capable of eliciting mediator release.[222] Lowenstein et al.[130] and Morel et al.[142] found that PA pressure increase after rapid protamine injection in three patients was associated with increases of thromboxane B_2 along with C5a.

Plasma histamine levels were unchanged in these patients. In contrast, a patient who developed a decrease in SVR and profound systemic hypotension without PA hypertension had a tenfold elevation in plasma histamine and no change in thromboxane B_2 or C5a levels. Thus, it appears likely that more than one mechanism may be responsible for the adverse reactions associated with protamine.[220]

Rubber (Latex)

Although rubber products have been used for many years, contact urticaria and systemic reactions to latex have only relatively recently been described.[91] It is possible that in the past, the connection to latex exposure and reactions was never made. It is more likely that the increased need for latex products, because the adoption of universal precautions, has resulted in some change in the manufacturing process that has led to increased antigenicity of latex products, particularly gloves.[79,80] The proteins that are present in natural rubber latex are considered to be the responsible antigens, and the hypersensitivity responses include contact and generalized urticaria, angioedema, rhinitis, conjunctivitis, bronchospasm, life-threatening anaphylaxis, and death. Latex present in various materials, especially surgical gloves, has become responsible for a dramatic change in the etiology of intraoperative anaphylactic shock, increasing in one series from 0.5% of anaphylactic shock in 1989 to 12.5% of cases in 1991.[155]

Natural rubber latex is a wound sealant for rubber trees. It is a milky cytoplasmic fluid produced by lactifer cells of the Hevea brasiliensis tree, which is indigenous to Brazil, but commercially cultivated mainly in Southeast Asia and West Africa. This harvested sap is ammoniated to prevent coagulation following collection, centrifuged to separate latex solids from liquids and cross-linked for stability during the manufacturing process by the application of heat (vulcanization) and addition of a variety of chemicals. These (primarily) sulfur-based antidegradants and accelerators impart deformability, elasticity, and tensile strength. Molds in the shape of the desired medical product (e.g., gloves) are then dipped into this latex liquid, and subsequently passed through a washing process (called leaching). A powder, often starch-based, is often added during the final phase to decrease friction and increase wearer comfort. The glove (or other dipped product) is then inverted (i.e., the inside becomes the outside) and packaged.[78]

Although the total amount of protein present in natural rubber latex concentrate is relatively constant at about 1.6 to 2.0% by weight, the amount of extractable protein in the latex product may be highly variable.[192] The total protein concentration of glove extracts ranges from 3 to 337 μg/g per glove.[157] It is possible to reduce glove allergenicity to almost zero by modifying the manufacturing process.[125]

Multiple latex proteins act as allergens. Accelerators present in the rubber of protective gloves remain the most frequent source of allergy, especially in healthcare workers. Thiurams cause oversensitivity in 52.9% of rubber-contact dermatitis patients, thiocarbamates in 41.2%, thiazoles in 35.3%, guanidine derivatives in 11.8%, and thiocarbamide in 9.8%. In general, allergy to thiocarbamates is concomitant with allergy and sensitivity to thiazoles.[102] Dithiocarbamate-type accelerators have also been found to be allergenic.[97] Amine compounds and quinoline derivatives are used in rubber mixtures to prevent rubber oxidation. Allergy to amine compounds was found in 58.8% of patients and to quinoline derivatives in 9.8% of rubber contact dermatitis patients.[103] The starch powder covering the finished gloves acts as an airborne carrier of the latex, resulting in bronchial asthma upon inhalation.

Although the chemicals added to latex have long been associated with contact dermatitis, it is only recently that major latex allergy and anaphylaxis have come to medical attention.[151] Infrequent contact dermatitis to latex was noted in healthcare workers, with systemic reactions rarely described[28,175,203] until shortly after the embracing of universal precautions, when alarming reports from around the world described generalized urticaria, angioedema, upper- and lower-respiratory obstructions, and cardiovascular collapse.[67,124,140,154,187] At times, these reactions have been fatal.[199] Patients who have suffered severe systemic reactions often have a history of contact urticaria or angioedema to rubber products such as gloves, rubber balloons, or atopy.[32,46,137,162,166,168,189,196] Occupational allergic rhinitis, with a positive skin-prick test specifically for IgE to latex, has been demonstrated, which seems to precede the onset of work-related asthma.[138]

Certain populations are at significantly increased risk for latex allergy. These include healthcare workers, who have had increased exposure to latex, usually in the form of gloves, patients with prolonged or frequent exposure to latex products such as urinary catheters, and latex factory

BOX 92-5
CHECKLIST FOR LATEX-ALLERGIC PATIENTS

Preoperative

Solicit specific history of latax allergy or risk for latex allergy
- History of chronic care with latex-based products
- History of spina bifida, urologic reconstructive surgery
- History of repeated surgical procedures (e.g., > 9)
- History of intolerance to latex-based products: balloons, rubber gloves, condoms, dental dams, rubber urethral catheters
- History of allergy to tropical fruits
- History of intraoperative anaphylaxis of uncertain etiology
- Healthcare workers, especially with a history of atopy or hand eczema

Consider Allergy Consultation
- *In vitro* testing
- *In vivo* testing

Minimize latex exposure for at-risk patients
- Latex alert—patients with significant risk factors for latex allergy but no overt signs or symptoms
- Latex allergy—patients with or without significant risk factors for latex allergy and positive history, signs, symptoms, or allergy evaluation

Carefully coordinate care between surgical anesthesia and nursing teams
- Have lists available of nonlatex product alternatives
- First case of the day is preferable to decrease aeroallergen concentration
- Diplay Latex Allergy or Latex Alert signs inside and outside operating room

Intraoperative

Anesthesia equipment
- Latex-free gloves, airways, endotracheal tubes
- Masks—polyvinylchloride if available, or old, well-washed, black rubber masks
- Rebreathing bags—neoprene if available, or old, well-washed black rubber masks
- Ventilator bellows—neoprene or silicone if available, or old, well-washed black rubber bellows
- Breathing circuit—disposable, polyvinylchloride, packaged separately from a latex rebreathing
- Remove rubber stoppers from multidose vials
- Beware of latex intravenous injection ports, penrose-type tourniquets, and rubber band; use nontoxic latex glove as tourniquet; tape latex inject ports, or use silicone injection ports or stopcock
- Blood pressure cuffs—if new latex, cover with soft cotton
- Ambu-type bag—assure that bag and valve do not have latex components
  - Alternative is silicone self-inflating bag
- Check syringe plungers; reconstitute medications every 6 hours
- Dilute concentration of epinephrine (0.01 mg/ml, or 1:100,000)

Surgical equipment
- Avoid latex surgical gloves
- Avoid latex drains (e.g. penrose)
- Avoid latex urinary catheters
- Avoid latex instruments mats
- Avoid rubber-shod clamps
- Avoid latex vascular tags
- Avoid latex-bulb syringes for irrigation
- Avoid rubber bands

Postoperative

- Medical Alert tage
- Warning sign posted on chart
- Warning sign posted on bed

(Reprinted with premission from Holzman RS, *Anesth Analg* 76:35–41, 1993.[91])

workers.[32] Patients with meningomyelocele or congenital urologic anomalies seem particularly susceptible, with an estimated incidence of latex allergy averaging 50%.[*] **Latex allergic patients are more likely to have a history of asthma, rubber-contact allergy, food allergy, rash caused by adhesive tape, daily rectal disimpaction, nine or more prior surgical procedures, latex-specific IgE, or increased total serum IgE levels. People of nonwhite race, rubber-contact allergy, history of food allergy, and nine or more surgical procedures are significant as independent risk factors.**[100]

Upwards of 6.5% of healthcare workers with latex exposure may be sensitized.[**] Serologic testing confirmed the suspected diagnosis in 62% of workers (15 of 24) with systemic symptoms but was only positive in 27% of workers (4 of 15) with symptoms limited to contact urticaria.[30] Dental students showed progression in latex allergy positivity from 2% in their second semester to 10.4% positive in their tenth semester. Atopic diseases and hand eczema are additional risk factors.[86] Hospital housekeepers regularly exposed to latex gloves had an 8% prevalence overall, with a 20% prevalence among atopic housekeepers.[195] Users of household and other protective gloves, although less extensively studied, form an even larger group with natural-rubber latex allergy, which often is work related. Eczema and atopy are again the most frequent risk factors for sensitization.[205,207]

IgE antibodies play a major role in the immunopathogenesis of latex-induced allergy and anaphylaxis. Incubation of extracts from latex or *Hevea brasiliensis* caused release of histamine from basophils of two patients who had previous systemic reactions attributed to rubber exposure.[182] Confirmation that IgE antibodies to latex were the cause of the reactions was obtained by passively sensitizing IgE antibodies from the reactor's serum onto normal control basophils. Incubation with latex-induced histamine release from the control basophils that had been sensitized with IgE from the reactor's serum. This response could be attenuated by heat treatment of the serum, which destroys IgE antibodies, and by absorption of IgE using anti-IgE antibodies.[182]

The diagnosis of latex allergy is made by a combination of medical history, physical examination, and reliable *in vivo* or *in vitro* tests. Although skin-prick testing is both sensitive (100%) and specific (99%),[137] this method should be restricted to patients with a compelling history and an inconclusive serologic test result because of possible systemic reactions.[49] RAST testing for latex-specific IgE is recommended, although it is less sensitive than skin-prick testing.[110] The FDA has recently approved a test system to measure circulating levels of latex-specific IgE with an accuracy rate reported at 85%.[62]

Serum tryptase levels in the immediate postanaphylaxis period may be helpful in confirming the diagnosis following a clinical episode.[9] A provocative challenge to latex has also been described. It involves placing a latex glove on a dampened hand for 15 minutes and comparing the response of the contralateral hand wrapped in a vinyl glove.[206,226] Provocation tests, however, should be avoided if severe, systemic reactions have occurred. Multiple allergies are often found in latex-allergic patients.[132,134,176] Cross-reactivity of latex with tropical fruits is not uncommon,[24] and such findings in the history may be used to heighten suspicion about a patient's potential for latex allergy as well.[7,33,109,115,131,139]

For patients who have had serious allergic reactions to latex and in patients at high risk (e.g., patients with meningomyeloceles), one should avoid contact with latex products. Because prophylactic drug protocols have proven ineffective, a latex-free environment is advocated.[89,152,201] Box 92-5 on page 2401 contains a checklist for handling patients with latex allergies. Moreover, patients in identified high-risk pediatric groups, such as children with urologic birth defects and myelomeningocele, should be offered latex-free exposure in the operating room from birth to avoid subsequent sensitization.[51] Box 92-6 contains recommendations of the Task Force on Allergic Reactions to Latex of the American Academy of Allergy and Immunology and should be followed.[8]

*References 15, 45, 52, 100, 124, 161, 182, 183, 189, 197, 229

**References 18, 90, 95, 111, 136, 168, 204, 208, 225, 228, 230

BOX 92-6
RECOMMENDATIONS OF THE TASK FORCE ON ALLERGIC REACTIONS TO LATEX OF THE AMERICAN ACADEMY OF ALLERGY AND IMMUNOLOGY

Patients in high-risk groups should be identified.

All patients, regardless of risk group status, should be questioned about a history of latex allergy.

All high-risk patients should be offered testing for latex allergy.

Procedures on all patients with spina bifida, regardless of history, should be performed in a latex-free environment.

Procedures on all patients with positive history, regardless of risk group status, should be performed in a latex-free environment.

A latex-free environment is one in which no latex gloves are used by any personnel. In addition, there should be no latex accessories (e.g., catheters, adhesives, tourniquets, anesthesia equipment) that come into direct contact with the patient.

Low-risk patients with negative histories are extremely unlikely to react to latex. At this time, routine testing is not recommended for persons with negative histories.

Patients identified as latex allergic by either history or testing should be advised to obtain a Medic Alert bracelet and self-injectable epinephrine. Medical records should be appropriately labeled.

KEY POINTS

- Anaphylaxis is an acute reaction leading to severe physiologic derangements of multiple systems. True anaphylaxis denotes an IgE-antibody–mediated reaction.
- Non–IgE-mediated reactions resembling true anaphylaxis also occur (radiocontrast media) and are commonly called *anaphylactoid reactions.*
- Known or suspected mediators of anaphylaxis include histamine, ECF-A, NCF, prostaglandin D_2, platelet-activating factor, and leukotrienes.
- Clinical symptoms of anaphylaxis include urticaria, flushing, nausea, vomiting, abdominal pain, laryngeal edema, bronchospasm, and cardiovascular collapse.
- Treatment of anaphylaxis consists of discontinuing the suspected initiating agent, securing the compromised airway, and establishing IV access. Bronchospasm and laryngeal edema are treated with epinephrine, and hypotension and cardiovascular collapse are treated with volume, epinephrine, and CPR if needed.
- Evaluation of an anaphylactic reaction starts with a detailed patient history and may include skin testing, RAST, and/or provocative challenge.
- Agents commonly used by anesthesiologists that are known to cause anaphylactic reactions include penicillin, cephalosporins, barbiturates, muscle relaxants, and latex products.
- Penicillin antibiotics constitute the most common medications causing allergic reactions. Anaphylaxis occurs in 0.004% to 0.015% of treatment cases and results in 400 to 800 deaths yearly.
- The most useful piece of information in assessing an individual's potential for an IgE-mediated reaction to penicillin is the skin-test response to major and minor penicillin determinants.
- Several commonly used anesthetic agents lead to nonimmunologic histamine release, including neuromuscular-blocking agents (curare and atracurium) and opiates (especially morphine and codeine).
- True allergic reactions to local anesthetics are exceedingly rare, and cases labeled as such are usually due to other causes (e.g., vasovagal response, IV injection).
- The exact mechanism of adverse reactions to protamine remains unclear, but the clinical syndrome includes rash, urticaria, bronchospasm, pulmonary vasoconstriction, and cardiovascular collapse.
- Diabetics exposed to protamine-containing insulin have a 40- to 50-fold increased risk for life-threatening reactions to protamine. Fish-allergic individuals and vasectomized men may also be at increased risk.
- Seven to 10% of healthcare workers regularly exposed to latex and 28% to 67% of children with spina bifida have a positive skin-test result to latex proteins. Life-threatening anaphylaxis can occur intraoperatively in highly sensitive patients because of mucosal absorption of latex protein allergens from a surgeon's gloves.
- The present treatment for latex allergy is careful avoidance of latex materials. Persons in high-risk groups should be referred for appropriate evaluation and testing, advised to avoid exposure to latex-derived products, and advised to carry self-injectable epinephrine.

KEY REFERENCES

Abraham GN, Petz LD, Fudenberg HH: Immunohaematological cross-allergenicity between penicillin and cephalothin in humans, *Clin Exp Immunol* 3:343, 1968.

Charpin D, Benzarti M, Hemon Y, et al: Atopy and anaphylactic reactions to suxamethonium, *J Allergy Clin Immunol* 82:356, 1988.

Fisher M: Intradermal testing after anaphylactoid reaction to anaesthetic drugs: practical aspects of performance and interpretation, *Anaesth Intens Care* 12:115, 1984.

Gottschlich GM, Gravlee GP, Georgitis JW: Adverse reactions to protamine sulfate during cardiac surgery in diabetic and non-diabetic patients, *Ann Allergy* 61:277, 1988.

Harle DG, Baldo BA, Fisher MM: Detection of IgE antibodies to suxamethonium after anaphylactoid reactions during anaesthesia, *Lancet* i:930, 1984.

Hirshman CA, Edelstein RA, Ebertz JM, et al: Thiobarbiturate-induced histamine release in human skin mast cells, *Anesthesiology* 63:353, 1985.

Hirshman CA, Peters J, Cartwright-Lee I: Leukocyte histamine release to thiopental, *Anesthesiology* 56:64, 1982.

Lasser EC, Berry CC, Talner LB, et al: Pretreatment with corticosteroids to alleviate reactions to intravenous contrast material, *N Engl J Med* 317:845, 1987.

Holzman RS: Latex allergy: an emerging operating room problem, *Anesth Analg* 76:635-641, 1993.

Weiss ME, Adkinson NF Jr, Hirshman CA: Evaluation of allergic drug reactions in the perioperative period, *Anesthesiology* 71:483, 1989.

Weiss ME, Nyhan D, Zhikang P, et al: Association of protamine IgE and IgG antibodies with life-threatening reactions to intravenous protamine, *N Engl J Med* 320:886, 1989.

REFERENCES

1. Abraham GN, Petz LD, Fudenberg HH: Immunohaematological cross-allergenicity between penicillin and cephalothin in humans, *Clin Exp Immunol* 3:343, 1968.
2. Abraham GN, Petz LD, Fudenberg HH: Cephalothin hypersensitivity associated with anti-cephalothin antibodies, *Int Arch Allerg Appl Immunol* 34:65, 1968.
3. Adkinson NF Jr: Penicillin allergy. In Lichtenstein LM, Fauci A, editors: *Current therapy in allergy, immunology and rheumatology,* Ontario, 1983, BC Decker.
4. Adkinson NF Jr: Tests for immunological drug reactions. In Rose NF, Friedman H, editors: *Manual of clinical immunology,* Washington, 1986, American Society for Microbiology.
5. Adkinson NF Jr, Wheeler B, Swabb EA: Clinical tolerance of the monobactam aztreonam in penicillin allergic subjects (abstract), 14th International Congress of Chemotherapy, (in Japan):1984.
6. Adourian UA, Fuches E, Adkinson NF Jr, et al: Incidence of anti-protamine antibodies in vasectomized males (abstract), *Anesthesiology* 73(A):1257, 1990.
7. Ahlroth M, Alenius H, Turjanmaa K, et al: Cross-reacting allergens in natural rubber latex and avocado, *J Allerg Clin Immunol* 96:167, 1995.
8. American Academy of Allergy and Immunology: Task force on allergic reactions to latex, *J Allerg Clin Immunol* 92:16, 1993.
9. Angelsioo L, Palmqvist P, Sandin R: A case report. Tryptase in serum indicated latex-induced anaphylaxis [in Swedish], *Lakartidningen* 92:1131, 1995.
10. Atkins PC, Norman M, Weiner H, et al: Release of neutrophil chemotactic activity during immediate hypersensitivity reactions in humans, *Ann Intern Med* 86:415, 1977.
11. Audicana M, Bernaola G, Urrita I, et al: Allergic reactions to betalactams: studies in a group of patients allergic to penicillin and evaluation of cross-reactivity with cephalosporin, *Allergy* 49:108, 1994.
12. Baldo BA, Fisher MM: Substituted ammonium ions as allergenic determinants in drug allergy, *Nature* 306:262, 1983.
13. Barnard JH: Studies of 400 Hymenoptera sting deaths in the United States, *J Allerg Clin Immunol* 62:259, 1973.
14. Beard K, Jick H: Cardiac arrest and anaphylaxis with anesthetic agents, *JAMA* 254:27, 1985.
15. Beaudouin E, Prestat F, Schmitt M, et al: High risk of sensitization to latex in children with spina bifida, *Eur J Pediatr Surg* 4:90, 1994.
16. Benjamin E, Oropello JM, Abalos AM, et al: Effects of acid-base correction on hemodynamics, oxygen dynamics, and resuscitability in severe canine hemorrhagic shock, *Crit Care Med* 22:1616, 1994.
17. Bennett MJ, Anderson LK, McMillan JC, et al: Anaphylactic reaction during anaesthesia associated with positive intradermal skin test to fentanyl, *Can Anaesth Soc J* 33:75, 1986.
18. Berky ZT, Luciano WJ, James WD: Latex glove allergy. A survey of the US Army Dental Corps, *JAMA* 268:2695, 1992.
19. Best N, Sinosich MJ, Teisner B, et al: Complement activation during cardiopulmonary bypass by heparin-protamine interaction, *Br J Anaesth* 56:339, 1984.
20. Bickell WH, Dice WH: Military antishock trousers in a patient with adrenergic-resistant anaphylaxis, *Ann Emerg Surg* 13:189, 1984.
21. Binkley K, Cheema A, Sussman G, et al: Generalized allergic reactions during anaesthesia, *J Allerg Clin Immunol* 89:768, 1992.
22. Bird AG: Severe drug reactions during anaesthesia [Review], *Adv Drug React Acute Poison Rev* 6:117, 1987.
23. Blanca M: Allergic reactions to penicillins: a changing world, *Allergy* 30:777, 1995.
24. Blanco C, Carrillo T, Castillo R, et al: Latex allergy: clinical features and cross-reactivity with fruits, *Ann Allergy* 73:309, 1994.
25. Boguniewicz M, Leung DY: Hypersensitivity reactions to antibiotics commonly used in children [review], *Ped Infect Dis J* 14:221, 1995.
26. Boileau S, Hummer-Sigiel M, Moeller R, et al: Reassessment of the respective risks of anaphylaxis and histamine liberation with anesthetic substances (Review) [in French], *Ann Fr Anesth Reanim* 4:195, 1985.
27. Bruce CA, Rosenthal RR, Lichtenstein LM, et al: Diagnostic tests in ragweed-allergic asthma. A comparison of direct skin tests, leukocyte histamine release, and quantitative bronchial challenge, *J Allerg Clin Immunol* 53:230, 1974.
28. Carrillo T, Cuevas M, Munoz T, et al: Contact urticaria and rhinitis from latex surgical gloves, *Contact Dermatol* 15:69, 1986.
29. Cavarocchi NC, Schaff HV, Orszulak TA, et al: Evidence for complement activation by protamine-heparin interaction after cardiopulmonary bypass, *Surgery* 98:525, 1985.
30. Charous BL, Hamilton RG, Yunginger JW: Occupational latex exposure: characteristics of contact and systemic reactions in 47 workers, *J Allerg Clin Immunol* 94:12, 1994.
31. Charpin D, Benzarti M, Hemon Y, et al: Atopy and anaphylactic reactions to suxamethonium, *J Allerg Clin Immunol* 82: 356, 1988.
32. Charpin D, Vervloet D: Epidemiology of immediate-type allergic reactions to latex (review), *Clin Rev Allerg* 11:385, 1993.
33. Cinquetti M, Peroni D, Vinco A, et al: Latex allergy in a child with banana anaphylaxis, *Acta Paediatr* 84:709, 1995.
34. Clarke RS, Watkins J: Drugs responsible for anaphylactoid reactions in anaesthesia in the United Kingdom, *Ann Fr Anesth Reanim* 12:105, 1993.
35. Craddock PR, Fehr J, Brigham KL, et al: Complement and leukocyte-mediated pulmonary dysfunction in hemodialysis, *N Engl J Med* 296:769, 1977.
36. Currie M, Webb RK, Williamson JA, et al: The Australian Incident Monitoring Study. Clinical anaphylaxis: an analysis of 2000 incident reports, *Anaesth Intens Care* 21:621, 1993.
37. Degges RD, Foster ME, Dang AQ, et al: Pulmonary hypertensive effect of heparin and protamine interaction: evidence for thromboxane $[\beta]_2$ release from the lung, *Am J Surg* 154:696, 1987.
38. deShazo RD, Nelson HS: An approach to the patient with a history of local anesthetic hypersensitivity: experience with 90 patients, *J Allerg Clin Immunol* 63:387, 1989.
39. DeSwarte RD: Drug allergy. In Patterson R, editor: *Allergic diseases: Diagnosis and management,* Philadelphia, 1989, JB Lippincott.
40. Didier A, Cador D, Bongrand P, et al: Role of the quaternary ammonium ion determinants in allergy to muscle relaxants, *J Allerg Clin Immunol* 79:578, 1987.
41. Dierich MP, Schulz T: Physiological and pathological effects of activated complement (review), *Haematologia* 17:3, 1984.
42. DiPiro JT, Hamilton RG, Adkinson NF Jr: Facilitation of penicilloation of proteins by serum cofactors, *J Allerg Clin Immunol* 85:192, 1990.
43. Dolovich J, Evans S, Rosenbloom D, et al: Anaphylaxis due to thiopental sodium anesthesia, *Can Med Assoc J* 123:292, 1980.
44. Doolan L, McKenzie I, Krafchek J, et al: Protamine sulphate hypersensitivity, *Anaesth Intens Care* 9:147, 1981.
45. Dormans JP, Templeton JJ, Edmonds C, et al: Intraoperative anaphylaxis due to exposure to latex (natural rubber) in children, *J Bone Joint Surg Am* 76:1688, 1994.
46. Dry J, Leynadier F, Pecquet C, et al: Immediate hypersensitivity to latex: a new problem. Future perspectives (review) [in French], *Bull Acad Natl Med* 173:913, 1989.
47. Dykewicz MS, McGrath KG, Davison R, et al: Identification of patients at risk for anaphylaxis due to streptokinase, *Arch Intern Med* 146:305, 1986.
48. Ebertz JM, Hermens JM, McMillan JC, et al: Functional differences between human cutaneous mast cells and basophils: a comparison of morphine-induced histamine release, *Agents Actions* 18:455, 1986.
49. Ebo DG, Stevens WJ and De Clerck LS: Latex anaphylaxis (review), *Acta Clin Belg* 50:87, 1995.
50. Eisen HN: Hypersensitivity to simple chemicals. In Lawrence HS, editor: *Cellular and humoral aspects of the hypersensitive states,* New York, 1959, PB Hoeber.
51. Ellsworth PI, Merguerian PA, Klein RB, et al: Evaluation and risk factors of latex allergy in spina bifida patients: is it preventable? *J Urol* 150:691, 1993.
52. Emans JB: Allergy to latex in patients who have myelodysplasia. Relevance for the orthopaedic surgeon (review), *J Bone Joint Surg Am* 74:1103, 1992.
53. Etter MS, Helrich M, Mackenzie CF:

Immunoglobulin E fluctuation in thiopental anaphylaxis, *Anesthesiology* 52:181, 1980.

54. Fearon DT, Ruddy S, Schur PH, et al: Activation of the properdin pathway of complement in patients with gram-negative of bacteremia, *N Engl J Med* 292:937, 1975.
55. Fisher AA: Allergic contact reactions in health personnel (review), *J Allerg Clin Immunol* 90:729, 1992.
56. Fisher M: Intradermal testing after anaphylactoid reaction to anaesthetic drugs: practical aspects of performance and interpretation, *Anaesth Intens Care* 12:115, 1984.
57. Fisher MM: Intradermal testing in the diagnosis of acute anaphylaxis during anaesthesia—results of five years experience, *Anaesth Intens Care* 7:58, 1979.
58. Fisher MM, Baldo BA: The incidence and clinical features of anaphylactic reactions during anesthesia in Australia, *Ann Fr Anesth Reanim* 12:97, 1993.
59. Fisher MM, Baldo BA: The diagnosis of fatal anaphylactic reactions during anaesthesia: employment of immunoassays for mast cell tryptase and drug-reactive IgE antibodies, *Anaesth Intens Care* 21:353, 1993.
60. Fisher MM, Hirshman CA: Hypersensitivity to drugs and other substances. In Scurr C, Feldman S, Soni N, editors: *Scientific foundations of anaesthesia: The basis of intensive care,* Chicago, 1990, Year Book Medical Publishers.
61. Fisher MM, More DG: The epidemiology and clinical features of anaphylactic reactions in anaesthesia, *Anaesth Intens Care* 9:226, 1981.
62. Food and Drug Administration: Latex sensitivity test, *FDA Med Bull* 25:2, 1995.
63. Foreman JC, Lichtenstein LM: Induction of histamine secretion by polycations, *Biochem Biophys Acta* 629:587, 1980.
64. Frank MM: Complement: a brief review (review), *J Allerg Clin Immunol* 84:411, 1989.
65. Galpin JE, Chow AW, Yoshikawa TT, et al: "Pseudoanaphylactic" reactions from inadvertent infusion of procaine penicillin G, *Ann Intern Med* 81:358, 1974.
66. Gell PGH, Coombs RRA: Classification of allergic reactions responsible for clinical hypersensitivity and disease. In Gell PGH, Coombs RRA, Hachmann PJ, editors: *Clinical aspects of immunology,* Oxford, 1975, Blackwell-Scientific Publications.
67. Gerber AC, Jorg W, Zbinden S, et al: Severe intraoperative anaphylaxis to surgical gloves: latex allergy, an unfamiliar condition, *Anesthesiology* 71:800, 1989.
68. Ghebrehiwet B: The complement system: mechanisms of activation, regulation, and biological functions. In Kaplan AP, editor: *Allergy,* New York, 1985, Churchill-Livingstone.
69. Gottschlich GM, Georgitis JW: Protamine-specific antibodies in protamine anaphylaxis. In American College of Allergists, editor: *Allergy changing for the future,* Boston, 1987, American College of Allergists.
70. Gottschlich GM, Gravlee GP, Georgitis JW: Adverse reactions to protamine sulfate during cardiac surgery in diabetic and nondiabetic patients, *Ann Allerg* 61:277, 1988.
71. Grammer LC, Patterson R: Proteins: chymopapain and insulin, *J Allerg Clin Immunol* 74:635, 1984.
72. Grant JA, Cooper JR, Albyn KC, et al: Anaphylactic reactions to protamine in insulin-dependent diabetics after cardiovascular procedures (abstract), *J Allerg Clin Immunol* 73:180, 1984.
73. Greenberger PA: Contrast media reactions, *J Allerg Clin Immunol* 74:600, 1984.
74. Greenberger PA, Patterson R: Beneficial effects of lower osmolality radiocontrast media in pretreated high risk patients, *J Allerg Clin Immunol* 85:229, 1990.
75. Grieco MH: Cross-allergenicity of the penicillins and the cephalosporins, *Arch Intern Med* 119:141, 1967.
76. Grillo JA, Gonzalez ER: Changes in the pharmacotherapy of CPR (review), *Heart Lung* 22:548, 1993.
77. Hagedorn HC, Jensen BN, Kraup NB, et al: Protamine insulin, *JAMA* 106:177, 1936.
78. Hamann C: Natural rubber latex protein sensitivity in review, *Am J Contact Dermat* 4:4, 1993.
79. Hamann CP: Latex hypersensitivity: an update (review), *Allerg Proc* 15:17, 1994.
80. Hamann CP, Kick SA: Allergies associated with medical gloves. Manufacturing issues (review), *Dermatol Clin* 12:547, 1994.
81. Hamilton RG, Adkinson NF Jr: Serological methods in the diagnosis and management of human allergic disease, *Crit Rev Clin Lab Sci* 21:1, 1984.
82. Hamilton RG, Rendell M, Adkinson NF Jr: Serological analysis of human IgG and IgE anti-insulin antibodies by solid-phase radioimmunoassays, *J Lab Clin Med* 96: 1022, 1980.
83. Harle DG, Baldo BA, Coroneos NJ, et al: Anaphylaxis following administration of papaveretum. Case report, implication of IgE antibodies that react with morphine and codeine and identification of an allergic determinant, *Anesthesiology* 71:489, 1989.
84. Harle DG, Baldo BA, Fisher MM: Detection of IgE antibodies to suxamethonium after anaphylactoid reactions during anaesthesia, *Lancet* 1:930, 1984.
85. Harle DG, Baldo BA, Smal MA, et al: Detection of thiopentone-reactive IgE antibodies following anaphylactoid reactions during anaesthesia, *Clin Allerg* 16:493, 1986.
86. Heese A, Peters KP, Stahl J, et al: Incidence and increase in type I allergies to rubber gloves in dental medicine students [in German], *Hautarzt* 46:15, 1995.
87. Hermens JM, Ebertz JM, Hanifin JM, et al: Comparison of histamine release in human skin mast cells induced by morphine, fentanyl, and oxymorphone, *Anesthesiology* 62:124, 1985.
88. Hirshman CA, Edelstein RA, Ebertz JM, et al: Thiobarbiturate-induced histamine release in human skin mast cells, *Anesthesiology* 63:353, 1985.
89. Hirshman CA, Peters J, Cartwright-Lee I: Leukocyte histamine release to thiopental, *Anesthesiology* 56:64, 1982.
90. Holm JO, Wereide K, Halvorsen R, et al: Allergy to latex among hospital employees, *Contact Dermatol* 32:239, 1995.
91. Holzman RS: Latex allergy: an emerging operating room problem, *Anesth Analg* 76:635, 1993.
92. Idsoe O, Guthe T, Willcox RR, et al: Nature and extent of penicillin side-reactions, with particular reference to fatalilities from anaphylactic shock, *Bull World Hlth Organ* 38:159, 1968.
93. Ishizaka T: Mechanisms of IgE-mediated hypersensitivity. In Middleton E, Jr, Reed CE, Ellis EF, et al, editors: *Allergy: Principles and practice,* St. Louis, 1988, Mosby–Year Book.
94. Jacobs RL, Rake GW Jr, Fournier DC, et al: Potentiated anaphylaxis in patients with drug-induced beta-adrenergic blockade, *J Allerg Clin Immunol* 68:125, 1981.
95. Jacobsen N, Hensten-Pettersen A: Occupational health problems among dental hygienists, *Comm Dent Oral Epidemiol* 23:177, 1995.
96. James LP, Austen KF: Fatal systemic anaphylaxis in man, *N Engl J Med* 270:597, 1964.
97. Kaniwa M, Isama K, Nakamura A, et al: Identification of causative chemicals of allergic contact dermatitis using a combination of patch testing in patients and chemical analysis. Application to cases from rubber gloves, *Contact Dermatol* 31:65, 1994.
98. Keller R: Interrelations between different types of cells. II. Histamine-release from the mast cells of various species by cationic polypeptides of polymorphonuclear leukocyte lysosomes and other cationic compounds, *Int Arch Allerg Appl Immunol* 34:139, 1968.
99. Kelly JF, Patterson R, Lieberman P, et al: Radiographic contrast media studies in high-risk patients, *J Allerg Clin Immunol* 62:181, 1978.
100. Kelly KJ, Pearson ML, Kurup VP, et al: A cluster of anaphylactic reactions in children with spina bifida during general anesthesia: epidemiologic features, risk factors, and latex hypersensitivity, *J Allerg Clin Immunol* 94:53, 1994.
101. Kettelkamp NS, Austin DR, Cheek DBC, et al: Inhibition of d-tubocurarine-induced histamine release by halothane, *Anesthesiology* 66:666, 1987.
102. Kiec-Swierczynska M: Occupational contact dermatitis induced by allergens present in rubber. I. Allergy to rubber accelerators [in Polish], *Medycyna Pracy* 45:303, 1994.
103. Kiec-Swierczynska M: Occupational contact dermatitis induced by allergens present in rubber. II. allergy to antioxidants [in Polish], *Medycyna Pracy* 45:393, 1994.
104. Kirklin JK, Chenoweth DE, Naftel DC, et al: Effects of protamine administration after cardiopulmonary bypass on complement, blood elements, and the hemodynamic state, *Ann Thorac Surg* 41:193, 1986.
105. Kishiyama JL, Adelman DC: The cross-reactivity and immunology of beta-lactam antibiotics (review), *Drug Safety* 10:318, 1994.
106. Knape JTA, Schuller JL, de Haan P, et al: An anaphylactic reaction to protamine in a patient allergic to fish, *Anesthesiology* 55:324, 1981.
107. Kurtz AB, Gray RS, Markanday S, et al: Circulating IgG antibody to protamine in

patients treated with protamine-insulins, *Diabetologia* 25:322, 1983.
108. Kurtz M, Laxenaire MC, Husson R: Severe anaphylactic complications during anesthesia induction. Survey of accidents reported to the Sou Medical Insurance Company from 1963 to 1983 [in French], *Cah Anesthesiol* 33:441, 1985.
109. Kurup VP, Kelly T, Elms N, et al: Cross-reactivity of food allergens in latex allergy, *Allergy Proc* 15:211, 1994.
110. Kwittken PL, Sweinberg SK, Campbell DE, et al: Latex hypersensitivity in children: clinical presentation and detection of latex-specific immunoglobulin E, *Pediatrics* 95:693, 1995.
111. Lagier F, Vervloet D, Lhermet I, et al: Prevalence of latex allergy in operating room nurses, *J Allerg Clin Immunol* 30: 319, 1992.
112. Lakin JD, Blocker TJ, Strong DM, et al: Anaphylaxis to protamine sulfate mediated by a complement-dependent IgG antibody, *J Allerg Clin Immunol* 61:102, 1978.
113. Laroche D, Dubois F, Lefrancois C, et al: Early biological markers of anaphylactoid reactions occurring during anesthesia [in French], *Ann Fr Anesth Reanim* 11:613, 1992.
114. Lasser EC, Berry CC, Talner LB, et al: Pretreatment with corticosteroids to alleviate reactions to intravenous contrast material, *N Engl J Med* 317:845, 1987.
115. Lavaud F, Prevost A, Cossart C, et al: Allergy to latex, avocado pear, and banana: evidence for a 30 kd antigen in immunoblotting, *J Allerg Clin Immunol* 95: 557, 1995.
116. Lawrence ID, Warner JA, Cohan VL, et al: Purification and characterization of human skin mast cells, *J Immunol* 139:3062, 1987.
117. Laxenaire MC: Drugs and other agents involved in anaphylactic shock occurring during anaesthesia. A French multicenter epidemiological inquiry, *Ann Fr Anesth Reanim* 12:91, 1993.
118. Levine BB: Immunochemical mechanisms involved in penicillin hypersensitivity in experimental animals and in human beings, *Fed Proc* 24:45, 1965.
119. Levine BB: Immunologic mechanisms of penicillin allergy. A haptenic model system for the study of allergic diseases of man, *N Engl J Med* 275:1115, 1966.
120. Levine BB, Redmond AP: Minor haptenic determinant-specific reagins of penicillin hypersensitivity in man, *Int Arch Allerg Appl Immunol* 35:445, 1969.
121. Levine BB, Redmond AP, Fellner MJ, et al: Penicillin allergy and the heterogenous immune responses of man to benzylpenicillin, *J Clin Invest* 45:1895, 1966.
122. Levy JH: *Anaphylactic reactions in anesthesia and intensive care,* Boston, 1992, Butterworth-Hanemann.
123. Levy JH, Kettelkamp N, Goertz P, et al: Histamine release by vancomycin: a mechanism for hypotension in man, *Anesthesiology* 67:122, 1987.
124. Leynadier F, Pecquet C, Dry J: Anaphylaxis to latex during surgery, *Anaesthesia* 44:547, 1989.
125. Leynadier F, Xuan T, Dry J: Allergenicity suppression in natural latex surgical gloves, *Allergy* 46:619, 1991.
126. Lichtenstein LM, Norman PS, Kagey-Sobotka A, et al: The immunologic basis for the efficacy of immunotherapy. In Kerr JW, Ganderton MA, editors: *XI International Congress of allergy and clinical immunology,* London, 1983, MacMillan.
127. Lichtenstein LM, Osler AG: Studies on the mechanisms of hypersensitivity phenomena. IX. Histamine release from leukocytes by ragweed pollen antigen, *J Exp Med* 120:507, 1964.
128. Loehr MM: Suit up against anaphylaxis, *Ann Emerg Med* 14:127, 1985.
129. Lorenz W, Doenicke A: H1 and H2 blockade: a prophylactic principle in anaesthesia and surgery against histamine-release responses of any degree of severity: Part II (review), *N Engl Reg Allerg Proc* 6:174, 1985.
130. Lowenstein E: Lessons from studying an infrequent event: adverse hemodynamic response associated with protamine reversal of heparin anticoagulation, *J Cardiothorac Anesth* 3:99, 1989.
131. Makinen-Kiljunen S: Banana allergy in patients with immediate-type hypersensitivity to natural rubber latex: characterization of cross-reacting antibodies and allergens, *J Allerg Clin Immunol* 93:990, 1994.
132. Masood D, Brown JE, Patterson R, et al: Recurrent anaphylaxis due to unrecognized latex hypersensitivity in two healthcare professionals, *Ann Allerg Asth Immunol* 74:311, 1995.
133. Mathews KP, Hemphill FM, Lovell RG, et al: A controlled study on the use of parenteral and oral antihistamines in preventing penicillin reactions, *J Allergy* 27:1, 1956.
134. McCormack DR, Heisser AI, Smith LJ: Intraoperative vecuronium anaphylaxis compounded by latex hypersensitivity, *Ann Allergy* 73:405, 1994.
135. Metzger H, Alcaraz G, Hohman R, et al: The receptor with high affinity for immunoglobulin E, *Annu Rev Immunol* 4:419, 1986.
136. Mizutari K, Kuriya N, Ono T: Immediate allergy to rubber gloves: a questionnaire study of hospital personnel, *J Dermatol* 22:19, 1995.
137. Moneret-Vautrin DA, Beaudouin E, Widmer S, et al: Prospective study of risk factors in natural rubber latex hypersensitivity, *J Allerg Clin Immunol* 92:668, 1993.
138. Moneret-Vautrin DA, Debra JC, Kohler C, et al: Occupational rhinitis and asthma to latex, *Rhinology* 32:198, 1994.
139. Moneret-Vautrin DA, Kanny G: Food-induced anaphylaxis. A new French multicenter study [in French], *Bull Acad Natl Med* 179:161, 1995.
140. Moneret-Vautrin DA, Laxenaire MC, Bavoux F: Allergic shock to latex and ethylene oxide during surgery for spinal bifida, *Anesthesiology* 73:556, 1990.
141. Morales C, Basomba J, Carreira, et al: Anaphylaxis produced by rubber glove contact. Case reports and immunological identification of the antigens involved, *Clin Exp Allerg* 19:425, 1990.
142. Morel DR, Zapol WM, Thomas SJ, et al: C5a and thromboxane generation associated with pulmonary vaso- and bronchoconstriction during protamine reversal of heparin, *Anesthesiology* 66:597, 1987.
143. Moscicki RA, Sockin SM, Corsello BF, et al: Assessing the predictive value of skin testing for general anesthetic agent hypersensitivity (abstract), *J Allerg Clin Immunol* 83:270, 1989.
144. Moscicki RA, Sockin SM, Corsello BF, et al: Anaphylaxis during induction of general anesthesia: subsequent evaluation and management, *J Allerg Clin Immunol* 86: 325, 1990.
145. Nagel JE, Fuscaldo JT, Fireman PL: Paraben allergy, *JAMA* 237:1594, 1977.
146. Nell LJ, Thomas JW: Frequency and specificity of protamine antibodies in diabetic and control subjects, *Diabetes* 37:172, 1988.
147. Neumar RW, Bircher NG, Sim KM, et al: Epinephrine and sodium bicarbonate during CPR following asphyxial cardiac arrest in rats, *Resuscitation* 29:249, 1995.
148. Norman PS: Skin testing. In Rose NR, Friedman H, Fahey JL, editors: *Manuel of clinical laboratory immunology,* Washington, 1986, American Society for Microbiology.
149. Norman PS, Lichtenstein LM, Ishizaka K: Diagnostic tests in ragweed hay fever. A comparison of direct skin tests, IgE antibody measurements, and basophil histamine release, *J Allerg Clin Immunol* 52:210, 1973.
150. North FC, Kettelkamp N, Hirshman CA: Comparison of cutaneous and *in vitro* histamine release by muscle relaxants, *Anesthesiology* 66:543, 1987.
151. Nutter AF: Contact urticaria to rubber, *Br J Dermatol* 101:597, 1979.
152. Occelli G, Amedeo J, Raucoules M, et al: Evaluation of the activities and value of allergo-anesthetic consultation at the University Hospital Center of Nice 1985–1991 [in French], *Therapie* 47:423, 1992.
153. Ong R, Sullivan T: Detection and characterization of human IgE to cephalosporin determinants, *J Allerg Clin Immunol* 81: 222, 1988.
154. Ortiz JR, Garcia J, Archilla J, et al: Latex allergy in anesthesiology (see comments) (review) [in Spanish], *Rev Esp Anestesiol Reanim* 42:169, 1995.
155. Oulieu S, Olivier J, Bourget P, et al: Therapeutic strategy in anaphylactoid shock during general anesthesia. Etiologic agents and diagnostic evaluation (review) [in French], *Therapie* 50:59, 1995.
156. Ovary Z: The history of immediate hypersensitivity, *Hosp Pract* 24:169, 1989.
157. Pailhories G: Reducing proteins in latex gloves. The industrial approach (review), *Clin Rev Allerg* 11:391, 1993.
158. Parker CW: The immunochemical basis for penicillin allergy, *Postgrad Med J* 40:141, 1964.
159. Patterson R, DeSwarte RD, Greenberger PA, et al: Drug allergy and protocols for management of drug allergies, *N Engl Reg Allerg Proc* 4:325, 1986.
160. Patterson R, Lucena G, Metz R, et al: Reaginic antibody against insulin: demonstration of antigenic distinction between native and extracted insulin, *J Immunol* 103:1061, 1969.
161. Pearson ML, Cole JS, Jarvis WR: How common is latex allergy? A survey of children with myelodysplasia, *Dev Med Child Neurol* 36:64, 1994.

162. Pecquet C, Leynadier F: IgE mediated allergy to natural rubber latex in 100 patients (review), *Clin Rev Allerg* 11:381, 1993.
163. Petz L: Immunologic cross-reactivity between penicillins and cephalosporins: a review, *J Infect Dis* 137:S74, 1978.
164. Pienkowski MM, Kazmier WJ, Adkinson NF Jr: Basophil histamine release remains unaffected by clinical desensitization to penicillin, *J Allerg Clin Immunol* 72:171, 1988.
165. Plaut M, Lichtenstein LM, Henney CS: Properties of a subpopulation of T cells bearing histamine receptors, *J Clin Invest* 55:856, 1975.
166. Rankin KV, Jones DL, Rees TD: Latex reactions in an adult dental population, *Am J Dent* 6:274, 1993.
167. Rent R, Ertel N, Elsenstein R, et al: Complement activation by interaction of polyanions and polycations I. Heparin-protamine induced consumption of complement, *J Immunol* 114:120, 1975.
168. Salkie ML: The prevalence of atopy and hypersensitivity to latex in medical laboratory technologists, *Arch Pathol Lab Med* 117:897, 1993.
169. Samuel T: Antibodies reacting with salmon and human protamines in sera from infertile men and from vasectomized men and monkeys, *Clin Exp Immunol* 30:181, 1977.
170. Sauder RA, Hirshman CA: Protamine-induced histamine release in human skin mast cells, *Anesthesiology* 73:165, 1990.
171. Saxon A, Beall GN, Rohr AS, et al: Immediate hypersensitivity reactions to beta-lactam antibiotics [clinical conference], *Ann Intern Med* 107:204, 1987.
172. Schatz M: Skin testing and incremental challenge in the evaluation of adverse reactions to local anesthetics, *J Allerg Clin Immunol* 74:606, 1984.
173. Schwartz LB, Metcalfe DD, Miller JS, et al: Tryptase levels as an indicator of mast-cell activation in systemic anaphylaxis and mastocytosis, *N Engl J Med* 316:1622, 1987.
174. Sciple GW, Knox JM, Montgomery CH: Incidence of penicillin reactions after an antihistamine simultaneously administered parenterally, *N Engl J Med* 261:1123, 1959.
175. Seaton A, Cherrie B, Turnbull J: Rubber glove asthma, *Bri Med J Clin Res Ed* 296:531, 1988.
176. Sethna NF, Sockin SM, Holzman RS, et al: Latex anaphylaxis in a child with a history of multiple anesthetic drug allergies, *Anesthesiology* 77:372, 1992.
177. Shapiro S, Siskind V, Slone D, et al: Drug rash with ampicillin and other penicillins, *Lancet* 2:969, 1969.
178. Sharath MD, Metzger WJ, Richardson HB, et al: Protamine-induced fatal anaphylaxis, *J Thorac Cardiovasc Surg* 90:86, 1985.
179. Sheffer AL: Anaphylaxis, *J Allerg Clin Immunol* 75:227, 1985.
180. Shibata K, Atsumi T, Horiuchi Y, et al: Immunological cross-reactivities of cephalothin and its related compounds with benzylpenicillin (penicillin G), *Nature* 212:419, 1966.
181. Siraganian RP: Histamine secretion from mast cells and basophils, *Trends Pharmaol Sci* 4:432, 1983.
182. Slater JE: Rubber anaphylaxis, *N Engl J Med* 320:1126, 1989.
183. Slater JE, Mostello LA, Shaer C, et al: Type I hypersensitivity to rubber, *Ann Allerg* 65:411, 1990.
184. Smith PL, Kagey-Sobotka A, Bleecker ER, et al: Physiologic manifestations of human anaphylaxis, *J Clin Invest* 66:1072, 1980.
185. Smith RM, Iwamoto GK, Richerson HB, et al: Trimethoprim-sulfamethoxazole desensitization in the acquired immunodeficiency syndrome, *Ann Intern Med* 106:335, 1987.
186. Sogn DD: Prevention of allergic reactions to penicillin, *J Allerg Clin Immunol* 78:1051, 1986.
187. Sondheimer JM, Pearlman DS, Bailey WC: Systemic anaphylaxis during rectal manometry with a latex balloon, *Am J Gastroenterol* 84:975, 1989.
188. Southorn PA, Plevak DJ, Wright AJ, et al: Adverse effects of vancomycin administered in the perioperative period, *Mayo Clin Proc* 61:721, 1986.
189. Spaner D, Dolovich J, Tarlo S, et al: Hypersensitivity to natural latex, *J Allerg Clin Immunol* 83:1135, 1989.
190. Stevenson DD: Adverse reactions to aspirin and nonsteroidal anti-inflammatory drugs, 12th International Congress of Allergy and Clinical Immunology, Washington, 1985.
191. Stewart WJ, McSweeney SM, Kellett MA, et al: Increased risk of severe protamine reactions in NPH insulin-dependent diabetics undergoing cardiac catheterization, *Circulation* 70:788, 1984.
192. Subramanian A, Yip E, Ng K, et al: Extractable protein content of gloves from prevulcanised natural rubber latex. In Latex Protein Workshop of the International Rubber Technology Conference, Kuala Lumpur, Malaysia, 1993,
193. Sullivan TJ: Facilitated haptenation of human proteins by penicillin, *J Allerg Clin Immunol* 83:255, 1989.
194. Sullivan TJ, Yecies LD, Shatz GS, et al: Desensitization of patients allergic to penicillin using orally administered beta-lactam antibiotics, *J Allerg Clin Immunol* 69:275, 1982.
195. Sussman GL, Lem D, Liss G, et al: Latex allergy in housekeeping personnel, *Ann Allerg Asthma Immunol* 74:415, 1995.
196. Swartz J, Braude BM, Gilmour RF, et al: Intraoperative anaphylaxis to latex (review), *Can J Anaesth* 37:589, 1990.
197. Swartz JS, Gold M, Braude BM, et al: Intraoperative anaphylaxis to latex: an identifiable population at risk, *Can J Anaesth* 37:S131, 1990.
198. Tan F, Jackman H, Skidgel RA, et al: Protamine inhibits plasma carboxypeptidase N, the inactivator of anaphylatoxins and kinins, *Anesthesiology* 70:267, 1989.
199. Tersegno MM: Recall of E-Z-EM balloon-retaining barium enema tips (letter), *Am J Roentgenol* 156:869, 1991.
200. Theissen JL, Zahn P, Theissen U, et al: Allergic and pseudo-allergic reactions in anesthesia. II: Symptoms, diagnosis, therapy, prevention (review) [in German], *Anasthesiol Intensivmed Notfallmed Schmerzther* 30:71, 1995.
201. Tobias JD, Kubos KL, Hirshman CA: Aminophylline does not attenuate histamine-induced airway constriction during halothane anesthesia, *Anesthesiology* 71: 723, 1989.
202. Tobin MC, Karns BK, Anselmino LM, et al: Potentiation of human basophil histamine release by protamine: a new role for a polycation recognition site, *Mol Immunol* 23:245, 1986.
203. Tosi LL, Slater JE, Shaer C, et al: Latex allergy in spina bifida patients: prevalence and surgical implications, *J Pediatr Orthop* 13:709, 1993.
204. Turjanmaa K: Incidence of immediate allergy to latex gloves in hospital personnel, *Contact Dermatol* 17:270, 1987.
205. Turjanmaa K: Update on occupational natural rubber latex allergy (review), *Dermatol Clin* 12:561, 1994.
206. Turjanmaa K, Reunala T, Rasanen L: Comparison of diagnostic methods in latex surgical glove contact urticaria, *Contact Dermatol* 19:241, 1988.
207. van der Walle HB, Brunsveld VM: Latex allergy among hairdressers, *Contact Dermatol* 32:177, 1995.
208. Vandenplas O, Delwiche JP, Evrard G, et al: Prevalence of occupational asthma due to latex among hospital personnel, *Am J Respir Crit Care Med* 151:54, 1995.
209. Verburg KM, Bowsher RR, Israel KS, et al: Histamine release by vancomycin in humans, *Fed Proc* 44:1247, 1985.
210. Vervloet D, Arnaud A, Senft M, et al: Leukocyte histamine release to suxamethonium in patients with adverse reactions to muscle relaxants, *J Allerg Clin Immunol* 75:338, 1985.
211. Vervloet D, Nizankowska E, Arnaud A, et al: Adverse reactions to suxamethonium and other muscle relaxants under general anesthesia, *J Allerg Clin Immunol* 71:552, 1983.
212. Volcheck GW, Li JT: Elevated serum tryptase level in a case of intraoperative anaphylaxis caused by latex allergy, *Arch Intern Med* 154:2243, 1994.
213. Vuitton D, Neidhardt-Audion M, Girardin P, et al: Epidemiologic characteristics of 21 peranesthetic anaphylactoid accidents observed in a population of 12,855 surgically treated patients [in French], *Ann Fr Anesth Reanim* 4:167, 1985.
214. Vyas GN, Perkins HA, Fudenberg HH: Anaphylactoid transfusion reactions associated with anti-IgA, *Lancet* 2:312, 1968.
215. Wasserman SI, Marquardt DL: Anaphylaxis. In Middleton E, Reed CE, Ellis EF, Adkinson NF, Yunginger JW, editors: *Allergy: Principles and practice,* St. Louis, 1992, Mosby–Yearbook.
216. Watkins J, Clark A, Appleyard TN, et al: Immune-mediated reactions to althesin (alphaxalone), *Br J Anaesth* 48:881, 1976.
217. Weiler JM, Gellhaus MA, Carter JG, et al: A prospective study of the risk of an immediate adverse reaction to protamine sulfate during cardiopulmonary bypass surgery, *J Allerg Clin Immunol* 85:713, 1990.
218. Weiss ME: Evaluation and treatment of patients with prior reactions to beta-lactam antibiotics (review), *Curr Clin Top Infect Dis* 13:131, 1993.
219. Weiss ME, Adkinson NF Jr: Immediate hypersensitivity reactions to penicillin and related antibiotics, *Clin Allerg* 18:515, 1988.
220. Weiss ME, Adkinson NF Jr: Allergy to protamine. In Vervloet D, editor: *Clinical reviews in allergy: Anesthesiology: anes-*

thesiology and allergy, New Brunswick, 1991, Humana Press.

221. Weiss ME, Adkinson NF Jr, Hirshman CA: Evaluation of allergic drug reactions in the perioperative period, *Anesthesiology* 71:483, 1989.
222. Weiss ME, Chatham F, Kagey-Sobotka A, et al: Serial immunological investigations in a patient who had a life-threatening reaction to intravenous protamine, *Clin Exp Allerg* 20:713, 1990.
223. Weiss ME, Nyhan D, Peng Z, et al: Association of protamine IgE and IgG antibodies with life-threatening reactions to intravenous protamine, *N Engl J Med* 320: 886, 1989.
224. Wickern GM, Nish WA, Bitner AS, et al: Allergy to beta-lactams: a survey of current practices, *J Allerg Clin Immunol* 94:725, 1994.
225. Wrangsjo K, Osterman K, van Hage-Hamsten M: Glove-related skin symptoms among operating theatre and dental care unit personnel (II). Clinical examination, tests and laboratory findings indicating latex allergy, *Contact Dermatol* 30:139, 1994.
226. Wrangsjo K, Wahlbert JE, Axelsson GK: IgE-mediated allergy to natural rubber in 30 patients with contact urticaria, *Contact Dermatol* 19:264, 1988.
227. Yancey KB, Hammer CH, Harvath L, et al: Studies of human C5a as a mediator of inflammation in normal human skin, *J Clin Invest* 75:486, 1985.
228. Yassin MS, Lierl MB, Fischer TJ, et al: Latex allergy in hospital employees, *Ann Allerg* 72:245, 1994.
229. Yassin MS, Sanyurah S, Lierl MB, et al: Evaluation of latex allergy in patients with meningomyelocele (abstract), *Ann Allerg* 69:207, 1992.
230. Zaza S, Reeder JM, Charles LE, et al: Latex sensitivity among perioperative nurses, *AORN J* 60:806, 1994.
231. Zeiss CR, Grammer LC, Levitz D: Comparison of the radioallergosorbent test and a quantitative solid-phase radioimmunoassay for the detection of ragweed-specific immunoglobulin E antibody in patients undergoing immunotherapy, *J Allerg Clin Immunol* 67:105, 1981.
232. Zucker-Pinchoff B, Ramanathan S: Anaphylactic reaction to epidural fentanyl, *Anesthesiology* 71:599, 1989.

CHAPTER 93

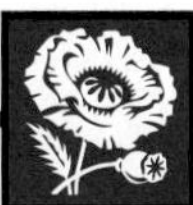

Blood Component Therapy: Indications and Risks

DAVID J. MURRAY

Clinical transfusion practice has changed dramatically over the past several decades. Fear of acquiring AIDS from blood led to reevaluation of prior indications for blood and new guidelines for transfusion.[37–39,44,60,86,113,100] Twenty years ago, indications for blood were based on the notion that allogeneic blood was both safe and effective therapy.[4,69,79] Over the last decade, most stringent guidelines and indications for blood and blood components have been implemented.[37–39] Now that the chance of acquiring an infectious disease from a blood transfusion has been markedly reduced,[45,46] current transfusion indications which proscribe blood and blood components until symptoms and signs indicate potential morbidity may need to be reevaluated. An assessment of risk, benefit, and efficacy and more recently cost efficacy will influence not only donor testing[31,76] but also the future role of allogenic as well as autologous transfusion practice.[11,16,50,60,73,101,110]

More than 50% of transfusions are administered in the perioperative period. Potential benefits should be weighed against delayed complications of transfusion when decisions are required about transfusion.[45,46,63,107,113,114,120] Frequently, rapid transfusion decisions are required, yet limited information is available to guide clinical judgement. The major morbidity from blood components are long-term complications primarily caused by infectious diseases, immunologic, and immunomodulatory effects of blood transfusion, such as alloimmunization and decreased immune surveillance.[20,124,125] Because these risks are the primary reasons for changes in indications for transfusion, anesthesia providers should have updated information about infectious disease prevalence and how newer clinical and laboratory screening methods improve the safety of blood. Indications for blood will continue to change as the balance between long-term risks of transfusion are weighed against lifesaving benefits of blood components. With increasing improvement in the sensitivity of donor testing methods for infectious disease, it is conceivable that transfusion transmitted infectious disease could all but be eliminated from the nation's blood supply.[31,76]

Less than 100 years ago, blood group antigens and antibodies were determined to be the cause of hemolytic reactions between donor and recepient.[75] Compatibility testing of blood between donor and recipient solved the major problems that prohibited allogeneic transfusion.[47,75] Refinements in cross-match and compatibility testing methods decreased the frequency of fatal hemolytic transfusion reaction, but transfusion risks were still recognized as greater with whole blood than with fractionated plasma derivatives.[47] Anticoagulants, blood preservatives, sterile collection systems, and small-bore needles for collection and administration of blood products led to the safe use of blood particularly during World War II as the modern blood bank evolved. Blood use during the perioperative period increased markedly with new surgical procedures. During the 1950s, 1960s, and 1970s, the introduction of cardiopulmonary bypass, renal transplant, and vascular surgical techniques led to marked increases in perioperative blood component use.[35,69] A concern about replacement of blood loss with large volumes of crystalloid resulted in the widespread use of whole blood to manage even small perioperative blood volume losses.[4] Owing to the apparent safety of blood, mild anemia during the perioperative period was not tolerated and allogeneic transfusion was used extensively. The infectious risks of transfusion brought an end to the liberal use of perioperative red cell and blood component transfusion.[113,114]

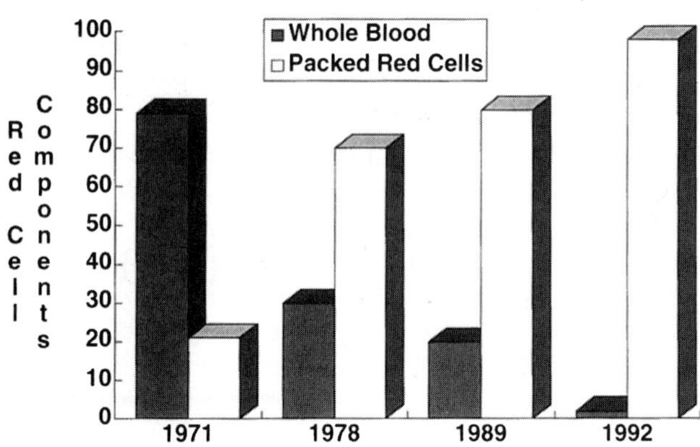

Fig. 93-1. The decline in whole blood use and increase in packed red cell use over the past 25 years. In the 1990s, less than 2% of red cell containing blood components are provided as whole blood.

COMPONENT THERAPY

During the same period that cardiac and vascular surgical techniques were introduced, fresh frozen plasma and fresh whole blood preparations were recognized as effective treatments for bleeding disorders, but the large volumes of plasma and blood required prevented effective long-term therapy. In 1964, Pool et al.[95] found that the precipitate formed when fresh frozen plasma was thawed at 4 to 8° C was rich in factor VIII activity. This protein-rich precipitate markedly improved hemophilia care and led to even greater demand for blood components, with consonant reduction in availablility of whole blood (Fig. 93-1).[79,103,104,109] Fresh frozen plasma and plasma exchange were used to treat a variety of clinical disorders which further increased the demand for plasma preparations.[22,27] A tenfold increase in plasma use was reported during the 1970s primarily because blood components were believed to be safe (Fig. 93-2).[89,114] Plasma was used not only for clotting factors, but also as a volume-replacement solution and a treatment modality for a variety of medical illnesses.[22,27,39,89] The transient benefits of plasma and increased awareness of transfusion risks have led to the abandonment of many such therapies.[22,27,39,89]

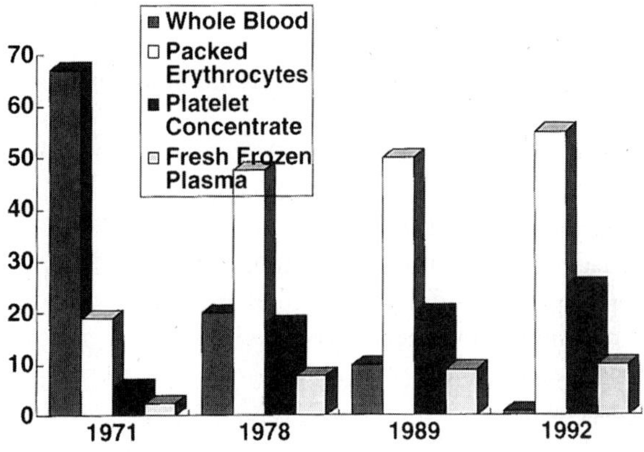

Fig. 93-2. Blood component use per 1000 operations based on data from the American Association of Blood Banks. Changes in whole blood, packed red cell, platelet, and fresh frozen plasma (FFP) use over the past 25 year period. Data from Rosen,[100] Surgenor,[114] and Wallace.[121]

At present, less than 2% of red cell containing blood components are provided as whole blood, primarily because of the need for plasma components (Fig. 93-1). Plasma derived immune globulin preparations are used for prevention of conditions such as Rh disease, tetanus, hepatitis A and B, cytomegalovirus (CMV), and herpes. Albumin, plasma protein preparations, platelets, and leukocytes prepared from human blood donors are currently the only source of these blood components and derivatives (Box 93-1). An increasing number of patients who have hematologic side effects from antineoplastic agents and from bone marrow and liver transplantation have also increased the demand for blood components. Heat treatment and chemical processing of donor plasma can provide purified specific factor VIII or IX preparations for persons with hemophilia, but the separation and processing to decrease infectious risks markedly decrease the yield of the protein preparation. As a result, the demand for donor blood to provide the raw material for these highly purified, extensively processed proteins has increased.[55]

Newer preservatives have increased the storage period for many blood components. More effective separation methods have improved the yield of components collected by blood donation (see Box 93-1 and Table 93-1). Blood components obtained by plasmapheresis of a single donor offer some hope of decreasing the infectious risks of platelets, plasma, and granulocytes.[61]

Erythropoietin to stimulate red cell production may help decrease red cell requirements of many patients with acute and chronic anemias[56,67,109,118,120] and increase the harvest of

BOX 93-1
THERAPEUTIC COMPOUNDS AND DERIVATIVES OBTAINED FROM BLOOD

Components (mechanical process separate from single whole blood donor unit centrifuge, freezing)

Whole blood
Packed red cells
Adsol preservative
Citrate phosphate dextrose and adenine preservative
Heparin preservative
Frozen red cells
Washed red cells
Single-donor plasma
Fresh frozen plasma
Cryoprecipitate
Platelets

Derivative (pooled plasma treated by heat chemical processes to derive prepartion)

Plasmanate
Albumin 5%
Albumin 25%
Immune globulin (intramuscular or intravenous)
(Hepatitis B, rabies, tetanus, lymphocyte, Rh antiglobulin, etc.)
Factor VIII concentrate
Factor IX concentrate

autologous predeposited red cells.[56] A synthetic factor VIII preparation derived from recombinant DNA synthesis would markedly improve the care and decrease the need for human donor-derived blood components for the hemophiliac. A stable hemoglobin preparation derived from recombinant DNA synthesis with a similar O_2 dissociation curve to intracellular hemoglobin may alter approaches to allogeneic transfusion.[97] These approaches may alter component therapy in the future but are not yet ready for approval and release.

PREVENTION OF TRANSFUSION PROBLEMS

Blood bank procedures continue to alter transfusion risk and as a result change indications for transfusion.[37–40,86,100,113] Answers to a variety of questions should help in understanding how risk changed indications for blood components:

- What procedures are followed to ensure donated blood is safe?
- What donor testing is performed before releasing blood components for recipients?
- What testing of the recipient is required to ensure a lesser incidence of side effects or complications?
- What are the immediate and long-term complications and side effects of transfusion?
- What changes occur because of storage and the use of preservatives?
- What components and derivatives of blood are in fact available? Do these components and derivatives have similar infectious risks?
- What special equipment and precautions are necessary when administering blood products?
- What preventive steps are available to decrease complications and side effects of transfusion?
- What therapy is required when a side effect or complication of transfusion occurs?

Donor Testing

Blood banks seek donor blood that will be safe and effective (Tables 93-2 and 93-3).[13,102,120] The initial step to ensure safe blood components is the donor history, which is later combined with a battery of serologic tests to confirm compatibility and the absence of infectious disease.[102] A careful history is needed not only to specifically exclude blood products that may be a risk to the recipient but also to prevent donor complications from blood donation.[13,91]

A confidential signed statement by blood donors that indicates the donated unit can be safely transfused may be one of the most important steps in excluding infectious disease from the donated blood.[13] Although many blood banks practiced these steps before widespread recognition of the viral risks of transfusion, the increased emphasis on donor health screening was not mandated until transfusion-related HIV transmission was recognized as a serious health risk for recipients.[33,40–42,52] Donors who may be at high risk for asymptomatic HIV infectious disease can be excluded from blood donation (e.g., parenteral drug abuse, homosexual activity, prostitution, as well as persons from countries having a high prevalence of HIV infection).[13,23,102] A population with increased prevalence of HIV infection also tends to have an increased prevalence of hepatitis B and hepatitis C infection.[23,70] For this reason, excluding donors with one viral disease has a positive impact in decreasing other transfusion-related viral diseases (Table 93-4).[1,7,68] At present, predonation history and signed attestations are important to prevent disease transmission from blood products; but the increasing prevalence of HIV and other viral diseases increases, in all segments of the population has led to an increasing reliance on blood screening tests to ensure safe blood.[13,131]

Viral and Bacterial Infection

A common feature of transfusion-related infectious disease is an asymptomatic, blood-borne carrier state in healthy appearing blood donors. Syphilis was an early example of a blood-borne infectious problem with a relatively asymptomatic carrier state.[98] The identification and elimination of potentially infectious donors from the blood supply should rely on donor history and sensitive health screening tech-

Table 93-1 Blood components

Product	Description	Volume hematocrit	Shelf life
Red cell components			
Whole blood		450 ml (40%)	35 days
Modified whole blood	Platelets and cryoprecipitate removed by centrifuge	350 ml (50%)	35 days
Packed red cells	Plasma and platelets removed by centrifuge		
CPD-A1	(Citrate Phosphate Dextrose adenine)	250 ml (70%)	35 days
Adsol	(Adenine, Dextose, Mannitol)	300 ml (60%)	49 days
Leukocyte-depleted red cells	Depth-filtered packed cells (99% leukocytes removed)	200 ml (70%)	24 hours (from preparation)
Washed red cells	(80% removal of leukocytes) 20% loss of red cells	200 ml (70%)	24 hours (from preparation)
Frozen red cells	Frozen with glycerol for protection	250 ml (70%)	5–10 years (12 hours after thaw and wash)
Plasma components			
Platelets, single-donor	Removed from whole blood (20°–24° C) by centrifuge	50 ml	3–5 days
Platelet pheresis unit	Pheresed from single donor (20°–24° C) (equal to 6–8 single units of platelets)	250 ml	3–5 days
Fresh frozen plasma	Plasma separated and frozen within 6 hours of collection (−18°)	250 ml	1 year from collection (24 hours after thawed)
Cryoprecipitate	Precipitate obtained after frozen plasma thawed at 4°–8° C	15 ml	1 year from collection (6 hours after thawed)
Leukocytes	Pheresed (20°–24°)		24 hours from collection

Table 93-2 Immunologic complications of transfusion

Problem	Etiology
Hemolytic transfusion reaction (immediate)	Donor red blood antigen reacts with antibody present in recipinet (complement activation)
(delayed)	Donor red blood cell antigen induces increase in undetected antibody in recipient (48–72 hr after transfusion)
Anaphylactic (uriticarial)	Recipient lacks IgA (protein differences between recipient and donor)
Febrile nonhemolytic	Donor leukocyte or platelet antigens cause febrile reactions in recipients
Noncardiogenic pulmonary edema	Recipient has antibody to donor plasma proteins or leukocyte
Graft versus host reaction	Donor lymphocyte engrafts in recipient, leading to rejection by recipient (immunocompromised recipient)
Post-transfusion purpura	Donor antigen produces recipient antibody to platelets
Isoimmunization	Donor antigen causes antibody formation in recipient that complicates future cross-match
Immune modulation	Decreased immune surveillance 1) cancer recurrence, 2) postoperative infection

niques. Methods currently employed by blood banks exclude many donated units from the donor pool by using sensitive but often nonspecific screening techniques. In the interest of maintaining highly sensitive screening methods, nonspecific tests are included in the screening programs (see Table 93-4).[102] Despite these rigorous standards, the infection risk of transfusion should be carefully considered when blood products are transfused.[120]

Transfusion-related HIV infection

The increased incidence and prevalence of HIV infection has focused attention on the steps blood donor centers use

Table 93-3 Complications of transfusion

Transfusion problems created by storage, preservatives, and infusion	
Citrate intoxication	Chelation of Ca^{++} leads to hypocalcemia
Hyperkalemia	Release of K^{++} by cells during storage
Microaggregates	Fibrin and platelet deposits (10–70 μm)
Hypothermia	Infusion of large volume of blood components store at low temperature
Hemoglobinemia	Free hemoglobin from damaged red cells
Hemolysis	Excessive pressure or overheating leads to destruction of red cells
Acidosis	Lactic acid production by red cells during storage
Decreased P50 of hemoglobin	Decreased 2,3 DPG levels

Table 93-4 Policies implemented to decrease viral infections risk from donor population

Policy	Date implemented
Screening HbSAg	1972
Voluntary exclusion of high-risk patients	1983
High-risk behavior exclusion of HIV	1984
ELISA screening for HIV	1985
Exclusion of high-risk for HIV	1985
Confidential donor self-exclusion	1986
Screen for alanine aminotransferase	1986
Antibody screening HbCAg	1987
Antibody to HLTV	1988
Antibody testing for hepatitis C	1990
Antibody testing to HIV I/II	1990
p24 antigen test	1995

to ensure safe blood products.[13,40,91,102,122,131] The specificity and sensitivity of current screening tests need to be clearly delineated before undue reliance is placed on the test result.[13,106,122,131] Previous screening tests for HIV detected antibody to the viral antigen rather than testing for the actual causative antigen.[13,122] Although the enzyme-linked immunoabsorbant antibody assay (ELISA) is sensitive to the presence of HIV antibody, antibody may not be present in the serum of carriers for weeks following exposure to HIV.[123] This false-negative problem may be solved by using an antigen marker rather than antibody testing, but, based on experience with sensitivity of antigen testing used for many years for hepatitis B, false negative testing still may occur.[5] One of the first HIV antigen tests, namely p24 HIV antigen, has been implemented to further increase the safety of blood.[31,76] This antigen testing may increase the sensitivity of blood screening for the HIV carrier state, although based on theoretical models, the added reduction in preventing potential HIV transmission is small because of the combined current high efficacy of the other measures to prevent the potential transmission of blood borne infectious disease. The HIV antigen also may be more difficult to interpret as a marker of infectivity, as the antigen may not be present during all stages of the disease.[13,41,102,123,131]

Based on current knowledge of disease prevalence and current testing techniques, the risk of a unit of blood carrying HIV antigen may now be less than 1:500,000/unit transfused. This frequency depends not only on effective blood screening but also primarily on the underlying frequency of HIV infection in the donor population and the quality and confidentiality of the donor self-exclusion program.[120,123,131] In 1996, if 18 million units of blood are transfused—based on the current prevalence of the HIV carrier state, donor self-exclusion, and newer HIV screening methods—it is predicted that less than 20 recipients would receive a transfusion of HIV antigen from a donor.[31,76] This assumes that HIV infection prevalence remains constant. If and when the HIV carrier state becomes more prevalent, the frequency of undetected HIV transmission in blood screened negative for HIV could increase.[13,102,120,123,131]

Transfusion-related hepatitis

Hepatitis B. Hepatitis B infection transmitted by donated blood has been all but eliminated by serologic testing.[5,13] HbSAg—the surface antigen to the hepatitis virus—appears early during hepatitis B infection and persists in those individuals who enter a carrier state for hepatitis B.[19] Screening for HbSAg excludes donors who potentially could transmit hepatitis B. The persistent asymptomatic carrier state for hepatitis B approaches 20% in developing countries, but is estimated to be 0.3% to 0.5% in the United States.[1,13,72] **Hepatitis B is still the most serious and frequent cause of fulminant and chronic hepatitis worldwide,**[72] and the threat of infection from parenteral exposure (intravenous [IV] drug abuse, needle sticks, sexual encounters) remains a major health risk. **Immunization for hepatitis B is an effective preventive program for decreasing the risk of infection,**

particularly in high-risk groups (health care workers), and offers hope of decreasing the prevalence of the carrier state as well as the incidence of serious hepatitis B acute infection.

Posttransfusion hepatitis. Ninety percent of posttransfusion viral hepatitis is caused by hepatitis C which, unlike hepatitis B, has until recently had no identified viral genome.[7] A serologic screening test has now been implemented to identify blood donors who may be carriers of this hepatitis C virus.[6,8,74] Because of the high prevalence of hepatitis C in the donor population (1% to 5% of donors), this has been of major benefit to transfusion recipients in reducing hepatitis risk.[1,3,45,46] Transfusion-acquired hepatitis, although less feared than HIV, in fact remains a greater morbidity and mortality threat to blood recipients.[1,3,7,13,63,120] In 1972, implementation of hepatitis B surface antigen testing markedly reduced hepatitis B from donated blood but had little impact on decreasing posttransfusion hepatitis.[5] Before the introduction of serologic screening for hepatitis C, liver enzyme and surrogate testing of donated blood were used to exclude potential carriers.[13,68,70] The latter two steps, introduced in 1986, decreased the prevalence of hepatitis C to less than 2% of all blood components.[7,13,14,68,70,102,109] The addition of the hepatitis C serologic test has eliminated an additional 90% of transfusion-related hepatitis in recipients and, as a result, the prevalence of blood components with the potential to transmit hepatitis C is currently less than 1 per 1000 donor units.[8,74,85]

Acute hepatitis C infection, which is asymptomatic in 70% of patients (and donors), is not cause for alarm, but progression of infection to chronic hepatitis and eventual liver failure or hepatocellular cancer over the course of years poses a considerable risk for blood recipients.[1,3,23,68,102,120] Although hepatitis C testing has reduced hepatitis from transfusion, if a 1% incidence of hepatitis occurred per 100 transfusion recipients (most recipients receive 3 units of blood), the risk of developing a form of progressive chronic hepatitis leading to liver failure or hepatocellular cancer has been estimated to be 1 for every 10,000 transfused patients.

Transfusion-related hepatitis is not clearly understood, particularly because hepatitis C cannot be traced to parenteral exposure in 60% of the patients. Development of hepatitis C in hospitalized patients who have not received any blood or blood products confounds estimates of transfusion-related "non-A," "non-B" (i.e., "C" hepatitis).[6,7] In addition, the number of components transfused and incidence of hepatitis C are not directly related, because large blood-volume transfusion does not appear to increase the risks of hepatitis C.

Cytomegalovirus

Disseminated CMV infection can be a serious or lethal disease in an immunocompromised host. This common viral illness in healthy patients has minimal symptoms, but the leukocytes of previously infected individuals may continue to carry the CMV for years following infection.[96] Transfusion-related CMV infection is a real possibility when blood products are administered to a CMV-negative patient.[96] The high prevalence of prior CMV infection in the donor population (20% to 80%) can be documented by testing for the presence of IgG and IgM antibodies, which indicate prior infection. Fortunately, the risk of seropositive donor blood or blood product transmitting the infectious agent to seronegative recipients is 2% to 3%.[127] A more specific method of identifying potentially infectious blood would make it easier to provide CMV-negative blood to CMV-negative recipients. In 70% to 80% of infected individuals, CMV infection is asymptomatic; in the remainder of patients, a viral syndrome associated with a 2- to 3-week period of lethargy and fatigue begins 2 weeks after transfusion. Serious disseminated CMV infection may occur in the immunocompromised patient (e.g., transplant recipient or patient with malignancy receiving chemotherapy) or neonate.[117,130] In these recipients, donor blood should be free of CMV infection or have leukocytes removed by filtration or washing.[80] This can be accomplished by providing blood from CMV-negative blood donors, using blood filters to remove leukocytes, extensively washing red cell preparations, or using frozen blood.[13,120]

Bacterial and protozoal infection

Similar to the transfusion-associated viral infectious risk, preventing transmission by bacterial and protozoal infection is based on excluding donors at risk.[102] Acute bacterial infections can be excluded based on history and physical examination, but chronic infectious processes with minimal symptoms and signs often cannot be excluded based on donor history alone. The American Association of Blood Banks requires that blood banks screen blood donors for syphilis, but most other latent bacterial or protozoal diseases, such as malaria, are excluded by no history of travel to endemic areas.[98,102] Transmission of parasitic infections such as Chagas disease, toxoplasmosis, and filariasis should be unlikely when a travel history is also included in the exclusion criteria for donors.[13,120]

Two North American tick–borne diseases that potentially can be transmitted by blood products include Babesosis, a tick-borne parasite prevalent in the northeastern United States,[13,120] and the spirochete which causes Lyme disease. Donor-transmitted Lyme disease has been reported in transfusion recipients, because this spirochete can survive blood storage.

Bacterial infection may also result from contamination of blood during or after collection.[26,88] Sterile, closed-collection systems have decreased the frequency of this occurrence, but blood is an excellent culture medium and serious systemic infection is possible.[88,120] Cryophilic bacteria that survive and grow at temperatures at which blood is stored, such as some *Pseudomonas yersinia* organisms, have caused morbidity and mortality in blood recipients.[88,120]

IMMUNOLOGIC PROBLEMS RELATED TO BLOOD TRANSFUSIONS

Virtually all of the elements in donor blood can be recognized as foreign by the recepient and lead to a variety of transfusion problems. In addition, in the immunocompromised host, donor lymphocytes can engraft in the recipient leading to a donor versus recepient (graft versus host) illness. Even in patients without immunologic compromise, allogeneic blood may cause decreased immune surveillance and potentially greater cancer recurrence and infection. With more than 400 antigens present on red cells alone, it is surprising that immunologic problems, such as the development of antibodies to foreign red cell antigens, develop in so few transfusion recipients (< 1%). The immunologic matching between donor and recipient red cells referred to as *compatibility testing* provides information about the presence or absence of three antigens (i.e., A, B, and the Rh D antigen). The remainder of standard compatibility testing is to determine whether additional alloantibodies are present in donor or recipient serum.[92] The compatibility assessment of donor and recipient provides a framework for understanding the cause and treatment of immunologic problems related to transfusion including the most serious problem, the hemolytic transfusion reaction (see Tables 93-2 and 93-3).[29,32,87]

Group and Type

Naturally occurring antibodies of the ABO system probably result when antigen exposure occurs via the gastrointestinal (GI) tract.[92] In a type O patient (absent A and B antigens on red cells), the alloantibodies A and B will be present in serum. Type AB patients (both A and B antigens on red cells) will have no alloantibodies in the serum (Table 93-5).[92] Additional antibodies to red cell antigens of other blood group systems do not develop unless the patient has had parenteral exposure to the absent antigen from transfusion or during pregnancy (Table 93-5).[59,77,92]

Antibodies to foreign antigens that result from exposure to the same species are referred to as *alloantibodies.* When the recipient is exposed to foreign antigens, an antibody response does not always occur; even when there is exposure to the D antigen of the Rh system.[59,77,92] A transfusion recipient who lacks the D antigen (Rh negative) and receives Rh-positive blood will have a 70% chance to develop antibody to the D antigen (i.e., become sensitized). The high prevalence of antibody formation to the Rh system is the reason that donor and recipient blood is typed to define the presence of the D antigen of the Rh system. For all other antigens of the red cell, such as the Kell, other Rh antigens, Duffy, Kidd, and Lewis, exposure to a foreign red cell antigen leads to a recipient becoming sensitized (developing antibodies) less than 1% of the time.[59,77] The ABO group and Rh type of donor and recipient, therefore, provide only an initial framework to establish compatibility between donor and recipient.[92]

Type and Screen Versus Type and Cross-Match

Screening of donor and recipient sera is effective to determine whether a patient has developed antibodies outside of the naturally occurring alloantibodies of the ABO system.[25] A commercially obtained red cell sample "kit" containing most major red cell antigens is screened against donor and recipient sera.[25,92] A negative screen indicates that the tested serum (either donor or recipient) does not contain antibody to the most common red cell antigen systems outside of the ABO system. Because the commercial red cell preparation used for screening contains almost all antigen systems known to be responsible for hemolysis, the transfusion of donor cells is unlikely to result in a hemolytic reaction (hemolytic reaction risk < 1:10,000).[25,92] As a final check, an *in vitro* test of donor cells with recipient serum and recipient cells with donor serum is performed to make sure no incompatibility exists. Because most recipients receive more than a single blood unit (average 3 to 4 units), the screening of blood also provides some assurance of compatibility among the multiple donors to whom the recipient will be exposed during the transfusion process (Table 93-6).[92]

If these prior screening tests are negative, a major hemolytic transfusion reaction is very unlikely. The traditional three-phase cross-match that entails room-temperature testing, an albumin and normal saline match at 37° F,

Table 93-5 ABO and Rh compatibility requirements

Recipient blood group	Frequency (%)	Antigens on red cells	Antibodies in serum	Donor blood groups compatible with* Recipient serum	Recipient red cells
A	35	A	Anti-B	A, O	A, AB
B	15	B	Anti-A	B, O	B, AB
AB	5	A and B	O	AB, A, B, O	AB only
O	45	—	Anti-A/Anti-B	O only	O, A, B, AB
Rh positive	85	D	—	Rh positive, Rh negative	
Rh negative	15	Anti-D, if sensitized	Anti-D, if sensitized	Rh negative	

Table 93-6 Donor compatibility transfusion*

Cross match	< 1:100,000	60 min
Rapid spin cross-match	< 1:100,000	45 min
Type and screen	< 1: 10,000	30 min
Type-specific	< 1: 1,000	5 min
O-negative	< 1: 500	0 min

*The table shows differences in potential transfusion reaction among various types of compatibility testing procedures. The frequency of transfusion reaction (immunologic) caused by atypical antibodies is based on estimates of the frequency in the transfusion recipient population. The total time required for appropriate laboratory testing is also estimated.

and a final Coombs test may not be required. The final cross-match procedure does provide further assurance that an incompatibility does not exist between donor and recipient, but many blood bank are reconsidering whether this test should be continued when blood is screened negative.[92]

Can a transfusion recipient receive blood or red cells outside his or her group and type? Based on the preceding, a type O individual will require type O red cells, but an A, B, or AB type individual may theoretically receive red cells from a donor who has no antigen (i.e., an O type individual). An Rh-positive patient may receive red cells without the Rh D antigen (i.e., from an Rh-negative donor). Donor red cells for an AB-positive recipient can theoretically be A, Rh-negative or B, Rh-negative, or O, Rh-negative. Based on an understanding of red cell antigen systems, the risk of antibody development, and limitations of blood bank inventories, recipients do sometimes receive compatible blood outside of their blood group and type.

Antibody develops to donor antigens in less than 1% of transfusions, but predicting which recipient and what alloantibody will develop following a homologous transfusion is not possible.[59,77] Certain antigens have greater potential for sensitization; the "K" of the Kell and "c" of the Rh system stimulate alloantibody formation more commonly than other antigens.[77,92,112] In recipients who have developed antibodies from prior red cell antigen exposure, cross-matching techniques, although more complicated, are invaluable. In this setting the antibody screen will be positive. Further compatibility testing is indicated.[112] The *in vitro* cross-match may be redundant in patients who have negative antibody screening, but in patients who screen positive for antibodies, the final stage *in vitro* cross-match becomes imperative. If the antibody the recipient carries is a very common antigen group on the red cell, attempts to identify the specific antibody by more sophisticated screening procedures can help identify potentially compatible donors. Without a clear indication of the antigen responsible for the positive antibody screen, the cross-match should be relied on to provide compatible blood. This may require cross-matches against large number of donor units. In some circumstances, the patient has antibodies that cause agglutination with all recipient blood. In this circumstance, special cross-matching may be required and occasionally an *in vivo* trial transfusion may be required before administering blood. These infrequent situations continue to be poorly understood by anesthesia and surgical teams, and the situation in the operating room may become difficult, even desperate, but a hemolytic transfusion reaction will be certain to compound all other difficulties. Communication among blood bank, anesthesia care team, and surgeons on how to proceed when compatible blood is difficult to obtain needs to be individualized and based on clinical circumstances.[92]

"O negative" blood and group- and type-specific transfusion

If immediate resuscitation dictates emergent restoration of oxygen-carrying capacity, then a reasonable alternative to the group, type, and cross-match is to provide red cells without A or B antigen (type O) and without the Rh "D" antigen (Rh-).[21] If more than two units of O-negative cells are given in an emergency setting, then O-negative cells will be needed throughout the resuscitation and immediate care of recipients.[92] A sample of blood should be drawn before the transfusion of O-negative cells, but repeated cross-matches may be required to follow changes in recipient group and type when O-negative blood has been used in this manner.[21] The small amount of plasma that contains A and B antibodies in multiple units of O-negative red cells may lead to high enough titers of anti-A and anti-B antibodies to result in hemolysis of the recipient's cells. Although use of O-negative cells can be life-saving, the procedure does have implications for later patient management. The presence of elevated titers of antibodies to A and B antigens from the (residual) sera of O-negative donor cell units may prevent use of appropriate grouped blood for a prolonged period after transfusion of O-negative cells. For this reason, group- and type-specific blood is much preferable in an emergency. This level of testing takes 5 to 10 minutes and will be less likely to create later problems in the patient's management. Less than 1 in 1000 patients who need blood in an emergency have antibodies outside the ABO blood group, and for this reason O negative and group- and type-specific blood are unlikely to have major consequences for the patient either during resuscitation or in the postresuscitation period. Also, since the demand for O-negative cells is likely to be greater than the supply, use of this modality should be restricted to the most dire of emergency indications.

Practical blood transfusion

A variety of formulae guide clinicians on how much blood is required to correct a hematologic abnormalities. The following information is based on the kinetics of blood, analogous to drug pharmacokinetics.

Red cell transfusion. Red cells are distributed only in the vascular space which, based on an average blood volume of 70 ml/kg, suggests that seven milliliters of transfusion per kilogram will increase hematocrit 10%. Red cell preparations have hematocrits between 60% and 70% (i.e., each ml of packed red cell preparation contains 0.7 milliliters of red cells). If 1 ml of red cell preparation are administered for each kilogram of body weight (assuming a blood volume of 70 ml per kilogram) the anticipated increase in hematocrit would be 1%.

For each unit of red cells, based on a donation hematocrit of 40% and a 450-ml volume of blood per unit, the yield of red cells is approximately 200 ml per unit. Preservatives used with the red cells add volume, producing a final red cell unit with a volume of 250 to 300 ml per unit and an hematocrit of 60% to 70%. Based on an average adult blood volume of 5000 ml each unit of red cells will increase the patient's hematocrit by 3% or 4%. This is consistent with rule of thumb that 1 ml of packed red cell per kilogram equals 1% increment in hematocrit.

Platelet. Dosage requirements for platelets are also based on principles used in drug kinetics and are similar to those discussed for red cell replacement. **The half-life of transfused platelets is approximately 24 hours.** A single transfusion timed in the period prior to operation should be adequate to prevent perioperative bleeding complications. Principles involved when determining platelet requirements are based on:

- Dose of platelets provided in a single unit;
- Distribution volume of platelets;
- Half-life of platelets.

Rough guidelines for platelet therapy indicate that a single unit of platelets will lead to a platelet count increment of 10,000/ mm^3. A single platelet unit derived from an adult whole blood donor unit contains approximately 5 to 7 $\times$ 10^{10} platelets [(150,000 platelets/ul^{-1} $\times$ 450 ml (4.5 $\times$ 10^6 ul)/unit of blood].

Platelets distribute primarily in the intravascular space (70 ml/kg) but sequestration in the spleen adds to the volume of distribution. Under ideal circumstances, platelet transfusion should precede surgery by two hours, so that a one-hour post-transfusion platelet measurement can be used to assure an increase in platelet count has occurred. In a patient who has had multiple prior platelet transfusions, an early sign of development of platelet antibody is failure of platelet count to increase following transfusion. When this occurs, frequently a larger platelet dose is indicated or occasionally plasmapheresis may be required to decrease platelet antibody level.

Fresh frozen plasma. The principal method to treat coagulation factor deficiency is with fresh frozen plasma. Similar pharmacokinetic principles can be applied to the kinetics of coagulation factors. Based on a plasma volume of 50 ml per kilogram, a dose of 10 to 15 ml per kilogram of fresh frozen plasma will increase coagulation factor levels approximately 20% to 30%. Effective surgical hemostasis can usually be acheived with coagulation factor levels of 30% to 50% of normal. Some coagulation factors have a larger volume of distribution than plasma Factor VIII, for example, is estimated to have a Vd of 100 ml per kilogram. A single unit of fresh frozen plasma with 250 ml of plasma is expected to increase coagulation factor levels by 7% to 8% (250 ml/3000 ml).

Cryoprecipitate. Cryoprecipitate is the primary source of von Willebrand factor, but this component also contains Factor VIII, plus fibronectin as well as fibrinogen. In the perioperative setting, the usual reason cryoprecipitate is considered is in settings of fibrinolysis and acute disseminated intravascular coagulopathy (DIC) to treat low fibrinogen levels as the cause of increased bleeding. A unit of cryoprecipitate contains approximately 50% of the fibrinogen in a unit of plasma; approximately 200 mg.

Fibrinogen levels less than 100 mg/dl are considered a potential cause of increased surgical bleeding. Based on a distribution in the blood volume, a single unit of cryoprecipitate will increase Fibrinogen levels by 20 to 30 mg per 100 ml. Three or four units of cryoprecipitate will increase fibrinogen levels by approximately 100 mg per 100 ml.

Factor VIII concentrate and Factor IX concentrate. Plasma components with active coagulation factor activity include Factor VIII concentrate and Factor IX concentrate. Specific factor concentrations provide replacement for patients with isolated congenital or acquired coagulation factor deficiencies. The indication and effective dosages are outlined in chapter 20. The goal of providing a specific coagulation factor has been realized for the congenital hemophilias. Cryoprecipitate, a fibrinogen- and factor VIII-rich preparation, provides replacement for von Willebrand factor and rare patients with congenital fibrinogen or fibronectin deficits.

Coagulation factor replacement may be required in patients with acquired coagulation factor deficits, such as liver disease, DIC, dilutional coagulopathy, or a coagulopathy after cardiopulmonary bypass. Multiple coagulation factor deficits may exist simultaneously, and the use of fresh frozen plasma is the most appropriate replacement. The coagulation factor replacement in one unit of fresh frozen plasma should increase coagulation factor levels by approximately 7% to 10% in a 70-kg man. If a reasonable goal of coagulation factor replacement is to achieve levels of 30%, a large volume of fresh frozen plasma may be required when coagulation factors are indicated.

Hemolysis during transfusion

With all steps properly taken to ensure blood compatibility, a hemolytic transfusion reaction should be a rare event. When hemolysis is detected, appropriate diagnosis and management should be promptly instituted. The most serious cause, namely hemolytic transfusion reaction, has severe consequences.[29,65,81,87,105,108,120] The most frequent sign of hemolysis during surgery is the presence of red urine that occurs unexpectedly during a major operation.[29]

Multiple other factors may lead to hemolysis during transfusion, including high pressure,[51] temperature,[10,90] outdated or previously frozen blood.[15,57] The presence of red or pink urine should immediately lead to the following questions:

- *Does the red urine indicate hemoglobin is present?* Specifically, is it an ultrafiltrate of plasma hemoglobin from intravascular lysis or is it a result of red cells added to urine from the renal collecting system or bladder secondary to trauma or surgery itself?
- *If intravascular lysis is likely, does a recheck of the donor units indicate appropriate labels?* This is critical to be done at the earliest moment, because there may be another patient at risk if labels have somehow been switched.
- *Are any other signs of hemolytic transfusion present?*

Hypotension and bronchospasm may develop secondary to complement activation and release of vasoactive substances.[53,54,63] Coagulation abnormalities can develop if the lysed cells act as a thromboplastin substance leading to consumption of coagulation factors and disseminated coagulation.[54]

Hemolytic transfusion reaction

The most catastrophic, and in many cases preventable, complication of blood transfusion is a hemolytic transfusion reaction.[29,32,65,87] The group and type of the donor when combined with screening of donor blood for the most common antibodies and cross-matching provides a donor population of red cells unlikely to create major reactions if given to an appropriate recipient.[92] Occasionally, antibody titers may be too low to be detected or an uncommon antibody may exist in recipient or donor blood, but these situations, although frequently the cause of a delayed hemolytic reaction, are an uncommon cause of an acute massive hemolytic transfusion reaction.[29,62,77,93] By far, the most common cause of acute hemolytic reaction is human error. A number of steps have been identified during the cross-match when human errors can occur:

- Labeling blood drawn from the recipient
- Laboratory testing of group and type
- Laboratory screening and cross-matching of recipient and donor
- Labeling the donor units tested for the recipient
- Matching the donor unit label with the intended recipient before transfusion.

All these steps can potentially result in the wrong blood being given to a recipient and a hemolytic transfusion reaction.[29,65,87] Three specific conditions should exist before an acute hemolytic transfusion reaction develops:[32,53,54]

- Donor cells should have antigen uncommon to recipient
- The recipient should have antibody present to the antigen
- The resulting antigen-antibody reaction should bind complement, leading to hemolysis of the donor cells.

The antibodies that develop to red cell antigen vary in their abilities to bind complement and produce the rapid lysis of transfused red cells leading to an acute hemolytic transfusion reaction (Table 93-7). The IgM antibody class is most likely to lead to intravascular hemolysis. The ABO antibodies are of this class and lead to acute, severe hemolytic reactions. Most other antibodies to the red cell antigens are IgG. Although some of these do bind complement and lead to the cascade of events that produce acute hemolysis, usually hemolytic reactions are less severe and are often delayed.[62,77,82,93]

Acute hemolytic transfusion reaction primarily occurs when a human error leads to administration of ABO-incompatible blood. The recipient antibodies to the foreign ABO antigens of the donor cells rapidly bind complement and lead to donor red cell lysis.[29,32,87] The appearance of free hemoglobin in the urine is frequently the first sign of this event during anesthesia and surgery.[58,71,78,81] Hypotension and a bleeding diathesis are frequently associated with the hemolytic event (Box 93-2).[32,54,58,115] The exact etiology of the hypotension and bleeding diathesis may relate to the effects of the red cell membrane, leading to the release of vasodilating substances and a thromboplastinlike action of the membrane rapidly followed by intravascular clotting and DIC.[17,32,53,54,71,78,81,115] The volume of red cells transfused during the event is a major factor in determining the severity of the hemolytic episode.[120] Via multiple mechanisms, the hemolytic event may cause renal impairment, either acute tubular necrosis caused by a generalized renal vasoconstriction from the release of vasoactive mediators or, less commonly, renal cortical necrosis resulting from DIC.[53,54,115] Considerable attention has been directed to therapy that "flushes" hemoglobin through the body; these steps have therapeutic impact primarily by increasing renal blood flow and maintaining urine output rather than preventing hemoglobin deposition in the renal tubule, despite the likelihood that the latter may not be the primary mechanism of

Table 93-7 Erythrocyte antibodies and hemolytic transfusion

Antibody class	Red cell antigen	Complement fixation	Hemolysis	Reaction
IgM	ABO	Yes	Intravascular	Acute, severe
IgG	Kidd, Duffy, Kell	Yes	Intravascular and extravascular	Variable severity
IgG	Rh, Duffy, Kell	No	Extravascular	Delayed

BOX 93-2
STEPS TO TAKE IN TRANSFUSION WHEN THERE IS INTRAVASCULAR HEMOLYSIS

1. Stop the transfusion
2. Confirm intravascular hemolysis — centrifuge urine and blood specimens to determine the presence of hemoglobin
3. Maintain tissue oxygenation:
   a. Provide volume replacement and inotropic support if needed
   b. Maintain urine output using Lasix, mannitol, or dopamine
4. Identify etiology — send recipient blood specimen to blood bank for recross-match
5. Return all used and unused donor units to the blood bank
6. Investigate and treat bleeding complications with platelet and coagulation factor replacement

Table 93-8 Causes of hemolytic transfusion reaction

Cause	Frequency (%)
Collection of recipient sample (patient care unit)	25
Sample drawn from wrong patient	
Misidentification of blood specimen	
Error in blood release form	
Blood center	20
Samples misidentified in blood bank	
Wrong donor unit released from blood bank	
Error in serologic testing	
Blood administration (patient care unit)	50
Blood given to wrong patient	
Serologic testing failed to identify antibody	< 5

renal damage.[17,97] For this reason, dopamine and Lasix may be more effective than osmotic diuretic therapy. Bicarbonate therapy to increase urine pH and prevent hematin deposition does not appear to have clinical merit.[53,54] The primary emphasis of treatment is immediate cessation of the primary cause of the problem (transfused blood) followed by support of the circulation, maintenance of renal perfusion as indicated by urine output, and treatment of any resultant disseminated coagulopathy, which may require use of multiple blood components to arrest surgical bleeding.[54,58,63,120]

Acute hemolytic transfusion reactions are most frequently iatrogenic errors. Prevention cannot be overemphasized, because only a tiny fraction of immediate hemolytic transfusion reaction cases can be traced to a failure of current compatibility testing techniques to detect incompatibility between donor or recipient (Table 93-8).[29,65,87,105]

Delayed hemolytic transfusion reaction

A type and screen test may not identify antibodies present in low titers in patients who have become sensitized to red cell antigens. Infusion of red cells may lead to a rapid increase in antibodies when a recipient is reexposed to the foreign antigen. When levels of antibody increase, a hemolytic reaction results.[68,82,92,93] Usually, the hemolysis occurs at extravascular sites and does not bind complement. Delayed instead of immediate hemolysis occur, usually a few days or even 1 to 2 weeks following transfusion, depending on the rapidity of the antibody titer increase (Box 93-3).[108,126] The donor red cells are sequestered and lysed in the spleen or liver rather than in the circulation. Antibodies to red cell antigens of the Rh (anti-D), Kell (anti-k), Duffy (anti-Fy^a, anti-Fy^b), Kidd (anti-Jk^a, anti-Jk^b), or Lewis (anti-Le^a, anti-Le^b) have been reported to cause delayed hemolytic reactions.[63,92]

BOX 93-3
CAUSES OF DELAYED TRANSFUSION REACTION

A low antibody concentration is undetected by the screen or cross-match of recipient blood
Increase in antibody level in recipient occurs after exposure
Extravascular or occasionally intravascular hemolytic reaction occurs 2 to 12 days after transfusion

Symptoms and signs of a delayed transfusion reaction can be particularly difficult to interpret in the postoperative period. Often the patient may be anemic, have a low-grade fever, and experience a precipitous decrease in hemoglobin level. These may easily be mistaken for other perioperative complications if delayed hemolytic transfusion is not considered in the differential diagnosis. Sensitization of the recipient from exposure to foreign antigens occurs in approximately 1% of transfusions and can greatly complicate later transfusion therapy.[120]

Additional immunologic transfusion reactions

The immunologic events surrounding hemolytic transfusion reactions can also be applied in understanding other immunologic problems with other formed elements of blood.[63,120] The erythrocyte constitutes 99% of the formed elements in blood, and major reactions are prevented by cross-match techniques. Fortunately, incompatibility reactions are usually less severe and self-limited with other formed elements in blood, but in a critically ill patient, these events can have profound cardiorespiratory consequences. When leukocytes are transfused to a sensitized patient (antibody-to-leukocyte antigens) the antigen-antibody reaction may lead to a variety of events, including fever, hypotension, flushing, and chills from release of vasoactive substances into the circulation.[43,63,120] In the awake patient, these self-limited reactions are unpleasant and are partially relieved by antihistamines. Severe reactions to leukocytes can lead not only to hypotension and bronchospasm but also to a noncardiogenic form of pulmonary edema.[43] Treatment is supportive, and prevention of these leukocyte reactions can be managed by removing most of the leukocytes with depth filters or by using washed red cells that are virtually leukocyte-free.[80] Repeated transfusions of blood frequently are followed by more severe leukocyte reactions, as 10% of recipients develop antileukocyte antibodies.

Problems with antibody formation to foreign antigens are particularly troublesome for patients who require repeated transfusions of platelets or, in the case of hemophilia, factor VIII replacement. Repeated transfusions of platelets or factor VIII preparations may lead to antibody formation against HLA antigens of the platelets or, in the case of hemophilia, antibody to the absent factor VIII. Platelet transfusion will be followed by rapid destruction of exogenous platelets. Frequently, the only effective therapy is transfusing platelets that are antigen matched with the recipient. In the hemophiliac patient with antibodies to factor VIII, the situation is far more difficult to manage, as almost all forms of factor VIII are recognized as foreign. This problem frequently requires steps to attempt to decrease the titer of the antibody to factor VIII such as plasmapheresis or the use of porcine or bovine factor VIII preparations.

Post-transfusion purpura, which is a delayed antibody response to platelets, may occur following transfusion.[48,63] The platelet-specific antibody stimulated by transfusion leads to transient thrombocytopenia, petechiae, and purpura in the recipient.

Anaphylactic reactions

Anaphylactic reactions associated with blood are most frequently related to IgA,[30] but in many patients with documented anaphylaxis to blood, the recipient lacked IgA antibody.[119,120] Approximately 1 in 600 patients lacks IgA antibody. Urticarial reactions may be caused by similar reactions, perhaps stimulated by donor plasma.[120] Release of biologic mediators such as leukotrienes, histamine, and complement, appears to occur more frequently when plasma preparations are administered and may represent immunologic differences between recipient and donor.[120]

Graft versus host disease: irradiated blood products

At the opposite immunologic extreme from recipient destruction of foreign cells, is the problem of failed recipient immunologic surveillance and engraftment of donor lymphocytes leading to graft versus host disease.[34,124] Graft versus host disease has been observed in bone marrow transplant recipients, immunodeficiency syndromes, Hodgkin's disease, and neonates.[28,34,124]

Graft versus host disease is also possible when directed blood donation from an HLA–matched relative engrafts in the recipient. Donor lymphocytes engraft in the recipient and lead to a syndrome of chronic rejection manifest in the skin, lung, and kidney. The lymphocyte can be prevented from mitotic activity by irradiation in a dose of 1500 to 5000 rads,[120,124] a simple process that adds 5 minutes to the preparation time for blood components and appears to have minimal effect on other formed elements of blood.[120]

Decreased immune surveillance-immunomodulation

Considerable attention has been directed to: (1) a possible increased recurrence of malignancy in patients who required perioperative blood transfusion;[18,20,107] and (2) greater frequency of postoperative infection following blood transfusion.[66,120] These observations suggest that blood transfusion may lead to reduced immune surveillance. The actual incidence of these problems and the cause require additional study. For the present, these observations need to be confirmed by a carefully controlled study, because conflicting results have been reported.[18,20,125]

Preoperative autologous donation

Prevention of donor-transmitted infectious disease and immunologic problems related to transfusion has led to a marked increase in autologous blood donation.[109,111,114,118] Collection of autologous units should begin at least 2 to 3 weeks before a planned operative procedure.[113] Collection in anticipation of surgery can be accomplished months ahead of time, if frozen storage of cells is available. The 72-hour period before surgery is the limit of preoperative collection to assure restoration of vascular volume before operation.[118] Successful programs have been reported in a variety of age groups of patients who participated in autologous donation before elective surgery.[12,111,116,129] The risks of donation are similar to those for age-related volunteer blood donors.[118] With the declining risk of infection from contaminated blood, several studies have reported the high cost of using autologous blood. These studies of cost effectiveness will undoubtedly influence clinical practice, although not all of the risks of transfusion are considered (or known) when assigning measures of effectiveness versus cost.[11,16,50,73]

Limitations of successful autologous donation primarily relate to early entry of patients who may require allogeneic transfusion and availability of predonation programs at local blood banks.[118] The trend toward increasing use of preoperative donation has been reported.[114,118] Once a patient is entered into a predonation program, successful collection of multiple units depends on an adequate reticulocyte response to prevent anemia and to allow maximal red cell yield of autologous units. Maximal erythropoiesis may not be stimulated by removal of autologous units; therefore, administration of iron is recommended to collect multiple donor units in patients over a 4- to 6-week period before operation.[56] The role of exogenous erythropoietin administration in allowing maximal blood collection before operation appears promising.[56]

The risk of infection is prevented by autologous donation, but the incidence of clerical errors, which account for

80% of hemolytic transfusion reactions, may not be decreased by use of autologous blood and in fact might even be increased because of the larger inventories of blood created by autologous donation.

TRANSFUSION PROBLEMS RELATED TO STORAGE, PRESERVATIVES, AND INFUSION

Preservatives and storage techniques for blood components maintain the longest *in vitro* storage period and the best *in vivo* survival of the blood product.[83,128] The donor collection system contains 64 ml of a solution containing citrate, phosphate, dextrose, and adenine in a sterile system (CPD-A). The citrate maintains anticoagulation, by chelating calcium to prevent coagulation activation.[83,104,128] A satellite bag system for plasma and platelet separation or one that includes an adenine, saline, mannitol, and dextrose solution (Adsol) to resuspend packed cells to further extend the storage period is used by blood donor centers to separate components from red cells.

Storage of blood in these preservative solutions leads to a variety of biochemical and metabolic changes in the plasma and blood.[83,128] The metabolic and biochemical changes occur because of anerobic metabolism of the red cell during storage, which leads to gradual loss of potassium from the red cell, as well as a combined metabolic and respiratory acidosis.[83]

Physical changes also occur because of the micro- and macroagglutination of red cells leading to the formation of microaggregates in stored blood.[99] Duration of storage also decreases the level of 2,3 DPG in the plasma, and shifts the hemoglobin O_2 dissociation curve of the erythrocyte to the left.[24,64] Although the physical, metabolic, and biochemical changes during whole blood and red cell storage are major, few, if any, of these changes impact the clinical care of patients, even those patients given large volumes of blood.[83]

Storage-related changes in blood components have been the focus of extensive investigation over the past 40 to 50 years. In many instances, theoretic concerns have not been confirmed by actual clinical practice.

Microaggregates and Blood Filtration

During red cell and whole blood storage, particulate matter results from lysis and crenation of red cells which in combination with fibrin filaments, other proteins, and platelets, form microaggregates. Even after relatively brief periods of storage, microaggregates develop varying in size from 10 to 170 μm.[99] Packed red cells with platelets and plasma removed contain fewer microaggregates than whole blood.[63,80,83,120] These microaggregates have been considered a cause of pulmonary dysfunction in the massively transfused patient.[14,49,84,95]

A cause-and-effect relationship between microaggregates and post-transfusion pulmonary dysfunction still remains inconclusive.[14,49,84,95] No disagreement or controversy exists regarding formation of microaggregates in blood or their presence in the pulmonary microcirculation of massively transfused patients,[99] but no conclusive answers have been provided about whether microaggregates—even in large quantities during massive transfusion—cause clinical respiratory abnormalities in the form of increased alveolar-arterial O_2 gradients, decreased lung compliance, or altered outcome following trauma.[14,49,84] At present, because packed red cells contain only one fifth the concentration of microaggregates when compared with whole blood preparations and 40 micron filter rather than 170 micron filter use, concern about microaggregates may be of academic interest only.[63,83,120] Neither microaggregate nor depth filters alter the function of plasma or coagulation proteins, but a screen filter should be used to administer platelet and leukocyte components. Use of microaggregate filters decreases the maximal infusion rate of blood products, which may be problematic in situations of massive blood loss.

An increasingly common role of filters is the removal of leukocytes for prevention of CMV transmission. CMV is a potentially lethal complication of transfusion in the transplant recepient who is CMV negative. These depth filters remove leukocytes from whole blood and red cells and decrease the possibility of CMV transmission, and may also be helpful in decreasing the incidence of febrile transfusion reaction. The filters remove 95% to 99% of leukocytes but considerably reduce the flow properties of red cell concentrates. In the situation of rapid massive blood loss, microfilters can prevent effective red cell replacement and jeopardize resuscitation efforts.

Acid-Base Changes During Storage of Red Cells

Hydrogen ion and CO_2 concentrations increase as duration of red cell storage increases as a result of anaerobic metabolism.[83] The pH of stored blood may decrease to 6.5 during 4 weeks of storage. Increased P_{CO_2} rapidly decreases when CO_2 is excreted via the lungs. Lactic acid accumulation is readily cleared when blood is reinfused. Citrate metabolism further counters the mild acidosis related to blood products, and metabolic alkalosis often is observed in the period following transfusion. In addition, red cells' buffering capacity for H^+ is rapidly restored upon reinfusion. For this reason, acidosis with red cell infusion is a less important concern than when large volumes of crystalloid solutions are infused (i.e., lactated Ringer's, pH = 5.5, normal saline, pH = 6.0).

The improved O_2 transport is another effect of blood transfusion that counters any detrimental effect whole blood or packed cells might have in contributing to acidosis. The presence of continuing metabolic acidosis during red cell or whole blood transfusion should lead to a careful evaluation of other more likely causes of acidosis, in particular, inadequate tissue perfusion. The cause is rarely related to exogenous blood infusion, and empiric or "formula" use of bicarbonate during blood transfusion is never indicated.

Red Cell Storage Changes in Oxygen-Dissociation Curve

Depletion of energy substrates can be documented during red cell storage.[24] Decreased 2,3 DPG levels leading to an increasing hemoglobin affinity for O_2 has been contended to be an important physiologic alteration potentially of clinical significance.[24,36,64,118] Levels of 2,3 DPG are not regenerated for 12 to 36 hours, and a left shift of the hemoglobin dissociation curve can be demonstrated. Patients who have marginal cardiovascular reserve appear to experience few, if any, clinical changes when the hemoglobin dissociation curve is shifted to the left. Increased tissue extraction of O_2 as a compensatory mechanism to meet a reduction in O_2 supply has a more limited role in meeting O_2 decreases than increased tissue blood flow. An increased capillary tissue blood flow is the primary compensatory mechanism for decreased O_2 supply. The left- and right-shifted hemoglobin dissociation curves are important in understanding uptake of O_2 by hemoglobin, but as a compensatory mechanism for improving tissue extraction of O_2, these changes are of limited clinical importance in the range of hematocrits frequently observed in perioperative patients (21% or greater).

Citrate Intoxication

The anticoagulant preservative solution citrate chelates Ca^{++}, which can lead to cardiovascular changes manifested as hypotension from decreased contractility and prolonged repolarization times.[83,120] **If transfusion is sufficiently rapid, and the volume of citrate infused is large, hypocalcemia can lead to electrocardiogram (ECG) changes and a disturbance in myocardial contractility leading to hypotension.** The increased use of packed red cell concentrates with smaller volumes of citrated plasma present have decreased the frequency of citrate intoxication. The infusion of greater concentrations of citrate with fresh frozen plasma and whole blood can lead to hypocalcemia more frequently, because the citrate can be administered very rapidly. Presence of liver disease, which delays metabolism of citrate, and frequent fresh frozen plasma use in patients during liver transplantation leads to more frequent episodes of hypocalcemia requiring treatment.

Hyperkalemia

Plasma K^+ content increases during storage as a result of impaired red cell metabolism and inadequate Na^+/K^+ ATPase function.[83,128] Reinfusion rapidly reverses this abnormality, corrects the acid-base abnormality, returns the metabolic integrity of red cells, and decreases serum K^+ levels.

Even without rapid correction of the metabolic function of the red cell, the amount of K^+ infused/unit of packed cells is small because little plasma is present (60 ml). If potassium concentrations in plasma are 80 mEq/l, less than 5 mEq K^+/unit of packed red cells would be present. For this reason, a major K^+ load would not be expected unless massive blood loss leads to rapid red cell administration. Potassium elevation from multiple units over an extremely brief time period occasionally can lead to symptomatic hyperkalemia. Therapy for hyperkalemia (e.g., calcium chloride, insulin and glucose, and bicarbonate) may be necessary, but because acidosis and hyperkalemia are infrequently directly attributable to blood transfusion, a search for other more common causes of these problems should be considered rather than attributing the cause to blood-product administration.

KEY POINTS

- Transfusion risk is the primary factor that has changed indications for blood components during the past decade.
- Infectious transfusion risks are rapidly changing as HIV disease prevalence changes and screening tests improve, for the present, infectious risk has markedly decreased with newer donor screening methods.
- Immunologic (alloimmunization) and immunomodulatory effects (e.g., cancer recurrence, increased infection) are increasingly recognized as risks of transfusion.
- The battery of serologic tests needed to assure the safety of blood components and increasing use of plasma components has all but eliminated whole blood and "fresh whole blood" from surgical practice.
- Studies that add measures of cost versus benefit in terms of disease prevention (i.e., cost-effectiveness) may change indications for autolgous blood and a variety of other procedures during the next decade.
- Familiarity with the ABO, Rh, and minor blood groups provides reasons why compatible donor red cells may differ from a recipient's blood group and type. In addition, recognizing the problems of type O-negative blood as a "universal donor."
- The root cause and therapy for acute hemolytic transfusion reaction will convince the anesthesia provider that therapy is mostly supportive and prevention by rigid adherence to proper procedures is critical in a busy operating room setting.
- Citrate toxicity, acid-base changes, and hyperkalemia are primarily problems of rapid transfusion of large quantities of blood. Treatment may be indicated in these situations but not as a "routine" therapy.

KEY REFERENCES

Aach RD, Stevens CE, Hollinger FB, et al: Hepatitis C virus infection in post-transfusion hepatitis. An analysis with first and second-generation assays, *N Engl J Med* 325: 1325–1329, 1991.

Busch MP, Alter HF: Will human immunodeficiency virus p24 antigen screening increase the safety of the blood supply and, if so, at what cost? *Transfusion* 35:536,1995.

Consensus Conference: Platelet transfusion therapy, *JAMA* 257:1777, 1987.

Consensus Conference: Perioperative red cell transfusion, *JAMA* 260:2700, 1988.

Consensus Conference: Fresh frozen plasma indications and risks, *JAMA* 253:551, 1985.

Capon SM, Sacher RA: Hemolytic transfusion reactions: a review of mechanisms, sequelae, and management, *J Int Care Med* 3:100, 1989.

Dodd RY: The risk of transfusion-transmitted infection, *N Engl J Med* 327:419–421, 1992.

Donahue JG, Munoz A, Ness PM, et al: The declining risk of posttransfusion hepatitis C virus infection, *N Engl J Med* 327:369–372, 1992.

Etchason J, Petz L, Keeler E: The cost effectiveness of preoperative autologous blood donations, *N Engl J Med* 332:719–724, 1992.

Heaton WAL: Changing Patterns of blood use, *Transfusion* 34:365–367, 1994.

Moroff G, Dende AM: Characterization of the biochemical changes during storage of red cells, *Transfusion* 23:484, 1983.

Stehling L, Luban NLC, Anderson KC, et al: Guidelines for blood utilization review, *Transfusion* 34:438–448, 1994.

Surgenor DM, et al: Changing patterns of blood transfusion in four sets of United States hospitals, 1980 to 1985, *Transfusion* 28:513, 1989.

REFERENCES

1. Aach RD, Kahn RA: Posttransfusion hepatitis. Current perspectives, *Ann Intern Med* 92:539, 1980.
2. Aach RD, Stevens CE, Hollinger FB, et al: Hepatitis C virus infection in post-transfusion hepatitis. An analysis with first and second-generation assays. *N Engl J Med* 325:1325–1329, 1991.
3. Aach RD, Szmuness W, Mosley JW, et al: Serum alanine aminotransferase of donors in relation to the risk of non-A, non-B hepatitis in recipients: the transfusion-transmitted viruses study, *Ann Intern Med* 92:539, 1980.
4. Adams RS, Lundy JS: Anesthesia in cases of poor surgical risk: some suggestions for decreasing the risk, *Surg Gynecol Obstet* 71:1011, 1941.
5. Ahtone J, Maynard JE: Laboratory diagnosis of hepatitis B, *JAMA* 249:2067, 1983.
6. Alter HJ, et al: Detection of antibody to hepatitis C virus in prospectively followed transfusion recipients with acute and chronic non-A, non-B hepatitis, *N Engl J Med* 321:1494, 1989.
7. Alter HJ, et al: Donor transaminase and recipient hepatitis. Impact on blood transfusion services, *JAMA* 246:630, 1981.
8. Alter HJ, Hadler SC, Judson FN: Risk factors for acute non-A, non-B hepatitis in the United States and association with hepatitis C virus infection, *JAMA* 264:2231, 1990.
9. American Red Cross Blood Services Reports, 1978–1979 Washington DC: American Red Cross, 1979.
10. Arens JF, Leonard GL: Danger of overwarming blood by microwave, *JAMA* 218: 1045, 1971.
11. Axelrod FB, Pepkowitz SH, Goldfinger D: Establishment of a schedule of optimal preoperative collection of autologous blood, *Transfusion* 29:677–680, 1989.
12. Bailey TE, Mahoney OE: The use of banked autologous blood in patients undergoing surgery for spinal deformity, *J Bone Joint Surg (Am)* 69A:329, 1987.
13. Barker LF, Dodd: Viral hepatitis, acquired immunodeficiency syndrome and other infectious transmitted by transfusion. In Petz LD, Swisher SN, editors: *Clinical practice of transfusion medicine,* ed 2, New York, 1989, Churchill-Livingstone.
14. Barrett J, Tahir AH, Litwin MS: Increased pulmonary arteriovenous shunting in humans following blood transfusion, *Arch Surg* 113:947, 1978.
15. Bechdolt S, Schroeder LK, Samia C, et al: *In vivo* hemolysis of deglycerolized red blood cells, *Arch Pathol Lab Med* 110:344, 1986.
16. Birkmeyer JD: Cost effectiveness of preoperative autologous blood donation for total hip and knee replacement, *Transfusion* 33:544–551, 1993.
17. Birndorf NI, Lopas H: Effects of red cell stroma-free hemoglobin solutions on renal function in monkeys, *J Appl Physiol* 29: 573, 1970.
18. Blair SD, Janvrin SB: Relation between cancer of the colon and blood transfusion (letter), *Br Med J* 290:1516, 1985.
19. Blumberg BS, Alter JH, Visnich S: A "new" antigen in leukemia sera, *JAMA* 191:541, 1965.
20. Blumberg N, et al: Further evidence supporting a cause and effect relationship between blood transfusion and earlier cancer recurrence, *Ann Surg* 207:410, 1988.
21. Blumberg N, Bove JR: Uncrossmatched blood for emergency transfusion, *JAMA* 240:2057, 1978.
22. Bove JR: International forum: which is the factual basis in theory and clinical practice of the use of fresh frozen plasma, *Vox Sang* 35:428, 1978.
23. Bove JR: Transfusion-transmitted diseases: current problems and challenges, *Prog Hematol* 14:123, 1986.
24. Bowen JC, Fleming WH: Increased oxyhemoglobin affinity after transfusion of stored blood, *Ann Surg* 180:760, 1974.
25. Boyd PR, Sheedy KC, Henry JB: Type and screen: use and effectiveness in elective surgery, *Am J Clin Pathol* 73:694, 1980.
26. Braude AI: Transfusion reactions from contaminated blood, *N Engl J Med* 258: 1289, 1958.
27. Braunstein AH, Oberman HA: Transfusion of plasma components, *Transfusion* 24: 281, 1984.
28. Brubaker DB: Human posttransfusion graft-versus-host disease, *Vox Sang* 45:401, 1983.
29. Brzica SM: Complications of transfusion, *Int Anesth Clin* 20:171, 1982
30. Burks AW, Sampson HA, Buckley RH: Anaphylactic reactions after gamma globulin administration in patients with hypogammaglobulinemia: detection of IgE antibodies to IgA, *N Engl J Med* 31:560, 1986.
31. Busch MP, Alter HF: Will human immunodeficiency virus p24 antigen screening increase the safety of the blood supply and, if so, at what cost? *Transfusion* 35:536, 1995.
32. Capon SM, Sacher RA: Hemolytic transfusion reactions: a review of mechanisms, sequelae, and management, *J Int Care Med* 3:100, 1989.
33. Centers for Disease Control: Possible transfusion-associated acquired immune

deficiency syndrome (AIDS)—California, *MMWR* 31:642, 1982.
34. Cohen D, Weinstein H, Mihm M, et al: Nonfatal graft-versus-host disease occurring after transfusion with leukocytes and platelets obtained from healthy donors, *Blood* 53:1053, 1979.
35. Cole WH, Zollinger RM: *Textbook of surgery,* New York, Appleton-Century-Crofts.
36. Collins JA, James PM, Bredenberg CE, et al: The relationship between transfusion and hyoxemia in combat casualties, *Ann Surg* 188:513, 1978.
37. Consensus Conference: Platelet transfusion therapy, *JAMA* 257:1777, 1987.
38. Consensus Conference: Perioperative red cell transfusion, *JAMA* 260:2700, 1988.
39. Consensus Conference: Fresh frozen plasma indications and risks, *JAMA* 253: 551, 1985.
40. Consensus Conference: The impact of routine HLTV-III antibody testing of blood and plasma donors on public health, *JAMA* 256:1178, 1986.
41. Curran JW, et al: Acquired immunodeficiency syndrome (AIDS) associated with transfusions, *N Engl J Med* 310:69, 1984.
42. Curran JW, et al: The epidemiology of AIDS: current status and future prospects, *Science* 229:1352, 1985.
43. deRie MA, van der Plas-van Dalen CM, Engelfriet CP, et al: The serology of febrile transfusion reactions, *Vox Sang* 49:126, 1985.
44. Despotis GJ, Grishaber JE, Goodnough LT: The effect of an intraoperative treatment algorithm on physicians transfusion practice in cardiac surgery, *Transfusion* 34:290–294, 1994.
45. Dodd RY: The risk of transfusion-transmitted infection, *N Engl J Med* 327:419–421, 1992.
46. Donahue JG, Munoz A, Ness PM, et al : The declining risk of posttransfusion hepatitis C virus infection, *N Engl J Med* 327: 369–372, 1992.
47. Drinker CK, Brittingham HH: The cause of the reactions following transfusion of citrated blood, *Arch Intern Med* 23:133, 1919.
48. Dunstan RA, Rosse WF: Posttransfusion purpura, *Transfusion* 25:219, 1985
49. Durtschi MB, Haisch CE, Reynolds L: Effect of micropore filtration on pulmonary function following massive transfusion, *Am J Surg* 138:8, 1979.
50. Etchason J, Petz L, Keeler E: The cost effectiveness of preoperative autologous blood donations, *N Engl J Med* 332:719–724, 1994..
51. Eurenius SM, Smith RM: Hemolysis in blood infused under pressure, *Anesthesiology* 39:650, 1973.
52. Evatt BL, Ramsey RB, Lawrence DH, et al: The acquired immunodeficiency syndrome in patients with hemophilia, *Ann Intern Med* 100:499, 1984.
53. Garratty G: The significance of complement in immunohematology, *CRC Crit Rev Clin Lab Sci* 20:25, 1984.
54. Goldfinger D: Acute hemolytic transfusion reactions. A fresh look at pathogenesis and considerations regarding therapy, *Transfusion* 17:85, 1977.
55. Gomperts ED: Procedures for the inactivation of viruses in clotting factor concentrates, *Am J Hematol* 23:295, 1986.
56. Goodnough LT, et al: Increased preoperative collection of autologous blood with recombinant human erythropoietin therapy, *N Engl J Med* 321:1163, 1989.
57. Gossinger H, Laggner A, Druml W, et al: Hemodynamic, pulmonary, and renal reactions to inadvertent transfusion of outdated blood, *Crit Care Med* 14:70, 1986.
58. Greenwalt T: Pathogenesis and management of hemolytic transfusion reactions, *Semin Hematol* 18:84, 1981.
59. Grobbelaar BG, Smart E: The incidence of isosensitization following blood transfusion, *Transfusion* 7:152, 1967.
60. Heaton WAL: Changing Patterns of blood use, *Transfusion* 34:365–367, 1994.
61. Herman JH, Kamel HT: Platelet transfusion: current techniques, remaining problems, and future prospects, *Am J Pediatr Hematol/Oncol* 9:272, 1987.
62. Hewitt PE, Macintyre EA, Devenish A, et al: A prospective study of the incidence of delayed haemolytic transfusion reactions following peri-operative blood transfusion, *Br J Haematol* 69:541, 1988.
63. Holland PV: The diagnosis and management of transfusion reactions and other adverse effects of transfusion. In Petz LD, Swisher SN, editors: *Clinical practice of transfusion medicine,* ed 2, New York, 1989, Churchill-Livingstone.
64. Holsinger JW, Salhany JM, Eliot RS: Physiologic observations on the affect of impaired blood oxygen release on the myocardium, *Adv Cardiol* 9:81, 1973.
65. Honig CL, Bove JR: Transfusion associated fatalities: review of Bureau of Biologics reports, *Transfusion* 20:653, 1980.
66. Kaplan J, Sarnaik S, Levy J: Transfusion-induced immunologic abnormalities not related to the AIDS virus, *N Engl J Med* 313:1227, 1985.
67. Kickler TS, Spival JL: Effect of repeated whole blood donations on serum immunoreactive erythropoietin levels in autologous donors, *JAMA* 260:65, 1988.
68. Kline JA, et al: Hepatitis B core antibody (anti-HBc) in blood donors in the United States: implications for surrogate testing programs, *Transfusion* 27:99, 1987.
69. Kowalyslym TJ, Prager D, Young J: A review of the present status of preoperative hemoglobin requirements, *Anesth Analg* 51:75, 1972.
70. Koziol DE, et al: Antibody to hepatitis B core antigen as a paradoxical marker for non-A, non-B hepatitis agents in donated blood, *Ann Intern Med* 104:488, 1986.
71. Krevans JR, Jackson DP, Conley CL, et al: The nature of the hemorrhagic disorder accompanying hemolytic transfusion reactions in man, *Blood* 12:834, 1957.
72. Krugman S, et al: Viral hepatitis, type B. Studies on natural history and prevention re-examined, *N Engl J Med* 300:101, 1979.
73. Kruskall MS, Yomtovian R, Dzik WH: On improving the cost-effectiveness of autologous blood transfusion practices, *Transfusion* 33:544–551, 1993.
74. Kuo G, Chuo QL, Alter JH, et al: An assay for circulating antibodies to a major etiologic virus of human non-A, non-B hepatitis, *Science* 244:362, 1989.
75. Landsteiner K: Zur Kenntnis der antifermentativen, lytischen und aggutinierenden Wirkungen des Blutserums und des Lymphe, *Zentralbl Bakteriol Mikrobiol Hyg* 27:357, 1900.
76. Le Pont F, Costagliola C, Rouzioux C, et al: How much would the safety of blood transfusion be improved by including p24 antigen in the battery of tests, *Transfusion* 35: 542, 1995.
77. Lostumbo MM, Holland PV, Schmidt PJ: Isoimmunization after multiple transfusions, *N Engl J Med* 275:141, 1966.
78. McKay DG, Hardaway RM, Wahle GH, et al: Alterations in blood coagulation mechanism after incompatible blood transfusion, *Am J Surg* 89:583, 1955.
79. Mead JH, Anthony CD, Sattler M: Haemotherapy in elective surgery, *Am J Clin Pathol* 74:223, 1980.
80. Meryman HT, Hornblower M: The preparation of red cells depleted of leukocytes. Review and evaluation, *Transfusion* 26: 101, 1986.
81. Moore JM: Uncontrollable post-operative haemorrhage after incompatible blood transfusion, *Br Med J* 2:1201, 1958.
82. Moore SB, Taswell HF, Pineda AA, et al: Delayed hemolytic transfusion reactions, *Am J Clin Pathol* 74:94, 1980.
83. Moroff G, Dende AM: Characterization of the biochemical changes during storage of red cells, *Transfusion* 23:484, 1983.
84. Moseley RV, Doty DB: Death associated with multiple pulmonary emboli soon after battle injury, *Ann Surg* 171:336, 1970.
85. Mosley JW, Aach RD, Hollinger FB, et al: Non-A, non-B hepatitis and antibody to hepatitis C virus, *JAMA* 263:77, 1990.
86. Mozes B, Epstein M, Ben-Bassat I, et al: Evaluation of the appropriateness of blood and blood product transfusion using preset criteria, *Transfusion* 29:473, 1989.
87. Myhre BA: Fatalities from blood transfusion, *JAMA* 244:1333, 1980.
88. Myrhe BA: Bacterial contamination is still a hazard of blood transfusion, *Arch Pathol Lab Med* 109:982, 1985.
89. Oberman HA: Inappropriate use of fresh frozen plasma, *JAMA* 255:556,1985
90. Opitz JC, Baldauf MC, Kessler DL, et al: Hemolysis of blood in intravenous tubing caused by heat, *J Pediatr* 112:111, 1988.
91. Peterman TA, Jaffe HW, Feorino PM, et al: Transfusion-associated acquired immunodeficiency syndrome in the United States, *JAMA* 254:2913, 1985.
92. Petz LD: Red cell compatibility tests: clinical significance and laboratory methods. In Petz LD, Swisher SN, editors: *Clinical practice of transfusion medicine,* ed 2, New York, 1989, Churchill-Livingstone.
93. Pineda AA, Taswell HF, Brzica SM: Delayed hemolytic transfusion reaction. An immunologic hazard of blood transfusion, *Transfusion* 18:1, 1978.
94. Pool JG, Herschgold EJ, Pappenhagen AR: High potency anti-hemophiliac factor concentrate prepared from hemoglobin precipitate, *Nature* 203:312, 1964.
95. Popovsky MA, Moore SB: Diagnostic and pathogenetic considerations in transfusion-related acute lung injury, *Transfusion* 25: 573, 1985.
96. Prince AM, Szmuness W, Millian SJ, et al:

A serologic study of cytomegalovirus infections associated with blood transfusion, *N Engl J Med* 284:1125, 1971.

97. Rabiner SF, Helbert JR, Lopas H, et al: Evaluation of stroma-free hemoglobin solution for use as a plasma expander, *J Exp Med* 126:1127, 1967.
98. Ravitch MM, Farmer TW, Davis B: Use of blood donors with positive serologic tests for syphilis—With a note on the disappearance of passively transferred reagin, *J Clin Invest* 28:18, 1949.
99. Reynolds LO, Simon TL: Size distribution measurements of microaggregates in stored blood, *Transfusion* 20:669, 1980.
100. Rosen NR, Bates LH, Herod G: Transfusion therapy: improved patient care and resource utilization, *Transfusion* 33:341–347, 1993.
101. Rutherford CJ, Kaplan HS: Autologous donation: can we bank on it. *N Engl J Med* 332:740–742, 1995.
102. Sandler SG, Aubachon JP: Qualifications and management of blood donors. In Petz LD, Swisher SN, editor: *Clinical practice of transfusion medicine,* ed 2, New York, 1989, Churchill-Livingstone.
103. Sarma DP: Use of blood in elective surgery, *JAMA* 243:1536, 1980.
104. Schmidt PJ: Red cells for transfusion, *N Engl J Med* 299:1411, 1978.
105. Schmidt PJ: Transfusion mortality, with special reference to surgical and intensive care facilities, *J Fla Med Assoc* 67:151, 1980.
106. Schorr JB, et al: Prevalence of HTLV III antibody in American blood donors, *N Engl J Med* 313:384, 1985.
107. Schriemer PA, Longnecker DE, Mintz PD: The possible immunosuppressive effects of perioperative blood transfusion in cancer patients, *Anaesthesiology* 68:422, 1988.
108. Seyfried H, Walewska I: Immune hemolytic transfusion reactions, *World J Surg* 11:25, 1987.
109. Sherman L: The implications of trends in transfusion, *Transfusion* 28:511, 1988.
110. Silberstein LE, Kruskall MS, Stehling LC, et al: Strategies for the review of transfusion practices, *JAMA* 262:1993–1997, 1989.
111. Silvergleid AJ: Safety and effectiveness of predeposit autologous transfusion in preteen and adolescent children, *JAMA* 257: 3403,1987.
112. Spielmann W, Seidl S: Prevalence of irregular red cell antibodies and their significance in blood transfusion and antenatal care, *Vox Sang* 26:551, 1974.
113. Stehling L, Ellison N, Gotta A: A survey of transfusion practices among anesthesiologists, *Vox Sang* 52:60, 1987.
114. Surgenor DM, et al: Changing patterns of blood transfusion in four sets of United States hospitals, 1980 to 1985, *Transfusion* 28:513, 1989.
115. Tanaki A, Kato H, Takeda S, et al: The role of disseminated intravascular coagulation in shock induced by transfusion of human blood in dogs, *Transfusion* 19:404, 1979.
116. Thomson JD, et al: Prior deposition of autologous blood in elective orthopedic surgery, *J Bone Joint Surg (Am)* 69:320, 1987.
117. Tolkoff-Tubin NE, Rubin RH, Keller EE, et al: Cytomegalovirus infection in dialysis patients and personnel, *Ann Intern Med* 89:625,1978.
118. Toy PTCY, et al: Predeposited autologous blood for elective surgery, *N Engl J Med* 316:517 1987.
119. Vyas GN, Holmdahl L, Perins HA, et al: Serological specificity of human anti-IgA and its significance in transfusion, *Blood* 34:573, 1969.
120. Walker RH: Award Lectures and Special Reports. Special report: transfusion risks, *Am J Clin Pathol* 88:374, 1987.
121. Wallace EL, Surgenor DM, Hao HS, An J, et al: Collection and transfusion of blood and blood components in the United States, 1989, *Transfusion* 33:139–144, 1993.
122. Ward JM, et al: Laboratory and epidemiologic evaluation of an enzyme immunoassay for antibodies to HTLV-III, *JAMA* 256:357, 1986.
123. Ward JM, et al: Transmission of human immunodeficiency virus (HIV) by blood transfusions screened as negative for HIV antibody, *N Engl J Med* 318:473, 1988.
124. Weiden P: Graft-vs-host disease following blood transfusions, *Arch Intern Med* 144: 1557, 1984.
125. Weiden PL, Bean MA, Schultz P: Perioperative blood transfusion does not increase the risk of colorectal cancer recurrence, *Cancer* 60:870, 1987.
126. Whitehead PJ: Blood transfusion, *Anaesthesiology* 2:236, 1989.
127. Wilhelm JA, Matter L, Schopfer K: The risk of transmitting cytomegalovirus to patients receiving blood transfusions, *J Infect Dis* 154:169, 1986.
128. Wolfe LC: The membrane and the lesions of storage in preserved red cells, *Transfusion* 25:185, 1985.
129. Woolson ST, Marsh JS, Tanner JB: Transfusion of previously deposited autologous blood for patients undergoing hip replacement surgery, *J Bone Joint Surg (Am)* 69:325, 1987.
130. Yeager AS, Grumet FC, Hafleigh EB, et al: Prevention of transfusion-acquired cytomegalovirus infections in newborn infants, *J Pediatr* 98:281, 1981.
131. Zuck T: Transfusion-transmitted AIDS reassessed (editorial), *N Engl J Med* 318:511, 1988.

CHAPTER 94

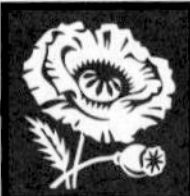

Hyperthermia and Hypothermia

STEVEN M. KARAN
EDWIN W. LOJESKI
SHEILA M. MULDOON

Hyperthermia and hypothermia are two complications of special significance to anesthesiologists. These complications have little in common except abnormal body temperature. **Hyperthermia during an anesthetic may be the result of sepsis, central nervous system (CNS) injury, transfusion or drug reaction, environmental conditions, equipment malfunction, disease states such as pheochromocytoma and thyrotoxicosis, or malignant hyperthermia (MH).** All of these conditions, with the exception of MH, are discussed in detail in other chapters. Therefore only MH will be discussed in this section.

New developments presented in this chapter include the discovery of a single-point mutation in the pig model, genetic heterogeneity in human MH, standardization of *in vitro* contracture testing, and further decline of MH mortality.

In contrast to MH, inadvertent hypothermia is an almost inevitable accompaniment of modern anesthesia and surgery. Air-conditioned operating rooms, application of cold solutions to the skin, exposure of body cavities, infusion of room-temperature fluids, and cutaneous vasodilation can all contribute to heat loss in anesthestized patients. Further, induction of general anesthesia causes vasodilatation and a redistribution of heat from the core to the periphery, lending to a decline of core temperature. Failure to maintain normothermia intraoperatively is usually of little physiologic consequence provided the core temperature is greater than 35° C. Nonetheless, any loss of body heat that occurs during surgery must be regained in the postoperative period by shivering and vasoconstriction. Shivering results in large increases in whole-body O_2 consumption that imposes severe demands on the cardiovascular reserve of critically ill patients. This chapter reviews what has been reported concerning the ability of humans to regulate temperature during anesthesia and the treatment of hypothermia in the perioperative period.

MALIGNANT HYPERTHERMIA

Historic Perspective

Since 1900, rare, fatal, hyperpyrexic episodes have been reported in the medical literature after the administration of potent inhalation anesthetics. Although the clinical descriptions of some of these "pyrexic episodes" suggest MH, in retrospect, it is impossible to determine whether these were MH episodes or whether they were related to either excessive heat in operating rooms or other complications of anesthesia and surgery. The MH syndrome and the genetic basis for that syndrome were not described until the early 1960s, when a case report was published describing the anesthetic complications sustained by a 21-year-old man.[22] The man had a compound fracture of his right leg and was extremely apprehensive about receiving general anesthesia. The anesthesiologist reassured him that there was no need to worry because he planned to use a new inhalation anesthetic—

halothane. Ten minutes after induction of anesthesia, tachycardia, hot sweaty skin, peripheral mottling, and cyanosis developed. The anesthetic was stopped, and the patient was packed in ice and survived. An internist was asked to investigate the family history and found that 10 of the patient's family members had died during anesthesia. The anesthetic agents administered were either diethyl ether or ethyl chloride. Hyperpyrexia was a common feature of the deaths that had occurred. Denborough and Lovell[21,22] concluded that this anesthetic-induced hyperpyrexia was the result of an unrecognized error in metabolism inherited as a Mendelian dominant characteristic. This report was followed by documentation of affected families in South Africa, North America, and other parts of the world.

Understanding of MH was greatly enhanced by the discovery of an animal model. Pig farmers have long known that the stresses of shipping, separation, and fighting could lead to death in their stock. These deaths resulted in pale, soft, exudative pork (PSE). Breeding patterns designed to produce greater muscle mass and rapid growth increased the incidence of PSE and led to the term porcine stress syndrome (PSS). Topel et al.[115] confirmed that PSS was a disorder of muscle and, in 1966, Hall et al.[42] reported abnormal reactions to halothane and succinylcholine in pigs from the same litter. The reaction was characterized by acidosis, extreme rigidity, hyperthermia, and death. In 1970, Berman et al.[7] described the clinical, metabolic, and biochemical course of MH in the susceptible pig and demonstrated that the metabolic changes occurred before the physiologic changes. Together these discoveries provided the important connection between PSS and human MH.

Early workers assumed that the hyperpyrexia in humans was either of central origin or related to uncoupling of oxidative phosphorylation. Lesions of hypothalamic nuclei, endocrinopathies of various types, or unknown pathologic events were also considered. These hypotheses were more difficult to support because, following administration of succinylcholine, many patients developed prolonged muscle fasciculations, rigidity, hypercapnia, metabolic acidosis, and hyperkalemia before any detectable rise in temperature. Myoglobinuria and elevation in creatine-phosphokinase (CK)—an enzyme normally confined to skeletal or cardiac muscle—provided further support that the syndrome was primarily a disorder of skeletal muscle. Satnick's[92] case report of a patient who developed MH with increased muscle tone everywhere except distal to a tourniquet provided more data that skeletal muscle was the target tissue. Although this report is often cited as providing definitive proof that MH is of peripheral origin, it does not rule out the possibility that MH might be induced by the release of some centrally mediated factor or factors. The enhanced contracture response of *in vitro* muscle strips from patients with MH to halothane and caffeine[25,55] focused investigations on skeletal muscle as the primary target tissue and provided a laboratory diagnostic test for MH. These *in vitro* halothane-caffeine studies led to the hypothesis that a derangement in calcium regulation was the cellular mechanism responsible for MH. This hypothesis was further supported when Lopez et al.[68] demonstrated that intracellular calcium concentrations were increased in muscle from MH-susceptible (MHS) swine and humans.[68] The possibility that uncoupling of oxidative phosphorylation might be the mechanism for development of hyperthermia was discarded when thermodynamic studies showed that even if all mitochondria were uncoupled, the increased production of heat could not account for the dramatic rise in temperature in patients with MH.[123] In addition, several investigators showed that mitochondria isolated from either MHS humans or swine were more highly coupled than normal and that the addition of halothane produced metabolic changes similar in direction and degree to those seen in normal mitochondria.[13]

A major advance in the management of MH occurred in 1979 with the approval of dantrolene for clinical use by the Food and Drug Administration. Dantrolene decreases intracellular calcium concentrations and, in combination with a greater awareness of MH and a reliable clinical test, has helped to reduce the rate of mortality associated with MH.

Another major advance was the discovery that a single-point mutation in the porcine ryanodine receptor gene segregated with the MH phenotype in over 450 MHS pigs, spanning 6 different breeds. Unfortunately, identifying the genetic defect(s) in human MH has proven more complex because of genetic heterogeneity.

Organization, education, and dissemination of information have expanded understanding of MH and improved the survival of patients. This effort has been enhanced through multiple international symposiums on MH and the formation of both the European and North American MH registries. The registries are designed to help physicians identify patients with MH, provide standardization of testing among the diagnostic centers, and build a data base of patients with MH. This information will also provide a data base for future molecular biology and genetic studies on MH.

Incidence

The prevalence of MH in the population is unknown; however, based on data collected from Children's Hospital in Toronto, an acute MH event has been estimated to occur once in every 14,000 potent inhalational anesthetics. In 1977, the Danish MH registry was established to collect MH episodes reported from Danish anesthesiologists.[80] The Danish registry reported one suspicious MH event for every 6167 administrations of potent inhalation anesthetics. Because not all patients received triggering anesthetic drugs, the actual incidence is likely to be greater than that reported.

Diagnosis of MH susceptibility is made with certainty only after a fulminant MH episode occurs. Fulminant episodes are now rare since new monitoring modalities permit early detection of nonspecific metabolic changes that may indicate early signs of an MH episode. Once early therapeutic intervention is made during a suspected MH episode, a definitive diagnosis of MH susceptibility cannot be made on clinical grounds.

Genetics

When Denborough and Lovell[22] first reported MH, there seemed to be little question of its pattern of autosomal dominant inheritance. The family in the report met four criteria for autosomal dominant inheritance: (1) the trait appeared in every generation, with no skipping; (2) the trait was transmitted by an affected person to an average of half the children; (3) unaffected persons did not transmit the trait to their children; and (4) the occurrence and transmission of the trait was not influenced by gender.

As more cases of MH were reported, however, this pattern of inheritance could no longer explain the genetics of all MH families. McPherson and Taylor's review of 93 kindreds demonstrated autosomal dominant inheritance in approximately 50% of the families, but in others, MH appeared to be an isolated event or of recessive or multifactorial inheritance.[74] The inheritance of MH will not be resolved without further advances in the molecular genetics of MH.

Clinical Syndrome

A broad spectrum of clinical presentations have been reported for MH. The time of onset is unpredictable and does not determine the rate of progression which varies from minutes to hours. The most common scenario that comes to mind for MH may be the fulminant episode that occurs at anesthetic induction, however this presentation accounts for only 50% of fulminant episodes. Episodes that first present in the postanesthesia care unit are rare, and on further work-up, often represent more common processes (sepsis, hypoventilation, hypoperfusion, etc.). Patients exhibiting masseter muscle rigidity (MMR) can progress to fulminant MH, but it is impossible to predict which ones will progress. Unexpected hyperkalemic pediatric cardiac arrest following succinylcholine, anesthetic-induced myoglobinuria, and neuroleptic malignant syndrome (NMS) have all been considered variant forms of MH but current evidence does not support a direct relationship with MH (Table 94-1). Stress-induced malignant hyperthermia is less well defined and documented in humans than the porcine model.

All potent inhalation anesthetics and succinylcholine are capable of triggering an MH reaction in susceptible humans (Box 94-1), but an MH episode does not always occur with each exposure. **Approximately 50% of all human MH episodes have been preceded by one or more uneventful anesthetics.** The patient's genetic predisposition or expression of their genetic defect may affect the course of the episode. Despite recent genetic advances, however, the extent of the genetic contribution in humans is still unknown. Other factors that may delay the onset or progression of an MH episode include the choice and dosage of volatile anesthetic,[126] a barbiturate induction, some nondepolarizing muscle relaxants,[38] and hypothermia.[79]

Myoglobinuria is a clinical sign that is common to MH, MMR, NMS, unexpected hyperkalemic pediatric cardiac arrest, and anesthetic-induced myoglobinuria. Elevations of serum myoglobin and CK can range from modest to severe and gross myoglobinuria may be present or absent. Both myoglobin and CK are used as markers of muscle destruction. Myoglobinemia is detectable prior to CK elevation (30 to 60 minutes versus 6 to 12 hours). Myoglobin's lower molecular weight (17,500 versus 70,000) allows it to leak out of muscle cell membranes that have altered permeability more easily than CK. The normal serum myoglobin range is 5 to 80 ng/ml and can be as high as 5000 ng/ml in patients with myopathies. The normal urine myoglobin range is less than 12 ng/ml. Chemical sticks designed to detect hematuria will react positively to myoglobinuria at levels between 300 to 500 ng/ml while cola colored urine does not usually appear until the urine myoglobin concentration is greater than 250 μg/ml. In normal patients, the administration of succinylcholine has been reported to increase serum myoglobin up to 5000 ng/ml (normal range 5 to 80 ng/ml) and serum CK up to 3000 IU.[17] The increases are dependent on the sequence and type of drugs used with succinylcholine (i.e., inhalation agent, defasciculating dose of non-depolarizing neuromuscular blocking agent) and on the type of surgical procedure. The degree of fasciculations does not correlate with enzyme elevations.

Fulminant episode

Increased skeletal muscle metabolism is the hallmark of MH. CO_2 production, O_2 consumption, and lactic acid release from skeletal muscle are all increased and result in a decrease in venous pH and an increase in venous CO_2 content (Box 94-2).[39] An unexplained rise in end-tidal CO_2 provides the earliest, most sensitive, and specific sign of an MH episode. The sympathetic nervous system responds to the increasing metabolic demand by releasing catecholamines which increase cardiac output. Minute ventilation also increases, but tachypnea will be masked if controlled ventilation and neuromuscular blockade are employed. Without end-tidal CO_2 monitoring, an unexpected increase in heart rate may be the most valuable early sign. Tachycardia may be more prominent than blood pressure elevations early in the course of the episode. Core temperature begins to rise when the body is no longer able to dissipate the heat generated from the increased skeletal muscle metabolism. Increases in temperature of 1° C every 15 minutes have been reported, however this rate will vary depending on conditions such as the ambient temperature, site and size of the surgical incision, the patient's baseline temperature, and heat preservation techniques employed for the patient.

Rigidity is the most unique sign of MH, but it is not the most consistent. In an early series, muscle rigidity was reported in 70% of the patients.[12] Rigidity is seen less frequently now, probably due to the ability to diagnosis and treat MH earlier in its course. The progression of body and limb muscle rigidity usually parallels the progression of the

Table 94-1 Malignant hyperthermia and associated diseases

	Malignant hyperthermia	Masseter muscle rigidity	Unexpected cardiac arrest in children	Anesthetic-induced myoglobinuria	Neuroleptic malignant syndrome
Underlying defect	Abnormal calcium regulation in skeletal muscle	Unknown vs. physiologic response to succinylcholine	Undiagnosed myopathy in children	Undiagnosed myopathy vs. normal variant	Central dopamine receptor blockade
Key event	Increased skeletal muscle metabolism	Increased jaw tension	Hyperkalemic cardiac arrest	Postoperative myoglobinuria	Fever following neuroleptic therapy
Common signs	Elevated $ETCO_2$ Acidosis Tachycardia Tachypnea Hyperkalemia Hyperthermia Muscle rigidity Myoglobinuria Increased CK	Myoglobinuria Increased CK Can progress to MH	Hyperkalemia Acidosis Myoglobinuria Increased CK	Myoglobinuria Increased CK	Hyperthermia Muscle rigidity Tachycardia Myoglobinuria Increased CK
Differences	Usually reponds promptly to dantrolene therapy	Usually does not progress to MH Dantrolene therapy may limit CK elevation	Presents as severe bradycardia or cardiac arrest Majority of patients are diagnosed with a subclinical myopathy postop Dantrolene may limit muscle damage	Apparently normal anesthetic course No evidence of myopathy on exam	Induced by neuroleptic drugs Not triggered by anesthetics No pattern of inheritance Altered consciousness Dantrolene has no effect on outcome but may decrease length of episode
Relationship with MH		May progress to MH	Unlikely	Unlikely	None

MH—malignant hyperthermia; CK—creatine kinase; $ETCO_2$—end-tidal CO_2.

clinical syndrome and can interfere with perfusion and with ventilation. Less frequently, severe total body rigidity occurs immediately after the administration of succinylcholine. This total body rigidity is distinct from MMR which is detected at intubation, usually limited to the jaw muscles, and does not develop into a fulminant MH episode in most cases (MMR is discussed in a later section). Alterations in skeletal muscle membrane permeability lead to elevations in serum potassium, sodium, calcium, phosphate, myoglobin, and CK.[45]

Ultimately, the clinical signs are a reflection of the body's inability to respond to an extraordinary increase in metabolic demand. When the metabolic demand can no longer be sustained, the syndrome accelerates and organ system failure occurs. Ventricular arrhythmias result from hypoxia, hyperkalemia, severe acidosis, or increased catecholamine release. Although patients can appear cyanotic, mottled, or have dark blood on the surgical field, arterial blood gas analysis rarely identifies gross hypoxia. Muscle damage can lead to myoglobinuria, acute renal failure, and disseminated intravascular coagulation. Peripheral vasoconstriction and decreasing cardiac function probably account for regional hypoperfusion, which compounds the metabolic disorder. Without prompt treatment, death is inevitable. Even after treatment, the patient is at risk for recrudescence of the syndrome for up to 24 hours.[72]

The ability to recognize the clinical syndrome is complicated by its rare occurrence, nonspecific signs, lack of a noninvasive screening test, and by the fact that susceptible patients may not trigger with every exposure to triggering agents. Laboratory signs useful in diagnosing MH include elevated Pa_{CO_2} or Pv_{CO_2}, acidosis, hyperkalemia, myoglobinuria, and elevated CK. In a retrospective review, Larach et al.[65] found that only patients with two or more adverse anesthetic signs or abnormal laboratory findings were MH susceptible via muscle contracture testing. Hypercapnia, acidosis, arrhythmia, tachycardia, myoglobinuria, or fever alone did not add significantly to the probability of diagnosing MH susceptibility. Prior to capnographic monitoring, routine anesthetic monitoring could not easily detect small or slowly progressive increases in metabolism. Malignant hyperthermia episodes would progress

BOX 94-1
TRIGGERING AND NONTRIGGERING ANESTHETIC AGENTS OF MALIGNANT HYPERTHERMIA

Triggering agents

All volatile anesthetic agents
Succinylcholine

Nontriggering agents

Nitrous oxide
Barbiturates
Etomidate
Propofol
Ketamine*
Local anesthetics (amide and esters)
Nondepolarizing muscle relaxants
Benzodiazepines
Narcotics
Catecholamines*
Calcium
Vasoactive drugs*

*Pharmacologic response may mimic MH (i.e., increased heart rate and blood pressure).

BOX 94-2
CLINICAL SIGNS OF MALIGNANT HYPERTHERMIA

- Increased metabolism
  - Increased CO_2 production
    - Increased minute ventilation
    - Elevated end-tidal CO_2 and $Paco_2$
  - Increased oxygen consumption
    - Decreased Pvo_2
    - Hypoxia, cyanosis, mottling
  - Acidosis (respiratory and metabolic)
- Tachypnea (only with spontaneous ventilation)
- Tachycardia (may lead to other dysrhythmias)
- Rigidity
- Fever/profuse sweating
- Muscle damage
  - Myoglobinuria/myoglobinemia
  - Creatine kinase elevation
  - Hyperkalemia, hypercalcemia, hyperphosphatemia

unchecked until the metabolic imbalance became pronounced enough to be detected by other signs, thus making treatment more difficult. With routine capnographic monitoring, however, clinicians can detect increasing CO_2 production by either a rising end-tidal CO_2 or an increasing minute ventilation requirement with a stable end-tidal CO_2.

BOX 94-3
DIFFERENTIAL DIAGNOSIS OF MALIGNANT HYPERTHERMIA

Sepsis
Iatrogenic hyperthermia
Hypoventilation
Light anesthesia
Hyperkalemic cardiac arrest
Myotonic reaction
Thyroid storm
Pheochromocytoma
Hypoxia
Hypoxic encephalitis
Intracranial trauma
Neuroleptic malignant syndrome
Cocaine toxicity
Drug reaction
Factitious

Increasing minute ventilation early in an episode provides only supportive treatment and can mask other confirmatory signs. In a slowly developing episode, small, intermittent increases in minute ventilation may be the only clinical indication of MH.[57] Therefore, end-tidal CO_2 and minute ventilation must be evaluated together to detect increased CO_2 production.

The differential diagnosis of MH is extensive and outlined in Box 94-3. Pheochromocytoma[4] and thyroid storm[111] can be difficult to differentiate from MH (Table 94-2). Although an elevated end-tidal CO_2 is most frequently associated with MH, it can be seen in all three conditions. Hypertension and tachycardia are the most prominent signs of pheochromocytoma, whereas atrial dysrhythmias and tachycardia are more prominent for thyroid storm. There is no rapid diagnostic test for any of these conditions. Nonetheless, MH usually responds dramatically to dantrolene therapy, whereas the response to dantrolene in pheochromocytoma and thyroid storm is limited.

Masseter muscle rigidity

Trismus, masseter muscle spasm, and MMR all describe rigidity of the jaw muscles that prevents the patient's mouth from being opened following the administration of succinylcholine. This rigidity is a transient phenomenon that usually lasts less than 10 minutes and occurs despite flaccid paralysis of the extremities. Mask ventilation is usually not impaired. Tachycardia, ventricular arrhythmias, and elevations in end-tidal CO_2 are common. Discontinuation of the triggering agents usually results in an uneventful recovery. The incidence of MMR progressing to a fulminant MH episode is unknown. Progression to a fulminant episode can begin immediately, but is more likely to develop 20 to 30 minutes after the resolution of MMR. Serum CK levels can be

Table 94-2 Comparison of the clinical signs of malignant hyperthermia, thyroid storm, and pheochromocytoma

	Malignant hyperthermia	Thyroid storm	Pheochromocytoma
Increased $ETCO_2$	+ + +	+ +	+ +
Tachycardia	+ + +	+ + +	+ + +
Hypertension	+	+ +	+ + +
Rigidity	+ +	+ / −	−
Acidosis	+ + +	−	+
Diagnostic test	Muscle biopsy	Free T4, TSH	Urinary VMA, Plasma catecholamines
CK	+ + +	−	+ / −
Myoglobinuria	+ +	−	−
Response to dantrolene	+ + +	+ / −	−

(Adapted from Weglinski MR, Wedel DJ: Differential diagnosis of hyperthermia during anesthesia and clinical import. In Levitt RC, editor: *Anesthesiology Clinics of North America,* Philadelphia, 1994, WB Saunders).
$ETCO_2$—end-tidal CO_2; CK—creatine kinase; TSH—thyroid stimulating hormone; VMA—vanillylmandelic acid.

markedly elevated, especially if a second dose of succinylcholine has been administered. The serum CK peaks at 8 to 12 hours after induction. Patients should be monitored postoperatively for the resolution of myoglobinuria to decrease the risk of renal complications. The differential diagnosis for MMR includes inadequate skeletal muscle relaxation, abnormal physiologic response to succinylcholine, temporomandibular joint dysfunction, and myotonic reactions.

When MMR was first described, the mortality of an MH episode was approximately 30% and no other signs were available to predict the occurrence of an MH episode. Since that time, capnographic monitoring and dantrolene therapy have become available for the early diagnosis and treatment of MH. Contracture test results have shown that only 50% of pediatric patients and 25% of adult patients with MMR test positive for MH.[2,24,87] In addition, succinylcholine has been shown to transiently increase the basal tension of masseter muscles.[117,119] Finally, the incidence of MMR in children receiving an inhalation induction followed by intravenous (IV) succinylcholine was found to be at least tenfold greater than the incidence of MH.[67] For these reasons, the role of MMR as a predictive sign of MH has been questioned. The lack of a standard, widely accepted definition of MMR has also added confusion. Recently, Kaplan[56] proposed a practical guideline for increased jaw tension following succinylcholine administration (Table 94-3). Patients are placed in one of three groups based on the ability to open the patient's mouth and perform laryngoscopy. A clinical response is also suggested for each group.

The incidence of MMR following an IV induction with barbiturates is greatly reduced when compared to an induction with volatile anesthetics. Thus, the routine use of IV succinylcholine following induction with a potent inhalation agent should be avoided.[20] Until the relationship between MH and MMR is better understood, we recommend that succinylcholine be used only when required for children.

Unexpected hyperkalemic pediatric cardiac arrest following succinylcholine

Patients with muscular dystrophy are known to be susceptible to hyperkalemic cardiac arrest following the use of succinylcholine (see Chapter 15). In early reports, many of these patients exhibited signs that resembled MH and an association between muscular dystrophy and MH was postulated. More recently, an association has been identified in apparently healthy infants and children between succinylcholine administration and hyperkalemic ventricular dysrhythmias leading to cardiac arrest.[88,93] These cases were identified by reports to the MH hotlines in the United States and Germany. Several of these patients have subsequently been found to have a previously undetected myopathy, such as Duchenne's muscular dystrophy, without obvious clinical signs. **Therefore, when a healthy appearing infant or child develops cardiac arrest soon after administration of succinylcholine, not believed to be caused by inadequate ventilation, oxygenation, or anesthetic overdose, immediate treatment for hyperkalemia should be instituted. Extraordinary and prolonged resuscitative efforts have been effective.**[66] In most cases, these events are more likely the result of the interaction between succinylcholine and a subclinical myopathy rather than MH. Nevertheless, dantrolene therapy may be useful by stabilizing muscle membranes and limiting muscle damage.

Anesthetic induced myoglobinuria

Anesthetic induced myoglobinuria has been used to describe reports of gross myoglobinuria with serum CK elevations up

Table 94-3 Clinical approach to increased jaw tension

	Clinical signs		Clinical response		
	Mouth opening	Intubation	Anesthetic	Surgery	Malignant hyperthermia workup
Normal jaw stiffness	Fully opens with firm pressure	No difficulty with laryngoscopy	Continue planned anesthetic	Continue surgery	No
Jaw tightness	Incompletely opens with firm pressure	Laryngoscopy difficult	Switch to nontriggering anesthetic	Continue surgery	Yes
Masseter muscle rigidity	Cannot be opened	Laryngoscopy impossible	Stop anesthetic	Stop surgery	Yes

to 150,000 IU after uneventful anesthetics in which succinylcholine was administered (no masseter muscle rigidity, dehydration, extremes of positions, signs of increased metabolism, etc.).[8,9,31] These patients usually present with gross myoglobinuria on the first postoperative void and have no other complaints. Rarely, myoglobinuria has been reported when only potent inhalation agents have been administered, but these patients were later found to have muscular dystrophy.[18,89] **The differential diagnosis for postoperative myoglobinuria includes genetic metabolic disorders, nonanesthetic drugs, toxins, infection, and neuroleptic malignant syndrome.** Bernhardt and Hörder[8] reported an incidence of anesthetic-induced myoglobinuria at approximately 1 in 250 in a series of 1704 consecutive patients (4 to 16 years of age) that received succinylcholine following an anesthetic induction with halothane. He suggested a possible relationship with MH in this subgroup of patients. In two other reports, *in vitro* contracture testing was performed and found to be positive in one case and negative in the other.[9,31] Given our current understanding of MH as a metabolic event that may result in muscle destruction, variable *in vitro* contracture results for patients with myopathies, and the recent discovery that subclinical myopathies can result in severe muscle destruction when succinylcholine is administered, it appears that anesthetic induced myoglobinuria is more closely related to a subclinical myopathy rather than MH. These patients should be monitored to prevent renal complications, be advised to avoid succinylcholine for future anesthetics, and receive a thorough neurologic examination to rule out undiagnosed myopathies and other sources of myoglobinuria.

Neuroleptic malignant syndrome

Neuroleptic malignant syndrome usually develops 24 to 72 hours after psychotropic drug therapy is started and is characterized by akinesia, muscle rigidity, hyperthermia, tachycardia, cyanosis, autonomic dysfunction, altered consciousness, diaphoresis, and raised serum CK concentration. The defect in NMS is believed to be related to dopamine receptor blockade. Nigrostriatal system blockade is responsible for inducing rigidity and heat generation. Haloperidol is the most commonly implicated neuroleptic drug but has the lowest mortality.

Although there appears to be many clinical similarities between MH and NMS (hyperthermia, rigidity, muscle destruction, first described in the 1960s, initial mortality approached 80% but sharply declined to 20% with greater awareness and supportive care), experimental evidence indicates that their pathogenesis does not overlap. NMS has a central origin, whereas MH originates in skeletal muscle. In addition, unlike MH, there is no genetic link with NMS. *In vitro* contracture test results have been variable in NMS patients, similar to contracture test results from patients with neuromuscular diseases.[16] There have been no reports of MH in patients with a history of NMS.[60] Given that MH susceptible patients are not immune to coexisting diseases, it is likely that NMS will eventually occur in a MHS individual. **Nonetheless, current clinical and experimental evidence does not justify avoiding anesthetics that trigger MH in patients with a history of NMS.**

Treatment of NMS consists of drug withdrawal and symptomatic measures, such as cooling, correction of dehydration, and management for cardiovascular, renal, and respiratory complications. Dantrolene and bromocriptine may shorten the duration of the NMS episode, but they have had no effect on outcome. Electroconvulsive therapy has been used successfully in patients that do not respond to conservative care and drug therapy.[16]

Stress-induced MH

In MH-susceptible swine an MH crisis can be triggered by environmental stresses that include exercise, heat, hypoxia, apprehension, and excitement. Whether these same factors can trigger an MH crisis in a susceptible human is uncertain. These stresses have occasionally been implicated in humans, but convincing and complete data is hard to obtain.[11,37,40,128] Patients identified as MH susceptible, either by clinical episode or by contracture testing, that have no prior history of an adverse reaction to stress are very unlikely to experience an adverse reaction to stress in the future. Limitation of activity is unnecessary in this group. If a susceptible patient has experienced a reaction to stress, that stress and similar stresses should be approached with caution, if not avoided.

Site of Defect in Skeletal Muscle

In skeletal muscle, the contraction process is initiated by an action potential that originates at the neuromuscular junction and spreads rapidly over the muscle surface and down the transverse tubular (T) system.[26] This electrical signal, on reaching the T system, triggers a rapid and massive release of Ca^{++} from the sarcoplasmic reticulum (SR). The signal transduction mechanism from the T system to SR is referred to as excitation-contraction (E-C) coupling and occurs at junctional locations where T system and SR membranes are in close proximity (Fig. 94-1). The nature of the signal or signals between the T system and the SR remain controversial.[63]

Recently, a calcium-release channel has been identified that bridges the space between the T system and the SR. This channel is called the ryanodine receptor because of its high binding affinity for ryanodine, a plant alkaloid. Three separate genes encode ryanodine receptors and each is pre-

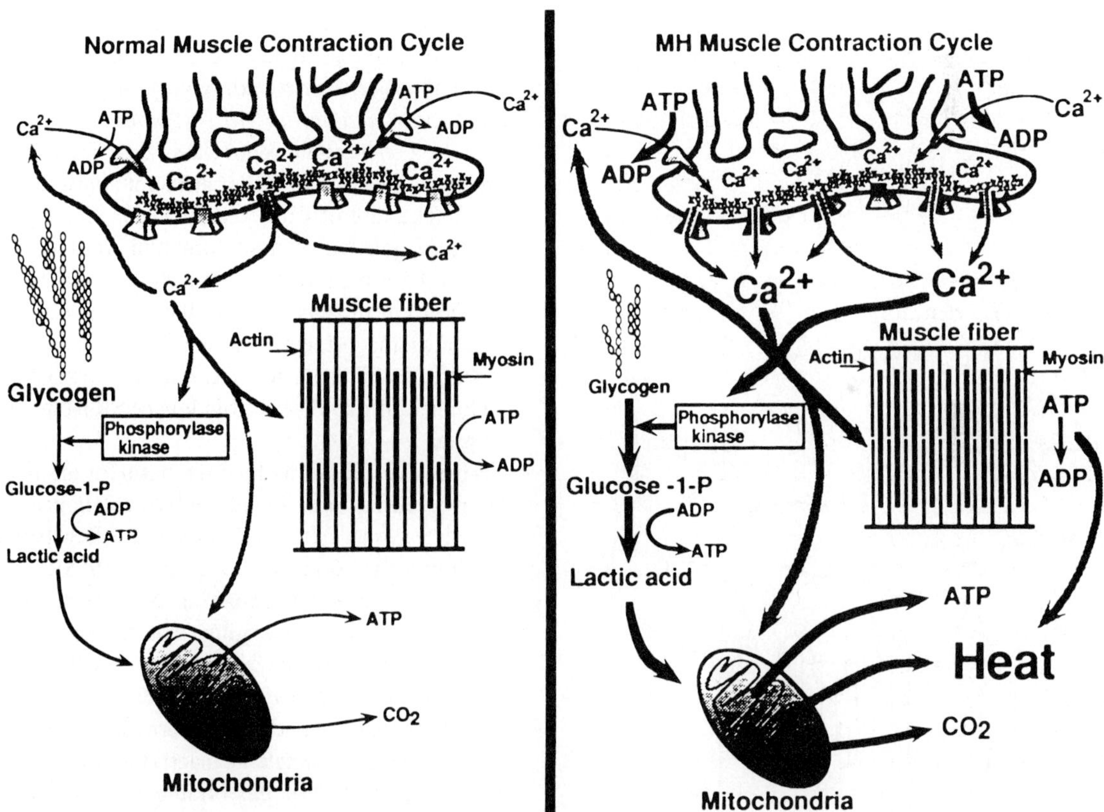

Fig. 94-1. A proposed mechanism for induction of malignant hyperthermia caused by abnormalities in the Ca^{2+}-release channel of skeletal muscle sarcoplasmic reticulum. Muscle contraction, glycolysis, and mitochondrial function are regulated by cytoplasmic Ca^{2+} concentrations. In a normal relaxation-contraction cycle (left), Ca^{2+} is pumped into the sarcoplasmic reticulum by Ca^{2+} ATPase to initiate relaxation, stored within the lumen in association with calsequestrin, and released through a Ca^{2+}-release channel to initiate contraction. Glycolytic and aerobic metabolism proceed only rapidly enough to maintain the energy balance of the cell. The Ca^{2+}-release channel can be regulated by Ca^{2+} itself, ATP, Mg^{2+}, and calmodulin and even when stimulated, has a relatively short open time. The abnormal malignant hyperthermia Ca^{2+}-release channel (right) is sensitive to lower concentrations of stimulators of opening, releases Ca^{2+} at enhanced rates, and does not close readily. The abnormal channel floods the cell with Ca^{2+} and overpowers the Ca^{2+} pump that ordinarily lowers cytoplasmic Ca^{2+}. Sustained muscle contraction accounts for rigidity, and sustained glycolytic and aerobic metabolism accounts for the generation of lactic acid, CO_2, heat, and enhanced O_2 uptake. Damage to cell membranes and imbalances of ion transport can lead to the life-threatening systemic problems that appear during a malignant hyperthermia episode. (From MacLennan DH, Phillips MS: Malignant hyperthermia, *Science* 256:789, 1992).

dominantly expressed in a specific tissue: (1) RYR1—skeletal muscle; (2) RYR2—cardiac muscle; and (3) RYR3—brain. The RYR1 receptor is a tetrameric protein complex constructed from four identical 565 kDa subunits. The $-$COOH end of the protein spans the SR membrane and forms a central transmembrane ion channel while the $-NH_3$ end forms a footlike structure in the cytoplasmic space between the SR and the dihydropyridine receptors of T system membrane (Fig. 94-2).[110] The footlike structure resembles a four-leaf clover with a depression or hole at the center of each leaf.[120]

Triadin and FK-506 binding protein are other structural proteins that have been identified near the foot region of the ryanodine receptor. Their function is still unclear, but may be important in modulating the Ca^{++} release channel.

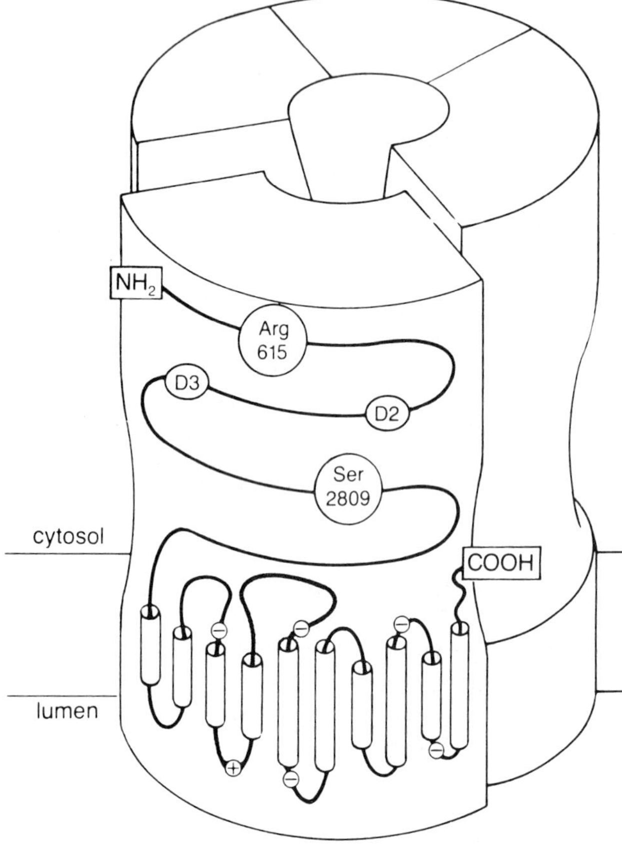

Fig. 94-2. Schematic model of the ryanodine receptor. The large N-terminal domain (approximately 4000 amino acids) extends into the cytoplasm. The transmembrane segments that anchor the molecule to the membrane of the Ca^{2+} stores are localized in the last fifth of the molecule; the C-terminal of the molecule is also located in the cytoplasm. Thus, only a relatively small part of this large molecule is intraluminal. The functional channel is believed to have a tetrameric structure. Arg614 site represents the human MH mutation that corresponds to the Arg615 site in swine. Ten transmembrane domains are represented here; this differs from other models that propose only four transmembrane domains (shown in a larger size). (Adapted from Sorrentino V, Volpe P: Ryanodine receptors: How many, where and why? *TiPS* 14:95, 1993).

There is general agreement that the immediate cause of the acute MH crisis is a sudden rise in the concentration of myoplasmic calcium, and that this increase is caused by the effect certain anesthetic agents have on the Ca^{++} release channel. In swine, a single-point mutation of the RYR1 gene, Arg615 to Cys, has been identified in all breeds that exhibit reactions to triggering agents.[30] How this defective translates to abnormal cellular function is not completely understood. Most work has focused on Ca^{++}-induced Ca^{++} release (CICR) as the mechanism to explain the increased rate of calcium release from the SR in MH, although it does not normally play a direct role in excitation-contraction coupling in skeletal muscle.

Prior to the discovery of the genetic RYR1 pig defect, Michelson and colleagues[75] reported that pigs, homozygous for halothane sensitivity, exhibited a distinct phenotype with regard to *in vivo* and *in vitro* response of muscle to halothane. In a subsequent report, they described the properties of SR fractions isolated from different strains of susceptible pigs.[108] The rate of Ca^{++} release from SR of homozygous MHS pigs was twice that of normal pig muscle, whereas SR Ca^{++} ATPase activity, a marker for myoplasmic Ca^{++} uptake, was not different among the various pig phenotypes. Further, in the presence of free Ca^{++}, the binding of ^{3}H-ryanodine to SR isolated from homozygous MHS pigs was of a higher affinity than the binding of SR isolated from normal pigs.

Fill et al.[27] further defined the basis for an increased rate of Ca^{++} release and altered Ca^{++} regulation using normal and MHS swine.[27] In agreement with Michelson's studies, they found that Ca^{++} efflux from MHS SR was two- to threefold larger than from normal SR over a wide range of myoplasmic Ca^{++}, indicating that CICR is much more prominent in MHS. They also found that the ryanodine receptor channel remained in an open state for a significantly longer time than channels from normals, indicating a failure of Ca^{++}-release channels to inactivate at physiologic Ca^{++} gradients. Nonetheless, this finding could also be explained by two distinct ryanodine receptor channels in the SR. The most likely conclusion from the work of Michelson and Fill is that the higher rate of Ca^{++} efflux observed in MHS SR is the result of failure of the MHS channels to be inactivated by physiologic Ca^{++} concentrations.

This conclusion is in agreement with the molecular genetic data of a single-point mutation in porcine RYR1. Support for the causal nature of the point mutation was provided by experiments in which suitably mutated rabbit cDNA was expressed in muscle cells. When treated with halothane or caffeine, these mutated cells showed a hypersensitive Ca^{++}-release response. It has been suggested that the Arg615 to Cys mutation may lead to the suppression of an inhibitory binding site of the CICR mechanism, an event consistent with the alteration of the equilibrium between open and closed states of the channel and with the idea that the $-NH_3$ terminal portion of the molecule is involved in the suppression of the Ca^{++}-induced Ca^{++}-release activity.

The results of studies with MHS human Ca^{++}-release channels have some similarities with the swine data but are not as consistent. This is not unexpected, given that there is strong evidence for multiple genetic loci for human MH and that MHS humans are rarely found to have the corresponding RYR1 swine mutation (human genetics will be addressed later in this section). Nelson[78] examined the effects of low concentrations of halothane on normal and MH human skeletal muscle Ca^{++}-release channels. The experimental approach was similar to that used in the MHS swine studies. Single Ca^{++}-release channels from SR membrane vesicles were incorporated into planar lipid bilayers. The release of Ca^{++} by this mechanism requires a critical threshold Ca^{++} load for CICR to occur. The effect of halothane on the conductance and gating properties was measured by electrophysiologic techniques. In 7 MHS patients, 7 of 13 channels responded to halothane by increasing the probability that the channel was changed from the inactive closed state to the active, open state. Halothane had no measurable effect on channels from normal subjects. Nelson concluded that halothane's effect was to lower the threshold Ca^{++} concentration for Ca^{++} channel opening, supporting a defect in the RYR sensitive Ca^{++}-release channel in human MH muscle. Three of the seven MHS individuals did not respond, however, suggesting the existence of another predisposing defect in these individuals.

Fill et al.[28] investigated normal and MHS human SR Ca^{++}-release channels by examining the properties of conductance, open state probability, channel gating, and the action of ryanodine. These characteristics were not significantly different between MHS and normal subjects. Further, the gating of MHS channels corresponded well to the averages of normal human muscle. Because abnormal myoplasmic Ca^{++} dependence was described in pig SR Ca^{++} channels, they also looked for this abnormality in the human muscle, but were unsuccessful. The apparent lack of a Ca^{++} regulation defect in MHS human channels was felt to reflect subtle genetic differences between MH in humans and swine. The caffeine sensitivity of human Ca^{++} channels was also explored because human diagnostic testing is in part based on abnormal contractile response to caffeine, and because caffeine is a potent modulator of the channel. Human skeletal muscle biopsies were divided into two portions, one for diagnostic contracture testing and the other to prepare microsomes for single-channel experiments. Channels prepared from subjects with normal contracture test results were not significantly affected by a 1-mM caffeine concentration. Nevertheless, channels prepared from subjects with positive or equivocal contracture results were significantly activated by a 1-mM caffeine concentration. These results suggest an abnormal sensitivity to caffeine and support the hypothesis that abnormalities exist in the Ca^{++}-release channel of MH subjects.

Molecular genetic studies in pigs and humans

On the basis of genetic studies in MH susceptible pigs linking halothane sensitivity to the glucose phosphate isomerase (GPI) locus on chromosome 6, a homologous MHS locus on human chromosome 19q12-13.2 was identified.[73] In the same year, the gene encoding the Ca^{++}-release channel (RYR1) was cloned, mapped to chromosome 19q13.1, and proposed as a candidate for the molecular defect in humans.[71] A base transition in the RYR1 gene, C1840T, resulting in a substitution of cysteine for arginine in position 614 of the human RYR protein has been suggested as the causative mutation for MH in the human. The evidence supporting a causal role for a MH mutation in RYR1 gene of the MHS swine is very strong. A single mutation was found in the Ca^{++}-release channel (RYR1) Arg615 to Cys ruling out the need to distinguish between the mutation and a polymorphism that might have occurred on the same chromosome. This mutation has now been identified in more than 600 pigs representing six breeding strains and all MHS pigs can be traced to a common ancestor. Experiments in which suitably mutated rabbit cDNA was expressed in muscle cells or in COS-7 cells showed an enhanced Ca^{++} release when the transfected cells were exposed to halothane and caffeine.[116] Nonetheless, in humans this mutation was found in 1 of 35 pedigrees with MH,[32] and in 1 of 62 kindreds.[46] In an investigation of German pedigrees, Deufel et al.[23] found the mutation in 10 of 120 independent MH pedigrees. Thus, the frequency of this mutation is estimated as ranging between 5% and 10%. This mutation has not been found in several hundred MHN subjects and has not been detected in any patient in whom chromosome 19 has been excluded as a locus. Seven other mutations have been identified in the RYR1 gene (Table 94-4) but four of these are considered to be rare independent mutations or occurring in Central Core Disease families.[70]

Of the three remaining mutations found in the RYR1 receptor, one included a Gly341-Arg substitution reported by Quane et al.[84] This mutation was found in 10 of 95 unrelated Caucasian MHS patients making it the most common mutation identified. Quane stated that this mutation is not likely to be a coincidental polymorphism as it was clearly linked to MHS phenotype in the pedigrees investigated and has not been detected in 500 normals tested. Keating et al.[59] undertook a further systematic screening of the RYR1 gene in 104 unrelated MHS individuals. She found a GLY2433-Arg mutation in 4 of 104 MH individuals which was not present in normal population. Finally, Gillard et al.[33] found an Gly248-Arg substitution in 1 of 45 MH susceptible families. Further screening and identification of this defect in susceptible

Table 94-4 Genetic mutations of the RYR1 gene and disease association in humans

Mutation	Association
Glycine 248 to arginine	MH
Glycine 341 to arginine	MH
Arginine 614 to cysteine	MH
Glycine 2433 to arginine	MH
Arginine 163 to cysteine	MH/CCD
Isoleucine 403 to methionine	MH/CCD
Tyrosine 522 to serine	MH/CCD
Arginine 2434 to histidine	MH/CCD

MH — malignant hyperthermia; CCD — central core disease.
(Adapted from MacLennan DH: Discordance between phenotype and genotype in malignant hyperthermia, *Curr Opin Neurol,* 8:397, 1995).

families is required to determine if this is a private mutation or a casual mutation for MH.

Genetic heterogeneity of human MH has been demonstrated by exclusion of linkage to the RYR1 gene on chromosome 19 thus prompting the search for other MHS genes in man. Linkage studies have identified three other candidate genes. One of these is the gene for the dihydropyridine receptor (DHP) on chromosome 7q21.1,[51] another is on chromosome 3 but sequencing of this gene has not been completed.[114] Finally, Vita et al.[119] proposed that a locus on chromosome 17 was associated with MMR. Nonetheless, this defect, a Gly-Ala mutation in the sodium channel α-subunit gene, is also believed to be causal for myotonia fluctuans.[50,86] The increased jaw tension that is commonly seen when anesthetics are administered to these patients may represent their response to anesthetics rather than the possibility of an association with MH.

Evaluation of Malignant Hyperthermia Susceptibility

No simple screening test or minimally invasive diagnostic test exists to identify patients susceptible to MH. Although physical examination can identify loosely associated abnormalities that are common in the general population, the syndrome lacks a distinct physical sign to identify susceptible patients. Numerous tests have tried to identify susceptible patients. These include serum CK, serum cholinesterase levels, chemiluminescence, human leukocyte antigen (HLA), platelet nucleotide depletion test, erythrocyte fragility, phosphorus nuclear magnetic resonance spectroscopy, and the calcium uptake test in muscle. Although some of these tests may be useful under restricted conditions, they have not been successful when applied to a larger population of patients. **The only test to reliably identify patients that have exhibited the clinical syndrome of MH is the *in vitro* contracture test that measures the response of skeletal muscle strips to either halothane or caffeine.**[64]

Genetic research provides hope for a simpler and more accurate diagnostic test for the future. To date, four mutations of the RYR1 gene have been described and proposed as casual for MH. Several recent reports have used either linkage to the RYR1 gene or identification of a known casual mutation of the RYR1 gene, in conjunction with the *in vitro* contracture testing to determine the status of MH susceptibility in large families.[23,94,121] Nonetheless, this approach is only applicable in very selected families with our current understanding of the genetics of MH. The likelihood is low of a practical genetic screening test or tests being available in the next 10 years.

Clinical assessment of the MHS patient

A variety of physical findings have been reported to be associated with MHS. Most commonly observed are increased muscle bulk, hyperextensible joints, strabismus, scoliosis, and other spinal abnormalities. The clinical utility of such observations is limited because many of the abnormalities cited occur with some frequency in the general population and because these physical abnormalities have a higher likelihood of requiring surgical intervention and anesthesia. A history of muscle cramps and heat intolerance increases the index of suspicion of MHS but has no predictive value. Abnormalities have been identified in MHS patients with electrodiagnostic tests but these tests alone are not diagnostic for MHS. **The only diseases/syndromes that have been definitely associated with MH to date are King-Denborough syndrome[62] and central core disease.**

Halothane and caffeine contracture tests

In 1970, Kalow and Britt[55] reported that isolated strips of human muscle demonstrated enhanced contracture response to caffeine when obtained from patients who had muscle rigidity during their MH episode. The following year, Ellis et al.[25] reported that muscle strips from patients with MH developed contractures when exposed to halothane *in vitro* (Fig. 94-3). Since that time, many pharmacologic agents have been shown to induce contracture in muscle from MHS patients, but only halothane and caffeine have been accepted as reliable testing agents. Unlike halothane, caffeine has never been reported to trigger MH. Both normal and MHS muscle contract when exposed to caffeine, however MHS muscle contracts at a lower dose. A standard testing protocol was adopted by European diagnostic centers in 1984 and by North American diagnostic centers in 1987 so that patients and test results from the various diagnostic centers could be pooled for further investigation. The two protocols are slightly different. The North American protocol uses a single dose of halothane (3%) and an incremental dose of caffeine (0.5, 1, 2, 4, 8, and 32 mM) while the European protocol uses incremental doses of halothane (0.5, 1, 2, and 3%) and caffeine (0.5, 1, 1.5, 2, 3, 4, and 32 mM). The interpretation of the results also dif-

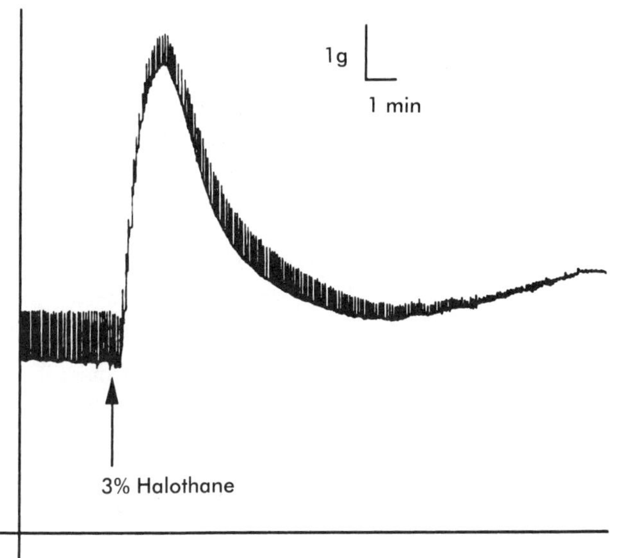

Fig. 94-3. Abnormal contracture response of human skeletal muscle to 3% halothane. The response was obtained in the presence of transmural electrical stimulation. Tension is on ordinate and time is on the abscissa.

fer. A patient is reported as MH susceptible by the North American protocol if any muscle strip exhibits a positive response to either halothane or caffeine, whereas the European protocol requires a positive response from both agents. If the patient's muscle responds to only one agent, they are labeled as MH equivocal by the European protocol. The North American MH Registry database has been used to determine the sensitivity and specificity of the North American Protocol, 97% and 78% respectively. The Registry was established to create a database of MH case reports and contracture test results and currently contains more than 2500 contracture test results.

Contracture testing cannot be used as a routine screening test because of its invasiveness, complexity, limited access, and cost. Six viable muscle strips (25 to 30 mm in length and 2 to 3 mm in diameter) are required for diagnostic testing and can only be obtained via open muscle biopsy. Less than a dozen medical centers have the experience and resources required to provide diagnostic contracture testing in North America. Because muscle viability standards require that testing be completed within 5 hours, patients are required to travel to a diagnostic center for testing.

Like the majority of laboratory tests, there may be some overlap between a positive and negative response in contracture testing. In the North American Protocol, interpretation of the responses favor false-positive errors rather than false-negative errors. Nonetheless, this is no guarantee against the occurrence of false-negative errors. Currently, there is one report of false-negative results using the European Protocol.[52] Although no false-negative results have been reported using the North American Protocol, few reports exist of patients with negative contracture results and subsequent exposure to triggering agents.[2,14]

Who should be tested and when should it be done

Laboratory testing serves two functions: to help in the management of the disease and to aid in its diagnosis. Clearly, contracture test results are not essential to conduct a safe anesthetic for patients that might be MHS. Nevertheless, many of cases reported to the MH Hotline are being diagnosed and treated before the traditional clinical signs can confirm the diagnosis. In these cases, contracture testing is useful in confirming the diagnosis. Contracture testing is also useful to rule out the diagnosis in the case of patients with a questionable history and incomplete or missing documentation. Likewise, many patients are not satisfied with the prospect of an uncertain diagnosis and request contracture testing to help define their status regarding MH susceptibility. Finally, phenotyping susceptible families by contracture test results is crucial in the ongoing search for a simpler, noninvasive screening test.

Every patient labeled as MHS should be counselled as to how contracture testing may effect them and their family so that informed decisions can be made. Contracture testing is elective, so testing can be scheduled to best fit the needs of the individual or family. The Malignant Hyperthermia Association of the United States (607-674-7901) is a valuable resource for details of contracture testing and can also provide a list of diagnostic centers for referral.

Management of Malignant Hyperthermia

Successful treatment of MH relies on prompt recognition of the clinical situation (see Box 94-2), quick access to supplies necessary for treatment (MH Cart, Box 94-4), and initiation of appropriate therapeutic measures. This combination can result in a mortality rate near zero. The MH Hotline (U.S. and Canada: 1-800-MH-HYPER/1-800-644-9737; all others: 1-315-428-7924) is available 24 hours a day and is a valuable resource to assist all practitioners in the management of suspected cases. This section discusses the management of fulminant episodes, patients with a documented history of MH, patients with a questionable history of MH, and patients with MMR. It is assumed that routine noninvasive monitors (i.e., electrocardiogram [ECG], blood pressure cuff, pulse oximetry, capnography, and electronic temperature monitoring) are in use or readily available.

Patient with a fulminant episode

Although the current management of MH focuses on dantrolene, it is not the only course of action in treating MH (Box 94-5). Early supportive care plays a vital role when dantrolene is being prepared for administration, and successful

BOX 94-4
MALIGNANT HYPERTHERMIA CART

1. Dantrolene — 36 vials
2. Sterile water for injection — 3 l (for reconstitution of dantrolene — 60 ml per vial)
3. 5 to 10 50-ml syringes and 16-gauge needles to mix dantrolene
4. Lidocaine — bolus and continuous infusion
5. Procainamide — bolus and continuous infusion
6. Sodium bicarbonate — 10 ampules
7. Dextrose 50% — 4 ampules
8. Lasix — 200 mg
9. Mannitol 25% — 100 g (8 ampules)

Plan for rapid access of:

1. Refrigerated normal saline solution for infusion and irrigation
2. Ice maker or crushed ice
3. Central pressure catheters, transducers, and monitors
4. Blood collection tubes/laboratory processing of samples — blood gas analysis/electrolytes/glucose
5. Cooling blanket
6. Rectal tube/irrigating Foley catheter

BOX 94-5
MANAGEMENT OF PATIENT WITH FULMINANT EPISODE OF MALIGNANT HYPERTHERMIA

Discontinue all potent inhaled anesthetic agents and hyperventilate with 100% O_2.

Obtain assistance and inform the surgeon to expedite or abort the procedure if possible.

Administer dantrolene, 2.5 mg/kg intravenous. Be prepared to repeat this dose until the patient responds with a decreased in end-tidal CO_2, ventilatory requirement, rigidity, or heart rate.

Monitor acidosis using blood gas analysis to determine if bicarbonate therapy is indicated. Consider central or intra-arterial catheter placement for serial measurements.

Hyperkalemia is common and should be treated with insulin and glucose (10 units regular insulin in 1000 ml of $D_{10}W$). Serum potassium and glucose levels should be monitored.

Efforts to cool the patient should correspond to the extent of temperature elevation. Patients can be cooled by decreasing the room temperature, infusion of cold solutions, surface cooling with ice, or using cold solutions for gastric, bladder, and rectal lavage.

treatment of MH before the discovery of dantrolene therapy supports this viewpoint.[85] Assistance from medical personnel is a necessity because many of the actions discussed later should occur simultaneously. Prioritizing tasks is critical in the management of the fulminant episode. When anesthesia-trained personnel are unavailable, the professional skills and assistance of the operating room nurse, the operating room technicians, and the surgeon are invaluable. The tasks should be prioritized in the following order. First, discontinue the triggering agents (potent inhalation agents and succinylcholine) and hyperventilate with 100% oxygen at high-flow rates. This action will limit the patient's exposure to the agent(s) and assist in their elimination from the body stores while providing maximal oxygenation. Vigorous manual ventilation is often attempted to correct the rising end-tidal CO_2 but is usually unsuccessful. Changing the anesthesia machine to a noncontaminated one is no longer necessary or desirable. Likewise, removal of the vaporizers and replacing the circuit, fresh gas hose, and ventilator bellows only increases the risk of inadequate ventilation. Second, dantrolene should be obtained, prepared, and administered. Malignant Hyperthermia Association of the United States (MHAUS) recommends that each hospital or freestanding outpatient surgery center stock 36 vials of dantrolene (20 mg per vial). If the facility does not stock dantrolene or only stocks a limited amount, aggressive supportive care, as outlined in Box 94-5, must be instituted until dantrolene is available.

The initial dose of dantrolene is 2.5 mg/kg and should be given as an IV bolus into a large vein. A decrease in end-tidal CO_2 is the first sign that the therapy is effective and is followed by a decrease in temperature. If there is no response, the initial dantrolene dose should be repeated until the therapeutic effect is achieved. Muscle rigidity may continue and heart rate may remain elevated despite a decrease in end-tidal CO_2 and temperature. Continued elevation of the heart rate may be related to emergence from the discontinued anesthetic and may respond to small doses of narcotics or benzodiazepines. Reports have shown that, in severe cases, the patient may not awaken for several hours. Continued respiratory support is determined on a case-per-case basis. After the episode is controlled, dantrolene should be continued at 1 mg/kg every 6 hours for at least 24 hours. During this time, clinical signs and laboratory results indicate if further dantrolene is necessary. Strict vigilance must be maintained at all times for recrudescence of MH, which is managed with the urgency of a new episode of MH.

Dantrolene is packaged in lyophilized form at 20 mg/vial and is reconstituted with 60 ml of sterile water in which it is relatively insoluble. A 70-kg patient will require 9 vials of dantrolene and 540 ml of sterile water to prepare the initial treatment dose. Sodium hydroxide and 3 g of mannitol are added to the vial to allow the dantrolene to dissolve in 2 to 3 minutes. The resulting pH of the solution is 9.5, so care must be taken to prevent extravasation and to monitor for thrombophlebitis. Mannitol is an osmotic diuretic and therefore central venous pressure (CVP) monitoring may be necessary to manage volume status. A novel dantrolene preparation, lecithin-coated dantrolene microcrystals, is currently under investigation and offers significant advantages over the currently available dantrolene preparation.[58] The new preparation has a neutral pH and enough dantrolene (200 mg) is contained in a single 10-ml vial to treat an 80-kg adult. The preparation has been successfully used to treat MH episodes in susceptible swine but further investigation is required before human trials can begin.

The objective of cooling the patient is to decrease core temperature and thereby lower O_2 consumption, decrease the rate of metabolism, and limit temperature related brain injury. Core cooling is superior to surface cooling and is accomplished by cold gastric and rectal lavage, cold wound irrigation, and refrigerated IV solution. Surface cooling can be used effectively if peripheral vasoconstriction is avoided. Ice packs to the groin and axilla help accomplish this task. Decreasing the room temperature or packing the patient in ice may induce peripheral vasoconstriction and actually be counterproductive. The patient's temperature needs to be continuously monitored to detect hypothermia from overaggressive cooling or to detect recrudescence of MH. Dysrhythmias result from the byproducts of the hypermetabolic state, which include hypoxia, hypercapnia, acidosis, and hyperkalemia in combination with an increased sympathetic tone. Treatment of the primary condition should control the dysrhythmias, but if they persist or become life-threatening, lidocaine (1 to 2 mg/kg), or procainamide (2 to 3 mg/kg), should be administered IV and repeated as needed. Currently there is no evidence that procainamide is more or less effective than lidocaine in controlling dysrhythmias during an MH episode. If heart rate is unresponsive to the previously described measures, short-acting beta blockers such as esmolol should be used instead of calcium channel blockers. In both humans and swine, the combination of dantrolene and verapamil resulted in cardiovascular collapse secondary to hyperkalemia.[90,91] The same result has been reported in swine administered dantrolene and diltiazem. Hyperkalemia was not observed when dantrolene and nifedipine were administered, but mild hyperkalemia was noted in one case in humans.[90]

Blood gas analysis (arterial, venous, and central) is the most useful laboratory evaluation to assess the effectiveness of therapy. Capnography does not eliminate the need for blood gas assays for several reasons. First, rapid ventilation can produce an end-tidal CO_2 that is falsely low because a stable plateau phase at end-expiration may not be reached. Second, even if a stable plateau phase is present, the calibration must be verified to validate the continued use of the end-tidal CO_2 trend. Third, acidosis, another marker in assessing the effectiveness of therapy, cannot be detected by capnography and may still be present even when the end-tidal CO_2 has returned to baseline. Further, bicarbonate therapy for the correction of evolving acid-base disorder cannot be managed without repeated blood gas analysis. Empiric bicarbonate therapy risks severe alkalosis and adds to the burden of additional CO_2 elimination since bicarbonate is excreted via the lung as CO_2. Finally, blood gas analysis can assess the adequacy of O_2 delivery more precisely than pulse oximetry. If a central venous access is present, mixed venous O_2 measurements allow calculation of O_2 consumption.

Serum abnormalities include potassium, calcium, sodium, and glucose and serial measurements are necessary. Hyperkalemia results from the acidosis that shifts K^+ out of the cell in exchange for H^+ ion and from the leakage of K^+ out of the damaged muscle cells. The most effective therapy for hyperkalemia is treatment of the underlying MH with dantrolene, but if it persists or results in dysrhythmias, intravenous glucose and insulin (10 units regular insulin in 1000 ml $D_{10}W$), and bicarbonate should be administered slowly. Potassium-binding agents may be useful after cold gastric or rectal lavage has been completed. Slow correction of hyperkalemia is recommended because it is usually followed by hypokalemia. Calcium therapy may be used to control life-threatening hyperkalemic dysrhythmias or for inotropic support. Variations in serum calcium levels are reflected on the ECG as a shortening or prolongation of the QT interval. Hypocalcemia is more common and is treated with incremental doses of calcium. Sodium values can be increased as a result of the large sodium load contained in mannitol or decreased because of a dilutional effect from fluid therapy. The risk of hypoglycemia or hyperglycemia increases if insulin and glucose therapy are used to treat hyperkalemia.

Late laboratory evaluations include CK, myoglobin, and coagulation studies, and in cases resistant to therapy, catecholamine levels and thyroid function tests. Serum CK and myoglobin should be followed every 6 to 8 hours until the CK approaches baseline and the myoglobin has been cleared from the urine. This action defines the at-risk period for myoglobinuric renal failure and the need for renal protective measures. These tests also identify a smoldering case if the values do not return to baseline. Disseminated intravascular coagulation (DIC) has been reported following fulminant MH episodes. Factors contributing to DIC include hemolysis, cellular edema with increased release of tissue thromboplastins, and inadequate tissue perfusion. A high level of suspicion combined with serial laboratory evaluation of the coagulation system aids in this diagnosis. There are no special considerations for treating DIC in this setting. If the clinical situation appears to be MH but the patient continues to only partially respond to appropriate therapy, continue current therapy but consider other processes (Box 94-3). Catecholamine levels and thyroid function tests may help to identify thyroid storm or a pheochromocytoma, which may mimic MH. When the episode has been reversed and the patient's status has stabilized, arrangements should be made for intensive care unit care for at least 24 to 48 hours. The major areas of concern include recrudescence of the initial episode, renal protection therapy to prevent myoglobinuric renal failure, the occurrence of DIC, delayed awakening possibly related to cerebral edema, and the patient's underlying medical condition that warranted surgical intervention.

Patient with a documented history of malignant hyperthermia

The goal for patients with histories of documented MH is preparation and administration of a safe anesthetic. Regardless of the surgical procedure or anesthetic technique, additional time is required to prepare the anesthetic machine, check the monitors, and inspect the MH cart (Box 94-6). Some departments maintain an anesthesia machine without vaporizers for use only with MH patients. This practice is unnecessary because of the ease of preparing an uncontaminated machine. Although it is impossible to define a background level of inhalation agent that may trigger an MH episode, a practical goal can be defined by adopting the National Institute of Occupational Safety and Health (NIOSH) standard for waste gas exposure. The NIOSH standard is 2 parts per million (ppm) concentration of a halogenated agent and is an acceptable level because this concentration may be present in the operating room or recovery room ambient air. Levels of inhalation agent below this standard can be obtained for both the circle system and the Mapleson D system. In either case, it is recommended to seal or remove the vaporizers, replace the old fresh gas outlet hose with a new one, use a new disposable circuit, and flush the machine with a fresh gas flow of 10 l/min for 5 minutes.[5] Necessary monitoring equipment includes capnography with real-time display, pulse oximetry, electronic temperature probe, ECG, and a noninvasive blood pressure device. The MH cart should be inspected to ensure that the medications have not expired.

Our practice includes scheduling the procedure as the first case of the day to allow time for preparation and to avoid contamination of the room by waste anesthetic gas. Extended observation in the recovery room (4 to 6 hours) is arranged and the intensive care unit is alerted in anticipation of any signs of an MH episode. These patients can undergo outpatient surgery as long as the above conditions are met.

Currently, most experts do not recommend the administration of dantrolene preoperatively. Nonetheless, close examination of both approaches reveals that each position has merit. Arguments for no pretreatment with dantrolene include the possibility of masking or delaying an MH episode, depletion of a limited supply of the drug, and avoiding the risk of morbidity from the drug. Arguments in favor of pretreatment with dantrolene are based on preventing MH through prophylactic measures and in preventing stress-induced MH. If pretreatment is chosen, an IV dose of 2.5 mg/kg just before the start of the anesthetic is recommended to achieve therapeutic serum levels. A Foley catheter is also required because of the osmotic diureses caused by the use of mannitol. Oral dantrolene, 5 mg/kg, in 3 or 4 divided doses every 6 hours with the last dose 4 hours preoperatively has also been shown to be effective.[1] **Pretreatment with dantrolene does not eliminate the need for a nontriggering anesthetic technique.**

Anxiety and stress have been implicated in predisposing a patient to MH. Preoperative sedation may be ben-

BOX 94-6
ANESTHETIC MANAGEMENT OF THE PATIENT WITH A DOCUMENTED HISTORY OF MALIGNANT HYPERTHERMIA

Equipment

1. A "clean" anesthesia machine should be prepared by removing or sealing the vaporizers, replacing the fresh gas hose, and using a new disposable circuit. Next, flush the machine with a fresh gas flow of 10 l/min for 5 minutes. Prepare the anesthetic machine even if a regional technique or monitored anesthesia care is planned in case of failed technique or emergency.
2. Capnography with real-time display, electrocardiogram, blood pressure, and electronic temperature monitoring are required.
3. Malignant hyperthermia cart must be checked for expired medications.

Scheduling

1. First case of the day.
2. Observation in recovery room for 4 to 6 hours.
3. Outpatient surgery is acceptable if the patient can be observed in the recovery room for 4 to 6 hours and intensive care support is readily available.

Premedication

1. Dantrolene prophylaxis is at the discretion of the anesthesiologist.
2. Sedation is at the discretion of the anesthesiologist.

Technique

1. Monitored anesthesia care.
2. Regional anesthesia (peripheral or central axis).
3. Nontriggering agents for general anesthesia.

Postoperative Care

1. Monitoring — respiratory rate, blood pressure, heart rate, and temperature.
2. Laboratory — if the clinical course remains uneventful, tests are not necessary.
3. Health care providers in the recovery room should be alerted to the patient's malignant hyperthermia status.

eficial and can be accomplished by administering appropriate doses of narcotics, benzodiazepines, barbiturates, or antihistamines.

The anesthetic technique depends on the patient, procedure, and anesthesiologist and may include monitored care, regional anesthesia, or use of a nontriggering technique for general anesthesia. Administration of a nontriggering anesthetic may be routine in some centers, but it is not always easily applied as highlighted in the following two case histories:

A 4-year-old girl with a history of MH and severe asthma for bilateral myringotomy tube placement.

A 3-year-old boy with acute epiglottis requiring intubation, who has a cousin with a documented history of MH.

In the first case, an inhalation induction with no IV placement is unacceptable. N_2O/O_2 alone does not provide sufficient analgesia. Intramuscular (IM) or IV ketamine can be used in combination with N_2O; however, the sympathetic response to ketamine may invalidate tachycardia and hypertension as early clinical signs for MH in a situation when capnography may not be reliable (a child who is not intubated). Continuous IV anesthesia (e.g., propofol, alfentanil, or methohexital) requires IV access before induction.

The second case contrasts two possibly fatal complications, loss of a tenuous airway and a fulminant MH episode. The possibility exists that the patient may not be susceptible. In this situation, securing the airway takes precedence. Before the inhalation induction begins, however, IV access must be established and dantrolene should be dissolved. Pretreatment with dantrolene is not recommended because of the possibility of muscle weakness severe enough to precipitate respiratory arrest. After the patient has been intubated, the clinical situation determines the use of dantrolene.

No special precautions are necessary for obstetric patients. The stress of labor has not been shown to predispose patients to MH, and MH is not a contraindication for epidural or spinal anesthesia. We recommend avoiding pretreatment of obstetric patients with dantrolene for emergency cesarean section under general anesthesia. If an episode is triggered during the anesthetic, however, dantrolene should be administered immediately. To date, dantrolene appears to have little or no adverse effect on the fetus or newborn.[76]

In the postoperative period, the patient should be monitored for signs of MH for at least 4 to 6 hours. To ensure early detection of postoperative MH, recovery room/intensive care unit staff must be alert and educated regarding MH. If the procedure was uneventful, no special laboratory analysis is indicated. If dantrolene was given prophylactically, it need not be continued in the postoperative period.

Patient with a questionable history of malignant hyperthermia

When MH is suspected, patients must be treated as though they have MH, until either a chart review or a negative contracture test proves otherwise (Box 94-7). If the diagnosis is still in question following chart review, contact MHAUS for the nearest MH diagnostic center for consultation. Even when the diagnosis is inconsistent with MH, provide documentation and counseling to the family regarding the findings; this helps to eliminate confusion for the family and their future health care providers. Elective surgery can proceed as scheduled (follow guidelines in Box 94-6) without the results of contracture test as long as a nontriggering technique is administered. The patient and family members should be advised to be identifiable with a Medic-Alert tag stating that they are MHS until proven otherwise.

Patients with masseter muscle rigidity

When a patient develops MMR the conservative approach has been to abort the anesthetic and surgical procedure and closely monitored the patient for other signs of MH (Box 94-8). In the case of emergency surgery, the surgeon should be informed and surgery should be expedited. All potential triggering agents should be discontinued and replaced by nontriggering agents (propofol/barbiturates/opiates, N_2O, and nondepolarizing muscle relaxants). End-tidal CO_2, arterial blood gases, and core temperature should be monitored continuously. Dantrolene should be available in the operating room. More recently, it has been suggested that even elective cases need not be stopped immediately. If end-expired CO_2, arterial blood gases, blood pressure, pulse rate, temperature, serum CK, urine color, and muscle tone are

BOX 94-7
PATIENT WITH A QUESTIONABLE HISTORY OF MALIGNANT HYPERTHERMIA

1. Treat the patient as malignant hyperthermia susceptible (MHS).
2. Elective surgery may proceed following preparations listed in Box 95-6. However, if contracture testing is indicated/desired, a second anesthetic will be required.
3. Identify susceptible family members and provide information for Medic-Alert indentification. If the diagnosis is found to be negative, the Medic-Alert tags can be discarded.
4. Verify the diagnosis to rule out mislabeled patients.
   a. If a patient or family member in question has been registered, calling the North American MH Registry (717) 531-6936 can confirm the history or contracture test results.
   b. Obtain and review records of the event in question.
   c. If the diagnosis is still unclear, consult with the nearest MH diagnostic center, which is available through MHAUS (607) 674-7901.
5. Provide documentation and counseling for the patient and affected relatives.

BOX 94-8
PATIENT WITH MASSETER MUSCLE RIGIDITY

1. Avoid the use of succinylcholine following an inhalation induction.
2. When masseter muscle rigidity is diagnosed (see Table 94-3):
   a. Discontinue potent inhaled anesthetic agent and continue to ventilate by mask with 100% O_2.
   b. Do not give a second dose of succinylcholine
   c. Call for assistance and the malignant hyperthermia cart.
   d. Continue to monitor end-tidal CO_2, electrocardiogram, blood pressure, and temperature.
   e. Obtain blood gas analysis if the situation does not rapidly improve.
3. The decision whether to proceed or abort must consider the anesthesiologist's experience, the urgency and length of the surgical procedure, the human and treatment resources available, monitoring capabilities, and the patient's increased risk to progress to a fulminant malignant hyperthermia episode.
4. If the procedure is aborted, it can be rescheduled after the creatine kinase has returned to normal.
5. If the procedure is continued, a nontriggering anesthetic technique should be used and end-expired CO_2, arterial blood gases, blood pressure, pulse rate, temperature, serum creatine kinase, urine color, and muscle tone should continue to be monitored for signs of malignant hyperthermia.
6. Postoperative management:
   a. Institute intensive care unit/overnight recovery room observation for 24 hours to monitor urine output and signs of increased metabolism (increased heart rate, blood pressure, respiration, acidosis, and temperature).
   b. Obtain serial creatine kinase measurements every 8 hours for 24 hours or until the creatine kinase has peaked.
   c. Test urine for the presence of myoglobin:
      (1) If positive, maintain urine output above 1 ml/kg/hr until clear.
      (2) If negative, continue to monitor until creatine kinase has peaked.

monitored and remain stable, the procedure may be continued with a nontriggering anesthetic technique. In all cases the urine should be tested for myoglobinuria. Serum CK should be measured at the time and at 6 to 8 hour intervals over the next 24 hours. The patient should be labeled as MHS and nontriggering techniques should be administered for future anesthetics unless a negative contracture test proves otherwise. If the procedure is aborted, it can be rescheduled after the CK has returned to normal. The decision whether to proceed or abort must consider the anesthesiologist's experience, the urgency and length of the surgical procedure, the human and treatment resources available, monitoring capabilities, and the patient's increased risk of progressing to a fulminant MH episode.

HYPOTHERMIA

Homeothermic animals such as birds and mammals require an almost constant internal body temperature to maintain normal metabolic and physiologic function. Significant deviation in internal temperature can result in deterioration of metabolic and physiologic functions, and death may result. The human body has developed an elaborate system to maintain core temperature usually within 0.2° C of its target temperature. Anesthetics profoundly affect these control mechanisms and impair thermoregulation. Perioperative hypothermia is common and may result in a number of complications (Table 94-5). An understanding of normal and anesthetic-effected thermoregulation will facilitate prevention and treatment of these complications.

Normal Thermoregulation

Like other physiologic systems, the thermoregulatory system has at least three major components: (1) sensory receptors (an afferent limb); (2) a central integrator or controller; and (3) an effector organ system (an efferent limb). The sensory receptors provide information from thermosensitive sites in the skin and other body structures (spinal cord and viscera) to a central controller that compares this information with a standard reference or set-point. On the basis of the difference between the receptor input and the set-point, the controller provides information to effector systems controlling heat production or loss. Most authorities agree that the hypothalamus is the most likely part of the nervous system to sense body temperature, compare the result with a set-point, and institute an appropriate neural response. Central thermoregulatory control appears to be intact even in premature infants but thermoregulatory failure is common in the elderly. Investigations by neuroanatomists and neurophysiologists have greatly increased understanding of how the three components of the thermoregulatory system function to maintain a thermal balance; details concerning these experimental studies are the subject of numerous books and review articles.[6,29,43,44]

Adults regulate heat exchange with their environment by: (1) cutaneous vasomotor adjustments; (2) sweating; (3) shivering; and (4) environmental behavioral adjustments. It is also agreed that nonshivering thermogenesis is not a significant source of heat in adult humans. Normothermia is generally accepted to be an oral temperature of 36° to 37.5° C. Diurnal variations occur, with temperature being lowest in the morning during sleep and highest in the early afternoon. Sublingual, skin, and axillary temperatures are shell temperatures and relate poorly to core

Table 94-5 Consequences of mild (2°–3° C) hypothermia

Consequence	Effect
Advantages	
Cerebral ischemia and hypoxia	Decreases cerebral metabolic rate approximately 8% for each °C reduction in temperature Possibly other mechanisms (i.e., decreased release of excitatory amino acids)
Malignant hyperthermia	May decrease the likelihood of triggering May slow the progression of an episode
Wound infection	Directly impairs immune function Decreases blood flow and therefore O_2 delivery Induces protein wasting and decreases collagen synthesis
Disadvantages	
Blood loss	Blood loss increases 0.5 unit for each °C decrease in core temperature Significantly increases blood loss and transfusion requirements during hip arthroplasty
Coagulation	Reduces platelet function Decreases activation of the coagulation cascade
Drug metabolism	Vecuronium duration of action doubles at 34.5° vs. 36.5° C MAC of halothane reduced roughly 5% per °C reduction in core body temperature Propofol concentration during constant infusion increases approximately 30% with a 3° C decrease in core temperature
Patient discomfort	Often considered the most unpleasant aspect of surgery by patients
Shivering	Can increase O_2 consumption by more than 200% Possible cause of myocardial ischemia Exacerbates postoperative pain

temperature. Core temperature, which is widely used by anesthesiologists, is not a precisely defined entity, but it is accepted that it reflects mean temperature of the well-perfused organs (i.e., brain, heart, kidney, and lungs). The different sites used to measure body temperature during anesthesia and the advantages/disadvantages of each site are listed in Table 94-6.

Mechanisms of Heat Conservation

Hypothermia triggers efferent responses to maintain core temperature by increasing metabolic heat production (shivering and nonshivering thermogenesis) or decreasing environmental heat loss (active vasoconstriction and behavioral patterns). Energy-efficient responses, such as vasoconstriction, are generally maximized before metabolically costly responses, such as shivering, are initiated. In conscious humans, behavioral regulation (dressing appropriately, modifying environmental temperature) is the most important mechanism of heat conservation.

Cutaneous vasoconstriction

This is usually the first and most consistent thermoregulatory response to hypothermia. In a cold environment, cutaneous vasoconstriction raises thermal insulation provided by skin and can decrease entire body heat loss by 25% to 50%.[98,107] If heat loss continues and core temperature falls, shivering and the associated increase in heat production must be initiated to restore core temperature.

Shivering

This response is the primary mechanism for heat production, and is dependent on central neuronal coordination and normal neuromuscular function. Shivering is initiated only after maximal vasoconstriction, nonshivering thermogenesis and behavioral adjustments have proven inadequate to maintain body temperature. **Shivering is an energy-inefficient means of heat production and can cause a twofold to fivefold increase in whole-body O_2 consumption.** Although maximum heat production from shivering can increase eightfold, sustained shivering rarely increases heat production more than two- to threefold, and thermal equilibrium in unprotected individuals cannot be attained during prolonged severe cold stress. Newborn and premature infants do not shiver but can increase metabolic heat production by nonshivering thermogenesis.

Nonshivering thermogenesis

This response increases metabolic heat production without producing mechanical work. Brown adipose tissue is an important site of nonshivering heat production in the neonate.

Table 94-6 Sites of temperature measurement

Site	Advantages	Disadvantages
Tympanic membrane	Close to hypothalamus	Rare risk of perforation and bleeding
Nasopharyngeal	Close to hypothalamus	Probe is affected by the temperature of inspired gases; displacement can occur easily
Esophageal	Convenient, close to great vessels and heart	Probe needs to be placed in the lower quarter of the esophagus to avoid effect of inspired anesthetic gases
Rectal	Traditional site	Variable reflector of core temperature; is affected by feces, peritoneal lavage, and cystoscopy
Bladder	Better reflector of core temperature than rectum; temperature sensors are now incorporated into urinary drainage catheter	Affected by rate of flow; cannot be used in genitourinary procedures
Oral	Convenient	Not practical during anesthesia
Axillary	Convenient	Must be placed over axillary artery; affected by blood pressure cuff, intravenous solutions, and patient movement
Skin	Provides index of peripheral vasoconstriction	Cutaneous temperature correlates poorly with core temperature
Pulmonary artery	Provides temperature of mixed venous blood	Probe can be affected by temperature of inspired gases; cannot be used during thoracic surgery

The brown fat is rich in mitochondria and is distributed over the neck, back, viscera, and great vessels. The metabolism of brown fat is stimulated by beta-adrenergic effects of norepinephrine. Although the exact mechanism of heat production is not known, it is suggested that it is either related to an uncoupling of oxidative phosphorylation of the brown fat mitochondria in the presence of fatty acids or results from lipolysis-lipogenesis coupled with ATP utilization and heat production.

Mechanisms of Heat Loss

There are two main mechanisms of heat loss.

Sweating

This is the most effective method of heat loss. Benzinger reported that an increase in temperature of 0.5° C produces a sevenfold increase in sweat rate and body conductivity.[6] Sweating is mediated by cholinergic sympathetic fibers and can be nearly abolished by even small doses of atropine.

Vasodilation

This response is important in the transfer of heat from the core to the periphery, which supplies the sweat mechanism with heat for evaporation. Sweating and vasodilation responses work synchronously to counter any increase in core temperature.

Hypothermia under General Anesthesia

It has long been known that anesthetized patients become hypothermic, and numerous studies document the incidence and severity.[47,77,100,104] **Hypothermia which develops during general anesthesia typically follows a predictable pattern: (1) an initial rapid decrease in core temperature of between 0.5° and 1.5° C during the first hour after induction, believed to be the result of internal redistribution of heat;[97] (2) a more gradual linear decline in core temperature; usually lasting 2 to 3 hours that apparently results from cutaneous heat loss exceeding metabolic heat production (typically 0.5° to 1° C/hr);[49] and (3) a plateau phase when core temperature stabilizes after 3 to 4 hours and which results from thermoregulatory compensation.[100]**

In unanesthetized patients, tonic thermoregulatory vasoconstriction maintains a significant core to peripheral temperature gradient. Induction of general anesthesia causes vasodilation which results in redistribution of heat from the core to the periphery. The result is a markedly decreased core temperature, but mean body temperature and heat content remain unchanged.[97] Although internal redistribution of heat is believed to be the major reason core body temperature decreases soon after the induction of general anesthesia, several other factors affect the patient's heat balance. These factors include: (1) decreased metabolic heat production under general anesthesia; (2) heat loss from the patient to the environment; and (3) the effects of anesthetic agents on thermoregulation. Induction of anesthesia decreases metabolic heat production by approximately 20% by limiting muscular activity, reducing the metabolic rate, and diminishing the work of breathing.[10,112] Evaporation of surgical skin preparation solutions,[106] anesthetic-induced vasodilation and impairment of central thermoregulatory control,[97,113] and cold operating room temperatures all increase cutaneous heat loss, although not enough to be the major cause of hypothermia during surgery.

Effect of Anesthetic Agents on Thermoregulation

General anesthesia profoundly impairs the body's ability to regulate temperature. Behavioral regulation is not relevant during general anesthesia, because patients are unconscious, and shivering is often prevented because of muscle relaxants. Therefore, vasoconstriction is the major thermoregulatory response available to anesthetized, paralyzed, hypothermic adult patients. Clinically relevant doses of general anesthetics decrease the activation threshold (temperature triggering a response) for hypothermia by 2° to 4° C.[99,113,124] Activation thresholds for responses to hyperthermia are also affected, but to a lesser degree than those for hypothermia (approximately 1° C).[102] The result is an increased interthreshold range (temperature range over which no regulatory response occurs) over which patients are poikilothermic, and core temperature changes are passively determined by redistribution of heat within the body and environmental heat loss.

The exact central temperature which triggers thermoregulatory vasoconstriction is agent and dose dependent and may vary depending on the age of the patient and the intensity of surgical stimulation. Patients who become sufficiently hypothermic during surgery eventually reach the vasoconstriction threshold and trigger the response. Once triggered, the gain and maximum intensity of the thermoregulatory response remains near normal.[69,95,125] **Markedly altered thermoregulatory thresholds with preserved gain and maximal intensities characterize the effect of general anesthetics on the thermoregulatory system.**[101]

Postanesthesia tremor has been reported to occur in up to 40% of patients postoperatively, although the more frequent use of narcotic agents may have caused the incidence to decrease.[19,81] The cause of spontaneous postanesthesia tremor has been variously attributed to uninhibited spinal reflexes, pain, decreased sympathetic activity, pyrogen release, adrenal suppression, respiratory alkalosis, and most commonly to a normal thermoregulatory response to intraoperative heat loss. Sessler et al.[96] compared electromyograms (EMGs) of patients during emergence from isoflurane with those of nonanesthetized patients who experienced thermoregulatory shivering and with those patients having pathologic clonus secondary to spinal cord injury. Two distinct EMG patterns were seen after isoflurane anesthesia: (1) a tonic pattern resembling normal shivering, typically having a 4 to 8 cycle/min waxing and waning component; and (2) a phasic, 5- to 7-Hz bursting pattern resembling pathologic clonus. These results lead the authors to postulate that the tonic pattern was usually caused by normal shivering, whereas the EMG clonus was a spinal reflex facilitated by the presence of residual isoflurane. Nonetheless, this study was unable to address the thermoregulatory contribution to the observed tremor patterns because all patients were hypothermic. A subsequent study by Sessler[105] established that the tonic and clonic patterns were thermoregulatory (i.e., always preceded by central hypothermia and vasoconstriction). It is likely that the more common tonic pattern (which resembles normal shivering) is a simple thermoregulatory response to hypothermia. The relatively rare clonic pattern is not a normal component of thermoregulatory shivering and appears specific to recovery from volatile anesthetics. Although the precise etiology of this tremor pattern remains unknown, it likely results from anesthesia-induced disinhibition of spinal reflexes.[105]

Postanesthetic tremor can be prevented in most patients by maintaining normothermia. If tremor occurs, skin-surface warming may be effective therapy. Pharmacologic treatments include meperidine (25 mg IV), clonidine (75 ug IV), and ketanserin (10 mg IV).[41,53] The mechanism(s) by which these drugs abolish shivering is unknown.

Central thermoregulation remains intact during regional anesthesia but hypothermia frequently occurs because: (1) regional anesthetics depress regional thermal afferent input and efferent responses, such as vasoconstriction and shivering; (2) patients lose heat to the operating room environment; and (3) redistribution of heat within the body occurs.

Traditionally, hypothermia during regional anesthesia was believed to primarily result from increased heat loss to the environment secondary to sympathetic blockade–induced vasodilation. Recently, Hynson et al.[48] investigated the importance of different etiologic factors in causing hypothermia during epidural blockade. In healthy, nonpregnant, normal volunteers, core and skin temperature, heat loss and O_2 consumption were measured before and after epidural blockade to an approximate T4 level was induced. They found that during epidural anesthesia, skin temperature increased, core temperature decreased, and heat loss to the environment increased only slightly. Most subjects shivered during the epidural block, so heat production increased during the study. This data suggest that heat loss to the environment cannot account for the fall in core temperature seen during regional anesthesia. The authors concluded that **redistribution of heat within the body is the primary factor responsible for the development of central hypothermia during epidural blockade.** A subsequent study by Glosten et al.[34] supports this hypothesis.

Hypothermia during regional anesthesia is often accompanied by tremor. The incidence of shivering during regional anesthesia has been reported in 0% to 70% of patients.[36] Numerous clinical studies have failed to demonstrate a consistent relationship between core temperature and shivering during major regional anesthesia. Absence of a consistent relationship between hypothermia and tremor during epidural anesthesia raises the question of whether this response was thermoregulatory or of some other etiology.

Investigations using nonsedated, normal volunteers have

defined the nature of this tremor. Studies show: (1) that the tremor is thermoregulatory (preceded by central hypothermia and central vasoconstriction above the block);[103] (2) that it does not result from stimulation of neuraxial thermoreceptors;[83] and (3) that it is not caused by systemic absorption of local anesthetics.[35] EMGs recorded from shivering subjects during epidural anesthesia have the 4 to 8 cycle/min waxing-and-waning pattern observed in shivering, unanesthetized subjects.[112] These findings indicate that tremor during regional anesthesia is normal thermoregulatory shivering, triggered by a decreased core temperature.

The tremor seen in pregnant patients undergoing regional anesthesia may have a different etiology. A number of studies have shown an increased incidence of shivering in pregnant patients when cold solution is injected epidurally.[82,122] This response is not seen in nonpregnant volunteers or patients, suggesting that thermosensitive tissue within the spinal canal contributes to the shivering observed with extradural anesthesia in parturients.[36]

Shivering that occurs with regional anesthesia can be prevented if normothermia is maintained.[103] Cutaneous warming of patients for two hours prior to inducing epidural anesthesia helps prevent hypothermia and prevents shivering.[34] Pharmacologic treatment is the same as for postanesthetic tremor with general anesthesia.

Prevention and Treatment

Control of ambient temperature

Increasing the room temperature has been repeatedly shown to be an effective method of preventing heat loss in surgical patients.[29] At operating room temperatures greater than 24° C, most adult patients will maintain normothermia.[77]

Insulation

Applying insulation to the skin is the easiest way to decrease cutaneous heat loss. An enveloping cover of plastic wrap, space blanket, or steridrape can decrease heat loss by convection and radiation. Most of the benefit in reducing heat loss is provided by the layer of air trapped beneath the covering which decreases heat loss by convection. Radiant heat loss is also decreased, although the benefit may be lost when the covering warms itself to skin temperature.[109]

Warm solutions

Warming skin preparation solutions and irrigation fluids prevents evaporative heat loss. When rapid transfusion of cold bank blood is required, the use of blood warmers decreases the degree of hypothermia. One unit of blood at 4° to 8° C, or 1 l of colloid or crystalloid at 16° to 20° C, can decrease core temperature approximately 0.25° C.[109]

Heat and humidification

Only 10% of metabolic heat is lost from the respiratory tract. Thus, although heating and humidifying inspired gases can prevent all of this heat loss, they have minor effects on core temperature.[49] Inspired anesthetic gases can be passively warmed and humidified to a state similar to that induced by the nasopharynx. Devices such as a Humidvent placed in the airway to trap the heat and humidity of the patient's expired air are effective in maintaining humidity and minimizing heat loss. Nonetheless, such devices cannot add significant heat to an already hypothermic patient. Active (i.e., electrical) devices provide artificial heating and humidification. Advantages include conservation of heat, prevention of shivering, and decreased drying of pulmonary secretions. Disadvantages, such as problems with condensation and rain-out, contamination, water overload and rarely, thermal burns, can occur.

Heating mattresses

Heating mattresses (40° to 41° C) work well when placed on top of the patient but have been shown not to be effective when placed under the patient because only one third of the body surface area is in contact with the mattress. Overall, heating mattresses are less effective than increasing the temperature in the operating room.

Forced-air heating system

Forced-air convection systems are the most effective active warming system. Lennon et al.[66a] compared the efficiency of a forced-air heating system (Bair Huggar, Augustine Medical Inc, Eden Prairie, MN) with covering patients with cotton blankets warmed to 37° C. After application of the forced-air heating system, patients were warmer at all time intervals. Numerous other studies have evaluated forced-air systems and found them to maintain normothermia, even during extensive procedures.[15,54,61]

KEY POINTS

- Malignant hyperthermia was first described in the early 1960s in a case report that also suggested a genetic basis for the syndrome.
- Skeletal muscle is the primary target tissue in MH. A laboratory diagnostic test for MH was derived using the enhanced contracture response of *in vitro* muscle strips from MH patients. Studies using these tests suggest that the cellular mechanism responsible for MH is a derangement in calcium regulation.
- No convenient laboratory test for MH susceptibility is yet available. Halothane and caffeine contracture tests are the most reliable indicators.

- Genetic research provides hope for a simpler and more accurate diagnostic test for the future. To date, four mutations of the RYR1 gene have been described and proposed as casual for MH.
- The immediate cause of an MH crisis appears to be a sudden rise in the concentration of myoplasmic calcium; this rise is believed to follow from the action of certain anesthetic agents on the sarcoplasmic reticulum (SR).
- All potent volatile anesthetics are capable of triggering an MH reaction, but an MH episode does not always occur with each exposure to an inhalation agent, even in persons known to be susceptible.
- Time of onset of a fulminant episode of MH is unpredictable, varying from within minutes to within several hours of induction; it may even occur in the recovery room.
- The earliest, most sensitive, and most specific sign of an MH episode is an unexplained rise in end-tidal CO_2.
- Laboratory signs in MH include hypercapnia, a respiratory and metabolic acidosis, hyperkalemia, hypercalcemia, elevated CK, and myoglobinuria.
- In 1979 dantrolene, a drug that decreases intracellular calcium concentrations, was approved for clinical use by the Food and Drug Administration; this was a major advance in the management of MH.
- A near-zero mortality rate from MH can result from prompt recognition of the clinical situation, ready access to supplies necessary for treatment, and initiation of appropriate therapeutic measures.
- Neuroleptic malignant syndrome usually develops 24 to 72 hours after psychotropic drug therapy is started. It is characterized by akinesia, muscle rigidity, hyperthermia, tachycardia, cyanosis, autonomic dysfunction, altered consciousness, diaphoresis, and raised serum CK concentration.
- Adults regulate heat exchange with their environment by cutaneous vasomotor adjustments, sweating, shivering, and environmental behavioral adaptation (dressing appropriately, modifying environmental temperature).
- Heat loss occurs via sweating and cutaneous vasodilation. Heat conservation results from cutaneous vasoconstriction and behavioral adaptation. Heat generation occurs secondary to shivering.
- In neonates, who do not shiver, nonshivering thermogenesis occurs.
- Although not precisely defined, core temperature reflects mean temperature of the well-perfused organs (e.g., brain, heart, kidney, and lungs).
- Hypothermia which develops during general anesthesia typically follows a predictable pattern: (1) an initial rapid decrease in core temperature of between 0.5° and 1.5° C during the first hour after induction, believed to be the result of internal redistribution of heat;[97] (2) a more gradual linear decline in core temperature, usually lasting 2 to 3 hours that apparently results from cutaneous heat loss exceeding metabolic heat production (typically 0.5° to 1° C/hr);[49] and (3) a plateau phase when core temperature stabilizes after 3 to 4 hours and which results from thermoregulatory compensation.[100]
- Normal thermoregulatory response to heat loss is the most common cause of spontaneous postanesthesia tremor.
- During regional anesthesia, central thermoregulation remains intact but hypothermia occurs frequently. Hypothermia during regional anesthesia is caused by depression of regional thermal afferent input and efferent responses, such as vasoconstriction and shivering, loss of heat to the operating room environment, and redistribution of heat within the body.
- Hypothermia during anesthesia may be prevented or treated by control of ambient temperature, insulation, warm IV solutions, heating and humidifying inspired gases, heating mattresses placed on top of the patient, and application of a forced-air heating system.

KEY REFERENCES

Beebe J, Sessler DI: Preparation of anesthesia machines for patients susceptible to malignant hyperthermia, *Anesthesiology* 69:395,1988.

Caroff SN, Mann SC, Campbell EC: Hyperthermia and neuroleptic malignant syndrome. In Levitt RC, editor: *Anesthesiology Clinics of North America,* Philadelphia, 1994, WB Saunders.

Glosten B: Thermoregulation and regional anesthesia, *Prob Anesth* 8:99, 1994.

Hammel HT: Anesthetics and body temperature regulation, *Anesthesiology* 68:833,1988.

Kaplan RF: Clinical controversies in malignant hyperthermia susceptibility. In Levitt RC, editor: *Anesthesiology Clinics of North America,* Philadelphia, 1994, WB Saunders.

Karan SM, Crowl F, Muldoon SM: Malignant hyperthermia masked by capnographic monitoring, *Anesth Analg* 78:590,1994.

Keck PE, Caroff SN, McElroy SL: Neuroleptic malignant syndrome and malignant hyperthermia: End of a controversy? *J Neuropsych* 7:135,1995.

MacLennan DH, Phillips MS: Malignant hyperthermia, *Science* 256:789,1992.

Lee G, Antognini JF, Gronert GA: Complete recovery after prolonged resuscitation and cardiopulmonary bypass for hyperkalemic cardiac arrest, *Anesth Analg* 79:172,1994.

Littleford JA, Patel LR, Bose D: Masseter muscle spasm in children: implications of continuing the triggering anesthetic, *Anesth Analg* 72:151,1991.

Rosenberg H, Gronert GA: Intractable cardiac arrest in children given succinylcholine, *Anesthesiology* 77:1054, 1992.

Sessler DI: Perianesthetic thermoregulation and heat balance in humans, *FASEB J* 74:638,1993.

Wallace AJ, Wooldridge W, Kingston HM, et al: Malignant hyperthermia—a large kindred linked to the RYR1 gene, *Anaesthesia* 51:16,1996.

REFERENCES

1. Allen G, Cattran CB, Peterson RG, et al: Plasma levels of dantrolene following oral administration in malignant hyperthermia-susceptible patients, *Anesthesiology* 69: 900, 1988.
2. Allen GC, Rosenberg H: Malignant hyperthermia susceptibility in adult patients with masseter muscle rigidity, *Can J Anaesth* 37:31, 1990.
3. Allen CG, Rosenberg H, et al: Safety of general anesthesia in patients previously tested negative for malignant hyperthermia susceptibility, *Anesthesiology* 72:619, 1990.
4. Allen GC, Rosenberg H: Phaeochromocytoma presenting as acute malignant hyperthermia—a diagnostic challenge, *Can J Anaesth* 37:593, 1990.
5. Beebe J, Sessler D: Preparation of anesthesia machines for patients susceptible to malignant hyperthermia, *Anesthesiology* 69: 395, 1988.
6. Benzinger TH: Heat regulation: homeostasis of central temperature in man, *Physiol Rev* 49(4):671, 1969.
7. Berman MC, Harrison HH, Bull AB: Changes underlining halothane-induced malignant hyperpyrexia in Landrace pigs, *Nature* 225:653, 1970.
8. Bernhardt D, Hörder MH: CK isoenzyme bei anaesthesie-induzierter myoglobinurie (AIM), *Anaesthesist* 30:131, 1981.
9. Birmingham PK, Stevenson GW, Uejima T, Hall SC: Isolated postoperative myoglobinuria in a pediatric outpatient: a case report of malignant hyperthermia, *Anesth Analg* 69:864, 1989.
10. Bissonette B, Nebbin S: Hypothermia during anesthesia, *Anesth Clin North Am* 12:3, 1994.
11. Britt BA: Combined anesthetic- and stress-induced malignant hyperthermia in two offspring of malignant hyperthermic-susceptible parents, *Anesth Analg* 67:393, 1988.
12. Britt BA, Kalow W: Malignant hyperthermia: a statistical review, *Can Anaesth Soc J* 17:293, 1970.
13. Britt BA: Metabolic aspects of anesthesia. In Cohen PJ, editor: *Clinical anesthesia: Metabolic aspects of anesthesia,* Philadelphia, 1975, FA Davis.
14. Britt BA: The clinical aspects of hyperthermia. In Felipe MA, Gottmann S, Khambatta HJ, editors: *Malignant hyperthermia: current concepts,* Darmstadt, 1989, Normed Verlag.
15. Camus Y, Delva E, Just B, et al: Thermal balance using a forced air warmer (Bair Hugger) during abdominal surgery, *Anesthesiology* 75:A491, 1991.
16. Caroff SN, Mann SC, Campbell EC: Hyperthermia and Neuroleptic malignant syndrome. In Levitt RC, editor: *Anesthesiology Clinics of North America,* Philadelphia, 1994, WB Saunders.
17. Casella ES, Soule MA, Blanck JJ: Creatine kinase activity and temperature in children after cardiac surgery, *J Cardiothorac Anesth* 2:156, 1988.
18. Chalkiadis GA, Branch KG: Cardiac arrest after isoflurane anaesthesia in a patient with Duchenne's muscular dystrophy, *Anaesthesia* 45:22, 1990.
19. Cohen M: An investigation into shivering following anesthesia: Preliminary report, *Proc Royal Soc Med* 60:752, 1967.
20. Delphin E, Jackson D, Rothstein P: Use of succinylcholine during elective pediatric anesthesia should be reevaluated, *Anesth Analg* 66:1190, 1987.
21. Denborough MA, Forster JFA, Lovell RR, et al: Anesthesia deaths in a family, *Br J Anaesth* 34:395, 1962.
22. Denborough MA, Lovell RH: Anesthesia deaths in a family, *Lancet* 2:45, 1960.
23. Deufel T, Sudbrak R, Feist Y, et al: Discordance, in a malignant hyperthermia pedigree, between *in vitro* contracture-test phenotypes and haplotypes for the MHS1 region on chromosome 19q12-13.2, comprising the C1840T transition in the RYR1 gene, *Am J Hum Genet* 56:1334, 1995.
24. Ellis FR, Hallsall PJ: Suxamethonium spasm: a differential diagnostic conundrum, *Br J Anaesth* 56:381, 1984.
25. Ellis FR, Harriman DGF, Keaney NP, et al: Halothane-induced muscle contracture as a cause of hyperpyrexia, *Br J Anaesth* 43: 721, 1971.
26. Endo M: Calcium release from the sarcoplasmic reticulum, *Phys Rev* 57:71, 1977.
27. Fill M, Coronado R, Mickelson JR, et al: Abnormal ryanodine receptor channels in malignant hyperthermia, *Biophys J* 50:471, 1990.
28. Fill M, Stefani E, Nelson TE: Abnormal human sarcoplasmic reticulum Ca^{2+} release channels in malignant hyperthermic skeletal muscle, *Biophys J* 59:1085, 1991.
29. Flacke JW, Flacke WE: Inadvertent hypothermia: frequent, insidious, and often serious, *Semin Anesth* 2:3, 1983.
30. Fujii J, Otsu K, Zorzato F: Identification of a mutation in porcine ryanodine receptor associated with malignant hyperthermia, *Science* 233:448, 1991.
31. Gibbs JM: A case of rhabdomyolysis associated with suxamethonium, *Anaesth Intens Care* 6:141, 1978.
32. Gillard EF, Otsu K, Fujii J: A substitution of cysteine for arginine 614 in the ryanodine receptor is potentially causative of human malignant hyperthermia, *Genomics* 11:451, 1991.
33. Gillard EF, Otsu K, Fujii J, et al: Polymorphisms and deduced amino acid substitutions in the coding sequence of the ryanodine (RYR1) gene in individuals with malignant hyperthermia, *Genomics* 13: 1247, 1992.
34. Glosten B, Hynson J, Sessler DI, et al: Preanesthetic skin-surface warming reduces redistribution hypothermia caused by epidural block, *Anesth Analg* 77:488, 1993.
35. Glosten B, Sessler DI, Ostman CG, et al: IV lidocaine does not cause shivering-like tremor or alter thermoregulation, *Reg Anesth* 16:218, 1991.
36. Glosten B: Thermoregulation and regional anesthesia, *Prob Anesth* 8:99, 1994.
37. Grinberg R, Edelist G, Gordon A: Post-operative malignant hyperthermia episodes in patients who received "safe" anaesthetics, *Can Anaesth Soc J* 30:273, 1983.
38. Gronert GA, Milde JH: Variations in onset of porcine malignant hyperthermia, *Anesth Analg* 60:499, 1981.
39. Gronert GA, Theye RA: Halothane-induced porcine malignant hyperthermia: metabolic and hemodynamic changes, *Anesthesiology* 44:36, 1976.
40. Gronert GA, Thompson RL, Onofrio BM: Human malignant hyperthermia: awake episodes and correction by dantrolene, *Anesth Analg* 59:377, 1980.
41. Guffin A, Girard D, Kaplan JA: Shivering following cardiac surgery: Hemodynamic changes and reversal, *J Cardiothorac Vasc Anesth* 1:24, 1987.
42. Hall LW, Woolf N, Bradley JW, et al: Unusual reaction to suxamethonium chloride, *Br Med J* 2:1305, 1966.
43. Hammel HT: Anesthetics and body temperature regulation, *Anesthesiology* 68:833, 1988.
44. Hammel HT: Regulation of internal body temperature, *Ann Rev Physiol* 30:641, 1968.
45. Harrison GG: Porcine malignant hyperthermia. In Britt BA, editor: *International Anesthesiology Clinics: Malignant Hyperthermia,* Boston, 1978, Little, Brown.
46. Hogan K, Couch F, Powers P, Gregg R: A cysteine-for arginine substitution (R614C)

in the human skeletal muscle calcium release channel cosegregates with malignant hyperthermia, *Anesth Analg* 75:441, 1992.
47. Holdcroft A, Hall GM: Redistribution of body heat during anaesthesia, *Anaesthesia* 34:758, 1979.
48. Hynson J, Sessler DI, Glosten B, et al: Thermal balance and tremor patterns during epidural anesthesia, *Anesthesiology* 74:680, 1991.
49. Hynson J, Sessler DI: Intraoperative warming therapies: a comparison of three devices, *J Clin Anesth* 4:194, 1992.
50. Iaizzo PA, Lehmann-Horn F: Anesthetic complications in muscle disorders, 82: 1093, 1995.
51. Iles DE, Lehmann-Horn F, Scherer SW, et al: Localization of the gene encoding the alpha subunits of the L-type voltage dependent calcium channel to chromosome 7q and analysis of the segregation of flanking markers in malignant hyperthermia susceptible families, *Hum Mol Genet* 3:969, 1994.
52. Isaacs H, Badenhoust M: False negative results in contracture testing for malignant hyperthermia, *Anesthesiology* 79:5, 1993.
53. Joris J, Banache M, Bonnet F, et al: Clonidine and ketanserin both are effective treatments for post anesthetic shivering, *Anesthesiology* 79:532, 1993.
54. Just B, Delva E, Camus Y, et al: Prevention of hypothermia by skin-surface warming during liver transplant: Effects of bypass and liver reperfusion, *Anesthesiology* 77: A565, 1992.
55. Kalow W, Britt JA, Terreau ME, et al: Metabolic error of muscle metabolism after recovery from malignant hyperthermia, *Lancet* 2:895, 1970.
56. Kaplan RF: Clinical controversies in malignant hyperthermia susceptibility. In Levitt RC, editor: *Anesthesiology Clinics of North America,* Philadelphia, 1994, WB Saunders.
57. Karan SM, Crowl F, Muldoon SM: Malignant hyperthermia masked by capnographic monitoring, *Anesth Analg* 78:590, 1994.
58. Karan SM, Lojeski EW, Haynes DH, et al: Intravenous lecithin-coated microcrystals of dantrolene are effective in the treatment of malignant hyperthermia: investigation in rats, dogs, and swine, *Anesth Analg* 82: 1996.
59. Keating KE, Quane KA, Manning BM, et al: Detection of a novel RYRI mutation in four malignant hyperthermia pedigrees, *Hum Mol Genet* 3:1855, 1994.
60. Keck PE, Caroff SN, McElroy SL: Neuroleptic malignant syndrome and malignant hyperthermia: end of a controversy? *J Neuropsych* 7:135, 1995.
61. Kelley JD, Prager MC, Sessler DI, et al: Forced air warming minimizes hypothermia during orthotopic liver transplant, *Anesthesiology* 73:A433, 1990.
62. King JD, Denborough MA: Anesthetic-induced malignant hyperpyrexia in children, *J Pediatr* 83:37, 1973.
63. Lai FA, Meissner G: The muscle ryanodine receptor and its intrinsic Ca^{2+} channel activity, *J Bioenerg Biomembr* 21:227, 1989.
64. Larach MG, for the North American Malignant Hyperthermia Group: Standardization of the caffeine halothane muscle contracture test, *Anesth Analg* 69:511, 1989.
65. Larach MG, Rosenberg H, Larach DR, Broennle AM: Prediction of malignant hyperthermia susceptibility by clinical signs, *Anesthesiology* 66:547, 1987.
66. Lee G, Antognini JF, Gronert GA: Complete recovery after prolonged resuscitation and cardiopulmonary bypass for hyperkalemic cardiac arrest, *Anesth Analg* 79:172, 1994.
66a. Lennon RL, Hosking MP, Conover MA, et al: Evaluation of a forced-air system for warming hypothermic postoperative patients, *Anesth Analg* 70:424, 1990.
67. Littleford JA, Patel LR, Bose D: Masseter muscle spasm in children: implications of continuing the triggering anesthetic, *Anesth Analg* 72:151, 1991.
68. Lopez JR, Medina P, Alamo L, et al: Dantrolene sodium is able to reduce the resting ionic [Ca^{2+}] in muscle from humans with malignant hyperthermia, *Muscle Nerve* 10:77, 1987.
69. Lopez M, Ozaki M, Sessler DI, et al: Physiologic response to hyperthermia during epidural anesthesia and combined epidural/enflurane anesthesia in humans, *Anesthesiology* 78:1046, 1993.
70. MacLennan DH: Discordance between phenotype and genotype in malignant hyperthermia, *Curr Opin Neurol* 8:397, 1995.
71. MacLennan DH, Duff C, Zorzato F, et al: Ryanodine receptor gene is a candidate for predisposition to malignant hyperthermia, *Nature* 343:559, 1990.
71a. MacLennan DH, Phillips MS: Malignant hyperthermia, *Science* 256:789, 1992.
72. Mathieu A, Bogosian AJ, Ryan JF: Recrudescence after survival of an initial episode of malignant hyperthermia, *Anesthesiology* 51:454, 1979.
73. McCarthy TV, Healy JM: Localization of the malignant hyperthermia susceptibility locus to human chromosome 19q12-13.2, *Nature* 343:562, 1990.
74. McPherson EW, Yaylor CA Jr: The genetics of malignant hyperthermia: evidence for heterogeneity, *Am J Med Genet* 11:273, 1982.
75. Mickelson JR, Gallant EM, Rempel KM, et al: Effects of the halothane-sensitivity gene on sarcoplasmic reticulum function, *Am J Physiol* 257:C787, 1989.
76. Morison D: Correspondence: placental transfer of dantrolene, *Anesthesiology* 59: 265, 1983.
77. Morris RH: Operating room temperature and the anesthetized paralyzed patient, *Arch Surg* 102:95, 1971.
78. Nelson TE: Halothane effects on human malignant hyperthermia skeletal muscle single calcium-release channels in planar lipid bilayers, *Anesthesiology* 76:588, 1992.
79. Nelson TE: Porcine malignant hyperthermia: critical temperatures for *in vivo* and *in vitro* responses, *Anesthesiology* 73:449, 1990.
80. Ording H: Incidence of malignant hyperthermia in Denmark, *Anesth Analg* 64:700, 1985.
81. Pauswasdr S, Umpornpukd S: Post-anesthesia shivering, *J Med Assoc Thail* 66: 212, 1983.
82. Ponte J, Collett B, Walmsley A: Anaesthetic temperature and shivering in epidural anesthetics, *Acta Anaesthesiol Scand* 30: 584, 1986.
83. Ponte J, Sessler DI: Extradurals and shivering: effects of cold and warm epidural saline injections in volunteers, *Br J Anaesth* 64:731, 1990.
84. Quane KA, Keating KE, Manning BM, et al: Detection of a novel common mutation in the ryanodine receptor gene in malignant hyperthermia; implications for diagnosis and heterogeneity studies, *Hum Mol Genet* 3:471, 1994.
85. Relton JE, Creighton RE, Conn AW, et al: Generalized muscular hypertonicity associated with general anaesthesia: a suggested anaesthetic management, *Can Anaesth Soc J* 14:22, 1967.
86. Ricker K, Moxley RT, Heine R, Lehmann-Horn F: Myotonia fluctuans: a third type of muscle sodium channel disease, *Arch Neurol* 51:1095, 1994.
87. Rosenberg H, Fletcher JE: Masseter muscle rigidity and malignant hyperthermia susceptibility, *Anesth Analg* 65:161, 1986.
88. Rosenberg H, Gronert GA: Intractable cardiac arrest in children given succinylcholine, *Anesthesiology* 77:1054, 1992.
89. Rubiano R, Chang J, Carroll J, et al: Acute rhabdomyolysis following halothane anesthesia without succinylcholine, *Anesthesiology* 67:856, 1987.
90. Rubin A, Zablocki A: Hyperkalemia, verapamil, and dantrolene, *Anesthesiology* 66: 246, 1987.
91. Saltzman L, Kates R, Corke BC, et al: Hyperkalemia and cardiovascular collapse after verapamil and dantrolene administration in swine, *Anesth Analg* 63:473, 1984.
92. Satnick JH: Hyperthermia under anesthesia with regional muscle flaccidity, *Anesthesiology* 30:472, 1969.
93. Schulte-Sasse VU, Dbdrlein HJ, Schumucker I, et al: Should the use of succinylcholine during pediatric anesthesia be reevaluated? *Anesthesiol Reanim* 18:13, 1993.
94. Serfas KD, Bose D, Patel L, et al: Comparison of the segregation of the RYR1 C1840T mutation with segregation of the caffeine/halothane contracture test results for malignant hyperthermia susceptibility in a large manitoba mennonite family, *Anesthesiology* 84:322, 1996.
95. Sessler DI, Hynson J, McQuire J, et al: Thermoregulatory vasoconstriction during isoflurane anesthesia minimally decreases heat loss, *Anesthesiology* 76:670, 1992.
96. Sessler DI, Israel D, Pozos RS, et al: Spontaneous post-anesthetic tremor does not resemble thermoregulatory shivering, *Anesthesiology* 68:843, 1988.
97. Sessler DI, McGuire J, Moayeri A, et al: Isoflurane-induced vasodilation minimally decreases cutaneous heat loss, *Anesthesiology* 74:226, 1991.
98. Sessler DI, Moayeri A, Stoen R, et al: Thermoregulatory vasoconstriction decreases cutaneous heat loss, *Anesthesiology* 73:656, 1990.
99. Sessler DI, Olofsson CI, Rubinstein EH, et al: The thermoregulatory threshold in humans during halothane anesthesia, *Anesthesiology* 68:836, 1988.
100. Sessler DI, Olofsson CI, Rubinstein EH:

The thermoregulatory threshold in humans during halothane anesthesia, *Anesthesiology* 68:836, 1988.
101. Sessler DI: Perianesthetic thermoregulation and heat balance in humans, *FASEB J* 74:638, 1993.
102. Sessler DI: Perioperative temperature regulation, *ASA Refresher Course* 265, 1995.
103. Sessler DI, Ponte J: Shivering during epidural anesthesia, *Anesthesiology* 72: 816, 1990.
104. Sessler DI, Rubinstein E, Eger EI II: Core temperature changes during N_2O fentanyl and halothane/O_2 anesthesia, *Anesthesiology* 67:137, 1987.
105. Sessler DI, Rubinstein E, Moayeri A: Physiologic responses to mild perianesthetic hypothermia in humans, *Anesthesiology* 75:594, 1991.
106. Sessler DI, Sessler AM, Hudson S, et al: Heat loss during surgical skin preparation, *Anesthesiology* 78:1055, 1993.
107. Sessler DI: Sweating threshold during isoflurane anesthesia in humans, *Anesth Analg* 73:300, 1991.
108. Shomer NH, Mickelson JR, Louis CF: Caffeine stimulation of malignant hyperthermia-susceptible sarcoplasmic reticulum Ca^{2+} release channel, *Am J Physiol* 267:C1253, 1994.
109. Sladen RN: Temperature regulation and anesthesia, *Lecture 243, ASA Refresher Course,* 1990.
110. Sorrentino V, Volpe P: Ryanodine receptors: how many, where and why? *TiPS* 14:95, 1993.
111. Stevens JJ: A case of thyrotoxic crisis that mimicked malignant hyperthermia, *Anesthesiology* 59:263, 1983.
112. Stevens W, Cromwell T, Halsey M, et al: The cardiovascular effects of a new inhalational anesthetic, Forane, in human volunteers at constant arterial carbon dioxide tension, *Anesthesiology* 35:8, 1971.
113. Stoen R, Sessler DI: The thermoregulatory threshold is inversely proportional to isoflurane concentration, *Anesthesiology* 72:822, 1990.
114. Stoen R, Sessler DI: The thermoregulatory threshold is inversely proportional to isoflurane concentration, *Anesthesiology* 72: 822, 1990.
115. Sudbrak R, Procaccio V, Klausnitzer M, et al: Mapping of a further malignant hyperthermia susceptibility (MHS) locus to chromosome 3q13.1, *Am J Hum Genet* 56:684, 1995.
116. Topel DG, Bicknell EJ, Preston KS, et al: Porcine stress syndrome, *Mod Veterin Pract* 49:40, 1968.
117. Treves S, Larini F, Menegazzi P, et al: Alteration of intracellular Ca^{2+} transients in COS-7 cells transfected with the cDNA encoding skeletal-muscle ryanodine receptor carrying a mutation associated with malignant hyperthermia, *Bichem J* 301:661, 1994.
118. Van Der Spek AF, Fang WB, Ashton-Miller JA, et al: The effects of succinylcholine in mouth opening, *Anesthesiology* 67:459, 1987.
119. Van der Spek AF, Fang WB, Ashton-Miller JA: Increased masticatory muscle stiffness during limb muscle flaccidity associated with succinylcholine administration, *Anesthesiology* 69:11, 1988.
120. Vita GM, Olckers A, Jedlicka AE, et al: Masseter muscle rigidity associated with glycine[1306]-to-alanine mutation in the adult muscle sodium channel α-subunit gene, *Anesthesiology* 82:1097, 1995.
121. Wagenknecht T, Grassucci R, Frank J, et al: Three-dimensional architecture of the calcium channel/foot structure of sarcoplastic reticulum, *Nature* 338:167, 1989.
122. Wallace AJ, Wooldridge W, Kingston HM, et al: Malignant hyperthermia—a large kindred linked to the RYR1 gene, *Anaesthesia* 51:16, 1996.
123. Walmsley AJ, Giesecke AH, Lipton JM: Contribution of extradural temperature to shivering during extradural anaesthesia, *Br J Anaesth* 58:1130, 1986.
124. Wang JK, Moffitt EA, Rosevear JW: Oxidative phosphorylation in acute hyperthermia, *Anesthesiology* 30:439, 1969.
125. Washington DE, Sessler DI, McQuire J, et al: Painful stimulation minimally increases the thermoregulatory threshold for vasoconstriction during enflurane anesthesia in humans, *Anesthesiology* 77:286, 1992.
126. Washington DE, Sessler DI, Moayeri A, et al: Thermoregulatory response to hyperthermia during isoflurane anesthesia in humans, *J Appl Physiol* 74:82, 1993.
127. Wedel DJ, Gammel SA, Milde JH, Iaizzo PA: Delayed onset of malignant hyperthermia induced by isoflurane and desflurane compared with halothane in susceptible swine, *Anesthesiology* 78:1138, 1993.
128. Weglinski MR, Wedel DJ: Differential diagnosis of hyperthermia during anesthesia and clinical import. In Levitt RC, editor: *Anesthesiology Clinics of North America,* Philadelphia, 1994, WB Saunders.
129. Wingard DW: Malignant hyperthermia-acute stress syndrome of man? In Henschel EO, editor: *Malignant hyperthermia: Current concepts,* East Norwalk, 1977 Appleton-Century-Crofts.

CHAPTER 95

Dental Complications

KIRK L. FRIDRICH
GERALD KIRK

The practice of anesthesia requires the anesthesia provider to work daily in the oral cavity. Airway management involves use of instruments and equipment that can potentially damage teeth, as well as materials or appliances used to restore the dentition. Although all anesthesia providers are aware of the potential for dental injury, few have more than a superficial knowledge of oral pathology and prosthetic restorations. This chapter will provide the anesthesia provider with a basic understanding of normal and abnormal oral structures to aid in the prevention of dental injury.

SCOPE OF DENTAL INJURY IN ANESTHESIA

Dental damage is the most commonly reported complication of general anesthesia. A survey of U.S. teaching hospitals published in 1986 indicated that approximately 1 dental injury per 1000 anesthetics occurs involving oral endotracheal intubation.[28] We have no reason to believe that the situation is much (if any) better today.

Retrospective studies conducted separately at two university hospitals revealed similar complication rates.[13,28] Many of these injuries occur during laryngoscopy. Injuries also occur during emergence from anesthesia when patients bite down on oropharyngeal airways or grind their teeth. More than 50% of these incidents are reported to occur during intubations later classed as difficult or emergent, and most involve teeth that were diseased or previously restored.[8,28]

Over a seven-year period, the Harvard Risk Management Foundation found that dental damage was the most frequent injury associated with malpractice claims (i.e., 29% of case files reviewed).[22] An 11-year review of malpractice claims in Washington state also indicated that dental damage was the most commonly reported complication. Malpractice claim data most likely underrepresent the incidence of dental damage because anesthesia providers may choose to pay for the damages themselves, rather than report the problem to their insurer.[35] The current trend toward more stringent risk management and quality assurance programs may help provide more complete data on the incidence of anesthesia-related dental injury (see Chapter 98).

Although dental injury is neither life threatening (although aspiration of a broken tooth can lead to lung abscess and major problems) nor as costly as more catastrophic mishaps, it represents a major source of patient dissatisfaction with anesthetic care. At times anesthetic injuries to teeth may be unavoidable, but relevant dental knowledge can aid in reducing patient inconvenience.

BASIC DENTAL ANATOMY

The tooth is divided into two parts, crown and root, each consisting of three layers.[38] The hard outer layer is enamel, which is brittle if not properly supported by dentin. Dentin is the second layer, yellowish in color, which provides the basic structure of the tooth. The innermost layer consists of blood vessels and nerve tissue and is known as the pulp.[10]

Cementum is found on the root surface as the outermost layer and is softer than enamel.[5]

The periodontium is a collective term for the structures that support the tooth. Its components include alveolar bone, the periodontal membrane that anchors the tooth from cementum to bone, and the overlying, protective gingiva.[9]

DEVELOPMENT OF DENTITION AND PEDIATRIC CONSIDERATIONS

Teeth are the only structures in the body replaced entirely during a person's life span. From birth to 6 months of age, infants are edentulous, but unerupted tooth buds lying below the mucosa of the gums are at risk for damage by airway manipulation during this period. Laryngoscopy and prolonged intubation have been implicated in developmental defects of primary dentition in infants. Relative mandibular hypoplasia in addition to macroglossia in neonates and infants makes laryngoscopy more difficult.[19] Excessive pressure of a laryngoscope blade or an oral airway on the alveolar ridge has been suggested as a cause of damage to developing dentition. This theory is supported by data that show a greater incidence of defects in the dentition of intubated and mechanically ventilated infants than in nonintubated infants. Anterior maxillary teeth are most commonly involved, further implicating laryngoscopy as a cause of injury. Defects described include enamel hypoplasia and angulation of the root or crown of a tooth (dilaceration).[2,6,29,32]

Eruption of the 20 primary or deciduous teeth begins at 6 months and is complete by 2 years of age. Because of their slender root structures, these teeth are prone to fracture during laryngoscopy. Although they are not permanent structures, premature loss of deciduous teeth can cause abnormal development and eruption of secondary teeth.[18,31]

At approximately 5 years of age, a transition phase begins in which primary teeth are lost and are replaced by permanent or adult teeth. This mixed dentition period continues until approximately 11 years of age. Primary teeth are shed by progressive resorption of their underlying root structure. Eventually the crown is held in place only by soft tissue attachment. This is followed by eruption of the adult teeth into the oral cavity.[20] Dental accidents in children occur most frequently during the mixed dentition phase. Children of this age group should be questioned about loose teeth, if possible; if this is not possible, palpation may identify mobile teeth. **Teeth with more than several millimeters of lingual-labial movement should be considered for extraction to prevent the risk of aspiration.**[18] Loose deciduous teeth can be removed by grasping the tooth with a gauze pad or forceps and pulling it out with a twisting motion. This can be performed either preoperatively or after induction of anesthesia (but before laryngoscopy). To prevent aspiration, a pack should be placed in the mouth whenever a tooth is to be removed during general anesthesia.[15] The removed tooth will consist only of a crown, as a result of root resorption. Parents should be informed if a child's tooth is to be removed intraoperatively, and the tooth should be saved and given to the child postoperatively (remember the tooth fairy).

PERMANENT OR ADULT TEETH

The primary teeth are replaced by permanent teeth that are larger in size. The maxilla and mandible enlarge to allow space for them. Full adult dentition consists of 32 teeth, but for many individuals, some or all of the third molars (wisdom teeth) erupt late or never appear in the oral cavity. There are various schemes for numbering teeth that are useful for noting in the medical record. One of the simplest is to divide the dental arches into four quadrants and number from the midline (Fig. 95-1). However, many dentists use the progressive numbering method shown in Fig. 95-2. Each tooth is numbered from 1 to 32, beginning with the upper-right third molar.[24] An alternative to numbering teeth is to use name and position to identify teeth (e.g., upper-left central incisor) (Fig. 95-3). Whatever method is chosen, it is important for the anesthesiologist to precisely identify and chart diseased or missing teeth.

DENTAL CARIES AND PERIODONTAL DISEASE

Because many injuries occur to diseased teeth, a basic summary of dental disease should be considered. The most common disease affecting the tooth is dental caries. Bacteria ad-

	Right								Left							
MAXILLA	8	7	6	5	4	3	2	1	1	2	3	4	5	6	7	8
MANDIBLE	8	7	6	5	4	3	2	1	1	2	3	4	5	6	7	8

Fig. 95-1. Method of numbering teeth.

	Right								Left							
MAXILLA	1	2	3	4	5	6	7	8	9	10	11	12	13	14	15	16
MANDIBLE	32	31	30	29	28	27	26	25	24	23	22	21	20	19	18	17

Fig. 95-2. Alternative method for numbering teeth.

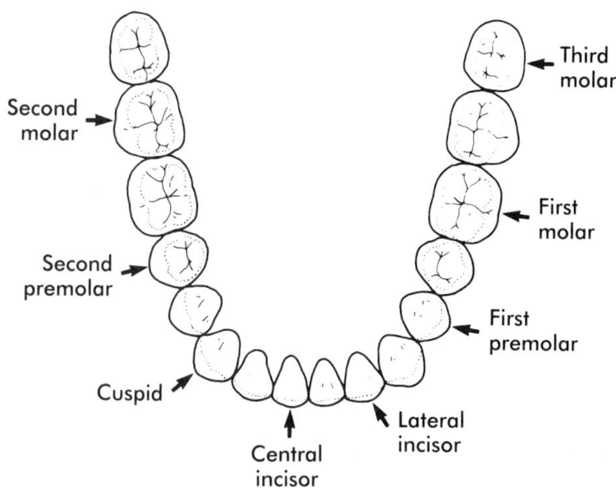

Fig. 95-3. Dental nomenclature. (Modified from Dornette WHL: Care of the teeth during endoscopy and anesthesia. In Dornette WHL, editor: *Legal aspects of anesthesia,* Clinical Anesthesia Series, vol 8, Series, Philadelphia, 1972, FA Davis.)

here to the tooth surface and produce acids that decalcify and/or dissolve the enamel to involve the dentin and eventually undermine the enamel.[33] Treatment of caries involves removal of the decayed portion of the tooth and the placement of a dental restoration (filling).[4,10] The most common restoration is an amalgam or silver filling. Composite or tooth-colored restorations are commonly used for anterior teeth. Restorations do not usually strengthen the tooth and likely weaken it. Gingival (gum-line) caries and large anterior restorations render teeth prone to breakage. Advanced dental caries involving the pulp requires endodontic (root canal) therapy. Replacement of the vascular and nerve components (pulp) with gutta percha (a rubber-like material) desiccates the tooth leaving a brittle remnant that often requires a full-coverage crown for support.

Periodontal disease is a painless, irreversible dissolution of supporting dental structures, including alveolar bone and periodontal ligaments.[9] The etiologic agents are proteolytic bacteria. Tooth loss after 30 years of age is most often caused by periodontal disease; in fact, the latter is probably the most widespread chronic human disease in the world. Treatment is limited to stabilizing or slowing the disease via meticulous oral hygiene, mechanical curettage, or surgery. **Most teeth avulsed in adults during general anesthesia exhibit advanced periodontal disease before loss.** Preoperative examination that reveals receding gingiva, tooth mobility, and calculus deposits (tartar) should alert the anesthesia provider to the risk of dental damage.[31]

FRACTURE, SUBLUXATION, AND AVULSION

Traumatic fracture of teeth may involve enamel, dentin, pulp, or root structure. The prudent anesthesia provider who observes or is consulted about the possibility of such a fracture preoperatively should obtain dental consultation before proceeding with elective anesthesia. Enamel fracture usually requires only smoothing of sharp edges or bonding with a tooth-colored material.[4] Fracture into the yellowish dentin layer usually gives rise to thermal sensitivity. This requires more extensive restoration.[10] Fracture into the pulp is very painful and may ultimately require an endodontic (root canal) procedure and a full-coverage restoration, such as a crown, for support.[12,34] Root fracture is difficult to detect and is invariably associated with compromised periodontal support; treatment often involves extraction of the tooth.[1]

Subluxation is partial displacement of a tooth within the alveolar bone. Treatment involves replacement of the tooth to its original position,[1] but dental consultation is advised because stabilization and endodontic therapy may be required.

Avulsion is complete removal of a tooth from its socket. Maxillary incisors are at greatest risk for avulsion, especially those with advanced periodontal disease. **The anesthesia provider must make all reasonable effort to locate any avulsed tooth and/or fragments as rapidly as practical to prevent aspiration.**[37] Radiographs of the head, neck, chest, and abdomen may be necessary to locate the tooth. Because aspiration of a tooth can cause lung abscess, bronchoscopy or even thoracotomy may occasionally be necessary to retrieve the tooth.[18] The nasopharynx should also be considered as a potential site. Once the tooth is located and retrieved, it should be considered a candidate for possible reimplantation. It should be held only by the crown, avoiding contact with the root. Any periodontal ligament remaining on the root may enhance reimplantation. Gentle rinsing with normal saline may be used to remove debris.[25] Returning the tooth to the socket within 20 minutes is associated with the best prognosis.[1]

If not reimplanted immediately, the tooth should be saved in a saline-moistened gauze. Although such a reimplanted tooth may be relatively stable, the anesthesia provider should weigh the potential risk for repeated avulsion and possible aspiration during patient emergence and recovery from anesthesia against the potential benefits of salvaging a tooth. If reimplanted, dental consultation should be obtained for stabilization splinting.

PROSTHETIC RESTORATIONS

Replacement of a missing tooth or teeth in the dental arch may involve one of four basic techniques[10]: (1) removable partial denture; (2) conventional fixed bridgework; (3) acid-etched or butterfly bridge; or (4) osseointegrated implants (Fig. 95-4).

The removable partial denture has retaining hooks anchoring the replacement teeth to the natural dentition. It can be readily removed before induction of anesthesia. Damage to abutment teeth may render the entire prosthesis unusable.[31]

Fixed bridgework is a combination of cemented crowns on adjacent remaining teeth, with a tooth replacement called a "pontic" soldered between. Although "permanently" cemented, the conventional bridge can be dislodged, especially those placed anteriorly or if recurrent decay has undermined the abutment teeth. If dislodged, retrieval is

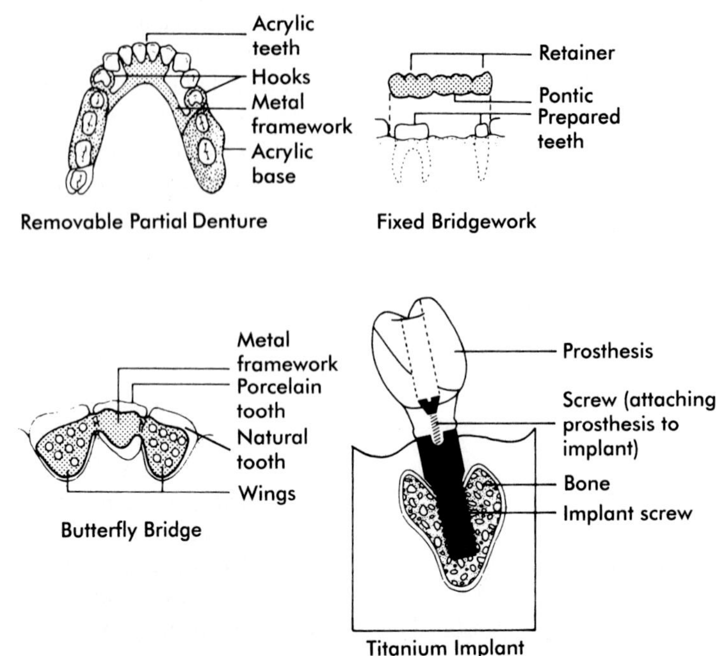

Fig. 95-4. Types of dental restorations. (Modified from Clokie C, Metcalf I, Holland A: Dental trauma in anaesthesia, *Can J Anaesth* 36:675, 1989.)

mandatory, and should be followed by protection of exposed abutments with petroleum jelly. The crown or bridge can be recemented postoperatively.

The acid-etched (butterfly) bridge has become increasingly popular for replacement of teeth, especially in the anterior region of the mouth. Primary advantages include minimal damage to adjacent teeth and ease of fabrication.[21,27,36] The wings on the bridge are bonded to adjacent teeth and may be easily dislodged; therefore the acid-etched bridge lacks the inherent strength of a conventional fixed bridge.[10] Recognition of its presence permits a heavy suture to be tied around one of the wings if desired, to aid in retrieval if the bridge is accidentally dislodged.[10]

Osseointegrated titanium implants can be used to replace single or multiple missing teeth or an entire dental arch. Because the bone-implant interface is inherently strong,[7] fracture and dislodgement will likely occur at the prosthetic-implant interface or within the prosthesis itself. Once again, recognition of the presence of an implant is important. If a difficult intubation is anticipated, this expensive appliance can be unscrewed by a dentist and replaced postoperatively.

DENTURES

Complete dentures are commonly used to replace entire dental arches in the edentulous patient. They are processed acrylic bases with plastic or porcelain teeth and are brittle and prone to fracture.[31]

As a general rule, they should be removed preoperatively and placed in water; potential airway obstruction can occur during anesthetic induction because such dentures are easily removable and not secure within the mouth. Sensitive patients occasionally conceal the fact that they wear dentures. If excessive mandibular atrophy has occurred, a good mask seal may be difficult to attain without the dentures to support the perioral musculature and maintain the vertical dimension of the face. In this instance, the dentures may be left in place during induction to enhance facial contours and facilitate mask fit, keeping in mind their inherent instability.[31] Before intubation, the dentures should be removed. With excessive alveolar bone loss, mandibular fractures have occurred during vigorous airway management.[18]

COSMETIC RESTORATIONS

Dental bonding using porcelain laminate veneer is becoming increasingly popular.[23] Natural enamel thickness is first reduced by approximately one half, after which a thin (0.70 mm) porcelain laminate veneer is bonded to the tooth.[10,23] This restoration is not prone to dislodgement but may be chipped, cracked, or crazed.[21] Special care to avoid damaging such restorations is important because they are typically found on the maxillary anterior incisors and in patients who are very much concerned about appearance. Porcelain-fused metal crowns are also found in aesthetic-oriented patients. Although "permanently cemented," they are prone to the same types of damage as porcelain laminate veneer.

ORAL APPLIANCES

Numerous oral appliances may be encountered by the anesthesia provider. Most of these appliances are seen during the period of mixed dentition and in adolescence,[31] although adult orthodontia is increasing and related appliances are seen in this population as well. Appliances include braces for correcting malocclusion, space maintainers to retain spaces caused by premature loss of primary teeth, and devices designed to prevent thumb-sucking or tongue-thrusting.[31] Such appliances may be fixed or removable and should be evaluated preoperatively. Removable appliances may become obstructive hazards and should be removed before induction of general anesthesia.[31] Fixed appliances may have small hooks with elastics (rubber bands) attached. Elastics are easily broken and aspirated and should be removed before induction of anesthesia.[24]

DISLOCATION OF THE MANDIBLE

Dislocation of the lower jaw during anesthesia has been reported.[36] This can occur if the jaw is opened widely for laryngoscopy in the anesthetized, relaxed patient. The temporomandibular joint is the articulation of the mandibular condyloid process with the glenoid fossa of the temporal bone. Usually, the condyloid process moves somewhat forward on opening the mouth but is limited by the articular eminence of the temporal bone. Dislocation results from subluxation of the condylar process anterior to the articular eminence (Fig. 95-5). The dislocation may not be apparent when the patient is anesthetized but may manifest first during recovery as temporal pain, and by the fact that the patient will be unable to bring the upper and lower teeth together. Treatment of the dislocation after anesthesia involves: (1) placing the patient's head against a firm surface when standing at the side of the supine patient; (2) placing the thumbs of each hand in the mouth over the mandibular molars with the fingers of each hand curling under the mandible; and (3) applying downward pressure with the thumbs to slip the condyle inferior to the eminence and into the fossa (Fig. 95-5). A bite-block should be put in place to prevent the jaws from snapping together on the treater's thumbs.[24,31,36]

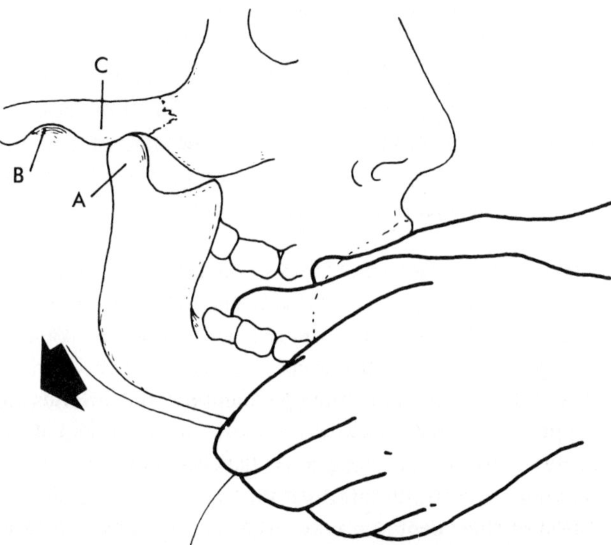

Fig. 95-5. Dislocated mandible. The mandibular condyle **(A)**, which normally lies in the glenoid fossa **(B)**, has moved anterior to the articular eminence **(C)**. Reduction requires displacing the mandible inferiorly and posteriorly (large arrow) to restore the condyloid process to the fossa. (Modified from Klein SL: A dental primer for anesthesiologists, *Anesthesiol Rev* 3:25, 1980; Sosis M, Lazar S: Jaw dislocation during general anesthesia, *Can J Anaesth* 34:407, 1987.)

PREVENTION OF DENTAL INJURY

Proper evaluation includes evaluation of the patient's dental condition. **Decay, state of repair, mobility, and prosthetic restorations should be mentioned in the preanesthetic note. Dental consultation should be obtained preoperatively in elective cases in which risk of dental injury is believed to be high.** Each patient should be informed that dental injury is a known but infrequent complication of anesthesia. Patients should be warned if they are at greater risk for damage because of poor dentition or repair. Accurate documentation of preexistng dental problems and an informed patient may aid in prevention of postoperative medicolegal difficulties.[19,28]

Attention should be paid to factors known to make laryngoscopy more difficult, such as retrognathia, protruding maxillary incisors, and conditions limiting neck extension and/or mouth opening.[31] Proper technique for laryngoscopy and intubation has been described elsewhere. Care should be taken to avoid any contact between the laryngoscope blade and the anterior maxillary teeth during laryngoscopy. It has been suggested that increased use of nondepolarizing muscle relaxants instead of succinylcholine may result in less complete relaxation for intubation and thus greater risk for dental damage.[8] Alternative techniques, such as regional anesthesia or nasal fiberoptic intubation, may be considered if the patient is believed to be at high risk for dental damage,[19] but intubation should not be avoided if it is necessary for patient safety.[17] Poor dentition alone is generally not considered sufficient indication alone to perform fiberoptic intubation.

Attempts have been made to modify the laryngoscope blade in order to prevent dental trauma, but these modifications have not gained widespread use in practice. Modifications proposed for the Macintosh blade include replacing the posterior half of the flange with rubber[30] or attaching a strip of polyfoam along the existing flange.[26]

Tooth protectors also have been advocated to prevent dental trauma during laryngoscopy and anesthesia.[28] One group reported that prefabricated tooth guards unfortunately made laryngoscopy and intubation more difficult, especially for inexperienced trainees.[3] Because they are made of thinner materials, custom-made plastic guards may be better than generic rubber tooth guards.[13] The disadvantage is that they require dental laboratory fabrication. These guards may protect enamel from being chipped or crazed, but they do

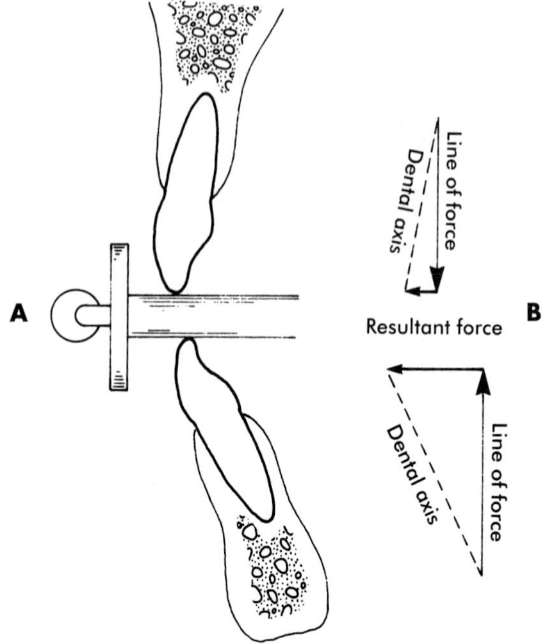

Fig. 95-6. **A**, Oral airway used as a bite-block distributes force along the anterior teeth of the dental arch. **B**, Axes of the incisors are not aligned with the applied biting force, so the resultant anterior force places these teeth at risk for fracture or avulsion. (Modified from Dornette WHL, Hughes BH: Care of the teeth during anesthesia, *Anesth Analg* 38:206, 1959.)

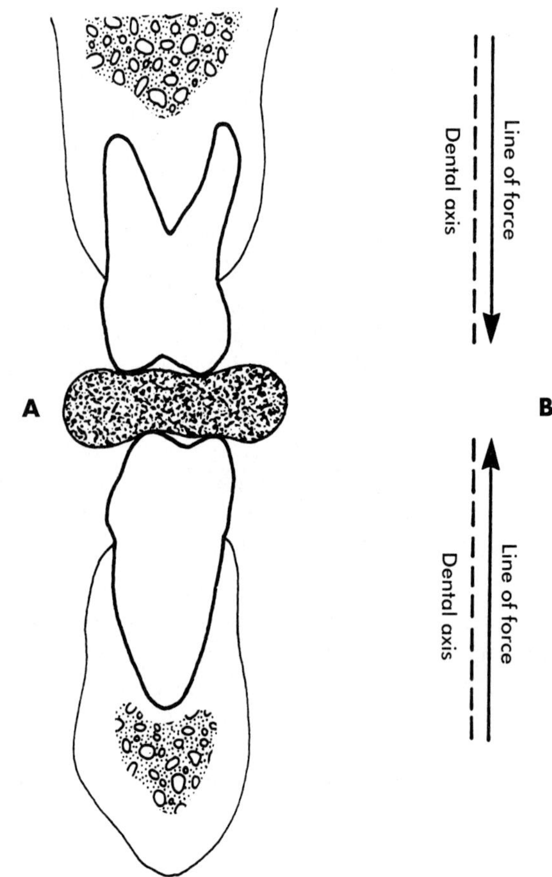

Fig. 95-7. **A**, Adhesive tape–covered gauze mouth prop is used as a bite-block over the molar and premolar teeth. **B**, The dental axes and biting force are aligned and thus the teeth are not subject to forces that predispose to displacement or avulsion. (Modified from Dornette WHL, Hughes BH: Care of the teeth during anesthesia, *Anesth Analg* 38:206, 1959.)

not protect against tooth avulsion because they are not sufficiently rigid enough to distribute pressure from the laryngoscope blade.[16]

Most damage to teeth during the recovery phase of anesthesia is caused by using oropharyngeal airways as bite-blocks. The oral airway distributes bite force along the anterior teeth of the dental arch. The incisor and cuspid teeth are thin, monorooted, and not well aligned with the biting forces (Fig. 95-6). If a patient bites down on an oral airway, fracture or avulsion of the anterior teeth is possible (especially if they are mobile or diseased). The molar and premolar teeth, in contrast, are multirooted, designed for grinding food, and have dental axes aligned with the biting force (Fig. 95-7).[14,15] An adhesive tape–covered gauze mouth prop placed posteriorly over the sturdy molars and premolars makes a safer bite-block if one is needed to prevent compression of an endotracheal tube during emergence (Fig. 95-8).[15,19] Nasopharyngeal airways are an alternative to the oral airway for overcoming airway obstruction, but these airways carry with them the risk of major bleeding from that highly vascular region.

CONCLUSION

Ability to recognize potential dental problems preoperatively is important in preventing dental injury during administration of anesthesia. Appropriate knowledge of anesthesia-related dental risk, as well as careful attention to details, can permit the anesthesia provider to reduce the risk of these complications.

When a dental complication occurs, the anesthesia provider should make a notation in the record detailing the injury. Dental consultation should be obtained as soon as possible, and the patient should be informed of the complication.[39] Decisions concerning payment for such injuries are best guided by risk-management policies of individual insurance carriers and institutions. Patients with poor dentition who are tactfully informed that specific further deterioration of their dentition may result during anesthesia and surgery and that care will be taken to prevent or treat injuries will likely be reasonable if, indeed, dental damage does occur.

A

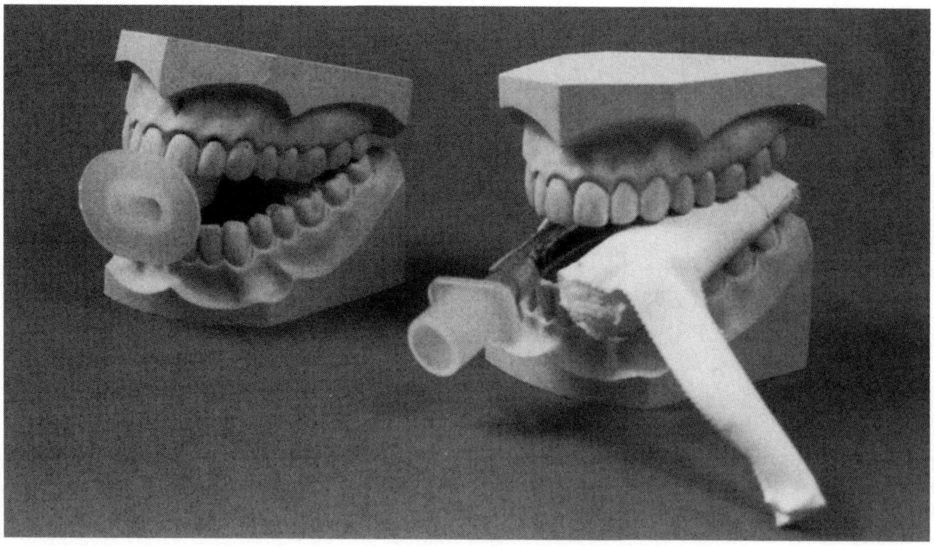

B

Fig. 95-8. **A**, Oral airway used as a bite-block is undesirable (see Fig. 95-6 and text). **B**, Adhesive tape–covered gauze mouth prop placed posteriorly distributes the biting force over the sturdy molars and premolars but still prevents compression of the endotracheal tube during emergence. (Modified from Dornette WHL, Hughes BH: Care of the teeth during anesthesia, *Anesth Analg* 38:206, 1959.)

KEY POINTS

- Dental damage is a common, nonlethal, but definitely irritating problem both for the anesthesia provider and the patient. Although anesthesia providers seldom focus much attention on dentition, they should consider that instruments and equipment can potentially damage teeth as well as the materials and appliances used to restore them.
- Understanding the nature of partial removable versus nonremovable bridgework is important in anticipating problems associated with damage to these appliances during anesthesia.
- Unrecognized mandibular dislocation during and especially immediately following anesthesia can occur. This has resulted in allegations that it resulted in severe temporomandibular joint problems later on.
- Laryngoscopy is made more difficult by retrognathia, protruding maxillary incisors, and any condition that limits neck extension and mouth opening.
- Modifications to the laryngoscopic blade may help prevent dental trauma, but prefabricated tooth guards probably make laryngoscopy and intubation more difficult.
- When a tooth is noted to be damaged or broken off, the anesthesia provider should make reasonable attempts to find all the pieces, including those that may have been swallowed or aspirated, including use of x-ray and bronchoscopy if indicated. When such a complication occurs, complete and full disclosure in the medical record and to the patient and/or family should take place. Dental consultation should then also occur as well as risk-management decisions regarding patient compensation.

KEY REFERENCES

Andreason JO: *Traumatic injuries of the teeth,* Toronto, 1981, WB Saunders.

Burton JF, Baker AB: Dental damage during anaesthesia and surgery, *Anaesth Inten Care* 15:262, 1987.

Clokie C, Metcalf I, Holland A: Dental trauma in anaesthesia, *Can J Anaesth* 36:675, 1989.

Gallagher DM, Milliken RA: Dental considerations in clinical anesthesia, *Anesthesiol Rev* 6:30, 1979.

Lockhart PB, Feldbau EV, Gabel RA, et al: Dental complications during and after tracheal intubation, *J Am Dent Assoc* 112:480, 1986.

Rosenberg MB: Anesthesia-induced dental injury, *Int Anesthesiol Clin* 27:120, 1989.

REFERENCES

1. Andreason JO: *Traumatic injuries of the teeth,* Toronto, 1981, WB Saunders.
2. Angelos GM, Smith DR, Jorgenson R, et al: Oral complications associated with neonatal oral tracheal intubation: a critical review, *Pediatr Dent* 11:133, 1989.
3. Aromaa U, Pesonen P, Linko K, et al: Difficulties with tooth protectors in endotracheal intubation, *Acta Anesthesiol Scand* 32:304, 1988.
4. Baum L, Lund MR, Phillips RW: *Textbook of operative dentistry,* Toronto, 1981, WB Saunders.
5. Bhaskar SN: *Oral histology and embryology,* St Louis, 1976, CV Mosby.
6. Boice JB, Krous HF, Foley JM: Gingival and dental complications of orotracheal intubation, *JAMA* 236:957, 1976.
7. Branemark PI: *Tissue integrated prostheses,* Chicago, 1985, Quintessence.
8. Burton JF, Baker AB: Dental damage during anaesthesia and surgery, *Anaesth Inten Care* 15:262, 1987.
9. Carranza FA: The tissues of the periodontium; the gingiva. In Carranza FA, editor: *Glickman's clinical periodontology,* Toronto, 1984, WB Saunders.
10. Clokie C, Metcalf I, Holland A: Dental trauma in anaesthesia, *Can J Anaesth* 36: 675, 1989.
11. Cohen MM, Duncan PG, Pope WD, et al: A survey of 112,000 anesthetics at one teaching hospital (1975-83), *Can J Anaesth* 33:22, 1986.
12. Cohen RC, Burns RC: *Pathways to the pulp,* St Louis, 1980, CV Mosby.
13. Davis FO, DeFreece AB, Shroff FB: Custom-made plastic guards for tooth protection during endoscopy and orotracheal intubation, *Anesth Analg* 50:203, 1971.
14. Dornette WHL: Care of the teeth during endoscopy and anesthesia. In Dornette WHL, editor: *Legal aspects of anesthesia,* Clinical Anesthesia Series, vol 8, Philadelphia, 1972, FA Davis.
15. Dornette WHL, Hughes BH: Care of the teeth during anesthesia, *Anesth Analg* 38: 206, 1959.
16. Dunnett IA, Goodman NW, Hall CR, et al: Anaesthesia, teeth, and litigation (letter), *Lancet* 2:1400, 1987.
17. Fisher TL: Teeth-and the anesthetist, *Can Med Assoc J* 106:602, 1972.
18. Gallagher DM, Milliken RA: Dental considerations in clinical anesthesia, *Anesthesiol Rev* 6:30, 1979.
19. Garber JG, Herlich A: Dental complications. In Orkin F, Cooperman L, editors: *Complications in anesthesiology,* Philadelphia, 1983, JB Lippincott.
20. Gorski DW, Rao TL, Hartman J: Deciduous teeth and root resorption, *Anesthesiol Rev* 9:37, 1982.
21. Highton R, Caputo AA: A photoelastic study of stress on porcelain laminate preparations, *J Prosthet Dent* 58:157, 1987.
22. Holzer JF: Current concepts in risk management, *Anesthesiol Clin North Am* 22:91, 1984.
23. Jordan RE: *Esthetic composite bonding: techniques and materials,* Toronto, 1986, BC Decker.
24. Klein SL: A dental primer for anesthesiologists, *Anesthesiol Rev* 3:25, 1980.
25. Lind GL, Spiegel EH, Munson ES: Treatment of traumatic tooth avulsion, *Anesth Analg* 61:469, 1982.
26. Lisman SR, Shephard NJ, Rosenberg MB: A modified laryngoscope blade for dental protection, *Anesthesiology* 55:190, 1981.
27. Livadits GJ: A chemical etching system creating micromechanical retention in resin bonded retainers, *J Prosthet Dent* 56:181, 1986.
28. Lockhart PB, Feldbau EV, Gabel RA, et al: Dental complications during and after tracheal intubation, *J Am Dent Assoc* 112:480, 1986.
29. Moylan FM, Sedlin EB, Shannon DC, et al: Defective primary dentition in survivors of neonatal mechanical ventilation, *J Pediatr* 1:106, 1980.
30. Nique TA, Bennett CR, Altop H: Laryngoscope modification to avoid perioral trauma due to laryngoscopy, *Anesth Prog* 2:47, 1982.
31. Rosenberg MB: Anesthesia-induced dental injury, *Int Anesthesiol Clin* 27:120, 1989.
32. Seow KW, Brown JP, Tudehope DI, et al: Developmental defects in the primary dentition of low birthweight infants: adverse effects of laryngoscopy and prolonged endotracheal intubation, *Pediatr Dent* 6:28, 1984.
33. Shafer WG, Nine MK, Levy BM: *Oral pathology,* Toronto, 1983, WB Saunders.
34. Shillingburg T, Hobo S, Whitsett LD: *Fundamentals of fixed prosthedontics,* Chicago, 1981, Quintessence.
35. Solazzi RW, Ward RJ: The spectrum of medical liability cases, *Int Anesthesiol Clin* 22:43, 1984.
36. Sosis M, Lazar S: Jaw dislocation during general anesthesia, *Can J Anaesth* 34:407, 1987.
37. Wasmuth CE: Legal problems in the practice of anesthesiology: problem overview, *Int Anesthesiol Clin* 11;1, 1973.
38. Wheeler RC: *Dental anatomy, physiology and occlusion,* Toronto, 1974, JB Lippincott.
39. Wright RB, Manfield FF: Damage to teeth during the administration of general anaesthesia, *Anesth Analg* 53:405, 1974.

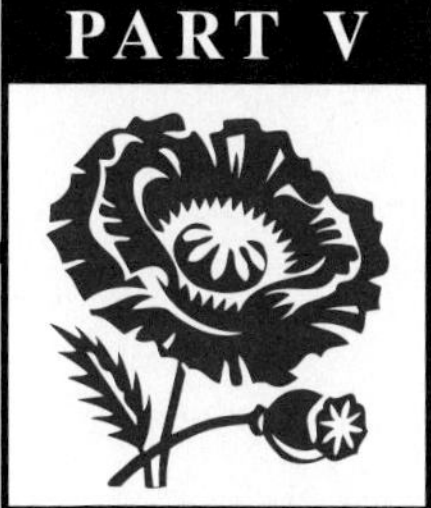

Practical Issues for the Anesthesiologist

CHAPTER 96

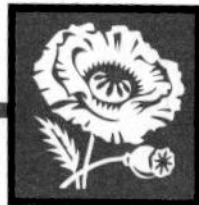

Legal Issues in Anesthesiology

JOHN H. TINKER
WILLIAM W. HESSON

Doctors cut, burn, and torture the sick, and then demand an undeserved fee for such service.

Heraclitus, circa 500 BC

SITUATIONS IN WHICH A LAWSUIT MAY RESULT

Although there are always exceptions, it is the case that several situations exist in which a lawsuit should be considered a reasonable possibility by caregivers. One reason the possibility of litigation exists is that the field of medicine has never provided performance bonding for what is done medically. A new car comes with a new car warranty. If problems develop with the car within the limits and conditions of a (very carefully written) warranty, the purchaser is entitled to return it and have it fixed free. When, for example, a total hip replacement is performed on a patient, the physician never tells the patient, "If it breaks, falls out, or becomes infected within 1 year, come back and we'll fix it for free."

The near-universal rejection of performance bonding by physicians may lead naturally to the scenario that **when results of surgery are poor, patients can become angry to the point of undertaking litigation.** The patient may indeed have been injured, permanently or temporarily, or may have died. In describing anesthetic and surgical procedures to patients and/or their families, anesthesia and surgical caregivers are certainly not motivated to present the situation in starkly negative terms. The complications a patient might suffer are (hopefully) presented, but in a relatively optimistic light, except for the highest-risk situations. Physicians perhaps delude themselves into thinking that the point is to avoid scaring patients, but for whatever reasons, this upbeat manner is generally used in presenting the case for anesthesia or surgery to patients. There is nothing inherently wrong with this approach, but physicians should not be surprised, after a poor result, if patients become angry and/or disappointed. Expectations of excellence have been created. Indeed, our organized medical associations continually extol the preeminence of American medical care. When something goes awry, some patients naturally assume that somebody was negligent either by omission or commission. This same view is held by the consumer when purchasing goods. The consumer may be filled with righteous indignation when something is not as advertised, but at least there often is a warranty to fall back upon. In view of all this, anesthesiologists and other caregivers should understand why patients may seek legal remedies when poor results occur.

Not only can legal action be expected if poor results occur during or after anesthesia or surgery, but there is also the same possibility after unexpected results. After total hip surgery, a patient may be able to walk fairly well without pain, but no one may have mentioned that there might be some numbness down the leg. A patient who has had a successful arthroscopy only to have an ulnar nerve injury can be expected to become angry and perhaps litigious. These unexpected results of surgery or anesthesia do not necessarily need to be related to the site of operation. The patient who wakes up with a broken tooth is a good example of thissituation.

Although it is accepted in medicine that complications do indeed occur, it is also true as practitioners gain experience, over time, complication rates may decrease. Paradoxically, as a particular procedure becomes associated with lower and lower complication rates, the patient who experiences a major complication may be more likely to assume negligence precisely because of the known low complication rate. Although physicians may believe this is unrealistic, they should remember that, although medicine has been traditionally quick to take credit for decreased complication rates and excellent outcomes, when complications occur, a common attitude is: "it just happened." One result of this attitude can be litigation, and the practitioner should be prepared, whenever there are poor results or complications—expected or unexpected, rare or not rare, occurring to informed or less-than-well-informed patients—for this eventuality.

INFORMED CONSENT

One might ask, "How can anyone who is not board certified in anesthesiology give completely informed consent for any anesthesiologic procedure?" This question has troubled many practitioners, the concern arises because the phrase "informed consent" is a short-hand description of the practitioner's potential liability for negligent nondisclosure. The *duty* of the clinician is clear—it is *process* and *disclosure.* The anesthesia provider must present in clear detail to the patient the anesthetic procedures to be performed and then proceed with an *interactive process* whereby the patient and the anesthesia provider agree that all relevant questions have been addressed. Medical jargon should be avoided and the procedure should be explained in lay terms; realistically possible complications should be delineated as objectively as possible, including ones of most concern to the patient and family with cogent explanations of relative risks, insofar as they are known. In many states, there is a specific obligation to inform the patient that death is a possibility. The often-stated idea that "informing a patient that death is a possibility will unduly scare the patient" is not supportable. Neither is the occasionally heard statement, "I'm required to tell you that you might die during anesthesia, but the risk of that is much, much lower than the risk you took driving to the hospital." That statement is simply a misleading perversion of the requirement that an honest discussion of this possibility be carried out.

Informed consent is a process which should involve a truly compassionate interaction between physician and patient, and as such, it is a powerful tool in the care of patients, not just as a part of risk management strategies. In our experience, once practitioners genuinely accept informed consent as a process—not some document or some obstacle or governmental interference—patient care improves.

LEGAL EXPOSURE FOR THE ANESTHESIA CARE PROVIDER

Anesthesia practitioners can be sued for abandonment or battery, but usually are sued for negligence. Abandonment can occur in the practice of anesthesia. The caregiver who can be shown to have left the operating room without being relieved by another qualified person can be sued for abandonment. In the case of a longer-term relationship, such as in a pain clinic, the physician who intends to relinquish a patient's care may do so at any time but must give reasonable notice and should make at least a reasonable attempt to provide an appropriate referral.

It is also possible to sue a physician for battery. Battery is unauthorized touching of a person, and, in the context of anesthesia and surgery, the allegation usually results when a procedure is performed without appropriate consent. A breast biopsy that turns into a mastectomy when consent had only been given for the former may be a battery. A patient who signs an operative consent but is under the influence of premedicants might make this allegation. If consent is given only for the removal of a gallbladder but the surgeon proceeds to do an unrelated procedure, particularly an elective one, this may be considered battery. Adult Jehovah's Witnesses who preoperatively refuse the transfusion of blood but then are transfused anyway may allege battery.

Although a patient may claim abandonment or battery, by far the most common allegation in a lawsuit for malpractice is *negligence.* This allegation will be explored in considerable detail, particularly the evidence required by a plaintiff to make a negligence claim. Even if a patient's case has elements of abandonment and/or battery, the lawsuit will most likely be based on proving negligence.

Early Activity by the Plaintiff

A former patient, now a possible plaintiff, who believes he or she has been injured by a medical caregiver, begins by contacting an attorney. The latter will listen carefully to the case presented by the potential plaintiff. Anesthesia caregivers should understand what is at stake in initial conferences between potential plaintiffs and attorneys. In most cases, the attorney must decide either to take the case on a contingency basis or decline. The contingency fee basis on which most attorneys operate provides that approximately one third of any monetary settlement or judgment plus accumulated expenses can be collected by the attorney after the case. In turn, the attorney agrees to absorb the cost for pursuit of the case up to the point of judgment or settlement. If the judgment or settlement is against the plaintiff, the attorney will recover nothing for his or her investment of time and may have difficulty recouping any expenses advanced on behalf of the client. This means, in essence, that the potential plaintiff must convince the attorney to invest time and effort and accept financial risk to take the case.

Physicians who do not appreciate the risks involved in the contingency fee method have argued that the contingency fee should be abandoned because it takes such a large percentage of any resulting settlement or judgment on their behalf. If a patient's injury is inconsequential or relatively minor, or if the potential for recovery of damages is low, the patient (no matter how angry or disgruntled), may have a difficult time retaining an attorney on a contingency fee. This process, in turn, tends to limit litigation to cases that are not "nuisances" (i.e., cases in which permanent disabling injury or death has occurred).

In the next step in the litigation process, the plaintiff's attorney obtains medical records and waivers so consultants can examine them. Consultants are employed by the plaintiff's attorney and usually have nursing or medical backgrounds. Caregivers and institutions who are asked to provide medical records are obliged to provide full and complete records under these circumstances. Records must not be "doctored" or tampered with in any way. On receipt of these records and after the consultants' review, the plaintiff's attorney must decide whether or not to "invest" in the case. This is a critical aspect of medical malpractice litigation as it is practiced in the United States. At this early stage, plaintiffs' attorneys may encounter considerable difficulty finding sufficient evidence in the medical record to support an allegation of negligence. Sometimes a plaintiff's attorney obtains advice from a consultant that is less than valid in this regard. For example, if the advising consultant is biased in hopes of later testifying and earning money, the attorney may be convinced to pursue an insubstantial case that can result in an unfortunate expenditure of time, money, and emotional resources by all parties involved. The quality of the early advice given to the plaintiff's attorney is crucial to the subsequent pursuit of the case. There is often "no turning back" once major amounts of time, money, emotions of family, plaintiffs, and physician defendants are invested.

In some communities, physicians who are competent and qualified may agree to review cases for plaintiffs' attorneys but will not agree to testify, even if they advise that grounds for negligence do exist. Such individuals are not held accountable for the advice they have given, but should be. Successful plaintiffs' attorneys carefully maintain a network of competent senior physicians and other caregivers who review possible cases, advise whether or not to proceed with a lawsuit, based on the evidence, and testify on behalf of the plaintiff if they believe the case is valid. In the absence of evidence, the wise attorney will decline cases he or she is advised against, even though he or she may be sympathetic to the plaintiff and even if injury is severe or death has occurred.

If the attorney decides to proceed with the case, a lawsuit is filed, often against a large number of defendants, because the anesthetized patient cannot know exactly who did what or when at this stage of the process. After that, the process of discovery begins.

Early Activity by the Defendant

Once notified of the lawsuit, the physician or other caregiver (defendant) notifies his or her insurance carrier, whose job it is to provide competent legal representation. **These early defendant-attorney conferences are critically important, because the defendant and attorney *evaluate one another.* The importance of full and complete disclosure cannot be overemphasized; the defendant must relate to his or her attorney every detail of the procedure performed, along with interpretation of the medical record in an honest and forthright manner. Provision of medical literature relevant to the case is also helpful.** Obviously there will be areas of concern in the defendant's case; it is extremely important that the facts about the defendant physician's role in the case not "dribble out" over months between the defendant's attorney and the defendant (i.e., surprises can be extremely problematic).

After these conferences, the process of discovery for the defendant's side also begins.

Discovery

Discovery* is a collective process during which each side has the right to find out, as completely as possible before trial, *the content of the other's case. Each party has the right to know, in detail, what the other's witnesses, both material and expert, intend to offer under oath at the trial.

The process of discovery—which may take months or years—includes the recording of *depositions.* A deposition is usually given at the office of the attorney or the person being deposed (i.e., both parties' attorneys should be present if possible). A court reporter is present, who records the witnesses' answers given under oath. Motions by both attorneys are made for the record to be considered later by a judge. Sometimes, depositions may be given by teleconference or videotaped.

Several key points regarding depositions should be kept in mind by physicians and other caregivers. First, the atmosphere in which they are taken may be relatively informal (i.e., attorneys may know each other, arrive together, talk, even laugh and joke together, and express familiarity with each other). The witness to be deposed—whether a defendant, material witness, or expert witness—must not be misled by this camaraderie. This is serious business. All information provided under oath at these depositions will be closely examined and can be used at the trial.

Each party is trying to discover what the other will say at trial, but parties are not necessarily trying out strategies of impeachment against any individual witness. Sometimes—especially when expert witnesses are being deposed—a party may try its "plan of attack" on the scenario. In these cases, the deposition atmosphere may suddenly turn quite hostile. More often, however, the atmosphere is informal and almost exaggeratedly polite. In the latter circumstance, inexperienced expert witnesses may be led to believe that their testimony is uncritically accepted by the other side, only to receive a "rude awakening" during the trial.

An answer to a question at a deposition should be specific to that question, exactly as asked, and should not be expanded upon. Amplified or defensive answers can often be exploited by attorneys, resulting in unhappy consequences for the party being questioned. The defendant or witnesses should never answer a question that requires referral to the medical record, other documents, or literature references without taking the time to look up those facts, wherever they may be, including paging through piles of records or previous depositions.

There are strategies used by attorneys during the discovery process and later at the trial. Some of these will be discussed in the section on trial testimony later in this chapter.

The national practitioner data bank and its influence on medical malpractice actions

An unpleasant point must be made about a defendant's interactions with his/her attorneys. Since January 1, 1991, any money that has changed hands via settlement or adjudication from defendant to plaintiff, must be noted to the Federal Practitioner Data Bank. Prior to this time, insurance companies often asked caregivers to agree to small dollar settlements of cases that could have cost more to defend than to settle. Defendant physicians often agreed to this or even signed agreements in advance that permitted insurors to do so without their consent. With the emergence of the Federal Practitioner Data Bank, this situation has become more problematic (i.e, greater pressure in some cases to go to trial, despite expense and emotional distress). Data obtained from this Data Bank are used in various licensure and credentialling processes.

Finding Expert Witnesses

In almost every case, it will be necessary for the plaintiff to present evidence detailing care provided by the responsible caregivers was below the existing (i.e., the date of the care given) national *standard of care*. Another way this is often stated is that the care provided was below the standard expected of a well-trained practitioner of that specialty. This means that qualified experts are needed to testify on both sides. Finding truly qualified experts tends to be easier for the defendant than for the plaintiff. Many jurisdictions have attempted to verify the expertise of such witnesses, often with mixed results. This process will be discussed in the section on tort reform. These experts are deposed before trial so that their opinions may be discovered and impeachment strategies planned.

Building the Case, Maneuvering, and Developing Strategies

As the lawsuit progresses, it may not appear to the principals on either side that much is happening. In fact, things are happening, albeit slowly sometimes. Opposing attorneys confer. Each side may make motions to be ruled on by the judge—motions dealing with inclusion or suppression of evidence, dismissal of various defendants or experts, and other technical matters. Settling the case before trial may also be discussed—a solution almost always favored by the judge. Finally, a trial date is set. The judge may mandate vigorous efforts at settlement as the trial date draws near. Demands and offers of settlement may more rapidly approach each other as the trial date approaches.

Basic Workings of a Trial

Although a medical lawsuit can be tried before a judge alone, this seldom happens in the case of medical malpractice lawsuits, because a substantial part of the plaintiff's case is to appeal, on behalf of an injured (or dead) patient, to the sympathies of a jury. Because each side is committed to use every legal means to win its case, the defendant physician should not be disturbed by the apparently prejudicial nature of this.

At the end of the trial, the jury is, in essence, presented with two sets of "facts" or "proofs" introduced into evidence by each side. It is imperative that the *content* of each set of "facts" introduced into evidence address certain key elements, or the case will not be allowed to go to the jury. Once these separate sets of "facts" are admitted into evidence, the jury's job is to choose one of three options: (1) the jury can rule for the plaintiff; (2) for the defendant; or (3) it can declare itself unable to decide (i.e., a "hung" jury). The jury's role is difficult because laypersons are asked to understand a remarkable amount of complex medical facts and opinions in reaching a verdict. Their role is also starkly simple; if they are not to be a "hung" jury, they must accept one set of facts and make their decision based on them. Guidelines vary as to numbers of jurors and as to size of the majority required for a ruling.

Defendant physicians, unfamiliar with the workings of the court, also may not understand the critical role of the judge. **One of the many important roles of the judge is to *interpret the rules of evidence.* In so doing, the judge has considerable control over the content of what is admitted to each set of "facts" presented to the jury.** If an objection to a particular question is made by an opposing side, this is a motion before the court and the judge. This motion, if overruled by the judge, allows the question to be asked and answered, and the answer to be entered into that party's set of "facts." If the motion is sustained, however, the jury is not permitted to take that statement into account and will not hear the witness's answer (or is instructed to disregard what may have been said). Many key issues on admissibility of evidence are decided pretrial by the judge. Watching the workings of a trial carefully, one immediately notices that the judge must make quick decisions which must be justified by the law.

Another role of the judge is to instruct the jury at the end of the presentation of evidence about the law pertaining to the case. These instructions may be the most important element of the trial. The witnesses for both sides are likely to present conflicting facts or opinions, and it is the role of the jury to choose between them. Having done so, however, the jury is required to apply the law to those facts as that law is explained to them by the judge. In many cases, disputes between the lawyers over the content of these instructions are often the most hotly contested issues in the trial.

Testimony

There are various forms of testimony: (1) that given in deposition versus that given at trial; (2) testimony given by plaintiffs versus that given by defendants; and (3) testimony given by material witnesses (e.g., operating room nurses not named as defendants who were present during the incident) versus that given by expert witnesses for each side. These different kinds of testimony are all given under oath and must be factual and truthful. Testimony is generally not given in narrative form, but rather in response to closed-ended questions posed by attorneys. This method is foreign and often offensive to most medical personnel, and therefore, poses difficulties in the way attorneys direct the testimony. Sticking to the facts—not trying to *interpret* or put "*spin*" on them, not trying to "select" them—and directly answering each question carefully are the best guidelines to follow to get through the process. Witnesses who try to figure out an attorney's "direction" in a line of questioning or who take long pauses before answers to simple questions will have credibility problems before the jury.

Numerous strategies are used by attorneys when questioning physicians, especially in front of juries, although these methods are also used occasionally at depositions. The attorney's tone of voice, inflection, and choice of words may lead a witness to assume a defensive attitude, to become angry, or to respond unwisely. All of these tactics are designed to create doubt about the scenario descripted by the witness or to shake the confidence of the witness in his or her testimony. **A key point to remember is the legal term *within a reasonable degree of medical certainty*—a phrase that is oft-used, but rarely defined. This term is intended to convey the recognition that there is little in medicine that is certain but physicians must nevertheless make life-and-death decisions. The law considers sufficiently reliable that level of certainty that a physician accepts as a basis for decision-making in medical practice. Often, this means "more likely than not."**

An expert witness must truly believe in the testimony he or she is offering and in the facts presented by their retaining party and the medical records. The expert witness must believed that the scenario and explanation occurred "with a reasonable degree of medical certainty." The attorney may try to provoke the expert witness or defendant to "hedge" by asking if there are other possible explanations for the alleged incident. The answer to that question is complex. One possible reply would be "of course there are other possible explanations, but I believe within a reasonable degree of medical certainty that my explanation is what actually happened." Competent expert witnesses must completely espouse the scenario they have developed and should not be trapped into "hedging." The phrase "within a reasonable degree of medical certainty" is important to remember and use at this critical juncture. Health care professionals do not typically work in "either/or" adversarial situations. Many find the necessity for strong advocacy distasteful, but it must be forceful.

Attorneys often produce "learned treatises" that appear to disagree with the expert witness' testimony. A common question is "Doctor, is this text [or paper] authoritative?" If the expert witness agrees that the text in question is an authoritative reference source, then his or her prior testimony may be successfully impeached in the eyes of the jury. A reasonable answer to the question is, "This textbook was written by a multitude of authors, some of whom I agree with and some of whom I may not. Texts are often given some but not necessarily exhaustive peer review."

Preparation for testimony

It is important to emphasize that many people are not as able to express their knowledge or competence orally. Anesthesia caregivers, in particular, work by thinking about differential diagnoses and performing minute-to-minute corrections and therapies in the operating room, and are seldom required to verbalize their decisions. It can be difficult to explain in words how an anesthetic is administered relative to the act itself; yet, this procedure is required in the courtroom. Testimony should be verbally practiced by witnesses. This practice builds confidence in oral answers to such questions. Each witness should have detailed information about the questions that will likely be asked. It is prudent to practice answering them.

Caregivers must not allow a lawsuit to adversely affect current and future practice, except in the sense of correcting errors. Each new patient deserves the best possible care, not a caregiver who is morose, depressed, cynical, or otherwise unduly affected by ongoing legal proceedings. Anesthesia practitioners must not allow themselves to feel "persecuted," embittered, or paranoid. Such attitudes can interfere with the quality of patient care given. This is not a frivolous or idle possibility; during depositions, plaintiff experts may have severely criticized a defendant's care. This criticism must be absorbed by the defendant in the context of the adversarial nature of the legal proceeding.

Defendants should not try to dictate legal strategy to their attorneys. As mentioned previously, the attorney should not have to drag the facts or weaknesses of the case out of the defendant. Once these problems are carefully considered, the defendant should avoid self-castigation and should not a priori believe in the scenario detailed by the plaintiff's expert witnesses. For example, the caregiver who was certain that he or she was properly attentive and vigilant and that the cause of cardiac arrest lies elsewhere should not now become convinced of otherwise just because a glib, or even "famous," plaintiff expert insists that he or she is "certain" that the defendant did not meet the standard of care. It is always painful to hear that your actions harmed a patient, but the anesthesia provider must adhere to his or her beliefs regarding the facts.

In some cases, competent expert witnesses for the defendant can find an alternative explanation, well supported by the facts of the case, and believe in it "to a reasonable degree of medical certainty." This alternative may not involve negligence on the part of one of the defendants and (hopefully) does not implicate other defendants, either. Often this situation is difficult, but as a general principle, defendants "finger-pointing" is counterproductive.

Testifying as an expert witness

If asked by either a defendant's or a plaintiff's attorney to review the records in a medical malpractice case, an anesthesiologist, nurse anesthetist, physician's assistant should subject the records to the following "tests." Before reading the records, the practitioner should not allow the attorney to wield undue influence. Attorneys can be very convincing about the merits of their cases. The anesthesia provider must study the records and make an independent judgment. Objectively, the following questions are pertinent:

- Am I competent by virtue of my training and (recent) expertise to actually testify and become involved in this case?
- Would I have performed the procedure this way?
- If I would not have performed the procedure this way, would "my way" necessarily and "within a reasonable degree of medical certainty" have prevented or ameliorated the negative outcome that occurred?

Many times, clinical methods other than those chosen by the defendant practitioner involved can be used. There is seldom only one way "within a reasonable degree of medical certainty" to perform a procedure. It is often extraordinarily difficult to prove, or even provide a convincing argument, that "my way" would have prevented the poor result. This is a critical distinction with respect to accepting a plaintiff's or a defendant's case. If "my way" is not provably superior to the defendant's way, and the evaluation could provide testimony for a defendant, the expert probably *can* provide testimony on behalf of the defendant. If "my way" is not the method use by the defendant and the anesthesia professional is asked to review the case for possible testimony on behalf of a plaintiff, *the same test should be applied:* Would "my way," "within a reasonable degree of medical certainty," have prevented the negative outcome? If so, the expert can testify on behalf of a plaintiff. **If the professional reacts with anger at: (1) the way the case was performed; (2) the quality of record keeping; (3) because of personal bias; or (4) because of suspicion that the defendant is not telling the truth, but there is no solid evidence in either record or deposition testimony, the potential expert *should not testify* on behalf of the plaintiff. If the expert believes that the defendant performed below the standard of care for the case's circumstances at that time and that this substandard conduct directly or indirectly led to the negative outcome, a qualified expert can testify against the defendant and should not suffer castigation from fellow professionals for doing so.** Although an expert's evaluation may be based on whether the care provided was consistent with "my way," an expert's testimony must be based on expert knowledge of the prevailing standard of care.

Critical Points in a Case of Negligence Against an Anesthesia Caregiver

Duty

The plaintiff must provide evidence that the anesthesia caregiver (defendant) did have a duty to the patient, arising from an actual patient-physician relationship. This duty is an obligation of due care—a requirement that the caregiver exercise the skill and knowledge common to his or her profession. The law does not require the very best of this care, although the expert witnesses may!

Breach of duty

The plaintiff must prove that the defendant breached the duty. Although this is a relatively straightforward process of comparing the defendant's actual acts to the previously established standard, it can become more complicated when more than one caregiver is involved. For example, if there was a nurse anesthetist present in the operating room at the time of the incident, but the nurse anesthetist was medically directed by an anesthesiologist, then both are likely involved in the lawsuit. The individual who performed the negligent act will be liable, but the anesthesiologist may also be liable for the acts or omissions of the nurse anesthetist. Resolution of this issue will revolve around the employment relationship (if any) between the two, the supervisory responsibility (if any) of the anesthesiologist, and the nature of the alleged negligent act.

Consider this scenario:

- Patient scheduled for elective open-eye procedure.
- Anesthesiologist/nurse anesthetist successfully induced anesthesia and intubated trachea aided by succinylcholine.
- Anesthesiologist leaves operating room to prepare other room for which he is responsible.
- Ten minutes later, with the eye open, patient begins to move. Nurse anesthetist administers additional dose of succinylcholine.
- Vitreous is vigorously extruded.

Who is liable in this case?

If there is even the slightest question about who was responsible for a given act, judges generally leave all named parties in the lawsuit.

Establishment of causation of injury

Testimony must establish that there was an "act" (of omission or commission) or possibly several acts. Next, it must be established that the act caused the plaintiff's injury. In some cases, such as delayed nerve injury, the injury may not have become apparent for several weeks after hospitalization. Much effort will be spent litigating whether or not the act(s) actually caused the patient's injuries. This is a critical point often minimized or overlooked by plaintiff's experts. The defendant's "way" may have been outdated, or record keeping poor, even abysmal, but did any of these factors actually *cause* the plaintiff's injury?

Establishment of standard of care with respect to the act

Qualified experts must testify that the act(s) of omission or commission done (or not done) by the defendants actually caused the injury—directly or indirectly—and that these acts were below the then-existing standard of care in the United States for a reasonable and prudent practitioner with reasonable training, skill, and knowledge in that same specialty. "Qualifications" of an expert is a prescribed process formally described with the jury present. The other side has the opportunity to try to impeach not only the expert's testimony, but also his or her credentials. The practitioner does not need to be "board certified" in anesthesiology to be held to a national standard of care. Indeed, family practitioners who perform anesthesia "occasionally" would do well to understand this point.

Many times, two physicians serving as expert witnesses, who are both board certified, and who attended respected medical schools, residencies, and so forth, testify to almost opposite conclusions. Key for the jury is the credibility of these expert witnesses. During their testimony, expert witnesses may use graphics, charts, slides, movies, and other visual aids. They may or may not introduce references, but in the end, it is these experts' credibility that often determines the weight the jury gives to such testimony.

Summary of required evidence

For the judge to submit the plaintiff's case to the jury for a decision, the plaintiff must have established:

- There was an act or omission.
- The act or omission breached the prevailing standard of care.
- The act or omission actually caused injury.
- The injury is permanent or disabling and has monetary value; if the injury is not permanent, it nonetheless has monetary value (e.g., "loss of consortium" or "pain and suffering").

These are the elements that must be present for the plaintiff's case to go to the jury. Contradicting testimony on as many points as possible will be presented in the defendant's case. If the defendant's attorney believes that the plaintiff has not provided sufficient testimony about one of these key elements, the attorney can move for *summary judgment* or a *directed verdict.* Such a motion, if granted, removes the case from the jury. In medical malpractice cases, these motions are usually sustained only when the plaintiff has failed to offer expert testimony concerning the standard of care.

PROBLEMS WITH THE CURRENT SYSTEM AND TORT REFORM

Medical malpractice cases come under the general category of "tort law." A *tort* is a civil, not a criminal, action. The "law" involved in such cases is usually "common law" as opposed to "statutory law." *Common law* means the weight and preponderance of previous decisions, especially those rendered by appellate courts, state supreme courts, and of course, the U.S. Supreme Court. Statutory law means laws that are "on the books" (i.e., passed by law-making bodies). After a verdict is rendered, it can often be appealed. If appealed, the appellate court begins a laborious process of deciding what it believes the "law" says pertinent to the case. This involves thorough and painstaking search for precedent. **The whole process from the initial filing of the lawsuit through appellate decisions can be quite lengthy—a major problem with the current system.** People's memories blur and change. Massive expenses may be incurred. There can be an injured patient (plaintiff) who really does need continuing care. If the case regarding such a patient takes years, who pays for the care of that patient during those years? Does the care of that injured person devolve to the taxpayer? Does the resultant jury award or settlement go toward the care of the injured person?

In our view, it is unethical for physicians to procrastinate or deliberately delay needed medical diagnosis or therapy. If the patient suffered at the beginning of this lawsuit, it is fair to say that such suffering probably continues throughout the ordeal of the case. In some jurisdictions, there are efforts made to speed up medical malpractice trials. One such effort (which has by and large failed), is that of empowering "panels" to prejudge these cases and to decide whether or not they should continue. The "panel" system fails when the hearings become trials themselves and subject those involved to two trials.

Plaintiff's attorneys usually receive, as a contingency fee, approximately one third of any settlement or judgment that results, plus expenses. If the jury finds for the plaintiff, that part of the settlement designated for continued care of the injured party may be paid to the family of the injured plaintiff in a lump sum. For example, if the plaintiff requires continued care in a nursing facility, but the family spends the money elsewhere, the plaintiff could eventually become a ward of the state without having received the full intended benefit of the settlement. **To address this problem, *structured settlements* are strongly advocated. In a structured settlement, funds earmarked for actual care of the injured plaintiff may be set aside and managed by a court-appointed trustee.** If experts estimate that the patient will likely live a long time and a large amount of patient care money is set aside for that purpose, but the plaintiff dies "early," leftover funds may be returned to an insurance pool instead of the family of the plaintiff in some structured settlement. In many jurisdictions, the plaintiff or his or her family is also entitled to recover damages for "pain and suffering" or "loss of consortium." Structured settlements should, in our opinion, have strong support from state and county medical societies and legislatures as well as both plaintiff and defense bar associations.

In many states, legislative battles have been fought over "capping" maximum awards for "pain and suffering," "loss of consortium," or other "non-economic damages." These efforts are more likely to be successful and survive constitutional challenge, if they are applied to tort law in general, rather than being limited to medical malpractice. Recently, judges and attorneys have developed greater sophistication regarding testimony from "experts" who are not qualified by *recent* expertise, skill, and up-to-date knowledge.

Regarding the qualifications for expert witnesses, many agree that the expert witness testifying in a medical malpractice case should: (1) be qualified in the specialty in question in the case; (2) be actively practicing in that specialty (i.e., not retired); and (3) not earn a substantial portion of his or her income from expert testimony. Unfortunately, beyond these relatively simple requirements, things become complex. For example, should a "cardiac anesthesiologist" testify in a case involving an obstetric anesthetic? What if the case involving the obstetric anesthetic was actually an intraoperative cardiac arrest? Is the cardiac anesthesiologist then qualified to testify? It is necessary to appreciate the complexity of determining qualifications for expert witnesses and to permit flexibility in the system.

Each time an expert witness is "qualified" by his or her party's attorney, the other party has the opportunity to impeach that witness. Contentions by either party that an expert witness is not "truly an expert" must be carefully brought into evidence during the trial. Impeachment of improperly or poorly qualified expert witnesses is still the best protection currently available against this problem. Testimony of expert witnesses at previous trials is discoverable and can often be introduced into evidence to impeach current testimony. The qualifications of an expert witness is a major problem because of the paramount importance of this expert testimony in most medical malpractice cases.

LEGAL ISSUES OTHER THAN MALPRACTICE

Contracts

Today, many "business" arrangements used by anesthesia providers are covered (or not covered) by contracts. Hospitals that have competitive institutions within a reasonable distance can issue exclusive contracts to individuals or groups of anesthesia practitioners to provide all (or portions of) anesthesia services. "Open" staffs of hospitals are rapidly declining, especially for "hospital-based" specialists. (Anesthesiology, radiology, and pathology have been considered "hospital-based" by HCFA and many others, whether or not their professional organizations agree.) Details and advice regarding such contracts are beyond the scope of this chapter, except to note that anesthesia practitioners *should attend personally and in considerable detail to such matters.* Legal and business professionals are nearly mandatory advisors today, but it is unwise to "leave all the details" of contracting, privileging, bylaws, group formation, and incorporation of contracts for payment from individual payors to others.

Government Rules and Regulations

Despite the fact that the U.S. Healthcare Financing Administration is not a legislative body and that the organization operates under laws that are often nonspecific, it appears to have force of law. In this chapter, we have *not* discussed *criminal* legal jeopardy for anesthesia professionals, but there is exactly that kind of jeopardy in the myriad of rules and local or regional "carrier" interpretations of these rules that are frequently "revised." Violations of these rules, such as "concurrency" (e.g., billing for supervising a nurse anesthetist while directly performing an anesthetic in another operating room), can be a criminal act. Professionals who practice anesthesia should not consider in-depth knowledge of these rules to be "beneath" them or someone else's responsibility.

Conflicts of Interest and Discrimination

Because health care professionals are more often employees or subcontractors, conflicts of interest are also of concern, especially to employers. An anesthesia professional who is administratively responsible for purchasing drugs or equipment for an anesthesia department should know and understand institutional or corporate "conflict of interest" rules.

Discrimination takes many forms, and the "private" practitioner or "private" institution is not exempt from federal, state or local laws regarding gender, religious, or age-based discrimination in hiring and laws against sexual harassment. Breaches of patient, colleague, or employee confidentiality or defamation are also areas in which physicians, in the past, tended to be cavalier.

With all this potential jeopardy, why continue to render professional anesthesia care? Why enter this specialty in the first place?

A short, but valid answer to this is: There still are sick and suffering patients who will benefit enormously from our care. Competent, up-to-date practice performed with care, attention, and vigilance and coupled with earnest and open attempts to communicate with patients and families are quite successful in protecting caregivers and clearly remain professionally satisfying.

KEY POINTS

- Anesthesia practitioners can expect legal problems if poor results occur from anesthesia or surgery, whether or not these results are expected or unexpected.
- *Informed consent* does not mean educating the patient to the level of a board-certified anesthesiologist. It means talking to the patient frankly and reasonably about the major risks of the procedure, including the possibility of death, and frankly and openly answering every question. It is nothing more or less than a process—a truly compassionate interaction between a physician and a patient.
- It is sometimes difficult for the plaintiff's attorneys to receive legitimate advice about proceeding with a lawsuit.
- The process of discovery means that each party is entitled to find out all the elements of the other's case.
- "Expert witnesses" must be expert in anesthesiology.
- A critically important role of the judge in a medical malpractice case is to interpret the rules of evidence so that they may be used to determine the eventual content of each side's testimony to be considered by the jury.
- A competent expert witness for the defendant must develop an alternative scenario which he or she can believe and which is supported by the facts of the case, including the written record and the sworn testimony.
- Most important, the caregiver (defendant) must not let any aspect of the case interfere with his or her provision of quality anesthesia care to current or future patients.
- One must not agree to become a plaintiff's expert witness because the defendant performed anesthesia via a method of which one does not approve. If, however, the anesthesia care delivered was considerably below the standards of care known to exist at the time the activity occurred, competent expert witness testimony should be provided.
- The essential elements in a case of negligence involve: (1) establishing duty to the patient; (2) responsibility for the patient; (3) causation of an injury by an act of omission or commission; and (4) proving that the standard of care provided by the physicians involved fell below the national standard of care.
- The essential elements of tort reform involve: (1) achieving structured settlements; (2) determining better expert witness qualifications; and (3) establishing reasonable levels of compensation for pain and suffering.

SUGGESTED READINGS*

Annas GJ, Law SA, Rosenblatt RE, et al: *American health law,* Boston, 1990, Little Brown.

This is a provocative discussion of the medical malpractice system as a form of quality assurance.

Havighurst CC: *Health care law and policy,* New York, 1988, The Foundation Press.

This is a recent discussion of various tort reform initiatives and their fate when analyzed under constitutional and/or common law scrutiny.

Fifty-six American law reports, Second Series 696, Rochester, 1956, Lawyers Cooperative Publishing.

See also updates published yearly entitled "Later Case Service" in this series. These are cases involving allegations of battery.

Pegalis SE, Wachsman HF: *American law of medical malpractice,* Rochester, 1981, Lawyers Cooperative Publishing.

This contains several cases illustrating the contrasting theories articulated by the plaintiff and defendant in anesthesia malpractice cases.

Southwick AF: *The law of hospital and health care administration,* ed 2, New York, 1988, Health Administration Press. Also see the following cases: *Cobbs vs. Grant,* 8 Cal. 3rd 229, 104 Cal. Rptr. 505, 502 P. 2nd 1 (1972); *Canterbury vs. Spence,* 464 F. 2d 772 (D.C. App. 1972).

Chapter 10 contains a thorough discussion of the doctrine of informed consent. The cases cited are the leading underpinnings of the modern legal theory of informed consent.

*These readings have been annotated because the reader may not be familiar with legal texts and/or citation methodology. They are included for those who wish to pursue these issues from a legal perspective. Note also that the anecdotes used in this chapter are specifically not referenced. Some did not even become legal cases. All are cases either from authors' experiences or were related to the authors by professionals involved.

CHAPTER 97

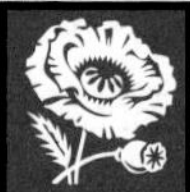

Substance Dependence and Abuse by Anesthesia Care Providers

ROBERT P. FROM

Psychoactive substances (e.g., legal and illegal drugs, medications, and toxic chemicals) affect the mind and mental processes. Inappropriate use of psychoactive drugs by those who provide anesthesia may significantly impair vigilance (e.g., decreased reaction time, altered perception, and affected judgment) and place patients at risk.[111] If such use increases and achieves the level of a psychoactive substance abuse disorder, personal, physical, and psychologic damage and legal problems can affect friends, family, colleagues, and co-workers. If left untreated, the disease will progress and often will be fatal. It should be recognized that early intervention, therapy, and subsequent careful monitoring can be used to rehabilitate the impaired individual.[34] If unaffected anesthesia providers can achieve a reasonable understanding of these disorders, then appropriate, rapid, and safe action can be taken to facilitate treatment and save the life of a fellow anesthesia care team member when realistic concerns or evidence surfaces.

DEFINITIONS

Psychoactive drugs are not "good" or "bad"; they have multiple effects, which, in turn, depend on the amount taken and the individual's expectations or resultant effects.[72] At issue is the behavior—impairment of social or occupational functioning—that results from drug seeking and use and the conflict that arises when attempting to define "abuse."[17,27] For instance, "use" of certain chemicals to depress or influence feelings or mood is often encouraged by sociocultural convention, but some would argue and sincerely believe that using substances in such a manner is a disguised form of "abuse" and that such practices should not be socially accepted.[20,112] Psychomotor stimulant drugs, such as caffeine, have been shown to improve vigilance in humans under conditions of fatigue.[15] Such effects are viewed as positive and their use is encouraged in many cultures. In other words, what is "use" to one group of people may be "abuse" to another. The behavior that results from the "use" of a substance may be accepted and even encouraged depending on the sociocultural reference point. In an attempt to deal with this ever-changing bias, the American Psychiatric Association (APA) has created the fourth edition of the *Diagnostic and Statistical Manual of Mental Disorders*

BOX 97-1
CRITERIA FOR SUBSTANCE DEPENDENCE

A maladaptive pattern of substance abuse, leading to clinically significant impairment of distress, as manifested by three (or more) of the following factors, occurring at any time in the same 12-month period:

1. Tolerance, as defined by either of the following:
   (a) A need for markedly increased amounts of the substance to achieve intoxication or desired effect
   (b) Markedly diminished effect with continued use of the same amount of the substance
2. Withdrawal, as manifested by either of the following:
   (a) The characteristic withdrawal syndrome for the substance (refer to criteria A and B of the criteria sets for withdrawal from the specific substances)
   (b) The same (or a closely related) substance is taken to relieve or avoid withdrawal symptoms
3. The substance is often taken in larger amounts or over a longer period than was intended
4. There is a persistent desire or unsuccessful efforts to cut down or control substance abuse
5. A great deal of time is spent in activities necessary to obtain the substance (e.g., visiting multiple doctors or driving long distances), use the substance (e.g., chain-smoking), or recover from its effects
6. Important social, occupational, or recreational activities are given up or reduced because of substance abuse
7. The substance abuse is continued, despite knowledge of having a persistent or recurrent physical or psychologic problem that is likely to have been caused or exacerbated by the substance (e.g., current cocaine use despite recognition of cocaine-induced depression or continued drinking despite recognition that an ulcer was worsened by alcohol consumption)

Criteria for Substance Abuse

A. A maladaptive pattern of substance use leading to clinically significant impairment or distress, as manifested by one (or more) of the following, occurring within a 12-month period:
   1. Recurrent substance use resulting in a failure to fulfill major role obligations at work, school, or home (e.g., repeated absences or poor work performance related to substance abuse; substance-related absences, suspensions, or expulsions from school; neglect of children or household)
   2. Recurrent substance abuse in situations in which it is physically hazardous (e.g., driving an automobile or operating a machine when impaired by substance abuse)
   3. Recurrent substance-related legal problems (e.g., arrest for substance-related disorderly conduct)
   4. Continued substance abuse, despite having persistent or recurrent social or interpersonal problems caused or exacerbated by the effects of the substance (e.g., arguments with spouse and consequences of intoxication, physical fights)

B. The symptoms have never met the criteria for Substance Dependence for this class of substance.

Modified from: American Psychiatric Association: *Diagnostic and statistical manual of mental disorders*, ed 4, Washington, 1994, American Psychiatric Association.

(DSM IV).[3] The manual attempts to assign behavioral definitions by describing the activity or symptoms a patient will exhibit if the disease is present. Disorders created by use of psychoactive substances are divided into four categories each of which includes behavioral, psychologic, and cognitive symptoms: (1) substance dependence; (2) abuse; (3) intoxication; and (4) withdrawal.[68] These categories are placed under the heading of "Substance-Related Disorders." By using this latter definition standard, it is possible to assign diagnostic criteria and recognize distinct forms of the disease process.

Both dependence and abuse are described as patterns of substance use that are maladaptive and lead to clinically significant impairment or distress. Substance dependence is more severe abuse of a drug often accompanied by a physiologic dependence with associated tolerance and withdrawal symptoms.[27] The criteria for substance dependence and substance abuse are listed in Box 97-1. These terms replace older definitions such as addict, addiction, alcoholism, physiologic dependence, impairment, and drug misuse.[68,74]

PREVALENCE* AND INCIDENCE** IN MEDICINE AND ANESTHESIOLOGY

It has been argued that no one knows or will ever know precisely how many practicing physicians are having alcohol and drug abuse problems.[16] Data that estimate the number of physicians with a substance abuse–related disorder come from three main sources: (1) medical licensing boards; (2) surveys; and (3) treatment programs. The sources are vulnerable to criticism due to inadequate or nonrepresentative samples confined to physicians in a single medical center, state, or treatment program.[46] Also, physicians may tend to

*The total number of cases of a disease in a given population at a specific time; at one point in time.

**Extent or frequency of occurrence; the rate at which an event occurs.

select particular types of treatment.[16] Physicians have often been considered more likely to succumb to drug misuse than the general population. A statement in 1957 by the first Commissioner of the Bureau of Narcotics suggested that, whereas 1 in 100 physicians was a substance abuser, only 1 in 3000 in the general population suffered a similar problem.[4] This statement appears to be the source of the many reports contending that psychoactive substance abuse disorders among physicians may be 30 times greater than those of the general population. These estimates, based on information from the 1950s, have questionable relevance today.[33]

With the above caveats in mind, it is still worthwhile to discuss the likely rates of substance abuse disorders in physicians both in training and in practice, and to compare rates among different specialties. Medical students report a 3.4% lifetime alcohol dependence rate, and 1.6% believe they currently need help with substance abuse.[8] Heavy substance abuse patterns are seldom seen in resident physicians.[48] Less than 0.2% of resident physicians reported dependence on any substance (except tobacco) in the preceding year.[46] A number of studies examined training programs by specialty. Psychiatric training programs reported a substance abuse problem of 1%.[77] Surgical residents reported use of alcohol, marijuana, and cocaine within the last 30 days at a prevalence of 73.5%, 3.2%, and 0.4%, respectively.[50] A survey of oral and maxillofacial surgery training programs reported a 1.2% incidence rate of substance abuse.[76] Emergency medicine residency program directors suspected or identified 1% of their residents as being substance dependent.[65] **Surveys of anesthesia training programs report an incidence of confirmed substance abuse of 0.4% to 2%.**[6,41,66,105,110] Almost 8% of physicians reported having substance-abuse or dependence problems at some point in their lives.[47] In contrast, the reported lifetime rate of abuse in the general population is estimated at 16%.[47,73] Disciplinary actions for substance-abuse disorders range from 0.9% to 3% for all physicians.[47]

Anesthesiologists, compared with other medical specialists, appear to be at high risk for substance-related disorders.[35,79,88] Treatment programs report a disproportional number of anesthesiologists in treatment compared with other medical specialists.[42,94] It has been stated that anesthesiologist's risk of nonalcohol chemical abuse is as much as four times greater than that of the general physician population.[52] In addition, death from suicide is reported as higher among anesthesiologists than among age- and socioeconomically matched control groups in the years 1947 to 1976.[18,19,59] Anesthesiologists are considered to suffer losses from suicide at a rate that is the second or third highest among specialty groups.[19] There is speculation that this increased suicide rate may, at least in part, be the result of substance-related disorders.[7,11,26]

On the other hand, the American Society of Anesthesiologists (ASA) is one of the most progressive medical-specialty societies. In fact, of the 16 Societies, Colleges, and Academies listed as sponsoring organizations for their corresponding Residency Review Committees in the Graduate Medical Education Directory,[40] only the American College of Surgeons and the ASA have specific descriptive information regarding substance abuse disorders in physicians (e.g., booklets, videotape) available for its members (Appendix 97-1 on page 2482).[7,24,31,49,71,109]

Nonetheless, there is some good news. It may be that the efforts to look for, find, and treat impaired physicians is being rewarded. More recent studies using a survey format and studying only rates of substance abuse have found no significant difference in the use of psychoactive substances between anesthesiologists in training or in practice compared with other peer groups.[47,60] Results of a study in progress indicate that rates of substance-abuse disorders in anesthesia training programs have declined since 1986.[6] The incidence rate for new substance abuse in the 1994-1995 training years is estimated at 0.4% per year for residents and 0.1% per year for attending physicians.[6]

Even with these encouraging developments, it should not be assumed that the problem has been mitigated. It could be argued that the ASA report is likely to be more complete than other medical specialties, that the specialty looks for the problem and finds it, and that this may be one reason why anesthesiologists *appear* to be at greater risk for substance-related disorders; contending that substance abuse is not a serious threat to our specialty is not in the best interest of anesthesiologists or their patients.[35,79,95,104,107] Increased education with respect to identification of victims and knowledge that treatment is available may cause a greater proportion of afflicted anesthesiologists to seek and receive treatment.

DISEASE CONCEPT OF ADDICTION

In the past, a psychoactive substance-abuse disorder was considered a "disease of the will."[10] It is now understood that this type of disorder *causes* emotional or physical afflictions or aggravates those that already exist.[5] A psychoactive substance-related disorder is now considered not to be secondary to other psychiatric diseases but rather is considered a primary affliction. Genetic, neurobiologic, and environmental factors are proposed as etiologic mechanisms that cause this disease.

Genetic Factors

Over the past 80 years, more than 100 studies have shown that alcohol abuse is three to five times as frequent in the parents, siblings, and children of alcoholics as in the general population.[25] Family, twin, and adoptive studies suggest that alcoholism is a genetically influenced disorder.[39,64,97] Some research has focused on specific genes that may carry an increased vulnerability for the disease.[9] Increased frequency of substance-abuse disorders for other substances also has been shown to be genetic.[21]

Neurobiologic Factors

A great deal of investigational research has focused on alcoholism, and theories that explain this disorder may be applicable to other psychoactive substances. These theories include the possibilities: (1) that alcoholics are seeking relief from hypoglycemia; (2) that they have various allergies to alcohol; or (3) that some sort of differential brain responsiveness to alcohol exists in alcoholics.[83] It is possible that alcohol produces morphinelike substances in the brains of those susceptible to alcoholism.[36]

Differences in the concentration of certain blood metabolites between alcoholics and nonalcoholics have been demonstrated. For instance, inhibition of monoamine oxidase (MAO) by ethanol is higher, and stimulation of platelet adenylate cyclase by specific chemical mediators is lower in platelets of alcoholics than those in control groups.[93] Also, there is less change in cortisol and prolactin blood levels following alcohol challenge in subjects with a positive family history of alcoholism than in subjects with no family history.[81]

These reports suggest that some individuals may be prone or susceptible to alcoholism because they tolerate large quantities of alcohol. The ability to tolerate alcohol may be a genetically inheritable trait that allows the victim to drink large quantities of alcohol without suffering adverse effects.[38] For instance, some populations suffer unpleasant reactions to even small quantities of alcohol (e.g., approximately 75% of persons of Asian descent undergo cutaneous flush), whereas the lack of response to alcohol in susceptible individuals may allow them to consume large quantities without experiencing unpleasant symptoms.[38] Unlike opiates, it appears that large quantities of alcohol must be consumed for a psychoactive substance-related disorder to develop.

Environmental Factors

Within a particular culture, rates of alcoholism have been reported to be influenced by age, social class, subcultural and religious affiliation, and occupation.[29] The influences of specific environmental risk factors within the medical community have been proposed to explain the incidence of psychoactive substance-abuse disorders among physicians.

For physicians, in general, the following risk factors have been proposed:

- Self-deception on the part of the impaired physician.[94]
- Self-medication by physicians as means of dealing with stress, anxiety, or physical discomfort.[32,88]
- The "stressful" lifestyle of physicians, with little attention devoted to personal health maintenance and the inability to recognize needs for mental or physical help.[88]

The following risk factors have been proposed for anesthesiologists:

- Accessibility to potent drugs that, in very small quantities, over short time periods, are rapidly addictive.[35,98]
- Many of the drugs used for anesthesia are unique to the specialty.[35]
- Diverting small amounts of such drugs without getting caught may be easier in anesthesiology than in other specialties.[35]
- Drug handling and access for anesthesiologists is greater than for any other specialty.[35]
- In anesthesia, unlike other specialties, the provider is directly in the controlled-substance chain of custody from the pharmacy to the patient.[66]

It has been contended that fentanyl, parenterally and perhaps even orally administered, is the substance most likely to be misused by anesthesiologists.[35,43,58,66,75,85,87] This last factor has been used to suggest an additional risk specific to anesthesiologists.[98] The theory is that it is not uncommon for adolescents and young adults to experiment with psychoactive substances. Curiosity, impulse, and the urge to rebel lead to risk-taking behavior that, in turn, may lead to experimentation with drugs during these early life periods. This early experimentation can perhaps be thought of as the "minor leagues." The person may "succeed" in that he or she does not become physiologically or psychologically addicted to the substances most readily available to persons in those age groups (e.g., alcohol, marijuana.) The person then believes he or she can "win" the game and avoid a substance-related disorder. If that person later enters anesthesiology training and if the risk-taking behavioral urges are still present, the drugs now "available" can be termed "major league." When curiosity leads to experimentation with powerful substances used for anesthesia (e.g., fentanyl), the "game" is lost from the outset and a psychoactive substance-abuse disorder begins. Personality traits peculiar to individuals who enter anesthesiology may also contribute to the problem. A study of graduate nursing students, using a standard personality inventory, found that those specializing in anesthesiology exhibited a greater tendency for excitement-seeking and had a greater number of positive additive-tendency scores than those pursuing general nursing graduate degrees.[63]

This kind of theorizing about anesthesiology trainees (residents and student nurse anesthetists) who become addicted to fentanyl or other substances used for anesthesia is perhaps radical in that it tends to refute the formerly held belief that the training programs for the profession produced such stress that some trainees were almost "driven" to drug abuse. This newer concept also implies that some trainees enter anesthesiology at least partly (perhaps subconsciously) *because* of the easier availability of drugs. Fentanyl seems particularly suited to this kind of abuse—many addicted anesthesia care providers have reported that use of fentanyl allowed them to remain "high" but also awake and alert (at least in their opinions). Self-identified fentanyl users distinguish the "nod" (i.e., the long plateau phase of intoxication characterized by a sleepy, painless euphoria) from fentanyl as longer and "better" than that obtained with heroin use.[55]

IDENTIFICATION

Diagnosis is the act or process of identifying or determining the nature and cause of a disease or injury through evaluation of patient history, examination, and review of laboratory data. Early diagnosis is critical to increase the salvage rate.[23] The process of identifying a substance-abuse disorder among anesthesia care providers is analogous to diagnosis and should not be considered a confrontation with a "criminal." Every individual who works in the anesthesiology profession can and should attempt to identify victims of a substance-related disorder. Indeed, professional practitioners are "mandatory reporters"; laws which have as their primary intent removal for treatment of substance abusers.

What if you attempt to intervene when in fact your colleague or co-worker is *not* suffering from the disease? What is your liability? There are several layers of protection: (1) if the intervention is carried out in a closed forum, it is unlikely that a defamation case could be supported; and (2) it is unlikely that the patient would publicize the case with a lawsuit.[106] There is greater liability for not taking action.[106] In some states, identification of a psychoactive substance-related disorder in a health care professional is free from legal discovery if treatment is undertaken voluntarily. Many states have mandatory reporting laws, which require suspicion that a licensed professional is abusing a psychoactive substance, to be reported either to the state medical or nursing society or to any existing licensing or disciplinary bodies.[101] These laws identify the parties who have an affirmative duty to report, including physician colleagues and health care providers with whom the impaired physicians serve on staff.[103] The law clearly places responsibility for handling these issues on the medical profession and the hospitals.[89] Failure to report an incident as required by law may result in disciplinary action against a particular designated individual or hospital who knew (or reasonably should have known) of an individual's impairment.[1,103] In most states, as long as reports are provided in good faith, reporters are protected from liability under a legal doctrine known as "qualified privilege." The Health Care Quality Improvement Act of 1986 provides immunity from lawsuits for reporters and sanctions for failure to report.[44] There are numerous ways in which an afflicted anesthesia care provider may be identified.

Signs and Symptoms of the Disease

A person's acute intoxicated state depends on what, when, and how much of a substance has been consumed. Age, weight, metabolic activity, and tolerance level affect the disposition of drugs. Signs and symptoms of stimulants (e.g., cocaine) suggest sympathetic nervous system overactivity, whereas evidence of depressants (e.g., barbiturates, opiates) suggests sympathetic nervous system depression. Most tragically, among anesthesia care providers, death or anoxic brain injury may be the very first presenting symptom.[66]

Often, signs and symptoms of an acute intoxicated state are too vague or nonspecific for a definitive diagnosis to be possible. Professional performance may remain above reproach in the early stages.[23] In fact, poor patient care is rarely the factor that establishes the disorder.[51] More commonly, identification occurs when the characteristic changes of a substance-related disorder are recognized in multiple areas of a professional's life (i.e., when a constellation of symptoms and activities suggests a problem.) The signs of a psychoactive substance-abuse disorder in six significant dimensions of a physician's life are summarized in Box 97-2.

Specific warning signs of a psychoactive substance-abuse disorder for anesthesia care providers include the following:

- Early arrival and late departure from the operating room area
- Preference for isolation (e.g., at lunch and coffee breaks)[51]
- Desire to work alone and undisturbed
- Heavy "wastage" of controlled drugs
- Inappropriate drug requests
- Refusal of work relief
- Sloppy anesthetic records
- Unexplained drowsiness or inattentiveness
- Unusually high percentage of use of narcotic techniques[7]
- Frequent requests for bathroom relief

In addition, other suspicious changes that may be seen include: (1) wide mood swings; (2) periods of depression, anger, and irritability, alternating with periods of euphoria; (3) insistence on personally administering narcotics in the recovery room; (4) he or she is difficult to find between cases; and (5) weight loss, tremors, pale skin, pinpoint pupils, diaphoresis.[31]

It is unlikely that an anesthesiologist will be the first health care worker to ask questions about a colleague's behavior.[107] Operating room nurses, who are in positions to constantly observe anesthesia providers administering anesthesia, are often the first to question behavior.[107]

Controlled Substance Dispensing and Accountability

No clinically practical system for drug accountability can prevent misuse of controlled substances by a determined anesthesia care provider.[54,56,78] Multiple psychoactive substances are readily available in all anesthesiology departments, and most hold potential for misuse,[66] although the most commonly abused substance, even for anesthesia providers, is still alcohol.[32] If a system of control and accountability of potentially abusive drugs is in place, then identification of individuals who divert controlled substances for personal use will be enhanced.[2]

There are five generic dispensing methods used: (1) traditional nurse dispensing (41.7%); (2) satellite pharmacy (34%); (3) anesthesia-controlled locked box (11.9%); (4)

BOX 97-2
SIGNS OF PSYCHOACTIVE SUBSTANCE ABUSE DISORDER IN SIX DIMENSIONS OF A PHYSICIAN'S LIFE

Community

- Arrests for driving while intoxicated
- Embarrassing behavior at social functions
- Unpredictable behavior (e.g., inappropriate spending)
- Unreliability/unpredictability in community and social functions
- Withdrawal from community and leisure activities, hobbies, church

Employment

- Complicated and elaborate medical history
- Frequent hospitalizations
- Indefinite or inappropriate references
- Numerous job changes
- Reluctance to let spouse/children be interviewed

Office

- Absence from office, unexplained or due to frequent illness
- Complaints by patients to staff about doctor's behavior
- Disruption of appointment schedule
- Excessive ordering of supplies for drugs from local druggist by mail
- Hostile, withdrawn, unreasonable behavior to staff and patients
- "Locked-door" syndrome

Hospital

- Inappropriate orders or over prescription of medications
- Lateness for rounds or inappropriate behavior during rounds
- Desire to work alone
- Decreasing quality of performance (e.g., in staff presentations, writing in charts)
- Excessive drinking at staff functions
- Presence on the job when not on duty
- Refusing work relief

Family

- Delinquent behavior by children
- Domestic violence
- Separation from family unit
- Sexual problems (e.g., impotence, extramarital affairs, contract sex)
- Withdrawal from family activities

Physical status

- Frequent visits to physicians and dentists
- Multiple physical signs/complaints
- Numerous prescriptions and drugs
- Accidents
- Deterioration in personal hygiene

Modified from Talbott GD, Benson EB: The impaired physician: The dilemma of identification, *Postgrad Med* 68:56, 1980.

central pharmacy locked-box control (7.3%); and (5) dispensing machine (4.4%).[54] The latter method may be efficacious in smaller departments.

Although any system will require modification for specific institutions, basic elements of a practical system have been proposed.[2] First, use of a "locked box" in a visible, secured location, in or immediately adjacent to the operating room suite, as the initial storage area for unopened vials or ampules is important. Drugs should not be predrawn into syringes in the central pharmacy.[61] Frequent audits of supplies by two or more people should be done (e.g., at shift change.) Second, the controlled-substance register must contain the times and dates of transactions, patient name and hospital number, and signatures of the anesthesia care provider and the person from whom the supplies were obtained. A master and an individual register makes this system efficient. Individual registers with multiple copies allow the original to remain at the central dispensing location when copies are taken to anesthesia-use locations. Following administration of the substances, unused, discarded, returned, or "lost" drugs must be listed. Operating room policies that mandate disposal of controlled substances in front of witnesses are also helpful, but witnessing clear liquid leaving a syringe does not assure verification.[107] (A recent "ploy" is for the user or resident to substitute a dilute solution of esmolol in an attempt to fool the supervising physician into believing the syringe to contain fentanyl, because of the resultant bradycardia, thus placing the patient in serious jeopardy.) It may be necessary to randomly determine the contents of syringes that are supposed to contain undiluted drugs. Analysis of use trends by individuals should be performed and audits ordered when trends are not easily explained.[2] Finally, personal responsibility for all controlled substances should be emphasized.

Drug Testing

A careful clinical correlation is required to evaluate the connection between the presence of a drug in a person's urine or blood and its relation to suspected or reported impairment.[22] Urine testing for drugs is subject to legal, technical, and procedural constraints, is expensive, and does result in occasional false-positive readings.

Legal considerations

Preemployment drug screening by urinalysis is practiced by a large number of companies in the U.S.[102] Federally regulated industries and agencies practice postaccident evaluation and random unannounced drug testing.[102] These practices have been accepted as reasonable by the courts as long as the policies are in place before the request for a specimen is made, and the policies are applied to all employees in an equitable and uniform manner. Demands for individual urine or blood samples based on specific objective facts have thus far withstood legal challenges that were argued on the principle of unreasonable search and seizure. Random or scheduled screening for monitoring recovery progress during rehabilitation as a condition of reemployment is also valid. "Suspicionless" testing of physicians is more problematic.[84] In one survey, 60% of physicians believed that testing infringed on the physician's right to privacy (although, 87% said they would submit to testing if required by a hospital).[57] It may be expected that such testing will result in litigation over false-positive test results, privacy interference, breach of confidentiality, defamation, or interference with career and income.[103]

Technical considerations

Immediate on-site urine testing for some common substances of abuse is available with a number of simple-to-use diagnostic kits. They are popular in the criminal justice system, hospital emergency departments, the military and private industry. They can simultaneously test for multiple drugs or drug metabolites without handling of laboratory reagents or urine specimens. They are becoming more convenient and results are available in less than 5 minutes. They provide only preliminary results. More specific alternate chemical methods must be used to confirm the analytical results.[12,70] If an initial screening assay shows a sample as being positive, a second assay should be employed to confirm the initial results.[102] The second or confirmatory assay include gas chromatography or mass spectrometry. These confirmatory assays are quite specific and provide a documented data record suitable for review and interpretation by outside experts.[102]

Metabolites of meperidine and morphine can be detected in urine up to 72 hours and 3 days, after administration, respectively.[91] Detection of fentanyl in biologic samples by radio immunoassay (RIA) has been available since at least 1974.[45] Urine screening has been more difficult, but reliable tests are now available.[90,99,108] It is estimated that regular users will have detectable fentanyl in urine for 3 to 5 days after cessation.[86] After small doses (e.g., 100 μg) of fentanyl, the fentanyl metabolite norfentanyl can be detected in urine for up to 96 hours using gas chromatographic/mass spectral analysis.[86] Urine testing for norfentanyl, rather than fentanyl, may yield a higher frequency of positive results in suspected users.[86] Alfentanil and sufentanil can be detected in the urine of race horses, so screening for these drugs in humans should be possible through urinalysis.[99]

Procedural considerations

The validity of the results of a urine drug test depends on the integrity of the specimen.[62] There are many ways for a specimen to be invalidated: (1) water from a commode will dilute urine; (2) detergent from soap dispensers can destroy drugs or affect the specimen and generate a false-negative analysis; and (3) a pinhole in the bottom of the urine container can be created that results in a leak that might not be detected at the collection site, but during shipping such urine can leak out.[62] There is lyophilized (freeze-dried) drug-free human urine allegedly for sale "on the street" along with a wearable rubber penis connected to a bag, worn like a shoulder holster, which holds and warms the "urine." These extreme measures are noted only so that the reader will understand the depth of this problem. Direct observation of the specimen being given is critically important. Someone unfamiliar with these and several other deceptive practices may allow the victim of a substance-related disorder to provide the specimen privately, avoiding embarrassment to both parties, but also allowing the test to be defeated.[62] A chain-of-custody must be demonstrable if the urine is to be used as "evidence." The sample is kept in constant view until sealed and labeled, then a chain-of-custody form is signed by both the person releasing the specimen and the person accepting it.[87]

Poppy seeds used on bagels can contain sufficient amounts of opiate to produce detectable concentrations of morphine and codeine in urine, although the amount of ingested morphine is insufficient to cause behavioral effects.[30,92] This is not exactly a technical problem because a positive urine test resulting from poppy seeds is not a false-positive outcome because the drug is actually present.[102] Caution must be exercised in interpreting such a positive result as an indicator of opiate misuse, but this is a frequently used excuse when a positive test for opiates is reported.

Phenylpropanolamine and ephedrine available in diet pills and cold remedies can produce an apparent positive assay for amphetamines in immunoassay screens. Ibuprofen was reported to have interfered with one older screening test and caused apparent positive screens for a marijuana metabolite.[102] This problem has been corrected. False positive are very unlikely if confirmatory assays are properly carried out because the latter techniques identify agents specifically.[102]

INTERVENTION

Denial is the hallmark of substance-related disorders.[23,87] Denial is such a potent and malignant facet of the disease that outside help is often lifesaving.[13,14,67] Any process that effectively halts the progressive and destructive effects of chemical dependency is called "*intervention*."[53] Experts recommend that an intervention team be assembled consisting of friends, relatives, and co-workers. Individual confrontations are discouraged, because they may be dangerous. Left alone with the knowledge that his or her colleagues are suspicious, the victim may increase drug use, resulting in an overdose or intentional suicide.[51] The selection of team members and preparation for the intervention may take several days. In an anesthesiology department, suspicion should be enough to prompt an intervention, with or without mandatory reporting laws, because patients' safety must be placed above all other considerations.

Identification and Treatment of the Victim of Substance Use Disorder Using Fentanyl as a Model

At some point during fentanyl use, requirements for the drug exponentially increase. Why or when this occurs is unknown and unpredictable. Before this occurs, a user may not be detected if he or she carefully attends to record-keeping and diverts only small quantities. Although it may be true that some providers "get away" with "chronic" fentanyl use for long periods of time, the exponential increase in requirement is the time during which the individual is most likely to be suspected or positively identified. It is during this phase that record-keeping may begin to indicate large wastage, may not add up, may involve inordinate "breakage" reports, or ampoules or vials of fentanyl may simply be reported as missing. Responsible departmental authorities must assume if these events happen that there is an individual within the department suffering a substance-abuse disorder and *must* audit, scrutinize, question, and be alert to suspicious behavior. If this routine is not completed, the next "event" may be discovery of a colleague's death! **The importance of responsible, prompt, and thorough behavior by departmental personnel and authorities at that level cannot be overemphasized.**

Most often, after a death has occurred, retrospective analysis will show that there were subtle or not-so-subtle behavioral signs that were recognized but dismissed or even excused or covered up. Personnel must be educated that documenting and reporting suspicious behavior to responsible authorities is not considered "snitching," it can easily be lifesaving. Virtually every anesthesiology training program and many, if not most, anesthesiology departments of any size at all, in both private and public hospitals, have had a substance-abuse disorder affect them. When that event is accompanied by tragedy, the collective guilt, blame-taking, blame laying on others, and even legal entanglement with the victim's family may last years.

If there are reports of excess or suspicious wastage, breakage, or "nodding off" in the operating room, or the suspected individual is around when not on call, or there is a relief individual administering liquid from syringes labeled as "narcotic" without apparent effect on the patient, the departmental chair or chief of anesthesia (residency program or private hospital) *must* take action. In legal terms, "probable cause" now exists. A demand, on the spot, for a witnessed sample of blood or urine (given the caveats noted previously) is now justified and entirely proper. At this point, the hospital's attorney may advise caution or actually advise against a demand for a sample. To repeat, the departmental chair must consider the patient's safety above all other considerations. The hospital's attorney may speak of liability for defamation or unreasonable search. However, if the behavioral reports are documented with the records from cases or controlled substance records or audits, the departmental chair should act in the best interests of the patients and demand a sample or confession, or, in the absence of either, exercize his or her authority to suspend the individual from practice immediately and refer the matter to the state licensing board or other authorities.

The suspected user has several options: (1) agree to provide the sample; (2) refuse to provide the sample and refuse to acquiesce to a voluntary suspension from clinical duties; (3) admit to drug abuse and agree to immediate admittance to a rehabilitation program; or (4) resign from the hospital staff or residency program. If the suspected user demands that his or her attorney be present when a sample is taken, and, if that will take sufficient time so that the suspected substance may no longer be present, then the departmental chair should consider this response a refusal to provide a timely sample and should immediately suspend the individual from clinical duties. There must be "probable cause" before this action is taken.

If the individual refuses to provide a sample, his or her suspension must begin immediately, and the suspension as well as the circumstances must be reported to the appropriate state authorities, usually the state board of medical or nursing examiners. The same reporting is required if the provider resigns from the hospital staff or confesses to the abuse and asks for a referral to rehabilitation. In many states, if a sample is voluntarily given and is negative, no reporting to state authorities is required, although this should be individually checked by the departmental chair. If a sample is voluntarily given, it is usually up to the discretion of the departmental chair as to whether the individual is permitted to return to the operating room pending results of testing. The hospital administration obviously also has in this decision.

If a provider tests positive or admits to drug abuse, an immediate referral should be made to a rehabilitation program, although the departmental chair or hospital cannot mandate that the provider actually seek rehabilitation (the mandatory reporting of this situation to the state authorities will almost always assure that rehabilitation is at least attempted). During rehabilitation, most treatment center authorities will try to convince the provider to keep the departmental chair or hospital informed about his or her progress. The state authorities also are kept informed; usually it is state law to do so.

TREATMENT

There are approximately 7500 inpatient chemical-dependency treatment programs throughout the United States.[113] Questions to determine the characteristics of a good treatment program are summarized in Box 97-3. Treatment referrals can be obtained from a reliable list of resources (Appendix 97-2 on page 2483).

BOX 97-3
QUESTIONS TO ASK A TREATMENT PROGRAM

1. Are you accredited? By which organizations?
2. What kind of services do you offer families? Do you provide services for children?
3. Do you follow a "twelve-step" orientation? Do you offer other kinds of support groups?
4. What is your philosophy about the nature and causes of addiction?
5. What are the goals of recovery?
6. Do all patients receive the same treatment? How do treatment plans vary? What kind of treatment would you recommend for the patient?
7. What are the costs? Are costs insurance reimbursable? How much will the patient be required to pay? Will the patient need to make a cash deposit?
8. Does this program often treat people with this particular addiction?
9. Do you prescribe drugs to patients? Under what circumstances? Over what period of time?
10. How much time do you devote to assessing the patient? What kinds of things do you assess the patient for?
11. How many counselors are on staff? What disciplines do they represent? How many are in recovery? How much training do recovering counselors receive?
12. How many caseloads does each counselor carry at any given time?
13. How much time each day is devoted to therapy and education? How much free time are patients given?
14. How much time is devoted to group therapy versus individual therapy?
15. Do you offer nutritional counseling? How much time each day is spent on physical exercise?
16. When did this program first begin operating? How long has this particular treatment team been working together? How many employees are on staff? How many employees have gone to work for other companies in the past year?
17. Do you publish materials for patients or professionals?
18. What does the program do for women, ethnic groups, adolescents, the elderly, and other special populations?
19. How much time do you devote to relapse prevention planning? What tools do you offer to develop relapse prevention skills?
20. How do you help patients plan for ongoing recovery after treatment?
21. How long does your aftercare program last? What kind of services do you provide?
22. What activities do you offer alumni?

Modified from Yoder B: *The recovery resource book,* New York, 1990, Simon & Schuster.

Discussion of specific treatment modalities are beyond the scope of this chapter. It is critical that a psychoactive substance-abuse disorder receive the same full-time, expert attention that any other serious, lethal, and complex disease receives.[88] In general, three basic goals should be accomplished:

(1) Maximize the physical and mental health of the care provider, because a person will find it difficult to achieve abstinence if chronic medical problems have not been adequately treated.
(2) Enhance motivation toward abstinence through educating the care provider and his or her family about the usual course of the disorder, employing appropriate medications to stop the individual from returning to substance misuse (e.g., naltrexone) and using behavior modification to maintain abstinence.
(3) Help the care provider rebuild a life without the substance, through vocational and avocational counseling, family counseling, and help him or her develop a substance-free peer group.[80,82] This decision often involves a new specialty of medicine or nursing.

Options

Treatment options include inpatient and outpatient programs. The Georgia Disabled Doctors Program encourages at least an initial 96-hour triage in a diagnostic detoxification unit.[95] There is flexibility with respect to the length of inpatient therapy. In general, the typical length of stay for chemical-dependency treatment is 4 weeks, followed by 1 to 2 years of outpatient aftercare.[113] Although initial inpatient therapy is preferred, 4 to 12 weeks of therapy may cost from $12,000 to $25,000.[87] This cost may be covered by the individual's health insurance. Many policies typically will cover cost for substance-abuse treatment, but may require payment of a deductible and have limitations with respect to the specific facility and the duration of the treatment. Rehabilitation typically takes at least 6 months before the individual is judged remotely ready to return to medical practice.

The question always arises: "Should this anesthesia provider return to anesthesiology, with the relatively easy availability of drugs?" Many rehabilitation center authorities counsel against such a return, exploring alternative types of medical practice, especially if the individual has suffered a relapse.

It is the policy of the ASA to treat substance-abuse disorders as a disease.[5,7] As such, the organization recommends that anesthesiology departments give rehabilitating (it is never-ending) victims *one further chance* in practice with monitoring (see following discussion). To take such an individual back during monitored rehabilitation is often difficult, yet such individuals may be better motivated and more productive than ever before in their lives. To be sure, there is a relapse risk (its true percentage is unknown), but there are real success stories.

In addition, the Americans With Disabilities Act (ADA) of 1992 contains some protections for individuals who have completed a rehabilitation program, or who are currently in rehabilitation and no longer engaged in the illegal use of drugs. The ADA does not prohibit policies or procedures, such as drug testing, to ensure that the individual continues to be drug free.[100] Monitoring of such a provider during rehabilitation *must:* (1) be frequent at first, although it can be tapered considerably; (2) be randomized; (3) involve urine/blood samples that are visually observed and signed for by a designated monitoring individual; and (4) provide testing paid for by the provider, not by the hospital or the department. Many monitors prefer to demand frequent samples, actually sending only a few per month for testing, especially after an initial period. A carefully drawn contract (reentry contract) needs to be signed by the provider, the hospital, and the department chair that specifies all the provisions for testing and guarantees that the rehabilitated user agrees to the release of the drug-test results to the responsible authorities, plus any other stipulations deemed necessary. Often the provider will be required to agree in advance that this is his or her "last chance" (i.e., that no further reentry contracts will be forthcoming). If a relapse occurs, grounds for dismissal from the hospital staff usually exist as well as grounds for suspension or loss of medical license.

Letters of recommendation to other anesthesiology departments concerning individuals known (i.e., proved) to have had problems with substance or alcohol abuse *must* contain factual information about that problem. The practice of allowing such individuals to skip from locality to locality must be condemned and stopped.[28]

Outcomes

A relapse in alcohol abuse in men is rare after 5 years of abstinence.[101] Treatment outcomes have been favorable in 65% to 83% of physicians.[37,69] Experts have stated that "physicians [anesthesiologists] who continue in treatment have an excellent prognosis,[88] and the ASA concurs that prognosis for long-term recovery is good."[7]

However, the relapse rate of anesthesiology residents with a history of opioid substance abuse, who are allowed to reenter a training program, has been reported to be 66%, with 25% of relapses resulting in death from either overdose or suicide.[66]

Although the fate of those residents who did not immediately reenter a residency program is not indicated,[66] this alarming statistic suggests that, at least for anesthesiologists in training, reentry into the specialty following opioid abuse may be both extremely hazardous and unwise.

Members of the anesthesiology community must realize that a psychoactive substance-abuse disorder is simply not compatible with continuing practice in this specialty, in particular, and perhaps medicine in general. Other useful and productive occupations may allow such an individual to lead a much happier life. In any case, we must not avoid our responsibilities to our colleagues and to our patients.

KEY POINTS

- It should be recognized that early intervention, therapy, and subsequent monitoring often can be used to rehabilitate the impaired individual. If an understanding of these disorders exists, appropriate, rapid, and safe action can be taken to facilitate treatment when realistic concerns or reasonable evidence surface.
- Psychoactive drugs are neither good nor bad; they have multiple effects, which, in turn, depend on the amount taken and the individual's expectations of those effects.
- It has been argued that no one really knows or will ever know precisely how many practicing physicians have problems with alcohol and other drugs. Data that tally the number of physicians with a substance-related disorder come from three main sources: (1) medical licensing boards; (2) surveys; and (3) treatment programs. The sources are vulnerable to criticism because of inadequate or nonrepresentative samples confined to physicians in a single medical center, state, or treatment program. Also, physicians may tend to select particular types of treatment.
- It is highly doubtful that an anesthesiologist will be the first health care worker to ask questions about a colleague's behavior. Operating room nurses, who actually observe anesthesiologists' work in progress, are often the first to question behavior.
- Anesthesiologists, compared with other specialists, appear to be at high risk for substance-related disorders.
- It may be that the efforts to look for, find, and treat impaired physicians is being rewarded. More recent studies using a survey format and looking only at rates of substance use have found no significant difference in the use of psychoactive substances between anesthesiologists in training or in practice compared with peer groups. Results of a study in progress report that rates of substance-abuse disorders in anesthesia training programs have declined since 1986. The incidence rate for new substance abuse in the 1994-1995 training years is estimated at 0.4% per year for residents and 0.1% per year for attending physicians.
- It has been contended that fentanyl, parenterally and perhaps orally administered, is the substance most likely to be misused by anesthesiologists. The process of identifying a substance-abuse disorder among anesthesia care providers is analogous to diagnosis and should not be

considered a confrontation with a "criminal." Every individual who works in the anesthesiology profession can and should attempt to identify victims of a substance-related disorder.

- No clinically practical system for drug accountability can prevent misuse of controlled substances by a determined anesthesia care provider. Multiple psychoactive substances are readily available in all anesthesiology departments, and almost all hold potential for misuse. The most commonly abused substance, even for anesthesia providers, is still alcohol, which is available outside the department.
- Immediate on-site urine testing for substance abuse is available with a number of simple-to-use devices. These devices are popular in the criminal justice system, hospital emergency departments, the military, and private industry. They can simultaneously test for multiple drugs or drug metabolites without handling of laboratory reagents or urine specimens.
- Denial is the hallmark of substance-related disorders. It is such a potent and malignant facet of the disease that outside help is lifesaving.
- It is the policy of the ASA to treat substance-abuse disorders as a disease. As such, the organization recommends that anesthesiology departments give rehabilitating (it is never-ending) victims one further chance in their medical practice with monitoring. In addition, the AWDA of 1992 protects individuals who have completed a rehabilitation program, or who are currently in rehabilitation and no longer engaged in the illegal use of drugs. The ADA does not prohibit policies or procedures, such as drug testing, to ensure that the individual continues to be drug free.
- A relapse in alcohol abuse in men is rare after 5 years of abstinence. Treatment outcomes have been favorable in 65% to 83% of physicians. Experts have stated that "physicians [anesthesiologists] who continue in treatment have an excellent prognosis, and the ASA concurs that prognosis for long-term recovery is good."

KEY REFERENCES

American Psychiatric Association: *Diagnostic and statistical manual of mental disorders,* ed 3, Washington, 1987, American Psychiatric Association.

Davison GC, Neale JM: Psychoactive substance use disorders. In *Abnormal psychology,* ed 6, New York, 1996, John Wiley & Sons.

Demos MP: What every physician should know about the national practitioner data bank, *Arch Intern Med* 151:1708, 1991.

Gordis E: Alcohol Research: at the cutting edge, *Arch Gen Psych* 53:199, 1996.

Gravenstein JS, Kory WP, Marks RG: Drug abuse by anesthesia personnel, *Anesth Analg* 62:467, 1983.

Klein RL, Stevens WC, Kingston HGG: Controlled substance dispensing and accountability in United States anesthesiology residency programs, *Anesthesiology* 77:806, 1992.

Menk EJ, Baumgarten RK, Kingsley CP, et al: Success of reentry into anesthesiology training program by residents with a history of substance abuse, *JAMA* 263:3060, 1990.

Ray O, Ksir C: *Drugs, society, and human behavior,* ed 7, St. Louis, 1996, Mosby–Year Book.

Silverstein JH, Silva DA, Iberti TJ: Opioid addiction in anesthesiology (review), *Anesthesiology* 79:354, 1993.

Ward CF: Substance abuse (editorial), *Anesthesiology* 77:619, 1992.

Yoder B: *The recovery resource book,* New York, 1990, Simon & Schuster.

REFERENCES

1. Aach RD, Girard DE, Humphrey H, et al: Alcohol and other substance abuse and impairment among physicians in residency training, *Ann Intern Med* 116:245, 1992.
2. Adler GR, Potts FE III, Kirby RR, et al: Narcotics control in anesthesia training, *JAMA* 253:3133, 1985.
3. American Psychiatric Association: *Diagnostic and statistical manual of mental disorders,* ed 4, Washington, American Psychiatric Association, 1994.
4. Ansliger HJ: Quoted by Green RC, Carroll GJ, Buxton WD: *Drug addiction among physicians, JAMA* 236:1372, 1976.
5. Arnold WP III: Substance abuse and chemical dependence in anesthesiology, *News Am Soc Anesthesiol* 55:4, 1991.
6. Arnold WP: 1995 substance abuse survey in anesthesiology training programs: a brief summary, *News Am Soc Anesthesiol* 59:12, 1995.
7. American Society of Anesthesiology Committee on Occupational Health of Operating Room Personnel: *Questions and answers about chemical dependence and physician impairment,* pp. 1–13, 1986.
8. Baldwin DC, Hughes PH, Conrad SE, et al: Substance use among senior medical students, *JAMA* 256:2074, 1991.
9. Ball DM, Murray RM: Genetics of alcohol misuse, (review), *Br Med Bull* 50:18, 1994.
10. Berridge V: Drug Policy: should the law take a back seat? *Lancet* 347:301, 1996.
11. Blachly PH, Osterud HT, Josslin R: Suicide in professional groups, *N Engl J Med* 268:1278, 1963.
12. Blanke RV: Accuracy in Urinalysis. In Hawks RL, Chiang CN, editors: *Urine testing for drugs of abuse,* Rockville, 1988, National Institute on Drug Abuse Research Monograph Series.
13. Blondell RD: Impaired physicians, *Prim Care* 20:209, 1993.
14. Bohigian GM, Croughan JL, Sanders K:

Substance abuse and dependence in physicians: an overview of the effects of alcohol and drug abuse, *Miss Med* 91:233, 1994.
15. Bonnet MH, Avand DL: The use of prophylactic naps to maintain performance during a continuous operation, *Ergonomics* 37:1009, 1994.
16. Brewster JM: Prevalence of alcohol and other drug problems among physicians, *JAMA* 255:1913, 1986.
17. Brown LS: Federal drug policy and terminology: Foes or allies? *J Natl Med Assoc* 72:575, 1980.
18. Bruce DL, Eide KA, Linde HW, et al: Causes of death among anesthesiologists: a 20-year survey, *Anesthesiology* 29:565, 1968.
19. Bruce DL, Eide KA, Smithe NJ, et al: A prospective survey of anesthesiologist mortality, 1967–1971, *Anesthesiology* 41:171, 1974.
20. Bullis RK: Swallowing the scroll: legal implications of the recent supreme court peyote cases, *J Psych Drugs* 22:325, 1990.
21. Cadoret RJ, Troughton E, O'Gorman TW, et al: An adoptive study of genetic and environmental factors in drug abuse, *Arch Gen Psych* 43:1131, 1986.
22. Canavan DI: Screening: urine drug tests, *Md Med J* 36:229, 1987.
23. Centrella M: Physician addiction and impairment-current thinking: a review. *J Addict Dis* 13:91, 1994.
24. *Chemical Dependence Guidelines for Departments of Anesthesiology,* Washington, 1991, American Society of Anesthesiologists.
25. Cotton NS: Cited by Cloninger CR: Neurogenetic adaptive mechanisms in alcoholism, *Science* 236:410, 1987.
26. Crawshaw R, Bruce JA, Eraker PL, et al: An epidemic of suicide among physicians on probation, *JAMA* 243:1915, 1980.
27. Davison GC, Neale JM: *Abnormal psychology,* ed 6, New York, 1996, John Wiley & Sons.
28. Demos MP: What every physician should know about the national practitioner data bank, *Arch Intern Med* 151:1708, 1991.
29. Donovan JM: An etiologic model of alcoholism, *Am J Psych* 143:1, 1986.
30. Eisohly HN, Eisohly MA: Poppy seed ingestion and opiates urinalysis: a closer look, *J Anal Toxicol* 14:308, 1990.
31. Farley WJ, Arnold WP III: *Unmasking addiction: Chemical Dependency in Anesthesiology,* Titusville, 1991, Janssen.
32. Farley WJ, Talbott GD: Anesthesiology and addiction (editorial), *Anesth Analg* 62:465, 1983.
33. Flaherty JA, Richman JA: Substance use and addiction among medical students, residents, and physicians, *Psych Clin North Am* 16:189, 1993.
34. Fleming MF: Physician Impairment: options for intervention, *Am Fam Phys* 50:41, 1994.
35. Gallegos KV, Browne CH, Veit FW, et al: Addiction in anesthesiologists: drug access and patterns of substance abuse, *QRB* 14:116, 1988.
36. Gianoulakis C, Kirshnan B, Thavundayil J: Enhanced sensitivity to pituitary β-endorphin to ethnologic in subjects at high risk of alcoholism, *Arch Gen Psych* 53:250, 1996.
37. Goby MJ, Bradley NJ, Bespalec DA: Physicians treated for alcoholism: a follow-up study, *Clin Exp Res* 3:121, 1979.
38. Goodwin WD: Alcoholism and heredity, *Arch Gen Psych* 36:57, 1979.
39. Gordis E: Alcohol Research: at the cutting edge, *Arch Gen Psych* 53:199, 1996.
40. *The Graduate Medical Education Directory,* Chicago, 1995, American Medical Association.
41. Gravenstein JS, Kory WP, Marks RG: Drug abuse by anesthesia personnel, *Anesth Analg* 62:467, 1983.
42. Gualtieri AC, Cosentino JP, Becker JS: The California experience with a diversion program for impaired physicians, *JAMA* 249:226, 1983.
43. Hays LR, Stillner V, Littrell R: Fentanyul dependence associated with oral ingestion, *Anesthesiology* 77:819, 1992.
44. The Health Care Quality Improvement Act of 1986, 45 US Code § 11101-11152.
45. Henderson GL, Frincke J, Leung CY, et al: Antibodies to fentanyl, *J Pharmacol Exp Ther* 192:489, 1974.
46. Huges PH, Baldwin DC, Sheehan DV, et al: Resident physician substance use, by specialty, *Am J Psych* 149:1348, 1992.
47. Huges PH, Brandenburg N, Baldwin DC, et al: Prevalence of substance use among us physicians, *JAMA* 267:2333, 1992.
48. Huges PH, Conard SE, Baldwin DC, et al: Resident physician substance use in the United States, *JAMA* 265:2069, 1991.
49. Hyde GL, Miscull BG: *The impaired surgeon,* 1995, American College of Surgeons.
50. Hyde GL, Wolf J: Alcohol and drug use by surgery residents, *J Am Coll Surg* 181:1, 1995.
51. *The impaired practitioner* (videotape 12), ASA Patient Safety Videotape Series. ASA Committee on Patient Safety and Risk Management
52. Jackson SH: Humanism and anesthesia safety. In Miller ED, editor: *Current reviews in clinical anesthesia,* Miami, 1988, Current Reviews.
53. Johnson VE: *Intervention,* Minneapolis, 1986, Johnson Institute Books.
54. Klein RL, Stevens WC, Kingston HGG: Controlled substance dispensing and accountability in United States anesthesiology residency programs, *Anesthesiology* 77:806, 1992.
55. Labarbera M, Wolfe T: Characteristics, attitudes and implications of fentanyl use based on reports from self-identified fentanyl users, *J Psych Drugs* 15:293, 1983.
56. Lecky JH, Aukburg SJ, Conahan TJ III, et al: A departmental policy addressing chemical substance abuse, *Anesthesiology* 65:414, 1986.
57. Lemon SJ, Sienko DG, Alguire PC: Physicians' attitudes toward mandatory workplace urine drug testing, *Arch Intern Med* 152:2238, 1992.
58. Lerner WD: Treatment of narcotic dependence. In Lerner WD, Barr MJ, editors: *Handbook of hospital-based substance abuse treatment,* New York, 1990, Pergamon Press.
59. Lew EA: Mortality experience among anesthesiologists 1954–1976, *Anesthesiology* 51:195, 1979.
60. Lutsky I, Hopwood M, Abram SE, et al: Use of psychoactive substances in three medical specialties: anaesthesia, medicine and surgery, *Can J Anaesth* 41:561, 1994.
61. Maki DG, Klein BS, McCormick RD, et al: Nosocomial *Pseudomonas pickettii* bacteremias traced to narcotic tampering, *JAMA* 265:981, 1991.
62. Manno JE: Specimen collection and handling. In Hawks RL, Chiang CN, editors: *Urine testing for drugs of abuse,* Rockville, 1988, National Institute on Drug Abuse Research Monograph Series.
63. McDonough JP: Personality, addiction and anesthesia, *JAANA* 58:193, 1990.
64. McGue M, Pickens RW, Svikis DS: Sex and age effects on the inheritance of alcohol problems: a twin study, *J Ab Psych* 101:3, 1992.
65. McNamara RM, Margulies JL: Chemical dependency in emergency medicine residency programs: perspective of the program directors, *Ann Emerg Med* 23:1072, 1994.
66. Menk EJ, Baumgarten RK, Kingsley CP, et al: Success of reentry into anesthesiology training programs by residents with a history of substance abuse, *JAMA* 263:3060, 1990.
67. Miller NS: *Addiction psychiatry,* New York, 1995, Wiley-Liss.
68. Morrison J: *DSM-IV made easy,* New York, 1995.
69. Morse RM, Martin MA, Swenson WM, et al: Prognosis of physicians treated for alcoholism and drug dependence, *JAMA* 251:743, 1984.
70. OnTrak TesTcup™ Product Insert, Roche Diagnostic Systems, 1995, U.S. Order No. 47226, Art No. 07 5561 3.
71. *Out of control* (videotape), American College of Surgeons, 1995.
72. Ray O, Ksir C: *Drugs, society, and human behavior,* ed 7, St. Louis, 1996, Mosby–Year Book.
73. Regier DA, Farmer ME, Rae DS, et al: Comorbidity of mental disorders with alcohol and other drug abuse: results from the epidemiologic catchment area study, *JAMA* 264:2511, 1990.
74. Rinaldi RC, Steindler EM, Wilford BB, et al: Clarification and standardization of substance abuse terminology, *JAMA* 259:555, 1988.
75. Robb N: University acknowledges special risks, introduces drug program for anesthetists, *Can Med Assoc J* 153:449, 1995.
76. Rosenberg M: Drug abuse in oral and maxillofacial training programs, *J Oral Maxillofac Surg* 44:458, 1986.
77. Russell AT, Pasnau RO, Taintor ZC: The emotionally disturbed psychiatric resident, *Am J Psych* 134:59, 1977.
78. Schmidt KA, Schlesinger MD: A reliable accounting system for controlled substances in the operating room, *Anesthesiology* 78:184, 1993.
79. Schmidt KA: Reply to letter to the editor by Woods GM: Anesthesiologists and substance abuse, *Anesthesiology* 79:190, 1993.
80. Schuckit MA, Cahalan D: Evaluation of alcoholism treatment programs. In Filstead WJ, Rossi JJ, Keller M, editors: *Alcohol and alcohol problems: New thinking and new directions,* Cambridge, 1976, Ballinger.

81. Schuckit MA, Gold EO: A simultaneous evaluation of multiple markers of ethanol/placebo challenges in sons of alcoholics and controls, *Arch Gen Psych* 45:211, 1988.
82. Schuckit MA: Drug and alcohol abuse: a clinical guide to diagnosis and treatment. In Woods SM, editor: *Critical issues in psychiatry,* New York, 1995, Plenum Medical.
83. Schuckit MA: Etiologic theories on alcoholism. In Estes N, Heinemann E, editors: *Alcoholism,* St Louis, 1986, CV Mosby.
84. Scott M, Fisher KS: The evolving legal context for drug testing programs, *Anesthesiology* 73:1022, 1990.
85. Silsby HD, Kruzich DJ, Hawkins MR: Fentanyl citrate abuse among health care professionals, *Milit Med* 149:227, 1984.
86. Silverstein JH, Rieders MF, McMullin M, et al: An analysis of the duration of fentanyl and its metabolites in urine and saliva, *Anesth Analg* 76:618, 1993.
87. Silverstein JH, Silva DA, Iberti TJ: Opioid addiction in anesthesiology (review), *Anesthesiology* 79:354, 1993.
88. Spiegelman WG, Saunders L, Mazze RI: Addiction and anesthesiology, *Anesthesiology* 60:335, 1984.
89. Springer EW: Peer Review/Hospital Privileges/Credentialling, *Leg Med* p. 57, 1994.
90. Stiller RL, Scierka AM, Davis PJ, et al: A brief technical communication: detection of fentanyl in urine, *Forens Sci Int* 44:1, 1990.
91. Stoelting RK: *Opioid agonists and antagonists, pharmacology and physiology in anesthetic practice,* Philadelphia, 1987, JB Lippincott.
92. Struempler RE: Excretion of codeine and morphine following ingestion of poppy seeds, *J Anal Toxicol* 11:97, 1987.
93. Tabakoff B, Hoffman PL, Lee JM, et al: Differences in platelet enzyme activity between alcoholics and nonalcoholics, *N Engl J Med* 318:134, 1988.
94. Talbott GD, Benson EB: Impaired physicians: the dilemma of identification, *Postgrad Med* 68:56, 1980.
95. Talbott GD, Gallegos KV, Wilson PO, et al: The Medical Association of Georgia's Impaired Physicians Program, *JAMA* 257:2927, 1987.
96. Talbott GD, Richardson AC, Mashburn JS, et al: The Medical Association of Georgia's Disabled Doctors Program: a 5-year review, *J Med Assoc Ga* 70:545, 1981.
97. Thacker SB, Veech RL, Vernon AA, et al: Genetic and biochemical factors relevant to alcoholism, *Clin Exper Res* 8:375, 1984.
98. Tinker JH: *Personal communication,* March, 1991.
99. Tobin T, Kwiatkowski S, Watt DS, et al: Immunoassay detection of drugs in racing horses. XI. ELISA and RIA detection of fentanyl, alfentanil, sufentanil and carfentanil in equine blood and urine, *Res Commun Chem Pathol Pharmacol* 63:129, 1989.
100. United States Department of Justice, Civil Rights Division: *The Americans with Disabilities Act,* Title III Technical Assistance Manual, III 2.3000 Drug addiction as an impairment. November, 1993.
101. Vaillant GE: A long-term follow-up of male alcohol abuse, *Arch Gen Psych* 53:243, 1996.
102. Walsh JM: *Employee drug screening,* National Institute on Drug Abuse, 1986, US Department of Health and Human Services, (ADM) 88-1442.
103. Walzer RS: Impaired physicians: an overview and update of the legal issues, *J Leg Med* 11:131, 1990.
104. Ward CF, Newman LM: Report of scientific meeting, *Anesthesiology* 68:979, 1988.
105. Ward CF, Ward GC, Saidman LJ: Drug abuse in anesthesia training programs, *JAMA* 250:922, 1983.
106. Ward CF: Quoted by Polk SL: Substance abuse in anesthesia: patient safety among issues, *Anesth Pat Safe Found News* 6:1, 1991.
107. Ward CF: Substance abuse (editorial), *Anesthesiology* 77:619, 1992.
108. Watts VW, Caplan YH: Evaluation of the Coat-A-Count 1251 fentanyl RIA: comparison of 125I RIA and GC/MS-SIM for quantification of fentanyl in case urine specimens, *J Anal Toxicol* 14:266, 1990.
109. Wearing Masks: *The potential for drug addiction in anesthesia,* Chicago, 1993, Rainbow Production.
110. Weeks AM, Buckland MR, Morgan EB, et al: Chemical dependence in anaesthetic registrants in Australia and New Zealand, *Anaesth Intens Care* 21:151, 1993.
111. Weinger MB, Englund CE: Ergonomic and human factors affecting anesthetic vigilance and monitoring performance in the operating room environment, *Anesthesiology* 73:995, 1990.
112. Wiedman D: Big and little moon peyotism as health care delivery systems, *Med Anthropol* 12:371, 1990.
113. Yoder B: *The recovery resource book,* New York, 1990, Simon & Schuster.

APPENDIX 97-1

INFORMATIONAL MATERIAL AVAILABLE TO PHYSICIANS FROM MEDICAL SOCIETIES

Item	Where available
1. *The Impaired Surgeon*[49] 2. *Out of Control*[71] (video tape)	American College of Surgeons 55 East Erie Street Chicago, IL 60611-2797 (312) 664-4050 ext. 310
3. *Questions and Answers About Chemical Dependence and Physician Impairment*[7] 4. *Chemical Dependence Guidelines for Departments of Anesthesia*[24] 5. *Unmasking Addiction*[31] (video tape) 6. *Wearing Masks: The Potential for Drug Addition in Anesthesia*[109] (video tape)	American Society of Anesthesiology Executive Office 520 North Northwest Highway Park Ridge, IL 60068-2573 (708) 825-5586 ext. 27

APPENDIX 97-2

SERVICES FOR IMPAIRED PHYSICIANS AND HEALTH CARE WORKERS BY STATE

Alabama

Physicians Recovery Network
Medical Association of Alabama
Director: Gerald Summer, MD
19 South Jackson Street
PO Box 1900
Montgomery, AL 36102
(334) 263-6441

Alaska

Alaska State Medical Association
Executive Secretary: Pam Ventgan, CMA
4107 Laurel Street
Ankorage, AK 99508-9301
(907) 562-2662 or (907) 349-9301

Alaska Practitioner Recovery Program
Alaska Nurses Association
Kate Morris, RN
237 East 3rd Avenue
Anchorage, AK 99501-2532
(907) 274-0827 (8:30AM – 2:00PM)

Arizona

Director: David Greenberg, MD
Physicians Health Program
400 West Camelback Road
Phoenix, AZ 85013
(602) 263-0665

Impaired Nurse Committee
Arizona Nurses Association
Sara Withgott, RN, MS
1850 East Southern Avenue, Suite 1
Tempe, AZ 85282
(602) 831-0404

Arkansas

Physicians Health Committee
Arkansas Medical Society
Director: Joseph Martindale, MD
302 West South
Benton, AR 72015
(501) 778-4511

Recovery for Nurses Council
Arkansas Nurses Association
Charlene Bradham, RN, MNSc
Department of Nursing
University of Arkansas-Little Rock
2801 South University Avenue
Little Rock, AR 72204
(501) 569-8084 (daytime)
(501) 562-2444 (evening)

California

Committee on Well-Being of Physicians
California Medical Association
Director: Sandra Bressler
221 Main Street, 2nd Floor
PO Box 7690
San Francisco, CA 94120-7690
(415) 541-0900

Well Being Committee
California Nurses Association
Director: Rose Anne DeMoro
1145 Market Street, 11th Floor Suite 1110
San Francisco, CA 94103
(415) 864-4141

Colorado

Colorado Physician Health Program
Director: Stephen Dilts, MD
899 Logan Street, Suite 505
Denver, CO 80203
(303) 860-0122
(800) 927-0122

Connecticut

Physician Health Committee
Connecticut State Medical Society
160 Saint Ronan Street
New Haven, CT 06511-2390
(203) 865-0587
(800) 635-7740 (hotline)

Delaware

Physicians' Health Committee
Medical Society of Delaware
Director: Mark A. Meister, MD
1925 Lovering Avenue
Wilmington, DE 19806
(302) 652-6512

District of Columbia

Physicians Health Committee
Director: Barbara Allen
2215 M Street, Northwest
Washington, DC 20037
(202) 466-1800

Florida

Impaired Physician Program
Florida Medical Association
Director: Roger Goetz, MD
PO Box 1881
Fernandina Beach, FL 32035-1881
(904) 277-8004
(800) 888-8776

Georgia

Physician Well-Being Program
Director: John D. Lenton, MD
PO Box 279
Hinesville, GA 31310
(912) 884-2686

Hawaii

Hawaii Health Committee
Director: Leonard Jacobs, MD
1360 South Beretania Street, 2nd
Honolulu, HI 96814
(808) 536-7702

Idaho

Physician Recovery Network
Director: Richard W. Gerber, MD
1512 12th Avenue Road
Nampa, ID 83651

Program Coordinator: John Southworth, CADC
224 Arrow Rock Lane
Boise, ID 83706
(800) 486-4372

Illinois

Physician Assistance Program
Illinois State Medical Society
Chairman: Dale Sysert, MD
Director: Susan Wagner
20 North Michigan Avenue, #700
Chicago, IL 60602
(312) 580-2499

Indiana

Physician Assistance Program
Indiana State Medical Association
322 Canal Walk
Indianapolis, IN 46202-3252
(317) 261-2060

Iowa

Impaired Physician Program
Iowa Medical Society
1001 Grand Avenue
West Des Moines, IA 50265
(515) 223-1401
(800) 747-3070 (helpline)

Kansas

Medical Advocacy Program (MAP)
623 West 10th Avenue
Topeka, KS 66612
(913) 235-2383
(800) 332-0156

Kentucky

Impaired Physician Program
Kentucky Medical Association
301 North Hurstboume Parkway, Suite 200
Louisville, KY 40222-8512
(502) 426-7761

Louisiana

Impaired Physician Program
Louisiana State Medical Society
Director: Dave Tarver
3501 North Causeway Boulevard, Suite 800
Metairie, LA 70002
(504) 832-9815
(800) 375-9508

Louisiana State Board of Nursing
150 Baronne Street, Suite 912
New Orleans, LA 70112
(504) 556-9867

Maine

Committee on Physician Health
Maine Medical Association
PO Box 190, Association Drive
Manchester, ME 04351
(207) 623-9266

Maryland

Physician Rehabilitation Program
Medical & Chirurgical Faculty of Maryland
Michael C. Llufrio CCDC, NCAC II
1204 Maryland Avenue, 2nd Floor
Baltimore, MD 21201
(800) 992-7010

Board of Physician Quality Assurance
(410) 764-4777

Massachusetts

Physicians Health Services
Massachusetts Medical Society
1440 Main Street
Waltham, MA 02154
(617) 893-4610

The Massachusetts Nurses Association Peer Assistance Program
Massachusetts Nurses Association
Department of Nursing Staff
340 Turnpike Street
Canton, MA 02021
(617) 821-4625 (daytime)

Michigan

Impaired Physicians Program
Michigan State Medical Society
120 W. Saginaw, PO Box 950
East Lansing, MI 48826-0950
(517) 337-1351

Michigan Impaired Professional Funding Committee
Michigan Nurses Association
Sheila Abood
2310 Jolly Oak Road
Okemos, MI 48864
(517) 349-5640

Minnesota

Physicians Support Services
3433 Boardway Street, Northeast, Suite 300
Minneapolis, MN 55413
(612) 378-1875
Fax (612) 378-3875

The Minnesota Nurses Association
Peer Assistance Program for Nurses
Minnesota Nurses Association
1295 Bandana Boulevard, North, Suite 140
St. Paul, MN 55108
(612) 646-4807

Mississippi

Caduceus Club of Mississippi
Director: Kay Gatewood
2600 River Ridge Road, Suite 203
Jackson, MS 39216-0513
(601) 981-3408

The Mississippi Nurses' Foundation's
Educational Resource Committee
Mississippi Nurses Association
Betty Dickson
135 Bounds Street
Jackson, MS 39206
(601) 982-9183

Missouri

Missouri Physicians Health Program
Missouri State Medical Association
113 Madison Street, PO Box 1028
Jefferson City, MO 65102
(573) 636-5151

Montana

Montana Medical Association
Director: Brian Zins
2021 11th Avenue, Suite 1
Helena, MT 59601
(406) 443-4000

Nebraska

Physician Advocacy Committee
Nebraska Medical Association
1512 FirsTier Bank Building
Lincoln, NE 68508
(401) 474-4471

Licensee Assistant Program
Director: Malcolm Head
Division of Alcohol & Drug Abuse and Addiction Services
Department of Public Institutions
PO Box 94728
Lincoln, NE 68509-4728
(402) 471-2851

Nevada

Impaired Physician Program
Nevada State Medical Association
3660 Baker Lane, #101
Reno, NV 89509
(702) 825-6788
Washoe City Medical Society–Reno
(702) 825-0278
Clark City Medical Society–Las Vegas
(702) 739-9989

Disability Advisory Committee
Nevada Board of Nursing
1755 East Plum Lane #260
Reno, NV 89502
(702) 786-2778

New Hampshire

Physician Effectiveness Committee
New Hampshire Medical Society
7 North State Street
Concord, NH 03301
(603) 224-1909

Nurses Peer Assistance Group
New Hampshire Nurses Association
48 West Street
Concord, NH 03301
(603) 224-3632 (hotline)

New Jersey

Impaired Physicians Program
Medical Society of New Jersey
2 Princess Road
Lawrenceville, NJ 08648
(609) 896-1766

Peer Assistance Committee
New Jersey State Nurses Association
Dorothy Flemming, RN, MSN
320 West State Street
Trenton, NJ 08618
(609) 392-4884 (daytime)
(609) 662-0108 (hotline)

New Mexico

Physicians Aid Committee
New Mexico Medical Society
Director: Randy Marshall
7770 Jefferson Northeast
Albuquerque, NM 87109
(505) 828-0237

Committee to Assist Nurses Recover
New Mexico Nurses Association
Marie McMillian, RN
909 Virginia N.E., Suite 101
Albuquerque, NM 87108
(505) 268-7744

New York

Committee for Physicians Health
Medical Society of the State of New York
16 The Sage Estate, Suite 302
Albany, NY 12204
(581) 436-4723

The Committee on Impaired Nursing Practice
New York State Nurses Association
Miriam Aaron MPA, CEAP, RN
46 Cornell Road
Latham, NY 12110
(518) 782-9400

North Carolina

North Carolina Physician Health Program
Six Forks Center One
4700 Six Forks Road, Suite 220
Raleigh, NC 27609
(919) 881-0585

North Carolina Nurses Association Peer Assistance Program
North Carolina Nurses Association
Hazel Browning-Moore
PO Box 12025
Raleigh, NC 27605
(919) 821-4250

North Dakota

Committee on the Impaired Physician
North Dakota Medical Association
PO Box 1198
Bismarck, ND 58502
(701) 223-9475
(800) 732-9477 (hotline)

Ohio

Physician Effectiveness Program
Director: Robert C. Erwin, DO
635 Park Meadow Road, Suite 203
Westerville, OH 43081
(614) 891-0080

Ohio Nurses Association
Peer Assistance Program for Nurses
Ohio Nurses Association
Zandra Ohri, RN, MA, MS
4000 East Main Street
Columbus, OH 43213-2983
(614) 237-5414 ext. 143

Oklahoma

Physician Recovery Program
Oklahoma State Medical Association
Director: Darrell Smith, MD
6704 West Tucumseh
Norman, OK 73072
(405) 360-4535

Oklahoma Association of Nurse Anesthetists
Chemical Dependency Program
Chairman: Dolores V. Pasierb, CRNA
609 Broad Lane
Norman, OK 73069
(405) 321-0849

Oregon

Oregon Health Professionals Program
6950 Southwest Hampton, Suite 220
Tigard, OR 97223-8331
(503) 620-9117

Nurse Assistance Network
Oregon Nurses Association
Chris O'Neill, RN
616 East 16th Street
Eugene, OR 97401
(503) 687-1110

Pennsylvania

Physicians' Health Programs
Pennsylvania Medical Society
777 East Park Drive
PO Box 8820
Harrisburg, PA 17105-8820
(717) 558-7750
(717) 558-7817 (hotline)

Pennsylvania Nurses Association
Christine Filipovich, MSN, RN
Administrator, Nursing Practice Program
2578 Interstate Drive
Harrisburg, PA 17110
(717) 657-1222
Fax (717) 657-3796

Rhode Island

Physicians' Health Services Committee
Rhode Island Medical Society
Director: William Mocoair, RN
106 Francis Street
Providence, RI 02903
(401) 331-3207

Rhode Island State Nurses' Association
Peer Assistance Program
Rhode Island State Nurses Association
Sharon Goldstein, RN, CD, CADAC, CEAP
c/o Rhode Island Employee Assistance Program
120 Centerville Road
Warwick, RI 02886
(800) 445-1195

South Carolina

Physicians Advocacy & Assistance
South Carolina Medical Association
Director: High V. Coleman, MD
PO Box 11188
Columbia, SC 29211
(803) 798-6207

Peer Assistance Program for Impaired Nurses
South Carolina Nurses Association
Sarah Forbes, RN
1821 Gadsden Street
Columbia, SC 29201
(803) 252-4781

South Dakota

Physicians HELP Program
South Dakota State Medical Association
1323 South Minnesota Avenue
Sioux Falls, SD 57105
(605) 336-1965

Tennessee

Impaired Physicians Program
Tennessee Medical Association
2301 21st Avenue South
PO Box 120909
Nashville, TN 37212-0909
(615) 385-2100
(615) 385-3319 (hotline)

Peer Assistance Program for Chemically Dependent Nurses
Tennessee Nurses Association
Director: Diana Kulas
545 Mainstream Drive, Suite 414
Nashville, TN 37228-1201
(615) 254-0350

Texas

Committee on Physician Health and Rehabilitation
Texas Medical Association
Director: Linda Kuhn
401 West 15th Street
Austin, TX 78701-1680
(512) 370-1300
(800) 880-1640 (hotline)

Texas Peer Assistance Program for Nurses
Texas Nurses Association
Michael VanDoren, RN, MSN
7600 Burnet Road, Suite 440
PO Box 9877
Austin, TX 78766-9877
(512) 467-7027
(800) 288-5528

Utah

Physicians Health Committee
David W. Feigal, MD
PO Box 17354
Salt Lake City, UT 84117
(801) 355-7477

Nurses Assisting Nurses with Substance Abuse
Utah Nurses Association
Alice Parkinson
University of Utah College of Nursing
25 South Medical Drive, Room 449
Salt Lake City, UT 84112
(801) 581-8244

Vermont

Vermont Recovering Professionals Program
Director: Suzanne Parker
118 Pine Street
Burlington, VT 05401
(802) 864-6595

Virginia

Physicians' Health & Effectiveness Program
Medical Society of Virginia
Director: Bette Bois
4205 Dover Road
Richmond, VA 23221
(804) 353-2721

Virginia Nurses' Association's Peer Assistance for Chemically Dependent Nurses
Virginia Nurses Association
7113 Three Chop Road, Suite 204
Richmond, VA 23226
(800) 868-6877

Washington

Washington Physicians Health Program
Director: Lynn Hankes, MD
720 Olive Way, Suite 525
Seattle, WA 98101
(206) 583-0127

West Virginia

Physician Health & Well Being Committee
Director: Thomas Haymond, MD
4307 MacCorkle Avenue, Southeast
PO Box 4106
Charleston, WV 25364
(304) 925-0342

Wisconsin

Director: David G. Benzer, DO
State Medical Society Statewide Physician Health Program
PO Box 1109
Madison, WI 53701
(608) 257-6781

Impaired Professionals Procedure (PP)
Department of Regulation & Licensure
Attention: Lee Ann Cooper
PO Box 8935
Madison, WI 53708
(608) 267-9883

Wyoming

Physicians' Wellness
Director: Richard W. Johnson, Jr.
PO Drawer 4009
Cheyenne, WY 82003
(307) 635-2424

In addition, the National Institute on Drug Abuse maintains a toll-free number:
National Institute on Drug Abuse: Drug Information
Treatment and Referral Hotline, 11426
Rockville Pike, Suite 410
Rockville, MD 20852
(800) 662-HELP (English)

CHAPTER 98

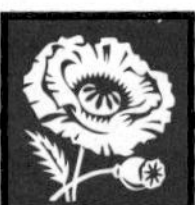

Quality Improvement in Anesthesiology

DENNIS D. DOBLAR
R. GILBERT RITCHIE

Patient outcome has been the traditional focus of quality-related activities for individual practitioners and anesthesia departments. **Previously, assessment of outcome was focused on the individual provider as the one responsible for the outcome. In contrast, the modern quality improvement (QI) paradigm focuses on the process used to deliver care rather than the individual provider.** The approach is based on evidence that most adverse outcomes result from process failures. **An effective QI program sets goals and objectives, selects indicators, identifies the causes for the problems, implements corrective action, and monitors the effect of those actions on the quality of care.** Indicators may be critical events, complications, or process variables that represent how well the process works. Peer review occurs during review of critical events identified by the QI system. Process review occurs during analysis of variations in process variables. Education and dissemination of information directed at improvements in the process result from the peer and process review activities. The pressures on physicians and healthcare organizations to measure, trend, improve quality of care, and document improvement have been steadily increasing in parallel with activities in healthcare reform, managed care initiatives, increasing competition and regulatory pressures.

This chapter will review the regulatory and competitive pressures for development of QI programs, a brief history of the development of the QI process, highlight the components of a QI system and discuss approaches to the development and implementation of a QI program. Anesthesiologists may use the information to structure their own programs to benefit their patients, which will ultimately serve to improve their practice and contribute to the professional advancement of the specialty.

SOURCES OF PRESSURE FOR QUALITY IMPROVEMENT SYSTEM IMPLEMENTATION

The motivating force behind quality improvement activities has historically been provided by the Joint Commission for

Accreditation of Healthcare Organizations (JCAHO). In the present healthcare market, pressure to improve and document quality of care arises from JCAHO, managed care organizations, the media, the public, industry seeking less expensive employee healthcare coverage, and third-party payors. Prior to 1986, the focus of JCAHO was on organizational structure, personnel, equipment, record keeping, and the physical facilities of hospitals.[3,8] In 1987, JCAHO made "Performance Improvement" a central theme for their "Agenda for Change."[8] Most recently, JCAHO has developed perioperative indicators to be used as performance measures in comparing institutions; however, schemes for risk-adjusting outcomes have not been disclosed by the JCAHO. Media attention to rising healthcare costs and expensive technological advances has made employers receptive to healthcare cost reduction strategies offered by managed care organizations that demand documentation of quality of care, cost effectiveness, and outcome data. Managed care and private payors use practice parameters or clinical pathways—systematically developed guidelines that direct physician decision making to specified algorithms of care that are of "proven" clinical efficacy—to reduce variations in practices that drive costs, to standardize payments, to predict costs of care, and to compare costs of care among institutions.[15] Mandating adherence to practice parameters by linking payment to compliance is similar to the current utilization review process. Private insurers have already introduced plans forcing compliance with practice parameters.[15] The American Society of Anesthesiologists (ASA) is actively developing practice parameters; the most recent pertains to transesophageal echocardiography (TEE). QI is a component of this practice guideline.[18]

Anesthesiology groups that do not conduct effective QI programs may find themselves "data poor" in contract negotiations, both from the perspective of practice and income protection and from the perspective of patient advocacy in an environment of cost-containment efforts. Comprehensive QI programs represent one of the few safeguards against inappropriate cost reductions achieved by withholding care, restricting access to care, avoiding the use of expensive technologies and specialists, or shortened, less intensive hospital stays. Efforts directed toward quality of care are essential to the status of anesthesiology regardless of the current or future diversity of the specialty.[11]

CURRENT JOINT COMMISSION FOR ACCREDITATION OF HEALTHCARE ORGANIZATIONS STANDARDS

The JCAHO is the primary regulatory agency forcing hospitals to develop their QI efforts. Performance improvement has been fundamental to the JCAHO "Agenda for Change" since its inception in 1987. The "Dimensions for Performance" create the framework supporting the JCAHO performance improvement guidelines. Two major areas are emphasized: (1) "doing the right thing," which addresses the efficacy of producing the desired outcomes and the appropriateness of the care delivered; and (2) "doing the right thing well," which addresses issues such as availability of care, timeliness of delivery, continuity of care, effectiveness, efficiency, patient safety, and respect and caring demonstrated toward patients. Based on these guidelines, standards are published in the JCAHO Accreditation Manual for Hospitals, which is updated and issued annually. Hospitals undergoing JCAHO inspection are scored on how well they meet these standards. The current guidelines relevant to this chapter are listed in Table 98-1; those guidelines directly relating to anesthesia are in bold typeface. The first

Table 98-1 JCAHO performance improvement standards relevant to anesthesia

Paragraph	JCAHO standard (1996)
PI.1/1.1	The hospital has a planned, systematic, hospital-wide approach to process design and performance measurement, assessment, and improvement, *and* these activities are collaborative and interdisciplinary.
PI.3.2/3.2.1	The important processes or outcomes on which the hospital collects data include at least: **operative, other invasive, and noninvasive procedures that place patients at risk.**
PI.4.1	The assessment process uses appropriate statistical qualilty control techniques.
PI.4.2	The hospital makes internal comparisons of its performance of processes and outcomes over time.
PI.4.3	The hospital compares performance data about its process with information from up-to-date sources.
PI.4.4	The hospital compares performance data about its process and outcomes with other hospitals, including through the use of reference databases.
PI.4.5.2	**Adverse events or patterns of adverse events during anesthesia use are intensively assessed.**
PI.4.7	When assessment findings relate to the performance of an individually licensed independent practitioner, the medical staff determines their use in peer review, ongoing monitoring, and periodic evaluations of the individuals' competence.
PI.5.1	When improvement activities lead to a determination that an individual with performance problems is unable or unwilling to improve, the hospital modifies the person's clinical privileges or job assignment or takes other appropriate action in accordance with the relevant standards in this manual.

two letters of the paragraph number indicate the section where the guideline can be found in the manual; "PI" stands for the Performance Improvement section.[9]

In addition to scoring conformance to standards, JCAHO has developed clinical indicators for measuring a hospital's performance and comparing performance among institutions (Box 98-1). Although participation in a indicator-based performance measurement system is optional in 1996, it will be mandatory in the future.[9] JCAHO has also developed a computer-based indicator measurement system—the IMSystem—which enables hospitals to submit indicator data regularly and receive quarterly performance reports based on data submitted.[9] The IMSystem perioperative indicators are the first five indicators listed in Box 98-1. The other seven indicators are recommended by JCAHO but are not part of their IMSystem indicators. Use of IMSystem is not mandatory; JCAHO states that hospitals may choose alternative, approved measurement systems.

Each indicator in Box 98-1 is intended by JCAHO to be represented as a rate. The numerator is the number of patients triggering the indicator; the denominator for indicators 1 through 5—the IMSystem indicators—is all patients undergoing procedures involving anesthesia and an inpatient stay. JCAHO does not specifically indicate the denominator for the other indicators; presumably, it is all patients undergoing procedures involving anesthesia, whether or not there was an associated inpatient stay.

Given the performance improvement guidelines, standards, and performance indicators, how does an anesthesia department support the hospital in complying with JCAHO expectations? The following steps may be considered:

1. Develop a departmental QI plan and, where appropriate, collaborate with other departments, such as perioperative nursing or surgery. Involving the hospital administration in the QI plan will facilitate compliance with standard PI1./1.1.
2. Ensure that the plan includes the systematic collection of data for operative procedures. This will facilitate the administration's compliance with PI3.2/3.2.1.
3. Ensure that the plan includes peer review of all cases in which a perioperative performance indicator was triggered. This satisfies PI4.5.2. Such case-by-case peer review should be documented. If peer review reveals avoidable anesthesia-related problems, appropriate action should be taken to prevent their recurrence, and such action should be documented.

Scoring guidelines for PI3.2.1 indicate that hospitals should review the following processes for operative, invasive, or noninvasive procedures that place the patient at risk: (1) selection of the appropriate procedure; (2) patient preparation for the procedure; (3) performance of the procedure and patient monitoring; (4) postprocedure care; and (5) postprocedure patient education. If the average number of cases per quarter is more than 600, at least 5% of the cases should be reviewed. If the average per quarter is less than 600, at least 30 cases should be reviewed. If there are fewer than 30 cases per quarter, then 100% of the cases should be reviewed. For procedures involving anesthesia, the review should indicate whether a preoperative assessment was performed, consent for anesthesia was obtained, the risk versus benefits of the anesthesia were discussed with the patient, and the patient was appropriately prepared. This satisfies processes (1) and (2) mentioned previously.

Performance indicators should be collected for every anesthetic in order to satisfy the previous process (3) and the soon-to-be mandatory indicator monitoring system require-

BOX 98-1
1996 JCAHO PERIOPERATIVE INDICATORS

1. Patients developing a CNS complication within two postprocedure days of procedures involving anesthesia administration
2. Patients developing a peripheral neurological deficit within two postprocedure days of procedures involving anesthesia administration
3. Patients developing an acute myocardial infarction within two postprocedure days of procedures involving anesthesia administration
4. Patients with a cardiac arrest within two postprocedure days of procedures involving anesthesia administration
5. Intrahospital mortality of patients within two postprocedure days of procedures involving anesthesia administration
6. Patients with discharge diagnosis of fulminant pulmonary edema developed during procedures involving anesthesia administration or within one postprocedure day of conclusion
7. Patients diagnosed with an aspiration pneumonitis occuring during procedures involving anesthesia administration or within two postprocedure days of conclusion
8. Patients developing a postural headache within four postprocedure days following procedures involving spinal or epidural anesthesia administration
9. Patients experiencing a dental injury during procedures involving anesthesia care
10. Patients experiencing an ocular injury during procedures involving anesthesia care
11. Unplanned admission of patients to the hospital within two postprocedure days following outpatient procedures involving anesthesia
12. Unplanned admission of patients to an intensive care unit within two postprocedure days of procedures involving anesthesia administration and with intensive care unit stay greater than one day

ments. The data to be collected should include at least the IMSystem performance indicators (indicators 1 through 5 in Box 98-1), although all indicators listed in Box 98-1 should be considered. Additional indicators may also be appropriate. A distinction should be made between "sentinel events," which are rare events requiring intensive peer review, and rate-based indicators, which occur more frequently and therefore may be subjected to statistical analysis. For example, in-hospital death within two postprocedure days is a sentinel event indicator, whereas postoperative nausea and vomiting that requires treatment may be an appropriate rate-based indicator.

Peer review of each case triggering a sentinel event indicator satisfies PI4.5.2 and enables each occurrence to be "risk adjusted." Although JCAHO has stated that IMSystem will risk-adjust indicators using patient characteristics,[10] the course of action is not revealed in the 1996 JCAHO Manual of Accreditation for Hospitals. Risk adjustment of outcomes will enable hospitals to better track performance, especially when the comparisons among hospitals are conducted (per PI4.4). This is particularly true for anesthesia, because external risk adjustment by the JCAHO is likely to use ICDM-9 codes. There are no codes for many anesthesia risk factors, such as the diagnosis of the difficult airway or refusal of blood-product transfusion, yet adverse perioperative outcome or escalation of care could be linked to either factor.

Review of the evolution of the JCAHO perioperative indicators reveals that their focus has changed significantly over time. In 1987, JCAHO convened an Anesthesia Care Task Force, which was composed of anesthesiologists and certified registered nurse anesthetists (CRNAs) to develop clinical indicators for anesthesia care.[8] In 1989, the task force recommended eight anesthesia indicators, which later were termed *perioperative indicators,* to reflect the scope of care beyond anesthesia. Three were rate-based: (1) perioperative unintentional respiratory arrest; (2) unplanned postanesthesia hospital admission; and (3) unplanned postoperative intensive care unit admission. Five were sentinel events requiring peer review: (1) perioperative CNS complication; (2) perioperative peripheral neurologic deficit; (3) perioperative acute myocardial infarction (MI); (4) perioperative unintentional cardiac arrest; and (5) perioperative death. The task force intended that the indicators serve as "flags" or "screens" highlighting the need for problem analysis and peer review as appropriate, not as measures of performance. During field testing, the three rate-based indicators were considered less reliable than the others and were discontinued in 1993. Around that time, JCAHO developed the IMSystem to provide comparative performance data using the indicators. Therefore, indicators that were originally intended to highlight the need for problem analysis and peer review (where risk adjustments could be made) evolved into performance indicators that are not peer reviewed and for which risk adjustment is unclear.[8] JCAHO standards and indicators have changed significantly over time; therefore, annual review of the JCAHO Accreditation Manual for Hospitals and the departmental QI program is advisable to ensure conformance to changing JCAHO standards. The responsibility for QI activities remains with the hospital (although this, too, is evolving with the development of health systems rather than free-standing hospitals), but it cannot execute this responsibility without the participation of the physicians, especially in the perioperative area.

HISTORICAL FOUNDATIONS OF MEDICAL QUALITY IMPROVEMENT

The underlying principles for QI find their roots in the work of W. Edwards Deming who developed a method for correcting deficiencies in quality that is now incorporated in QI programs.[4,23,21] Avedis Donabedian and Ernest Codman[5] applied these techniques to medicine.

W. Edwards Deming

Deming learned about employee motivation, efficiency, and quality in the workplace at a Western Electric assembly plant in Chicago. His statistical expertise prompted his recruitment for overseeing the 1951 census in Japan and subsequently his involvement with Japanese industrial quality and productivity. He taught the Japanese to design quality into their products at the onset and that dependence on "quality assurance" inspections at the end of the assembly line was an inefficient and expensive way to operate. In the early 1980s, Deming's methods were adopted by American manufacturers.

The primary convictions held by Deming were that workers generally desire to produce quality products and that poor quality is usually the fault of the process and not the individual worker. Involvement of the worker in the QI process is essential in his approach to QI. Deming identified common dysfunctional patterns of organization and management that must be eliminated before quality and efficiency could be obtainable goals. These dysfunctional patterns are referred to as "Deming's deadly diseases," and they include: (1) lack of constancy of purpose; (2) emphasis on short-term gain; (3) annual performance ratings; (4) job hopping; (5) management with visible figures only; (6) excessive medical costs; and (7) excessive costs of litigation.[4] He also identified numerous "Barriers and Obstacles" to the implementation of a successful QI system and cautioned that simple endorsement of the business's plan to implement a QI system does not guarantee success (Box 98-2).[4] The steps required for implementation of the QI system were similar across different businesses to establish efficiency and quality output. From this experience, Deming developed the "Fourteen Points" for QI (Box 98-3). All are applicable to the development of a medical QI system.

Application of the Deming Technique to the Healthcare Industry

Japanese, and subsequently American industrial management leaders, vigorously adopted these management recommendations into everyday business operation. The American health care industry is beginning to recognize the need to adopt the same techniques. The translation of Deming's deadly diseases, fourteen points, and barriers and obstacles into the modern healthcare industry is remarkably direct. Strong leadership is needed to direct the changes. Education of all department members to the principles of QI and how these principles relate to department objectives is essential.

Application of the Deming principles to medicine: Avedis Donabedian

The principles and focus of Deming in the pursuit of industrial QI were applied to the healthcare industry in the 1960s by Avedis Donabedian and Ernest Codman. Donabedian's framework for QI process includes three inter-related areas:

BOX 98-2
DEMING'S BARRIERS AND OBSTACLES TO IMPLEMENTATION OF A QUALITY IMPROVEMENT SYSTEM

1. The assumption that new technology and automation will transform the business
2. The assumption that "our problems are different"
3. Poor understanding of statistical tools
4. Quality improvement is not my job; it is handled by the quality improvement department
5. Our troubles lie entirely in the workforce
6. The assumption that it is only necessary to meet specification
7. The fallacy of "Zero Defects"
8. Anyone who tries to help must understand our business

1. Structure—This category includes facilities, equipment, policies, anesthesia and ancillary personnel, credentialing, finances, and the overall departmental organization. Components of this category must be carefully developed at the departmental level.
2. Process—This is defined by the JCAHO as "a goal-directed, inter-related, series of actions, events, mechanisms, or steps" for patient care.[9] It has also been defined as "what is done for and by individual patients."[19] It is likely the most important of the three components of this QI model because the process may be changed in search of techniques that yield improved outcomes. The "process" encompasses a myriad of issues ranging from operating room scheduling to implementation of practice parameters for case management. The process includes the techniques used for the acquisition of QI data and educational activities directed at changes in the process. Educational goals are developed and continuously evolve based on analysis of data from the QI activities.
3. Outcome—This is defined by the JCAHO as "the result of performance (or nonperformance) of a function or process(es)."[9] It has also been defined as "what is accomplished for and by individual patients."[19] The components of outcome are related to process through the management of the anesthetic and the patient's perioperative care. The relationship between outcome, delivery of care, and complications is complex.

These QI techniques have been applied recently to the study of hospital mortality associated with coronary artery bypass graft (CABG) procedures.[1,12] A consortium of physicians, administrators, and scientists in all five hospitals that perform CABG surgery in Maine, New Hampshire, and

BOX 98-3
DEMING'S FOURTEEN POINTS FOR ESTABLISHMENT OF A QUALITY IMPROVEMENT SYSTEM

1. Create constancy of purpose. Resources must be committed to accomplish these goals and leadership must vigorously support the long-range plans.
2. Adopt a new philosophy: intolerance of poor workmanship and sullen service. Things must be done right the first time by proper design of the process.
3. Cease dependence on mass inspection. This mandates the shift from quality assurance to quality improvement activities. Some quality assurance will be necessary but is not used for process improvement.
4. Do not award business contracts based on price. Price can only be evaluated in the light of quality.
5. Implement continual quality improvement. The process is not static and the system used must incorporate flexibility in order to provide useful information and keep up with change.
6. Institute on the job training. All personnel should receive training in the quality improvement system.
7. Institute leadership. Leaders must support quality improvement.
8. Drive out fear. The assumption should be made that the process failed and not the individual. This will rarely be proven false.
9. Break down barriers between staff areas.
10. Eliminate slogans, targets, and exhortations for the work force.
11. Eliminate numerical quotas.
12. Remove barriers to pride of workmanship to include work evaluations.
13. Institute programs for education and retraining. Self improvement is important for advancement, self-esteem, and improving quality.
14. Take action to implement the transformation.

Vermont applied three interventions to the problem of QI: (1) feedback of outcome data; (2) training in continuous QI; and (3) site visits to other medical centers for first-hand observation of patient care delivered by others. One result was the combined hospital mortality rate decreased by 24% for 6488 cases. Many aspects of a medical QI system were successfully employed in this endeavor. Using similar study design, patient-specific risk factors contributed more to cardiovascular events in the postanesthesia care unit than did differences in anesthetic management.[13]

OUTCOME ANALYSIS IN MEDICINE

Outcomes Defined

The belief that "good" outcomes provide evidence that individuals and institutions provide quality care is only partly true. There may be more sensitive, albeit more difficult-to-document, measurements to establish that quality care was delivered. In two studies involving a total of 79,146 patients, complications (adverse events) were predicted primarily by patient factors. The "failure to rescue from complications" was found to be a better measure of the contribution of the provider to the quality of care.[16,17] Because the intermediate steps in patient care are largely unknown, complications caused by human error may occur without discovery because they may be corrected without sequellae.[14] Based on these studies, it may be advantageous to focus QI data analysis on the anesthesiologist's ability to "rescue" patients from complications. The self-reporting of *all* complications encountered during patient care is important to the success of the QI system because in the vast majority of cases rescue will have occurred without adverse outcome. The care providers, by contributing accurate information to the QI system, will develop a rescue database that will provide evidence of their ability to prevent adverse outcomes despite the occurrence of complications during care. Complications resulting from poor judgment or lack of vigilance are more likely to be discovered in the peer review stage of chart review.

The most intangible but important outcome indicator, "patient satisfaction," is receiving increased attention, particularly in managed care and in highly competitive environments. Patients may experience adverse or less than optimal outcomes and report no dissatisfaction with their care. The results of carefully designed telephone or patient-administered satisfaction questionnaires may be appended to the QI database for subsequent analysis.

Risk Adjustment of Outcomes

In the peer review process, the medical record is examined to identify preexisting conditions or treatment decisions that predisposed the adverse outcome. Although it is impossible to mimic precisely the intangibles of peer review, it is possible to devise algorithms to link adverse outcomes and associated risk factors in the database, thus facilitating rapid review of numerous cases. Risk-adjusting outcomes serve two functions. Within the institution, they focus QI efforts on process problems that may be related to preexisting conditions (e.g., the absence of a difficult airway cart for a patient at risk). If data are compared across institutions, risk adjustment allows comparison of outcomes via normalization of the data set (i.e., correcting for differences in risk of adverse outcome). Risk adjustment should mimic peer review when unexpected outcomes or outcomes not correlated to preoperative risk prompt chart review.

THE SCOPE OF THE ANESTHESIOLOGY QUALITY IMPROVEMENT SYSTEM

The anesthesiology QI system should encompass all aspects of anesthesia care. The work flow includes the following: (1) data acquisition; (2) data verification; (3) appending data to the database; (4) periodic query of the database for generation of reports for the QI committee; (5) selection of charts for review; and (6) the QI committee meeting during which peer review takes place. Educational or process change recommendations are made to the department or individuals based on the analysis of QI data. Documentation of the peer review proceedings should be appended to the database to complete the process. Subsequent QI activities should include assessment of the effect of education and process change on problems discovered and acted upon in the course of QI activities.

Indicators

The system should provide secure, efficient, inexpensive data entry and validation, flexible administrative functions, a well-designed and flexible indicator selection and reporting mechanism, and it should incorporate feedback from peer review activities of the QI committee. System flexibility is paramount to the design, to accommodate ongoing changes in JCAHO or managed care demands, and changing clinical practice standards. The QI system should provide data for at least ten areas in anesthesia practice (Box 98-4). Each will require a means of data acquisition, sets of unique indicators, procedures, responses, administrative data. One form used at The University of Alabama at Birmingham (UAB) will serve as an example. All QI solutions will require the definition of anesthesia indicators that will be reported as critical events, occurrences, or risks. Discussions of each area are illustrative and not intended to be comprehensive.

Patient interview and risk factor documentation

At UAB, approximately 80 preoperative risk factors are documented by completion of the preoperative scanner sheet. These risk factors are applicable to the QI system for all anesthesia activities previously listed and are important in outcomes analysis and peer review.

Intraoperative anesthesia indicators

Intraoperative anesthesia indicators are the descriptions of critical events or complications of care that need not be

BOX 98-4
SPECIFIC AREAS IN ANESTHESIOLOGY REQUIRING QUALITY IMPROVEMENT ANALYSIS

1. Preoperative patient evaluation and interview with risk factors
2. Intraoperative indicators and procedures
3. Postoperative indicators and procedures
4. Obstetrics epidural service, operative procedures
5. Acute pain service indicators and procedures
6. Chronic pain service indicators and procedures
7. Ambulatory anesthesia services
8. Consultation services, monitoring, and resuscitation
9. Patient satisfaction survey
10. Research projects

anesthesia-specific. The choice of indicators will be influenced by financial, regulatory, local, and competitive pressures in the evolving marketplace and will, therefore, change. Indicators may be added when the QI system is being used to acquire data for a clinical study of cost effectiveness of therapy, the evaluation of practice parameters, or for clinical research.

The UAB intraoperative indicators are found in Fig. 98-1. Administrative data (surgical location, type of anesthesia, surgical service, special procedures, ASA category) permit correlation of events with services performed. The indicators include major intraoperative events or complications that would merit detailed review if they were to occur in isolation, and other events with higher frequency of occurrence but lesser impact on outcome. All current JCAHO anesthesia requirements are covered on the UAB forms. The addition of procedure times will allow the statistical determination of procedure duration and will be used to identify delays caused by the process.

Postoperative anesthesia indicators

The UAB postoperative indicators are contained on a third form, which is completed by the physician, the postanesthesia care nurse, the resident, or CRNA. Postanesthesia care unit nursing QI indicators have been added to the form to efficiently acquire data for their area of responsibility using the same technology. Similar additions of nursing QI data will likely occur in obstetrics, the preoperative holding area, and the operating room in some applications.

Obstetric anesthesia indicators

Data acquisition in obstetrics is needed for epidural analgesia and anesthesia for operative delivery or procedures. Indicators peculiar to obstetrics must include complications of epidural analgesia; failure of equipment used in conjunction with the epidural such as the infusion pump and catheter; failed blocks; and intraoperative indicators (Fig. 98-1). Documentation of patient satisfaction as an outcome is included.

Acute pain service indicators

Complications of procedures performed for the relief of pain, such as nausea and vomiting, urinary retention, puritis, respiratory depression, as well as positive indicators such as pain scale assessment, patient satisfaction, length of stay, ventilator weaning rates, and time to ambulation, and equipment failure, will comprise the bulk of the QI efforts in this clinical area.[7] Compliance with Acute Pain Service Guidelines for patient care and monitoring are assessed and include: (1) identification of the medications used; (2) vital signs; (3) level of sensory and/or motor blockade if appropriate; (4) condition of the catheter and dressing; (5) documentation of respiratory rates and level of sedation at specified intervals.

Chronic pain service indicators

The complications of invasive procedures (e.g., cervical, thoracic, and lumbar epidurals, nerve blocks, plexus blocks, neural ablation procedures) and should be included in the QI data set for clinical practice in addition to many of the indicators mentioned in the previous paragraph on acute pain.

Outpatient anesthesia services indicators

Regulatory bodies regarding outpatient surgery include the JCAHO and the Accreditation Association for Ambulatory Health Care (AAAHC), which was incorporated in 1979. It is recognized by several surgical societies, and the AAAHC has published guidelines for QI activities. The JCAHO is involved primarily with ambulatory surgery centers that are hospital-based or hospital-affiliated. Anesthesia indicators are essentially the same as for inpatient procedures, with expansion in the area of unanticipated admission to the hospital or prolonged stay in recovery.[20]

Consultation indicators

The code and resuscitation consultation is an area that receives little attention in the QI process, but it is associated with substantial risk to patients and is an area that many hospitals assume direct responsibility for monitoring. Resuscitation committees are usually multidisciplinary and, as such, serve as an example of the ideal composition of a comprehensive QI review panel. The committee develops the indicator list for tracking.

Patient satisfaction

This area of anesthesia QI is receiving increased attention for inpatient and outpatient surgery, primarily as the result of competitive pressures. The patient's perception of the "quality of the medical care" and the patient's postoperative functionality are very important indicators of quality care.

54057

UAB Dept. of Anesthesiology
Intra-op QI Data Form
Confidential

Shade circles like this: ● Not like this: ⊗ ✓

Use all caps and block style letters

MedRec# [| | | | | |]

Mo [|] / Day [|] / Year [9|6]

Use 1st 6 letters of last name

Anesthesiologist [| | | | |]

Resident/CRNA [| | | | |]

Pt's 2nd operation today? No ○ Yes ○

Location	Anesthesia	Surgical Service		Procedures Performed by Anesthesia	ASA
○ Main OR	○ General	○ GS	○ Neuro	○ A-line	○ 1
○ CV OR	○ SAB/Epid	○ GU	○ Vasc	○ Central line	○ 2
○ L&D	○ Gen/Epid	○ CV	○ ObGyn	○ Swan-Ganz	○ 3
○ Cath lab	○ Regional	○ Transplant	○ Ortho	○ Fiberoptic	○ 4
○ Radiology	○ MAC	○ ENT	○ ECT	○ EEG/TCD/EP	○ 5
○ ECT/Cardio	○ CPR/Intub	○ Plastics	○ Rad/Onc	○ TEE	○ E
○ Code/ER	○ Mask	○ Other		○ Jet ventilation	
○ Other	○ Other				

Miscellaneous

○ Pre-anesthetic assessment performed　○ Equipment Checklist performed pre-op　○ Post-procedure status documented　○ Not recovered in PACU　○ Case postponed　○ Case delayed

Cardiac Events

○ Death
○ Cardiac arrest
○ Hypotension - MAP<20%NL for >5 min
○ Hypertension - MAP>20%NL for >5 min
○ Dysrhythmia requiring treatment
○ Ischemia requiring treatment
○ Other cardiac event requiring treatment

Regional Events

○ Unsatisfactory regional anesthesia requiring supplemental intervention
○ Technical complications w/regional requiring supplemental intervention
○ Unintentional dural puncture
○ Other regional event requiring treatment

Airway/Pulmonary Events

○ Unable to mask ventilate
○ Failed intubation with direct laryngoscopy
○ Intubation req'd >3 tries over >10 min
○ Unable to intubate by any technique
○ Aspiration
○ Unexpected hypoxemia causing SpO2 < 90% for > 3 min
○ Unplanned reintubation
○ Laryngospasm or bronchospasm
○ Pulmonary edema
○ Unexpected delayed extubation
○ Pneumothorax
○ Other airway/respiratory event requiring treatment

Miscellaneous Events

○ Non-drug allergic or anaphylactoid reaction
○ Adverse drug reaction requiring treatment or altering therapy

○ PRBC > 10 units
○ Dental injury
○ Unintentional hypothermia: <35C
○ Hyperthermia: >38C
○ Machine/equipment failure
○ Peripheral neurologic deficit
○ CNS event
○ Ocular injury
○ Positioning injury
○ Transfusion error
○ Invasive monitor event
○ Unplanned ICU admit
○ Other events requiring QI review (document in chart)

Anesthesiologist's Signature: ____________________

Fig. 98-1. The University of Alabama intraoperative computer data sheet. Data entered on this form are appended to the QI database when the form is optically scanned. (From University of Alabama at Birmingham Research Foundation.)

Managed care plan administrators are particularly attentive to patient satisfaction data.

Peer review, Vitez mthodology, and the quality improvement meeting

In 1990, the Vitez technique for analysis of QI data was developed and subsequently adopted by the ASA.[22] The Vitez method completes the QI process by a standard chart review and provides a uniform reporting tool for discussion and disposition of the case. The reviewer is expected to:

1. Decide whether the event is related to anesthesia care;
2. Determine the nature of the incident (systems, mechanical, judgmental, vigilance);
3. Identify the management area (airway, circulation, pulmonary, positioning, etc.);
4. Assign an outcome score: determine whether escalation of care, organ injury, or death resulted;
5. Make recommendations to decrease occurrence of the same or similar errors.

The Vitez score results are retained in the QI database for documentation and tracking purposes. The indicator is followed in the future to determine if educational intervention or process change reduced the incidence of the complication.

The QI meetings are greatly facilitated by the QI system and a database with flexible query structure. Charts for review are selected by querying the database for indicators that the committee has selected to follow, and for any indicators previously studied that may require follow-up. Members arrive at the meeting with their peer review conclusions based on chart review documented on the Vitez form. The case findings are discussed and recommendations for education, process changes, or referral to or collaboration with other departments are made. Completion of the process is documented by appending the results to the QI database.

Quality Improvement and Credentialing

The QI data may be used for credentialing, because physician-specific QI data, or profiles, are easily extracted from the QI database. Such information is protected as confidential peer review information under the Federal Health Care Quality Improvement Act of 1986. These data provide the leader(s) of the practice group accurate, complete data on procedures, complications, peer review decisions based on review of the complications, and documentation of resulting educational activities directed at QI. Inequities in practice experience among physicians may be discovered, such as case complexity, age extremes, or special procedures and may be adjusted by changes in subsequent case assignments. The issue of procedure-specific credentialing or recredentialing is complex; using the QI database for credentialing will be an individual departmental decision.

It is clear, however, that use of the QI database as a source of information for punitive action will quickly be discovered by all care providers and will likely result in total failure of the system. Change in the process of healthcare delivery is the primary goal of the QI process, not punishment of individuals. The QI system should be designed to encourage participation on the part of the practitioners, rather than encourage fear or resistance of the system.

TOOLS FOR QUALITY IMPROVEMENT

Manually tracking perioperative indicators for all anesthetics is too labor intensive for all but the smallest practices; therefore, some tools are required to make the task manageable. Several options exist: (1) an anesthesia information system (AIS) with integrated preoperative evaluation, intraoperative record-keeping, postoperative modules, and QI reporting mechanisms; (2) a paper-based system using scannable forms and an associated database; (3) manual data entry to a database from existing hospital documents; and (4) manual chart review of cases in which indicators are triggered and independently reported. Manual data entry[3] is cost prohibitive for larger departments. Manual chart review[4] is unlikely to work except in the small departments. All are acceptable if 100% of the cases with triggered indicators are reported.

Anesthesia Information Systems

Anesthesia information systems (AIS) have the advantage of capturing most indicators as part of routine documentation of patient care. Extracting the indicators from the AIS database is dependent upon database design and database interrogation tools (i.e., query and reporting software). The support of QI activities by AIS is usually insufficient justification for the capital cost. However, the cost of AIS may be justified by other advantages, such as electronic intraoperative record keeping and automatic patient charge capture. AIS may not provide QI data capture for nonsurgical obstetrics and anesthesia pain services; QI activities in these areas will require a separate system.

Paper-based QI systems that use page scanner technology for data entry can reduce data entry costs associated with manual methods. They also provide efficient acquisition and analysis of data when coupled with a well-designed database without the capital outlay for computerized network solutions.

Anesthesiology QI systems, including computer-based systems, should support an indicator monitoring system, such as the JCAHO IMSystem. The AIS should be designed to interface with the hospital information system also. Although commercial software is available that may meet these needs, expertise is often required to produce a flexible database and reporting system that meets local needs.

If the data collection depends on paper forms, a mechanism for securing and processing the completed forms is required. At UAB, page images are stored digitally and then the forms are shredded. Computer-based QI systems will require security measures to prevent unauthorized access because of the confidential data. Reports generated from any QI system need to be labeled as "Confidential QI Data," and a statement about the privileged nature of the information should be printed on each sheet in an effort to protect the data from discovery.

Turning Data into Information

One purpose of a QI system is to decrease variation. Sentinel events should be peer reviewed on a case-by-case basis, because their infrequent occurrence prevents the application of statistical process control methods to these data. However, valuable QI information may be gained from analysis of rate-based indicators using such methods.

Modern QI techniques focus on processes. An important tool in monitoring and improving processes is the control chart.[2,21] Control charts track the variation associated with the process and are used to reduce variation to improve quality. To construct a control chart, a variable or set of variables that indicate how well the process works are measured and plotted over time. For example, the average daily postanesthesia care unit length of stay on consecutive days may be tracked by recording admission and discharge times. Over the course of approximately 40 days, the variation in average daily postanesthesia care unit time may be analyzed. Upper and lower control limits are derived statistically from the data using standard statistical formulas.[2] Data points above the upper control limit or below the lower control limit indicate that the process is "out of control." The intent is to identify a "special cause" for the change, because there is less than a 0.3% chance that normal process variation would account for such a variation. If a "special cause," is identified, it should be eliminated to improve the process. In our example, suppose that a data point for average daily postanesthesia care unit stay was above the upper control limit because of the inability to move a number of inpatients to hospital beds in a timely manner. Once "special causes" are eliminated and the process is within control, then the mean value of the process variable may then be reduced by analyzing the process and making the appropriate changes.

Testing the System

The process by which the department or group tracks QI data must be subjected to QI itself. Validation of data entry, the accuracy and completeness of self-reporting of complications, uniform interpretation of the quality indicators, and the case review process all require validation. Occasional random manual chart review can determine the accuracy. Definitions of the indicators should be distributed to all departmental care providers to improve uniformity in reporting. Verification of accuracy may also be accomplished using automated acquisition of physiologic data during anesthesia.

Interfacing with the Hospital

Adding nursing QI indicators to the anesthesia QI system enhances the value of the system for the hospital and encourages better documentation of postanesthesia care unit anesthesia QI indicators. Education of nurses is also an important feature of a successful QI program. Routine reporting of nonsensitive data to physicians and nurses involved in QI data acquisition and use of the QI system for clinical research also increases interest in the QI process. The hospital benefits from an efficient QI program because workforce requirements for 100% sampling are reduced drastically. Fractional sampling fails to provide data required by the JCAHO and the rate of complications remains unknown. Periodic query of the database for reports on indicators can provide a list of medical record numbers for which chart review is necessary. With automated QI, chart review is focused on problem solving and far fewer staff-hours are needed to investigate all the events that occur monthly.

SUMMARY

An effective QI system is critical for the advancement of anesthesiology departments. Leaders must encourage compliance with application of the system and the education that results from QI activities. With improvement in outcome and reduction in complications, the overall cost of care delivery will decrease. Practice parameters will play an important role in the QI process because they decrease variability. They may also be refined using a QI system. This concept extends to benchmarking[6] of QI information among institutions, a process which is being driven by individual departments that seek a point of reference for their group. Information-rich anesthesiology departments will be in a position to negotiate more effectively with managed care entities and to advance the specialty through improved approaches to patient care.

KEY POINTS

- A quality improvement system should provide a means of data acquisition to enable analysis and improvement of the process of delivery of medical care, education of providers and staff, and improvement in patient outcome and satisfaction.
- The QI system should be based on the philosophy proven effective in other industries by Deming and in medicine by Donabedian.
- Strong supportive leadership is needed to propagate an effective QI system. Use of QI data for personnel actions or punitive measures will rapidly destroy compliance with self-reporting and cause the failure of the system.

- Similar attention to QI activities in areas outside the operating room may preempt criticism of anesthesiologists involved in the delivery of critical care, pain, obstetrics, or consultative services as the marketplace changes.
- Attention to the JCAHO's Agenda for Change is appropriate, but compliance with the minimum requirements of the JCAHO will be inadequate for response to competitive pressures outside the JCAHO.

KEY REFERENCES

Deming WE: *Out of the crisis,* ed 2, Cambridge, 1986, Massachusetts Institute of Technology Center for Advance Engineering Study.

Donabedian A: Promoting quality through evaluating the process of patient care, *Med Care* 6:181–202, 1986.

Joint Commission on Accreditation for Healthcare Organizations: *1996 Comprehensive Accreditation Manual for Hospitals,* Oakbrook Terrace, 1995, Joint Commission for Accreditation of Healthcare Organizations.

Van Matre JG: *Foundations of TQM: a readings book,* San Antonio, Texas, 1995, Harcourt Brace.

Vitez TS: A model for quality assurance in anesthesiology, *J Clin Anesth* 2:280, 1990.

REFERENCES

1. Berwick DM: Harvesting knowledge from improvement (editorial), *JAMA* 275:877, 1996.
2. Carey RG, Lloyd RC: *Measuring quality improvement in healthcare: a guide to statistical process control applications,* New York, 1995, Quality Resources.
3. Cheney FW: Quality assurance—peer review, *Clin Anesth Up* 3:1, 1992.
4. Deming WE: *Out of the crisis,* ed 2, Cambridge, 1996, Massachusetts Institute of Technology Center for Advance Engineering Study.
5. Donabedian A: Promoting quality through evaluating the process of patient care, *Med Care* 6:181, 1986.
6. Eagle CJ, Davies JM: Current models of "quality"—an introduction for anesthetists, *Can J Anesth* 40:851, 1993.
7. Flemming BM, Coombs DW: A survey of complications documented in a quality-control analysis of patient-controlled analgesia in the postoperative period, *J Pain Symp Manage* 7:463, 1992.
8. Gabel RA: Evolution of Joint Commission Anesthesia Clinical Indicators, *Am Soc Anesthesiol News* 58:24, 1994.
9. Joint Commission on Accreditation of Healthcare Organizations: *1996 Comprehensive Accreditation Manual for Hospitals,* Oakbrook Terrace, 1995, Joint Commission for Accreditation of Healthcare Organizations.
10. Koss R, Nadzam D, Loeb JM: From The Joint Commission on Accreditation of Healthcare Organizations (letter to editor), *JAMA* 273:99, 1995.
11. Longnecker DE: Planning the future of anesthesiology (editorial), *Anesthesiology* 84:495, 1996.
12. O'Connor GT, Plume SK, Olmstead EM, et al: A regional intervention to improve the hospital mortality associated with coronary artery bypass graft surgery, *JAMA* 275:841, 1996.
13. Rose DK, Cohen MM, DeBoer DP: Cardiovascular events in the postanesthesia care unit. Contribution of risk factors, *Anesthesiology* 84:772, 1996.
14. Schroeder SA, Kabcenell AI (editorial): Do bad outcomes mean substandard care? *JAMA* 265:1995. 1991.
15. Shoemaker S: Practice policies in anesthesia: a foretaste of practice in the 21st century, *Anesth Analg* 80:388, 1995.
16. Silber JH: Comparing the contributions of groups of predictors: which outcomes vary with hospital rather than patient characteristics? *J Am Stat Assoc* 90:7, 1995.
17. Silber JH, Williams SV, Krakauer H, et al: Hospital and patient characteristics associated with death after surgery. A study of adverse occurrence and failure to rescue, *Med Care* 30:615, 1992.
18. Thys DM, Abel M, Bollen BA, et al: Practice guidelines for perioperative transesophageal echocardiography, *Anesthesiology* 84:986, 1996.
19. Tinker JH, Jensen NF: CQI—continuous quality improvement, *Intern Anesth Res Soc Rev Course Lec,* 40, 1993.
20. Twersky RS: How to assess quality in ambulatory surgery, *J Clin Anesth* 4:25S, 1992.
21. Van Matre JG: *Foundations of TQM: a readings book*, San Antonio, Texas, 1995, Harcourt Brace.
22. Vitez TS: A model for quality assurance in anesthesiology, *J Clin Anesth* 2:280, 1990.
23. Walton M: *The Deming management method*, ed 1, New York, 1986, Putnam Publishing Group.

CHAPTER 99

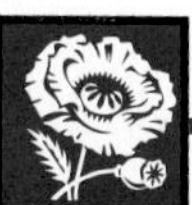

Cost-Effective Anesthetic Practice

G. EDWARD MORGAN, JR.

Cost control has become the number one health care priority in the United States. The statistics defy exaggeration. National health care expenditures in 1994:

- exceeded 1 trillion dollars
- represented 15% of the gross domestic product (GDP)
- amounted to $4000 per person
- were paid in large part (50%) from federal and state government sources[39]

In fact, health care costs continue to rise faster than the overall economy, and health economists predict they will exceed 18% of the GDP by the year 2000 and a staggering 25% by the year 2010. This compares with an average of 8% in other industrialized nations. Not surprisingly, the cost of anesthesia in the United States has been estimated to be up to 660% greater than some other countries because of the use of more expensive drugs, disposable equipment, and ancillary supplies, and access to modern technology.[19,84]

Although demographic factors (i.e., an increasing and aging population with increasingly severe illnesses), structural anomalies (e.g., government tax subsidies to employers and the aged that shield the consumer from the true cost of care), advances in medical technologies, new diseases (e.g., AIDS), and administrative costs (24 cents of every health care dollar is spent on administrative services such as insurance marketing, billing, claims processing, and utilization review)[144,145] may explain a large portion of the increased expenditures, legislative attention continues to focus on the cost of clinical services—specifically on the cost of medical care providers.

Anesthesiologists can directly impact at least three resource-intense areas of clinical practice: (1) the operating room; (2) the intensive care unit[91]; and (3) the pain clinic. The operating room has been estimated to account for one third[76] and the intensive care unit up to one fourth[15,88,125] of all inpatient hospital costs. Anesthesia costs have been estimated to comprise approximately 6% of total hospital costs.[76]

Several strategies for cost containment have been explored including:[42,43]

- controlling price inflation with price controls (e.g., limiting physician, hospital, or pharmaceutical company reimbursement) or competitive strategies (e.g., managed care)
- minimizing administrative "waste" (administrative costs have increased 30% more rapidly than the overall rate of

health care inflation), but many of these costs may actually be increasing the efficiency of medical delivery
- developing and promoting new technologies that provide cost savings (e.g., percutaneous transluminal coronary angioplasty) and at the same time hindering more expensive technologies
- emphasizing preventative medicine (e.g., prenatal care)
- eliminating ineffective care with utilization controls (e.g., inappropriate cesarean sections) or limiting access to medical services (e.g., increasing patient cost sharing)
- prioritization based upon cost-effectiveness analysis

This last strategy provides the primary focus for discussion in this chapter.

BASIC PRINCIPLES OF CLINICAL ECONOMICS

Important Definitions

Categorization of costs

Understanding cost-effectiveness requires a basic knowledge of economic theory and jargon.[32] The first question that must be answered is "Whose cost?" Unless otherwise specified, this discussion will focus on hospital costs, as opposed to societal, patient, or payor (e.g., insurance company) costs. *Fixed costs* remain constant in the short term, regardless of the volume of goods produced or services provided. For example, a hospital mortgage would not typically vary with its average daily census. On the other hand, *variable costs* change with the amount of goods produced or services provided. Anesthetic drugs would be considered a variable cost because the amount used varies with the volume of surgery. Most strategies aimed at reducing medical costs deal with decreasing variable costs. The *incremental (or marginal) cost* describes the cost of producing one additional item. Thus, the incremental cost of adding a fourth lipotripsy case to the operating room schedule might depend on whether the additional case would result in overtime pay or whether it could be completed during regular hours. *Acquisition costs* reflect the actual prices paid. The acquisition cost of a drug is the price the hospital pharmacy paid for a single unit of the drug and does not take into account other facets of cost (e.g., wastage, dispensing costs). Costs can also be categorized as *direct costs* which are those easily identified and linked to an individual patient's care (e.g., the acquisition cost of an antiemetic medication and the labor cost involved in administering it) or *indirect costs* which tend to be more obscure, difficult to quantitate, and not directly related to an individual patient (e.g., administrative overhead). Some indirect costs are almost impossible to quantitate because they deal with nonfinancial intangibles (e.g., the emotional cost of experiencing postoperative pain) or because they represent a cost to society as a whole (e.g., the loss of productivity resulting from a additional inpatient day).

Cost analysis studies

The costs described above can be analyzed in different ways (Table 99-1). *Cost-identification* (also known as *cost-minimization) studies* measure costs without considering differences in outcomes. These studies usually attempt to identify the lowest cost treatment alternative, such as the least expensive induction agent (i.e., lowest acquisition cost) and assume outcomes (e.g., side-effects) are equivalent. The weakness of these types of studies can be described as "knowing the cost of everything and the value of nothing."[68] In contrast, traditional medical research assumes unlimited resources and investigates the effectiveness of a medical intervention without any consideration of costs. Likewise, individual clinicians treating individual patients typically search for the most effective clinical course, regardless of cost. In today's environment of society's decreasing willingness and ability to pay for any and all health care, alternative treatments must compete for available resources. Some decisions are easier than others. The decision to adopt a less expensive but more effective modality, and the decision to refute a more expensive but less effective alternative are intuitive. But if a more expensive treatment is also considered to be more effective, cost-effectiveness studies may prove useful.

Table 99-1 Cost analysis studies are categorized by how they measure clinical outcomes

Type of study	Outcomes measured
Cost-identification (cost-minimization)	None
Cost-benefit	Monetary
Cost-effectiveness	Biologic
Cost-utility	Quality

Cost-effectiveness analysis is a collection of methods (health production functions) that help solve the problem of allocating limited resources (i.e., rationing health care dollars).[31] *Cost-effectiveness* can be used as a generic term describing studies that balance the net costs (expenditures minus savings) with the clinical outcomes associated with competing strategies. Stated differently, cost-effectiveness studies assess efficiency by considering both the effectiveness of therapy and the resources required for delivery of therapy. Thus, drug A may be more cost-effective than drug B, despite having a higher acquisition cost if it provides a benefit (e.g., less postoperative nausea) that can be demonstrated to have a greater cost saving consequence (e.g., less antiemetic usage in the recovery room) or that is valued more by the patient than the additional expense. **The most cost-effective alternative is that which achieves the maximal incremental health benefit for a fixed amount of resources.**[24]

A *cost-benefit analysis* expresses the clinical outcome in monetary units such as dollars, whereas *cost-effectiveness analysis* (in the technical use of the term) measures outcome in biologic or clinical terms that coincide with the treatment objective such as "years of life saved" or "millimeters of blood pressure reduction achieved." *Cost-utility analysis* additionally considers the quality of life or usefulness (e.g., quality-adjusted life years). An advantage of cost-benefit studies is that because costs and benefits are both expressed in dollars, the net cost can be determined by subtracting treatment costs from treatment benefits. Converting the clinical benefits demonstrated by a cost-effectiveness study into dollars (e.g., the value of avoiding postoperative nausea) may require difficult value judgments. One test estimates the population's "willingness-to-pay." Likewise, placing a monetary value on the quality of life or the value of life measured in a cost-utility study is not an easy task.

Sometimes cost-effectiveness analyses are expressed as a ratio which measures the amount of benefit provided for a specified amount of cost. For example, a cost-benefit ratio would express some outcome per dollar, whereas a cost-effectiveness ratio would measure the outcome per some natural unit. Ideally, the ratios of alternative treatments can then be ranked in order of their cost-effectiveness, with priority given to the alternatives that produce the greatest benefit per unit of cost.

Poor estimates of benefits or cost can easily discredit cost-effectiveness studies. Although quantitating costs may be difficult, defining benefits usually proves to be harder. Specifically, whereas this chapter deals with hospital costs, the benefits point-of-view could be either society or the individual patient (Figure 99-1). Is society defined in a way to include future generations or citizens of other countries?[122] A *sensitivity analysis* can evaluate the effect of varying these assumptions upon the conclusions of the analysis. There are also practical problems with this type of analysis. Treatments can have multiple alternatives, each with its own benefits and harms that need to be weighted. Outcomes can be difficult to measure, particularly in a field such as anesthesiology, which lacks specific diseases and cures.[16–18] It is important to keep in mind that although cost-effectiveness studies deal with providing the maximum benefit to a population of patients, clinicians have to manage providing the maximum benefit to an individual patient.

The Cost-Quality Relationship

The relationship between quality of care and cost is complex. Medical cost-quality relationships are often considered to have an upward but diminishing slope (Figure 99-2). In other words, large improvements in quality would be expected by small initial investments in cost (e.g., polio vaccination). Eventually, the allocation of resources reaches a point where large investments return a small incremental improvement in outcome (i.e., the law of diminishing returns). This decreasing marginal return describes the marginal cost-effectiveness of an additional investment. One difficulty in analyzing the cost-quality relationship lies in determining when an incremental increase in quality is no longer worth its additional cost. A second difficulty is that the cost-quality relationship may not always be positively related. In other words, there is little evidence that high-cost medical practice renders better care or achieves better outcomes or higher patient satisfaction than low-cost practice.[50,114,131] At some point, additional medical services may even have a negative effect on patient outcome because of

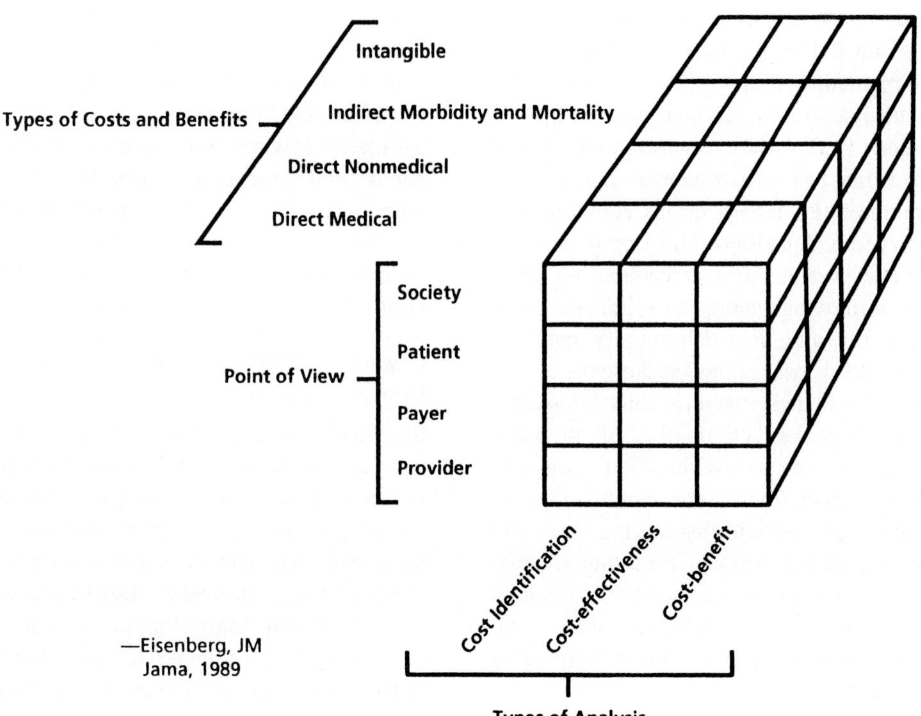

Fig. 99-1. Economic analysis can vary tremendously based upon the type of cost measured, the point of view of the study, and the type of analysis performed. (From Eisenberg JM: Clinical economics: A guide to the economic analysis of clinical practices, *JAMA* 262:2879, 1989.)

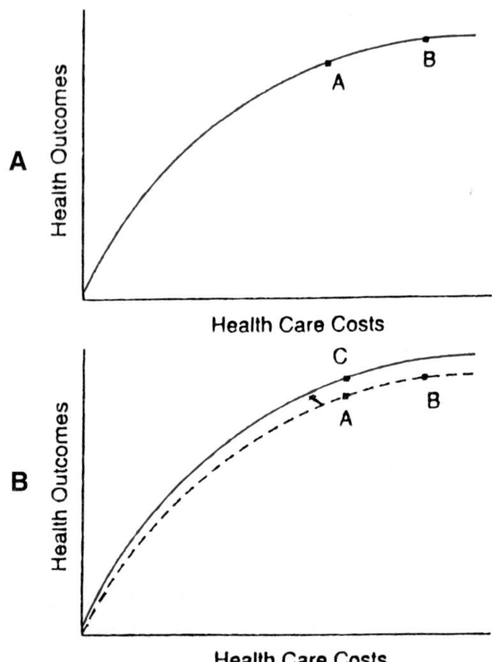

Fig. 99-2. A theoretical model of health care costs and health outcomes. **A,** Moving from point A to point B is associated with higher costs and better health outcomes. **B,** Elimination of waste shifts the curve to a more efficient relationship between costs and health outcomes. (From Grumbach K, Bodenheimer T: Painful vs. painless cost control, *JAMA* 272:1458, 1994.)

the complications associated with its use. An example is the use of low-yield screening laboratory tests. The corollary of this is also true: costs fall as quality improves.[54] The cost-benefit curve can be shifted to a more favorable position if those interventions with flat or negative (i.e., inappropriate care) effects are eliminated.

Waste due to poor quality may account for 25% to 40% of all hospital costs.[1,144] Eliminating wastage is a cost-minimization practice that has no detrimental effects on patient care. For example, eliminating serious complications after high-risk surgery (e.g., lung lobectomy or coronary bypass) could reduce the cost of those procedures by up to 30%.[27,118] However, improving quality to eliminate infrequent complications following low-risk surgery may not produce significant (< 2%) cost savings, because the cost of these complications contributes insignificantly to overall hospital costs.[27,62] Further, even elimination of all waste would only provide a one-time cost savings; the long-term rate of increase of health care expenditures would not be affected. It should not need to be said that cutting costs will not necessarily improve quality. Simply instituting all cost-minimization strategies would be unacceptable, because these strategies do not take into account quality of care, and patient safety must continue to be an overriding priority in anesthetic management.

The Concept of Value-Based Anesthesia

In 1994, the American Society of Anesthesiologists (ASA) established the Task Force on Value-Based Anesthesia. Value-based care has been succinctly defined as "essentially the best patient outcome achievable at a reasonable cost."[92] Outcome includes patient satisfaction in addition to medical result. **Increased value can be achieved by: (1) maintaining or increasing quality while reducing costs; or (2) increasing quality to a greater degree than costs. Thus, the pursuit of value-based care relies upon the knowledge of two parameters: clinical outcomes (quality) and true costs.** Unfortunately, few studies in the anesthesia literature deal with both of these issues, and it is difficult to convert to dollars the value of an increase in quality. Further, generalizing even a well-performed study to different clinical environments may introduce false assumptions or different values that invalidate the study's conclusions. For example, the results of a study that analyzes anesthetic costs and outcomes at an academic medical center with surgical and anesthesia residency training programs may be not be applicable to a private practice environment located in a different part of the country with a very different patient population.[147] Therefore, customizing the delivery of value-based anesthesia needs to be adopted to some degree by individual provider groups and facilities. One strategy that addresses this need is the development of institution-specific practice guidelines (see following paragraphs).

MEASURING ANESTHETIC COSTS

Cost-effective decision-making requires accurate measurements of cost and outcome. The first step in cost analysis is the identification of all significant cost components: fixed, variable, direct, and indirect costs. A complete analysis of hospital anesthetic costs includes the costs of anesthetic drugs, intravenous (IV) fluids, disposable supplies, capital equipment (nondisposable equipment), labor, laboratory tests, and any other costs incurred as a result of providing anesthetic services.[10] Evaluation of cost-effectiveness depends upon comparing the cost of anesthesia determined by these methods with measurements of clinical outcome (i.e., side effects, complications, benefits). Accurate cost accounting allows the rational development of departmental protocols and clinical pathways.

Common Errors in Measuring Anesthetic Costs

Cost-to-charge ratios

It is vitally important, but ofttimes quite difficult, to obtain accurate cost information. Historically, hospital accounting systems were designed to track hospital revenue (i.e., patient charges) as opposed to actual hospital costs. Further, these revenue-based financial systems were organized by a department (e.g., pharmacy) instead of by a clinical process (e.g., cholecystectomy) that might span many departments. Hospitals originally generated this charge data based upon "what the market could bear" as opposed to their actual internal cost structure. **Many hospitals still have information systems that are incapable of providing true cost data. Instead, they rely upon a conversion factor (the cost-to-charge ratio) which is applied to patient charges**

in an attempt to estimate hospital costs. This method of "guess-timating" costs has many problems. For one, different cost centers within the hospital (e.g., the pharmacy versus respiratory therapy) have different margins (Table 99-2) and there may be great variation, even within one department.[76] For example, the percent mark-up of inexpensive disposables by the hospital central supply department is usually much greater than for more expensive items (Fig. 99-3). Also, because the gross margin of the hospital includes many indirect costs that do not generate a specific patient charge (e.g., the mortgage on the building), those direct costs that are chargeable (e.g., drugs) tend to be overestimated (i.e., cost shifting). Charges typically vary depending upon the negotiating power of the purchaser (Medicare rates versus self-pay charges). Finally, hospital information systems often artificially group fixed and variable costs together, creating large categories of charges that cannot be effectively analyzed (e.g., a blanket charge for 1 hour of operating room time ignoring actual staffing requirements).

Average wholesale price

Another common pitfall in measuring anesthetic costs is relying upon the average wholesale price (AWP) for drug costs. The AWP is listed for each drug in a pharmaceutical industry reference (e.g., the Red Book), which is published by the same company that publishes the Physicians' Desk Reference (i.e., Medical Economics Data). Although the AWP is purported to be the average U.S. hospital cost of a drug, it almost always exceeds the price that most hospitals pay (Fig. 99-4). For example, although the AWP of droperidol is $5.31, a typical actual hospital cost would be approximately $0.50 (the patient charge may exceed $25.00). Beware of pharmaceutical salespeople that compare the actual hospital cost of their company's drug with the AWP of their competitor's product. One study that measured the accuracy of information presented to physicians by pharmaceutical sales representatives found that 11% of the statements made were inaccurate and contradicted information readily available to the salesperson. Not surprisingly, all of the inaccurate statements were favorable toward the promoted drug.[146]

Table 99-2 The cost-to-charge ratio varies between hospital departments and thus charge should not be considered a reliable indicator of hospital cost

Hospital department	Cost-to-charge ratio
Surgery admission unit	0.92
Radiology	0.63
Postanesthesia care unit	0.54
Blood bank	0.53
Patient ward	0.52
Laboratory	0.50
Miscellaneous	0.48
Operating room	0.44
Pharmacy	0.41
Intensive care unit	0.37
Anesthesia	0.29

Adapted from Macario A, et al: Where are the costs in perioperative care? Analysis of hospital costs and charges for inpatient surgical care, *Anesthesiology* 83:1138, 1995.

Measurement of Specific Components of Anesthetic Costs

Inhalational anesthetic cost

Some components that comprise total anesthetic cost are more difficult to measure than others. For example, most drug costs and the cost of disposable supplies (e.g., a face mask) are fairly straightforward and can usually be obtained with the cooperation of the pharmacy and central supply departments.[140] The cost of inhalational anesthetic agents is more difficult to assess because current vaporizers do not quantify the amount of volatile anesthetic vaporized during a single case.

A precise formula for calculating the cost of volatile anesthetics has been described[96]:

$$\text{COST} = (P)(F)(T)(M)(C) / (24.12)(d)(100)$$

In this equation:

P = percent delivered by vaporizer (%)
F = fresh gas flow (l/min)
T = time (min)
M = molecular weight of agent (g)
C = cost of agent per milliliter liquid ($)
d = density of agent (g/ml)
24.12 = liter volume of 1 mole of gas at 21° C

Fortunately, this formula can be simplified. The amount of volatile anesthetic expended is directly proportional to flow rates:

anesthetic vapor expended = (fresh gas flow rate) × (percent inspired concentration)

The amount of gaseous anesthetic agent expended during an anesthetic can be estimated by measuring O_2, N_2O, and air flow rates and vaporizer settings at 15-minute intervals. The conversion from vapor to liquid depends upon molecular weight and density, but can be approximated by a simple rule of thumb:

1 ml volatile anesthetic liquid = 200 ml volatile anesthetic vapor

Thus, the rate of liquid anesthetic expended can be approximated:

liquid volatile anesthetic (ml) consumed per minute = (flow rate, l/min) × (concentration agent, %) / 200

Alternatively, liquid agent consumed per hour can be quickly estimated as three times the product of fresh gas flow and percent concentration. The cost of bulk O_2 and N_2O is a relatively minor contributor to total anesthetic cost in the U.S., and can be ignored.

Comparing the cost of volatile anesthetics requires con-

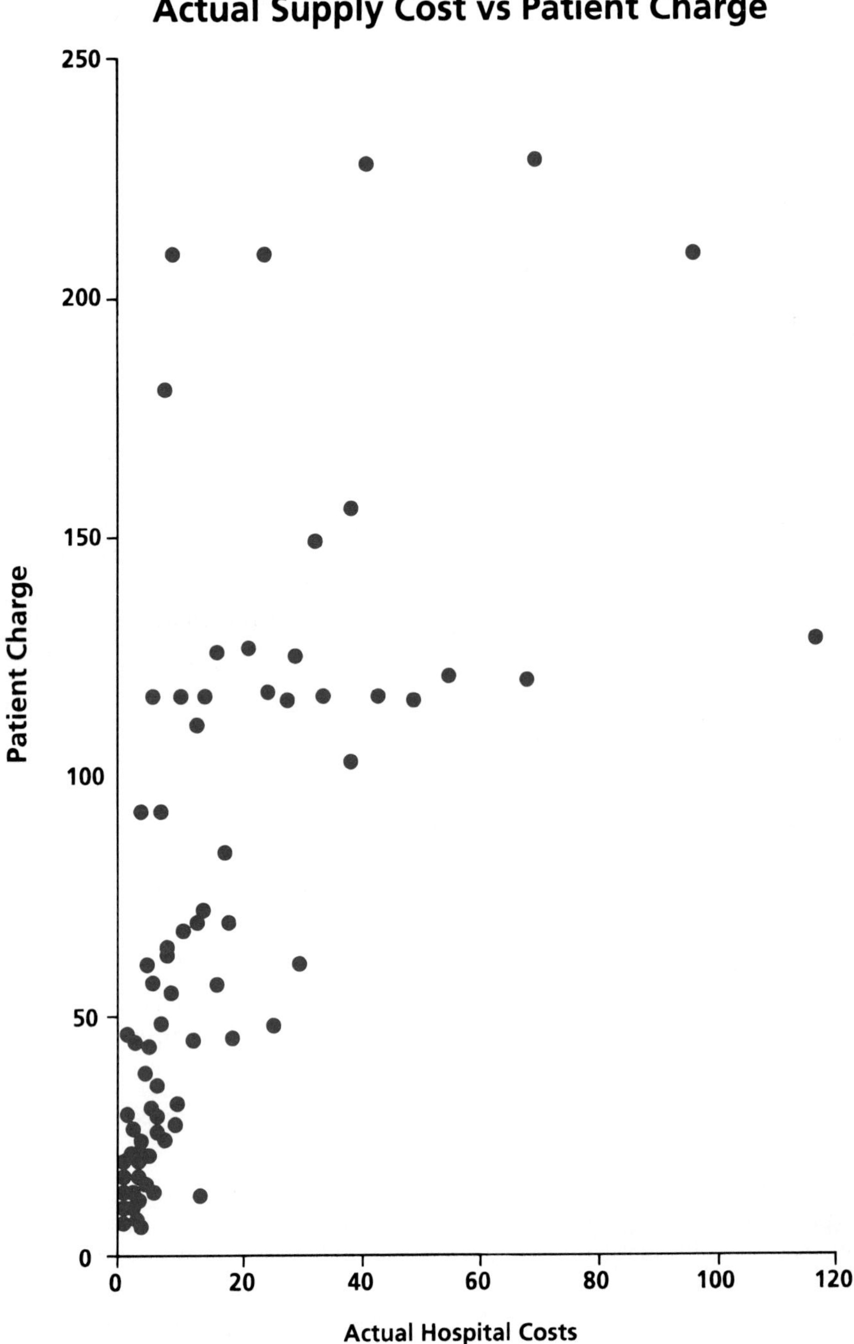

Fig. 99-3. At most hospitals there is a very poor correlation between the amount a patient is charged for disposable supplies and the actual hospital cost. Thus, a cost-to-charge ratio can not accurately convert patient charges to hospital costs.

sideration of four factors: (1) the cost per milliliter of liquid anesthetic (i.e., acquisition cost); (2) the volume of vapor that results from each milliliter of liquid; (3) the effective potency of the anesthetic; and (4) the background flow of gases chosen (i.e., total fresh gas flow rate).[135] Although halothane has the lowest acquisition cost of any volatile anesthetic agent, concerns regarding its hepatotoxicity have greatly limited its use in the U.S. and to a lesser extent in the U.K.[7,70] Directly comparing the cost of volatile anesthetics must account for differences in potency (minimum alveolar concentration [MAC]) and solubility (anesthetic uptake). Highly soluble agents require more anesthetic to replace the amount taken up. The interplay between MAC and solubility determines the *effective* potency. For example, the fivefold increased potency (MAC) of isoflurane compared with desflurane is partially offset by the former's threefold greater solubility.[135] Thus, anesthetic solubility influences the amount of time required before

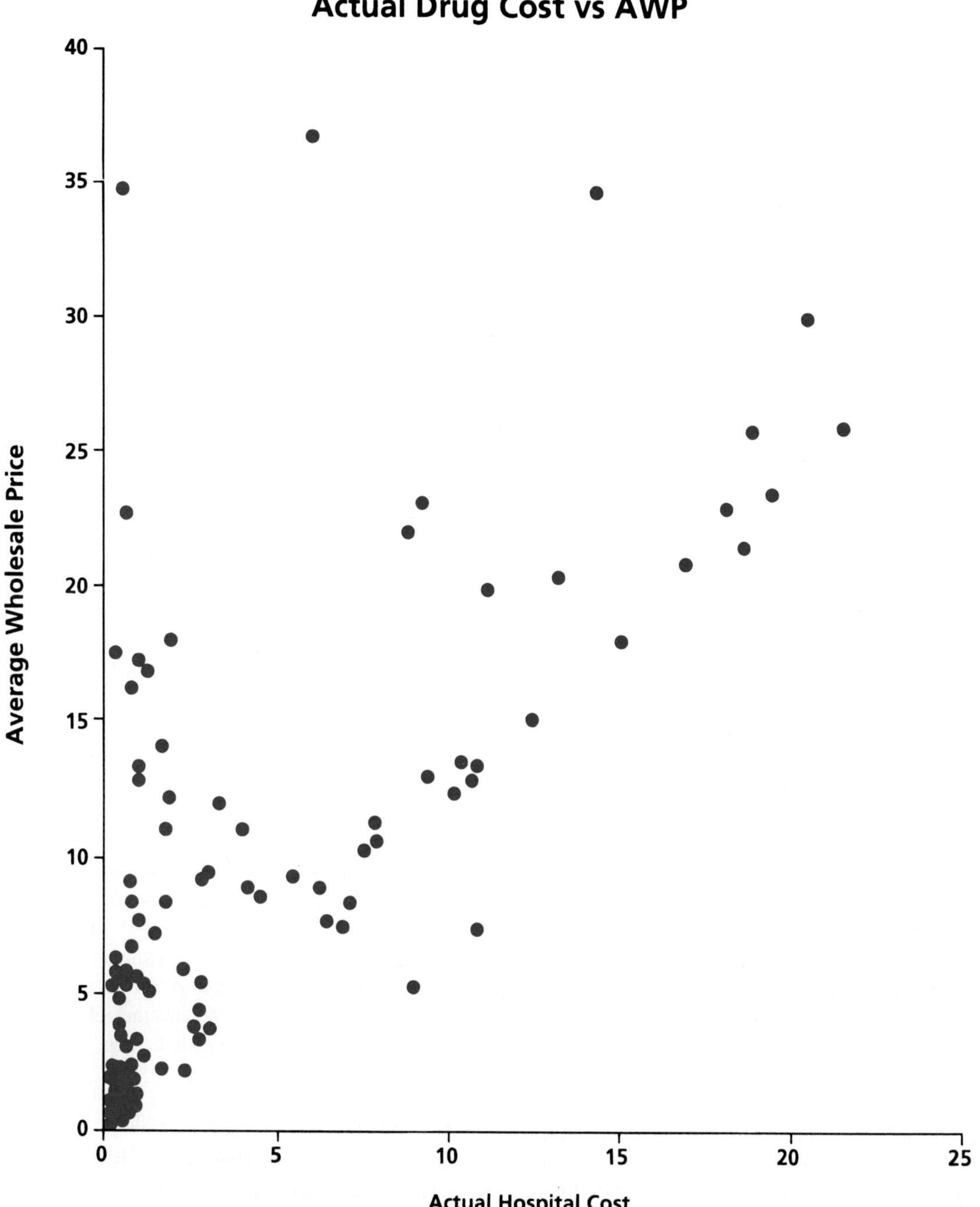

Fig. 99-4. The average wholesale price does not usually approximate actual hospital costs.

achieving a state of equilibrium, the fresh gas flow rates required for a given level of anesthesia, and the amount of time required for awakening. All of these factors can affect cost calculations.

Nondisposable equipment cost

The cost of nondisposable equipment (e.g., an anesthesia machine) can be estimated for each case if the initial purchase price and life expectancy of the product are known. Life expectancy is not necessarily equivalent to the depreciation guidelines used by hospital finance departments for taxation and accounting purposes. Rather, it should reflect the product's expected years of clinical life. The cost of each nondisposable item can then be amortized over its expected life span using a straight-line depreciation method (SLN):

SLN = (unit cost × quantity) / (lifespan)

The resulting total annual cost can be converted to a cost per minute of anesthesia time by extrapolating operating room utilization data.

Labor costs

Utilization of operating room personnel and recovery room personnel is directly affected by the efficiency of anesthesia services. Specifically, four periods of time that are influenced *primarily* by anesthesiologists can be identified, two of which directly involve the operating room:

- **Preoperative time**—the time between the placement of invasive lines by the anesthesiologist (e.g., monitoring and epidural catheters) in the preoperative holding room and transport of the patient to the operating room (only applicable if a preoperative holding room is used for line placement);
- **Induction time**—the time between when the patient enters the operating room and when the patient is ready for surgical positioning;
- **Extubation time**—the time between repositioning the patient at the end of surgery and the patient leaving the operating room;
- **Recovery time**—the time between the patient arriving in the recovery room and the patient being discharged from the recovery room.

These four time intervals can be measured and entered into a spreadsheet that calculates the associated labor costs based upon the hourly wage (including benefits) of preoperative, operative, and recovery room personnel. Typically, a preoperative area requires a nurse who can simultaneously assist multiple anesthesiologists during line placement. For example, if nursing policies allow care for up to three patients, this nurse's hourly cost per case would be reduced by a factor of at least 0.5 (0.33 would assume maximum utilization which is rarely achievable). Likewise, recovery time requires a recovery room nurse who can care for, at most, two patients and recovery cost per hour can be adjusted by a factor of 0.66 (0.5 would assume maximal utilization).

The logic for labor cost allocation during induction time is more involved. Consider for example a hospital that uses two circulating nurses and one scrub technician for hip arthroplasty surgery. One circulating nurse is essentially dedicated to assisting with patient transfer and positioning, noninvasive monitor placement, and other tasks as requested by the anesthesiologist. Thus, this individual's labor cost during induction time should be considered an anesthetic cost. In contrast, the second circulating nurse and the scrub technician are involved in surgical activities such as instrument preparation. However, these surgical activities are usually completed within 20 to 30 minutes, after which these individuals are essentially waiting for the patient to be positioned and prepped. Thus, the labor costs of the second circulating nurse and scrub technician become anesthesia costs whenever induction time exceeds 25 minutes. Extubation time could be considered in an analogous manner.

A teaching hospital may pay the salary of anesthesia residents, but not anesthesia faculty. Assume a hospital pays 14 resident salaries to provide coverage for 11 operating rooms. Annual operating room utilization data can be used to calculate the adjusted cost of anesthesia residents per minute of anesthesia time. The rationale for using an adjusted cost per minute is that it captures the labor costs associated with resident time outside the operating room (e.g., preoperative clinic, recovery room, vacation time, and sick leave) without requiring specific measurement of this time. Therefore, the total hospital cost related to the resident's salary for a given case can be estimated by multiplying the operating room time by the resident's adjusted cost per minute. Operating room time includes induction time, extubation time, and the time interval between patient positioning after induction and repositioning before extubation.

The hospital costs associated with salaried anesthesiologists, nurse anesthetists, or anesthesia technicians could be similarly considered. For example, total annual anesthesia technologist's labor cost including benefits divided by total operating room time produces an adjusted cost per minute.

Laboratory costs

The hospital cost of perioperative laboratory studies can be estimated by determining three basic components: (1) the depreciated cost of initial equipment purchased; (2) the cost of reagents and controls; and (3) the labor costs associated with performing the tests. It could be argued that most preoperative and postoperative laboratory tests, although important contributors to hospital cost, are *primarily* surgical costs and not principally a consequence of anesthetic management. However, because *intra*operative test ordering is primarily determined by the anesthesiologist, it should definitely be considered an anesthetic cost.

An example: The cost of anesthesia at a university hospital

The comparative contributions of drugs, fluids, disposable supplies, nondisposable equipment, labor, and lab tests to the overall anesthetic cost of hip and knee arthroplasty surgery at the University of Southern California University Hospital are summarized in Figure 99-5. Labor and disposable equipment are responsible for 70% of the anesthetic cost. The cost of resident salaries represent the majority of labor expenses (Figure 99-6), whereas monitoring supplies (e.g., central venous pressure kits) are the largest component of disposable supply costs. Capital equipment and intraoperative lab studies contribute little to overall cost. Midazolam, vecuronium, atracurium, and isoflurane account for the largest share of drug costs. Inhalational agents represent approximately 20% of total drug cost. The cost of N_2O contributes approximately 5% of the cost of inhala-

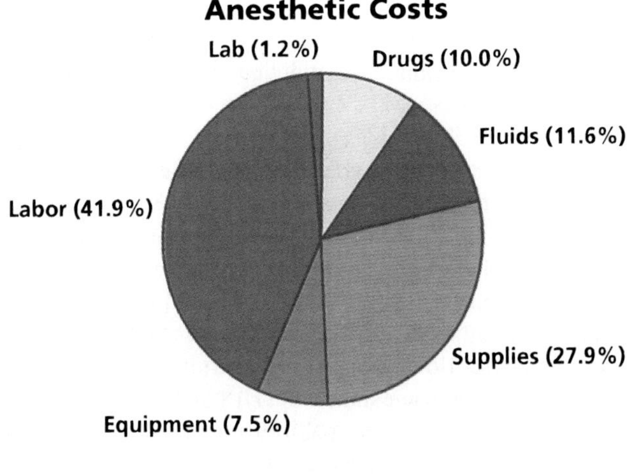

Fig. 99-5. Breakdown of anesthetic costs for hip arthroplasty surgery at a university hospital.

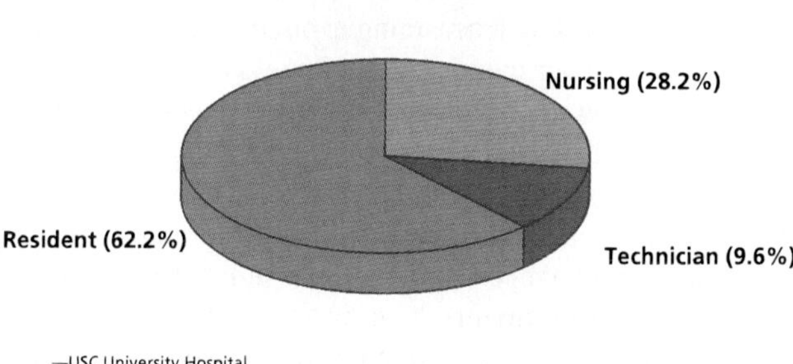

Fig. 99-6. Components of anesthetic related labor costs during hip arthroplasty surgery at a university hospital.

tional anesthetics and 1% of total drug cost. Albumin administration is an important determinant of fluid cost.

A REVIEW OF THE ANESTHETIC LITERATURE DEALING WITH COST

In 1991, fewer than 10% of the clinical investigations in the journal *Anesthesiology* mentioned costs, and only 2 of 700 contained information useful to judge cost-effectiveness.[60,123] Since then, articles regarding the economic aspects of anesthesiology have received more attention, but the area of cost-effectiveness must still be considered to be in its infancy. Thus, the reader should consider the results of the studies summarized below with a degree of skepticism. Most, if not all, of the studies have design flaws which prevent them from providing true cost-effective analysis.[130] Nonetheless, they provide a starting point for discussion and ideas for future critical study.

Preoperative Laboratory Testing

It has been estimated that from $1.3 billion to $12 billion per year is spent on unnecessary preoperative laboratory testing and its consequences[75,87,102] and that 60% to 75% of all preoperative tests could be eliminated without adversely affecting the quality of care.[75,87] The low positive predictive value of most preoperative tests adds virtually nothing to an adequate preoperative history and physical examination, and certainly does not warrant their aggregate cost.[125] It has been further estimated that in 96% of cases, a patient history and physical examination can determine the patient's fitness for surgery.[142] In fact, a healthy patient undergoing 30 tests—each with a 95% probability of producing a normal result—has an 80% chance of having one abnormal test result. Even when a patient is found to have a laboratory abnormality, it is unlikely that anesthetic management will be altered.[125] Thus, the routine ordering of batteries of lab tests in healthy patients has undergone intense scrutiny in recent years, and recommendations for rationale lab testing have been proposed.[87,101,102] These risk stratification strategies suggest specific testing parameters depending upon patient gender, age, and results of his or her medical history (sometimes computerized) and physical examination.[126] Although such early assessment of outpatients often requires an extra patient visit and additional facility resources, these costs are presumably offset by savings associated with better preoperative control of underlying medical conditions, fewer delays and cancellations on the day of surgery, and omission of unnecessary screening laboratory tests.[139] In addition to directly adding cost, unnecessary testing introduces the possibility of harming patients during the pursuit of false-positive or borderline abnormalities. Further, not recording or pursuing an abnormality in an ordered test result could introduce a degree of medical-legal risk.

Preoperative evaluation of vascular surgery patients can be especially expensive. Although dobutamine stress echocardiography and dipyridamole thallium scintigraphy have similar utility in predicting cardiac outcomes, the former may be more cost-effective.[34] Depending upon the selection criteria used for testing, the cost per life saved has been estimated to range from $250,000 to more than $1,000,000.

Pharmaceuticals

Drug costs have received a disproportionate share of attention in studies of the cost of anesthesia, particularly when compared with the larger costs associated with labor[51,70,73] or to the overall cost of a surgical procedure.[123] In fact, pharmaceuticals only account for approximately 5% of hospital costs.[46,140] Nonetheless, anesthesia drug sales in the U.S. exceeded $1 billion in 1992, and are expected to reach $2.1 billion by 1999 (a 9.2% compound annual growth rate).[36] Much of the growth can be attributed to the development and release of a growing number of more expensive short-duration drugs, spurred by the growth in outpatient surgery (Fig. 99-7).

Premedication

The cost-effectiveness of premedication has received little attention. IV midazolam is a significant budgetary item for

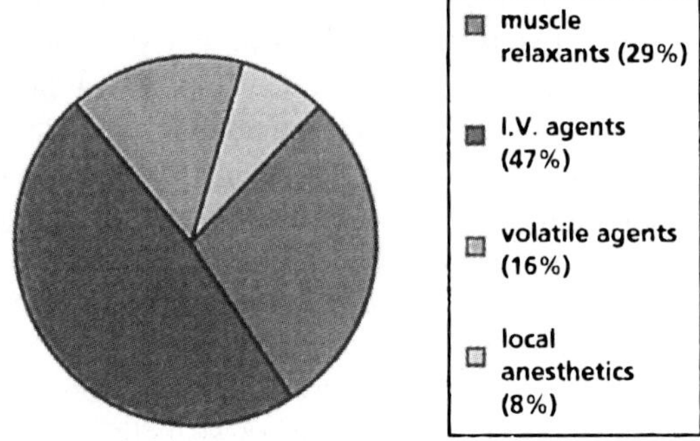

Fig. 99-7. Estimated market share (1999) by type of anesthetic drug. (From Gannon K: Anesthesia drug market climbing through 1999, *Hosp Pharm Rep,* 7:32-35, 1993.)

many hospital pharmacies. The worth of sedation to the patient prior to being taken to the operating room is difficult to estimate and probably varies greatly among individuals. One less costly alternative to midazolam is diazepam. However, diazepam has a much longer duration of action (particularly in elderly patients), frequently causes pain on injection, and has been associated with venous phlebitis. The use of an new emulsified preparation of diazepam (Dizac) appears to avoid these last two complications.

Muscle relaxants and reversal agents

The cost of muscle relaxants has received considerable attention. As with other categories of pharmaceuticals, generic medications no longer protected by patents (i.e., succinylcholine, curare, or pancuronium) have much lower acquisition costs than the newer alternatives which generally possess fewer side effects. Compared with dramatic cost differentials, the differences in side effects usually appear subtle. The most obvious distinction between muscle relaxants is probably their duration of action.[44] Factors that need to be considered in addition to acquisition cost include potency, duration of action, and patient outcome. Two drugs with similar unit costs (cost per vial) and duration of action may differ in overall cost because of differences in potency or packaging (milligrams per vial).[41]

Pancuronium appears to be an obvious choice for facilitating mechanical ventilation both in the intensive care unit[121] and for longer surgical procedures, particularly in patients without significant heart, renal, or hepatic disease. To be cost-effective, its use cannot be associated with a high incidence of residual paralysis in the recovery room requiring reintubation or prolongation of mechanical ventilation. Some have questioned whether the greater cardiovascular stability (i.e., less heart rate increase) seen with doxacurium or pipecuronium justifies their tenfold greater cost compared with pancuronium, even for cardiac surgery.[98] Combining two nondepolarizing muscle relaxants that potentiate each other leads to a reduction in the total amount of drug required and has been advocated as a novel method of cost reduction.[22] Furthermore, the cost and side effects (e.g., postoperative nausea and vomiting) of muscle-relaxant reversal should be considered. This additional factor might particularly favor mivacurium, a short-acting muscle relaxant.[28]

Inhalation and intravenous anesthetics

The key to controlling volatile anesthetic agent cost is minimizing fresh gas flow rates.[3,20,77,95,129,141] Low gas flows (< 1 lpm) also minimize the difference and can even reverse the relationship between the cost of various volatile anesthetic agents.[135] For example, compared with the much greater cost of desflurane at high flows (3 to 6 l/min), at closed circuit flow rates (300 ml/min) the cost of desflurane and isoflurane are similar ($11.18 and $13.57, respectively for an anesthetic lasting 169 minutes).[47] The longer the duration of the case, the greater the cost advantage of low solubility. Using the extreme example of closed-circuit flow rates may be unrealistic in many practices,[52,56] but illustrates the complex interplay of multiple factors on cost determinations.

Although low flow rates will result in greater soda lime exhaustion caused by rebreathing expired gas, this increased cost is insignificant compared with the savings in volatile agent. Low flow rates will also decrease the cost of O_2,[9] but the use of bulk liquid O_2 makes this savings negligible. Minor considerations in the cost of volatile anesthesia include the cost of monitoring (i.e., analyzing end-tidal concentrations) and the cost of delivery (e.g., desflurane requires a special vaporizer).

Like other areas of cost analysis, the costs of using volatile anesthetics may vary depending upon locale. For example, in the Caribbean, the savings accrued by replacing N_2O with compressed air-O_2 exceeds the cost of the additional halothane required.[83] Although in the U.S. the cost of N_2O contributes little to overall anesthetic drug costs, it was found to be the largest anesthetic drug cost for a London teaching hospital as recently as 1982.[2]

Documenting cost-effectiveness requires more than merely determining the least costly alternative. For example, in a comparison of sevoflurane and halothane for pediatric outpatient surgery, the cost of the inhalation agents was less for halothane ($0.25) than sevoflurane ($5.45) for a 25-minute operation.[132] However, sevoflurane anesthesia contributed to a 5.8-minute savings in operating room turn-around time, potentially allowing one additional surgical case during an 8-hour shift of 30-minute cases.[132] Likewise, desflurane has been associated with faster eye opening than isoflurane,[89,112] but with no change in actual outpatient discharge time.[37] The determination of cost-effectiveness relies on so many interrelated factors that subtle differences may depend upon a specific clinician's practice habits (e.g., induction agent, flow rates, adjuvant drugs, use of antiemetics, etc.).

The combination of propofol (induction and maintenance) with N_2O (maintenance) compared with thiopental (induction) and isoflurane-N_2O (maintenance) has been repeatedly shown to be associated with a shorter recovery time and a lower incidence of nausea and vomiting following short surgical procedures.[29,115,137] Likewise, propofol offers some minor advantages in response time, ambulation time, vomiting, and drowsiness during recovery compared with methohexital for induction and maintenance during brief (< 30 minutes) gynecologic surgery.[12] These subtle differences in outcome become harder to justify after long procedures because the cost of propofol becomes prohibitive. Further, whether or not the advantages attributed to propofol translate into actual monetary savings depends on several other factors. For instance, the conclusion that quicker awakening or reduced nausea and vomiting result in faster discharge, less recovery room use, and lower labor costs has been questioned.[26,48] Any difference in length of recovery room stay between anesthetic maintenance with desflurane or propofol is probably small and represents insignificant cost savings.[127] The possibility of societal savings based upon earlier return to work and resumption of normal activities is even less clear and harder to quantify.[139]

The effect of an anesthetic agent upon patient outcome could easily outweigh any differences in acquisition costs. However, neurosurgical patients anesthetized with either fentanyl-N_2O, propofol-fentanyl, or isoflurane-N_2O demonstrated only minor outcome differences (the fentanyl-N_2O group had a higher incidence of vomiting).[120] There were no detectable differences in brain conditions (e.g., swelling, postoperative neurologic deficits) or time to awakening, despite a three- to tenfold greater drug cost in the propofol-fentanyl group. This difference in cost became inconsequential when compared with the total cost of the procedure.

Anesthetic adjuvants

The cost-effectiveness of routine antiemetic therapy has been investigated. Although less than 50% of postoperative patients experience nausea within 24 hours of general anesthesia, the resulting delay in discharge and occasional need for unplanned admission of outpatients may warrant the routine administration of some antiemetic. The cost of managing postoperative nausea and vomiting at an outpatient surgery center (including personnel, supply, and drug costs) has been estimated at $14.94 per patient.[14] Affected patients also spent an average of 24 additional minutes in the recovery room, adding another $7.00 of nursing labor to the overall facility cost. Further, the psychologic cost to the patient of avoidable nausea or vomiting can not be easily assigned a monetary value, yet this factor could overshadow the acquisition cost of any antiemetic drug. Metoclopramide and droperidol are inexpensive drugs, which when given in proper dosages, have been shown to be effective and possess few side effects. Ondansetron may be even more effective, but its much higher cost has relegated its use to patients at a high risk of emesis or patients who experience symptoms despite initial, less costly therapy. One cost-effectiveness study that relied upon average wholesale price (AWP) instead of actual hospital cost (AHC) found ondansetron (AWP = $20.75; AHC = 17.05) and droperidol (AWP = 5.31; AHC = 0.46) to be more cost effective than metoclopramide (AWP = 2.35; AHC = 0.25). Prophylactic administration of ondansetron became cost effective in populations with a risk of emesis greater than 33%, whereas the cost-effective risk threshold for droperidol prophylaxis was only 10%. As the authors point out, the conclusions of studies such as this depend heavily upon the accuracy of direct cost data and the assumptions regarding indirect cost.[133]

Ketorolac—a nonsteroidal anti-inflammatory drug available in parenteral form—has been shown to be an effective postoperative pain medication. However, its use has not been consistently shown to prevent symptoms traditionally blamed on opioid therapy (e.g., nausea, vomiting, respiratory depression) or to improve overall quality of life parameters (e.g., time to resumption of normal activities).[143] As with so many other agents, any small gain in discharge time probably would not translate into significant cost savings. Indomethacin, while not available in a parenteral form, has been shown to provide equally effective relief of minor postoperative pain at less than one half the cost of ketorolac.[82] The rather high cost of flumazenil, a specific benzodiazepine antagonist, should be compared with its ability to decrease recovery room time and eliminate unnecessary hospitalization of oversedated outpatients.[38]

Fluid Management

The cost of blood transfusion includes the procurement costs of blood products (e.g., compatibility testing, overhead expenses), the equipment (e.g., blood warmer) and supplies (e.g., blood filter) required for transfusion and the possibility of transfusion-related complications. The procurement costs of several blood components has been determined (Table 99-3).[35] The use of blood salvage equipment (e.g., Cell-Savers) to reduce the need of banked blood probably only becomes cost effective if two or more units can be re-infused,[5] but would depend upon the cost of the required disposables and labor costs (i.e., whether or not a dedicated technician is needed). This analysis does not include the potential cost savings of autologous transfusion associated with its decreased risk of disease transmission, compatibility reactions, and immunologic compromise (i.e., cancer recurrence, postoperative infections).

Table 99-3 Base cost of blood components

Cost	Erythrocytes	Pooled platelets	Fresh frozen plasma	Cryoprecipitate
Variable	80.81	424.98	60.61	311.86
Fixed	26.45	116.16	21.24	20.32
Total	107.26	541.14	81.85	332.18

*Pooled platelets were from seven donor units; cryoprecipitate was pooled from ten donor units. Data excludes administrative costs, delivery supplies, and blood products ordered but not transfused. Data from Gan TJ, et al: *Anesth Analg* 82:5123, 1996

The hospital cost of an allogeneic erythrocyte transfusion at a university hospital has been determined to be $151.20.[72] This analysis included associated costs, such as handling costs and the cost of possible transfusion-related complications. **The cost-effectiveness of autologous blood transfusion depends upon the cost savings attributable to avoidance of complications associated with homologous transfusion and the wastage of overcollection.** Thus, it may prove cost-effective for a high blood loss procedure (e.g., bilateral hip arthroplasty) but not for a low blood loss procedure (e.g., unilateral knee arthroplasty).[6] Because the average gain in life expectancy by avoiding allogeneic blood transfusion with the preoperative donation of autologous blood is only 0.05 to 0.07 days, the cost per quality-adjusted year of life gained translates into between $0.5 and $2.1 million.[40] If the rate of autologous blood wastage (i.e., preoperative donation without perioperative transfusion) is high, the cost per life-year gained can swell to $14 million.[63] Intraoperative blood collection has been advocated as being more cost-effective than preoperative blood donation of autologous blood for patients with a low probability for transfusion yet who request autologous blood.[107]

Disposable Supplies

Continuously measuring mixed venous O_2 saturation could be cost-effective if patient outcomes were improved or if the cost of the catheter was offset by savings elsewhere (e.g., fewer cardiac output determinations or venous blood gas determinations). One study of cardiac surgery patients confirmed the higher charges associated with mixed venous O_2 monitoring, but could not demonstrate any differences in outcome or other cost savings.[94] A study of critical care patients did not demonstrate a decrease in adverse hemodynamic events, length of intensive care unit stay, or mortality attributable to continuous measurement of mixed venous O_2 saturation.[55] Similarly, the cost-effectiveness of pulmonary artery (PA) catheters has been questioned.[4,53,124] Despite a greater cost compared with central venous catheters, PA catheters provided no significant advantages in terms of mortality, morbidity, or length of stay. These studies do not necessarily prove that measurement of mixed venous O_2 saturation or PA pressure is worthless, but any potential benefits were too subtle for the studies' design.

Forced-air warming blankets have been repeatedly shown to effectively prevent intraoperative hypothermia. Nonetheless, to be cost-effective, some savings must be demonstrated to offset the cost of the disposable warming blanket. Following their use in one study during outpatient arthroscopic knee surgery, patient shivering decreased, but no reduction in recovery room stay could be demonstrated.[113]

Spinal needles vary in cost with the Quincke (26 g) being the least expensive, the Whitacre (25 g) intermediate, and the Sprotte (24 g) costing the most. Quincke needles tend to have a higher incidence of postdural puncture headache, whereas the Sprotte design has been associated with an increased need for intraoperative supplementation. This has lead one group of authors to recommend the Whitacre needle as a cost-effective alternative.[13]

Even the reuse of disposable syringes after injection through a Y-port extension set containing a back-check valve has been examined as a method to decrease drug wastage between patients.[65] The collection, decontamination, and reuse of undamaged disposable supplies can significantly affect the cost of wastage.[108] Patients receiving prolonged mechanical ventilation had no increase in ventilator-associated pneumonia rates when ventilator circuits were changed at 7-day intervals compared with 48-hour intervals.[49]

Capital Equipment

The cost of nondisposable supplies depends upon their initial purchase price, use rate (i.e., reuse rate), and potential salvage value at the time of their replacement. For instance, a nondisposable item (i.e., the laryngeal mask airway [LMA]) could potentially save money if it replaced the use of a less expensive disposable supply (i.e., endotracheal [ET] tube) several times during its lifespan, indirectly altered the use of other resources, or lowered the cost of treating complications. Compared with maintaining an airway with a face mask or ET tube, one study found the LMA became cost-effective for use in cases lasting longer than 40 minutes if it is reused 40 times before being discarded.[74] Most of the cost savings in this study came from elimination of neuromuscular-blocking drugs and decreased volatile anesthetic requirements. Thus, the cost advantage of the LMA became greater with increased reuse rate or increased anesthetic duration. The attenuated hemodynamic response and lesser incidence of sore throat following LMA insertion compared with ET intubation may or may not justify its routine use. However, its contribution to difficult airway management and the associated costs of potentially devastating hypoxemic complications, at least make its availability cost-effective.

Monitoring equipment can be cost-effective if it decreases the rate of costly complications (including the cost of legal claims) or replaces other more expensive monitoring techniques. The former rationale has been used to promote many currently available monitors including the pulse oximeter, capnograph, spirometer, agent-specific analyzer, noninvasive blood pressure monitor, O_2 analyzer, stethoscope, electrocardiograph monitor, and temperature monitor.[138] An example of the latter would be a demonstration of reduced use of arterial blood gas determinations after the introduction of pulse oximeters and capnographs. In fact, the savings achieved more than pay for the cost of the equipment, without even considering any improvement in the quality of patient care.[103] Pulse oximetry use in the recovery room has been touted as a means of cost savings by determining which patients required O_2 supplementation as evidenced by a SpO_2 of less than 94%.[30] However, the "savings" accrued from withholding supplemental O_2 to patients not apparently needing it ($100 per patient, or an amazing $623,272 per year in the author's hospital) was based upon patient charges, not hospital cost (which amounted to only $4.48 per patient). These cost savings may even be lower in other hospitals ($0.58 per patient)[106] and would certainly seem insignificant if this practice was associated with an increased rate of perioperative complications such as myocardial infarction.[58,93] New technology assessment must focus on not only the technical capabilities of a piece of equipment but also its clinical, economic, and social consequences.[33]

Labor

Labor costs are the single largest component of anesthetic costs.[2,10] As mentioned earlier, anesthesiologists influence operating room use during at least two periods of time: (1) the time interval between the patient entering the operating room and the beginning of positioning or skin preparation (induction time); and (2) the interval between the application of the surgical dressing and the patient leaving the operating room (extubation time). Efforts to shorten these time intervals are cost-effective only if they result in a increase in the number of cases performed during a shift (typically 8 hours), in turn decreasing overtime pay and increasing revenues. In fact, depending upon the average length of cases, even decreasing these time intervals to zero may not generate enough operating room time to schedule one additional case.[25] Shortening the turnover time between cases will effectively increase the amount of elective operating room time only if the facility is already near capacity.[78] Further, as most anesthesiologists are well aware, operating room delays are usually caused by other factors such as scheduling delays, surgeons arriving late, or inadequate patient preparation.[90,100,117]

Anesthetic technique can also affect the time a patient spends in the recovery room. Because labor costs are the largest component of recovery room costs, decreasing recovery room time might be expected to favorably affect recovery room costs. The two areas receiving the most attention have been earlier patient awakening and prevention of postoperative nausea and vomiting. Although both of these options can affect recovery room time, it is unlikely that improving either would create significant cost savings.[26] This apparent paradox can be explained by examination of the factors determining recovery room staffing levels:

- the patient-to-nurse ratio usually exceeds 1:1, therefore early discharge of one patient may not eliminate the need for one nurse
- many hospitals require a minimum of two recovery room nurses, even if only one patient is in the recovery room
- the recovery room does not "close" after a single patient is discharged, nor can small changes in staffing needs be easily anticipated
- factors outside the control of the anesthesiologist affect the use of the recovery room (e.g., surgical complications such as postoperative bleeding, mandated minimum recovery room stays, unavailability of transport personnel)

In contrast, it has been suggested that arranging the operating room schedule to optimize recovery room use could affect the number of nurses required.[26]

Another area of labor cost-effectiveness concerns the relative cost to society, as opposed to the hospital, of physician versus nurse anesthesia providers. It has been proposed that the lower salary costs of nurse anesthetists along with their ability to serve as "close substitutes" make them an attractive alternative to higher-cost physician services.[21,80,105] Not surprisingly, the veracity of these assumptions have been challenged.[136] Because mortality and morbidity rates with differing providers have not been adequately defined by outcome studies, the total cost of any particular provider arrangement can not be accurately determined. It has been proposed that the very fact that a free market places a premium on physician services may be an indicator of their intrinsic value.[57] Teaching is another labor cost. One study found that 10.5% ($3000) of the total cost of intensive care patients was related to teaching activities. This was explained by increased intensity and frequency of monitoring, testing, and treatment (but not prolonged intensive care unit stays).[147]

Regional Versus General Anesthesia

Regional anesthetic techniques tend to cost less than general anesthetic techniques.[97] This is particularly true for minor surgical procedures under local anesthesia with or without monitored anesthesia care (e.g., bunionectomy, inguinal hernia repair, tonsillectomy, genioplasty).[99,128] Cost reductions are typically demonstrated in the areas of pharmaceuticals and disposable supplies.[97] These savings become proportionately less important in surgeries requiring postoperative hospitalization. Nonetheless, even major surgical procedures (e.g., carotid endarterectomy, total knee arthroplasty) may prove to be less costly when performed under regional anesthesia if this results in less intensive care unit use, a shorter total hospital length of stay, or fewer postoperative complications.[85]

Although postoperative IV patient-controlled analgesia may have lower direct costs than epidural analgesia,[61] if the epidural was also used for intraoperative anesthesia its maintenance costs should be very low. Further, the labor costs associated with postoperative patient-controlled analgesia may account for up to 89% of its total cost.[81] The possible benefits of preemptive analgesia should also be considered for valuing a regional technique for some surgical procedures. The advantages of regional or general anesthesia may not apply uniformly for all patient populations, so the most cost-effective anesthetic technique for healthy patients may not be appropriate for patients at risk for a specific complication. Likewise, not all regional techniques have equal cost-efficacy. Spinal anesthesia for cesarean section has been shown to result in shorter operating room time (an average of 17 minutes less per case) as a result of a shorter interval between arriving in the operating room and skin incision, and thus less indirect hospital costs than epidural anesthesia.[100]

COST-EFFECTIVE ANESTHESIA PRACTICE GUIDELINES

An Overview of Clinical Practice Guidelines

Clinical practice guidelines, also known as protocols, pathways, or care maps, are a set of specifications which are systematically developed to help standardize medical

practice to repeatedly obtain the best possible outcome. The philosophy underlying their adoption contends two important tenets: (1) there is one "best way" to treat patients; and (2) that unnecessary variation from this "best way" usually increases waste and decreases quality. Therefore, identifying and minimizing *inappropriate* differences in physician practice habits should improve the quality and efficiency of care patients receive. These guidelines should be distinguished from practice standards, which are a more rigidly applied minimum requirement.[111] Useful guidelines should be scientifically valid, reliable, clinically relevant, flexible, clear, periodically monitored, and documented. Clinical practice guidelines have been demonstrated to offer many advantages including lower liability risk, reduced unnecessary treatment, lower hospital costs, more efficient use of resources, better documentation of care rendered, and standardized physician behavior.[11] The actual process of developing guidelines forces one of their greatest benefits: a critical reexamination of medical cost and outcome data to formulate a set of idealized medical decisions. Clinical practice guidelines are not meant to eliminate appropriate variation in care to individual patients, or to replace physician judgment with a form of "cookbook medicine." Quite the contrary, they promote critical medical decision-making by allowing the clinician to focus on the unique aspects of a particular patient's disease instead of wasting time with routine management. Guidelines encourage similar patients to be treated similarly, not all patients to be treated the same.

Developing practice guidelines in sufficient detail to be clinically useful can be an arduous task. A few of the steps involved include:

- identifying a process to be studied (e.g., anesthesia for hip arthroplasty)
- fractionating the process into a series of functional steps (e.g., preoperative evaluation, induction of anesthesia, pain control, etc.)
- isolating those steps where interpractioner variation exists (e.g., lab tests ordered, induction agents, epidural versus IV analgesia)
- reviewing the scientific literature and other sources of outcome studies (e.g., benchmark data)
- analyzing the costs involved
- reaching a consensus of opinion of what is the "best way" for each step
- implementing the resulting guidelines
- monitoring compliance and updating the guidelines

Standardization of medical practices has been repeatedly shown in other specialties to improve patient care and decrease cost.[8,67,79,104] The development of clinical pathways must consider patient outcome measurements in addition to hospital costs. For example, possible outcome parameters of hip surgery that could be monitored include estimated blood loss, postoperative physical therapy and pain management scores, time in the recovery room and the intensive care unit, time until discharge from the hospital, and the occurrence of perioperative complications (e.g. deep vein thrombosis, infection, and dislocation).

Development of Clinical Practice Guidelines in Anesthesiology

Only approximately 50% of the total costs of anesthesia are under the control of the anesthesiologist (e.g., drugs, lab work, fluids, supplies).[76] The remaining 50% represent fixed costs (e.g., equipment depreciation) or are determined by the duration of the surgical procedure (e.g., anesthesia resident labor cost). The clinical decisions under the control of the anesthesiologist that may result in a high-cost event (e.g. albumin administration) can be easily identified once accurate cost information has been obtained. Potential less costly alternatives or substitutions for each high cost event can then be considered (Box 99-1).

After identifying potential cost-saving alternatives, a group of anesthesiologists can jointly decide which, if any, of the alternatives are acceptable to them as clinicians. Specifically, the justification for the choice (e.g., substituting a crystalloid solution for albumin) should be examined considering current knowledge as reflected in the medical literature and the outcome parameters being monitored at that hospital. Two questions can be asked:

- If this is the preferred choice, why isn't the entire group using it?
- If there is no preferred choice, why not choose the least costly alternative?

Conclusions for each high-cost event can be summarized in a suggested protocol (Box 99-2) for anesthetic management for a specific type of surgery (process management). **It is important to keep in mind that there will still be *considerable* differences between the manner in which patients will be anesthetized. Further, these guidelines are *not* meant to be followed in all cases, because no guideline could account for all patient variants.** In fact, an 80% compliance rate would be exceptional. Compliance with the suggested protocol must be intermittently monitored by retrospective chart review, episodes of noncompliance reviewed by the group, and modifications to the suggested protocol considered. Costs of anesthetic management can be compared before and after adoption of the suggested protocol.

Implementation of Clinical Practice Guidelines

Successful implementation of clinical practice guidelines begins with their development, through the involvement of the entire group of physicians affected by the guidelines. The seriousness of the problem being addressed must be understood and appreciated, a common goal of improving patient care must be accepted, and physician consensus must be constantly sought. Physician control over the guidelines is essential for their long-term commitment, because physicians place a high value on their professional autonomy.[66] The best approach to altering physician behavior has been described as one that provides credible up-to-date information, encourages group decisions, and rewards positive be-

BOX 99-1
HIGH COST ANESTHETIC EVENTS AND POSSIBLE ALTERNATIVES

Drug savings

Fentanyl ($0.38) for alfentanil ($10.72)
Pancuronium (1.71) for vecuronium (18.70)
Diazepam (0.30) for midazolam (13.23)
Pentothal (3.35) for propofol (10.26)
Bupivacaine (1.77) for lidocaine (7.89)
Inhalational anesthetics account for a very small part of total drug costs, assuming low (2 l) flows are used.

Total possible savings based upon current actual usage: $35.14 per case out of average drug cost of approximately $70.00.

Fluid savings

Substituting 2 l of normal saline ($0.66/l) or lactated Ringer's solution ($0.81/l) for 500 ml of albumin.

Total possible savings: $78.33 per case out of average fluid cost of approximately $85.00 per case.

Supply savings

Argon central venous pressure kit (17.75) instead of the Arrow double lumen kit (54.60) or introducer kit (38.95)
20-g IV catheter (0.55) instead of the Arrow radial arterial kit (7.50)
Single transducer (12.50) for double transducer (25.00)
Blood hand-pump IV set (2.48) instead of blood warming sets (25.00)
Omit blood transfusion filter (8.35) in cases with two or less units transfused
Primary vented IV tubing (0.82) instead of Dial-a-Flow (9.30)

Total possible savings of $68.58 out of average supply cost of approximately $250.00.

Labor savings

The only method available to the anesthesiologist to lower labor costs would be to place the epidural or other lines in the recovery prior to surgery.

Total possible savings of $150 or $5.55 per case out of a total labor cost of approximately $375.00 per case.

Conclusion

Out of a total hospital cost of $870.00 to provide anesthetic services per hip case, a maximum savings of $187.60 (22%) could potentially be achieved. A per-case savings of $131.32 assumes a 70% compliance rate with all cost-reduction guidelines and represents a 15% overall savings in the cost of anesthesia.

havior.[45] Physicians alter their behavior when exposed to compelling, scientifically convincing data; when subjected to the pressure of peer review; or when given direct financial incentives. After adoption of the guidelines, continuous or intermittent monitoring provides clinicians with feedback on guideline compliance, patient outcomes, and cost savings. Variations from the guidelines can be classified as appropriate (e.g., caused by patient variance or a guideline that needs modification) or as inappropriate. Minimizing the latter depends upon clear communication to the physicians involved.

BOX 99-2
PRACTICE GUIDELINES FOR THE ANESTHETIC MANAGEMENT OF HIP AND KNEE ARTHROPLASTY AT A UNIVERSITY HOSPITAL

Drugs

Avoid alfentanil — use fentanyl.
Avoid vecuronium — use pancuronium.
Avoid midazolam — use Dizac (an emulsified diazepam).
Avoid propofol — use thiopental.
Avoid high flow rates (> 2 lpm).

Fluids

Avoid albumin and Hespan — use crystalloid solutions.

Supplies

Avoid placing central venous pressure catheters in healthy, primary hip and knee patients.
Avoid placing a-lines in healthy knee patients.
Avoid doulbe-lumen central venous pressure and introducer kits — use the Argon Blitt central venous pressure kit.
Avoid using Arrow a-line kits — use 20-g angiocatheters.
Avoid using double transducers — use a single transducer with a male-to-male connector and a stopcock for the central venous pressure line.
Avoid using the Level-1 blood warming sets — use a hand blood pump. (You can still use pressure chambers for rapid transfusion — to warm fluids, place tubing under Warm-Touch blanket.)
Avoid blood transfusion filters (Pall) in cases where two or less units of blood are transfused.
Avoid disposable Dial-a-Flow sets — use the nondisposable Sigma pump.

The Efficacy of Clinical Practice Guidelines

The development and implementation of clinical practice guidelines in anesthesiology is in its infancy.[64] One study investigated the influence of an anesthetic regimen on outcome and hospital charges for patients undergoing gastric reservoir reduction at two hospitals. Invasive monitoring and postoperative ventilation were associated with prolonged intensive care stays, longer hospitalization, increased hospital charges, and no improvement in patient outcome.[69] Other studies have implemented practice guidelines for coronary artery bypass graft surgery which specifically address the timing of postoperative extubation. These studies demonstrated that altering anesthetic technique could promote more rapid extubation, a reduced length of patient stay, and decreased hospital charges.

A study focusing on practice guidelines for drug use (e.g., pancuronium for cases > 90 minutes; propofol for outpatients only; etomidate for ASA IV patients only; lower usage of colloids; opioid use limited to fentanyl) demonstrated a decline by 40% in drug costs. Measured indicators of clinical outcome included the interval from the end of surgery to recovery room arrival, postoperative nausea and vomiting, mechanical ventilation, and length of recovery room stay. The only detrimental finding was a clinically insignificant increase in the interval from the end of surgery to recovery room arrival.[71,109]

The effects of traditional educational efforts to promote cost containment have been mixed. Such tactics have included distributing lists and spreadsheets of drug costs to providers, lecturing on low-flow anesthetic techniques, making expensive drugs more difficult to access, providing cost data on test requisition forms, and discussing cost issues at case conferences and departmental meetings.[23,86,116,140] Although some cost savings may be initially achieved,[116,134] the effects are often short-lived because of a perceived lack of reward, extraordinary activities by drug representatives, and the lack of an ongoing educational program.[59,119] In general, physician education alone does not appear to be an effective hospital cost containment strategy,[110] however the way the message is presented may be an important differentiating factor.[45]

CONCLUSION

As providers accept more risk, their knowledge of costs becomes critical for optimal decision-making. As profit margins narrow, the risks of capitation increase. Without accurate cost figures, bidding for contracts promising future health services can quickly produce catastrophic financial losses. Further, cost information can influence marketing decisions and internal program development. Programs with large profit margins can be heavily marketed and expanded, whereas those with marginal or negative margins should be scrutinized for cost savings and their functional value to the institution reassessed. One method to decrease costs and improve quality of care is the development, monitoring, and continual updating of clinical pathways.

KEY POINTS

- Anesthesiologists can directly impact at least three resource-intense areas of clinical practice: (1) the operating room; (2) the intensive care unit; and (3) the pain clinic. The operating room has been estimated to account for one third and the intensive care unit up to one fourth of all inpatient hospital costs. Anesthesia costs have been estimated to comprise approximately 6% of total hospital costs.
- The most cost-effective alternative is that which achieves the maximal incremental health benefit for a fixed amount of resources.
- It is important to keep in mind that although cost-effectiveness studies deal with providing the maximum benefit to a population of patients, clinicians have to manage providing the maximum benefit to an individual patient.
- Many hospitals still have information systems that are incapable of providing true cost data. Instead, they rely upon a conversion factor (the cost-to-charge ratio) which is applied to patient charges in an attempt to estimate hospital costs. This method of "guess-timating" costs has many problems.
- Another common pitfall in measuring anesthetic costs is relying upon the average wholesale price (AWP) for drug costs. Although the AWP is purported to be the average U.S. hospital cost of a drug, it almost always exceeds the price that most hospitals pay.
- It has been estimated that from $1.3 to $12 billion per year is spent on unnecessary preoperative laboratory testing and its consequences, and that 60% to 75% of all preoperative tests could be eliminated without adversely affecting the quality of care.
- The key to controlling volatile anesthetic agent cost is minimizing fresh gas flow rates.
- Labor costs are the single largest component of anesthetic costs.
- Regional anesthetic techniques tend to cost less than general anesthetic techniques.
- Clinical practice guidelines, also known as protocols, pathways, or care maps, are a set of specifications which are systematically developed to help standardize medical practice to repeatedly obtain the best possible outcome. The philosophy underlying their adoption contends two important tenets: (1) there is one "best way" to treat patients; and (2) that unnecessary variation from this "best way" usually increases waste and decreases quality.
- Standardization of medical practices has been repeatedly shown in other specialties to improve patient care and decrease cost. Successful implementation of clinical practice guidelines begins with their development: involvement of the entire group of physicians affected by the guidelines.
- After adoption of the guidelines, continuous or intermittent monitoring provides clinicians with feedback on guideline compliance, patient outcomes, and cost savings.

KEY REFERENCES

Becker KE: Practical methods of cost containment in anesthesia and surgery, *J Clin Anesth* 6:388, 1994.

Broadway PJ, Jones JG: A method of costing anaesthetic practice, *Anaesthesia* 50:56, 1995.

Detsky AS, Naglie IG: A clinician's guide to cost-effectiveness analysis, *Ann Intern Med* 113:147, 1990.

Dexter F, Tinker JH: The cost efficacy of hypothetically eliminating adverse anesthetic outcomes from high-risk, but neither low—nor moderate—risk, surgical operations, *Anesth Analg* 81:939, 1995.

Eddy DM: Cost-effectiveness analysis: a conversation with my father, *JAMA* 267:1669, 1992.

Eisenberg JM: Clinical economics: a guide to the economic analysis of clinical practices, *JAMA* 262:2879, 1989.

Fuchs VR, Garber AM: The new technology assessment, *N Engl J Med* 323:673, 1990.

Grumbach K, Bodenheimer T: Mechanisms for controlling costs, *JAMA* 273:1223, 1995.

Grumbach K, Bodenheimer T: Painful vs. painless cost control, *JAMA* 272:1458, 1994.

Johnstone RE, Martinec CL: Costs of anesthesia, *Anesth Analg* 76:840, 1993.

Lubarsky DA, Glass PSA, Ginsberg B, et al: The successful implementation of pharmaceutical practice guidelines, *Anesthesiology* 86:1145, 1997.

Macario A, Vitez TS, Dunn B, et al: Where are the costs in perioperative care? Analysis of hospital costs and charges for inpatient surgical care, *Anesthesiology* 83:1138, 1995.

Sperry RJ: Principles of economic analysis, *Anesthesiology* 86:1197, 1997.

Turnbull JM, Buck C: The value of preoperative screening investigations in otherwise healthy individuals, *Arch Intern Med* 147:1101, 1987.

Watcha MF, White PF: Economics of anesthetic practice, *Anesthesiology* 86:1170, 1997.

White PF, White LD: Cost containment in the operating room: Who is responsible? *J Clin Anesth* 6:351, 1994.

REFERENCES

1. Anderson CA, Daigh RD: Quality mind-set overcomes barriers to success, *Health Finan Man* 45:21, 1991.
2. Astley BA, Walker JS: Cost of anesthesia, *Br Med J* 285:189, 1982.
3. Bailey CR, Ruggier R, Cashman JN: Anaesthesia: cheap at twice the price? Staff awareness, cost comparisons and recommendations for economic savings, *Anaesthesia* 48:906, 1993.
4. Bashein G, Johnson PW, Davis KB, et al: Elective coronary bypass surgery without pulmonary artery catheter monitoring, *Anesthesiology* 63:451, 1985.
5. Becker KE: Practical methods of cost containment in anesthesia and surgery, *J Clin Anesth* 6:388, 1994.
6. Birkmeyer JD, Goodnough LT, AuBuchon JP, et al: The cost-effectiveness of preoperative autologous blood donation for total hip and knee replacement, *Transfusion* 33:544, 1993.
7. Blogg CE: Halothane and the liver: the problem revisited and made obsolete, *Br Med J* 292:1691, 1986.
8. Bowen J, Yaste C: Effect of a stroke protocol on hospital costs of stroke patients, *Neurology* 44:1961, 1994.
9. Briscoe CE: Halving the cost of anaesthetic agents, *Br Med J* 1:488, 1970.
10. Broadway PJ, Jones JG: A method of costing anaesthetic practice, *Anaesthesia* 50: 56, 1995.
11. Burda D: Changing physician practice patterns: quality improves and so do profits, *Mod Health,* 2:18-26, 1989.
12. Cade L, Morley PT, Ross W: Is propofol cost-effective for day-surgery patients? *Anaesth Intens Care* 19:201, 1991.
13. Campbell DC, Douglas MJ, Pavy TJG, et al: Comparison of the 25-gauge Whitacre with the 24 gauge Sprotte spinal needle for elective caesarean section: cost implications, *Can J Anaesth* 40:1131, 1993.
14. Carroll NV, Miederhoff PA, Cox FM, et al: Costs incurred by outpatient surgical centers in managing postoperative nausea and vomiting, *J Clin Anesth* 6:364, 1994.
15. Cerra FB: Healthcare reform: the role of coordinated critical care, *Crit Care Med* 21:457, 1993.
16. Cohen MM, Duncan PG, Tweed WA, et al: The Canadian four-center study of anaesthetic outcomes: I. Description of methods and populations, *Can J Anaesth* 39:420, 1992.
17. Cohen MM, Duncan PG, Pope WDB, et al: The Canadian four-center study of anaesthetic outcomes: II. Can outcomes be used to assess the quality of anaesthesia care? *Can J Anaesth* 39:430, 1992.
18. Duncan PG, Cohen Mm, Tweed MA , et al: The Canadian four-center study of anaesthetic outcomes: III. Are anaesthetic complications predictable in day surgical practice? *Can J Anaesth* 39:440, 1992.
19. Cooper JO: The relative costs of anesthesia drugs in New Zealand versus the United States (letter), *Anesth Analg* 80:848, 1995.
20. Cotter SM, Petros AJ, Dore CJ, et al: Low-flow anaesthesia: practice, cost implications and acceptability, *Anaesthesia* 46: 1009, 1991.
21. Cromwell J, Rosenbach M: The impact of nurse anesthetists on anesthesiologist productivity, *Med Care* 28:159, 1990.
22. Cruz JC: Reducing the cost of using neuromuscular relaxants (letter), *Anesth Analg* 65:315, 1986.
23. Cummings KM, Frisof KB, Long MJ, et al: The effects of price information on physicians' test-ordering behavior: ordering of diagnostic tests, *Med Care* 20:293, 1982.
24. Detsky AS, Naglie IG: A clinician's guide to cost-effectiveness analysis, *Ann Intern Med* 113:147, 1990.
25. Dexter F, Coffin S, Tinker JH: Decreases in anesthesia-controlled time cannot permit one additional surgical operation to be reliably scheduled during the workday, *Anesth Analg* 81:1263, 1995.
26. Dexter F, Tinker JH: Analysis of strategies to decrease postanesthesia care unit costs, *Anesthesiology* 82:94, 1995.
27. Dexter F, Tinker JH: The cost efficacy of hypothetically eliminating adverse anesthetic outcomes from high-risk, but neither low—nor moderate—risk, surgical operations, *Anesth Analg* 81:939, 1995.
28. Ding Y, Fredman B, Newson C, et al: Use of mivacurium for laparoscopy: effect of eliminating succinylcholine and reversal agents on recovery, *Anesthesiology* 79: 125, 1993.
29. Doze VA, Shafer A, White PF: Propofol-nitrous oxide versus thiopental-isoflurane-nitrous oxide for general anesthesia, *Anesthesiology* 69:63, 1988.
30. DiBenedetto RJ, Graves SA, Gravenstein N: Pulse oximetry monitoring can change routine oxygen supplementation practices

in the postanesthesia care unit, *Anesth Analg* 78:365, 1994.

31. Eddy DM: Cost-effectiveness analysis: a conversation with my father, *JAMA* 267: 1669, 1992.
32. Eisenberg JM: Clinical economics: a guide to the economic analysis of clinical practices, *JAMA* 262:2879, 1989.
33. Fuchs VR, Garber AM: The new technology assessment, *N Engl J Med* 323:673, 1990.
34. Foss JF, Mantha S, Ellis JE, et al: A decision analysis of the cost-effectiveness of dobutamine stress echo and dipyridamole thallium scan in the evaluation of vascular surgery patients, *Anesth Analg* 80:SCA42, 1995.
35. Gan TJ, Lubarsky D, Robertson K, et al: The hospital cost of perioperative transfusion of a unit of red blood cells and other blood products, *Anesth Analg* 82:S123, 1996.
36. Gannon K: Anesthesia drug market climbing through 1999, *Hosp Pharm Rep,* 7:32–35, 1993.
37. Ghouri AF, Bodner M, White PF: Recovery profile following desflurane-nitrous oxide versus isoflurane-nitrous oxide in outpatients, *Anesthesiology* 74:575, 1991.
38. Ghouri AF, Ramirez-Ruiz M, White PF: Flumazenil after midazolam sedation decreases outpatient recovery times, *Anesthesiology* 77:A11, 1992.
39. Ginzberg E: A cautionary note on market reforms in health care, *JAMA* 274:1633, 1995.
40. Goodnough LM, Grishaber JE, Birkmeyer JD, et al: Efficacy and cost-effectiveness of autologous blood predeposit in patients undergoing radical prostatectomy procedures, *Urology* 44:226, 1994.
41. Gratz I, Larijani GE, DeCastro N, et al: A cost comparison of atracurium (A) and vecuronium (v) when used for maintenance of neuromuscular blockade (NMB) for elective surgical procedures, *Anesthesiology* 77:A1121, 1992.
42. Grumbach K, Bodenheimer T: Mechanisms for controlling costs, *JAMA* 273:1223, 1995.
43. Grumbach K, Bodenheimer T: Painful vs. painless cost control, *JAMA* 272:1458, 1994.
44. Hampel K, Schanbacher M, Dugan D, et al: Can the anesthesiologist reliably decide which muscle relaxant he is using? *Anesthesiology* 77:A941, 1992.
45. Harris JS: Why doctors do what they do: determinants of physician behavior, *J Occup Med* 32:1207, 1990.
46. Hawkes C, Miller D, Martineau R, et al: Evaluation of cost minimization strategies of anesthetic drugs in a tertiary care hospital, *Can J Anaesth* 41:894, 1994.
47. Hendrickx J, De Wolf AM: Costs of administering desflurane or isoflurane via a closed circuit, *Anesthesiology* 80:240, 1994.
48. Hertz CM, Glass PSA, Gan TJ, et al: Nausea and vomiting-a costly anesthetic complication? *Anesthesiology* 83:A1036, 1995.
49. Hess D, Burns E, Romagnoli D, et al: Weekly ventilator circuit changes: a strategy to reduce costs without affecting pneumonia rates, *Anesthesiology* 82:903, 1995.
50. Hickson GB, Altemeier WA, Perrin JM: Physician reimbursement by salary or fee-for-service: effect on physician practice behavior in a randomized prospective study, *Pediatrics* 80:344, 1987.
51. Hudson RJ, Friesen RM: Health care "reform" and the costs of anaesthesia, *Can J Anaesth* 40:1120, 1993.
52. Humphrey D, Downing JW, Brock-Utne JG: Cost of anesthesia, *Br Med J* 286:800, 1983.
53. Isaacson IJ, Lowdon JD, Berry AJ, et al: The value of pulmonary artery and central venous monitoring in patients undergoing abdominal aortic reconstructive surgery: a comparative study of two selected, randomized groups, *J Vasc Surg* 12:754, 1990.
54. James BC: Improving quality can reduce costs, *QA Rev* 1:4, 1989.
55. Jastremski MS, Chelluri L, Beney KM, et al: Analysis of the effects of continuous on-line monitoring of mixed venous oxygen saturation on patient outcome and cost-effectiveness, *Crit Care Med* 17:148, 1989.
56. Johnstone RE: Costs of inhaled anesthetics: II, *Anesthesiology* 80:1404, 1994.
57. Johnstone RE: Market costs of short-term physician and nurse anesthesia services, *J Clin Anesth* 6:129, 1994.
58. Johnstone RE: Studies of cost savings require cost measurements (letter), *Anesth Analg* 79:816, 1994.
59. Johnstone RE, Jozefczyk KG: Costs of anesthetic drugs: experiences with a cost education trial, *Anesth Analg* 78:766, 1994.
60. Johnstone RE, Martinec CL: Costs of anesthesia, *Anesth Analg* 76:840, 1993.
61. Joshi GP: Epidural analgesia versus IV-PCA: a cost-benefit analysis, *Anesth Analg* 82:S208, 1996.
62. Kapur PA: Cost containment: at what expense? *Anesth Analg* 81:897, 1995.
63. Kattan MW, Easthman JA, Yawn DH, et al: A decision analysis of the cost effectiveness of preoperative autologous blood donation prior to radical prostatectomy for clinically localized prostate cancer, *Med Dec Mak* 15:429, 1995.
64. King K, Dear G, Ginsberg B, et al: Cost analyses to develop practice guidelines for muscle relaxants, *Anesth Analg* 82:S233, 1996.
65. Kroll H, Mandell S, Brown M: The reuse of syringes with a Y-port extension set: Is it safe? *Anesth Analg* 80:S254, 1995.
66. Ku L, Fisher D: The attitudes of physicians toward health care cost-containment policies, *Health Serv Res* 25:1, 1990.
67. Kuperman G, James B, Jacobsen J, et al: Continuous quality improvement applied to medical care: experiences at LDS hospital, *Med Dec Mak* 11:S60, 1991.
68. Lanier WL, Warner MA: New frontiers in anesthesia research: assessing the impact of practice patterns on outcome, health care delivery, and cost, *Anesthesiology* 78:1001, 1993.
69. Ledgerwood AM, Harrigan C, Saxe JM, et al: The influence of an anesthetic regimen on patient care, outcome, and hospital charges, *Am Surg* 58:527, 1992.
70. Lethbridge JR, Walker JS: Cost of anaesthetic drugs and clinical budgeting, *Br Med J* 293:1587, 1986.
71. Lubarsky DA, Gan TJ, Glass PSA, et al: PACU clinical outcomes and financial savings following a pharmaceutical cost containment program in anesthesia using practice guidelines, *Anesth Analg* 82:S285, 1996.
72. Lubarsky DA, Hahn C, Bennett DH, et al: The hospital cost (fiscal year 1991/1992) of a simple perioperative allogeneic red blood cell transfusion during elective surgery at Duke University, *Anesth Analg* 79:629, 1994.
73. Lubarsky DA, Smith LR, Glass PSA: A comparison of maintenance drug costs of isoflurane, desflurane, sevoflurane, and propofol with OR and PACU labor costs during a 60 minute outpatient procedure, *Anesthesiology* 83:A1035, 1995.
74. Macario A, Chang PC, Stempel DB, et al: A cost analysis of the laryngeal mask airway for elective surgery in adult outpatients, *Anesthesiology* 83:250, 1995.
75. Macario A, Roizen MF, Thisted RA, et al: Reassessment of preoperative laboratory testing has changed the test-ordering patterns of physicians, *Surg Gynecol Obstet* 175:539, 1992.
76. Macario A, Vitez TS, Dunn B, et al: Where are the costs in perioperative care? Analysis of hospital costs and charges for inpatient surgical care, *Anesthesiology* 83:1138, 1995.
77. Matjasko J: Economic impact of low-flow anesthesia, *Anesthesiology* 67:863, 1987.
78. Mazzei WJ: Operating room start times and turnover times in a University Hospital, *J Clin Anesth* 6:405, 1994.
79. Metcalf E: The orthopaedic critical path, *Orthop Nurs* 10:25, 1991.
80. Michels KA: AANA testifies before PPRC on federal healthcare reform, *JAANA* 61:549, 1993.
81. Moote CA: Pharmacoeconomics of patient-controlled analgesia, *Persp Pain Man* 3:7, 1994.
82. Morley-Forster P, Newton PT, Cook MJ, et al: Ketorolac and indomethacin are equally efficacious for the relief of minor postoperative pain, *Can J Anaesth* 41:1126, 1994.
83. Moseley H, Kumar AY, Bhanvani Shankar KB, et al: Should air-oxygen replace nitrous oxide-oxygen in general anaesthesia? *Anaesthesia* 42:609, 1987.
84. Nagasandra VR, Cable E, Reddy M: A comparative study of the costs of anesthesia in U.S.A. and overseas, *Anesth Analg* 80:S335, 1995.
85. Narbone RF, Hopkins EM, McCarthy RJ, et al: Cost-effectiveness analysis of anesthetic usage patterns for total knee replacement, *Anesthesiology* 79:A1065, 1993.
86. Narbone RF, McCarthy RJ, Tuman KJ, et al: Selectivity in drug utilization: Impact on anesthetic drug costs, *Anesth Analg* 80: S341, 1995.
87. Narr BJ, Hansen TR, Warner MA: Preoperative laboratory screening in healthy Mayo patients: cost-effective elimination of tests and unchanged outcomes, *Mayo Clin Proc* 66:155, 1991.
88. National Center for Healthcare Statistics: Health, United States 1991, Hyattsville, 1992, Public Health Services 266.
89. Natonson RA, Ampel LL, Gilbert HC, et al: Comparisons of cost and recovery following desflurane or isoflurane anesthesia, *Anesthesiology* 83:A50, 1995.

90. Newson CD, White LD, White PF: Operating room delays: inpatient versus ambulatory procedures, *Anesth Analg* 76: S297, 1993.
91. Norris C, Jacobs P, Rapoport J, et al: ICU and non-ICU cost per day, *Can J Anaesth* 42:192, 1995.
92. Orkin FK: Moving toward value-based anesthesia care, *J Clin Anesth* 5:91, 1993.
93. Orkin FK, Cohen MM, Duncan PG: The quest for meaningful outcomes, *Anesthesiology* 78:417, 1993.
94. Pearson KS, Gomez MN, Moyers JR, et al: A cost/benefit analysis of randomized invasive monitoring for patients undergoing cardiac surgery, *Anesth Analg* 69:336, 1989.
95. Pedersen FM, Nielsen J, Ibsen M, et al: Low-flow isoflurane-nitrous oxide anaesthesia offers substantial economic advantages over high-and medium-flow isoflurane-nitrous oxide anaesthesia, *Acta Anaesthesiol Scand* 37:509, 1993.
96. Peter D: The cost of anaesthetic vapours, *Can J Anaesth* 39:633, 1992.
97. Podugu R, Morscher A, Smith CE, et al: Influence of anesthetic technique and agent on cost of ambulatory anesthesia, *Anesthesiology* 83:A49, 1995.
98. Rathmell JP, Brooker RF, Prielipp RC, et al: Hemodynamic and pharmacodynamic comparison of doxacurium and pipecuronium with pancuronium during induction of cardiac anesthesia: does the benefit justify the cost? *Anesth Analg* 76:513, 1993.
99. Reinhart DJ, Wang WP: Cost and resource utilization for foot surgery: General vs. MAC anesthesia, *Anesth Analg* 82:S376, 1996.
100. Riley ET, Cohen SE, Macario A, et al: Spinal versus epidural anesthesia for cesarean section: a comparison of time efficiency, costs, charges, and complications, *Anesth Analg* 80:709, 1995.
101. Roizen MF: Cost-effective preoperative laboratory testing, *JAMA* 271:319, 1994.
102. Roizen MF: Preoperative evaluation. In Miller RD, editor: *Anesthesia,* ed 3, New York, 1990, Churchill Livingstone.
103. Roizen MF, Schreider B, Stin W, et al: Pulse oximetry, capnography, and blood gas measurements: reducing cost and improving the quality of care with technology, *J Clin Monit* 9:237, 1993.
104. Romito D: A critical path for CVA patients, *Rehab Nurs* 15:153, 1990.
105. Rosenbach MA, Cromwell J, Pope GC, et al: Study of nurse anesthesia manpower needs, *JAANA* 59:233, 1991.
106. Rosenberg MK: The cost of oxygen therapy in the postanesthesia care unit (letter), *Anesth Analg* 79:808, 1994.
107. Rosenblatt MA, Cantos EC, Mohandas K: Intraoperative collection of blood is more cost-effective than preoperative donation, *Anesthesiology* 83:A1031, 1995.
108. Rosenblatt WH, Silverman DG: Cost-effective use of operating room supplies based on the remedy database of recovered unused materials, *J Clin Anesth* 6:400, 1994.
109. Sanderson IC, Gilbert WC, Lubarsky DA: Cost containment using an automated anes thesia record keeper, *Anesth Analg* 82: S391, 1996.
110. Schroeder SA, Myers LP, McPhee SJ, et al: The failure of physician education as a cost containment strategy: report of a prospective controlled trial at a University Hospital, *JAMA* 252:225, 1984.
111. Shomaker TS: Practice policies in anesthesia: a foretaste of practice in the 21st century, *Anesth Analg* 80:388, 1995.
112. Smiley RM, Ornstein E, Matteo RS, et al: Desflurane and isoflurane in surgical patients: comparison of emergence time, *Anesthesiology* 74:425, 1991.
113. Smith I, Newson CD, White PF: Use of forced-air warming during and after outpatient arthroscopic surgery, *Anesth Analg* 78:836, 1994.
114. Starfield B, Powe NR, Weiner JR, et al: Costs vs. quality in different types of primary care settings, *JAMA* 272:1903, 1994.
115. Sung YF, Reiss N, Tillette T: The differential cost of anesthesia and recovery with propofol-nitrous oxide anesthesia versus thiopental sodium-isoflurane-nitrous oxide anesthesia, *J Clin Anesth* 3:391, 1991.
116. Szocik JF, Learned SW: Impact of a cost containment program on the use of volatile anesthetics and neuromuscular blocking drugs, *J Clin Anesth* 6:378, 1994.
117. Taylor E, Ghouri AF, White PF: Identifying causes of operating room delays: first case vs. to follow cases, *Anesth Analg* 76:S428, 1993.
118. Taylor GJ, Mikell FL, Moses HW, et al: Determinants of hospital charges for coronary artery bypass surgery: the economic consequences of postoperative complications, *Am J Cardiol* 65:309, 1990.
119. Tierney WM, Miller ME, McDonald CJ: The effect on test ordering of informing physicians of the charges for outpatient diagnostic tests, *N Engl J Med* 322:1499, 1990.
120. Todd MM, Warner DS, Sokoll MD, et al: A prospective, comparative trial of three anesthetics for elective supratentorial craniotomy: propofol/fentanyl isoflurane/nitrous oxide and fentanyl/nitrous, *Anesthesiology* 78:1005, 1993.
121. Tobias JD, Lynch A, McDuffee A, et al: Pancuronium infusion for neuromuscular block in children in the pediatric intensive care unit, *Anesth Analg* 81:13, 1995.
122. Trumbull WN: Who has standing in cost-benefit analysis? *J Polic Anal Man* 9:201, 1990.
123. Tuman KJ, Ivankovich AD: High-cost, high-tech medicine: are we getting our money's worth? *J Clin Anesth* 5:168, 1993.
124. Tuman KJ, McCarthy RJ, Spiess BD, et al: Effect of pulmonary artery catheterization on outcome in patients undergoing coronary artery surgery, *Anesthesiology* 70:199, 1989.
125. Turnbull JM, Buck C: The value of preoperative screening investigations in otherwise healthy individuals, *Arch Intern Med* 147:1101, 1987.
126. University Hospital Consortium Technology Assessment: Routine preoperative diagnostic evaluations, Oak Brook, 1994, University Hospital Consortium.
127. Van Hemelrijck J, Smith I, White PF: Use of desflurane for outpatient anesthesia. A comparison with propofol and nitrous oxide, *Anesthesiology* 75:197, 1991.
128. Van Sickels JE, Tiner BD: Cost of a genioplasty under deep intravenous sedation in a private office versus general anesthesia in an outpatient surgical center, *J Oral Maxillofac Surg* 50:687, 1992.
129. Vinik HR: Practical comparison of the cost of desflurane and isoflurane with 1 and 2L flow rates, *Anesth Analg* 82:S468, 1996.
130. Vitez TS: Principles of cost analysis, *J Clin Anesth* 6:357, 1994.
131. Wagner EH: The cost-quality relationship do we always get what we pay for? *JAMA* 272:1951, 1994,
132. Watcha MF: Cost comparisons of halothane and sevoflurane for pediatric outpatient surgery, *Anesth Analg* 82:S477, 1996.
133. Watcha MF, Smith I: Cost-effectiveness analysis of antiemetic therapy for ambulatory surgery, *J Clin Anesth* 6:370, 1994.
134. Weiner S, Carter J: Cost containment in the operating room: the role of physician education, *Anesthesiology* 79:A533, 1993.
135. Weiskopf RB, Eger EI: Comparing the costs of inhaled anesthetics, *Anesthesiology* 79:1413, 1993.
136. Weiss JB: Perspective: an anesthesiologist, *Health Affairs,* 3:20-25, 1988.
137. Wetchler BV, Alexander CD, Kondragunta RD: Recovery from the use of propofol for maintenance of anesthesia during short ambulatory procedures, *Semin Anesth* 11:20, 1992.
138. Whitcher C, Ream AK, Parasons D, et al: Anesthetic mishaps and the cost of monitoring: a proposed standard for monitoring equipment, *J Clin Monit* 4:5, 1988.
139. White PF, Smith I: Impact of newer drugs and techniques on the quality of ambulatory anesthesia, *J Clin Anesth* 5:3S, 1993.
140. White PF, White LD: Cost containment in the operating room: who is responsible? *J Clin Anesth* 6:351, 1994.
141. Williams MJ, Leighton BL: A simple method to reduce anesthetic delivery cost, *Anesth Analg* 82:S494, 1996.
142. Wilson ME, Williams NB, Baskett PJF, et al: Assessment of fitness for surgical procedures and the variability of anaesthetists' judgements, *Br Med J* 1:509, 1980.
143. Wong HY, Carpenter RL, Kopacz DJ, et al: A randomized, double-blind evaluation of ketorolac tromethamine for postoperative analgesia in ambulatory surgery patients, *Anesthesiology* 78:6, 1993.
144. Woolhandler S, Himmelstein D: The deteriorating administrative efficiency of the US health care system, *N Engl J Med* 324:1253, 1991.
145. Woolhandler S, Himmelstein DU, Lewontin JP: Administrative costs in U.S. hospitals, *N Engl J Med* 329:400, 1993.
146. Ziegler MG, Lew P, Singer BC: The accuracy of drug information from pharmaceutical sales representatives, *JAMA* 273:1296, 1995.
147. Zimmerman JE, Shortell SM, Knaus WA, et al: Value and cost of teaching hospitals: a prospective multicenter, inception cohort study, *Crit Care Med* 21:1432, 1993.

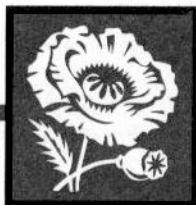

Appendix A: Formulary

MAGED S. MIKHAIL
G. EDWARD MORGAN, JR.

To calculate drug dose as μg/kg/min:

$$\frac{\text{drug (mg)} \times 1000\ \mu\text{g} \times \text{rate (ml)} \times 1\ \text{hour} \times 1}{\text{drug volume (ml)} \times 1\ \text{mg} \times 1\ \text{hour} \times 60\ \text{minutes} \times \text{patient weight (kg)}}$$

To calculate drug infusion rate as ml/hour:

$$\frac{\text{desired dose } (\mu\text{g}) \times \text{patient weight (kg)} \times 60\ \text{minutes}}{\text{kg} \times \text{minute} \times \text{drug concentration } (\mu\text{g/ml}) \times 1\ \text{hour}}$$

Table A-1 Analgesic agents

Drug	Route	Usual dose	How supplied	Form	Cost*†
Oral analgesics nonopioid					
Acetaminophen	PO	325–1000 mg	325 mg	Tablet	$0.01
Acetylsalicylic acid	PO	325–1000 mg	325 mg	Tablet	$0.01
Choline magnesium trisalicylate	PO	500–1000 mg	500 mg	Tablet	$0.10
Diflunisal	PO	500–1000 mg	500 mg	Tablet	$0.30
Ibuprofen	PO	200–800 mg	200 mg	Tablet	$0.01
Indomethacin	PO	25–50 mg	25 mg	Tablet	$0.01
Ketorolac	PO	10 mg	10 mg	Tablet	$1.00
Naproxen	PO	250–500	550 mg	Tablet	$0.15
Propoxyphene	PO	100 mg	65 mg	Tablet	$0.10
Sulindac	PO	150 mg	150 mg	Tablet	$0.10
Tramadol	PO	50–100 mg	50 mg	Tablet	$0.50
Opioid					
Codiene	PO	30–60 mg	30 mg	Tablet	$0.25
Codiene/acetaminophen	PO	30–60 mg	30 mg/300 mg	Tablet	$0.05
Hydrocodone	PO	5–7.5 mg	5 mg	Tablet	$0.10
Hydrocodone/acetaminophen	PO	5–7.5 mg	10 mg/650 mg	Tablet	$0.50
Hydromorphone	PO	2–4 mg	2 mg	Tablet	$0.50
Levorphanol	PO	2 mg	2 mg	Tablet	$0.40
Methadone	PO	20 mg	5 mg	Tablet	$0.10
Oxycodone	PO	5–10 mg	5 mg	Capsule	$0.20

*Cost reflects the cost to a hospital that is part of a large drug-purchasing consortium.
†Costs have been rounded off as follows: $0.02 to $0.05 rounded to nearest $0.05; $0.06 to $0.99 rounded to nearest $0.10; $1.01 to $4.99 rounded to nearest $0.50; $5.01 and greater rounded to nearest $1.00.

Continued

Table A-1 Analgesic agents — cont'd

Drug	Route	Usual dose	How supplied	Form	Cost*†
Transdermal opioids					
Fentanyl	Transdermal	25–100 mcg/hr	25 mcg/hr	Patch	$8.00
			100 mcg/hr		$23.00
Parenteral analgesic/nonopioid					
Ketorolac	IM	30–60 mg	30 mg 1 ml	Injection	$7.00
	IV	15–30 mg	60 mg 2 ml		$7.00
Parenteral opioids					
Alfentanil	IV	8–100 mcg/kg	1000 mcg/2 ml	Injection	$6.00
		0.3–3.0 mcg/kg/min	2500 mcg/5 ml		$11.00
			10000 mcg/20 ml		$32.00
Codiene	IV	30–60 mg	30 mg 1 ml	Injection	$0.50
Fentanyl	IV	0.5–1.5 mcg/kg	50 mcg/ml 2 ml	Injection	$0.20
		1.5–150 mcg/kg	50 mcg/ml 5 ml		$0.35
		0.3–1 mcg/kg/min	50 mcg/ml 20 ml		$1.50
Hydromorphone	IV	0.5–2 mg	2 mg 1 ml	Injection	$2.00
Levorphanol	IV	1–3 mg	2 mg 1 ml	Injection	$2.50
Meperidine	IM	0.5–1.0 mg/kg	100 mg 1 ml	Injection	$0.40
	IV	0.2–0.5 mg/kg			
Morphine sulfate	IM	0.05–0.2 mg/kg	10 mg 1 ml	Injection	$0.40
	IV	0.03–0.15 mg/kg			
		0.1–1.0 mg/kg			
Oxymorphone	IV	1–1.5 mg	1.5 mg/ml 10 ml	Injection	$35.00
Remifentanil	IV	0.5–1 mcg/kg	1 mg 3 ml	Injection	$10.00
		0.05–1.0 mcg/kg/min			
Sufentanil	IV	0.25–30 mcg/kg	50 mcg 1 ml	Injection	$5.00
		0.075 mcg/kg/min	50 mcg/ml 2 ml		$14.00
			50 mcg/ml 5 ml		$27.00
Epidural opioids					
Alfentanil	Epidural	250–1000 mcg	1000 mcg/2 ml	Injection	$6.00
Fentanyl	Epidural	50–100 mcg	50 mcg/ml 2 ml	Injection	$0.20
Hydromorphone	Epidural	0.75–1.5 mg	2 mg 1 ml	Injection	$2.00
Meperidine	Epidural	25–75 mg	50 mg 1 ml	Injection	$0.20
Methadone	Epidural	1–5 mg	10 mg/ml 20 ml	Injection	$11.00
			10 mg 5 ml		$0.40
Morphine sulfate	Epidural	2–5 mg	1 mg/ml 10 ml	Injection	$1.50
Sufentanil	Epidural	20–50 mcg	50 mcg 1 ml	Injection	$5.00
Intrathecal opioids					
Fentanyl	Intrathecal	10–25 mcg	50 mcg/ml 2 ml	Injection	$0.20
Meperidine	Intrathecal	10–20 mg	100 mg 1 ml	Injection	$0.40
Morphine sulfate	Intrathecal	0.25–0.6 mg	1 mg/ml 10 ml	Injection	$1.50
Sufentanil	Intrathecal	3–10 mcg	50 mcg 1 ml	Injection	$5.00
Opioid agonist/antagonists					
Buprenorphine	IV	0.3 mg	0.3 mg 1 ml	Injection	$2.00
Butorphanol	IV	0.5–2 mg	2 mg/ml 2 ml	Injection	
Nalbuphine	IV	10 mg	10 mg 1 ml	Injection	$0.30
Opioid antagonists					
Naloxone	IV	0.5–1 mcg/kg	0.4 mg 1 ml	Injection	$0.30
		Increments			
		4–5 mcg/kg/hr			
Naltrexone	PO	50 mg	50 mg	Tablet	$4.00

Table A-2 Sedative, hypnotic, and general anesthetic agents

Drug	Route	Usual dose	How supplied	Form	Cost*†
Barbiturates					
Methohexital	PR	25 mg/kg	500 mg 10 ml	Injection	$6.00
	IV	1–2 mg/kg			
	IV	0.2–0.4 mg/kg			
Pentobarbital	PO	150–200 mg	30 mg 1 ml	Injection	$1.50
	PR	2–4 mg/kg			
	IM				
Secobarbital	PO	150–200 mg	100 mg 2 ml	Injection	$2.00
	PR	2–4 mg/kg			
	IM				
Thiamylal	IV	3–6 mg/kg	1 g	Injection	$2.00
	IV	0.5–1.5 mg/kg			
Thiopental	PR	25–30 mg/kg	500 mg	Injection	$2.50
	IV	3–6 mg/kg	1 g	Injection	$3.00
	IV	0.5–1.5 mg/kg			
Benzodiazepines					
Diazepam	PO	0.1–0.5 mg/kg	10 mg	Tablet	$0.01
	IV	0.04–0.2 mg/kg	10 mg 2 ml	Injection	$0.30
		0.3–0.6 mg/kg			
Diazepam (Dizac)	IV	2–20 mg	5 mg/ml 3 ml	Injection	$3.00
Lorazepam	PO	0.05 mg/kg	2 mg	Tablet	$0.02
	IM	0.03–0.05 mg/kg	2 mg 1 ml	Injection	$2.50
	IV	0.03–0.05 mg/kg			
Midazolam	IM	0.07–0.15 mg/kg	5 mg/ml 2 ml	Injection	$15.00
	IV	0.01–0.1 mg/kg	1 mg/ml 5 ml		$8.00
	IV	0.1–0.4 mg/kg			
Phenothiazines					
Droperidol	IM	0.04–0.07 mg/kg	5 mg/2 ml	Injection	$0.40
	IV	0.01–0.07 mg/kg			
Haloperidol	IM	2–5 mg	5 mg 1 ml	Injection	$0.45
Chlorpromazine	IV	25–50 mg	25 mg/ml 2 ml	Injection	$0.60
Antihistamines					
Diphenhydramine	PO	50–100 mg	25 mg	Tablet	$0.10
	IM	50–100 mg	50 mg 2 ml	Injection	$0.50
	IV	25–100 mg	50 mg 1 ml	Injection	$0.50
Hydroxyzine	PO	25–100 mg	50 mg	Tablet	$0.01
	IM	25–100 mg	50 mg/ml 10 ml	Injection	$0.50
Promethazine	PO	12.5–50 mg	25 mg	Tablet	$0.30
	IM	12.5–50 mg	25 mg 1 ml	Injection	$0.40
	IV	12.5–50 mg			
Other agents					
Chloral hydrate	PO	500 mg	500 mg/ml 5 ml	Syrup	$2.00
		50–100 mg/kg	500 mg	Capsule	$0.10
Etomidate	IV	0.2–0.5 mg/kg	2 mg/ml 20 ml	Injection	$19.00
Ketamine	IM	3–5 mg/kg	50 mg/ml 10 ml	Injection	$11.00
	IV	1–2 mg/kg			

*Cost reflects the cost to a hospital that is part of a large drug-purchasing consortium.
†Costs have been rounded off as follows: $0.02 to $0.05 rounded to nearest $0.05; $0.06 to $0.99 rounded to nearest $0.10; $1.01 to $4.99 rounded to nearest $0.50; $5.01 and greater rounded to nearest $1.00.

Continued

Table A-2 Sedative, hypnotic, and general anesthetic agents — cont'd

Drug	Route	Usual dose	How supplied	Form	Cost*†
Other agents—cont'd					
Propofol	IV	1–2.5 mg/kg	10 mg/ml 20 ml	Injection	$11.00
	IV	25–200 mcg/kg/min			
Halogenated volatile anesthetics					
Desflurane	Inhalation	6.0% MAC	240 ml	Bottle	$73.00
Enflurane	Inhalation	1.7% MAC	250 ml	Bottle	$60.00
Halothane	Inhalation	0.75% MAC	250 ml	Bottle	$19.00
Isoflurane	Inhalation	1.2% MAC	250 ml	Bottle	$69.00
Methoxyflurane	Inhalation	0.16% MAC	125 ml	Bottle	$471.00
Sevoflurane	Inhalation	2.0% MAC	250 ml	Bottle	$180.00

Table A-3 Muscle relaxants and reversal agents

Drug	Route	Usual dose	How supplied	Cost*†
Depolarizing				
Succinylcholine	IM	4–6 mg/kg	20 mg/ml 10 ml	$0.40
	IV	1–2 mg/kg		
Nondepolarizing				
Atracurium	IV	0.5 mg/kg	10 mg/ml 10 ml	$43.00
Cis-atracurium	IV	0.1–0.15 mg/kg	2 mg/ml 10 ml	$14.00
Doxacurium	IV	0.05 mg/kg	1 mg/ml 5 ml	$15.00
Gallamine	IV	3 mg/kg	20 mg/ml 10 ml	$20.00
Metocurine	IV	0.3 mg/kg	2 mg/ml 20 ml	$22.00
Mivacurium	IV	0.15–0.2 mg/kg	2 mg/ml 20 ml	$22.00
Pancuronium	IV	0.08–0.12 mg/kg	1 mg/ml 10 ml	$1.50
Pipecuronium	IV	0.06–0.1 mg/kg	10 mg 10 ml	$38.00
Rocuronium	IV	0.45–0.6 mg/kg	10 ml/ml 5 ml	$15.00
			10 ml/ml 10 ml	$29.00
Tubocurarine	IV	0.5–0.6 mg/kg	3 mg/ml 10 ml	$2.50
Vecuronium	IV	0.08–0.12 mg/kg	10 mg 10 ml	$15.00
Reversal agents				
Edrophonium	IV	0.5–1 mg/kg	10 mg/ml 15 ml	$10.00
Edrophonium/atropine	IV	0.5–1 mg/kg	10 mg/ml 15 ml	$10.00
Neostigmine	IV	0.04–0.8 mg/kg	1 mg/ml 10 ml	$0.05
Pyridostigmine	IV	0.1–0.4 mg/kg	5 mg/ml 5 ml	$3.00

*Cost reflects the cost to a hospital that is part of a large drug-purchasing consortium.
†Costs have been rounded off as follows: $0.02 to $0.05 rounded to nearest $0.05; $0.06 to $0.99 rounded to nearest $0.10; $1.01 to $4.99 rounded to nearest $0.50; $5.01 and greater rounded to nearest $1.00.

Table A-4 Local anesthetic agents

Drug	Usual dose	How supplied	Form	Cost*†
Topical				
Benzocaine	3–4 times/day	20% 2 oz	Spray	$3.00
Cetocaine	200 mg (1 second)	56 g bottle	Spray	$40.00
Cocaine	3 mg/kg maximum	10% 10 ml	Topical	$47.00
		4% 10 ml		$13.00
Dibucaine	1 mg/kg maximum	0.5% 1.5 oz	Cream	$3.00
EMLA cream	2.5 g	2.5% 30 g	Cream	$27.00
		2.5% 5 g	Cream	$6.00
Lidocaine	4.5 mg/kg maximum	2% 20 ml	Jelly	$6.00
Injections				
Bupivacaine	3 mg/kg maximum	0.5% 30 ml	Injection	$1.50
Chloroprocaine	12 mg/kg maximum	2% 30 ml	Injection	$13.00
Etidocaine	4 mg/kg maximum	1% 30 ml	Injection	$14.00
Lidocaine	4.5–7 mg/kg maximum	0.5% 50 ml	Injection	$2.00
		1% 30 ml		$0.50
		2% 20 ml		$0.80
		2% w/epi 20 ml		$1.50
		4% 5 ml		$2.00
Mepivacaine	4.5–7 mg/kg maximum	2% 20 ml	Injection	$4.00
Prilocaine	8 mg/kg maximum	4% 1.8 ml	Injection	$0.30
Procaine	12 mg/kg maximum	2% 30 ml	Injection	$0.50
Ropivacaine	3 mg/kg maximum	0.5% 30 ml	Injection	$10.00
Tetracaine	3 mg/kg maximum	1% 2 ml	Injection	$4.50

*Cost reflects the cost to a hospital that is part of a large drug-purchasing consortium.
†Costs have been rounded off as follows: $0.02 to $0.05 rounded to nearest $0.05; $0.06 to $0.99 rounded to nearest $0.10; $1.01 to $4.99 rounded to nearest $0.50; $5.01 and greater rounded to nearest $1.00.

Table A-5 Cardiovascular drugs

Drug	Route	Usual dose	How supplied	Form	Cost*†
Anticholinergic agents					
Atropine	IV	0.5–2 mg	1 mg/10 ml	Injection	$1.00
		0.01–0.02 mg/kg	0.4 mg 1 ml	Injection	$0.20
Glycopyrolate	IV	0.2–1 mg	0.2 mg/ml 2 ml	Injection	$0.25
		5–10 mcg/kg	0.2 mg/ml 5 ml	Injection	$2.00
Scopolamine	IV	0.2–0.6 mg	0.4 mg 1 ml	Injection	$0.80
Antiarrhythmics					
Adenosine	IV	6–12 mg	12 mg 4 ml	Injection	$41.00
		0.1–0.2 mg/kg	6 mg 2 ml	Injection	$21.00
		60–120 mcg/kg/min			
Amiodarone	IV	5–10 mg/kg	150 ml 3 ml	Injection	$58.00
Bretylium	IV	5–10 mg/kg	50 mg/ml 10 ml	Injection	$1.50
Digoxin	PO	0.125–0.25 mg	0.25 mg	Tablet	$0.01
	IV	0.125–0.5 mg	0.5 mg 2 ml	Injection	$0.80
		0.007–0.015 mg/kg			

*Cost reflects the cost to a hospital that is part of a large drug-purchasing consortium.
†Costs have been rounded off as follows: $0.02 to $0.05 rounded to nearest $0.05; $0.06 to $0.99 rounded to nearest $0.10; $1.01 to $4.99 rounded to nearest $0.50; $5.01 and greater rounded to nearest $1.00.

Continued

Table A-5 Cardiovascular drugs—cont'd

Drug	Route	Usual dose	How supplied	Form	Cost*†
Antiarrhythmics—cont'd					
Isoproterenol	IV	0.5–4 mcg 1–10 mcg/min 0.1–1 mcg/kg/min	0.2 mg 5 ml	Injection	$8.00
Lidocaine	IV	1–2 mg/kg 1–3 mg/min 20–50 mcg/kg/min	1% 10 ml 2% 5 ml 1 g	Injection Injection Injection	$3.00 $0.80 $3.00
Phenytoin	IV	5–15 mg/kg	50 mg/ml 5 ml	Injection	$0.30
Procainamide	IV	5–17 mg/kg	100 mg/ml 10 ml	Injection	$2.00
Inotropes and vasopressors					
Amrinone	IV	0.5–1.5 mg/kg 5–10 mcg/kg/min	5 mg/ml 20 ml	Injection	$49.00
Dobutamine	IV	2–20 mcg/kg/min	250 mg 250 ml	Injection	$6.00
Dopamine	IV	2–20 mcg/kg/min	400 mg 10 ml 400 mg 250 ml	Injection Injection	$1.50 $15.00
Ephedrine	IV	5–25 mg 0.1 mg/kg	50 mg 1 ml	Injection	$0.30
Epinephrine	IV	1–10 mcg 0.01–0.2 mg/kg 1–10 mcg/min 0.1–1 mcg/kg/min	1:10000 10 ml 1:1000 1 ml	Injection Injection	$1.00 $0.20
Metaraminol	IV	100 mcg 40–400 mcg/min	1% 10 ml	Injection	$8.00
Methoxamine	IV	2–10 mg	20 mg 1 ml	Injection	$19.00
Milrinone	IV	50 mcg/kg 0.375–0.75 mcg/kg/min	10 mg 10 ml	Injection	$51.00
Norepinephrine	IV	2–16 mcg/min 0.1–1 mcg/kg/min	1 mg/ml 4 ml	Injection	$6.00
Phenylephrine	IV	50–100 mcg 1–2 mcg/kg 10–50 mcg/min	1% 1 ml	Injection	$0.50
Antihypertensive agents					
Clonidine	PO	0.2 mg	0.1 mg	Tablet	$0.01
Enalaprilat	IV	0.625–1 mg	1.25 mg	Injection	$10.00
Hydralazine	IV	5–20 mg	20 mg 1 ml	Injection	$24.00
Methyldopa	IV	250–100 mg	50 mg/ml 10 ml	Injection	$0.80
Phenoxybenzamine	PO	10–20 mg	10 mg	Tablet	$0.50
Phentolamine	IV	1–5 mg	5 mg	Injection	$24.00
Beta Blockers					
Esmolol	IV	0.5 mg/kg	100 mg/ml 10 ml	Injection	$12.00
Labetalol	IV	2–20 mg	5 mg/ml 20 ml	Injection	$10.00
Metoprolol	IV	5–10 mg	1 mg/ml 5 ml	Injection	$3.00
Propranolol	IV	1–3 mg 0.01 mg/kg	1 mg 1 ml	Injection	$3.50

Table A-5 Cardiovascular drugs—cont'd

Drug	Route	Usual dose	How supplied	Form	Cost*†
Calcium channel blockers					
Diltiazem	IV	0.25–0.35 mg/kg	50 mg/ml 10 ml	Injection	$18.00
Nicardipine	IV	0.25–0.5 mg	2.5 mg/ml 10 ml	Injection	$17.00
Nifedipine	SL	10 mg	10 mg	Capsule	$0.05
Nimodipine	PO	60 mg	30 mg	Capsule	$4.50
Verapamil	IV	2.5–5 mg 0.1–0.3 mg/kg	2.5 mg/ml 4 ml	Injection	$0.40
Vasodilators					
Nitroglycerin	SL	0.4	0.4 mg	Tablet	$0.05
	Transdermal	1 inch	2% 30 g	Ointment	$2.50
	IV	25–100 mcg 0.5–10 mcg/kg/min	50 mg 10 ml	Injection	$0.50
Nitroprusside	IV	25–100 mcg 0.5–10 mcg/kg/min	50 mg 5 ml	Injection	$0.80
Prostaglandin E1	IV	0.05–0.4 mcg/kg/min	500 mcg 1 ml	Injection	$143.00

Table A-6 Intravenous fluids and electrolytes

Drug	How supplied	Cost*†
Albumin 25%	50 ml	$40.00
Albumin 5%	250 ml	$40.00
Dextrose 10%	1000 ml	$0.90
Dextrose 5%	1000 ml	$0.80
Dextrose 5%	250 ml	$0.70
Dextrose 5%/sodium chloride 0.45%	1000 ml	$0.90
Dextrose 5%/sodium chloride 0.45%/KCl 20 meq	1000 ml	$1.50
Hetastarch 6%	6% 500 ml	$31.00
Lactated Ringer's solution	1000 ml	$0.90
Plasmalyte A	1000 ml	$2.00
Sodium chloride 0.9%	1000 ml	$0.70
Sodium chloride 0.9%	250 ml	$0.60
Calcium chloride	10% 10 ml	$1.00
Calcium gluconate	10% 10 ml	$1.00
Magnesium sulfate	50% 10 ml	$0.40
Potassium chloride	20 meq 10 ml	$0.20
Sodium bicarbonate	7.5% 50 ml	$1.00
Tromethamine (THAM)	500 ml	$83.00

*Cost reflects the cost to a hospital that is part of a large drug-purchasing consortium.

†Costs have been rounded off as follows: $0.02 to $0.05 rounded to nearest $0.05; $0.06 to $0.99 rounded to nearest $0.10; $1.01 to $4.99 rounded to nearest $0.50; $5.01 and greater rounded to nearest $1.00.

Table A-7 Anesthetic adjuncts

Drug	Route	Usual dose	How supplied	Form	Cost*†
Diuretics					
Acetazolamide	IV	250 mg	500 mg	Injection	$13.00
Bumetadine	IV	0.5–2 mg	0.25 mg/ml 2 ml	Injection	$1.00
Ethacrynic acid	IV	50–100 mg	50 mg	Injection	$16.00
Furosemide	IV	10–40 mg 0.2–1 mg/kg	10 mg/ml 4 ml	Injection	$0.50
Mannitol	IV	0.25–1 g/kg	20% 500 ml	Injection	$33.00
			25% 50 ml	Injection	$2.00
Metolazone	IV	5–20 mg	5 mg	Tablet	$0.50
Antacid and aspiration prophylaxis					
Cimetadine	PO	300 mg	300 mg	Tablet	$0.20
	IM	300 mg	300 mg 2 ml	Injection	$1.00
	IV	300 mg			
Famotidine	PO	20 mg	20 mg	Tablet	$1.50
	IV	20 mg	10 mg/ml 2 ml	Injection	$3.00
Ranitidine	PO	150 mg	150 mg	Tablet	$1.50
	IM	50 mg	150 mg 10 ml	Injection	$4.50
	IV	50 mg			
Metoclopramide	PO	10–20 mg	10 mg	Tablet	$0.01
	IV	10–20 mg	5 ml/ml 2 ml	Injection	$0.20
Omeprazole	PO	20 mg	20 mg	Tablet	$3.00
Sodium citrate 0.3 M	PO	15–30 ml 0.3 M	30 ml	Solution	$0.20
Sucralfate	PO	1 g	1 g 10 ml	Suspension	$1.00
Bronchodilators					
Albuterol	Inhalation	2.5–5 mg	0.5% 20 ml	Solution	$5.00
Ipratropium	Inhalation	0.5 mg	0.02% 2 ml	Aerosol	$1.00
Isoetharane	Inhalation	2.5–5 mg	1% 0.5 ml	Aerosol	$0.40
Metaproterenol	Inhalation	2.5 mg	5% 10 ml	Solution	$11.00
Terbutaline	Inhalation	0.25–0.5 mg	7.5 ml	Aerosol	$8.00
	SC	0.25 mg	1 mg 1 ml	Injection	$0.70
Aminophyline	IV	5 mg/kg 0.5–0.9 mg/kg/min	250 mg 10 ml	Injection	$9.00
Antibleeding agents					
Aminocaproic acid	IV	4–5 g	5 g 20 ml	Injection	$13.00
Aprotinin	IV	280 mg 70 mg/hr	10 mu/ml 200 ml	Injection	$300.00
Desmopressin	IV	0.3 mcg/kg	4 mcg 1 ml	Injection	$16.00
Protamine	IV	25–250 mg	50 mg 5 ml	Injection	$0.60
Tranexamic acid	IV	10 mg/kg 1 mg/kg/min	100 mg 10 ml	Injection	$13.00
Anticonvulsants					
Carbamazepine	PO	200–1200 mg/day	200 mg	Tablet	$0.10
Clonazepam	PO	1–18 mg/day	1 mg	Tablet	$0.80
Gabapentin	PO	900–1800 mg/day	100 mg	Tablet	$0.30
Phenytoin	PO	200–600 mg/day	100 mg	Tablet	$0.05
Valproic acid	PO	750–1250 mg/day	250 mg	Tablet	$0.05

*Cost reflects the cost to a hospital that is part of a large drug-purchasing consortium.
†Costs have been rounded off as follows: $0.02 to $0.05 rounded to nearest $0.05; $0.06 to $0.99 rounded to nearest $0.10; $1.01 to $4.99 rounded to nearest $0.50; $5.01 and greater rounded to nearest $1.00.

Table A-7 Anesthetic adjuncts — cont'd

Drug	Route	Usual dose	How supplied	Form	Cost*†
Antidepressants					
Amitriptyline	PO	25–300 mg/day	150 mg	Tablet	$0.05
Desipramine	PO	50–300 mg/day	100 mg	Tablet	$0.20
Doxepine	PO	75–400 mg/day	100 mg	Tablet	$0.90
Fluoxetine	PO	20–80 mg/day	20 mg	Tablet	$2.00
Imipramine	PO	75–400 mg/day	100 mg	Tablet	$0.01
Nortriptyline	PO	40–150 mg/day	10 mg	Capsule	$0.05
Trazodone	PO	150–400 mg/day	100 mg	Tablet	$0.05
Intravenous dyes					
Fluorescein	IV	500 mg	10% 5 ml	Injection	$6.00
Indigo carmine	IV	400 mg	0.8% 5 ml	Injection	$7.00
Methylene blue	IV	10 mg	1% 1 ml	Injection	$3.00
Glucocorticoids					
Triamcinolone	Infiltration	3–48 mg	40 mg/ml 5 ml	Injection	$5.00
Dexamethasone	IV	2–10 mg	4 mg/ml 5 ml	Injection	$0.50
Hydrocortisone	IV	50–100 mg	100 mg 2 ml	Injection	$1.00
Methylprednisolone	IV	20–40 mg to 30 mg/kg	20 mg/ml 10 ml	Injection	$3.00
	PO	4–48 mg	60 mg	Tablet	$1.00
Prednisone	PO	5–60 mg	20 mg	Tablet	$0.05
Other hormones					
Fludrocortisone	PO	0.1 mg	0.1 mg	Tablet	$0.40
Glucagon	IV	0.5–1.0 mg	1 mg	Injection	$26.00
Insulin (human)	IV	5–20 units	1.5 ml	Injection	$2.00
		0.02–0.1 units/kg/hr			
Levothyroxine	PO	10–15 mcg/kg	0.2 mg	Tablet	$0.01
	IV	1 mcg/kg	0.2 mg 1 ml	Injection	$4.00
Immunosuppressants					
Azothioprine	IV	3–5 mg/kg	100 mg 20 ml	Injection	$58.00
Cyclosporine	IV	5–6 mg/kg	50 mg/ml 5 ml	Injection	$23.00
Tacrolimus	IV	0.05–0.1 mg/kg/day	5 mg 1 ml	Injection	$925.00
Nutritional supplements					
Aminosyn 8.5%	IV		500 ml	Injection	$8.00
Dextrose 25%	IV		10 ml	Injection	$2.00
Dextrose 50%	IV		50 ml	Injection	$2.50
Fat emulsion 20%	IV		100 ml	Injection	$9.00
Freamine 6.9%	IV		1000 ml	Injection	$43.00
Nephramine 5.4%	IV		250 ml	Injection	$18.00
Thiamine	IV	50–100 mg	100 mg 1 ml	Injection	$1.50
Vitamin K	IV	10 mg	10 mg 1 ml	Injection	$2.00
Vitamin C	IV	250–1000 mg	500 mg 1 ml	Injection	$0.80
Miscellaneous agents					
Acetyl cysteine	Inhalation	250 mg	20% 30 ml	Solution	$20.00
Alcohol, 98% ethyl	Infiltration		5 ml	Injection	$9.00
Baclofen	PO	5–20 mg	10 mg	Tablet	$0.10
	Intrathecal	12.5–50 mcg	10 mg/5 ml	Injection	
Caffiene sodium benzoate	IV	250–500 mg	250 mg 2 ml	Injection	$6.00
Capsaicin	Topical	3–4 times daily	0.025% 42.5 g	Cream	$8.00
Dantrolene	PO	25 mg	50 mg	Capsule	$0.90
	IV	1–10 mg/kg	20 mg	Injection	$48.00

Continued

Table A-7 Anesthetic adjuncts — cont'd

Drug	Route	Usual dose	How supplied	Form	Cost*†
Miscellaneous agents—cont'd					
Dextroamphetamine	PO	5–60 mg	5 mg	Tablet	$0.20
Doxapram	IV	0.5–1 mg/kg 1.3 mg/min	20 mg/ml 20 ml	Injection	$18.00
Epinephrine, racemic	Inhalation	5–15 mg	0.5 oz	Aerosol	$6.00
Ethyl chloride	Topical		3.5 oz	Spray	$8.00
Flumazenil	IV	0.6–1 mg 0.5 mg/hr	0.1 mg/ml 5 ml	Injection	$25.00
Granisetron	IV	10 mcg/kg	1 mg 1 ml	Injection	$103.00
Heparin	IV	5000–25000 units	1 mu/ml 10 ml	Injection	$0.50
Hyaluronidase	Infiltration	150 u	150 u/ml 1 ml	Injection	$5.00
Methergine	IM	0.2 mg	0.2 mg	Injection	$2.50
Mexilitine	PO	150–250 mg	200 mg	Tablet	$0.40
Octreotide	SC	50 mcg	0.1 mg 1 ml	Injection	$8.00
Ondansetron	IV	4 mg	2 mg/ml 2 ml	Injection	$17.00
Oxytocin	IV		10 u/ml	Injection	$0.20
Papavarine	IV		30 mg/ml 2 ml	Injection	$3.00
Phenol	Infiltration		16 oz	Crystals	$18.00
Physostigmine	IV	0.01–0.03 mg/kg	2 ml	Injection	$2.00
Sodium nitrite	IV	300 mg	500 g	Crystals	$20.00
Sodium thiosulfate	IV	12.5 g	10% 10 ml	Injection	$3.50

Table A-8 Antibiotics

Drug	Route	Usual dose	How supplied	Form	Cost*†
Acyclovir	IV	5 mg/kg	1000 mg	Injection	$87.00
Amikacin	IV	7.5 mg/kg	500 mg/2 ml	Injection	$11.00
Amoxicillin	PO	1.5–3 g 50 mg/kg	500 mg	Tablet	$0.10
Amphotericin B	IV	0.3–1.5 mg/kg	50 mg	Injection	$55.00
Ampicillin	PO	250–500 g	250 g	Tablet	$0.05
	IV	1–2 g 50 mg/kg	500 mg 6 ml	Injection	$0.30
Ampicillin/sulbactam	IV	3 g	3 g	Injection	$10.00
Cefazolin	IV	0.5–1 g	1 g 10 ml	Injection	$1.50
Cefotaxime	IV	2–3 g	10 g 100 ml	Injection	$70.00
Cefoxitin	IV	2 g	2 g	Injection	$13.00
Ceftazidime	IV	2 g	2 g	Injection	$17.00
Ceftizoxime	IV	2–4 g	2 g	Injection	$14.00
Ceftriaxone	IV	1–2 g	2 g	Injection	$49.00
Cefuroxime	IV	0.75–1.5 g	1.5 g	Injection	$6.00
Chloramphenicol	IV	12 mg/kg	1 g	Injection	$3.00
Ciprofloxacin	IV	200–400 mg	200 mg 100 ml	Injection	$13.00
Clindamycin	IV	600–900 mg	600 ml 50 ml	Injection	$3.50
Erythromycin	PO	0.5–1 g	500 mg	Tablet	$0.10
	IV	20 mg/kg	500 mg	Injection	$1.00
Gancyclovir	IV	5 mg/kg	500 mg 10 ml	Injection	$29.00
Gentamicin	IV	1.5–2 mg/kg	80 mg 50 ml	Injection	$1.50
Imipenem	IV	0.5–1 g	500 mg	Injection	$21.00
Metronidazole	IV	7.5 mg/kg	500 mg 100 ml	Injection	$1.50
Mezlocillin	IV	3 g	3 g	Injection	$8.00
Nafcillin	IV	2 g	1 g 10 ml	Injection	$1.50
Oxacillin	IV	2 g	1 g 50 ml	Injection	$3.00
Penicillin G	IV	1–3 million units	1 mu 50 ml	Injection	$0.60
Penicillin VK	PO	250 mg	250 mg	Tablet	$0.01
Pipercillin	IV	3 g	2 g	Injection	$7.00
Pipercillin/taxobactam	IV	4.5 g	2.25 g	Injection	$8.00
Tetracycline	PO	250–500 mg	250 mg	Capsule	$0.05
Ticarcillin	IV	3 g	3 g 50 ml	Injection	$8.00
Ticarcillin/clavulonic acid	IV	3.1 g	3.1 g	Injection	$10.00
Tobramycin	IV	2 mg/kg	80 mg 8 ml	Injection	$3.00
Trimethoprim/sulfmethoxazole	IV	10–20 mg/kg	80 mg/400 mg 5 ml	Injection	$0.40
Vancomycin	IV	15–20 mg/kg	1 g	Injection	$5.00

*Cost reflects the cost to a hospital that is part of a large drug-purchasing consortium.
†Costs have been rounded off as follows: $0.02 to $0.05 rounded to nearest $0.05; $0.06 to $0.99 rounded to nearest $0.10; $1.01 to $4.99 rounded to nearest $0.50; $5.01 and greater rounded to nearest $1.00.

Index

D

E

F

I

J

K

U

V